SEVENTH EDITION

COMPANION TO PSYCHIATRIC STUDIES

EDITED BY

Eve C. Johnstone CBE MD FRCP (Glasgow and Edinburgh) FRCPsych
Professor of Psychiatry and Head of the Department of Psychiatry, University of Edinburgh, UK

D. G. Cunningham Owens MD(Hons) FRCP FRCPsych
Reader in Psychiatry and Honorary Consultant Psychiatrist, University Department of Psychiatry, Royal Edinburgh Hospital, Edinburgh, UK

S. M. Lawrie MD(Hons) MRCPsych MPhil
Senior Research Fellow, University Department of Psychiatry, Edinburgh, UK

M. Sharpe MA MD FRCP MRCPsych
Professor of Psychological Medicine and Symptoms Research, University of Edinburgh Division of Psychiatry, Royal Edinburgh Hospital, Edinburgh, UK

C. P. L. Freeman MB ChB MPhil FRCPsych
Consultant Psychotherapist, Royal Edinburgh Hospital; Senior Lecturer, Department of Psychiatry, University of Edinburgh, UK

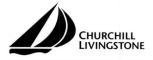

CHURCHILL LIVINGSTONE

EDINBURGH LONDON NEW YORK OXFORD PHILADELPHIA ST LOUIS SYDNEY TORONTO 2004

CHURCHILL LIVINGSTONE

First edition 1973
Second edition 1978
Third edition 1983
Fourth edition 1988
Fifth edition 1993
Sixth edition 1998
Seventh edition 2004

ISBN 0443 072639

British Library Cataloguing in Publication Data
A catalogue record for this book is available from the British Library

Library of Congress Cataloging in Publication Data
A catalog record for this book is available from the Library of Congress

Note
Medical knowledge is constantly changing. Standard safety precautions
must be followed, but as new research and clinical experience broaden
our knowledge, changes in treatment and drug therapy may become
necessary or appropriate. Readers are advised to check the most current
product information provided by the manufacturer of each drug to be
administered to verify the recommended dose, the method and duration
of administration, and contraindications. It is the responsibility of the
practitioner, relying on experience and knowledge of the patient, to
determine dosages and the best treatment for each individual patient.
Neither the Publisher nor the editors assumes any liability for any injury
and/or damage to persons or property arising from this publication.
The Publisher

 your source for books,
journals and multimedia
in the health sciences
www.elsevierhealth.com

The
publisher's
policy is to use
**paper manufactured
from sustainable forests**

Printed in China

Preface

The *Companion* has now truly come of age with this, its seventh edition, which in publishing terms makes it an old friend. It was born, in two volumes covering basic sciences and clinical material separately, in 1973 under the editorship of the late Drs Alistair Forrest and James Affleck, and rapidly acquired a following. Through four subsequent editions, over 20 years, its guiding influence was, however, Professor Robert Kendell, and it was with particular sadness that the present editors noted his sudden death in December 2002. It was typical of Bob Kendell's meticulousness that his contribution to the present volume was delivered only one week before his death and a reflection of his clear and stylish writing that it required very little modification. His erudition and support will be greatly missed.

With Cochrane reviews and the internet, there are some who argue that the days of textbooks are over, that those seeking information in their chosen field are better served by primary sources, that expertise is a debased commodity. We would adopt a different position. While primary source material represents an important tool in life-long learning, the role of the textbook is about context. For those starting out in psychiatric practice from whatever angle (specialist, general practitioner, nurse etc.) the field can seem strange and intimidating, a perception to which the mature practitioner is not immune! The role of a competent general text is to provide the reader with bearings – a map of the landscape, a guide to what the specialty is 'about', traditionally as well as currently. Thus, a general text is more to do with breadth than depth. And while the one thing the world is hardly short of nowadays is knowledge, the role of contributors to a text such as this is less about displaying that knowledge than it is about prioritising the facts and presenting to the reader what, in their judgement, is essential, what is important, what is new, what is currently irrelevant and what frankly has been proved wrong. This is what expertise is about.

Thus, in the present volume we try to present an overview of the psychiatric 'terrain' as it is currently perceived by a wide range of specialists with acknowledged expertise. With this edition, the Companion retains its claim to the shorthand name by which it has become affectionately known – the 'Edinburgh' textbook, as the majority of contributors are still clinicians and researchers working in Edinburgh. We are particularly grateful however to those with only tenuous (or no) links to the city who nonetheless willingly agreed to participate – such as David Cooke, Else Guthrie, Phil Harrison-Read, Stephen Hart, Peter McKenna, Anne Rogers and Peter Tyrer. However, the contents and sources of the book have no geographic or national boundaries, and the material should be of interest throughout the English language world. The book should be of particular value to those starting off in psychiatric practice and especially to students studying for the Membership examination of the UK Royal College of Psychiatrists. We would be disappointed, however, if this were its only audience, for we believe it should be of value to others interested in clinical psychiatry, including clinical psychologists, neuroscientists, clinical pharmacists and psychiatric nurses – and trust it will also provide a useful up-to-date source for those more mature psychiatrists confronting a moment of professional intimidation!

Those familiar with previous editions will notice that this one has received a bit of a facelift. This has resulted from a wish to enliven the presentation, to focus where possible, while keeping costs low. The burden of editorship has also been more widely spread, reflecting an increasing need to harness the varied expertise of the broad church psychiatry now is. Inevitably some shift of emphasis will also be evident from the previous edition, as psychiatry is more than ever a specialty on the move. We have reintroduced several topics omitted from the sixth edition (such as Sociology and Social Influences and Sleep Disorders) and have dropped some given an airing previously (e.g. Disorders Specific to Women). In line with the zeitgeist, evidence-based principles have been introduced along with a number of appropriate web links. We are grateful to those contributors to the previous edition who have, with good grace, redone their efforts for the present one and welcome several contributing for the first time.

As the preface to the previous edition noted, the latest advances tend to seem more exciting than those viewed from a distance, but once again we can (we think!) genuinely present areas where our knowledge base has extended since the last edition six years ago – in basic neuroscience, in genetics, and perhaps especially in neuroimaging, particularly functional imaging, where developments in analysis are allowing us to unlock ever more information about some of our most challenging disorders. In other areas things have perhaps been more static, a comment that might most pertinently apply to psychopharmacology, where distance is now allowing a more measured appraisal of the past decade's developments. But psychiatry is a specialty in which practice innovation tends anyway to be evolutionary rather than revolutionary and although much of our increasing knowledge remains to be adapted into practical innovations in patient care, our greatest wish is that the reader will find in the following pages examples of those tried and tested practice principles that form the foundations of good clinical care. For it is in this that the true mark of psychiatric expertise should be found.

The present volume tends to the use of the male pronoun, unless otherwise stated. This merely reflects ease of presentation rather than any systematic editorial bias.

Edinburgh, 2004

E.C.J.
D.G.C.O.
S.M.L.
M.S.
C.P.L.F.

Contributors

Neil H Anderson MB ChB MRCPsych
Consultant Psychiatrist, Royal Edinburgh Hospital; Honorary Senior Lecturer, Dementia Services Development Centre, University of Stirling, Stirling, UK

Gordon Arbuthnott BSc PhD
Honorary Professor, Division of Neuroscience, University of Edinburgh, Edinburgh, UK

Jeanne E Bell MD FRCPath FRSE FMed Sci
Professor of Neuropathology, Division of Pathology, Western General Hospital, Edinburgh, UK

Douglas Blackwood MB ChB PHD FRCP FRCPsych
Professor of Psychiatric Genetics and Honorary Consultant Psychiatrist, University of Edinburgh, Edinburgh, UK

Tom Brown MB MPhil MRCP MRCPsych
Consultant Liaison Psychiatrist, Trust Headquarters, College of Nursing, Stobhill Hospital, Glasgow, UK

Malcolm Bruce MB ChB FRCPsych PhD
Consultant Psychiatrist in Addiction, Royal Edinburgh Hospital, Edinburgh, UK

Roch Cantwell MB MRCPsych
Consultant Perinatal Psychiatrist and Honorary Senior Lecturer, Section of Psychological Medicine, University of Glasgow, Gartnavel Royal Hospital, Glasgow, UK

Alan J Carson MB ChB MPhil MRCPsych MD
Consultant Neuropsychiatrist, Royal Edinburgh Hospital and Western General Hospital; Part-time Senior Lecturer, University of Edinburgh, Edinburgh, UK

Jonathan Cavanagh MB ChB MPhil MD MRCPsych
Senior Lecturer in Psychiatry and Honorary Consultant Psychiatrist, University of Glasgow, Glasgow, UK

Derek Chiswick MB MPhil FRCPsych
Consultant Forensic Psychiatrist, Royal Edinburgh Hospital; Honorary Clinical Senior Lecturer, University of Edinburgh, Edinburgh, UK

David J Cooke BSc MSc PhD FBPsS FRSE CPsychol (Clinical & Forensic)
Professor of Forensic Psychology, Glasgow Caledonian University; Consultant Clinical Psychologist, Douglas Inch Centre, Glasgow, UK

John H M Crichton BMedSci BM BS PhD MRCPsych
Consultant Forensic Psychiatrist, Royal Edinburgh Hospital; Honorary Fellow in Law, University of Edinburgh, Edinburgh, UK

David G Cunningham Owens MD(Hons) FRCP FRCPsych
Reader in Psychiatry and Honorary Consultant Psychiatrist, University Department of Psychiatry, Royal Edinburgh Hospital, Edinburgh, UK

Richard J Davenport DM FRCP(E)
Consultant Neurologist, Royal Infirmary of Edinburgh and Western General Hospital, Edinburgh, UK

Christopher P L Freeman MB ChB MPhil FRCPsych
Consultant Psychotherapist, Royal Edinburgh Hospital; Senior Lecturer, Department of Psychiatry, University of Edinburgh, UK

John R Geddes MD FRCPsych
Professor of Epidemiological Psychiatry, Department of Psychiatry, University of Oxford, Oxford, UK

Guy M Goodwin MA DPhil BM MCh FRCPsych
W A Handley Professor of Psychiatry, University Department, Warneford Hospital, Oxford, UK

Elspeth Guthrie MB ChB MSc MD MRCPsych
Professor of Psychological Medicine and Medical Psychotherapy, University of Manchester, Manchester Royal Infirmary, Manchester, UK

Phil Harrison-Read BSc MB BS PhD FRCPsych
Consultant Psychiatrist, North Camden Mental Health Service, Royal Free Hospital, London, UK

Stephen D Hart PhD
Professor, Department of Psychology, Simon Fraser University, Burnaby, Canada, and Faculty of Psychology, University of Bergen, Bergen, Norway

Peter Hoare DM FRCPsych
Senior Lecturer, University of Edinburgh; Honorary Consultant Psychiatrist, Royal Hospital for Sick Children, Edinburgh, UK

Alan Jacques BSc MB BCh FRCPsych
Formerly Medical Commissioner, Mental Welfare Commission for Scotland, Edinburgh, UK

Eve C Johnstone CBE MD FRCP (Glasgow and Edinburgh) FRCPsych
Professor of Psychiatry and Head of the Department of Psychiatry, University of Edinburgh, UK

Robert E Kendell CBE MD FRCP FRCPsych (deceased)
Formerly Chief Medical Officer, Scottish Office Home and Health Department; Formerly Professor of Psychiatry, University of Edinburgh, Edinburgh, UK

Stephen M Lawrie MD(Hons) MRCPsych MPhil
Senior Research Fellow, University Department of Psychiatry, Edinburgh, UK

Siobhan MacHale MB MRCP(I) MPhil MRCPsych
Consultant Liaison Psychiatrist, Department of Psychological Medicine, Royal Infirmary of Edinburgh, Edinburgh, UK

Andrew M McIntosh BSc MB ChB MPhil MRCPsych
MRC Research Fellow, Division of Psychiatry, University of Edinburgh, Royal Edinburgh Hospital, Edinburgh, UK

Peter J McKenna MD (Oxon) MB ChB MRCPsych
Consultant Psychiatrist, Fulbourn Hospital, Cambridge, UK

George Masterton MSc MD FRCPsych FRCP(Edin)
Consultant Psychiatrist, Royal Infirmary of Edinburgh, Edinburgh, UK

Walter J Muir BSc (Hons) MRCPsych
Reader in the Psychiatry of Learning Disability, Division of Psychiatry,
School of Molecular and Clinical Medicine, University of Edinburgh;
Honorary Consultant Psychiatrist, Royal Edinburgh Hospital,
Edinburgh, UK

Ronan O'Carroll BSc MPhil PhD
Professor of Psychology, University of Stirling, Stirling, UK

Stephen Potts MA BM BCh MRCPsych
Consultant in Liaison Psychiatry, Department of Psychological
Medicine, Royal Infirmary of Edinburgh; Honorary Senior Clinical
Lecturer, Department of Psychiatry, University of Edinburgh,
Edinburgh, UK

Michael J Power BSc DPhil MSc
Professor of Clinical Psychology, University of Edinburgh; Consultant
Clinical Psychologist, Royal Edinburgh Hospital, Edinburgh, UK

Ian C Reid MB ChB BMed Biol PhD MRCPsych
Head of Psychiatry Department, University of Dundee, Dundee, UK

Bruce Ritson MD FRCP(E) FRCPsych
Honorary Fellow, Department of Psychiatry, University of Edinburgh;
Former Senior Lecturer and Clinical Director, University of Edinburgh,
Royal Edinburgh Hospital, Edinburgh, UK

Anne Rogers BA(Hons) Social Science MSc(Econ) Sociology as applied to medicine
PhD (Sociology and Social Administration)
Professor of the Sociology of Health Care, School of Primary Care,
University of Manchester, Manchester, UK

Peter Sandercock MA DM FRCPE FMed Sci
Professor of Medical Neurology and Honorary Consultant Neurologist,
Department of Clinical Neurosciences, Western General Hospital,
Edinburgh, UK

David M Semple MB ChB MRCPsych
Lecturer in Psychiatry and Honorary Specialist Registrar, University of
Edinburgh, Royal Edinburgh Hospital, Edinburgh, UK

Michael Sharpe MA MD FRCP MRCPsych
Professor of Psychological Medicine and Symptoms Research, University
of Edinburgh Division of Psychiatry, Royal Edinburgh Hospital,
Edinburgh, UK

Douglas Steele MB ChB BSc PhD MIPEM MRCPsych
Lecturer in Psychiatry, University of Edinburgh; Honorary Specialist
Registrar in Psychiatry, Royal Edinburgh Hospital, Edinburgh, UK

Gary Scot Stevenson BSc MB ChB MRCPsych MPhil DipFMSA
Consultant Psychiatrist, Stratheden Hospital, Cupar, Fife, UK

Lindsay D G Thomson MB ChB MRCPsych MPhil MD
Senior Lecturer in Forensic Psychiatry, University of Edinburgh;
Honorary Consultant Forensic Psychiatrist, The State Hospital,
Carstairs, UK

Peter Tyrer MD FRCP FRCPsych FFPHM FMedSoc
Professor of Community Psychiatry, St Mary's NHS Trust, London, UK

Adam Zeman MA BM BCh MRCP DM
Consultant Neurologist and Part-time Lecturer, Division of Clinical
Neurosciences, Western General Hospital, Edinburgh, UK

Contents

1

A brief introduction to the history of psychiatry

Eve C Johnstone

EARLY CONCEPTS

Psychiatric disorders have a long history. Early Egyptian papyri contain references to mental disturbances, and cases of mental disorder (affecting, for example, Saul, David and Nebuchadnezzar) are recorded in the Old Testament. Mental disorders received extensive discussion in Ancient Greek medical texts, and authors such as Hippocrates (Jones 1972) and Aretaeus (Adams 1856) appeared to regard mental illnesses as having bodily causes and as requiring medical treatment. The concept of melancholia as described by Aretaeus has obvious similarities to our current concept of severe depressive illness, and the link between morbid depression and morbid elevation of mood was clearly appreciated at that time:

> And yet in certain of these cases there is mere anger and grief and sad dejection of mind . . . those affected with melancholy are not every one of them affected according to one particular form but they are either suspicious of poisoning or flee to the desert from misanthropy or turn superstitious or contract a hatred of life. Or if at any time a relaxation takes place, in most cases hilarity supervenes. The patients are dull or stern, dejected or unreasonably torpid. . . . They also become peevish, dispirited and start up from a disturbed sleep.

Nonetheless, while it is possible, and perhaps appealing, to link such descriptions over gaps of centuries, it is important to recognise that the conceptual framework within which psychopathological descriptions have been set has changed greatly over the years. The meanings ascribed to terms used for describing diagnostic concepts and behaviours may vary considerably from time to time, so that the assumption that terms such as 'mania', 'melancholia' and 'hypochondria' mean the same now as they did even two centuries ago may not be justified and any parallel with more ancient times is appropriately the work of professional historians (Berrios & Porter 1995).

Whether or not the syndromes that were described in the ancient world closely resemble those which we see now, it is evident that mental disorders have been studied since Graeco-Roman times. The work ascribed to Hippocrates (4th century BC) was followed by that of Celsus, Aretaeus and Galen, writing in the 1st and 2nd centuries AD. The heritage of Graeco-Roman times was developed by Arab scientists, notably Avicenna, the Persian physician who, in the 11th century, developed Galen's ideas in his *Canon of Medicine*. A brief summary of what is known of Indo-European understanding of psychiatry from ancient times until the 18th century is given in Table 1.1.

THE MIDDLE AGES TO THE MODERN ERA

Universities in which medical subjects were taught were set up in Europe from the 13th century, and some development of these ideas continued. However, ideas that mental disorder was a spiritual rather than a medical problem were prominent throughout the Middle Ages, the mentally ill being thought of as possessed by the Devil or practitioners of witchcraft (Sprenger & Kramer 1486). Lunacy legislation in England dates from 1320, when it was enacted during the reign of Edward II that the property of lunatics should be vested in the Crown. Bethlem, the first hospital in the British Isles to care for the insane, was founded in 1247 as a priory of the Order of the Star of Bethlem. The humoral tradition of the Greeks was maintained in Europe, and detailed accounts from this point of view were written in French and in English, most notably by Robert Burton in his *Anatomy of Melancholy* (Burton 1621).

Sydenham's (1696) work was a turning point on the road towards modern psychiatry, as well as to modern medicine as a whole. In the ancient world symptoms and signs, e.g. fever, asthma, rashes, joint pains, were themselves regarded as diseases to be studied separately, and it was really only with Sydenham's work that the idea of disease as a syndrome or constellation of symptoms having a characteristic prognosis became established. This laid the foundation for the rational diagnosis and classification of disease.

As far as psychiatry in Britain was concerned, the recurrent mental disorder suffered by King George III in the 18th century had the benefit of arousing public interest. The controversies provoked by the differences of opinion between those called upon to treat the King led to the decision by the House of Lords to appoint a committee to institute a detailed enquiry. This provided consideration not only of the treatment of the King's illness but also of the care of the mentally ill throughout the country (Henderson & Batchelor 1962).

THE MODERN ERA — THE 18TH CENTURY TO THE PRESENT DAY

The main developments in psychiatry in the Western world from the 18th century until the present time are summarised in Table 1.2.

The first major development was the period of humane reform. Philippe Pinel working at the Bicêtre Hospital in Paris wrote extensively on psychiatric subjects (Pinel 1801, 1806) and

Table 1.1   Ancient times until 18th century

Time period	State of knowledge	Notable relevant events	Individuals of note
1500 BC until 2nd century BC	Reference to mental disorders in Egyptian papyri 1500 BC and in Old Testament Greek physicians 4th century BC → 2nd century AD classify mental disorders and consider them to be bodily conditions requiring medical treatment Relationship between melancholia and elevated mood described by Aretaeus		Hippocrates (Greek) 4th century BC Aretaeus (Cappadocian) 2nd century AD
2nd → 12th century AD	Graeco-Roman ideas developed by Arab scientists, notably Avicenna author of *Canon of Medicine*		Avicenna (Persian) 11th century; Trotula of Salerno (Italian) 12th century
13th → 18th century AD	Ideas that mental disorder was a spiritual rather than a medical matter prominent throughout the middle ages (Sprenger & Kramer 1486) Arguments of a medical kind were used against these ideas (Weyer 1564)	Universities in which medical subjects were taught set up in Europe from 13th century Bethlem 1st hospital in Britain to care for the insane founded 1247 1st Lunacy legislation in England in 1320 (property of lunatics to be vested in the Crown)	
	Idea of disease as a constellation of symptoms with a characteristic prognosis became established (Sydenham 1696)		Sir Thomas Sydenham (English) 17th century
		Recurrent mental disorder suffered by King George III and controversies surrounding his treatment led to appointment of Committee by House of Lords to consider the case not only of the King but of the mentally ill in general	Francis Willis (English) 18th century clergyman and provider of care for King George III when he was mentally ill

popularised methods of treatment involving non-restraint. So-called 'moral treatment' of the insane began in Britain in the Retreat at York, opened by the Quaker, William Tuke in 1796, and similar programmes of care were put into practice in the new lunatic asylums that were being built in the first half of the 19th century to replace the private madhouses, which had, until then, provided care for the mentally disordered. In Scotland in 1792, Andrew Duncan, Professor of Medicine at the University of Edinburgh, sponsored an appeal for funds to establish the Royal Edinburgh Mental Hospital which was opened in 1813.

The reforms begun by Tuke were followed by the introduction in 1808 of a Bill for the purpose of providing 'better care and maintenance of lunatics being paupers or criminals in England'. A series of amendments of the subsequent Act in 1811, 1815, 1819 and 1824 was followed by the established in 1845 of the Lunacy Commission, which later, in 1913, became organised as the Board of Control. The powers of this Board were dissolved in England at the time of the introduction of the Mental Health Act 1959, but were resurrected in 1983 in the form of the Mental Health Act Commission.

The development of academic psychiatry

European academic psychiatry began in France with the work of Pinel, who published his *Traité de la Manie* in 1801. It was in Germany, however, that psychiatry first became established as a subject for academic study in universities. Griesinger was appointed first Professor of Psychiatry and Neurology in Berlin in 1865 and developed a department for the study of mental disorders. This work involved clinical and pathophysiological research based upon the hypothesis that 'mental illness is a somatic illness of the brain' (Griesinger 1861).

With the development of academic departments, the study of psychiatric disorder began to flourish in Germany. The first important theme was the natural course of mental disorders as studied by Kahlbaum and Kraepelin. It was largely on the basis of these outcome studies that Kraepelin developed his comprehensive classification of mental illness which is the foundation of the schemes now in use throughout the world, such as ICD-10 (WHO 1992). Kraepelin, Professor of Psychiatry in Heidelberg, and later in Munich, wrote nine editions of his *Lehrbuch der*

Table 1.2 The modern era — 18th century until the present day

Time period	Areas of interest	Specific events or advances	Individuals of note
1790s–1830	Introduction of ideas of humane reform	Popularisation of methods of treatment involving non-restraint	Philippe Pinel (1801, 1806)
		Development of moral treatment of insanity notably in the Retreat in York	William Tuke (opened Retreat in 1796)
	Development of textbooks on psychiatry, lecture courses in psychiatry and the setting up of academic departments of psychiatry	Pinel's initial work developed by Esquirol who set up series of lectures in psychological medicine which formed model for lecture course set up in Edinburgh 1823	Jean Esquirol Sir Alexander Morison
		Chair of Mental Therapy set up in Leipzig 1811	
1830–1914	Development of the view that psychiatric illnesses are somatic disorders of the brain	Demonstration of pathology of general paralysis of the insane (Bayle 1822)	Wilhelm Griesinger (1861)
	Study of neuropathology in relation to progress of particular psychotic symptoms and signs	Pathological description of Wernicke's encephalopathy	Carl Wernicke (1881)
		Report of neurofibrillary tangles and plaques in 51-year-old woman with cognitive impairment	Alois Alzheimer (1897)
	Hereditary issues and developmental theories	Idea that mental illness affecting one generation could be passed on to the next in ever worsening degree (degeneration theory)	Benedict A Morel (1860)
		Such ideas influenced Sir Thomas Clouston and led on to his ideas of developmental insanity	Sir Thomas Clouston (1891)
	Development of psychoanalytic theories	Initially studying cases of hysteria using hypnosis, Sigmund Freud began to develop the technique of psychoanalysis which was later used to explain the psychological causes of symptoms	Sigmund Freud (Breuer & Freud 1895, Freud 1915, 1916) Carl Jung (1916) Alfred Adler (1912) Pierre Janet (1903)
		Emphasis given to the unconscious mind and to sexual motives.	
		Formed International Psychoanalytic Association with members, including Adler, Jung, Bleuler & Ferenczi. Adler & Jung later formed their own movements	
	Study of the natural course of psychiatric illness leading to coherent classifications on which modern classifications are based	Descriptive accounts of syndromes, e.g. of hebephrenia by Hecker (1871), catatonia by Kahlbaum (1874), folie circulaire by Falret and Baillarger (Sedler 1983) led to coherent system of classification devised by Kraepelin and developed in nine editions of his textbook *Lehrbuch der Psychiatrie* (1883–1927)	Emil Kraepelin, Professor of Psychiatry in Heidelberg & Munich
	First interest in issue that exposure to untoward events could cause nervous symptoms, developed in relation to compensation claims following railway accidents	Controversy between those holding that the complaints had a physical cause (e.g. possible pin-point haemorrhage (Erichsen 1866, Oppenheim 1889) and those who considered that the symptoms resulted from the effects on the mind. This was the background against which later controversies over 'shell shock' developed	
1914–1947	The First World War and issues relating to shell shock	157 cases of shell shock diagnosed among 523 cases of functional nervous disorder by December 1914 but this became much more common by 1916	William H R Rivers (1923) of Craiglockhart War Hospital
		Controversy as to whether there was an organic basis for this (Mott 1916) or was a form of malingering (War Office 1922).	
		Military authorities considered distinction between intentional and non-intentional symptoms of vital importance (Myers 1915).	

(Continued)

Table 1.2 Continued

Time period	Areas of interest	Specific events or advances	Individuals of note
		Cowardice and desertion were capital offences in British Army during First World War. The numbers (16 138 cases of functional nervous disorder in the 6 months following the Battle of the Somme) meant that the distinction between neuropathologically and emotionally based disorders was not tenable (Brown 1995). Neurasthenia and related conditions were accepted as disorders for which military pensions could be drawn (Macpherson et al 1923). Psychological illness was recognised, and it was appreciated by the general public as well as military and medical authorities that stress could produce such disorders (Riggs 1922)	
	Early development of neuroimaging	Pneumo-encephalography developed by American neurosurgeon, Dandy, in 1919 and used first to investigate patients with schizophrenia by Jacobi & Winkler (1927)	
	Expansion of psychiatric facilities and development of their services and standards	Opening of Maudsley Hospital. Development of academic departments of psychiatry, first in Britain opened in Edinburgh in 1919. The views of Adolph Meyer, who emphasised the need for an eclectic approach combining physical, social and psychological aspects, were influential	Sir Aubrey Kewis (London) Sir David Henderson (Edinburgh)
	Development of new forms of physical treatment	Insulin coma introduced (Sakel 1938) initially for drug addiction, but later widely used for schizophrenia (Sakel 1952, Ackner et al 1957). Convulsive treatment introduced by Cerletti & Bini (1938) initially for schizophrenia, but more widely used for severe depressive illness. Psychosurgery introduced by Moniz in 1935	
1948–present day	Setting up of the National Health Service in Britain	This provided a comprehensive system of general practice allowing early treatment and permitting many milder cases of psychiatric disorder to be treated entirely in general practice. In addition it enabled large cohort studies to be conducted and provided a background for the conduct of investigations in biological and social psychiatry	John Wing (Institute of Psychiatry)
	Development of the antipsychiatry movement	Antipsychiatry is essentially the belief in the sociogenesis of severe mental illness, particularly schizophrenia. It had some popularity in Europe and in the USA in 1960s and early 70s	Ronald D Laing (1960) UK Thomas Szasz (1961) USA Franco Basaglia (1979) Italy
	Development of effective psycho-pharmacological agents and methods of understanding their mechanisms of action	Lithium, the first effective mood stabiliser, was introduced into psychiatric practice in 1949. Antipsychotic effects of chlorpromazine appreciated in early 1950s. MAOIs introduced in 1957 and tricyclics in 1958. Mechanisms of action of antidepressants and antipsychotics understood in 1960s	John Cade Delay & Deniker (1952) Arvid Carlsson (1963)
	Development of non-invasive methods of brain imaging	Structural imaging (CT & MRI) emission tomography and later functional MRI could be used to compare subjects and controls, demonstrating the biology of psychiatric disorders and, with fMRI, of psychological processes	Godfrey Hounsfield (1973)

Psychiatrie, published between 1883 and 1927. He was concerned to move away from the earlier 19th-century nosological concepts which he criticised as unreliable from a clinical, and especially prognostic, point of view (Hoff 1995). In the fifth and sixth (Kraepelin 1883–1927) editions he developed the concept of dementia praecox (later more commonly known by Eugen

Bleuler's term of schizophrenia) and its separation, with a poor prognosis, from manic–depressive insanity, with a good, or at least a better, prognosis. In defining dementia praecox he had drawn together hebephrenia as described by Hecker (1871), catatonia as described by Kahlbaum (1874) and his own dementia paranoides, regarding them as manifestations of the same disorder which typically had its onset in early adult life and had a poor outcome.

A further major theme concerned the relationship of mental disorder to brain pathology. Griesinger's ideas had stimulated this area of work, but it was greatly encouraged by the progress that was being made in identifying pathological lesions in neurological disorders: for example, general paralysis of the insane which had been described by Bayle (1822) under the title 'arachnitis chronique'. Neuropathological approaches to dementia were also successful. In 1881, Wernicke published a description of the encephalopathy which was named after him, and Alzheimer in 1907 reported neurofibrillary tangles, plaques and other changes in a 51-year-old woman with cognitive impairment and psychotic features.

A further theme of early research concerned hereditary issues. This developed from the work of Morel (1860), who proposed what came to be known as the theory of degeneration. He had suggested an aetiological rather than a symptomatic classification, and emphasised hereditary issues. Although hereditary taint had been mentioned in relation to insanity before this time, it was highlighted by Morel's work. His degeneration theory involved the idea that mental illness affecting one generation could be passed on to the next, in ever worsening degree. Two mechanisms were thought to be involved: transmission and degradation of the tainted seed (Berrios & Bear 1995). As the hereditary taint was thought not only to be behavioural but also physical, stigmata of degeneration, such as deformed teeth, ears, head, etc. were assessed (Talbot 1898). The notion that behaviours such as alcohol abuse and masturbation could promote degeneration was included in the general theory.

These ideas influenced Sir Thomas Clouston (1890), who in addition put forward the concept of developmental insanity and considered that the results of his investigations of palatal structure in adolescent insanity (which he saw as being part of Kraepelin's disease entity of dementia praecox) demonstrated that this disorder represented a form of developmental defect of ectodermal tissue (Clouston 1891).

The moral and religious overtones of the degeneration theory seemed increasingly inappropriate by the end of the 19th century. It was partly as a reaction to the pessimistic and unsympathetic view of the mentally ill put forward by the degeneration theories that an increasing interest in psychological causes of mental disorder developed from the end of the 19th century.

Psychoanalytic theories

Sigmund Freud began his career in neurological research and visited Charcot in Paris with a view to learning about the use of hypnotism in cases of hysteria. He developed the alternative method of free association in which patients were encouraged to speak without distraction about what was in their mind. Although initially intended as a treatment, Freud used this technique to develop an understanding of the psychological causes of these disorders. He went on to develop his own theories, which included ideas concerning the importance of childhood experience in the behaviour of adults and the part played by the unconscious and irrational parts of the mind in influencing behaviour. He gave emphasis to sexual motives as determinants of symptomatology. Other prominent figures in this field at that time were Karl Jung, Alfred Adler and Eugen Bleuler. The French psychiatrist Pierre Janet was also concerned with psychological causes of mental disorder and shared with Freud concepts of the unconscious mind and of mental forces, but saw recent rather than childhood experiences as important in the causation of neurotic illness.

The effects of the first world war

Interest in the idea that exposure to untoward events could cause nervous symptoms developed during the second half of the 19th century in relation to compensation claims following railway accidents. There was controversy as to whether the complaints of affected individuals had a physical cause with resultant effects upon the mind. It was against this background that cases of 'shell shock' began to be diagnosed in the First World War. Details are given in Table 1.2. The importance of these events from the point of view of the generality of the population over the last 90 or so years, has been that these circumstances led to a recognition of psychological illness and to the acceptance in the general public as well as among military and medical authorities of the idea that overwhelming stress could produce illness, even in soldiers whose bravery had been recognised by military decorations. Psychological explanations of war neurosis were accepted to such a degree that they were used as a paradigm for the explanation of neurosis in general in popular work (Riggs 1922).

The 1920s to the present day

After the First World War, there was an expansion of psychiatric facilities and a broadening of their scope. The Maudsley Hospital, with its emphasis on teaching, research and early treatment, was opened. Academic Departments of Psychiatry were set up and began to develop outpatient clinics for the treatment of milder disorders, and child guidance clinics were set up. The development of pneumoencephalography in 1919 meant that it became possible to examine the brain during life. In the 1920s and 1930s, physical treatments which were believed to be effective were introduced. The first of these, malarial treatment for neurosyphilis, for which Julius Wagner-Jauregg received the Nobel Prize in 1927, was superseded by the introduction of antibiotics. Insulin coma too has fallen out of use but was, up until 1950, believed to be the treatment of choice for schizophrenia. Electroconvulsive therapy continues in use to a lesser extent, as does psychosurgery. After 1948, the pace of progress increased. The setting up of the National Health Service in Britain provided a comprehensive system of general practice. This meant that it was possible for illnesses to be detected at an early stage, so that many milder cases of psychiatric disorder could be treated entirely in general practice. In addition, the data collection systems set up in relation to the health service provided a background for the conduct of investigations in both biological and social psychiatry. Social psychiatry flourished at this time but was followed by the development of the antipsychiatry movement. Antipsychiatry is essentially the belief in the sociogenesis of severe mental illness, especially schizophrenia. This had some popularity in the UK, in other parts of Europe, especially Italy, and in the USA in the

1960s and early 1970s, but its influence thereafter waned against the background of developments of effective pharmacological agents and methods of investigating brain structure and function.

The 1950s are sometimes described as the 'golden decade' for psychopharmacology because it was at that time that the first effective mood stabilisers (in the form of lithium salts), the first effective antipsychotic drugs (the prototype being chlorpromazine) and the first effective antidepressants (both MAOIs and tricyclics) were introduced. All of these treatments were introduced on an empirical basis, but their effects on patient care have been far reaching. In addition, the fact that pharmacological treatments, which have measurable modes of action in physiological terms, can have effects upon psychiatric illness may be taken as evidence that these disorders do have a basis in physiological dysfunction. It is clearly possible that understanding of the mode of action of an effective treatment will give information about the biological basis of the condition that it relieves. Much research in this area has been conducted over the past 40 years, and well-accepted theories of the pathogenesis of both schizophrenia and depressive illness initially relied heavily on the known pharmacological actions of effective treatment for these disorders (Schildkraut & Kety 1967, Snyder et al 1974). Increasingly sophisticated methods of examining receptor function and other indices of neurotransmission have further clarified the way in which these drugs provide the benefits that they have been clearly shown to have.

Pneumoencephalography, introduced by Dandy in 1919, is unpleasant and potentially dangerous, which meant that it could not be used in normal controls. The introduction by Hounsfield of computed tomography in 1973 meant that it became possible to examine the structure of the brain repeatedly in patients with psychiatric disorder and compare this with normal controls. In brain imaging, computed tomography has now been replaced by structural magnetic resonance imaging (MRI), while function can be examined by both emission tomography and, more recently, functional magnetic resonance imaging (fMRI). fMRI does not involve ionising radiation and thus can repeatedly be used.

The introduction of these methods, in particular of fMRI, has meant that it is possible to study mental events in health as well as in disease. The physiological reality of thoughts and actions can now clearly be demonstrated. This has meant that the search for an underlying morbid physical state for psychiatric disorders which was such a problem in diagnostic categorisation until the recent past (Schneider 1958, Kendell 1975) can pass into history (Weinberger 1995). These elements of progress were noted in the last edition. It is difficult at present to determine just exactly what progress there may have been since 1997. The increasingly clear findings from functional imaging seem important, although we await the judgement of time.

Another important step perhaps relates to 'evidence-based' medicine, though the techniques of meta-analyses and systematic review can only provide so much help in psychiatry. As yet, there simply is not adequate evidence. One clear benefit of these techniques, however, is the fact that idiosyncratic and uneven analyses of the available evidence should no longer be acceptable. Clear information about the basis upon which plans of management are suggested is more widely available, not only to health service staff, but also to the patients themselves.

This brief account is intended to provide a historical setting for the chapters which follow. Further information can be found in the detailed scholarly works listed below.

FURTHER READING

Berrios G E, Porter R 1995 A history of clinical psychiatry: the origin and history of psychiatric disorders. Athlone Press, London
Porter R 2002 Madness: a brief history. Oxford University Press, Oxford
Shorter E 1997 A history of psychiatry: from the era of the asylum to the age of prozac. John Wiley, New York

REFERENCES

Ackner B, Harris A, Oldham AT 1957 Insulin treatment of schizophrenia: a controlled study. Lancet i: 607–611
Adams F 1856 The extant works of Aretaeus the Cappadocian. Sydenham Society, London
Adler A 1912 The nervous character. J F Bergmann, Wiesbaden
Alzheimer A 1897 Beitrage zur pathologischen Anatomie der Hirnrinde und zur anatomischen Grundlage der Psychosen. Monatsschrift für Psychiatrie und Neurologie 2: 8–120
Alzheimer A 1907 Uber eine eigenartige Erkrankung der Hirnrinde. Allegemeine Zeitschrift für Psychiatrie und Psychisch-Gerichtlich Medizine 64: 146–148
Basaglia F 1979 A psiquiatria alternativa: contra o pessimismo da razao, o otimismo da pratica: conferencias no Brasil. Brasil Debates, San Paulo
Bayle A L J 1822 Recherches sur les maladies mentales. Medical thesis.
Berrios G, Porter R 1995 Introduction. In: Berrios G, Porter R (eds) A history of clinical psychiatry. Athlone Press, London
Berrios G E, Bear D 1995 Unitary psychosis concept. In: Berrios G, Porter R (eds) A history of clinical psychiatry. Athlone Press, London
Breuer J, Freud S 1895 Studien über Hysterie. Franz Deuticke, Leipzig
Brown E M 1995 Post-traumatic stress disoder and shell shock. In: Berrios G, Porter R (eds) A history of clinical psychiatry. Athlone Press, London
Burton R 1621 The anatomy of melancholy: what it is. Henry Cripps
Carlsson A, Lindqvist M 1963 Effect of chlorpromazine and haloperidol on formation of 3-methoxy-tyramine and normetanephrine in mouse brain. Acta Pharmacologica et Toxicologica 20: 140–144
Cerletti U, Bini L 1938 L'elettroshock. Archives of General Neurology & Psychiatry, Psychoanalysis 19: 266
Clouston T S 1890 Clinical lectures on mental diseases, 6th edn. Churchill, London
Clouston T S 1891 The neuroses of development being the Morison Lectures for 1890. Oliver & Boyd, Edinburgh
Dandy W E 1919 Roentgenography of the brain after injection of air into the cerebral ventricles. American Journal of Roentgenography 6: 26
Delay J, Deniker P 1952 Le traitment des psychoses par une méthode neuroleptique derivée de l'hibernothérapie. In: Delay J, Deniker P (eds) Congrès de Médecines Aliénistes et neurologistes de France. Masson Editeurs Libraires de L'Academie de Médecine, Paris
Erichsen J E 1866 On railway and other injuries of the nervous system. Lea, Philadelphia
Freud S 1915 Introductory lectures on psycho-analysis (Parts I & II) 1915–1916. Trans by James Strachey 1963. Hogarth Press, London
Freud S 1916 Introductory lectures on psychoanalysis (Part III) 1916–1917. Trans by James Strachey 1963. Hogarth Press, London
Griesinger W 1861 Die Pathologie und Therapie der psychischen Krankheiten, 1st edn 1845. Krabbe, Stuttgart
Hecker E 1871 Die Hebephrenie: Ein Beitrag zur klinischen Psychiatrie. Archiv für pathologischen Anatomie und Physiologie und für klinische Medizin 52: 394–429
Henderson D, Batchelor I R C 1962 Henderson & Gillespie's textbook of psychiatry. Oxford University Press, London
Hoff P 1995 Kraepelin. In: Berrios G, Porter R (eds) A history of clinical psychiatry, Athlone Press, London
Hounsfield G N 1973 Computerized transverse axial scanning (tomography), 1: Description of system. British Journal of Radiology 46: 1016–1022
Jacobi W, Winkler H 1927 Encephalographische studien an chronisch schizophrenen. Archiv für Psychiatrie und Nervenkrankheiten 81: 299–332

Janet P 1903 Obsessive behaviour: neurasthenia. Félix Alcan, Paris

Jones W (trans) 1972 Works of Hippocrates. Loeb Classical Library. Heinemann, London

Jung C G 1916 Psychology of the unconscious: a study of the transformations and symbolisms of the libido; a contribution to the history of the evolution of thought. Moffat, Yard & Co, London

Kahlbaum K L 1874 Die Katatonie onder das Spannungirresein: Eine Klinische Form psychischer Krankheit. Hirschwald, Berlin

Kendell R E 1975 The role of diagnosis in psychiatry. Blackwell, Oxford

Kraepelin E 1883–1927 Lehrbuch der Psychiatrie, nine editions. Abel, Leipzig (1883, 1887, 1889, 1893); Barth, Leipzig (1896, 1899 2 vols; 1903, 1904 2 vols; 1909, 1910, 1913, 1915 4 vols; 1927 2 vols)

Laing R D 1960 The divided self: a study of sanity and madness. Tavistock, London

Macpherson W G, Herringham W P, Elliott T R, Balfour A 1923 History of the great war medical services. Diseases of war. HMSO, London

Morel B A 1860 Traité des maladies mentales. Masson, Paris

Mott F W 1916 Special discussion on shell shock without visible signs of injury. Proceedings of the Royal Society of Medicine part III (suppl 9):1–44

Myers C S 1915 A contribution to the study of shell shock. Lancet i:316–320

Oppenheim H 1889 Die traumatischen Neurosen. Hirschwald, Berlin

Pinel P 1801 Traité medico philosophique sur l'alienation mentale ou la manie. Caille & Ravier, Paris

Pinel P 1806 A treatise on insanity. Davis D D (trans). Cadell & Davies, Sheffield

Riggs A F 1922 Just nerves. Houghton Mifflin, Boston

Rivers W H R 1923 Conflict and dream. Kegan Paul, London

Sakel M 1952 Insulinotherapy and shock therapies. Congress on Psychiatry 1950, 4: 163

Sakel M 1938 The pharmacological shock treatment of schizophrenia. Nervous and mental diseases monograph series no 62. Nervous & Mental Disease Publication Co, New York

Schildkraut J J, Kety S S 1967 Biogenic amines and emotion. Science 156: 21–37

Schneider K 1950 Die psychopathischen Personlichkeiten. Hamilton MW (trans). 9th edn 1958. Cassell, London

Sedler M J 1983 Falret's discovery: the origin of the concept of bipolar affective illness. American Journal of Psychiatry 140: 1127–1133

Snyder S H, Banerjee S P, Yamamura H I, Greenberg D 1974 Drugs, neurotransmitters and schizophrenia. Science 184: 1243–1253

Sprenger J, Kramer H 1486 Malleus maleficarium – the hammer of witchcraft, second part, question two, chapter V, Prescribed remedies for those who are obsessed owing to some spell. Summers M. (trans) 1968. Folio Society, London

Sydenham I 1696 The whole works of that excellent physician Dr Thomas Sydenham. Pechy J (trans). Richard Wellington & Edward Castle, London

Szasz T S 1961 The myth of mental illness: foundations of a theory of personal conduct. Harper & Row, New York

Talbot E S 1898 Degeneracy: its causes, signs and results. Walter Scott, London

War Office 1922 Report of the War Office committee on enquiry into 'shell shock'. HMSO, London

Weinberger D R 1995 Schizophrenia: from neuropathology to neurodevelopment. Lancet 346: 552–557

Wernicke C 1881 Lehrbuch der Gehirnkrankheiten für Arzte und Studierende I. Fischer, Berlin

Weyer J 1564 De praestigiis daemonium (On the trickery of demons). Cited in Trillat E 1995 Conversation disorder and hysteria. In: Berrios G, Porter R (eds) A history of clinical psychiatry. Athlone Press, London, p 433–450

World Health Organization 1992 The ICD-10 classification of mental and behavioural disorders: clinical descriptions and diagnostic guidelines. World Health Organization, Geneva

2 | Functional neuroanatomy

J Douglas Steele, Ian C Reid

INTRODUCTION

Neuroanatomy analyses the structure of the nervous system. The three-dimensional organisation of the central nervous system (descriptive anatomy) and its development during the individual's lifespan (developmental anatomy) provide the substrate for its function. Functional neuroanatomy needs to combine such structural knowledge with behavioural data. It puts anatomy into the context of the living organism, by asking not only 'How?', but also 'Why?' and 'To what purpose?' This chapter cannot give a systematic overview as would be provided by an anatomy atlas or a standard undergraduate textbook. We will rather try to focus on aspects of functional anatomy that are of relevance to the psychiatrist. We will use the more detailed discussion of a limited number of topics to illustrate important principles of the organisation of the central nervous system (CNS).

- For an introduction, we will discuss the research methods employed to link the anatomical substrate with behaviour. This will, we hope, allow the reader to see the inherent limitations of established 'knowledge'.
- The second part of the chapter will deal with the visual system, which is the most important sensory system in most humans. It will serve to illustrate the principles of neuronal organisation in achieving complex information processing.
- The third part will deal with the important frontosubcortical circuits underlying movement, cognition and affect. The emphasis is here on the circular nature of connections, which lead to the interaction of such diverse structures as the basal ganglia, the cerebellum and the frontal cortex.
- Part four deals with the limbic system, which is generally thought to be associated with motivations and emotions. The close interconnection of cognitive function, such as memory, with emotion, autonomic responses and automatic behavioural sequences will be demonstrated by pointing to the common anatomical substrates for these functions.
- The final section of the chapter will use a hybrid approach to anatomy, combining the pharmacology of transmitter substances with the anatomical distribution of these transmitter systems throughout the CNS in order to localise function.

It should be apparent by now that we are concerned with the investigation of brain–behaviour relationships, an exciting, fast-growing area that in our mind represents the essence of psychological medicine. It is just over 100 years ago that Fritsch and Hitzig, and a little later Herrick and Tite, electrically stimulated the brains of animals to demonstrate movements, much to the amazement of their peers. Today, the assumption that CNS function is specifically localised is a commonly held belief, that receives further growing support by new methods of investigation such as functional magnetic resonance imaging (fMRI) and transcranial magnetic stimulation.

THE METHODS OF FUNCTIONAL NEUROANATOMY

In order to relate CNS structure with function, clear and objective methods have to be developed to identify both the anatomical substrate and the functional correlate. The first task has been tackled in a variety of ways, using macroscopic anatomy, histology, pharmacology and neurochemistry. One system, that is still valid after 90 years, is Brodmann's classification of cortical areas according to the architecture of their cell layers. Primary sensory cortex, for example, receives large inputs from the thalamus, which end in layer 4, so that this layer is disproportionately thick. In primary motor cortex, layer 4 is relatively underdeveloped. Cortical architecture thus reflects functional variety, and Brodmann's system is still widely used, for example by researchers employing functional neuroimaging methods (Fig. 2.1).

Behavioural measures are generally more subjective, more difficult to quantify and to elicit in a reliable way. We are talking here of animal behaviour, reward driven learning or the performance of neuropsychological tests in humans. The localisation of function in humans has for a long time only been possible by examining patients with focal CNS lesions. The characterisation of such lesions was only possible postmortem. Recent advances in in vivo imaging methods have made it possible to pinpoint the site of such lesions within the millimetre range. Nevertheless, lesion studies have a number of limitations that make firm conclusion about brain–behaviour relationships difficult. The CNS is characterised by a high degree of connectivity. Any lesion is likely to affect function in remote areas, which can seriously limit the localising power of any clinical observations. Discrete subcortical lesions, for example, can result in widespread cortical underactivity and be associated with clinical depression or dementia (Grasso et al 1994, Tatemichi et al 1995). The natural history of lesions can further exaggerate (post-traumatic oedema) or reduce (plasticity) the impact of a focal disturbance at different times. Using a purely logical approach, focal lesions may identify structures necessary for a specific function, but these structures need not be sufficient for the performance of the function; in fact, they may only constitute a small link in the causal chain. The concepts of dissociation and double dissociation are often used to support

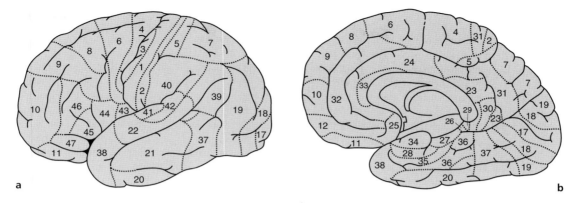

Fig. 2.1
The cytoarchitectural map of the cerebral cortex after Brodmann: (a) lateral surface; (b) medial surface.

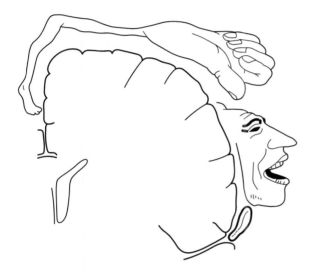

Fig. 2.2
The motor homunculus. (After Penfield & Rasmussen 1954.)

specific brain–behaviour relationships between certain localised lesions and psychological impairments. A *dissociation* between two types of psychological deficits is said to exist if one is associated with a particular lesion, but the other is not. *A double dissociation* is then found if two separate psychological deficits are each associated with their own specific lesion sites, and are not affected by lesions at the other site.

A more fine-grained method of localisation was used by Penfield & Rasmussen (1954), who used electrodes to stimulate the cortex of epileptic patients undergoing neurosurgery for the treatment of their illness. Their research resulted in the famous homunculi for the primary motor and sensory cortices (Fig. 2.2). While direct electrical stimulation gives meaningful results over primary sensorimotor cortex, the effects of stimulation over association or limbic cortex are more difficult to interpret. A further drawback of this method is that the subjects examined are of necessity epileptic patients, whose brain disease may have already resulted in functional changes. Finally, even contemporary criticism was based on the possibility of current spread to related pathways (Phillips et al 1984). As a major advance on intracranial stimulation, for the last 10 years it has been possible to stimulate superficial cortex,

using strong magnetic fields generated by a coil held over the head. This allows us to examine healthy volunteers (or indeed any patient group) and map primary sensorimotor function over the pre- and postcentral gyri with a spatial resolution of several millimetres. Such studies can, for example, track changes in the size of responsive neuronal areas in motor cortex with learning, and thus give a first-hand demonstration of neuronal plasticity. During the repeat performance of a complex serial reaction time task in one study, subjects performed faster with time (implicit learning), with motor cortical output maps for the muscles involved in the task covering an increasingly larger area. Once subjects became aware of the 'rules' of the task (explicit learning), motor output maps shrank to the original size (Pascual-Leone et al 1994).

The new methods of functional neuroimaging have revolutionised the investigation of brain–behaviour correlations (Ch. 5). Three strategies have been employed to quantify this relationship. Experiments can be designed in a modular manner; for example a verbal memory task is compared with a control task that contains all components, such as sensory input and motor response, except the memory task itself. The principle of this approach is that, by subtracting the two brain activity states, it is possible to isolate the anatomical substrate linked with memory function. Studies using this paradigm have generated a number of intriguing findings, such as deactivations of certain brain regions during tasks and reciprocal changes between certain regions (e.g. frontal and temporal cortex). A more sophisticated approach uses factorial designs, such as different drug treatments (or placebo) crossed with several different activation tasks, so that interactions between task and treatment can be observed. A further interesting example of such a factorial design involves the effect of time on cerebellar activation during a finger apposition task. During this task, which is used by pianists or guitarists as a finger exercise, all fingers of one hand have to touch the thumb of the same hand in succession. In untrained subjects, motor learning takes place over repeated trials. It is, in fact, the interaction between task and repeat performance that demonstrates the effect of learning. Such an effect can be observed in the cerebellum, i.e. with increasing practice the cerebellar activation becomes less pronounced. This may be caused by long-term depression, which has been observed in animals during motor learning and may involve synapses on apical dendrites of Purkinje cells in the neocerebellar cortex (Friston 1994). If the behaviour under study is quantifiable, a parametric design can be employed, which correlates, for example, performance measures during a task, or psychiatric symptom scores with brain activity. This assumes a linear relationship between symptoms or performance and brain activity, although all or nothing (modular), or other non-linear relationships can be modelled in principle. In addition to factorial and parametric designs, it is possible to examine the correlation between the activity of different brain areas during several activation procedures. Such inter-regional correlations can be interpreted as evidence of coordinated activity in functional neuronal networks. An example for this approach is given by Friston (1994). Principal components analysis of brain activity during a sequence of 12 alternating word generation and word shadowing tasks produced two main components. The first accounted for the experimentally introduced variability in brain activity (71% of the variability over the time of the experiment) and involved increases in anterior cingulate, left dorsolateral prefrontal cortex, Broca's area, thalamus and cerebellum, with decreases in both temporal lobes and posterior cingulate. The second component reflected change over time (maybe attentional change) and mainly involved anterior cingulate activity. Time series of scans with changing task conditions, therefore, provide a most powerful tool to unravel the co-operation of remote structures in the brain for achieving the tasks. Functional MRI, which can be repeated many times over, is likely to be the standard method used in such studies in the future.

The methods described so far have in common the fact that they can be applied to human subjects. Animal studies, particularly in other mammals, have provided and still do provide essential information on functional neuroanatomy, which cannot be generated from human studies. Among the most informative approaches in neuroscience have been in-vivo recording techniques. Electrodes are implanted very precisely into an area of interest, and spontaneous (single cell) neuronal activity during animal behaviour can be recorded. The spatial resolution of this method combined with postmortem confirmation of the electrode location is higher than any imaging mode has achieved so far, and information in the time domain is naturally superior. Recording, rather than stimulation, techniques avoid the problem of current spread (see above). Single-cell recording in frontal cortex can, for example, identify neurons that fire during a delay after presentation of a stimulus, which has to be compared with other stimuli later on. This method can therefore identify the 'neuronal working memory trace'. Some neurons fire depending on the spatial localisation of the stimulus, others depending on its shape or colour (Goldman-Racic 1995). Local neurotransmitter concentrations can be measured with an implanted probe that is equally able to deliver pharmacologically-active agents to a small region in the brain. Mechanical, chemical and thermal lesioning and ablation techniques have played an important part in identifying the functional roles of different brain regions. In contrast to clinical studies, the size and location of the lesion can be rigorously controlled, so that many of the limitations discussed earlier can be circumvented. Kainic acid is used as a non-specific neurotoxin to create localised lesions. For some transmitter systems, very specific toxins that are taken up only into one type of neuron and destroy it selectively, are available. An example is 1-methyl-4-phenyl-1,2,3,6-tetrahydropyridine (MPTP), a specific toxin of the nigrostriatal dopaminergic system, that has been used as a model of Parkinson's disease.

Postmortem, many methods are now available to explore the functional role of brain structures and systems. Brain slice preparations are used for electrophysiological and pharmacological experiments. Neurons belonging to specific transmitter systems can be tracked in their projections by certain neurochemical reactions, such as fluorescence of catecholaminergic and serotoninergic neurons. Immunohistochemistry provides in vitro markers for neurotransmitters, enzymes and other proteins; in-situ hybridisation allows for the localisation of specific mRNA. Axon transsection in vivo results in anterograde (Wallerian) degeneration; postmortem their course can be followed, for example using myelin staining. Locally applied markers, such as amino acids, fluorescent dyes or neurotoxins, are taken up into the axon and are transported in anterograde (proline/leucine) or retrograde (pseudorabies virus) directions. Some markers also bridge the synaptic cleft and allow for the tracing of projections beyond the original neuron (Cooper et al 1996). Receptor distributions can be mapped by radioactively labelled receptor ligands. After labelling, the brain is sectioned in a microtome, thin sections are apposed to sensitive film, and maps of radioactivity patterns are generated, which can be compared with the histology of the original brain slice (Fig. 2.3). Similar to positron emission tomography (PET) and single photon emission computerised tomography (SPECT), cerebral blood flow and metabolism can be measured and mapped by autoradiographic methods, which allow for the localisation of specific pharmacological effects.

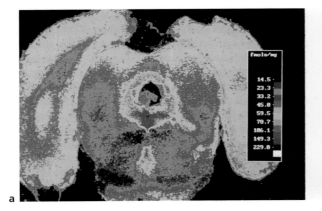
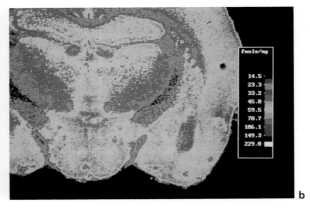

Fig. 2.3
Autoradiography of paroxetine-binding areas in the rat brain. High transporter binding in (a) central raphe and (b) hippocampus. (Reproduced with kind permission of Dr Judith K McQueen, MRC Brain Metabolism Unit, and Dr John Sharkey, Fujisawa Institute of Neuroscience.)

The most recent addition to the armamentarium of the functional anatomist is the generation of transgenic animals with specific localised abnormalities in brain proteins, such as receptors. 'Knockout' mice have been created, which miss the gene for the R1 subunit of the *N*-methyl-D-aspartate (NMDA) receptor specifically in CA1 pyramidal neurons of the hippocampus. These mice appear to show abnormalities in spatial memory (Morris & Morris 1997, Wilson & Tonegawa 1997).

Functional neuroanatomy is thus increasingly based on a large variety of complex analytic methods, which need to be integrated with clinical observation in order to achieve a balanced appreciation of brain function. It is self-evident that this chapter cannot be comprehensive: it reflects the clinical and scientific biases of the current and previous authors (since this chapter is an update of that in the previous edition). We hope, however, that our subjective selection will give the reader an appreciation of the principles involved in functional neuronal organisation and transmit some of the excitement of modern neuroscience.

PRINCIPLES OF FUNCTIONAL NEURAL ORGANISATION

This section considers the functional anatomy of information processing in the brain, using sensory systems in general and the visual system in particular as examples. We begin with a brief overview of the cortex and the general functional properties of sensory systems, and then turn in more detail to visual processing. Functionally relevant anatomical features are described, but the emphasis here is on how cellular arrangements process information, rather than on detailed discussion of structural anatomy. Some basic knowledge of neuroanatomy is assumed, but is not essential in order to follow the principles embodied in the aspects of neural processing described below. Structural anatomical detail can be found in relevant undergraduate textbooks. Although much of the information which follows has been derived from the study of the brains of cats and monkeys, it is likely that the principles described apply also in the human brain.

The cortex

The cerebral hemispheres consist of two large, thin, wrinkled sheets of cell bodies and their associated dendritic processes (cortex — grey matter) overlying myelinated (white matter) tracts. The hemispheres are connected by a white-matter tract, the corpus callosum. The wrinkles in the cortical sheet — sulci and gyri — indicate the extensive folding necessary to contain the remarkable processing power of the cortex within the limited confines of the skull. The gyral and sulcal pattern provides the basis of the division of the cortex into anatomical lobes, which in turn show some degree of functional specialisation. Folded under the neocortex and within the temporal lobe are important grey-matter structures, such as the hippocampus and amygdala, which will be discussed later when considering the limbic system.

Focusing in on the cortex, the cortical sheet is seen to have a laminar structure, consisting of six layers, numbered (top to bottom) from 1 to 6 — essentially a stack of six sheets (laminae), on average 2 mm thick, with layer 1 below the pial meningeal covering, and layer 6 above the white-matter tracts. The layers are made distinct by their variable composition of different cell types and cell processes, and the relative proportions of cells

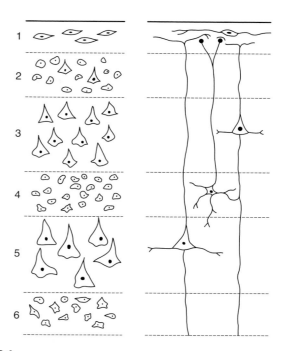

Fig. 2.4
Cellular layers in the neocortex. The right of the figure shows the connections between pyramidal and stellate cells.

and processes. The thickness and composition of individual laminae varies across the cortical sheet (Fig. 2.4), and provides the basis for a more detailed 'cytoarchitectural' classification of cortical divisions proposed by Brodmann, mentioned above. Though Brodmann's classification is still used, insight into the functional and anatomical complexity of the microstructure of the cortex has led to a more fine-grained subclassification — as we shall see later when considering the structure and function of the visual cortex.

Superimposed over this laminar (horizontal) organisation of the cortex are vertical aggregations of cylinders or columns of cells with rich interconnections, which share functional properties. These properties vary with the overall function of the cortical areas that the columns inhabit, and are determined by the input which they receive and process. It may help to imagine the columns as many regularly spaced buildings arranged into many city blocks (individual cortical areas), which in turn make up an entire city (the cortex). Each building has six floors — each representing one of the six laminae — though the floors must be numbered in reverse to follow cortical convention, such that the bottom floor is the sixth floor, and the top floor is the first floor. As described earlier, the lamina vary in size depending on the function of the cortical area in which they are located: the fourth floor (layer 4, which receives input) in a sensory area (or city block) will be larger than the fourth floors of buildings in a motor output 'district', where floor 5 (layer 5, concerned with output) is bigger.

Sensory systems

All sensory systems follow a similar general plan. In functional terms, sensory receptors in each system transduce the energy of stimuli (mechanical, thermal, chemical or electromagnetic) into electrochemical energy and, by means of a variety of neural coding strategies, detect the modality, intensity, duration and location of stimuli. Sensory systems conduct, transform and integrate neural impulses actively in a variety of ways to allow us to perceive our environment. In order to achieve this, sensory systems are organised in a hierarchical, parallel and topographic fashion. They are hierarchical in the sense that successive stages extract increasingly complex features from the sensory environment; their parallel nature ensures that different kinds of information are processed separately; and their topographic organisation reflects the spatial relationship of stimuli from adjacent parts of the sensory field and their ability to affect each other. Neurons belonging to a particular sensory system, therefore, respond specifically to more or less complex stimuli, to particular aspects of sensory events, and to a specific locality within the sensory field — depending on their position within the chains of information processing. In the visual system there are cells which respond only to points of light from a highly restricted portion of the visual field, no matter to which gestalt this point belongs. In contrast, other cells respond to complex stimuli, such as faces, located anywhere in the visual field. These are manifestations of the hierarchical and topographical aspects of processing. Parallel processing, on the other hand, segregates information about movement from information about colour and shape. Thus, the visual system makes a neurological distinction between 'where' something is as opposed to 'what' it is (Macko et al 1982). It is important to remember that cells within sensory systems have a 'projective field', as well as a receptive field. This determines how information received is subsequently transformed.

The visual system — complex information processing

Visual processing begins in the retina

The receptor organ of the visual system is the retina. Light is absorbed and transduced into electrochemical energy by photoreceptor cells — the rods and cones. Information collected by these receptors passes into a network of four further types of retinal cell: horizontal cells, bipolar cells, amacrine cells and ganglion cells. The cells are arranged such that final retinal output is from the ganglion cells, modified by the precise, regular network of connections between the various cell types. In this way, the network confers specific receptive field properties on to the ganglion cells (Tessier-Lavigne 1991). Ganglion cells have circular receptive fields, with a central circular portion surrounded by a concentric outer area which operates as 'antagonistic surround'. This means that stimuli in the centre of the receptive field have the opposite effect to stimuli falling within the more peripheral area of the receptive field of any individual cell. The 'effect' of a stimulus is to alter the firing rate of a ganglion cell. There are 'on-centre' cells and 'off-centre' ganglion cells. Cells with an 'on-centre' field fire more vigorously when a point of light falls on the central portion of the field, and less vigorously when the antagonistic, surrounding area is illuminated. 'Off-centre' cells have the opposite property: increased firing is encouraged by a stimulus within the outer portion, while firing is dampened down when the central portion of the field is activated. If illumination falls evenly across the receptive fields of either cell type, there is very little change in firing rate. The receptive fields of ganglion cells are therefore interested in contrasts and movement in their small portions of the visual field: even at this very early stage in visual processing, active computational processes are abstracting features of the electromagnetic environment by segregating information into parallel ('on-centre' and 'off-centre') streams.

A further, parallel division of information also occurs at this level. There are two types of ganglion cell, each type including cells with 'on-centre' fields and with 'off-centre' fields. One type, called M cells (magnocellular — large cells), respond mainly to rapid changes in the visual field and are primarily interested in movement. The other type, P cells (parvocellular — small cells), are more numerous and respond more to contrast changes and wavelength in their portions of the visual field. In some of these cells, the centre and 'antagonistic surround' areas of their receptive fields are responsive in an oppositional way to different wavelengths of light (such as red versus green light) — so called 'single-opponent' cells — in addition to the presence or absence of light; these cells are interested in colour. Other P cells are more interested in achromatic contrast and thus fine detail.

Leaving the retina

Information from the retina projects to a variety of brain areas: to the pretectal area in the midbrain, where pupillary reflexes are controlled; to the superior colliculus to provide information for the control of eye muscles; and to the lateral geniculate nuclei — the thalamic relay of the visual perception system. Retinal ganglion cell axons form the optic nerves, which course through the optic chiasm to become the optic tracts and terminate in the lateral geniculate nucleus (LGN). A further set of parallel information streams must be considered at this point: visual information is coming, of course, from each of two eyes. The nasal halves of each retinal projection decussate in the optic chiasm, the temporal halves do not. The left half of each retina (the left visual 'hemifield') projects to the left LGN; the right half of each retina (right 'hemifield') to the right LGN. Therefore, each nucleus receives input from both eyes.

In general, sensory systems project along a chain of neurons from their receptor sheet through peripheral sensory nerves to the spinal cord and then, via a relay in the thalamus, to their individual 'primary' sensory cortex and beyond. The olfactory system, however, has no thalamic relay, and the visual system has no 'peripheral' nerve — the optic nerve strictly speaking is a central neuronal pathway heading for the thalamus.

The thalamus is an egg-shaped structure which constitutes the largest part of the diencephalon. It acts as a gateway to the cortex for sensory information — its output to the cortex can be modified by the reticular activating system in the brainstem, for example. In view of its massive, widespread projection to (and back projection from) the cortex, the thalamus exerts considerable influence on cortical processing: it has been described as a 'brain within the brain'. The thalamus is divided up into several regions in terms of the cortical areas to which it projects. The parts of the thalamus concerned with visual information are the left and right lateral geniculate nuclei.

The lateral geniculate nucleus

The lateral geniculate nucleus has six layers, receiving highly ordered ganglion cell projections. The most ventral two layers have larger cells than the more rostral four layers. Each of the ventral, large-cell layers are contacted by projections from the retinal ganglion M cells — one layer from M cells responding to stimuli activating the right eye's retinal contribution to the hemifield, the other responding to the left eye contribution. The four smaller cell layers receive P cell input, alternately segregated into left and right eye projections, two layers for each eye. Pathways carrying P cell (colour, detail) information remain separate from, but run parallel to, M cell (movement, flicker) projections. Information from the left and right eyes within a hemifield is similarly segregated, again illustrating the parallel nature of neural processing. Relationships between elements of the visual field are preserved at this level, following the principle of topographic organisation. Cells responding to adjacent portions of the visual field in the retina project to adjacent cells in the LGN. The LGN is said to possess a 'retinotopic' map, or rather several retinotopic maps, layer by layer. The receptive fields of the LGN cells are therefore similar to those observed in the corresponding retinal ganglion cells — circular, with a central portion and an antagonistic surround — and they too respond best to points of light falling on the retina.

There are few collateral connections or cross-talk between cells within the LGN; the information they obtain from the retina therefore appears to pass on to visual cortex with little modification. In this sense, the LGN may seem to act as a rather 'dumb', though highly ordered, relay. However, more than 80% of synaptic contacts within the LGN come not from the retinal ganglion cells but from cortical back-projections, and from the reticular formation in the brainstem. Higher order processing can therefore exert a profound influence on the LGN's activities, as can different arousal states. The details of these back-projections, and indeed cortical back-projections in general, are poorly understood. Therefore we have to await new insights into such arrangements before a fuller understanding of LGN function becomes available.

Visual cortex — 'V1'

The first stage of cortical processing takes place in the striate cortex surrounding the calcarine sulcus of the occipital lobe and extending over the occipital pole at the back of the brain. Much of the visual cortex is hidden from view because it is folded into the depths of the calcarine sulcus. Again, it is more helpful to think of the visual cortex unfolded and laid out as a sheet. The striate cortex is so named because of its prominent striations or stripes of myelinated axons running parallel to the cortical sheet in layer 4. Brodmann classified striate cortex as area 17, and contiguous 'extrastriate' visual areas as 18 and 19. More detailed analysis and understanding of visual cortical areas has led to further subdivisions. At least 20 distinct cortical areas have been identified, with still more having partial visual properties. They are designated by number (striate cortex is now area V1) or by anatomical designation and number (such as area MT, middle temporal area; V5, located on the posterior edge of the superior temporal sulcus). Not all visual areas will be described here, but the structure and function of important examples will be considered.

V1 is relatively thin, six-layered cortex. From a vertical perspective, taking each lamina in turn, layer 1 (the outermost layer, nearest the pial surface) contains many cell processes, such as the apical dendrites from cells in lower layers, but few cell bodies. Some input from other cortical areas arrives here. Layers 2 and 3 contain many pyramidal cells, which project to cells in other cortical areas. Layer 4 has spiny, stellate cells and few pyramidal cells. This is the main input layer of V1, where axons from cells in the LGN terminate. The cells here contact cells in other layers of V1, principally in layers 2 and 3. Layers 5 and 6 have many pyramidal cells. Cells in layer 5 receive some of their input from layer 3 and project beyond the cortex. Cells in layer 6 both receive input from and project back to the thalamus, in addition to

receiving input from layer 5. It also sends a (negative) feedback loop to layer 4. To return to our city block analogy, the foregoing describes activities on the six floors of one of the buildings. To grossly simplify, the fourth floor receives information from the LGN, passes it up to floors 2 and 3 (remember that the floors are numbered in reverse!). From there it is sent out to other city blocks and districts (other cortical areas) and also down to the fifth floor some information is then sent to the sixth floor, and some right out of the city to 'other lands' (to non-cortical areas, such as the spinal cord). The sixth floor sends inhibitory signals back to the fourth (input) floor — in this case, completing a negative feedback loop (Lund 1988). While this analogy does little justice to the complexity of cortical processing (and is somewhat inaccurate, as it does not take account of the fact that there is enormous information transfer among layers between vertical elements — between floors in different buildings — and that cells in lower layers have dendrites in upper layers and are thus influenced by inputs to other floors), it is intended to convey the idea that complicated but orderly integration of information is going on.

Input to V1 from the LGN

As noted in the preceding section, projections from the LGN terminate principally in layer 4 of V1. The M (magnocellular, concerned with flicker and movement) and P (parvocellular, concerned with fine contrast detail and colour) cell projections terminate, however, in different sublaminae of layer 4, preserving parallel but segregated information streams. Topographic mapping is also maintained, but the map is transformed, or distorted, such that there is increased representation of cells responding to stimuli closer to the centre of gaze. The receptive fields of the cells directly receiving input from the LGN in layer 4 are, of course, otherwise similar to the LGN cells themselves: circular, and responding to points of light. However, presumably as a consequence of the complex integration within V1 described above, cells above and below layer 4 have very different receptive field properties altogether.

Orientation columns

These cells do not respond preferentially to points of light, but to linear stimuli — bars or lines of light excite the cells. Furthermore, individual cells respond to bars with specific orientations: some cells to vertical bars, some to horizontal bars, some to transverse bars. These response characteristics are similar to those encountered earlier, in that the receptive field consists of an area which, when 'stimulated', enhances cell activity, and a surrounding area, which inhibits it — except that rather than concentric circles, the central area consists of a linear strip with a particular orientation. It is believed that the integration of overlapping, circular centre/surround fields in layer 4 generates these new, higher order receptive fields. Indeed, there are cells which respond individually to each orientation around the central axis of a bar stimulus through 360°. Moving horizontally across the V1 cortex, cells are found which respond to an orderly progression of bar orientations. The first cell may respond to a vertical bar. The next cell to a bar tipped 15° from vertical. The next cell to a bar 30° from vertical, and so on, until, over a distance of about 1 mm, we reach cells again responding to vertical bars. From a vertical perspective, cells, one above the other, tend to respond to the same orientation — while, moving horizontally, the next 'column' of cells all respond to a slightly different orientation (e.g. Hubel & Wiesel 1979).

Returning to our analogy, it is as if we were walking down a street in a cortical city, passing buildings (columns of cells), each specialising in dealing with different orientations of bars of light. Each floor (layer) within any one building deals with the same orientation, but the next building along deals with the next 15° rotation of the bar, and the next building a further rotation and so on. By the time we reach the end of the street (a distance of about a millimetre), we will have passed one building for each orientation — right around the clock. The first building of the next block we meet starts again at the first orientation we encountered, and the orderly progression continues. Each vertical column of cells (building) dealing with one orientation is known as an 'orientation' column, and the entire block with each orientation represented is considered to be part of a 'hypercolumn' (see below). Each cell in a hypercolumn (a whole city block) contributes to the same part of the retinal map, and each cell in one of the component columns has a different line orientation sensitivity from all the cells in the other columns of the hypercolumn, so in essence every portion of the visual field has an element dedicated to every line orientation. Thus the next block, in which all the buildings are concerned with a different, adjacent part of the visual field, also has a full set of orderly arranged buildings dealing with each line orientation. The discovery of orientation columns — amongst other work — earned David Hubel and Torsten Wiesel the Nobel prize.

Within VI there are cells with more complex receptive fields still — sensitive to linear stimuli throughout the visual field rather than in specific portions, or linear stimuli moving in a particular direction across the visual field, or to lines of particular length, and so on. Presumably, these more complex fields are abstracted from integration of output from cells with simpler receptive field characteristics. Given that, as we have been, fields tend to be responsive to changes in contrast and movement, it seems likely that the linear preoccupation of V1 cells is concerned with the detection of edges at different angles, and thus the construction of static and moving outlines in the visual field from short line segments with a variety of orientations.

Ocular dominance columns

What of the input from each eye? Remember that the left hemifield is conducted to the right hemisphere and the right hemifield to the left, such that each visual area has parallel input from each eye. The six layers of the LGN maintain separation of right and left eye contributions to hemifield input: the two ventral layers receiving M cell input, one for right, one for left; the four upper layers receiving P cell input, left and right eye information alternately. These left and right eye contributions are projected separately to another set of columns in V1 — the ocular dominance columns. The ocular dominance columns thus contain vertical aggregations of cells, which all tend to respond to stimuli falling on a small portion of the field of view of one eye, either right or left. The columns are arranged such that right eye and left eye responsive columns alternate as we move horizontally across the cortical sheet. It is likely that this arrangement plays an important role in stereoscopic vision (Hubel et al 1978).

The 'horizontal' route, which reveals the orderly left/right responsiveness alternation, is orthogonal to the orientation column axis, which we encountered earlier. To make this clearer, we can

employ again our city map analogy. Imagine that we have just walked one 'block', say east to west, past each of the 'buildings' responsible for each orientation of a strip of light (see above). If we turn 90°, and head north, we are now passing buildings alternately responsible for left eye input and right eye input. If we consider a complete 'block' as bounded east–west by a row of buildings comprising a complete set of line orientation columns, and bounded north–south by a left eye building and a right eye building, then our whole block contains the parallel distributed information for a single hemifield portion — a 'hypercolumn'. It is tempting to think of such units as individual cortical processing 'modules'. The principle of topographic mapping is sustained by finding that the next block in the city deals with an adjacent portion of the visual hemifield, and so on.

The features of this arrangement are not unique to the visual system. Auditory cortex, for example, has a topographic 'cochleotopic' map, which receives ordered input, preserved through the many way stations from the cochlea, in terms of the sound frequency spectrum (analogous to the parallel processing of information from the visual field of the visual system). Each hemisphere also receives input from both ears, such that blocks in the 'auditory city' have a frequency dimension and a 'binaural' dimension: thus enabling the identification and localisation of sound.

Blobs and interblobs in V1

A further aspect of V1 structure must now be considered. Situated above and below layer 4 in the centre of the cortical visual 'blocks' are small peg-like regions called 'blobs' (the larger surrounding area of the block is sometimes described as the 'interblob' region). The blobs can be identified on the basis of their particular staining characteristics on histological examination. Cells within the blob regions are responsive to colour information, rather than the orientation of linear stimuli. They receive information initially generated by the 'single-opponent' P (parvocellular) cells described earlier, when considering the retina. Information from the other P cells, which are concerned with fine (but colourless) contrast detail, eventually arrives in the interblob regions, where cells do respond selectively to the orientation of stimuli. Therefore, we can distinguish two parallel pathways: the M (magnocellular) pathway originating with the M ganglion cells in the retina and concerned with detection of movement; and the P pathway, initiated by the P ganglion cells. The P pathway can be subdivided into a P-blob pathway, concerned with colour vision, and a P-interblob pathway concerned with detail and shape.

A parallel distributed system

Drawing these aspects of V1 together, we can see that this cortical area identifies line segments in the visual field, maintains and processes parallel pathways for colour, form and movement, and takes part in the ordering of information from both eyes for depth perception. Various elements across the visual field are, unsurprisingly, interconnected — such that cells concerned with a particular linear orientation (or a particular colour characteristic) from one part of the visual field talk to cells with similar colour or orientation interests, but with receptive fields serving a different part of the visual field.

Why does the cortex process information in this parallel, distributed way? There are certainly advantages to the arrangement. Multiple distributed modules might solve wiring problems: to mangle an analogy of Crick's (Crick 1994), and give it a psychiatric flavour, the existence of distributed modules may be similar to the convenience to the population of many community resource centres — rather than having to travel some distance to a central asylum. (Crick thought more in terms of many convenience stores versus one large supermarket in a city.) Distributed networking is also 'damage resistant'. Losing a single resource centre is not as catastrophic as losing the whole asylum. The mathematical neural network models beloved by theoretical neurobiologists demonstrate the principle of 'graceful degradation' in response to damage — just as small lesions to portions of V1 reduce visual acuity rather than causing complete blindness.

Extrastriate cortex — beyond V1

As noted above, there are many distinct cortical visual areas. In general, as we move in the direction of information flow, the size of individual cellular receptive fields increases, and the stimuli eliciting a response become more complex (Tanaka 1993). Nonetheless, parallel information streams carrying specific kinds of information continue. The pathway originating in the M cells in the retina, initially responding to changes in contrast, and later orientation and movement in V1, projects via area V2 (part of Brodmann's area 18) to the middle temporal (MT) area or V5 (part of Brodmann's area 19). Here, more complex features are constructed, such as speed and direction of movement. Further projections terminate in parietal regions, where a complex analysis of position and motion is carried out. It is in this sense that the visual system makes a neurological distinction between 'what' and 'where' — the M pathway terminating in parietal cortex is the 'where' pathway. The P pathway, arising from the parvocellular ganglion cells in the retina, and eventually dividing into blob (colour) and interblob (detail and form) streams in V1, projects via area V2 to area V4, where a great deal of colour processing occurs. Recordings from cells receiving information via the P-blob stream in area V4 show that they do not simply respond to wavelength, but to perceived colour — which, despite invariant wavelength, can be changed by altering the background colour against which a coloured cue is placed. Cells in the P-interblob pathway are sensitive initially to edges, and ultimately to outlines and therefore shapes. Their projection from area V4 along with the P-blob stream to the inferotemporal visual area represents the end of the 'what' pathway. A small proportion of cells in this area respond uniquely to some very complex stimuli indeed, such as any orientation of a hand, anywhere in the visual field; or to faces. The 'what' and 'where' streams finally merge in the entorhinal and frontal cortices. Complex polysensory information is believed to be processed and constructed into memories in the hippocampus and the related entorhinal cortex (see limbic system, below); while the integration of 'what' and 'where' information may take place in the 'working memory' systems of the prefrontal cortex (Rao et al 1997).

Perception, attention and consciousness

Where then, is visual awareness in the brain? There is ample evidence that there is no 'homunculus' sitting inside the brain watching information about shape, colour and movement arriving on a monitor (Dennett 1991). This raises the question of how consciousness arises in the brain, a topic of interest to philosophers for millennia. There are many texts discussing the issue of consciousness; Zeman, for example, has recently provided a good introduction (Zeman 2002). Over the past two decades, a number of scientists have additionally become involved in the debate. A few of these scientific theories will be discussed here (see, for extensive references, Zeman 2002), with most detail being on Zeki's theory.

Edelman and Tononi's theory proposes that the neural correlate of consciousness (NCC), is a 'shifting coalition of strongly interacting elements', which is also referred to as the 'dynamic core'. They argue that this core is responsible for consciousness of perceived events, information passing between functionally segregated (specialised) brain regions. Essentially, they emphasise the importance of interactions between regions of the cortex and thalamus. Crick and Koch advance a similar theory, but additionally suggest that the NCC will 'comprise a sparse but widespread network of neurones' and suggest it can be identified on the basis of neuronal firing pattern and other features such as anatomy; e.g. the 'bursty' pyramidal cells in layer 5 of the cortical visual areas. Damasio suggests that consciousness occurs only when the brain represents the effects of sensory data by 'second order mapping', a process that transforms the sensations to make them 'explicit', which he specifically locates in the somatosensory cortex, thalamus, basal ganglia and upper brainstem.

Zeki and Bartels propose a theory of visual consciousness (Bartels & Zeki 1998, Zeki & Bartels 1998, 1999, Zeki 2001). Although confining the theory to the visual system, nonetheless they suggest that it may be applicable to other brain regions, which may include those of more relevance to the study of psychiatric disorders (see below). They note that anatomical and physiological studies indicate that the primate visual system consists of many distributed processing systems acting in parallel. They emphasise psychophysiological studies and interpret them as demonstrating that neural activity in each of the parallel systems reaches its perceptual endpoint at a slightly different time, leading to 'perceptual asynchrony in vision'. They argue that this, combined with clinical and imaging evidence, suggests that the processing systems are also perceptual systems, with each system acting in a semi-autonomous manner (Bartels & Zeki 1998). Additionally, they argue that such activity can have a conscious correlate (microconsciousness) without necessarily involving activity in other systems, and conclude that visual consciousness is itself modular, reflecting the basic modular organisation (functional specialisation or segregation) of the brain. Zeki and Bartels cite a substantial amount of experimental evidence as consistent with their theory.

Having argued for a fundamentally 'fractionated' basis of visual consciousness, they then consider the issue of integration of microconsciousness to form a perceptual unity (Zeki 2001). As part of this 'theory of multistage integration', they begin by distinguishing three categories of anatomical connection between functionally specialised areas. First, they recognise 'forward' connections: e.g. from V1 to V5 (motion), or from V1 to V4 (colour). Next, they identify 'reverse' connections in the opposite direction. Finally, they identify 'parallel' connections between stages of different processing streams (e.g. between V4 and V5). They note that timing creates a problem, with different nodes reaching a perceptual end-point at different times, and ask whether there is any 'third area', besides a general 'enabling' system in the brainstem.

Citing various imaging studies (see Zeki 2001), they argue for the presence of 'transient' cortical areas allowing parallel binding: e.g. the superior parietal lobe. Thus subjects viewing motion alone, or colour alone, do not activate the parietal cortex. But in the case of perception of objects constructed from *both* colour and motion, the parietal cortex becomes active, as if a temporary connection between V4, V5 and the fusiform gyrus had been formed (Zeki 2001). These connections are temporary from a functional and not an anatomical perspective. (See also the discussion on Volterra formulations in Ch. 5). They speculate that 'thought processes' may involve such temporary areas. Finally, they argue that we are not conscious of the activity in such putative temporary areas, but only of the final result.

Zeki and Bartels's theory is important because it explicitly argues that segregation of function in the brain may be associated with a corresponding conscious correlate. Currently, there is much interest in attempting to identify functionally-segregated regions of the prefrontal and temporal cortices, since dysfunction in localised regions might begin to explain some symptoms of psychiatric illness (see Ch. 5). It is well known that some regions of the prefrontal and temporal lobe may have direct conscious correlates: i.e. direct electrical stimulation 'feels like something'; for example, see evidence for the medial temporal lobe (Heath 1964, Aggleton 1992) and anterior cingulate (Heath 1964, Talairach et al 1973). By contrast, stimulation of the dorsolateral prefrontal cortex (e.g. with transcranial magnetic stimulation) is not associated with a conscious correlate. Could such areas correspond to similar conscious and transient regions, respectively? Additionally, there is considerable interest in studying patterns of normal and abnormal connectivity between functionally segregated brain regions in psychiatric disorders (see Ch. 5), particularly with regard to schizophrenia and mood disorder. Could a theory of multistage integration shed light on reported disconnectivity in psychiatric disorders? Only further work will clarify these issues.

FRONTOSUBCORTICAL LOOPS — CONTROLLING MOVEMENT AND COGNITION

Frontal cortex not only has an important role in the execution of movements, in cognition, social and motivated behaviour; it also appears to be implicated in psychiatric illness. Abnormalities in frontal lobe function have been described in the dementias, in depression and schizophrenia, and in obsessional disorder. The anatomical organisation of the frontal lobe and its functional implications are therefore of great interest to psychiatrists. As an important organisational principle, the parallel arrangement of neural loops connecting cortex with subcortical structures, such as striatum, pallidum and thalamus, has emerged over the last 15 years. These loops appear to be mutually exclusive, i.e. they connect clearly-separated compartments in frontal cortex with similarly separate areas in basal ganglia (Alexander et al 1990). Of these, the 'motor circuit' has been characterised in most detail (Fig. 2.5). Before describing this circuit in greater detail a few more general observations on motor function are necessary to put the corticobasal-ganglia–thalamic circuit into a wider functional context.

Motor function

Movement is essential for the expression of language, planned action, learning with practice and instinctive activity. Output from primary motor cortex (area 4) is a final common anatomical pathway for such behaviour. Area 4 projects to motor neurons in the anterior horn, directly and indirectly via spinal interneurons. There is also output to nuclei of the dorsal columns, the reticular

formation, the pons and the inferior olive, the centromedian nucleus of the thalamus, and the putamen. Input to area 4 converges directly from other cortical areas, e.g. the parietal association cortex, or more indirectly from the basal ganglia and cerebellum via the thalamus. The motor function of the cerebellum has long been appreciated by the clinical effects of cerebellar lesions, which result in disturbances of fine coordination, posture and walk, depending on the site of the lesion. The cerebellum receives input from vestibular, ascending sensory and descending pontine fibres. The pontine nuclei have input from the contralateral cerebral hemispheres, mainly primary motor (area 4), premotor (area 6), primary sensory (areas 1, 2, 3) and somatosensory association cortex (area 5). The cerebellum is thus equipped with a wealth of sensorimotor information. It projects via the dentate nucleus to the somatotopically organised ventral lateral thalamus and from there back to areas 4 and 6, closing the functional loop and enabling the cerebellum to act as a parallel processor to modulate movement and be involved in motor learning (see above). The ventrolateral portion of the dentate nucleus in fact projects to prefrontal association cortex and may be involved in cognitive processes (Martin 1996). A shorter loop courses from the dentate nucleus to the red nucleus, to the inferior olivary nucleus and via climbing fibres back to the cerebellum. The internal circuitry of the cerebellum is relatively simple (Fig. 2.6). Granule cells are the only excitatory (glutamatergic) neurons in the cerebellum; all other cells are inhibitory, using γ-aminobutyric acid (GABA) or taurine (stellate cell) as a transmitter (Martin 1996). The output of Purkinje cells to the dentate nucleus is inhibitory as well. The detailed functional significance of this simple, relatively orderly arrangement of negative feedback is not yet clear, but its potential as a modulating circuit parallel to the neocortical motor centres is obvious.

The motor circuit

The terminology describing the basal ganglia is somewhat confusing. Figure 2.7 summarises the structures involved, grouped by their connection with input, output and internal structures. Putamen and pallidum are sometimes combined under the name lenticular nucleus. Similar to the cerebellum, the putamen receives motor input from area 4, but also from the supplementary motor cortex (medial area 6), the premotor cortex (lateral area 6), and sensory input from areas 1, 2, 3 and 5 (Fig. 2.5). This input is somatotopically organised, so that the leg zone lies dorsolateral, the orofacial zone ventromedial, and the arm zone in between. Neurons with GABA and substance P as transmitters project from putamen to the internal segment of the globus pallidus, as well as to the pars reticulata of the substantia nigra, while neurons with GABA and enkephalin project to the external segment of the pallidum. There is thus a direct and an indirect pathway from putamen to thalamus. A short direct path leads via the internal segment of the pallidum or the substantia nigra back to the ventral lateral, ventral anterior and the centromedian nucleus of the thalamus (Fig. 2.5). An indirect pathway links the external segment of the globus pallidus with the subthalamic nucleus, and hence with the internal segment of the globus pallidus or substantia nigra and the thalamus. These two paths have opposite effects on the internal segment of the pallidum or the substantia nigra: excitatory glutamatergic input from cortex to putamen activates GABAergic cells in the putamen, which in turn inhibit GABAergic cells in the internal segment of the globus pallidus projecting to the thalamus.

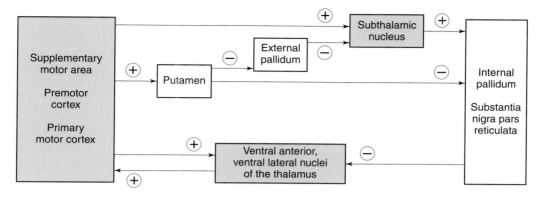

Fig. 2.5
The motor circuit (+, activation; –, inhibition). (After Alexander et al 1990 and Martin 1996.)

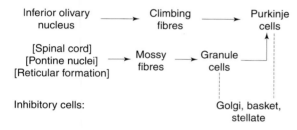

Fig. 2.6
Internal circuitry of the cerebellum. (After Martin 1996.)

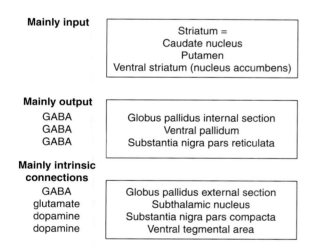

Fig. 2.7
Basal ganglia structures and neurotransmitters. (After Martin 1996.)

The net result is an activation of the thalamus, which itself has an activating input to cortex (and striatum). The indirect path involves inhibition of the external segment of the globus pallidus by GABAergic putamen cells; their output to the subthalamic nucleus is GABAergic too, whereas the output from the subthalamic nucleus to the internal segment of the globus pallidus or substantia nigra is excitatory. The net result is an inhibition of the thalamus. Moreover, there seems to be a differential effect of dopamine on striatal cells projecting to the external (GABA/enkephalin, inhibitory) and the internal (GABA/substance P, excitatory) globus pallidus. The depletion of dopaminergic input from the substantia nigra (pars compacta) to the striatum would, therefore, result in reduced thalamic excitation via the direct path and increased thalamic inhibition via the indirect path, both consistent with thalamic and consequently cortical underactivity. This additive effect explains the akinesia observed in parkinsonism. Recent results have qualified this simple model somewhat; in particular the straight linear connections within the indirect path are probably more complex than described (Chesselet & Delfs 1996, Feger 1997). Lesions of the subthalamic nucleus result in hemiballismus. A reduced excitatory input to the internal pallidum leads to decreased inhibition of the thalamus and consequent motor over-activity. Similarly, in Huntington's chorea there is a reduction of inhibitory enkephalinergic input from putamen to the external pallidum. This causes increased inhibition of the subthalamic nucleus by the external pallidum, reduced excitation of the internal pallidum by the subthalamic nucleus, and reduced inhibition of the thalamus by the internal pallidum, thus again causing increased movement. Finally, pallidotomy has been employed in the treatment of Parkinsonism. Stereotactic lesions of the internal pallidum result in reduced thalamic inhibition and consequent reversal of the akinesia.

A similar circuit subserving oculomotor function exists but will not be discussed here in any detail. The corticobasal-ganglia–thalamic circuits are described here in a simplified manner. A diversity of inputs to all stations of the circuits exists; there may also be links between the parallel loops.

The prefrontal circuit

The other parallel but mainly separate circuits linking dorsolateral prefrontal, orbitofrontal and anterior cingulate cortex with basal ganglia and thalamus (Figs 2.8 and 2.9) are not as well characterised as the motor circuit. The dorsolateral prefrontal cortex has long been implicated in cognitive function based on animal (Goldman-Racic 1995) and human studies (Petrides 1995, Stuss et al 1995). It receives input from a loop that includes the head of the caudate, the substantia nigra and the globus pallidus via the ventral anterior and medial dorsal nuclei of the thalamus. Both posterior parietal association cortex and premotor cortex project into this circuit via the head of the caudate. The most convincing interpretation of neuronal function in this circuit is that it subserves working memory. Working memory requires the active manipulation of a number of items within a memory store. Such a function is required during delayed matching-to-sample tasks: the

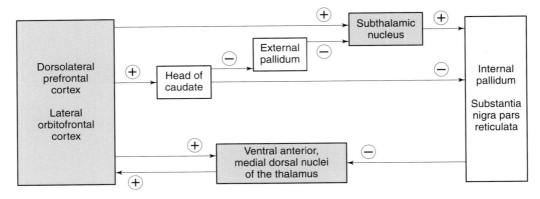

Fig. 2.8
Prefrontal circuit. (After Alexander et al 1990 and Martin 1996.)

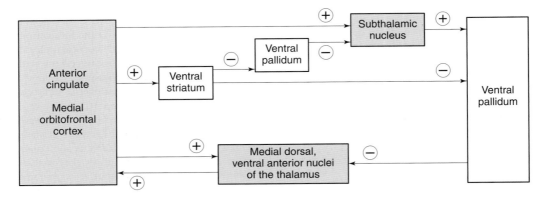

Fig. 2.9
Limbic circuit. (After Alexander et al 1990 and Martin 1996.)

subject has to select stimuli after evaluating their similarity in shape, colour or position with a previously presented sample. Similarly, self-ordering tasks require the retention and manipulation of a number of items, for example numbers. The word generation or verbal fluency task also requires the remembering of self-generated words in order to avoid repetition of the same word. There is now some evidence that spatial properties are processed separately from object properties in working memory. In non-human primates this may involve different regions within each hemisphere, whereas in humans the equivalent distinction between verbal and visuospatial properties likely maps on to different hemispheres. Closely associated with working memory are the concepts of the articulatory loop and the visuospatial scratch pad, where verbal and non-verbal information is held, and the central executive or supervisory attentional system, which is responsible for the manipulation of verbal and visuospatial information (Shallice 1982, Baddeley 1986). It has been suggested that these storage and processing functions of working memory in fact map onto different parts of the lateral prefrontal cortex (Goldman-Racic 1995), but there may also be a common area (area 46) that is involved in working memory of any type (Wickelgreen 1997).

So-called frontal dementias have been described in connection with a variety of illness processes, with an overactive, disinhibited presentation in association with orbitofrontal, and an apathetic presentation with dorsolateral prefrontal atrophy (Neary 1995). The basal ganglia are said to be invariably involved. In fact, prima-rily subcortical diseases, such as Huntington's disease, are occasionally associated with a 'subcortical' dementia of a frontal type. A similar explanation has been suggested for the cognitive abnormalities associated with severe depression, which often shows functional basal ganglia as well as prefrontal cortex underactivity. The hypofrontality associated with cognitive impairment in schizophrenia mainly affects the dorsolateral prefrontal cortex, possibly after an initial hyperactivity of this region (Wiesel et al 1987, Ebmeier 1995).

The limbic circuit

The limbic circuit receives cortical input from lateral and medial temporal lobe structures such as the temporal cortex, amygdala and hippocampus. As with other prefrontal cortical areas, the anterior cingulate and orbitofrontal cortices are part of a re-entrant subcortical circuit (Fig. 2.9).

The ventral striatum, which includes the nucleus accumbens and olfactory tubercle, is known to be linked to reward mechanisms, in that manipulations alter the incentive effects which learned rewarding stimuli (e.g. light associated with food) have on behaviour (Rolls 1999 p. 54). For example, dopamine depletion in the ventral striatum abolishes the effects on feeding, which result from stimulus–reinforcement learning. Rolls notes that electrophysiological studies in primates indicate that the majority of ventral striatal neurons do not respond to unconditional rewarding stimuli. Instead, neuronal responses depend on memory for whether the stimulus was recognised or associated with reinforcement.

Although it has been known for some time that the ventral striatum is involved in stimulus–reinforcement learning, a recent interesting development has been the linking of classical conditioning concepts with predictive models (e.g. Dayan et al 2000). This is based on experimental evidence that dopamine neuronal activity codes errors in the prediction of rewarding events (Schultz et al 1997). Such experimental evidence provides the basis for quantitative (and testable) models of neuronal function: e.g. the temporal difference model and Kalman filter models (Dayan et al 2000). Based on such work, it has been suggested that the ventral striatum forms part of a system, together with the ventral tegmental area and substantia nigra (see below), which reports ongoing reward prediction errors.

Older models of basal ganglia function do not consider the possibility of neuronal activity coding for predictions and focus on imbalances between direct and indirect pathways. Reflecting this, there have been some theories of basal ganglia dysfunction in psychiatric disorders. For example, Baxter and colleagues have advanced a theory of basal ganglia dysfunction in obsessive–compulsive disorder (Baxter et al 1996). They suggest that obsessive–compulsive disorder is associated with an increase in the tone of the direct pathway resulting in thalamic and therefore cortical activation. They further speculate that such increased activity may be reflected in symptoms such as ruminations and compulsions. There are various problems with this theory, not the least being only limited evidence for the limbic circuit having identifiable direct and indirect pathways (Alexander et al 1990).

In summary, although progress continues to be made in understanding the functions of the frontal subcortical loops, much remains to be done. Nevertheless, recent developments are promising. Dysfunction in a mechanism which predicts reward and punishment, plus errors in such prediction, may clearly form the basis of new and testable theories of loop dysfunction in psychiatric disorder. Further discussion of the evidence for the brain's acting in a predictive manner will follow, before more detailed discussion of the limbic system.

Behavioural neurophysiology — neural optimal control theory

Neural optimal control theory has been specifically applied to the frontal–subcortical loops (Baev et al 2002), but it is a general theory of neuronal function (Baev 1998) and possibly much more besides. Alternatives to the theory will be discussed followed by the theory itself. Experimental studies, which appear consistent with Baev's theory will also be discussed; however, it is important to note that these, although similar, differ in scope and emphasis. The origin of Baev's theory lies in extensive experimental work on spinal 'central pattern generators' (CPGs).

The oldest alternative is the classical reflex theory, which has its origins about 350 years ago with Descartes (see Baev 1998 p. 7). It suggests that the nervous system acts according to deterministic 'stimulus–reaction' principles and that understanding brain function requires a knowledge of numerous reflexes inherent in a given species. The behaviour of an animal can be understood if the reflex arcs are known, and the interactions of such arcs are balanced by excitatory and inhibitory influences. This theory is reflected by current clinical thinking. It is conventionally held that

(neurological) 'primitive reflexes' are tonically inhibited by higher brain regions and 'released' by damage to these regions (as in concepts of behavioural disinhibition resulting from prefrontal cortical damage).

The problems with reflex theory are well known. Only simple reflexes appeared explainable with this approach; tracing cause–effect relationships for complex behaviours proved impossible (Baev 1998). An influential attempt to extend the reflex theory was the 'program control' theory. The notion was of a 'fixed action pattern'; a series of complex stereotyped acts (i.e. programs) triggered by internal or external stimuli. Such concepts remain central to ethological theories of behaviour. The realisation of each program, in the form of behaviour, is assumed to result from activity in different neural circuits. This approach is very similar to that adopted generally in experimental neurobiology. Inborn automatic movements such as locomotion, breathing, swallowing, chewing and scratching are the most extensively studied. Such behaviours are generated by corresponding neural centres or CPGs. Complex behaviours are assumed to result from activity in CPGs and the interaction between these centres.

Again there are problems. For example, how do the CPGs initially become programmed? How does a CPG modify its behaviour or rhythm during ontogenesis? CPGs appear to share common neuronal regions. How is it possible to approach the relationship between structure and function? The answer, argues Baev, is that a more sophisticated theory of behavioural neurophysiology is needed. He proposes a hierarchy of semi-autonomous 'neural optimal control systems' (NOCSs).

The theory can be considered to have two closely related components. First, there is the concept of a *predictive* control system, a mathematical theory borrowed from engineering science. The control system acts on a 'controlled object' (e.g. musculoskeletal system and environment). However, the system plus object are continually subject to disturbances which would result in the controlled object deviating from the instructions of the control system. Therefore, the control system comprises two parts: a controller and a predictive model. The model receives the same instructions from the controller as does the controlled object and predicts the sensory or other feedback to the controller. The real sensory feedback to the controller is always incomplete and subject to ambiguity (since the controlled objects are only partly observable), and the job of the model is to 'fill in the gaps', adapting (learning) to a changing environment (as in concepts of 'top-down' processing in perception). The discrepancy between actual and predicted feedback gives rise to an error signal. The objective of adaption is to minimise the error signal through an 'error distribution system'. Second, there is the concept of an ordered hierarchy of such NOCSs with error and control signals passing between them. The controlled objects for higher NOCSs comprise lower NOCSs.

This brief discussion leaves out much detail, and the reader is referred to the original texts. Essentially though, it addresses problems such as learning and adaptation, which are features of a system that attempts to optimise responses in the face of changing environmental circumstances and damage to the system. The concept of physiological control systems is not new. Simpler (non-stochastic) control models have been developed for many physiological systems: e.g. respiratory control, aortic flow, neuronal dynamics such as Hodgkin–Huxley and Bonhoffer–van der Pol theories, sleep apnoea, the pupillary reflex loop, blood glucose regulation, etc. (Khoo 2000). Such control system models reflect far older physiological concepts for achieving 'homeostasis' (Walter Cannon) and the 'fixity of the milieu interior' (Claude Bernard) in the face of disturbances to the organism (Khoo 2000).

It was the physiologist Cannon who first recognised that the sympathetic and parasympathetic nervous systems have distinct functions: the sympathetic system 'fight or flight' behaviour, the parasympathetic 'rest and digest' behaviour. Cannon further proposed that the autonomic nervous system, under the control of the hypothalamus, is a component of a negative feedback control system (see quote by Cannon in Kandel et al 2000 Ch. 49). There is clearly some relationship between the sympathetic nervous system and brain behavioural defence systems (e.g. Gray's theory, see below), also the parasympathetic nervous system and brain appetitive reward systems (see below).

Of relevance to psychiatric disorders, Kupferman and colleagues argue that motivational states arising from internal stimuli (e.g. thirst, hunger, etc.) can be modelled by control systems (Kandel et al 2000 Ch. 51). This suggests that emotional states arising as a consequence of the presence or absence of reinforcers (e.g. water in the case of thirst; see Roll's theory of emotion, below) might also be modelled using control theory. Consequently, it is interesting that Solomon originally formulated his 'opponent-process' theory of normal emotion, drug addiction and motivation, as being an adaptive control system, which aims to restore euthymic homeostasis (Solomon & Corbit 1974 Fig. 3). More recently, Gray's theory of septo-hippocampal function (and anxiety) could be regarded as describing a form of control system involving selection of goals through behavioural inhibition (Gray & McNaughton 2000).

Baev's theory represents an advance, emphasising as it does the predictive nature of biological control systems (plus potential dysfunction), and the propagation of error and control signals through the hierarchy. The presence of predictive signals in biological systems is demonstrated by animal experimental work on the ventral striatum and ventral tegmental area as discussed above (e.g. Dayan's work), plus the orbitofrontal cortex (see below). Additionally, it may be supported by recent electroencephalographic work on humans. A component of the human event-related potential, termed the error-related negativity (ERN) (Scheffers & Coles 2000), which some workers have localised to the anterior cingulate, occurs in response to perceived behavioural errors. This clearly implies the presence of a neural mechanism that predicts and monitors performance. Schultz & Dickinson provide a good general review of neuronal coding of prediction errors (Schultz & Dickinson 2000). Predictive control system theory, in the form of Kalman filters, has been applied to the study of human motor (Wolpert et al 1995) and visual sensory systems (Rao & Ballard 1999) with some success.

Baev argues that each frontosubcortical loop is an NOCS, which includes a model of object behaviour (mostly within the basal ganglia) plus an error distribution system (which includes dopaminergic neurons), the latter being necessary to tune the model to the controlled object. He then applies the model to consideration of medication, lesioning and deep brain stimulation, used in the treatment of Parkinson's disease. A detailed discussion of the application of the theory to the limbic loop is also provided, further emphasising the potential relevance of the theory to the study of psychiatric disorders.

In summary, there is diverse experimental evidence that the brain may function as a hierarchy of partially autonomous, self-optimising, predictive control systems. The frontosubcortical loops may function in this manner, just as the rest of the brain. Nevertheless, considerable work is required to test this theory and clarify details of prefrontal behavioural physiology. From the perspective of psychiatry, the usefulness of the theory will be reflected by the extent to which it sheds new light on disordered brain function in psychiatric illness. In that context, it is interesting to note that abnormal ERN has been reported in obsessive–compulsive disorder (Gehring et al 2000).

THE LIMBIC SYSTEM: BORDER OF COGNITION AND EMOTION

The limbic system is essentially a collection of interconnected cortical and subcortical structures, described and defined in a variety of ways, and generally implicated in aspects of emotion, learning and memory (see limbic loop above). The concept of the limbic system can be confusing because both anatomical and functional considerations have determined its components over the years, and our understanding of brain and behaviour relationships has evolved over this time.

Historical background and conceptual overview

Paul Pierre Broca, a 19th-century French surgeon and anthropologist (perhaps best known for describing the motor speech centre of the brain), first used the term 'limbic lobe' to delineate the tissues constituting the border (L. *limbus*, border) between neocortex and diencephalon. Although Broca himself regarded the limbic lobe as representing 'the seat of the lower faculties which predominate in the beast' and the extralimbic mass (neocortex) as 'the seat of superior faculties' — thus anticipating some later conceptualisations — neuroanatomists in the succeeding decades ascribed incorrectly a sensory (largely olfactory, hence rhinencephalon) role to the lobe. The early history of the limbic lobe is succinctly reviewed by Corsellis (Corsellis & Janota 1985).

The concept of a limbic system involved in emotional function developed later, from the speculations of Papez (1937) and the subsequent theorising of Paul McLean (1949). On largely theoretical grounds, and drawing on the work of physiologist Walter Cannon, Papez proposed that a specific circuit (encompassing the hypothalamus, anterior thalamic nuclei, cingulate cortex and hippocampus) was responsible for the apprehension and expression of emotion. In the same year, Klüver & Bucy (1937) rediscovered the emotional effects of temporal lobe lesions which included limbic structures, originally described by Brown & Schaefer (1888). In the preceding year, Egas Moniz had begun treating pathological anxiety and agitation using the neurosurgical procedure of prefrontal leucotomy, and it became increasingly appreciated that damage to frontal white matter had a marked effect on emotion and feeling — amongst other effects. In 1949, McLean extended the Papez circuit to include the prefrontal cortex, septum and amygdala and thus invented the original version of the limbic system (see Fig. 2.10). Reprising Broca's notions, McLean elaborated the concept of the limbic system as the visceral brain, the presumed source of basic emotions. It is easy to see the analogies being made in the minds of early investigators between the central tenets of Freudian psychoanalysis and non-cortical brain structure.

In 1957, Scoville & Milner reported that bilateral neurosurgical resection of the medial temporal lobes, including the hippocam-

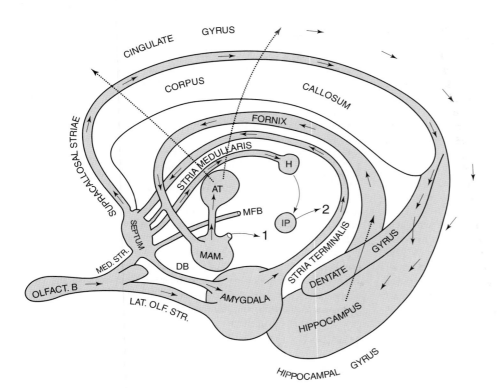

Fig. 2.10
Internal connections within the limbic system: OLFACT B, olfactory bulb; LAT OLF STR, lateral olfactory stria; MED STR, medial olfactory stria; AT, anterior nucleus of the thalamus; MFB, medial forebrain bundle; MAM, nucleus of the mamillary body (1, connection to midbrain reticular formation); DB, diagonal band of Broca; H, habenular nucleus; IP, interpeduncular nucleus (2, connection to midbrain reticular formation). (After MacLean 1949.)

pus and amygdala, resulted in a severe impairment in memory function. Their now famous case (known in the literature as patient HM) had suffered from intractable temporal lobe epilepsy, and the lesions had been made in an effort — which was largely successful — to relieve the disorder. The role of limbic structures in memory function has been extensively studied in the years since. Further diencephalic structures, such as the mamillary bodies of the hypothalamus and the dorsomedial nucleus of the thalamus, earn their place in the limbic system both on grounds of anatomical considerations and the fact that they are implicated in the memory dysfunction which occurs in Korsakoff's syndrome.

Limbic structures thus play a role in memory and emotional function, and this overlap underscores the potential for confusion generated by the naive assumption that psychological concepts need to relate in any simple way to brain structure. Part of the problem in defining the limbic system is simply a reflection of the way in which research has developed: structures have come to be defined both in terms of crude gross anatomy (the original limbic lobe, for example) and in terms of function (such as those structures, which, when compromised or stimulated, are observed to interfere with emotional behaviour or memory function). These provisional approaches to classification do not map easily one to another. They are provisional in the sense that psychological constructs such as emotion or memory are subject to continuous conceptual refinement. Memory function, for example, is no longer considered a unitary entity and is at present better characterised as a series of dissociable subsystems, each of which may have its own structural substrate (see below). The same is true of emotion. Ultimately, the distinction between memory and emotion is likely to be modified: structural and functional concepts have mutually co-evolved in the light of new findings, and continue so to do. The term 'limbic' therefore now fails to

serve a variety of masters (not least the ingenious MCQ authors of the Royal College of Psychiatrists), but, though there have been calls for its abolition, it has not yet been removed from office.

Here, the functional neuroanatomy of selected major limbic structures is described: the limbic (or paralimbic) cortex (orbitofrontal and anterior cingulate cortices), the hippocampal formation (with a brief note regarding the role of the dorsomedial nucleus of the thalamus in memory function), the hypothalamus and the amygdaloid complex. The role of limbic structures in emotional and cognitive behaviour is the focus of each review.

The orbitofrontal cortex

In animals and humans the orbitofrontal cortex (OFC) receives already highly processed unimodal and polymodal, exteroceptive and interoceptive information from every sensory modality. For example, the primary somatosensory cortex projects directly (and also indirectly via the anterior insula) to the OFC. Signals from the visual cortex are processed through multiple stages along the temporal lobe, which projects to the OFC. Taste and olfactory pathways project via the thalamus and olfactory cortex respectively to the OFC (Rolls 1999).

Primate electrophysiological studies and human imaging studies provide evidence that the rewarding and aversive qualities of the sensations are represented in the OFC (and other areas such as the amygdala and hypothalamus), in contrast to earlier processing stages (Rolls 1999). Reward is defined as anything an animal will work for, punishment anything an animal will work to avoid (Rolls 1999). For primary reinforcers, representation of reward value occurs only after several stages of processing; e.g. in the taste system, reward (the emotional component of the taste) is decoded in the OFC but not in the primary taste cortex, which represents what the taste is (Rolls 1999). In the somatosensory system, the primary reinforcer of pleasantness of touch is represented in the OFC, whereas intensity and location of sensation is represented in the primary sensory cortices (Rolls 1999). Although pain appears to be decoded early in sensory processing, some affective representations appear to be located in the OFC, since damage to this structure reduces affective responses to pain in humans (Rolls 1999).

For secondary reinforcers, which includes sight of particular persons or objects, initial sensory processing in the inferior temporal lobe proceeds to the stage of invariant object representation (neurons that respond to a given object regardless of orientation) before reward and punishment representation in the OFC, and other regions such as amygdala (Rolls 1999). If these later stages are damaged, then the Kluver–Bucy syndrome can result. The OFC also implements a mechanism which evaluates whether a reward is expected, and, if not received, generates a mismatch signal comprising a firing of non-reward neurons (Rolls 2000 p. 186). According to Rolls, the representations of rewards and punishments in the OFC constitute various 'goal states' for potential behavioural responses. Electrophysiological studies in primates indicate that regions such as the OFC allow rapid stimulus–reinforcement learning.

Closely linked to the above work on the OFC is a theory of emotion based on response to rewards and punishments (Rolls 1999). Essentially, Rolls proposes that emotions can be usefully seen as states produced by instrumental reinforcing stimuli. A wide range of emotions can be accounted for by considering a number of factors, including the reinforcement contingency (whether reward or punishment is given or withheld), the intensity of the reinforcer, the context in which a reinforcer is given (e.g. whether active or passive behavioural response is possible), etc. There is considerable scope for cognitive influences affecting the perception of whether a reinforcer is rewarding or aversive. Only a brief discussion of Roll's theories can be provided here, and the reader is referred to the original texts.

Given evidence of structural and functional abnormalities in the OFC in a variety of psychiatric disorders (see Ch. 5), Rolls's work has important implications. If the OFC mechanisms of reward and punishment, representation and prediction were not to function correctly, it might account for some psychiatric symptoms. Additionally, the normal physiological function of neuromodulators such as serotonin and dopamine appears to include direct effects on synaptic plasticity via changes in long-term potentiation and depression (Reid & Stewart 2001) and stimulus–response learning (Rolls 1999). These same neuromodulators are influenced by antidepressants and antipsychotics.

The above work does not address the issue of large-scale segregation of function in the OFC. However, Zald notes that, in primate studies, the medial orbitofrontal cortex (MOFC) and lateral orbitofrontal cortex (LOFC) appear to play complementary and dissociable roles (Zald & Kim 1996 p. 252). LOFC lesions result in behavioural deficits, particularly when it is appropriate to inhibit a previously rewarded response. Elliott and colleagues have reviewed a series of their functional imaging studies in humans, arguing that they demonstrate MOFC and LOFC dissociation of function consistent with animal studies (Elliott et al 2000). The MOFC was activated when subjects had to monitor the reward value of previous stimuli and weigh up the possible reward value of future responses. In contrast, the LOFC was activated when the tendency to select previously rewarded responses had to be suppressed.

The anterior cingulate cortex

Detailed reviews of cingulate structure and connections are available (Vogt and Gabriel 1993, Devinski et al 1995). There is evidence that the anterior cingulate (AC) supports executive behaviours and that the posterior cingulate (PC) supports evaluative function (Vogt et al 1992). Human functional imaging studies have consistently reported PC activation in memory tasks. In contrast to the PC, the AC is implicated in psychiatric disorders (see Ch. 5), and so it will be discussed further.

Animal studies emphasise a general tripartite segregation of functional anatomy in the rostral to caudal direction supporting emotion, cognition and motor function. It has been argued that the emotion and cognition divisions reflect different cytoarchitecture (Devinski et al 1995): emotion comprising Brodmann areas (BA) 25, 24 and 32 and the cognitive division predominately 24' and 32'. The boundary between the two areas is best described by a (quite precisely defined) supragenual line. The motor division of the AC comprises its most caudal area adjacent to the more superior supplementary motor area. The distinction between the emotional division and the rest of the cingulate can be traced to trends in evolutionary development. Specifically, a phylogenetically older orbitofrontal–amygdala-centred region extends throughout the emotional division of the AC, temporal polar and anterior insular regions. Additionally, a more recent hippocampal-centred region extends throughout the rest of the AC and the PC (Mega & Cummings 1997).

In addition to these three broad AC divisions, other authors, on the basis of animal studies, have proposed subregions: e.g. a vocalisation control region within the emotional division, and a nociceptive cortical region within the caudal AC (Devinski et al 1995). Regarding the putative nociceptive region, in the rabbit, area 24 responds to noxious stimuli in various modalities, such responses having no specific spatial localisation information (i.e. represent the punishment quality of pain). Midline thalamic nuclei contain nociceptive neurons in the rabbit and monkey, and these project to the anterior cingulate. Application of lidocaine to midline thalamic nuclei blocks anterior cingulate activation with noxious stimuli. Cingulate lesions in rats, monkeys and humans significantly reduce pain sensitivity and associated affective response (Vogt & Gabriel 1993 Ch. 10).

Bush and colleagues have reviewed a number of functional imaging studies demonstrating that the more rostral area is activated in tasks involving emotion, whereas the more caudal anterior cingulate is activated with cognitive-motor tasks (Bush et al 2000). That review provides good evidence that many functional imaging studies are consistent with animal and anatomical studies in regard to segregation of emotional and cognitive function. In a further link between human and monkey literature, Bush and colleagues described an imaging study demonstrating significant activation of the dorsal AC (cognitive and motor region) in response to a task involving reward reduction (Bush et al 2002). The pattern of activation matched an earlier study in monkeys using electrophysiological single-unit recording. Imaging studies of patients with mood disorder and schizophrenia have reported abnormal structure and function of the AC (see Ch. 5). Given that depressive illness is associated with anhedonia and anxiety, it is interesting that there is evidence that the usual function of the anterior cingulate may be as part of an executive response selection system for some emotional states, perhaps especially when they are aversive (Rolls 1999 p. 136), and that the AC responds to reduced reward.

The hippocampal formation

Structural anatomy and information-processing pathways

The hippocampus and related structures are known collectively as the hippocampal formation (fancifully compared in shape to a seahorse = hippocampus). The structures are bilateral. The formation comprises the subiculum, hippocampus proper (sometimes called Ammon's horn — cornu Ammonis) and the dentate gyrus. Together, they represent a fold of three-layered evolutionarily ancient cortex which projects into the floor of the lateral ventricle in each hemisphere. The three layers are designated in terms of their cellular characteristics, with an inner polymorphic cell layer, a prominent pyramidal cell layer in the middle, and an outer molecular layer, consisting of fine nerve fibres and small neurons, which is continuous with the outermost layer of neocortex. The pyramidal cells of the hippocampus proper are replaced by smaller granule cells in the transition to the dentate gyrus. The formation is continuous with the six-layered entorhinal neocortex, the transition from six to three layers occurring at the subiculum. The entorhinal cortex merges with perirhinal cortex anteriorly and forms part of the parahippocampal gyrus posteriorly. These cortical areas merge laterally with the cortex of the inferior edge of the temporal lobe, and medially meet the subiculum and dentate gyrus where the fold of cortex turns in on itself.

The hippocampal formation and associated entorhinal cortex occupies an important nodal point in the processing of polysensory information. As a result, the structure has been very intensively investigated. The formation has reciprocal connections via the entorhinal cortex, with polysensory associational neocortical regions in the frontal, temporal and parietal lobes and the paralimbic cortex of the cingulate gyrus and prefrontal cortex (see above). Highly processed information is thus passed to entorhinal cortex, from there to the hippocampus proper, and then back to cortex. Information is passed around a circuit or loop within the hippocampus prior to projection back to cortical areas. This internal circuit starts in the dentate gyrus, where projections from the entorhinal cortex synapse on granule cells. These in turn project in series to subdivisions within the hippocampus, distinguished by their cytoarchitectural features. The granule cells of the dentate gyrus project to the pyramidal cells of area CA3 (cornu Ammonis), which themselves project in turn to pyramidal cells in area CA1. The axons of the CA1 cells then project to the subiculum, which projects back to the entorhinal cortex, completing the loop. This circuit (dentate–CA3–CA1–subiculum) is known as the trisynaptic loop. Damage to any component within the circuit essentially disables the entire loop. The hippocampus has a lamellar organisation, with the lamellac in transverse orientation to the long axis of the structure. Each lamella contains a complete hippocampal circuit loop, an arrangement which is exploited in the study of hippocampal function. Individual living lamellar slices can be isolated after dissection of the hippocampus from experimental animals, and the trisynaptic loop examined electrophysiologically in vitro.

Significant output from the hippocampus and subiculum is also carried via a structure known as the fornix. Axons arising from the pyramidal and polymorphic cell layers stream together on the ventricular surface of each hippocampus (forming the alveus), developing into increasingly substantial tracts (the fimbriae) as fibres accumulate together posteriorly. The fimbriae continue from each hippocampal formation as the crura of the fornix, merging together as the body of the fornix which loops up and anteriorly over the thalamus and underneath the corpus callosum, to curve down and largely (mainly subicular output) terminate in the mamillary bodies of the hypothalamus (see below). Though predominantly an output pathway, the fornix also carries cholinergic connections from the septal area back to the hippocampus. The fornix link between hippocampus and hypothalamus is a prominent component of Papez's original circuit.

Further inputs from locus coeruleus (noradrenergic system) and the raphe nuclei (serotonergic system) modulate hippocampal activity. The hippocampal formation also communicates extensively with the amygdala, with principal projections from the lateral and basal nuclei of the amygdala (both via entorhinal cortex and directly to the hippocampus proper). Reciprocal projections from the hippocampus back to the amygdala appear to be more rare, though the basal nucleus of the amygdala receives input from CA1, the subiculum and entorhinal cortex.

The hippocampal formation and memory

From a functional point of view, the hippocampus has been most extensively implicated in memory function. Though entorhinal cortex and other medial temporal lobe structures degenerate early and extensively in Alzheimer's disease, accounting for the prominent memory impairment which characterises the disorder, specific evidence for the role of the hippocampal formation in memory function comes from the neuropathology of a more rare and circumscribed disorder of memory, the amnesic syndrome. The syndrome is characterised by an anterograde memory impairment of varying severity (an inability to learn and remember new material), usually accompanied by a variable degree of retrograde amnesia (failure to recall events occurring prior to the onset of amnesia), in the setting of a clear sensorium with preserved intellectual and language function. In contrast to the anterograde amnesia, certain forms of learning remain conspicuously intact, and this apparent dissociation between spared and impaired learning capacities has proved of particular interest in the development of current concepts of the neurobiology of memory, in implying the existence of at least two (and perhaps multiple) memory systems.

The amnesic syndrome may occur for a variety of reasons. Herpes simplex encephalitis, for example, is a rare but severe form of acute necrotising encephalitis which shows a predilection for medial temporal lobe structures. Postmortem and radiological studies reveal extensive lesions in hippocampus, amygdala and uncus, while diencephalic structures are left intact (Parkin 1987). Such patients therefore share similar pathology to those unfortunate enough to have undergone bilateral temporal lobe surgery, described above. Scoville & Milner's (1957) post-temporal lobectomy series suggested, following analysis of operative procedures, that all amnesic subjects had both hippocampus and amygdala removed. However, there is evidence that amygdalectomy alone does not cause amnesia (Parkin 1987), while the amnesic case RB, described by Zola-Morgan (Zola-Morgan et al 1986), was shown to have damage restricted to a bilateral lesion of the CA1 cell field of the hippocampus (demonstrated by an extensive postmortem neuropathological survey — the lesion in this case was caused by an ischaemic episode). Unfortunately, the study of brain damage leading to human amnesia in an effort to elucidate the biology of memory will always be hampered by the vagaries of 'uncontrolled' illness, varieties of clinical presentation and deficits additional to postulated 'core' or 'critical' damage. Animal models of the amnesic syndrome have permitted some of these difficulties to be overcome.

Animal models of amnesia. Efforts to produce a non-human analogue of amnesia have been dominated by two important considerations: the kinds of test required to demonstrate impaired learning and memory in animals; and the nature of brain damage required to produce such deficits. While early attempts to localise memory function in animals were unsuccessful, later studies consistently demonstrated, initially in primates and later in other mammals, that specific cortical damage could cause deficiencies in the acquisition and performance of discrimination tasks. Such tasks involved the discrimination of simultaneously presented cues, one of which was consistently associated with reward. Lesions were initially made in the inferotemporal cortex (non-primary, visual association areas), and the deficit produced was specific to visual discrimination learning. Subsequent studies demonstrated analogous isolated deficits in tactile and auditory modalities, placing lesions in the relevant cortical association areas. Control tasks used in these studies demonstrated that the deficits were associative in nature, and not due to impaired sensory or motor function. While the studies generally supported the principle that specific brain areas might subserve aspects of learning and memory, the findings did not mirror the pattern of global, multi-sensory deficit seen in human amnesia. Efforts to produce a global amnesia in primates and lower mammals, by destroying the limbic areas to which the cortical association areas project (and which are damaged in some amnesic humans), were initially disappointing, as the kinds of discriminative tasks used were largely, although not entirely, unaffected.

Significant progress was made, however, following the development of new types of memory task. These new tasks, initially developed by Gaffan (1992), differed from the earlier tasks in employing trial-unique visual stimuli, necessitating single-trial acquisition of information. A version of this new class of task, 'delayed non-match to sample' (DNMS), was found to be sensitive to limbic lesions (Mishkin 1978). The task consists of two phases. In the first ('sample') phase, the monkey is presented with a distinctive object, under which it finds a reward. The object is then removed and, after a variable interval, the second phase ('choice') begins. The animal is now confronted with two objects, one of them the object seen earlier, the other an unfamiliar object. The food is now concealed under the new object and the monkey must choose to displace it rather than the familiar object to obtain reward. Each trial makes use of a new pair of objects, such that the information needed to perform successfully changes from trial to trial, with none of the cues repeatedly associated with reward.

Normal monkeys performed the task with greater than 90% accuracy over an interval of 1–2 minutes between the sample and non-match phases of the trial, while animals with combined amygdalohippocampal lesions performed almost at chance. Importantly, however, the impairment does not occur in lesioned animals when the delay between sample and non-match phases is short (less than 20 seconds), indicating not only that sensory and motor systems are intact but also that the 'rule' of choosing the unfamiliar object is successfully learned and remembered. The effects of limbic damage on this task (Mishkin 1978) are not restricted to the visual modality. Similar impairments have been observed in tactile versions of the task (Murray & Mishkin 1984), suggesting that the learning deficit is global. In sharp contrast, and

in confirmation of the earlier work discussed above, repeated-trial visual discrimination learning (where cues are repeatedly presented and consistently associated with reward) is largely unimpaired in lesioned monkeys, even at long delays between individual trials.

In interpreting these findings, Mishkin and colleagues (Murray & Mishkin 1984) have proposed the operation of two learning systems, only one of which is impaired by limbic lesions. The impaired system is considered to subserve both recognition memory (as measured by the DNMS task) and associative recall (for example, one-trial object–reward association). The spared system is viewed as 'involving the gradual development of a connection between an unconditioned stimulus object and an approach response, as an automatic consequence of reinforcement by food' (Murray & Mishkin 1984). Mishkin designated this particular capacity as 'habit formation', which he described as a 'non-cognitive' form of learning operating independently of limbic structures and therefore unaffected by limbic lesions. Contemporary formulations draw an analogy between explicit memory in humans and the function impaired by limbic lesions in the DNMS task in monkeys.

The nature of the critical limbic lesion has, however, been disputed. In Mishkin's original report (Mishkin 1978), combined bilateral damage to both the amygdala and hippocampus was required to produce a severe delay-dependent deficit in the DNMS task, the degree of impairment being significantly greater than that produced by damage to either structure alone. This result was taken to indicate that circuits through both the hippocampus and amygdala contribute to those aspects of recognition memory which are assessed by the DNMS task. However, in the creation of the combined hippocampus and amygdala lesion, periallocortex ventrally adjacent to both structures was removed. Interpretation of the experiment was therefore confounded by damage to additional tissue.

In an effort to determine the relative contributions of these various structures to the memory impairment, Murray & Mishkin (1986) compared the effects of damage to the cortical tissue subjacent to both hippocampus and amygdala combined with either bilateral hippocampal lesions or bilateral amygdala lesions. They found impairment after both lesion combinations, with greater impairment seen in the condition involving the amygdala. The finding was taken to support the notion that damage to both amygdala and hippocampus was necessary, given that removal of the cortical tissue in the condition involving the amygdala would have effectively deafferented the hippocampus.

Zola-Morgan and his colleagues have conducted a series of studies examining the performance of monkeys with a variety of more selective lesions on the DNMS task (reviewed by Zola-Morgan et al 1991). They developed a useful notation to indicate the nature of the various lesions: 'H' refers to the hippocampus, 'A' to the amygdala, and the optional suffix '+' to adjacent cortical damage, such that Mishkin's original combined lesion would be designated 'H+A+'. The lesion 'H+' includes, for example, the hippocampal formation and much of the parahippocampal gyrus but excludes the most anterior portions of the entorhinal cortex. This lesion caused a significant delay-dependent impairment on the DMNS task, but less severe than that seen with the 'H+A+' lesion, consistent with Murray & Mishkin's (1986) result. The 'A' lesion constitutes a lesion of the amygdaloid complex, sparing the surrounding cortex (periamygdaloid, entorhinal and perirhinal cortices), while the 'A+' lesion includes all of these structures.

Monkeys with the selective 'A' lesion performed normally on the DNMS task, while monkeys with the 'H+A' lesion were significantly impaired, but no more so than monkeys with the 'H+' lesion alone. Further studies examining the effects of lesions restricted to perirhinal ('PR') cortex and perihippocampal ('PH') gyrus alone resulted in performance deficits apparently as severe as those seen in the 'H+A+' lesion, but could not be directly compared as the monkeys required a modification of the DMNS procedure in which the sample stimulus was presented twice in succession prior to the choice phase of the trial. The same subjects performed normally in pattern discrimination. Taking these findings together, Zola-Morgan and his colleagues suggest that the deficit seen following the 'H+A+' lesion results from damage to the hippocampal formation and related cortex, rather than to the hippocampus and amygdala as proposed by Mishkin's group. Furthermore, because the 'PRPH' lesion may cause a greater deficit than the 'H+' lesion, Zola-Morgan has concluded that the impairment cannot simply represent a hippocampal disconnection phenomenon, and suggests that these cortical areas are implicated in aspects of normal memory function in their own right (Zola-Morgan et al 1991).

Effects of diencephalic and medial temporal lesions. It should be noted that diencephalic limbic structures are also implicated in memory function. The most common form of human amnesia is seen in the Wernicke–Korsakoff syndrome, most frequently a sequel to chronic alcoholism, though the syndrome may result from any situation in which thiamine deficiency occurs, such as chronic malnutrition or malabsorption. Neuropathological surveys of such subjects consistently reveal damage to diencephalic structures, particularly the dorsomedial nucleus of the thalamus and the mamillary bodies, rather than temporal lobe structures such as the hippocampal formation and amygdala. There is disagreement as to which of these structures is critical to the disorder of memory function. Victor et al (1971) suggest that the most consistent factor is disorganisation of the dorsomedial nucleus of the thalamus. On the other hand, Kahn & Crosby (1972, in a review by Parkin 1987) describe two patients rendered amnesic following tumour resection largely restricted to the region of the mamillary bodies, while Squire & Moore (1979) detail the amnesic effects of a stab wound destroying (as far as can be determined on the basis of radiological evidence) the left dorsomedial nucleus of the thalamus in the patient NA. (More recent functional imaging studies suggest, however, that NA may have had additional temporal lobe dysfunction).

Although superficially similar, the neuropsychological consequences of medial temporal and diencephalic damage have been suggested to differ in detail (Parkin 1987). This is likely to be due, in part, to the variable sequelae of additional damage incurred dependent upon precise aetiology. In herpes simplex encephalitis, for example, damage can be so extensive that the Klüver–Bucy syndrome supervenes — deficits never seen after diencephalic damage. Similarly, patients suffering from the Wernicke–Korsakoff syndrome following prolonged alcohol abuse are frequently found to have widespread cortical atrophy (presumably as a consequence of the toxic effects of prolonged alcohol consumption, and not specific to the Wernicke–Korsakoff syndrome) and occasionally evidence of repeated head injury, these factors conspiring to extend neuropsychological deficits beyond the 'core' amnesic syndrome and exaggerating perceived neuropsychological differences between diencephalic and medial temporal syndromes. In particular, deficits on frontal tasks are frequently reported in Korsakoff patients. Despite these potential confounds, there is some evidence that differences exist. Parkin (1987) reviews a series of studies bearing on this issue and draws particular attention to the fact that patients with diencephalic amnesia often have a less well-circumscribed retrograde amnesia, and that temporal lobe amnesics may forget new information more rapidly than diencephalic amnesics. Squire (1986) reviews studies showing cognitive deficits in Korsakoff patients rarely found in bitemporal amnesics (such as impaired 'metamemory skills', failure to release from proactive interference, disproportionately large impairments of judgement of temporal order, and 'source' amnesia) which do not correlate with the degree of anterograde amnesia, and are therefore perhaps unrelated to the 'core' amnesic syndrome. These differences may reflect different aspects of cognitive function processed by separate limbic circuit components.

Connective plasticity and neurogenesis. Studies of the internal physiology of the hippocampus in both whole animals and isolated slices have provided clues as to how the hippocampus may form memories. An electrophysiological phenomenon known as long-term potentiation (LTP) — the ability of neurons to change their strength of connection with one another — is readily demonstrated in the hippocampus. The changes in connection strength occur rapidly and are long lasting — important properties for a candidate memory mechanism. The process is mediated by a subclass of excitatory amino acid receptor, the (NMDA) receptor complex, which (though distributed throughout the brain) is found in greatest density in the hippocampus. Pharmacological blockade of the receptor, or genetic manipulation using knockout techniques (Morris & Morris 1997), results in memory impairment in rats and mice.

Morphological studies of the hippocampus implicate the structure in schizophrenic disorder. Quantitative in-vivo structural imaging techniques, such as MRI, demonstrate significant reductions in medial temporal lobe grey matter, most pronounced in amygdala and anterior hippocampus (reviewed by Roberts 1991). Neurohistological studies conducted postmortem suggest that pyramidal cell number (Falkai & Bogerts 1986) and orientation (Kovelman & Scheibel 1984) may be abnormal in the hippocampus of some schizophrenic subjects. Though such studies have by no means been replicated consistently, they imply a neurodevelopmental pathology in schizophrenia, and may account for some of the neuropsychological abnormalities observed. On-going longitudinal studies of subjects 'at risk' for the development of schizophrenia may ultimately clarify this issue (see Ch. 5).

The hippocampus and associated structures demonstrate important plastic capacities. In addition to the changes in connectivity mediated by the excitatory amino acid systems described above, the dentate gyrus of the hippocampus also produces new neurons throughout adulthood in a variety of species, including humans (Eriksson et al 1998). This property of continuous neurogenesis is poorly understood, but may play an important role in affective disorder. Studies in infrahuman primates and other mammalian species have established that psychological stressors reduce markedly the rate at which new neurons are formed, and may, in concert with stress-related elevation in corticosteroid production, promote cell death (Gould et al 1998). The resultant net reduction in neural tissue observed experimentally may account for the reductions in hippocampal volume described in patients with chronic depression (Shah et al 1998) and other stress-related conditions such as post-traumatic stress disorder. It is possible that antidepressant treatments may act to protect against, or even reverse, these changes. Antidepressant treatments from different classes, including electroconvulsive stimulation and lithium, enhance neurogenesis rates in rats (Reid & Stewart 2001). The antidepressant tianeptine has been shown to protect against stress-induced neurogenesis impairment (Czeh et al 2001), while electroconvulsive stimulation prevents steroid-induced reductions in neurogenesis (Hellsten et al 2002) in animal models.

The hypothalamus

The hypothalamus has been considered a minor station between the cognitive and the visceral, communicating on the one hand with higher structures such as the thalamus and limbic cortex, and on the other with the ascending fibre systems from the brainstem and spinal cord. It represents a major centre for control of the autonomic nervous system, and responds not only to neural information but also to chemical information in the circulating blood. The hypothalamus is a bilateral structure, bounding the third ventricle on each side, below the thalamus. It extends posteriorly to the mamillary bodies and anteriorly to the optic chiasm. Below, attached by the stalk of the infundibulum, is the pituitary gland. The hypothalamus consists of a number of important nuclei with diverse functions related to the maintenance of homeostasis, such as the regulation of food and water intake, and plays an important role in sleep, and sexual and defensive function. The hypothalamic–pituitary–adrenal axis, controlling corticosteroid activity, plays an important role in affective disorder (see Ch. 20).

The passage of the fornix to the mamillary bodies divides the hypothalamus into medial and lateral sections. The lateral region consists mainly of lateral hypothalamic nucleus and fibre tracts, including the medial forebrain bundle carrying, among others, monoaminergic pathways from brainstem nuclei to neocortex. The medial component contains several well-defined nuclei, including the supraoptic and paraventricular nuclei in the anterior portion, which produce the neurohormones vasopressin and oxytocin.

The hypothalamus has long been believed to play an important role in basic emotional expression. Primitive rage responses appear to be coordinated by the hypothalamus: stimulation of the lateral hypothalamus in cats results in reactions analogous to anger, while lesions of the region render animals placid and poorly responsive to threatening stimuli. Decortication has similar effects to stimulation, resulting in non-specific, non-directed, but coordinated defensive responses, described as sham rage by Walter Cannon in his studies conducted in the 1920s. If decortication is combined with hypothalamic damage, sham rage does not occur. These early findings led to the idea that higher structures, and input from higher limbic structures in particular, provided the analytical, directive components of emotional reactions and inspired the speculations of Papez, McLean and later theorists. Extensive projections from the amygdala to the hypothalamus (via the stria terminalis and the ventral amygdalofugal pathway), and from the hippocampus via the fornix, convey descending neocortical influence; while connections from the hypothalamus to prefrontal cortex and from mamillary bodies, via the anterior thalamic nucleus to the cingulate gyrus, complete McLean's modified view of the Papez circuit.

More selective, chemical stimulation and lesion techniques are refining understanding of the role of the hypothalamus as an emotional output station. Using microinjection of excitatory amino acids to destroy cell bodies, but to spare fibres of passage,

it is becoming clearer that older, less specific electrical stimulation or more extensive mechanical destruction has produced some misleading findings. Effects ascribed to damage to, or stimulation of, the hypothalamus itself may be due instead to the interruption or stimulation of fibres passing through the structure. Contemporary findings emphasise the involvement of projections from the amygdaloid complex (see below) through the hypothalamic area to other brain regions (such as the central grey region) in defensive behaviours, though autonomic responses to threatening situations do indeed appear to be mediated by the hypothalamus itself (reviewed by LeDoux 1998).

The amygdaloid complex

The amygdaloid complex (AC) is an almond-shaped (L. *amygdala*, almond) collection of subcortical nuclei which lie in the anterior pole of each temporal lobe, above the tip of the inferior horn of the lateral ventricle. The anatomy of the AC is indeed complicated: the various nuclei and areas are a heterogeneous group, each distinguished by specific cytoarchitectural, histochemical and internal and external connectivity features. Classification of the various elements has become increasingly sophisticated: contemporary surveys (e.g. Amaral et al 1992) recognise at least 12 major subdivisions comprising nuclear and cortical structures. There are three main groups: the deep nuclei (including lateral and basal nuclei); superficial nuclei and areas, including cortical elements (such as the periamygdaloid cortex); and the central nucleus. The lateral nucleus is an important input station in the amygdala, while the central nucleus has output functions.

The amygdaloid complex has widespread interconnection with subcortical and cortical areas. Subcortical projections range across autonomic and visceral centres in the diencephalon and brainstem, while there are numerous reciprocal neocortical–amygdaloid connections via the external capsule.

Two major extrinsic fibre systems project from the central nucleus of the amygdala to the hypothalamus and the dorsomedial nucleus of the thalamus (the stria terminalis and ventral amygdalofugal pathway respectively). The deep nuclei have important projections to the nucleus accumbens and striatum proper; and both superficial and deep nuclei have interconnections with the hippocampal formation, directly with the hippocampal subfields (CA1 and CA3) and also via the entorhinal cortex and subiculum. Neocortical areas have an extensive reciprocal connection with the amygdaloid complex: the superficial nuclei receive higher-order uni- and polymodal sensory information from widespread cortical areas, in addition to input from prefrontal and cingulate paralimbic cortex. The amygdaloid complex in turn projects back even more widely to cortical areas, including, for example, those subserving the very early stages of visual processing in the occipital lobe. The cells in the amygdaloid complex receiving information from the cortex are not the same cells that project back; the amygdala therefore appears to take part in a processing loop, receiving highly processed sensory information, performing further computation, and then modulating the earlier stages of cortical sensory input.

This brief anatomical overview clearly indicates that the amygdaloid complex must play an important role in cognitive and emotional function. It has been known since the late 19th century that bilateral damage to the anterior portion of the temporal lobes, including the amygdala, results in gross behavioural (emotional, cognitive and perceptual) abnormalities. This syndrome was formally described by Klüver and Bucy in monkeys in 1937. It now bears their names, and consists of visual agnosia (inability to recognise objects by sight: psychic blindness); strong oral tendencies (the inappropriate oral investigation of objects); loss of fear and aggressiveness; and hypersexual and misdirected sexual behaviour). Aspects of the syndrome have been described following a variety of neurological disorders affecting the temporal lobes in humans (e.g. meningitis, temporal lobe surgery).

Subsequent, more refined neurobiological investigations in non-human primates indicated that damage to the amygdala was critical to the development of the syndrome (e.g. Weiskrantz 1956), though temporal cortical lesions are also necessary. A remarkable experiment conducted by Downer (1961) clarified the role of the amygdala in processing emotional features in visual input. He restricted input from each eye to its ipsilateral hemisphere (by division of the optic chiasm and forebrain commissures) in monkeys with unilateral amygdala damage. In this way, one eye projected exclusively to its ipsilateral hemisphere with an intact contribution from the amygdala to visual processing; while the other eye projected exclusively to the other hemisphere without amygdala input. Threatening stimuli presented to the intact system elicited normal fearful and defensive reactions, while the same stimuli presented to the other eye, though detected, did not elicit an emotional response. The idea that the amygdala contributes to the processing of the emotional significance of sensory input thus developed, and begins to explain aspects of the Klüver–Bucy syndrome, such as lack of fearfulness.

Recent studies indicate that the amygdala makes important and specific contributions to fear responses and anxiety. Joseph LeDoux and his colleagues (reviewed LeDoux 1998) have examined the role of the amygdala in fear conditioning in rats, in which formerly neutral stimuli come to evoke fear responses (such as 'freezing' in rats) after repeated pairing with aversive events. Using a combination of anatomical, lesion and physiological techniques, they have tracked the processing of auditory stimuli in the development of fear conditioning from the earliest stages of auditory input in the brainstem, via the amygdala, through to the initiation of fearful motor responses. There are at least two pathways to the amygdala. There is a relatively direct route from the auditory thalamic relay (medial geniculate nucleus) to the lateral nucleus of the amygdala, which bypasses primary auditory cortex, and a longer route via auditory cortex to the lateral nucleus. Simple auditory stimuli paired with aversive experience can thus be rapidly processed and associated, while more complex stimulus discrimination may require the contribution of the cortical route. LeDoux (1998) has suggested that the direct pathway provides a fast rough representation of threatening stimuli, which may prepare the amygdala to receive and evaluate more detailed information from the cortex. The central nucleus of the amygdala then orchestrates motor responses to the conditioned stimulus, activating autonomic systems via the lateral hypothalamus, and fear responses via the central grey matter.

Using a rather different experimental paradigm, Michael Davis and his colleagues (Davis et al 1987) have studied the role of the amygdala in the development of the increased startle response in rats which occurs in the presence of cues previously associated with aversive events. They suggest that the amygdala represents a critical integrative brain site where neural activity produced by conditioned and unconditioned stimuli converge, and is essential for the expression of the startle response via connections with the brainstem nuclei, which mediate startle. Interestingly, there is evidence that NMDA receptor-mediated synaptic plasticity

(encountered above in the hippocampus) is essential for the acquisition of the startle response, though not for its expression once acquired (Miserendino et al 1990).

These findings in rats relating to aversive experiences may shed light on the neural basis of human anxiety disorders. There is also a body of evidence implicating amygdala function in reactions to rewarding stimuli, which may in turn relate to the neural substrates of affective disorder. Such studies (e.g. Everitt & Robbins 1992) emphasise projections from the basolateral amygdala to the ventral striatum, and the nucleus accumbens in particular, in the expression of voluntary responses to reward. The nucleus accumbens has been considered a 'limbic–motor' interface, modulated by dopaminergic input from the ventral tegmental area (see below). Electrical stimulation of such brain areas is innately rewarding, and they may play an important role in the appreciation and expression of hedonic tone in concert with the amygdala. Amygdalostriatal interactions may thus represent an alternative limbic output pathway, operating in parallel with amygdala–hypothalamic pathways, but more concerned with voluntary aspects of emotional response (Everitt & Robbins 1997) rather than the reflexive fear responses discussed above.

The amygdaloid complex has also been specifically implicated in explicit memory function. Though the relative contributions of amygdala and hippocampus have been much debated, as we have seen, they may in fact make independent contributions to different aspects of memory. For example, amygdala, but not hippocampal, lesions have been shown to impair a cross-modal DNMS task (Murray & Mishkin 1985). In the sample phase of this task, cues are presented in the tactile modality (by presenting the cues in the dark), but in the choice phase the same cues are presented in the visual modality. The monkey must therefore use information gained via touch in the recognition of a visually presented object in order to perform successfully. This impairment of cross-modal association may explain elements of the visual and oral abnormalities observed in the Klüver–Bucy syndrome. Conversely, the hippocampus plays an important role in tasks requiring the use of spatial information, but the amygdala does not. Monkeys trained preoperatively to associate objects with locations, performed at near chance levels following hippocampectomy, whereas their amygdalectomised counterparts performed as well as they had on the task prior to surgery (Parkinson et al 1988).

The amygdala is also thought to play a crucial role in social behaviour in primates (Kling & LA 1992, Brothers 1996). Single-unit recordings from the amygdala of monkeys indicate that specific neural responses are tuned to individual social stimuli, such as faces and their expressions, aversive and arousing events and so on. Direct stimulation of the amygdala in monkeys results in patterned social displays, and in humans may elicit subjective feelings of fear or pleasure. It seems likely that the amygdala subserves aspects of the reception of, and response to, social signals.

Studying aspects of social behaviour in adult macaque monkeys, Amaral and his colleagues (Amaral 2002) have shown that selective, bilateral lesions of the amygdala result in a lack of the usual fear response to novel inanimate objects and socially 'disinhibited' behaviour. In contrast, amygdala lesions created in neonatal macaques result in more fearful behaviour in social situations after weaning (compared with age-matched normal macaques), though fear of inanimate objects was reduced, in a similar manner to the pattern observed in animals lesioned in adulthood. These results are difficult to interpret at present, but imply that fear in social situations may be mediated separately in the brain from fear of inanimate objects, and that there is an important developmental aspect to the psychological expression of amygdala damage.

Recent PET studies in humans indicate that neural responses in the amygdala may be modulated by photographs showing varied intensities of emotional facial expressions, such as happiness and fearfulness (Morris et al 1996). Given the implication that the amygdala is involved in the 'neural representations of the dispositions and intentions of others' (Kling & LA 1992), it is hardly surprising that dysfunction of the amygdala has been implicated in schizophrenic disorder, particularly paranoid states, anxiety disorders and depression. Frodl et al (2003), for example, have reported that among brain structures, the amygdala may be the only neural region which is enlarged (rather than atrophic) in depressive states. They studied inpatients during their first episode of major depressive disorder using morphometric MRI imaging and suggest that the change may be a 'state' rather than a 'trait' phenomenon consequent on increased vascular volume, or enhanced dendritic branching. These findings are, however, by no means consistent — as ever, much more research needs to be done.

Summary

Put crudely, the various components of the limbic system can be thought of as working together to generate important elements of the emotional and cognitive basis of everyday normal mental life: memories, fears, hopes and feelings. The hippocampal formation appears to produce explicit records of events, the amygdala provides emotional tone and responses, the hypothalamus directs neuroendocrine and autonomic output, while the frontal lobes monitor, control and plan activities on a moment by moment basis. Clearly, an evolving understanding of the detailed functions of limbic structures promises a rich and sophisticated scientific psychopathology (see Andreasen 1997).

CHEMICAL NEUROANATOMY

In understanding brain–behaviour relationships, we are only beginning to grasp the complexities of the pattern of neurochemical brain function. The notion that there may be a simple relationship between single neurotransmitter systems and psychiatric disorders, by analogy with the relatively successful analysis of Parkinson's disease, is likely to be too optimistic. This is exemplified by the increasing uncertainties surrounding the dopamine hypothesis of schizophrenia. In developing comprehensive theories or descriptions of the biological basis of normal brain function and dysfunction, a number of conceptual dimensions or levels must be considered and eventually synthesised. These range from the analysis of molecular aspects of receptor function, through patterns of synaptic connectivity and computational aspects of information processing, to functional macroanatomy and ultimately neuropsychology. A crucial piece of this jigsaw lies in the anatomy of neurotransmitter systems. The range and specific functional properties of neurotransmitters and modulators are considered in Chapter 3. Here, we provide a brief survey of the anatomy of classical neurotransmitter systems of special relevance to psychiatric disorder: dopaminergic (DA), noradrenergic (NA), serotonergic (5HT, 5-hydroxytryptamine) and cholinergic (ACh, acetylcholine) systems. It is important to be aware that, despite their prominence in the psychiatric literature, these 'classical'

systems account for only a fraction of the synaptic activity in the brain: most of the work is done by the amino acids glutamate and GABA, to say nothing of the efforts of a bewildering array of other transmitters and neuromodulators.

In anatomical overview, each 'classical' system consists of defined nuclei or groups of cell bodies, mostly in the brainstem, with associated projection targets throughout the central nervous system. For monoamine-containing systems, the cell body group designations in the brainstem follow the convention established by Dahlström & Fuxe (1964) (for example, A1–A15 for catecholamine-containing neurons; B1–B9 for serotonergic neurons). The brainstem will be discussed next, followed by each neurotransmitter system in turn.

Brainstem anatomy and physiology

Antidepressants and antipsychotics have actions on all the main classical neuromodulator systems: serotonin, noradrenaline, dopamine and acetylcholine. The nuclei of cells, which synthesise these chemicals, are located in the brainstem. These cells project widely to terminal fields in the rest of the brain via axonal connections, which include the medial forebrain bundle.

Figure 2.11 shows a sagittal view of the brain together with a transverse section through the brainstem at the level of the midbrain–pons junction. The nuclei are elongated along the axis of the brainstem and extend well into the pons, in some cases further into the medulla. The bilateral substantia nigra cell bodies project mostly to basal ganglia motor nuclei (e.g. putamen). Blockade of dopaminergic projections from these nuclei with antipsychotic medication results in striatal dysfunction which is manifested clinically as extrapyramidal motor signs (e.g. parkinsonism and dystonic reactions). The corticospinal, or pyramidal (voluntary movement) motor tracts run anterior to the substantia nigra forming the cerebral peduncles.

The ventral tegmental area (VTA) is medial to these areas, though it is now recognised to overlap with the substantia nigra. The VTA is a major source of dopamine for non-motor areas of the brain: e.g. limbic system and prefrontal cortex. The beneficial effects of antipsychotic medication may be partly due to blockade of dopamine synthesised in VTA cells. The VTA is preferentially activated in animals and humans receiving substances such as amphetamines, cocaine, opiates and alcohol (see Ch. 5). These substances all release dopamine to some extent.

In animals, the periaqueductal grey (PAG) matter in the brainstem has been reported to be functionally segregated along the axis of the brainstem with regard to behaviour (Bandler & Keay 1996). The lateral PAG is associated with active defensive behaviour (fight and flight), hypertension, tachycardia and non-opioid analgesia. Within this region, there is evidence of further segregated function: the rostral region is associated with fight, the caudal region with flight. The ventrolateral PAG is associated with passive behaviour, hypotension, bradycardia and opioid analgesia (Bandler & Keay 1996). Direct electrical stimulation of the PAG has long been known to be aversive (Olds & Olds 1964). More recently, Gray has described a hierarchical behavioural defence system with the PAG at the lowest level (Gray & McNaughton 2000).

Lateral to, and partially overlapping with the PAG, are the paired locus coeruleus nuclei (Afshar et al 1978). In the midline, anterior and also overlapping with the PAG, lie the dorsal and median raphe nuclei (Baker et al 1990). The locus coeruleus cells

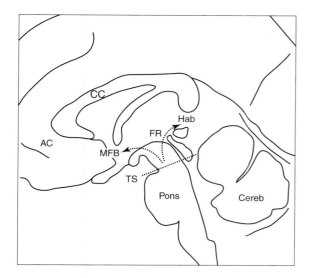

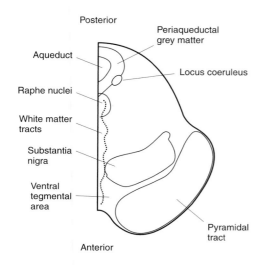

Fig. 2.11
Sagittal and transverse view of brainstem. TS indicates the location of the transverse slice through the inferior midbrain. AC, anterior cingulate; CC, corpus callosum; MFB, medial forebrain bundle; FR, fasciculus retroflexus; Hab, habenular nucleus; Cereb, cerebellum. 'White-matter tracts' include the MFB and FR.

synthesise noradrenaline, the raphe serotonin for the limbic system and the rest of the brain. Virtually all empirically derived antidepressants increase the brain levels of both these neurotransmitters by various mechanisms. Large reductions in $5HT_{1A}$ receptor numbers in the brainstem of unmediated depressed patients have been reported by Drevets and colleagues (see Ch. 5). In the anterior midbrain PAG and lateral posterior pons lie the pedunculopontine and lateral dorsal tegmental nuclei (Mesulam et al 1989), which synthesise ACh. These nuclei do not conform to the usual cytoarchitectonic boundaries and so have not been represented in Figure 2.11. Most antidepressants and antipsychotics block ACh transmission as a side-effect.

Reviews of the normal physiological role of these monoamines and ACh have been published. Dopamine is strongly implicated in motor and behavioural reward mechanisms, noradrenaline in non-specific arousal and selective attention, and ACh in cognitive

function including memory formation (Robbins & Everitt 1995). In the case of serotonin, however, the role is less clear. One theory specifically implicates serotonin in the mediation of defensive behaviour and anxiety (Graeff 1993) and is included as such in Gray's behavioural inhibition theory of septo-hippocampal function (Gray & McNaughton 2000). However, in general it is difficult to ascribe a single unitary role for serotonin, and there is significant evidence for serotonin acting in opposition to the other major neuromodulators (Robbins & Everitt 1995). This emphasises the fact that all neurotransmitters do not act in isolation but instead interact. From a behavioural viewpoint, appetitive rewarded behaviours are associated with anterior brainstem regions and the medial forebrain bundle, defensive behaviours with the posterior periaqueductal (and periventricular) regions (Olds & Olds 1964). All four classical neuromodulator systems are components of the more general reticular activating system (Robbins & Everitt 1995).

The fibre tracts connecting these nuclei to the rest of the brain pass mostly along the midline (Lang 1993). One tract, the medial forebrain bundle, then runs anteriorly through the lateral hypothalamus and ventral striatum to more distant prefrontal cortical regions implicated as structurally and functionally abnormal in imaging studies of psychiatric disorders (see Ch. 5). Another, the fasciculus retroflexus, passes posteriorly to the habenular nucleus in the dorsal diencephalon. It has long been known that direct electrical stimulation of the medial forebrain bundle in animals is rewarding (i.e. animals will work to repeat the stimulation) (Olds & Olds 1964) and, more recently, that this is specifically due to stimulation of the dopaminergic fibres (Rolls 1999). Rolls argues that stimulation (whether by electricity or drugs) of this tract (and projection sites such as orbitofrontal cortex) is rewarding because it comprises part of the system controlling appetitive behaviour (e.g. food ingestion, sexual activity, etc.) (Rolls 1999). In animals, the fasciculus retroflexus degenerates in response to sustained high levels of various drugs, including stimulants and nicotine, which may mimic the effects of human binge use (Ellison 2002). This tract is involved in the regulation of brainstem neurotransmitter activity and has been reported as exhibiting abnormal connectivity in a tryptophan depletion study of depressive illness relapse (see Ch. 5). The 'white matter tracts' shown in Figure 2.11 have been reported to be structurally abnormal in various studies of unipolar depressive illness (see Ch. 5).

In summary, the brainstem is clearly of interest in the study of psychiatric disorders. However, the region is comparatively small and lies deep within the brain, so it poses particular problems. Methods for studying the brainstem non-invasively in humans are consequently only now being developed. Each of the four major neurotransmitter systems will now be discussed in more detail.

Anatomy of the dopamine neurons

Groups of dopamine-containing neurons have been described and classified anatomically in a number of ways: in terms of distinct cell body groups, designated A8–A17; in terms of their efferent projection length characteristics — ultrashort, intermediate and long — (Cooper et al 1996); and in terms of the course of their projections through the brain (e.g. mesolimbic, nigrostriatal).

Cellular groups A16 and A17 represent 'ultrashort' projection systems found in the olfactory bulb and retina, respectively. These dopamine-containing cells act as intrinsic neurons (hence the designation 'ultrashort') in both olfactory bulb and retina. They thus form part of the networks of neurons involved in initial sensory processing. In the retina, for example, the cells represent a subclass of amacrine cell, a cell type we encountered when considering visual processing above. It is conceivable that dopamine deficiencies in the retina and olfactory bulb account for some of the visual and olfactory abnormalities encountered in Parkinson's disease.

The cell bodies of the 'intermediate length' projection systems (A11–A15) lie in the diencephalon. The majority of axons from this group remain within the diencephalic region (hence 'intermediate length'; an exception is the efferent fibres from A11 to the spinal cord). Principal cell groups include the ventromedial and arcuate hypothalamic nuclei (sometimes termed the tuberohypophyseal cells) projecting to the intermediate lobe of the pituitary and the median eminence; and the incertohypothalamic neurons which bridge dorsal posterior and anterior hypothalamus. Prolactin release from the anterior pituitary is inhibited by dopamine release from hypothalamic dopaminergic neurons; blockade of postsynaptic dopamine receptors here by antipsychotics raises serum prolactin levels, which may result in such adverse effects as breast enlargement, galactorrhoea and amenorrhoea.

Dopamine cell bodies located in the mesencephalon constitute the 'long length' projection system. Three cell groups are recognised: A8 (the retrorubral nucleus); A9 (the pars compacta of the substantia nigra); and A10 (the ventral tegmental area). The projections from these cells make up three important 'long' dopaminergic tracts: the nigrostriatal pathway; the mesolimbic pathway; and the mesocortical pathway. The relationship between cell body group and tract is not straightforward, with cell groups contributing heterogeneously to the main projections. There is however a degree of topographic organisation, such that adjacent cell bodies tend to project to adjacent target sites.

The nigrostriatal tract, mainly carrying fibres from the A8 and A9 groups, projects to the caudate and putamen of the neostriatum and plays a major role in motor control. Parkinson's disease results from a loss of dopaminergic cells from substantia nigra, with a consequent reduction in striatal dopamine — though dopaminergic projection loss in the condition is not exclusive to the nigrostriatal tract. Neuroleptic-induced pseudoparkinsonism and other adverse motor effects of antipsychotic drugs are mediated by effects on this system.

The mesolimbic and mesocortical projections arise from all three mesencephalic cell groups, with a principal contribution from A10 neurons. Limbic projection targets include the nucleus accumbens, the central nucleus of the amygdala and the hippocampus. Cortical targets include the medial prefrontal and anterior cingulate cortices, and the piriform and entorhinal cortices. Frontal activation abnormalities observed in schizophrenia may partly be mediated by dysfunction in the mesocortical dopamine system, while projections from the ventral tegmental area to the nucleus accumbens — increasingly implicated in rewarded behaviour — may play an important role in affective disorder.

The mesencephalic dopaminergic systems are functionally heterogeneous, with electrophysiological, biochemical and metabolic factors distinguishing the mesocortical, mesolimbic and nigrostriatal projections. Indeed, functional differences are described even between mesoprefrontal and mesocingulate systems. Differing dopaminergic system responses to classical and atypical neuroleptics may explain the variations in side-effect profile and efficacy observed among these drugs (Cooper et al

1996). It is likely that continuing study of such heterogeneity will prove a potent stimulus to the development of safer and perhaps more effective antipsychotic agents.

Anatomy of the noradrenergic neurons

The cell bodies of the noradrenergic neurons lie in the brainstem, designated A1 to A7. They form two main cell groups: a rostral group at the level of the midbrain–pons junction known as the locus coeruleus (A6, LC) forming a prominent dark patch in the floor of the fourth ventricle; and a diffusely scattered medullary/medullopontine group found more caudally throughout the ventral lateral tegmentum. The LC itself contains 50% of the central noradrenergic neurons. Though major input to the central noradrenergic system is highly restricted, both groups of neurons have very widespread efferent ascending projections to higher centres, in addition to descending projections to the spinal cord.

The ascending LC neurons (sometimes called the dorsal noradrenergic bundle) project widely to midbrain structures, the thalamus, limbic system and branch diffusely throughout the entire cortex. A further projection innervates cerebellar cortex. The descending projections course down through the mesencephalon, sending collaterals to motor nuclei in the brainstem, and then into the spinal cord (the coerulospinal pathway), innervating the ventral horn and basal part of the dorsal horn. Ascending projections from the diffuse tegmental cells (the ventral noradrenergic bundle) innervate brainstem, hypothalamic and some limbic cortical targets. Descending projections terminate in the grey matter of the spinal cord. In overview, though there is a degree of overlap, LC neurons contribute the main noradrenergic input to the cortex, while the tegmental group provide principal noradrenergic innervation to the brainstem and spinal cord.

LC neurons appear to play a role in the detection of suddenly changing or aversive sensory input. In such circumstances, the neurons increase activity in a rapid and coordinated way (Role & Kelly 1991), and abnormalities in central noradrenergic systems may play an important role in anxiety disorders (Brawman-Mintzer & Lydiard 1997). LC neurons respond in a similar way to novel sensory input. This in turn appears to increase cell excitability in subfields of the hippocampus via limbic noradrenergic projections, and may thus influence memory processing (Kischka et al 1997).

Anatomy of the serotonergic neurons

The cell bodies of serotonergic neurons are also found in the brainstem (cell groups B1 to B9). They constitute the most extensive monoaminergic system, with larger cell numbers than either noradrenergic or dopaminergic systems. The most caudal cell groups (B1–B4) have descending projections to the spinal cord, where they modulate spinal sensory and motor neurons. There are small, separate projections of serotonergic cell groups to the cerebellum and the LC. The raphe nuclei of the midbrain and pons (B7 and B8) play an important role in psychiatric neurobiology. The two main nuclei, the dorsal raphe nucleus (DRN) and median raphe nucleus (MRN) have ascending projections to striatum, limbic system and cortex. The DRN is found at a similar level in the brainstem to the dopamine-containing neurons of the ventral tegmental area, and has similar projection targets: the basal ganglia, nucleus accumbens, amygdala, and frontal cortex; while the MRN is located near the LC, with projection targets in thalamus, anterior temporal neocortex and hippocampus.

Deakin (1996) has suggested that the MRN and DRN serotonergic systems mediate different coping responses to acute and chronic aversive events, consistent with the long-held view that serotonergic systems play an important part in the genesis of depressive disorder. It is proposed that DRN neurons modulate forebrain circuits concerned with evaluative and motor aspects of avoidance behaviour, while MRN neurons modulate sensory and memory processing of aversive events. Dysfunction of these putative normal serotonergic activities is hypothesised to result in depressive disorder, which is in turn corrected by scrotonin reuptake inhibition by chemical antidepressants.

Appreciating the anatomical distinction between groups of cell bodies in the brainstem and their distant widespread projection fields is essential in understanding contemporary formulations of the action of specific scrotonin reuptake inhibitors (SSRIs). These drugs act at reuptake sites both at cell bodies and terminals, but with different effects over time. It has been suggested that $5HT_{1A}$ autoreceptors at the cell body shut down cell firing in the short term, acting against expected increases in synaptic 5HT in the projection field. Once the cell body autoreceptors desensitise in the face of chronic reuptake blockade, and cell firing increases again, then the effect of reuptake inhibition at the terminals now results in an increase in synaptic 5HT availability (Goodwin 1996). This may explain the delay in response to antidepressants seen in clinical practice, and informs recent attempts to accelerate antidepressant action using $5HT_{1A}$ autoreceptor blockers.

There are morphologically distinct serotonergic axon types: fine axons with small varicosities project from the DRN; while beaded axons, with large spherical varicosities, originate in the MRN. While the functional significance of the different types remains speculative (see Deakin 1996), they have a differential sensitivity to the neurotoxic effects of MDMA (Ecstasy), such that the fine axons may be permanently damaged (Green et al 1995).

Anatomy of the cholinergic neurones

Central cholinergic neurons fall into two principal groups: those that do not project from the regions in which they are located (i.e. local circuit cells like the ultrashort projection dopaminergic neurons described above); and projection neurons which link different brain regions.

Local circuit cells are represented by the cholinergic interneurons of the caudate and putamen, and those found in the nucleus accumbens and olfactory tubercle.

Projection neurons fall into two main groups of nuclei: a more caudal pontine group (the pontomesencephalotegmental cholinergic complex); and the more rostral basal forebrain cholinergic complex. The pontine group have both ascending projections (to the thalamus, basal ganglia and ventral diencephalic structures) and descending projections to the reticular formation, cerebellar nuclei, vestibular nuclei and cranial nerve nuclei. It is believed that these neurons have a role in arousal processes, amongst other activities.

The basal forebrain cholinergic complex consists of a group of nuclei, including the medial septal nucleus, the diagonal band nucleus, the substantia innominata, the magnocellular preoptic field and the nucleus basalis. Cells from these nuclei have a very widespread projection throughout limbic and neocortical targets.

Cholinergic neurotransmission has long been implicated in memory function in general, and in the pathology of Alzheimer's disease in particular, including the suggestion that there is a specific degeneration of the nucleus basalis. Reductions in concentrations of acetylcholine and choline acetyltransferase (an important enzyme involved in the synthesis of acetylcholine) have been observed at postmortem examination in brains from patients with Alzheimer's disease. However, neurotransmitter deficits in Alzheimer's disease are not restricted to the cholinergic system, and the notion that the cholinergic system has a specific role in learning and memory has been increasingly challenged. The use of more recently available neurotoxins which selectively destroy cholinergic neurons in studies of animal memory indicate that the nucleus basalis projections are probably more concerned with visual attentional processes (reviewed by Wenk 1997). Nonetheless, there is some evidence that hippocampal cholinergic projections from the medial septal nucleus may be more specifically involved in short-term working memory, while basalis–amygdala projections may influence affective learning. Projections from the diagonal band nuclei to the cingulate cortex may also contribute to learning processes (Everitt & Robbins 1997).

REFERENCES

Afshar F, Watkins E S, Yap J C 1978 Stereotaxic atlas of the human brainstem and cebellar nuclei: a variability study. Raven, New York

Aggleton J P 1992 The amygdala: neurobiological aspects of emotion, memory, and mental dysfunction. Wiley-Liss, New York

Alexander G E, Crutcher M D, DeLong M R 1990 Basal ganglia-thalamocortical circuits: parallel substrates for motor, oculomotor, "prefrontal" and "limbic" functions. In: Uylings H B M, Van Eden G C, De Bruin J P C et al (eds) Progress in brain research. Elsevier Science, New York

Amaral D G 2002 The primate amygdala and the neurobiology of social behavior: implications for understanding social anxiety. Biological Psychiatry 51: 11–17

Amaral D G. Price J L, Pitkänen A et al 1992 Anatomical organisation of the primate amygdaloid complex. In: Aggleton J P (ed) The amygdala. Wiley, New York

Andreasen N C 1997 Linking mind and brain in the study of mental illnesses: a project for a scientific psychopathology. Science 275: 1586–1593

Baddeley A 1986 Working memory. Oxford University Press, London

Baev K V 1998 Biological neural networks: the hierarchial concept of brain function. Birkhauser, Boston

Baev K V, Greene K A, Marciano F F et al 2002 Physiology and pathophysiology of cortico-basal ganglia-thalamocortical loops: theoretical and practical aspects. Progress in Neuropsychopharmacology & Biological Psychiatry 26: 771–804

Baker K G, Halliday G M, Tork I 1990 Cytoarchitecture of the human dorsal raphe nucleus. Journal of Comparative Neurology 301: 147–161

Bandler R, Keay K A 1996 Columnar organization in the midbrain periaqueductal gray and the integration of emotional expression. Progress in Brain Research 107: 285–300

Bartels A, Zeki S 1998 The theory of multistage integration in the visual brain. Proceedings of the Royal Society of London Series B: Biological Sciences 265: 2327–2332

Baxter L R Jr, Saxena S, Brody A L et al. 1996 Brain mediation of obsessive-compulsive disorder symptoms: evidence from functional brain imaging studies in the human and nonhuman primate. Seminars in Clinical Neuropsychiatry 1: 32–47

Brawman-Mintzer O, Lydiard R B 1997 Biological basis of generalized anxiety disorder. Journal of Clinical Psychiatry 58(suppl 3): 16–25; discussion 26

Brothers L 1996 Brain mechanisms of social cognition. Journal of Psychopharmacology 10: 2–8

Brown S, Schaefer E A 1888 An investigation into the functions of the occipital and temporal lobe of the monkey's brain. Philosophical Transactions of the Royal Society of London Series B: Biological Sciences 179: 303–327

Bush G, Luu P, Posner M I 2000 Cognitive and emotional influences in anterior cingulate cortex. Trends in Cognitive Science 4: 215–222

Bush G, Vogt B A, Holmes J et al 2002 Dorsal anterior cingulate cortex: a role in reward-based decision making. Proceedings of the National Academy of Sciences of the USA 99: 523–528

Chesselet M F, Delfs J M 1996 Basal ganglia and movement disorders: an update. Trends in Neuroscience 19: 417–422

Cooper J R, Bloom F E, Roth R H 1996 The biochemical basis of neuropharmacology, 7th edn. Oxford University Press, New York

Corsellis J A N, Janota I 1985 Neuropathology in relation to psychiatry. In: Shepherd M (ed) The scientifc foundations of psychiatry. Cambridge University Press, Cambridge

Crick F H C 1994 The astonishing hypothesis. Simon & Schuster, London

Czeh B, Michaelis T, Watanabe T et al 2001 Stress-induced changes in cerebral metabolites, hippocampal volume, and cell proliferation are prevented by antidepressant treatment with tianeptine. Proceedings of the National Academy of Sciences of the USA 98: 12796–12801

Dahlström A, Fuxe K 1964 Evidence for the existence of monoamine-containing neurones in the central nervous system, I: Demonstration of monoamines in the cell bodies of the brain stem neurones. Acta Physiologica Scandinavica Supplement 232: 1–55

Davis M, Hitchcock J M, Rosen J B 1987 Anxiety and the amygdala: pharmacological and anatomical analysis of fear potentiated startle. In Bower G H (ed) The psychology of learning and motivation. Academic Press, San Diego

Dayan P, Kakade S, Montague P R 2000 Learning and selective attention. Nature Neuroscience 3(suppl):1218–1223

Deakin J F W 1996 5HT, antidepressant drugs and the psychosocial origins of depression. Journal of Psychopharmacology 10: 31–38

Dennett D C 1991 Consciousness explained. Penguin, London

Devinski O, Morrell M, Vogt B A 1995 Contributions of anterior cingulate cortex to behaviour. Brain 118: 279–306

Downer J D C 1961 Changes in visual gnostic function and emotional behaviour following unilateral temporal lobe damage in the 'split-brain' monkey. Nature 191: 50–51

Ebmeier K P 1995 Brain imaging and schizophrenia. In: Den Boer J A, Westenberg H G M, van Praag H M (eds) Advances in the neurobiology of schizophrenia. Wiley, Chichester, p 131–155

Elliott R, Friston K J, Dolan R J 2000 Dissociable neural responses in human reward systems. The Journal of Neuroscience 20: 6159–6165

Ellison G 2002 Neural degeneration following chronic stimulant abuse reveals a weak link in brain, fasciculus retroflexus, implying the loss of forebrain control circuitry. European Neuropsychopharmacology 12: 287–297

Eriksson P S, Perfilieva E, Bjork-Eriksson T et al 1998 Neurogenesis in the adult human hippocampus. Nature Medicine 4: 1313–1317

Everitt B J, Robbins T W 1992 Amygdala-ventral striatal interactions and reward-related processes. In: Aggleton J P (ed) The amygdala: neurobiological aspects of emotion, memory, and mental dysfunction. Wiley, New York, p 401–429

Everitt B J, Robbins T W 1997 Central cholinergic systems and cognition. Annual Review of Psychology 48: 649–684

Falkai P, Bogerts B 1986 Cell loss in the hippocampus of schizophrenics. European Archives of Psychiatry & Neurological Sciences 236: 154–161

Feger J 1997 Updating the functional model of the basal ganglia. Trends in Neurosciences 20: 152–153

Friston K J 1994 Statistical parametric mapping. In: Thatcher R W, Hallett M, Zeffro T et al (eds) Functional neuroimaging: technical foundations. Academic Press, San Diego, p 79–93

Frodl T, Meisenzahl EM, Zetzsche T et al 2003 Larger amygdala volumes in first depressive episode as compared to recurrent major depression and healthy control subjects. Biological Psychiatry 53: 338–344

Gaffan D 1992 Amygdala and the memory of reward. In: Aggleton J P (ed) The amygdala: neurobiological aspects of emotion, memory, and mental dysfunction. Wiley, New York, p 471–483

Gehring W J, Himle J, Nisenson L G 2000 Action-monitoring dysfunction in obsessive-compulsive disorder. Psychological Science 11: 1–6

Goldman-Racic P S 1995 Architecture of the prefrontal cortex and the central executive. Annals of the New York Academy of Sciences 769: 71–84

Goodwin G M 1996 How do antidepressants affect serotonin receptors? The role of serotonin receptors in the therapeutic and side effect profile of the SSRIs. Journal of Clinical Psychiatry 57 (suppl 4):9–13

Gould E, Tanapat P, McEwen B S et al 1998 Proliferation of granule cell precursors in the dentate gyrus of adult monkeys is diminished by stress. Proceedings of the National Academy of Sciences of the USA 95: 3168–3171

Graeff F G 1993 Role of 5-HT in defensive behavior and anxiety. Reviews in the Neurosciences 4: 181–211

Grasso M G, Pantano P, Ricci M et al 1994 Mesial temporal cortex hypoperfusion is associated with depression in subcortical stroke. Stroke 25: 980–985

Gray J A, McNaughton N 2000 The neuropsychology of anxiety: an enquiry into the functions of the septo-hippocampal system, 2nd edn. Oxford University Press, Oxford

Green A R, Cross A J, Goodwin G M 1995 Review of the pharmacology and clinical pharmacology of 3,4-methylenedioxymethamphetamine (MDMA or "Ecstasy"). Psychopharmacology (Berlin) 119: 247–260

Heath R G 1964 Pleasure response of human subjects to direct stimulation of the brain: physiologic and psychodynamic considerations. In: Heath R G (ed) The role of pleasure in behaviour. Hober, New York, p 219–243

Hellsten J, Wennstrom M, Mohapel P et al 2002 Electroconvulsive seizures increase hippocampal neurogenesis after chronic corticosterone treatment. European Journal of Neuroscience 16: 283–290

Hubel D H, Wiesel T N 1979 Brain mechanisms of vision. Scientific American 241: 150–162

Hubel D H, Wiesel T N, Stryker M P 1978 Anatomical demonstration of orientation columns in macaque monkey. Journal of Comparative Neurology 177: 361–380

Kandel E R, Schwartz J H, Jessell T M 2000 Principles of neural science. McGraw-Hill, New York

Khoo M C K 2000 Physiological control systems: analysis, simulation and estimation. IEEE Press, Piscataway

Kischka U, Spitzer M, Kammer T 1997 [Frontal-subcortical neuronal circuits]. Fortschritte der Neurologie-Psychiatric 65: 221–231

Kling A S, LA B 1992 The amygdala and social behaviour. In: Aggleton J P (ed) The amygdala. Wiley, New York

Klüver H, Bucy P C 1937 'Psychic blindness' and other symptoms following bilateral temporal lobectomy in rhesus monkeys. American Journal of Physiology 119: 352–353

Kovelman J A, Scheibel A B 1984 A neurohistological correlate of schizophrenia. Biological Psychiatry 19: 1601–1621

Lang J 1993 Surgical anatomy of the brain stem. Neurosurgical clinics of North America 4: 367–403

LeDoux J 1998 The emotional brain. Phoenix, London

Lund J S 1988 Anatomical organization of macaque monkey striate visual cortex. Annual Review of Neuroscience 11: 253–288

Macko K A, Jarvis C D, Kennedy C et al 1982 Mapping the primate visual system with [2–14C]deoxyglucose. Science 218: 394–397

McLean P D 1949 Psychosomatic disease and the 'viseeral brain': recent developments bearing on the Papez theory of emotion. Psychosomatic Medicine 11: 338–353

Martin J H 1996 Neuroanatomy — text and atlas. Prentice-Hall, London

Mega M S, Cummings J L 1997 The cingulate and cingulate syndromes. In: Trimble M R, Cummings J L (eds) Contempory behavioural neurology. Butterworth-Heinemann, Oxford

Mesulam M M, Geula C, Bothwell M A et al 1989 Human reticular formation: cholinergic neurons of the pedunculopontine and laterodorsal tegmental nuclei and some cytochemical comparisons to forebrain cholinergic neurons. Journal of Comparative Neurology 283: 611–633

Miserendino M J, Sananes C B, Melia K R et al 1990 Blocking of acquisition but not expression of conditioned fear-potentiated startle by NMDA antagonists in the amygdala. Nature 345: 716–718

Mishkin M 1978 Memory in monkeys severely impaired by combined but not by separate removal of amygdala and hippocampus. Nature 273: 297–298

Morris J S, Frith C D, Perrett D I et al 1996 A differential neural response in the human amygdala to fearful and happy facial expressions. Nature 383: 812–815

Morris R G, Morris R J 1997 Neurobiology. Memory floxed. Nature 385: 680–681

Murray E A, Mishkin M 1984 Severe tactual as well as visual memory deficits follow combined removal of the amygdala and hippocampus in monkeys. Journal of Neuroscience 4: 2565–2580

Murray E A, Mishkin M 1985 Amygdalectomy impairs crossmodal association in monkeys. Science 228: 604–606

Murray E A, Mishkin M 1986 Visual recognition in monkeys following rhinal cortical ablations combined with either amygdalectomy or hippocampectomy. Journal of Neuroscience 6: 1991–2003

Neary D 1995 Neuropsychological aspects of frontotemporal degeneration. Annals of the New York Academy of Sciences 769: 15–22

Olds J, Olds M E 1964 The mechanisms of voluntary behaviour. In: Heath R G (ed) Role of pleasure in behaviour. Harper and Row, New York

Papez J W 1937 A proposed mechanism of emotion. Archives of Neurology and Psychiatry 38: 725–743

Parkin A J 1987 Memory and amnesia: an introduction. Blackwell, Oxford

Parkinson J K, Murray E A, Mishkin M 1988 A selective mnemonic role for the hippocampus in monkeys: memory for the location of objects. Journal of Neuroscience 8: 4159–4167

Pascual-Leone A, Grafman J, Hallett M 1994 Modulation of cortical motor output maps during development of implicit and explicit knowledge. Science 263: 1287–1289

Penfield W, Rasmussen T 1954 The cerebral cortex of man: a clinical study of localization of function. Macmillan, New York

Petrides M 1995 Functional organization of the human frontal cortex for mnemonic processing. Evidence from neuroimaging studies. Annals of the New York Academy of Sciences 769: 85–96

Phillips C G, Zeki S, Barlow H B 1984 Localization of function in the cerebral cortex: past, present and future. Brain 107(Pt 1):327–361

Rao R P, Ballard D H 1999 Predictive coding in the visual cortex: a functional interpretation of some extra-classical receptive-field effects. Nature Neuroscience 2: 79–87

Rao S C, Rainer G, Miller E K 1997 Integration of what and where in the primate prefrontal cortex. Science 276: 821–824

Reid I C, Stewart C A 2001 How antidepressants work: new perspectives on the pathophysiology of depressive disorder. British Journal of Psychiatry 178: 299–303

Robbins T W, Everitt B J 1995 Arousal systems and attention. In: Gazzaniga M S (ed), The cognitive neurosciences. MIT Press, Cambridge, Mass

Roberts G W 1991 Temporal lobe pathology and schizophrenia. In: Kerwin R (ed) Neurobiology and psychiatry, vol 1. Cambridge University Press, Cambridge

Role L W, Kelly J P 1991 The brain stem: cranial nerve nuclei and the monoaminergic systems. In Kandel E R, Schwartz J H, Jessel T M (eds) Principles of neural science, 3rd edn. Elsevier, New York

Rolls E T 1999 The brain and emotion. Oxford University Press, Oxford

Rolls E T 2000 Precis of The brain and emotion. Behavioral & Brain Sciences 23: 177–191; discussion 192–233

Scheffers M K, Coles M G 2000 Performance monitoring in a confusing world: error-related brain activity, judgments of response accuracy, and types of errors. Journal of Experimental Psychology: Human Perception & Performance 26: 141–151

Schultz W, Dickinson A 2000 Neuronal coding of prediction errors. Annual Review of Neuroscience 23: 473–500

Schultz W, Dayan P, Montague P R 1997 A neural substrate of prediction and reward. Science 275: 1593–1599

Scoville W B, Milner B 1957 Loss of recent memory after bilateral hippocampal lesions. Journal of Neurology, Neurosurgery and Psychiatry 20: 11–21

Shah P J, Ebmeier K P, Glabus M F et al 1998 Cortical grey matter reductions associated with treament-resistant unipolar depression: controlled magnetic resonance imaging study. British Journal of Psychiatry 172: 527–532

Shallice T 1982 Specific impairments of planning. Philosophical Transactions of the Royal Society of London Series B: Biological Sciences 298: 199–209

Solomon R L, Corbit J D 1974 An opponent-process theory of motivation, 1: Temporal dynamics of affect. Psychological Review 81: 119–145

Squire L R 1986 Mechanisms of memory. Science 232: 1612–1619

Squire L R, Moore R Y 1979 Dorsal thalamic lesion in a noted case of human memory dysfunction. Annals of Neurology 6: 503–506

Stuss D T, Shallice T, Alexander M P et al 1995 A multidisciplinary approach to anterior attentional functions. Annals of the New York Academy of Sciences 769: 191–211

Talairach J, Bancaud J, Geier S et al 1973 The cingulate gyrus and human behaviour. Electroencephalography and Clinical Neurophysiology 34: 45–52

Tanaka K 1993 Neuronal mechanisms of object recognition. Science 262: 685–688

Tatemichi T K, Desmond D W, Prohovnik I 1995 Strategic infarcts in vascular dementia: a clinical and brain imaging experience. Arzneimittelforschung 45: 371–385

Tessier-Lavigne M 1991 Phototransduction and information processing in the retina. In: Kandel E, Schwartz J H, Jessel T (eds) Principles of neural science, 3rd edn. Elsevier, New York

Victor M, Adams R D, Collins G H 1971 The Wernicke-Korsakoff syndrome. Blackwell, Oxford

Vogt B A, Gabriel M 1993 Neurobiology of cingulate cortex and limbic thalamus. Birkhauser, Boston

Vogt B A, Finch D M, Olson C R 1992 Functional heterogeneity in cingulate cortex: the anterior executive and posterior evaluative regions. Cerebral Cortex 2: 435–443

Weiskrantz L 1956 Behavioural changes associated with ablation of the amygdaloid complex in monkeys. Journal of Comparative and Physiological Psychology 49: 381–391

Wenk G L 1997 The nucleus basalis magnocellularis cholinergic system: one hundred years of progress. Neurobiology of Learning a Memory 67: 85–95

Wickelgreen I 1997 Getting a grasp on working memory. Science 275: 1580–1582

Wiesel F A, Wik G, Sjogren I et al 1987 Regional brain glucose metabolism in drug free schizophrenic patients and clinical correlates. Acta Psychiatrica Scandinavica 76: 628–641

Wilson M A, Tonegawa S 1997 Synaptic plasticity, place cells and spatial memory: study with second generation knockouts. Trends in Neurosciences 20: 102–106

Wolpert D M, Ghahramani Z, Jordan M I 1995 An internal model for sensorimotor integration. Science 269: 1880–1882

Zald D H, Kim S W 1996 Anatomy and function of the orbital frontal cortex, II: function and relevance to obsessive compulsive disorder. Journal of Neuropsychiatry and Clinical Neurosciences 8: 249–261

Zeman A 2002 Consciousness: a users guide. Yale University Press, New Haven

Zeki S 2001 Localization and globalization in conscious vision. Annual Review of Neuroscience 24: 57–86

Zeki S, Bartels A 1998 The autonomy of the visual systems and the modularity of conscious vision. Philosophical Transactions of the Royal Society of London Series B: Biological Sciences 353: 1911–1914

Zeki S, Bartels A 1999 Toward a theory of visual consciousness. Consciousness & Cognition 8: 225–259

Zola-Morgan S, Squire L R, Amaral D G 1986 Human amnesia and the medial temporal region: enduring memory impairment following a bilateral lesion limited to field CA1 of the hippocampus. Journal of Neuroscience 6: 2950–2967

Zola-Morgan S, Squire L R, Alvarez-Royo P et al 1991 Independence of memory functions and emotional behavior: separate contributions of the hippocampal formation and the amygdala. Hippocampus 1: 207–220.

3 Neuropharmacology

Gordon Arbuthnott

INTRODUCTION

Neuropharmacological studies contribute extensively to the evaluation of drug treatments in psychiatry and have provided useful insights into the neurobiology of mental illnesses. The fact that mental illnesses cannot be fully understood from a pharmacological perspective is in part attributed to their complexity but is to some extent related to the present stage of development of neurobiology as a science. Molecular mechanisms, especially those involving drug–receptor interaction and the control of genetic expression in the brain, form the focus of much current research in neuropharmacology. It is to be expected that as these studies progress the source of symptoms in psychiatric disorders will be understood and rational treatment will become possible, in the same way as understanding the cause of peripheral diseases such as diabetes made the symptoms accessible to rational therapy.

BRAIN METABOLISM

The first attempts to apply chemical methods to the study of brain function were made several hundred years ago, and information concerning the inorganic constituents of the brain was obtained as early as 1719. With the development of suitable chemical fractionation techniques in the 19th century, detailed investigations of the organic constituents of neural tissue became feasible. Julius Schlossberger in his *General and Comparative Animal Chemistry* devoted 135 of its 616 pages to the chemistry of neural tissues. This work stimulated a number of more extensive studies of the nervous system by the methods of organic chemistry, culminating in the most comprehensive of 19th century studies of brain composition: Thudichum's *Treatise on the Chemical Constitution of the Brain*, published in 1884 (see McIlwain 1990). As early as 1833 attempts were being made to relate mental disorders to alterations in the chemical composition of the brain.

The emphasis on studies of brain constituents in the early phase of the development of neurochemistry was due in part to the widely held, but erroneous, view that brain metabolism was a very slow process. Subsequently, with the advent of isotopic tracer techniques, it became apparent that the brain had one of the highest metabolic rates of any tissue and that most cerebral constituents are in a dynamic state, undergoing rapid changes in association with changes in cerebral functioning. Knowledge of the chemical composition of the brain does not, therefore, in itself, afford much understanding of cerebral function. Although

the composition of the brain is altered significantly in a number of conditions (such as some of the inborn errors of lipid and amino acid metabolism), most present-day research on the neurochemistry of mental disorders concentrates on dynamic processes such as synthesis, turnover, release, uptake and transport of neurotransmitters. Formidable practical obstacles still exist, including the structural and functional complexity of the brain, its cellular heterogeneity and the enormous range of time-scales over which reactions can occur.

There are, for example, two major cell types in the brain — neurons and glia — and the difference in their functional roles is reflected in their very different chemical composition and metabolic properties. However, even small samples of brain tissue will contain several types of neuron and glia, usually in close juxtaposition, and it is extremely difficult to separate the contributions of each cell type to the metabolism of the tissue as a whole. A further complication is that the intracellular concentrations of many chemicals within brain cells are not uniform. Each cell is composed of many types of organelle, each having a different chemical composition and different metabolic properties. The existence of different metabolic 'pools' within cells is known as *compartmentation* and is particularly pronounced in the brain. Many brain constituents, e.g. amino acids such as glutamate, are found in several intracellular pools that differ in size and turnover rate.

For these reasons classical biochemical methods for studying metabolism (for example, the use of tissue slices and homogenates in vitro) can, when applied to the brain, yield data that are extremely difficult to interpret. Although some of the problems can be overcome by use of such techniques as histochemistry (to assist in precise localisation of substances), it has been necessary to develop fractionation and analytical techniques to enable the study of the metabolism of different cell types in isolation and the study of metabolism at the subcellular level. The successful development of such methods, particularly micromethods of single-cell analysis and fractionation methods that permit the study of isolated nerve endings ('synaptosomes'), has contributed greatly to progress in neurochemistry.

The tasks performed by the cells of the brain are less conspicuously energy consuming than those of many other cells, since they do not involve mechanical work, osmotic work or significant external secretory activity. There are, nevertheless, many functions of brain cells that are energy intensive: the maintenance of membrane potentials, active transport and the synthesis and axoplasmic transport of cellular materials. It is not surprising, therefore, that, with its organisational complexity and wide range of endergonic activities, the brain has a high metabolic rate. Although it comprises a mere 2% of body weight it accounts for approximately 10% of the energy expenditure and 20% of the oxygen consumption of the body at rest. In children this percentage is even higher; the brain of a 5-year-old accounts for approximately 50% of the resting total body oxygen consumption. The oxygen consumption of a typical neuron is between 10 and 100 times greater than that of a glial cell.

Energy metabolism is not responsible for absolutely all the oxygen consumption of the brain, as the brain contains a variety of oxidases and hydroxylases that have a role in the synthesis and metabolism of a number of neurotransmitters. However, important though these are, they account for a negligible proportion of the total oxygen consumption of the brain.

As a consequence of its high energy requirement the brain is extremely sensitive to disturbances in the supply of its energy sources, and many clinical conditions associated with disturbances of brain function can often be traced back to a deficiency in the production or utilisation of energy. Furthermore, in view of the poor regenerative abilities of nerve cells, an energy deficiency of any duration can have long-term implications for both functional and structural integrity.

Primary energy sources

The brain, like the rest of the body, obtains its chemical energy by the oxidation of foodstuffs. The energy derived from this oxidation is stored in a utilisable form as high-energy phosphate in molecules of adenosine triphosphate (ATP). The primary energy source of the central nervous system (CNS) is glucose, and in this the brain differs from other tissues which are able to utilise lipids and, to a lesser extent, protein. There is little storage of either lipid or glycogen. The glycogen content of brain is only 2–4 μmol/g and therefore the metabolism of the brain cannot be sustained by its carbohydrate reserves. Consequently, it is dependent on a constant blood-borne supply of glucose. Under normal conditions, the brain utilises approximately 16–20 μmol of glucose per gram of brain per hour, and cessation of the blood supply of glucose and oxygen results in loss of consciousness within less than 10 seconds (the time taken to consume the oxygen within the brain and its blood) and irreversible brain damage within minutes.

In nutritional studies, a commonly used index for estimating the proportion of fat and carbohydrate being utilised is the respiratory quotient (RQ; calculated by dividing the volume of carbon dioxide produced by the volume of oxygen consumed). The RQ for fat oxidation is 0.71 and the RQ for carbohydrate oxidation is 1.00. The RQ calculated for the adult brain is 0.99. Under normal conditions, the amount of oxygen consumed in the brain is equivalent to that of the glucose removed from the blood (McIlwain & Bachelard 1985).

The normal arterial blood glucose concentration is approximately 80 mg/100 ml. When hypoglycaemia occurs, brain glucose consumption is reduced more than its oxygen utilisation and the total carbon dioxide produced by the brain can be increased to twice the basal level. Isotope experiments have shown that this increased carbon dioxide production is due to the oxidation of non-carbohydrate substrates, probably amino acids and lipids. As a result, hypoglycaemia may be associated with marked neurological manifestations, including convulsions. In insulin-induced hypoglycaemia the blood glucose concentration may fall as low as 8 mg/100 ml and coma can result because, under these condi-

tions, the reduced production of ATP is inadequate for normal brain function. The pre-eminence of glucose as the substrate supporting the energy-requiring activities of the mammalian brain was first established over fifty years ago and remains unchallenged by more modern research. For review, see Sokoloff (1989).

Nervous tissue contains all the enzymes and metabolic intermediates of anaerobic and aerobic carbohydrate metabolism and is also able to utilise lipid and protein in vitro. The brain depends on glucose as its primary energy source in vivo because the availability of other substrates is severely limited by the set of diverse homeostatic mechanisms known as the blood–brain barrier. Whereas glucose has an unimpeded entry from the blood into the brain and rapidly reaches tissue levels adequate for maintaining normal metabolism, the entry of fructose, lactate, pyruvate, succinate and glutamate is restricted and tissue levels comparable to those achieved by glucose are not reached.

Glucose metabolism

The manner in which the potential chemical energy of glucose is captured and utilised for the synthesis of ATP in the brain is broadly similar to that in other tissues. It is achieved in three main stages. First, glucose is converted to pyruvic acid by the glycolysis (Embden–Meyerhof) pathway in the cell cytoplasm. Although this glycolytic pathway is the main pathway of glucose utilisation, the pentose phosphate pathway is also functional and accounts for approximately 1% of the metabolic flux of glucose in human brain. Its primary role is to generate reduced coenzymes for use in biosynthetic pathways, but the pentose phosphates it produces are also important for local nucleotide synthesis, as, in the adult, there is a restricted entry of nucleotides from the blood to the brain. In the second stage of glucose breakdown, pyruvic acid is oxidised in the mitochondria to carbon dioxide via acetyl coenzyme A (acetyl-CoA) and the Krebs (or tricarboxylic) acid cycle. In the third stage, the electrons produced by the Krebs cycle enter the electron transport chain (avoprotein–cytochrome system) where they are used in the reduction of oxygen. This process is coupled with the generation of ATP and is known as oxidative phosphorylation. A summary of glucose metabolism in brain is shown schematically in Figure 3.1.

ATP production

During glycolysis, direct transfer of high-energy phosphate from 1,3-diphosphoglyceric acid and phosphoenolpyruvate to adenosine diphosphate (ADP) results in the formation of two ATP molecules. Under anaerobic conditions, therefore, there is a net synthesis of two ATP molecules as glucose breaks into two triose molecules, and two ATP molecules are used in the formation of glucose 6-phosphate and fructose 1,6-diphosphate. Under aerobic conditions, however, the reduced coenzyme nicotinamide-adenine dinucleotide (NAD) produced in the oxidation of glyceraldehyde phosphate is re-oxidised through the avoprotein cytochrome system, with the formation of three ATP molecules. Further oxidation of each pyruvate molecule to carbon dioxide and water via the tricarboxylic acid cycle yields a further 15 molecules of ATP, i.e. a further 30 molecules per molecule of glucose. This ATP is produced by the re-oxidation of reduced NAD, NAD phosphate (NADP) and flavin-adenine dinucleotide (FAD) by the electron transport chain, but ATP is also produced by reaction of ADP and guanosine triphosphate (GTP) formed in the conversion

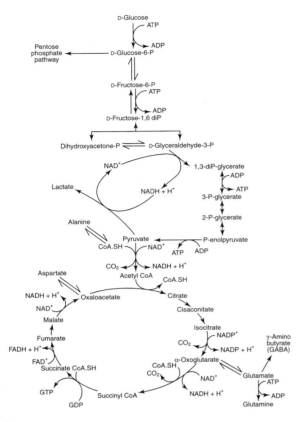

Fig. 3.1
Principal metabolic pathways of the brain.

Cerebral carbohydrate metabolism exhibits considerable flexibility to supply energy according to functional need. For example, during anaesthesia glucose utilisation is of the order of 0.15 mmol $kg^{-1}min^{-1}$ but during convulsions utilisation can increase to more than 10 mmol $kg^{-1}min^{-1}$. Such flexibility in the cerebral metabolic rate is possible because cerebral glucose metabolism is regulated at a number of different levels: by changes in cerebral circulation; by changes in glucose transport from the blood; and by changes in the rate of individual enzyme reactions brought about by environmental influences on the activity of key regulatory enzymes such as the glycolytic enzymes, hexokinase and phosphofructokinase. Energy output and oxygen consumption in the brain are associated with high levels of enzyme activity in the Krebs cycle. The actual flux through the cycle depends on a number of factors. For example the rate of glycolysis and acetyl-CoA production can 'push' the cycle, while the activity of the pyruvate dehydrogenase complex controls the rate of pyruvate entering the cycle. In addition, the local ADP level, which is the prime activator of oxidative phosphorylation to which the cycle is linked, is likewise important. Another factor contributing to the flexibility in metabolic rate is the fact that the substrate levels found under normal physiological conditions are generally well below those required for maximum enzyme activities. For example, under normal conditions only half of the brain pyruvate dehydrogenase is active.

The γ-aminobutyrate (GABA) shunt

The metabolism of the adult brain is characterised by a high rate of incorporation of glucose carbon into free amino acids. In this respect the brain differs markedly from other organs such as the liver, kidney, lung, muscle and spleen. The explanation of this phenomenon is that the metabolism of certain glucose metabolites is closely related to that of the 'glutamate group' of amino acids. Members of this group (glutamate, aspartate and GABA) have a special role in the CNS and account for 75% of the free amino acids in the brain. They are found primarily in the grey matter and are associated with neuronal mitochondria. Glutamate, by its energy-dependent conversion to glutamine, plays an important role in the detoxification of ammonia in the brain, and both glutamate and GABA function physiologically as transmitters.

Aspartate and glutamate are glycogenic since they are readily and reversibly converted into oxaloacetate and α-oxoglutarate by transamination reactions. These reactions allow the extensive synthesis of non-essential amino acids from Krebs cycle intermediates and aid in regulating the concentration of metabolites entering this cycle. Another possible regulator of the Krebs cycle in the CNS is the metabolic sequence known as the 'GABA shunt' shown in Figure 3.2. This is a bypass around the cycle from α-oxoglutarate to succinate and accounts for approximately 10% of the total glucose turnover. Although this pathway is found at extremely low levels in some other tissues such as kidney, heart and liver, it is, by far, most active in the brain. This is due to the relatively high levels in the CNS of the enzyme responsible for catalysing the decarboxylation of glutamate to GABA. This enzyme, glutamate decarboxylase, in common with the transaminase enzyme, requires vitamin B_6 phosphate (pyridoxal phosphate) as a cofactor. The importance of these interrelationships between the glutamate group of amino acids and glucose metabolism is illustrated by the deleterious effects of vitamin B_6 deficiency. Glutamate decarboxylase and transaminase inhibition

of succinyl-CoA to succinate. Thus during the complete oxidative breakdown of glucose to carbon dioxide and water there is a net production of 38 molecules of ATP. This represents a theoretical efficiency of 42% in capturing the energy latent in the glucose. However, in practice, approximately 15% of brain glucose is converted from pyruvate to lactate and does not enter the Krebs cycle, and therefore the net gain of ATP is nearer 33 molecules per molecule of glucose utilised (Clarke et al 1989).

Regulation: metabolism in relation to functional state

Anaerobic metabolism of glucose, yielding as it does a mere two molecules of ATP, cannot supply the energy requirements of normal cerebral function, and as a result the brain is very dependent on the efficient working of the Krebs cycle. This dependence is reflected in the neurological dysfunction that can ensue as a consequence of interference with its normal operation. Deficiency of thiamine, a cofactor in the conversion of pyruvate to acetyl-CoA, has profound effects on the CNS, as does a deficiency of niacin (required for NAD synthesis). However, carbohydrate metabolism in brain is relatively insensitive to a number of factors that have pronounced effects on other organs. Thyroid hormones have been shown to have no effect on the cerebral respiration rate in the adult human, although the development of the adult pattern of cerebral glucose metabolism is retarded after neonatal thyroidectomy. There is even doubt whether insulin affects glucose transport and utilisation in nervous tissue directly, although there have been reports that insulin does facilitate the entry of glucose in nervous tissues.

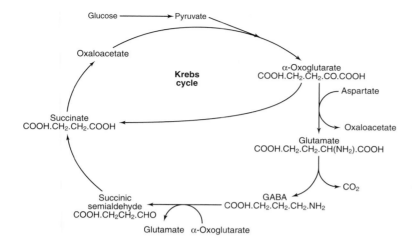

Fig. 3.2
The GABA shunt, a minor but important metabolic route in brain cells.

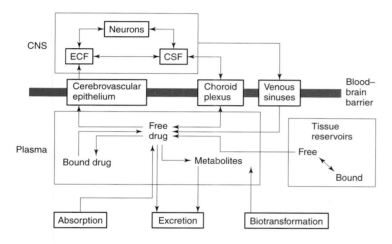

Fig. 3.3
Pharmacokinetics of drug entry into the central nervous system. (CSF, cerebrospinal fluid; ECF, extracellular fluid.)

caused by such a deficiency results in seizures. These seizures may be alleviated by the administration of GABA, suggesting that they are primarily due to the dysfunction of glutamate decarboxylase.

Metabolic imaging

The powerful dependence of brain metabolism on glucose and on oxygen supply has advantages for those who want to study the activity of areas of brain. There are methods for the direct study of both blood flow and glucose utilisation in animal brain. The animals are treated with 2-deoxyglucose, which enters the brain on the glucose uptake pathways but is not metabolised normally, so that, if it is suitably radioactively tagged, the amount of radioactivity in a brain area reflects the metabolic activity in the area. Similarly iodo-^{14}C-antipyrine follows the blood into brain and can be detected autoradiographically (Sokoloff 1989). It is extremely unusual for these two markers to be discordant, and both usually mark areas of brain active during the drug application. Recent human brain imaging studies have used these principles to detect the areas of human brain active during various sensory, motor or cognitive tasks. Results from these methods are presented in greater detail in Chapter 5.

PHARMACOKINETICS

The effective concentration reached by any applied substance in the relevant tissues depends upon its absorption, distribution, biotransformation and excretion, and those in turn depend upon its movement across cell membranes. This is determined by a substance's physical characteristics and the presence or absence of specific mechanisms to facilitate its passage across membranes. Passive movement of water-soluble substances of low molecular weight (less than 200 Da) is by filtration through aqueous channels, but these are too narrow (less than 0.4 nm) for most drugs, which must pass through the cell membrane to enter a cell. Many drugs are organic electrolytes and are weak acids or bases. The extent to which a drug is ionised is determined by the pH of its solution and the dissociation constant (K_d) of the drug. The un-ionised portion is usually 10^4 times more lipid soluble than the ionised portion and consequently much more soluble in the lipid bilayer of the cell membrane. The pharmacokinetics of drug entry into the CNS are complex and are summarised in Figure 3.3. The fraction labelled 'free' in this diagram is available to pass into the brain, and its rate of movement is proportional to its concentration gradient from plasma to the extracellular fluid of the nervous system. The effective concentration in brain is also controlled by active mechanisms of both accumulation into, and elimination from, the cerebrospinal fluid (CSF).

Absorption and distribution

The passage of drugs into the brain is governed by the general principles of drug absorption and also by the specific 'active' properties of the blood–brain barrier. One important general principle is that drugs given in aqueous solution are absorbed more quickly than those dissolved in oils or given as solids. Most drugs are given by mouth, and the wide pH range encountered in the gastrointestinal tract influences absorption. Oral ingestion is the most convenient and economical method of administration and, because drugs are absorbed relatively slowly from the gut, is also relatively safe because adverse effects also develop slowly. Intravenous administration rapidly produces the desired plasma concentration of a drug, but, because the effects are immediate, so are adverse reactions. Table 3.1 summarises the properties of common routes of drug administration. After a drug is absorbed into the bloodstream, it is distributed between extracellular and intracellular fluids. At rest, distribution is determined by the relative blood flow to the various regions of the body, so that highly perfused organs can reach peak concentrations within the first few minutes. Except in the brain, capillary endothelial membranes are highly permeable, allowing molecules as large as albumin (67 000 Da) to pass through intercellular aqueous channels.

The most immediate reservoir for drugs is formed by binding to plasma proteins, particularly albumin. Binding is relatively non-selective, so drugs compete for these binding sites. Drugs can also accumulate in other reservoirs such as muscle, fat or bone, and as the plasma concentration of a drug falls, it may be released from body compartments, which would allow its action to be sustained. Many drugs are highly lipid soluble and so they can be stored in body fat. In obese persons, this is an important drug reservoir.

The blood–brain barrier

The brain and CSF are separated from the blood by the blood–brain barrier, which regulates the movement of substances into and out of the nervous system. It is represented structurally by the capillary endothelium of the brain, and functionally by a complex set of active transport mechanisms. The cells of cerebral vessel walls are so tightly bound together that diffusion between cells is negligible and the cells function as a single continuous sheet, behaving like a lipid membrane. Lipid-soluble substances pass readily through this membrane, whereas non-lipid-soluble substances and proteins enter the brain much more slowly.

In some specialised areas of brain the capillary endothelium is permeable — in the subfornical organ, the area postrema in the medulla, and in the region of the median eminence — and these areas are often said to be outside the blood–brain barrier. These high-permeability areas may allow transfer of compounds such as peptides that cannot cross into brain elsewhere.

The permeability of the blood–brain barrier to drugs (when there is no specific mechanism of entry) is determined by the general principles set out above. A ready guide to a drug's entry into the nervous system is provided by the 'pH partition hypothesis'. This states that the permeability of a cell membrane to a drug is proportional to that drug's partition coefficient, which is the ratio of the fractional concentrations of un-ionised drug at equilibrium in two immiscible media — lipid and water. The latter is usually measured as the optimal lipid/water partition coefficient. The pH of CSF can be regulated independently of plasma pH because un-ionised carbon dioxide passes across the blood–brain barrier much more readily than bicarbonate ions. CSF pH is usually 0.1 of a unit lower than plasma pH and, at equilibrium, concentrations of weak electrolytes may differ on either side of the blood–brain barrier, so that weak bases tend to accumulate in the CSF whereas weak acids tend to be excluded. The pH gradients between plasma and CSF can, therefore, produce concentration gradients at equilibrium for dissociated compounds. Figure 3.4 illustrates these principles by showing the relationship between the uptake by the brain of radiolabelled substances and their lipid/water partition coefficients. When a drug has a partition coefficient greater than 0.03, it is almost completely cleared from the blood after carotid artery injection during a single brain passage.

A group of substances is enclosed within a box in Figure 3.4, and these exceptions to the general rule show high clearance yet have very low partition coefficients. Specific carrier transport systems unrelated to lipid affinity are available for these substances. Amino acids, essential for brain function, are not usually synthesised in the brain and so need to be transported from the blood. For example, the rate of entry of tryptophan into the brain is directly dependent on the ratio of its plasma concentration to the sum of the concentrations of phenylalanine, leucine, valine and isoleucine. These other amino acids all compete with tryptophan for the same transport system. Amino acid transport mechanisms are stereospecific, preferring the laevo- to the dextro-isomer.

Table 3.1 Properties of common routes of drug administration			
Route	Absorption	Advantages	Problems
Oral	Variable	Convenience Safety	Drugs of low solubility or high hepatic clearance have low oral availability
Subcutaneous	Quick in aqueous solution	Useful for some insoluble drugs and pellets	Pain, local necrosis Unsuitable for large volumes
Intramuscular	Quick in aqueous solution	Useful for low to medium volumes and some preparations of irritating drugs	Slow from depot Contraindicated during anticoagulant therapy
Intravenous	Often immediate	Useful in emergency and suitable for large volumes	Can have immediate adverse reactions Unsuitable for oily or insoluble preparations

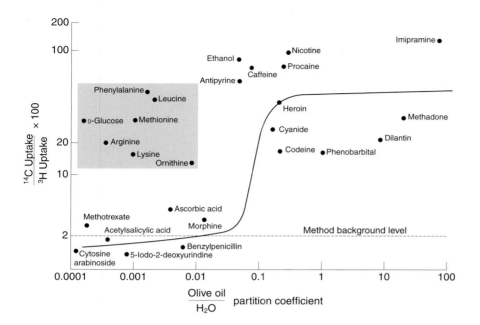

Fig. 3.4
Percentage clearance of radiolabelled substances plotted against their lipid/water coefficients during a single brain passage following carotid arterial injection. Drugs with a partition coefficient greater than about 0.03 show nearly complete clearance. The substances inside the box have very low lipid affinity but penetrate the blood–brain barrier by virtue of specific carrier transport systems. (After Oldendorf 1974 and Bradbury 1979.)

Active transport can operate in both directions and against concentration gradients, either from the brain to the blood or from the blood to the brain. This carrier which removes drugs and metabolites from brain has many properties in common with the acid transporter in the kidney, and may be a closely related mechanism. Some nervous system metabolites do not have specific mechanisms to clear them from CSF, and so are only removed when CSF passes back into the blood.

Biotransformation and excretion

Biotransformation of most drugs takes place in hepatic microsomal enzyme systems, though other systems — including plasma, gut, lung or kidney — may be involved. Lipid-soluble drugs are more readily metabolised by hepatic microsomes because of their ease of entry into the cell. Considerable individual variation in biotransformation can be related to genetic factors, the effects of age, hepatic disease or induction of microsomal enzymes by other drugs or environmental agents. The processes of biotransformation can lead to activation or inactivation of a drug and may involve numerous drug metabolites. Unchanged drugs or their metabolites are removed from the body by excretory organs such as the kidney or lung. Substances with high lipid solubility are not readily excreted until they have been metabolised to more polar compounds. The kidneys remove most drugs or their metabolites by renal excretion involving glomerular filtration, active tubular secretion and passive tubular reabsorption. Like all cell membranes, kidney tubular cells are less permeable to the ionised portion of drugs, and more permeable to lipid-soluble compounds. Excretion of drugs in other body fluids is relatively unimportant, with the exception of breast milk.

Clearance

In psychiatric practice, the usual aim is to maintain the concentration of a drug within its presumed therapeutic range. 'Steady-state' concentrations are attained when the rate of drug elimination (clearance) equals the rate of drug administration. When complete bioavailability of a drug can be assumed, the rate of drug administration is therefore determined by its clearance. For most drugs used in psychiatry, clearance is typically constant within the range of concentrations seen in clinical practice. This arises because clearance mechanisms are not usually saturated and drug clearance is observed to be a linear function of the drug's blood concentration. A constant fraction of most drugs is cleared per unit of time, and when this happens the drug is said to follow *first-order kinetics*. When clearance systems for a drug are saturated, the pharmacokinetics of the drug becomes *zero order* and a constant amount of that drug is cleared per unit of time. Clearance is calculated as the total volume of blood (or other body fluid) from which a drug must be completely removed, not as the total amount of drug removed. Total clearance represents the sum of clearance by each organ of elimination (kidneys, liver, lung, etc.).

In some circumstances, clearance of a drug by a specific organ becomes a matter of clinical concern, for example the renal elimination of lithium. Clinical investigation of renal function of a patient on long-term lithium therapy might, therefore, use an alternative definition of clearance. Clearance can be defined by the blood flow to the organ under investigation (Q), arterial concentration (C_A) and venous concentration (C_V). The difference between the products of blood flow and blood concentration gives the clearance by an organ (CL_{organ}):

$$\text{elimination} = QC_A - QC_V = Q(C_A - C_V)$$
$$CL_{organ} = Q(C_A - C_V)/C_A$$
$$= QE$$

The expression $(C_A - C_V)/C_A$ defines the *extraction ratio* (E) for a drug by a specific organ.

Some drugs show dose-dependent clearance that varies with drug concentration in blood:

$$\text{total blood clearance} = V_M/(K_M + C_B)$$

where K_M is the blood concentration at which 50% of the maximum rate of elimination is reached (in units of mass/volume) and V_M is the maximum rate of elimination (in units of mass/time). Dosing schemes for these drugs can be difficult.

Drugs such as chlorpromazine and imipramine are mostly cleared by the liver. Hepatic clearance is largely determined by hepatic blood flow, i.e. the rate at which the drug can be transported to hepatic sites of biotransformation and/or excretion in bile. Although changes in drug binding to blood components and other tissues (Fig. 3.1) may influence hepatic or renal clearance, in present circumstances, when a drug's extraction ratio (E) is high, changes in protein binding due to disease or competitive processes should have little effect on drug clearance. However, when the extraction ratio is low, changes in protein binding and intrahepatic functions will substantially alter drug clearance, but changes in hepatic blood flow will have little effect. Because a drug bound to blood proteins is not filtered and thus not subject to active glomerular secretion and/or reabsorption, renal clearance is substantially influenced by protein binding and thus by those diseases that affect protein binding.

NEUROTRANSMISSION

More than fifty years ago, intracellular recording techniques established beyond reasonable doubt the neurochemical nature of synaptic transmission in most of the mammalian CNS. The small number of specialised electrical connections between central neurons is probably of little interest to neuropharmacology. Chemical neurotransmitters were shown to produce inhibition or excitation of neurons by briefly and rapidly increasing neuronal membrane permeability to specific ions. Box 3.1 shows the 'classical' criteria for the identification of neurotransmitters that were once widely accepted. Later, studies on single neurons identified noradrenaline (norepinephrine), acetylcholine, serotonin, dopamine, γ-aminobutyric acid (GABA), glycine and glutamate as transmitters at synapses in the CNS. A major development in understanding the function of neurotransmitters in neural networks was provided by Yamamoto & McIlwain (1966), who demonstrated the feasibility of recording from slices of brain in vitro. The most popular structure for this method is the transverse slice of the hippocampus, since it contains numerous neurotransmitters and their receptors and since electrophysiological preparations preserve the precise laminar structure and much of the neuronal circuitry of the hippocampus. Many accounts of neuropharmacology present information in terms of a single synapse (the functional unit of the nervous system). The data summarised in such accounts have often been obtained and characterised in model neuronal systems, which, like the hippocampal slice preparation, preserve particular sets of synaptic connections in vitro (Bloom 1990). Of course in the intact brain such simplifications may be misleading because of 'emerging' properties of more complicated neuronal networks, but they form the basis from which models of such properties may be derived.

Neurotransmitters may open or close ion channels in the pre- or postsynaptic neuronal membrane and can do this either directly or by activating adjacent proteins. Initially, it was inferred that neurotransmitters caused a brief hyperpolarisation or depolarisation of the postsynaptic membrane. Now, it is known that neurotransmitters may have a much longer time-course of action produced by their altering the properties of voltage-sensitive (or 'voltage-gated') ion channels that are involved in the regulation of neuronal excitability. This is especially important in the case of K^+ and Ca^{2+} ion channels.

The release of neurotransmitters represents the 'final common pathway' of all neuronal functions. Table 3.2 summarises the properties of substances active at synapses. Neurotransmitters stored in presynaptic vesicles fuse with the presynaptic membrane at the nerve terminal. Synaptic vesicles are coated on their cytoplasmic face by synapsins, a particularly abundant group of extrinsic membrane proteins (Südhof 1995). The synapsins appear to connect synaptic vesicles to each other and to the neuronal cytoskeleton and probably regulate vesicular position in the nerve terminal. Synapsins share many common structural features and seem likely to comprise a single family of proteins with a common ancestor. Careful study of the molecular biology and physiology of synaptic transmission has provided a complex life history of synaptic vesicles (Fig. 3.5).

Calcium channels

Neurotransmitter release is Ca^{2+} dependent, and study of entry of Ca^{2+} across surface membranes is of intense interest to neuropharmacologists. In part this interest stems from technological developments and the availability of specific agents with which to study Ca^{2+} channels. The interest is also based on the ubiquitous nature of neuronal Ca^{2+} and its clinical relevance. Ca^{2+} channels open in response to membrane depolarisation and generate electrical and chemical responses. Ca^{2+} entry into the neuron carries a depolarising charge that contributes to paroxysmal phenomena such as epileptiform or pacemaker activity. It also causes the intracellular Ca^{2+} concentration to rise, and this in turn alters Ca^{2+}-dependent mechanisms involved in neurotransmitter release from synaptic vesicles, enzyme activation, Ca^{2+}-sensitive ion channels, and intracellular Ca^{2+} stores which are themselves sensitive to cytosolic Ca^{2+}. Thus, many diverse aspects of neuronal metabolism can be changed by Ca^{2+} entry. Indeed it has been suggested that the final common factor in neuronal death may be the cataclysmic increases in intracellular Ca^{2+} that follow the release from intracellular stores in response to extensive Ca^{2+} influx through

---

Box 3.1 Criteria for identification of neurotransmitters

1. The transmitter must be shown to be present in the presynaptic terminals of the synapse and in the neurons from which those presynaptic terminals arise
2. The transmitter must be synthesised in the presynaptic neuron
3. The transmitter must be stored in an inactive form in the presynaptic terminal
4. The transmitter must be released from the presynaptic nerve concomitantly with presynaptic nerve activity
5. The effects of the putative neurotransmitter when applied experimentally to the target cells must be identical to those of the presynaptic pathway
6. The amount released by nervous activity (4) should be comparable to that required to produce postsynaptic action (5)
7. A method for control of the postsynaptic concentration which is capable of terminating the action of the transmitter is required, e.g. a presynaptic uptake system or an enzymatic degradation at the synapse

Table 3.2 Substances active in neuronal signalling

Substance	Properties	Example
Neurotransmitter	A substance found in neuron type A, secreted from it and acting on target neuron type B	Acetylcholine
Neurohormone	Peptide secretions from neurons directly into the blood that also act on other neurons as neurotransmitters	Corticotrophin-releasing factor (CRF)
Neuromodulator	A substance that influences neuronal activity and originates from non-synaptic sites	Steroid hormones
Neuromediator (second messenger)	Postsynaptic compounds that participate in generation of postsynaptic responses	Cyclic adenosine monophosphate (cAMP)
Neurotrophin	Substances released by postsynaptic structures which 'maintain' presynaptic neuronal structure	Nerve growth factor

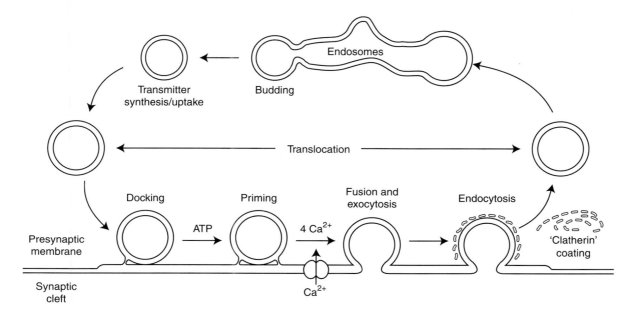

Fig. 3.5
Life history of synaptic vesicles. Synapsins are involved in every phase of vesicle function shown. (After Südhof 1995.)

voltage and transmitter gated Ca^{2+} channels. Since such extensive entry of Ca^{2+} can be the result of excitatory neurotransmitter action, it is often referred to as 'excitotoxicity'.

Multiple types of Ca^{2+} channel exist in neurons, and it is important to distinguish them in order to understand neuronal function and its modification by drugs and neurotransmitters. Early electrophysiological studies demonstrated two classes of Ca^{2+} channel: 'low-voltage activated' (LVA) and 'high-voltage activated' (HVA). Subsequently, the HVA Ca^{2+} channel was found to comprise N and L subtypes, yielding three subtypes designated T (or LVA), N and L. These acronyms should not be taken too literally but do have some mnemonic value: T for 'transient', L for 'long-lasting' and N for channels that are 'neither T nor L' (Tsien et al 1988). At present, none of the subtypes of Ca^{2+} channel is assigned an exclusive physiological role. However, T channels are important in pacemaker depolarisation in heart cells and are the primary voltage-sensitive entry points for Ca^{2+} on contraction of certain smooth muscle cells. Ca^{2+} entry by L channels is associated

with heart muscle contraction and substance P and noradrenaline release in the CNS. Only L channels are sensitive to blockade by the dihydropyridine Ca^{2+} channel-blocking drugs (nicardipine, nimodipine, diltiazem, nifedipine and verapamil). In brain the list of Ca^{2+} channels is expanded by two (at least): the P channel that was first described in Purkinje cells and seems to be common on many other central neurons, and a 'residual' or R channel (or channels) that has been proposed to explain current carried by none of the channels so far described. The complexity of the regulation of Ca^{2+} entry into neurons is not surprising in view of the central importance of intracellular Ca^{2+} in so many aspects of neuronal function. The fact is that there are multiple types of voltage-sensitive Ca^{2+} channel and, as will be described later, multiple types of receptor-operated Ca^{2+} channel. This very variety indicates the adaptability available to the neuron in 'fine-tuning' intracellular Ca^{2+} concentrations.

Pharmacological studies of the Ca^{2+} channel blockers have shown that each binds to a different recognition site on a single protein–receptor complex. Although these drugs do not influence neurotransmitter release, their diverse chemical structures resemble many other clinically useful compounds (Snyder 1989). The antipsychotic drugs comprise several chemical classes: phenothiazines, butyrophenones and diphenylbutylpiperidines. This last class is a Ca^{2+} channel antagonist equipotent with the Ca^{2+}-blocking drugs listed above. Ca^{2+} channel blockade probably also accounts for some side-effects of antipsychotics. Electrocardiogram (ECG) changes produced by thioridazine are similar to those produced by the Ca^{2+} channel blocker verapamil. Impaired vas deferens contraction and ejaculation observed in experiments using Ca^{2+}-blocking drugs probably explains a common side-effect of thioridazine that is rarely encountered with other phenothiazines or butyrophenones. Cardiac and ejaculatory side-effects of thioridazine may well be caused by thioridazine-induced Ca^{2+} channel blockade.

Phosphatidylinositol (PI) metabolism

Protein kinase C (PKC) is a Ca^{2+}-dependent enzyme concentrated at synapses. It is activated by diacylglycerol (DAG), a cleavage product of a group of membrane lipids called phosphatidylinositols. PKC activation in turn potentiates neurotransmitter release. These events are important components of the regulation of neurotransmission and are affected by lithium. Initially, in response to extracellular signals, lipases including phospholipase C (PLC) degrade phosphatidylinositols into precursors of two intracellular 'second messengers'. These are inositol phosphates (IPs) and DAG. Inositol 1,4,5-triphosphate (IP_3) synthesis is the major product of phosphatidylinositol degradation. The PLC enzyme that initiates this cascade of events in fact comprises a group of at least five structurally dissimilar enzymes. This highly conserved diversity of enzyme structure is poorly understood but probably allows distinct pathways (e.g. through IP_3 and arachidonic acid) to respond selectively to specific extracellular signals and to be negatively influenced by products of these pathways. PKC activation by phorbol esters mimics the action of DAG and is blocked by lithium. Since PKC activation also potentiates serotonin and noradrenaline release, this effect of lithium at therapeutically relevant concentrations suggests a possible mode of its action in the treatment of mania and prophylaxis of manic–depressive illness (Wang & Friedman 1989).

PHARMACODYNAMICS

Pharmacodynamics concerns the mechanism of action of drugs. Knowledge of drug pharmacodynamics in psychiatry is basic to their clinical use. Studies of drug action aim to identify chemical and physical interactions between drug and neuron. A proper understanding of the temporal order and scale of drug–neuron interactions provides the basis for understanding drug effects. It can be used to help design improved drugs, and potentially may provide information of relevance to understanding neurobiological components of psychiatric disease.

RECEPTORS

Receptors are conceptualised as large, functional molecules that, in response to binding with endogenous or pharmacological molecules (ligands), change cellular activity. The physical and chemical features of receptor molecules may vary substantially. Some are protein constituents of the cellular membrane, others are proteins that are important in the maintenance of subcellular architecture, and some are intracellular enzymes or proteins concerned with cellular transport. Likewise, interactions between drugs and receptors are of multiple types and include covalent, ionic, hydrophobic, and van der Waals binding. Covalent binding tends to be of long duration, while non-covalent high-affinity binding is usually reversible. The physical configuration of the receptor largely determines the structural requirements of a drug designed to interact with that receptor. Several clinically important drugs in psychiatry have been developed from deliberate chemical changes to the structure of the endogenous ligand (*physiological agonists*). (Additionally, small changes of structure can alter the pharmacokinetic properties of drugs.) Neural receptor mechanisms include recognition of the neurotransmitter (usually by a cell surface protein) and transduction of the message into alterations of cellular activity that may involve changes in ionic permeability and the formation of intracellular *second messengers*, such as cyclic adenosine monophosphate (cAMP), IP_3, or immediate early genes (IEG).

Drugs that bind to receptors and initiate a response in neuroeffector tissue are *agonists*. Drugs that produce a maximal response are *full agonists*, and those producing less than the maximal response are *partial agonists*. Drugs that have no intrinsic pharmacological activity but produce effects by preventing an agonist initiating a response are *antagonists*. Some antagonists can produce a partial pharmacological response ('partial agonist activity') at receptor binding sites where they compete with endogenous ligands. Some drugs combine both agonist and antagonist properties as *mixed agonist–antagonists*, and understanding these properties may have therapeutic potential. For example, a mixed opiate agonist–antagonist might have the advantage of providing relief of pain with much less risk of addiction than a full agonist such as morphine. Pharmacological antagonism is distinct from physiological antagonism produced by substances initiating an opposing response in neuroeffector tissue. For example, noradrenaline can act as a physiological antagonist of acetylcholine but has negligible action at acetylcholine receptors.

Classical receptor theory assumes that the effect of a drug is proportional to the number of receptors with which that drug interacts. The ease with which a drug attaches to a receptor is termed the affinity of the drug for that receptor. Receptors for neurotransmitters are components of the neural membrane. They are able to recognise specific neurotransmitters and produce physiological responses in neuroeffector tissues. Receptors can, therefore, be defined both in terms of their ability to recognise specific ligands and by the physiological responses they initiate (Box 3.2).

Receptor sensitivity

Drug–receptor interactions may be modified by changes in receptor sensitivity. The sensitivity of receptors is influenced by complex regulatory and homeostatic factors. When receptor sensitivity changes, the same concentration of a drug will produce a greater or lesser physiological response. Changes in sensitivity occur, for example, when, after prolonged stimulation of cells by agonists, the cell becomes refractory to further stimulation. This is also termed 'desensitisation' or 'downregulation'. Underlying mechanisms of desensitisation may involve receptor changes (e.g. phosphorylation), or the receptor may be concealed within

Box 3.2   Criteria for identification of receptors

- 'Possible':   Radioligand binding sites
  - — Saturability and reversibility of radioligand binding
  - — Homogeneous population of sites
  - — Regional and species variation
  - — Pharmacological properties
- 'Probable': Functional correlates
  - — Identification of special messenger links
  - — Delineation of physiological effects on membranes
  - — Behavioural or other models of action
- 'Definite':   Structural identification
  - — Unique amino acid sequence
  - — Cloned sequences mimic actions of natural receptor

After Peroutka (1988).

Table 3.3   Examples of 'superfamilies' of receptors

Superfamily	Neuroreceptor ion channel
G-protein-coupled receptors	Visual pigments
	Adrenergic
	Muscarinic cholinergic
	Serotonergic
Ligand-gated ion channel receptors	Nicotinic cholinergic
	$GABA_A$
	Glycine
	Glutamate
Tyrosine-kinase-linked receptors	NGF
	Neurotrophins
	BDNF
	CNTF
	GDNF

NGF, nerve growth factor; BDNF, brain-derived neurotrophic factor; CNTF, ciliary neutrophic factor; GDNF, glial cell-derived neurotrophic factor.

the cell so that it is no longer exposed to the ligand. Long-term desensitisation may involve negative-feedback mechanisms that inhibit new receptor synthesis or cause a structurally modified receptor to be synthesised. In the nicotinic receptor, desensitisation involves at least two distinct 'closed' states. Both 'closed' states display a higher affinity for acetylcholine than does the resting (or 'active') conformation. Structural studies show that a specific segment of the lumen-facing part of the ion channel is crucial in the process of desensitisation in response to prolonged agonist exposure (Revah et al 1991). This segment of the ionic channel is highly conserved in other receptor types (e.g. $GABA_A$ and glycine receptors) where it may play a similar role.

Supersensitivity ('upregulation' or 'hypersensitivity') was first described after removal of the presynaptic element but often follows prolonged receptor blockade. This may involve synthesis of new receptors so that an increased number of receptors is exposed on the cell surface to their physiological ligands. In the case of supersensitivity following the destruction of the presynaptic terminal the loss of mechanisms that terminate transmitter action (e.g. uptake, enzymatic degradation) also contribute to the increase in response to agonist.

Receptor families

Historically, there has been considerable debate about criteria for the characterisation of receptor subtypes. Practically, the identification of new receptor types has quickly followed the development of specific, potent agonists and/or antagonists that selectively bind to the new receptor. Molecular, biochemical and physiological techniques indicate the existence of several 'superfamilies' (probably less than 10) of receptor macromolecules (Table 3.3). Molecular biological techniques have provided the best classification of subtypes within receptor superfamilies. Progress in this field has consistently led to revision of classification systems based on biochemical and physiological studies. Within each superfamily of receptor types there can be considerable structural diversity of their endogenous ligands. Receptors within each receptor family, however, have many structural similarities with other members of the same family and share common mechanisms of signal propagation.

Table 3.4   Neurotransmitter ligands acting through G-protein-coupled receptors

Neurotransmitter	Receptor subtypes	Examples of effectors
Catecholamines	$\alpha_1, \alpha_2, \beta_1, \beta_2, \beta_3$	Adenylate cyclase;
Cholinergic	M_1, M_2, M_3	PLC; phospholipase A_2;
Dopamine	D_1, D_2	phosphodiesterases;
Serotonin	$5HT_{1A-F}, 5HT_2$	Ca^{2+}, K^+ channels;
Histamine	H_1, H_2, H_3	guanylyl cyclase;
GABA	$GABA_B$	PKC
Glutamate	$mGLUr(1-5)$	
Angiotensin	$A_1\ A_{2A}\ A_{2B}$	

PKC, protein kinase C; PLC, phospholipase C.

G-protein-coupled receptors

A family of cellular proteins called 'G proteins' — guanine triphosphate (GTP)-binding — link cell surface receptors to a variety of enzymes and ion channels. By far the largest known class of receptor (summarised in Table 3.4) functions by stimulating membrane-bound G proteins. Members of this large family of G proteins are composed of three homologous subunits: α, β and γ. Figure 3.6 shows the likely organisation of receptors, G proteins and effectors (such as ion channels, adenylate cyclases, and enzymes involved in phosphatidylinositol metabolism). Receptors coupled to G proteins have similar structures that include seven transmembrane helices (Fig. 3.6a). Sequence homology among the G-protein-coupled receptors is found largely in the membrane-spanning regions. The cytoplasmic regions and loops between spans 5 and 6 show minimal sequence homology (Ross 1989). Neurotransmitter and hormonal ligands bind to G-protein-coupled receptors in the pocket formed by the seven helices as illustrated in Figure 3.6b. The G proteins are located on the intracellular surface of the plasma membrane, and it is likely that part of the receptor which regulates G proteins is also on the intracellular face. Binding of the ligand to the extracellular part of

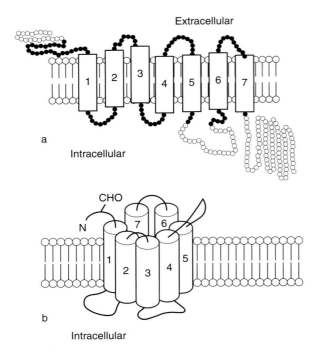

Extracellular

a

Intracellular

CHO

N

Intracellular

b

Fig. 3.6
(a) The peptide chains of the β-adrenergic receptor (and
G-protein-coupled receptors in general) are assumed to span the
extracellular membrane as shown. (b) A three-dimensional array of
the seven membrane-spanning helices shown in (a).

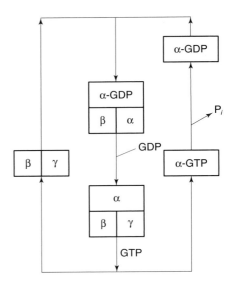

Fig. 3.7
The G protein cycle of activation in transmembrane signalling. The
αβγ complex is stable only with GDP bound to the α subunit.
Binding GTP to the α subunit dissociates the complex, which can
only reassociate after dephosphorylation of GTP to GDP. The free
βγ complex acts on many cellular subsystems, including ion
channels and intracellular signalling pathways. (After Sternweis &
Pang 1990.)

the receptor distorts the binding site to an extent sufficient to alter
the cytoplasmic part of the receptor and to transform it from its
passive to active state. The cytoplasmic loop between spans 5 and
6 is probably the G protein regulation site, as G protein regulation
is sensitive to mutations in this region.

The β-adrenoceptor is a G-coupled receptor whose ligand-
binding domain lies within the core of the receptor molecule.
Structure–activity analyses of adrenoceptor ligands and the amino
acid sequences in the receptor core have been greatly helped by
the synthesis of 'mutant' receptors. These studies point the way
toward the development of new drugs. They are also important in
understanding molecular mechanisms of receptor desensitisation
(Strader et al 1989).

Figure 3.7 shows the process of signal transduction by G
proteins. A ligand binds at its receptor and produces a change in
receptor–G-protein interaction. This change allows GTP (in the
presence of Mg^{2+}) to replace guanosine diphosphate (GDP) on
the α subunit of the G protein. Now activated, the α-GTP subunit
dissociates from the βγ subunit allowing one or both subunits to
interact with an effector (e.g. adenylate cyclase). The α subunit
possesses intrinsic GTPase activity and hydrolyses GTP to GDP,
releasing inorganic phosphate (P_i), and the cycle is terminated by
α-GDP recombining with a βγ subunit. Throughout this cycle,
the βγ subunit remains a single functional unit and all phases of
the cycle take place in the cytoplasmic compartment. βγ subunits
released in the cycle can interact with other effectors such as phospholipase A_2 (PLA_2) in some cell systems. The α subunit is
thought to remain attached to the inner surface of the plasma
membrane throughout this cycle (Neer & Clapham 1988).

There are very many G proteins, and they can be subdivided
by their susceptibilities to bacterial toxins. There are subtypes
specific for:

- cholera toxin only;
- pertussis toxin only;
- both toxins;
- neither toxin.

Cholera toxin-susceptible G proteins were initially thought to
stimulate adenylate cyclase (G_s) and the pertussis toxin-susceptible
G proteins to inhibit adenylate cyclase (G_i). These toxins modify
different types of α subunit ($α_i$ and $α_s$) which then act upon a wide
range of effectors. Structural analysis of the α and β subunits has
revealed more subtypes than there are presently known functions.
The $α_i$ subtype alone is divisible into $α_0$, $α_i$-1, $α_i$-2 and $α_i$-3. These
are highly conserved and their individual genes probably derive
from a common ancestor. The β and γ subtypes are also heterogeneous, and the overall picture is of a loose spatial organisation of
receptors, G proteins and their effectors. Receptors can interact
with a single G protein, and the same G protein can interact with
several receptors or effectors. Probably up to 15 distinct kinds of
receptor can stimulate adenylate cyclase through G_s. Interactions
between G proteins and effectors, however, seem to be much
more specific, so that, for example, only G_s and not G_i or G_o can
stimulate the most common of the adenylate cyclases found in
neurons. This capacity of G proteins to interact with multiple
effectors underlies the advantages of G proteins as signal trans-
ducers. Multiple receptors, G proteins and effectors make up
a complex signalling network. These networks sort extracellular
signals and integrate incoming information (Birnbaumer 1990).
The effector enzyme, adenylate cyclase, can be stimulated or
inhibited by numerous hormones or transmitters either directly or

along the G protein pathway. Structural studies have revealed multiple forms of adenylate cyclase that, surprisingly in view of its intracellular functions, contain numerous transmembrane spans. The structure has many features shared with G protein-regulated Ca^{2+} channels and transporter molecules. These structural similarities probably relate to hitherto unrecognised functions of adenylate cyclase. The 10 cyclases cloned (so far) differ in their sensitivity to calcium and to G proteins, so that they too will eventually need to be specified in the description of the action of any receptor, G protein, adenyl cyclase cascade. Molecular cloning has isolated many proteins with good homology to this family of seven-transmembrane-segment receptors, but their ligands remain unknown. These 'orphan' receptors may represent a source of future drugs for psychiatry as their expression patterns and pharmacology are elucidated.

Ligand-gated ion channels

Many of the best-known transmitter actions are mediated by this superfamily of receptors. Acetylcholine acts at the neuromuscular junction on just such a receptor, and the major receptors for glutamate and for GABA in brain are also of this type. The nicotinic acetylcholine receptor, because of the ease of its purification from the electroplax of fish, was the first to be isolated, and its molecular structure is now described in some detail. Elucidation of the molecular biology of this receptor allowed the investigation of the other receptors of this class. They all have ion channels formed from several subunits (usually five), and the pentamer may be formed of many combinations of the individual subunits — thus perhaps conferring a variety of subtle properties on the receptors formed with different combinations.

The pentameric structure of the nicotinic receptor formed of two α, two β and one γ subunit is shown in Figure 3.8. It is thought that as acetylcholine binds to the α subunits the channel opens wider and allows the passage of cations, thus depolarising the membrane. The resulting excitatory postsynaptic potential (EPSP) may reach threshold for the voltage-sensitive Na^+ channel to open and an action potential to be generated.

Not all the receptor-operated ion channels are excitatory, however, and although the structure of the receptor shares many features in common with the nicotinic channel, the GABA receptor tetrameric channel opens to allow K^+ and Cl^- to pass through, with the consequence that the membrane resting potential is 'clamped' at Cl^- equilibrium potential. In most neurons this means that it is harder to change the membrane potential and the generation of action potentials is inhibited. One note of caution is perhaps warranted at this stage: since each of the subunits of the receptor exists in many forms, it seems likely that there may be some combinations which never occur in vivo, otherwise the numbers of different GABA receptors, for example, would be astronomical! Finally, some ligand-gated ion-channel receptors may have a major effect intracellularly, in spite of the fact that the agonist opens an ion channel. This is particularly the case if the ion channel allows the entry of Ca^{2+}. This Ca^{2+} is just as able as the Ca^{2+} liberated by phosphatidylinositol breakdown to initiate cascades of intracellular signalling pathways, and indeed it seems likely that the potency of the *N*-methyl-D-aspartate (NMDA) glutamate receptor depends on just such a cascade. Indeed, recent proteomic analysis of the postsynaptic density in central synapses suggests that several signalling possibilities are 'packaged' with the NMDA receptors within the postsynaptic region of the cell.

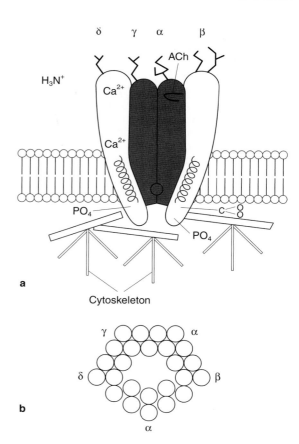

Fig. 3.8
Model of the ion channel of the nicotinic acetylcholine receptor. (a) Longitudinal section (ACh, acetylcholine). (b) Cross-section of the narrowest part of the channel. (After Guy & Hucho 1987.)

Steroid and thyroid hormone-like receptors

Receptors for steroid and thyroid hormones, vitamin D and the retinoids are all part of a single family of receptor macromolecules (Evans 1988). The receptors are highly ligand-specific, so that each type mediates the effect of a specific hormone or other ligand on its 'target' gene. The receptors comprise a ligand-binding domain and a part that couples the receptor to intracellular metabolic processes. The latter, in turn, has two components which bind DNA. In the better-understood of these, the DNA-binding regions are soluble proteins that, in their inactivated state, inhibit transcription of the related gene. Binding of the endogenous ligand to its receptor removes this inhibitory effect. Removal of the ligand-binding domain from the receptor also activates the remaining fragment, making it almost as effective in the regulation of genetic transcription, when applied intracellularly, as the natural ligand-bound receptor. The third part of the receptor binds to regulatory sites on nuclear DNA. Its function is ill understood, but it probably serves to promote the regulatory activity of the receptor macromolecule.

Tyrosine-kinase-linked receptors

The receptors for nerve growth factor (NGF) have long been a puzzle, but the recent description of the receptors for NGF and for a range of neuronal growth and survival factors called *neurotrophins* has revealed a family of receptors which are rapidly growing to become another superfamily. In this case the molecular structure is unlike any of the above receptors and usually includes a tyrosine kinase region as well as a membrane attachment domain. The receptors are relatively specific to their neurotrophin agonist and have been imaginatively named *trk* (for tyrosine kinase) A, B and C. Some recent animal studies seek to explain the long time taken for antidepressant drugs to have a therapeutic action by involving a neurotrophin in the long-term response to the drugs. Animal studies suggest that the antidepressants imipramine and fluoxetine may need intact trkB and brain-derived neurotrophic factor (BDNF) signalling for the standard Porsolt forced swimming response to the drugs to be observed. Along with an apparent antidepressant action of intracerebral injections of BDNF in rats the authors suggest that these experiments support an antidepressant action independent of the short-term actions on monoamine release for which the drugs were designed.

AMINO ACID NEUROTRANSMISSION

Inhibitory amino acid neurotransmission (IAA)

GABA and the amino acid glycine are the major inhibitory neurotransmitters. GABA receptors are more abundant at inhibitory synapses in the brain, whereas glycine receptors are more numerous in the brainstem and spinal cord. Postsynaptic inhibition is mediated by the opening of ion channels in the postsynaptic membrane. These are selectively permeable to Cl^- and small monovalent cations. Electrophysiological studies show that glycine and GABA receptors have similar properties, but distinct pharmacology.

Glycine receptors

Recent pharmacological and molecular biological studies of receptors for GABA and glycine have established that several receptor macromolecules are involved. The postsynaptic glycine receptor (GlyR) is a member of the ligand-gated ion channel superfamily of receptors (Betz 1987). Like other ligand-gated ion channels GlyR is composed of a core made up of four subunits, two of which are the same (Fig. 3.9). Although these receptors were among the earliest inhibitory mechanisms discovered and are widely distributed in the CNS, beyond the antagonism by strychnine, the neuropharmacology of glycine remains poorly understood. Strychnine (a potent neurotoxic convulsant) is believed to have its own specific binding site on GlyR close to the integral ion channel. The amino acids taurine and β-alanine are effective agonists at GlyR, but alanine, proline and serine are less effective. No non-amino-acid agonists at GlyR have been detected, and GABA has little effect at GlyR at physiological concentrations.

GABA receptors

GABA is the main cortical inhibitory neurotransmitter. Its inhibitory actions are Cl^- dependent and are blocked by the plant alkaloid bicuculline. Some effects of GABA are, however, insensitive to bicuculline, indicating the existence of two different types of GABA receptor. The classical $GABA_A$ receptor is a ligand-gated ion channel that has an integral transmembrane Cl^- channel that

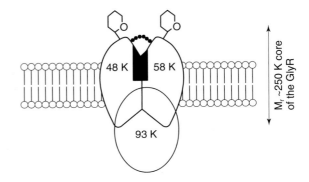

Fig. 3.9
The postsynaptic glycine receptor (GlyR). The core of the receptor is likely to be made up of four subunits, but only one copy of each subunit is shown here. (After Betz 1987.)

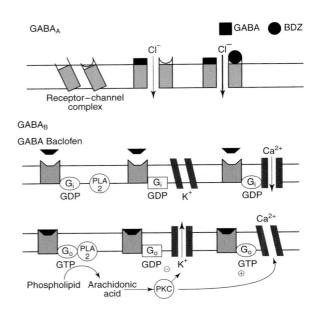

Fig. 3.10
$GABA_A$ and $GABA_B$ receptors. The $GABA_A$ receptor complex with its central Cl^- ion channel is modulated by benzodiazepine binding (BDZ), which may increase Cl^- currents (shown by a thicker arrow). $GABA_B$ receptors are coupled to two G proteins affecting K^+ (G_i) and Ca^{2+} (G_o) permeabilities in opposite directions.

mediates inhibitory transmission by opening and allowing Cl^- entry. $GABA_B$ receptors are coupled to G proteins and linked to Ca^{2+} or K^+ channels (Fig. 3.10).

The $GABA_A$ receptor The $GABA_A$ receptor is present on most brain neurons, exists in several forms, and has at least four different sites at which ligands may bind (Fig. 3.10). The sites bind:

- the GABA agonist/antagonist;
- picrotoxin (where agents that block GABA transmission may bind);
- benzodiazepine drugs;
- many CNS depressant drugs that prolong activation of the integral channel by GABA.

Each of these sites may be occupied simultaneously by their respective ligands, implying that each is a physically distinct part of the same receptor molecule. A group of molecular biologists led by Eric Barnard achieved the first purification and then sequenced the GABA$_A$ receptor protein. The purified protein contains subunits of the types α (about 53 kDa) and β (about 57 kDa). The receptor is composed of four subunits, two of which are of type α and two of type β. The combination of subtypes of α and β varies from receptor to receptor (i.e. it is a heterotetrameric protein). Electrophysiological studies show that occupation of both of the two binding sites for GABA is necessary to open the integral Cl⁻ channel. These sites are on the two β subunits, and binding sites for benzodiazepine drugs are on the two α subunits. Receptor complementary DNA (cDNA) cloning and functional expression of full-length α and β subunits provide conclusive evidence that the α and β subunits constitute the receptor and its chloride channel. The genes for α_1, α_2, α_3, and β_2 subunits of the GABA$_A$ receptor have been cloned and expressed in cell lines to produce reconstituted ion channels. These have been made up of combinations of single GABA$_A$ receptor subunits and have characteristics (ion permeability and ligand binding) of the native receptor (Blair et al 1988), which suggests that these characteristics are determined by structural motifs that are shared by all subunits. The gene encoding the α_3 subunit of the GABA$_A$ receptor is on the X chromosome in a region previously linked to susceptibility to manic–depressive illness. The GABA$_A$ α_3 gene is a possible candidate gene for this group of disorders (Bell et al 1989). The constituent amino acid segments of the receptor comprise parts that are sufficiently large to span the membrane and are also hydrophobic. Both α and β subunits contain four such parts and have a cytoplasmic loop. The β subunit loop is longer and probably serves to modulate receptor function. The entire receptor thus contains 16 transmembrane subunits (α_2, β_2), and these crowd around the integral ion channel of 51 nm diameter. Five α subunits could make up the necessary diameter, but the likeliest solution is that one helix from each of four different subunits together form a single ion channel (Barnard et al 1987). Expression of recombinant subunits produces functional receptors. When variants of the α subunit are co-expressed with standard β subunits the receptors produced are differentially distributed in the CNS.

Benzodiazepine drugs are widely used as anxiolytics and anticonvulsants. They bind with high affinity to sites at the GABA$_A$ receptor and potentiate the actions of GABA. Pharmacological studies of benzodiazepine binding show that variants of α subunits of the GABA$_A$ receptor may differ in their binding characteristics for these agents.

Inverse benzodiazepine receptor agonists of the β-carboline type decrease GABA$_A$ receptor-induced Cl⁻ flow through the central channel. Epileptogenic agents like picrotoxin and *t*-butyl bicyclophosphorothionate (TBPS) block the Cl⁻ channel by binding at a site close to the channel (Fig. 3.10). The convulsant actions of penicillin G and pentylenetetrazole involve blocking GABA$_A$ receptor function by an unknown mechanism. Barbiturates prolong GABA$_A$ receptor channel burst duration but neither affect conductance nor directly activate Cl⁻ channels. The synthetic steroid, alphaxalone has similar actions to barbiturates and points to the possibility that endogenous steroid metabolites may modulate GABA$_A$ receptor function. The regulation of GABA$_A$ receptor function by intracellular mechanisms is little understood. GABA$_A$ receptor sensitivity is substantially reduced after a rapid increase in intracellular Ca²⁺ concentration, and this suggests that Ca²⁺ may alter GABA$_A$ receptor function in vivo. The cytoplasmic loops of the α and β subunits contain phosphorylation sites for cAMP-dependent protein kinase, and their presence indicates interactions between the GABA$_A$ receptor and protein phosphorylation of a second messenger system.

The GABA$_B$ receptor GABA$_B$ receptors are pharmacologically differentiated from GABA$_A$ receptors. They are unaffected by bicuculline and are not stimulated by GABAergic drugs such as isoguvacine. GABA binds at both GABA$_A$ and GABA$_B$ receptors, but only GABA$_B$ receptors are selectively stimulated by (−)-baclofen (β-*p*-chlorophenyl GABA). There is, however, a paucity of specic antagonists at GABA$_B$ receptors with which to explore its pharmacology.

The GABA$_B$ receptor is not associated with an integral Cl⁻ channel. Instead, it is coupled to adjacent Ca²⁺ channels by G proteins, and its structure shows it to be a member of the superfamily of receptors characterised by seven helical membrane-spanning domains. Binding between GABA or the agonist baclofen at the GABA$_B$ receptor selectively opens K⁺ channels and closes Ca²⁺ channels (Deisz & Lux 1985). The GABA$_B$ receptor activates two membrane-bound G proteins. There are thus two likely routes along which the GABA$_B$ receptor can modify K⁺ and Ca²⁺: one involves G$_i$ protein and the other involves G$_o$. G$_i$ inhibits adenyl cyclase, which opens K⁺ channels, while the activation of G$_o$ results in the closing of the Ca²⁺ channels.

Roles of the two types of GABA receptor. GABA$_A$ and GABA$_B$ receptors share inhibitory functions in the CNS. They represent distinct receptor populations whose physiological functions are as yet poorly understood. The GABA$_B$ receptor may be more important in the regulation of Ca²⁺ entry and has been shown to have a role in the modulation of Ca²⁺-dependent neurotransmitter release, and to be present presynaptically. GABA$_A$ receptors are more widely distributed than GABA$_B$ receptors; they appear to be mainly postsynaptic in location. Thus, like many other transmitters, GABA has receptors that are members of both of the major superfamilies, whose locations in brain are different.

Excitatory amino acid neurotransmitters

Excitatory amino acid neurotransmitters (EAAs) are the focus of considerable current research. There is extensive evidence that EAAs provide the CNS with many useful functions that are essential in learning and memory, in the structural and functional organisational changes (plasticity) that occur in neural development and in neurodegeneration. The most abundant EAAs are glutamate and aspartate, and these are the most frequently encountered excitatory neurotransmitters in the brain.

EAA effects are mediated through at least four different receptor systems. The first three are ligand-gated ion channels and the fourth is coupled to G proteins and stimulates the IP–Ca²⁺ intracellular signalling pathway. The properties of some of these receptors are shown in Table 3.5, and the receptors are pharmacologically defined as:

- *N*-methyl-D-aspartate (NMDA)
- AMPA
- kainate
- the metabotropic glutamate receptor family (mGluR 1–7).

AMPA receptors are widely distributed. They are highly concentrated in the cerebellum, and elsewhere in the brain their

Table 3.5 Ionotrophic excitatory amino acid receptor subtypes

Receptor type	Agonists (most selective)	Competitive antagonists	Non-competitive antagonists	Allosteric agonist	Ions involved in ionotropic functions	Second messengers
NMDA	NMDA IBO	APV APH CPP	Ketamine MK-801, PCP SKF 10047 Mg^{2+}	Glycine	Ca^{2+} K^+ Na^+	Ca^{2+}(***) 1,4,5-IP_3(**)/ cGMP?(**)
Kainate	K Domoate	γDGG, GDEE, GAMS, FG9065	JSTX		Na^+, K^+	Ca^{2+}(*) 1,4,5-IP_3(*)
AMPA	AMPA Quinolinate	γDGG, GDEE, GAMS, FG9065	JSTX		Na^+, K^+	1,4,5-IP_3(?) Ca^{2+}(?)

APH, D-2-amino-4-phosphorobutyrate; PCP, phencyclidine; AMPA, α-amino-3-hydroxy-5-methylisoxazole-4-propionic acid; cGMP, cyclic guanosine monophosphate. (*,**,***), level of efficiency in producing second messengers.
After Sladeczek et al (1988).

density is markedly different from that of NMDA receptors. AMPA receptors are the synaptic effectors at most glutamatergic junctions. They act to depolarise the postsynaptic membrane by opening non-specific anion-carrying channels. The NMDA receptor channel is normally blocked by the binding of a Mg^{2+} ion, and so it seems likely that it is normally silent and that the normal signalling function of glutamate must take place via the other receptor types. In cells with both AMPA and NMDA receptors, the depolarisation due to AMPA receptor activation may reach levels where the Mg^{2+} is released from the NMDA receptor and its activation follows. The consequent influx of Ca^{2+} ions leads to the intracellular cascade already described above, whose final action may be either to change the sensitivity of the cell to excitatory transmission for a very long time (long-term potentiation or LTP) or, in less physiological conditions, the death of the cell.

Because of this potential for good or evil the NMDA receptors have been the subject of extensive study. They are made from at least one NR_1 subunit and a selection from NR_{2A-D}. The time-course of action is determined by which of the NR_2 subunits contribute to the receptor confirmation. Receptors with NR_{2D} subunits (common during development but less common in the adult) have a half-time for closing of many seconds whereas the NR_{2A} subunits confer a much more conventional time-scale in the tens of milliseconds.

It has also been shown that NMDA receptors are linked in the postsynaptic membrane to a very large (> 600) group of cytoskeletal and signalling molecules whose functional significance is still to be fully explored but which may allow different routes of intracellular signalling downstream from the receptors in different circumstances.

NMDA receptors include a binding site for glycine and also for phencyclidine (PCP). Interactions between these receptor sites and the ion channels they regulate may prove as complex as the GABA–benzodiazepine ion channel. Although initially introduced as an anaesthetic, PCP is a potent psychotomimetic ('angel dust'), and its drug-induced psychosis has been advanced as a useful model of schizophrenia. A similar psychosis can be induced by benzomorphan drugs, which are synthetic opiates (such as cyclazocine) that activate σ opiate receptors. PCP and σ opiate receptor activation antagonises the excitatory effects of NMDA activation but does not affect AMPA receptors (Sonders et al

1988). Since many glutamate-releasing nerve terminals also have presynaptic mGLuRs whose activation reduces glutamate release, drugs that are agonists at mGLuRs are also suggested to be antipsychotic, and have been shown to reduce the effects of NMDA activation in animals.

Glutamate and its analogues are potent neurotoxins (Olney 1989). Exogenous NMDA agonist compounds are established neurotoxins. The legume *Lathyrus satirus* contains β-*N*-oxalylamino-L-alanine (BOAA) which, if ingested chronically, causes neuronal degeneration by excessive excitatory neuronal stimulation. This model of excitatory neurotoxicity by exogenous compounds (as in lathyrism) or endogenous compounds (as proposed for Huntington's disease) has been extended to include other neurodegenerative disorders, including Alzheimer's disease, head trauma, brain ischaemia and epilepsy (Olney 1989). Anti-excitotoxic agents are currently in development, and the NMDA antagonist memantine is now licensed for the treatment of moderate to severe Alzheimer's disease. Others may soon enter clinical trials of their value in selected neuropsychiatric disorders.

Kainate receptors also mediate excitatory neurotransmission and are present on both neuronal and glial membranes, especially in the cerebellum. Their pharmacological and structural characteristics are those of the superfamily of ligand-gated ion channels. Antagonists able to differentiate between AMPA and kainate channels are becoming available.

CHOLINERGIC NEUROTRANSMISSION

Acetylcholine is a widely distributed neurotransmitter present in many regions of the brain and spinal cord. It is present in the neostriatal interneurons and septal–hippocampal pathway as well as in all motor neurons. Some central effects of acetylcholine can be mimicked by muscarine and antagonised by atropine. These are termed 'muscarinic effects'. Other effects of acetylcholine are mimicked by nicotine, not antagonised by atropine but selectively blocked by tubocurarine. The two types of cholinergic effect are mediated through two classes of cholinergic receptor: muscarinic and nicotinic. Cholinergic neuropharmacology is summarised in Table 3.6.

Table 3.6 Muscarinic pharmacology

Presynaptic

Site of action	Effect	Drug	Use
Synthesis	Increases	Choline	Experimental
	Decreases	Hemicholinium	Experimental
Storage	Inhibits acetylcholine vesicle transport	Vesamicol	Experimental
Release	Increases	Black widow spider venom	Experimental
	Blocks	Botulinum toxin	Treatment of Aystonias Cosmetic use

Postsynaptic

Receptor	Tissue	Agonist responses	Agonist	Antagonist	Molecular mechanisms
M_1	Cerebral cortex	?	Oxotremorine	Atropine	↑PLC
	Sympathetic ganglia	Depolarisation		Pirenzepine	↑Ca^{2+}
M_2	Heart	Slowed depolarisation		Atropine	↑K^+ channels
	Sinoatrial node	Hyperpolarisation			↓Adenylate cyclase
	Atrium	Shortened action potential			
	Atrioventricular node	Decreased contractile force			
	Ventricle	Decreased conduction velocity			
M_3	Smooth muscle				↑PLC
	Secretory glands				↑Ca^{2+}

Degradation

Cholinesterase inhibitors (e.g. physostigmine, donepezil, rivastigmine, galantamine); PLC, phospholipase C.

Nicotinic receptors are ligand-gated ion channels and, when activated by ligand binding, produce a rapid increase in cellular permeability to Na^+ and K^+. Muscarinic receptors are G-protein-coupled and are not necessarily only linked to ion channels. The structures of nicotinic and muscarinic receptors show that they belong to two distinct superfamilies of receptor types. The channel of the nicotinic cholinergic receptor is composed of five homologous subunits (Guy & Hucho 1987). The neuromuscular nicotinic receptor contains four distinct subunits (α, β, δ, γ) arranged as a pentamer (the γ subunit is replaced by an ε subunit in adult muscle). Nicotinic receptors in the CNS are also pentamers but comprise only two subunits (α and β). Brain nicotinic receptors are open to complex variation, as there are multiple forms of both α and β subunits, and it appears that different parts of the brain contain different combinations of α and β subtypes. The structure of the nicotinic receptor is shown in Figure 3.8. The four genes encoding the $α_2$, $α_3$, $α_4$ and $β_2$ subunits of the nicotinic cholinergic receptor are differentially distributed in vertebrate brain. All four mRNAs are present in the cerebellum, whereas only $α_2$ and $β_2$ mRNAs are found in lateral spiriform nuclei of chicken brain. This indicates that neurons are capable of differential expression in vivo of nicotinic receptor subunits and points to nicotinic receptor heterogeneity in the CNS. The mRNAs for these subunits also show different temporal patterns of expression during brain development.

Muscarinic cholinergic receptors also exist as various subtypes. Pharmacological studies had supported the subdivision of muscarinic receptors into M_1, M_2 and M_3. Structural studies have determined three corresponding receptor subtypes termed m_1, m_2 and m_3. Two further molecules termed m_4 and m_5 have also been detected. Like all other G-protein-coupled receptors, there are seven transmembrane domains; the characteristics of muscarinic receptors are shown in Table 3.7 (Bonner 1989).

Muscarinic receptors M_1 and M_3 activate a G protein that stimulates PLC activity. PLC stimulates hydrolysis of phosphatidylinositol phosphates to IP_3, which can release intracellular Ca^{2+}. DAG is also produced by PLC and this leads to PKC activation. Ligand binding to M_2 and M_4 receptors activates G_i proteins, which inhibit adenylate cyclase, and open K^+ and close Ca^{2+} channels.

Drugs affecting cholinergic neurotransmission

Drugs affecting acetylcholine synthesis

Acetylcholine is synthesised in a single step from acetyl coenzyme A (produced in neuronal mitochondria) and choline (from the liver), which is catalysed by choline acetyltransferase. Synthesis of acetylcholine can be increased by choline administration because the synthetic enzyme is not fully saturated.

Drugs affecting acetylcholine release

Newly synthesised acetylcholine is preferentially released on stimulation from storage in presynaptic cholinergic terminals. Black widow spider venom produces a rapid release of acetylcholine and also causes morphological changes in the presynaptic storage vesicles.

Drugs affecting nicotinic receptors

Nicotinic receptors are excitatory and function by opening ionic channels. They are specifically blocked by α-bungarotoxin.

Table 3.7 Properties of cloned muscarinic receptors

Property	m_1	m_2	m_3	m_4	m_5
Molecular weight	51 387	51 681	66 085	53 014	60 120
Pirenzepine affinity	High	Low	←——————— intermediate ———————→		
Phosphatidylinositol response	Stimulates	None	Stimulates	None	Stimulates
cAMP response	Stimulates	Inhibits	Stimulates	Inhibits	Stimulates
Arachidonic acid response	Stimulates	None	Stimulates	None	Stimulates
Ca^{2+}-dependent K_A^+ channel	Opens	No effect	Opens	No effect	opens
mRNA distribution	Brain	Brain	Brain	Brain	Brain
	Glands	Heart	Smooth muscle		
		Smooth muscle			

After Bonner (1989).

Nicotinic receptors are present in the brain, particularly in the thalamus and cerebellar cortex. Outside the brain, the cholinergic input from the spinal cord synapses on to nicotinic receptors at the neurotransmitter junction. Most nicotinic receptor antagonists have profound effects at the neuromuscular junction. The best known agent is (+)-tubocurarine, which does not easily cross the blood–brain barrier. Decamethonium and succinylcholine are also nicotinic receptor antagonists but, instead of competing with acetylcholine for the receptor site, they bind to the receptor for a long period, making it insensitive to acetylcholine. Like (+)-tubocurarine, decamethonium and succinylcholine have almost no central effects. Agonists at nicotinic receptors include nicotine, dimethyl-phenylpiperazinium (DMPP) and phenyl-trimethylammonium (PTMA).

Nicotine is present in tobacco (*Nicotiana tabacum*), and most smokers identify 'stress reduction' as a major determinant of their habit, saying that smoking helps them to relax. Small, repeated injections of nicotine, similar to those received while smoking, produce increased cortical release of acetylcholine and electrocortical arousal. Adrenergic blockade has no effect on this action of nicotine, but both muscarinic and nicotinic blockade prevent nicotine from activating the cortex. Lesion studies suggest that tobacco smoking increases electrocortical arousal by acting at sites of the cholinergic projections to the cortex. On the other hand the habit-forming nature of smoking may be related to nicotinic receptors present on dopamine neurons in substantia nigra and the ventral tegmental area in the brainstem. Low doses of nicotine produce stimulation in the periphery, while higher doses block nicotinic receptors and cause paralysis of neuromuscular junctions. One explanation for the 'stress reduction' claimed by smokers is that mild blockade of peripheral neuromuscular junctions is associated with feelings of 'relaxation' and well-being.

Drugs affecting muscarinic receptors

M_1 receptors are concentrated in the sympathetic ganglia, stomach and corpus striatum. They are selectively antagonised by pirenzipine and are closely associated with K^+ channels. M_2 receptors are concentrated in the hindbrain, cerebellum and heart. They are regulated by gallamine and GTP and inhibit adenylate cyclase. Muscarinic receptor antagonists therefore have both central and peripheral actions. Atropine and scopolamine are the best known and, in the periphery, they decrease secretion from the gut, nasopharynx and respiratory tract and increase the heart rate.

Their central effects include confusion, lassitude and drowsiness, and higher doses can cause delirium ('atropine psychosis'). Agonists at muscarinic receptors include muscarine, pilocarpine, arecoline, methacholine and carbachol.

The tricyclic antidepressants commonly cause anticholinergic side-effects. These include dry mouth, excessive sweating, blurring of vision and urinary retention, which may be especially troublesome in the elderly. It is important, therefore, to know the relative potencies at muscarinic receptors of antidepressant drugs to guide prescribing, for example, in patients with glaucoma or prostatism. Amitriptyline has about 5% of the anticholinergic potency of atropine, but, as it is used in much greater doses (100–150 mg daily) than the well-known anticholinergics (0.6 mg), its therapeutic administration can produce an extensive blockade of cholinergic receptors.

Anticholinergic drugs in parkinsonism

Until the introduction of L-dopa and decarboxylase inhibitors, anticholinergic drugs formed the mainstay of treatment for parkinsonism. These drugs remain useful for patients in the early stages of Parkinson's disease, for patients unable to tolerate L-dopa, and in addition to L-dopa in selected patients. They can be especially useful in drug-induced parkinsonism.

The anticholinergic drugs used to treat drug-induced parkinsonism are tertiary amines (benztropine, trihexyphenidyl and procyclidine). Their extra-CNS antimuscarinic effects are much weaker than those of atropine. Diphenhydramine is an antihistamine drug that has slight anticholinergic properties and is especially well tolerated by old people.

Anticholinesterases

Anticholinesterase drugs cause acetylcholine to accumulate at cholinergic synapses. These drugs inhibit the enzyme acetylcholinesterase, and the prototype drug is physostigmine. Others were developed as insecticides and investigated for use in chemical warfare. These latter types cause irreversible inhibition of acetylcholinesterase. The mechanism of action of anticholinesterases (including physostigmine) is based on their binding with the enzyme and, in the case of physostigmine and neostigmine, hydrolysing slowly. The terms 'reversible' and 'irreversible' as applied to anticholinesterases are only relative and refer to the speed at which the enzyme recovers function. In psychiatry, the main use of physostigmine is experimental in Alzheimer's disease, where it may transiently produce a modest improvement in mental functions. Rarely, intravenous physostigmine may be used to reverse a brief psychosis induced by antimuscarinic drugs. Physostigmine does not reverse the anticholinergic cardiotoxic effects of tricyclic antidepressants. In recent years acetylcholinesterase inhibition has reached clinical fruition with the introduction of compounds effective in the treatment of early dementias, especially Alzheimer's type. Currently these comprise donepezil, rivastigmine and galantamine (see Ch. 15).

NORADRENERGIC NEUROTRANSMISSION

Adrenoceptors

An understanding of the classification and properties of the different types of adrenoceptor is essential to understanding the diverse effects of catecholamines and the neuropharmacology of this system. Physiological studies by Ahlquist (1948) supported the distinction between two types of adrenoceptor, termed α and β. This initial distinction was supported by observations on adrenergic antagonists at α adrenoceptors (e.g. phenoxybenzamine) and β adrenoceptors (e.g. propranolol). Subsequently, β receptors were subdivided into β_1 and β_2, and later structural studies identi-

fied a third type, termed β_3. The relative number of each of these subtypes varies with tissue type. Alpha adrenoceptors are present in the iris, where they stimulate contraction of the radial muscle, thus producing dilatation. They are also present in the eyelid where their stimulation raises the lid. The heart contains β_1 receptors, which mediate increases in both the rate and force of cardiac contractions. All β receptors are coupled through G proteins to the enzyme adenylate cyclase.

Drugs affecting noradrenergic neurotransmission

Table 3.8 summarises the sites of action, effects and uses of drugs that act on noradrenergic neurotransmission. Some drugs act specifically at noradrenergic synapses, whereas others affect several monoamines. Tricyclic antidepressants are believed to have mood-elevating actions because of their inhibition of uptake of monoamines, particularly noradrenaline and serotonin, from the synaptic cleft. These actions of antidepressants have led to the 'monoamine hypothesis of affective disorders'. Simply stated, the hypothesis postulates that in depressive illness there is reduced efficiency of neurotransmission at noradrenergic and/or serotonergic synapses and that this may involve abnormalities in the affinity of monoaminergic receptors for their endogenous ligands (see Ch. 20).

Table 3.8   Noradrenergic pharmacology

Presynaptic

Site of action	Effect	Drug	Use
Synthesis	False transmitter	α-Methyldopa	Hypotensive
	Decreased	α-Methyl-p-tyrosine	Experimental
Storage	Decreased (irreversible)	Reserpine	Hypotensive
	Decreased (reversible)	Tetrabenazine	Chorea
	Increased	Monoamine oxidase Inhibitors (MAOIs)	Antidepressant
Release	Increased	Amphetamine	Euphoriant
	Increased	Tyramine	Experimental
	Decreased	Debrisoquine	Hypotensive

Postsynaptic

Receptor	Tissue	Agonist responses	Agonist	Antagonist	Molecular mechanisms
α_1	Vascular smooth muscle	Contracts	Isoprotenerol Phenylephrine	Prazosin	$\uparrow$PLC $\uparrow$IP$_3$ $\uparrow$K$^+$ channels $\uparrow$Intracellular Ca^{2+}
α_2	Heart Neural	Increased contractile force $\downarrow$Noradrenaline release	Clonidine	Yohimbine	$\downarrow$Adenylate cyclase $\uparrow$K$^+$ channels $\downarrow$Ca^{2+} channels
β_1	Vascular smooth muscle Heart	Contracts Increased contractile force			$\uparrow$Adenylate cyclase $\uparrow$Ca^{2+} channels
β_2	Smooth muscle	Relaxation	Salbutamol		$\uparrow$Adenylate cyclase

Degradation

Site of action	Effect	Drug	Use
Reuptake	Inhibits	Desipramine	Antidepressant
	Inhibits	Amitriptyline	Antidepressant
	Inhibits	Cocaine	Euphoriant

Drugs inhibiting noradrenaline synthesis

Noradrenaline is synthesised from L-tyrosine by the following steps: L-tyrosine is hydroxylated to L-dopa (by tyrosine hydroxylase), L-dopa is decarboxylated to dopamine (by aromatic-L-amino-acid decarboxylase), and dopamine is then hydroxylated to noradrenaline (by dopamine β-hydroxylase). Tyrosine hydroxylase is inhibited by α-methyl-*p*-tyrosine, and this drug is used experimentally to prevent the synthesis of dopamine, noradrenaline and adrenaline. Carbidopa inhibits aromatic-L-amino-acid decarboxylase at sites outside the CNS and can be given at the same time as L-dopa, when it will prevent enhancement of dopamine synthesis outside the CNS. Dopamine β-hydroxylase is inhibited by disulfiram and by FLA63. Synthesis of noradrenaline can also be disrupted by the structurally similar precursor α-methyldopa. This is synthesised to α-methylnoradrenaline, which then acts as a 'false neurotransmitter' — that is, it is released by the usual mechanisms involved in noradrenaline release but it is much less effective at noradrenaline receptors.

Drugs affecting the storage of noradrenaline

Most noradrenaline is stored in a presynaptic complex of noradrenaline, adenosine triphosphate (ATP), metallic ions of magnesium, calcium, copper and proteins called chromogranins. Dopamine β-hydroxylase is present in noradrenergic storage vesicles, probably in association with the vesicular limiting membrane. Noradrenaline is taken up into storage by an active transport mechanism that is magnesium dependent and requires ATP, although a little noradrenaline is available in the cytoplasm. The *Rawalfia* alkaloids (e.g. reserpine and tetrabenazine) disrupt noradrenaline storage and inhibit noradrenaline uptake into storage vesicles; reserpine causes irreversible damage to granules, whereas tetrabenazine has reversible effects. These processes can be relatively slow, so that noradrenaline released from storage may be degraded by intracellular monoamine oxidase before it can bind with postsynaptic receptors. Reserpine can initially produce postsynaptic adrenoceptor stimulation by releasing noradrenaline, and in the presence of monoamine oxidases it releases the relatively large storage pool onto the postsynaptic receptors.

Drugs affecting the release of noradrenaline

Noradrenaline is released along with the contents of the storage vesicles by a calcium-dependent process involving fusion of the vesicles with the presynaptic membrane and also involving prostaglandins (PGE_2 inhibiting and PGE_{2a} facilitating release). Release may be regulated by prostaglandins and other local hormones acting on noradrenergic nerve terminals. Presynaptic catecholamine receptors (autoreceptors) are important in the regulation of impulse-induced noradrenaline release, but presynaptic receptors may be sensitive not only to the local concentration of noradrenaline but also to acetylcholine, cAMP, prostaglandins and neuropeptides like thyrotrophin-releasing hormone.

Drugs that release noradrenaline quickly enough to bind with postsynaptic receptors are called 'indirectly acting sympathomimetic amines'. Examples are amphetamine, tyramine and ephedrine. Some drugs inhibit noradrenaline release from storage, for example antihypertensive agents such as debrisoquine, bethanidine and guanethidine. These drugs do not readily cross the blood–brain barrier (their lipid solubility is low), and they therefore have few psychotoxic effects.

Drugs acting on adrenergic receptors

There are two main types of receptor for noradrenaline: α and β adrenoceptors. The existence of these two types was deduced from studies on smooth muscle where catecholamines produce both excitatory and inhibitory effects. Later studies of the binding of drugs to adrenoceptors supported the original division into α and β receptor types. Phenoxybenzamine produces selective blockade of α receptors, and propranolol blocks β receptors. The development of more selective antagonists and agonists allowed these receptors to be further subdivided into β_1, β_2, α_1 and α_2 receptors. The relative number of the various subtypes of adrenoceptor varies with each tissue. Stimulation of α adrenoceptors in blood vessels causes vasoconstriction. Additionally, the pilomotor muscles and salivary glands are stimulated through their α adrenoceptors. The gastrointestinal tract has both α and β adrenoceptors, and the smooth muscle in the tract relaxes in response to stimulation of either receptor type. Sphincter muscles, however, contract in response to excitation of α adrenoceptors.

The heart contains β_1 receptors, which mediate increases in both rate and force of cardiac contraction. Stimulation of β_2 receptors in bronchial smooth muscle produces bronchodilatation. They are also present in the gastrointestinal tract, uterus and bladder, where their stimulation produces smooth muscle relaxation. Beta receptors are also involved in the regulation of certain metabolic processes such as increasing lipolysis or gluconeogenesis and reducing insulin release. All β receptors are linked to the enzyme adenylate cyclase, so that stimulation of β receptors increases the synthesis of cAMP from ATP. Phosphodiesterases degrade cAMP to non-cyclic 5'-AMP. Drugs that inhibit phosphodiesterases (such as caffeine, aminophylline and theobromine) enhance the physiological responses to β adrenoceptor stimulation.

Alpha adrenoceptor agonists include noradrenaline and adrenaline. Noradrenaline acts mostly through α adrenoceptors and adrenaline largely through β adrenoceptors. Phenylephrine and clonidine are directly acting α adrenoceptor agonists with few β adrenoceptor effects, and their actions are therefore similar to those of noradrenaline. Isoprenaline is a synthetic catecholamine acting only on β receptors, where it is more potent than either adrenaline or noradrenaline. Salbutamol is a selective β_2 adrenoceptor agonist and has been used as an antidepressant. The rationale leading to this application is derived from the 'amine hypothesis of depression', where a postulated reduction in the functional efficiency of neurotransmission at synapses involving monoamines concerned with the regulation of mood is accompanied by increased postsynaptic sensitivity to those monoamines. Administration of a selective monoaminergic receptor antagonist such as salbutamol might therefore allow re-establishment of more efficient neurotransmission. Alpha adrenoceptor antagonists are used mostly in experimental work, though phentolamine (a reversible α adrenoceptor antagonist) is useful in the emergency treatment of hypertension and the diagnosis of phaeochromocytomas.

Some β adrenoceptor antagonists may have local anaesthetic-like activity on membrane fluidity as well as actions at adrenoceptors. These drugs are used mostly in the control of hypertension and the relief of angina. Their exact mode of action in the control of hypertension is unknown. Non-selective β adrenoceptor antagonists include propranolol and atenolol. Atenolol and metoprolol are selective β₁ adrenoceptor antagonists that in large doses affect all β receptors. These drugs act at both pre- and postsynaptic adrenoceptors. Presynaptic β₁ receptors facilitate noradrenaline release, whereas presynaptic β₂ receptors are inhibitory. These receptors may be involved in the pathogenesis of affective symptoms, and effective antidepressants could exert some or all of their effects at these sites.

Antidepressants and adrenergic receptors

There is a close relationship between the potencies of tricyclic antidepressants to occupy postsynaptic α₁ adrenoceptors and their sedative–hypotensive effects. The tertiary amines (e.g. amitriptyline) are more potent at these sites than secondary amines (e.g. nortriptyline) and are only slightly less potent than the better-known α adrenoceptor antagonist phentolamine. Chronic administration of antidepressants, but not short-term treatment, reduces noradrenaline-coupled adenylate cyclase activity and also reduces the number of β receptors in brain tissue. These effects do not seem to be limited to one type of antidepressant treatment but are found with tricyclic drugs, mianserin, iprindole, monoamine oxidase inhibitors and also in an animal model of electroconvulsive therapy (ECT). Some antidepressants may act therefore by initially increasing the synaptic concentration of noradrenaline, which in turn reduces the sensitivity and/or number of β adrenoceptors. The initial increase of noradrenaline may be caused by inhibition of noradrenaline uptake, blockade of presynaptic inhibitory autoreceptors, or actions at other sites.

Drugs affecting noradrenaline uptake

Antidepressants and euphoriants such as cocaine and amphetamine act rapidly on the presynaptic reuptake of noradrenaline. The structure of the noradrenaline transporter is known and has much in common with other members of the superfamily of neurotransmitter transporters. Distribution of the transporter matches the localisation of noradrenaline neurons in the CNS (Pacholczyk et al 1991). The transporter may be important in neurodegenerative diseases. Potent neurotoxins (such as 1-methyl-4-phenylpyridinium (MPP⁺) and 6-hydroxydopamine (6-OH-DA)) can be actively taken up by the noradrenaline transporter and, if allowed to accumulate in neurons, cause selective neuronal death. The transporter is an important site of action of mood-affecting drugs, and its further study (e.g. binding to novel, potentially antidepressant compounds) may facilitate new drug development. It may also prove relevant to understanding the genetic contribution to affective disorders.

Uptake of noradrenaline from the synaptic cleft is an energy-consuming process that is sodium dependent and involves ATP. Some drugs inhibit the uptake of monoamines from the synaptic cleft, and this is thought to be the principal action of tricyclic antidepressants. These drugs affect both noradrenaline and serotonin uptake (see Ch. 15) but have little effect on dopamine. The tertiary amines imipramine and amitriptyline, in contrast, mostly affect the uptake of serotonin. Secondary amines like desipramine and nortriptyline largely affect noradrenaline. Many tertiary amines are metabolised to secondary amines, so in reality the tertiary amines often affect both noradrenaline and serotonin uptake. A number of drugs have been developed to act selectively on serotonin or noradrenaline uptake, but there are no clear differences in antidepressant activity between the two. Inhibition of uptake is evident

from pharmacological studies within 24 hours of administration of the drug, but clinical effects are not typically seen for about 10–20 days. Because the tricyclic drugs and their related compounds were derived from the phenothiazines, they share several pharmacological properties with them. In particular, they have anticholinergic and antihistaminergic effects. The anticholinergic effects are evident within hours of first administering the drug, and tolerance usually develops before the onset of the antidepressant effect. For these reasons, the anticholinergic effects of the tricyclic antidepressants are probably not relevant to their antidepressant action. Further, the incidence of anticholinergic side-effects does not differ between patients who respond and those who do not respond to a tricyclic. The antihistaminergic effects of tricyclic drugs may prove relevant to their antidepressant actions.

Drugs affecting degradation of noradrenaline

Noradrenaline that is not taken up by the presynaptic terminal from the synaptic cleft can be fused into the postsynaptic membrane, where it is degraded by the enzymes monoamine oxidase and catechol-O-methyl-transferase (COMT). Monoamine oxidases are a group of enzymes that are present in a wide variety of tissues in which their substrate specificity and physical properties may differ. There are two types, known as A and B. Type A is more effective in the degradation of noradrenaline, serotonin and dopamine. Tyramine (a naturally occurring amino acid present in many foods) is a substrate for both forms, and the use of a monoamine oxidase inhibitor is associated with the hazard of toxic reactions to excessive amounts of tyramine (see Ch. 15). The antidepressant actions of monoamine oxidase inhibitors such as tranylcypromine, pargyline, phenelzine and clorgyline (a selective type A inhibitor) are produced largely by their inhibition of monoamine oxidase. They also affect aromatic-L-amino-acid decarboxylase and various other oxidases and inhibit uptake of noradrenaline and serotonin, but the clinical relevance of these effects is not known. The metabolism of concomitantly administered drugs may also be affected by monoamine oxidase inhibitors, so that the action of barbiturates may be prolonged and the effect of amphetamine exaggerated.

Monoamine oxidase inhibitors also reduce the 'first-pass' presystemic degradation of tyramine after its intestinal absorption. Tyramine is selectively taken up into adrenergic neurons (by a high-affinity system), where it releases stored noradrenaline. Monoamine oxidase inhibitors thus potentiate the effects of tyramine and other indirectly acting sympathomimetic agents. New monoamine oxidase inhibitors have been developed that are selective for monoamine oxidase A, and there are claims that these do not potentiate the tyramine response and are also effective antidepressants. Moclobemide is a recent reversible inhibitor of monoamine oxidase A. Since it spares the monoamine oxidase A present in the gut as a defence against ingested amines, it is potentially a useful antidepressant.

DOPAMINERGIC NEUROTRANSMISSION

The modern era of pharmacotherapy in psychiatry began with the introduction of phenothiazine antipsychotics in 1952 and was quickly followed by the development of phenothiazine-derived tricyclic antidepressants. At first, the mode of action of these drugs was unknown, but during the past forty years the effects of antipsychotic drugs on central dopaminergic transmission have

Table 3.9   Dopaminergic pharmacology

Presynaptic

Site of action	Effect	Drug	Use
Synthesis	Inhibits	α-Methyltyrosine	Occasionally in phaeochromocytoma
	Increases	L-Dopa	Parkinson's disease
Storage	Inhibits	Tetrabenazine	Chorea
		α-Methyltyrosine	As above
		Reserpine	Occasionally in treatment of refractory psychoses
Release	Increases	Amphetamine	Experimental
	Inhibits	γ-Hydroxybutyrate	Experimental

Postsynaptic

Receptor	Tissue	Agonist	Antagonist	Molecular mechanisms
D$_1$	Renal, mesenteric and coronary vessels (vasodilatation) Pituitary-hypothalamic axis Cell bodies and presynaptic terminals of intrinsic striatal neurons	Pergolide SKF 38393	Lisuride SCH 23390	↑cAMP ↑Adenylate cyclase
D$_2$	Neuronal cell bodies of striatum and presynaptic terminals of dopaminergic striatal neurons	Bromocriptine Pergolide Lisuride Apomorphine	Butyrophenones Sulpiride	↓Adenylate cyclase or no effect

Degradation

Site of action	Effect	Drug	Use
Uptake	Inhibits	Benztropine	Parkinson's disease
		Nomifensine	Experimental (clinically withdrawn)
		Cocaine	Experimental
		Amitriptyline	Antidepressant

been established as an important component of their antipsychotic actions. The neuropharmacology of dopaminergic neurotransmission is summarised in Table 3.9.

Dopamine synthesis, storage and release

Dopamine synthesis Dopamine is synthesised from the amino acid L-tyrosine by the following steps: L-tyrosine is hydroxylated to L-dopa (by tyrosine hydroxylase) and then decarboxylated (by aromatic-L-amino-acid decarboxylase) to form dopamine. Oral administration of L-dopa increases dopamine synthesis. In Parkinson's disease, dopaminergic neurons are damaged and have a much-reduced capacity to synthesise dopamine. Adjacent glial cells retain dopamine synthetic capacity, and, during L-dopa therapy, dopamine may leak out from these glial cells to stimulate surviving supersensitive dopamine receptors. Alternatively the serotonin nerve terminals in the basal ganglia contain a closely related decarboxylase which could also supply dopamine from applied L-dopa.

Dopamine storage. Dopamine is stored in presynaptic complexes of dopamine, ATP, magnesium, calcium, copper and chromogranins. Drugs that disrupt the storage of noradrenaline, like *Rawolfia* alkaloids and tetrabenazine, also disrupt dopamine storage complexes, and many of the behavioural sequelae of their administration may be related to the action on dopamine storage rather than on that of noradrenaline.

Dopamine release. Dopamine is released from central dopaminergic terminals by two discrete mechanisms that differ in their sensitivity to dopamine uptake inhibitors (Raiteri et al 1979). An energy-dependent transport mechanism for dopamine uptake is inhibited by nomifensine, benztropine and cocaine. A second carrier-independent mechanism for dopamine release is dependent upon extracellular Ca^{2+} concentrations and involves fusion of dopamine-containing vesicles with the presynaptic membrane upon the Ca^{2+} influx that follows action potentials. This type of release is facilitated by amphetamine at concentrations much lower than those required for amphetamine to stimulate postsynaptic catecholaminergic receptors. Amphetamines stimulate rapid release of dopamine, inhibit its uptake from the synaptic cleft and also inhibit its degradative enzyme monoamine oxidase.

The dopamine hypothesis of schizophrenia

The 'dopamine hypothesis of schizophrenia', simply stated, postulates that certain dopaminergic pathways are overactive in schizophrenia and so cause the symptoms of an acute schizophrenic episode. Clinical studies indicate that drugs like L-dopa or amphetamine, which potentiate dopaminergic activity, may induce or exacerbate schizophrenic symptoms.

When the antipsychotic drugs were first introduced, their mode of action was unknown. At first, studies in the peripheral nervous system suggested that the anti-adrenergic effects of chlorpromazine probably explained its antipsychotic action, perhaps by reducing arousal. However, the fact that potent anti-adrenergic agents had no antipsychotic benefit clearly did not support this hypothesis. Carlsson & Lindqvist (1963) first suggested that dopamine receptor blockade was the basis of antipsychotic effects. The low activity of butyrophenone antipsychotics at dopamine receptor sites linked to adenylate cyclase stimulation was seen as evidence against this idea. It was supported, however, by the recognition of two types of dopamine receptor. One (called D_1) was linked to adenylate cyclase stimulation, and another, higher affinity one (called D_2) was sometimes associated with adenylate cyclase inhibition and exhibited preferential binding of butyrophenones.

Neuropharmacological studies provide virtually all the evidence to support the 'dopamine hypothesis of schizophrenia'. Although some of the newer 'atypical' antipsychotic agents are weak dopamine receptor antagonists, all effective antipsychotics are believed to share the ability to impair dopaminergic neurotransmission. Postmortem studies of schizophrenic brains have demonstrated increased dopamine receptor (D_2) densities, but these densities are probably considerably influenced by antemortem drug treatments. Positron emission tomographic studies of D_2 receptor binding in antipsychotic-naive schizophrenic patients have provided conflicting results.

The CNS location of the site of antipsychotic drug action is unknown. Dopamine receptors are present in the basal ganglia, the mesolimbic system, the tuberoinfundibular region and, to a much lesser extent, in the cerebral cortex. Studies on the effects of dopaminergic transmission of psychotomimetic agents such as amphetamine, PCP and benzmorphan point to a possible common mechanism of psychotic action. Carlsson (1988) has proposed that 'information overload' and 'hyper-arousal' are integral features of many psychotic illnesses. He postulates that these features arise because of impairment of the protective effects on cortical function of the mesolimbic system. In health, Carlsson argues that mesolimbic glutamate-releasing neurons oppose mesolimbic dopaminergic pathways and maintain this protective function. It is true that drug-induced psychoses are caused by blocking glutamatergic function (e.g. by PCP or benzmorphan) or by increasing dopaminergic activity (e.g. amphetamine). Recent anatomical investigations show that dopamine synapses are present on, or close to, the necks of spines on dendrites in the basal ganglia, where glutamate synapses are present on the heads of the same spines. This close anatomical association may well be the substrate for the dopamine–glutamate interactions which many authors associate with psychotic symptoms.

Dopamine receptors

Pharmacological studies show that there are at least two types of dopamine receptor: D_1 and D_2. There is very good agreement between the affinity of a standard antipsychotic drug for D_2 receptors and the average daily dose of that drug used to treat schizophrenia. The structures of D_1 and D_2 receptors are now established and, when expressed in cell lines, are seen to possess the pharmacological properties predicted in earlier studies.

Blockade of D_2 receptors is the likely cause of unwanted extrapyramidal system effects, and therefore, if blockade of the D_2 receptor is also the site of antipsychotic action, all effective antipsychotics should be equipotent in the induction of extrapyramidal side-effects (EPS) and in antipsychotic efficacy. Some newer drugs used to treat schizophrenia (sometimes termed 'atypical') are reported to have a lower tendency to produce EPS than older drugs such as haloperidol. (Atypical antipsychotic drugs include thioridazine, sulpiride and clozapine, and many newer drugs in various stages of development (see Ch. 15).) Pharmacological studies have not detected differences between postsynaptic D_2 receptors located in the striatum (where EPS arise) and in the mesolimbic system (where the antipsychotic action is presumed to be located).

Structural analysis of dopamine receptor types has revealed a family of at least five similar G-protein-coupled molecules (Sunahara et al 1990). The mRNA for D_1 is most abundant in the caudate, nucleus accumbens and olfactory tubercle, with little in the substantia nigra. Structurally, D_1 receptors are most like the β adrenoceptor (Sunahara et al 1990) and are functionally coupled to adenylate cyclase. Subsequently, similarities between the known structures of G-protein-coupled receptors helped to isolate and characterise the D_2 receptor. Structural studies also identified two D_2 receptor isoforms: one predicted by pharmacological studies but the other probably an alternative product of a single D_2 gene (Monsma et al 1989). The D_2 receptor isoforms are termed $D_2(414)$ or D_{2short} and $D_2(443)$ or D_{2long}. Discovery of D_2 isoforms suggests a means by which different dopaminergic neuronal populations might adjust responses to stimuli (such as chronic exposure to antipsychotics) or be a source of genetically determined receptor variability of possible relevance to the aetiology of schizophrenia. However, no abnormalities of D_2 isoform structure in schizophrenia have been described, though linkage between the D_2 receptor gene (located in the q22–q23 region of human chromosome 11) has been reported in alcoholism (Blum et al 1990).

Using in-situ hybridisation, it has been shown that the spiny output cells of the caudate/putamen are in two classes. In one, the mRNA for D_1 receptors predominate and they also make enkephalin and project to the globus pallidus and thence to the output nuclei of the basal ganglia (substantia nigra and the globus pallidus interna). The other class of spiny neurons makes D_2 receptors and substance P and dynorphin and project directly to the substantia nigra. The balance between these two output pathways is vital for the normal expression of movement, and loss of dopamine increases synthetic activity in the enkephalin-containing cells and reduces the activity of the others.

Further subtypes of dopamine receptor have been revealed by structural analysis. The D_3 receptor is located in the limbic system. It is present on both postsynaptic and presynaptic membranes and may mediate the therapeutic effects of antipsychotics drugs (Sokoloff et al 1990). The neuropharmacology, CNS localisation and, possibly, connections with intracellular signalling systems of the D_3 receptor subtype, all differ from D_1 and D_2. For example, butyrophenones are 10–20 times more potent at D_2 than at D_3 receptors, but sulpiride, thioridazine and clozapine are only 2–3 times more potent at D_2 than D_3. These observations probably account for differences between antipsychotic drugs in their ability to induce EPS. The D_3 receptor forms the basis of current attempts to design new antipsychotic drugs with fewer EPS and to develop new drugs for Parkinson's disease. The novel antipsychotic clozapine has a markedly reduced liability to cause 'tardive dyskinesia', a particularly difficult form of EPS common in patients treated for long periods with older, more conventional antipsychotics.

A further subtype of dopamine receptor termed D_4 has been described and found to bind clozapine preferentially (Van Tol et al 1991). It is structurally related to other members of the G-protein-coupled receptor 'superfamily', and, as for D_3, understanding of its structure and functions may facilitate development of novel antipsychotic drugs. Sunahara et al (1991) have also described a further subtype of dopamine receptor (termed D_5 or D_{1b}) that is also primarily located in the limbic system and may be involved in D_2 regulation by D_1 activation, which has been reported in vivo. On the other hand a recent report of its localisation in hippocampus suggests as yet unknown actions. D_5 receptors are not always co-expressed with D_1. The D_5 form of the receptor is the one found in cholinergic neurons in the basal ganglia and in cortex. In globus pallidus and in the subthalamic nucleus the firing pattern of the neurons may be dependent on D_5 receptor activation.

Administration of dopamine-receptor-blocking drugs can produce supersensitivity of dopamine receptors. The mechanism(s) underlying supersensitivity following chronic administration of antipsychotics are largely unknown. In some patients (postmenopausal women seem most susceptible) continuous administration of antipsychotics can cause a syndrome of involuntary movements to emerge ('tardive dyskinesia') (See Ch. 15).

Drugs affecting dopaminergic neurotransmission

Drugs affecting dopamine uptake

Amphetamine and other drugs which release dopamine also inhibit its uptake and so potentiate the action of dopamine. Nomifensine and cocaine are also well-established dopamine uptake inhibitors. Benztropine and to a lesser extent benzhexol and orphenadrine inhibit the uptake of dopamine and also block cholinergic receptors, actions that contribute to the effects of these anticholinergic drugs in the treatment of parkinsonism. The action of cocaine has been localised to the dopamine system in the

basal ganglia (Volkow et al 1997). The number of dopamine receptors (estimated from positron emission tomography of antagonist binding) was shown to be reduced in chronic cocaine users, and the extent of the 'high' obtained by cocaine doses closely correlated to the binding of cocaine to the dopamine uptake sites in the brains of the users. Such data reinforce the idea that dopamine receptors have an action in the control of drug-taking behaviour, although the relationship to therapeutic actions of dopamine blockers is less clear.

Drugs affecting degradation of dopamine

Monoamine oxidase inhibitors like tranylcypromine reduce the degradation of dopamine by monoamine oxidase. Tranylcypromine also reduces uptake of dopamine, but this is probably not relevant to its antidepressant action because drugs such as benztropine (a potent dopamine uptake inhibitor) are not effective antidepressants. In contrast the actions of the monoamine oxidase B inhibitor selegeline seems to be less on the metabolism of amines and more on the reduction of oxidative stress and its concomitant neurotoxicity. A large multicentre trial suggested strongly that pre-treatment with selegeline slows the progression of symptoms of Parkinson's disease.

Parkinsonism

There is a substantial reduction of dopaminergic innervation of the basal ganglia in Parkinson's disease. The loss of dopamine leads to parkinsonian signs and symptoms, and restoration of dopaminergic neurotransmission is the aim of all effective treatments. A simplified summary of the neural connections of the basal ganglia is shown in Figure 3.11. The pathways that connect the caudate-nucleus–putamen to the substantia nigra are of most importance in parkinsonism. Dopamine-containing cell bodies in the pars compacta of the substantia nigra degenerate in Parkinson's disease. The efferents of these cell bodies in normal

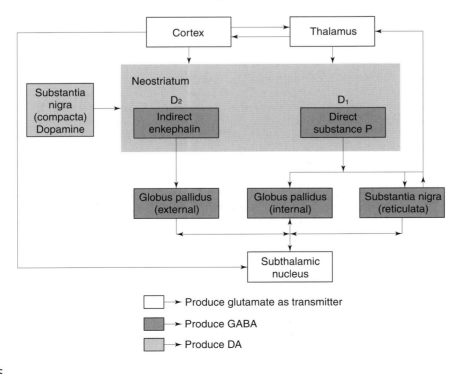

Fig. 3.11
Neural connections of the basal ganglia. Dopaminergic, and cortical and thalamic (glutamatergic), inputs reach all of the cells in the neostriatum, although the spiny output cells form at least two output pathways from neostriatum. Dopamine D_1 receptors predominate on the direct pathway, while the indirectly projecting cells make D_2 receptors.

brain synapse on all types of output cell in the caudate–putamen. The effect of dopaminergic inputs to the caudate–putamen is the modification of its output to other structures. In particular, loss of dopamine results in the reduction of the synthesis of substance P in those cells which make D_1 receptors and project directly to the substantia nigra, and in an increase in the synthesis of enkephalin in the indirectly projecting, D_2 receptor-synthesising cells. Current surgical treatment in parkinsonian patients aims to redress the imbalance in the two pathways by surgically reducing the activity of the indirect pathway with a lesion in the globus pallidus interna, or by chronic high-frequency stimulation of the subthalamic nucleus which interrupts its normally excitatory actions. Reserpine and phenothiazines can produce parkinsonism, the first by depletion of dopamine storage granules and the second by blocking dopamine receptors. Both these treatments also produce the expected changes in synthesis in the two output pathways.

In health, dopaminergic and excitatory cholinergic activity in the caudate–putamen is balanced, and because cholinergic cells are spared in Parkinson's disease there is a relative excess of cholinergic activity. Blockade of cholinergic activity has therefore been used in the treatment of parkinsonism. Anticholinergic drugs (muscarinic antagonists) are commonly used in psychiatry to relieve drug-induced parkinsonism. Currently they are regarded as less effective than L-dopa in idiopathic Parkinson's disease but can often be usefully combined with L-dopa in patients who have not fully responded. Restoration of dopaminergic transmission by oral supplementation of L-dopa, a dopamine precursor, is also effective. Dopaminergic agonists that are useful in parkinsonism are mostly ergot derivatives: bromocriptine (often used as an adjunct to L-dopa), lisuride, and pergolide mesylate. In experimental animals, selegiline (a selective inhibitor of monoamine oxidase B) can prevent neurotoxin-induced parkinsonism by preventing the conversion of MPTP (1-methyl-4-phenyl-1,2,3,6-tetrahydropyridine) to its toxic metabolite MPP^+ by monoamine oxidase B.

SEROTONERGIC NEUROTRANSMISSION

Serotonin (5-hydroxytryptamine, 5HT) is present in the enterochromaffin granules of the intestines and in blood platelets. Less than 2% of the total body serotonin is in the CNS. Early studies of serotonin indicated that disturbances of its physiology could produce abnormal behaviour, at times strongly suggestive of mental illness. Substances with marked structural similarities to serotonin possess considerable pharmacological potency. Examples are N,N-dimethyltryptamine (DMT) and bufotenine (both present in the cahobe bean). Mexican hallucinogenic mushrooms also contain serotonin-related substances such as psilocybin. All three have a long history of abuse.

Serotonin, like noradrenaline and dopamine, is localised within specific neuronal pathways in the brain, and serotonin-containing cell bodies are found in discrete brain nuclei, especially the midbrain and brainstem raphe nuclei.

Serotonin synthesis, storage and release

Serotonin synthesis Serotonin is synthesised from L-tryptophan, being first hydroxylated to 5HTP (by tryptophan hydroxylase), which is then decarboxylated to 5HT (by aromatic-L-amino-acid decarboxylase). The capacity of the brain to synthesise serotonin is greatly in excess of requirements. Serotonin synthesis can be increased by oral tryptophan and takes place in neurons in both somata and nerve terminals.

Serotonin storage Serotonin is transported to the terminals of axons, where it forms a readily releasable pool. It is stored in presynaptic complexes comparable to those storing catecholamines. The *Rauwolfia* alkaloids and tetrabenazine reduce serotonin stores by disrupting these granules. When serotonin storage is disturbed, large quantities of serotonin are released, and outside the CNS this causes side-effects such as diarrhoea and abdominal cramps.

Serotonin release Serotonin release is a Ca^{2+}-dependent process, and there is some evidence, as with dopamine, that release takes place by two separate mechanisms. The amphetamines and some tricyclic antidepressants release serotonin from storage granules. Amphetamine analogues containing halogen atoms (e.g. fenfluramine) are more effective in stimulating serotonin release than those without.

Serotonin receptors

Receptors for serotonin are found in the CNS as part of a diffuse serotonergic network. There are multiple 5HT receptors (currently at least a dozen and rapidly heading for 20), and the neuropharmacological study of 5HT receptor function in the CNS is a rapidly expanding field.

Subtypes of serotonergic receptors

Physiological responses to serotonin are mediated through multiple serotonin receptor subtypes. Individual serotonin receptor subtypes activate different intracellular signalling systems. $5HT_{1A}$ and $5HT_{1B}$ receptors regulate adenylate cyclase or couple to G proteins that directly activate ion channels. $5HT_{1C}$ and $5HT_2$ receptors activate PLC and stimulate phosphoinositol metabolism. 5HT receptor classification is shown in Table 3.10. Continuing problems in receptor classification arise because of a lack of compounds with sufficient specificity to demonstrate differences between putative receptor subtypes. The $5HT_{1A}$ receptor is specifically activated by 8-hydroxy-2-(di-N-propylamino)tetralin (8-OH-DPAT). $5HT_{1A}$ receptor density is highest in the CA1 region and dentate gyrus of the hippocampus and in the raphe nuclei. Clinically useful drugs that are selective partial agonists at the $5HT_{1A}$ receptor are buspirone and ipsapirone, both effective antianxiety agents. $5HT_2$ receptors probably mediate excitatory effects; $5HT_3$ receptors may act similarly, but their exact functions are unknown although the combination of antagonism of these receptors with D_2 antagonism is the profile of newer antipsychotic drugs. The distinct ligand-binding properties of each subtype of serotonin receptor are based on important structural differences between them. Julius et al (1988) cloned the $5HT_{1C}$ receptor. This receptor shares much in common with other members of the G-protein-coupled superfamily of receptors. There are seven membrane-spanning regions, the amino terminus is located on the extracellular side of the membrane and the carboxyl terminus is intracellular.

The $5HT_2$ receptor has also been characterised by Julius et al (1990). It is homologous with the $5HT_{1C}$ receptor and is also a member of the G-protein-coupled superfamily. About 50% of the amino acid sequences are common to both $5HT_{1C}$ and $5HT_2$

Table 3.10   Serotonergic pharmacology

Presynaptic

Site of action	Effect	Drug	Use
Synthesis	Increases	Tryptophan	Antidepressant
	Blocks	p-Chlorophenylalanine	Experimental
	Blocks	5-Fluotryptophan	Experimental
Storage	Depletes	Reserpine	Experimental
	Depletes	Tetrabenazine	Chorea
Release	Increases	Amphetamine	Experimental
	Increases	Tricyclic antidepressants	Antidepressant
	Increases	Fenfluramine	Experimental

Postsynaptic

Receptor	Tissue (example)	Agonist responses	Agonist	Antagonist	Molecular mechanisms
$5HT_{1A}$	Postsynaptic 5HT neurons	Inhibits neuronal firing	LSD (partial) 8-OH-DPAT	Pindolol Metergoline Methysergide	↓Adenylate cyclase
$5HT_{1B}$	Presynaptic 5HT autoreceptor	Inhibits 5HT release	RU 24969	Methysergide Metergoline	↓Adenylate cyclase
$5HT_{1C}$	Choroid plexus and brain	Induction of specific behaviours (e.g. feeding)	TFMPP ICI 169369	Ritanserin	↑Phosphoinositol
$5HT_2$	Postsynaptic 5HT neurons	Induces slow wave sleep	LSD (partial)	Metergoline Ritanserin	↑Phosphoinositol
$5HT_3$	Area postrema Limbic system	Emesis Modulation of dopamine and acetylcholine release	2-Methyl 5HT	Ondansetron Granisetron Raclopride Zacopride	Via ionic channels

Degradation

Site of action	Effect	Drug	Use
Uptake	Inhibits	Zimelidine	Experimental (withdrawn clinically)
		Clomipramine	Antidepressant
		Fluoxetine	Antidepressant
		Fluvoxamine	Antidepressant
		Paroxetine	Antidepressant
		Citalopram	Antidepressant

Monoamine oxidase (A and B) inhibition, clorgyline, selegiline

receptors. These two receptors are further examples of the evolution of receptor subtypes within families that bind the same ligand (5HT) and are coupled to the same signalling system (G proteins). However, the distinct structural differences between family members may provide the means for selective activation of intracellular pathways by different concentrations of the endogenous ligand or may be relevant to a comprehensive understanding of the genetic regulation of neurotransmitter function. Because the many CNS effects of serotonergic drugs are mediated through subtypes of 5HT receptors, these structural studies are required in order to clarify individual differences in response to psychotomimetic drugs (e.g. LSD or other 5HT agonists) and may in turn lead to a better understanding of some psychotic illnesses.

Chronic treatment with a wide range of antidepressant drugs (including the tricyclics, monoamine oxidase inhibitors and atypical antidepressants such as mianserin) is known to reduce the number of $5HT_1$ and $5HT_2$ receptors. Electroconvulsive shocks

also decrease $5HT_{1A}$ receptors but increase $5HT_2$ receptor numbers. This difference may possibly explain why some depressive illnesses do not respond to a therapeutic course of oral antidepressant therapy but later respond to ECT.

Antidepressant drugs produce substantial decreases in $5HT_2$ receptor numbers after long-term treatment, and these effects may be greater than their actions in catecholaminergic systems. For example, amitriptyline and imipramine reduce β adrenoceptor binding by about 20% but reduce $5HT_2$ binding even more, by about 40%. Monoamine oxidase inhibitors also reduce serotonin binding site numbers after chronic treatment, selective monoamine oxidase A inhibitors being most effective.

Abnormalities in serotonin receptor function have been put forward as part of the pathophysiology of depressive illness. Limited support for this hypothesis has been found in studies of [³H] serotonin binding to platelets and [³H] serotonin and [³H] spiroperidol binding to cortical tissue in suicide victims. The hypothesis has been extended to involve increased release of serotonin acting upon hypersensitive postsynaptic serotonin receptors, and this has been suggested as a possible cause of depressive illness.

Cyproheptadine and methysergide are commonly used serotonergic antagonists. Structurally, cyproheptadine resembles the phenothiazines and also blocks histaminergic (H_1) and cholinergic (M_1) receptors. Methysergide is structurally similar to LSD, which can stimulate some serotonergic receptors and, especially in the periphery, be an antagonist at others. The physiological and biochemical actions of serotonergic receptors appear complex, and study of their properties has been hindered by lack of specific antagonists or agonists. The recent development of such drugs is certain to add substantially to knowledge of the serotonergic system and will probably lead to better understanding of the mode of action of antidepressants as well.

Drugs affecting serotonergic neurotransmission

Drugs affecting serotonin uptake

The reuptake systems for serotonin resemble those for the catecholamines and are influenced by many antidepressant drugs. These may differ markedly in their relative affinities for serotonergic and catecholaminergic reuptake mechanisms. The structure of the serotonergic transporter is known (Blakely et al 1991) and has much in common with other members of the superfamily of neurotransmitter transporters. The tricyclic antidepressant clomipramine was the first drug to inhibit serotonergic without also inhibiting noradrenergic reuptake, although its metabolite (desmethylclomipramine) is a strong inhibitor of noradrenergic reuptake. The first truly specific serotonergic uptake inhibitor was zimelidine which, though an effective antidepressant, was withdrawn because of its toxic effects.

The currently available inhibitors of serotonin uptake comprise a class of antidepressants known as 'selective serotonin reuptake inhibitors' (SSRIs). Table 3.11 summarises potency and relative selectivity data. These show paroxetine to be the most potent inhibitor of serotonin reuptake and citalopram to be the most selective. In vivo, the pharmacological profile of each of these drugs is changed by the formation of active metabolites, which may possess pharmacokinetic properties that differ markedly from their parent compound. For example, fluoxetine is metabolised to

norfluoxetine with a half-life of 7–15 days. Since norfluoxetine is equipotent with fluoxetine and is equally selective, it probably contributes importantly to the antidepressant effects of fluoxetine. However, the metabolites of sertraline, fluvoxamine and paroxetine are considerably less active than their parent compounds and probably do not affect their clinical actions.

These drugs also interact with monoaminergic receptors (Table 3.12) but have considerably fewer effects on histaminergic, adrenergic and muscarinic cholinergic receptors than the tricyclic antidepressants.

Drugs affecting serotonin degradation

Most serotonin is oxidised by monoamine oxidase to 5-hydroxyindoleacetaldehyde and then to 5-hydroxyindoleacetic acid (5HIAA) by aldehyde dehydrogenase. 5-Hydroxyindoleacetaldehyde is also reduced by alcohol dehydrogenase to 5-hydroxytryptophol. 5HIAA is the major metabolite of 5HT degradation. Monoamine oxidase inhibitors are the principal drugs to modify serotonin degradation, although it is likely that serotonin's synaptic actions are restricted more by the uptake system than by catabolism.

Table 3.11 Relative potencies of antidepressants after oral administration to rats for inhibition of noradrenaline and serotonin uptake (Concentration required for inhibition)

Drug	Inhibition of serotonin uptake (ED_{50}, mg/kg)	Inhibition of noradrenaline uptake (ED_{50}, mg/kg)
Paroxetine	0.4	—
Citalopram	2	>10
Fluoxetine	8	>100
Fluvoxamine	5	>30
Sertraline	—	—
Clomipramine	15	30
Imipramine	50	7
Amitriptyline	120	50
Desipramine	180	3

After Maitre et al (1982)

Table 3.12 Inhibition of radioligand binding in rat brain membranes in vitro by different types of antidepressant

Antidepressant	Receptor subtype / radioligand							
	α_1/prazosin	α_2/clonidine	β/DHA	D_2/spiperone	$5HT_1$/5HT	$5HT_1$/ketanserin	Histamine H_1/mepyramine	Muscarinic/ QNB
Paroxetine	>10 000	>10 000	>5 000	>7 700	>10 000	>1 000	>1 000	89
Citalopram	4 500	>10 000	>5 000	>10 000	>10 000	>1 000	>1 000	2 900
Fluvoxamine	>10 000	>10 000	>5 000	>10 000	>10 000	>1 000	>1 000	>10 000
Fluoxetine	>10 000	>10 000	>5 000	>10 000	>10 000	>1 000	1 000	1 300
Amitriptyline	170	540	>5 000	1 200	1 000	8.3	3.3	5.1
Imipramine	440	1 000	>5 000	2 400	8 900	120	35	37
Clomipramine	150	3 300	>5 000	430	5 200	63	47	34
Desipramine	1 300	8 600	>5 000	3 800	2 500	160	370	68

QNB, quinuclidinylbenzilate; DHA, dihydroalprenolol.
After Thomas et al (1987).

PEPTIDERGIC NEUROTRANSMISSION

Advances in neurobiology have demonstrated that the neural and endocrine systems are closely linked. Previously, differences between the systems were apparent from a structural standpoint and seemed supported by the distinctive means of communication between the component parts of each system. Patterns of release following electrical activity in the nervous system were clearly not the same as the release of chemicals by endocrine tissue to act on distant target organs. The neural regulation of endocrine function is now seen to provide important insights into the working of the brain that are relevant to psychiatry. This view is based upon the following lines of evidence.

- There is extensive evidence showing that the neurotransmitter systems preferentially modified by effective psychotropic drugs (e.g. the dopaminergic and noradrenergic pathways) are also intimately involved in the limbic–hypothalamic integration and regulation of pituitary function. Putative abnormalities of these transmitter systems may extend from sites in the brain involved in the pathogenesis of mental illness to the hypothalamic–pituitary system and may therefore be detected in abnormal endocrine functioning.
- The hypothalamus regulates the anterior pituitary by synthesising and secreting releasing factors into the pituitary portal vessel system to act upon anterior pituitary cells. These releasing factors are synthesised and released at sites elsewhere in the nervous system without any obvious endocrine function, and there is experimental evidence that they may function as neurotransmitters or neuromodulators and thereby play important roles in the neural regulation of certain behaviours. The abnormalities characteristic of severe mental illnesses may therefore be caused by pathological changes in the non-endocrine functions of the releasing factors.
- The hormones released by the pituitary regulate hormone production of target endocrine glands. These peripheral hormones can, in turn, act upon many aspects of neural function, for example by affecting neural development and classical neurotransmitters like noradrenaline. The actions on the brain of hormones such as testosterone, thyroxin and cortisol may be relevant to sex differences in the incidence of mental illnesses such as depression and the increased prevalence of psychological symptoms in endocrinopathies such as thyroid or adrenal cortical disease.
- Releasing factors and 'classical neurotransmitters' can coexist in the same nerve terminal (e.g. serotonin and thyrotrophin-releasing factor, TRF). In this circumstance, the releasing factor may modify (or 'modulate') the actions of the neurotransmitter, and this may be of relevance, for example, to the serotonergic hypothesis of the mode of action of some antidepressant treatments.
- Stress responses to threatening or noxious stimuli include activation of the hypothalamic–pituitary system. These patterns of endocrine responses to stress are specific to the type of stressful stimulus. Since there is abundant evidence from clinical studies implicating stressful stimuli in the pathogenesis of mental illnesses, study of the neural regulation of endocrine responses to stress might elucidate important individual differences relevant to variations in vulnerability to mental illnesses.

Molecular biology of peptidergic transmission

Most regulatory substances released by the nervous system are peptides, i.e. they consist of amino acids joined by peptide bonds. Unlike classical neurotransmitters, these compounds are synthesised as parts of larger molecules that are cleaved by proteolysis and carboxylation into active fragments of amino acid chains at the point of release. Local tissue-specific differences in the activity of processing enzymes can yield important topographical variations in the proportions of peptide fragments derived from a single precursor. However, with the exception of pro-opiomelanocortin (POMC), the specific degradative, cleavage and post-translational processing enzymes involved are usually unknown. Fundamental questions relevant to proper understanding of the actions of drugs on the brain arise from this uncertainty. Neuropeptide fragments may be cleaved from widely available precursor molecules by enzymes specific to that cleavage site and/or general-purpose enzymes that are locally regulated.

The chromosomal locations of neuropeptide genes are distributed widely throughout the human genome. Although some neuropeptides are close members of structurally related families, with the single exception of oxytocin and vasopressin, genes for these related family members are located on different chromosomes (Sherman et al 1989).

Neural regulation of neuropeptide synthesis and release

The hypothalamus controls the release of pituitary hormones in two ways, both of which involve neurons that synthesise and release neuropeptides. In the first, specialised neurons in the hypothalamus synthesise and secrete releasing factors. In the second, the magnocellular neurons of the hypothalamus synthesise precursor molecules (preprovasophysin and preproxyphysin) that are processed and transported to terminals in the posterior pituitary, from which vasopressin, oxytocin and their related neurophysins are stoichiometrically released. The neuroendocrine neurons of the hypothalamus are influenced by many types of neurotransmitter. Releasing-factor-producing neurons are richly supplied with noradrenergic, dopaminergic and serotonergic connections.

Co-transmission of neuropeptides

Neuropeptides are present in the central nervous system in concentrations between 10^{-12} and 10^{-15} mol/mg of protein. These are much lower than the concentrations of the 'classical neurotransmitters', which vary from 10^{-9} to 10^{-10} mol/mg of protein. High concentrations of neuropeptides in the brain are found in the hypothalamic–pituitary system but some neuropeptides (e.g. cholecystokinin and vasoactive intestinal peptide) have their highest concentrations in the cortex. Other neuropeptides (e.g. oxytocin and vasopressin) are present in cell bodies only in the hypothalamus, and their presence in other brain or spinal cord areas is accounted for by the long projections of these cells into those areas. Some widely distributed neuropeptides (e.g. TRF and substance P) are found in neurons in numerous areas.

Hökfelt et al (1987) have demonstrated the coexistence of neuropeptides and 'classical neurotransmitters' within the same neuron at many sites in the nervous system. The physiological importance of coexistence is not yet known, but a number of models have been put forward, some of which may prove to be of relevance to hypotheses concerning changes in receptor sensitivity in mental illness. In one model, a nerve terminal containing serotonin, substance P and TRF responds to low-frequency electrical stimulation by releasing serotonin. The released serotonin attaches to the postsynaptic receptors, where it generates a small postsynaptic potential. Some serotonin also attaches to the presynaptic serotonergic receptors (autoreceptors) which inhibit further serotonin release. As electrical stimulation is increased, TRF and substance P are also released. TRF and serotonin then act synergistically on the postsynaptic serotonin receptor to generate an increased postsynaptic potential, while substance P blocks the serotonergic autoreceptors, preventing inhibition of serotonin release. The three substances thus combine to produce prolonged postsynaptic activation without inducing compensatory responses at a presynaptic level. These interactions between a monoamine neurotransmitter and neuropeptides may be relevant to long-term changes in homeostatic mechanisms, neural learning and long-term potentiation of synaptic activity. They have also been related to the mode of action of antidepressant treatments (including ECT) and pathological alterations in receptor sensitivity that may occur in affective disorders and schizophrenia.

Peptidergic receptors

The receptors for most neuropeptides are less well studied but almost certainly will yield as many variations as are seen for the 'classical' transmitters. The products of the preprotachykinin genes (substance P, neurokinin A, neuropeptide K) seem to act on a group of at least three related receptors, all of which respond to substance P and which are labelled NK1, NK2 and NK3. The relationships between these receptors and the central actions of the tachykinins are still being elaborated. However, it seems certain that, as a group, neuropeptides appear to act on G-protein-coupled receptors. Opioid receptors appear linked to G_i and G_o proteins (Wong et al 1989).

Neuropeptides can function as:

- neurotransmitters released by one neuron at a presynaptic terminal to act on the adjacent postsynaptic membrane;
- neuromodulators that act by modifying the turnover, release or action of classical neurotransmitters;
- neurohormones released by one neuron to act at a site distant to the point of release.

The most detailed understanding of a peptidergic receptor system currently available is provided by the pharmacology of opioid receptors. There is good evidence for the existence of three subtypes of opioid receptor.

Endorphins and enkephalins

The endorphins (literally 'endogenous morphine') are the endogenous ligands for the opioid receptors. Their study is a rapidly expanding field of research and has given rise to a confusing terminology. The term 'opiate' is used to describe drugs derived from the juice of the poppy *Papaver somniferum*. The word 'opioid' describes all substances with morphine-like actions. The word 'narcotic' is no longer used in pharmacology, although originally it described drugs that induced sleep and was later applied to morphine-like analgesics. The sites of action of opioid drugs in the nervous system appear to be the receptors for a number of endogenous ligands, which include the pentapeptides,

leucine-enkephalin (Leu-enkephalin) and methionine-enkephalin (Met-enkephalin). The amino acid sequence of Met-enkephalin is the same as the sequence contained in amino acid residues 61–65 in the pituitary hormone β-lipotrophin (β-LPH). Other opioid peptides are represented in fragments of the β-lipotrophin amino acid sequence. The carboxyl terminus of amino acid residues 61–91 is called β-endorphin. Sequences of amino acid residues 61–76 are called α-endorphin and amino acid residues 61–77 are called γ-endorphin. The enkephalins and endorphins derived from β-lipotrophin probably belong to separate physiological systems. β-Endorphin is present in the hypothalamic pituitary system, where it is derived from a larger precursor molecule, POMC, containing the amino acid sequences for both β-lipotrophin and adrenocorticotrophic hormone (ACTH). The enkephalins are not derived from POMC but are produced by cleavage of a separate precursor molecule.

The physiological role of endogenous ligands for opioid receptors is still unknown, but they appear to be involved in the perception of pain and the neural control of certain aspects of endocrine function, the regulation of movement, mood and some aspects of behaviour. A large number of drugs are agonists at opioid receptor sites. Opioid agonist drugs appear to act largely at the μ receptor, with a few actions mediated at the κ receptor. Opioid agonists include morphine, heroin (diacetylmorphine), dihydromorphine, codeine, pethidine, methadone, pentazocine and levorphanol. Many of these agonists are structurally related to morphine but some, like meperidine and methadone, are chemically quite dissimilar. Naloxone, naltrexone and nalorphine are antagonists at opioid receptor sites. Pentazocine has both opioid agonist actions and weak antagonist activity. All the compounds listed above have clinical applications, and their specific use has been determined by their pharmacokinetics, pharmacodynamics and liability to produce dependence. All opioid drugs, when regularly administered, appear able to induce tolerance and dependence. Tolerance may be innate or acquired. Innate tolerance is subject to wide individual variation, determined presumably by genetic factors and the age and reproductive status of the individual. Acquired tolerance is observed as the need to increase the dose of the opioid drug if the same effects are to be obtained with repeated administration. The mechanisms underlying the development of tolerance are ill understood but may include the proliferation of new receptor sites or reduction in sensitivity of opioid receptors to their agonists. There is extensive cross-tolerance between opioid drugs. When they are administered regularly, tolerance frequently develops, but this must not be taken to imply that withdrawal symptoms will always occur if the drug is removed. The manifestation of withdrawal symptoms (which may be either physical or psychological) demonstrates that an individual has become dependent (physically or psychologically) on the drug. Symptoms that can follow opioid withdrawal include insomnia, restlessness, anxiety, nausea and vomiting, abdominal cramps, sweating, piloerection and rhinorrhoea. These symptoms may persist for several days and may be accompanied by a craving for the drug to be reintroduced. Tolerance may also develop to alcohol, barbiturates and hypnotic drugs. The withdrawal symptoms observed following prolonged administration of these substances are primarily rebound effects in the systems most affected by the drug. Depressant drugs tend to be followed by rebound hyperexcitability, and mood-elevating drugs like the amphetamines by lethargy and depressed mood. Epileptic seizures may be seen in withdrawal from drugs that raise the seizure threshold.

Theories of drug dependence and withdrawal usually attempt to explain withdrawal symptoms in terms of some form of rebound phenomenon. Pharmacological explanations have included modification of receptor sensitivity, change in numbers of receptors, the utilisation of otherwise redundant neural pathways and the induction of enzymes involved in the synthesis of neurotransmitters.

Peptide regulatory factors

CNS peptide regulatory factors are not the same as neuropeptides. They act through a different class of receptor and are important in the normal development of the nervous system, when they are usually called neurotrophins. These trophic substances are also important in neurodegenerative diseases, where they are necessary for the restoration of neural circuits and the co-ordination of glial responses to damage.

Nerve growth factor (NGF) is the best known trophic factor. It is a neurotrophic factor and influences the synthesis of neurotransmitters, cytoskeletal proteins and neuropeptides whose actions have been worked out in most detail in the autonomic nervous system. The survival and functional maintenance of neurons depends upon the presence of specific neurotrophins; Cholinergic neurons damaged in Alzheimer's disease contain high concentrations of mRNA for NGF receptor, and it is hypothesised that cholinergic loss in this condition may be reversed by NGF treatment (Perry 1990). Other neurotrophins include neurotrophins 2 and 3 (NT2, NT3), brain-derived neurotrophic factor (BDNF), glial cell-derived neurotrophic factor (GDNF, which may be important in Parkinson's disease), neuroleucin, glial nexin, insulin-like growth factors, platelet-derived growth factor and epidermal growth factor. Since the cellular mechanisms that regulate neurotrophin metabolism can be manipulated by noxious factors, study of psychological stress in humans has been extended to include effects on functions influenced by trophic factors. Animal studies of electroconvulsive stimulation (ECS) which are of possible relevance to the mode of action of ECT have included direct measures of neurotrophin metabolism. Repeated ECS probably alters the expression of many neural genes along a time-course that is relevant to the actions of ECT (Leviel et al 1990). Interleukins 1 and 2 also have trophic actions and can be produced by the brain when stressed. Their functions may include integration of neural and immune responses to injury, studied in psychoneuroimmunology.

NEURONALLY PRODUCED GASES

The most recent puzzle in neurochemistry is the discovery that some neurons possess the enzymatic machinery to produce gases. The best-studied example is the enzyme called nitric oxide synthase (NOS). This is one of a family of NOS enzymes, which occur in various sites in the body. The best known is perhaps the NOS of macrophages that may be involved in cell killing in the immune system. Why would neurons have evolved such a potentially lethal cargo? It seems that there are soluble GTPases in neurons that are appropriate receptors for NO formed when arginine is converted to citrulline by NOS. The NO is implicated in the control of NMDA receptor sensitivity, and by some is held responsible for the action of LTP-producing stimuli on presynaptic release. Endothelial cells also generate a NOS which is thought to provide a vasodilator tone in the CNS. The possibility

for independent control of these three enzymes exists, but at present there are few NO receptor antagonists of any specificity and so the functional signicance of these potentially toxic substances in neuropharmacology is still obscure. The fact that the cells in the caudate–putamen which produce NO are the last to die in Huntington's disease has led to the suggestion that they may cause at least some of the neurotoxic damage in that condition.

A suggestion that a heamoxygenase might be present in nerve cells which could then produce carbon monoxide (Dawson & Snyder 1994) is just one of the many challenges facing us in the continued battle to understand enough of the neurochemistry and neuropharmacology of the brain to be able to help alleviate the symptoms of mental disease.

REFERENCES

Ahlquist R P 1948 A study of the adrenotropic receptors. American Journal of Physiology 153: 586–600

Barnard E A, Darlison M G, Seeburg P 1987 Molecular biology of the GABA$_A$ receptor: the receptor/channel superfamily. Trends in Neurosciences 10(12): 502–509

Bell M V, Bloomeld J, McKinley M et al 1989 Physical linkage of the GABA$_A$ receptor subunit gene to the DX5374 locus in human Xq28. American Journal of Human Genetics 45: 882–888

Betz H 1987 Biology and structure of mammalian glycine receptor. Trends in Neurosciences 10(3): 113–117

Birnbaumer L 1990 G proteins in signal transduction. Annual Review of Pharmacology and Toxicology 30: 675–705

Blair L A, Levitan E S, Marshall J et al 1988 Single subunits of the GABA$_A$ receptor form ion channels with properties of the native receptor. Science 242: 577–579

Blakely R D, Berson H E, Fremeau R T Jr et al 1991 Cloning and expression of a functional serotonin transporter from rat brain. Nature 354: 66–70

Bloom F E 1990 Neurohumoral transmission and the central nervous system. In: Goodman A G, Rall T W, Nies A S, Taylor P (eds) The pharmacological basis of therapeutics. Pergamon Press, New York, p 244–268

Blum K, Noble E P, Sheridan P J et al 1990 Allelic association of human dopamine D$_2$ receptor gene in alcoholism. Journal of the American Medical Association 263: 2055–2060

Bonner T I 1989 The molecular basis of muscarinic receptor diversity. Trends in Neurosciences 12(4): 148–151

Bradbury M 1979 The concept of the blood–brain barrier. Wiley, London

Carlsson A 1988 The current status of the dopamine hypothesis of schizophrenia. Neuropsychopharmacology 1: 179–186

Carlsson A, Lindqvist M 1963 Effect of chlorpromazine or haloperidol on formation of 3-methoxytyramine and normetanephrine in mouse brain. Acta Pharmacologica et Toxicologica 20: 140–144

Clarke D D, Lathja A L, Maker H S 1989 Intermediary metabolism. In: Siegel G J, Alberto R W, Agranoff B W, Molinoff P B (eds) Basic neurochemistry: molecular, cellular, and medical aspects, 4th edn. Raven, New York, p 541–564

Dawson T M, Snyder S H 1994 Gases as biological messengers: nitric oxide and carbon monoxide in the brain. Journal of Neuroscience 14: 5147–5159

Deisz R A, Lux H D 1985 Gamma-aminobutyric acid-induced depression of calcium currents of chick sensory neurons. Neuroscience Letters 14;56(2): 205–210

Evans R M 1988 The steroid and thyroid hormone receptor superfamily. Science 240: 889–895

Guy H R, Hucho F 1987 The ion channel of the nicotine acetylcholine receptor. Trends in Neurosciences 10(8): 318–321

Hökfelt T, Millhorn D, Seroogy K et al 1987 Coexistence of peptides with classical neurotransmitters. Experientia 43: 768–780

Julius D, McDermott A B, Axel R, Jessell T M 1988 Molecular characterization of a functional cDNA encoding the serotonin 1c receptor. Science 241: 558–564

Julius D, Huang K N, Livelli T J et al 1990 The 5HT2 receptor defines a family of structurally distinct but functionally conserved serotonin receptors. Proceedings of the National Academy of Sciences of the USA 87: 928–932

Leviel V, Fayada C, Guibert F et al 1990 Short- and long-term alterations of gene expression in limbic structures by repeated electroconvulsive-induced seizures. Journal of Neurochemistry 54: 899–904

McIlwain H 1990 Biochemistry and neurochemistry in the 1800s: their origins in comparative animal chemistry. Essays in Biochemistry 25: 197–224

McIlwain H, Bachelard H S 1985 Metabolism of the brain in situ. In: Biochemistry and the central nervous system, 5th edn. Churchill Livingstone, Edinburgh, p 8–32

Maitre L, Baumann P A, Jaekel J 1982 5-HT uptake inhibitors: psychopharmacological and neurochemical criteria of selectivity. In: Ho B T (ed) Serotonin in biological psychiatry. Raven, New York, p 229–246

Majerus P W, Connolly T M, Bansal V S et al 1988 Inositol phosphates: synthesis and degradation. Journal of Biological Chemistry 263: 3051–3054

Monsma F J Jr, McVittie L D, Gerfen C R et al 1989 Multiple D_2 dopamine receptors produced by alternative RNA splicing. Nature 342: 926–929

Neer E J, Clapham D E 1988 Roles of G protein subunits in transmembrane signalling. Nature 333: 129–134

Oldendorf W H 1974 Lipid solubility and drug penetration of the blood–brain barrier. Proceedings of the Society of Experimental Biological Medicine 147: 813

Olney J W 1989 Excitatory amino acids and neuropsychiatric disorders. Biological Psychiatry 26: 505–525

Pacholczyk T, Blakely R D, Amara S G 1991 Expression cloning of a cocaine- and antidepressant-sensitive human noradrenaline transporter. Nature 350: 350–354

Peroutka S J 1988 5-Hydroxytryptamine receptor subtypes: molecular, biochemical and physiological characterization. Trends in Neurosciences 11: 496–500

Perry E K 1990 Hypothesis linking plasticity, vulnerability and nerve growth factor to basal forebrain cholinergic neurons. International Journal of Geriatric Psychiatry 5: 223–231

Raiteri M, Cerrito F, Cervon A M, Levi G 1979 Dopamine can be released by two mechanisms differentially affected by the dopamine transport inhibitor nomifensine. Journal of Pharmacology and Experimental Therapeutics 208: 195–202

Revah F, Bertrand D, Galzi J-L et al 1991 Mutations in the channel domain alter desensitization of a neuronal nicotinic receptor. Nature 353: 846–849

Ross E M 1989 Signal sorting and amplication through G protein-coupled receptors. Neuron 3: 141–152

Sherman T G, Akil H, Watson S J 1989 The molecular biology of neuropeptides: neuropeptide genetics. In: Magistretti P J (ed) Discussions in neuroscience. Elsevier, Amsterdam, vol VI, No 1

Sladeczek F, Récasens M, Bockaert J 1988 A new mechanism for glutamine receptor action: phosphoinositide hydrolysis. Trends in Neurosciences 11(12): 545–549

Snyder S H 1989 Drug and neurotransmitter receptors: new perspectives with clinical relevance. Journal of the American Medical Association 261: 3126–3129

Snyder S H 1991 Vehicles of inactivation. Nature 354: 187

Sokoloff L 1989 Circulation and energy metabolism of the brain. In: Siegel G J, Alberto R W, Agranoff B W, Molinoff P B (eds) Basic neurochemistry: molecular, cellular, and medical aspects, 4th edn. Raven, New York, p 565–590

Sokoloff P, Giros B, Martres M-P et al 1990 Molecular cloning and characterization of a novel dopamine receptor (D_3) as a target for neuroleptics. Nature 347: 146–151

Sonders M S, Keana J F W, Weber E 1988 Phencyclidine and psychotomimetic sigma opiates: recent insights into their biochemical and physiological sites of action. Trends in Neurosciences 11: 37–40

Sternweis P C, Pang I-H 1990 The G protein-channel connection. Trends in Neurosciences 13(4): 122–126

Strader C D, Sigal I S, Dixon R F 1989 Structural basis of β-adrenergic receptor function. FASEB Journal 3: 1825–1832

Südhof T C 1995 The synaptic vesicle cycle: a cascade of protein–protein interactions. Nature 375: 645–646

Sunahara R K, Niznik H B, Weiner D M et al 1990 Human dopamine D_1 receptor encoded by an intronless gene on chromosome 5. Nature 347: 80–83

Sunahara R K, Guan H-C, O'Dowd B F et al 1991 Cloning of the gene for a human dopamine D_5 receptor with higher affinity for dopamine than D_1. Nature 350: 614–619

Thomas D R, Nelson D R, Johnson A M 1987 Biochemical effects of the antidepressant paroxetine a specific 5-HT uptake inhibitor. Psychopharmacology 93: 193–200

Tsien R W, Lipscombe D, Madison D V, Bley K R, Fox A P 1988 Multiple types of neuronal calcium channels and their selective modulation. Trends in Neurosciences 11(10): 431–438

Van Tol H H M, Bunzow J R, Guan H-C et al 1991 Cloning of the gene for a human dopamine D_4 receptor with high affinity for the antipsychotic clozapine. Nature 350: 610–614

Volkow N D, Wang G -J, Fischman M W et al 1997 Relationship between subjective effects of cocaine and dopamine transporter occupancy. Nature 386: 827–833

Wang H-Y, Friedman E 1989 Lithium inhibition of protein kinase C activation-induced serotonin release. Psychopharmacology 99: 213–218

Wong Y H, Bemoliou-Mason C D, Barnard E A 1989 Opioid receptors in magnesium-digitonin-solubilized rat brain membrane are tightly coupled to a pertussis toxin-sensitive guanine nucleotide-binding protein. Journal of Neurochemistry 52: 999–1009

Yamamoto C, McIlwain H 1966 Electrical activities in thin sections from the mammalian brain maintained in chemically-defined media in vitro. Journal of Neurochemistry 13(12): 1333–1343

4 Neuropathology

Jeanne E Bell

INTRODUCTION

This chapter describes the neuropathological findings in a spectrum of psychiatric conditions, including the dementias. Neuropathology constitutes that branch of the clinical neurosciences which has traditionally achieved diagnoses of brain diseases by means of macroscopic and microscopic examination of the brain. It is currently a rapidly expanding discipline in which neuropathologists are beginning to implement molecular pathological methods in routine diagnosis, as well as maintaining active participation in research. These developments are providing new insights into the aetiology and pathogenesis of many brain diseases, particularly the dementias. Despite this evidence of progress, some of the major psychoses continue to present a major challenge to neuropathology in that it has so far proved impossible to identify a cellular basis of disease.

It may be difficult to achieve a precise clinicopathological correlation for an individual patient with psychiatric symptoms, for a variety of reasons. First, although most dementing illnesses are associated with characteristic pathological lesions in the brain, a minority of demented patients may show very little in the way of specific pathology. It is also puzzling to note that other individuals who have retained normal cognitive function until the end of life are found at postmortem examination to display remarkably advanced pathology of a type usually associated with dementia. Added to this are the complexities which emerge as a consequence of the frequent occurrence of mixed pathology in older patients. Several different diseases of the brain may apparently coexist in a single individual, and current thinking is forcing a reappraisal of the comorbidity of neurodegenerative conditions. Rather than merely coincidental coexistence, it is now held that some mixed pathology may represent synergy between particular neurodegenerative diseases.

It is undoubtedly true that there have been considerable advances in the neuropathological definition both of well-defined conditions such as Alzheimer's disease and of newer entities identified among the movement disorders. This progress in neuropathology could not have happened in isolation. Developments in cell- and tissue-based methods in histopathology have occurred alongside major advances in neuroimaging, neurochemistry, neuropharmacology and molecular genetics as well as insights gained from the study of transgenic animals. These combined approaches have certainly highlighted certain disorders which appear to blur the conventional distinctions between diagnostic categories in the psychiatric disease spectrum. They also point to the possibilities of new approaches to the assessment and classification of diseases of the brain. The lessons of history suggest that present dogma will surely change in the light of expanding knowledge. This applies to neuropathology particularly in those challenging areas of psychiatry in which neuropathology has had so little to offer. This chapter describes the current state of knowledge of neuropathological abnormalities which may be detected in patients with psychiatric diseases.

RELATIONSHIP OF NEUROPATHOLOGY WITH PSYCHIATRY AND OTHER ALLIED DISCIPLINES

In examining the nature of these relationships, it is pertinent to ask what has been the contribution of neuropathology to the understanding of psychiatric diseases up to the present time and which challenges remain outstanding at the outset of the 21st century. The potential division between these two disciplines is embodied in the view that neuropathology focuses on diseases of the brain while psychiatry is concerned with diseases of the mind. This notion has been explored recently by Lishman (1995), who came to the conclusion that neuropathology does indeed have much to offer in the field of psychiatry. The connection is both historic and contemporary. Neuropathology is based firmly in the traditions of classic neuroanatomy and first evolved during the 19th century. The latter end of the 1800s saw the first clear delineation of some of those disorders which present with dementia, including general paralysis of the insane which was still common at that time. However, it was not until the start of the 20th century that neuropathology began to contribute significantly to the understanding of brain diseases. Alzheimer first described in the 1920s the neuropathology of the dementing illness now known by his name. Parkinson's disease and Creutzfeldt–Jakob disease (CJD) were examined and characterised in the first half of the 20th century. However, other major disorders such as dementia with Lewy bodies (DLB) were recognised only quite recently.

As more and more brain diseases were subjected to microscopic scrutiny by neuropathologists, this kind of analysis came to be seen as a standard of diagnosis against which others had to be measured. Inevitably neuropathology has fallen short of this high expectation in some significant areas of psychiatry but has had most to offer in the field of organic brain disease, where there has been considerable and accelerating progress in the last two decades. Specialised techniques have been developed which are able to identify and localise specific proteins and DNA sequences within tissues and cells, thus generating a much more detailed view of brain pathology than that obtained through more traditional staining methods. A multidisciplinary approach has ensured that

Abbreviations	
AB, βA4	— β amyloid
AD	— Alzheimer's disease
ADC	— AIDS dementia complex
AIDS	— acquired immune deficiency syndrome
ApoE	— apolipoprotein E gene and protein
APP	— amyloid precursor protein
CA	— cornu ammonis
CBD	— corticobasal degeneration
CERAD	— Consortium to Establish a Registry for Alzheimer's Disease
CJD	— Creutzfeldt–Jakob disease
CNS	— central nervous system
CT	— computerised tomography
DLB	— dementia with Lewy bodies
FDTP-17	— frontotemporal dementia with parkinsonism-chromosome17
GABA	— γ aminobutyric acid
GFAP	— glial fibrillary acidic protein
GPI	— general paralysis of the insane
HAD	— HIV-associated dementia
HD	— Huntington's disease
HIV/AIDS	— human immunodeficiency virus / acquired immunodeficiency syndrome
IL1	— interleukin 1 α and β
LRP	— lipoprotein receptor-related protein
kDa	— kilodaltons
MRI	— magnetic resonance imaging
NFT	— neurofibrillary tangle
PSP	— progressive supranuclear palsy
TNF	— tumour necrosis factor
vCJD	— variant Creutzfeldt-Jakob disease

on the one hand molecular genetics has informed recent neuropathology searches while on the other the identification of novel pathological features has sometimes prompted the discovery of new brain proteins or has initiated developments in genetic research. A genuine explosion of knowledge has resulted which points the way to appropriate treatment strategies, particularly in the field of dementias.

Extension of research studies beyond the confines of hospitals and into the community has focused attention more than ever before on the apparent continuum, in terms of neuropathology, between simple ageing of the brain and the earliest stages of pathology of disease (Neuropathology Group of MRC CFAS 2001). While it is not possible with present knowledge to separate the two states, the identification of the earliest changes which truly signal the onset of disease and of the events which initiate those changes presents an important challenge, particularly with respect to defining a process of healthy ageing. The difficulties are compounded when the time interval between the aetiological event and the onset of symptomatic illness is very protracted. There are a number of diseases of the brain, both genetic and acquired, which are characterised by a long prodromal phase and by slow progression. Multidisciplinary research which exploits a variety of neuroscience expertise is required to solve these and other outstanding problems, as has occurred for variant Creutzfeldt–Jakob disease (vCJD) (Brown et al 2001). The establishment in the last few decades of brain banks which aim to collect and store a resource of clinically and neuropathologically well-characterised brains has proved to be a very useful investment

for further study and has led directly to significant progress. Patient support groups and lay organisations have been highly significant in furthering these efforts, not least through promoting with the general public the cause of brain donation.

Schizophrenia and other psychoses remain an outstanding challenge to which neuropathology must rise. If a pathological substrate could be established for the ventricular enlargement so consistently observed on neuroimaging, this would represent a significant step forward in understanding these disorders. However, any defining neuropathology for this group of disorders may be at best subtle and difficult to establish, and for the present remains elusive.

DEVELOPMENT AND AGEING OF THE BRAIN — PRESYMPTOMATIC PATHOLOGY

Development

The brain and spinal cord are formed in the embryo largely from cells derived from the progenitor neuroectoderm of the neural tube. Neuroectodermal cells give rise to neurons, astrocytes and oligodendroglia. The process of orderly cell division, migration, differentiation and outgrowth of processes is orchestrated by a variety of growth factors, notably platelet-derived growth factor A & B, transforming growth factor alpha and insulin-like growth factor. Bone-marrow-derived microglia invade the neural tube during early fetal life, and blood vessels grow into the developing nervous system from the surrounding mesoderm. Vascularisation of the developing nervous system provides the opportunity for hormones and other blood-borne proteins to modulate differentiation. Many cells fail to complete the maturation process successfully and are removed by a process of programmed cell death or apoptosis. Mature neurons are of many different varieties and functions, characterised by their location, connections and transmitters. Astrocytes and oligodendroglia are also sophisticated cells which turn over slowly in normal circumstances. The process of development of the CNS continues in post-natal life, and only in late adolescence or early adult life can brain development be considered complete. There are some aspects of development which are directly relevant to the state of the central nervous system (CNS) in later life and particularly in relation to neurodegenerative diseases. Among these are the putative role of growth factors in ongoing neurotrophic support for ageing nerve cells and the possibility that the recently recognised stem cells still present in the adult brain may retain full differentiation capability. The implications of these findings for repair and regeneration in the mature brain are far from clear but will become so with future research (Armstrong & Barker 2001, Steindler & Pincus 2002).

Ageing changes

Neurodegenerative diseases which target particular subsets of nerve cells within the brain and spinal cord are devastating in their effect precisely because fully differentiated neurons are post-mitotic cells which, according to current thinking, are not replaced when lost. However, ageing of the individual and of the brain does not invariably result in evidence of neurodegenerative diseases even though the brain does display shrinkage or atrophy with increasing age. Although this has been attributed in the past to neuronal loss, a more likely basis is now thought to be white-matter shrinkage. Neuronal counts appear to be generally well preserved in the cortex in simple ageing, although neuronal loss does occur in the substantia nigra of the brainstem. However, more subtle changes of neuronal atrophy and reduced functional integrity, combined with a loss in plasticity, may contribute significantly to declining brain function (Mirra & Hyman 2002).

Most aged brains display changes in the vascular system which include atheroma of the major vessels and small vessel hyalinisation (Neuropathology Group of MRC CFAS 2001). These vascular abnormalities are frequently associated with loss of brain substance, particularly in the white matter, and with small and large infarcts, which contribute to cognitive impairment in old age. However, minor degrees of vascular pathology in the brain should probably be considered as part of normal ageing (Mirra & Hyman 2002). Neuronal changes associated with ageing include increasing accumulation of lipofuscin and ubiquitin. The expression of lipofuscin, a lysosomal associated pigment, is associated with cellular ageing for reasons which are unclear. While it may partly reflect the metabolic waste disposal systems of long-lived cells, the fact that lipofuscin may appear during childhood in certain neuronal groups such as the olivary nucleus of the brainstem suggests that the causes may be more complex. Nerve cells and their processes also accumulate a protein known as ubiquitin during ageing. As its name suggests, ubiquitin is a protein expressed in many cell types but which is not normally detectable in any significant amount in individual cells. Ubiquitin expression is certainly increased in normal ageing but this process is accentuated in a number of neurodegenerative diseases, particularly in the form of ubiquitin positive inclusions which may be intranuclear or intracytoplasmic (Glickman & Ciechanover 2002). Astrocytes also show ageing changes and upregulate their expression of glial fibrillary acidic protein (GFAP). Corpora amylacea are round amorphous basophilic bodies consisting largely of glycoprotein, which accumulate within the processes of astrocytes, particularly at the interface of brain tissue with the pia mater and ependyma, and around blood vessels. Microglial cells also display increasing activation in older subjects.

The concept has been advanced that ageing changes may represent a step towards symptomatic neurodegenerative disease because they erode the so-called brain reserve, coupled with the notion that diseases become clinically evident when there is a decline below a certain critical functional threshold. It is likely that a number of different insults might combine to accelerate this process towards the emergence of symptoms. The likely contribution of genetic factors to age-related phenotypic expression of disease is well illustrated by the observation that in Huntington's disease the greater the deviation from normal in the Huntington gene the earlier the disease becomes apparent in the affected individual. More generally, mRNA transcription is likely to become less reliable with ageing such that proteins are generated which are less amenable to normal degradation and turnover.

Presymptomatic neurodegeneration or simple ageing?

More problematic is the appearance within the ageing brain of features which are usually seen in association with the neurodegenerative diseases. These may include amyloid deposits, neurofibrillary tangles and Lewy bodies. Each of these lesions may be identified in the brains of aged individuals who had been assessed as cognitively intact until the time of death (Neuropathology Group of MRC CFAS 2001). Careful analysis suggests that most of the amyloid plaques seen in such individuals are diffuse and made up of non-fibrillary amyloid. There is considerable debate as to whether the presence of small numbers of neuritic plaques or of Lewy bodies is merely a feature of ageing or whether these lesions are always pathological (Mirra & Hyman 2002). Weight of opinion has now swung towards considering that these lesions do represent a presymptomatic phase of one or other of the common neurodegenerative diseases.

Although the brain may atrophy somewhat with increasing age, the onset of specific pathology is not an inevitable consequence of ageing. There are some individuals who remain cognitively intact and who display no neurodegenerative pathology even in extreme old age. As presently understood, these individuals are genetically well endowed to resist the onslaught of neurodegenerative diseases and have escaped, or have endured successfully, those environmental triggers which also predispose to these disorders. A better understanding of the factors which promote healthy brain ageing could make a substantial contribution to the well-being of old age.

ANATOMY AND PATHOLOGY OF THE DEMENTIAS

Definition and prevalence of dementia

The many definitions of dementia have in common the notion that affected individuals suffer deterioration of higher intellectual function while consciousness is preserved, and that the condition is relentlessly progressive. The deterioration encompasses a number of cognitive deficits including memory impairment and impaired executive functioning and may be allied with specific problems such as aphasia, apraxia and agnosia. The dementing illnesses are largely conditions of later life occurring in middle and old age. In large surveys based both in hospital and in the community, the prevalence of dementia rises from between 5% and 10% of the population aged 65 and over to nearer 30% of those who have reached the age of 85 and over (Hofman et al 1991, Palmer et al 2003). Recent studies confirm that diagnosis of the early stages of dementia remains difficult, although memory impairment appears to be the most sensitive early marker (Palmer et al 2003). Given that individuals with dementia often survive for up to 10 years, the burden on families and on society is clearly very large. The encouraging fact is that a much larger proportion of elderly people remain relatively cognitively intact and are able to lead an independent life so far as their mental faculties are concerned.

The causes of dementia are many and include not just the common neurodegenerative diseases such as Alzheimer's disease (AD), but also infections, neoplasms, metabolic and other derangements of the CNS (Box 4.1). Conversely, not all neurodegenerative diseases are necessarily accompanied by cognitive impairment. For instance many individuals with Parkinson's disease or motor neuron disease remain intellectually intact.

Regional brain involvement in the dementing illnesses

No part of the brain is entirely exempt from involvement in one or other of the dementias, reflecting the range of causes and of the

Neurodegenerative
- AD (15% familial)
- DLB
- Pick's
- CBD
- PSP

Genetic
- Huntington's disease
- Familial AD
- Familial prion diseases

Developmental

Trauma
- Head injury, particularly repetitive (e.g. boxing)

Vascular
- Multi-infarct dementia and stroke
- Chronic subdural haematoma
- Binswanger's disease
- Amyloid angiopathy

Infective
- HIV/AIDS
- Prion diseases, including CJD (15% also genetic)
- Progressive multifocal leucoencephalopathy (JC virus)
- General paralysis of the insane (syphilis)

Metabolic
- Alcohol abuse
- Drug misuse
- Hepatic encephalopathy

Neoplastic
- Frontal lobe tumours benign or malignant

AD, Alzheimer's disease; CBD, corticobasal degeneration; CJD, Creutzfeldt–Jakob disease; DLB, dementia with Lewy bodies; HIV/AIDS, human immunodeficiency virus / acquired immune deficiency syndrome; PSP, progressive supranuclear palsy.

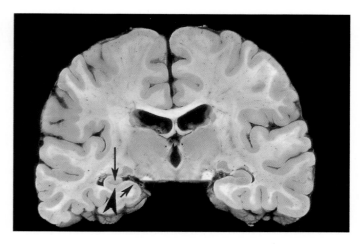

Fig. 4.1
Coronal slice through the brain of a cognitively unimpaired elderly patient showing slight dilatation of the ventricular system but no other significant abnormality. Regions of the hippocampal formation are highlighted by arrows: the cornu ammonis (long arrow), subiculum (arrow head) and entorrhinal cortex (short arrow).

Diagnosis of dementia and underlying proteinopathies

Careful review of the clinical and family history, with the help of someone close to the patient if cognitive impairment is pronounced, usually leads to a likely diagnosis when the results of a full physical examination are taken into account. Neuroimaging may pinpoint focal lesions such as tumours, subdural haematomas and infarcts, as well as providing information on less specific but no less significant conditions such as brain atrophy. Atrophy is reflected in ventricular enlargement and sulcal widening, or diffuse white matter shrinkage. History of the progression of cognitive impairment will reveal whether this has been a steady or stepwise decline. Other significant factors in the history include the occupation and level of education, previous head injury, alcohol or drug intake, and infections of the CNS, while general examination may reveal a likely predisposing factor for, or symptom of, neurodegeneration. These signs would include vascular disease and high blood pressure, liver disease and the presence of any abnormal movements. However, the definitive diagnosis may be problematic in a proportion of cases even as the disease progresses and may remain so until the postmortem examination. More than one pathology may be present in the brain, giving rise to a potentially confusing clinical picture. The pathological diagnosis of dementias has evolved considerably in recent years (Lowe 1998). Comprehensive sampling of the brain, with exploratory immunocytochemistry as well as routine staining, is required to establish the diagnosis. Neuropathologists have come to realise that what for them may be a single diagnosis with a particular range of microscopic abnormalities may present with a wide variety of clinical signs and symptoms, rendering an exact diagnosis extremely difficult in life. A good example of this is the condition known as corticobasal degeneration.

It is now clear that many of the major neurodegenerative diseases actually represent disorders of protein metabolism in which the neurodegeneration is associated with the accumulation

attendant signs and symptoms. Given the extent of grey matter which is involved in cognitive functions, and the white matter tracts which connect the different centres, it is hardly surprising that many different pathological conditions in the brain interfere with cognitive function. Inspection of the intact brain clearly identifies the involvement of the frontal and temporal lobes in certain diseases, while in others the occipital and parietal lobes may also appear atrophic, leading to a globally shrunken brain. The neuroanatomical features of the brain are considered elsewhere in this volume but in the present context, it is useful to confirm that while the major dementing illnesses result from pathology in the neocortex, in others the most obvious pathology is within the basal ganglia or thalami or even in the brainstem. It is not surprising that in basal ganglionic diseases, dementia is frequently accompanied by movement disorders reflecting the functional implications of damage to deep grey matter. Bilateral pathology in any component of the limbic system, including the hippocampus, temporal and entorhinal cortex (Fig. 4.1), dentate gyrus, fimbria, mamillary bodies, thalamus, amygdala and the cingulate cortex, will lead to significant cognitive impairment. Even the cerebellum, which may show significant pathology in many of the prion diseases, has been implicated in cognitive function (Middleton & Strick 1994).

of insoluble deposits of protein within and between cells (Lowe 1998, Mirra & Hyman 2002). Growing knowledge of these proteins has significantly advanced the understanding of neurodegenerative disorders, and is not merely of theoretical interest but also has implications for therapy. The major proteins to be deposited in the brain in this context are β amyloid (BA4), phosphorylated tau, α synuclein and prion protein. Because ubiquitin binds to proteins scheduled for degradation, many insoluble deposits are also ubiquitinated. Immunocytochemistry using antibodies specific for each of these accumulating proteins is a standard method for protein identification and localisation in cells and tissues and is now indispensable in the neuropathological categorisation of disease (Lowe 1998). Disorders in which an abnormal protein is deposited are known as proteinopathies and include the amyloidopathies, tauopathies, synucleinopathies and prion disorders (Table 4.1). Not all of these disorders result in cognitive impairment, depending on which neuronal systems are maximally affected.

β amyloidopathies

BA4 is derived from a normal transmembrane protein, β amyloid precursor protein (APP), coded from the corresponding gene on chromosome 21 (Bayer et al 2001). Figure 4.2 shows a diagrammatic representation of the APP molecule. The normal processing of APP involves cleavage by an α secretase which releases that portion of APP which is external to the cell in a secreted form of APP. The β amyloidogenic fragment of APP straddles the cleavage site at which α secretase operates. By definition therefore, the cleavage of APP produced by α secretase prevents the formation of an intact β amyloid fragment. In contrast, two further enzymes known as β and γ secretase target respectively the N-terminal and C-terminal ends of the β amyloidogenic fragment. The β secretase is preferentially expressed in neurons. The amyloidogenic fragment of APP gives rise to Aβ1-40 or Aβ1-42, depending on the site cleaved by γ secretase. These fragments form the basis of the β amyloid deposits seen in AD and are preferentially formed within the Golgi apparatus during intracellular trafficking of the APP molecule (Wilson et al 1999). The β amyloidopathies include not only AD but also the associated vascular disorder of amyloid angiopathy.

Tauopathies

Hyperphosphorylated tau is another important insoluble protein deposited not only in AD but also in a wider spectrum of neurodegenerative diseases now defined as tauopathies (Tolnay & Probst 1999). Most diseases in this group display only tau positive inclusions, but AD is unusual in showing both tau and βA4 amyloid positive inclusions and deposits, thus qualifying as both a tauopathy and an amyloidopathy. Tau protein is one of the cytoplasmic microtubule-associated proteins which function to stabilise and bind microtubules within neuronal cytoplasm. Consequently, tau is intimately concerned with the function of axonal transport and stabilisation of neuronal shape and structure, and is found in axons throughout the nervous system. Other functions, including signal transduction, have been ascribed to tau recently. Six isoforms of normal tau are known to exist, normally derived by alternative splicing from a gene on chromosome 17 and ranging in molecular weight from 45 to 65 kDa. These vary in their distribution around the brain. The normal tau subtypes are

further characterised by the presence or absence of inserts in the N-terminal and a repeat within the C-terminal. Phosphorylation of these normal tau isoforms is a key step associated with neurodegeneration. Hyperphosphorylation of all six isoforms is characteristic of AD, but in other tauopathies the reasons for tau aggregation are less well understood. Abnormally accumulating tau may be detected in neurites, neuritic plaques, and in neurofibrillary tangles. In some diseases it is found also in glial cells. The different phosphorylated tau proteins are easily distinguished by Western blots, and the six isoforms found in AD form characteristic triplets (Table 4.1). These aggregate into paired helical filaments which form the basis of neurofibrillary tangles (NFTs). Other tauopathies, including Pick's disease, display a phosphorylated tau doublet of 60 and 64 kDa on Western blots, whereas corticobasal degeneration (CBD) and progressive supranuclear palsy (PSP) are both characterised by a doublet of 64 and 68 kDa. The differing tau molecular sequences form the background to the abnormal phosphorylation pattern seen in the different conditions included here. They also give rise to slightly different aggregated paired helical filaments which form the major component of the neuronal inclusions. These paired helical filaments are straight in PSP but are twisted in CBD.

Synucleinopathies

Alpha synuclein is a presynaptic protein encoded by a gene on chromosome 4 and maximally expressed in the grey matter. The role of α synuclein is normally associated with transfer of neurotransmitter vesicles to synapses, but its contribution to the generation of disease is poorly understood as yet (Hashimoto & Masliah 1999). Certainly, α synuclein accumulates in the form of neuronal inclusions known as Lewy bodies which are found in Parkinson's disease and DLB. Lewy bodies are probably not in themselves neurotoxic, and smaller aggregates of α synuclein are more likely than the classic inclusions to be harmful to neurons. Apart from Lewy body diseases, those disorders which form variants of multiple system atrophy display widespread α synuclein inclusions, particularly in glial cells (Dickson et al 1999). Diseases which display α synuclein positive inclusion bodies have been designated the synucleinopathies.

Disorders manifesting as dementia
Alzheimer's disease

This condition is characterised by a dementia of insidious onset and slow progression ultimately leading to death 10 years or more after the onset of the disorder. Although usually found in elderly individuals and of late onset, the characteristic neuropathological features of this condition were first described by Alzheimer in a woman in her fifties. Subjects who develop AD generally display a period of memory impairment preceding the onset of unambiguous dementia. AD is the most frequent cause of dementia, although its prevalence is variable, the estimates being sometimes confounded by methodological problems. Best estimates of the prevalence of AD are up to 10% of the population over 65 years, which clearly represents the vast majority of those affected by dementia overall. Autopsy investigations suggest that 80% of demented individuals show AD pathology, either with other brain pathology or in isolation (Neuropathology Group of MRC CFAS 2001). Approximately 10% of cases of AD are familial. While AD

Table 4.1 The major dementias — pathology, proteins and genes

Protein conformation abnormality	Disease	Major pathological findings	Disease-associated protein	Gene/chromosome (no mutation present unless stated)
Amyloidopathies	Sporadic AD	βA4 plaques (mainly AB1-42) NFTs	βA4, tau, APP, ApoE, ubiquitin (tau triplet 60, 64 & 68 kDa)	*APP* (Ch21) *ApoE* ε4 (Ch19) *Tau* (Ch17) *IL-IA* 2/2 (Ch2)
	Familial AD	βA4 plaques (mainly AB1-42) NFTs	βA4, tau, APP, ApoE, ubiquitin (tau triplet 60, 64 & 68 kDa)	Mutations in *APP* (Ch21) Mutations in *Presenilin 1* (Ch14) Mutations in *Presenilin 2* (Ch1)
	Down syndrome (trisomy 21)	βA4 plaques (& NFTs) appearing prematurely	βA4, tau, APP, ApoE, ubiquitin (tau triplet 60, 64 & 68 kDa)	Triple gene *APP* (Ch21)
	Amyloid angiopathy	βA4 in vessel walls (AB1-40)	βA4	*APP* (Ch21) *ApoE* ε2 (Ch19)
Tauopathies	Sporadic & familial AD	As above	As above	As above No *tau* mutations in familial AD
	Pick's disease	Pick bodies: some spongiform change	Tau, ubiquitin (tau doublet 60 & 64 kDa)	*Tau* (Ch17)
	PSP	NFTs & glial tau inclusions	Tau straight filaments (doublet 64 & 68 kDa)	*Tau* polymorphisms (Ch17) Mutations in tau-modulating genes
	CBD	Ballooned neurons; tau positive neurites in white matter	Tau twisted filaments (doublet 64 & 68 kDa)	*Tau* (Ch17)
	FTDP-17	NFTs & glial tau inclusions	Tau twisted filaments (doublet 64 & 68 kDa)	Mutations in *tau* (Ch17)
Synucleinopathies	PD	Lewy bodies in brainstem	α synuclein, ubiquitin, parkin	*α synuclein* (Ch4) *parkin* (Ch6)
	Familial PD	Lewy bodies in brainstem	α synuclein, ubiquitin, parkin	Mutations in *α synuclein* (Ch4) Mutations in *parkin* (Ch6)
	DLB	Lewy bodies in brain stem & cortex Some spongiform change	α synuclein, ubiquitin, parkin	*α synuclein* (Ch4)
	MSA	Inclusions in glial & neuronal cells	α synuclein, ubiquitin	*α synuclein* (Ch4)
Polyglutamine disorders	Huntington's disease	huntingtin positive intranuclear inclusions	huntingtin	Mutations in *huntingtin* (Ch4)
Prion disorders	Sporadic CJD	Variable spongiform change and prion deposition	PrP^sc	*PRNP* (Ch20) (codon 129 methionine or valine homozygous)
	Familial prion diseases	Variable spongiform change and prion deposition	PrP^sc	Mutations in *PRNP* (Ch20)
	vCJD	Consistent florid plaques & heavy prion deposition	PrP^sc	*PRNP* (Ch20) (codon 129 methionine homozygous)

AD, Alzheimer's disease; APP, amyloid precursor protein; ApoE, apolipoprotein E; βA4 & AB1-42 & AB1-40, β amyloid varieties; Ch, chromosome; CJD, Creutzfeldt–Jakob disease; DLB, dementia with Lewy bodies; FTDP-17, frontotemporal dementia with parkinsonism associated with chromosome 17; kDa, kilodaltons; IL-1A, interleukin 1A; MSA, multiple system atrophy; NFT, neurofibrillary tangle; PD, Parkinson's disease; PRNP, prion gene; PRP^sc, disease-associated prion protein; PSP, progressive supranuclear palsy; vCJD, variant CJD.

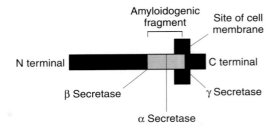

Fig. 4.2
Diagram of the structure of amyloid precursor protein. This transmembrane protein has N-terminal extracellular and C-terminal intracellular domains. The amyloidogenic fragment is potentially split by α secretase but is cleaved as an entire fragment by β and γ secretases acting together.

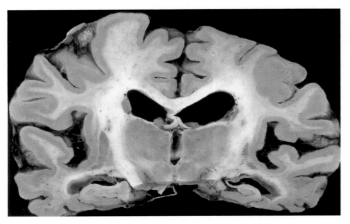

Fig. 4.3
Coronal brain slice from a patient with Alzheimer's disease, age-matched with that in Figure 4.1. The brain shows generalised atrophy with ventricular dilatation, opening of the subarachnoid spaces and particularly marked loss in the medial temporal lobe.

is said to be uncommon in African and Asian populations this may be more to do with decreased life expectancy in less affluent societies than with genuine ethnic differences in prevalence (Ritchie & Lovestone 2002).

In AD the brain shows generalised atrophy with compensatory dilatation of the ventricular system. Atrophy is most pronounced in the frontal and temporal lobes (Fig. 4.3). Microscopic evidence of pathology may be maximal in the medial temporal lobes but certainly involves the neocortex in other lobes of the brain, including the occipital lobes (although those display less overt atrophy). At the microscopic level, the lesions of AD characteristically comprise amyloid plaques, neurofibrillary tangles (NFTs), neuronal and synaptic loss, astrocytosis and microgliosis (Mirra & Hyman 2002). These lesions are found at greatest density in a characteristic distribution involving the medial hippocampus, including the entorhinal cortex, the amygdala, and the neocortex of the occipital, frontal and temporal lobes. Amyloid deposits and NFTs may also be conspicuous in the basal ganglia, thalami and even in the substantia nigra, although the amyloid deposits in this location are of a more diffuse form than the complex neuritic plaques found in the neocortex in AD. Diffuse plaques are made up of non-fibrillary amyloid whereas neuritic plaques contain a high proportion of amyloid fibrils.

While conventional staining with haematoxylin and eosin may be strongly suggestive of the presence of AD lesions (Fig. 4.4), special stains are required to demonstrate the full burden of amyloid deposits and of NFTs. Traditionally a silver stain has been used to demonstrate these lesions, and AD pathology has generally been assessed on the basis of Bielschowsky staining (Fig. 4.5). Alternative silver methods include Gallyas and Bodian stains. Thioflavine staining is useful since the reagent fluoresces at the site of amyloid deposition, as does congo red (Fig. 4.6). Latterly, immunocytochemical techniques have been used for the specific demonstration of amyloid deposits (antibody to βA4 amyloid) and of NFTs (antibody to phosphorylated tau).

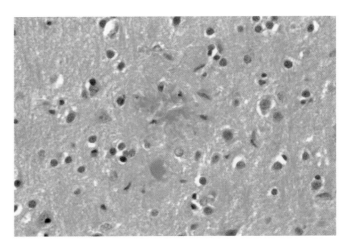

Fig. 4.4
Cerebral cortex from a patient with Alzheimer's disease showing deposition of eosinophilic amyloid material in the grey matter, forming an amyloid plaque. Haematoxylin and eosin. Original magnification × 200.

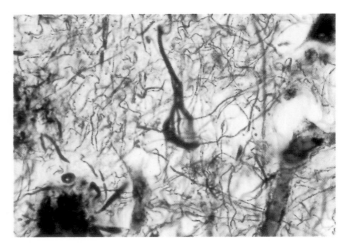

Fig. 4.5
Cortex from a brain displaying the features of Alzheimer's disease and stained with a silver technique to display neuropil threads throughout the cortex, a centrally placed, vertically arranged neurofibrillary tangle and two extracellular plaques shown in part at the left and lower borders of the frame. A small capillary traverses the section in the lower right hand corner. Bielschowsky stain. Original magnification × 400.

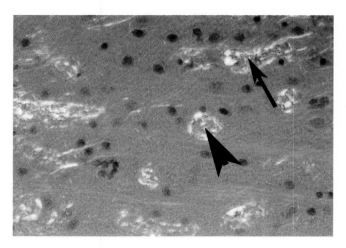

Fig. 4.6
Section of the cortex from a patient with Alzheimer's disease and viewed in a fluorescent microscope. The brightly fluorescing lesions mark the deposition of β amyloid in the walls of small grey-matter vessels (arrow) and in extracellular amyloid plaques (arrow head). Congo red staining. Original magnification × 200.

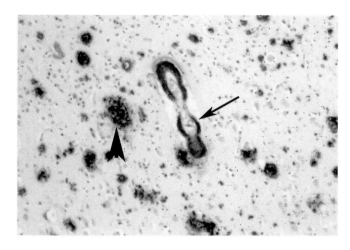

Fig. 4.7
Immunocytochemical preparation showing the cortex of a patient with Alzheimer's disease, stained for β amyloid. The immunopositive lesions include the walls of a small blood vessel (arrow) and numerous large and small amyloid plaques (arrow head). Original magnification × 40.

Amyloid plaques are extracellular accumulations of insoluble fibrillary and non-fibrillary material composed of βA4 amyloid. These microscopic deposits are of several different types. Neuritic plaques are composed of amyloid aggregates, often with a compact amyloid core, which are interspersed with, and surrounded by, expanded and damaged neuritic processes with associated astrocytic and microglial reactions. Diffuse plaques consist only of amorphous deposits of non-fibrillary amyloid lacking the neuritic and glial elements. Fluffy deposits of amyloid may also be seen in a subpial location. Blood vessels within the grey matter and in the subarachnoid space may also accumulate βA4 within their walls, particularly if the burden of amyloid plaques is high in the neocortex (Fig. 4.7). Occasionally only the dense amyloid core persists, and this lesion has been classified as a burnt out plaque. It is generally supposed that amyloid deposits evolve from the diffuse to the neuritic form with advancing disease.

The question of whether amyloid plaques are always a pathological lesion or may be found incidentally in ageing brains has been addressed earlier in this chapter. The current consensus is that their presence always indicates a pathological event.

All amyloid plaques are visualised by immunocytochemical techniques which employ antibodies to βA4, and the AB42–43 molecular form of amyloid is particularly prevalent in plaques. Although β amyloid is predominant, other molecules also accumulate in plaques, including APP, alpha-1 antichymotrypsin, apolipoprotein E (ApoE), complement and ubiquitin, as well as molecules associated with neurites, including tau protein, neurofilaments, synaptophysin and neurotransmitters. Amyloid promotes the deposition of ubiquitin. Neuritic plaques are more characteristically found in the neocortex than in subcortical grey matter in AD, but those seen in the basal ganglia are generally diffuse. Vascular amyloid deposition is largely restricted to the cortex and subarachnoid space, sparing the white matter, and is present in the majority of cases of AD but may also occur in individuals who lack the other pathology of AD. This isolated pathology of blood vessels constitutes the condition known as cerebral amyloid angiopathy, which is associated with an increased

risk of cerebral haemorrhage. The amyloid which is laid down in vessels is AB1-40.

Neurofibrillary tangles are intraneuronal aggregations of paired helical filaments largely composed of insoluble tau protein. Failure of normal tau to bind to microtubules may lead to hyperphosphorylation, and this in turn is associated with the development of paired helical filaments made up of protein strands of between 10 and 20 nm in diameter displaying regular constrictions which contribute to the twisted appearance of the helical strands. Unlike amyloid plaques, NFTs are often laminar in distribution in the neocortex. In AD, NFTs probably appear first in the CA1 sector of the cornu ammonis, subiculum and entorrhinal cortex of the medial temporal lobe. The amygdala is also involved. As AD progresses, NFTs involve more and more of the temporal cortex. The insular cortex and the cingulate gyri display NFTs in the large neurons of layer two as well as in deeper cortical layers in the worst affected areas. Glutamatergic neurons appear to be more vulnerable to NFTs than those using γ aminobutyric acid (GABA) or calbindin. NFTs may also be found in neurons within the basal ganglia, thalami and substantia nigra in advanced AD. Well-formed NFTs are visible with conventional staining and are generally flame shaped in the cytoplasm of pyramidal neurons in the cortex (Fig. 4.8) whereas those in the midline structures, including the brainstem, are less angular in form. NFTs are rather basophilic on conventional H&E staining.

The presence of NFTs within neuronal cytoplasm indicates a profound derangement of neuronal function. Many affected neurons die and disappear in advanced stages of disease, leaving the insoluble tangle as the only visible residue of the neuron it occupied previously (Fig. 4.9). These ghost tangles may be very numerous in the hippocampus. NFTs and neuritic plaques are both highlighted by tau immunocytochemistry (Fig. 4.10). Individual tau positive neuritic threads become increasingly prominent in late stages of AD. NFTs are not specific for AD, being found in aged non-demented subjects as well as in other neurodegenerative diseases detailed below. However, if NFTs are present predominantly in the neocortex, and are accompanied by

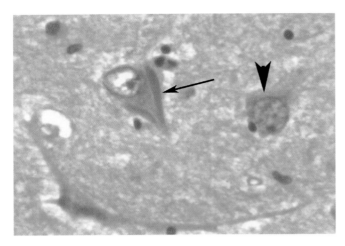

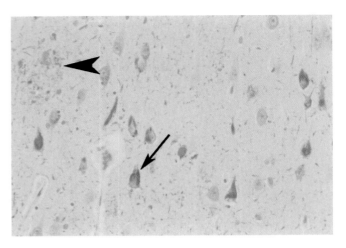

Fig. 4.8
Cornu ammonis from a patient with Alzheimer's disease showing an intraneuronal neurofibrillary tangle (arrow) and a neighbouring apparently normal neuron with no such inclusion (arrow head). Haematoxylin and eosin. Original magnification × 400.

Fig. 4.10
Immunocytochemical preparation from the subiculum of a patient with Alzheimer's disease, showing the presence of numerous tau-positive neurofibrillary tangles (arrow) and the tau positive neurites of a neuritic plaque (arrow head). Immunocytochemical staining for tau protein (AT8). Original magnification × 200.

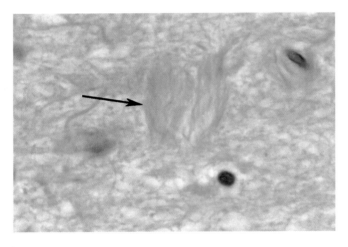

Fig. 4.9
Cornu ammonis from the same patient as that shown in Figure 4.8, displaying a residual 'ghost' tangle which marks the former position of a neuron which has disappeared. Haematoxylin and eosin. Original magnification × 400.

a heavy burden of β amyloid plaques, these lesions together are a sufficient neuropathological substrate to substantiate a clinical diagnosis of AD. There is considerable evidence to suggest that the burden of NFTs is a better correlate for dementia than the number of amyloid plaques. Rare dementias are characterised by the presence of NFTs virtually in isolation in a form of tangle predominant dementia. Dementia pugilistica, associated with a history of boxing, displays a preponderance of NFTs, although diffuse plaques and evidence of cerebrovascular disease may be present.

Neuronal loss is a prominent feature in late-stage AD, and the neocortex frequently shows astrocytosis and many activated microglia, particularly in association with amyloid plaques. The mode of neuronal death is unclear. Beta amyloid is known from in-vitro experiments to be neurotoxic. Neuronal apoptosis has been implicated in AD following the demonstration of caspase 3 activation in response to the presence of amyloid both in vitro and in animal models. Caspase 3 activation is an important stage on the apoptotic pathway and marks an irreversible commitment to the process of cell death. However, its demonstration in human AD cortex has not been well validated, and the contribution of apoptotic neuronal death to the atrophy seen in AD remains to be determined. Neuronal dysfunction and synaptic loss are more likely to be the key events underlying cognitive decline, and actual neuronal death may well be a late event. Understanding the pathogenesis of this process, particularly the initial trigger events, is vital for devising effective treatment strategies.

Hirano bodies are brightly eosinophilic rod-shaped neuronal inclusions composed of actin together with other proteins. They are seen best in the hippocampus along with granulovacuolar degeneration which may represent lysosomal accumulations within neuronal cytoplasm. The clinical significance of these two microscopic features is not clear. Their distribution is considerably more limited than that of NFTs and amyloid deposits, and it is the latter two lesions which are used to grade the severity of the pathology in AD.

The loss of cholinergic neurons in AD, particularly in the temporal cortex, is confirmed by a measurable decline in acetylcholine in the cortex and by the clinical response, at least in some patients, to anticholinesterase agents given therapeutically. Cholinergic neurons are also lost in the nucleus of Meynert in the basal forebrain. Adrenergic neurons within the locus coeruleus in the brainstem are also likely to be depleted in AD.

The pathological diagnosis of AD depends crucially on assessment of a variety of brain sections for the presence of NFTs and amyloid plaques. The fact that these may be present in small numbers in non-demented aged subjects can cause diagnostic difficulty. Various histological staging schemes have been devised to address this problem and to ensure greater uniformity. The first of these was devised by Khachaturian (1985), based on a quantitative assessment of amyloid plaques in the

Box 4.2   CERAD (Consortium to Establish a Registry for Alzheimer's Disease) criteria for diagnosis of Alzheimer's disease

- Brain weight
- Distribution of atrophy
- State of vessels
- Ventricular dilatation
- Lacunar and large infarcts
- Pallor of substantia nigra
- Assessment of amyloid plaque density (various cortical areas including hippocampus, entorrhinal cortex and midbrain)
- Other features: neurofibrillary tangles and Lewy bodies

brain. From 1988, the Consortium to Establish a Registry for Alzheimer's Disease (CERAD) (Mirra et al 1991) sought to refine the Khachaturian criteria. In a study of 142 demented patients thought to be suffering from AD, and 8 non-demented controls, CERAD assessed the number of neuritic plaques based on the examination of five areas of the cortex, namely the middle frontal gyrus, the superior and middle temporal gyri, the inferior parietal lobule, the hippocampus and the entorhinal cortex, as well as the midbrain, including the substantia nigra. The CERAD criteria are listed in Box 4.2. The Bielschowsky silver stain was chosen for the comparative study since this method displayed neuritic plaques particularly well. Antibodies to β amyloid were also used but, because this immunocytochemical technique decorated both diffuse and neuritic plaques, there was some difficulty in distinguishing between the two. While the clinical significance of the two types of plaque is not thoroughly understood, and diffuse plaques may be very widespread in advanced AD, the scoring system sought to assess neuritic plaques, which were coded as sparse, moderate or frequent. When the age of the patient and the clinical history of dementia were taken into account, the investigators were able to stratify the diagnosis for an individual patient as definite, probable or possible AD based on the neuropathological findings.

In 1991, Braak & Braak published a study of 83 neuropathologically assessed brains from aged individuals who were not primarily ascertained on the basis of dementia, although a significant proportion were demented. In this study NFTs were used as the basis of a grading system according to their number and localisation. Braak & Braak described six stages of increasingly severe NFT pathology which reflected the spreading involvement of the entorhinal cortex, the CA1 sector of the hippocampus and lastly the wider neocortex. Cases with severe NFT changes consistently showed widespread amyloid plaques although the converse was not always true in that some brains which had a heavy amyloid burden were not affected by NFTs. This study found that grading of NFTs correlated better with dementia than did the presence of amyloid deposits. Several very elderly individuals were identified, including one 85 year old, who had neither amyloid deposits nor NFTs despite very wide sampling of all brain areas. They concluded that the presence of even sparse numbers of NFTs was pathological.

In 1999 the National Institute of Ageing, in collaboration with the Reagan Institute, revisited the classification of AD pathology and chose to formally include both amyloid deposits and NFTs in their assessment (Newell et al 1999). From the starting point of a neuropathological examination which included a subjective assessment of the number and distribution of neuritic plaques together with an assessment of the Braak staging, the study judged the likelihood of AD to be high, intermediate or low. The NIA–Reagan study included some demented patients who were not suffering from AD, and the conclusion which was reached was that an assessment based on both amyloid and NFT burden proved to be a highly significant correlate of AD. Overall the Bielschowsky staining technique was recommended because of the difficulty of distinguishing plaque types by means of antibodies to amyloid. Braak & Braak found little difference in reliability between routine silver stains and antibody techniques for tau so far as the demonstration of NFTs was concerned. It has been suggested that the CERAD approach should be recommended for the diagnostic assessment of AD, while Braak staging is deemed particularly appropriate for AD research projects (Hyman & Trojanowski 1997).

In current routine practice, neuropathologists who use these staging tools achieve a high degree of interobserver consistency for probable and definite AD, as shown in a recent Australian study (Halliday et al 2002). However, that study revealed that opinions proved diverse on cases of possible AD, illustrating once more the difficulty of separating early or mild AD pathology from normal or the 'control' population.

Pathogenesis   The causes of AD are not known, although a number of risk factors have been recognised which are of help in understanding the pathogenesis. Among the factors linked to an increased risk of developing AD are older age, certain genetic factors such as *ApoE* ε4, a history of head injury, and a poorer level of education. There is some evidence of gender imbalance in that women generally survive longer with AD than do men, and hormone replacement therapy is emerging as potentially protective for the development of AD. A protective effect has been shown in patients on long-term anti-inflammatory treatment, in whom the risk of developing AD appears to be halved (McGeer & McGeer 1999). This protective effect of anti-inflammatory drugs has focused attention on the possible role of inflammation in the genesis of AD. Microglial activation and pro-inflammatory cytokine production are both characteristic of AD. Certain alleles of the interleukin 1 (IL-1) polymorphism, particularly IL-1A 2/2, appear to be linked to an increased risk of sporadic AD (Mrak & Griffin 2000).

Subjects with Down syndrome show precocious development of AD-type pathology and tend to develop widespread amyloid deposits by their fourth decade (Teller et al 1996), which has been attributed to a triple gene dose effect for *APP*, since this gene is found on chromosome 21. For reasons that are less clear, subjects with Down syndrome also have a tendency for premature development of NFTs. Apart from trisomy 21, mutations in the *APP* gene are associated with some familial cases of AD. Other genes which have been linked to early-onset familial AD are *presenilin 1* (on chromosome 14) and *presenilin 2* (on chromosome 1). Mutations are not present in the more common sporadic cases but these are influenced by the different alleles of the *ApoE* polymorphism (on chromosome 19). The *ApoE* ε4 allele is associated with an increased risk of late-onset AD, being overrepresented in cohorts of AD patients (Saunders 2000), whereas the most common allele, ε3, and the least common, ε2, do not show this association. In fact *ApoE* ε2 may be protective in regard to vulnerability to AD. It seems likely that possession of *ApoE* ε4 hastens the onset of AD in individuals who are susceptible for other reasons. However *ApoE* ε4 is not necessarily predictive for AD, in that some individuals reach advanced old age while remaining cognitively intact despite having an ε4/4 genotype. The function of ApoE in the brain is not completely understood, although there is clearly some interaction with APP. Individuals possessing one or more *ApoE* ε4 alleles are more likely than those without to form amyloid deposits, and this has been well shown following head injury. Head injury is a known risk for AD, and the mechanism may be linked to deposition of β amyloid following APP upregulation, particularly in individuals with *ApoE* ε4 genotype. In contrast to AD, investigation of subjects with amyloid angiopathy appears to show overrepresentation of *ApoE* ε2. A link between *ApoE* genotype and a propensity for developing amyloid plaques is supported by studies of NFT-rich dementia occurring in very elderly subjects. Affected individuals have very few amyloid deposits and show a correspondingly low prevalence of *ApoE* ε4 allele (Jellinger & Bancher 1998).

Other pathogenetic mechanisms which have been implicated in AD include oxidative damage and withdrawal of neurotrophic factors, but the evidence for these mechanisms is not yet well substantiated. Cerebral hypoperfusion associated with vascular disease has been proposed as a common pathogenetic mechanism for AD (De La Torre 2002).

Dementia with Lewy bodies

Patients with DLB display a fluctuating cortical dementia, usually but not always with some features of parkinsonism, which tends to be accompanied by hallucinations. This condition may be confused in life with multi-infarct dementia and indeed may coexist with it (Lishman 1995, Lowe 1998). Autopsy studies have established the presence of cortical Lewy body pathology in up to 25% of elderly demented patients (McKeith et al 1996) with or without coexisting AD pathology. The causes of both Parkinson's disease and DLB remain elusive.

Lewy bodies are intracytoplasmic inclusions which were first identified in substantia nigra neurons in Parkinson's disease (Fig. 4.11a) but are also present in other neuronal collections within the brainstem (Ince et al 1998). However, approximately 10% of Parkinson's disease patients also develop increasing cognitive impairment amounting to dementia. When such patients come to autopsy a wider search in the cortex reveals the presence of neuronal cytoplasmic inclusions which are similar to, although not as obvious as, those in substantia nigra neurons, and these rounded inclusions are known as cortical Lewy bodies (Fig. 4.11b). Cortical Lewy bodies distend the cytoplasm and distort the nucleus, resulting in neuronal degeneration, but individual neurons are not markedly swollen. A major contribution to the understanding of Parkinson's disease was made with the discovery that these inclusions are largely composed of α synuclein, a presynaptic protein normally expressed in neurons (Dickson 2002). Cortical Lewy bodies are generally found in the deeper cortical layers of the temporal and cingulate gyri of the temporal and frontal lobes, often with associated spongiform change. Lewy bodies may be found in the amygdala and less commonly in the parietal and occipital cortex. Lewy bodies also stain positively with ubiquitin since this protein is involved in the degradation of α synuclein and of parkin, another protein contributing to the pathogenesis of familial Parkinson's disease.

Small numbers of cortical Lewy bodies are frequently found in association with Parkinson's disease but appear to be subclinical.

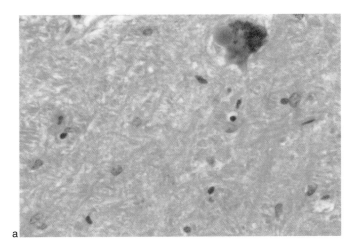

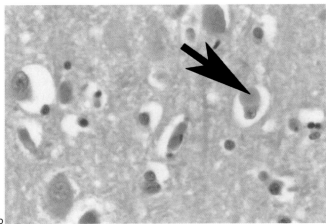

Fig. 4.11
Routinely stained preparations from the brains of patients with Lewy body disorders. In (a), a pigmented neuron of the substantia nigra contains a darkly eosinophilic inclusion in a patient with Parkinson's disease. In (b), a cortical Lewy body (arrow) distends the cytoplasm of a neuron in a patient with dementia with Lewy bodies. Haematoxylin and eosin. Original magnification of each × 400.

The dementing illness known as dementia with Lewy bodies is associated with large numbers of cortical Lewy bodies. There is an intriguing association with AD. The coexistence of AD and DLB has suggested to some that DLB is no more than one form of AD. Alternatively the two conditions may occur together coincidentally in ageing individuals. They may even be synergistic and each may promote the progression of the other. The exact nature of the relationship between the two pathologies remains to be elucidated (Hamilton 2000).

Vascular dementias

Individuals with evidence of vascular disease may display a stepwise deterioration of cognitive function in old age which in the absence of other neurodegenerative disease constitutes a vascular dementia.

Dementia associated with cerebrovascular disease is not generally associated with deposition of abnormal protein, with the exception of amyloid angiopathy. In terms of prevalence of the condition, vascular dementia is similar in importance to AD and DLB. Evidence of white-matter pathology associated with small-vessel disease is common and has been reported in up to half of all patients with AD (Lishman 1995). The exact prevalence of vascular dementia is difficult to determine. A recent study revealed cerebrovascular pathology in 78% of 209 community-based autopsies in 85-year-old individuals (Neuropathology Group of MRC CFAS 2001). The presence of cerebrovascular disease significantly enhanced the likelihood of dementia occurring in patients with early Alzheimer pathology (Esiri et al 1999). The notion that AD may be primarily a vascular disorder has also been advanced (De La Torre 2002). In practice, some degree of vascular disease is frequently found together with the pathology of these two primary neurodegenerative diseases (Jagust 2001).

Atheroma of larger cerebral vessels is common in ageing, leading to luminal narrowing and erosion of their smooth lining, with a consequent increased tendency for mural or occlusive thrombosis. Another common change is hyalinisation of the walls of smaller vessels, which renders them inelastic. These vascular conditions separately or together may significantly compromise the blood supply to the brain. Occlusion of a major vessel supplying the brain can result in a clinical episode of stroke due to infarction of brain tissue. Sometimes this sudden clinical event is followed by the appearance of overt dementia. It is supposed that the dementia represents the cumulative result of the immediately preceding brain injury and previous episodes of minor brain damage. In some individuals diagnosed with multi-infarct dementia there may be no recollected episode of clinical stroke. Any condition which gives rise to multiple emboli to the brain, for example atrial fibrillation, may contribute to the onset of significant cognitive impairment. Vascular disease leads to significant loss of the white matter due to perivascular degeneration of tissue amounting to small lacunar infarcts (Fig. 4.12). This is thought to be a sufficient substrate for dementia even in the absence of AD pathology, although there are as yet no agreed criteria for quantifying the extent and severity of vascular abnormality in the CNS.

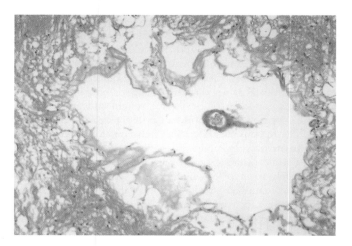

Fig. 4.12
Deep central white matter from a patient with cerebrovascular disease. A small vessel with a thickened wall consistent with arteriolosclerosis is surrounded by rarified white matter, amounting to a lacunar infarct. Haematoxylin and eosin. Original magnification × 100.

Binswanger's disease is a form of vascular brain damage which is not well understood. It appears to involve greater myelin loss in the cortical white matter than may be accounted for simply as a result of micro-infarction, but some do regard it as an extensive form of lacunar infarction. Both lacunar infarcts and Binswanger's disease are associated with hypertension and result in loss of white matter with compensatory dilatation of the ventricular system.

Rarer dementias

In this category are included a number of neurodegenerative conditions which have been characterised much more recently and are less common than AD. Most of these conditions are associated with the deposition of abnormal tau protein (Lee et al 2001). Although tau inclusions are found most commonly in AD within NFTs and tau-positive neuritic plaques, the pathology of AD is also characterised by heavy deposits of β amyloid as described previously. In the group of disorders considered in this section, tau inclusions are prominent in the absence of β amyloid deposition (Lowe & Leigh 2002). The disorders include Pick's disease, progressive supranuclear palsy (PSP), corticobasal degeneration (CBD) and frontotemporal dementia with parkinsonism associated with chromosome 17 (FTDP-17). PSP has been known in the past as the Steele Richardson Olszewski syndrome (Trojanowski & Dickson 2001). Although each of these conditions may display characteristic and distinctive pathological appearances there is in practice a spectrum of pathology and clinical symptomatology spanning the tau-associated neurodegenerative diseases (tauopathies), which may make exact diagnosis difficult.

Recent developments in genetic analysis and characterisation of the tau subtype which is expressed in the individual brain have proved to be of the utmost importance in clarifying the nature of the neurodegenerative condition in an individual patient. The different tau-associated neurodegenerative conditions may be distinguished on Western blots. Pick's disease is characterised by bands of 60 and 64 kDa phosphorylated tau, whereas PSP and CBD display bands of 64 and 68 kDa. In contrast, the phosphorylated tau of AD has a characteristic triplet pattern of 60, 64 and 68 kDa.

Pick's disease was first described more than a hundred years ago, preceding the description of AD, and characterised by frontal lobe signs in the context of progressive dementia. This disorder may have come to attention relatively early in the study of dementias because its onset is at a somewhat younger age, usually in early middle life, and because of the characteristic extreme degree of brain atrophy. Most cases are sporadic and display a very striking frontal and temporal lobar atrophy which contrasts markedly with the apparent macroscopic preservation of the remaining cortical structures (Dickson 1998). On closer examination the cerebral hemispheres may be asymmetric, with the atrophy affecting one side more than the other and with variable involvement of the basal ganglia leading to atrophy in these structures. The pathology of Pick's disease is characterised by the presence of swollen cortical neurons containing round inclusions or Pick bodies. The presence of Pick bodies is frequently associated with spongiform change in the cortex and astrocytosis. These inclusions stain positively with silver stains and with antibodies to ubiquitin and most particularly to tau. Pick bodies are detectable in the cornu ammonis of the temporal lobe both in the granule and in the pyramidal cells. As well as the neocortex, Pick bodies may also be present in the neurons of basal ganglia and periaqueductal grey matter. Neuronal loss may be found in the substantia nigra. Occasional tau-positive inclusions are also noted in glial cells in Pick's disease.

A familial form of Pick's disease has been described which also displays typical Pick inclusions but which has intriguing links to FTDP-17 (Lee et al 2001, Lowe & Leigh 2002). Both diseases show marked frontal and temporal lobar atrophy and are familial, but the microscopic pathology in FTDP-17 is of intraneuronal NFTs rather than Pick bodies. FTDP-17 commonly displays asymmetrical atrophy of the frontal lobe with corresponding loss of frontal lobe functions, language deficits and parkinsonism. Mutations of the tau gene have been detected in association with this condition, and the resulting tau deposits are widely distributed through the brain. Although this familial form of frontotemporal dementia is rare, it is of great interest in helping to elucidate the role of phosphorylated tau in neurodegenerative conditions. Mutated tau has an impaired ability to interact normally with microtubules, and NFTs are found in neurons while tau-positive inclusions are found in glial cells.

Progressive supranuclear palsy (PSP) presents as a movement disorder with cognitive impairment together with some rigidity and poverty of movement but without tremor. Supranuclear gaze palsy is usually present. Although lobar atrophy is not seen macroscopically, there may be visible degeneration of the globus pallidus, periaqueductal grey matter, substantia nigra and lower brainstem nuclei (Bergeron et al 1998), where neuronal loss and gliosis are also detected. The tau positive NFTs in the stem tend to be spherical or non-angulated, and are known as globose tangles (Fig. 4.13). Tau-positive inclusions are characteristically prominent in glial cells, whose processes takes on a tufted appearance. Microscopic involvement of the neocortex usually underlies the observed cognitive impairment. The tau of PSP displays a 64 and 68 kDa doublet on Western blot, and mutations of the tau gene are not generally detected. Coexistent pathology including that of AD and Parkinson's disease, as well as infarcts, may be present more often than expected (Lowe & Leigh 2002).

Corticobasal degeneration (CBD) is primarily a pathological diagnosis which may underlie a range of symptomatology which includes cognitive impairment and movement disorder resistant to levodopa. Asymmetric cortical atrophy is generally present, and there may be white-matter and basal ganglionic degeneration as well as brainstem involvement (Bergeron et al 1998, Dickson et al 2002). The substantia nigra is usually pale. The characteristic microscopic feature is the presence of very swollen or ballooned neurons with granular tau-positive inclusions in neurons and in neuritic threads. These are so abundant as to impart a brownish hue to the white matter on naked-eye inspection. The Western blot pattern for tau protein is similar to that in PSP in that a 64 and 68 kDa doublet is seen. The condition may be sporadic or familial.

The subclassification of rarer dementias continues to evolve. Cognitive impairment may be associated with motor neuron disease and characterised by ubiquitin-positive inclusions in cortical neurons and neurites not only in the motor cortex, brainstem and anterior horn of the spinal cord but also more widely in the neocortex and basal ganglia. The inclusions are found particularly in the hippocampus and dentate granular cells and in frontotemporal cortex, often with superficial grey matter vacuolation. In some cases the dementia, with associated cortical changes, may be present without motor impairment (Jackson et al 1996). Tau inclusions are not generally found in this condition.

In a small minority of patients with dementia, there may be no distinctive histology or the pathological lesion may be manifested only as small deposits within neuronal processes which stain positively with silver stains and with antibodies to hyperphosphorylated tau. This condition has been designated argyrophilic grain disease (Braak & Braak 1989) with a relative paucity of associated β amyloid deposition despite the presence of cognitive impairment. Intriguingly, this condition has been associated with the *ApoE* ε2 allele in contrast with AD, which is more generally linked to *ApoE* ε4.

A familial dementia has been described in association with myoclonus and with mutations in the gene encoding the neuronal protein neuroserpin. The underlying neuropathology includes neuronal inclusions which stain positively with anti-neuroserpin antibodies, and the condition has been labelled a neuroserpinopathy (Lomas & Carrell 2002).

Acquired dementias are seen in some patients who are addicted to alcohol, and these include Korsakoff's psychosis. Apart from the focal lesions of Wernicke's encephalopathy, which are induced in the mamillary bodies and hypothalamus and which are preventable by thiamine, there is evidence for more widespread cortical atrophy and white matter loss in some alcoholics, which is reflected in ventricular dilatation. The mamillary bodies are an important component of the limbic system and are reduced in size in AD as well as in Wernicke's encephalopathy (Sheedy et al 1999). The reasons for differences between alcoholics in cortical and white matter vulnerability, such that some become cognitively impaired while others escape unscathed, are poorly understood but are likely to involve genetic factors. Astrocytes in the basal ganglia and brainstem grey matter may display characteristically enlarged, pale and irregular nuclei, the change being known as Alzheimer II astrocytosis and associated with hepatic dysfunction causing encephalopathy.

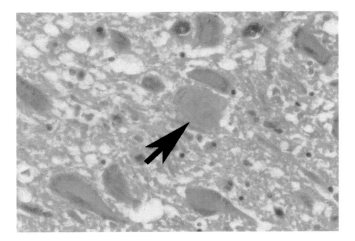

Fig. 4.13
Periaqueductal grey matter from the brainstem of a patient with progressive supranuclear palsy. A globose tangle distends the cytoplasm of a degenerate neuron (arrow). Haematoxylin and eosin. Original magnification × 400.

Overlapping and coexisting pathology

A significant number of individuals with cognitive impairment or frank dementia may display not only a mixed and potentially confusing clinical picture but also reveal a non-typical picture on neuropathological examination (Mirra & Hyman 2002). Although the pathology of the individual conditions described above is rather characteristic, there may be overlap between the different conditions or these may coexist. While there is no difficulty in diagnosing the cause of severe and long-standing dementia in an aged patient displaying numerous amyloid plaques and NFTs in the characteristic distribution, difficulties surrounds the accurate diagnosis of subjects with less obvious pathology. Clinicopathological anomalies are well known in ageing subjects, including those with severe dementia of frontal lobe type in whom little or no AD pathology is found nor any other very obvious cause. Conversely some subjects with well documented intact cognitive function are found to have quite widespread Alzheimer type pathology on examination of the brain. Current consensus among neuropathologists is that the presence of NFTs and/or amyloid deposits always constitutes a pathological lesion and is not merely a sign of advancing age. The younger the patient at death the greater the significance attached to these two lesions, however sparse they may be.

Attempts to classify and grade the pathology of AD are fraught with difficulty not only because patients die at different stages of the disease due to other fatal conditions but also because the pathology of AD may be complicated by other lesions in the brain. These include vascular lesions such as infarcts and small-vessel disease which affect predominantly the white matter. Other neurodegenerative diseases may apparently coexist with AD. Lewy bodies are present in up to 60% of AD patients, most commonly in the amygdala, and it is currently unclear whether this dual pathology constitutes a pathogenetically distinct subset of AD or merely the concurrence of two different diseases: AD and DLB (Hamilton 2000). Dementias that are not quite characteristic of AD may display cortical Lewy body pathology together with Alzheimer pathology below the diagnostic threshold on formal staging. Since both these conditions may give rise to dementia in their own right, it is not surprising that the corresponding clinical picture may be rather different from that of pure AD. While the presence of more than one neurodegenerative disease of the brain in an individual patient may simply reflect increasing vulnerability with age, there is increasing suspicion that an active synergy may be operating which promotes one or other or both pathologies when they coexist. The nature of this putative association is poorly understood at present. Examples of commonly occurring coexisting dementing conditions are AD with vascular disease or AD with DLB. Progressive supranuclear palsy may show coexisting pathology of Parkinson's disease or AD, and infarcts appear to occur more commonly than expected in all of these conditions. Apart from these examples where two pathologies are clearly present, the pathology of individual conditions such as FTDP-17 displays overlapping pathology not only with Parkinson's disease but also with a familial form of Pick's disease.

These complexities present challenges for conventional neuropathology and serve not only as an incentive for further research but pinpoint the need for additional genetic and biochemical information in achieving a diagnosis. They also require the introduction of standardised assessment systems for categorising and grading pathology. These are now quite well formulated for the common neurodegenerative diseases, including the CERAD (Mirra et al 1991) and Braak (Braak & Braak 1991) systems for AD, but are less well worked out for the rarer dementias. Particularly important are the implications for developing treatment for patients with combined or atypical dementia. For instance the symptoms of parkinsonism may reflect a range of different underlying pathologies in the brain, and not all of these will be responsive to levodopa. Finally, accurate clinicopathological correlations in large cohorts of dementing and ageing patients may lead to new thinking on causation and vulnerability, which has the potential for varied and new strategies for prevention and treatment.

Prion diseases

Since the first description of Creutzfeldt–Jakob disease (CJD) in the 1920s, this group of disorders has attracted attention to a degree which appears disproportionate to their prevalence of approximately 1 case per million of the population worldwide. The preoccupation with prion disorders is justified in that these dementing disorders may be both transmitted and inherited, although up to 90% are in fact sporadic with no evidence for either factor being the cause (De Armond et al 2002). The clinical features of sporadic CJD characteristically include rapidly progressive dementia, myoclonus and periodic spikes in the electroencephalogram, in patients almost always over 50 years. However, the clinical diagnosis of CJD is frequently suspected in individuals who subsequently prove to have AD, DLB, Pick's disease, paraneoplastic syndrome or almost any other dementing condition.

Prion disorders are classified according to whether they are sporadic, dominantly inherited or acquired (Box 4.3), and similar diseases are encountered in animals, notably scrapie in sheep. Most prion diseases are characterised by the presence of immunocytochemically demonstrable prion protein which accumulates as an insoluble amyloid product within brain tissue. Resulting nerve cell loss and astrocytosis may be profound and give rise to spongiform degeneration within the grey matter (Fig. 4.14). The disease-associated prion protein (PrP^{sc}) is derived from the normal form (PrP^c) by a post-translational conformational change. PrP^c is a cell surface protein encoded by a gene on chromosome 20 and expressed at high level in neurons but whose function is not yet understood. In the inherited prion disorders one or other mutation in the prion gene results in a protein which is more easily subverted to the insoluble form. The fact that these diseases are also transmissible has been appreciated in scientific circles for many decades. Brain tissue from individuals suffering from prion disorders is capable of transmitting the disease if injected into, or ingested by, a secondary host of the same or other susceptible species. Investigation of this phenomenon has ruled out the presence of any conventional micro-organism, and the transmissible

---

Box 4.3	**Classification of prion diseases**

Sporadic
- Creutzfeldt–Jakob Disease (CJD)
- Sporadic fatal insomnia

Inherited
- Familial CJD
- Gerstmann Sträussler Scheinker Syndrome
- Fatal familial insomnia

Acquired
- Kuru
- Iatrogenic (growth hormone & dural/corneal transplants)
- variant CJD

Adapted from Dearmond et al (2002).

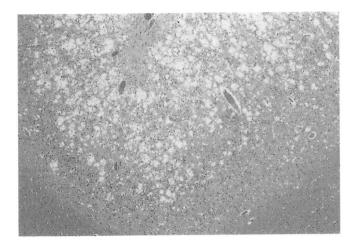

Fig. 4.14
Cerebral cortex from a patient with sporadic Creutzfeldt–Jakob disease, displaying spongiform change throughout the layers of the cortex. Haematoxylin and eosin. Original magnification × 25.

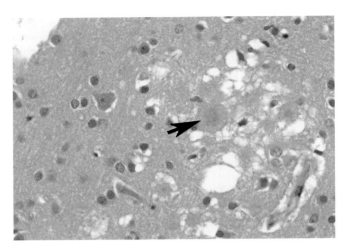

Fig. 4.15
Cerebral cortex from a patient with variant Creutzfeldt–Jakob disease, displaying florid plaques surrounded by spongiform change (arrow). Haematoxylin and eosin. Original magnification × 400.

agent appears to be largely, if not entirely, made up of prion protein.

Prion disorders, and particularly CJD, came to widespread public attention with the appearance of variant CJD (vCJD) in the wake of the UK epidemic of bovine spongiform encephalopathy. The total number of vCJD cases has remained less than originally feared (Brown et al 2001). Affected individuals have generally become symptomatic at a younger age than patients with the sporadic form and have presented with a vague history of psychiatric and emotional disturbance prior to deterioration into a state of akinetic mutism. The reasons for the differences in clinical presentation between sporadic CJD and vCJD are not entirely clear, although the slower progression and the psychiatric presentation in the latter may reflect the more consistent involvement of basal ganglionic structures and the different form of the prion agent involved.

While the pattern of spongiform pathology and prion distribution is variable in sporadic CJD the histological appearances of vCJD are uniformly predictable and consist of widespread florid prion plaques in the cortex (Fig. 4.15). The cerebellum shows a particularly heavy load of prion protein (Fig. 4.16). Reliable laboratory methods to detect PrP^{sc} in tissues include immunocytochemistry, histoblots and Western blots (De Armond et al 2002). These are useful in distinguishing CJD from other dementias which may be associated with cortical spongiform change, including DLB and motor neuron disease with dementia. There is no reliable clinical test for detecting vCJD in the early stages, when mild personality changes may be reported, and it remains a matter of urgency to develop such diagnostic tools. Increased signal in the thalamic pulvinar on magnetic resonance imaging is now used as one of the criteria of vCJD, but this is not always present early in the disease and is not a feature of sporadic CJD. Brain biopsy may be useful in confirming vCJD, which predictably involves all of the cerebral cortex, in contrast to sporadic CJD, in which the focal nature of the cortical changes renders biopsy unreliable. Biopsy may also exclude a treatable cause of dementia. However, surgical instruments have to be destroyed after the biopsy procedure because of the danger of transmitting infection. Detection of

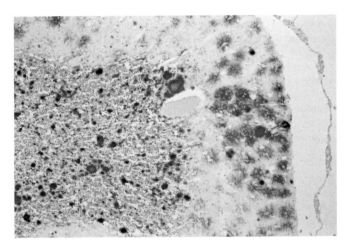

Fig. 4.16
Immunocytochemical staining of the cerebellar cortex from a patient with variant Creutzfeldt–Jakob disease, displaying the heavy load of disease-related prion protein in the molecular and granular layers. Anti-prion protein antibody 3F4. Original magnification × 40.

the 14-3-3 protein in cerebrospinal fluid is helpful but is not specific. Tonsillar tissue and gut-associated lymphoid tissue probably contain detectable prion protein before the onset of symptoms, but biopsy of these tissues is not a practicable option in all young people with new onset of psychiatric symptoms. Development of a suitable clinical test would have the advantage of identifying patients who pose a possible risk to other individuals. While there is no evidence in sporadic CJD that the agent is present in the blood, this remains a possibility in vCJD. Blood donations and contaminated surgical instruments represent the chief concerns for the transmission of human prion diseases during healthcare. As yet there are no effective treatments for these conditions.

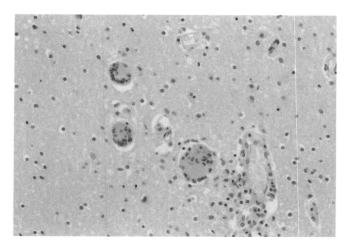

Fig. 4.17
Central white matter from a patient with HIV encephalitis, showing three giant multinucleated cells with hypercellular inflammatory foci made up of microglia, macrophages and lymphocytes. Haematoxylin and eosin. Original magnification × 100.

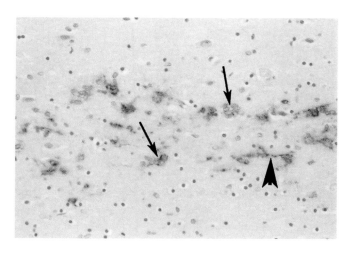

Fig. 4.18
Immunocytochemical staining of grey-matter / white-matter junction in a patient with HIV encephalitis, showing positivity for HIV p24 protein in small giant cells (arrows) and in morphologically normal microglial cells (arrow head). Original magnification × 100.

Mutations in the *PrP* gene, best known at codons 102, 178 and 210, are important factors in inherited prion diseases, but no mutation is present in sporadic CJD or vCJD. The natural valine/methionine polymorphism at codon 129 influences the phenotype of the disease as well as having an apparent effect on vulnerability. All patients with vCJD have been methionine homozygotes up to the present time, and homozygosity at codon 129 is overrepresented among patients with sporadic CJD.

HIV / AIDS

Soon after the onset of the AIDS epidemic, it became apparent that cognitive impairment often amounting to dementia was a prominent complication of HIV/AIDS. The combination of a dementing illness with motor problems was designated the AIDS dementia complex (ADC) in the early 1980s (McArthur 2000). The pathological substrate for this was partially characterised in 1985 when giant cells were identified as the pathognomonic feature of HIV-related infection of the brain (HIV encephalitis, Fig. 4.17). However, the advancing immune suppression which characterises HIV/AIDS also predisposed to a variety of opportunistic infections and CNS lymphoma. Before the advent of effective combination chemotherapy which can halt the decline into advanced immunosuppression, HIV encephalitis was present in up to 40% of subjects with AIDS and frequently accompanied by opportunistic conditions in the brain. Some of these, particularly cytomegalovirus encephalitis, progressive multifocal leukoencephalopathy and CNS lymphoma, could give rise to cognitive impairment in their own right.

The exact relationship between HIV encephalitis and dementia remains poorly understood despite considerable research (Anderson et al 2002). The two conditions may be discordant but, in general, dementia is fairly closely correlated with the presence of HIV encephalitis and a high viral burden within brain tissue. HIV targets microglial cells and macrophages within the CNS through CD4 and chemokine cell surface receptors. Infected microglia probably give rise to giant cells (Fig. 4.18). There is no general agreement that neurons, oligodendrocytes or endothelia can regularly support HIV infection, although there is increasing evidence that astrocytes are restrictedly infected. Considerable neuronal loss is found in AIDS dementia, with evidence of synaptic, dendritic and axonal damage in HIV encephalitis, all leading to brain atrophy. Since neurons are not thought to be a direct target for HIV infection, neurotoxicity in HIV encephalitis may result from viral proteins (gp120 and tat), glutamate, free radicals or nitric oxide, but the favoured theory is exposure to pro-inflammatory cytokines (TNFα and IL-1β) released by activated microglial cells and macrophages. Deprivation of neurotrophic factors and toxic molecules leaking across a deficient blood–brain barrier have also been implicated.

Combined antiretroviral therapy including protease inhibitors is effective in ameliorating or preventing HIV-associated dementia (HAD). However, it is clear that subtle neuropsychological impairment may still occur in treated subjects (Sacktor et al 2002). Whether this relates to lingering inflammation within the brain is not known at present.

Huntington's disease

This autosomal-dominant condition was first described by George Huntington at the end of the 19th century. The prevalence varies between 4 and 7 per 100 000 population. The initial presentation is usually with abnormal choreiform movements, which are followed by dementia. However, younger patients may first present with poverty of movement and rigidity, or an early disturbance of neuropsychological functions. The hyperkinetic form has been linked to maternal transmission, whereas the akinetic form is associated with paternal transmission. The disease is characterised neuropathologically by mild generalised cortical atrophy and much more marked atrophy of the basal ganglia (Fig. 4.19) (Lowe & Leigh 2002). Neuronal loss is detectable in the cerebral cortex but is maximal in the caudate nucleus and

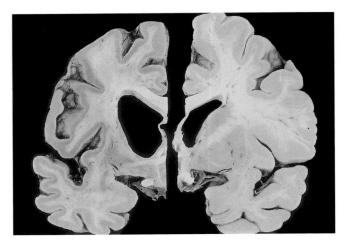

Fig. 4.19
Montage of two half brain slices, comparing the cerebral hemisphere from a patient with Huntington's disease on the left with an age-matched, cognitively normal subject on the right. In Huntington's disease the lateral ventricle is dilated and there is generalised cortical atrophy with specific and severe atrophy in the basal ganglia, such that the lateral margin of the lateral ventricle is no longer convex.

putamen, where microglial activation and severe astrocytosis are also found. The loss of GABA-containing spiny neurons in the caudate and putamen, which project to the lateral globus pallidus, results in decreased inhibitory control of the thalamic nuclei (via subthalamic nuclei, medial globus pallidus and substantia nigra reticularis), which in turn increase their glutamatergic output to the cerebral cortex, leading to choreiform movements.

Following the identification of the *huntingtin* gene on the short arm of chromosome 4, the inherited abnormality has been traced to a variable expansion in a trinucleotide triplet sequence, this expansion leading to accumulation of polyglutamine within the brain. Longer repeats are linked to earlier onset of the disease. The way in which this genetic abnormality is translated into brain-specific cellular pathology is unknown despite intensive study and the development of transgenic mouse models. While it is clear that abnormal huntingtin gives rise to ubiquitin-positive intranuclear inclusions, the presence of these inclusions is not clearly linked to maximal neuronal damage, in that the cortex may show rather numerous inclusions whereas they are sparse in the badly affected basal ganglia. It is also unclear why the systemic expression of huntingtin does not lead to disruption of cellular function in other tissues.

PATHOLOGY OF PSYCHOSES

Schizophrenia

Although there may be diagnostic overlap between schizophrenia and bipolar disorder, the diagnostic criteria are sufficiently distinctive at the two ends of the spectrum to allow for separate investigation of the epidemiology, causation and neuropathology of these two disorders (Esiri & Crow 2002). Each of these disorders has a prevalence of about 1% of the population.

The pathological basis of schizophrenia has been singularly difficult to study. The disease has its onset in young adult life, and

affected individuals are likely to have had symptoms, and been treated with appropriate drug therapy, for a number of years before death and neuropathological analysis. However, detailed neuroimaging studies have clearly identified ventricular dilatation as an early and consistent finding in affected individuals, which is present not only prior to the onset of treatment, but which may also antedate the onset of symptoms (Harrison 1999). The ventricular dilatation is accompanied by cortical diminution, particularly in the medial temporal lobe. Early stages of the disease correlate with decreased brain weight (Johnstone et al 1994).

The identification of families with several affected individuals points to likely genetic factor(s) predisposing to the condition and has allowed detection of at-risk individuals in the preclinical state. Although the responsible genetic factors are only now becoming clearer, this has not prevented longitudinal clinical and neuroimaging studies of the at-risk family members, which have established the presymptomatic characteristics. Some neuroimaging work also reveals that the two hemispheres are usually less asymmetrical than usual. This curious finding appears to represent a loss of the asymmetry which normally exists between cerebral hemispheres and which first appears during fetal life and suggests a very early onset for the structural abnormality which underlies the later appearance of schizophrenia. Pathology studies, insofar as they have contributed to understanding, have been supportive of a fetal origin in that no gliotic reaction has been found in affected brains despite the reduced cortical size. Neuronal arborisation abnormalities rather than reduced neuronal number may underlie the cortical changes. The dorsal thalamus is also smaller than normal. Cortical cytoarchitectural abnormalities have been reported, but further studies are needed to substantiate these. Whether the primary defect is of genetic origin or the result of in-utero environmental influences remains controversial (Weinberger 1995). Recent findings suggest that further neuroimaging abnormalities may be added to the earlier changes as the disorder progresses (Pantelis et al 2003). Susceptibility loci for schizophrenia have been reported on chromosomes 6, 8, 12, 13 and 22, and there is increasing evidence pointing to an association with some specific genes (Harrison & Owen 2003). Although the idea that retroviruses may be involved in schizophrenia has lately tended to be discounted, some recent work has suggested a possible role for reactivated endogenous retroviruses at the onset of disease (Karlsson et al 2001), but this has yet to be replicated.

Bipolar disorders

Ventricular dilatation with accompanying sulcal widening is also present in individuals presenting with mood disorder (Elkis et al 1995, Muller-Oerlinghausen et al 2002). Studies of untreated patients with bipolar disorder suggest reduced levels of serotonin metabolites in the raphe nuclei and the limbic system, implicating the serotonergic system in the pathogenesis, although results have been contradictory (Esiri & Crow 2002). Abnormalities in the size of the amygdala have been reported on neuroimaging (Muller-Oerlinghausen et al 2002). Identification of susceptibility genes for bipolar disorder which were different from those implicated in schizophrenia would support the view that these are independent entities. Borna virus is reportedly detected more commonly in brain tissue of patients with major depression than in control healthy populations, but these findings may represent technical artefacts and await confirmation.

Autism

There have been very few neuropathological studies of this male-predominant psychiatric condition which usually presents in childhood. The ventricles do not appear to be enlarged in this condition and the brain has been variously reported as normal or as enlarged, while there may also be focal atrophy in the parietal lobe and in the cerebellum. The number of brains examined precludes a reliable view of the neuropathological basis of such images. Further study is needed urgently, but the availability of tissue from patients with disorders such as these which arise in childhood is obviously problematic.

CURRENT DEVELOPMENTS IN NEUROPATHOLOGY

Correlation with neuroimaging

Although sophisticated neuroimaging is an almost routine part of the investigation of cognitive decline in current times, it is important to remember that none of these benefits were available just over two decades ago. Before that time, accurate estimation of ventricular size or brain tissue volume was rarely possible in life. The clinical benefits of computerised tomography (CT), magnetic resonance imaging (MRI) and functional imaging have been enormous, and their potential in further research is by no means exhausted. It is salutary to note, however, that while MRI can instantly differentiate an ischaemic from a haemorrhage stroke the images still contain elements which have not yet yielded to neuropathological correlation. These include the hyperintense white-matter foci seen on T2-weighted images in a wide variety of brain disorders.

Neuroimaging both serves and challenges the discipline of neuropathology. While imaging may confirm the global and lobar atrophy which is an expected element of many neurodegenerative conditions, it may also generate condition-specific results which are consistently present and which require investigation. One example of this is the high signal seen on MRI in that part of the posterior part of the thalamus known as the pulvinar, in cases of vCJD. Although this sign is now recognised as part of the diagnostic criteria, the exact pathological substrate remains to be determined; however, astrogliosis is a characteristic feature. The neuroimaging abnormalities in schizophrenia and bipolar disorders are also evolving in that longitudinal studies of individuals who are at risk for these disorders display new features at the time of presentation which are added to the pre-existing abnormalities (Pantelis et al 2003). A loss of the normal asymmetry between cerebral hemispheres, particularly in the temporal lobes, is now well known in schizophrenia. An interesting recent development in AD research is the discovery that ApoE variants influence not only the hippocampal volume (Lehovirta et al 1995) but also the degree of asymmetry (Geroldi et al 2000), according to the different alleles. Functional imaging also provides insights into the pathogenesis of brain disorders. Using cell- and receptor-specific ligands, it is possible to highlight particular brain cell subsets. This approach has revealed that activated microglia appear early in the AD disease process and may not be a merely reactive phenomenon (Cagnin et al 2001).

There are of course limitations to the diagnostic capabilities of neuroimaging. For instance, although ventricular dilatation and reduced periventricular white-matter signal intensity have been attributed to HIV encephalitis, these appearances are actually non-specific and may be present in individuals with opportunistic infections or lymphoma.

Molecular diagnostics

Psychiatric diseases are occasionally the result of a single gene exerting an effect in isolation, and studies of families with many affected members have identified mutations which direct attention to a likely role for particular gene–protein combinations in the causation of disease. Examples include *APP* and *presenilin* mutations in familial early-onset AD. Much more frequently, genes of small effect increase or decrease only slightly the vulnerability of an individual to a particular disorder. The best known example of this phenomenon is the ε4 allele of the *ApoE* gene. While there has been huge progress and a significant number of important gene discoveries in respect of AD, it is now clearer than ever that sporadic AD results from the interaction of a number of different genes which certainly include *APP*, *presenilin-1* and *presenilin-2* and *ApoE* ε4. Others for which there is mounting evidence include *interleukin-1* (IL-1α) and α1 *macroglobulin*. A number of different mutations have been described in the *presenilin-1* gene on chromosome 14. *Presenilin-2* was subsequently located to chromosome 1, and mutations in this gene are a less common cause of autosomal-dominant AD. Research in the molecular biology of AD suggests that the presenilins may equate with γ secretase, which generates amyloid peptide from APP (Selkoe 1999). Very rarely, mutations in the *APP* gene give rise to familial AD. In each of these cases the plaques are largely composed of AB42. With respect to the more common late-onset AD, individuals who are destined to develop AD and who possess *ApoE* ε4 alleles appear to develop the disease at an earlier age than those with non-*ApoE*-ε4 genotypes (Meyer et al 1998). Well over half the population may live to an extreme old age without developing AD, possibly reflecting the relative frequency of *ApoE* ε3 alleles in the population. Conversely not all individuals with an *ApoE* ε4/4 genotype develop AD, which suggests that other gene(s), as yet undiscovered, may be as important for disease susceptibility.

Beta amyloid appears to be central to the pathogenesis of AD. It is now known that the amyloidogenic peptide AB is produced under normal circumstances and is present in serum and CSF but is normally catabolised by an endopeptidase, inhibition of which accelerates AB4 deposition (Selkoe 1999). The normal processing and degradation of proteins is the focus of much current research, with emphasis on extracellular proteases and intracellular proteasomal and aggresomal pathways. It is certainly possible that abnormal protein accumulation is the result of poor degradation as much as overproduction. Molecular neuropathology has made great strides in the field of tau metabolism, and tau immunocytochemistry has widened the focus in neurodegenerative disease beyond neuronal pathology. Tau-positive glial inclusions should not be regarded purely as an adjunct to the pathological subclassification of the tauopathies, and the contribution of glial pathology to the dementing and neurodegenerative illnesses requires urgent further investigation.

The significant developments in molecular pathology in all domains of neurodegenerative disease augur well for similar progress in psychotic illness, although it is difficult to predict when this will happen.

Characterisation of animal models

For some diseases that affect the human nervous system, a naturally occurring animal model has long been known. Scrapie in sheep is a well-known prion disease which displays similar neuropathology to that of affected humans. Animals have also been used in transmissibility and pathogenesis studies in prion diseases and other infective diseases caused by retroviruses resembling HIV. However it is the development of transgenic animals which has made the most significant contribution to the understanding of CNS disease processes. For instance, ubiquitin-positive nuclear inclusions were first identified in transgenic models of Huntington's disease which lead to their discovery in human diseases and the identification of related trinucleotide repeat disorders. Transgenic animal models have been used to elucidate not only the role of genetic mutations in AD and the metabolic relationships of β amyloid and tau protein but also to investigate the therapeutic possibilities. Immunisation of human *APP* transgenic mice with human AB peptide has been shown to lead to clearance of the β amyloid burden in the brain and to reduction in behavioural impairment (Janus et al 2000). Remarkably, antibodies to amyloid peptide administered peripherally to transgenic mice can enter the brain and also induce clearance of β amyloid (Bard et al 2000). Current and future research is likely to solve the remaining uncertainties regarding the exact relationship between β amyloid and tau pathology in AD.

CONCLUSION

The last two decades have seen major advances in the neuropathology of psychiatric disease, particularly in the dementing illnesses. Neuropathology encompasses both a diagnostic and a research role, which is responsive to progress in other disciplines or itself provides the lead. Careful clinicopathological correlation will continue to be a cornerstone of further development in the endeavour to understand why on the one hand a single neuropathological entity such as the pathological lesions of corticobasal degeneration may have diverse clinical symptoms, while on the other hand two different pathological conditions such as AD and frontotemporal dementia may lead to the same cognitive impairment syndrome. Studies of this kind will help to elucidate the proximate cause of cognitive decline in patients who have pathology in their brains.

New approaches are challenging long-held concepts of particular pathogenetic pathways. The recognition that AD is less common in individuals who have been treated long-term with anti-inflammatory drugs raises the possibility that inflammation is a key pathogenetic factor, possibly through activation of microglia and perivascular macrophages, with consequent upregulation of cytokine release within the brain (McGeer & McGeer 1999). This cascade is remarkably reminiscent of HIV-associated dementia. Similarly, reclassification of AD as a vascular dementia may be an unexpected development but, in questioning current thinking, may open fresh lines of enquiry (Vagnucci & Li 2003). Other long-held concepts being challenged include the dogma that neuroregeneration is extremely limited in adult life. The discovery of stem cells holds out the hope for regeneration of functional neuronal circuits possibly by transplantation but also by recruitment from an endogenous source. Before that can occur the effects of deleterious genes and of environmental insults

on the CNS stem cell population will require further study. Dedifferentiation and functional transformation of already committed cells might also be a future goal. Closer to realisation should be the proper understanding of disease processes which still present gaps in knowledge, for example the accumulation and intracellular processing of huntingtin in Huntington's disease. On a wider front, if it became clear that the presence of one pathology such as AD influenced or accelerated the development of another neurodegenerative condition, for instance DLB, this would be significant information in the quest for effective strategies to prevent or halt the progression of neurodegenerative diseases. Symptomatology may be further complicated by comorbid systemic diseases affecting the brain, such as thyrotoxicosis, underlining the requirement to assess the whole patient.

Comparison between different neurodegenerative disorders may also yield insights. It is instructive to compare prion diseases with other amyloidopathies such as AD, although transmissibility of β amyloid, unlike prions, has not been confirmed. Both disorders are commonly sporadic but are familial in 10–15% of cases; both are amyloidopathies, although the amyloid is made up of prion protein in the one and βA4 in the other, and both are associated with microglial inflammation. In each case the insoluble amyloid material is derived from a normal cell surface precursor protein whose function is not yet understood. The difference appears to be that APP gives rise to βA4 far more readily than the corresponding change from PrP^c to PrP^{sc}. However, both events probably occur within the endosome system after internalisation of the relevant cell surface molecule.

Developing classifications of dementia will legitimately be based on disorders of protein metabolism (Table 4.1) at least in part because of implications for therapy. Carefully planned pathology investigation of transgenic animals and of in-vitro models enables the stages of disease progression to be established and may throw light on the earliest stages of many human brain diseases, which remain largely speculative at present. Understanding the steps in the pathway offers a real opportunity for devising new therapies which may ameliorate symptoms or prevent further deterioration. Prevention would allow healthy brain ageing to be achieved. This may be seen as a goal which is relevant only to societies which are sufficiently affluent to be troubled by the diseases of old age. In fact the burden of psychiatric disease is very heavy worldwide, and comparative studies are needed particularly with respect to ethnic and environmental influences which are likely to have an important influence. The genetics of psychiatric disease will remain a major research focus (Owen & Cardno 1999). The point has been made that if the onset of AD could be delayed by 10 years, most of the problem would be eliminated through death from other causes while AD is held at bay by the use of neuroprotective drugs.

In summary, we have moved on from the era when 'the relationship between psychiatry and neuropathology has often tended to be one of frustration bordering on despair' (Lishman 1995), and the future looks bright.

ACKNOWLEDGEMENTS

I acknowledge with gratitude the assistance of colleagues and staff in the Neuropathology Unit in the preparation of this chapter, particularly Ms Angela Penman. Ms Jan Macleod provided invaluable assistance with the illustrations.

REFERENCES

Anderson E, Zink W, Xiong H, Gendelman H E 2002 HIV-1-associated dementia: a metabolic encephalopathy perpetrated by virus-infected and immune-competent mononuclear phagocytes. Journal of AIDS 31: S43–S54

Armstrong R J E, Barker R A 2001 Neurodegeneration: a failure of neuroregeneration? Lancet 358: 1174–1176

Bard F, Cannon C, Barbour R et al 2000 Peripherally administered antibodies against amyloid beta-peptide enter the central nervous system and reduce pathology in a mouse model of Alzheimer disease. Nature Medicine 6(8): 916–919

Bayer T A, Wirths O, Majtenyi K et al 2001 Key factors in Alzheimer's disease: β-amyloid precursor protein processing, metabolism and intraneuronal transport. Brain Pathology 11: 1–11

Bergeron C, Davis A, Lang A E 1998 Corticobasal ganglionic degeneration and progressive supranuclear palsy presenting with cognitive decline. Brain Pathology 8: 355–365

Braak H, Braak E 1989 Cortical and subcortical argyrophilic grains characterize a disease associated with adult onset dementia. Neuropathology & Applied Neurobiology 15(1): 13–26

Braak H, Braak E 1991 Neuropathological stageing of Alzheimer-related changes. Acta Neuropathologica 82: 239–259

Brown P, Will R G, Bradley R et al 2001 Bovine spongiform encephalopathy and variant Creutzfeldt-Jakob disease: background, evolution and current concerns. www.cdc.gov/ncidod/EID/vol7no1/brown.htm; 7(1)

Cagnin A, Brooks D J, Kennedy A M et al 2001 In-vivo measurement of activated microglia in dementia. Lancet 358: 461–467

De Armond S J, Kretzschmar H A, Prusiner S B 2002 Prion diseases. In: Graham D I, Lantos P L (eds) Greenfield's neuropathology. Arnold, London, p 273–323

De La Torre J C 2002 Vascular basis of Alzheimer's pathogenesis. Annals of the New York Academy of Science 977: 196–215

Dickson D W 1998 Pick's disease: a modern approach. Brain Pathology 8(2): 339–354

Dickson D W 2002 Dementia with Lewy bodies: neuropathology. Journal of Geriatric Psychiatry & Neurology 15(4): 210–216

Dickson D W, Liu W, Hardy J et al 1999 Widespread alterations of alpha-synuclein in multiple system atrophy. American Journal of Pathology 155(4): 1241–1251

Dickson D W, Bergeron C, Chin S S et al 2002 Office of Rare Diseases Neuropathologic Criteria for Corticobasal Degeneration. Journal of Neuropathology & Experimental Neurology 61(11): 935–946

Elkis H, Friedman L, Wise A, Meltzer H Y 1995 Meta-analyses of studies of ventricular enlargement and cortical sulcal prominence in mood disorders: Comparisons with controls or patients with schizophrenia. Archives of General Psychiatry 52: 735–746

Esiri M M, Crow T J 2002 Neuropathology of psychiatric disorders. In: Graham DI, Lantos PL (eds) Greenfield's neuropathology. Arnold, London, p 431–470

Esiri M M, Nagy Z, Smith M Z et al 1999 Cerebrovascular disease and threshold for dementia in the early stages of Alzheimer's disease. Lancet 354: 919–920

Geroldi C, Laakso M P, DeCarli C et al 2000 Apolipoprotein E genotype and hippocampal asymmetry in Alzheimer's disease: a volumetric MRI study. Journal of Neurology, Neurosurgery & Psychiatry 68: 93–96

Glickman M H, Ciechanover A 2002 The ubiquitin-proteasome proteolytic pathway: destruction for the sake of construction. Physiology Review 82(2): 373–428

Halliday G, Ng T, Rodriguez M et al 2002 Consensus neuropathological diagnosis of common dementia syndromes: testing and standardising the use of multiple diagnostic criteria. Acta Neuropathologica 104(1): 72–78

Hamilton R L 2000 Lewy bodies in Alzheimer's disease: a neuropathological review of 145 cases using α-synuclein immunohistochemistry. Brain Pathology 10: 378–384

Harrison P J, Owen M J 2003 Genes for schizophrenia? Recent findings and their pathophysiological implications. Lancet 361: 417–419

Harrison P J 1999 The neuropathology of schizophrenia: A critical review of the data and their interpretation. Brain 122: 593–624

Hashimoto M, Masliah E 1999 Alpha-synuclein in Lewy body disease and Alzheimer's disease. Brain Pathology 9: 707–720

Hofman A, Rocca W A, Brayne C et al 1991 The prevalence of dementia in Europe: a collaborative study of 1980–1990 findings. Eurodem prevalence research group. International Journal of Epidemiology 20(3): 736–748

Hyman B, Trojanowski J Q 1997 Editorial on consensus recommendations for the post mortem diagnosis of Alzheimer disease for the National Institute on Aging and the Reagan Institute Working Group on diagnostic criteria for the neuropathological assessment of Alzheimer disease. Journal of Neuropathology & Experimental Neurology 56(10): 1095–1097

Ince P G, Perry E K, Morris C M 1998 Dementia with Lewy bodies: A distinct non-Alzheimer dementia syndrome? Brain Pathology 8: 299–324

Jackson M, Lennox G, Lowe J 1996 Motor neurone disease-inclusion dementia. Neurodegeneration 5(4): 339–350

Jagust W 2001 Untangling vascular dementia. Lancet 358: 2097–2098

Janus C, Pearson J, McLaurin J et al 2000 Aβ peptide immunization reduces behavioural impairment and plaques in a model of Alzheimer's disease. Nature 408: 979–985

Jellinger K A, Bancher C 1998 Senile dementia with tangles (tangle predominant form of senile dementia). Brain Pathology 8: 367–376

Johnstone E C, Brunton C J, Crow T J et al 1994 Clinical correlates of postmortem brain changes in schizophrenia: decreased brain weight and length correlate with indices of early impairment. Journal of Neurology, Neurosurgery & Psychiatry 57(4): 474–479

Karlsson H, Bachmann S, Schroder J et al 2001 Retroviral RNA identified in the cerebrospinal fluids and brains of individuals with schizophrenia. Proceedings of the National Academy of Sciences of the USA 98(8): 4634–4639

Khachaturian Z S 1985 Diagnosis of Alzheimer's disease. Archives of Neurology 42(11): 1097–1105

Knopman D S, Mastri A R, Frey W H et al 1990 Dementia lacking distinctive histologic features: a common non-Alzheimer degenerative dementia. Neurology 40(2): 251–256

Lee V M, Goedert M, Trojanowski J Q 2001 Neurodegenerative taupathies. Annual Review of Neuroscience 24: 1121–1159

Lehovirta M, Laakso M P, Soininen H et al 1995 Volumes of hippocampus, amygdala and frontal lobe in Alzheimer patients with different Apolipoprotein E genotypes. Neuroscience 67(1): 65–72

Lishman W A 1995 Psychiatry and neuropathology: the maturing of a relationship. Journal of Neurology, Neurosurgery & Psychiatry 58: 284–292

Lomas D A, Carrell R W 2002 Serpinopathies and the conformational dementias. Nature Reviews Genetics 3(10): 759–768

Lowe J S 1998 Establishing a pathological diagnosis in degenerative dementias. Brain Pathology 8: 403–406

Lowe J S, Leigh N 2002 Disorders of movement and system degenerations. In: Graham D I, Lantos P L (eds) Greenfield's neuropathology. Arnold, London, p 325–430

McArthur J C 2000 HIV-associated dementia. In: Davis L E, Kennedy P G E (eds) Infectious diseases of the nervous system. Butterworth-Heinemann, Oxford, p 165–213

McGeer P L, McGeer E G 1999 Inflammation of the brain in Alzheimer's disease: implications for therapy. Journal of Leukocyte Biology 65: 409–415

McKeith I G, Galasko D, Kosaka K et al 1996 Consensus guidelines for the clinical and pathologic diagnosis of dementia with Lewy bodies (DLB): report of the consortium on DLB international workshop. Neurology 47(5): 1113–1124

Meyer M R, Tschanz J T, Norton M C et al 1998 ApoE genotype predicts when – not whether – one is predisposed to develop Alzheimer disease. Nature Genetics 19: 321–322

Middleton F A, Strick P L 1994 Anatomical evidence for cerebellar and basal ganglia involvement in higher cognitive function. Science 266: 458–461

Mirra S S, Hyman B T 2002 Ageing and dementia. In: Graham D I, Lantos P L (eds) Greenfield's neuropathology. Arnold, London, p 195–271

Mirra S S, Heyman A, McKeel D et al 1991 The consortium to establish a registry for Alzheimer's disease (CERAD). Part II: Standardisation of the neuropathologic assessment of Alzheimer's disease. Neurology 41: 479–486

Mrak R E, Griffin W S 2000 Interleukin-1 and the immunogenetics of Alzheimer disease. Journal of Neuropathology & Experimental Neurology 59(6): 471–476

Muller-Oerlinghausen B, Berghofer A, Bauer M 2002 Bipolar disorder. Lancet 359: 241–247

Neuropathology Group of the Medical Research Council Cognitive Function & Ageing Study (MRC CFAS) 2001 Pathological correlates of late-onset dementia in a multicentre, community-based population in England and Wales. Lancet 357: 169–175

Newell K L, Hyman B, Growdon J H, Hedley-Whyte E T 1999 Application of the National Institute on Aging (NIA)–Reagan Institute criteria for the neuropathological diagnosis of Alzheimer disease. Journal of Neuropathology & Experimental Neurology 58(11): 1147–1155

Owen M J, Cardno A G 1999 Psychiatric genetics: progress, problems, and potential. Lancet 354: 11–14

Palmer K, Backman L, Winbald B, Fratiglioni L 2003 Detection of Alzheimer's disease and dementia in the preclinical phase: population based cohort study. British Medical Journal 326: 245–247

Pantelis C, Velakoulis D, McGorry P D et al 2003 Neuroanatomical abnormalities before and after onset of psychosis: a cross-sectional and longitudinal MRI comparison. Lancet 361: 281–288

Ritchie K, Lovestone S 2002 The dementias. Lancet 360: 1759–1766

Sacktor N, McDermott M P, Marder K et al 2002 HIV-associated cognitive impairment before and after the advent of combination therapy. Journal of Neurovirology 8: 136–142

Saunders A M 2000 Apolipoprotein E and Alzheimer disease: an update on genetic and functional analyses. J Neuropathol Exp Neurol 59(9): 751–758

Selkoe D J 1999 Translating cell biology into therapeutic advances in Alzheimer's disease. Nature 399: A23–A31

Sheedy D, Lara A, Garrick T, Harper C 1999 Size of mamillary bodies in health and disease: useful measurements in neuroradiological diagnosis of Wernicke's encephalopathy. Alcoholism, Clinical & Experimental Research 23(10): 1624–1628

Steindler D A, Pincus D W 2002 Stem cells and neuropoiesis in the adult human brain. Lancet 359: 1047–1054

Teller J K, Russo C, De Busk L M et al 1996 Presence of soluble amyloid β-peptide precedes amyloid plaque formation in Down's syndrome. Nature Medicine 2: 93–95

Tolnay M, Probst A 1999 Review: Tau protein pathology in Alzheimer's disease and related disorders. Neuropathology & Applied Neurobiology 25: 171–187

Trojanowski J Q, Dickson D W 2001 Update on the neuropathological diagnosis of frontotemporal dementias. Journal of Neuropathology & Experimental Neurology 60(12): 1123–1126

Vagnucci A H, Li W W 2003 Alzheimer's disease and angiogenesis. Lancet 361: 605–608

Weinberger D R 1995 From neuropathology to neurodevelopment. Lancet 346: 552–557

Wilson C A, Doms R W, Lee V M-Y 1999 Intracellular APP processing and Aβ production in Alzheimer disease. Journal of Neuropathology & Experimental Neurology 58(8): 787–794

FURTHER READING

Dickson D (vol ed) 2003 Neurodegeneration: The molecular pathology of dementia and movement disorders. IARC Press, Lyon

Esiri M M, Morris J H 1997 The neuropathology of dementia. Cambridge University Press, Cambridge

Farrer L A, Cupples L A, Haines J L et al 1997 Effects of age, sex, and ethnicity on the association between apolipoprotein E genotype and Alzheimer disease: a meta-analysis. ApoE and Alzheimer Disease Meta Analysis Consortium. Journal of the American Medical Association 278(16): 1349–1356

Graham D I, Lantos P L (eds) 2002 Greenfield's neuropathology, 7th edn. Arnold, London

Greicius M D, Geschwind M D, Miller B L 2002 Presenile dementia syndromes: an update on taxonomy and diagnosis. Journal of Neurology, Neurosurgery & Psychiatry 72: 691–700

McNaught K St P, Shashidharan P, Perl D P et al 2002 Agresome-related biogenesis of Lewy bodies. European Journal of Neuroscience 16(11): 2136–2148

Prusiner S B (ed) 1999 Prion biology and diseases. Cold Spring Harbor Laboratory Press, Cold Spring Harbor

5 | Neuroimaging

J Douglas Steele, Stephen M Lawrie

INTRODUCTION

Psychiatric disorders are increasingly recognised as being associated with disturbances of brain structure and function. This view has received considerable support over the past thirty years from an increasing array of sophisticated and complementary neuroimaging methods. There is now a substantial imaging literature on many psychiatric disorders, which has generated several replicated findings. Refinements of techniques and their application to particular populations may provide further insight into the pathophysiology of these disorders in the coming years. Additionally, they are likely to help in the delineation of endophenotypes, facilitating the application of molecular biological techniques.

The first section of the present chapter describes briefly the principles of the main methods of neuroimaging currently used, their limitations, applications and potential, as well as methods of image analysis. The second section summarises the main findings obtained by applying these techniques to the study of particular psychiatric disorders and identifies some important questions to be addressed in the future.

Structural techniques — computerised tomography (CT), structural magnetic resonance imaging (sMRI) and magnetic resonance spectroscopy (MRS) — are reviewed first; followed by an account of the main functional imaging methods — single photon emission (computed) tomography (SPECT), positron emission tomography (PET), functional MRI (fMRI) and some of the relevant electrophysiological methods.

Only an introduction to these techniques can be provided here. For a more detailed discussion the reader is referred to other texts (George et al 1991, Toga & Mazziotta 1996, Webb 1996, Frackowiak et al 1997, Mitchell 1999, Moonen & Bandettini 2000).

PRINCIPLES OF NEUROIMAGING

STRUCTURAL IMAGING

The first attempts at imaging brain structure in vivo were conducted using pneumoencephalography. After lumbar puncture, cerebrospinal fluid (CSF) was withdrawn and replaced with a gas, usually air, to outline the cerebral ventricles and cortical surface using X-ray roentgenography. The technique was first applied to psychiatric patients by Jacobi & Winkler in 1927, who described an apparent loss of brain tissue in schizophrenia. Enlarged lateral and third ventricles, as well as widened cortical sulci, proved to be widely replicated findings (Haug 1982), but the risks and discomfort involved in pneumoencephalography meant that it could not be used extensively.

X-ray computerised tomography (CT)

Principles

Compared with pneumoencephalography, CT is a relatively safe and non-invasive method of imaging the brain, and it has presented clinicians and researchers with many new opportunities. X-rays are detected using various methods, e.g. sodium iodide crystals and photomultiplier tubes. CT images are obtained from the reconstruction of X-ray transmission from multiple projections around the object of interest.

Limitations

A major limitation of CT scanning arises from the absorption of lower-energy X-ray photons as they pass through tissue, so that the beam becomes composed of higher-energy rays ('beam hardening'). The effect is loss of contrast next to bony structures, such as the petrous bones surrounding the posterior fossa. An additional limitation of CT is the relatively poor spatial resolution it affords for tissues such as brain. For these reasons, most authorities have concluded that CT does not provide sufficiently detailed information on regional brain abnormalities, particularly for research studies. Nevertheless, CT remains a commonly used technique, since it is readily available.

Utility

CT was developed in 1971 (Hounsfield 1973), and clinical studies began soon after. The first use of the technique in patients with schizophrenia followed, when the outline of the ventricles and the brain were traced onto graph paper and the ventricle:brain ratio (VBR) was calculated (Johnstone et al 1976).

CT continues to be useful in detecting space-occupying lesions and in the differential diagnosis of stroke. Any calcification, for example, in the basal ganglia is easily observed. The extent of atrophy and ventriculomegaly in dementia overlap with that in the general population, but some treatable causes of dementia can be identified.

A number of macroscopic abnormalities (e.g. usually benign tumours, cysts, vascular malformations) are occasionally found in psychotic patients — with a prevalence of approximately 5–10%.

Table 5.1 Comparison of X-ray CT and structural MRI		
	CT	MRI
Maximum number of examinations	Limited by radiation dose	No limit
Soft tissue contrast	1–2%	100–200%
Spatial resolution	> 1 mm	< 1 mm
Imaging plane	As patient position	Any
Bone signal	Strong	Low
Posterior fossa visibility	Poor	Good

However, these appear to have no specific relationship to particular disorders, are as often developmental as acquired and rarely change medical management (Lawrie et al 1997).

The considerable methodological problems associated with CT mean that this technique is now of limited research value in comparison with structural magnetic resonance imaging (see Table 5.1).

Structural magnetic resonance imaging (sMRI)

Principles

MRI uses signals from protons — usually the hydrogen nucleus in water. An isolated proton can be considered as a charge rotating about a randomly orientated axis (Fig. 5.1a). When an external magnetic field (B_0) is applied, the axis of rotation (p) aligns along the axis of the field but rotating about it (Fig. 5.1b). This rotation is termed *precession* or *resonance*. The resonance frequency is the product of the magnetic field strength (B_0) and the 'gyromagnetic ratio'.

When many protons are present, there is a net alignment along the magnetic field. The effect of this alignment is that the magnetic fields from the protons add up to produce a measurable signal (M). Only the component of M at right angles to B_0 (in the transverse xy plane) is measurable, so to measure M it is necessary to temporarily tilt (or flip) M away from B_0 (Fig. 5.1c). The magnitude of this effect is referred to as the flip angle. It is achieved by brief application of a resonant radio-frequency (RF) pulse.

T1 image contrast Following the RF pulse, transverse magnetisation returns towards the longitudinal plane (axis of B_0) over a period of time known as the T1 relaxation time (Fig. 5.2a). This period is also known as the *spin-lattice* or longitudinal relaxation time. T1 differs between tissues, such differences being exposed by choice of image acquisition parameters, leading to image contrast.

To obtain an image, it is usually necessary to repeatedly apply RF pulses. The reason is that spatial information is encoded using magnetic gradients in three dimensions. RF pulses have to be applied in a series, each with different values of the encoding gradients. The time between each pulse is called the repetition time (TR). For any two tissues with different T1s, there is an optimal TR that produces best image contrast. Additionally, for any given TR there is an optimal flip angle, which maximises signal strength.

Clinically, T1 images provide good grey–white matter contrast and therefore anatomical information.

T2 image contrast Tilting M results in a rotational component in the xy plane, which is measurable and termed an *echo*. Initially, all the proton axes are essentially rotating together (in phase) but begin to rotate at different speeds (dephasing), result-

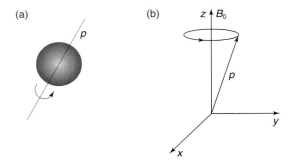

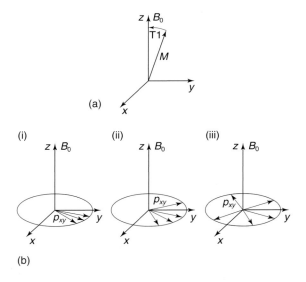

Fig. 5.1
(a) Proton represented as a spherical rotating charge with axis p; (b) precession of p about z due to B_0; (c) tilt of p by external radio-frequency pulse.

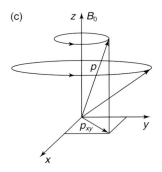

Fig. 5.2
(a) T1 relaxation time: time for M to realign with z axis; (b) T2 relaxation time: dephasing of p_{xy} from (i) to (iii), causing loss of signal M_{xy}.

ing in a loss of transverse M and therefore signal over a period termed T2 or the 'transverse magnetisation time' (Fig. 5.2b). This period is also known as the *spin–spin* relaxation time. Note that T2 is less than or equal to T1. The interval between the creation of transverse magnetisation and its measurement is the echo time (TE). Not all tissues exhibit differences in T2 but, for those that do so, an optimal TE exists and provides the best image contrast.

T2-weighted images are particularly useful for imaging pathological processes in the brain. Such processes include white matter hyperintensities, demyelination, infarction or haemorrhage.

T2* images If the applied magnetic field varies from proton to proton, protons exposed to higher magnetic fields resonate faster, and vice versa. This causes dephasing and accelerated loss of transverse magnetisation (and therefore signal). Such magnetic field variation can be due to air-containing cavities in the head, such as frontal sinuses and ear canals. As the head has different magnetic properties to air, the cavities create magnetic fields (such creation being termed 'susceptibility') in adjacent brain tissue.

The consequence is signal loss and displacement in regions such as the orbitofrontal cortex and inferior temporal lobe: this is known as the 'susceptibility artefact'. The combined decay of transverse magnetisation from T2 relaxation and magnetic field heterogeneity is termed T2* relaxation.

Diffusion tensor imaging (DTI) Water is ubiquitous in biological tissue and is constantly in random Brownian motion. Such random movement is constrained by anatomical structures such as fibre tracts. Using MRI, it is possible to measure water molecule diffusion along three orthogonal dimensions in each voxel (volume element). This 'diffusion tensor imaging' (DTI) technique produces summary measures of mean diffusion and anisotropy, which can be presented as images, allowing inferences about the integrity of structural connections.

Different graphical methods can be used for display. One method is an 'ellipsoid plot', where the extent and direction of diffusion at each voxel is shown. Other methods allow 'surface rendering' of fibre tracts, i.e. viewing tracts constructed as solid objects in relevant parts of the brain. While these techniques are visually appealing, any structural abnormalities of connections relevant to psychiatric research are likely to be subtle and require quantitative analysis. Only now are such methods being developed (see e.g. Burns et al, 2003).

Magnetic resonance spectroscopy (MRS) In a molecule, nuclei are shielded from an external applied magnetic field (B_0) by the electron cloud of other atoms. This shielding also creates small additional magnetic fields characteristic of an atom's position in the molecule. This difference in magnetic field causes a shift in resonance frequency, which can be measured and presented as a magnetic resonance spectrum (Fig. 5.3), allowing identification of certain biochemicals.

Table 5.2 lists some of the more commonly used nuclei in MRS and their biological significance. Current limitations of MRS include relatively poor spatial resolution with consequent partial volume effects, long data acquisition times and the susceptibility artefact. Nevertheless it remains a promising technique.

Limitations

MRI is sensitive to subject movement, and this can cause image blurring (such sensitivity being a reflection of relatively long image acquisition times). Various methods have been developed to reduce this movement, including head restraint, and cardiac and respiratory 'gating' of image acquisition (i.e. only acquiring images at the same point in the cardiac or respiratory cycle). T2* weighted images are subject to signal loss in brain regions of particular interest to psychiatric research: orbitofrontal and adjacent subgenual

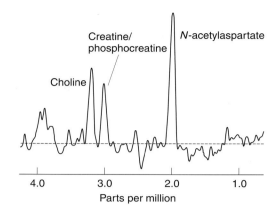

Fig. 5.3
Magnetic resonance spectrum. (Courtesy of Dr I Marshall, Western General Hospital, Edinburgh.)

Table 5.2 Some nuclei commonly used in magnetic resonance spectroscopy	
Nucleus	**Use**
^{19}F	Labelled drugs
^{1}H	Glutamate, lactate, choline, creatine
^{7}Li	Allows monitoring of lithium treatment
^{23}Na	Intra- and extracellular measurement
^{31}P	ATP/ADP energy measurement

anterior cingulate, temporal lobe and perhaps brainstem. Methods are available, however, to reduce the signal loss (Lipschutz et al 2001)

Subjects must be excluded from any MRI studies if they have any implanted metallic objects, such as a cardiac pacemaker, cerebral aneurism clips or metallic fragments from an accident.

Utility

MRI is the structural imaging modality of choice because of its high spatial resolution, improved soft tissue contrast and absence of ionising radiation. MRI has replaced X-ray CT for research work and is preferred for most routine clinical work, although CT continues to be used (see comments above).

FUNCTIONAL IMAGING

Kety and Schmidt were the first to develop, in the 1940s, a feasible method of in-vivo examination of putative 'metabolic derangements' of the brain. They used invasive measures with nitrous oxide, as a diffusible inert index of arterial and venous blood flow (brain uptake being the difference between the two), but could only examine global cerebral blood flow and oxygen consumption and did not find any differences between patients with schizophrenia and normal controls. Many years were to pass before technological advances allowed a greater exploitation of the potential of functional imaging in psychiatric disorders.

This section begins with a discussion of neuroenergetics — the study of the physiological basis of the functional imaging signals.

Following this, the main functional imaging techniques themselves will be discussed.

Neuroenergetics

PET and functional MR images are assumed to reflect neuronal activity, but do so indirectly, through measurement of blood flow and metabolism. Generally it is assumed that increased blood flow itself is a response to increased metabolic demand of active neurons. However, the molecular mechanisms associated with these demands remain unclear, and are consequently a source of some controversy. *Neuroenergetics* is defined here as the study of these issues and their effects on functional imaging signals. Only a brief introduction can be presented. For further discussion the reader is referred to other texts (Moonen & Bandettini 2000, Frackowiak et al 2001).

PET and fMRI are based on different physics (see below): PET on radioactive decay, fMRI on dynamic radio-frequency pulses in a static magnetic field. Using different isotopes, PET allows measurement of the following physiological cerebral indices:

- blood flow (CBF);
- oxygen extraction fraction (OEF);
- blood volume (CBV);
- glucose metabolic rate (CMR_{gluc}).

The rate of oxygen metabolism ($CMRO_2$) is derived from CBF, OEF and CBV. The commonest method of fMRI is blood oxygen level dependent (BOLD) contrast (see later) which measures the differential properties of deoxygenated and oxygenated haemoglobin. The amount of the former depends on arterial CBF, $CMRO_2$ and CBV (Frackowiak et al 2001).

This coupling between neuronal activity and energy metabolism is the basis of PET and fMRI image interpretation. Fortunately, although both imaging techniques are only *indirect* measures of neuronal activity, *very similar results* have been obtained when similar questions have been addressed (Frackowiak et al 2001).

The point of the above discussion is to emphasise that there is not a simple relationship between 'brain activation' and underlying neuronal activity. Perhaps the single most important practical implication of this complex relationship is as follows. Many different aspects of brain function, such as synaptic excitation, synaptic inhibition, neuronal soma action potentials and subthreshold depolarisation, are translated into just one dimension of metabolic and haemodynamic response according to energy need. Both inhibitory as well as excitatory events may induce increased energy need (Moonen & Bandettini 2000).

Thus, functional brain images are ambiguous with regard to the underlying neurophysiological events. A region of a functional image that is 'activated' may reflect inhibitory and/or excitatory neuronal events. 'Deactivation' of a region reflects a lack of both categories of neuronal events, relative to the comparison condition.

Single photon emission (computed) tomography (SPECT)

Principles

Image acquisition For SPECT imaging, a radioactive tracer substance is administered, with minimal environmental stimulation (sometimes with ears and eyes patched) and subjects are asked to remain physically inactive during the equilibration period. Most research studies now include some type of sensory, motor or cognitive activation paradigm, or pharmacological stimulation, as the main purpose of the study. For routine clinical studies, such paradigms or stimulation are not usually used.

Radiopharmaceuticals for SPECT scanning are of four main types. In all cases however, the radioisotopes emit a single gamma ray per nuclear disintegration. (In contrast, positron emission tomography (see later) involves the use of different radioisotopes which emit positrons, leading to the creation of pairs of gamma rays.)

Dynamic or *diffusible* indicators, such as inhaled [133]Xe (10 mCi/minute), are relatively cheap and can give absolute or quantitative regional cerebral blood flow (rCBF) values (in ml/min/100 g brain tissue) as long as tracer input is measured. However, their low energy (80 keV) limits resolution. This is further limited by SPECT's tendency to overestimate high blood flows (especially in white matter) and an insensitivity to small activity differences at high perfusion, leading to limited grey–white matter resolution. Inferior frontal regions can also be contaminated by inhaled gas in the nasal passages and cause a false 'hyperfrontality'.

[123]*I-labelled lipophilics*, such as IMP ([123]I N-isopropyl p-iodoamphetamine), generate high-energy gamma rays (159 keV) with enhanced photopeak detection and resolution, but may only accurately reflect rCBF for 60 minutes after injection, because of redistribution (despite radioactive half-lives of 13 hours). They perform better at high rCBF than hexamethylpropyleneamine oxime (HMPAO) but are no longer widely used, as iodination requires a cyclotron and equilibration of the 3–5 mCi (111–185 MBq) dose takes longer.

Thirdly, [99m]*Tc-labelled lipophilics*, such as ^{99m}Tc-HMPAO (technetium-hexamethylpropyleneamine oxime/exametazime), are widely available and extensively used as they have a similar distribution but are less expensive than ^{123}I lipophilics. The 10–20 mCi (370–740 MBq) dose needs only 1–2 minutes for uptake, and the half-life is only 6 hours. The main problem with HMPAO is pronounced back-diffusion in high flow regions, which, combined with higher extraction in low flow areas, can result in poor contrast.

Finally, [123]*I-labelled neuroreceptor* ligands (see Table 5.3) have limited availability and are expensive as they require a cyclotron for their manufacture.

Instrumentation Contemporary machines use a rotating gamma camera with multiple detectors, which can generate contiguous brain sections with good resolution. Gamma cameras are composed of a lead collimator with a sodium iodide crystal. The origin of the single gamma rays emitted by the radiotracer is calculated from their trajectory through parallel holes in the collimator, which only lets photons from a certain direction

Table 5.3 Commonly used receptor ligands for SPECT	
Receptor	Ligand
Muscarinic	[123]I Quinuclidinyl-iodobenzilate
GABA	[123]I Iomazenil
Dopamine D_1/D_2	[123]I Iodobenzamide (IBZM)
5HT/DA transporter	[123]I 2-β-carbomethoxy-3-β-(4-iodophenyl)-tropane (β-CIT)

through, absorbing the others and thereby 'focusing' the detection. The sodium iodide crystal scintillates (produces small flashes of light) on contact with gamma rays; the light signals are then amplified by photomultiplier tubes and recorded.

Image processing After acquisition, the data are processed with a 'filtered back-projection' technique. Excessive or inadequate filtering will reduce image resolution. Signal attenuation is corrected by reference to a model, which assumes scatter is homogenous within an ellipsoid brain. Reconstructed axial sections can then be displayed, which can be qualitatively (visually) assessed, but further processing is necessary for quantitative analysis (see below).

Limitations

Methodological artefacts may arise as a result of differences in scanning protocol. Even having the eyes open or closed may alter rCBF symmetry and reproducibility, in that the more 'physiological' condition of eyes open may give more reproducible results, with less variability, as long as stimulation is minimised. The spatial resolution with SPECT is typically about 8–12 mm (though better than this for the most modern systems). Spatial resolution is to some extent limited, compared with PET, by scattering and collimator performance.

Utility

The latest SPECT systems have a resolution approaching that of PET; and ligand studies of neuroreceptor binding remain of great research interest. Clinically, SPECT is particularly sensitive to some pathology, including epileptic foci and arteriovenous malformations, which are associated with altered blood flow and metabolism. SPECT can usefully inform the differential diagnosis of dementia, particularly in differentiating dementia and depression in old age. Qualitative visual inspection of scans is unreliable except in the most dramatic cases, but clinical applications of quantitative methods show much potential (see below).

The SPECT image reflects the blood flow distribution at the time of radioactive tracer injection, not scanning (cf. PET and fMRI later). This is because the tracer acts like a tag delivered to brain tissue and remains there for some time. This can be a considerable advantage in situations where it would be otherwise impossible to do PET or fMRI scanning, e.g. during active physical exercise.

Positron emission tomography (PET)

Principles

As discussed earlier, PET allows measurement of the following physiological cerebral indices: CBF, OEF, CBV and CMR_{gluc}. In addition, the technique can also be used to investigate various types of receptor binding and occupancy. A PET scanner uses a ring of radiation detectors to produce images of the distribution of radio-isotopes in the brain. The isotopes are usually labelled with one of four radionuclides — ^{11}C, ^{13}N, ^{15}O or ^{18}F — which are unstable, have an excess of protons and emit positrons during radioactive decay.

Positrons travel a distance of 1–3 mm before losing kinetic energy and colliding with an electron, with the consequent emission of two 511 keV gamma ray photons at 180 degrees to each other. Coincidence detectors respond to two simultaneous

(within 5–20 ns) photons travelling in opposite directions. In fact, due to conservation of momentum, the photons do not quite travel at 180 degrees, but for practical reasons it is necessary to make this assumption. The consequence is a finite limit on the ultimate spatial resolution of PET — to about 2–3 mm.

The brain image is reconstructed from a filtered back-projection algorithm of all these coincidence lines, with filtering ('smoothing') chosen to balance spatial resolution against statistical noise and edge effects. PET measurements of metabolism depend on the observation that the functional capacity of the adult brain is almost entirely dependent on oxidative glucose consumption (see Ch. 3). It should be noted though that the usual tight coupling between regional cerebral blood flow (rCBF) and oxygen extraction is loosened in some acute diseases and by acute physiological stimulation.

Limitations

The PET signal is very sensitive to various activation effects. This is a strength of the technique but easily becomes a limitation if tasks are poorly designed and applied in small numbers of unmatched subjects. There is an age-related decline in blood flow to grey matter, frontal metabolism appears to decrease from an early age, and dopamine receptor numbers fall by approximately 10% per decade. The greatest limitations of PET are: (i) the tracers and ligands require an on-site cyclotron for their manufacture, which is expensive to run, and (ii) patients are exposed to radioactivity, thus limiting the total number of scanning sessions for each subject. Of course, the significance of the latter consideration depends on other factors such as reproductive status and age of patient. Despite this, PET is likely to remain a research tool.

Utility

Particular nuclides are incorporated into specific compounds for use in different techniques for determining metabolism. ^{15}O has a half-life of only 2 minutes — which makes it ideal for activation studies, by allowing multiple scans and sequential activations in the same session. Specific functional anatomy in adjacent brain areas can be discerned by appropriate subtractions from baseline activity.

In addition, PET can be employed to determine neurotransmitter turnover, by administering a radioactive substrate such as fluorodopa, and receptor quantification by a variety of techniques involving labelled ligands (see Table 5.4). In-vivo receptor density measurement can be undertaken by either single-dose tracer kinetics or saturation analysis at equilibrium.

Table 5.4	Commonly used receptor ligands for PET
Receptor	Ligand
Muscarinic	^{11}C-scopolamine
Benzodiazepine	^{18}F-flumazenil
Dopamine D_2/D_3	^{11}C-raclopride
Dopamine $D_2/D_3/D_4$	^{11}C-3*N*-methylspiperone (NMSP)
5HT$_2$	^{11}C-ketanserin and ^{18}F-setoperone
Presynaptic dopamine synthesis	^{18}F-fluorodopa

Table 5.5 Comparison of SPECT and PET methods

	SPECT	PET
Running costs	Low (radiopharmacist)	High (cyclotron)
Repeatable	Once or twice per session	Up to 12 times per session
rCBF quantifiable	Some tracers	Yes
Scattered photons	Removed with energy filter	Do not produce coincidence events
Attentuation correction	Modelled	Empirical
Resolution	8–12 mm, limited by Compton scatter and collimator performance	3–4 mm, limited by distance between positron emission and annihilation reaction
Radiation energy	Lower (75–160 keV)	Higher (511 keV)
Tracer half-lives	Long (6–13 hours)	Short (2–110 mins)

In studies of dopamine receptors, kinetic studies use ^{11}C-N-methylspiperone (NMSP) or one of its analogues, while saturation experiments use ^{11}C-raclopride. These techniques can also be employed to estimate the receptor occupancy of different medications as used in clinical practice. A comparison of PET and SPECT methods is summarised in Table 5.5.

Functional MRI (fMRI)

Principles

Blood oxygen level dependent (BOLD) fMRI Brain function is anatomically segregated. As discussed earlier, fMRI can detect metabolic and haemodynamic changes secondary to alterations in neuronal activity. The coupling between neuronal activity and haemodynamic change is tight but slow (seconds) compared with neuronal events (tens of ms). BOLD fMRI uses the endogenous contrast agent deoxyhaemoglobin as a source of contrast, since the ferrous iron has different magnetic properties depending on whether it is bound to oxygen or not. This difference can be detected by T2* imaging (although susceptibility artefacts may be present).

As previously discussed, fMRI images are ambiguous with regard to the underlying neurophysiological events. However, other knowledge, such as from depth electrode studies in animals, may be used to assist interpretation of human fMRI studies and help resolve such ambiguity (Moonen & Bandettini 2000).

Arterial spin labelling (ASL) fMRI. Arterial spin labelling is a promising alternative to BOLD fMRI. The ASL signal results from the delivery of magnetically tagged water to the region of brain being imaged. Exchange of arterial water with neuronal tissue is rapid but, because of the large tissue compartment, clearance is slower. As the ASL signal is localised to neuronal tissue of interest, in contrast to the predominantly venous BOLD signal, ASL may theoretically provide better maps of functional brain activity. However, multislice ASL imaging is significantly slower than BOLD fMRI, and so the latter currently remains the fMRI technique of choice (Moonen & Bandettini 2000).

Limitations

fMRI has few general limitations additional to those already mentioned for structural MRI. However BOLD fMRI does appear to be particularly sensitive to subject movement. For various reasons, ASL should be much less sensitive to movement artefact (Moonen & Bandettini 2000) than BOLD; however, this

has not yet been achieved in practice. One major limitation of fMRI is that it is not possible to study ligand binding effects directly. PET or SPECT remain the techniques of choice for such studies.

A further limitation of fMRI is that scanners tend to have particularly enclosed spaces, and there is considerable noise generated by the pulse sequences. The acceptability of this environment to the patient is therefore an important consideration in research studies.

Utility

Functional brain imaging is time consuming and expensive. Consequently the number of subjects in many published studies is relatively small. This leads to low study power and an increased risk of missing an effect which is really present (increased type 2 error). On the other hand, as it does not use ionising radiation, fMRI allows the repeated presentation of baseline and activation stimuli, potentially hundreds of times, for each subject. This allows sufficient data to be acquired to detect statistically-significant brain activation or deactivation, in a single subject. The consequence is reduced type 2 error, but a difficulty in the interpretation of the wider significance of results in the context of the general population of interest.

QUANTITATIVE IMAGE ANALYSIS

Structural and functional brain abnormalities of interest in psychiatric research tend to be subtle, requiring quantitative analyses of imaging data obtained from groups of patients and carefully matched controls. There are two general methods. The first uses pre-specified regions of interest (ROIs), the second is voxel-based image analysis. These methods, which allow identification of regional brain abnormality, will now be briefly discussed. Following this, the complementary measurement of brain connectivity will be mentioned.

Functional images

Region of interest method

Quantitative analysis of functional images can be conducted by placing outlines of regions on pre-specified (often transverse) brain slices. Figure 5.4 gives an example of such outlines. The average signal within each region of a functional scan (reflecting

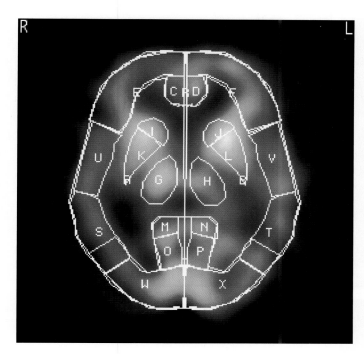

Fig. 5.4
SPECT axial slice with region of interest (ROI) mask superimposed. ROIs include anterior cingulate gyrus (C and D), dorsolateral prefrontal cortex (R and F), basal ganglia (J and K), occipital cortex (W and X). (Courtesy of Professor K Ebmeier, Royal Edinburgh Hospital, Edinburgh.)

local brain metabolic demand and therefore activity) can be calculated and analysed statistically. In SPECT and PET imaging, as the amount of radioactivity taken up by the brain is variable, these averaged counts are usually each divided by the total brain counts (to form normalised counts).

As an example of such analysis, it might be hypothesised in advance that the rostral anterior cingulate is more active in depression compared with matched controls. Averaged normalised counts for a group of depressed patients and another from controls could then be obtained from ROIs and directly compared with a t-test. Additionally, it might be hypothesised that such anterior cingulate activity correlates with Hamilton depression rating. Calculating the correlation between average normalised counts and depression score is straightforward.

One of the main limitations of ROI-based analysis is 'partial volume effects'. This results from the need to pre-specify the location of the ROI. Functional activation may occur in only part of an outlined anatomical structure, and even if uniform activation occurs, the estimated position of the ROI might be slightly in error. The consequence of this mismatch is the same for both situations: reduced power of the statistical tests. If however, the ROI matches the functional activation well, ROI methods may be more powerful than voxel-based methods.

Voxel-based methods (VBM)

Problems with partial volume effects, and the need for fully automated (objective) analyses have resulted in the development of voxel-based methods of image analysis. The most popular method is statistical parametric mapping (SPM, see http://www.fil.ion.

bpmf.ac.uk/spm/), developed by Friston and colleagues, (Frackowiak et al 1997). SPM analysis typically follows a standard processing sequence. Only some of the main principles underlying the simplest analyses will be discussed here.

The first stage may be realignment of each scan in an imaging time series to one another. This is because there tends to be small but significant movement of the head during scanning in even the most co-operative subjects. Such movement can result in spurious activation effects (i.e. signal distortion which could be misinterpreted as brain activation) unless correction is made. Co-registration of the functional image to a structural image may sometimes follow.

The next stage is typically spatial normalisation. This involves deforming the brain images from each subject so that the size of each conforms to a standardised (template) brain image. Images will otherwise differ because each person's brain is a slightly different size, and there will be small differences in orientation of each subject's head during scanning. It is important to note that the aim of this procedure is to remove global differences from the size and orientation of each image, but to retain local differences. After spatial normalisation, it can be reasonably assumed that the same anatomical regions in each image occupy the same voxels; with attendant benefits of reduced statistical variance and increased power. Note that since the template images approximate to the Talairach Atlas (Talairach & Tournoux 1988), there is a direct correspondence between voxels (with three-dimensional coordinates x,y,z) and anatomical structures. (In fact, the templates are based on the Montreal Neurological Institute standard, which differs significantly from the Atlas, but there are methods to transform coordinates from MNI to Talairach space and back (see http://www.mrc-cbu.cam.ac.uk/Imaging/).

The next stage may be spatial smoothing (blurring) of the image. This might seem at first sight counterintuitive since it will reduce the spatial resolution of the image. However, there are a number of reasons for smoothing the data (Friston (2002), http//www.fil.ion.ucl.ac.uk/spm/papers/spm-chapter.pdf), which include maximising the probability of signal detection, and ensuring validity of subsequent statistical methods. Images are not always smoothed; it depends on the extent of existing image blurring.

The next stage is statistical analysis of the data, e.g. in the comparison of two groups, to calculate a t-test statistic for each voxel. As before, it is necessary to take account of variations in global brain functional activity. In practice, the general linear model is used (actually, multiple linear regression) with global counts as a covariate of no interest and dummy variables to indicate group membership. The resultant three-dimensional map of t-values (all at identifiable locations in the Talairach Atlas) is a 'statistical parametric map'. (Note that SPM is not the only way of producing such maps.)

A final stage is necessary in the interpretation of this map: correction for multiple testing. As there are typically several hundred thousand voxels, the statistical tests are repeated many times, and the likelihood that some tests will be found significant, simply by chance, is high. A straightforward Bonferoni correction is, however, too conservative as adjacent voxels are not independent measures, because of image blurring. SPM currently uses the method of random gaussian fields to correct for multiple testing (Friston 2002).

Figure 5.5 shows increased cingulate activation in controls relative to patients with schizophrenia, when performing a task

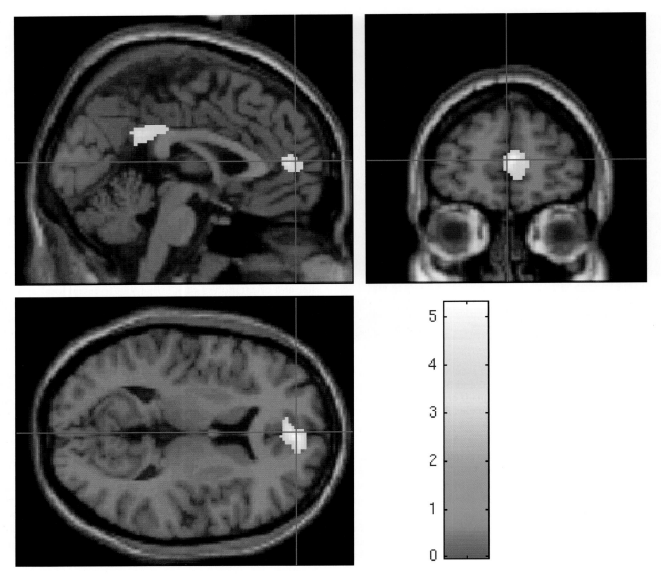

Fig. 5.5
Statistical parametric maps showing two regions of increased activity in controls relative to patients with schizophrenia.

in the scanner. The yellow coloured region indicates a collection of voxels where brain activity differs significantly between the two groups. This region has been superimposed onto a structural T1 scan to assist interpretation.

Structural images

Region of interest methods

Volumetric ROI methods are still frequently employed in the analysis of structural brain images. Typically, a detailed protocol for identifying anatomical landmarks will be developed and then applied by one or more experienced operators to outline structures of interest, blind to subject details. The method is very operator intensive and slow, but it remains the 'gold standard' for structural analysis. It is relatively straightforward to examine reproducibility by tests of inter- and intra-rater reliability.

Variations of this approach may be used to examine the gyrification pattern of the cortex, or to 'parcellate', i.e. outline, very small regions in three dimensions simultaneously.

Voxel-based methods

SPM can be applied to the study of local structural abnormalities. For example, T1 structural images can be spatially normalised in the same manner as functional images. The images can then be partitioned or 'segmented' into grey and white matter and CSF using automated (e.g. Bayesian) methods. A t-statistic can be calculated at each voxel of two groups of normalised grey matter images and correction made for multiple testing as before.

Note that voxel-based methods (VBM) detect changes in the surfaces or boundaries between different parts of the brain (e.g. grey–white matter interfaces), and any group differences are differences in the probability of e.g. grey matter at a particular voxel. By contrast, ROI methods are used to detect changes in the volume of outlined structures.

Functional integration

The image-processing methods discussed above are useful for identifying functional segregation, i.e. functional specialisation within a localised brain region. Complementary methods are used to investigate functional integration or connectivity. (Note that DTI is used to measure structural connectivity.)

Two concepts are relevant: functional and effective connectivity. *Functional* connectivity is defined as the temporal correlations between remote neurophysiological events; *effective* connectivity as the effect one neuronal region has on another. Functional connectivity does not provide direct insight into how the observed correlations are mediated. Effective connectivity, in contrast, is closer to the intuitive notion of a neuronal connection and depends on two models: an anatomical model describing *which* (functionally segregated) regions are connected, and a mathematical model describing *how* regions are connected (Friston 2002).

Statistical methods used to measure functional connectivity include eigenimage analysis and canonical variates analysis (see Friston 2002 and Ch. 11). Functional connectivity will not be discussed further here — the rest of this section focuses on the measurement of effective connectivity.

Effective connectivity

To illustrate the concept of effective connectivity, consider Figure 5.6. This shows a simplified diagram of the limbic basal ganglia thalamocortical loop (Alexander et al 1990). The cortex and thalamus are reciprocally connected, and a corticofugal unidirectional projection exists from cortex to thalamus via the basal ganglia. Using ROI methods, it is possible to determine brain activity for each of the regions shown in Figure 5.6. These values can then be used to calculate an observed covariance matrix.

Next, a mathematical model of the connections shown in Figure 5.6 can be defined using structural equation modelling (SEM) techniques (also referred to as path analysis). Using such methods, a set of connection strengths (path values) between each region can be specified and used to predict an observed covariance matrix. (Each path value might be considered analogous to a regression coefficient.) This is compared with the observed matrix to determine the discrepancy. A different set of connection strengths is then specified and the comparison repeated. By systematically testing different connection strengths such that the discrepancy is minimised, an optimum set can be defined which best predicts the observed covariance matrix. This calculation has been implemented in various computer programs.

The influence of one neuronal system on another is thus estimated by the optimal set of path estimates. If one optimal set is obtained, e.g. from a group of depressed patients, and another from a group of matched controls, then methods are available to determine whether the sets are significantly different. If so, this would indicate that one or more connections differ between the depressed and non-depressed subjects. This would be of interest since dysfunction in such loops has been predicted to occur in depressive illness, using different methods.

Anatomical modelling issues

It should be noted that the anatomical model shown in Figure 5.6 is necessarily simpler than that described previously (Alexander et al 1990) as it is not possible to measure brain activity in sufficiently small voxels, because of the limited spatial resolution of the imaging techniques. While the various subcortical regions may be considered functionally homogeneous units due to limited spatial resolution, there is evidence of segregation of function within the regions (Alexander et al 1990). Clearly this makes interpretation of the results more difficult. The cortical regions referred to in Figure 5.6 are quite large and may similarly exhibit segregation of function. Consequently, sampling from one part of the cortical region may produce quite different results from sampling from another. These problems are of course examples of partial volume effects.

In many connectivity studies, the anatomical model is not so explicitly defined a priori. Instead, voxel-based analysis is first undertaken to identify interesting regions. Once the regions are identified, connections between the regions are decided upon and path values calculated. The effect is to increase the likelihood of finding significant results. Arguably though, it is more difficult to interpret the results because of a lack of clear a-priori hypotheses.

Pitfalls of structural equation modelling

SEM can encompass many different statistical techniques and is therefore a very general method. However, there are a number of potential problems with path analysis that every study should address in order that the reported connectivity values can be considered valid (http://www.gsu.edu/~mkteer/semfaq.html discusses some of the issues, and provides references to relevant books and publications).

Non-linear methods

The methods discussed so far are linear and cannot deal with connections expressed in one context but not in another. Such non-linearity of response is believed to occur in the brain, and to take account of this 'Volterra formulations' can be used (Friston 2002). Figure 5.7 illustrates the concept of the Volterra formulation. The influence on one brain region has two components. First, there is a direct influence from a hierarchically lower region (R1) on a higher region (R2). Second, there is a modulatory influence from a brain region (R3), hierarchically higher than the

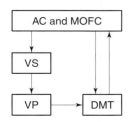

Fig. 5.6
Limbic/basal ganglia/thalamocortical loop. AC, anterior cingulate; MOFC, medial orbitofrontal cortex; VS, ventral striatum; VP, ventral pallidum; DMT, dorsal medial nucleus of thalamus.

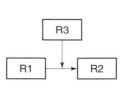

Fig. 5.7
Volterra formulation. Three brain regions: R1, R2 and R3. R1 is lower in hierarchy than R2, the former 'driving' the latter. R3, higher in hierarchy than other regions, modulates the influence of R1 on R2.

other two regions, on the effects of R1 on R2. By introducing 'moderator' variables, which reflect interaction between two regions producing activity in a third region, SEM can accommodate Volterra formulations.

Summary

Quantitative image analysis techniques are of two main types: ROI and VBM. (Note that this is a simplification as VBM can incorporate ROI methods; see e.g. Job et al 2002.) SPM is an example of a popular VBM method. Various statistical approaches to functional imaging data can be used to investigate 'functional' and effective connectivity, whereas DTI can provide an index of structural connectivity.

Finally, it was mentioned earlier that functional imaging techniques are unable to distinguish different neurophysiological events. The consequence for measurement of brain connectivity is that, for example, a high positive path value between two brain regions cannot be simply identified as 'excitatory', nor a negative value as 'inhibitory'.

ELECTROPHYSIOLOGICAL METHODS

Principles

Electroencephalography (EEG). In conventional EEG, electrodes are placed on the scalp, making it a safe non-invasive procedure. Electrodes can also be placed on the surface of the brain and within it using, for example, transphenoidal routes. Scalp recording uses the International 10–20 System of electrode placement.

Scalp-recorded EEG measures the summed electrical activity of many neurons discharging at the same time (in phase), allowing detection of the well-known alpha, beta, delta and theta rhythms. Evoked potentials (EP) represent much slower activity and, to detect them, it is necessary to apply repeated sensory stimuli, measure the EEG, then average the EEG over all measurements.

Brain electrical activity mapping (BEAM) is a method of forming images from EEG or EP data. Such imaging techniques continue to be developed — see, for example, a recent report of pretreatment increased theta activity in the subgenual anterior cingulate being associated with better antidepressant response (Pizzagalli et al 2001).

Magnetoencephalography (MEG). The development of superconducting quantum interference devices in the 1980s allowed non-invasive measurement of the small magnetic fields caused by neuronal discharge. Unlike EEG, MEG requires electrostatic shielding and head immobilisation.

Limitations

The objective of EEG and MEG imaging is to identify the locations of the sources of the electromagnetic activity. This is done by (software) postulating the location of various sources of activity and calculating a predicted pattern of recorded EEG or MEG data. The predicted pattern which best matches the observed pattern defines the best estimate of neuronal discharge (sometimes called the solution of the inverse problem).

The main limitation of both EEG and MEG imaging is that it is only possible to image structures close to the scalp. It was

pointed out some time ago (Fenwick 1987) that if both methods were ever to have much impact on psychiatric research, better detection of deeper signals from orbitofrontal cortex, limbic structures and brainstem would be required. Progress thus far appears limited. Both techniques have relatively poor spatial resolution, and MEG is expensive. However, there is much current interest in multimodal imaging to combine the advantages of, for example, EEG and fMRI.

Utility

The main advantage of EEG and MEG techniques is their excellent temporal resolution. MEG is an optimal technique for detecting electromagnetic sources parallel to the scalp, while EEG is optimal for detecting perpendicular sources. Thus, pooling EEG and MEG data allows better source localisation, although this is rarely done. Given cost considerations, if the measurement of fast electromagnetic activity near the scalp is of interest, EEG imaging may be the method of choice.

PSYCHIATRIC IMAGING STUDIES

In this section, some of the most recent and significant findings obtained from imaging studies of various psychiatric disorders will be discussed. As an introduction, it is worthwhile attempting to put this discussion into context.

- While there are now a substantial number of psychiatric imaging studies published per year, this degree of research effort has developed comparatively recently, i.e. over the past decade. The basis for the early work was the hypothesis that the major psychiatric disorders were biologically based — that it might be possible to detect structural and functional brain abnormalities in the brains of patients. Perhaps of necessity, there was often little refinement of the prior hypothesis, such as where such abnormality might be found.
- Early studies used methods only able to detect abnormality with relatively poor spatial resolution, compared with later techniques. Such studies particularly implicated the prefrontal and temporal lobes. More recent studies, using better analysis methods, appear to implicate quite specific regions of the prefrontal and temporal lobes. However, many authors have noted that there is a significant degree of inconsistency in the psychiatric imaging literature. As a consequence, far more attempts at replication at a subregional level are required.
- Brain function is anatomically segregated in the primary motor and sensory cortices. Localised damage to such regions produces neurological deficits understandable on the basis of loss of normal function. Brain function is also likely to be segregated in the prefrontal and temporal lobes, and psychopathology may in part reflect localised structural and/or functional abnormality. However, despite a great deal of non-imaging animal work studying these brain regions, only a very limited understanding of normal prefrontal and temporal functional segregation has been obtained. Human imaging studies have begun comparatively recently.
- Although replicated imaging abnormalities are emerging in various psychiatric disorders, it will always be difficult to understand their significance, as long as normal brain function remains poorly understood. The study of normal functional

segregation (and integration) may be useful to help clarify such issues.

- The study of functional segregation is not sufficient, in itself, to determine the fundamental principles of brain function. Nevertheless such mapping, or cartography, is a necessary prelude to other types of studies (Friston 2002), for example, of functional connectivity using Volterra formulations.

DEMENTIA

As the neurobiology of dementia has become clearer, the clinical differentiation of underlying aetiologies has, if anything, become more complex. This is not just because of an increasing recognition of disorders other than Alzheimer's disease and vascular dementia, but also because different pathophysiological processes can have similar phenotypic expressions depending on the part of the brain affected. For example, Alzheimer's disease typically presents with a temporoparietal predominance, but can present as a frontotemporal dementia. This has important implications for the study of disorders such as schizophrenia and depression.

Alzheimer's disease — structural abnormalities

Despite the above, there are consistent findings in neuroimaging of the different dementias, which often show reasonably strong correlations with neuropathology (especially in Alzheimer's) and clinical characteristics such as cognitive impairment. There is even a remarkably consistent association between temporal lobe pathology and psychotic features. CT and structural MRI have a role in detecting the 5–10% of demented patients with gross abnormalities (Burns 1990), and the 1–2% with treatable causes such as normal pressure hydrocephalus and subdural haematomas.

More sophisticated applications of these techniques may soon have clinical utility in early diagnosis. Early CT studies were unable to discriminate dementia of Alzheimer type (DAT) from normal ageing, probably because of lack of sensitivity and difficulties in reliable imaging of the hippocampus. The Oxford project to investigate memory and ageing (OPTIMA) conducted longitudinal temporal lobe oriented CT scans at yearly intervals from 1988 and found that a simple calliper measurement of the medial temporal lobe minimum width at the level of the brainstem was substantially lower in subjects with pathologically confirmed Alzheimer's disease (AD). Although controls showed an estimated age-related decline of about 1% of medial temporal lobe thickness each year, the sensitivity and specificity of the finding was 93% and 81%, respectively (Smith & Jobst 1996). Initial longitudinal analyses also found a 10-fold increase in the rate of ventricular dilatation in AD cases, of approximately 15% per year.

These findings has been pursued with MRI studies. In particular, voxel-based automated studies have shown that the disease process begins in and around the hippocampus, with progressive atrophy in the medial temporal lobe and the temporoparietal cortex — and that the frontal lobes are usually only affected at a much more advanced stage (e.g. Scahill et al 2002). These measures do not, as yet, discriminate different types of dementia or improve diagnostic precision over the careful application of clinical criteria. Further studies are also required to see if hippocampal volumes can discriminate the elderly with mild cognitive impairment from those without. However, improved detection can be expected with the development and increasing use of disease-specific probabilistic brain atlases (e.g. Thompson et al 2001), perhaps using them in tandem with apolipoprotein-E genotyping and other imaging techniques.

Other dementias — structural and spectroscopic abnormalities

Discrimination between Alzheimer's disease and vascular or multi-infarct dementia can often be made on the overall appearance of brain structure (see Table 5.6). However, dementia with Lewy bodies (DLB) is less distinct from both diagnoses on these measures (McKeith 2002).

Automated analyses of MRI white-matter segments, and diffusion tensor imaging (DTI) of white-matter tracts, are relatively new research tools, but preliminary results suggest that reductions in white-matter connectivity may underly age-related cognitive decline and may have a role in the early detection of Alzheimer's dementia. Structural MRI and DTI may also be able to detect early changes in Creutzfeldt–Jakob disease (CJD) and the location of gliotic epileptic foci.

Spectroscopy, of both the phosphorous and protein varieties, suggests early alterations in decreasing phosphomonoester/increasing phosphodiester level and reduced N-acetylcholine/increased myoinositol, respectively, that may be more sensitive than MRI; but very similar patterns are evident in a range of disorders, including epilepsy and CJD.

Table 5.6 Discriminating dementia with imaging			
Investigation	Alzheimer's disease	Vascular/multi-infarct dementia	Dementia with Lewy bodies
CT/MRI	Generalised atrophy, particularly in medial temporal lobes initially (10–15% progression/year)	Multifocal infarcts (usually bilateral) and atrophy (<5% progression/year)	Relative sparing of medial temporal lobes in majority
Deep white-matter lesions on MRI	Moderate increase	Extensive	Moderate increase
Periventricular lucencies on MRI	Frequent	Extensive	Frequent
SPECT HMPAO scan (blood flow)	Global reduction, especially posterior parietotemporal	Variable, multifocal deficits	Global reduction, especially occipital. Medial temporal lobes relatively preserved
HMPAO, hexamethyl propyleneamine oxime.			

Alzheimer's disease — functional abnormalities

The clinical potential of imaging techniques in the differential diagnosis of dementia has been most studied with SPECT in Alzheimer's disease, although the very first such study was conducted with PET in 1981 (Geaney & Abou-Saleh 1990). Characteristic SPECT findings in AD are bilateral reductions in cerebral blood flow in the parietal and temporal lobe, with relative sparing of the frontal and occipital lobes at least in the early stages of the disease. In contrast, patients with depression (and Korsakoff's psychosis) usually have more pronounced frontal deficit (Goodwin 1996). SPECT in multi-infarct dementia shows a variable pattern depending on the location of infarcts (for which SPECT may be more sensitive than structural imaging techniques).

The OPTIMA study found that parietotemporal perfusion below the 5th percentile for controls, together with a similar degree of abnormality on CT of the medial temporal lobe width, had a sensitivity of 83% and a specificity of 91% for Alzheimer's disease (Smith & Jobst 1996). Recent studies have shown that voxel-based analyses of SPECT data may be able to discriminate Alzheimer's disease from healthy ageing and depression (Ebmeier et al 1998), and that the changes in DLB are more prominent in posterior regions. PET and fMRI may be able to detect very early changes in the entorhinal cortex in particular and be able to identify patients who will develop dementia. For example, excessive memory-related activation of the hippocampus, parietal and frontal regions in subjects at high genetic risk (presumably compensating for some premorbid cognitive difficulties) can perhaps predict who will develop dementia over 2 years (Bookheimer et al 2000).

Finally, there are suggestions that it may be possible to identify DLB by means of dopamine ligand studies, because such patients show a relatively low uptake in basal ganglia regions (similar to what is observed in patients with Parkinson's disease).

SCHIZOPHRENIA

Generalised structural abnormalities

Demonstration of ventriculomegaly in schizophrenia (Johnstone et al 1976) was greeted with scepticism, but has been convincingly replicated many times over (Lewis 1991). A number of studies also showed that a similar degree of abnormality was present in first-episode cases (Lewis 1991), in keeping with a developmental rather than a degenerative cause. However, CT studies of cerebral 'atrophy', and lateral and third ventricular enlargement, failed to find consistent associations with aetiological factors or disease characteristics. Although a meta-analysis of these studies found a statistical association between lateral ventricular enlargement and cumulative hospitalisation, this could not clarify cause or effect (Raz & Raz 1990). Moreover, ventricular enlargement presumably reflects tissue loss in (several) neighbouring brain regions.

The first MRI study in schizophrenia was published in 1984, but it was several years before researchers took full advantage of the technique in measuring regional brain volumes. There are now well over 100 controlled MRI studies of various regional volumes in schizophrenia, and although they find a slightly different pattern of significant differences, two systematic and quantitative analyses have confirmed volume reductions of approximately 3% in the whole brain, 5% in the frontal and temporal lobes and 5–10% in temporal subregions (Lawrie & Abukmeil 1998, Wright et al 2000). Neuropathological studies suggest that neuronal numbers are preserved, i.e. it is neuropil that is reduced (Harrison 1999) (cf. mood disorder later).

As with CT, MRI studies have found similar abnormalities in first-episode cases and no apparent relation to treatment (with the exception of antipsychotic-related enlargement of parts of the basal ganglia). There are, however, a number of well-conducted studies that suggest there may be some progressive reduction in frontal and temporal lobe volumes in the early years after onset, and possibly even during the initial development of psychotic symptoms (Lawrie et al 2002).

Other structural imaging techniques have delivered complementary findings. There is a consistent MR spectroscopy literature, which finds reduced concentrations of some phospholipids and N-acetylaspartate in frontal and temporal lobes, although it is unclear whether this reflects structural or functional abnormalities. Similarly, the emerging technique of DTI suggests abnormalities in frontal areas, perhaps specifically those that are part of white-matter tracts connecting the frontal and temporal or parietal lobes (e.g. Burns et al, 2003).

Localised structural abnormalities

Prefrontal cortex (PFC)   The volume of the PFC is reduced by about 5% in schizophrenia (Lawrie & Abukmeil 1998, Wright et al 2000). A small number of parcellation studies suggest particular reduction in orbitomedial cortex and the anterior cingulate, with mixed reports on specific frontal gyri and the dorsolateral PFC. These findings are, however, very much in keeping with a similar number of VBM studies (e.g. Job et al 2002). There are also some intriguing suggestions of morphological disturbances, particularly of altered gyral complexity. A final point of great potential relevance is the increasing evidence that some of these frontal reductions are related to genetic liability to the disorder (e.g. Lawrie et al 2001), which may explain why so few consistent clinical associations of PFC volumes have been found.

Temporal lobe   The overall volume reductions from ROI studies are similar to those for the PFC, with possibly greater decrements and asymmetry abnormalities in parts of the superior temporal gyrus. The medial limbic structures are however reduced in volume by as much as 10%. While such findings have not always been replicated in macroscopic postmortem work (Harrison 1999), there is an emerging consensus from these and VBM studies that the parahippocampal gyrus may be the most structurally abnormal region of the brain in schizophrenia. Methodological differences may explain the apparent inconsistencies in the literature on the amygdala–hippocampus complex (AHC), particularly given the likelihood that these structures are more variable in shape and size in patients with schizophrenia. There is nevertheless good evidence that reduced AHC volumes are found in the healthy relatives of patients (Lawrie et al 2001) and that these may be attributable to an interaction between genetic risk and environmental factors such as obstetric complications (Shenton et al 2001). Wider temporal lobe volume losses may be associated with the development of positive psychotic symptoms (Lawrie et al 2002) and may even progress in the early stages of the illness.

Basal forebrain   There is an impressive degree of agreement between ROI and postmortem studies that the thalamus, and the mediodorsal nucleus in particular, is smaller in schizophrenia than one would expect from global tissue reductions. This also appears to be true of high-risk populations. There are also intriguing, albeit inconsistent findings that the adhesio interthalamica (or massa intermedia) is more frequently absent in people with schizophrenia. This midline structure is formed in the first trimester, and similar qualitative abnormalities — such as the increased prevalence of a cavum septum pellucidum between the frontal horns of the lateral ventricles — suggest early disruption of brain development (Shenton et al 2001).

The basal ganglia, on the other hand, are increased in volume, and this appears to be the only structural abnormality in schizophrenia that can be attributed to antipsychotic medication. The increases are maximal, approaching 20%, in the globus pallidus (Wright et al 2000).

Other regions There are suggestions that the parietal lobes may be structurally abnormal and the occipital lobes essentially normal in schizophrenia, but further studies — particularly of the parietal subregions — are required (Shenton et al 2001). The few studies suggesting cerebellar 'atrophy' but an increased amount of cerebellar white matter also require wider replication.

Functional abnormalities

Prefrontal cortex The first widely replicated functional imaging finding in schizophrenia was that of 'hypofrontality', a relative underactivation of specifically the dorsolateral prefrontal cortex, particularly on cognitive activation (Weinberger et al 1986). However, such studies could not ensure that the patients were doing the tasks, let alone doing them as well as the controls. Pacing the task, for example by asking subjects in the scanner to produce a response every 5 seconds, tends to remove hypofrontality (Frith et al 1995) and suggests, if anything, a 'hyperfrontality' while patients are able to do the task, and a progressive loss of frontal activity as the task becomes more difficult and performance fails (Fletcher et al 1998). The issue is further complicated by frequent suggestions of an association between negative symptoms and hypofrontality, and possible subregional effects (see the subsection on mood disorders, below).

Temporal Resting SPECT and PET studies tended to find, if anything, a 'hypertemporality'. Subsequent studies have shown, with remarkable consistency, that increased activation of (frontal and) temporal language areas is associated with auditory hallucinations. This work has been replicated with sophisticated fMRI studies (Shergill et al 2000). In contrast, there are very few studies that have specifically addressed and found functional abnormalities of medial structures. This is, however, a focus of much current research.

Other regions There are a number of reports of abnormal activations in patients with schizophrenia even on simple sensory and motor tasks, which suggest a generalised difficulty in cerebral organisation. This is compatible with increasing reports of parietal lobe abnormalities and suggestions of abnormal frontostriatal and fronto-thalamo-cerebellar networks.

Dysconnectivity Following on from these observations, and the work of Frith and colleagues in particular (Frith et al 1995), there is a rapidly increasing literature directly implicating dysconnectivity in schizophrenia. The best evidence at present is for reduced frontotemporal connectivity, which may be related to auditory hallucinations in particular (Lawrie et al 2002), but other intra- and inter-regional disconnections are likely. Moreover, there is strongly suggestive evidence, albeit as yet not replicated, that

this may be modulated by dopaminergic neurotransmission (Fletcher et al 1996).

Ligand studies Although the literature is inconsistent, overviews of PET ligand studies strongly suggest an increase in dopamine D_2 receptor numbers (Laruelle 1998). Further, amphetamine challenge studies and, in particular, studies using fluorodopa binding as an index of presynaptic dopaminergic activity (Meyer-Lindenberg et al 2002), almost unanimously indicate abnormally high dopamine turnover and sensitivity in the disease. Studies with other ligands are rare.

Summary

Imaging studies in schizophrenia have provided new insights into the pathophysiology of schizophrenia. Structural deficits are likely to be partly genetic and partly related to the expression of the phenotype. Functional imaging is making progress in identifying the neurobiological substrates of particular symptoms. However, structure/function/clinical relationships need to be much more accurately determined — and distinguished from other disorders — before any of these techniques can have sufficient sensitivity or specificity for clinical use.

LEARNING DISABILITY

It is surprising that arguably one of the most 'organic' areas of psychiatric practice has, until recently, been a relatively neglected area for imaging researchers. There is now a rapidly increasing literature on specific disorders, but there is only space here to mention a few replicated findings and those of particular interest.

Disorders of known aetiology

Patients with *Down syndrome* have a generalised reduction in brain volume, changes in sulcal/gyral morphology, and more specific deficits of the amygdala and hippocampal formation that are likely to further change with the development of dementia (Krasuski et al 2002). Most studies of children and adults with *fragile X syndrome* show reductions in the volume of the cerebellar vermis, particularly lobules VI and VII, and may fail to activate frontal and parietal cortex on working memory tasks. The latter has been related to gene expression (Reiss et al 2000, Kwon et al 2001). In contrast, subjects with *Williams' syndrome* may have an enlarged cerebellum, volume reductions in the parietal and occipital lobes, and reduced cerebral curvature, when compared with age- and gender-matched controls (Reiss et al 2000). A recent flurry of structural MRI studies in *velocardiofacial syndrome (VCFS)* have consistently identified whole brain volume reductions of approximately 10% with relative sparing of the frontal lobes, prominent white-matter hyperintensities and a high prevalence of cavum septum pellucidum (Reiss et al 2000), although there may also be specific ageing and genomic imprinting effects. As yet, there is a rather limited and poorly replicated literature on *sex chromosome aneuploidies*, but there are replicated reports of parietal lobe reductions in *Turner's syndrome* (Reiss et al 2000).

It is tempting to speculate that the reports of cerebellar hypoplasia in *VCFS*, *fragile X* and *autism* (see below) may be related to the withdrawn, hyposocial behaviour evident in these disorders, as compared with the hypersociality observed in people with *Williams' syndrome*. However, it is important to note that such findings are not particularly consistent, and the specific behaviours differ between conditions; e.g. fragile X and autism.

Idiopathic disorders

Attention deficit hyperactivity disorder (ADHD) and *autism* have been relatively well studied. Whilst both conditions can be associated with learning disability, equally they may not, and so are only included in this section for convenience. Structural imaging studies in *ADHD* have shown reduced prefrontal and caudate volumes, while functional imaging studies suggest hypoperfusion and hypometabolism in the same regions (Hale et al 2000). Cognitive activation studies also suggest abnormal responses in these regions to attention and executive tasks. However, results of dopaminergic ligand studies are, as yet, inconclusive. There is an increasing interest in *autism* and *Asperger's disorder*, which fairly consistently show abnormalities of the frontal lobes, amygdala and cerebellum — particularly on functional imaging studies, which suggest that global feature rather than specific item information processing is abnormal.

Summary

Imaging in these and related disorders is likely to be a growth area in the next few years, for several reasons. These studies are of direct clinical interest, as they may help in differentiating particular diseases. More generally, imaging the range of phenotypes associated with known genetic abnormalities, within and across disorders, is likely to have relevance to the study of other psychiatric disorders. Additionally, it will be useful to use serial imaging to study the natural history of these neurodevelopmental disorders.

MOOD DISORDERS

Traditionally, there is believed to be complete recovery between episodes of depression or mania. Consequently, it might seem pointless to search for structural brain changes in patients with a mood disorder. However, as is often forgotten, there are a number of common episodic medical disorders caused by permanent structural abnormalities, such as some cases of epilepsy, the early stages of multiple sclerosis and exercise-induced cardiac arrhythmia secondary to coronary artery disease. Although a neglected topic of research (Jeste et al 1988), there is significant evidence of structural abnormalities in the brains of patients with unipolar and bipolar mood disorders. Only a brief discussion of the main findings can be presented here. For more detailed discussion of some of these issues, the reader is referred to other texts (Ebmeier & Kronhaus 2002).

General structural abnormality

A large meta-analysis concluded that radiological signs of ventricular enlargement and sulcal prominence in unipolar and bipolar mood disorder patients were highly significant, with an effect size only slightly less than in patients with schizophrenia (Elkis et al 1995). Similarly, another recent review concluded that there was clear evidence of cerebral and also cerebellar atrophy (Videbech 1997).

Signal hyperintensities are punctate lesions with reduced myelination and neuropil atrophy, which are best visualised on T2 images. When coalescent, these lesions are also known as subcortical leucoencephalopathy. A recent meta-analysis concluded that such hyperintensities occurred more frequently than expected in both unipolar and bipolar disorder (Videbech 1997). Late-onset unipolar patients in particular tend to have many lesions, mostly periventricularly but also in the thalamus, in deep white matter and basal ganglia. This pattern suggests dysfunction in the prefrontal basal ganglia thalamocortical loops (Alexander et al 1990).

Localised structural abnormality

Prefrontal cortex   Studies have reported generalised reduction in prefrontal lobe volume in patients with major depression (Videbech 1997). Specific reductions in grey matter of the subgenual anterior cingulate have been reported (Drevets 2000) and in the medial orbitofrontal gyrus of patients with mood disorder. Postmortem studies have also reported reduction in grey matter glia and neurons in the subgenual anterior cingulate and orbitofrontal cortex of such patients (Drevets 2000) (cf. schizophrenia).

Imaging studies reporting rostral anterior cingulate grey matter loss are not specific to depression. Several VBM studies of schizophrenia have found such differences — including a recent study of first episode schizophrenia patients and those at high genetic risk of schizophrenia (Job et al 2002). It is noteworthy that Drevets and colleagues specifically recruited subjects with strong family histories of mood disorders, and all these studies excluded confounders such as alcohol misuse.

Temporal lobe   A few studies have reported generalised reduction in temporal lobe volume, although others have not found this (Videbech 1997). There have been a few reports of specific reduction in hippocampal volume in mood disorder patients (Sheline et al 1996, Shah et al 1998). In the first study, it was found that such changes occurred only in the most treatment-resistant patients. In the second study, volume reduction correlated with the duration of illness. Following animal work, it has been speculated that these changes may relate to hypercortisolaemia. Again, however, volume reductions in the medial temporal lobe are not specific to mood disorder, as they are also reported in schizophrenia and Alzheimer's dementia.

Basal forebrain   Several studies involving patients with unipolar depression have reported reduction in basal ganglia volume. This is in contrast to studies of bipolar disorder, where either no change in size has been reported or increased size has been found (Videbech 1997). In studies of patients with schizophrenia, increased basal ganglia volume, apparently secondary to antipsychotic drug treatment, is typical. Such an effect may also confound studies of mood disorder.

Endocrine abnormalities such as dexamethasone non-suppression have often been reported to occur in mood disorder, but are not specific to it, and it is known that pituitary size may change with endocrine status. Despite this, structural studies of pituitary size in mood disorder are rare; however, one has reported an increased volume, and another abnormal signal intensity (Videbech 1997).

Brainstem   Significant reductions in brainstem, cerebellar vermis and medulla size occurring in patients with depressive illness are occasionally reported. A common mode of action of virtually all empirically derived antidepressants is to increase serotonin and noradrenaline (norepinephrine) levels, and to a lesser extent dopamine. Antidopaminergic antipsychotics are often used to treat mania. The nuclei supplying these monoamines to the rest of the brain are located in the midbrain. Of interest therefore is a series of studies using transcranial ultrasound and MRI in unipolar depressed patients, reporting a structural abnormality in the midbrain raphae (Becker et al 2001). It has been argued that the imaging abnormalities in unipolar mood disorder are consistent with a relative loss of medial forebrain bundle fibres. These fibres connect the monoaminergic nuclei to the rest of the brain. It is tempting to speculate that antidepressant drug action might compensate for such a loss in patients predisposed to episodes of unipolar depression.

General functional abnormalities

Many functional imaging studies of mood disorder have been undertaken over the past decade. These tend to be of depressed patients, as manic patients are often unable to comply with study protocols. Imaging techniques have improved greatly over the same period. One noticeable aspect of early work is that the spatial resolution of such images was relatively poor, and often there was only a limited attempt to localise abnormal findings, such that reports of 'prefrontal hypoactivity' (or hyperactivity) were not uncommon.

Despite this, reviews of a number of imaging studies which did achieve better localisation of functional abnormality are available (Drevets 2000). Studies of the resting state (i.e. without a task being done by the subjects during scanning) tend to report dorsolateral hypoactivity, and ventromedial hyperactivity.

More recent studies often focus on abnormalities within specific brain regions. These will now be discussed.

Localised functional abnormalities

Ventromedial prefrontal area   This is taken to mean the rostral anterior cingulate and orbitofrontal cortex, although the boundaries of the area are unclear. A number of studies have reported abnormal metabolic activity in the subgenual anterior cingulate and adjacent supragenual anterior cingulate in depressive illness (Drevets 2000). Such increased regional activity is not specific to depressive illness, occurring with numerous emotion induction imaging paradigms (Bush et al 1998), and in various anxiety disorders. However, two studies have reported right subgenual anterior cingulate activity correlating with depression severity (Drevets 2000). Abnormal activity of the orbitofrontal cortex is also frequently reported, but is not specific to mood disorder, occurring in various anxiety disorders and normally on tasks involving a combination of emotional and cognitive processing (e.g. gambling tasks).

Dorsolateral prefrontal area   This is taken to mean the dorsolateral prefrontal cortex and caudal anterior cingulate, although the boundaries of the area are again unclear. The region, whilst often appearing hypoactive in resting studies of depressive illness, tends to be active when subjects engage in diverse cognitive-attentional tasks (Bush et al 1998). Dorsolateral hypoactivity is again not specific to depressive disorder, also being reported in schizophrenia and being associated with negative symptoms.

It has been suggested that reciprocal activation–deactivation in brain regions involved in emotional and cognitive function is a general finding in imaging studies, whether subjects are depressed or not (Drevets & Raichle 1998). This suggests the existence of a normal mechanism by which strong emotion, such as severe depression or anxiety, might interfere with cognitive function in a reversible manner. It also suggests a means by which cognitive methods (i.e. distraction) might reduce the experience of unpleasant emotion (Drevets & Raichle 1998).

Temporal lobe   Higher resting amygdala activity in unipolar and bipolar mood disorder patients, relative to controls, has been reported and this correlates with depression severity (Drevets 2000). Antidepressant treatment has been found to reduce amygdala activity in animals and humans. Medicated mood disorder patients in remission, who relapse on tryptophan depletion, have been reported to have higher resting amygdala activity. It has been claimed that high resting amygdala activity may be specific to mood disorder (Drevets 2000).

Basal forebrain   Reports of abnormal activity in basal ganglia structures also occur but appear somewhat inconsistent. Studies have more often reported results for the dorsal striatum (which is implicated in motor and cognitive function), rather than the ventral striatum, which is implicated in motivated behaviour and reward (Rolls 1999) and therefore might be more relevant. The latter area presents more difficulties in imaging, although methods are currently being developed.

Abnormal thalamic activity has been reported on several occasions. It has been speculated (Drevets 2000) that such cortical and subcortical abnormalities represent dysfunction in basal ganglia thalamocortical re-entrant loops (Alexander et al 1990), which are a prominent feature of prefrontal lobe structure. The motor loop is believed to be functionally abnormal in Parkinson's and Huntington's diseases (Alexander et al 1990), and the limbic loop may be abnormal in an analogous manner in mood disorder.

Brainstem   For reasons discussed above, this region is of interest in mood disorder because of the presence in the midbrain of the raphe nucleus, locus coeruleus and ventral tegmental area. However, the brainstem presents particular imaging problems because of its relatively small size. Various studies have reported brainstem activation or deactivation though no consistent results are yet available.

ANXIETY DISORDERS

Most of the anxiety disorders have been studied but much less so than mood disorders.

Structural abnormalities

Two recent reviews of *post-traumatic stress disorder (PTSD)* concluded that there was evidence of decreased hippocampal volume and increased numbers of white-matter intensities (Pitman et al 2001), and that the evidence for the former appeared relatively consistent (Villarreal & King 2001). One study of Vietnam veterans found hippocampal volume decreases that correlated with months of combat exposure, and speculated, on the basis of animal studies, that this decrease may be related to cortisol excess.

Obsessive–compulsive disorder (OCD) has been consistently associated with structural abnormalities of the basal ganglia and orbitofrontal cortex in a number of studies (Zald & Kim 1996, Saxena et al 2001). Two studies of *panic disorder* patients found evidence of reduced temporal lobe volume (Fontaine et al 1990, Vythilingam et al 2000). In contrast, a review of *social phobia* concluded that there was no evidence of structural brain abnormalities (Argyropoulos et al 2001).

Functional abnormalities

Functional imaging studies of *PTSD* tend to report increased activation of the amygdala and some limbic structures, together with deactivation of various cortical regions implicated in cognitive functioning (Pitman et al 2001). Failure of anterior cingulate activation in the context of amygdala activation has been noted (Pitman et al 2001, Villarreal & King 2001). In *OCD*, overactivity of the orbitofrontal cortex has been reported on a number of occasions, as has increased or decreased basal ganglia activity (Saxena et al 2001), leading to speculation about dysfunction in basal ganglia thalamocortical loops.

Anxiety disorder may represent dysfunction in brain regions implicated in healthy subjects experiencing anxiety or fear as a normal transient emotion. A meta-analysis of 55 functional imaging studies of healthy subjects experiencing emotion induction has been published (Phan et al 2002). Activation loci from these studies were plotted onto a spatially normalised brain volume, and regional patterns were studied quantitatively. A strong association was found between the amygdala and fear induction particularly when visual induction methods were used. By contrast, induction methods involving memory tended to activate the anterior cingulate.

SUBSTANCE MISUSE

Substances discussed here include those associated with harmful excessive use — such as alcohol, stimulants and opiates. Animal work over decades has explored the site of brain action of addictive substances. Whilst in many ways these drugs are very different, it is interesting to note that they all (except benzodiazepines) have a common property of promoting dopamine release in subcortical structures such as the ventral tegmental area and ventral striatum (Bardo 1998, McBride et al 1999), a factor robustly linked to their power to promote self-administration in animal studies. Although misused by humans because of their immediately rewarding properties, in regular high dosage they are all associated with an increased prevalence of depressive illness (McIntosh & Ritson 2001), although cause and effect continue to be debated.

Although hallucinogens are not usually studied in self-administration animal models of addiction, and indeed may not support such behaviour, the dopaminergic system is again implicated. For example, ketamine may have indirect effects via glutamate (see below), and LSD may inhibit midbrain serotonergic activity, which inhibits ventral tegmental dopaminergic activity. Cannabis might similarly act via effects on acetylcholine, which has well-known interactions with dopamine. Hallucinogens, by definition, have a tendency to cause psychotic symptoms in otherwise healthy subjects, and may exacerbate psychotic symptoms in patients with schizophrenia. In both cases, antidopaminergic drugs are useful treatments.

It is important to note that these substances have many clinically significant non-dopaminergic actions (e.g. cognitive deficits secondary to structural brain change in alcohol dependency). The aim of the above discussion is thus to highlight a common mode of action of diverse drugs, which are associated with similar behavioural problems. This is to suggest a possible association, and to provide a context for the interpretation of (mostly functional) imaging studies.

Structural abnormalities

Alcohol Brain shrinkage in alcohol misuse has been reported from the earliest pneumoenecephalography studies. This has subsequently been confirmed by many CT and MRI studies, which also report partial reversibility of abnormalities with abstinence (Kril & Halliday 1999). Confounds to such measurements are present — including the negative correlation between brain weight and age, due to a secular increase in brain size during the 20th century and a small reduction in brain size with age. Recognition of such problems has led to the introduction of correction methods.

Neuropathological studies have identified shrinkage of the white matter, which has been confirmed with radiological studies. This has included quantification of reduction in corpus callosum sagittal area, which has been found more marked in anterior brain areas. Marked generalised reduction in prefrontal white-matter volume has been found in other studies. While it has been suggested that white-matter shrinkage is a result of dehydration and its reversibility due to rehydration, both neuropathological and radiological studies have presented evidence that this is not the mechanism (Kril & Halliday 1999). Correlations between brain atrophy and memory impairment have been reported.

Grey-matter reductions have been reported in dorsolateral prefrontal, subcortical grey matter, and medial temporal lobes. There is the suggestion that atrophy is most pronounced in the dorsolateral regions. Since this region has also been reported to demonstrate the most age-related atrophy, a combination of both alcohol and age effects may account for the findings in alcohol misuse (Kril & Halliday 1999).

Medial temporal lobe atrophy affecting grey and white matter has been reported, with the suggestion that the anterior hippocampal region is selectively damaged. Patients with seizures may, however, account for the majority of such findings. Basal ganglia atrophy appears in proportion to atrophy in other areas. Neuropathological studies in humans confirm neuronal loss in the dorsolateral cortex but not hippocampal regions (Kril & Halliday 1999). This is in contrast to animal models of alcohol misuse, where hippocampal neuronal loss is frequently found.

Deficits in executive functions, including planning and working memory, may be attributable to structural prefrontal and perhaps temporal lobe damage. The exact mechanism of such damage remains unknown. Partial recovery suggests neurochemical involvement, while neuronal loss from regions other than the hippocampus (which has some capacity for neuronal regeneration) suggests irreversible brain damage (Kril & Halliday 1999).

Cannabis The relatively limited imaging literature in cannabis users has recently been reviewed. Contrary to one high-profile CT study, there is no consistent evidence of structural abnormalities. However, xenon inhalation SPECT and some PET studies have consistently found global reductions in cerebral blood flow that may be most marked in frontal and cerebellar lesions in users. This abnormality probably normalises on abstinence. Administration of tetrahydrocannabinol, with or without cognitive activation, seems to produce differential effects depending on the experience of the subjects. Generalised activations of frontal cortex, limbic regions and the cerebellum, are likely to relate to the effects of the drug; while heavy or dependent users appear to show additional activations of orbitofrontal cortex and the basal ganglia, similar to those seen in studies of cocaine and alcohol dependence.

Stimulants   By contrast, *Ecstasy* is known to be neurotoxic in animals. The very inconsistent imaging literature does not, however, clarify if this is also the case in humans. A recent study of *cocaine*-addicted subjects found localised grey-matter reductions in medial orbitofrontal cortex, anterior cingulate and superior temporal cortices (Franklin et al 2002).

Functional abnormalities

Stimulants   In a functional imaging study on *cocaine*-addicted subjects, cocaine infusion was associated with increased activity in the ventral tegmental area, which correlated with ratings of euphoria (Breiter et al 1997). In contrast, post-euphoria rating of craving was correlated with increased ventral striatal activity. Another functional imaging study on *amphetamine*-addicted subjects reported that administration of amphetamine increased activity in the ventral striatum, which correlated with euphoria rating (Drevets et al 2001). There is replicated evidence of alteration in striatal dopamine receptor and transporter density in ecstasy and cocaine users (Reneman et al 2002, Volkow and Fowler 2000), which in the latter case was related to orbitofrontal cortex activity.

Hallucinogens   Such studies are generally rare. We do not know of any imaging studies of the effects of *LSD*, but there are three PET studies of *psilocybin*, the active ingredient of 'magic mushrooms' — with replicated findings of increased metabolism in frontotemporal regions and the anterior cingulate in particular (Vollenweider et al 1997). There are quite a number of imaging studies of the effects of *ketamine*, a handful of which include patients with schizophrenia. Ketamine, which may precipitate psychotic symptoms in adults, activates frontocingulate regions and deactivates the hippocampus in healthy volunteers and patients with schizophrenia. It probably does so by reducing glutamate and indirectly increasing dopamine neurotransmission in the striatum (cf. stimulant challenge studies in schizophrenia), but the effects are short-lived (usually less than 2 hours) and not found to be distressing (Carpenter 1999).

EATING DISORDERS

Structural abnormalities

There are comparatively few structural imaging studies of anorexia nervosa and hardly any in bulimia. Early CT studies in anorexia found enlarged ventricles that were partially reversible after weight gain (Herholz 1996). MRI has confirmed this and suggests that white-matter 'atrophy' and ventriculomegaly may be related to weight loss and gain, while grey-matter and wider CSF abnormalities may be persistent (Hendren et al 2000). This could reflect trait or uncorrected state factors such as mood or hormonal disruption — or even acquired grey-matter loss secondary to prolonged malnutrition.

Functional abnormalities

There is a far greater functional imaging literature in both disorders, but this has to deal with issues of comorbidity (with e.g. depressive and obsessive symptoms) as well as the unknown effects of eating disorders on glucose metabolism in the brain. Initial PET

studies were essentially negative (Herholz 1996), but there are larger and better-analysed (especially SPECT) replicated reports of a generalised hypoperfusion and 'hypofrontality' in particular, as well as a 'hypertemporality' related to food cues — but the replications are rather inconsistent. Far more impressive is the consistent evidence implicating the serotoninergic system in bulimics and obese binge-eaters, and especially the reductions noted in the availability of the 5HT transporter in (hypo)thalamus (Tauscher et al 2001) and midbrain (Kuikka et al 2001) respectively (cf. depression).

CONCLUSIONS AND FUTURE DIRECTIONS

The principles of the main imaging techniques used in psychiatry, and the main findings obtained using these techniques, have been discussed. Quantitative imaging methods have established that structural and functional brain abnormalities are associated with most psychiatric disorders. Patterns of abnormality are beginning to emerge for what were once thought to be purely 'functional' disorders (see Table 5.7). It should be emphasised however that there is much overlap between patients and controls, and abnormalities that have been replicated are demonstrable only at the group, and not at the individual level. This may change with time.

Certain brain regions are implicated in various disorders. A major challenge is the better understanding of normal function in these particular regions, in order to understand dysfunction in disease. Study of normal functional segregation within the brain may be useful in this context. Connectivity studies are arguably best used when functional segregation is well established.

Regions where it is important to establish functional segregation include anterior cingulate, orbitofrontal and dorsolateral cortices. Medial temporal lobe structures such as amygdala and hippocampus, together with temporal cortical regions such as the superior temporal gyrus, are equally important. A major organising principle of the prefrontal cortices comprises the basal ganglia thalamocortical re-entrant loops. Much evidence implicates disordered function in various psychiatric disorders, and detailed information on structure and some aspects of function are available. Despite this, understanding of normal integrated function (what the loops do in the context of the rest of the brain) is almost completely lacking.

Earlier, it was mentioned that functional mapping is an important prelude to other types of studies. It is currently being argued that the inherent function of any cortical region (and even individual neurons) is dynamic and context sensitive. Interactions between brain systems involve driving (lower in hierarchy, forward projections) and modulatory (higher in hierarchy, backward projections) components that mediate regional specialisation. Specific specialisation is therefore not an intrinsic property of any region, but depends on the context defined by the connections. If correct, this requires a significant modification to the classical view of neuronal receptive fields (Friston 2002), and clearly needs to be taken account of in functional imaging studies of psychiatric disorders.

Finally, functional imaging methods are fundamentally ambiguous as to the underlying neurophysiological events. Given this ambiguity, arguably it is more important that a difference in brain activity occurs in a specific region, than the direction of the change. Linking work on animals to human imaging studies may

Table 5.7 Summary of replicated findings in various psychiatric disorders

Disorder	Findings
Dementia	• Alzheimer's type: medial temporal lobe atrophy • Multi-infarct: patchy perfusion deficits, SPECT may be more sensitive than CT or structural MRI
Schizophrenia	• Ventriculomegaly and cerebral atrophy—non-progressive • Largest and most consistent volume reductions in medial temporal lobes; however, some evidence for smaller reductions in prefrontal lobe volume. • Reduced concentrations of phospholipids and *N*-acetylasparate in frontal and temporal lobes using MRS
Learning disability	• Few studies available.
Mood disorders	• Ventriculomegaly and cerebral atrophy—non-progressive. Similar to schizophrenia but smaller effect size • Subcortical leucoencephalopathy associated with late-onset illness and treatment resistance • Better evidence for prefrontal than temporal volume reductions (cf. schizophrenia) • Most consistent pattern of functional abnormality is ventromedial overactivity and dorsolateral underactivity
Anxiety disorders	• Few studies available
Substance misuse	• Few studies available • Possible link between functional imaging studies and extensive animal work
Eating disorders	• Few studies available

These are localised structural abnormalities in prefrontal and temporal lobes in many disorders, but with different detailed patterns. The most recent work apparently implicates quite specific regions of the medial temporal lobe and anterior cingulate. Structural imaging results appear more consistent than those obtained using functional imaging. With the possible exception of dementia, abnormalities are demonstrable at the group but not at an individual level.

assist the interpretation of such work with regard to underlying neurophysiological function. These and other approaches may deliver information of direct diagnostic and therapeutic relevance in the next decade.

REFERENCES

Alexander G E, Crutcher M D, DeLong M R 1990 Basal ganglia-thalamocortical circuits: Parallel substrates for motor, oculomotor, "prefrontal" and "limbic" functions. In Uylings H B M, Van Eden G C, De Bruin J P C et al (eds) Progress in brain research. Elsevier Science, New York

Argyropoules S V, Bell C J, Nutt D J 2001 Brain function in social anxiety disorder. Psychiatric Clinics of North America 24: 707–722

Bardo M T 1998 Neuropharmacological mechanisms of drug reward: beyond dopamine in the nucleus accumbens. Clinical Reviews in Neurobiology 12: 37–67

Becker G, Berg D, Lesch K P et al 2001 Basal limbic system alteration in major depression: a hypothesis supported by transcranial sonography and MRI findings. International Journal of Neuropsychopharmacology 4: 21–31

Bookheimer S Y, Strojwas M H, Cohen M S et al 2000 Patterns of brain activation in people at risk for Alzheimer's disease. New England Journal of Medicine 343: 450–456

Breiter H C, Gollub R L, Weisskoff R M et al 1997 Acute effects of cocaine on human brain activity and emotion. Neuron 19: 591–611

Burns A 1990 Cranial computerised tomography in dementia of the Alzheimer type. British Journal of Psychiatry Supplement: 10–15

Burns J, Job D, Bastin M E et al 2003 Structural disconnectivity in schizophrenia: a diffusion tensor magnetic resonance imaging study. British Journal of Psychiatry 182: 439–443

Bush G, Whalen P J, Rosen B R et al 1998 The counting Stroop: an interference task specialised for functional neuroimaging — Validation study with functional MRI. Human Brain Mapping 6: 270–282

Carpenter W T Jr 1999 The schizophrenia ketamine challenge study debate. Biological Psychiatry 46: 1081–1091

Drevets W C 2000 Functional anatomical abnormalities in limbic and prefrontal cortical structures in major depression. In: Uylings H B M, Van Eden C G, De Bruin J P C et al (eds) Progress in brain research, vol 126. Elsevier Science, London

Drevets W C, Gautier C, Price J C et al 2001 Amphetamine-induced dopamine release in human ventral striatum correlates with euphoria. Biological Psychiatry 49: 81–96

Drevets W C, Raichle M E 1998 Reciprocal suppression of regional cerebral blood flow during emotional versus higher cognitive processes: implications for interactions between emotion and cognition. Cognition and Emotion 12: 353–385

Ebmeier K P, Glabus M F, Prentice N et al 1998 A voxel-based analysis of cerebral perfusion in dementia and depression of old age. Neuroimage 7: 199–208

Ebmeier K P, Kronhaus D 2002 Brain imaging and mood disorders. In: D'haenen H, den Boer J A, Willner P (eds) Biological psychiatry Wiley, London

Elkis H, Friedman L, Wise A et al 1995 Meta-analyses of studies of ventricular enlargement and cortical sulcal prominence in mood disorders: comparisons with controls or patients with schizophrenia. Archives of General Psychiatry 52: 735–746

Fenwick P 1987 The inverse problem: a medical perspective. Physics in Medicine and Biology 32: 5–9

Fletcher P C, Frith C D, Grasby P M et al 1996 Local and distributed effects of apomorphine on fronto-temporal function in acute unmedicated schizophrenia. Journal of Neuroscience 16: 7055–7062

Fletcher P C, McKenna P J, Frith C D et al 1998 Brain activations in schizophrenia during a graded memory task studied with functional neuroimaging. Archives of General Psychiatry 55: 1001–1008

Fontaine R, Breton G, Dery R et al 1990 Temporal lobe abnormalities in panic disorder: an MRI study. Biological Psychiatry 27: 304–310

Frackowiak R S, Magistretti P J, Schulman R G et al 2001 Neuroenergetics: relevance for functional brain imaging. HFSP Workshop Report XI. Strasbourg

Frackowiak R S J, Friston K J, Frith C D et al 1997 Human brain function. Academic Press, London

Franklin T R, Acton P D, Maldjian J A et al 2002 Decreased gray matter concentration in the insular, orbitofrontal, cingulate, and temporal cortices of cocaine patients. Biological Psychiatry 51: 134–142

Friston K 2002 Beyond phrenology: What can neuroimaging tell us about distributed circuitry? Annual Review of Neuroscience 25: 221–250

Frith C D, Friston K J, Herold S et al 1995 Regional brain activity in chronic schizophrenic patients during the performance of a verbal fluency task. British Journal of Psychiatry 167: 343–349

Geaney D P, Abou-Saleh M T 1990 The use and applications of single-photon emission computerised tomography in dementia. British Journal of Psychiatry Supplement: 66–75

George M S, Ring H A, Costa D C et al 1991 Neuroactivation and neuroimaging with SPECT. Springer-Verlag, London

Goodwin G M 1996 Functional imaging, affective disorder and dementia. British Medical Bulletin 52: 495–512

Hale T S, Hariri A R, McCracken J T 2000 Attention-deficit/hyperactivity disorder: perspectives from neuroimaging. Mental Retardation & Developmental Disability Research Review 6: 214–219

Harrison P J 1999 The neuropathology of schizophrenia: a critical review of the data and their interpretation. Brain 122 (Pt 4): 593–624

Haug J O 1982 Pneumoencephalographic evidence of brain atrophy in acute and chronic schizophrenic patients. Acta Psychiatrica Scandinavica 66: 374–383

Hendren R L, De Backer I, Pandina G J 2000 Review of neuroimaging studies of child and adolescent psychiatric disorders from the past 10 years. Journal of the American Academy of Child & Adolescent Psychiatry 39: 815–828

Herholz K 1996 Neuroimaging in anorexia nervosa. Psychiatry Research 62: 105–110

Hounsfield G N 1973 Computerized transverse axial scanning (tomography), 1: Description of system. British Journal of Radiology 46: 1016–1022

Jeste D V, Lohr J B, Goodwin F K 1988 Neuroanatomical studies of major affective disorders: a review and suggestions for further research. British Journal of Psychiatry 153: 444–459

Job D E, Whalley H C, McConnells et al 2002 Structural gray matter differences between first-episode schizophrenics and normal controls using voxel-based morphometery. Neuroimage 17: 880–889

Johnstone E C, Crow T J, Frith C D et al 1976 Cerebral ventricular size and cognitive impairment in chronic schizophrenia. Lancet 2: 924–926

Krasuski J S, Alexander G E, Horwitz B et al 2002 Relation of medial temporal lobe volumes to age and memory function in nondemented adults with Down's syndrome: implications for the prodromal phase of Alzheimer's disease. American Journal of Psychiatry 159: 74–81

Kril J J, Halliday G M 1999 Brain shrinkage in alcoholics: a decade on and what have we learned? Progress in Neurobiology 58: 381–387

Kuikka J T, Tammela L, Karhuncn L et al 2001 Reduced serotonin transporter binding in binge eating women. Psychopharmacology (Berlin) 155: 310–314

Kwon H, Menon V, Eliez S et al 2001 Functional neuroanatomy of visuospatial working memory in fragile X syndrome: relation to behavioral and molecular measures. American Journal of Psychiatry 158: 1040–1051

Laruelle M 1998 Imaging dopamine transmission in schizophrenia: a review and metaanalysis. Quarterly Journal of Nuclear Medicine 42: 211–221

Lawrie S M, Abukmeil S S 1998 Brain abnormality in schizophrenia: a systematic and quantitative review of volumetric magnetic resonace imaging studies. British Journal of Psychiatry 172: 110–120

Lawrie S M, Abukmeil S S, Chiswick A et al 1997 Qualitative cerebral morphology in schizophrenia: a magnetic resonance imaging study and systematic literature review. Schizophrenia Research 25: 155–166

Lawrie S M, Byrne M, Miller P et al 2001 Neurodevelopmental indices and the development of psychotic symptoms in subjects at high risk of schizophrenia. British Journal of Psychiatry 178: 524–530

Lawrie S M, Buechel C, Whalley H C et al 2002 Reduced frontotemporal functional connectivity in schizophrenia associated with auditory hallucinations. Biological Psychiatry 51: 1008–1011

Lewis S 1991 Computerised tomography in schizophrenia. British Journal of Psychiatry 159: 158–159

Lipschutz B, Friston K J, Ashburner J et al 2001 Technical Note: Assessing study-specific regional variations in fMRI signal. NeuroImage 13: 392–398

McBride W J, Murphy J M, Ikemoto S 1999 Localization of brain reinforcement mechanisms: intracranial self-administration and intracranial place-conditioning studies. Behavioural Brain Research 101: 129–152

McIntosh C, Ritson B 2001 Treating depression complicated by substance misuse. Advances in Psychiatric Treatment 7: 357–364

McKeith I G 2002 Dementia with Lewy bodies. British Journal of Psychiatry 180: 144–147

Meyer-Lindenberg A, Miletich R S, Kohn P D et al 2002 Reduced prefrontal activity predicts exaggerated striatal dopaminergic function in schizophrenia. Nature Neuroscience 5: 267–271

Mitchell D G 1999 MRI principles. W B Saunders, London

Moonen C T W, Bandettini P A 2000 Functional MRI. Springer-Verlag, Berlin

Phan K L, Wagner T, Taylor S F et al 2002 Functional neuroanatomy of emotion: a meta-analysis of emotion activation studies in PET and fMRI. NeuroImage 16: 331–348

Pitman R K, Shin L M, Rauch S L 2001 Investigating the pathogenesis of posttraumatic stress disorder with neuroimaging. Journal of Clinical Psychiatry 62 (suppl): 47–54

Pizzagalli D, Pascual-Marqui R D, Nitschke J B et al 2001 Anterior cingulate activity as a predictor of degree of treatment response in major depression: evidence from brain electrical tomography analysis. American Journal of Psychiatry 158: 405–415

Raz S, Raz N 1990 Structural brain abnormalities in the major psychoses: a quantitative review of the evidence from computerized imaging. Psychological Bulletin 108: 93–108

Reiss A L, Eliez S, Schmitt J E et al 2000 Brain imaging in neurogenetic conditions: realizing the potential of behavioral neurogenetics research. Mental Retardation & Developmental Disability Research Review 6: 186–197

Reneman L, Booij J, Lavalaye J et al 2002 Use of amphetamine by recreational users of ecstasy (MDMA) is associated with reduced striatal dopamine transporter densities: a B-CIT SPECT study. Psychopharmacology 159: 335–340

Rolls E T 1999 The brain and emotion. Oxford University Press, Oxford

Saxena S, Bota R G, Brody A L 2001 Brain–behavior relationships in obsessive–compulsive disorder. Seminars in Clinical Neuropsychiatry 6: 82–101

Scahill R I, Schott J M, Stevens J M et al 2002 Mapping the evolution of regional atrophy in Alzheimer's disease: unbiased analysis of fluid-registered serial MRI. Proceedings of the National Academy of Sciences of the USA 99: 4703–4707

Shah P J, Ebmeier K P, Glabus M F et al 1998 Cortical grey matter reductions associated with treatment-resistant unipolar depression: controlled magnetic resonance imaging study. British Journal of Psychiatry 172: 527–532

Sheline Y I, Wang P W, Gado M H et al 1996 Hippocampal atrophy in recurrent major depression. Proceedings of the National Academy of Sciences of the USA 93: 3908–3913

Shenton M E, Dickey C C, Frumin M, McCarley R W 2001 A review of MRI findings in schizophrenia. Schizophrenia Research 49: 1–52

Shergill S S, Brammer M J, Williams S C et al 2000 Mapping auditory hallucinations in schizophrenia using functional magnetic resonance imaging. Archives of General Psychiatry 57: 1033–1038

Smith A D, Jobst K A 1996 Use of structural imaging to study the progression of Alzheimer's disease. British Medical Bulletin 52: 575–586

Talairach J, Tournoux P 1988 Co-planar stereotaxic atlas of the human brain. Thieme, Stuttgart

Tauscher J, Pirker W, Willeit M et al 2001 [^{123}I] beta-CIT and single photon emission computed tomography reveal reduced brain serotonin transporter availability in bulimia nervosa. Biological Psychiatry 49: 326–332

Thompson P M, Mega M S, Woods R P et al 2001 Cortical change in Alzheimer's disease detected with a disease-specific population-based brain atlas. Cerebral Cortex 11: 1–16

Toga A W, Mazziotta J C 1996 Brain mapping: the methods. Academic Press, London

Videbech P 1997 MRI findings in patients with affective disorder: a meta-analysis. Acta Psychiatrica Scandinavica 96: 157–168

Villarreal G, King C Y 2001 Brain imaging in posttraumatic stress disorder. Seminars in Clinical Neuropsychiatry 6: 131–145

Volkow N D, Fowler J S 2000 Addiction, a disease of compulsion and drive: involvement of the orbitofrontal cortex. Cerebral Cortex 10: 318–325

Vollenweider F X, Leenders K L, Scharfetter C et al 1997 Positron emission tomography and fluorodeoxyglucose studies of metabolic hyperfrontality and psychopathology in the psilocybin model of psychosis. Neuropsychopharmacology 16: 357–372

Vythilingam M, Anderson E R, Goddard A et al 2000 Temporal lobe volume in panic disorder—a quantitative magnetic resonance imaging study. Psychiatry Research 99: 75–82

Webb S 1996 The physics of medical imaging. Institute of Physics, London

Weinberger D R, Berman K F, Zec R F 1986 Physiologic dysfunction of dorsolateral prefrontal cortex in schizophrenia, I: Regional cerebral blood flow evidence. Archives of General Psychiatry 43: 114–124

Wright I C, Rabe-Hesketh S, Woodruff P W et al 2000 Meta-analysis of regional brain volumes in schizophrenia. American Journal of Psychiatry 157: 16–25

Zald D H, Kim S W 1996 Anatomy and function of the orbital frontal cortex, II: function and relevance to obsessive compulsive disorder. Journal of Neuropsychiatry & Clinical Neurosciences 8: 249–261

6 Fundamentals of psychology

Michael J Power, Ronan E O'Carroll

INTRODUCTION

The case can be made that of all the disciplines that are essential for the study of psychiatry, knowledge of psychology is the most important. However, until recently, psychology (or behavioural science) has represented a very small component of the general medical curriculum. Most psychiatrists on commencing higher training have therefore had relatively little exposure to psychology, yet have elected to specialise in the medical discipline whose essence is the study and treatment of abnormal experience and behaviour. Such individuals will enter higher training with a good background in anatomy, physiology and pharmacology, yet may have relatively little knowledge and understanding of the scientific basis of perception, emotion, cognition and personality.

It is clearly impossible to provide even a cursory overview of psychology in one brief chapter; however, in the sections that follow, we attempt to present some basic psychological principles and theories that are particularly relevant for psychiatry. A separate chapter is provided on neuropsychology, and this material will therefore not be covered here.

What is 'psychology'? The definition depends on the view of psychology to which you subscribe. The behavioural approach, which we will consider later in detail, has traditionally defined psychology as the 'study of behaviour' because behaviour is observable and measurable. In contrast, cognitive psychologists have offered definitions of psychology along the lines of 'the science of mental life'. It may be possible of course to incorporate all of these elements and offer an integrated definition such as 'the science of behaviour and mental life . . .'. Although the focus of the present book is on psychiatry and its disorders, the different views about psychology are reflected in the different approaches to and models of these disorders. However, for most disorders there has as yet been no one particular model that has been sufficient in itself, but a number of models may need to be integrated eventually in order to provide a full account of the problem.

In order to examine the question of 'What is psychology?', we must first ask 'What is science?' in order to understand some of the associated disagreements. In so doing, we will see that two views of science can be identified: first, the traditional view which emphasises fact, experiment and measurement and which has had a strong influence on behavioural psychology, and, second, a modern view of science which emphasises subjectivity, unpredictability and non-deterministic processes. This modern view is more compatible with cognitive psychology.

The traditional view of science

The traditional view of science emphasises a number of basic principles which have proven of great value in the history and development of science. In fact, 19th-century scientists thought that all the major problems of science had been answered by the development of grand theories such as Newton's mechanics, thermodynamics and Darwin's theory of evolution, and that only the details were left to be filled in. The basic principles on which these developments were considered to depend are as follows.

Observation and fact Facts are observable measurable properties of the world: tigers are indigenous to India; the eye is sensitive to light: water freezes at 0°C. A large part of any science therefore is the routine accumulation of facts and observations; the modern computer can store a vast number of facts about weather conditions, star positions, activity in a bubble chamber, or amino acid sequences in proteins. Of course, even traditional science was aware that 'facts' do not always turn out to be what they appear to be. The Earth was originally thought to be flat because it looked flat, besides which if it wasn't flat you would fall of the edge; then astronomers discovered that the Earth was round. Later on we learned that the Earth was not perfectly round but flattened at the poles; finally, science told us that in fact the Earth is geoid-shaped (i.e. the fact is the Earth turns out to have been 'earth-shaped' all along!). In medicine of course observation of signs plays a crucial role in diagnosis; the collation of such signs and other symptoms is then used to provide descriptive classification systems such as that used in the American Diagnostic and Statistical Manual (DSM-IV) and the World Health Organization's International Classification of Diseases system (currently ICD-10), as we shall discuss next.

Description and classification If science only consisted of observation and fact, it would turn out no better than Dickens's character Mr Gradgrind, 'Give me the facts'. Instead, the next step is finding the appropriate level of description which can be meaningfully included in a classification system. For example, Linnaeus's classification of living things provided a magnificent taxonomy that helped to advance biology; the appropriate level of description seems relatively straightforward in that individual plants or animals provide the lowest level of description, which, in turn, can be grouped together at more general levels (species, phyla, etc.). Classification systems may nevertheless contain surprises that are counter to common sense, such as 'whales are mammals' and 'chillies are fruit'. It is precisely these 'surprises' to common sense that are generated by theoretically based rather than simply consensus-based classification systems.

A second example of a classification system that has powerful predictive properties is Mendeleev's periodic table, which provides a meaningful classification of the chemical elements. The original Greek classification of the four 'elements', earth, air, fire and water proved to be an inappropriate one for science in that each of these so-called 'elements' was divisible into more basic elements. The power of Mendeleev's system, which classified elements by their atomic weight, was that it revealed gaps or missing elements which had not been discovered at that time, but which have subsequently been discovered.

To return to the medico-psychiatric classification systems such as DSM-IV and ICD-10, these systems of diagnosis and classification are not theoretically based systems, but, instead, are systems agreed by committees who change their minds every few years. In fact, it is more accurate to state that the systems contain a mish-mash of theories, as powerful individuals on the committees horse-trade their favourite diagnoses with each other. Hardly the way to do science! Until psychiatry therefore has a theoretically based and empirically supported diagnostic and classification system, it will remain at a the level of mere descriptive science.

Theory and hypothesis Theories group together facts and descriptions in a way that provides an overall working model relevant to the domain in question. A good theory, as the philosopher Karl Popper stated, is both useful and falsifiable; that is, a good theory should generate hypotheses which may be novel and surprising and which can be tested in man-made or 'natural' experiments. One of the classic examples is that of Einstein's theory of relativity, which predicted that light would bend in a gravitational field, a prediction that was dramatically upheld when the light from a distant source was shown to bend as it passed the sun.

Popper and others used his notion of falsifiability to argue that certain 'theories' such as psychoanalysis are not scientific theories at all, because they are not falsifiable. Whatever happens in the rest of science, theories in psychology are rarely if ever rejected because of evidence to the contrary, but rather they go out of fashion. We will see later in the chapter, however, that Popper's antagonism towards psychoanalysis may have been misdirected and that there is a continuing interest in a number of psychoanalytic ideas.

Experiment Hypotheses derived from scientific theories may be tested in man-made and natural experiments in order to decide whether or not the experimental outcome is that predicted by the hypothesis. Experiments have to be carefully designed in order for us to be sure that the variable that the experimenter manipulates (the independent variable) is truly the one that leads to differences in the variable that is measured (the dependent variable). If the experimental outcome is due to some other confounding variable rather than the one that is manipulated, then the experiment is invalid. Psychology experiments on human subjects are notoriously difficult because what the *subject* thinks the experiment is about can often be more important that what the *experimenter* thinks the experiment is about. In addition, many of the advances in psychology and medicine come not from experiments in which the experimenter manipulates one or more variables, but rather from 'experiments of nature' such as road traffic accidents, strokes, life events and natural disasters, the tragic consequences of which can provide insights into how the mind works. Such single-case studies have always provided major advances in medicine, psychiatry and psychology; these studies can also move beyond the merely descriptive, and sophisticated single-case quasi-experi-

mental designs are now available to use as appropriate (e.g. see Barker et al 2002).

The modern view of science

The modern view of science does not reject the role of facts, measurement, observation, hypothesis, classification and experiment, but it does point to some severe limitations which draw modern science and modern psychology closer together. To begin with, let us take the building blocks of science: that is, 'facts' or 'observations'. These sacred objects have the status of absolute truths in traditional science, but modern science has emphasised their possible subjective nature and the role that inference as well as observation plays in making a fact a fact. For example, our sensory experience tells us the 'fact' that the Sun rises in the East and sinks in the West. The fact is, however, that it is not the Sun that rises and falls, but the Earth that rotates on its axis. Every schoolchild knows about the existence of electrons, protons and neutrons, but nobody has ever observed these particles directly. Instead, it is both useful and necessary to infer their existence from other observations such as pathways in a bubble chamber.

Traditional science has emphasised prediction and control in deterministic systems: that is, the idea that outcomes are always knowable if all of the initial conditions are known. In contrast, modern science emphasises unpredictability and non-deterministic systems. Even at the atomic level, Heisenberg's uncertainty principle tells us that we cannot know both the position of an electron and its momentum, because the measurement of one affects the other; at best all we can do is make probabilistic statements about what might or might not happen. In a similar manner in psychology and psychiatry we can study the rules that people use to construct sentences and participate in conversations but we can never determine what any speaker will say on any particular occasion. The problems faced by the complex systems that meteorologists and psychologists study is that very small differences in initial conditions can make a considerable difference to outcome: the developments in so-called 'chaos' or 'catastrophe theory' in the physical sciences demonstrate vividly how even simple systems can have unpredictable outcomes (see e.g. Gleick 1988). The moral of this tale for psychology is that both the traditional and the modern views of science have their advantages and disadvantages. Behavioural and experimental psychologists have focused typically on observation and measurement and, as we shall discuss, have made considerable contributions to our understanding of the laws of learning and the acquisition and treatment of a range of behavioural disorders. However, psychoanalytic and cognitive psychologists have come to emphasise the importance of subjective factors and how they influence an individual's thoughts, emotions and actions. The aim of this chapter is to demonstrate how each approach to psychology has something to offer for our understanding of psychological disorders. The chapter will focus on seven main areas of psychology: behaviourism, psychoanalysis, cognitive psychology, personality, emotion, psychobiology and developmental psychology.

BEHAVIOURISM

Behaviourism was a reaction against the 'introspectionist' approach to psychology, where armchair psychologists sat and recorded their own mental processes. The American psychologist

J B Watson was the leading figure of the behavioural approach to psychology. Watson argued that the study of the mind was a scientific irrelevance because the mind is unobservable, and indeed he subsequently focused primarily on the environment. He argued that only behaviour is observable and therefore that a science of psychology must be a science of behaviour. Behaviourists drew on the work of the Russian physiologist Ivan Pavlov. Pavlov was awarded the Nobel Prize for his work on the physiology of digestion. In the course of subsequent work on salivation in the dog, he noticed that the dogs began to salivate on seeing the attendant who normally fed them. Pavlov made those observations the basis for his subsequent study of the conditioned reflex (or 'conditional reflex' in Pavlov's own terms). His most famous studies were of bell-ringing and salivation in dogs.

Two other significant figures in behavioural psychology were Edward Thorndike and B F Skinner. Thorndike became famous for his study of how cats learned to escape from puzzle boxes; over a number of trials the cats were found through trial-and-error learning to escape more quickly from the boxes. Thorndike's so-called *law of effect* stated that responses were either more likely or less likely to occur according to the consequences that they produced. B F Skinner continued Thorndike's study of learning based on the consequences of behaviour. Many behaviourists accepted that thoughts and feelings had a causal role to play in our behaviour, but because they were unobservable were not within the domain of science. In contrast to these 'methodological behaviourists', Skinner espoused a so-called 'radical behaviourist' philosophy which stated that, although such private events existed, they played no causal role in behaviour but were merely by-products of internal physiological processes. Skinner stated that the true determinants of behaviour were the environment and the organism's genetics and learning history, which were both represented neurophysiologically.

Classical conditioning

This type of learning was originally identified by Pavlov, and hence is also known as Pavlovian conditioning. The basic paradigm is shown in Figure 6.1. The figure shows that an unconditioned stimulus (UCS) such as food leads to an unconditioned response (UCR) such as salivation. The pairing of an initially neutral stimulus such as a bell with the UCS eventually leads the bell to become a conditioned stimulus (CS) for the conditioned response (CR) of salivation. Pavlov demonstrated that conditioning occurs optimally if the CS occurs just prior to the UCS, that conditioning will generalise to other stimuli that are similar to the original CS, and that the CR will gradually extinguish over a number of

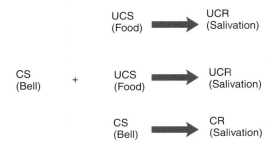

Fig. 6.1
An outline of classical (Pavlovian) conditioning. (U)C, (un)conditioned; S, stimulus; R, response.

trials if the CS is presented on its own without the UCS. Pavlov originally thought that any stimulus could be paired with any other stimulus, though subsequent research has questioned this idea. For example, Seligman (1971) suggested the concept of *preparedness*, that evolutionarily significant stimuli or 'prepared stimuli' may be more conditionable than others in fear reactions; thus, it is far more common for people to develop snake phobias than to develop sheep phobias, even though they may never have had any direct experience with a snake. However, the evidence for Seligman's proposal is still unclear (Rachman 1990).

One of the main applications of classical conditioning to adult psychological disorders has been through an analysis of 'conditioned emotional responses'. The idea is that the pairing of a neutral stimulus with an aversive or traumatic UCS which produces an unpleasant emotional response will lead the neutral stimulus to produce conditioned emotional responses. A famous early demonstration of this sequence was carried out by Watson & Rayner (1920) with a 1-year-old child named Little Albert. The child was happily playing with a white rat (the CS) when a loud noise (the UCS) behind him produced a startle reaction and considerable distress (the UCR). After a few such pairings of the white rat and the noise, the white rat eventually produced an unpleasant emotional reaction (the CR) on its own. This reaction generalised to other similar objects such as white rabbits (and even to Santa's beard!). This type of conditioning has been incorporated into learning models for the development of clinical phobias, for example a child traumatised by being bitten or frightened by a dog may develop a phobia of dogs.

Operant conditioning

Both Skinner and Thorndike emphasised that classical conditioning was one type of learning that applied in the main to more reflex-like or autonomic nervous system behaviour. In contrast, they argued that voluntary behaviour is dependent on its *consequences* for whether or not it is likely to be repeated. More formally, Skinner stated that operant (or 'instrumental') conditioning is based on the three-term contingency of *discriminative stimulus, response*, and *outcome*. A discriminative stimulus indicates whether or not a particular contingency applies: for example, a green light might indicate that any pressing of a lever in a Skinner box would lead to a food reward. The outcome can be positive (e.g. food) and therefore the likelihood of the response increases — that is, it is positively reinforcing — or it can be punitive (e.g. electric shock) in which case the response is punished and is less likely to occur again under those stimulus conditions.

Other key concepts in operant conditioning are *negative reinforcement, schedules of reinforcement*, and *shaping*. In contrast to the punishment procedure described above in which a response is less likely to occur because the outcome is unpleasant, in negative reinforcement the response is *more* likely to occur because it switches off an aversive stimulus such as shock or loud noise. For example, a rat that learns to avoid a section of its cage because it has received mild foot shock in the past has learned via negative reinforcement: moving away terminated the aversive experience. The term 'schedule of reinforcement' refers to the fact that in many situations not every response is reinforced; for example, people are typically rewarded with money for their work once a week or once a month (a 'fixed-interval' schedule), though some individuals on piecework are rewarded for the amount that they produce (normally a 'fixed-ratio' schedule). One of the properties of these partial rather than continuous reinforcement schedules is that the behaviour is more resistant to extinction; thus, if reinforcement is no longer presented, an individual who has been rewarded for every response will normally stop responding sooner than someone who has received partial reinforcement. The term 'shaping' refers to the technique whereby the organism is initially rewarded for responses that only vaguely resemble the desired response, but gradually the reinforced response approximates closer the desired response. For example, a performing dog in a circus is unlikely to pirouette three times and then roll over straight away, but through *shaping by successive approximations* to the desired behaviour, the dog could be trained to do so. A clinical example of the use of shaping procedures is in skill acquisition training for individuals with learning disabilities.

Escape and avoidance are two further important types of operant conditioning. In escape learning, the organism receives an aversive stimulus such as an electric shock, which a particular response such as pressing a lever will remove. In avoidance learning, an initial discriminative stimulus signals that if the appropriate response does not occur, then the aversive stimulus will be presented. One well-known variant on escape/avoidance learning is Seligman's (1975) 'learned helplessness'. In learned helplessness tasks, the organism initially receives non-contingent punishment, that is, the aversive stimulus is received whatever response the animal makes. The contingency is then changed such that a response would lead to escape from the aversive stimulus, but the typical finding is that the animal remains helpless and does not find the escape response. Seligman proposed that learned helplessness could provide a model for the acquisition and maintenance of depression in humans.

Behaviour therapy

A classic demonstration of behaviour therapy was carried out by Mary Cover Jones (1924). Following in the Little Albert tradition, she successfully treated a young boy's fear of rabbits by having him eat in the presence of a rabbit, while gradually bringing the rabbit closer to him over a number of occasions. The basic idea of the encouragement of a response such as eating which is incompatible with fear was further elaborated by Joseph Wolpe (1958). Wolpe first taught phobic adults a muscle relaxation technique, which they then used whilst imagining increasingly fearful stimuli — a technique that Wolpe called *systematic desensitisation*. Although sometimes still used, behaviour therapists now generally prefer to use actual exposure to the feared object or situation when this is possible rather than just working in imagination (e.g. Marks 1987). This technique is termed *graded exposure*; the phobic individual gradually works through a hierarchy towards the feared stimulus. For example, a dog phobic may work through a hierarchy from a photograph of a puppy, photograph of a larger dog, video of a puppy, video of a larger dog, puppy through a oneway mirror, etc. The phobic individual and therapist work as a team in a collaborative relationship, and the patient only moves on to the next stage of the hierarchy when he feels ready to do so. Exposure-based treatments have proved particularly effective in the treatment of anxiety disorders.

Two-factor learning theory

One of the classic theories on which behaviour therapy was based was Mowrer's (1939) two-factor theory of the acquisition and maintenance of fear. Mowrer proposed that both classical and operant conditioning were involved. The first step was that an originally neutral stimulus acquired fearful properties by being paired with a frightening or painful event, that is, through a classical conditioning procedure (e.g. as in the case of Little Albert). The second step is that through a process of operant conditioning, the individual learns to reduce the fear by avoidance of the relevant object or situation, and hence avoidance behaviour is reinforced. Much of the focus of behavioural interventions in anxiety and obsessional disorders has therefore included exposure to the feared object or situation, a procedure that is repeated until the fear response reduces substantially. However, it is now well recognised that not all fears are acquired in accordance with the two-factor theory (e.g. Rachman 1990) and that not all so-called fears or phobias are based on anxiety but that some are based on disgust reactions (Power & Dalgleish 1997). Most people with a fear of flying have never actually flown, so their fear could not have been acquired by classical conditioning in the situation itself. Conversely, not everybody who has experienced a traumatic event while flying (e.g. a hijack) develops a phobia. Instead, the observation of someone else (e.g. a parent) being fearful about an object or situation (known as *'vicarious'* or *'observational'* learning) is also a common source of fears and phobias.

PSYCHOANALYSIS

Psychoanalytic theory has been important historically in informing views concerning personality, consciousness and psychological interventions. However, psychoanalysis, the treatment developed by Sigmund Freud based on psychoanalytic theory, lost popularity largely because of criticisms regarding its efficacy (e.g. Eysenck 1969). Furthermore, many critics have suggested that psychoanalysis is not scientific, as it is not open to refutation by experimentation. More recently, psychoanalytic theory has undergone somewhat of a renaissance. Two main factors have contributed to this renewed interest. First, there has been a huge amount of attention devoted to the phenomenon of 'recovered memories' in adult survivors of child sexual abuse (Conway 1997, Davies & Dalgleish 2002). This has focused research attention to the issue of whether or not it is possible to have no memory of an experience for many years, only for it to resurface in later life. Recent studies within the domain of cognitive psychology have shown that repression can be induced in the laboratory (Conway 2001). Findings such as this have forced a re-examination of basic psychoanalytic concepts. Secondly, recent advances in our understanding of how unconscious processes can influence overt behaviour (e.g. studies of 'blind-sight' patients, studies of the effects of subliminal perceptual priming, and the study of explicit versus implicit memory systems) have made some of Freud's proposals on the role of the unconscious appear more plausible and, critically, empirically testable.

The unconscious

Freud did not simply see the unconscious as an inactive storehouse of past memories, but rather as a system of wishes, fantasies, impulses and memories that actively influenced our thoughts, actions, symptoms, dreams, mistakes, accidents and emotions. He proposed that the unconscious was derived from innate drives of which we could never become directly conscious, and repressed material which was typically of an unpleasant personal nature. One of the key points Freud proposed about the unconscious was that it defied time and logic and was not constrained by reality. For example, painful memories could be recalled from many years past as if they were happening now and had lost none of their emotional impact. (This phenomenon is observed in descriptions of the re-experiencing of traumatic memories in post-traumatic stress disorder.) In a similar manner, opposite and contradictory thoughts and impulses can be held in the unconscious; the same person can be both loved and hated at the same time.

Psychic energy

Freud believed that the mind was fuelled by psychic energy very much in the way that physical energy is needed to fuel a physical machine. This energy, or 'libido' as it was called, he initially considered to be derived from the life-preserving drives, 'Eros'. Freud added a second set of life-destroying drives, 'Thanatos', which typically manifested themselves as aggression towards the self or towards others.

The comparison that Freud made between psychic energy and physical energy led to him adopting the so-called 'principle of constancy'; namely, that by analogy with the laws of thermodynamics, psychic energy can never be created nor destroyed, but can only be changed from one form to another. For example, if sexual energy is blocked from being expressed through the normal channels, then it has to be expressed in other forms. In milder cases these forms could be disguised in dreams, in symptoms such as headaches, or in excessive intellectual activity, and so on. However, in more extreme cases Freud suggested that severe psychological disorders including anxiety, depression and obsessional disorders resulted from the blocking of sexual energy.

Repression

Freud used the term 'repression' in various ways in his writings in order to refer to either the conscious or the unconscious avoidance of painful or unwanted information — in particular, information about the self or the self in relation to significant others. Freud used repression as a general term therefore to refer to almost any defence mechanism. However, his daughter, Anna Freud, in 1937 provided a systematic list that, along with repression (in the specific sense of an *unconscious* avoidance of an unacceptable impulse or idea), included a number of other defence mechanisms such as reaction formation, sublimation and projection. Recently, Anderson & Green (2001) provided an elegant demonstration of experimentally induced memory repression in the laboratory. They showed that if a memory that is associated with something familiar is actively avoided every time that familiar object is seen, then the memory becomes repressed and the avoided item is later difficult to remember.

Developmental stages

Freud proposed that the child passes through a series of developmental stages labelled the oral, anal, phallic, latency and genital phases. The main sources of pleasure in the oral, anal and phallic stages are the mouth, the anus and the genitals, respectively. One of the additional proposals is that fixation can occur at different stages of development which can either be apparent as personality traits, or revealed at times of stress. Typical oral characteristics are talkativeness, greed, gullibility and generosity, whereas typical anal characteristics include obstinacy, orderliness and miserliness.

Transference and countertransference

Freud's early collaborator, Josef Breuer, found that one of his hysterical patients, Anna O, developed very strong feelings towards him in the course of his treatment of her. Breuer was unable to cope with the strength of her feelings and terminated her treatment. The feelings that the patient has for the therapist are called transference. Originally, therefore, transference was seen as a nuisance that impeded the therapeutic process, but Freud later recognised the therapeutic potential of transference. He believed that transference was a re-enactment in the relationship with the therapist of earlier significant relationships and provided an opportunity to examine their nature via the exploration of fantasies and feelings in the transference relationship. In fact, the exploration of transference is considered to be the key therapeutic tool in psychoanalytic work, because it provides insight into past and present relationships and allows the working through of related conflicts and problems. The intimate situation in which the therapist and patient are placed and the fact that the psychoanalyst sits behind the patient are methods which encourage transference. The technique of free association, whereby the patient is meant to say whatever comes into his or her mind, also allows the patient to dwell on fantasies about the therapist which the more directive therapies such as behaviour therapy and cognitive therapy would typically steer the patient away from.

The fact that patients have strong reactions to their therapists does not preclude the fact that therapists may have strong reactions, both positive and negative, to their patients. Such reactions are called counter-transference and again can either be seen as nuisance phenomena that have no relevance to the treatment process or can be used in the course of therapy as a source of important information about the therapeutic relationship.

COGNITIVE PSYCHOLOGY

The general area of cognitive psychology is a broad one that overlaps with other disciplines such as linguistics, philosophy, artificial intelligence and anthropology, and indeed a new discipline of 'cognitive science' has emerged from this overlap. There is as yet no one grand theory in cognitive psychology, but, instead, there is a general agreement that, whatever form they might take, internal mental states play important causal roles in the generation of action (e.g. Bolton & Hill 1996). Beyond this, there is agreement that the system must process information from a range of sensory inputs, that this information needs to be transformed in various ways so that, for example, meaningless sequences of sounds can be interpreted meaningfully, and that there must be an overall system that co-ordinates these multiple functions. Most of this information processing occurs outside of awareness, and we only become aware of the extent to which it is automatic when we put our foot on the 'brake' while sitting in the passenger seat, or drive home to the flat that we used to live in rather than the one that we've just moved to. In the remainder of this section an outline will be provided of a number of key areas from cognitive psychology that are relevant to adult psychiatric disorders.

Perception and attention

The German physicist and physiologist Hermann von Helmholtz is considered to be the father of the science of perception. Long before Freud had developed his ideas on the dynamic unconscious, Helmholtz, in the 1860s, had argued that perception must be based on 'unconscious inferences' (Power 1997). For example, when we look at an object at different distances it looks the same size, even though the physical size of the object on the retina is very different (so-called 'object constancy'); the same object can be looked at from different angles yet appears to preserve its shape (so-called 'shape constancy'); and an object can be viewed under different lighting conditions and appear the same colour (so-called 'colour constancy'). Although the unconscious perceptual processes which give rise to these constancies have clear advantages, the fact that processing necessarily distorts the incoming information can under other circumstances lead to disadvantages which, at one extreme can produce mildly amusing perceptual illusions, and at the other extreme can lead the individual to perceive life-threatening danger where there is none.

One of the central questions in the perception and attention literature has been the extent to which sensory information is analysed prior to conscious awareness. Broadbent (1958) argued that this input is analysed at a superficial physical level and that only input that reaches awareness is analysed for its meaning. Subsequent work on attention, however, has suggested that the sensory input can be analysed for meaning without the individual having to be aware of the input; in the so-called 'cocktail party phenomenon' an individual can be attending to one conversation, but suddenly become aware of his or her name being spoken in another conversation. This phenomenon demonstrates that the unattended information must have been analysed for meaning for the switch of attention to happen.

Memory

One of the questions that cognitive psychology has addressed is the form that internal representation of the world takes. Do we remember visual scenes as if they were video-recorded sequences? Or conversations as if they were tape-recorded? Given the arguments that couples have about who said what to whom and when, it might seem unlikely that memory is in any way veridical in the manner of tape and video-recorders. The question then is to what extent is memory a reconstruction, one part truth to nine parts fiction? This question has bedevilled recent debates about the possibility of repressed traumatic memories versus the possibility of false memories in cases of sexual abuse (see Davies & Dalgleish 2002).

In his classic book on cognitive psychology, Ulric Neisser (1967) took an extreme constructivist view that the process of remembering is like the palaeontologist who, on the basis of a couple of small bones, constructs a whole dinosaur. More recently, Neisser has stepped back from this extreme view in the recognition that memory can sometimes be surprisingly accurate. We must recognise too that in the development of childhood vulnerability for later adult disorders, the child may be given conflicting information that is difficult to integrate in memory; for example, a mother may repeatedly insist to the child that she loves him above all else, though her actions may clearly contradict her statements. There is no reason, of course, why there could not be more than one memory (or group of memories) of a particular event or person; a number of current views of memory would be consistent with such a possibility. In such cases some of the aims of therapy may be to help the adult identify such discrepancies, to work through the consequent emotions, and to reintegrate the memories into a more realistic overall representation of the person or the event (e.g. Power & Dalgleish 1997).

A further question that cognitive psychologists ask about memory is what the basic psychological units are. To this question there have been numerous answers and few if any conclusions. One of the types of internal representation that has played a significant role, from the work of Bartlett early in the 20th century onwards, is the *schema*. Piaget also used the term 'schema' in his studies of child development, and Beck in his account of cognitive therapy. Although there is considerable variation in the use of the term (see Power & Champion 1986), schemata refer to unitary representations of regularly encountered objects, events and situations, and activation of one part of a schema leads automatically to activation of all other parts. To give an example, if subjects are shown a picture of a car which does not show the wheels, they may make the schematic error later in recall and include wheels which were not originally shown, because cars normally have wheels. Schema theory therefore predicts that processes such as memory and perception are prone to schema-congruent errors. It must be noted that in certain clinical conditions these schemata are less than benign and may, of course, lead the depressed individual to perceive or to recall loss even where none is present objectively, or the anxious person to perceive or to recall life-endangering threat. It must be remembered that despite their widespread use, schemata constitute only one of panoply of units that have been proposed for the representation of knowledge.

Reasoning

An assumption made by many philosophers and psychologists is that people use formal logical rules in reasoning. Perhaps the clearest account of such a system was provided by Jean Piaget in his studies of child development (see section on developmental psychology, below). However, there is now a considerable body of research that demonstrates the limits of the adult capacity for reasoning, though the debate still continues over whether errors are the result of performance limitations (e.g. working memory being limited in processing capacity) or whether there is no such thing as 'mental logic'.

Three main types of reasoning task are *deduction*, *induction*, and *probability judgement*. Deduction is the drawing of a conclusion from a set of premises; induction is the drawing of a general rule on the basis of one or a limited number of instances; and probability judgements involve a statement about the likelihood of an event occurring. As an example of deductive reasoning, for the premises:

If I pass my exams I'll study medicine at university.

If I fail my exams I'll go into politics and become Prime Minister.

I've passed my exams.

the valid and perhaps fortunate conclusion is that I will study medicine at university. As an example of the problems that can arise with inductive reasoning, Wason and Johnson-Laird (e.g. see Johnson-Laird 1988) presented subjects with the series of digits '2 4 6' and asked them to discover the underlying rule through the production of additional examples. Most subjects set about *confirming* the possible rule 'even numbers increasing by two' by generating large numbers of positive instances of the rule, instead of attempting to *disconfirm* the rule by generating negative instances such as '7 8 9'. Had they done so, they would have eventually discovered that the rule was 'any three increasing numbers'. This confirmatory bias is one of the many biases that are evident from studies of reasoning. Other biases have been examined in an elegant series of studies by Kahneman and Tversky (e.g. Kahneman et al 1982). For example, the availability bias leads subjects to say that more words begin with the letter 'R' than have 'R' in the third letter, because it is easier to generate words beginning with 'R'. In a similar manner to the influence of biases introduced by schemata in memory, these reasoning biases can be quite benign in their effects and even on occasion lead us to be blissfully ignorant of our faults. However, under other circumstances the same biases can lead depressed individuals to conclude that they are insignificant and that life is not worth living, or paranoid individuals to conclude that their neighbours really are against them.

Cognitive therapy

Unlike psychoanalysis and behaviourism, where theory and therapy are very closely connected, cognitive therapy and cognitive psychology have developed almost independently of each other. Thus, it would be feasible to derive a cognitive-based therapy from current cognitive science that contrasted with current cognitive therapy on most points; or, more optimistically, it may be possible to bring cognitive therapy closer to cognitive science (Power 2001).

The details of cognitive therapy are given elsewhere, so they will only be summarised here. The theory has been developed by Beck (e.g. 1976) and is based on the idea that dysfunctional schemata arise in childhood typically in problematic parental relationships. These schemata normally remain dormant until later in life when a negative life event or stress occurs which activates them. For example, if the schemata focus on the need to feel loved by everybody and the first serious relationship goes wrong, the individual is vulnerable to becoming depressed. As a consequence of these activated schemata, the individual becomes overwhelmed with negative automatic thoughts such as 'I am unlovable', 'Nobody has ever really loved me', and so on, thoughts which lead the individual into a state of depression.

The therapy itself has four main components:

- *Education.* The depressed or anxious individual may have little information about depression or anxiety, or may have mistaken information such as a belief that a panic attack is the same as a heart attack. One of the useful features of cognitive therapy is the fact that individuals are provided with information about the condition they are experiencing and about the procedures used in cognitive therapy.
- *Goal-setting and graded activities.* Many depressed individuals withdraw from their normal activities, and the resultant inactivity may help to maintain the state of depression (e.g. reduced opportunity to experience reward). One of the key strategies of both cognitive therapy and behaviour therapy is the identification of what these activities might be, and then setting activities or homework to be carried out between clinical sessions. The activities typically begin with easier ones

and then gradually build up to more difficult ones in order to lessen the chance of failure early on in therapy.

- *The identification of negative automatic thoughts.* A key step in cognitive therapy is helping the individual to identify the negative automatic thoughts that are intimately connected with feelings of depression and anxiety. These may be identified in the clinical sessions themselves — for example, by asking the individual to role-play a difficult encounter — or they can be identified as homework by asking the individual to keep a diary of such thoughts in the situations in which they arise. Once identified, the individual is then encouraged to test their validity, to question them, and to check for the evidence for and against them.
- *Challenging dysfunctional schemata.* The identification and challenging of negative automatic thoughts leads into the final phase of cognitive therapy, which is challenging the dysfunctional schemata that underlie the negative thoughts. In depression, these core beliefs typically centre on the need to be loved or the need to do well at all costs. The depressed individual tends to take a one-sided view of past achievements in love and work and may feel hopeless about the possibility of any future success; although some of these views may well be realistic, the problem for the therapist is to disentangle the genuine failures from the imagined ones, so that individuals can take a more balanced view of themselves and their future.

PERSONALITY

Personality is the term used to describe consistency in peoples' behaviour, from one time to the next and from one situation to another. This is based on a fundamental assumption that certain behaviours characterise a person in a wide variety of situations. Critically, this view involves the belief that knowledge of an individual's personality will allow the prediction of how a given person will behave, even in situations in which the individual has never been observed before. Examples of the use of this predictive approach include personality assessment used in officer selection in the Second World War, and in selecting individuals for particular occupations, e.g. the sales force.

Nomothetic versus idiographic approaches

It has been traditional to categorise personality models into *nomothetic* or *idiographic* approaches. The nomothetic approach encompasses theories that portray personality in terms of shared attributes, i.e. there are a limited number of variables on which people differ. Within the nomothetic approach there are two main categories: *type* or *trait* approaches. Type theories are categorical in nature, i.e. are non-continuous. An example of the type approach within psychiatry is the use of diagnostic categories for specific personality disorders: you either have an antisocial personality disorder or you do not (see Ch. 25). The trait approach also advocates that there are a limited number of personality variables on which people differ; however, the critical difference is the notion that these variables are *continuous* in nature (akin to individual variation in height and weight). An example of the trait approach is Eysenck's three dimensions of personality: neuroticism, extraversion and psychoticism (Eysenck & Eysenck 1975). Theorists who favour the idiographic approach argue that the nomothetic type/trait method loses the individuality of the person. For example, two people could have the same scores on each of Eysenck's three dimensions of personality, but be viewed by others as quite different people. The idiographic approach considers each individual as unique. Psychodynamic and social learning theories are examples of nomothetic approaches.

Measuring personality

If personality is to be assessed, then one needs a measuring instrument that is both valid and reliable. The type of instrument that is developed clearly depends on the underlying theoretical model favoured.

Projective personality tests were developed from an idiographic, psychodynamic perspective, in particular that deeper layers of an individual's personality contain repressed wishes, impulses and desires that are not always accessible by conscious self-report. The essence of projective techniques is that they can bypass the individual's defence mechanisms by presenting stimuli which are ambiguous or unstructured. The examinee then has to impose some structure on the stimuli, and in doing so, reveals his own wishes, desires, impulses, etc. The two most widely used instruments are the Rorschach inkblots and the Thematic Apperception Test (TAT). The Rorschach inkblots were developed by a Swiss Psychiatrist, Herman Rorschach in 1921. The stimuli consist of 10 symmetrical ink blots, some coloured, some black and white. Examinees are asked to report what they 'see' in the ambiguous ink blots. The examinees' responses are thought to reflect their deep personality structure. By way of example, focusing on the small details of the ink blots can suggest compulsive rigidity. The TAT was developed by Morgan & Murray (1935) and consists of 30 pictures of various scenes; the examinee is asked to tell a story about each picture. As with the Rorschach, the product is thought to reflect the examinee's motives, conflicts, etc.

Attempts to evaluate the validity of the projective techniques have produced disappointing results. Several studies have compared projective test scores from psychiatric groups and healthy individuals, and have shown little if any difference between the groups in pattern of responding. Defenders of projective techniques argue that such studies are irrelevant, that the projective techniques are a means of facilitating communication between clinician and examinee, and that when used as part of a comprehensive clinical evaluation, they help to provide a richer understanding of the person (see Semeonoff 1976 for a detailed discussion of projective measures). Projective techniques are not widely used by clinical psychologists in the UK, largely because of concerns over reliability and validity.

Dimensions of personality

From a nomothetic perspective, if one believes that individuals can be described on a limited number of personality traits, how many traits are required? Allport & Odbert (1936) identified 18 000 words referring to personality traits in the unabridged English dictionary. It is clear that many of these words have similar meanings, and many attempts have been made to try to identify the core number of traits that are required in order to provide a full yet economic description of an individual's personality.

Cattell (1957) used the technique of factor analysis to reduce trait names to 16 personality factors, expressed as dimensions, e.g. tense versus relaxed, outgoing versus reserved. Cattell's factors

can be measured using his 16-PF self-report questionnaire (Cattell et al 1970). Further workers have proposed that a smaller number of dimensions can be used, and that each individual's personality can be described in terms of relative location on each of these dimensions.

Eysenck initially proposed a two-dimensional model: *neuroticism–stability* and *extraversion–introversion*. High neuroticism scorers would generally be described as anxious, prone to guilt, having low self-esteem and mood lability. High extraversion scorers tend to sociable, lively and assertive. Eysenck subsequently added a third dimension: *psychoticism* (P) or 'tough-mindedness'; a high P scorer would tend to be cold and lacking in empathy. Eysenck proposed that any individual's personality could be described by their relative placement on a 3-dimensional axis using his core three dimensions of personality. Eysenck's personality dimensions are assessed using self-report questionnaires such as the Eysenck Personality Questionnaire (EPQ) (Eysenck & Eysenck 1975).

The 'big five'

More recently, a number of investigators have conducted extensive factor-analytic studies and proposed that five dimensions are required in order to accurately describe an individual's personality structure (Norman 1963, Costa & McCrae 1992a) (Table 6.1). It is proposed that the richness of each individual's personality can be described in terms of relative placement on each of these five major dimensions of personality. Many studies using many different methods and questionnaires, conducted across different cultures, have generally found these same basic dimensions of personality. There has been a growing consensus that these five dimensions provide an economic method for describing a wide variety of individual differences. The 'Big Five' dimensions of personality can be measured using questionnaires such as the NEO Personality Inventory (Costa & McCrae 1992b). (A useful website which provides free measures and scoring keys for 'Big Five' instruments is the International Personality Item Pool – a Scientific Collaboratory for the Development of Advanced Measures of Personality Traits and Other Individual Differences: http://ipip.ori.org./ipip/new_home.htm).

Table 6.1 The 'Big Five' personality dimensions	
Factor name	**Scale dimensions**
Extroversion	Talkative / silent
	Adventurous / cautious
	Sociable / reclusive
Agreeableness	Good-natured / irritable
	Not jealous / jealous
	Co-operative / negativistic
Conscientiousness	Fussy, tidy / careless
	Responsible / undependable
	Scrupulous / unscrupulous
Neuroticism	Poised / nervous, tense
	Calm / anxious
	Composed / excitable
Openness to experience	Artistically sensitive / artistically insensitive
	Intellectual / unreflective, narrow
	Imaginative / simple, direct

The situational approach

Personality, by definition, is thought to be a stable phenomenon across situations and time. However, critics argue that refining instruments in order to perfect prediction of how individuals behave is a fruitless exercise as there is no such thing as stability in how people behave, i.e. people behave differently according to the situation in which they find themselves. Mischel (1968) is the most famous proponent of this viewpoint. He argued that studies which measured the behaviour of individuals across situations reported correlations which were not particularly impressive (e.g. $r = 0.3$). Mischel proposed that this is because human behaviour is largely determined by the characteristics of the situation itself rather than by stable characteristics of the person. A compromise position is that behaviour is determined by the *interaction* between the individual's personality traits and a particular situation. More recent research using more refined constructs of personality (such as the 'Big Five') has found impressive stability over time, e.g. 10-year stability for extraversion 0.7–0.8 and for neuroticism 0.6–0.7 (Costa & McCrae 1977).

EMOTION

Emotion lies at the very heartland of psychiatry. Many psychiatric disorders are characterised by abnormalities of emotional states, e.g. sadness in depressive disorders, fear in anxiety disorders, disgust in obsessive–compulsive disorder and some eating disorders. However, for many years emotional experience was considered to be outwith the domain of respectable scientific enquiry in psychology, as emotions were not overt, quantifiable behaviours. However, with the development of cognitive psychology, there have been significant advances in our understanding of the perception and experience of emotional states, and how cognition, emotion and behaviour interact.

How many emotions are there?

As with personality traits, there have been disagreements as to the number of core emotions. The work of Paul Ekman has proved hugely influential in showing that six basic facial expressions are apparently universally recognised across cultures: happiness, sadness, anger, surprise, disgust and fear (Ekman 1980) (Fig. 6.2). However, some authors have argued against treating 'surprise' as a basic emotion. Therefore, a number of authors now propose that there are five basic emotions (e.g. Oatley & Johnson-Laird 1987, Power & Dalgleish 1997). Facial expressions of human emotion are clearly key communication signals. Recent studies have shown that certain clinical disorders are characterised by a recognition deficit for specific emotions, e.g. people with Huntington's disease and people suffering from obsessive–compulsive disorder show severe deficits in recognising facial expressions of disgust, whereas people with lesions restricted to the amygdala are especially

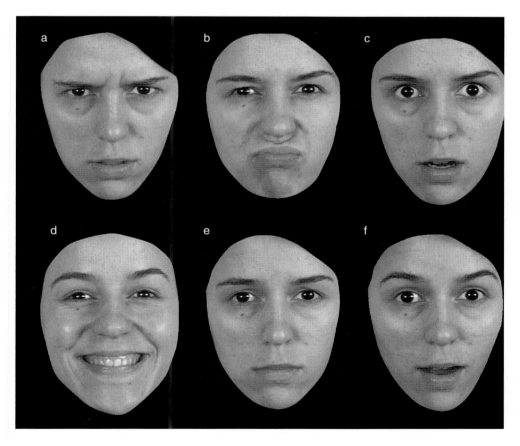

Fig. 6.2
An individual posing the six basic emotional expressions of (a) anger, (b) disgust, (c) fear, (d) happiness, (e) sadness and (f) surprise. (Figure kindly supplied by D M Burt, University of St Andrews.)

impaired in recognising facial expressions of fear (Calder et al 2001).

Theories of emotion

An influential early theory of emotion, the James–Lange theory, stated that physiological responses are central *and precede* the experience of emotion. William James (1884) stated that 'Common sense says . . . we meet a bear are frightened and run . . . The hypothesis to be defended here is that the order of the sequence is incorrect . . . the more rational statement is we feel afraid because we tremble'. James thus focused on the experience of emotion as a *consequence* of perception of body state. A contrasting model of emotional experience was proposed by Walter Cannon (1927). He manipulated peripheral feedback in animals and noted that surgical isolation of the viscera did not impair emotional behaviour and that artificial induction of visceral changes did not appear to produce emotional behaviour. Cannon also pointed out that, in general, sympathetic reactions to arousing stimuli are too slow to account for the speed of subjective emotional reactions. Cannon proposed that emotional stimuli produced two parallel effects in the brain: one that produced emotional experience and one which produced the somatic changes that readied the organism to respond ('fight or flight'). Thus, in this model, physiological changes were viewed as a consequence, not the cause, of emotional experience.

More recently the role of *cognitive appraisal* has been recognised as crucial in the perception and experience of emotion. In a widely cited (though much criticised) experiment, Schachter & Singer (1962) recruited healthy participants who were injected with either saline or noradrenaline (norepinephrine), and were then placed in a social situation designed to elicit euphoria or anger. In one condition a confederate acted in a playful manner, e.g. played with a hula-hoop, threw paper planes out of the window. In the other condition the confederate appeared sullen and irritable before storming out of the room. Critically, participants were either informed fully about the physiological effects of the drug, told nothing, or were misinformed (that it was a vitamin supplement). Those participants who were told nothing, or thought they had received vitamins experienced more extreme emotional reactions than those who were warned that the drug would induce arousal. The misinformed participants tended to describe their emotional state as similar to that of the confederate whose behaviour they witnessed. Schachter & Singer concluded that subjectively experienced emotion is the result of a cognitive evaluation process in which the participant interprets his own bodily reactions *in light of the given situation*. The role of peripheral feedback in influencing cognition has recently received considerable attention as a result of Damasio's Somatic Marker Hypothesis, where it is proposed that somatic feedback (e.g. 'gut feelings') influences decision-making processes in man, often in the absence of conscious awareness (Damasio 1994).

PSYCHOBIOLOGY

Psychobiology is the branch of psychology that concerns itself with the interface between biological processes and behaviour. The range of topics under this umbrella term is huge, including the study of nerve transmission, behavioural genetics, hormones and behaviour, psychopharmacology, biological bases of memory and learning and neuropsychology. Several of these areas are discussed in detail in Chapters 2, 3, 8 and 9.

A basic psychobiological tenet is that psychological disorders can result from pathogenic physical processes of external or internal origin. External pathogens include invasive agents such as harmful organisms and toxins which, when introduced into the body, can cause disease and temporary or permanent physical damage. Physical trauma may also cause temporary or permanent damage to the organism, e.g. closed head injury leading to changes in cognition, affect and personality. A number of psychiatric conditions are clearly the result of pathogenic physical processes of external or internal origin. For example, in multi-infarct dementia, a series of small strokes lead to the increased death of brain matter and consequent general intellectual and personality impairments in the sufferer. External agents include psychoactive drugs taken either deliberately or accidentally which can clearly lead to a wide range of psychological problems, e.g. drug-induced psychosis. However, it is critical to note that psychobiology posits *bidirectionality*, i.e. that while biology can clearly affect behaviour, it is equally the case that environment and experience can significantly impact upon biology. As discussed in the Developmental section below early environmental enrichment markedly affects neuronal development (Rosenweig & Bennett 1972). Also, recent advances in functional neuroimaging have clearly established that there is far greater plasticity in the adult human nervous system than was previously believed. For example, Karni et al (1995) have shown that during motor skill learning, a slowly evolving, long-term, experience-dependent reorganisation of the adult primary motor cortex occurs, and this may underlie the acquisition and retention of the motor skill.

Diathesis–stress models

It is clear that there is considerable individual variation in the development of psychiatric disorder. For example, following extreme stress or trauma, some individuals may develop conditions such as PTSD, whereas others who have experienced exactly the same stressor do not. How is this explained? The diathesis–stress model posits that a pre-existing vulnerability (diathesis) renders an individual more susceptible to particular diseases. Diathesis–stress models have been proposed for a number of psychiatric conditions, including psychosomatic disorders such as gastric ulcer, myocardial infarctions and eczema, and conditions such as schizophrenia and certain types of severe depression. In these disorders, the interaction between a vulnerability and some form of physical or psychosocial stress forms the central part of the model.

Diathesis–stress models are now commonplace, not only in the biomedical approach, but in a range of psychological and social models also, though the diathesis or vulnerability factor is expressed at a psychological (e.g. sensitivity to the experience of loss) or social level (e.g. a lack of social support from other individuals) rather than at a physical level. A good illustration of this is the work of Brown & Harris (1978) in relation to social factors and risk of depression. They proposed that certain *vulnerability factors* (lack of a confiding relationship, loss of mother before age 11, 3+ children aged < 15 years old at home, unemployed status) rendered women particularly at risk of depression in the face of certain severe *provoking factors* (life events) such as deaths, illness/accidents to significant others, job or residence change, etc. (Fig. 6.3).

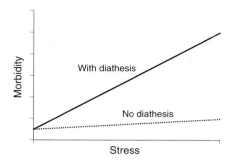

Fig. 6.3
Diathesis–stress model. Individuals who have the diathesis, or vulnerability, show greater morbidity in the presence of stress than those who have not.

Genes and behaviour

The relative contribution of genetic versus environmental factors to various psychological attributes (e.g. intelligence) has been vigorously debated for many years. Twin studies have been used extensively to try to inform the debate. The typical study compares the intelligence quotient (IQ) of monozygotic (MZ, identical) twins reared together with dizygotic (DZ, non-identical twins) reared together. Generally the correlation between the IQs of the MZ twins is significantly higher than that of the DZ twins. However, the greater similarity in IQ may not be simply attributable to genetic factors; MZ twins may have more similar environments than DZ twins. MZ twins clearly look alike (and sometimes are dressed alike), and this may encourage others to treat them more similarly than non-identical twins. Importantly, significant adults (parents and teachers) may develop the same expectations for MZ twins. Thus there may be strong environmental pressures that contribute towards the similarity in the measured intelligence of MZ twins. In order to try and tease apart the relative contribution of genetic from environmental factors, several studies have capitalised on occasions where MZ twins have been reared apart (e.g. given up for adoption soon after birth). In one study MZ twins who were reared apart during their formative years showed strong similarities in IQ: about 70% of the variance in IQ was found to be associated with genetic variation, not substantially less than that observed in MZ twins reared together (Bouchard et al 1990). Evidence such as this indicates that identical genotypes lead to highly similar IQs even when the identical twins grow up in different environments. Critics of such studies argue, however, that the allocation of environments to adopted twins is not truly random, and that twins often are raised in similar types of environments, and that the case for the relative genetic contribution towards IQ has been overstated. With recent developments in the 'new genetics' and the mapping of the human genome, a plethora of studies have emerged which aim to identify the relative genetic contribution to a number of psychiatric disorders (see Ch. 9).

Motivation

Pressure of space prevents a detailed review of the psychobiology of motivation; however, two topics which have particular relevance for psychiatry will be briefly presented: threat and reward.

Threat Human evolution required the development of an effective series of mechanisms to quickly perceive and respond to

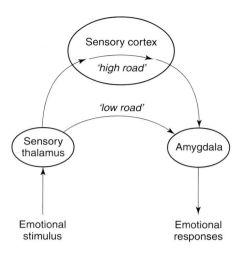

Fig. 6.4
LeDoux's model of the 'low' and 'high' roads to the amygdala. The low road is proposed as a 'quick and dirty' processing pathway.

threatening stimuli. Cannon (1927) proposed that the perception of threat triggers intense sympathetic arousal which mobilises the individual for 'fight or flight'. Physiological changes which occur include heart acceleration, inhibition of intestinal peristalsis, pupillary dilatation and the opening of respiratory passages. It has become increasingly clear that the limbic system, in particular the amygdala, plays an important role in the perception and appraisal of threat. LeDoux (1996) has proposed that two parallel neural pathways are activated when a potentially threatening stimulus is encountered: the 'low road' and the 'high road'. The stimulus is first processed in the sensory regions of the thalamus, and a 'glimpse' of information about the stimulus is shuttled down a short, 'quick and dirty' route to the amygdala. This triggers the amygdala to start to respond to the possible danger/threat. A slower route involves more detailed processing of the stimuli by the cortex (Fig. 6.4). If this cortical analysis confirms that genuine threat exists, additional signals for action are passed down to the amygdala. However, if the analysis indicates that the stimulus is not a threat, then the 'fight or flight' response is terminated. The amygdala is thus seen as playing a central role in the perception of threat. Recent neuroimaging studies have confirmed that the amygdala is activated in threatening situations, e.g. when patients with post-traumatic stress disorder are exposed to trauma reminders (Liberzon et al 1999). The amygdala also appear to play a critical role in memory formation for emotional experience (Cahill et al 1995).

Reward In a pioneering experiment, Olds & Milner (1954) chronically implanted electrodes in various brain regions of rats. They discovered that the rats would learn to press a lever if rewarded with a brief burst of electrical stimulation in certain regions of the hypothalamus and limbic system. The rewarding effect of this electrical stimulation was remarkable. The rats pressed the lever at rates as high as five thousand times per hour. They pressed for 15–20 hours until they fell asleep exhausted, and, on awakening, immediately restarted lever pressing. When forced to choose between food and self-stimulation, hungry rats often opted for self-stimulation. One interpretation of these findings was that the brain stimulation mimicked the natural reward system. Self-stimulation was most effective when applied to the medial forebrain bundle, which connects the ventral tegmental area with the nucleus accumbens. This pathway utilises dopamine as a neurotransmitter, and it has been established that dopamine plays a crucial role in the physiology of reward. This has clear relevance for psychiatry in that the dopaminergic system is thought to be implicated in the pathophysiology of a variety of psychiatric disorders (e.g. schizophrenia), and dopaminergic agonists and antagonists are widely used treatments in psychiatry. (Anhedonia, for example, may reflect a dysfunction of an endogenous reward system.)

DEVELOPMENTAL PSYCHOLOGY

In this brief section, the main Piagetian development stages will be outlined and criticised in light of more recent evidence. Then two specific developmental topics of particular relevance for psychiatry will be discussed: *attachment* and *theory of mind*.

Piagetian theory

Developmental psychology has been hugely influenced by the work of the Swiss psychologist Jean Piaget. Piaget proposed that the mental life of the child is qualitatively different from that of the adult. He believed that children were active contributors to their own learning. By acting on the environment a child constructs internal structures, and it is these structures, and not the environment, that controls the way a child thinks. He proposed that all children go through a fixed series of developmental stages: sensori-motor; concrete operational (including pre-operational) and formal operational.

Sensori-motor stage This stage extends from birth to roughly 18 months. Initially, the infant utilises reflex responses such as sucking and grasping, before gaining more motor control and progressing to initiating his own behaviour. In the first few months of life, in the mind of the infant, an object only exists as long as it is actively perceived, e.g. a toy dropped out of sight no longer exists. However, at around 12 months the object becomes permanent and the child will look for it (e.g. if it is hidden under a blanket). Active experimentation with objects then commences, e.g. pressing a toy to make it squeak.

Concrete operational stage This stage is thought to extend from about 2 to 12 years of age. Piaget proposed that this stage marks the transition between the literalness of perception and the ability for abstract thinking that characterises the next developmental stage. Between 18 months and 7 years a child is in the pre-operational period. During this stage a child begins to represent actions with symbols, which is illustrated by their rapid progress in acquiring language. Similarly, at about two years of age children begin to engage in symbolic play, e.g. a chair being ridden as a horse. During this period the child is *egocentric*, e.g. the child can only describe things from his own perspective. At around age 7 years the child begins to see the perspective of other people and also master the principle of *conservation*. Between 7 and 12 years the child enters the full concrete operational stage. For example, in demonstrating the principle of number conservation, an experimenter lays out a row of six red and a row of six blue counters side by side on a table, and asks the child 'are there more red counters or blue counters on the table?'; most children will say that there are the same number of red and blue counters. Next the researcher performs a transformation, e.g. pushing the red counters closer to each other to destroy the

one-to-one alignment with the blue counters (the row of red counters is now shorter than the blue row). The child is now asked the same question as previously. Children younger than 7 years of age typically respond 'There are more blue counters', those over 7 typically reply 'There are the same number of each'. Piaget interpreted this kind of finding as illustrative of the younger child's inability to reason logically, because of lack of understanding of general principles such that the number of objects in a set is independent of their spatial layout (but see criticisms below). By 7 years, the child is able to solve problems related to concrete events but has difficulty with abstract thought.

Formal operational stage This last developmental stage is thought to extend from 12 years onwards. During this phase the child begins to apply concrete operations to hypothetical situations, thus showing abstract thought. The adolescent develops the ability to form hypotheses to explain unfamiliar phenomena. During this developmental stage the individual can think logically and can do so with respect to abstract objects, and is considered to have reached cognitive maturity.

Criticisms of Piagetian theory

Many developmental psychologists would agree with several of Piaget's general claims, e.g. that cognitive development is influenced by an interaction between biological and environmental factors, that children play an active role in acquiring knowledge and making sense of their world, and that children's thinking is sometimes qualitatively different from adults. However, some researchers, notably Margaret Donaldson, have challenged some of Piaget's views. Donaldson (1978) argued that Piaget underestimated (a) young children's logical competence and conceptual understanding, (b) the influences of contextual factors on children's performance, and (c) the extent to which children's performance depends on their familiarity with the specific contents of the particular task. By way of illustration, the conservation of number task described above was repeated by Donaldson (1978), however, on this occasion, the transformation (pushing the row of red counters closer together) instead of being carried out by an adult experimenter, was carried out by 'naughty teddy who likes to mess up games'. With this modification, many more 4–6 year olds responded correctly that there were still equivalent numbers of red and blue counters. Donaldson (1978) argued that in Piaget's original version of the task the deliberate nature of the transformation misleads the children into inferring that the action is relevant to the question which immediately follows it, and the child misinterprets the question as referring to length. Donaldson proposed that the young child actively attempts to make sense of the total situation by attending not only to what is said, but also to how it is said, and that the child also makes inferences about other people's intentions (see section on theory of mind, below). Donaldson argued that young children are capable of logical reasoning, but they are more likely to be able to demonstrate this in circumstances where the task make sense to the child. Several other critics have argued that Piaget seriously underestimated the capabilities of infants. For example, Gibson & Walk (1960) showed that infants as young as 6 months of age could utilise perceptual clues in order to perceive depth. A visual cliff was created using a glass table with an apparently solid half (tiling immediately below the glass) and a 'cliff' (tiling several feet below the glass on the floor). When mothers were asked to entice their infants over the visual cliff, very few infants ventured over the apparent precipice, suggesting that they had a representation of depth. Further work also suggests that babies are born with a predisposition to look at human faces. Johnson & Morton (1991) showed that newborns preferentially look longer at a schematic face compared with a scrambled face or a blank pattern. Studies such as these suggest that infants are far more cognitively competent than Piaget initially proposed.

Attachment

A safe, secure and loving bond between parent and child is clearly an important foundation for optimal development. We largely learn how to be parents by our own experience as children and by observing others. What type of mothers do motherless mothers make? Harlow and colleagues in Wisconsin conducted a widely cited experiment using rhesus monkeys. The experimental monkeys were permitted no contact with their own mothers from birth. These motherless monkeys gave birth to their own babies at 4 years of age. The majority of these monkeys were totally inadequate as mothers, avoiding and refusing to nurse the newborns, and intensive care was required by the researchers in order to keep the babies alive. In many cases the mothers were extremely abusive to their babies, biting and hitting them. Despite this treatment, the infants persisted in attempting to cling to the abusive mothers, sometimes hanging on the mother's back where they would be safe from attack, rather than clinging in front (the normal position for infant monkeys). In a further experiment, Harlow and colleagues gave newborn rhesus monkeys the choice of two surrogate mothers; one constructed of wire mesh which mechanically provided milk, and the other covered with cloth but providing no nutrition. The infant monkeys dramatically preferred contact with the cloth mother; the wire mother was only intermittently visited for nutrition. The cloth surrogate mother was especially sought when fear-provoking stimuli were brought into or near the cage. Further experimental manipulations revealed that rocking cloth mothers were preferred to stationary ones, and warm cloth mothers were preferred to cool ones (Harlow & Harlow 1966). These animal experiments indicate that maternal neglect and abuse can be 'learned' and passed on to the next generation, and that warmth and tactile contact are critical components of the early mother–child bond.

Subsequent research with human infants has largely supported the view that neglect can lead to significant problems in the later life of the neglected child. Bowlby (1973) has been a strong advocate of the view that disturbance of a child's initial attachment to the mother will leave the child less secure in later life. Follow-up studies of children reared in inadequate institutional care (e.g. orphanages which provided nutrition but very little social, physical or emotional care) have shown that many developed significant social impairments, e.g. constantly craving attention or, in contrast, showing marked apathy towards others (Provence & Lipton 1962). While early environment is clearly critical in terms of learning and socialisation, animal studies also indicate that quality of the early environment directly influences brain development. Rosenweig & Bennett (1972) studied rats who were either reared in bare surroundings or in a cage that was environmentally enriched (running wheels, apparatus to climb on, etc.). After 80 days in the enriched environment, rats had developed 23% more neural interconnections than control rats raised in bare conditions. Evidence such as this indicates that the developing brain is markedly influenced by environmental stimulation.

Theory of mind

As stated above, Piaget proposed that in the concrete operational stage of development, children are initially egocentric and only at about 7 years can they appreciate the difference between another person's point of view and their own. More recently, 'theory of mind' studies have suggested that children can take the perspective of another person at about 4 years of age. A theory of mind is the ability to appreciate that minds contain mental states, e.g. beliefs, desires, intentions, and to use this knowledge to predict another person's actions. Theory of mind is commonly assessed using tests which evaluate a child's understanding of false beliefs. For example, two dolls, Sally and Anne, act out a scene: Sally puts a marble in a basket before leaving a room and Anne then moves it into a box. A child, who watches the scene, is asked where Sally will look for the marble when she returns? Young children (3-year-olds and younger) commonly respond 'in the box', i.e. they refer to the true location of the marble. Older children (4-year-olds and above) typically respond 'in the basket', i.e. they appreciate that Sally has a false belief about the marble's true location (Frith 1997). This finding has been interpreted as showing that young children assume that their beliefs are inevitably shared by others, not that beliefs can be true or false and that different people can have different beliefs. Recently, theory of mind deficits have been implicated in psychological models which attempt to explain disorders such as autism and schizophrenia (see Chs 27 and 21, for example).

SUMMARY AND CONCLUSIONS

In this chapter we have attempted to provide a brief overview of some of the major areas of psychology that have particular relevance for the study of psychiatric disorder. We hope we have managed to convey the breadth of topics that fall within the domain of psychology, from the study of schemas to the synapse. We began by suggesting that most psychiatrists on commencing higher training have had relatively little exposure to psychology. We hope to have gone some way in convincing the reader that an understanding of basic psychological principles is essential for the study of psychiatry. The ultimate scientific challenge for psychiatry is to explain key features of psychiatric disorder in psychological terms; for example, delusions and hallucinations are clearly abnormalities of belief and perception, fundamental psychological constructs. Far too often 'explanations' of psychiatric disorder are presented at an inappropriate level, e.g. hallucinating patients show abnormal brain structure in region X, therefore region X is implicated in hallucinatory experience. This does not *explain* the auditory perception whereby an individual clearly hears the voice of the devil speaking to him. A genuine explanation must be framed in psychological terms. However, we must be wary of replacing neurotransmitter or structural lesion-based explanations of psychopathology with seductive 'black-box' cognitive models. Demonstrating that a particular patient or patient group has a specific cognitive abnormality is of interest, but it does not necessarily provide a causal explanation of abnormal behaviour or experience. In most instances we still await truly convincing psychological explanations of psychopathological states.

REFERENCES

Allport G W, Odbert H S 1936 Trait-names: a psychological study. Psychological Monographs 47 (Whole No 211)

Anderson M C, Green C 2001 Suppressing unwanted memories by executive control. Nature 410: 366–369

Barker C, Pistrang N, Elliott R 2002 Research methods in clinical psychology, 2nd edn. Wiley, Chichester

Beck A T 1976 Cognitive therapy and the emotional disorders. Meridian, New York

Bolton D, Hill J 1996 Mind, meaning and mental disorder: the nature of causal explanation in psychology and psychiatry. Oxford University Press, Oxford

Bouchard T J Jr, Lykken D T, McGue M et al 1990 Sources of human psychological differences: the Minnesota Study of Twins Reared Apart. Science 250(4978): 223–228

Bowlby J 1973 Separation and loss. Basic Books, New York

Broadbent D E 1958 Perception and communication. Pergamon, Oxford

Brown G W, Harris T 1978 Social origins of depression. Tavistock, London

Calder A J, Lawrence A D, Young A W 2001 Neuropsychology of fear and loathing. Nature Reviews Neuroscience 2(5): 352–363

Cahill L, Babinsky R, Markowitsch H J, McGaugh J L 1995 The amygdala and emotional memory. Nature 377: 295–296

Cannon W B 1927 The James–Lange theory of emotions: a critical examination and an alternative theory. American Journal of Psychology 39: 106–124

Cattell R B 1957 Personality and motivation: structure and measurement. Harcourt, Brace and World, New York

Cattell R B, Eber H W, Tatsuolca M M 1970 Handbook for the Sixteen Personality Factor Questionnaire (16 PF). Institute for Personality and Ability Testing, Illinois

Conway M A 1997 Recovered memories and false memories. Oxford University Press, Oxford

Conway M A 2001 Repression revisited. Nature 410: 319–320

Costa P T, McCrae R R 1977 Age differences in personality structure revisited: studies in validity, stability and change. Aging and Human Development 8: 261–275

Costa P T, McCrae R R 1992a Four ways five factors are basic. Personality and Individual Differences 13: 653–655

Costa P T, McCrae R R 1992b Revised NEO Personality Inventory (NEO-PI-R) and NEO Five-Factor Inventory (NEO-FFI) Professional Manual. Psychological Assessment Resources, Odessa, Fl

Damasio A R 1994 Descartes' error. Papermac/Macmillan, London

Davies G M, Dalgleish T (eds) 2002 Recovered memories: seeking the middle ground. Wiley, Chichester

Donaldson M 1978 Children's minds. Fontana, Glasgow

Ekman P 1980 The face of man: expressions of human emotions in a New Guinea village. Garland STPM, New York

Eysenck H J 1969 The effects of psychological therapy. Science House, New York

Eysenck H J, Eysenck S B G 1975 Handbook of the Eysenck Personality Questionnaire. Hodder & Stoughton, London

Freud A 1937 The ego and the mechanisms of defence. Tavistock, London

Frith U 1997 The neurocognitive basis of autism. Trends in Cognitive Sciences 1: 73–77

Gibson E J, Walk R D 1960 The "visual cliff". Scientific American 202: 64–71

Gleick J 1988 Chaos: making a new science. Heinemann, London

Harlow H, Harlow M 1966 Learning to love. American Scientist 54: 244–272

James W 1884 What is an emotion? Mind 9: 188–205

Johnson M, Morton J 1991 Biology and cognitive development: the case of face recognition. Blackwell, London

Johnson-Laird P N 1988 The computer and the mind: an introduction to cognitive science. Fontana, London

Jones M C 1924 A laboratory study of fears: the case of Peter. Pediatric Seminars 31: 308–315

Kahneman D, Slovic P, Tversky A 1982 Judgement under uncertainty: heuristics and biases. Cambridge University Press, Cambridge

Karni A, Meyer G, Jezzard P et al 1995 Functional MRI evidence for adult motor cortex plasticity during motor skill learning. Nature 377(6545): 155–158

LeDoux J 1996 The emotional brain. Simon & Schuster, New York

Liberzon I, Taylor S F, Amdur R et al 1999 Brain activation in PTSD in response to trauma-related stimuli. Biological Psychiatry 45(7): 817–826

Marks I 1987 Fears, phobias and rituals. Oxford University Press, Oxford

Mischel W 1968 Personality and assessment. Wiley, New York

Morgan C D, Murray H A 1935 A method for investigating fantasies: the thematic apperception test. Archives of Neurological Psychiatry 34: 289–306

Mowrer O H 1939 A stimulus-response analysis of anxiety and its role as a reinforcing agent. Psychological Review 46: 553–565

Neisser U 1967 Cognitive psychology. Appleton-Century-Crofts, New York

Norman W T 1963 Toward an adequate taxonomy of personality attributes: replicated factor structure in peer nomination personality ratings. Journal of Abnormal and Social Psychology 66: 574–583

Oatley K, Johnson-Laird P N 1987 Towards a cognitive theory of emotions. Cognition and Emotion 1: 29–50

Olds J, Milner P 1954 Positive reinforcement produced by electrical stimulation of septal area and other regions of rat brain. Journal of Comparative Physiological Psychology 47: 419–427

Power M J 1997 Conscious and unconscious representations of meaning. In: Power M J, Brewin C R (eds) The transformation of meaning in psychological therapies. Wiley, Chichester

Power M J 2001 Integrative therapy from a cognitive-behavioural perspective. In: Holmes J, Bateman A (eds) Integration in psychotherapy: models and methods. Oxford University Press, Oxford

Power M J, Champion L A 1986 Cognitive approaches to depression: a theoretical critique. British Journal of Clinical Psychology 25: 201–212

Power M J, Dalgleish T 1997 Cognition & emotion: from order to disorder. Psychology Press, Hove, W Sussex

Provence S, Lipton R 1962 Infants in institutions. International Universities Press, New York

Rachman S J 1990 Fear and courage, 2nd edn. Freeman, New York

Robertson I H, Murre J M 1999 Rehabilitation of brain damage: brain plasticity and principles of guided recovery. Psychological Bulletin 125(5): 544–75

Rorschach H 1921 Psychodiagnostik. Bircher, Berne

Rosenweig M, Bennett E 1972 Cerebral changes in rats exposed individually to an enriched environment. Journal of Comparative & Physiological Psychology 80: 304–313

Schacter S, Singer J 1962 Cognitive, social and physiological determinants of emotional state. Psychological Review 769: 379–399

Seligman M E P 1971 Phobias and preparedness. Behaviour Therapy 2: 207–220

Seligman M E P 1975 Helplessness. W H Freeman, San Francisco

Semeonoff B 1976 Projective techniques. Wiley, London

Watson J B Rayner R 1920 Conditioned emotional reactions. Journal of Experimental Psychology 3: 1–14

Wolpe J 1958 Psychotherapy by reciprocal inhibition. Stanford University Press, Stanford

7 | Sociology, psychiatry and mental health

Anne Rogers

This chapter[1] explores the following:

- sociological orientations towards psychiatry and mental health;
- the three dominant social perspectives used to understand and explain the relationship between society, mental health and psychiatry: social causationism; social reaction; and social contructionism;
- mental health in society.

SOCIOLOGICAL ORIENTATIONS TOWARDS PSYCHIATRY AND MENTAL HEALTH

Sociological contributions to psychiatry have tended to reflect divergent theoretical and methodological orientations: social causation, interpretive micro-sociology, structuralism and post-structuralism. *Social causationism*, which is the oldest tradition, focuses on the social causes of mental illness and accepts the legitimacy of psychiatric nosology (treating diagnostic categories like 'depression' or 'schizophrenia' and the scientific method as unproblematic). A close association between sociology and medicine is evident within this tradition, traceable to 19th-century social medicine. The approach has largely spawned epidemiological surveys of community populations or hospital admissions.

The social causation thesis peaked in popularity in the 1950s. During the 1960s, versions of *micro-sociology* appeared, which challenged the methodological dominance of epidemiology and structural-functionalism (which tended to view society as a functional whole made up of interlocking and compatible subsystems). Its theoretical roots were to be found mainly in symbolic interactionism and social phenomenology which focused on interpreting phenomena in the social world (Goffmann 1961, Lemert 1967, Scheff 1966). The methodological emphasis was on ethnographic or naturalistic studies of institutional life and everyday rule enforcement. This approach allowed sociologists access to the fine grain of the life of the mentally ill, beyond what could be described by epidemiology. Symbolic interactionism allowed a perspective to emerge from the 'underdog'. In particular, a voice could be given to the 'unofficial' side of the hospital and being 'mentally ill' which countered uncritical structural-functionalist accounts of medical life (e.g. Parsons 1951). This interpretive sociology also subsumed the emergence of ethnomethodology. This described how individuals make sense

---

[1] Much of the content of this chapter is elaborated in more detail in Pilgrim & Rogers (1999) and Rogers & Pilgrim (2003)

of social situations, and at times it shaded into philosophical inquiry. Contra the social causationists, the focus turned towards the relativity of concepts of mental health and illness and the notion that both are socially negotiated.

During the 1970s doubts began to emerge about sociology settling into an interpretive scheme. In particular Marxian critiques tried to set the organisation and activities of psychiatry into a macro-economic context. For example, Scull (1979) was guided in the main by economic notions, backed up by documentary evidence analysing the emerging social control role of psychiatry in the 19th century and the functional value it held for the capitalist state. Scull (1977) also sought to explain the emergence of de-institutionalisation in response to fiscal pressures after the Second World War. A political economy approach to evaluating schizophrenia and its treatment also started to emerge in the work of some social psychiatrists (e.g. Warner 1985).

Over the past three decades the influence of Foucault on psychiatry has been apparent. Overall Foucauldian work stands separately from both micro-sociology and structuralism in relation to psychiatry. At the outset, in the 1960s, Foucault's own work centred on the emergence of the asylum (Foucault 1965). The methodological implications of Foucauldian research are novel — empirical knowledge claims are of interest not (only) to produce knowledge in itself but also to read and re-read or deconstruct that knowledge. This task is near to interpretive sociology (both can be placed in a hermeneutic framework) but focuses on discourses rather than social actors. Moreover, it does not accept the presuppositions of humanism, such as a coherent or stable subjectivity, nor does it privilege individual agents in sociological enquiry; instead it opposes or seeks to transcend the 'personalistic' or 'homocentric' features of the older interpretive tradition. On a second front, the over-determining role of the state or political economy is rejected. While this influence or role is conceded, stable or predictable causal patterns are not.

In the 1980s sociology in this post-structuralist mode issued a set of discourses on discourses. It opened up the inevitability of plural social realities regarding the precarious nature of knowledge claims. Foucault's own work on institutional psychiatry was categorised by his followers as scene setting — documenting the pre-history of the discipline or the conditions which made it possible. New formations of psychiatric work were subsequently the focus of de-constructionists. Twentieth-century psychiatry was described as eclectic, and its ambit was now seen to extend beyond the boundaries of both the asylum and madness. In particular, psychological as well as bio-deterministic features of psychiatry were highlighted. For example, the deconstruction of the emergent 'shell shock' problem of the First World War by Stone (1985) shows the eugenic discourse about 'England's finest blood'—officers and gentlemen and working class volunteers were breaking down under the strain of a war of unprecedented attrition and stalemate.

Post-structuralists also rejected the antipsychiatric emphasis on the destructive and oppressive features of modern psychiatry. Miller & Rose (1988) put this succinctly: 'We argue that it is more fruitful to consider the ways that regulatory systems have sought to promote subjectivity than to document the way in which they have crushed it'. Consequently their focus has been on new psychological discourses in contemporary society rather than on the legacy of Victorian biological psychiatry. A similar emphasis on the changing discursive forms of psychiatry can be found in the recent work of de Swaan, who draws attention to the particular features associated with neurosis and psychological therapies. de Swaan (1990) talks of clients now being proto-professionalised because they develop a cognitive set within which to see their personal difficulties in professional terms. Thus, it can be seen that recently an eclectic sociology has emerged, which embraces both the causal emphasis of Durkheim and Marx and the hermeneutic or interpretive emphasis from Weber. These have been supplemented further by deconstruction.

Having provided a general overview of dominant sociological positions in relation to psychiatry, we now explore in more detail the way in which society and mental health can be understood. The relationship between society and mental health can be broadly understood in three ways by sociologists, each with a different notion of the 'social':

- The mental health of people is partially or wholly caused by societal influences (*social causationism*).
- The mental health of people is socially negotiated (*labelling theory*).
- Mental health and illness are socially constructed (*social constructionism*).

THE THREE PERSPECTIVES OF THE SOCIAL

Social causationism

Mental health is *socially patterned*, and there is a large body of knowledge about the various ways in which membership of particular social groups makes people vulnerable to mental health problems. A groundbreaking example of this approach was Durkheim's scientific approach to the study of sociology, which, to a significant extent, was based on his exploration of the type of social conditions which could be expected to generate high rates of suicide. Durkheim (1952) argued that the type of explanations of suicide which focused only upon inner emotional experiences or personal reasons were inadequate. Since suicide rates remained relatively stable in any given society from year to year, he concluded that suicide had an existence external to any one instance of it. It was therefore possible to think of suicide as a 'social fact' which needed to be explained in terms of other social facts.

Other more recent examples of the social causationist approach, which have used key social variables, include:

- *Social class.* Mental health is positively correlated with social class. The poorer people are, the greater the chances that they

> ### Box 7.1 Key terms
>
> **Biodeterminism / biological determinism** The view that mental health problems result from biological abnormalities within individuals.
> **Deconstruction** The critical reading of texts or practices to study how reality is socially constructed.
> **Deviance (primary)** This refers to rule breaking in society, which can arise from biological, psychological or social causes.
> **Deviance (secondary)** This refers to the maintenance and amplification of primary deviance by the reactions of others.
> **Labelling (or societal reaction) theory** The study of the interaction between deviants and non-deviants to establish the processes of transition from primary to secondary deviance.
> **Social causationism** The view that mental health problems are caused by stressors impinging upon individuals in their social context.
> **Social constructionism** The view that all human knowledge is a product of communal exchange and that reality cannot be understood without reference to the representations created by this exchange.

will be diagnosed as being mentally ill. The correlation indicates the increased probability of mental health problems with decreasing socio-economic status. The direction of causality in this association between poverty and severe mental health problems has been the subject of particular controversy. Social causationists argue that greater exposure to the environment and social stressors associated with poverty increases the incidence of mental health problems. By contrast, the *social selection* theory suggests that social class is affected by mental disorder. That is, mentally ill people 'drift' into poverty because their illness makes them socially incompetent. Some evidence suggests that the validity of the different causal explanations may vary according to the type of mental health problem under investigation. Social causation may be stronger than social selection in explaining the inverse association of socio-economic status to severe depression in women, substance abuse and antisocial personality in men; but, for those who carry a diagnosis of schizophrenia, social selection may be a more relevant explanation (Dohrenwend et al 1992).

- *Gender.* The findings of community studies have been used to suggest that women experience relatively high rates of depression and other psychiatric disorders compared with men. Walter Gove and his colleagues focused on the higher rates among married women than men, and a number of studies since have identified differences in female rates compared with male (Kessler et al 1994). Gender differences have been attributed to a range of social, familial, personal and measurement artefact explanations. One of the most consistent findings is of a greater female prevalence of depressive disorder and 'non-specific' psychological distress which has been explained with reference to adverse experiences in childhood and adolescence, sociocultural roles and psychological attributes which predispose individuals to negative life events (Nazroo et al 1998).
- *Race.* Mental health is racially patterned. Estimates from the UK suggest that the annual prevalence of hallucinations is higher in Caribbean than south Asian or White populations.

This variation is accounted for with reference to cultural differences in experience and is not seen as invariably associated with psychosis (Johns et al 2002). In general terms, the racialisation of psychiatric provision reflects continuing disadvantages that were rooted in slavery, enforced migration, colonialism and racial discrimination. For example in Australia aboriginal people are over-represented in psychiatric populations. In the USA Black, Hispanic and Native American groups are over-represented. In England, Irish and Afro-Caribbean people are more likely to have mental health problems.

- *Age*. Certain problems emerge at different points in the lifespan. In old age, dementia increases in probability with time. A greater problem, though, is depression. Twice as many old people are depressed than are dementing. The raised incidence of dementia is generally deemed to reflect an amplification of neurological deterioration that occurs with the ageing process. However, social factors are also implicated. The severity of symptoms in dementia is correlated with both social stimulation and with earlier educational experience. With regard to depression in old age, this has been accounted for by one or more combination of the following stressors: poverty; the distress of multiple physical illness; aggregating grief as peers die around survivors; under-stimulating living conditions; and loss of control of the latter with enforced moves to hospitals, nursing homes or residential facilities. Severe mental health problems are also more likely to occur in young adulthood and late adolescence than in childhood and middle and later adulthood.
- *Victims of trauma*. People who have been sexually abused (in either childhood or later years) are more likely to develop mental health problems than those who are not sexually assaulted. Problems can emerge both in the immediate wake of the abuse and many years later. The correlation with diagnosis is important to note here. The over-representation of survivors of sexual abuse in a psychiatric population is accounted for by all diagnoses except schizophrenia, manic-depression and obsessive–compulsive disorder. Other sources of trauma that increase the probability of suffering from mental health problems include warfare, domestic violence, being a victim of urban crime, physical injury from accidents, and bereavement.

Because the above social groupings are not mutually exclusive, the social causationist position inevitably leads to complex, multifactorial models of causation. Among other things, it would imply that the mental health of individuals and groups would be facilitated and maintained by interpersonal support throughout the lifespan and the avoidance of stressors such as poverty, sexism, trauma and racism.

Much of the research exploring social causes has focused on factors external to the individual which emanate from the environmental or social context. This body of knowledge has emphasised mental ill health as a product of various forms of social stress, pressure or trauma, which have been accounted for by tracing antecedent social conditions. There is also interest in the reverse of this — that is the type of social conditions which protect, enhance or maintain positive mental health. Thus, the social causationist position provides a framework for understanding the promotion of mental health in society, which is discussed in more detail below.

Structural levels of analysis in social causation

Causal factors and their relevant mechanisms are seen to operate at different levels. The more common analytical method associated with social causationism is some version of social or psychiatric epidemiology. Populations or subpopulations (social groups) are studied in order to discover the distribution of first cases of mental ill health (incidence) and the aggregate of all diagnosed cases at a point in time (prevalence). In addition, the causal factors involved in variations in incidence or prevalence are proffered by researchers using this perspective.

Two broad conceptualisations have underpinned structural approaches to the study of social inequalities and mental health: social stratification and social class (Muntaner et al 2000). *Social stratification* studies use measures of inequalities, which focus on disparities in social resources such as years of education, occupation and income (Bartley et al 1998). *Social class* tends to refer to people's class locations originating from ownership and control over different types of assets (e.g. property organisation and credentials). Occupational status was originally based on the 1911 Registrar General's Classification of Occupations using a classification of:

   (i) Higher professional and managerial;
  (ii) lower professional, technical and managerial;
(iiin) skilled-non-manual workers and clerical workers;
(iiim) skilled manual workers;
 (iv) semi-skilled workers;
  (v) unskilled workers.

Traditional 'structural' approaches to mental health inequalities, such as the community studies of the impact of the environment on mental health conducted in the 1950s and 1960s (e.g. Hollingshead & Redlich 1958, Myers & Bean 1968) suggested links between social conditions and disadvantage (e.g. unemployment, poverty and racism) and psychiatric morbidity. At the outbreak of the Second World War, a prominent study based on social ecology (*Mental Disorders in Urban Areas*) was published by members of the Chicago School (Faris & Dunham 1939). In exploring the influence of poverty and deprivation, the authors contrasted the prevalence of manic–depressive psychosis, which appeared to be randomly distributed across the city of Chicago, with that of people diagnosed with schizophrenia, who were found predominantly in poorer areas.

More recent research has extended interest into exploring other dimensions and conditions produced by the social structure. The prevalence of mental disorder among women, and the impact of employment, unemployment and standard of living, point to the importance of macrostructural variables and environmental causes in determining mental health (Warner 1985, Thoits 1985, Paykel 1991, Lewis et al 1998). There is some evidence which demonstrates that improvements in mental health can be achieved by changing the socio-structural environment. One of the most obvious examples is the impact of employment and unemployment on mental health. Overall, unemployment has been shown to have a negative effect on mental health at least in terms of depression. Suicide rates are higher among the unemployed (Platt et al 1992). There is also some indication that the mental health of the population can be improved by improvements to housing and the local area. For example, re-housing on the grounds of mental health has been shown to impact favourably on anxiety and depression (Elton & Packer 1986). Provision of financial resources and reconstruction of housing has been found to make a critical difference to recovery from mental health emergencies that arise from major disruption to or destruction of living environments (Wang et al 2000).

Faris & Dunham (1939) focused on social isolation as a possible aetiological factor in explaining differential rates of mental disorder. Hollingshead & Redlich (1958) reflected the popular appeal of Freudian ideas, which were prevalent in the USA at that time, in suggesting the influence of social factors throughout the lifespan. However, the focus on the way in which individuals interacted with macrosocial changes was relatively crude, and one of the limitations of a focus on the wider structural and economic factors has been the tendency to treat individuals as the passive recipients of external events and circumstances. In this latter respect a psychosocial perspective on mental health has been more concerned with changes in and experience of life events, the social world of individuals and the way in which social environmental demands generate psychological stress (Dohrenwend & Dohrenwend 1982, Elstad 1998).

The psychosocial level of analysis

The psychosocial perspective refers to a number of related approaches which place greater emphasis on precipitating than on predisposing factors, and upon attempting a reduction of the prevalence rather than the incidence of mental health problems. The concept of stress provides a means of linking aspects of an individual's social situation with the occurrence or reoccurrence of mental ill health. The term 'stress' refers both to the characteristics of a person's circumstances (e.g. 'stressors', 'life events', 'stress situations') and responses that people make to those circumstances ('stress reactions'). Social stress theorists are also concerned with the distribution and deployment of coping resources (social support, self-esteem, a personal sense of control) and strategies (behavioural and cognitive devices to manage external and situational demands) among different groups in the population. Within this tradition it is possible to distinguish between approaches which examine direct influences on psychological distress versus those where the focus is more indirect, e.g. when stress is expressed in health-damaging behaviour such as violence or excessive consumption of alcohol and drugs (Elstad 1998). One of the most sophisticated developed theories of negative stressors is the life events model which encompasses the work of George Brown and his colleagues in relation to depression (Brown & Harris 1978). In mapping the social origin of depression, attention is drawn to three groups of interacting factors that produce depression: vulnerability factors, provoking agents and symptom formation factors.[2] This research focuses on ongoing circumstances which were stressful, and their model of depression incorporates the importance of both long-term difficulties and more temporary time-limited events.

While there has been a tendency in the past for researchers to focus on either the impact of macrostructural factors or the coping

and responses of individuals to adverse events, there is growing recognition of the need to view psychosocial influences as embedded in rather than separated out from material influences (Stansfield et al 1999). A link between agency and wider structural determinants of mental health is evident in a self-efficacy approach characterising the work of a number of social scientists interested in mental health (Mirowsky & Ross 1984, Pearlin 1989, Aneshensel 1992, Thoits 1995). Such studies have explored people's responsiveness to specific environmental opportunities and highlighted the effect of achievement of, or blocking of, personal goals on mental health. Thus, rather than viewing people as passive recipients of external circumstances, concepts such as 'mastery', 'goal seeking' and perceived control of the environment — and opposite notions such as fatalism and powerlessness — are viewed as important in relation to changing opportunity structures.

There is utility too in examining the interaction of structure and agency in relation to specific policy and environmental contexts. With regard to this latter point, there is some evidence that the contextual effects of neighbourhood disadvantage on adult psychological well-being are mediated by people's perceptions of localities (particularly urban ones) as chaotic and threatening places. People living in 'socially disorganised' localities are more likely to be exposed to 'ambient hazards' and experience psychological distress because of uncontrollable life events and psychosocial insults. They are more likely than others to be affected negatively by stresses such as unemployment, family disruption, violence and crime, and to have fewer supportive relationships. A study of Wythenshawe, an inner-city area of Manchester, found that higher symptoms scores are associated with less neighbourliness/security, fewer leisure opportunities, and a sense reported by residents that their area is in decline (Huxley & Rogers 2001)

Labelling theory

As mentioned above, most studies tracing the relationship between social disadvantage and mental illness implicitly accept the legitimacy of psychiatric knowledge, treating diagnostic categories, like 'depression' or 'schizophrenia', as unproblematic and focusing on their links to social conditions. Labelling theorists and social constructionists on the other hand emphasise that mental health is negotiated and thus cannot be understood simply in terms of cause and effect relationships. Labelling theorists have tended to ignore the issue of cause altogether, while the constructionists have explored the epistemological assumptions of bodies of scientific knowledge and linked them to the way in which knowledge is constructed and shaped by a number of social influences and factors.

Labelling theory emanates from a version of sociology called 'symbolic interactionism', which is concerned with mapping ways in which social reality is negotiated. Emphasis is placed on the roles people take up and the meanings that are exchanged with others when occupying different roles. A failure to act appropriately in a role then becomes a critical point of understanding for those involved. Labelling theory has been adapted and applied to a wide set of social situations and social groups (e.g. schooling and education, crime and criminology) but it was developed most fully in relation to mental illness by Thomas Scheff in his book *Being Mentally Ill* (1966).

Scheff argued that behaviour commonly thought of as symptomatic of mental illness should be seen as a form of deviance, and chronic mental conditions as a distinctive social role. According to

---

[2] Vulnerability factors refer to both personal and environmental influences: e.g. loss of mother before 11 years, lack of employment outside the home. Provoking agents are factors operating in women's contemporary everyday lives, include detrimental events such as loss through bereavement or marriage breakdown, or episodes of serious illness. Chronic difficulties as well as specific stressors are also included. Symptom formation factors refer to previous episodes of depression and personal characteristics such as low self-esteem.

Scheff, societal reaction to the breaking of 'residual rules', was 'the single most important cause of careers of residual deviance' (1966: 92–93). Residual rules were 'numerous and unnameable' acts that cannot be placed into clear-cut categories but were taken-for-granted unspoken rules of social interaction. Under most circumstances acts of residual deviance are ignored by others, and it is only under certain circumstances that they are noted publicly.

According to those emphasising societal reaction (labelling theorists), mental health can have a variety of influences, including biological, psychological and social factors. However, what labelling theorists are then keen to emphasise is that in certain situations rule breaking is accepted, ignored or 'normalised', whereas at other times it is labelled as deviant. Once action is taken in the wake of this labelling it sets in chain a process of negotiation about a deviant role. Under these circumstances, the labelled person starts to take on the role of being a mentally ill person. This role is maintained by the views of others and the new identity that the mentally ill person ascribes to herself.

The methodological emphasis of labelling theorists, as their name implies, is on investigating the process and consequences of labelling. Rather than what caused people to act oddly in the first place (*primary deviance*), their main interest is in how symptoms become diagnosed as mental illnesses so that the person takes on a deviant role (*secondary deviance*). The answer given is in terms of *contingencies*. That is, the same behaviour will be ignored in some circumstances, whereas in other circumstances it will provoke concerns and the need for expert help. The transition between these two sets of circumstances can be linked to either a one-off crisis or a series of gradual shifts.

Labelling theorists have pointed out that a deviant role can emerge either rapidly or following a lengthy period when oddity is present but a problem is denied. For example, in one study it was found that the partners of men eventually diagnosed as schizophrenic ignored or rationalised symptoms for varying periods of time before they sought professional help, in order to maintain the men in ascribed masculine roles (Yarrow et al 1955). This picture is consistent with the findings of community surveys that the prevalence of symptoms exceeds the incidence of formal diagnosis ('the clinical iceberg'). More recent evidence suggests that auditory hallucinations are widespread in community samples, and that voice hearers who have not been diagnosed as suffering from schizophrenia have various ways of living with the experience (Epstein et al 2002, Jones et al 2003).

Of great interest to labelling theorists are the circumstances under which primary deviance is confirmed and amplified by contact with professionals and lay people. Relatives or other 'significant others' change from tolerating, denying or ignoring problem behaviour and begin to acknowledge its existence. Those who are more relationally distant are more willing to identify and attach a label of mental illness. Mental illness is recognised in families before professionals are invited to rubber stamp this lay decision-making. The combination of labelling from professionals and significant others defines the deviant person in a new role: of psychiatric patient. The final phase of the process entails the labelled person accepting or internalising the ascribed deviant identity. Mental hospitalisation strips them of their old identity in what Goffmann calls a 'status degradation ceremony' and is replaced by a new identity and social role. Being a patient can then become a 'career'.

While generally a deviant role takes a while to emerge and to be confirmed and internalised, there has been some experimental evidence that it can occur very rapidly. For example, in one study, confederate 'pseudo-patients' were admitted to psychiatric facilities by presenting with isolated auditory hallucinations. In all other respects the confederates did not act oddly once admitted. Despite this, the psychiatric staff treated them as if they were mentally ill and reframed their actions in this light. For example, when the confederates were seen keeping field notes, their actions were recorded as 'indulges in writing behaviour' (Rosenhan 1973).

The popularity of labelling theory as propounded by sociologists such as Thomas Scheff has declined in part because supporting empirical evidence is weak and because of the ambiguity of key concepts upon which the theory rests. For example the way in which residual rules are defined lacks precision, and social reaction is applied in an overly deterministic way. Nonetheless, aspects of labelling theory still retain relevance in the arena of mental health. There is certainly strong evidence that being in an institutional setting both induces oddity and socially disables residents. Also, the ascription of psychiatric deviance is commoner in social groups that are relatively powerless. However, these findings need to be set against others. If lay people are so important in shaping the labelling process, we would expect their stereotypes of mental illness to mirror the patterning of psychiatric diagnosis in society. However, this is not the case. Lay people emphasise florid psychotic symptoms in their stereotypes and fail to describe depression. The latter is the commonest of all psychiatric diagnoses. Similarly, psychiatrists do not always concur with the ascriptions of deviance made by family members. Moreover, the confederates in the experiment noted above did not, once the study was over, continue to act oddly because they had taken on the role of a psychiatric patient and been confirmed in this role by the staff.

Modified labelling theory

A more recent derivative of these original ideas is modified labelling theory, which emphasises a causal role for stigma in the 'relapse' of episodes of mental distress, linked to negative outcomes in employment and social functioning. Stigma can be defined as constituting three elements:

- a label that separates a person from others;
- the linking of the marked person to undesirable characteristics;
- the rejection and avoidance of the stigmatised person by others.

Rejection may be experienced in a range of areas such as employment and housing, through to everyday slights and minor insults. Stigma has been found to be highly prevalent among people labelled with a serious mental health problem living in the community (Link et al 1997). The effects of labelling are mediated by social psychological mechanisms in which both former psychiatric patients and members of the general population internalise negative cultural conceptions and attitudes about people who have been diagnosed with a mental illness, leading to personal discrimination. For many former psychiatric patients a negative self-concept emerges from a combination of their primary disability and from the cumulative reaction of others. Social rejection is an ongoing and recursive experience in the community setting and a persistent form of social stress for discharged patients. Experiences of social rejection increase feelings of self-deprecation, which act to weaken a sense of mastery and self-control (Barham & Haywood 1991), and exposure to stigmatising everyday experiences from post-institutional living (e.g. negative or avoidance attitudes from others) constitutes a source of significant and recurrent stress. This has long-term implications for a person's ability to function fully in society. An ethnographic study has shown how the expectations and avoidance of stigma leads to restricted social networks among former psychiatric patients (Estroff 1981).

Whilst most of labelling theory has been concerned with the societal reaction of others (strangers, significant others, professionals) it is also the case that a significant amount of labelling of mental distress is self-labelling. Thoits (1985) has conceptualised this as 'emotional deviance' whereby people label on the basis of the breaking of 'feeling rules'. This is particularly the case in relation to conditions which are not seen as stigmatising (such as depression and anxiety). Whether or not people do in fact label on the basis of an internalised or explicit set of feeling rules is a moot point and is likely at least to be culturally contingent. A recent study of the experience of depression and help-seeking from primary care suggested that inchoate feelings characterised the onset of depression and that respondents struggled to articulate the nature of their problems. Additionally, it was conduct and not being able to fulfil previous role demands that led to help-seeking, rather than the self-labelling of emotions (Rogers et al 2001).

Social constructionism

One of the most influential theoretical positions evident in the sociology of health and illness in recent years has been social constructionism. Three main currents within social constructionism can be identified:

- The first approach has most affinity with labelling theory insofar as it is not concerned with demonstrating the reality or otherwise of social phenomena but with the social forces which *define* them. This might involve investigation of a social problem, such as drug abuse or mental illness, in terms of exploring the lived experience of social actors in 'deviant' communities or those working with and labelling them.
- The second approach is more influenced by the post-structuralism of Foucault and is concerned with deconstruction, which is the critical examination of language and symbols in order to illuminate the creation of knowledge, its relationship to power and the unstable varieties of reality which attend human activity — 'discursive practices'.
- The third approach is concerned with understanding the production of scientific knowledge and the pursuit of individual and collective professional interests (Latour 1987) or *interest work*. In contrast to the post-structuralist emphasis upon ideas, emphasis is placed more on action and negotiation.

Despite their differences, certain core themes can be detected across these three types:

- Reality is problematised to some degree.
- Scientific and other realities are viewed wholly or partly as a product of human activity.
- Power relationships are inextricably bound up with the ways in which reality is defined.

In relation to the field of mental health, the social constructionist position goes further than that put forward by the labelling theorists. It is also interested in the categories used to describe or account for primary deviance. It is concerned with understanding the ways in which concepts, constructs or representations about mental health emerge as products of communal exchange between social groups. There is a particular emphasis within this approach on analysing dominant professional representations and the interests that are served by them. Thus the method of investigation associated with social constructionism is *deconstruction* or *discourse analysis*. Accordingly, social constructionists emphasise that reality (about mental health or anything else) is socially constructed and thus bound up with the material and cognitive interests of social groups. This contrasts with the position of social causationists, which is that there is a stable reality that exists independently of the investigator (*realism* or *positivism*). The social constructionist is interested in examining how variations in human experience and conduct come to be represented as illness categories and how diagnoses *inscribe* a version of reality on some people but not others.

Some examples from social constructionism

Social constructionists researching mental health have made two main critical points. The first is that concepts (or constructs) that are fragile, incoherent, illogical or invalid may still survive or may even be actively promoted in society. The second point they make is that constructs serve the interests of the social groups utilising them (e.g. mental health professionals, relatives of identified patients, drug companies). Here are some examples from the field of mental health:

- Constructionists problematise the factual status of mental illness (e.g. Szasz 1961). They analyse the ways in which mental health work has been linked to the production of psychiatric knowledge. Schizophrenia has the status of an illness and yet the diagnosis lacks both conceptual validity and reliability. Two people with different symptoms can both be diagnosed as schizophrenic — it is a disjunctive construct. Despite large amounts of research funding over the past hundred years for investigations that have tested a variety of environmental and biological hypotheses, the aetiology of the disease remains highly contested.[3] There is no biological marker (analogous to a blood test to diagnose diabetes) for schizophrenia. One possible explanation for the continuation of a weak construct is the role it plays in supporting the mandate of psychiatry in society and the comfort it gives to the relatives of mad people.
- Agoraphobia emerged at the time when the social emancipation of women became a possibility. For this reason, the meaning of the condition can be understood as part of a context that problematised the use of public space, not just as a set of symptoms within its individual sufferers. Here de Swann (1990: 144) makes this point:

Women appearing in the streets alone had to be women who went to work out of necessity, women whose husbands could not provide for their families single handedly; such women could not possibly be decent. Once this line of demarcation had become established, it also came to imply a licence for men to allow themselves impertinence towards women who appeared in public

---

[3] Editorial note: These views are not held by all working in this field. See chapters 14 and 19.

unaccompanied. Thus, a woman could not afford to go out on those streets . . . .

- The way in which psychiatric knowledge about women is generated is, according to some feminist scholars, imbued with sexual role stereotypes and notions of female inferiority. These points are made contentiously in the work of Ehrenreich and English. Their key argument is that male doctors have historically defined women's problems as illness or sickness and have promoted a notion of femininity which itself is viewed as pathological. This combination has resulted in female dependence on male experts and in lives of inactivity.
- Like schizophrenia, the concept of psychopathy is incoherent because it covers so many people who have different symptoms but can share the same label and has no biological marker. The definition is inevitably circular. People are deemed to be psychopathic because of their antisocial acts and their antisocial acts are explained by the actor's psychopathy. As a consequence, there is no independent way of validating the diagnosis. It has the same explanatory value as the notion of evil. Given that evil has been medicalised, the deconstructionist would be interested in the social history of this professional interest in certain types of antisocial action.
- Depression seems to be a straightforward description of depressed mood. However, ascriptions of helplessness, powerlessness and worthlessness can only be made in relation to interpersonal processes. Thus depression cannot be understood simply as a set of affective and cognitive characteristics of suffering individuals — it is defined and constituted by social processes.

These are some specific examples of how psychiatric diagnoses might be understood within a social constructionist framework. Some deconstructionists, like Szasz, have argued that the whole body of knowledge that follows from a commitment to the notion of mental illness has arisen in order to ensure the individual and collective advancement of psychiatric professionals and to protect the social order. In this way, he argues, professional knowledge, professional advancement, and social control are intimately entwined. Other deconstructionists, such as Rose, extending the work of Foucault, go further and argue that voluntary therapies that are anxiously sought and gratefully received by clients also contribute to social order via self-surveillance and the individualisation of distress.

MENTAL HEALTH IN SOCIETY

Having outlined the three main perspectives on the social in discussions about mental health, we will now discuss some wider issues about mental health in society.

Mental health or mental illness?

Both professionals and lay people have a disproportionate interest in mental abnormality or illness. This in itself is a social phenomenon. The term 'mental health' in recent years has come to be used throughout Western societies as a substitute for its opposite (mental illness). For example, it is commonplace now to hear terms such as 'mental health policy' or 'mental health facilities', which are actually euphemisms that refer to the management of mental abnormality in society.

Difficulties in articulating mental healthiness

While the term 'mental health' has become a more acceptable substitute for 'mental illness' it has remained relatively underdeveloped as a concept (Jahoda 1958). Neither professionals nor lay people have a well-proven facility for discussing mental health. For example, all of the approaches described above refer to perspectives on mental abnormality — how it is determined, negotiated or constructed. There has until recently been comparatively little professional interest in positive notions of mental health. Moreover, much of this minority interest has been defined in relation to *preventing mental illness*. This rather lopsided interest in illness or abnormality reflects social processes that are common to professionals and lay people alike.

Sociologists point out that we are generally asked to produce accounts for others when things go wrong. We tend not to explain how things go *right*. For example, if a rule is broken, a convention breaks down, or a person acts out of character or out of role, explanations are expected. These explanations may be invited from the people acting in an odd way, those who witness the events, or those who are responsible for formally recognising and managing their consequences. By contrast, when life goes smoothly with no rule infraction and people acting in the way they expect of others and themselves, there are few calls for explanation. As a consequence of this difference between the two conditions, we become much more skilled at articulating reasons for abnormal than for normal phenomena in everyday life. It seems that people expect negative emotions to be part of everyday life, and separating the negative from the positive aspects of mental health does not relate easily to everyday experiences. Additionally, while the 'mind' is meaningful to people, it is not as readily described as the body (Rogers & Pilgrim 1997).

Traditionally the focus of health promotion policy has been predominantly on preventing physical ill health. Global and national policy statements about health promotion prevention have tended to cite only one mental health goal from the many identified for health in general, which is the reduction of the suicide rate, and have focused on the prevention of relapse of an existing mental health problem. Mental health promotion is informed by a different set of assumptions which underpin positive attempts to create or preserve mental health. In the past this has focused on the individual, whether in primary prevention (anticipation and pre-empting of the occurrence of mental health problems), secondary (intervention at an early stage) or tertiary mental health promotion strategies (minimising the effects associated with an existing mental health problem). In the UK, primary healthcare services have been targeted as agencies for the secondary prevention of mental health problems (Goldberg & Huxley 1980).

A more socially oriented model of health promotion or 'new' public health model underpins the quality standards of the National Service Framework for mental health. Importance has been placed on the notion of social capital, which refers to 'features of social life-networks, mores and trust that enable participants to act together more effectively to pursue shared objectives' (Putnam, cited in Wilkinson 1996:221). This notion implies that the quality of social relationships, and our perception of where we are relative to others in the social structure, are likely to be important psychosocial mediators in the aetiology of mental health problems.

This view of emotional and psychological health is aligned with an approach to addressing the causes of mental health problems which recognises that the effecting of positive changes in the lives of people who are recovering from mental health difficulties requires organisations and communities to challenge stigma and provide employment, financial and social opportunities — for example by improving the levels of access to mainstream adult community and further education (http://www.nimhe.org.uk/priorities/socialinclusion.asp).

Professionals and interprofessional relationships

Attempts to understand mental health professionals have drawn upon a number of theoretical strands from within the sociology of the professions.

Durkheimian tradition

Durkheim and structural functionalists (e.g. Talcott Parsons) have viewed professional groups as providing a disinterested and integrative societal function which counterbalanced the tendency of egotistical individuals to fragment society. From this perspective professions are a source of community for one another and stability for the wider society they serve. They regulate their own practices and practitioners (through, for example, 'peer review') and ensure good practice through the setting of codes of conduct and punishing errant colleagues. Followers of this approach to the sociology of professions have tended to take claims of special knowledge and altruism at face value and have focused on categorising professions in terms of traits and descriptions of their work.

Weberian tradition

The Weberian framework stresses the development of professional strategies to advance their own social status, persuade clients about the need for the service they offer and corner the market in a service sector in away that excludes competitors. From this perspective two aspects are particularly noteworthy: collective social advancement rests upon *social closure*, and professionals exercise power over others through *professional dominance*. Social closure refers to a situation where a monopoly is gained to work in a specialised way with a particular group so that other occupational groups seeking a similar role are excluded. In order for professionals to maintain their social status they must convince those outside their boundaries that they are offering a unique service, and as a consequence they develop various rhetorical devices to persuade the outside world of their unique and special qualities. To do this they need to justify a peculiar knowledge-base that has a technical rationality that is not easily understood or deployed by competitors.

Professional dominance refers to the exercising of power over others in three senses:

- Professions have power over their clients. An imbalance of specialised knowledge keeps the user in a state of ignorance, insecurity and vulnerability. This imbalance is reinforced by the tendency of professionals to operate within their own territory rather than that of their clients (e.g. treatment in hospital rather than in the client's own home).
- Professionals exercise power over their new recruits (e.g. trainees are dependent on their superiors for career progression).

- Professionals seek to establish a dominant relationship over other occupational groups working with the same client group.

Andrew Scull explains the rise and maintenance of psychiatry in terms of its functional value for economic order and efficiency under capitalism and in so doing draws on both neo-Marxian and Weberian frameworks. He points to the segregation of the mad in the 19th century and delegation by the State of powers to the medical profession to keep madness under control. The role of psychiatrists is seen as one of social control employed by the State to contain the threat of one section of a poor underclass — the mad. Scull also makes use of the notion of closure when explaining the dynamics of how doctors purged lay administrators from the asylums and sought upward mobility for themselves. Modern professions are not simply the dominant or most important providers of a particular service; instead they effectively monopolise a service market.

During the 19th century, mad-doctors manoeuvred to secure such a position for themselves and acceptance of their particular view of the nature of madness, seeking to transform their existing foothold in the marketplace into a cognitive and practical monopoly of the field, and to acquire for those practising this line of work the status 'owed' to professionals (Scull 1979:129).

Interprofessional relationships

The shifting location of mental health services has had a major impact on how professionals organise their work and the way in which they relate to patients and each other. The territorial base of the asylum and hospital has to a large extent been replaced by the need to negotiate one-to-one relationships in a domestic or community context. Mental health workers have been faced with the need to change their working practices and the way in which they interact. In particular, work outside the hospital has brought with it a philosophy of multidisciplinary working, which had already operated, in theory at least, in inpatient settings. The basic tenets of multidisciplinary working are:

- that each member of the mental health team has special skills to contribute to the management of patients;
- that these are contributed in co-operation and liaison with other mental health workers;
- that this leads to the establishment of corporate consensual goals in delivering a service.

One of the stated aims of multi- or interdisciplinary working is to produce a 'seamless' service across primary, secondary and community care sectors and is predicated on the ethos of effective communication and liaison. However, there are suggestions that rather than entailing mutuality and co-operation, interprofessional relations are characterised by defensiveness, lack of role clarity and conflict. Much of the conflict centres on bids for professional dominance or autonomy. Subordinate professionals have increasingly made attempts to counter the claims of uniqueness of skills made by psychiatrists as the dominant professional group. For example, clinical psychologists have developed a training and consultancy role, seeking higher levels of remuneration, adopting medical titles ('Consultant Psychologist') and accepting direct referrals from GPs. Threatened by deprofessionalisation, psychiatric nurses have been busy collecting more therapeutic skills which can be viewed as a means of countering claims of uniqueness of skills made by the other main groups of mental health workers.

Difficulties in ensuring multidisciplinary co-operation and corporate goal achievement stem from the differing secondary socialisation and training of mental health workers. Unidisciplinary groupings tend to emphasise the status, training levels and accreditation of their own group as their contribution to improving service quality, whereas multidisciplinary commitment to practice guidelines to standardise best practice and outcome tends to be less supported.

Team work poses a problem for professionals around role and identity once they have been fully socialised into distinct professional groupings, as suggested by Onyett et al (1994). The concentration of practitioners into teams places professional workers in a special dilemma. They become members of two groups: their profession and their team. As a result they may find themselves torn between the aims of a community mental health movement that explicitly values egalitarianism, role blurring and a surrender of power to lower status workers and service users on the one hand, and a desire to hold on to traditionally, socially valued role definitions and practices on the other (Onyett et al 1994). As well as competing professional interests, knowledge claims about mental health are varied and to some extent reflect different ideologies and values.

Social and cultural influences on models of illness and management of mental health problems

Cross-cultural and historical evidence suggests that notions of mental distress and madness are prevalent in all societies. The following points can be made to support this conclusion:

- In the pre-psychiatric times of ancient Rome and Athens, madness was documented as being associated with aimless wandering and violence.
- In more recent times, people living in societies such as Laos, which had neither mental hospitals nor psychiatric professionals, still provided accounts of madness.
- In localities without mental institutions, very clear conceptual distinctions are made by lay people about sanity and insanity.
- Whereas there are differences between cultures about how sadness, fear and madness are represented and explained, all societies, now and in the past, have provided descriptions of these emotional and behavioural phenomena. Put differently, anxiety, depression and psychosis may be products of modern Western psychiatry, but fear, sadness and madness are not.

Nonetheless, criteria used to judge both the cause and presence of mental illness can be rendered problematic if understood in their social context. Turning to mental health, social relativism appears immediately. Some notions in everyday use about mental health are only meaningful to people in cultures that contain and appreciate psychoanalysis or humanistic psychology. Resistance to stress is superficially appealing as a definition of mental health but what of those people who are unperturbed by stress? Many psychiatrists would describe these as 'primary psychopaths'. As for autonomy, what of people who are compulsively independent and avoid social relationships? Competence is not an invariant capacity but relies for its defini-tion on value judgments made in a specific social setting about conformity to expectations of roles and rules. The social context also determines whose judgement prevails about the competence of others. Finally judgements about accu-rate perception of reality are social judgements. Hearing voices, or seeing things others cannot, may be judged as signs of mystical powers in one culture or they may be deemed to be symptomatic of schizophrenia in another.

Even within the same culture or society there are competing professional discourses about abnormality. This is the case in relation to dominant Western norms, beliefs and models about mental illness (e.g. biodeterminism, psychoanalysis, behavioural psychology, humanistic psychology, legalism). As we have discussed above, whereas most studies tracing the relationship between social disadvantage and mental illness implicitly accept the legitimacy of psychiatric knowledge — treating diagnostic categories, like 'depression' or 'schizophrenia', as unproblematic and focusing on their links to social factors — the question of *what* is being identified has pervaded the contested nature of knowledge about mental health, both inside and outside of the psychiatric profession.

Some commentators have reflected on the influence of external social and economic factors on the content of explanatory models treating medical knowledge as an object of sociological inquiry. For example, Dohrenwend (1998:224) comments that:

> . . . [the] belief in the paramount role of genetic inheritance began to change especially in the United States, under the impact of two major events: the stock market crash of 1929 followed by the Great Depression, and the US entrance into World War II in 1941. The great depression made it clear that a person could become poor for reasons other than inherited disabilities and research conducted during World War II showed that situations of extreme environmental stress arising out of combat and imprisonment could produce serious psychopathology in previously normal persons, some of it long lasting.

The relativity of mental health knowledge is not just an abstracted object of philosophical interest but has practical and material consequences for those who find themselves the subject of a range of assumptions about behaviour and norms of behaviour. Such assumptions become rooted in the organisation and delivery of psychiatric services.

MENTAL HEALTH SERVICES IN THEIR SOCIAL CONTEXT

The discussion above has mainly focused on the relationship between society and forms of knowledge about mental health. Societal influences are also relevant when we come to understand the provision of mental health services. The notion of 'mental health services' is actually quite recent. Up until the first part of the 20th century there were only hospitals, clinics and asylums. The notion of 'services' has replaced these individual descriptions of facilities in the last fifty years.

The way in which the modern general hospital has been depicted provides a benchmark with which both the old asylum system and the new arrangements for delivering psychiatric services in a post-asylum era can be compared. The modern hospital, with its high-technology equipment, elaborate procedures and specialised skills, has frequently been viewed as an outcome of 'scientific developments' and medical progress over the last century (Tuckett 1976). This assumption has led a number of sociologists to comment that the modern hospital is an example of Max Weber's notion of a 'bureaucratic organisation'. Sociologists of organisations have identified characteristics of the 'typical' modern hospital that have been influenced by Weber's ideal type. Perrow (1965), a systems analyst, identified three factors which determine the way in which organisations function:

- the cultural system, which sets the legitimate or formal goals;
- technology, which is the means of achieving these goals (in the hospital this includes the types of therapeutic techniques in use);
- the structure of the organisation in which techniques are embedded and person-power is organised as a means of achieving the set goals.

Hospitals, like other complex organisations such as factories and schools, operate on the basis of an interdependence between technology and structure, are characterised by a highly specialised division of health labour (what Durkheim termed 'organic solidarity') and possess a complex authority and command system.

The asylum system

During the 19th century in western Europe and North America, most countries developed centrally regulated asylum systems. The emergence of large asylums in most localities was associated with the need to control non-productive deviance in increasingly urbanised and complex capitalist societies. In other words, economic life was disrupted or impaired by madness ('lunatics' or 'dements') and by those with learning difficulties ('aments'). Both of these groups were 'warehoused' in asylums to remove their negative impact on socio-economic order and efficiency, just as orphans, the physically sick and the elderly were placed in poorhouses. Professionals at that time took little or no interest in sane people who were frightened or sad (the neuroses). This changed after the First World War, when the 'shell shock' problem altered the focus of professional interest. Warfare ensured that stress-induced problems, later to be called 'battle neurosis' or 'post-traumatic stress disorder', recurringly shifted professional attention away from madness and toward neurosis during the 20th century. This also expanded the range of interventions offered or preferred by professionals to include talking treatments. As a result, psychiatric treatment became more eclectic, although it remained dominated by biomedical interventions.

During periods of peacetime, the focus on madness returned, along with biological treatments in institutional settings. After the Second World War, the old asylum system came into crisis for a number of reasons:

- The expansion of the remit of psychiatry and its associated professions to include talking treatments with neurotic patients in community settings, increased expectations that mental health services should shift away from biomedical treatments inside institutions.
- In the wake of the widespread cultural shock of the Nazi concentration camps, Western liberal democracies witnessed a popular disquiet about segregation. Also, lessons about the disabling impact of institutionalisation ('institutional neurosis') were drawn from observations in the camps of ritualised, rigid and stereotyped behaviour of their inmates.
- Large institutions were expensive and placed a large fiscal burden upon government budgets. Deinstitutionisation offered itself as a cost-cutting exercise.

- Doubts about institutional life were reinforced by research on its negative impact from social psychiatry, sociology, and from dissent within clinical psychiatry ('antipsychiatry').
- A new social movement of mental health service users that was critical of hospital-based biomedical regimens emerged internationally.

The above list does not contain any allusion to the so-called 'pharmacological revolution'. It is a commonly reported misconception that the increasing use of neuroleptic drugs (major tranquillisers) during the 1950s led to a process of deinstitutionalisation. In some countries, bed numbers began to drop before the introduction of the drugs. In others, bed numbers actually increased despite this introduction. The drugs also have been used on a variety of populations that were not deemed to be mentally ill (such as people with learning difficulties and older people). The drugs were only relevant in giving psychiatric staff more confidence in dealing with community-based patients; they do not explain the policy of deinstitutionalisation (Rogers & Pilgrim 2001).

The contemporary organisation of psychiatry

At the end of the 20th century, deinstitutionalisation had become a dominant mental health policy goal in most Western democracies. However, this formal goal has become clouded by evidence that the gradual reduction of large institutions has been replaced by a scattering of smaller ones 'in the community'. Also, most countries still have legal statutes to coercively remove madness from community settings. The extent of this continued coercive control varies from one country to another. For example, more conformist or authoritarian cultures such as Japan or Russia have higher rates of involuntary detention in psychiatric facilities. What is clear is that a policy of deinstitutionalisation and one of genuine community care are not the same. Currently, it may be more accurate to talk of 'reinstitutionalisation' as the actual outcome of large hospital closures rather than 'community care'.

There remains substantial confusion surrounding the meaning of the term 'community care', which reflects a lack of clarity over the ultimate goals of such a policy. In practice, community care refers to mentally disordered people receiving care in non-asylum settings. The main initiatives include the development of psychiatric units in District General Hospitals (DGH), psychiatric services in primary healthcare settings, the expanded use of community psychiatric nurses, the development of community mental health centres and teams, the development of residential daycare facilities and increased emphasis on voluntary services by friends and relatives, and the introduction of the case management and care programme approach.

There has been greater attention paid to considering the cause and solution of mental health problems within a public health context in which problem management stretches beyond the structural and organisational arrangements of traditional health services. A multi-sectoral approach to mental health is outlined in the Government's Green Paper *Our Healthier Nation* (1998) in which effective policy responses to mental health problems are viewed as implicating local and central players, community resources, the environment and individual action. Thus the focus has moved, at the level of policy at least, to incorporating aspects of employment, social, community and voluntary organisations in the prevention and management of mental health problems. New technologies and information systems have also led to fundamental changes and diversification in the availability of mental health technologies. For example, self-management for mental health problems is increasingly being seen as a means of making psychological therapies more widely available to those with 'mild' mental distress. A key aspect of the philosophy of such therapy relates to increasing the patient's self-efficacy, and the focus of facilitation is on increasing patients' feelings of confidence in using the technology of self-help. Much of self-management takes place within the person's own environment and is increasingly distanced from the place of professionally delivered services. One of the most important consequences of the use of new technologies such as the internet is the rapid increase it allows in mutual non-professional support. The anonymous helper in an electronic conference or the support group on the Web provides the basis of a revolution in mental health support that has emerged as an unpredicted and major element in the global organisation of mental healthcare. These emerging arrangements seem to bear little resemblance to the formal definitions of the hospital as an organisation discussed at the beginning of this section. Rather they are more consistent with the notion of postmodern organisational arrangements which are 'de-differentiated flexible niche marketed and have a multi-skilled works force held together by information technology networks and subcontracting' (Clegg 1990:53).

The gradient of coercion operating in mental health services

The growing eclecticism of psychiatric provision is accompanied by differentiation in levels of coercion. The coercive role of psychiatric services in response to certain types of social crisis and deviance has been a salient feature of sociological analysis about psychiatry (e.g. the work of Szasz, Laing, Scull and Goffmann). Collectively, this body of work suggests that the function of psychiatry is different from other branches of medicine. In psychiatric services, the over-representation of people from a lower social class and some ethnic minorities in coercive contexts is not about meeting need in the same way that health services respond to physical problems. In other words the assumptions of the 'inverse care law' (Tudor-Hart 1971) are not directly applicable. (The law is the notion that access to care has a tendency to increase with increasing class status, with the poorest people tending to get the poorest health care.)

In psychiatric services, involuntary detention and treatment are explicit and operational features. A proportion of patients are forcibly detained and treated by the use of therapeutic law; some are notionally voluntary but de facto detainees, and others are genuinely voluntary patients but are in a service context where the threat of coercion is ever present. In the light of these peculiar features about psychiatry, mental health management can be conceptualised as part of a wider State apparatus which controls the social problems associated with poverty and the underclass. Once conceived in this way, a unitary view of service contact as necessarily aiming for or achieving a gain in the mental health status of service recipients is rendered problematic.

Of course not all service provision is coercive to the same degree, but a graduated system of control operating in services is a relevant consideration in making judgements about the extent to which services meet need (Rogers & Pilgrim 2003). For example, some wards are locked in open psychiatric units ('intensive care units') and some hospitals hold patients in conditions of 'medium

security'. Others contain mentally disordered offenders in high-security conditions. Outside of acute inpatient provision and forensic services the coercive/social control function is lessened and the use of services is more akin to those for patients with physical conditions. However, even in primary care, the GP acts as a 'second opinion' medical practitioner in supporting applications for involuntary detention in hospital. This may mean that the possibility of compulsion and the stigma attached to secondary services may impact on the willingness to access and utilise primary-care services (Rogers et al 2001).

Nevertheless, overall, primary care is less coercive than other parts of the mental health system and is principally influenced by patients' decision-making about when and how to access services. It is also the area where the social contract in providing a national health service free at the point of need is most meaningful, given the direct access that it permits to citizens. The emergence of voluntary organisations, the increase of private practice and user-led services and self-management are significant changes in the pattern of service provision. The utilisation of non-State employees in the delivery of services also changes the nature of service delivery. The rise of self-employed primary-care counsellors trained outside mainstream State-provided higher education for health professionals is an example here. Users have taken on roles previously monopolised by mental health professionals both in the provision of user-led schemes (e.g. crises houses) and in increasingly using self-care options which, as discussed in the previous section, emphasise the centrality of self-efficacy and the patient as 'change agent'.

The impact of the entanglement of control and coercion in mental health care is compounded when psychiatric service contact with key marginal social groups is involved.

Racism and contact with psychiatry

Cultural analysis (analysis of differences in language, values, norms and beliefs) focuses on the individual or their culture and is concerned mainly with examining the role of prejudice and discrimination in determining differences in health behaviour and the use of services. 'Prejudice' implies a psychological concept in that it refers to a set of personal attitudes. Trans-cultural psychiatry, for example, is concerned with how different ethnic groups are treated by mental health workers socialised in the ways of the 'dominant culture' (Rack 1982, Fernando 1988). This position advocates initiatives aimed at challenging and changing prejudices through 'race awareness' training. This works on the premise of challenging the stereotypical and negative views about minority ethnic groups held by powerful individuals, like professionals. However what tends to be missing from analyses based on prejudice is a consideration of the impact of inequality — how the latter is manifested in mental illness rates, services and professional responses to black and other minority groups. In contrast to prejudice, racism implies a sociological rather than a psychological analysis and emphasises the roles of institutions in perpetuating disadvantage, and the need to combat institutional racism through anti-racism measures. A key focus of the debate about race and psychiatry relates to the type of contact that Afro-Caribbean young men have with mental health services.

Afro-Caribbean people are much more likely than white people to make contact with mental health services via the police, courts and prison, and, once contact has been made, there is evidence of their over-representation in compulsory admission and in receiving a diagnosis of schizophrenia compared with white people (Bhui et al 1995). At the other end of the spectrum there is evidence to suggest that black people are under-represented in outpatient and self-referred services and less likely than other groups to be referred by general practitioners (e.g. Harrison et al 1988).

The pathways by which young black men come to the attention of mental health services have led some commentators to suggests that the 'criminalisation' and medicalisation of black people are closely connected processes which implicate psychiatry as part of a larger social control apparatus which regulates and oversees the lives of black people (Francis 1988). The multiple contacts, judgements and processes which are involved in referral to psychiatric services may also imply a process of 'transmitted discrimination' in which contingencies and the subtle discriminatory acts and views may be transferred from one agency to another. Differences in the processes of referral, labelling and help-seeking are all likely to be implicated. Black people may express their distress at times in a culturally idiosyncratic way. Much of the psychiatric literature suggests that the manifestation of 'mental illness' predisposes Afro-Caribbeans towards police arrest because they present in a particularly disturbed way, and the place in which behaviour takes place is also deemed to be important. Bean (1986) suggests that if a greater part of young Afro-Caribbean social life takes place in public, then 'mad' behaviour is more likely to be detected and dealt with by agents such as the police, than is the case of white people, who have more of an 'indoor culture'. The tendency to label a person mentally ill increases with the cultural distance between the labeller and labelled, suggesting that members of minority ethnic groups are more likely to be labelled mentally ill than dominant indigenous groups by members of the public as well as by professionals.

Gender and sexuality

The psychiatric response to sexuality has changed according to changes in treatment philosophies and norms and values associated with homosexuality. In the 19th century the assumed biological determination of homosexuality led not to active physical intervention (as with other types of madness) but with fatalism to a 'problem behaviour' which prompted little therapeutic interest (Diamont 1987). It was only when psychoanalytical and the behavioural therapeutic methods were introduced during the 20th century that psychiatrists began to interfere with homosexuality and aspire to 'cure' the condition. The optimism of these newer environmental/psychological theories prompted professionals to be more interventionist. In relation to contemporary treatments and contact with services, a recent study of therapist attitudes to gay clients suggests that many therapists do not see social and gay and lesbian identity as relevant to the therapeutic process and that gay and lesbian mental health users may still encounter overt and covert bias which includes the pathologisation of homosexuality (Bartlett et al 2001).

It is likely that internalised stigmatised identities reinforce the biases of mental health professionals and therapies. For example, if gay and lesbian people have been socialised into accepting the bias in society against them, they may be more inclined to collude with ill-advised therapeutic efforts to modify sexual orientation. Negative stereotypes about sexuality may then be reinforced by therapists who share them and who fail to acknowledge them as indications of homophobia. However, it is also the case that changing norms about the acceptability of homosexuality in wider soci-

ety are also reflected in psychiatry. For example the Royal College of Psychiatrists established a Gay and Lesbian Mental Health Special Interest group in 2001 (http://www.rcpsych.ac.uk/college/sig/dayles.htm).

CONCLUSION

In this chapter different perspectives from inside and outside sociology about the topic of psychiatry and the identification and treatment of mental health and illness have been explored. It may seem at first reading that sociology is somehow a separate and recent commentator on mental health and illness. This is only partially true. Over the last fifty years sociologists have contributed to knowledge about psychiatry and the users of mental health services and have responded to the trends and practices coming from mental health workers. However, social science also has a history of being intertwined with medical research. The discipline of social psychiatry demonstrates this overlap, and some of the groundbreaking epidemiological works of the 1950s and 1960s discussed at the beginning of this chapter involved the collaboration of sociologists with psychiatrists. However, it is also true that more recent responses of sociologists have been seen as oppositional by those inside clinical psychiatry. During the late 1960s, sociologists become part of 'antipsychiatry', or 'critics of psychiatry' according to some commentators. Thus, sociologists are in an ambivalent relationship with psychiatry. On the one hand, they have contributed to an expanded theory of aetiology, in tracing the social causes of mental illness; on the other, they have set up competing ways of conceptualising mental abnormality. Finally, some version of critical realism (Bhaskar 1989) has been suggested as a means of maximising the advantages inherent in each of the sociological approaches to the study of mental health (Rogers & Pilgrim 2003). Critical realist thinking advocates a view in which it is not reality which is socially negotiated, but a way of conceptualising and investigating it. This necessitates that sociology as a practical project looks beyond the findings of individual projects and that a critical perspective be adopted, which unpicks professional interests, exposes the societal role of professional practice and draws into the frame of analysis knowledge-claims about services.

REFERENCES

Aneshensel C S 1992 Social stress theory and research. Annual Review of Sociology 18: 15–38

Barham P, Haywood R 1991 From the mental patient to the person. Routledge, London

Bartlett A, King M, Phillips P 2001 Straight talking: an investigation of the attitudes and practice of psychoanalysts and psychotherapists in relation to gays and lesbians. British Journal of Psychiatry 179: 545–549

Bartley M, Blane D, Davey-Smith G 1998 Beyond the Black Report. Sociology of Health and Illness 20(5): 563–577

Bean P 1986 Mental disorder and social control. Cambridge University Press, Cambridge

Bhaskar R 1989 Reclaiming reality. Verso, London

Bhui K, Christie Y, Bhugra D 1995 The essential elements of culturally sensitive psychiatric services. International Journal of Social Psychiatry 41(4): 246–256

Brown G W, Harris T O 1978 Social origins of depression: a study of psychiatric disorder in women. Tavistock, London

Clegg S R 1990 Modern organisations. Sage, London

de Swann A 1990 The management of normality. Routledge, London

Diamont L 1987 Male and female homosexuality: psychological approaches. Hemisphere, New York

Dohrenwend B P 1998 A psychosocial perspective in the past and future of psychiatric epidemiology. American Journal of Epidemiology 147(3): 222–229

Dohrenwend B P, Dohrenwend B S 1982 Perspectives on the past and future of psychiatric epidemiology. American Journal of Public Health 72: 1271–1279

Dohrenwend B P, Brice P, Levar I et al 1992 Socioeconomic status and psychiatric disorders: the causation selection issue. Science 255: 946–951

Durkheim E 1952 Suicide: a study in sociology. Routledge & Kegan Paul, London

Elstad J I 1998 The psycho-social perspective on social inequalities in health. Sociology of Health and Illness 20(5): 598–618

Elton P J, Packer J M 1986 A prospective randomised trial of the value of re-housing on the grounds of mental ill-health. Journal of Chronic Disease 39: 221–227

Ehrenreich B, English D 1978 For her own good: 150 years of the experts' advice to women. Pluto, London

Epstein R M, Bonell F, Visser A 2002 Hearing voices: patient centred care with diverse populations. Patient Education & Counselling 48: 1–3

Estroff S 1981 Making it crazy: an ethnography of psychiatric clients in an American community. University of California Press, Berkeley

Faris R E, Dunham H W 1939 Mental disorders in urban areas: an ecological study of schizophrenia and other psychoses. University of Chicago Press, Chicago

Fernando S 1988 Race and culture in psychiatry. Tavistock/Routledge, London

Foucault M 1965 Madness and civilization. Random House, New York

Francis E 1988 Black people, dangerousness and psychiatric compulsion. In: Brackx A, Grimshaw C (eds) Mental health care in crisis. Pluto, London

Goffmann E 1961 Asylums. Penguin, Harmondsworth

Goldberg D, Huxley P 1980 Mental illness in the community. Tavistock, London

Gove W 1972 The relationship between sex roles, marital status and mental illness: Social Forces 51: 33–44

Gove W, Tudor J F 1972 Adult sex roles and mental illness. American Journal of Sociology 78: 812–835

Harrison G, Owens D, Holton A et al 1988 A prospective study of severe mental disorder in Afro-Caribbean patients. Psychological Medicine 11: 289–302

Hollingshead A, Redlich R C 1958 Social class and mental illness. Wiley, New York

Huxley P, Rogers A 2001 Urban regeneration and mental health. Health Variations 7 (April): 8–9

Jahoda M 1958 Current concepts of positive mental health. Basic Books, New York

Johns L C, Nazroo J Y, Bebbington P, Kuipers E 2002 Occurrence of hallucinatory experiences in a community sample and ethnic variations. British Journal of Psychiatry 180: 174–178

Jones S, Guy A, Prmond J A 2003 A methodological study of hearing voices: a preliminary exploration of voice hearers and understanding of their experiences. Psychology & Psychotherapy 76: 189–209

Kessler R C, McGonagel K A, Zhai S et al 1994 Lifetime and 12-month prevalence of DSM-III-R psychiatric disorders in the United States. Archives of General Psychiatry 51: 8–19

Latour B 1987 Science in action: how to follow scientists and engineers through society. Cambridge, MA: Harvard University Press

Lemert E 1967 Human deviance, social problems and social control. Prentice-Hall, Englewood Cliffs, NJ

Lewis G, Bebbington P, Brugha T et al 1998 Socioeconomic status standard of living and neurotic disorder. Lancet 352: 605–609

Link B G, Struening E L, Rahav M et al 1997 On stigma and its consequences: evidence from a longitudinal study of men with dual diagnoses of mental illness and substance abuse. Journal of Health and Social Behavior 38: 177–190

Miller P, Rose N 1988 The Tavistock programme: the government of subjectivity and social life. Sociology 22(2): 171–192

Mirowsky J, Ross C E 1984 Mexican culture and is emotional contradictions. Journal of Health and Social Behavior 25(1): 2–13

Muntaner C, Eaton W W, Chamberlain C D 2000 Social inequalities in mental health: a review of concepts and underlying assumptions. Health 4(1): 89–109

Myers J, Bean L 1968 A decade later: a follow up of social class and mental illness. Wiley, New York

Nazroo J V, Edwards A C, Brown G W 1998 Gender differences in the prevalence of depression: artefact, alternative disorders, biology or roles? Sociology of Health and Illness 20(3): 312–330

Onyett S, Heppleston T, Bushnell D 1994 A national survey of community mental health team structure and process. Journal of Mental Health 3: 175–194

Parsons T 1951 The social system. Routledge & Kegan Paul, London

Paykel E S 1991 Depression in women. British Journal of Psychiatry 158(suppl 10): 22–29

Pearlin L I 1989 The sociological study of stress. Journal of Health and Social Behavior 30(3): 241–256

Perrow C 1965 Hospitals: technology, structure and goals. In: March J G (ed) Handbook of organisations. Rand McNally, Chicago

Pilgrim D, Rogers A 1999 A sociology of mental health and illness, 2nd edn. Open University Press, Milton Keynes

Platt S, Micciolo R, Tansella M 1992 Suicide and unemployment in Italy: description analysis and interpretation of recent trends. Social Science and Medicine 34(11): 1191–1201

Rack P 1982 Race, culture and mental disorder. Tavistock, London

Rogers A, Pilgrim D 1997 The contribution of lay knowledge to the understanding and promotion of mental health. Journal of Mental Health 6(1): 23–25

Rogers A, Pilgrim D 2001 Mental health policy in Britain, 2nd edn. Palgrave, Basingstoke

Rogers A, Pilgrim D 2003 Mental health and inequality. Palgrave, Basingstoke

Rogers A, May C, Oliver D 2001 Experiencing depression, experiencing the depressed: the management of depression in primary care. Journal of Mental Health 10(3): 317–333

Rose N 1990 Governing the soul. Routledge, London

Rosenhan D L 1973 On being sane in insane places. Science 179: 250–258

Scheff T 1966 Being mentally ill: a sociological theory. Aldine, Chicago

Scull A 1977 Decarceration: community treatment and the deviant — a radical view. Prentice-Hall, Englewood Cliffs, NJ

Scull A 1979 Museums of madness. Penguin, Harmondsworth

Stansfield S A, Fuhrer R, Cattell V et al 1999 Psychosocial factors and the explanation of socio-economic gradients in common mental disorders. Health variations 4: 4–5. ESRC, Lancaster

Stansfeld S A, Marmot M G 1992 Social class and minor psychiatric disorder in British Civil service: a validated screening survey using the General Health Questionnaire. Psychological Medicine 22: 739–749

Stone M 1985 Shell shock and the psychologists. In Bynum W F, Porter R (eds) The anatomy of madness. Tavistock, London

Szasz T S 1961 The uses of naming and the origin of the myth of mental illness. American Psychologist 16: 59–65

Thoits P A 1985 Self-labeling process in mental illness: the role of emotional deviance. American Journal of Sociology 91: 221–249

Thoits P A 1995 Stress, coping and social support processes: 'where are we — what next'. Journal of Health and Social Behavior (extra issue): 53–79

Tuckett D 1976 The organisation of hospitals. In: Tuckett D (ed) An introduction to medical sociology. Tavistock, London

Tudor-Hart J 1971 The inverse care law. Lancet (7696): 405–412

Wang X, Gao L, Shinfuku N et al 2000 Lontitudinal study of earthquake related PTSD in a randomly selected community sample in North China. American Journal of Psychiatry 157(8): 1260–1266

Warner R 1985 Recovery from schizophrenia. In: Psychiatry and political economy. Routledge, London

Wilkinson R G 1996 Unhealthy societies: the afflictions of inequalities. Routledge, London

Yarrow M J, Schwartz C, Murphy H, Deasy L 1955 The psychological meaning of mental illness. Journal of Social Issues 11: 12–24

8 Neuropsychology

Ronan E O'Carroll

INTRODUCTION

Neuropsychology is the study of brain–behaviour relationships, and has traditionally utilised the classical lesion-based approach — relating focal brain damage to patterns of preserved and impaired cognitive functioning. In the majority of psychiatric disorders, however, focal brain lesions are rare, and the real challenge of neuropsychology in relation to psychiatry is to understand abnormal behaviour in terms of dysfunctional processing of information. This is more likely to be related to abnormally functioning brain systems than to localised brain damage. Historically, within psychiatry, the role of the neuropsychologist was limited to an attempt to aid in the differential diagnosis of 'organic' versus 'functional' psychoses. However, in an overview of 34 studies, the mean 'hit rate' (classification accuracy) of patients with schizophrenia versus brain-damaged patients was 54%, prompting Green (1996) to state 'the contributions of clinical neuropsychology to the study of schizophrenia appear to be modest at best'.

Over the past decade, however, neuropsychology has led to considerable advances in the study of psychiatric disorder, to the extent that neuropsychology is now seen as an essential discipline for the study of psychiatric disorder. This progress has been achieved through reliable and precise quantification of discrete components of cognitive function and behaviour in relation to normal and abnormal mental states, e.g. study of cognitive function in 'high risk' individuals (Byrne et al 1999) and in the development of neuropsychological models of mental disorder (Frith 1992).

The determination of brain–cognition relationships is no easy undertaking in psychopathological states. Many neuropsychological studies in major psychiatric disorder are conducted on patients who are taking psychotropic medication, and such drugs may well have confounding effects on measures of cognitive functioning. Most psychiatric disorders involve affective status, therefore mood and motivation may also critically impact on neuropsychological test performance. In recent years greater attention has been placed on exploring specific syndromes or symptoms rather than 'illnesses'. For example, rather than trying to explain 'schizophrenia', attempts have been made to explain specific features (e.g. paranoid delusions) in neuropsychological terms.

Clinical neuropsychology also has an important role to play in the assessment of cognitive impairment in clinical practice. The development of neuropsychological measures allows for the valid and reliable assessment of treatment efficacy. This is particularly important as 'negative features' (including cognitive impairment) are becoming increasingly recognised as important targets for pharmacological treatment of psychiatric disorders.

Scope of the chapter

The study of brain–behaviour relationships in man is a huge area, therefore this chapter will focus on issues of particular relevance for psychiatry. Rapid progress in neuropsychology has occurred over the last decade via the use of functional brain imaging techniques (SPECT, PET and fMRI) as these techniques can be used to provide validation of localisation of function suggested by neuropsychological findings. These developments are covered in Chapter 5, on neuroimaging. The present chapter begins with a review of historically important single-case studies that were crucial in establishing the field of neuropsychology. The issue of localisation of function via neuropsychological instruments will be addressed. Major neuropsychological findings in relation to schizophrenia and depression will be summarised. The new field of 'cognitive neuropsychiatry' will be outlined. Recent findings on memory for emotional material will be presented. The chapter concludes with a brief overview of psychometric issues, followed by a summary of the most commonly used neuropsychological instruments in clinical research and practice.

SINGLE-CASE STUDIES

The traditional approach within neuropsychology has been the lesion approach, whereby inferences about brain–behaviour relationships are derived from the observations of behavioural abnormality in patients who have suffered selective brain damage. Historically, the field has been driven by key observations on single cases. Single-case studies avoid the *averaging artefact*, i.e. that data derived from group studies represent the average of a group, and may tell us little about particular individuals within the group. Advocates of the group-studies approach argue that the single-case approach violates the core assumption of the scientific method — *replicability* — in that the individual case is considered unique. In this section, some of the most influential of these single-case studies will be briefly reviewed.

Language function — the case of Tan

During the 19th century Gall and Spurzheim established the field of phrenology. Although later discredited, it is important historically in that it attempted to relate certain behaviours to specific brain areas. The relationships could be inferred by examination of the surface of the skull: a bump on the skull indicated a well-developed underlying region; for example 'selfish propensities' were thought to be located in the region above the right ear. In 1861 Broca published a landmark paper where he described the form of production aphasia which was later to bear his name. At postmortem, one of his patients, 'Tan' was shown to have sustained damage to the third convolution of the left frontal lobe. During his life, Tan could barely produce more than a few words; in fact his most common utterance was 'tan', hence his name. Broca concluded that damage to a specific brain region had led to a specific behavioural abnormality. This was a crucial observation, as at the time the notion of *equipotentiality* was popular, namely that it was not the site of brain damage that was important, rather it was the volume of damage that was critical. Wernicke later proposed that a particular type of receptive aphasia was associated with damage in an area in the left posterior temporal lobe. Thus the belief that certain aspects of behaviour were associated with discrete brain regions began to become established.

Executive function — the case of Phineas Gage

Seven years following Broca's publication describing Tan, JM Harlow published a paper in the *Publications of the Massachusetts Medical Society* with the graphic and descriptive title: 'Recovery from the passage of an iron bar through the head'. In it the case of Phineas Gage is described. (Damasio, 1994, provides an excellent, detailed description of the case.) The damage to Gage's brain occurred in 1848 when he was working for a railway company in Vermont. The workmen were using explosives to clear a path through rocks in order to lay the rail track. Gage was using a large iron bar (over 1 metre long and weighing over 13 pounds) as a tamping rod to pound down on a protective layer of sand, placed over a layer of explosive powder containing a fuse, in a hole drilled in the rock. However, tragically on this occasion, Gage 'tamped' the explosive powder before the protective layer of sand had been inserted. The tamping caused a spark to ignite the powder, and the iron rod was blown upwards, through Gage's left cheek and through his brain, exiting at the top of his head before landing more than a hundred feet away. Gage was thrown to the ground, but apparently remained conscious. He spoke within a few minutes and his workmates sat him in a cart and drove him to a local hotel where the doctor was called. The doctor later related that Gage 'talked so rationally and was so willing to answer questions that I directed my enquiries to him in preference to the men who were with him at the time of the accident. . . . Gage then related to me some of the circumstances, as he has since done; and I can safely say that neither at the time nor on any subsequent occasion, save once, did I consider him to be other than perfectly rational' (Dr Williams' account, cited in Damasio 1994). Remarkably, Gage survived this major injury and was pronounced cured in less than 2 months. While the story is unusual, the case is particularly famous owing to Harlow's description of the resulting changes in Gage's behaviour, which has become established as a classical account of the behavioural sequelae of frontal lobe injury.

His physical health is good, and I am inclined to say that he has recovered. He has no pain in head, but says it has a queer feeling which he is not able to describe. Applied for his situation as foreman, but is undecided whether to work or travel. His contractors, who regarded him as the most efficient and capable

foremen in their employ previous to his injury considered the change in his mind so marked that they could not give him his place again. The equilibrium or balance, so to speak, between his intellectual faculties and animal propensities, seems to have been destroyed. He is fitful, irreverent, indulging at times in the grossest profanity (which was not his previous custom), manifesting but little deference for his fellows, impatient of restraint or advice when it conflicts with his desires, at times pertinaciously obstinate, yet capricious and vacillating, devising many plans for future operations, which are no sooner arranged than they are abandoned in turn for others. . . . His mind is radically changed, so that his friends and acquaintances said he was 'no longer Gage'.

Thus Gage became a changed man — he was 'no longer Gage' and was not considered employable in his previous position. He then took a variety of different jobs, including a position as a circus attraction at Barnum's museum in New York, showing his wounds and tamping iron. He died following a series of convulsions in 1861, 13 years after sustaining his brain injury. Gage exhibited marked changes in his social behaviour (as eloquently described by Harlow) in the face of apparently preserved other cognitive abilities, e.g. attention, perception, memory, language and intelligence. During his lifetime the exact location of the brain injury was clearly not known. However, following his death, Gage's skull and the tamping iron were placed in a medical museum in Harvard Medical School. Recently, Damasio et al (1994), in a paper entitled 'The return of Phineas Gage', photographed the skull from a variety of angles, measured the distances between the areas of bone damage and a variety of bone landmarks, and reconstructed the skull, brain and most likely trajectory route of the tamping iron (Fig. 8.1). The bar did not damage brain regions necessary for

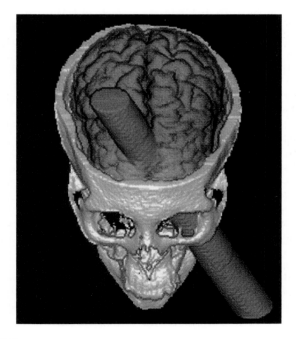

Fig. 8.1
When Gage died in 1861 no autopsy was conducted, but his skull was examined in 1994 and the trajectory of the iron bar was inferred. The reconstruction shows that the damage was largely in the ventromedial frontal brain area. (Reproduced, with permission, from Damasio 1994).

motor function or language, but appeared to have particularly destroyed the ventromedial prefrontal region, and this led to the marked changes in Gage's ability to plan for the future, conform to social conventions and to decide upon the most appropriate courses of action (Damasio 1994).

Memory function — the cases of HM and CW

The search for the 'engram', the brain location of the memory trace, has a long history. Lashley, working on monkeys, spent over thirty years carrying out selective ablations of different brain areas in an attempt to produce amnesia, and in 1951 he concluded that he had failed to find the location of the memory trace. Ironically, 2 years later, the neurosurgeon Scoville conducted a bilateral temporal lobectomy on the patient HM in an attempt to treat his intractable epilepsy. Unfortunately, the operation, though successful in reducing the frequency of seizures, caused a new form of devastating disability: it rendered HM amnesic (Scoville & Milner 1957).

HM has been investigated for the past fifty years, making his probably the most studied case in the history of cognitive neuroscience. He is unable to recall any new experiences, but he remains of above average intelligence level, and his perception, attention and short-term memory are intact. He also shows preserved procedural learning (such as mirror drawing), but with no conscious recollection of previous learning having occurred, thus he shows the classical dissociation between impaired explicit and preserved implicit memory. It is now widely accepted that the critical regions for the laying down of new explicit or declarative memories involve the hippocampus and hippocampal gyrus (Squire 1987). HM's case was particularly influential in establishing the critical role of temporal lobe structures in episodic or declarative memory functioning in man. To give a specific example of HM's deficit, when his father died, HM continued to ask where his father was, only to experience grief on each occasion of hearing of his father's death. This inability to lay down new explicit memories leads to the subjective experience for the amnesic as of a continual awakening from sleep or a dream, in a present without a past. As HM stated, 'Every day is alone, whatever enjoyment I've had, and whatever sorrow I've had.'

More recently the patient CW has been extensively studied since becoming amnesic. He was a world expert on Renaissance music, and tragically in 1985 the herpes simplex virus infected his brain. His life was saved with antiviral drugs, but the virus destroyed large regions of both temporal lobes (Wilson et al 1995). CW was left with devastating memory impairment as a result of this temporal lobe damage. Wilson et al (1995) claimed that CW has the most severe anterograde amnesia ever studied. CW's wife described his cognitive state in a TV documentary 'The Mind Machine' (BBC, 1988) as follows:

> CW's world now consists of a moment with no past to anchor it and no future to look ahead to. It is a blinkered moment. He sees what is right in front of him but as soon as that information hits the brain it fades. Nothing registers. Everything goes in perfectly well . . . he perceives his world as you or I do, but as soon as he's perceived it and looked away it's gone for him. So it's a moment-to-moment consciousness as it were . . . a time vacuum.

This moment-to-moment experience of consciousness is graphically depicted in the diary record which he has obsessively recorded for over 10 years (Fig. 8.2).

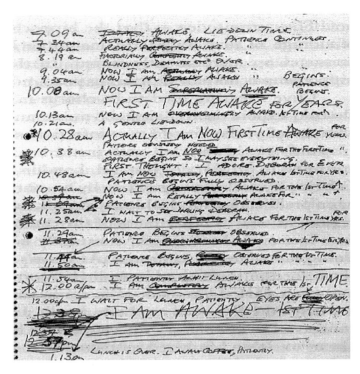

Fig. 8.2
Diary extract from CW reveals the horror of his constant sense of 'awakening' and his inability to lay down new conscious memories. (Reproduced, with permission, from Blakemore 1988.)

Box 8.1   Defining features of the amnestic syndrome

- Intact immediate memory
- Intact intelligence
- Intact semantic memory
- Severe and permanent anterograde amnesia (impaired memory for new information)
- A degree of retrograde amnesia (loss of memory of the period before brain damage)
- Intact procedural memory

Both HM and CW suffer from *amnestic disorder* (Box 8.1). The sufferer will often have clear recollection of episodes in their distant past, but will be unable to recall events that happened half an hour ago. There are a variety of possible causes of amnestic disorder. In some instances, notably in Korsakoff's syndrome, patients attempt to cover up their memory loss via confabulation, i.e. using their preserved language and intellectual abilities to create elaborate stories in an effort to compensate for the memories they have lost. The memory loss in amnestic syndrome is thought to be largely irreversible.

The essential features of amnestic syndrome are devastatingly impaired anterograde memory function, with a variable degree of impaired retrograde memory function (usually surrounding the time of the brain insult) in the presence of preserved other cognitive functions. This has often been demonstrated by the use of an intellectual minus memory quotient discrepancy. For example, a person who has a Wechsler intelligence quotient of 120 with a memory quotient of 70 would have a 50-point discrepancy, which

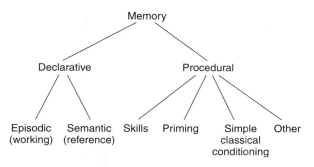

Fig. 8.3
A taxonomy of memory functioning. (After Squire 1987.)

would be consistent with an amnestic profile. Amnestic disorder can result from a variety of causes of cerebral pathology. Korsakoff's syndrome, a consequence of chronic alcoholism and thiamine deficiency, leads to selective atrophy of the mamillary bodies, and this can lead to the development of an amnestic syndrome. Many patients with alcohol-induced persisting dementia are misclassified as suffering from amnestic syndrome; however, they often do not have specific and isolated anterograde memory impairment, but rather have widespread cognitive impairments. A striking feature in amnestic syndrome is preserved implicit memory performance. For example, amnestic patients typically perform normally on implicit tasks such as the pursuit rotor or incomplete figures task, yet will have no explicit memory of having performed these tasks. Such evidence has been important in clarifying the neural substrates that subserve different components of memory function in man (Fig. 8.3) (Squire 1987).

LOCALISING MEASURES?

Case studies such as those outlined above were important in establishing the relationship between certain aspects of behaviour and localised brain damage. Subsequent work led to a crude 'mapping' of the brain in terms of neural substrate for psychological functions, e.g. left hemisphere dominance for speech and language, right hemisphere dominance for visuospatial abilities, right temporal lobe damage leading to visuospatial memory impairments, left temporal lobe damage impairing verbal memory functioning, and frontal lobe damage leading to problems in executive functioning. However, identifying lesion location using neuropsychological measures has largely fallen out of favour for three main reasons. First, most neuropsychological tests are extremely complex and tap a variety of cognitive functions, e.g. perception, attention, working memory, and require some motor response, thus activity in widely distributed brain regions is required for successful task completion. Second, developments in high-resolution structural and functional neuroimaging provide more accurate ways of determining localised brain damage or metabolic abnormality. Third, for many psychiatric disorders there has been no consensus over putative localised disturbance of the central nervous system. To take the example of schizophrenia, various authors have proposed that schizophrenia is characterised by cognitive test abnormalities indicative of either dysfunction of the frontal lobe, temporal lobe, left or right hemisphere, basal ganglia, etc. (Blanchard & Neale 1994). The extreme case is put by Meehl who stated 'I conjecture that whatever is wrong with the schizotaxic CNS is ubiquitous,

a functional aberration present throughout, operating everywhere from the sacral cord to the frontal lobes' (Meehl 1990, p. 14). Many current workers would surely agree with Shallice et al (1991) who proposed that from a neuropsychological perspective, the attempt to *understand* the nature of the information processing impairment in psychiatric disorder should precede the attempt to localise it.

'Frontal lobology'

Perhaps the most extreme example of attributing psychiatric disturbance to a localised brain region is the case of the putative involvement of the frontal lobes. David (1992) provocatively entitled this exercise 'frontal lobology' and described it as 'psychiatry's new pseudoscience'. He lists the psychiatric conditions which have been ascribed to frontal lobe dysfunction; the list includes personality disorders, obsessions, delusions, depression, mania, conduct disorder, schizophrenia, catatonia, thought disorder, anorexia nervosa and hysteria, 'All of psychiatry, not to mention human life is there' (David 1992, p. 244). As David points out, the frontal lobes are thought to be the seat of thought, intellect, creativity, etc., and as psychiatric disorders are, by definition, problems at the highest level of thought, it is an unhelpful tautology to state that such disorders are manifestations of frontal lobe pathology. Additionally, even if a particular disorder was shown to be associated with frontal lobe abnormality, how does this further our understanding, given that the frontal lobes constitute approximately one-third of the brain? 'Localising a disturbance to this region is rather like directing a visitor to an address marked Europe' (David 1992, p. 244).

NEUROPSYCHOLOGY IN MAJOR PSYCHIATRIC DISORDER

In the following sections some of the major contributions of neuropsychology to the understanding of schizophrenia and depression will be summarised

Schizophrenia

Schizophrenia has been described as perhaps the most devastating illness known to man, because it appears in early adolescence and can drastically impair the subsequent life of the sufferer and his or her family. In the 1960s, there was a widespread view that schizophrenia was a socially created disorder, and family dynamics, and in particular the 'schizophrenogenic mother', was often blamed. The finding of ventricular enlargement (Johnstone et al 1976) shifted the balance back to viewing schizophrenia as a brain/neuropsychological disorder. Prior to this time, it was widely believed that neuropsychological impairment was not an important feature of schizophrenia. (However, it must be emphasised that when differences have been found in brain morphology between patients with schizophrenia and matched controls, the degree of between-group overlap has usually been large.) Neuropsychological abnormalities are now widely reported in many patients diagnosed with schizophrenia. The most consistent findings are of impairments in learning, memory and executive functioning (Heinrichs & Zakzanis 1998). Importantly, these abnormalities are often observed in patients who are drug-free (Saykin et al 1994).

Palmer et al (1997) recently posed the question 'Is it possible to be schizophrenic yet neuropsychologically normal?'. They gave a comprehensive neuropsychological battery to 171 outpatients with schizophrenia and compared them with 63 healthy controls. Two experienced neuropsychologists conducted blind ratings of the test results. Only 27% of the patients were classified as neuropsychologically 'normal'. This indicates that significant cognitive impairment in schizophrenia is, in fact, the norm.

Pre-existing cognitive impairment?

Several studies have also confirmed that low intelligence and poor educational achievement precede early-onset schizophrenic psychosis. Jones et al (1994) used the subjects from the National Survey of Health and Development, a random sample of over 5000 births in England, Scotland & Wales during the first week of March 1946. Out of this sample, 30 cases of schizophrenia arose between ages 16 and 43. Children who developed schizophrenia in later life were significantly impaired on non-verbal and verbal intelligence tests from the age of 8 and on arithmetic/mathematic skills from the age of 11. This result clearly indicates the presence of detectable cognitive abnormalities in childhood, which pre-dated the development of the illness. David et al (1997) capitalised on a remarkable sample of 50 000 males conscripted to the Swedish Army between 1969 and 1970. Tests of cognitive functioning were recorded at conscription. In later life, 195 subjects were admitted to hospital with schizophrenia. Low IQ emerged as a clear risk factor for those later diagnosed with schizophrenia, and poor performance on verbal tasks and a mechanical knowledge test conferred a significantly increased risk of schizophrenia, even after taking into account general intellectual ability. In a more recent Swedish study, data were analysed from nearly 200 000 male conscripts, and over a 5-year period, 60 men developed schizophrenia. Poor intellectual performance at 18 was associated with elevated risk for schizophrenia, and importantly this increased risk was not attributable to prenatal adversity or childhood circumstances (Gunnell et al 2002).

Taken together, the results of these and other studies provide strong supportive evidence for the view that neuropsychological abnormalities pre-date the development of schizophrenia. It is tempting to interpret these findings as evidence of a neurodevelopmental abnormality in those individuals who develop schizophrenia in late adolescence / early adulthood. This association could be directly causal — i.e. with cognitive impairment leading to false beliefs and perceptions — or alternatively, could act via an indirect mechanism, with any factors which cause low IQ (such as abnormal brain development) increasing later risk for schizophrenia (David et al 1997). Individuals who are at high genetic risk of developing schizophrenia exhibit memory and executive impairments (Byrne et al 1999) together with reductions in hippocampal/amygdala complex volume (Lawrie et al 1999). Taken together, these findings add support to the view of schizophrenia as a neurodevelopmental disorder. However, it must be borne in mind that some individuals who develop schizophrenia, do so after a successful adolescence / early adulthood (e.g. attaining scholastic and academic excellence), therefore pre-existing cognitive impairment cannot explain all presentations of schizophrenia, and again this suggests that a variety of aetiologies may lie under the broad umbrella term of schizophrenia.

The myth of intellectual decline in schizophrenia?

While there is increasing evidence of the presence of cognitive impairments which precede illness onset, the evidence is not so clear regarding further cognitive deterioration following development of the illness. The published literature examining the subsequent course of impairment is inconsistent. Cross-sectional studies have provided evidence both for and against progressive deterioration but are, of course, vulnerable to cohort effects which produce differences which are not due to within-subject changes. Longitudinal studies are the best method for assessing the course of cognitive impairment over time. Early longitudinal studies showed no progressive deterioration, but were limited by a number of significant methodological weaknesses including the lack of an operationalised diagnosis of schizophrenia at a time when the diagnosis of schizophrenia was notoriously broad in the USA. More recently, well-designed longitudinal studies have again produced conflicting results, with some supporting the notion of progressive decline and others not. Russell et al (1997) in a paper entitled 'The myth of intellectual decline in schizophrenia' examined the childhood IQ of adult patients with schizophrenia (participants had IQ assessments on two occasions, with a 19-year interval between assessments). The authors reported that measured IQs were one standard deviation below the general population mean on both occasions, but there was no significant difference between child and adult IQs. The authors concluded that intellectual deficit observed in adult patients is lifelong and predates the onset of schizophrenia. However, in a recent 33-year follow-up of patients who had initially been assessed for intellectual function soon after illness onset, it emerged that patients with schizophrenia showed a highly significant intellectual deterioration over time compared with non-schizophrenic patient controls (Fig. 8.4) (Morrison et al 2004). This result suggests that while intellectual impairment may precede illness onset, in many patients with schizophrenia a further intellectual decline often occurs after the illness develops.

Are neuropsychological impairments in schizophrenia important?

Is impaired cognitive test performance in patients with schizophrenia an epiphenomenon, e.g. simply reflecting lack of motiva-

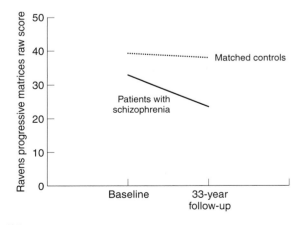

Fig. 8.4
Evidence of intellectual decline occurring in patients with schizophrenia after the onset of the disorder. (Adapted from Morrison et al 2004.)

tion or distraction by hallucinations? In order to convince sceptics that the neuropsychological impairment is important, one would have to demonstrate a clear relationship between cognitive test performance and 'real-life' functional outcome. Green (1996) reviewed studies that used cognitive measures as predictors of functional outcome. The most consistent finding to emerge was that verbal memory functioning was associated with all types of functional outcome. (Verbal memory was the cognitive domain which showed the greatest impairment in the recent meta-analysis by Heinrichs & Zakzanis 1998). Sustained attention/vigilance was also found to be related to social problem-solving and skill acquisition. Psychotic symptoms were *not* significantly associated with outcome measures in any of the studies that were reviewed. Green (1996) concluded that deficiencies in verbal memory and vigilance may prevent patients from attaining optimal adaptation and hence may act as rate-limiting factors in terms of rehabilitation. Thus the field has moved from a position where cognitive impairment was not considered to be particularly important in schizophrenia, to the current view, that it may be a central and rate-limiting feature in terms of rehabilitation. Recently, Addington & Addington (1999) used a novel videotaped measure of interpersonal problem-solving skills in outpatients with schizophrenia. They found that better cognitive flexibility and verbal memory were positively associated with interpersonal problem-solving ability. The evidence thus strongly supports the view that cognitive impairment in schizophrenia is important and is directly related to social deficits and functional outcome for many patients.

Can neuropsychology explain schizophrenia?

The ultimate challenge for neuropsychology is to provide convincing explanatory models for psychiatric disorders. False perceptions, beliefs and behaviours are psychological phenomena and must be explained in psychological terms. To date attempts to explain schizophrenia per se in neuropsychological terms have had limited success, possibly because of the heterogeneity of the disorder. Liddle & Morris (1991) assessed a group of chronic schizophrenic patients, using a battery of neuropsychological tests allegedly sensitive to frontal lobe dysfunction. Using factor analysis, signs and symptoms were clustered into three syndromes: psychomotor poverty, disorganisation and reality distortion. Scores for the disorganisation syndrome were associated with impairment on tests that required the subject to inhibit a well-established but inappropriate response. Ratings for the psychomotor poverty syndrome were found to be associated with slowness of mental activity. More recently, Baxter & Liddle (1998) confirmed that the psychomotor poverty syndrome was associated with psychomotor slowing and that disorganisation was associated with impaired performance on the Stroop attentional conflict task but not with other tests of cognitive inhibition. This led the authors to propose that the disorganisation syndrome might be associated with a specific difficulty in suppressing irrelevant verbal responses. This approach is appealing, because it attempts to use specific abnormalities of information processing to explain core features of schizophrenia. Pursuing this approach to a more detailed level would result in an attempt to explain specific signs or symptoms in terms of aberrant information processing; for example, McKenna (1991) proposed that delusions may arise as a consequence of a dysfunctional semantic memory system. Again, this hypothesis has intuitive appeal, as delusions by definition must represent false knowledge; however, one must be wary of tautological or untestable explanations.

Frith (1992) has been particularly influential in this area, by developing a model where internal stimuli (e.g. thoughts or intentions) are thought to be misclassified and misattributed to an external source. For example, he has proposed that auditory hallucinations in schizophrenia arise from a failure in the self-monitoring of speech processing. In this model, hallucinations are experienced as a result of a failure of the internal registration of the intention to generate inner speech, i.e. the hallucinating person's inner speech is perceived as alien, attributable to an external source. Blakemore et al (2000) investigated the ability of groups of psychiatric patients to differentiate perceptually between self-produced and externally produced tactile stimuli. They found that auditory hallucinations and passivity experiences were associated with an abnormality in the self-monitoring mechanism that normally allows individuals to distinguish self-produced from externally produced sensations, consistent with Frith's model.

Frith has extended his model to account for a variety of features of schizophrenia including thought broadcasting, insertion and withdrawal. An important element of his theory is that some key features of schizophrenia are due to an inability to monitor the beliefs and intentions of others. This is similar to the 'theory of mind' deficit in autism i.e. the inability to see the world from the perspective of another. Examples of Frith's description of features of schizophrenia as defects of self-awareness are given in Table 8.1. Frith proposes that there is one key difference in the theory of mind model in autism and schizophrenia:

> *The autistic person has never known that other people have minds. The schizophrenic knows that other people have minds, but has lost the ability to infer the contents of these minds: their beliefs and intentions. They may even lose the ability to reflect on the contents of their own mind. However, they will still have available ritual and behavioural routines for interacting with people, which do not require inferences about mental states.*
> (Frith 1992, p. 121)

Depression

Memory impairment

The only neuropsychological functions to feature in the DSM-IV diagnostic criteria for major depression are concentration and decision-making difficulties. However, many studies have reported a variety of neuropsychological impairments in depression, particularly deficits in memory, executive functioning and psychomotor functioning (Veiel 1997). Memory impairment in depression can be so severe that patients can be misclassified as having dementia — 'depressive pseudodementia'. Such a misdiagnosis can have catastrophic consequences in that a treatable, potentially fatal condition is missed. Lezak (1995) has described the separation of depression from dementia as perhaps the 'knottiest problem of differential diagnosis'.

Knopman & Ryberg (1989) suggested that elaborate encoding may provide a substantial benefit to non-demented subjects but not to patients with Alzheimer's disease and developed the Delayed Word Recall Test or DWR. This test involves presentation of 10 words individually; subjects are required to read each word and construct a sentence using each word; the process is then repeated and, after a 5-minute filled delay, memory (free recall) of the 10 words is tested. Both Knopman & Ryberg (1989) and Coen et al (1996) reported almost perfect separation of patients

Table 8.1   The signs and symptoms of schizophrenia described as defects of self-awareness

Level of awareness	Level of defect		
	Impaired content	Detached content	No content
Own goals *I must 'go to work'*	*I must 'become the boss'* Grandiose ability Grandiose identity Delusion of depersonalisation	*'Go to work'* Delusions of control Thought echo Voices commenting	*(No goals)* Lack of will Stereotyped behaviour Catatonia
Own intentions *I intend to 'catch the bus'*	*I intend to 'catch the plane'* Grandiose ideas Depersonalisation	*'Catch the bus'* Delusions of control Thought insertion Thought broadcast Voices commenting	*(No intentions)* Thought withdrawal Poverty of action Poverty of thought Loss of affect
Others' intentions *My boss wants of me 'you must be on time'*	*My boss wants of me 'you must die'* Delusions of reference Delusions of persecution Derealisation	*'You must be on time'* Voices talking to the patient Voices talking about the patient	*(No mentalizing)* Social withdrawal Autism

From Frith (1992), p. 127.

with early dementia from matched controls, using a < 3/10 cut-off. However, both studies used healthy participants as controls. When the comparison was repeated using dementia patients versus age-matched, clinically depressed patients, using the recommended < 3/10 cut-off, 44% of depressed patients would have been misclassified as having dementia (O'Carroll et al 1997). This finding highlights the degree of memory impairment that can exist in depression, and that extreme caution should be employed when considering categorical cut-off scores derived from studies that have compared patients with dementia with healthy controls.

Recently, Swainson et al (2001) have reported impressive findings using a computerised visuospatial paired associative learning test (PAL) which accurately distinguished Alzheimer patients from depressed and healthy control subjects. The measure also revealed a sub-group of questionable dementia patients who performed similarly to the Alzheimer patients. The performance of the 'questionable patients' correlated with the degree of global cognitive decline (as measured by the MMSE) over the next 8 months. At 32-month follow-up an equation based on initial PAL and graded naming test performance was used to predict those who would proceed to develop dementia, and the algorithm was 100% accurate. This is an impressive finding; however, the algorithm clearly has to be tested prospectively on new samples of patients.

Cognitive bias

Studies using affectively toned stimuli reveal that depressed patients have consistently shown a memory bias towards negative material. Lloyd & Lishman (1975) reported that when depressed patients were required to recall pleasant or unpleasant experiences from their past in response to cue words, the more severe the depression the quicker the patient recalled unpleasant relative to pleasant memories. Ridout et al (2003) have recently shown that this bias extends to memories for socially meaningful stimuli (emotional facial expressions): clinically depressed patients showed superior memories for sad faces, whereas non-depressed healthy

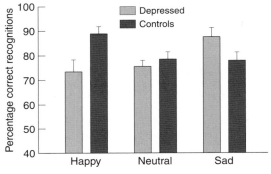

Fig. 8.5
Dissociation in memory bias for positive or negative facial expressions in depressed patients versus matched controls. Depressed patients show superior memory for sad faces whereas healthy controls show the opposite tendency. (From Ridout et al 2003.)

controls showed the opposite pattern, superior memory for happy expressions (Fig. 8.5).

Teasdale (1983) proposed that this mood-congruent memory bias may be an important mechanism in the maintenance of depression. If an individual is in a depressed state, a mood-congruent memory bias means that negative memories are more accessible, and recall of these memories may help maintain or exacerbate the depressed mood. This may then lead to recall of more negative memories, thus creating a self-perpetuating vicious circle. Williams et al (1996) have also described the phenomenon of overgeneral retrieval style in depression, where patients have marked difficulty in retrieving *specific* events from their past. This is seen where depressed patients have a significantly longer latency to produce a specific autobiographical memory in response to a positive cue word, e.g. 'happy' (Fig. 8.6).

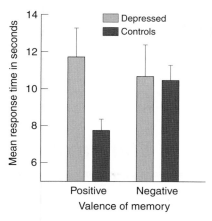

Fig. 8.6
Significant latency for positive specific autobiographical memories demonstrated by patients with clinical depression. (From Ridout et al 2003.)

It is commonly observed that patients tend to produce categorical memories, e.g. 'at weekends', rather than specific events, 'last Friday night at the party', despite repeated prompting. Williams et al (1996) propose that this difficulty in progressing beyond categorical to specific autobiographical memories — 'mnemonic interlock' — may serve the function of controlling affective state, in avoiding painful specific autobiographical memories, e.g. of a romantic dinner with a lover who has now left.

Effortful versus automatic processing in depression

Several authors have proposed that depressed patients experience particular difficulty on memory tasks that require elaborate or effortful organisation and processing of material to be remembered, but that they do not show problems in memory tasks on which 'automatic' memory processes are presumed to be involved. In line with this proposal, Weingartner (1986) reported that depressed patients demonstrate impairments on delayed free recall (effortful) with no impairment on recognition memory (relatively automatic), whereas demented patients perform poorly in both conditions. However, Lachner et al (1994) provided evidence which challenges the Weingartner model. They compared three groups (demented, depressed and healthy subjects) who were in their 70s on five verbal recall and two recognition memory tasks. They found that both delayed recall *and* recognition after long delay were the measures which best discriminated between the demented and the depressed patient groups. It is interesting to note that the recognition measure was more discriminating than free recall, selective reminding or serial learning, all presumably more 'effortful' than a recognition memory task. Lachner et al (1994) make the pertinent point that the labelling of some cognitive tasks as effortful versus automatic is often ambiguous: 'In future research, the tasks cognitive capacity requirements should be examined empirically to avoid inconsistencies by subjectively estimating capacity demands' (Lachner et al 1994, p. 10).

Is poor neuropsychological test performance in depressed patients an artefact of poor motivation?

Many writers have attributed observed neuropsychological impairment in depression to the non-specific effects of motivational deficits. Few studies have tested this hypothesis experimentally. Richards & Ruff (1989) randomly assigned two groups of subjects, depressed and non-depressed, to either motivation or non-motivation conditions; (motivation involved encouragement — a monetary incentive and performance feedback. The authors reported that performance (as measured by improvement on a simple card-sorting task) was significantly enhanced for the subjects in the motivation condition. Crucially, motivation did not significantly affect neuropsychological test performance, and the authors concluded that although depressed patients may be less motivated, this reduced motivation does not fully account for the observed neuropsychological impairments in depression.

What is the neurobiological substrate of memory impairment in depression?

Several studies have reported significant atrophy in medial temporal lobe structures in patients with chronic depression. It has been proposed that chronically raised cortisol levels in depression can facilitate hippocampal neuronal death, which in turn may cause dysregulation of the hypothalamo–pituitary–adrenal (HPA) axis. As well as showing temporal lobe atrophy in treatment-resistant patients (Fig. 8.7), Shah et al (1998) showed a significant positive correlation between left hippocampal density and performance in delayed verbal recognition in treatment-resistant, chronically depressed patients. Patients who had recovered from their depression had normal MRI scans.

Bipolar disorder

The neuropsychological study of bipolar disorder is in its infancy. Recent evidence suggests that while cognitive functioning is clearly impaired during illness episodes, some residual impairments can be observed in the euthymic state (Cavanagh et al 2002, Ferrier et al 1999). In addition, a more severe course of illness and a greater number of illness episodes are often associated with more impaired neuropsychological functioning, suggesting that repeated manic episodes may be neurotoxic. The pathophysiological mechanisms are not fully understood, though hypercortisolaemia may be implicated and may result in impaired neuropsychological functioning (McAllister-Williams et al 1998). Relatively few neuropsychological studies have been conducted on manic patients. Preliminary work suggests that both manic and depressed patients are impaired on tests of memory and planning, but differences have been noted in attentional shifting, with manic patients having difficulty with inhibition of behavioural response and attentional focus, and depressed patients impaired in their ability to shift the focus of their attentional bias (Murphy & Sahakian 2001). The same authors confirmed the affective bias for negative material in depression, but also demonstrated the opposite affective bias for positive stimuli in mania.

MEMORY FOR EMOTIONAL MATERIAL

Emotion lies at the heartland of psychiatry, and abnormalities of emotional processing are evident in a variety of disorders, perhaps most notably in post-traumatic stress disorder (PTSD). PTSD is a condition where exposure to an intense frightening emotional experience leads to lasting changes in behaviour, affect and cognition. Typically after a life-threatening incident (e.g. a violent assault, rape or wartime experience), the individual displays

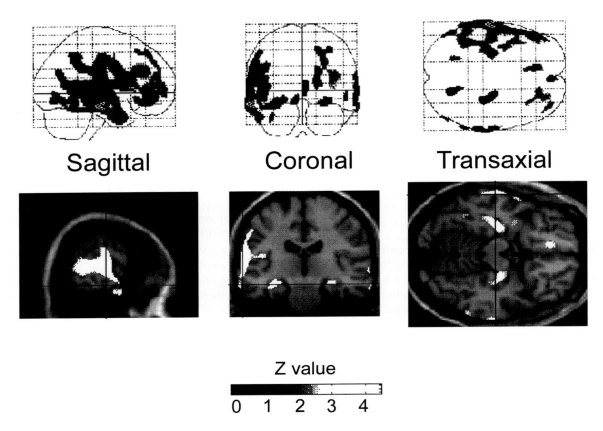

Fig. 8.7
Bilaterally reduced grey-matter density in medial temporal cortex in treatment-resistant, chronically depressed patients compared with 20 normal controls. The image is the result of subtracting values between depressed and healthy participants. The Z value represents the magnitude of the difference; lighter colour indicates greater difference. (Reproduced, with the permission of Elsevier Limited, from Doris A et al, *Lancet* 1999; 354: 1369–1375.)

re-experiencing of the event(s), e.g. via intrusive, distressing thoughts, images, 'flashbacks' or nightmares. The individual may exhibit phobic avoidance and/or physiological reactivity to reminders of the trauma. Increased arousal in terms of sleep disturbance, irritability and exaggerated startle response are common. In addition, the individual may exhibit a restricted range of affect, sense of a foreshortened future, and may lose interest in previously rewarding hobbies or activities. PTSD is characterised by intrusive distressing memories of the traumatic event. Paradoxically, it is also often associated with marked impairments in learning and memory for new material. Patients often complain that they remember what they do not want to, yet cannot remember what they now wish to. Heightened arousal at the time of encoding may result in modulation (strengthening) of the memory trace, possibly via noradrenaline (norepinephrine) release in the amygdala (Cahill & McGaugh 1998). Subsequent anterograde memory impairment may be due to the deleterious effects of stress hormones (e.g. long-term hypercortisolaemia) on the hippocampal function. Several MRI studies have now shown that PTSD is associated with reduction in volume of the hippocampus, a brain area critically involved in new learning and memory (e.g. Bremner 1999).

Dual representation theory of PTSD

Brewin (2001) has recently developed a dual representation theory of PTSD. Importantly, *PTSD is viewed as a failure of adap-*

tation, the inability to adapt following exposure to a traumatic event. Brewin proposes that two memory systems are critical for our understanding of PTSD: verbally accessible, declarative memory (VAM) and a situationally accessible, non-declarative memory (SAM). VAM memories are hippocampally dependent, whereas SAM memories are non-hippocampally dependent, and involve the amygdala. In PTSD, it is proposed that a considerable amount of trauma information resides solely in the SAM system, and these SAM memories are particularly vulnerable to reactivation by trauma cues, e.g. flashbacks in response to sight or smells of trauma reminders (Brewin 2001).

VAM memories can be retrieved either automatically or using deliberate, strategic processes, so that they can be edited and interact with the rest of the person's autobiographical memory. VAM memories are readily available for verbal communication with others and involve cognitive appraisals. SAM memories, in contrast, contain information from more extensive but lower level perceptual processing of the traumatic scene and the person's bodily responses. These SAM memories are difficult to communicate to others and are difficult to control, because people cannot always regulate their exposure to sights, sounds and smells that can act as reminders of the trauma. Brewin proposes that stress (possibly via effects of stress hormones such as cortisol) leads to an impairment of the hippocampus-dependent declarative (VAM) memory system. The resultant VAM memories are thus fragmented and incomplete. In contrast emotional and sensory information are encoded particularly well in the SAM system during times of stress, possibly via noradrenergic/amygdala effects acting to strengthen encoding (Cahill & McGaugh 1998). This results in detailed sensory memories which are not encoded for context, e.g. time, and when retrieved, they are re-experienced in the present.

It is proposed that during normal recovery from trauma, early flashbacks etc. lead to copying of extra information from non-declarative (SAM) to declarative systems (VAM). As this is a limited-capacity system, little information is transferred at any one time, but over time as the person attends to the images etc., information is recoded into a contextualised declarative memory, where the experience is clearly labelled as having occurred in the past. This leads to inhibition of the amygdala from responding inappropriately, as it is now recognised that threat is no longer present. Brewin (2001) proposes that in PTSD the declarative system (VAM) fails to make a good memory trace of the event and sensory information remains relatively isolated in the non-declarative memory system (SAM). These memories are re-experienced as in the present, and, with a failure of adaptation, progressive sensitisation over time occurs. The emotions that accompany SAM memories consist mainly of fear, helplessness, horror and shame. This leads to an overturning of basic assumptions, e.g. views of the world as benevolent and the self as worthy change to the world's being seen as a dangerous place with the self viewed as powerless, inferior and worthless. Brewin (2001) thus presents a theoretical model of PTSD (Fig. 8.8) that combines findings from cognitive psychology and neuroscience. It can inform therapeutic interventions, as it suggests that therapeutic procedures should aim to 'fill in the gaps' in VAM memory, e.g. via prolonged exposure, focusing on times of peak emotion during the trauma, and attempting to build up a detailed narrative. Over time, this process provides the declarative memory system with a retrieval advantage.

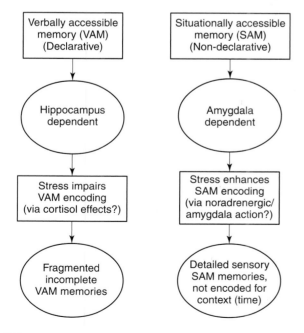

Fig. 8.8
Brewin's dual-representational model of post-traumatic stress disorder.

COGNITIVE NEUROPSYCHIATRY

Cognitive neuropsychiatry is a relatively new discipline which aims to further understanding of psychopathological states via careful analysis of information processing (Halligan & David 2001). One major thrust in this area is to focus on particular signs and symptoms (e.g. specific delusions) rather than attempt to explain broad illness categories. The following examples of delusional misidentification syndromes illustrate this approach.

The Capgras syndrome involves the belief that impostors have replaced people to whom the sufferer is emotionally close (e.g. a loved one or a relative). It is believed that the impostors have assumed the roles of the persons they impersonate and behave like them. Some patients who suffer from Capgras syndrome may threaten, harm or even kill the supposed impostor. Up to 40% of cases are associated with organic disorders, e.g. head injury and dementia. Right cerebral hemisphere dysfunction has also frequently been reported in patients suffering from Capgras syndrome. Ellis & Young (1990) presented a cognitive account of Capgras syndrome. They proposed two distinct routes to facial recognition: one for the actual identification of the face, and the other to give the face its emotional significance. They proposed that prosopagnosia results from a disruption of the first route, whereas Capgras syndrome is 'a mirror image' of prosopagnosia. Thus, they propose that Capgras patients have an intact primary route to face recognition but have a disconnection or damage within the route that gives the face its emotional significance. Ellis et al (1997) demonstrated that people with the Capgras delusion fail to show autonomic discrimination between familiar and unfamiliar faces. Their model proposes that to the person with Capgras syndrome, the impostor's face looks *identical but the emotional feelings associated with their face are abnormal*. Put another way, the patient receives a veridical image of the person they are looking at, which stimulates the appropriate semantic data about the person, but the patient lacks another set of confirmatory information which may carry the appropriate affective tone for a loved one. The patient then adopts a rationalisation strategy, i.e. the person looks the same but somehow does not *feel* the same, and therefore the person must be an impostor. The Capgras patient mistakes a change in themselves for a change in others. Recent work in this area is reviewed by Ellis & Lewis (2001).

PSYCHOMETRIC ISSUES — RELIABILITY AND VALIDITY

When evaluating a particular neuropsychological measure, one must pay particular attention to the test's reliability and validity. The *reliability* of a test refers to the accuracy, consistency and stability of test scores across situations. It is important to remember that a test score is always an *approximation* of an individual's hypothetical true score — i.e. the score an individual would receive if the test were perfectly reliable. The difference between this hypothetical true score and the obtained test score is termed the *measurement error*. A reliable test will have a small measurement error and consistent results should be obtained both within and between measurement sessions (e.g. *test–retest reliability*). While great care is taken in ensuring reliable measurement in many areas of biological psychiatry (e.g. neuroimaging, endocrine measurement), a surprisingly lax attitude is often taken towards the quantification of behaviour in neuropsychological assessment. Some researchers will cavalierly embark on a project with no or superficial training in neuropsychological test administration, often paying scant attention to the detailed administration instructions that are provided, with the result that substantial measurement error is introduced.

The *validity* of a test is the extent to which a test measures what it is supposed to measure, e.g. a prospective memory test should measure prospective memory! There are several forms of validity. *Construct validity* refers to the extent to which performance on a test fits into a theoretical schema about the attribute the test attempts to measure. *Predictive validity* refers to whether performance on the test accurately predicts some external criterion (e.g. final degree outcome). *Incremental validity* is the term used to describe what the test adds to the predictive validity already provided by other measures. *Criterion-related validity* is based on the test's correlation with a similar measure; if the related measure is administered at the same time, the degree of association is termed *concurrent validity*.

NEUROPSYCHOLOGICAL MEASURES

In this section, some commonly used neuropsychological measures in the broad domains of cognitive screening, current and premorbid intelligence, memory, language, visuospatial functioning, attention and executive functioning will briefly be presented. Finally, computerised neuropsychological assessment systems will be reviewed.

Cognitive screening measures

Mini Mental State Examination (MMSE)

The MMSE (Folstein et al 1975) is probably the most frequently used screening scale and is often used as part of a larger battery for a comprehensive assessment of dementia. It is a very brief and easily administered instrument and takes about 5–10 minutes in total. It tests orientation, information and visuoconstructive abilities; total scores can range between 0 and 30. In their original study, Folstein et al reported a high test–retest reliability of 0.83 when retesting was conducted by a different examiner, and 0.89 when the same examiner was used. High test–retest reliability has been confirmed by later studies. Caution is required when interpreting scores obtained from poorly educated individuals. Level of education has consistently been shown to be related to MMSE score.

CAMCOG

The CAMCOG (Roth et al 1986) contains the MMSE with the addition of some additional coverage of perception, memory and abstract thinking. The psychometric properties of the CAMCOG are satisfactory; the test–retest reliability of the scale as a whole is high (0.86), as is its internal consistency (coefficients range from 0.82 to 0.89). CAMCOG scores are, unsurprisingly, affected by age, sociocultural factors and hearing and visual deficits.

Measures of current intellectual ability

The Wechsler Adult Intelligence Scale, third edition (WAIS-III)

The WAIS tradition started with the publication of the Wechsler–Bellevue Intelligence Scale in 1939. This was revised and renamed the Wechsler Adult Intelligence Scale (WAIS) in 1955, which in turn was revised as the WAIS-R in 1981. Like its predecessors the recently published WAIS-III is likely to represent the 'gold standard' against which other measures of intellectual ability are gauged. The WAIS-III was developed and co-normed with the Wechsler Memory Scale, third edition (WMS-III) (see below). Wechsler originally described intelligence as the 'capacity of the individual to act purposefully, to think rationally, and to deal effectively with his environment'. The WAIS-III has normative data from 2450 individuals aged 16–89. The traditional Wechsler approach has been to administer a number of subtests, each tapping different aspects of intelligence, and then to reduce these to composite Verbal, Performance and Full-Scale IQ scores (VIQ, PIQ and FSIQ, respectively), each with an age-adjusted mean of 100 with a standard deviation of 15. This approach has been retained in the WAIS-III, Verbal IQ is calculated based on the sum of the following subtests: Vocabulary, Similarities, Arithmetic, Digit Span, Information and Comprehension. Performance IQ is calculated from the sum of the following subtests: Picture Completion, Digit Symbol coding, Block Design, Matrix Reasoning and Picture Arrangement. However, factor analytic studies have suggested that the subtests do not fall neatly into verbal and performance IQ; rather, four factors emerge: Verbal Comprehension, Perceptual Organisation, Working Memory and Processing Speed. With the addition of three further subtests (Symbol Search, Letter–Number Sequencing and Object Assembly) it is also possible to calculate scores on these four indices. The WAIS-III is a significant improvement on its predecessors, with better norms, improved artwork for visually presented items and impressive reliability coefficients for IQ scales and indexes (0.88–0.97).

Wechsler Abbreviated Scale of Intelligence (WASI)

The WASI is an abbreviated version of the full WAIS-III and thus is useful in cases where a brief measure of intellectual function is required. The WASI consists of four subtests: Vocabulary, Similarities, Block Design and Matrix Reasoning. The four-subtest form can be administered in 30 minutes and results in FSIQ, VIQ and PIQ scores. The PIQ score is obtained from the Matrix Reasoning and Block Design subtests. The Vocabulary and Similarities subtests compose the Verbal Scale and yield the VIQ. An estimate of general intellectual ability can be obtained from the two-subtest form, which can be given in about 15 minutes. This short form includes Vocabulary and Matrix Reasoning and provides only the FSIQ score. A particular strength of the WASI is that two parallel forms can be used, so that practice effects on repeated testing are avoided.

Raven's progressive matrices

The progressive matrices consist of a series of visuospatial problem-solving tasks, thought to tap general intelligence ('g') that is relatively independent of education or cultural influence. The standard progressive matrices have been most widely used in clinical practice and research and consist of 60 items. (Children's and advanced sets are also available.) The test is untimed but usually takes around 40 minutes to complete. Test–retest reliability is above 0.8 and internal reliability is above 0.7. An extremely useful feature of the matrices is the publication of a normative rate of decay profile (the normal pattern of failing more items as the test becomes progressively more difficult). This allows the detection of individuals who are faking poor performance, e.g. in compensation claims (Gudjonssen & Shackleton 1986). (A progressive matrices type subtest has now been included in the WAIS-III, entitled 'matrix reasoning', and of the performance subtests, has the highest correlation with overall full-scale IQ, $r = 0.69$).

Measures of premorbid intellectual ability

When one assesses an individual's cognitive ability, there is usually no record of that individual having been previously assessed; therefore one must infer whether cognitive deterioration has occurred. For example, if an individual's current full-scale intelligence quotient is measured at 85 (one standard deviation below the mean), is that a significant deterioration from a premorbid level, or has that individual always functioned at this level? Traditionally clinicians have used background information to help inform their opinion (e.g. based on occupation, years of full time education, etc.). However, over the last 20 years, measures have been developed which aim to formalise and improve the accuracy of this estimation of premorbid ability. These measures are largely based on the observation that reading ability is largely preserved in the face of organic impairment and is highly correlated with intellectual ability in the general population.

The National Adult Reading Test (NART)

To date the NART has been the test most widely used to estimate premorbid ability. The NART is a single-word, oral reading test consisting of 50 items. All the words are irregular, that is they violate grapheme–phoneme correspondence rules (e.g. *chord*). Because the words are irregular, intelligent guesswork should not provide the correct pronunciation, therefore the test taps *previous* word knowledge; as the test only requires the reading of single words, patients do not have to provide the word's meaning, and it is argued that the test therefore makes minimal demands on *current* cognitive ability (Nelson & Willison 1991). The development of the NART arose from the clinical observation that oral reading is commonly preserved in dementia (whereas reading for meaning is commonly impaired). However, the test is now used to estimate premorbid ability in a wide range of conditions.

To qualify for use as a measure of premorbid ability a test must fulfil three criteria. First, as with any psychological test, it must possess adequate reliability. The NART has high split-half reliability/internal consistency, test–retest reliability and inter-rater reliability (Crawford 1992). Second, it must have high criterion validity. The NART is normally used to provide an estimate of general premorbid IQ against which current performance is compared. Thus to meet the second requirement the NART must be capable of predicting a substantial proportion of IQ variance. In most studies using the WAIS or WAIS-R as the criterion variable the NART predicted well over 50% of IQ variance. The final criterion for a putative measure of premorbid ability is that test performance be relatively resistant to the effects of neurological or psychiatric disorder. NART performance appears to be largely

resistant to the effects of many neurological and psychiatric disorders, e.g. depression, acute schizophrenia, alcoholic dementia, closed head injury and Parkinson's disease (Crawford 1992, O'Carroll 1995). Mixed findings have been found in samples with probable dementia of the Alzheimer type. It is becoming increasingly clear that NART performance can be substantially impaired in many cases of moderate to severe dementia. There is a danger associated with the indiscriminate use of measures such as the NART in a variety of conditions where it is not clear that oral pronunciation is preserved. For example, both Crawford et al (1988) and O'Carroll et al (1992) found evidence of marked impairment in NART performance in patients with Korsakoff's syndrome, suggesting that it is inappropriate to estimate premorbid ability in Korsakoff's syndrome using the NART. Despite this, a number of studies have since been published using the NART in this patient group to estimate premorbid ability. The NART can be seen as a quick and easy way of estimating intellectual ability for subject matching in research studies. If the condition under investigation impairs reading/pronunciation ability, such subject matching is inevitably flawed.

The Cambridge Contextual Reading Test (CCRT)

It has been proposed that asking elderly demented individuals to read aloud a list of 50 irregular words is not the best way of maximising their performance, in that the unusual words are not presented in context. In the CCRT the NART words are embedded in sentences to provide a meaningful context for the examinee, e.g. 'the bride bought a beautiful bouquet' (Beardsall 1998). This results in improved accuracy of pronunciation by patients with dementia. Unfortunately, the CCRT has not been normed against current measures of intelligence (e.g. WAIS-III) so that it is not possible to readily use the CCRT to estimate premorbid intelligence level.

The Spot The Word test (STW)

Most of the premorbid estimate measures involve accuracy of oral pronunciation. These methods are clearly inappropriate for people with articulation/pronunciation difficulties. Additionally, it has been proposed that highly intelligent self-educated people who are well read, may well be familiar with a word (and its meaning) yet may make pronunciation errors. In order to overcome these difficulties the STW test was developed (Baddeley et al 1993). The STW is a lexical decision task in which the examinee has to identify 'real' words from a series of word/pseudo-word pairs (e.g. stamen/floxid). This is an interesting development; however, use of the STW is currently mainly limited to research applications, as (a) regression equations have yet to be developed to provide estimates of premorbid ability, and (b) there is insufficient evidence on the STW's relative sensitivity in cases of acquired cognitive impairment.

The Wechsler Test of Adult Reading (WTAR)

The WTAR is a NART equivalent, a 50-item word pronunciation test, developed to provide an estimate of premorbid intellectual functioning of adults aged 16–89, with the particular advantage of having been developed and co-normed with the WAIS-III and WMS-III. Thus, one can directly compare WTAR-predicted scores with those obtained from WAIS-III and WMS-III. The

WTAR provides tables of statistical significance in interpreting predicted minus obtained values. For example, a 68-year-old woman produced a WTAR-predicted IQ of 85, which compared with an obtained IQ score of 60. This 25-point discrepancy is considered to be statistically significant at the 1% level. The correlation between WTAR and WAIS-III Verbal IQ across the standardisation age groups ranged from 0.66–0.80, and for full scale IQ from 0.63–0.80, with an expected lower correlation with Performance IQ (0.45–0.66). The WTAR correlates well with other measures of reading (including the NART), range 0.73–0.90. In the UK the WTAR was also completed by 80% of the participants in the WAIS-III UK standardisation study. Given this co-norming procedure, it is likely that the WTAR will become widely used to estimate premorbid intellectual ability.

Measures of memory

The Wechsler Memory Scale, 3rd edition (WMS-III)

The WMS-III builds upon the success of its predecessors, the original Wechsler Memory Scale (WMS) and the Wechsler Memory Scale Revised (WMS-R) and is generally considered to be a considerable improvement. As stated above, the WMS-III was developed and co-normed with the WAIS-III. Normative scores for the WMS-III were obtained from 1250 adults, age range 16–89 years. Eleven subtests are presented and eight memory indices are calculated, each with an age-normed mean of 100 and a standard deviation of 15. The memory indices are: Auditory Immediate, Visual Immediate, Immediate Memory, Auditory Delayed, Visual Delayed, Auditory Recognition Delayed, General Memory and Working Memory. It is therefore possible to obtain accurate quantification of various components of memory functioning. However, a major limitation of the WMS-III is the lack of a matched, parallel version. In neuropsychological practice, it is common to reassess an individual in order to determine the extent of deterioration, treatment efficacy, etc. However, when one re-administers the same memory test, considerable savings occur. Indeed the WMS-III technical manual reports that when the test was re-administered within 2–12 weeks, the mean index scores increased by roughly 0.33–1 standard deviation from first to second testing.

The Auditory Verbal Learning Test (AVLT)

The AVLT is one of the most widely used word-learning tests in clinical research and practice (Rey 1964). Five presentations of a 15-word list are given, each followed by attempted recall. This is followed by a second 15-word interference list (list B), followed by recall of list A. Delayed recall and recognition are also tested. A key feature of the AVLT (and its successor, the California Verbal Learning Test) is that it affords the opportunity to measure rate of learning, as opposed to recall of a single stimulus, or series of stimuli. An equivalent form of AVLT has been provided by Crawford et al (1989).

The California Verbal Learning Test (CVLT)

In an attempt to expand upon the assessment of learning and retrieval strategies, the CVLT evolved from the AVLT and was developed in an attempt to provide an instrument 'reflecting the multifactorial ways in which examinees learn, or fail to learn, verbal material. The CVLT's assessment of learning strategies, processes and errors is designed for use in both clinical and research practice' (Delis et al 1987). A variety of memory measures are obtainable from this measure, including short-term and long-term free recall and recognition, serial learning curves, learning strategy (i.e. semantic versus serial clustering), etc. The CVLT also has the added advantage of presenting the stimuli in an everyday, relatively non-threatening manner, e.g. learning two shopping lists. The reliability data for the principal measures appear to be adequate, although some of the scores which are derived from them have poor reliability. The normative database consists of 273 neurologically intact individuals, with a mean age of 58.9 (15.4) years. This mean age for controls is considerably higher than that normally employed for psychometric test development. A computerised scoring procedure is also available (Delis et al 1987).

The Rivermead Behavioural Memory Test (RBMT)

The RBMT was specifically designed to try and detect impairment of everyday memory function by providing test items that resembled activities in everyday life, e.g. remembering to deliver a message, remembering to retrieve a personal belonging after an interval. The RBMT has the important advantage of having four matched parallel versions, thus allowing for repeated assessment to determine the effects of disease progression and/or clinical intervention. An additional important advantage of the RBMT is the careful work the authors have undertaken in order to ensure the measure's validity. They assessed validity in three ways: (a) by demonstrating a high correlation between the RBMT and other standard memory tests, (b) by demonstrating a high correlation between RBMT scores and subjective ratings of memory impairment, and (c), most importantly, by demonstrating a high correlation between RBMT score and observer ratings of memory lapses (Wilson et al 1989). In general, the RBMT is well tolerated on account of its 'everyday feel' and the fact that it consists of a number of brief, relatively non-threatening subtests. The initial normative data were provided from 118 subjects aged 16–69 years. Cockburn & Smith (1989) recruited additional normative data from 119 people aged 70–94 years, with a mean age of 80.5 years. A limitation of the RBMT is that it may be rather insensitive to mild impairments of memory. In order to improve the sensitivity of the test, the extended RBMT (RBMT-E) was developed. Versions A and B of the original RBMT were combined to make version 1 of the RBMT-E, and versions C and D were combined to make version 2 of the RBMT-E. The RBMT-E is useful in separating out those individuals who scored at the upper range of the original RBMT.

The Rey Complex Figure Test (CFT)

This test has been widely used, particularly because of the dearth of adequate visuospatial memory tests. A complicated figure is presented and the subject is requested to copy it. The original and copy are then removed and the subject is asked to draw the figure again from memory, after varying delay intervals. There have been many variants on administration and scoring criteria, e.g. immediate, 3-minute or 30-minute delay. Spreen & Strauss (1998) provide useful normative data up to 93 years of age. Test–retest reliability following a retest interval was reported as 0.76 for immediate recall and 0.89 for delayed recall.

The Recognition Memory Test (RMT)

The RMT is a widely used instrument, particularly in amnesia research. It consists of two subtests: recognition memory for 50 words and recognition memory for 50 faces. Following the presentation of the words and faces, the testee is required to perform an immediate two-choice recognition task; this is generally considered to be less stressful and anxiety provoking than many other memory measures (taking approximately 15 minutes to complete). The original normative data consists of 310 control inpatients without cerebral disease, aged 18–70 years (Warrington 1984); however, additional norms are provided in D'Elia et al (1995).

The Doors and People Test

The Doors and People Test was devised in order to provide comparable measures of visual and verbal memory that test both recall and recognition, that do not provide floor or ceiling effects and that include both learning and forgetting measures. The test consists of four sections: a doors test, where single doors have to be recognised against three competing distracters; a shapes test, where diagrams have to be reproduced from memory; a names test, which is a verbal recognition test; and finally, the peoples test, where the subject is required to learn an association between a series of photographs and names. Normative data from 238 subjects is provided, aged from 16 to 97 years. One of the stated aims of the authors was that Doors and People should 'provide an unstressful test that is acceptable to a wide range of subjects, extending from patients suffering from dementia or dense amnesia to healthy young normal subjects' (Baddeley et al 1994, p. 4). However, some elderly, cognitively impaired subjects find this test quite demanding.

Measures of language dysfunction

Naming

The Boston Naming Test (BNT) is one of the most widely used measures of naming. The original version of this test included 85 items; however, the shortened version produced in 1983 is used more frequently (Kaplan et al 1983). This test consists of 60 line drawings of objects of graded difficulty, ranging from very common objects (e.g. a tree) to less familiar objects such as an abacus. Although the original normative data are scanty, several studies have provided supplementary norms; these studies have been comprehensively reviewed recently by D'Elia et al (1995).

Vocabulary

The most widely used instrument for the assessment of vocabulary ability is the Vocabulary subtest of the WAIS-III scales. Performance on this test is greatly influenced by education and sociocultural factors rather than age. Vocabulary is the subtest of the WAIS-III and has the highest correlation with total IQ scores: Verbal IQ $r = 0.83$, Performance IQ $r = 0.65$ and Full scale IQ $r = 0.80$.

Verbal comprehension

The most widely used test of verbal comprehension is the Token Test. The original version of this test consists of 62 items, but a 36-item short-form is more commonly used in clinical practice

(De Renzi & Faglioni 1978). The materials consist of tokens which differ in colour, shape (squares and circles) and size (large and small). The examinee has to follow verbal instructions which increase in complexity from simple commands (e.g. 'Touch a circle'; 'Touch the red circle') to commands such as 'Before touching the yellow circle, pick up the red square'. The test authors recommend that scores be adjusted for years of education. Adjusted scores of between 25 and 28 are regarded as indicating mild comprehension problems, and 17–27 moderate problems; scores below this are classified as severe, or very severe.

Visuoconstructional ability

The Block Design subtest of the WAIS-III is widely used for assessing visuospatial constructional abilities. Block Design is often administered in its own right (rather than as part of the complete WAIS-III), and can be interpreted with reference to an age-controlled standard score of 10 with a standard deviation of 3. Visuoconstructional abilities can also be assessed by means of copying or free drawing. The Rey Complex Figure (described above) is the most widely used copying test.

Assessment of attention

The Test of Everyday Attention (TEA)

The TEA consists of eight subtests (standardised in a similar way to the WAIS-III and WMS-III to have an-age adjusted mean of 10 with a standard deviation of 3) which measure sustained, selective and divided attention (Robertson et al 1996). For example, in the Map Search subtest, which was designed as a measure of visual selective attention, the examinee has to search for symbols (e.g. a knife and fork representing eating facilities) on a tourist map of a city. The Elevator Counting subtest, which was designed to measure sustained attention, is a tone counting task in which the examinee is asked to imagine they are in an elevator in which the floor-indicator has failed (thus counting the tones is the only way to establish which floor the elevator is on). A related subtest, designed to measure auditory selective attention, requires the examinee to ignore distracter tones which are of a higher pitch.

The TEA was normed on 154 healthy participants aged between 18 and 80. In addition to reflecting current thinking on the fractionation of attention it is designed to be ecologically valid, i.e. many of the subtests are designed to mimic everyday activities. Another advantage is that it has three parallel versions; this avoids the interpretative problems encountered when attempting to measure change using the same test materials. Selected subtests from the TEA have been used in their own right to test specific hypotheses in research studies: e.g. if one is interested in distractibility, the elevator counting task with distraction may be a useful measure.

Behavioural Inattention Test (BIT)

This is a comprehensive battery for testing visual neglect (Wilson et al 1987). The BIT includes conventional tests (star cancellation, letter cancellation, figure copying, line crossing, line bisection, and representational drawing) and behavioural subtests (picture scanning, telephone dialling, menu reading, article reading, telling and setting the time, coin sorting, address and sentence copying, map navigation, and card sorting). The test manual reports impressively high coefficients for inter-rater reliability (0.99), test–retest reliability (0.99) and parallel form reliability (0.91). Among the six conventional tests included in the battery, star cancellation has substantially greater sensitivity than the other tests.

Executive functioning

The term 'frontal lobe' test is unsatisfactory as it implies a simple relationship between cognitive task and neural substrate, which is often not the case (e.g. see section, above, on localising measures). Cognitive measures should be described in psychological, not anatomical terms. Executive functions describe higher-order cognitive processes including initiation, planning, hypothesis generation, cognitive flexibility, decision making, judgement and feedback utilisation that are necessary for effective and socially appropriate behaviour (Spreen & Strauss 1998). For patients who have problems in these areas the term 'dysexecutive syndrome' is preferred as it stresses the psychological nature of the difficulties the patients experience rather than the putative area of the brain that has been damaged.

Verbal fluency

Verbal fluency tests, and in particular initial letter fluency, are widely used as tests of executive dysfunction. Initial letter fluency, also referred to as the Controlled Oral Word Association Test (COWAT), requires the generation of words from initial letters (normally F, A and S) under time constraints, normally 60 seconds per letter (Benton & Hamsher 1978). Fluency tests are reliable, quick to administer, and even patients with quite severe deficits can understand the task requirements. In an area replete with failures to replicate, studies of initial letter fluency have been remarkably consistent in demonstrating impaired fluency following left or bilateral frontal lobe damage. Frith et al (1991) also reported that verbal fluency tasks activated left frontal brain regions during PET scanning.

Behavioural Assessment of the Dysexecutive Syndrome (BADS)

Many formal neuropsychological tests fail to detect executive problems because they are highly structured. Shallice & Burgess (1991) note, 'The patient typically has a single explicit problem to tackle at any one time. The trials tend to be very short, task initiation is strongly prompted by the examiner and what constitutes successful trial completion is clearly characterised' (pp. 727–728). The Behavioural Assessment of the Dysexecutive Syndrome (BADS) represents an ambitious and systematic attempt to capture the core elements of the dysexecutive syndrome (Wilson et al 1996). The BADS battery consists of six subtests and was normed on a sample of 216 healthy participants with an age range of 16 to 87. Subtests include the Rule Shifts Cards Test in which a previously established response set (responding 'yes' to red cards, 'no' to black) has to be inhibited in favour of responding in terms of whether or not a card matches the colour of the card immediately preceding it. The Action Program Test is a planning task in which the solution requires the client to utilise various everyday materials e.g. plastic, cork and wire. The Modified Six Elements Test assesses scheduling and time management by requiring clients to tackle three different tasks within the time limit; there are two versions of each task, and the rules prohibit tackling these contiguously (Shallice & Burgess 1991).

The inter-rater reliability of the BADS is excellent; correlations between raters ranged from a low of 0.88 on one index from the Modified Six Elements Test, to unity, or near unity, on most of the other tasks. A useful supplement to the formal BADS subtests is the Dysexecutive Questionnaire (DEX). The DEX covers dispositional and cognitive changes and comes in two forms: one for completion by the client the other by a relative or carer. Large discrepancies between client and carer reports of change are common when working with clients who have executive problems. The DEX provides one means of quantifying this lack of insight; DEX results can also form a basis for discussion when counselling patients and their families.

Wisconsin Card Sorting Test (WCST)

This is a widely used test of set-shifting ability, an ability that is thought to be compromised in patients who have suffered frontal lobe damage. There are several versions of the task. In the standard condition, four target cards are placed in front of the examinee: one showing one red triangle, one with two green stars, one with three yellow crosses and one with four blue circles. The examinee is then given 128 cards and asked to sort the cards under the target cards according to a set criterion (colour, form or number) and the examiner provides feedback as to whether the decision was right or wrong. For example, the examinee could turn over the first card which had two blue triangles on it, this could be placed under the target card with four blue circles (sorting by colour), under the target card with two green stars (sorting by number) or under the target card with one red triangle (sorting by form). The sorting 'rule' is not made explicit by the examiner, and the examinee learns via the feedback provided after each trial whether they are correct or incorrect. After ten consecutive correct responses, the rule is changed without the examinee's knowledge, and the examinee must now learn the new rule. It is normal practice to score performance in terms of number of correct categories attained (runs of ten consecutive correct responses) and also in terms of percentage of perseverative errors. While the WCST has been widely used (Spreen & Strauss 1998), several researchers have queried the task's sensitivity to frontal lobe pathology. Furthermore, some authors have reported finding the full test quite stressful for the failing examinee, who receives persistent feedback that they are making errors. Accordingly, Nelson developed the modified Wisconsin Card Sorting Test, a shorter task using 48 rather than 128 target cards (Nelson 1976). Nelson provided data indicating that this abbreviated measure was also sensitive to frontal lobe damage, a claim that was subsequently challenged by van den Broek (1993).

Stroop Test of Attentional Conflict

The Stroop test measures the ease with which a person can shift his/her perceptual set to changing demands, and critically, to suppress a habitual response in favour of an unusual one. There are several versions of the Stroop task, the most widely used being that developed by Trenerry et al (1988). In the neutral condition, the examinee is required to read aloud a list of colour name words. The conflict condition is provided by having colour words written in an incongruous colour of ink, e.g. the word green written in red ink. The examinee is required to inhibit the dominant, automatic tendency to read the word name, and instead name the incongruent colour of ink in which the word is written. The number of correct responses made in 120 seconds is recorded. (The difference between the neutral and conflict condition is often taken as a measure of interference.) The task is thought to tap the ability to inhibit well-established responses, an ability thought to be impaired in brain damage, particularly frontal brain damage. Trenerry et al (1988) provide limited normative data for two age bands — 18–49 year and 50+ — together with percentile scores and 'probability of brain damage estimates'. Clearly there are vast differences in speed of processing between 50 and 80 years of age, and further age-banded norms are required. The principle of the Stroop task is widely used in cognitive psychology research, e.g. the use of an 'emotional Stroop' paradigm, where particularly salient words interfere with the colour-naming task.

Hayling and Brixton tests

These two tasks were developed to tap particular behaviours that are commonly exhibited by patients following frontal lobe damage. The Hayling test provides a measure of initiation speed as well as performance on a response suppression task. In section 1 the examinee has to complete a sentence, e.g. 'The job was easy most of the . . .'. The appropriateness of the response and latency to respond are recorded. In section 2 the subject is asked to give a word which is *completely unconnected*, e.g. 'The dog chased the cat up the . . .' and an appropriate response could be 'kettle'. The Brixton test consists of a stimulus booklet with an array of 10 circles numbered from 1 to 10. One of the circles is filled in blue. The examinee turns the pages and is asked where the next blue circle is likely to appear, by trying to see a pattern or rule from what they have seen on previous pages. Thus the Brixton test measures concept or rule attainment.

Normative data for the Hayling and Brixton tests are available from 121 healthy controls. The raw scores are converted to scaled scores. Test–retest reliability for the Hayling and Brixton tests fall in the range 0.62–0.71. Patients with anterior lesions performed poorly on both tasks (Burgess & Shallice 1997).

COMPUTERISED NEUROPSYCHOLOGICAL ASSESSMENT

Neuropsychological assessment requires training, and a detailed evaluation can take several hours, after which the tests must be scored, and compared with reference norms, and a report written. Thus detailed neuropsychological assessment can be an extensive and time-consuming process. In addition, appropriately trained clinical neuropsychologists are relatively scarce. Traditional 'paper and pencil' neuropsychological testing always includes a degree of error (e.g. stop-watch recording of an examinee's performance invariably incorporates variability in the examiner's reaction time!). Additionally, such assessment is limited in terms of the temporal sensitivity of measurement possible. Computerised neuropsychological assessment solves many of the problems outlined above. The measures do not require a highly trained administrator, parallel forms are often available, and measurement of responses can be very precise, e.g. in milliseconds. This degree of measurement precision may be particularly advantageous in neuropsychological research on psychiatric disorders, where one may be interested in subtle changes in cognition and behaviour (e.g. biases in retrieval, quantification of the effects of interference or distracters).

A computerised method of test administration has several advantages: all the information is presented in a standardised and consistent manner, responses are accurately recorded and complex analysis and scoring may be undertaken quickly, eliminating examiner error. The Cambridge Neuropsychological Test Automated Battery (CANTAB) (Sahakian & Owen 1992) is an example of such a computerised assessment system. CANTAB consists of a series of tests tapping visual memory, attention, working memory, planning, set-shifting, simple and choice reaction time, using a touch-sensitive screen response format. In the parallel battery, four different versions of some of the tasks are available, thus allowing repeated testing of the same individual to assess change over time in order to track deterioration or evaluate treatment efficacy. The CANTAB measures have been used to study the pattern of neuropsychological impairment in a variety of conditions, including Parkinson's disease, Alzheimer's disease, frontal and temporal lobe damage, etc. The parallel forms have afforded the opportunity to examine within-subject change over time, e.g. the effects of diurnal mood variation on neuropsychological status in depression (Moffoot et al 1994). As described in the section on depression, Swainson et al (2001) used the CANTAB visuospatial associative learning test and reported it to be particularly useful in the early detection of Alzheimer's disease.

The limitations of computerised assessment include the fact that the software and hardware can be expensive. In addition the response format often requires selection from a number of multiple choices using a touch screen response. Verbal responses, e.g. in testing of free recall for long-term memory assessment, still require oral or written output. The issue of portability of computerised assessment has largely been solved via the use of laptop or notebook PCs. There was initial concern that the computerised format may be daunting, particularly for elderly patients. However, as computers have become so widely integrated into day-to-day activities in society, these concerns have lessened considerably. Furthermore, in studies where methods of assessment have been compared, no clear preference for the traditional paper and pencil approach has been found.

CONCLUSION

The neuropsychological study of psychiatric disorders is still in its infancy. Exciting novel attempts to explain abnormal behaviour in terms of dysfunctional information processing are rapidly being developed. However, it is critical that such models are explicitly amenable to experimental testing and refutation. Increasingly sophisticated sets of neuropsychological measures have been developed which allow for the sensitive, reliable and valid assessment of specific components of cognitive functioning. This affords the opportunity for rigorous testing of brain–behaviour relationships in man. The next decade should result in significant advances in our knowledge of the neuropsychological underpinnings of psychiatric disorder, as well as a more sophisticated understanding of the effects of treatments on cognition and behaviour.

REFERENCES

Addington J, Addington D 1999 Neurocognitive and social functioning in schizophrenia. Schizophrenia Bulletin 25: 173–182

Baddeley A, Emslie H, Nimmo-Smith I 1993 The Spot-the-Word Test: A robust estimate of verbal intelligence based on lexical decision. British Journal of Clinical Psychology 32: 55–65

Baddeley A, Emslie H, Nimmo-Smith I 1994 Doors and People – test manual. Thames Valley Test Company, Bury St Edmunds

Baxter R D, Liddle P F 1998 Neuropsychological deficits associated with schizophrenic syndromes. Schizophrenia Research 30: 239–249

Beardsall L 1998 Development of the Cambridge Contextual Reading Test for improving the estimation of premorbid verbal intelligence in older persons with dementia. British Journal of Clinical Psychology 37: 229–240

Benton A L, Hamsher K 1978 Multilingual aphasia examination manual – revised. University of Iowa, Iowa City

Blakemore C 1988 The mind machine. BBC Books, London

Blakemore S J, Smith J, Steel R et al 2000 The perception of self-produced sensory stimuli in patients with auditory hallucinations and passivity experiences: evidence for a breakdown in self-monitoring. Psychological Medicine 30: 1131–1139

Blanchard J J, Neale J M 1994 The neuropsychological signature of schizophrenia: generalized or differential deficit? American Journal of Psychiatry 151: 40–48

Bremner J D 1999 Alterations in brain structure and function associated with post-traumatic stress disorder. Seminars in Clinical Neuropsychiatry 4: 249–255

Brewin C R 2001 A cognitive neuroscience account of posttraumatic stress disorder and its treatment. Behaviour Research and Therapy 39: 373–393

Burgess P, Shallice T 1997 The Hayling and Brixton tests. Thames Valley Test Company, Bury St Edmunds

Byrne M, Hodges A, Grant E et al 1999 Neuropsychological assessment of young people at high genetic risk for developing schizophrenia compared to controls: Preliminary findings of the Edinburgh High Risk Study (EHRS). Psychological Medicine 29: 1161–1173

Cahill L, McGaugh J L 1998 Mechanisms of emotional arousal and lasting declarative memory. Trends in Neurosciences 21: 294–299

Cavanagh J T, Van Beck M, Muir W, Blackwood D H 2002 Case-control study of neurocognitive function in euthymic patients with bipolar disorder: an association with mania. British Journal of Psychiatry 180: 320–326

Cockburn J, Smith P T 1989 The Rivermead behavioural memory test – Supplement 3: Elderly people. Thames Valley Test Company, Titchfield

Coen R F, Swanwick G R J, Maguire C et al 1996 Memory impairment in Alzheimer's disease: replication and extension of the delayed word recall (DWR) test. Irish Journal of Psychological Medicine 13: 55–58

Crawford J R 1992 Current and premorbid intelligence measures in neuropsychological assessment. In: Crawford J R, Parker D M, MacKinlay W M (eds). Handbook of neuropsychological assessment. Taylor & Francis, London, p 21–49

Crawford J R, Parker D M, Besson J A O 1988 Estimation of premorbid intelligence in organic conditions. British Journal of Psychiatry 153: 178–181

Crawford J R, Stewart L E, Moore J W 1989 Demonstration of savings on the AVLT and development of a parallel form. Journal of Clinical and Experimental Neuropsychology 11: 975–981

Damasio A R 1994 Descartes' Error. Papermac/Macmillan, London

Damasio H, Grabowski T, Frank R et al 1994 The return of Phineas Gage: clues about the brain from the skull of a famous patient. Science 264: 1102–1105

David A S 1992 Frontal lobology – psychiatry's new pseudoscience. British Journal of Psychiatry 161: 244–248

David A S, Malmberg A, Brandt L et al 1997 IQ and risk for schizophrenia: a population-based cohort study. Psychological Medicine 27: 1311–1323

De Renzi E, Faglioni P 1978 Normative data and screening power of a shortened version of the Token Test. Cortex 3: 327–342

D'Elia L F, Boone K B, Mitrushina A M 1995 Handbook of normative data for neuropsychological assessment. Oxford University Press, New York

Delis D C, Kramer J H, Kaplan E, Ober B A 1987 California Verbal Learning Test – Adult version research manual. The Psychological Corporation, San Antonio

Ellis H D, Lewis M B 2001 Capgras delusion: a window on face recognition. Trends in Cognitive Sciences 5: 149–156

Ellis H D, Young A W 1990 Accounting for delusional misidentifications. British Journal of Psychiatry 157: 239–248

Ellis H D, Young A W, Quayle A H, De Pauw K W 1997 Reduced autonomic responses to faces and Capgras delusion. Proceedings of the Royal Society: Biological Sciences B264: 1085–1092

Ferrier I N, Stanton B R, Kelly T P, Scott J 1999 Neuropsychological function in euthymic patients with bipolar disorder. British Journal of Psychiatry 175: 246–251

Folstein M F, Folstein S E, McHugh P R 1975 Mini-Mental State: a practical method for grading the cognitive state of patients for the clinician. Journal of Psychiatric Research 12: 189–198

Frith C D 1992 The cognitive neuropsychology of schizophrenia. Lawrence Erlbaum, Hove

Frith C D, Friston K J, Liddle P F, Frackowiak R S J 1991 A PET study of word finding. Neuropsychologia 29: 1137–1148

Green M F 1996 What are the functional consequences of neurocognitive deficits in schizophrenia? American Journal of Psychiatry 153: 321–330

Gudjonssen G H, Shackleton H 1986 The pattern of scores on Raven's Matrices during "faking bad" and "non-faking" performance. British Journal of Clinical Psychology 25: 35–42

Gunnell D, Harrison G, Rasmussen F et al 2002 Associations between premorbid intellectual performance, early-life exposures and early-onset schizophrenia — cohort study. British Journal of Psychiatry 181: 298–305

Halligan P W, David A S 2001 Cognitive neuropsychiatry: towards a scientific psychopathology. Nature Neuroscience 2: 209–215

Heinrichs R W, Zakzanis K K 1998 Neurocognitive deficit in schizophrenia: A quantitative review of the evidence. Neuropsychology 12: 426–445

Johnstone E C, Crow T J, Frith C D et al 1976 Cerebral ventricular size and cognitive impairment in chronic schizophrenia. Lancet 2: 924–926

Jones P, Rodgers B, Murray R, Marmot M 1994 Child development risk factors for adult schizophrenia in the British 1946 birth cohort. Lancet 344: 1398–1402

Kaplan E F, Goodglass H, Weintraub S 1983 The Boston Naming Test, 2nd edn. Lea & Febiger, Philadelphia

Knopman D S, Ryberg S 1989 A verbal memory test with high predictive accuracy for dementia of the Alzheimer type. Archives of Neurology 46: 141–145

Lachner G, Satzger W, Engel R R 1994 Verbal memory tests in the differential diagnosis of depression and dementia: discriminative power of seven test variations. Archives of Clinical Neuropsychology 9: 1–13

Lawrie S M, Whalley H, Kestelman J N et al 1999 Magnetic resonance imaging of brain in people at high risk of developing schizophrenia. Lancet 353: 30–33

Lezak M 1995 Neuropsychological assessment, 3rd edn. Oxford University Press, Oxford

Liddle P F, Morris D L 1991 Schizophrenic syndromes and frontal lobe performance. British Journal of Psychiatry 158: 340–345

Lloyd G C, Lishman W A 1975 Effects of depression on the speed of recall of pleasant and unpleasant experiences. Psychological Medicine 5: 173–180

McAllister-Williams R H, Ferrier I N, Young A H 1998 Mood and neuropsychological function in depression: the role of corticosteroids and serotonin. Psychological Medicine 28: 573–584

McKenna P J 1991 Memory, knowledge and delusions. British Journal of Psychiatry 159: 36–41

Meehl P E 1990 Toward an integrated theory of schizotaxia, schizotypy and schizophrenia. Journal of Personality Disorders 4: 1–99

Moffoot A P R, O'Carroll R E, Bennie J et al 1994 Diurnal variation of mood and neuropsychological function in major depression with melancholia. Journal of Affective Disorders 32: 257–269

Morrison G, O'Carroll R E, McCreadie R G 2004 The long term course of cognitive impairment in schizophrenia: a view from Nithsdale, Scotland over 33 years. Submitted for publication

Murphy F C, Sahakian B J 2001 Neuropsychology of bipolar disorder. British Journal of Psychiatry 178:S120–S127

Nelson H E 1976 A modified card sorting test sensitive to frontal lobe defects. Cortex 12: 313–324

Nelson H E, Willison J R 1991 The revised National Adult Reading Test–test manual. NFER-Nelson, Windsor

O'Carroll R 1995 The assessment of premorbid ability — a critical review. Neurocase 1: 83–89

O'Carroll R E, Conway S, Ryman A, Prentice N 1997 Performance on the delayed word recall test (DWR) fails to differentiate clearly between depression and Alzheimer's disease in the elderly. Psychological Medicine 27: 967–971

O'Carroll R E, Moffoot A, Ebmeier K P, Goodwin G M 1992 Estimating pre-morbid intellectual ability in the Alcoholic Korsakoff Syndrome. Psychological Medicine 22: 903–909

Palmer B W, Heaton R K, Paulsen J S et al 1997 Is it possible to be schizophrenic yet neuropsychologically normal? Neuropsychology 11: 437–446

Rey 1964 L'examen clinique en psychologie. Presses Universitaires de France, Paris

Richards P M, Ruff R M 1989 Motivational effects on neuropsychological functioning: Comparison of depressed versus nondepressed individuals. Journal of Consulting and Clinical Psychology 57: 396–402

Ridout N et al 2003 The neuropsychology of major depression: moving towards ecological validity. Unpublished data

Ridout N, Astell A J, Reid I C et al 2003 Memory bias for emotional facial expressions in major depression. Cognition and Emotion 17: 101–122

Robertson I H, Ward T, Ridgeway V 1996 The structure of normal human attention: The Test of Everyday Attention. Journal of the International Neuropsychology Society 2: 525–534

Roth M, Tym E, Mountjoy C Q et al 1986 CAMDEX: A standardised instrument for the diagnosis of mental disorder in the elderly with special reference to the early detection of dementia. British Journal of Psychiatry 149: 698–709

Russell A J, Munro J C, Jones P B 1997 Schizophrenia and the myth of intellectual decline. American Journal of Psychiatry 154: 635–639

Sahakian B J, Owen A M 1992 Computerized assessment in neuropsychiatry using CANTAB: discussion paper. Journal of the Royal Society of Medicine 85: 399–402

Saykin A J, Shtasel D L, Gur R E et al 1994 Neuropsychological deficits in neuroleptic naive patients with first-episode schizophrenia. Archives of General Psychiatry 51: 124–131

Scoville W B, Milner B 1957 Loss of recent memory after bilateral hippocampal lesions. Journal of Neurology, Neurosurgery and Psychiatry 20: 150–176

Shah P J, Ebmeier K P, Glabus M F, Goodwin G M 1998 Cortical grey matter reductions associated with treatment-resistant chronic unipolar depression — Controlled magnetic resonance imaging study. British Journal of Psychiatry 172: 527–532

Shallice T, Burgess P W 1991 Deficits in strategy application following frontal lobe damage in man. Brain 114: 727–741

Shallice T, Burgess P W, Frith C D 1991 Can the neuropsychological case-study approach be applied to schizophrenia? Psychological Medicine 21: 661–673

Spreen O, Strauss E 1998 A compendium of neuropsychological tests, 2nd edn. Oxford University Press, New York

Squire L R 1987 Memory and brain. Oxford University Press, Oxford

Swainson R, Hodges J R, Galton C J et al 2001 Early detection and differential diagnosis of alzheimer's disease and depression with neuropsychological tasks. Dementia Geriatric Cognitive Disorders 12: 265–280

Teasdale J 1983 Negative thinking in depression, cause, effect or reciprocal relationship. Advances in Behaviour Therapy 5: 3–25

Trenerry M R, Crosson B, DeBoe J, Leber W R 1988 STROOP neuropsychological screening test manual. Psychological Assessment Resources, Odessa, Florida

van den Broek M D 1993 Utility of the modified Wisconson Card Sorting Test in neuropsychological assessment. British Journal of Clinical Psychology 32: 333–343

Veiel H O 1997 A preliminary profile of neuropsychological deficits associated with major depression. Journal of Clinical and Experimental Neuropsychology 19: 587–603

Warrington E K 1984 Recognition Memory Test. Nelson, Windsor

Weingartner H 1986 Automatic and effort-demanding cognitive processes in depression. In: Poon L W (ed) Handbook for clinical memory assessment of older adults. American Psychological Association, Washington, DC, p 218–225

Williams J M, Ellis N C, Tyers C et al 1996 The specificity of autobiographical memory and imageability of the future. Memory and Cognition 24: 116–125

Wilson B, Cockburn J, Haligan P 1987 Development of a behavioural test of visuospatial neglect. Archives of Physical Medicine and Rehabilitation 68: 98–102

Wilson B A, Cockburn J M, Baddeley A D, Hiorns R 1989 The development and validation of a test battery for detecting and monitoring everyday memory problems. Journal of Clinical and Experimental Neuropsychology 11: 855–870

Wilson B A, Baddeley A D, Kapur N 1995 Dense amnesia in a professional musician following herpes simplex virus encephalitis. Journal of Clinical and Experimental Neuropsychology 17: 668–681

Wilson B A, Alderman N, Burgess P W et al 1996 BADS Behavioural Assessment of the Dysexecutive Syndrome. Thames Valley Test Company, Bury St Edmunds

9 Genetics in relation to psychiatry

Douglas H R Blackwood, Walter J Muir

INTRODUCTION

The completed full sequence of the human genome has recently been announced, an astonishing achievement coming only two years after the publication of the draft sequence in 2001. We are now in the post-genomic age, and it is important to keep pace with the rapid advances in genetics as applied to psychiatry. The number of human genes has turned out to be surprisingly small at around 30 000, and the molecular diversity of created proteins is greatly increased by a variety of processing mechanisms beyond DNA transcription. The principal aim of genetics is to relate genotype to phenotype, and in the last ten years over 1200 genes that cause human illness have been identified. There are also complex general and tissue-specific regulatory mechanisms that control gene expression, and important inherited (epigenetic) control factors that are not directly coded by DNA. Our genetic inheritance influences almost all disease to a greater or lesser extent, and this is particularly true of psychiatric disorders. Some of the best-established findings in psychiatry relate to the role of genetic factors in determining the risk of developing a disorder. The aim of this chapter is not to give in detail the genetic findings for every psychiatric illness; this information is found in other chapters of this volume. Instead the focus is on the basic mechanisms that underpin these findings, and the approaches that psychiatrists can take to analyse the contribution of genetics to psychiatric disorder.

THE GENETIC CODE AND MECHANISMS OF ITS TRANSMISSION

Inheritance can be interpreted in several ways. Culture is transmitted from one generation to the next through the experience of a social environment that persists and changes more slowly than the generational period. Information can be passed on over generations through stable media — books, photographs, recordings, and other such artefacts. The inheritance of genetic factors is mediated by the generational passage of deoxyribosenucleic acid (DNA). DNA consists of four nucleotide bases, adenine (A), thymine (T), cytosine (C), guanine (G), arranged in two anti-parallel strands where phosphate bonds link individual bases and the strands bind through hydrogen bonds in according to the base-pairing rule — A with T, C with G — which is the basis of the copying mechanism that ensures DNA fidelity during replication. This vertical flow of information dictates the development and maintenance of the human form.

The structure of the chromosome

Long linear molecules of DNA exist in the cell nucleus in association with a variety of histones and other chromosome-associated proteins; the whole complex (called chromatin) forms a discrete structure, the chromosome. Chromatin is packed at several levels: the DNA duplex wraps around a protein complex (nucleosome) in a bead-on-string fashion, the beads coil into a 30-nm chromatin fibre, which in turn is formed into twisted loops that radiate from a protein scaffold (Fig. 9.1).

During cell division, further compaction occurs, rendering the chromosome visible under light microscopy. The structure shows differential staining patterns with certain chemicals, producing the classical banded appearance at metaphase. This has an underlying functional basis, with light staining areas (using Giemsa dye) being gene-rich and dark bands gene-poor. The phase of the cell cycle during which DNA replicates also differs between bands.

In humans, chromosomes exist as 22 matched autosomes and one heteromorphic pair of sex chromosomes. The autosomal pairs are numerically labelled depending on their size (1 being the largest); sex chromosomes are labelled as XX (females) and XY (males). Thus a normal complement in a woman can be described as 46,XX, the digit indicating total chromosome number or diploid count, the letters the sex chromosome status. Human chromosomes have an obvious macrostructure during certain stages of cell division. A primary constriction, the centromere, divides the chromosome into two arms: a short (termed 'p') and a long ('q'). The centromere contains a particular type of repeated DNA motif (alpha-satellite), hypo-acetylated histones and centromere-specific proteins, some of which may have motor functions to drive chromosomes along microtubules during cell division. At the ends of human chromosomes are other specialised structures called telomeres where a repeated sequence (TTAGGG) caps the free chromosome end, acting as a halt to replication. Telomeres are replicated themselves by a separate enzymatic mechanism involving telomerase. During any cell division there is loss of telomeric DNA which telomerase serves to correct in undifferentiated cells. In differentiated cells, however, telomerase is not expressed, and shortening of telomeres occurs with ageing, leading eventually to cellular malfunction.

The formation of gametes: meiotic division

The germ cells (ova and sperm) differ from other (somatic) cells in that they only contain one chromosome from each original pair (haploid count). This is the end product of meiotic division, a reduction mechanism that involves recombination and random

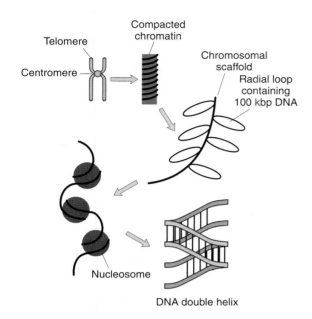

Fig. 9.1
The various levels of DNA compaction at metaphase: from the level of the whole chromosome (upper left), to the duplex DNA helix itself (lower right).

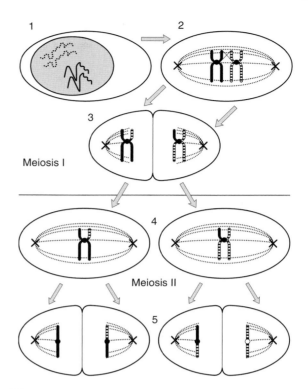

Fig. 9.2
Diagrammatic representation of the behaviour of one chromosome pair during meiosis. Stage 1: DNA replication. Stage 2: Nuclear membrane dissolves, spindle apparatus forms, duplicated chromosomes fuse at centromeres (forming bivalents) and move to equator, and recombination occurs. Stage 3: Homologous chromosomes move to poles, and cell divides in two. Stages 4 and 5: No further duplication, but a reduction division to form four haploid gametes.

chromosome assortment. It is a two-stage process. The first division involves chromosome doubling (during the prophase stage in which the chromosomes also condense and the nuclear membrane dissolves), each chromosome being linked at the centromere to its new partner. Each part of this doublet is now termed a sister chromatid, and the doublets of each chromosome of the pair appose each other so that the highly important process of recombination can occur. DNA segments (over 300 bp in length) are exchanged between the chromatids of the homologous chromosomes, a process (synapsis) that involves the formation of bridges (seen as chiasma under the light microscope) in a synaptonemal complex. Specific proteins (including human Rad51) can bind to a single strand of the DNA duplex and recognise a complementary strand in the DNA of the other homologous chromosome. In an energy-dependent step a heteroduplex junction is formed, with breakage, crossover and reunion of DNA between the homologues. Rearranged DNA is important in maintaining diversity within the genome, and hence its adaptability to differing and changing environments. Recombination can also act to repair DNA, preserving its fidelity; the template-scanning functions allow correction of damage caused by external (alkylating substances, radiation) and internal (reactive oxygen species) agents and errors due to the replication process itself.

Each paired sister chromatid unit has a specific protein-containing disk (kinetochore) at their fused centromere region which interacts and binds with a microtubule-based apparatus that radiates from two anchoring structures (poles) spaced apart within the cell. Through the addition or subtraction of molecular subunits to microtubules the spindle apparatus can 'pull' or 'push' chromosomes within the cell, either bringing them to the equator of the spindle (congression) as a prerequisite for recombination or separating them to opposite poles (segregation) prior to the formation of daughter cells. The kinetochores are orientated towards one pole or the other, and after recombination the individual members

of the homologous chromosome pair are drawn towards the poles. Such segregation is a random event introducing a mixture of paternal- and maternal-derived chromosomes into the germline, adding another element of adaptive variation into the transmitted genome. Meiosis I is completed, after the formation of two clusters of segregated chromosomes, by the disappearance of the spindle apparatus, the formation of new nuclear membranes, and finally by the ingression of the cell membrane in a closing purse-string fashion to separate into two daughter cells. The second meiotic division (meiosis II) does not involve DNA duplication — it is a reduction division, so that each gamete contains only half the original chromosomal material. The sister chromatids that were fused at the centromere during meiosis I are split and pulled (random orientation with respect to the poles ensuring random selection) to two new poles by the spindle apparatus of meiosis II. Four gametes are thus produced from each original cell, each containing only 23 chromosomes (normally either 23,X or 23,Y). The above description is simplified, and a large number of complex interactions occur involving molecular motors, checkpoint systems that control progress from one phase to the next, the spindle apparatus and kinetochores. In fact a significant proportion of all proteins produced by a cell are involved in the (seemingly simpler) process of somatic mitosis where there is neither recombination nor reduction division (Scholey et al 2003). Meiosis is illustrated in diagrammatic form in Figure 9.2.

In the male germline all four gametes are retained as sperm; however, in the formation of ova only one of the four gametes survives as an ovum, the others form polar bodies.

The gene

This is the basic unit of genetic information that lies within each chromosomal DNA sequence. Originally the term 'gene' was used in an abstract sense to explain why some traits seemed to be inherited. In fact the relationship between genes and proteins (Beadle's 1930s concept of 'one gene, one enzyme') was conceived well before the structure of DNA was known. The gene is now taken to mean a stretch of DNA that contains the information (genetic code, read as triplets of nucleotides) necessary to direct amino acids into the correct sequence order during protein assembly in the cytoplasm (using ribonucleic acid, RNA, intermediates), or to direct the formation of RNA molecules that are end-products in themselves. The products of so called RNA genes have structural, enzymatic or regulatory functions. Information in DNA is copied into messenger RNA (mRNA), which in turn acts as a template for polypeptide assembly through interaction with transfer RNAs (tRNAs) that are conjugated to specific amino acids. The emphasis is on functionality — a gene is that segment of the chromosome that directs the formation of a functional product. Many sequences within the genome bear great similarity to active genes but are either completely untranscribed, or their mRNAs are untranslated. Such pseudogenes produce no functional product. Within the gene the basic unit of information is the codon — a triplet of three nucleotide bases whose presence in a sequence will lead to a specific amino acid insertion into a protein. The genetic code maps DNA codons to amino acids, and the code has a degree of redundancy (degeneracy), with several different codons linked to individual amino acids (a triplet can be taken from four nucleotides in 64 different ways, but there are only 20 different amino acids). Some codons do not code for amino acids, but dictate operational events during protein formation such as initiation and termination of polypeptide chain assembly (start and stop codons; start codons also code for methionine, the initial amino acid in any polypeptide; Fig. 9.3).

An open reading frame (ORF) is a complete set of codons bracketed by start and stop codons. The fidelity of DNA is obviously of prime importance to cellular function, and a variety of mechanisms exist to preserve it. Ionising radiation or reactive oxidative molecules can induce double-stranded breaks. These can be repaired by homologous recombination (one key protein in this process BRAC1 is defective in an inherited breast cancer) or by a special repair mechanism (non-homologous end-joining). UV light exposure damage usually causes dimerisation of bases on a single strand, and a specific photoreactive enzyme system exists to reverse this. In some cases a bypass mechanism exists (sloppy copiers) which simply skips over damage and allows replication to continue but at the expense of introducing mutations into the protein. Cells are usually unable to cope with extensive DNA damage, however, and apoptotic mechanisms are activated to eliminate them from the healthy cell population (Friedberg 2003).

Transcription: DNA to mRNA

To describe transcription in relation to DNA sequence a nomenclature based on the sugar chemistry of DNA has developed. The fifth carbon of deoxyribose (the 5′-carbon; pronounced 'five

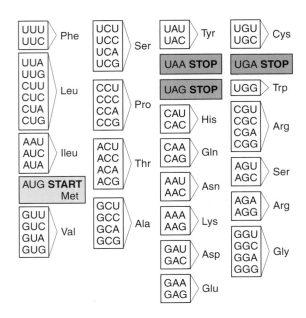

Fig. 9.3
The genetic code in mRNA. Left hand side of columns indicates the coding triplets. Columns are arranged by order of the second nucleotide in each triplet (U [uracil], C, A or G). The amino acid coded for is given on the right using the standard chemical abbreviations. Note the start (methionine) and stop codons. The code can easily be referred 'back' to DNA or 'forward' for tRNA triplets.

prime') is bound to a phosphate moiety, the third to a hydroxyl group. Diphosphate bonds are formed between the 3′ and 5′ of the first sugar leaving the first 5′ free (the '5′-end') and the last 3′ of the DNA free (the 3′-end). This gives a direction to the DNA sequence. Thus transcription of DNA into RNA begins at the 5′-end of DNA and proceeds in the 3′-direction. Normally a sequence of bases exists on either side of the ORF that is transcribed into mRNA but not translated into protein (untranslated regions; UTRs). RNA, normally single stranded, differs from DNA in its sugar backbone (ribose instead of deoxyribose) and the replacement of thymine with uracil bases. During transcription the duplex DNA is partly unwound to allow access to the key enzyme DNA-dependent RNA polymerase (RNApol). (There are three forms of RNApol in eukaryotes: RNApol I, which creates ribosomal or rRNA; RNApol II, which creates messenger or mRNA; and RNApol III, which creates transport or tRNA.) The initial event is binding of an initiation protein to a non-transcribed promoter sequence (normally containing a TATA nucleotide motif or box) near the 3′-end of the ORF. A complex of proteins that includes transcription factors (co-activators) and activator proteins that link to more distant enhancer elements in the DNA sequence itself help closely regulate transcriptional activity and also position RNApol correctly at the start of the ORF. Abnormalities in these regulatory proteins or the DNA motifs in the promoter and enhancer elements that they bind have been increasingly recognised as pathogenic in addition to direct alterations within gene sequence itself. In some cases the altered enhancer sequence (that up-regulates transcription) can be hundreds of kbp distant from the gene under regulation. Figure 9.4 summarises the gene unit and its regulatory elements. Not shown on this diagram are

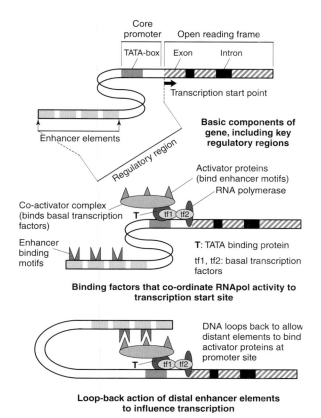

Fig. 9.4
The basic elements of eukaryotic gene structure and regulation.

silencer motifs that act to down-regulate transcription by binding specific proteins (repressors). Taken together this complex set of interacting proteins serves to position and stabilise RNApol at the transcription start site and to offer many targets for cellular fine-tuning of transcriptional activity.

Post-transcriptional modification and regulation of mRNA

All DNA within an ORF is initially transcribed into mRNA (primary transcript), but the sequence that codes for amino acids (exon) is usually interrupted by non-coding sequences (introns) that must be removed to form mature mRNA before translation into protein. RNA processing is a complex process involving at least three different mechanisms. A 7-methylguanosine cap structure is added to the 5'-end of mRNA during transcription, and immediately after transcription a polyadenylate tail (a sequence of repeated adenine nucleotides) is added at the 3'-end. These are essential to mRNA stability, protecting it from enzyme (exonuclease) attack as well as facilitating export from the nucleus and efficient translation. Introns are spliced out in the spliceosome, an assemblage of proteins and small nuclear ribonucleoproteins (snRNPs) that recognise terminal intronic sequences (largely conserved dinucleotides). The exons are often spliced together in different ways depending on up- and down-regulating protein- and tissue-specific signals. In this way the mammalian genome vastly increases its repertoire of protein types above the relatively limited number of human genes available. Neurons have a specific splicing regulatory system, dysfunction in which can lead to several disorders. Chromosome 17 linked frontotemporal dementia and parkinsonism is associated with mutations in the tau gene, leading to aberrant function of tau in microtubule assembly. Eleven exons are normally spliced into six different protein isoforms. Exon 10 has a number of repeated microtubule binding domains, and various mutations are associated with increased spliced-in copies of this exon leading to neurodegenerative disease. In spinal muscular atrophy there are mutations or small deletions at the exon splice sites, and the abnormal protein (called survival of motor neuron protein, SMN) may lead to a deficit in snRNP recycling essential to spliceosome function. Other neurological disorders (e.g. spinocerebellar ataxia 8 and amyotrophic lateral sclerosis) may also involve splicing dysfunction. NOVA proteins are a class of neuron-specific splice regulators that are produced from genes on chromosomes other than those harbouring the genes they act on (and are termed *trans*-acting, as opposed to *cis*-acting elements from elsewhere on the same DNA duplex as the gene). High levels of NOVA2, for example, seem restricted to cerebral cortex, hippocampus and dorsal spinal cord. They have KH-binding domains (cf. the similar domain in fragile-X-linked mental retardation protein described in Ch. 24) of a type implicated in splicing activity. NOVA1 is a similar splice regulator restricted to CNS regions controlling movement, and disruption leads to loss of inhibitory control of motor neurons (paraneoplastic opsoclonus myoclonus ataxia) (Dredge et al 2001).

mRNA is also modified by the process of RNA editing, which changes its coding function by converting cytosine residues to uracil, and adenine to inosine, using a series of specific editing enzymes (termed ADAR, APOBEC1 and ACF) (Keegan et al 2001). In mammals most of the ADAR-edited transcripts are expressed in the CNS, increasing again the amount of CNS protein diversity. Inosine-modified RNAs may act to target specific types of mRNA such as the brain-specific small nucleolar RNAs (snoRNAs) that are complementary to mRNA for the $5HT_{2c}$ receptor. Some (controversial) work suggests that $5HT_{2c}$ receptor mRNAs have reduced editing in schizophrenia or increased editing in those who have committed suicide. Editing changes in the GLUR-B gene (prefrontal cortex and striatum) have also been reported in Alzheimer's and Huntington's disease and in schizophrenia.

Finally, altering their decay rate regulates the levels of mRNAs. mRNAs are differentially stable and, although most mRNAs have a fixed half-life, there are a large number in which the levels change in response to environmental stimuli. Decay usually begins with shortening of the 3'-poly-A tail. An initial trimming in the nucleus is followed by a substantial deadenylation after movement of the processed mRNA into the cytoplasm via pores in the nuclear membrane. This is followed by rapid cleavage of the 5'-cap by a variety of factors. Decay of mRNA is tightly controlled by *cis*-acting elements, including some motifs in the 3'- and 5'-UTRs of genes. Signalling pathways can alter decay rate. Interleukin-2 mRNA has 3' and 5' elements that interact with extracellular stimuli such as calcium ionophores and phorbol esters. Aberrant stop codons in mRNA, that generate signals to stop synthesis prematurely, are also recognised and eliminated by rapid decay, helping maintain the fidelity of the RNA. This effect can help minimise the damage caused by premature stop codon abnormalities seen in many patients with diseases such as Duchenne muscular dystrophy (Wilusz et al 2001).

Translation: mRNA to polypeptide

Once mRNA has moved to the cytoplasm (stripped of splicing proteins and actively transported through nuclear pores), it associates with ribosomes in the final steps towards protein synthesis. Again the process is complex. Cytoplasmic translational factors must bind the mRNA to allow it to interact with the ribosome. In some cases inhibiting factors will prevent its translation (e.g. ferritin mRNA is usually inhibited by aconitase which binds with the initial 30 bp, forming a loop that cannot link to ribosomes; only in the presence of cellular iron which binds aconitase is this inhibition removed). Normally a large multi-protein initiation complex forms that positions the mRNA correctly in the ribosomal groove. Amino acids are shuttled to the ribosomal complex attached to tRNA molecules by genetic code-reading activating enzymes. Each tRNA molecule has one anticodon complementary to the codons on the template strand of duplex DNA and carries the amino acid dictated by the genetic code. There are three stages to translation:

- initiation, in which the leading strand of the mRNA is orientated exactly to the initiation protein complex and binds the initiation tRNA (carrying methionine); this is critical to correct reading of the transcribed open reading frame;
- elongation, in which the mRNA codon adjacent to the initiation codon is exposed to tRNA binding, selecting the correct tRNA codon to match and placing its amino acid directly next to methionine, with which it then bonds through a peptide linkage;
- conformational change in the ribosome, brought about by the first two steps, that releases the first tRNA from its amino acid and the ribosome itself and moves the second tRNA into its place, exposing a new codon of mRNA.

Thus the process moves stepwise linearly through the mRNA sequence to the termination step, the stop codon, at which time the polypeptide chain and mRNA are released from the complex again in the presence of specific protein (release) factors.

The control of gene expression from DNA to polypeptide can thus be seen as a complex and highly regulated pathway. The gene unit itself can vary tremendously in size from the very small genes for human tRNAs (around 100 bp long) to the very large genes of certain structural proteins such as dystrophin (2 Mbp and 79 exons; its disruption leads to Duchenne and Becker muscular dystrophies). Most genetic disorders involve disruption to the primary DNA sequence either as large-scale events such as chromosomal trisomies, monosomies and genomic disorders, or in the small scale as mutations within genes.

The genome outside genes

Chromatin is the term used to describe the nucleic-acid–protein complex that gives structure as well as function to the chromosome. As cells leave mitosis or meiosis, large stretches of chromatin become de-condensed and dispersed through the nucleus; Genes are embedded within this 'true' chromatin or euchromatin. Other areas do not de-condense but remain compacted at all stages of the cell cycle. This in general is termed heterochromatin (and classified as constitutive when it is present in all cell types and stages of differentiation; facultative when it is only heterochromatic in certain cells, such as the Barr body which represents the inactivated X-chromosome in females). Constitutive heterochromatin predominates around the centromeres and telomeres of the chromosome. The centromeres are bracketed by long stretches of large repeats of several hundred nucleotides length (satellite DNA), which form into dense heterochromatic noncoding regions (C-bands). This replicates at a different time of the cell cycle (late S phase) from euchromatin, and has large blocks of repeated DNA sequences. Although, historically, heterochromatin was considered inert, more recently it has been shown to have a host of regulatory functions, especially those related to epigenetic programming (see below). In general it contains very few genes but has the capacity to silence genes (a phenomenon called position-effect variegation) that are positioned within it by reason of a chromosomal rearrangement.

It is clear that histone proteins that package DNA are important in maintaining the distinct regional architecture of chromosomes. Histone methyltransferase enzymes (in humans Suv39h protein) selectively methylate histones (H3 histone) at lysine residues. This methylation acts as a signal for protein recruitment (HP1) to the 'chromodomain' on the histone's tail, and is vital for maintaining the transcriptional silence of the heterochromatin (Jenuwein & Allis 2001). It is now realised that a specific pericentromeric RNA species also interacts with the proteins at this site, similar to the situation that exists in the compacted X chromosome in females (see Ch. 24). Thus there seems to be a specific and complex system that maintains the state of heterochromatin (Maison et al 2002). This system may also play a role in epigenetic control of transcriptional activity. Histone methylation signalling motifs that can interact with HP1 are also present for some genes in euchromatin. The histone tail has other modifiable regions including a 'bromodomain' that interacts with de-acetylases, and hypoacetylated histone (H4) is another hallmark of heterochromatin. Histone modification is therefore a key modulator of transcriptional activity in eu- and heterochromatin, and is also crucial to the formation and maintenance of parental-sex-specific methylation that underlies the phenomenon of imprinting.

Much euchromatin is also transcriptionally inactive (90% at some loci) and is highly repetitive in sequence. The polymorphic nature of this DNA has made it useful in linkage studies and has attracted its own nomenclature. Small tandem DNA repeats of a few nucleotides long are termed microsatellites, of several tens of nucleotides minisatellites. Also present are transposable (and probably parasitical) elements (up to 45% of all DNA). Long interspersed nuclear elements (LINEs) are an ancient feature of around 6 kbp long that make up 20% of the genome and contain all the necessary information for self-transposition (including a DNA nickase and reverse transcriptase). Embedded within them are *Alu* sequences (10% genome; 300 bp) that seem to parasitise the LINEs moving with them. There are many other such elements: small interspersed nuclear elements (SINEs), long terminal repeats (LTRs or retroposons), DNA transposons (Prak & Kazazian 2000). One major role of the cell's methylation machinery may be to keep such elements transcriptionally silent. However, repeat sequences can also have other unwanted effects. Low-copy repeats (LCRs or segmental duplications) form over 5% of the genome, are 10–400 kbp long and show very high sequence identity. Their homology can lead to aberrant recombination at meiosis, resulting in segmental duplications and deletions, and their presence is now known to underlie a large number of chromosomal abnormalities such that a new class of conditions — the genomic disorders — has been created to contain them (Stankiewicz & Lupski 2002). They may underlie the complex chromosome 15 duplication events that have been found in Spanish families segregating for panic disorder (Gratacos et al 2001).

Gene mutations

At the simplest level, mutation can be taken to mean an alteration from normal in the DNA sequence of chromosomes. Various sizes of mutations can be delineated, ranging from duplications and deletions of whole chromosomes (trisomy and monosomy) through segmental changes involving short parts of chromosomes (partial monosomy and trisomy), to small deletions and duplications that only affect a few genes at a time (contiguous gene syndromes). These are covered in Chapter 24, and the focus here will be on those DNA changes that affect single gene units.

From the discussion of the genetic code it is clear that the ORF must be read correctly by the polymerase enzyme for the correct amino acids to be assembled into polypeptide. Any change in the sequence of base pairs of DNA within the ORF can lead to errors in reading, and such mutations usually involve one or a few bases (point mutations). If mutations occur in the germline they can be transmitted, and some will arise during the natural process of recombination. Others are caused by errors in the systems that preserve DNA fidelity or by external mutagenic agents (radiation, chemicals). Outside the ORF, mutation gives rise to the great variety of non-coding polymorphisms that are used as tools to study patterns of inheritance and co-segregation. Within the ORF, however, the results can alter transcription. Most changes involve the substitution of one base for another, and 50% of substitutions lead to *missense mutations* where a triplet coding for one amino acid is altered to one that codes for a different amino acid. Depending on the position of the amino acid within the polypeptide and the type of amino acid substituted, this can result in increased or decreased protein activity through to complete loss of function. *Nonsense mutations* (30%) arise when the substitution changes the codon to a stop signal; these are often pathological and usually lead to a decreased level or complete absence of any mRNA formed. The mechanism for silencing the production of the abbreviated mRNA is unclear. The exon position of the nonsense mutation is also important, those in the terminal exons have been sometimes found to have less effect. Nonsense mutations may also produce 'exon skipping' where the exon containing the stop codon is completely bypassed during transcription and an aberrant mRNA is formed. *Silent mutations* are those without phenotypic consequence. The redundancy built into the genetic code means that substitution may lead to an alternative triplet for the same amino acid (synonymous mutation). Insertions and deletions of bases, however, can lead to drastic consequences due to frameshift mutations. Here the entire downstream sequence of the reading frame is disrupted, resulting in a very aberrant mRNA. The disruption is maximal when the deletion or insertion is not a multiple of three (which leads to a resumption of correct frame reading after the mutation has been transcribed).

Mutations in Cytosine-*p*-Guanine dinucleotide pairs (CpG) account for up to a third of the total of single-base-pair mutations. The human genome is heavily methylated at CpG pairs except for specific CpG-dense clusters termed CpG islands that usually lie near or within actively expressed genes. However, all CpGs are very prone to mutation — the mechanism seems to be a conversion of methyl-cytosine to thymine on the coding DNA strand (when this occurs on the non-coding strand the cell mis-corrects the coding base to adenine, leading to G to A transition), and

although later unmethylated, CpG islands are heavily methylated in the early germline. The mutation rate here is much higher in male germline (oocytes are under-methylated), explaining some sex-biases in the origin of mutations (Antonarakis et al 2001).

Mutations can also cause differences in the way mRNA is spliced together. *Splice-junction mutations* as a source of human disorder are not rare (near 10% of all mutations). Failure of splicing may occur or mutations may lead to de novo splice site formation in aberrant positions. The cell may attempt compensation for loss of a splice site by splicing at a second illegitimate site (cryptic splice site), or by exon skipping (as in spinal muscular atrophy). Mutation in 5′ and 3′ UTRs can also be pathogenic. 5′ disruption can lead to disturbance of translational efficiency (as in Charcot–Marie–Tooth syndrome), and 3′ disruption to changed mRNA stability (Mendell & Dietz 2001). Finally, mutations in remote gene promoter and regulatory elements are increasingly recognised.

PATTERNS OF INHERITANCE

Complementary genes on both the paternally and maternally derived autosomes in a cell are normally both transcribed (bi-allelic expression), and a gene mutation on the chromosome derived from one parent usually leads to a reduction (haplo-insufficiency), not absence, of a gene product. The level of product may be sufficient for normal cell function, with no phenotypic consequences unless the complementary gene is also mutated. This situation would present as a classical recessive inheritance pattern. At the other extreme, when silencing or down-regulation of one gene of a pair is functionally uncompensated by the other, the resulting illness would show a dominant pattern (Fig. 9.5).

Mendel studied such phenotype patterns in plant breeding experiments, and suggested that quantal genetic factors were being inherited. Disorders due to the inheritance of a single mutated gene (monogenic disorders) are often said to be Mendelian. Recessive conditions rely on mutations in both genes of the pair — the affected person is usually *homozygous* for the same mutation. If the gene mutations in the paternally and maternally derived chromosomes differ, the offspring is said to be a compound *heterozygote*. The chances of inheriting rare gene mutations from both parents is increased if they are themselves closely related, and an increased rate of consanguinity is often found in recessive disorder. With more common recessive disorders such as cystic fibrosis (1:2500 live births) the frequency of mutations in the population is high. Either new mutation is frequent, or heterozygous carriage confers some reproductive advantage. If both parents carry one copy of the mutant gene then, on average, one in four of their children will be affected. No cases may occur in previous generations, the disease being apparent only in the children — '*horizontal*' inheritance.

Dominant disorders are more common than recessive (7:1000 live births as opposed to 2–3: 1000) and more likely to be associated with late-onset conditions. Fully dominant conditions result in a phenotype whether the person is heterozygous or homozygous for the mutant genes. Affected individuals are found in every generation ('*vertical*' inheritance), and around half of any sibship is affected. Fully dominant disorders are rare, and usually the clinical outcome is variable — especially in heterozygotes because of reduced *penetrance*, measured as the proportion of people heterozygous for the mutation who show any phenotypic feature.

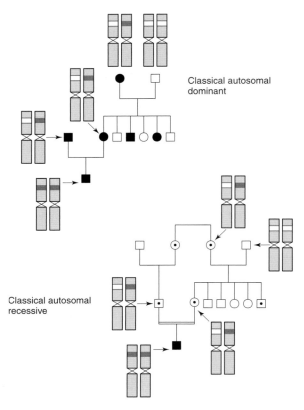

Fig. 9.5
Autosomal inheritance. Affecteds are in black. Chromosomes are given for certain individuals and show mutated (shaded) and wild-type alleles. Squares denote males and circles females. A central dot indicates an unaffected carrier. Consanguinity is shown by a double bar.

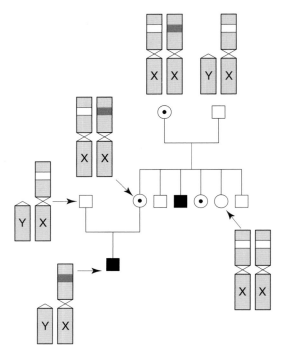

Fig. 9.6
Classical X-linked inheritance. In this case the inheritance is recessive. Affecteds are in black; they are all male. Females are either normal or disease-free carriers (the latter are shown with a central dot). The symbols follow the convention of Figure 9.5. Chromosomes are given for certain individuals and show mutated (shaded) and wild-type alleles on the X chromosomes. The Y chromosomes do not express the given allele.

Mutations in genes on the sex chromosomes form a third Mendelian group. Males can only pass on their Y chromosome to their sons, so that there will be no male-to-male vertical inheritance in X-linked conditions, but affected males are more common in X-linked pedigrees. The mothers of affected males will be carriers of the gene mutation, and either be unaffected (X-linked recessive) or affected (X-linked dominant). A typical presentation is shown in Figure 9.6, and various sex-linked disorders are considered in detail in Chapter 24.

Sometimes one gene may interact with another gene on the same or a different chromosome to influence the expression of a phenotype — a situation termed epistasis. In psychiatry an interesting example of this is shown by the effect on the risk of dementia of interactions between variations in the gene for apolipoprotein E, variations in the gene for amyloid protein, and variations at a separate gene locus on chromosome 10 (Lendon & Craddock 2001). Mutations in completely different genes may cause the same clinical picture (locus heterogeneity). Early-onset Alzheimer's disease provides an example, with mutations known in genes for presenilin I (chromosome 14), presenilin II (chromosome 1) and amyloid precursor protein (chromosome 21). Conversely some diseases may result from different pathogenic mutations within one single gene (allelic heterogeneity). Over 600 different mutations (mainly missense) resulting in cystic fibrosis are known in the cystic fibrosis transmembrane conductance regulator gene (*CFTR*).

Non-Mendelian inheritance

Quantitative trait loci (QTLs)

When the genetic contribution to a disorder is shared by several (oligogenic) or many (polygenic) genes the clinical phenotype is the result of the additive or interactive contributions at each locus. Variation in any single gene associated with a trait is neither necessary nor sufficient on its own to account for the phenotype, and the expression of the phenotype is best described under a liability/threshold model. Many aspects of psychopathology and descriptions of personality can be viewed as quantitative variables where clinical or pathological states represent extremes of a normal continuum of genetic and environmental variation found in the general population. This contrasts with the categorical approach we apply when classifying someone as being depressed or not, using standard criteria. Common conditions and attributes such as hypertension, obesity, cognitive abilities and personality dimensions are understood as quantitative traits, and it is likely that this model will best explain some aspects of common psychiatric conditions such as depression, anxiety and personality disorders. Quantitative trait loci (QTLs) are genes that contribute quantitatively to the variance of a continuous trait, as distinct from single gene mutations that may have a major effect on risk of disease. The methods of quantitative genetics have been widely applied to the analysis of complex heritable traits.

For example, linkage of a QTL for reading ability has been identified on chromosome 6, and it is predicted under this model that when a gene is identified it will be one of several with variants having small but significant effects on reading ability in good as well as poor readers, in other words across the whole spectrum of reading ability. Detecting genes with small effect in common disorders generally requires large, very well-defined study populations, and appropriate methods of linkage and association have been developed. (See pp. 160–162 for a description of these methods of analysis.) A QTL on chromosome 18 that influences the risk of developing dyslexia has been detected by genome scans of two large independent sets of families from the UK and USA and replicated in a further UK sample. This study used 401 polymorphic markers that covered the entire genome and used recent QTL-based variance component linkage analysis and deFries–Fulker regression-based linkage analysis statistical approaches (Fisher et al 2002).

Dynamic mutations

Most inherited disorders do not fall neatly into Mendel's classes. Partial penetrance is the commonest difference, but there are many others. Anticipation is said to occur when a disease has an earlier age-at-onset and increased severity in succeeding generations; it was originally proposed by Mott in 1910, who examined psychiatric illness in parent–offspring pairs. Since then it has been frequently described in psychiatric illness, especially bipolar disorder (Blackwood & Muir 2001). One possible cause is a dynamic mutation involving transgenerational expansion of repeat sequences that alter nearby gene expression dependent on their size. The classical dynamic mutation is the (non-coding) triplet repeat expansion associated with fragile X syndrome, fully described in Chapter 24. Over 20 neurological and developmental conditions are now known to be associated with expanded repeats of nucleotide triplets, but not all involve transgenerational repeat expansion. Those repeats that exist in the ORF of genes (coding dynamic mutations) often have CAG as the repeated triplet base, which then codes for a polyglutamine tract within the protein (Sugars & Rubinsztein 2003). This is the case in Huntington's disease, where the gene on the short arm of chromosome 4 has over 35 CAG triplets within the first exon, and the size of the repeat is related to age-at-onset of the disorder, explaining up to 60% of the variance. The aberrant protein (huntingtin) contains a polyglutamine sequence that alters its function (a gain of function effect). It may interact with nuclear transcription factors and similar proteins to disrupt the expression of other genes. It also forms abnormal complexes with cytoplasmic and nuclear proteins that may be toxic and play a role in neurodegeneration. In fact all eight known CAG expansion diseases have a clinical picture involving neurodegeneration (and all are also typically late-onset). The non-coding repeat in fragile-X syndrome is at the 5′ untranslated end of exon 1, and leads to methylation-driven gene silencing. Other non-coding repeats are known. The myotonic dystrophy type 1 repeat (CTG) is located at the 3′ UTR of the gene, and the pathology is thought to arise from accumulation of abnormal mRNA in the nucleus that then interferes with splicing and other functions. Myotonic dystrophy type 2 is associated with a tetranucleotide repeat (CCTG) in a completely different gene (*ZNF9* on chromosome 3), again untranslated but this time in the first exon. The strikingly similar clinical picture may result from similar patterns of mRNA accumulation leading to general effects on function of the cell nucleus (Ranum & Day 2002). Apart from the neurodegenerative conditions and disorders that are associated with learning disability such as myotonic dystrophy and fragile X syndrome, no convincing evidence has yet emerged for the involvement of repeat expansions in any form in general psychiatric illness.

Epigenetics, imprinting and parent-of-origin effects

Epigenetic mechanisms are those events occurring during development that lead to stable changes in the ability of cells to transcribe DNA. These alterations are heritable from parent to child without involving direct mutations in the DNA itself. There are at least three interacting routes by which such controls on expression are effected: chromatin remodelling, histone alteration and DNA methylation. The latter two may act sequentially to establish the stable state represented by the former. Thus DNA methylation may be the signal for histone modification that may then act to recruit other chromatin modelling proteins, which rearrange chromatin into a stable unexpressed state. DNA methylation occurs mainly at CpG sequences and follows a developmental route that differs between male and female genomes. Its main function seems to be as a signal that recruits cellular factors leading to the transcriptional silencing of associated coding regions of DNA. Originally it may have developed as a repressor of unwanted transcription of the widespread transposable elements that occur in mammalian genome, as well as to differentially regulate developmental gene expression. In the zygote the genome inherited from the father is actively stripped of methylation within hours of fertilisation, whereas methylation of the genome inherited from the mother passively decreases in later cleavage divisions. This de-methylation seems to be an essential 'slate-cleaning' process removing most (but importantly not all) of the inherited parental chromosomal DNA methylation patterns. An extensive de novo re-methylation follows, that then decreases in a tissue-specific fashion, releasing coding regions from their inactive states to produce the necessary proteins for cellular proliferation and differentiation. After methylation, erasure differences between the developmental routes in male and female embryos lead to sexually dimorphic methylation patterns in somatic cells. In germ cells, however, further reprogramming is needed to remove those methylation patterns that escaped the first general round of de-methylation. This is followed by sex-specific re-methylation, completed in developing sperm at a very early stage (pre-mitotic) but much later in ova (pre-meiotic stage). Thus methylation is one way in which the cell can 'mark' or 'imprint' its DNA in a sex-specific pattern.

It has been pointed out that DNA methylation is a system of 'cellular memory' that senses that a silent state is to be stabilised and invokes the mechanisms required for this (Jaenisch & Bird 2003). However, the actual primary marks that set this in play are still unclear. Both in somatic and germ cells the establishment of the correct methylation pattern is very important, and several disorders can result from its disruption. Some chromosomal regions that escape the first round of embryonic de-methylation end up with differential imprinting between loci inherited from mother or father. In such cases monoallelic gene expression is the normal outcome. Such genes usually come in clusters, and there is often a local DNA region that acts as a specific imprint control centre, as in the Prader–Willi/Angelman region (see Ch. 24).

Disruption of this specific imprinting pattern by deletions, uniparental disomy (both chromosomes of a pair originating from only one parent) or imprinting centre mutations can result in these syndromes. Other genes that are normally differentially imprinted include several important fetal growth factors (such as the insulin-related series). Disruption of epigenetic mechanisms may have a consequence for cognitive development (Reik & Walter 2001). More generally, such mechanisms (epimutations) may underlie many non-Mendelian features of psychiatric disorders: discordance in monozygotic twins, age-at-onset effects, sex-specific expression as well as parent-of-origin effects. In fact there is an abundance of parent-of-origin effects described for psychiatric disorders, including bipolar disorder and schizophrenia.

Mitochondrial (cytoplasmic) inheritance

The mitochondria contain DNA that resides outside the nucleus and thus does not segregate in meiosis. In man the mitochondrial DNA (mtDNA) is small (around 16.5 kb), has been entirely sequenced and contains genes particularly involved with oxidative phosphorylation. Since sperm have no mitochondria, inheritance is purely maternal. However, most cells have several copies of this genome, and mutations have been associated with a variety of human neurodegenerative diseases, including a form of deafness. The mutation may only occur in some of the copies, and the expression of the conditions can be very variable.

POPULATION GENETICS

Family, adoption and twin studies

Any disease with a significant genetic causation will tend to aggregate in families, and comparison of rates of illness in relatives with the general population rate will provide a measure of the strength and nature of the genetic contribution. Clustering of disease in families may be entirely the result of shared environment, for example when infections are related to poor living conditions, or shared genetic inheritance as in the case of Huntington's disease where all affected individuals in a family have inherited a mutated *huntingtin* gene. However, most psychiatric conditions are influenced by a mixture of genetic and environmental factors, and to dissect the relative contributions of nature and nurture on family members the two main strategies available are twin and adoption studies.

In general the association between a genetic risk factor and a disease in a population can be expressed as a relative risk (RR) defined as the ratio of the incidence of disease in an 'exposed' group and 'unexposed' groups and measured by studying the illness in population cohorts. To study aggregation of disease within families, it is useful to compare the relative risk of illness in specific groups of relatives with the general population risk. Data is often most easily obtained from siblings, and the relative risk (or risk ratio) for relatives (λr) or specifically for siblings (λs) is frequently used to evaluate the strength and significance of familial aggregation of a disease. λs is defined as the recurrence risk to siblings compared with the risk of the disorder in the general population. A high value of λs reflects a strong genetic effect: for example, in a single gene disorder with dominant inheritance such as Huntington's disease, λs is about 5000; and in cystic fibrosis, a recessive disorder, λs is around 500. Few psychiatric illnesses show

Table 9.1 Relative risk (λr) of common psychiatric conditions, derived from family studies	
	Relative risk in relatives
Attention deficit hyperactivity disorder	55
Autism	45
Schizophrenia	10
Bipolar disorder	7
Alcoholism	6
Generalised anxiety disorder	2–5
Anorexia	2–4
Unipolar depression	1.5–3
After McGuffin et al (2002).	

such clear-cut familial aggregation (Table 9.1). For schizophrenia λs is about 10, and in complex disorders λs greater than 2 is generally taken to indicate a significant genetic component. Caution is needed when evaluating λ because the value depends on the population prevalence of the disease and in general a strong genetic effect in a common disease will generate a smaller λ than the same effect in a rare disease.

Analysis of segregation

If a disease, measured as a discrete trait, is found to be heritable, it is often useful to know whether or not the disease follows Mendelian rules, or if more complex modes of inheritance need be considered. The laws of Mendelian inheritance allow precise predictions of the expected number of affected and unaffected offspring of affected parents, measured as segregation ratios. These ratios also allow prediction of the population frequencies of a disease, and the statistical methods of segregation analysis applied to data on the observed frequencies of a disease in families and the general population lead to predictions of whether the disease is caused by one or more loci.

Family and population data have been extensively studied to elucidate the mode of genetic transmission of schizophrenia. A highly influential book (Gottesman 1991) reviewing the results of several family studies in schizophrenia concluded that the risk of developing schizophrenia in relatives of probands with the disorder is significantly increased in all classes of relatives. In summary the life-time risk of developing schizophrenia and related illness was around 1% in the general population, 10% among first-degree relatives, dropping to about 3% in second-degree relatives. Offspring both of whose parents had schizophrenia had a 40–50% chance of becoming ill. A review of several more recent studies using strict diagnostic criteria (Kendler 2000) found rather similar rates of schizophrenia in these classes of relative, confirming that schizophrenia is a familial disease.

Segregation of illness in families is not consistent with a model of schizophrenia as a simple homogeneous condition caused entirely by a defect in a single major gene or even two or three genes. The mode of inheritance remains unclear, perhaps because schizophrenia is a heterogeneous group of conditions. Genetic findings to date suggest that several, perhaps many, genes are implicated and both Mendelian and non-Mendelian modes of inheritance are possible in different subgroups of the disorder. A multifactorial threshold model gave the best fit to observed family data (McGue & Gottesman 1989). However, in the absence of reliable biological markers, at-risk relatives who carry the genetic risk without developing symptoms cannot be reliably identified, so segregation studies in families based only on clinically defined cases may provide an incomplete picture. There is evidence from linkage studies to suggest that in some families the illness can be attributed to the effect of a single locus, though such families may be uncommon (Blackwood et al 2001).

Family and population studies in bipolar disorder using strict diagnostic criteria have confirmed an increased risk of bipolar disorder in relatives of bipolar probands, with an estimated relative risk in first-degree relatives of 5–10% (Craddock & Jones 1999). Similar studies of unipolar depression have reported relative risk of 1.5–3 for first-degree relatives, variation in results being due to differences in diagnostic criteria and varied estimates of the population prevalence of depression. Affective disorders are probably a heterogeneous group of conditions, and subgroups such as depression with onset early in adult life may show increased familiality. Because unipolar depression is common in the general population, heritability can be measured from large community-based twin registers, and estimates of heritability are in region 30–40% (Sullivan et al 2000). A further observation from the Virginia twin register was an almost complete correlation between generalised anxiety disorder and major depression, indicating that the same genetic factors contribute to depression and anxiety (Kendler et al 1992).

The mode of inheritance of mood disorders is not well understood, and it is probable that a variety of genetic, epigenetic and environmental factors contribute to the risk of illness. Some studies of the segregation of the disorder in families support a model in which single genes of relatively large effect cause illness in some families and different genes will be responsible for illness in different families (major genes with locus heterogeneity) (Rice et al 1987, Blackwood et al 1996). There is also evidence that, in many cases of the disorder, segregation is incompatible with a single major locus and illness may develop as the result of additive or interacting gene variants, each one alone being neither sufficient nor necessary for illness to develop (polygenic model) (Craddock et al 1997). Further complexity arises when we consider that other genetic and epigenetic effects may be important in some but not all families. Genomic imprinting mediated by DNA methylation was proposed as an explanation of an apparent parent-of-origin effect in linkage studies on chromosome 18p in bipolar disorder. Mitochondrial inheritance is another possible explanation of maternal inheritance in a subgroup of families. However, the mitochondrial hypothesis was not supported when the whole mitochondrial genome was sequenced in nine bipolar probands from families showing exclusively maternal transmission (McMahon et al 2000).

Adoption studies

Adoption studies are one of the most powerful ways to disentangle genetic from environmental influences on a disease. There are three main designs of adoption studies, and the choice of design will depend on the available methods of ascertainment.

- *Parent as proband.* One of the first studies of the adopted offspring of mothers diagnosed with schizophrenia was carried out in Oregon, where 47 individuals, adopted shortly after birth when their mothers were receiving institutional care,

were traced in adulthood (Heston 1966). Rates of illness among these adoptees were compared with those in 50 adopted offspring of mothers without psychiatric illness. The striking finding of the Oregon Adoption Study was a significant increase in schizophrenia in the adoptees whose mothers were schizophrenic: 5/47 compared with 0/50 in the control group. Similar findings have come from a much larger, more recent Finnish study of adopted offspring of mothers with schizophrenia (Tienari et al 2000).

- *Adoptee as proband.* In this approach, adopted children who become ill are ascertained and rates of illness are compared in their biological and their adoptive families. Studies carried out in Denmark, where national registers facilitate the tracing of adopted children, showed that 20% of 118 biological relatives and only 6% of 224 adoptive relatives had a diagnosis of schizophrenia. This difference between adoptive and biological relatives was significant (Kety et al 1994). To remove any doubts about the reliability of earlier diagnostic methods, Kendler et al (1994) re-analysed the data from the Danish study, applying strict DSM-III criteria and confirmed a diagnosis of schizophrenia in 8% of first-degree relatives of schizophrenic adoptees, contrasting with only 1% among relatives of control adoptees with no history of schizophrenia.

- *Cross-fostering design.* This compares the rate of illness in two groups of adoptees: one group has ill parents and after adoption has been raised by well parents, the second group has well biological parents but has been brought up in a family where a parent has become ill. Children adopted shortly after birth will still have experienced the pre- and perinatal environment provided by their biological mother and after adoption may suffer greater stress by virtue of being an adoptee. These potential limitations of adoption studies were addressed by the cross-fostering design. The possibility of strong shared environmental influences in utero was addressed by Kety (1976), who studied the rate of illness in a group of paternal half siblings of schizophrenic adoptees and demonstrated an increased incidence of schizophrenia in paternal half siblings that could not be attributed to pre- and perinatal effects. Also children adopted into a home where an adoptive parent becomes ill do not have an increased risk of illness.

Adoption studies in bipolar disorder have similarly confirmed increased rates of affective disorder in biological compared with adoptive relatives of adoptees.

Twin studies

Monozygotic (MZ) or identical twins result from a single fertilised ovum and therefore share all genes, whereas dizygotic (DZ) or fraternal twins are the result of the implantation of two separate fertilised ova and generally share about 50% of genes and are no more alike than other siblings. Since, in general, twins share a very similar cultural, family and educational environment, a comparison of MZ and DZ twins allows an estimate of genetic as well as environmental contributions to their phenotype. *Concordance* rate measures the similarity of phenotype between twins. If both members of a pair of twins develop a disease they are said to be concordant for that condition. For a fully genetic disease showing a dominant pattern of inheritance, concordance will be 100% in MZ twins and around 50% in DZ twins. In the case of a recessive disorder, DZ concordance will be about 25%. When a disease is entirely due to environmental causes we expect to find no difference in concordance rates in MZ and DZ twin pairs. Most psychiatric disorders are likely to be a result of both genetic and non-genetic factors, and concordance rates in MZ twins may be quite small, but a significant genetic contribution will be indicated by the comparison of MZ and DZ rates. The simplest way to measure this is pairwise concordance defined as the number of pairs of twins where both are affected divided by the total number of pairs studied. More commonly the probandwise concordance is quoted, and this is the number of affected co-twins with an affected proband divided by the total number of co-twins in the study. The mode of ascertainment of the sample of twins used in the study is very important and, unless an entire population has been systematically screened, probandwise concordance will be different from pairwise concordance because some twins will be counted twice if they have been independently ascertained for probandwise analysis.

In a classic twin study of schizophrenia, Gottesman & Shields (1972) found in their sample 11 concordant and 11 discordant pairs of MZ twins and 3 concordant and 30 discordant DZ pairs of twins. This gives a pairwise concordance rate of 11/22 = 50% for MZ and 3/33 = 10% for DZ twins. In the same sample, proband concordance was calculated to be 58% for MZ twins and 12% for DZ twins. The difference between the two methods of analysis arose because in 4/11 pairs of concordant MZ twins both of the twins were ascertained independently, so in effect counted twice, to calculate pairwise concordance. Similarly 1/3 pairs of concordant DZ twins were ascertained independently. This illustrates the importance of ascertainment in twin studies. Both analyses yielded significant differences between MZ and DZ concordance, proving a genetic effect. Early reports have been substantially supported by several more recent twin studies where probandwise concordance for MZ twins ranged between 40% and 65% compared with a range of 0–30% in DZ twin pairs (Cardno & Gottesman 2000). An important study of the offspring of MZ twins discordant for schizophrenia found that the children of unaffected co-twins inherited the same increased risk of schizophrenia as their cousins who were offspring of the affected twin (Kringlen & Cramer 1989). This suggests that the interpretation of 'environmental' risk in twin studies requires explanation because environment may include epigenetic risk factors that influence the expression of a gene in an individual but do not involve changes in the genome. Twin studies in schizophrenia report a concordance rate for MZ twins of around 50%, but it would be wrong to conclude that half of the variation in phenotype can be attributed to peri- or postnatal causes; the risk attributed to 'environment' includes non-transmitted biochemical effects on genes, for example the random variation that occurs in DNA methylation, a process that may alter gene expression but is not heritable.

In bipolar disorder, twin studies yield essentially similar findings as in schizophrenia. MZ concordance rates of 40–60% are significantly greater than DZ concordance rates, and the risk of bipolar illness in the offspring of MZ twins discordant for the disorder was the same among offspring of the affected and unaffected co-twins (Jones et al 2002).

MAPPING AND FINDING GENES

When family, adoption and twin studies have identified a substantial genetic contribution to a disease, different strategies can be followed for identifying genes. A 'functional' approach requires the selection of candidate genes to be directly examined for mutations. The selection of candidate genes is usually based on knowledge of the biology or pharmacology of the disease; but because, for most psychiatric conditions, we have no clear understanding of the underlying neurobiology, the range of possible candidates could include most of the 10 000 or more genes expressed in the brain. A 'positional' strategy aims to identify the approximate chromosomal location of genes using the methods of linkage analysis in families, association studies in populations, or mapping of cytogenetic anomalies in individuals. Regions of the genome thus identified are further examined by association studies, and candidates are selected from the genes known to reside within the region of linkage. A positional approach has been successful in identifying genes responsible for many single-gene disorders — including cystic fibrosis, Huntington's disease, muscular dystrophy and some familial cases of Alzheimer's disease—and does not rely on prior knowledge of the biology of the disease permitting the discovery of previously unknown genes.

Isolated populations that have low levels of out-breeding can be used to detect rare recessive conditions by examining regions inherited in common from shared ancestors (homozygosity mapping). This also reduces the problem of locus heterogeneity where several causal genes may give the same phenotype in a population admixture. Consanguinity has helped map over two hundred recessive genes in the last decade (Botstein & Risch 2003). Severity of disease also tends to correlate strongly with severity of the underlying gene mutation. For many diseases, identifying the mutation underlying the severe form has revealed other mutations that have milder outcomes (e.g. *Dystrophin* mutations in Duchenne muscular dystrophy and the milder Becker form). In fact it is such severe high-risk mutations that are selected for in most linkage studies, and subsequent gene cloning leads to identification of more frequent, but milder mutations. Single-gene mutational heterogeneity explains some clinical phenotypic variance; other modifier genes and environmental effects contribute to the rest.

Linkage analysis

Linkage studies look for the co-segregation of polymorphic DNA markers with disease in families. Studies on single large pedigrees, on many small two-generation families or on large numbers of pairs of affected siblings are widely adopted strategies.

The basis of linkage analysis is the recombination that takes place between pairs of homologous chromosomes during meiosis. On average, recombination takes place at two places on each chromosome during every meiosis, and the recombination fraction (denoted by θ) is the probability that a recombination event will occur between two markers or between a marker and a disease locus. Recombination fraction is a useful measure because over short distances it is a measure of the physical distance between two markers on a chromosome. When two genes are physically far apart on a chromosome they will usually become separated by recombination during meiosis and will assort independently of each other just as if they were on separate chromosomes (Mendel's Law of Independent Assortment). In general, the closer a polymorphic marker is to a disease locus, the more likely it is that the two will remain together from one generation to the next, because the chance of a recombination taking place between them is proportional to the physical distance that separates them. If two points are separated by a million base pairs of DNA (megabase Mb) then recombination will occur between them roughly once in every 100 meioses, which is 100 generations, and the statistical unit to describe this rate of recombination is termed the centimorgan (cM). The effect of recombination is analogous to cutting a pack of cards. The chance that two cards will be separated by the cut is proportional to how far apart they are in the pack and two consecutive cards are the least likely to be separated by repeated cutting. Genes far apart on the same chromosome co-segregate randomly and have a 50:50 chance of remaining on the same chromosome following meiosis. In a family linkage study the recombination fraction (θ) will therefore lie between 0 (indicating that a polymorphic marker is a physical part of the gene responsible for the disease so the marker and the gene never become separated) and 0.5 (completely independent assortment of marker and gene). For analysis of linkage the recombination fraction between a marker and disease locus can be measured directly in a family or group of families simply by counting the number of recombinant individuals, divided by the total number of offspring. Figure 9.7 illustrates the segregation of two markers in a family and the principles of linkage analysis. In large families calculation of

linkage is complex and the recombination fraction is estimated by the method of maximum likelihood and calculated using 'linkage' computer programs (Ott 1999). The conventional statistical method to test for linkage is to calculate the LOD (Log of the Odds) score from the recombination fraction. It is conventionally accepted that a LOD score of 3 (odds in favour of linkage of 1000:1) is considered proof of linkage and conversely a LOD score of –2 (odds against linkage of 100:1) is accepted as exclusion.

Linkage analysis is an important tool for the analysis of genetic loci, exploiting the immense amount of sequence variation found across the human genome. Typically a genome-wide screen for linkage in a group of families multiply affected by a disease will employ several hundred microsatellite markers or several thousand SNPs chosen to be evenly spaced at intervals of less than 10 cM across all chromosomes. Regions of interest may be further examined with a denser series of markers. Many independent linkage studies, including whole genome scans in large collections of multiply affected families or affected pairs of siblings, have been reported in schizophrenia and manic depressive illness with some encouraging convergence of results (Riley & McGuffin 2000, Baron 2002).

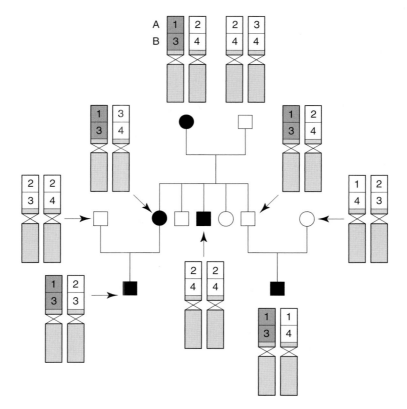

Fig. 9.7
The segregation of two polymorphic markers at two hypothetical points that lie close together on an autosome in a small family. Both markers are bi-allelic; for example, they might represent a single-nucleotide polymorphism (SNP). The allelotypes at locus A are (arbitrarily) labelled 1 and 2, and those at B are labelled 3 and 4. In this example the two loci are tightly linked together, and within this pedigree there are no examples of recombination between the homologous chromosomes. However, the presence of different allele combinations in those marrying into the pedigree suggests that this would not be the case if we could examine a considerable number of meioses. In addition to being close to each other on the chromosome, the markers have a combination of alleles (shaded 1,3) present in all individuals with the proposed disorder (the black pedigree symbols). Linkage analysis tests statistically whether such apparent segregation is likely to have occurred by chance. If this is unlikely, then a locus that increases the susceptibility of the diathesis lies close to the markers on the chromosome. Also note that, although apparently autosomal dominant, the disorder is not fully penetrant, and an unaffected individual who must carry the susceptibility locus occurs in the middle generation.

Some genes of apparently large effect have been detected in studies of extended families, although these may be relatively rare causes of illness in the general population. Large numbers of affected pairs of siblings are easier to recruit than large pedigrees, and if very large cohorts are studied the approach is suited to the detection of genes of small effects predicted under a polygenic model. However, if substantial locus heterogeneity is present, this approach requires unrealistically large samples. A large number of linkage projects using both strategies have been completed in the past two decades, and evidence for linkage, supported by more than one study, has emerged in several chromosomal regions. In a single family, carriers of a reciprocal translocation t(1;11)(q42.2;q21) which was stably inherited in a large Scottish pedigree were shown to have very high rates of major psychiatric illness when compared with non-carriers. The strongest evidence for linkage (LOD score of 7.1) was found with a phenotype that included both schizophrenia and affective psychosis, and linkage was also found at this region in families from the Finnish population (Blackwood et al 2001, Ekelund et al 2000). Candidate genes for schizophrenia, *Disrupted In Schizophrenia 1* (*DISC1*) and *Disrupted In Schizophrenia 2* (*DISC2*) were detected by cloning the translocation breakpoint (Millar et al 2000). Chromosome 22q11 is another region where a chromosomal abnormality has initially focused the search for genes. A small interstitial deletion at this location causes the velocardiofacial syndrome (VCFS), and patients with the disorder have characteristic congenital abnormalities in addition to carrying a substantially increased risk of psychosis. The deletion encompasses several candidate genes — including genes coding catechol-*O*-methyltransferase (COMT) and the G-protein-coupled receptor kinase 3 (GRK3), for which there is some evidence for association in schizophrenia and bipolar disorder. Linkage to a region on chromosome 6p was identified in Irish families, and evidence has been recently presented that a candidate gene in that region, *Dysbindin*, is associated with schizophrenia (Straub et al 2002). On chromosome 8p several groups have reported linkage, and the gene *Neuregulin-1* (*NRG1*) shows association with schizophrenia in the Icelandic and Scottish populations (Stefansson et al 2002, 2003). Other regions identified by linkage in families with schizophrenia include 13q, 6q, 2p, 5q, 6q, 10p and 13q. The focus is now to identify genes at these regions of interest and to study the expression patterns and biological functions of candidate genes in the regions.

Family linkage studies have identified several chromosome regions likely to harbour genes implicated in bipolar disorder. Recent results have been encouraging and chromosome regions identified in more than one linkage study include 1q, 4p, 6p, 10p, 10q, 12q, 13q, 18p, 18q, 21q, 22q and Xp. Further linkage studies may show that some of these are false positive findings, but it is likely that some are true linkages. The task of finding genes in these regions, using methods of linkage disequilibrium mapping and direct sequencing of candidate genes, is not trivial, because linkage typically has low resolution for locating genes and defines a broad chromosome region. For example the candidate region identified by linkage on chromosome 4 may contain around 50 genes, several of which are candidates for a role in mental disorders. At some chromosome regions linkage evidence has been consistently reported for both schizophrenia and bipolar disorders. A possible overlap of genetic risk of these conditions remains speculative, but the possibility of some genes contributing to increased risk of schizophrenia and affective disorders remains strong. At one such region on chromosome 13q

two novel linked genes, *G72/G30*, have been described (Hattori et al 2003).

Association studies

Linkage analysis is performed on families with more than one affected relative whereas association studies compare the frequency of alleles of a DNA marker in populations of patients and healthy controls. In the search for genes these two approaches are entirely complementary. The idea of association is simpler and is well known through the long-established association between HLA subtypes and some common diseases, including diabetes, rheumatoid arthritis and ankylosing spondylitis. When one allele of a DNA polymorphism, for example a SNP or a microsatellite marker, is found more commonly in a disease population than controls the marker and disease are said to be associated or in 'linkage disequilibrium'. This could occur because the polymorphic marker itself is a variant that directly influences the phenotype. One example is the association of late-onset Alzheimer's disease with ApoE4. The frequency of ApoE4 is about 0.4 in individuals with Alzheimer's disease compared with 0.15 in controls. This QTL increases the liability to develop dementia but is neither sufficient nor necessary to cause illness. Linkage disequilibrium may also occur between a disease and a polymorphic marker situated very close to the disease-related gene but not involved in causing the disease phenotype. When the marker and the disease gene are physically close on the genome they are less likely to become separated by recombination over many generations. In this situation, association between a disease and a polymorphic marker in a population can be explained by a founder effect when a significant proportion of people with the disease are the descendants of a single founder person who introduced the disease to the population many generations previously. Descendants with the disease will have inherited the disease-related gene together with the DNA sequence immediately surrounding that mutation. The more closely to the gene a DNA polymorphism is located the less it is likely to be separated by recombination, and the association of the polymorphism with disease will remain over many generations. The ideal setting for an association study would thus be a completely isolated island population where the disease had been introduced many generations previously by a single founder and all the people with the disease being studied were descended from that person. In practice, association studies are successfully carried out, for example in European populations, provided cases and controls are carefully matched for age and ethnic origin. Linkage disequilibrium typically extends over very short distances of a few hundred kilobases, giving much higher resolution for mapping genes than can be achieved by linkage strategies.

Candidate genes

Genes coding proteins related to neurotransmitter function, including dopamine, noradrenaline, serotonin, GABA and glutamate neurotransmission, have been extensively investigated in schizophrenia and bipolar disorder by association studies and directly for mutations by sequencing. Evidence that variants in neurotransmitter-related genes have a substantial causative role in schizophrenia remain unconfirmed, but studies on the gene on chromosome 22 coding for the enzyme COMT, which show significant association with schizophrenia, provide an illustration of the difficulties of establishing a link between a candidate gene and a complex disorder such as schizophrenia. The gene coding COMT is a strong candidate for a role in schizophrenia because of its biological function and its chromosomal location. COMT is one of the enzymes that degrades catecholamines, and the gene that codes it is located within the small region on chromosome 22 deleted in patients with velocardiofacial syndrome, a condition that carries an increased risk of schizophrenia. Numerous linkage and association studies around this region had produced conflicting results but very strong association was detected by Shifman et al (2002). In this study the important factors contributing to the detection of association were the large sample size (4800 controls and over 700 patients), a homogeneous study population and the use of several polymorphic markers in the association study (12 SNPs across the gene were genotyped), allowing analysis of association with individual markers and also with haplotypes made up of groups of these markers. The evidence from this study suggests that variants of the COMT gene are risk factors in schizophrenia.

Monoamine oxidase (MAO), another key enzyme in amine metabolism, has shown association with bipolar disorder in some studies, but the effects are small and not replicated. Specific serotonin reuptake inhibitors (SSRIs) are a mainstay of pharmacotherapy in the treatment of depression, and it is logical that their substrate, the human SErotonin Reuptake Transporter (hSERT), and its gene on the long arm of chromosome 17 have been the focus of intensive study. A polymorphism (a variable number tandem repeat or VNTR) affects the function of the gene, and there is evidence that the 12-repeat allele modestly increases the susceptibility to bipolar disorder in Caucasian populations. The primary function of aminergic neurotransmitters is to interact with a postsynaptic receptor to achieve their signalling actions. These membrane-bound receptor proteins are key candidates for dysfunction in psychiatric illness. The serotonergic receptor system has been examined both at the sequence level and by association analysis for seven of the 5HT receptor types, with very mixed results — with both positive and negative findings in abundance (Potash & DePaulo 2000).

Dopaminergic receptors have been more extensively studied in patients with schizophrenia than with bipolar disorder, and here again the results have been mixed. An example is DRD5 the gene encoding the type 5 dopamine receptor, which is found especially in the limbic and frontal cortex in human brain. This is strongly associated with schizophrenia but not bipolar disorder (Muir et al 2001) and yet lies within a region of linkage to bipolar disorder on chromosome 4. The confusing results that emerge from association studies of neurotransmitter systems may arise because studies are too small to detect genes that are components of a polygenic system.

Cytogenetic studies

Cloning disrupted genes from rare chromosomal rearrangements has been a very fruitful approach for a wide variety of inherited neurological conditions because — in contrast to linkage and association studies, where the results, even if positive, define broad areas at the molecular level — abnormalities of chromosomes can precisely pinpoint the position of disrupted genes (Evans et al 2001). Examples of the success of this approach are:

- the discovery of the novel genes DISC1 and DISC2 at the breakpoint of a translocation on chromosome 1 in a family with schizophrenia;

- the analysis of candidate genes including COMT, PRODH2 and the G-protein-coupled receptor kinase 3 (GRK3) in the region on chromosome 22 deleted in the velocardiofacial syndrome;
- the discovery of DIBD1 (Disrupted in Bipolar Disorder 1).

A small pedigree was described with a t(9;11)(p24;q23.1) translocation co-segregating with affective disorders. Five relatives who carried the translocation had bipolar disorder and one had early-onset recurrent major depression. A mannosyltransferase gene was shown to be disrupted by the chromosome 11 breakpoint (Baysal et al 2002) and labelled DIBD1 (Disrupted in Bipolar Disorder 1) a 15-exon brain-expressed gene that is possibly involved in protein N-glycosylation. This is one of the first novel genes described thought to have a role in bipolar disorder.

REFERENCES

Antonarakis S E, Krawczak M, Cooper D N 2001 The nature and mechanisms of human gene mutation. In: Scriver C R et al (eds) The metabolic & molecular bases of inherited disease. McGraw-Hill, New York, p 343–377

Baron M 2002 Manic-depression genes and the new millennium: poised for discovery. Molecular Psychiatry 7: 342–358

Baysal B E, Willett-Brozick J E, Badner J A et al 2002 A mannosyltransferase gene at 11q23 is disrupted by a translocation breakpoint that co-segregates with bipolar affective disorder in a small family. Neurogenetics 4: 43–53

Blackwood D, Muir W 2001 Molecular genetics and the epidemiology of bipolar disorder. Annals of Medicine 33: 242–247

Blackwood D H, He L, Morris S W et al 1996 A locus for bipolar affective disorder on chromosome 4p. Nature Genetics 12: 427–430

Blackwood D H, Fordyce A, Walker M T et al 2001 Schizophrenia and affective disorders — cosegregation with a translocation at chromosome 1q42 that directly disrupts brain-expressed genes: clinical and P300 findings in a family. American Journal of Human Genetics 69: 428–433

Botstein D, Risch N 2003 Discovering genotypes underlying human phenotypes: past successes for mendelian disease, future approaches for complex disease. Nature Genetics 33(suppl): 228–237

Cardno A G, Gottesman I I 2000 Twin studies of schizophrenia: from bow-and-arrow concordances to star wars Mx and functional genomics. American Journal of Medical Genetics 97: 12–17

Craddock N, Jones I 1999 Genetics of bipolar disorder. Journal of Medical Genetics 36: 585–594

Craddock N, Van Eerdewegh P, Reich T 1997 Single major locus models for bipolar disorder are implausible. American Journal of Medical Genetics 74: 18–20

Dredge B K, Polydorides A D, Darnell R B 2001 The splice of life: alternative splicing and neurological disease. Nature Reviews Neuroscience 2: 43–50

Ekelund J, Lichtermann D, Hovatta I et al 2000 Genome-wide scan for schizophrenia in the Finnish population: evidence for a locus on chromosome 7q22. Human Molecular Genetics 9: 1049–1057

Evans K L, Muir W J, Blackwood D H, Porteous D J 2001 Nuts and bolts of psychiatric genetics: building on the Human Genome Project. Trends in Genetics 17: 35–40

Fisher S E, Francks C, Marlow A J et al 2002 Independent genome-wide scans identify a chromosome 18 quantitative-trait locus influencing dyslexia. Nature Genetics 30: 86–91

Friedberg E C 2003 DNA damage and repair. Nature 421: 436–440

Gottesman I I 1991 Schizophrenia genesis: the origins of madness. Freeman, New York

Gottesman I I, Shields J 1972 Schizophrenia and genetics: a twin study vantage point. Academic Press, New York

Gratacos M, Nadal M, Martin-Santos R et al 2001 A polymorphic genomic duplication on human chromosome 15 is a susceptibility factor for panic and phobic disorders. Cell 106: 367–379

Hattori E, Liu C, Badner J A et al 2003 Polymorphisms at the g72/g30 gene locus, on 13q33, are associated with bipolar disorder in two independent pedigree series. American Journal of Human Genetics 72: 1131–1140

Heston L L 1966 Psychiatric disorders in foster home reared children of schizophrenic mothers. British Journal of Psychiatry 112: 819–825

Jaenisch R, Bird A 2003 Epigenetic regulation of gene expression: how the genome integrates intrinsic and environmental signals. Nature Genetics 33(suppl): 245–254

Jenuwein T, Allis C D 2001 Translating the histone code. Science 293: 1074–1080

Jones I, Kent L, Craddock N 2002 Genetics of affective disorders. In: McGuffin P, Owen M J, Gottesman I I (eds) Psychiatric genetics & genomics. Oxford University Press, Oxford, p 211–245

Keegan L P, Gallo A, O'Connell M A 2001 The many roles of an RNA editor. Nature Reviews Genetics 2: 869–878

Kendler K S 2000 Schizophrenia genetics. In: Sadock B J, Sadock V A (eds) Kaplan and Sadock's comprehensive textbook of psychiatry, 7th edn. Lippincott, Williams & Wilkins, Philadelphia, p 1147–1159

Kendler K S, Gruenberg A M, Kinney D K 1994 Independent diagnoses of adoptees and relatives as defined by DSM-III in the provincial and national samples of the Danish Adoption Study of Schizophrenia. Archives of General Psychiatry 51: 456–468

Kendler K S, Neale M C, Kessler R C et al 1992 Major depression and generalized anxiety disorder. Same genes, (partly) different environments? Archives of General Psychiatry 49: 716–722

Kety S S, Wender P H, Jacobsen B et al 1994 Mental illness in the biological and adoptive relatives of schizophrenic adoptees. Replication of the Copenhagen Study in the rest of Denmark. Archives of General Psychiatry 51: 442–455

Kety S S 1976 Studies designed to disentangle genetic and environmental variables in schizophrenia: some epistemological questions and answers. American Journal of Psychiatry 133: 1134–1137

Kringlen E, Cramer G 1989 Offspring of monozygotic twins discordant for schizophrenia. Archives of General Psychiatry 46: 873–877

Lendon C, Craddock N 2001 Susceptibility gene(s) for Alzheimer's disease on chromosome 10. Trends in Neurosciences 24: 557–559

Maison C, Bailly D, Peters A H et al 2002 Higher-order structure in pericentric heterochromatin involves a distinct pattern of histone modification and an RNA component. Nature Genetics 30: 329–334

McGue M, Gottesman II 1989 A single dominant gene still cannot account for the transmission of schizophrenia. Archives of General Psychiatry 46: 478–480

McGuffin P, Owen M J, Gottesman II 2002 Psychiatric genetics and genomics. Oxford University Press, Oxford

McMahon F J, Chen Y S, Patel S et al 2002 Mitochondrial DNA sequence diversity in bipolar affective disorder. American Journal of Psychiatry 157: 1058–1064

Mendell J T, Dietz H C 2001 When the message goes awry: disease-producing mutations that influence mRNA content and performance. Cell 107: 411–414

Millar J K, Wilson-Annan J C, Christie S et al 2000 Disruption of two novel genes by a translocation co-segregating with schizophrenia. Human Molecular Genetics 22: 1415–1423

Muir W J, Thomson M L, McKeon P et al 2001 Markers close to the dopamine D5 receptor gene (DRD5) show significant association with schizophrenia but not bipolar disorder. American Journal of Medical Genetics 105: 152–158

Ott J 1999 Analysis of human genetic linkage. Johns Hopkins University Press, Baltimore

Potash J B, DePaulo J R Jr 2000 Searching high and low: a review of the genetics of bipolar disorder. Bipolar Disorders 2: 8–26

Prak E T, Kazazian H H Jr 2000 Mobile elements and the human genome. Nature Reviews Genetics 1: 134–144

Ranum L P, Day J W 2002 Dominantly inherited, non-coding microsatellite expansion disorders. Current Opinion in Genetics & Development 12: 266–271

Reik W, Walter J 2001 Genomic imprinting: parental influence on the genome. Nature Reviews Genetics 2: 21–32

Rice J, Reich T, Andreasen N C et al 1987 The familial transmission of bipolar illness. Archives of General Psychiatry 44: 441–447

Riley B P, McGuffin P 2000 Linkage and associated studies of schizophrenia. American Journal of Medical Genetics 97: 23–44

Scholey J M, Brust-Mascher I, Mogilner A 2003 Cell division. Nature 422: 746–752

Shifman S, Bronstein M, Sternfeld M et al 2002 A highly significant association between a COMT haplotype and schizophrenia. American Journal of Human Genetics 71: 1296–1302

Stankiewicz P, Lupski J R 2002 Genome architecture, rearrangements and genomic disorders. Trends in Genetics 18: 74–82

Stefansson H, Sigurdsson E, Steinthorsdottir V et al 2002 Neuregulin 1 and susceptibility to schizophrenia. American Journal of Human Genetics 71: 877–892

Stefansson H, Sarginson J, Kong A et al 2003 Association of neuregulin 1 with schizophrenia confirmed in a Scottish population. American Journal of Human Genetics 72: 83–87

Straub R E, Jiang Y, MacLean C J et al 2002 Genetic variation in the 6p22.3 gene DTNBP1, the human ortholog of the mouse dysbindin gene, is associated with schizophrenia. American Journal of Human Genetics 71: 337–348

Sugars K L, Rubinsztein D C 2003 Transcriptional abnormalities in Huntington disease. Trends in Genetics 19: 233–238

Sullivan P F, Neale M C, Kendler K S 2000 Genetic epidemiology of major depression: review and meta-analysis. American Journal of Psychiatry 157: 1552–1562

Tienari P, Wynne L C, Moring J et al 2000 Finnish adoptive family study: sample selection and adoptee DSM-III-R diagnoses. Acta Psychiatrica Scandinavica 101: 433–443

Wilusz C J, Wormington M, Peltz S W 2001 The cap-to-tail guide to mRNA turnover. Nature Reviews Molecular Cell Biology 2: 237–246

10 | Epidemiology and research methods

Stephen M Lawrie, Peter Sandercock

INTRODUCTION

Epidemiology can be defined as 'the study of the distribution and determinants of health-related states or events in specified populations' (Last 1995) or simply as examinations of the frequency and associations of disease. It includes the study of causes, in terms of aetiological or risk factors, but does not include the study of pathophysiological mechanisms, which is the province of biomedical research. These two approaches, however, are obviously complementary, and the fundamental methods used are the same. Both 'psychiatric epidemiologists' and 'biological psychiatrists' pay close attention to case identification, control selection, accurate measurement and minimising bias in executing and interpreting research studies. Both can choose from a variety of research methods to study a particular issue, constrained by what is practicable.

Research — as simply 'the organized quest for new knowledge' (Last 1995) — has a long history, whereas epidemiology is generally regarded as having begun (in 1849!) with John Snow's famous localisation of an outbreak of cholera in London to a particular water pump. The methods that both employ have, however, been considerably developed since that time, particularly over the last fifty years or so, and continue to be refined. It is, for example, only comparatively recently that the case report and case series have been superseded by controlled studies of the causes and treatments of disease (Hennekens & Buring 1987). Much of contemporary medicine remains on comparatively shaky scientific foundations, and it is only through carefully conducted further study that we will be able to further improve on what we can currently offer our patients. Laboratory-based basic science ('blue skies research') and population-based epidemiology aim to deliver a greater understanding of the causes of disease, with the prospect of earlier detection, better treatment and even prevention. Therapeutic and health services research seeks to refine currently available treatments, optimise their delivery to those most likely to benefit, and be able to test any new therapies as and when they arise. Progress may seem frustratingly slow, but that is inevitable if the science is to be rigorously conducted and evaluated.

Epidemiology and research methods also underpin clinical practice in other ways. Several components of public health necessarily use such principles in determining disease prevalence and needs assessment for planning services, implementing and evaluating disease screening and assessing the population impact of causative factors with a view to prevention. The application of epidemiological and statistical principles to everyday clinical decisions used to be described as clinical epidemiology (Sackett et al 1991) and has, over the past 10 years or so, led to the development and implementation of evidence-based medicine. These statistics and their interpretation are discussed in the following two chapters. In this chapter, we shall briefly describe the three main classes of research study, before going over the principles, strengths and limitations of specific types. We shall then discuss the issues to be addressed in determining whether any observed association is causal, and conclude with a brief guide to conducting research studies and to the main interviews and rating scales currently used in psychiatric research. Before we go any further, we shall highlight the key ethical principles and some contemporary issues.

ETHICAL CONSIDERATIONS

The ethics of clinical research rest upon and are little different from the ethics of clinical practice. The fundamental principles of least harm, confidentiality and informed consent, which are the cornerstones of good clinical practice, are the same (Wing 1981). Clinicians and medical researchers both confront these issues daily. The principal difference between the two is that research does not aim to directly benefit an individual, although it may do so, whereas clinical practice does have this aim but may not. Even this distinction is muddied when one considers innovative clinical practice and audit.

Above all, do no harm   Most research does not lead to any harm to those involved. Indeed, there is some evidence that patient outcomes are better if treated within the disciplined context of a clinical trial than in routine clinical practice. Some procedures are physically or 'mentally' invasive, but usually lead only to transient discomfort or distress. This is also true of pharmacological evaluation studies. If a comparatively new product is being tested, then some insurance or indemnity agreement may be necessary for potentially serious adverse effects. Provided any risks are minimised and frankly acknowledged, so that truly informed consent is possible, these types of study do not pose any particular ethical issues.

There have, however, been extensive recent discussions about whether placebo-controlled trials are ethical in serious diseases, where there are standard treatments of proven efficacy, following the recommendation in the fifth revision of the Declaration of Helsinki (Vastag 2000) that they should no longer be conducted. This is a complex issue, as placebo-controlled trials provide their own check of internal validity – and trials comparing new and old drugs need to be much larger than these if they are to have enough power to show true equivalence rather than just no difference. It may not be ethically acceptable to compare any new antipsychotic or antidepressant drug against placebo, given that the evidence for the efficacy of the standard treatments is generally regarded as overwhelming, but it is definitely unethical to conduct research that cannot deliver a reliable answer. Many medical trials get round this problem by comparing a new treatment plus standard care versus standard treatment. At the very least, researchers clearly need to pay close attention to what kind of treatment participants are offered at the termination of a trial, particularly if they have been treated with placebo.

Maintain confidentiality   Research data are technically part of a person's medical record and are, therefore, confidential. Scientific data should generally be stored anonymously and in a locked facility. Issues of confidentiality rarely give rise to problems during research projects – if something of clinical relevance is discovered, it should be communicated to the patient's own doctor, and usually to the patient, as it is in the latter's best interests to do so. Following the UK Data Protection Act of 1998, however, there is some ambiguity and continuing debate about whether routinely collected clinical data can be used without the patients' explicit consent (Al-Shahi & Warlow 2000). This applies equally to clinical records, local case registers and national databases. Some have argued that the data can be used for audit but not for observational research, but this double-standard might well be against the public interest. Observational studies using this data have delivered important insights and clinical advances.

Obtain informed consent   Particular attention needs to be paid to the process of enrolling participants in any study. Potential subjects should be able to give 'fully informed consent' in that they fully appreciate the purpose and nature of the study, as well as the potential risks and benefits to them. This is an unarguable principle but easier said than done. Even people of above average IQ have difficulty understanding some scientific concepts (e.g. randomisation), cannot be expected to grasp subtle academic points, and can only be meaningfully informed about and retain the principal risks involved (cf. consent to clinical treatments). The information given obviously has to be selective, but there is no guidance on how. It is clear, however, that there is a potential for conflict of interest if patients' clinicians are seeking to enrol them in their own studies — if so, an independent clinician should be involved in seeking consent.

There may be particular issues about obtaining valid informed consent in people with psychiatric disorders and learning disabilities, but these are often overstated in a potentially prejudicial way (Roberts et al 2002). Patients who are detained (or imprisoned) are rarely included in, and often specifically excluded from, most research and clinical trials in particular. They may well still be capable of consenting to a study and are arguably worse served by a dearth or complete absence of relevant treatment information. Some recent reports, highlighted in a number of American and European newspapers, have suggested that even relatively stable psychotic patients may fail one or more of a number of criteria that establish whether somebody is able to give informed consent. Some work indicates that this problem is related more to cognitive impairment than psychotic symptoms, and can be overcome by spending more time with potential subjects (Carpenter et al 2000).

Ethical issues arise during the planning, conduct and analysis stages of any investigation. A worthwhile study needs to address a genuinely unresolved question with robust methods that are likely to provide a useful answer. It is therefore desirable to conduct a systematic review of the available evidence before any new study, both to check the question has not already been answered and to inform design. Studies which are poorly designed or likely to be inconclusive are unethical, as they expose patients to unnecessary and potentially dangerous interventions. If there is a sound rationale for doing a particular study, a research protocol needs to be submitted along with answers to standard questions to local Ethical Committees. Ethical Committee practices vary, however, from region to region and country to country. This has given rise to the unsatisfactory situation where an ethical application for a multicentre trial may be approved in one region, but rejected in another (Savulescu et al 1996). Research participants should not be paid for doing research, but they are entitled to receive compensation for, e.g., travel and subsistence expenses. It need hardly be said that fraudulent analyses or presentation of the results of a study are unethical, as they are at best misleading and could actually endanger lives. Fraud is rare, however; sloppy research and conclusions not supported by the data are much more common.

THE ARCHITECTURE OF CLINICAL RESEARCH

There are essentially three classes of clinical research study (Feinstein 1985):

- *Descriptive observational studies* — these usually describe the characteristics of a clinical population without a control group, and are, therefore, suitable only for hypothesis generation rather than testing. Examples include case reports and series, audit, qualitative studies and surveys.
- *Analytical observational studies* — these generally compare two subject groups, cases and controls, and are suitable for hypothesis testing. Ideally, the study and control groups are similar in all but the characteristic of main interest, i.e. demographically similar, but with and without disease (in case-control studies) or having been subject to a particular exposure or not (in cohort studies).
- *Experimental studies* — these can be used to directly infer causation or to assess the effect of treatment, as something is given or done to an experimental group but not to a control group (of patients). Controlled trials have similar strengths as experimental studies in laboratory settings, but efforts to minimise bias and measurement error are usually greater in trials, and random treatment allocation is rare in lab work.

These distinctions are not absolute. Some audits and surveys include control groups, while some cohort studies (e.g. of the prognosis of a disease) do not. Similarly, some so-called 'clinical trials' are not experimental and are merely uncontrolled case series.

There is also another type of research that does not fit easily into this scheme — so-called *secondary research* — that is, systematic reviews and meta-analyses of the existing literature. These can generate the most reliable results of all (see p. 176) and are increasingly used to inform the development of clinical guidelines (see Ch. 12).

DESCRIPTIVE STUDIES

Case reports and case series

These are simple descriptions of clinical observations, sometimes with results of investigations, in one or a small group of patients. The patients tend to be opportunistically identified from a single location, subject to all kinds of selection biases and hence unrepresentative. Any unusual constellation of features may be coincidental in the absence of a control group. For example, it was quite common 10 years or so ago to see reports of two or more 'specific' delusional syndromes in a particular patient when the patient may simply have had an unusual case of schizophrenia. Case studies are susceptible to misdiagnosis, bias and measurement error. This makes them unreliable (and often unrepeatable).

Nevertheless, case reports have had, and continue to have, an important role. Many of the clinical entities we still recognise were initially described in this way, and clues to the aetiology of some diseases and many genetic conditions first suggested. A description of the common features in a number of cases of a rare disease is likely to be the best available evidence on that problem. It is also possible to seek out particular cases to disprove general theories — if, for example, one or preferably more patients have a disease but not a putative risk factor, that factor can be ruled out as a general cause (Farmer 1999). Uncontrolled trials can obviate or demand further study. If trials to evaluate a new drug have included a total of 1000 patients, an adverse reaction which occurs in 0.1% of treated patients may well not have occurred at all by chance alone. Hence, uncommon adverse effects are more likely to be detected in uncontrolled post-marketing surveillance.

However, case reports and series should generally be regarded as means of only identifying priorities or hypotheses for further and more comprehensive study (see Box 10.1). Clinical experience is essentially a series of extended case series, in which one is most likely to remember the most dramatic successes and failures (recall bias).

Clinical audit

Audit, as the 'examination of the extent to which a condition, process or performance conforms to pre-determined standards or criteria' (Last 1995), is not strictly speaking a research method, but is included here as it typically uses research methods and arguably should be conducted routinely by every medical practitioner. The key distinguishing features include the measurement of clinical performance against a standard, some attempt to improve this performance and then a re-audit, to 'close the audit cycle', to assess any improvement. In a sense, if patients are studied before and after some initiative, they could be regarded as their own controls but 'historical controls' are notoriously prone to bias as there are so many influences on medical services, patients' well-being and outcomes over time. The same concerns are pertinent in so-called

'mirror image' studies of the effects of treatments in what are essentially uncontrolled trials.

Almost any aspect of clinical care can be audited, which can be conveniently classified as:

- *service structure*, e.g. personnel, equipment;
- *a process of care*, e.g. note-keeping, investigation use and utility, treatments;
- *clinical outcomes*, e.g. morbidity, mortality.

Clinical outcomes are arguably the most important, as they measure local clinical effectiveness, but can be difficult to define and measure. Outcomes are rarely systematically recorded in hospital records. Current drives to national bench-marking, hospital performance league tables and even routine outcome measurement are usually biased by the case mix, different practices in particular hospitals, and the difficulties in selecting appropriate assessment tools (see the last section of this chapter). It is, however, regrettable that more effort has not been made to systematically address these problems.

Audit has some potential to improve local services, but the evidence for its impact on clinical care is very limited and its effects are modest (O'Brien et al 2002a, b). Two national initiatives merit particular mention. The Royal College of Psychiatrists has audited the practice of electroconvulsive therapy in England and Wales over the past 20 years (Duffett & Lelliott 1998). As measured against Royal College Guidelines, some aspects of ECT administration have improved, but much greater improvement is desirable. In Scotland, the Clinical Standards Advisory Board (CSBS 2001) have devised standards for the management of schizophrenia and recently determined how Trusts have met these, with a generally acceptable proportion achieving the standards (http://www.clinicalstandards.org/schizo). Naylor & Guyatt (1996) have helpfully summarised the optimal, if somewhat stringent, criteria for assessing the quality of a clinical audit report (see Box 10.2). In the absence of any really good pragmatic guides

---

Box 10.1 Characteristics, strengths and limitations of case reports and series

Describe the clinical features or outcome in one or more patients

Strengths
- Arise from clinical practice
- Quick and easy
- May have important general implications

Limitations
- Apparent associations may be due to coincidence
- Non-systematic retrospective studies
- Unreliable results: misdiagnosis, measurement error, bias and confounding (see below)

Box 10.2 Critical appraisal of a clinical audit

I. Are the criteria (standards) valid?
- Was an explicit and sensible process used to identify, select, and combine evidence for the criteria?
- What is the quality of the evidence used in framing the criteria?
- Was an explicit and sensible process used to consider the relative values of different outcomes?
- Are the judgements of the experts who established the criteria reproducible?
- If the quality of the evidence used in originally framing the criteria was weak, have the criteria been prospectively evaluated and shown to improve patient outcomes?

II. Were the criteria applied appropriately?
- Did the process of applying the criteria meet scientific standards (e.g. auditors blind to practitioner or institution identity, admixture of index cases as accuracy checks, random or consecutive sampling, adequate sample size)?
- What is the impact of uncertainty associated with evidence and values on the criteria-based ratings of process of care?

III. Can you use the criteria in your own practice setting?
- Have the criteria been field-tested for feasibility of use in diverse settings?
- Are the criteria up-to-date?

to (psychiatric) audit, critical appraisal criteria can usefully highlight the chief issues to be considered in designing an audit project.

These criteria are however far from exhaustive. Other important issues to consider include the completeness of case ascertainment and data collection, and any bias in assessing case records/data extraction. Training, experience and support are required in audit study design, particularly for quality control of data collection and management, as with all research. It is therefore concerning that clinicians who might otherwise be hesitant to conduct observational research will attempt clinical audit without any methodological expertise or assistance.

Qualitative studies

Most medical research is quantitative, in that variables are 'objectively' measured in numerical terms and summarised or analysed statistically. Qualitative research of peoples' experiences, feelings, values and other types of opinion are seen as increasingly important. Complex issues and behaviours may not be easily amenable to quantitative approaches and may be better explored qualitatively. Qualitative studies may thus complement and even inform quantitative approaches by, for example, generating ideas and hypotheses for further testing and assisting in questionnaire development where relevant variables are not obviously apparent. They are often useful adjuncts to clinical trials, to identify why people might wish to participate or not, establish the feasibility of the trial and thus reduce difficulties in recruitment and follow-up.

Qualitative studies are not necessarily subjective or unscientific. Data are usually gathered with semi-structured interviews, in focus groups and/or through observation. Objectivity can be ensured by recording these observations, on audio or video-tape, and obtaining independent ratings by multiple trained observers. Common themes can be derived from the data by multiple passings through the recordings, and/or with a variety of increasingly sophisticated software programs. Direct quotations, addressing a clearly formulated initial question, a clear account of the researchers' perspectives and the explicit consideration of various explanations of the data all serve to improve the validity of a qualitative study. Each of the main approaches to data collection have their own advantages and disadvantages: individual interviews elicit specific opinions but may not generalise; a focus group can establish a group norm, but minority views may be obscured; and direct observation of behaviour (rather than just attitudes) in natural settings may give the strongest results, but may lose individual detail. The best methods depend upon the phenomenon under investigation, but as a general rule, it is desirable to collect data from more than one source. In addition, recent studies are increasingly adopting 'purposive sampling', to derive representative samples with desirable demographic characteristics. The essential features, strengths and limitations of qualitative studies are summarised in Box 10.3.

These approaches have, however, been largely neglected in psychiatry and medicine, although are likely to be increasingly used in the coming years. They might well, for example, shed light on prescribing behaviour, and the reasons for patients compliance, or non-compliance, with particular treatments. They could improve the acceptability of randomised trials of psychiatric interventions. In this way, they can potentially bridge the gap between medical science and clinical practice. There are, for example, already a handful of qualitative studies of patients' and relatives' experiences of psychotic disorders which relate the limitations of current

---

Box 10.3 Essential features, strengths and limitations of qualitative studies

Collect data on opinions, to generate ideas and hypotheses (i.e. inductive rather than deductive reasoning)

Strengths
- Offers insight when research is not well established or conventional theories seem inadequate
- Have validity, provided they are well-conducted
- Can inform and improve quantitative research

Limitations
- Prone to researchers' bias in the collection and analysis of data
- Without direct observation, attitudes do not necessarily equate to behaviour
- May lack reliability, particularly if only one rater analyses responses

---

psychiatric management, as well as the strengths, and even some perceived benefits of psychosis (Barker et al 2001).

There are, in addition, two qualitative approaches that habitually use quantitative techniques, particularly questionnaires, to deliver consensus in controversial areas, such as therapeutic approaches to particular disorders. The two most commonly used are the so-called *delphi or delphic process* and the *nominal group (or expert panel) technique*. Both approaches require the initial definition of a problem and the selection of 'experts'. Questionnaires elicit responses to a range of therapeutic options, which participants rate anonymously; that process continues or 'iterates', with participants receiving feedback on how their response compares with that of the group, and the opportunity to change their initial response, until consensus is achieved. There are slight differences in how the experts are selected, the questionnaires constructed and results fed back to participants; see Jones & Hunter (1995) for further details. These techniques have not been widely used, in psychiatry or medicine, but have already been used to assist in the development of clinical guidelines for the use of psychological therapies in the UK and the management of bipolar disorder in the USA. In all such uses, consensus-delivering techniques are complementary to, but should not replace, the systematic review of the literature and grading of recommendations desirable for valid clinical guidelines (see Ch. 12 and http://www.sign.ac.uk/guidelines/index.html).

Surveys

Survey is an ambiguous word, being merely 'the systematic collection of information' (Last 1995). Indeed, one sees at least three different uses of the word in the medical literature. It is relatively common to see the term 'questionnaire survey', particularly in accounts of often hastily cobbled together questions being sent out in the hope of eliciting opinions about medical training or practice, usually obtaining low, uninformative response rates. These are, in fact, simply poor qualitative studies or case series. The term survey is more accurately applied to *two-phase epidemiological surveys* (screening questionnaire then interview) to determine the prevalence of a disease and other types of cross-sectional study. These should not be confused with surveillance studies, e.g. the active or passive monitoring of adverse drug effects in phase IV 'clinical trials'. The key feature of *cross-sectional studies* is that they simultaneously ascertain the presence or absence of disease and the presence or absence of an exposure, at one particular point in time. They are, therefore, studies of prevalence or frequency and sometimes called so, and cannot reliably distinguish between cause and effect.

These studies need to pay particular attention to potential biases in population sampling. In an attempt to ensure that the population studied is representative, surveys tend to take a random sample from, for example, census data, the electoral roll or even a telephone directory. All of these are probably better than attempting to accost people in the street, but will, of course, miss those who move frequently, do not pay their 'community charge' or do not have a telephone — and psychiatric patients are probably over-represented in each category. Patients will be difficult to contact at home if they are currently hospitalised or in prison. Making false associations through 'sampling bias' is known as *Berkson's fallacy* (or bias). For example, the original description that hospitalised schizophrenic patients tended not to have epilepsy led to the introduction of ECT, whereas it is now clear that schizophrenics are, if anything, more likely to suffer from epileptic fits than the general population — the sampling bias presumably arising because epileptic schizophrenics were either unrecognised as schizophrenic or treated for epilepsy in different hospitals.

Close attention must equally be paid to how potential participants are approached. In large studies, such as two-phase epidemiological surveys of rare illnesses, it is standard to send out postal questionnaires because interviewing everybody would be too costly. Edwards et al (2002) systematically reviewed randomised controlled trials to compare methods of maximising response rates to postal questionnaires; they found that response was approximately doubled when questionnaires were sent out by recorded delivery, were short, were designed to be of interest to participants and when monetary incentives were offered. Response rates were also increased by such factors as personalising questionnaires and letters, using stamped returned envelopes, contacting participants before sending questionnaires, follow-up contact, providing non-responders with a second questionnaire and even using coloured ink. Questionnaires including sensitive questions were less likely to be returned. It is a general rule of clinical interviewing and questionnaire design that questions should be unambiguous and two questions should not be combined in one. Consideration of these issues is crucial to obtaining a response rate, in the region of 80–90%, which allows confidence in the results. Telephone or personal contact for a relatively brief interview may be more successful, particularly in a psychiatric population, as those affected with psychiatric disorders are known to be less likely to respond to questionnaires.

A particular type of cross-sectional survey, the *ecological or correlational study*, avoids the potential problems of response bias by examining pre-existing data on exposures and outcomes in populations rather than individuals. Usually, routinely collected data on disease rates is compared with data on the general level of exposure between particular geographical regions (or in regions over time in 'secular trend analysis' or 'time series studies'). If two or more computerised records are used, this is known as 'record linkage'. These approaches obviously have the additional advantages of being relatively cheap and quick, as well as the more dubious advantage of being able to examine an almost limitless range of potential associations. The price to pay is the inability to link exposure to outcome in individuals or to control adequately for confounding factors. In other words, any association discovered in an ecological study may not apply at an individual level and may arise from confounding by other factors. Incorrect conclusions from associations in ecological studies are called the 'ecological fallacy'. For example, deprived inner city areas have a high proportion of Afro-Caribbean residents and higher than average rates of suicide, but individual Afro-Caribbeans do not. Any association seems to arise because inner cities have more people from ethnic minorities and more people who live alone, but only the latter are at increased risk of suicide. These areas have more consultant psychiatrists, presumably relating to the location of teaching hospitals rather than more antipsychiatric interpretations. These false associations can sometimes be corrected statistically for potential confounding, but depend upon the pertinent information having been collected and available. Where it is not, and indeed in general, any such associations need to be confirmed in analytical studies.

In summary, descriptive observational research is comparatively quick and easy, and useful to develop new hypotheses, but cannot reliably test hypotheses or discern causal relationships. The main features of the individual types of study are summarised in Table 10.1. Those interested in further information are referred to excellent introductory (Hennekens & Buring 1987) or detailed (Feinstein 1985) epidemiology textbooks, a series of recent articles in the Lancet (Grimes & Schulz 2002) or Lawrie et al (2000).

ANALYTICAL STUDIES

Case-control studies

In a case-control study, individuals with a particular condition or disease (the cases) are selected and compared with individuals without the condition or disease (the controls). The case–control

Table 10.1 Summary features of descriptive observational studies

Type of study	Essential features	Advantages	Disadvantages
Case report	Observations in a single case	Cheap and easy way of generating hypotheses	Liable to coincidence, error, bias and confounding
Case series	Disease characteristics in a number of cases	May be the best information on very rare diseases	No comparison group, so cannot test hypotheses
Audit	Examines service provision and outcome	Gives information on service delivery	Unreliable estimate of effectiveness
Qualitative study	Elicits opinion	Can illuminate complex issues	May be unreliable
Cross-sectional study	Measures rates of disease	Identifies patterns of disease	Cannot distinguish cause and effect
Ecological study	Measures associations of disease	Can use pre-recorded data	Describes populations rather than individuals

> **Box 10.4   Case-control studies**
>
> Compare cases and controls on the relative frequencies of one or more exposure
>
> *Strengths*
> - Relatively quick and inexpensive
> - Suitable for rare diseases
> - Can evaluate distant and multiple exposures
>
> *Limitations*
> - Unsuitable for rare exposures
> - Susceptible, in particular, to selection bias
> - Susceptible to recall bias and reverse causality

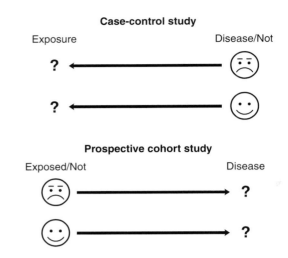

Fig. 10.1
In a case-control study disease status is established before exposure status; vice-versa in a cohort study.

comparison is the frequency of previous exposures or attributes potentially relevant to the development of the condition or disease under study. In essence, therefore, disease status is determined before exposure status (see Fig. 10.1). The development and increasing use of case-control studies, such that they are now the most common type of study published in medical journals, has largely followed their initial use in cancer epidemiology. Their relatively simple approach can identify important effects. They are particularly suitable in rare diseases or those that take a long time to develop, as in most psychiatric disorders. Many potential exposures can be investigated simultaneously (see Box 10.4).

They do, however, confront several potential problems. Paramount amongst these is the appropriate identification and recruitment of the cases and controls. Case-control studies are population based, and participants should be (but frequently are not) representative of their respective populations. All too often, patients are recruited as a 'convenience sample' of hospital-based patients who are prepared to participate. They are then compared with a similar convenience control sample of 'willing volunteers', e.g. hospital workers. The cases and controls will, therefore, differ in a very lengthy list of attributes and exposures (wealth, intelligence, adversity, etc.) and may falsely inflate any association or even lead to spurious ones. For example, early structural brain imaging studies in schizophrenia were particularly likely to find case–control differences because the patients tended to be male with relatively severe illnesses and hospital staff controls or indeed medical controls with normal brain scans were 'supernormal'. In such instances, case-control studies may find factors that relate to the severity of a disease rather than the causation. These types of selection bias can be minimised by true random sampling of e.g. all patients and controls in the community, or 'nesting' a case control study within a cohort study, but these make the study more difficult and expensive and begin to lose the attractions of the case-control approach. Sampling from cases in contact with medical services is the most practical and common method but demands that researchers pay careful attention to potential sources of bias (Lewis & Pelosi 1990). This selection bias can be compounded by response bias if only certain types of patients and controls participate.

Case-control studies also have to deal with various types of 'information bias' as the exposure is being assessed retrospectively. In particular, if subjects are asked whether or not they have been exposed, 'recall bias' commonly arises because those affected 'search after meaning' in seeking an explanation for their illness. This can apply equally to relatives or carers. Perhaps the best example of this in the psychiatric literature comes from studies of the association between life events and depression, where depressed mood may also influence the recall of particular events. For this reason, life events

researchers now focus on so-called 'independent events' such as bereavement, and especially those that can be verified as preceding the outcome, to avoid the possibility of 'reverse causality' (see p. 177). Similar difficulties can affect researchers, with 'observer bias' resulting from researchers not being blind to, or being able to guess, disease status and searching more rigorously for exposures in the cases. Some of these problems can be reduced, but not avoided entirely, by using pre-recorded exposure information.

One of the common methods to deal with selection bias is to match cases and controls on one or more important characteristics e.g. sex. This has the advantage of improving the power of the study, but runs the risk of seriously limiting the number of suitable subjects, over-matching and reducing associations, and makes it impossible to examine the effects of the matched variables statistically. It is usually better, therefore, to measure any potential confounder and to correct for it statistically unless the effect of a confounder is particularly large and can only be quantified with difficulty. Either approach, however, requires that the investigators know what the confounders are or might be.

For these reasons, exposures are, in general, more reliably related to particular diseases in prospective cohort studies. Shulz & Grimes (2002a) have, however, recently suggested five guidelines for investigators planning (or appraising) case-control studies:

- Explicitly define case diagnosis and eligibility criteria.
- Select controls from the same population as cases, independent of the exposure of interest.
- Blind the data gatherers to case or control status (or at least to the main hypothesis of the study).
- Train data gatherers to elicit exposure in a similar manner from cases and controls, e.g. using memory aids to facilitate and balance recall in both.
- Address confounding factors, either in the design stage or during analysis.

Cohort studies

Cohort studies first classify subjects according to whether or not they have been exposed to a suspected risk factor, or have a particular attribute, and then follow the exposed and non-exposed for a period of time (often years) to compare the frequency of an outcome such as disease (see Fig. 10.1). Prospective follow-up obviously needs to be sufficiently long and complete that enough subjects develop the condition of interest, without losing too much information from dropouts, to be able reliably to compare disease rates. The principal advantage of cohort studies is, therefore, that there is rarely any debate about whether or not the exposure predated the onset of disease, and this can be measured without any bias in relation to disease status. For this reason, it can be argued that poorly understood diseases should first be evaluated in cohort studies, and once potential confounders have been reliably identified, case-control studies can then proceed more economically (although the reverse is usually the case). Cohort studies also have the ability to study multiple possible outcomes of a single exposure. They are, however, expensive and time-consuming, usually include relatively few cases and are unsuitable for studying rare diseases (unless the outcome is very common amongst those exposed, i.e. the attributable risk percentage is high).

It should be noted that cohort studies do not necessarily need a control group. Even in aetiological studies, it is possible to follow-up exposed subjects (e.g. on the basis of genetic risk) with a plan to conduct a *nested case-control study* of those who do and do not develop the outcome of interest. This will, however, be unable to examine the effect of the selected exposure other than in a 'dose–response' analysis or as interactions with other putative risk factors. More commonly, the prognosis of a disease or the adverse events associated with a particular treatment have no need of a control group. Such studies do, however, have to be sufficiently large and lengthy to be of value, and in particular, they need to consist of representative samples of patients with a particular disorder or exposed to a particular treatment. It is also preferable that they commence from first onset or first treatment, respectively, to avoid selecting potentially atypical cases.

It is, in addition, possible to conduct retrospective cohort studies, where the cohort has already been exposed and developed the disease or not. These are particularly useful if the latent period between exposure and disease is long, where researchers would be likely to lose contact with large numbers of participants. This approach has been adopted to study neurodevelopment in children who go on to develop psychotic disorders, using data collected from national surveys of child development and linking them to registers of hospital admission. These studies are relatively easy, but obviously depend upon the existence of good quality data collected for other purposes, which may be incomplete and particularly deficient in information on potential confounders. This sort of research will, however, be much harder to do under the new data protection act.

Cohort studies are mainly liable to two types of bias. First, participants who drop out of the study or move away and become uncontactable are likely to differ from those that do not, often because they have developed the condition or disease of interest. As a general rule, follow-up rates of less than 80% are liable to deliver unreliable results. Second, the assignment of disease or outcome status can be subject to 'observer bias' unless such outcomes are rigorously defined and outcome assessors are blind to exposure status. In psychiatric studies, this demands at least a structured psychiatric interview. Cohort studies are less liable to the other main sources of bias because of the prospective collection of data (see Box 10.5).

EXPERIMENTAL STUDIES

It should already be apparent that, even in a medical sense, experimental studies are not synonymous with clinical trials. A clinical trial is any kind of study designed to establish the effects of a particular therapeutic intervention. This includes uncontrolled trials and phase I (development) and phase IV (surveillance) studies in evaluating new treatments — see Pocock (1983) or Lawrie (2002) for more details. Only (randomised) controlled trials are experimental. The randomised control trial (RCT) is the gold standard of medical experimentation, but there are an increasing number of variants which we will describe here (see Table 10.2) once we have considered some general issues.

Box 10.5	Summary of the essential features of cohort studies

Typically, those exposed or not are identified and then followed-up to compare frequency of subsequent disease

Strengths
- Ideal for rare exposures
- Can examine many outcomes of a single exposure
- Generally less liable to bias than other observational studies, particularly recall bias and reverse causality

Limitations
- Can be expensive and lengthy
- Usually unsuitable for rare diseases
- Losses to follow-up can affect validity

Table 10.2	Summary of the features of clinical trials		
Type of study	Essential features	Advantages	Disadvantages
Uncontrolled 'trials'	All subjects are given one treatment	Cheap and easy	No controls
Controlled trials	Two treatments are compared	Relatively straightforward	No randomisation
Randomised control trials	Random allocation of treatment	Randomisation reduces selection bias and confounding	Expensive and time-consuming
Cluster trials	Groups of individuals are randomised	Can assess the efficacy of certain health services	Often difficult to find enough clusters to give adequate power
Crossover trial	Subjects are their own controls	Can study treatment of rare, chronic disorders	Historical controls; order effects; carryover effects
N-of-1 trial	A single subject	Can establish effectiveness in an individual patient	As above, only applicable to certain types of chronic diseases

General issues

What is the aim of the study?

Clearly, the question has to be clinically relevant (i.e. the answer would help clinicians and their patients to make therapeutic decisions), ethically acceptable, and not have been satisfactorily answered already (e.g. in a systematic review or meta-analysis).

Which patients are to be studied?

A 'pure' highly selected group in an 'explanatory' trial may generate findings of little representativeness or generalisability. Broad inclusion criteria and minimal exclusions will serve to avoid the 'disappearing patient phenomenon', particularly when one allows for those who refuse to participate. For example, many psychiatric trials exclude patients with comorbid substance abuse, thus excluding about half of all potential participants, with the result that the study results may be inapplicable in approximately half of all patients that psychiatrists see and will probably overestimate the benefits of the new treatment (given that comorbid patients are notoriously reluctant to comply with medical interventions). Excluding those under the age of 16 to 18 or over the age of 60 to 65 means that child, adolescent and old-age psychiatrists are often obliged to prescribe drugs with little information from clinical trials and may actually have to prescribe a drug 'off licence'. Excluding involuntarily-detained patients has the effect that psychiatrists treating the most severely ill patients are often doing so in the absence of any reliable evidence.

Which interventions and how?

In a drug trial, one needs to consider the dose, type, formulation and route of administration of the medication. If comparing a new and a standard treatment, one can easily make the new drug look better (e.g. less toxic) by choosing a high dose of standard drug as the comparator (Geddes et al 2000). How the optimum dose of a drug is achieved and the dosing schedule require careful consideration. An important choice has to be made between allowing only fixed doses and allowing clinicians in the trial to tailor the dose to a particular patient. Fixed-dose trials generally give results that are easier to interpret, but they are obviously different from how a drug is used in clinical practice, and many patients will receive non-optimal doses. Flexible dosing is more clinically representative, but difficult if not impossible to achieve without unblinding the responsible clinicians. One must also decide what, if any, other drugs are permissible for participating patients. For example, antipsychotic trials usually permit the concomitant prescription of one or more anticholinergic drugs and 'rescue' medication for behavioural disturbance.

How long?

Many trials in psychiatry are short, lasting 6 weeks or less. This is simply because they are easier to do. Long trials are complex, expensive and liable to suffer from large numbers of people dropping out of the trial for various reasons. Clinical practice should, however, be informed by long-term clinical trials, particularly if we advise our patients to stay on a drug for a year or more, but trials which suffer from more than a 20% dropout over the duration of the study deliver results of dubious representativeness and reliability.

Is blinding possible?

Controlled trials may be open (if the doctors and patients both know what treatment is given), single-blind (if the patient is not told what treatment he is getting), double-blind (if the treating doctor does not know, or cannot work out, what treatment his patient is getting), or triple-blind (if, in addition, the outcome assessors do not know what treatment a patient has received). The purpose of single-, double- and triple-blinding is to improve the reliability of trial findings, by reducing observer bias. Single- and double-blinding also reduce placebo effects. Blinding is, however, rarely entirely complete. Patients and doctors can quite often guess whether that patient has received an active treatment according to whether they have responded or not and whether they have side-effects. Single- and double-blinding are also difficult, if not impossible, in psychotherapy trials. Even in comparative drug trials, particular side-effects can suggest that a specific drug has been administered: e.g. trials of the tricyclic antidepressants have commonly included anticholinergic compounds in the placebo, and trials which use this approach generally find less advantage of tricyclics over placebo than those which have not (Moncrieff et al 1998). Having independent outcome assessors can go some way to mitigating these problems, but suggestive information can still be given away by the patients or picked up by the observers. A useful method to quantify the success or otherwise of blinding in a trial is to simply ask patients, clinicians and/or outcome raters what treatment they think a particular patient has received — if blinding has been successful, they should score no better than chance (Even et al 2000). However, blinding is not as important (nor the same) as allocation concealment (see p. 173).

Which outcomes should be measured and how?

Clinical outcomes can be measured either categorically or continuously. Dichotomous categorical outcomes are probably the most clinically meaningful, as the doctor and patient can choose a particular treatment accordingly. 'Dead or alive' is the standard and least subject to bias outcome, but these events are too rare for practical use in psychiatric studies. Typical alternatives are 'readmitted or not', 'recovered or not', or 'relapsed or not', but it can be difficult to measure these. In many psychiatric trials, recovery or relapse have been determined from somewhat arbitrary cutoff points on symptom severity or behavioural scales. For example, recovery from acute illness is quite often measured as a 20% or 40% reduction in symptom severity. Not only are these unreliable and potentially invalid measures of benefit, they may be completely meaningless to patients. Psychiatric research has a surfeit of rating scales (many of dubious validity, reliability etc., which is why we mention so few later in this chapter), which can make it difficult to compare outcomes in different trials. For example, the first 2000 controlled trials in schizophrenia used 640 different scales (Thornley & Adams 1998). Further, researchers who devise their own scales for the purposes of particular study are more likely to report statistically significant effects than if they used standard pre-existing measures (Marshall et al 2000). This may be because it makes it easier to conceal the fact that only the items or subscales that showed benefit were reported. If an outcome measure requires rating by an observer, it should be shown to be reliably rated by two or more (preferably blind) observers and should ideally also be reliably sensitive to change. The best compromise may be to use re-hospitalisation as a proxy for relapse, despite all the local service and other determinants of whether someone is admitted or not.

Controlled trials

Uncontrolled trials are a means of establishing whether a treatment works at all and what sort of adverse effects are prominent, but an unreliable one. The absence of a control group means that some, or even all, of these apparent effects could be attributable to many different causes (the type of patient, severity of disease, a true treatment effect, placebo effect, etc.). If any treatment is given or taken with enough enthusiasm some people will benefit. James Lind, an 18th-century Scottish physician is generally credited with having completed the first controlled trial — of vitamin C for scurvy. The only Nobel prizes awarded in the field of psychiatry — to Wagner-Jauregg in 1927 for 'malaria therapy' and to Moniz in 1949 for the pre-frontal leucotomy — may never have been awarded if the importance of controls had been appreciated at the time. Controlled trials are obviously necessary if a particular treatment is to be evaluated against placebo or against a pre-existing treatment, but even controlled studies tend to overestimate therapeutic benefits. For example, there were numerous reports of apparent benefits from renal dialysis in schizophrenia until a series of randomised control trials found no beneficial effects (Carpenter et al 1983). The main potential problem with controlled trials is that patients getting the new treatment tend to be selected (consciously or not) to have a slightly less severe illness and/or better prognosis, so that the beneficial effects of the new drug or procedure are typically overestimated by 30% (Schulz et al 1995, Juni et al 2001). This is the main reason for the 'invention' of the randomised control trial by the English epidemiologist Bradford Hill.

Randomised control trials

Randomisation has two main purposes. First and foremost, it evenly distributes both the known and, more importantly, the unknown confounders (e.g. age, sex, prognostic factors) of the therapeutic effect in the two treatment groups. Secondly, it avoids the potential selection biases described above — this, however, depends on *allocation concealment*. To be properly randomised, a trial should use a randomisation schedule that is not predictable or known. For example, if patient treatment is allocated by dates of birth, days of admission to hospital, etc., it is possible for investigators to subvert the treatment allocation process by finding reasons to include or exclude particular patients.

Random numbers should therefore be generated to assign particular patients to a particular treatment (although tossing a coin is acceptable), the assignment should be sealed in opaque envelopes, kept in a locked cabinet and only opened by someone (preferably indifferent to the trial result) when a suitable patient has consented to participate. This may sound extreme, but Chalmers et al (1983) have shown that approximately 58% of published studies without randomisation find a significant treatment effect, and 24% with randomisation that allowed 'easy cheating' found a significant effect, whereas a significant effect was found in only 9% of studies in which subverting randomisation was judged to be difficult. Randomisation is not bona fide without allocation concealment. This is reflected in some 'trial quality scores', which award marks for randomisation but subtract them if the allocation is not convincingly concealed. It should be noted that phase II

('dose-ranging') and phase III ('comparative') trials, as part of drug development, may or may not be randomised.

People, even doctors, can cheat with sealed envelopes, however. Envelopes can also get lost or destroyed, thereby subverting the allocation sequence. Ideally, therefore, a 'central randomisation method' should be used. Once a patient has consented to participate, an investigator contacts a separate centre (by telephone, fax or computer), the patient's baseline data are entered, then a computer algorithm allocates the next treatment and the operator informs the investigator. This has the advantage that everyone involved knows who is in the trial immediately and baseline data collection is complete. It is more costly than using sealed envelopes, but touch-tone phone systems and the internet have made central randomisation more generally applicable and affordable. Indeed, a computer can operate the system 24 hours a day for global multicentre trials. A computer can also implement stratification or minimisation to ensure that prognostic factors are balanced between the treatment arms.

Various methods of randomisation are sometimes used to ensure that trial groups are balanced in terms of number and/or patient characteristics.

- *Blocked randomisation* simply randomises patients in groups (of four, six, etc.) to ensure that numbers are equal in the two groups.
- *Stratified randomisation* allocates patients on the basis of prognostic variables to ensure that these are evenly distributed, but requires an additional schedule for each stratum.
- An alternative is *minimisation (or adaptive) randomisation* in which each patient is allocated to a particular group by minimising any differences in important variables as each particular patient is entered into the trial (Pocock 1983).

The problem with all these procedures is that they can under some circumstances, if poorly designed or implemented, increase the chances of unblinding the allocation (Schulz & Grimes 2002b). They are, however, essential in small trials. In large trials, of say more than 500 patients, properly conducted simple randomisation will usually, but not always, generate sufficiently even groups by chance alone.

Cluster trials

One other important variant of randomisation is to randomise subjects in groups or clusters rather than as individuals. These so-called 'cluster trials' are most commonly used in evaluating more global aspects of health services than one particular treatment or where allocation of individual subjects is not practicable (Gilbody & Whitty 2002). For example, educating general practitioners about the detection and treatment of depression is ideally suited to cluster randomisation, as general practitioners tend to work in group practices and it would be difficult in practice to educate one partner without that being communicated to another. The main disadvantage of cluster randomisation is that the unit of randomisation should be the unit of analysis, so that large numbers of clusters are required to give the trial adequate power.

Explanatory versus pragmatic trials

The randomised control trial has given clinical therapeutics a sound scientific base but measures treatment efficacy rather than clinical effectiveness (i.e. whether a treatment works rather than whether it works in clinical practice). Randomisation generally increases the scientific quality or 'internal validity' of a trial, but can lead to problems with 'external validity' if patients who are included differ systematically from all potential participants. This is a type of selection bias which can limit the representativeness of the population being studied and the generalisability of the results. Pragmatic trials typically have less restrictive inclusion criteria and can therefore have greater generalisability. However, patients who are able to give informed consent and willing to be randomised may be just as likely, or even more so, to participate in an explanatory trial.

The distinction between explanatory and pragmatic trials is also not as clear as when the terms were introduced in 1967 (McMahon 2002). At that time, trials tended to exclude patients who violated the study protocol by, for example, not complying with their treatment. The pragmatic approach was to include all violators, as they had been part of the therapeutic programme (see 'intention to treat' analysis below), but this has now become standard. These days, an 'explanatory' trial is typically a small trial, with highly selective entry criteria, which focuses on one specific issue and often uses intermediate or surrogate outcome measures. A 'pragmatic' trial is usually larger, with broad entry criteria, in which the interventions can feasibly be provided in routine health care and the outcome is a major clinical event (Hotopf et al 1999). Both types of trial are desirable, as they address different information needs. There is a common tendency to regard pragmatic trials as 'good' and explanatory trials as unrepresentative, but treatment control is usually more careful in explanatory studies and no-one would argue that this is undesirable. Neither trial type will be truly representative, because only those prepared to be randomised will be included.

Indeed, the issue of generalisability is probably overplayed (McMahon 2002). Unless a treatment works in 100% of patients, there will be uncertainty about who will benefit. Doctors particularise, rather than generalise, trial results to their patients. The relevant question is therefore whether a patient is so different from those in a trial that the results do not apply (see Ch. 12). Extrapolating the results should also involve considering the biological mechanism of the treatment effect, as whether this mechanism is generalisable is more important than whether the patients are representative.

One 'pragmatic' approach to the representativeness issue is to conduct 'patient preference trials'. In these, patients who are not willing to be randomised, because they have a preference for a particular treatment, are given that treatment but otherwise followed-up as in the trial so that the results in these patients (who would otherwise not have participated) can be compared with those who were randomised; see Bedi et al (2000) for an example. The problem with this method is that although recruitment may be increased, and generalisablity possibly enhanced, the results are likely to be more biased and less reliable than if all eligible patients were randomised. Alternatively, a trial can be designed so that only patients in whom the clinician is uncertain as to which treatment should be prescribed are enrolled. If a particular patient's response to a particular drug is already known, then it makes little sense to run the risk of randomising them to a known ineffective treatment. The main advantage of this is that the trial addresses a definite area of clinical uncertainty. There are as yet few pragmatic trials in psychiatry, but examinations of the new antipsychotics and mood-stabilising drugs are currently in progress, and a study of psychological interventions for depression has recently been published (Dowrick et al 2000).

Crossover trials

These are trials in which all participants receive two or more interventions, one after the other, with the two groups receiving a different treatment first (Louis et al 1984). Patients may be randomised to receive a particular intervention first or second. Crossover trials are a real option in relatively rare diseases where the numbers of available participants may not permit a randomised parallel-group controlled trial. It is, however, probably preferable to attempt to conduct multicentre parallel-group trials in such instances. A second potential advantage of crossover trials is more apparent than real. If one of the treatment options is placebo, then a crossover trial gets round potential ethical concerns about not giving people effective treatment that may be required. There is, however, no reason, particularly in short-term trials, why all patients allocated to placebo cannot be offered active treatment after the cessation of the trial, and if there is a genuine need to test a new treatment against placebo then it cannot be unethical to conduct such a trial.

There are, however, several disadvantages of crossover trials. These amount to the difficulties in ensuring that the trial is long enough to ensure therapeutic effects are manifest in a reasonable number of participants, but short enough to avoid contaminating the results with natural fluctuations in a chronic disease. There are very few conditions in which disease activity is constant over time. There is also the problem of effects from one treatment carrying over into the second time period and the potential for drug interactions. It is possible to include a 'washout period' of no treatment, but this introduces new difficulties with sudden cessation of potentially effective treatments and in ensuring the washout period is long enough to be effective, but short enough to be ethical. The one type of crossover trial which is probably under-utilised is the *N-of-1 trial* in which a particular patient is given two treatments blind. This has some potential in individual patients in which it is simply not known which treatment they should receive, but obviously requires a consenting patient and co-operation from the hospital pharmacy (Guyatt et al 1986).

The need for large-scale trials in psychiatry

Most of the first 2000 controlled trials in patients with schizophrenia included less than 60 participants (see Thornley & Adams 1998 and Fig. 10.2). This sample size could only detect very, very large treatment effects. Trials comparing two active agents ('comparative studies') require much larger groups (as the difference in effects is generally much smaller). The main reason for larger trials is that very large effects are rare in medicine. Larger trials are needed chiefly to avoid missing a modest but clinically worthwhile benefit simply because the trial is underpowered. They also reduce random error and produce a more precise estimate of the treatment effect. The logical extension of this argument is to the so-called 'mega trial', in which thousands of patients are randomised to particular treatments (Peto et al 1993, Warlow 2002). This gives the best opportunity of reliably identifying moderate treatment effects. Such trials can benefit from computerised randomisation (which allows enrolment 24 hours a day worldwide), minimising data requirements and using simple objective outcome measures, but still require tremendous organisation. There is, however, no doubt that psychiatrists, like many medical specialists, are over-reliant on the pharmaceutical industry to evaluate new products and are years behind our colleagues in cardiology and

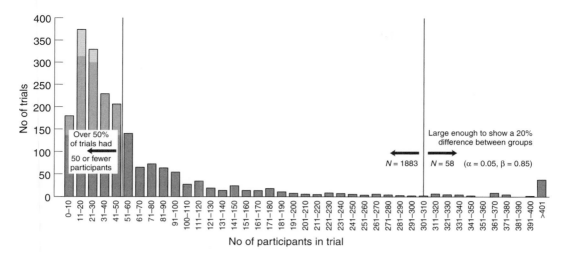

Fig. 10.2
Size of the first 1941 trials in schizophrenia. Most studies are very small; only 58 had enough power (β) to detect a 20% difference between groups with a P value (α) of 0.05. Reprinted with permission from the *British Medical Journal* (Thornley & Adams 1998).

neurology in carrying out large independent trials. Trials in psychiatry can be said to have particular problems, but large randomised 'sample trials have been conducted in comparably 'difficult' patients with epilepsy and traumatic brain injury.

Specific statistical issues

Multiple hypothesis testing in trials

A power calculation is necessary before any trial to determine how many participants will be required to detect a specific finding at a given level of statistical significance. One therefore needs a defined primary outcome measure and a means of estimating how many participants may develop it (for a dichotomous outcome) or the likely mean change in a continuous measure and some idea of its likely variance (in standard deviation units). There is, however, a drive to considering several outcomes, including those from the patient's point of view. These might include measures of adverse effect frequency, levels of functioning, or quality-of-life measures, as 'surrogate outcome measures'. Multiple outcome measures may be thought of as giving better coverage of therapeutic response, but increase the chances of finding statistically significant differences by chance alone.

Similarly, it is at best dubious and at worst fraudulent to attempt to define 'subgroups' of patients in trials who have responded particularly well or particularly badly to a treatment — unless there was a pre-specified hypothesis about this (Assmann et al 2000). Multiple hypothesis testing is acceptable if these were pre-specified hypotheses, but some sort of statistical correction for multiple testing should usually be made. Exploratory testing, sometimes known as 'data dredging', is unacceptable unless clearly acknowledged. Such analyses are and should be seen as hypothesis-generating (Pocock et al 2002). Hence they are, at most, a basis for further investigations, and cannot confirm or refute a particular hypothesis. Perhaps the best example of this problem comes from the ISIS-2 study, which found among other things that aspirin reduced mortality in acute myocardial infarction; an absurd (but educational) subgroup analysis by astrological sign showed a particularly strong effect for those born under Capricorn, and

no effect in Librans and Geminians (Peto et al 1993, Warlow 2002).

Intention-to-treat analysis

Generally speaking, using a continuous measure (e.g. a symptom severity score) gives more statistical power than using a dichotomous or categorical one, but less relevance. The latter has particular advantages when it comes to dealing with the results in participants who have dropped out of the trial before its completion. All trials should conduct *intention-to-treat analyses* of the results in all participants randomised to one treatment or another, regardless of whether they completed the trial — to include treatment failures and avoid overestimating the benefits of treatment (McMahon 2002). A standard approach with a continuous measure is to use the 'last observation carried forward' (LOCF), i.e. the last available measure for a particular subject is used as their final measure. This is, however, dubious for both statistical and clinical reasons. As most patients who drop out from a trial do so either because the drug has been ineffective and/or side-effects of the treatment cannot be tolerated, even allowing for those who drop out for other reasons, they should be regarded as treatment failures. Taking the LOCF, therefore, may over- or underestimate the benefits of the treatment depending on the treatment and condition evaluated. This may be trivial if dropouts are relatively few, but for example, most of the new 'atypical' antipsychotics have dropout rates of more than 30% in 6–12 weeks, and for one or two of the drugs the dropout rate is more than 50%. Employing a dichotomous outcome measure, on the other hand, allows one to (conservatively but correctly) assume that treatment dropouts are treatment failures and analyse them as such.

Checking randomisation

It is also briefly worth mentioning one statistical test that should not be conducted in clinical trials (or indeed most other studies). It makes little sense to statistically compare descriptive variables in two or more treatment groups 'to test the success of randomisation'. Not only is it inappropriate to conduct statistical tests for which there is no hypothesis, but if randomisation is truly random, then every now and then some descriptive variables will differ between allocated groups. Note, however, that it is necessary to check that the randomisation process has not been subverted, and important to detect and describe baseline imbalances. An imbalance in a major prognostic factor between the treatment and control groups may not reach 'statistical significance' but may still be enough to materially influence the outcome in the two groups and hence lead the trial to over- or underestimate the treatment effect. Thus, baseline statistical comparisons are overused, but tests of interactions between potential moderators and mediators of therapeutic effects are underused (Pocock et al 2002).

SYSTEMATIC REVIEWS AND META-ANALYSIS

Any one study — no matter how large or well conducted — needs independent replication. If, as is often the case, study results vary, systematic reviews and meta-analyses can help deliver consensus. These are examples of 'secondary research' in that they synthesise the available relevant evidence in a given research area. They are generally seen as increasingly important because, provided they are done well, they provide the single most reliable piece of evidence on a particular topic. Systematic reviews identify and cite studies in a pre-specified and reliable way; while meta-analyses provide an overall numerical effect across several studies. Although a systematic review has some value without an accompanying meta-analysis, the main advantage of a meta-analysis is that it is more precise and less biased than the estimate of effect from any one study. However, if the review has been flawed and collects only a biased selection of studies, this will yield a biased summary estimate of the true effect. Done properly, systematic reviews are important for two main reasons. First, as alluded to above, any individual study, no matter how rigorously conducted, analysed and interpreted, can only be an estimate of the true underlying effect and needs to be independently replicated; but subsequent studies often apparently disagree with the original for a wide variety of reasons. Second, the amount of literature in many areas is now so vast that doctors need access to high-quality review articles which reliably and conveniently provides an up-to-date summary. In addition, systematic reviews and meta-analyses are a crucial first step for planning future research and providing the evidence-base for valid clinical guidelines.

Raising awareness about the importance of these methods, and stimulating researchers to refine the techniques, has arguably been the greatest achievement of the evidence-based medicine 'movement' thus far. Traditional 'narrative' reviews, in journals or books, are generally based on a selective citation and/or reading of the literature, and books in particular tend to be out-of-date. A review is a study of studies and just as prone to selection bias. For example, thrombolysis for acute myocardial infarction could have been known to be beneficial about 10 years before textbooks were saying so if someone had done a systematic review and meta-analysis (see Ch. 12). There is no such dramatic example in psychiatry, but there are numerous treatments which are not routinely used despite good evidence for their efficacy (e.g. education and family interventions for schizophrenia). Reviewers with close financial ties to industry tend to have more favourable attitudes to new drugs in particular. Unfortunately, however, this applies equally to researchers and systematic reviewers – which is another reason for having a good grasp of valid research and reviewing techniques.

Perhaps most concerning of all, self-professed expertise is highly negatively correlated with adherence to systematic reviewing standards (Sackett et al 2000). So beware the conclusions of narrative, non-systematic reviews written by 'experts'.

Systematic reviews have the following key components:

- the formulation of a specific question;
- pre-specification of the types of article to be included and excluded;
- pre-specification of the outcome(s) of interest and important potential confounders or effect modifiers, and of any planned subgroup comparisons;
- use of several search strategies to identify articles from a number of sources (chiefly computerised databases), supplemented by searching through the references of included studies and preferably by contacting researchers for any published or unpublished studies of which they are aware; this is sometimes augmented by a hand search of key journals and/or by searching the 'grey literature' in e.g. textbooks, theses etc., and other unpublished studies;
- identifying the relevant articles and extracting the relevant data.

Properly conducted systematic reviews are, therefore, time-consuming, protocol-driven studies in their own right. The key feature is that such a review be repeatable, i.e. given your methods other researchers would identify the same articles and draw the same conclusions. Reliability is augmented if two or more researchers independently examine the (electronic) searches to identify papers for possible inclusion and search through such papers for data to be extracted. Oxman & Guyatt (1988) helpfully devised eight questions for assessing the quality of research reviews (see Box 10.6). The Department of Health (2001) psychotherapy guidelines, for example, included only reviews that met at least six of these eight criteria.

The desirability of contacting other researchers for any unpublished studies is that 'publication bias' is a large threat to the validity of a systematic review. *Publication bias* is the tendency for researchers to be more likely to write up, and (especially leading) journals to publish, positive than negative studies. As such, if one only searches for or finds published studies it is possible that the summary estimate will be biased — although this can be checked statistically (see Gilbody & Song 2000 and Ch. 11). Publication bias is more likely if one searches only one database (e.g. Medline is biased towards North American studies, whilst BIDS and Psychlit are more biased towards European studies). This is also

---

Box 10.6   Guidelines for assessing research reviews

- Were the questions and methods clearly stated?
- Were comprehensive search methods used to locate relevant studies?
- Were explicit methods used to determine which articles to include in the review?
- Was the validity of the primary studies assessed?
- Was the assessment of the primary studies reproducible and free from bias?
- Was variation in the findings of the relevant studies analysed?
- Were the findings of the primary studies combined appropriately?
- Were the reviewers' conclusions supported by the data cited?

the case if one extracts only English language articles ('language bias') as there are empirical examples of European researchers reporting negative results in their native languages and positive results in English (although the reverse has also been described). A tendency of researchers to *multiple publication bias* can have the same effect. It is alarming, but nevertheless true, that some researchers seem to adopt the strategy of conducting essentially one study and then serially publishing it over many years and sometimes even decades. The most dramatic example of this we are aware of is that one olanzapine trial has been published in one way or another in at least 83 separate publications (Gilbody & Song 2000). Indeed, we suggest that if systematic reviewers do not find examples of multiple publication bias, their search probably has not been detailed enough. Publication bias may, however, become less of a problem than it used to be, particularly for randomised control trials, as there are now a number of registers of completed and ongoing clinical trials (e.g. in the Cochrane Library), but it remains a particular problem for reviewers of observational research (Egger et al 2001). There are many other potential sources of bias in systematic reviews, and these must be very carefully addressed to minimise bias in estimating the overall effects (Egger et al 2001).

Meta-analyses mathematically combine the results of different studies to give one summary estimate of a given effect. Different studies may find apparently incompatible results for several reasons, including inadequate power, measurement error and different liabilities to bias and confounding. Simple 'vote-counting' summary techniques, comparing the number of positive studies to the number of 'negative' studies, are unreliable as they do not include an assessment of study size or quality and themselves have low power. Large studies tend generally to be of higher quality and provide more precise estimates of any given effect than smaller studies and should have relatively greater influence on a summary effect. This is achieved by 'weighting' studies according to their size and/or quality (see Ch. 11). The choice of techniques to perform and interpret meta-analyses is wide, and anyone undertaking a meta-analysis should have expert statistical advice and support. Under some circumstances, if there is substantial heterogeneity between studies, which cannot be explained, it may not be appropriate to generate an overall estimate of effect at all. In other cases, for example where the review combines a number of studies with poor methodology (e.g. trials with poor allocation concealment) and yields an apparent benefit of 20–30%, seemingly clinically worthwhile effects can merely be due to bias. In other words, the treatment may have no effect and the apparent effect could simply be due to poor methodology.

While no one can seriously challenge the desirability of systematic reviews, there remain many critics of meta-analysis. Meta-analysis certainly has its limitations, but not all of the most frequent criticisms are justified. Some 'authorities' state that meta-analysis is akin to 'combining apples and oranges' with the only result being a 'fruit salad'. Notwithstanding the fact that apples and oranges share many important similarities, there are now specific techniques which can and should be employed in any meta-analysis to assess whether studies can be meaningfully combined (tests for 'heterogeneity'; see Ch. 11). A more reasonable criticism, of 'rubbish in, rubbish out', is patently true but is not a reason for not doing meta-analyses. The result one gets from combining studies will depend on the quality of the originals, but it is far better to objectively assess study quality than to resort to the alternative of 'experts' citing the strengths of favoured studies, which are often

their own, and denigrating others. Indeed, there are a number of reliable ways of measuring study quality, and comparing the effects in high- and low-quality studies is an important part of a meta-analysis. It may, however, be best to focus on specific indices of quality (e.g. allocation concealment) rather than on generic quality scores (Juni et al 2001). This may even be the most important part of an observational meta-analysis in that clues to why studies find particular results can inform future studies of that issue.

More pertinent criticisms of meta-analyses include that they are unreliable if they include few outcome events and if there were only a small number of small studies. Importantly, since meta-analysis was devised to deal with the results from randomised control trials, there are still no ways of satisfactorily combining the results of randomised and non-randomised clinical trials, and the liabilities to bias in observational research require great caution in interpreting a meta-analysis of observational studies. A particular problem occasionally arises where a meta-analysis disagrees with the results from a large RCT or when two or more meta-analyses of the same issue find opposing results. Nonetheless, the advantages of meta-analysis generally outweigh the problems. Two recent articles have proposed standardised methods of reporting the results of observational and experimental meta-anlyses (Moher et al 1999, Stroup et al 2000) which are complementary to similar articles on the reporting of individual randomised control trials and serve as excellent introductions for potential reviewers. Particularly interested readers are referred to an excellent book (Egger et al 2001) that discusses all the foregoing in far greater detail.

CAUSAL INFERENCE

Factors to consider as possible explanations for research findings

Any association found in medical research could theoretically be attributable to one or more of the following explanations: chance, reverse causality, bias and/or confounding.

Chance

Chance or 'random error', and the related issues of study power and statistical significance, are discussed in Chapter 11. Suffice to say here that if a study is insufficiently powered, whether the result is positive or 'negative', chance remains a likely explanation. Further, studies which do not find a statistically significant association are, in fact, neutral rather than negative studies unless they have been specifically powered to be able to show 'non-equivalence', and this generally requires several hundreds of subjects in each group. In other words, a lack of evidence of an effect is not the same as evidence of a lack of effect.

Reverse causality

Reverse causality simply refers to the situation where a disease causes the apparent exposure rather than vice versa. This is particularly likely in case-control and descriptive studies. For example, the original descriptions of an association between schizophrenia and low social class have subsequently been attributed to social downward drift after the onset of the disorder (although there are now suggestions that living in a city or overcrowding may have an aetiological role). Similarly, non-independent life events can often follow depression rather than precede it.

Bias

Bias can be defined as 'any process at any stage of inference which tends to produce results or conclusions that differ systematically from the truth' (Sackett 1979). There are numerous subtypes of bias that can arise at any stage of research, and Sackett mentions 35, but there are two broad categories: selection (or recruitment) bias and information (measurement or observation) bias. These can be usefully subdivided according to whether they are primarily introduced by researchers or subjects themselves (see Box 10.7).

Selection bias stems from an absence of comparability between the groups being studied. This tends to arise either because researchers recruit from an unrepresentative population of subjects, e.g. hospital inpatients (*sampling bias*). The only way to avoid this is to randomly sample from population registers, but such attempts can always fail because of non-representative participation by subjects (*response bias*). Random samples are those in which every individual in a population has an equal chance of being included or excluded in a study, but non-response is far from random. As a rule, people are more likely to participate in research if they perceive a likely benefit for themselves or people like them, but the determinants of research participation have been poorly studied. These issues are particularly important in case-control studies as they do not have the advantage that surveys and cohort studies do of being able to identify a representative sample of controls from among large numbers of non-cases. Randomised control trials use the same patients as potential subjects and controls prior to randomisation. At least in such cases, it is possible to compare those who are identified and participate with those who do not in terms of possibly important confounders. An alternative to attempt random sampling in case-control studies is to use the 'snowball' technique to recruit subjects (ask those who do participate to nominate others they know of with the design characteristics who might also take part). Similarly, it is sometimes appropriate to recruit as controls genetic or non-genetic relatives or acquaintances of those who are affected.

Important sub-types of *sampling bias* include:

- admission (Berkson) bias — where hospitalisation rates differ for particular exposure/disease groups such that the relationship between exposure and disease is distorted in hospitalised patients;
- referral filter bias — when patient referrals from primary to secondary care increase the concentration of rare exposures and severe diseases;
- diagnostic purity bias — where the exclusion of comorbidity results in a non-representative sample;

- membership bias — where group affiliation is used to identify subjects, e.g. members of a patients' organisation, hospital staff controls;
- historical control bias — where secular changes in disease definition, exposures, treatments, etc. render such controls incomparable;
- ascertainment bias — where two groups of subjects are recruited in different ways and differ because of this.

Important sub-types of *response bias* include:

- non-respondent bias — as non-respondents are often those who are most ill — and the reverse situation of volunteer bias;
- unacceptable disease bias;
- missing data bias — e.g. on sensitive questions about sexuality, etc.

Information (measurement or observation) bias arises through the systematic misclassification of disease or exposure, or both, by researchers and the instruments they use or subjects themselves. If people know they are being observed, they tend to normalise their behaviour and minimise any perceived deviation from the norm ('attention bias'). Examples of this include the so-called 'Hawthorne effect'. Similar principles may at least partly underlie the often remarkably beneficial effects of simply asking patients, e.g. with eating disorders, to monitor certain aspects of behaviour.

Interviewer bias arises when researchers are not blind to exposure or disease status and tend to alter their approach, unconsciously or not. If the exposure is measured after disease, 'exposure suspicion bias' can influence both the intensity and the outcome of a search for exposures in affected subjects. Conversely, 'diagnostic suspicion bias' can arise if researchers strive harder to detect disease in those known to have been exposed. Generally, all observers, researchers and patients, tend to make observations that concur with their expectations ('expectation bias').

These problems can be reduced by using self-administered questionnaires and computerised assessments, but these are probably not suitable for illiterate and psychotic individuals. Highly structured interviews, searching for unambiguous or relatively 'hard' information, and blinding researchers to subject group membership are alternatives. Lay interviewers may be preferable to medical interviewers as they are more likely to follow instructions and less likely to use their own 'judgement' on deciding on exposure and disease, but this is obviously not possible if the information that is sought requires medical training to elicit.

Recall bias is the equivalent of interviewer bias, but introduced by subjects rather than researchers. Subjects generally tend to alter their responses in the direction they perceive is desired by the investigator ('obsequiousness bias'). Patients and their relatives are likely to 'search after meaning' for possible exposures to explain their disease (also called 'rumination bias'). A good psychiatric example is the maternal recall of obstetric complications in their schizophrenic children — although this can potentially be cross-checked with obstetric records. Conversely, if subjects know they have been exposed, they may be more likely to report symptoms of a disease.

In theory, any bias can increase or decrease the strength of an association, but the investigators' desire to find a positive result means that such biases tend to produce more false positives than negatives. As a rule, bias is introduced by poor research techniques and can be minimised, though probably not entirely avoided, by careful consideration of these issues in study design. It is difficult to measure bias and impossible to correct for it once it has occurred in a particular study. It is, however, sometimes possible to examine potential roles of bias in systematic reviews and meta-analyses of several studies combined.

Confounding

Confounding arises when the effects of two processes are not separated. It can be defined as 'the distortion of the apparent effect of an exposure brought about by the association with other factors that can influence the outcome' (Last 1995). Put another way, confounding mixes the effects between an exposure and a disease and a third factor associated with both. This can lead to a false association (positive confounding) or obscure a true association (negative confounding). A confounder is therefore an independent risk or protective factor for a disease that varies systematically with another exposure. Further, a confounder is in a triangular relationship with the other variables, rather than on the causal pathway (see Fig. 10.3). For example, there is increasing evidence that being born and raised in cities is a risk factor for schizophrenia. The social drift of previous generations of people with schizophrenia could, however, account for this association, i.e. genetic liability to schizophrenia and urban drift could positively confound the apparent association between urban upbringing and the disease. Age, sex and social class are common confounders. Confounders can, how-ever, only exert effects if they differ between study groups, and confounding can, sometimes, be reduced in the design stage or measured and controlled.

Controlling confounding The common methods for reducing confounding are:

- randomisation (as in RCTs);
- restriction;
- matching.

Restriction is done by selecting only subjects who have a particular range of values of a potential confounder, e.g. social class. *Matching*, on the other hand, at least in 'individual matching', selects case-control pairs with similar properties, e.g. age and sex. Rather confusingly, 'frequency matching' lies somewhere between restriction and individual matching, as the values of particular variables are 'balanced' overall between two groups. Matching reduces confounding and improves statistical power, but is not to be used lightly. Identifying potential subjects becomes more difficult; one cannot study the association between the disease and exposure on the matched variables (although this may be possible with balanced groups, and interactions with matched variables can be studied), and if one inadvertently matches on variables that are not confounders this will actually tend to reduce statistical power. In general, therefore, it is preferable to measure a potential confounder and control for it statistically. Matching is, how-ever, preferable if it is difficult to accurately measure or classify confounders (e.g. genetic liability to depression).

Statistical control of confounding involves two methods. The first is a 'stratified analysis' where a potential confounder such as age is treated by separating subjects into age groupings, or 'strata'. Standardised mortality rates are an example of this. The second, although related approach, is to conduct multivariate analyses using regression (see Ch. 11). As before, however, if it is difficult to measure a confounder accurately; attempted statistical control for it is likely to leave some 'residual confounding'. This is a particular problem when so-called proxy measures are used, e.g. using paternal social class as an index of childhood environment. If, as is common, adjustment for confounding reduces the association, residual confounding should be considered. On the other hand, confounding can be over-controlled if two variables are strongly related or if an apparent confounder actually lies on the causal pathway. This is a particular potential problem in psychiatric studies, as our knowledge of the mechanisms of most psychiatric disorders is rather limited. Statistical control for confounding should, therefore, always present both uncorrected and adjusted values of associations.

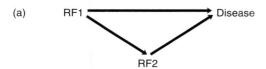

(a)   RF1 ────────────→ Disease
                   ↘   ↗
                    RF2

RF2 confounds the relationship between RF1 and the disease

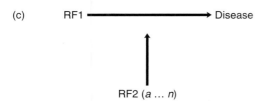

(b)   RF1 ──→ RF2 ──→ Disease

RF2 is the mediator between RF1 and the outcome

(c)   RF1 ────────────→ Disease
                   ↑
                  RF2 (a … n)

Different levels of RF2 modify the effect of RF1 on the likelihood or severity of the outcome

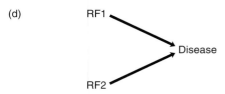

(d)   RF1 ↘
                      Disease
       RF2 ↗

RF1 and RF2 independently cause the outcome

Fig. 10.3
Schematic diagrams of (a) confounding, (b) intervening/mediator variable, (c) effect modifier/moderating variable, (d) independent risk factors (RF, risk factor).

The language of risk

A risk factor is 'an attribute or exposure that is associated with an increased probability of an outcome, such as disease' (Last 1995). The term is, however, rather loosely used and merits clarification and subdivision. Offord & Kraemer (2000) suggest that there are three different types of risk factor:

- a fixed marker — a risk factor that cannot be changed, e.g. sex;
- a variable marker — a risk factor that can be manipulated but, even so, does not change the risk of an outcome;
- a causal risk factor – which is both manipulable and changes the probability of an outcome.

For example, poverty is a risk factor for conduct disorder, but evidence thus far suggests that increasing income does not reduce the risk; whereas improving parenting practices does appear to reduce the incidence. This refinement of terms, which may seem rather abstract, has important implications. First, risk factors are not necessarily causal. Second, risk factors may differ in different populations and at different points in the history of a disease. Greater attention to these definitions might well help to shed further light on the aetiology and even pathogenesis of psychiatric disorder and is obviously required in considering the development of new therapeutic or preventative approaches. Aetiological research and screening programmes might best focus on fixed or variable (trait) markers, while pathophysiological and therapeutic studies should arguably focus on causal risk factors and state-related changes.

Similar complexities need to be appreciated about variables that potentially intervene between risk factors and outcomes (Kraemer et al 2001). Strictly speaking, intermediate or intervening variables are '*mediator variables*', which are caused to vary by independent variables and then cause variations in dependent variables (Last 1995). Distinguishing this from confounding clearly depends upon available biological knowledge. In contrast, 'effect modifiers' or '*moderators*' vary the exposure effect across different levels of that variable. Any distinction between mediators and moderators in many research reports is commonly ambiguous (but see Fig. 10.3). Kraemer et al (2001) suggest definitions of what they call proxy risk factors and overlapping risk factors (both of which are confounders), independent risk factors, mediators and moderators (which are not).

Criteria for causality

Establishing causation in multifactorial disorders is clearly complex and difficult. Old models, such as Koch's postulates and causes being 'necessary and sufficient', are inadequate. Bradford Hill proposed some criteria for deciding whether an exposure caused an outcome (see Box 10.8). Of these, perhaps the most important is that of establishing a temporal sequence, in demonstrating that the cause precedes the outcome, and that of an increase in the risk as the degree of exposure increases (a dose–response relationship). The strength of the association, i.e. size of the odds ratio or relative risk (see Ch. 12), is another important guide. Some authorities recommend that newly identified exposures or risk factors should only be taken seriously if the odds ratio is at least 3, at least until replication. Replication with different study designs and different methods is crucial. Finally, any observed association should have biological plausibility, based on what is known about pathophysiology.

DEVELOPING YOUR OWN RESEARCH IDEAS

Doing research is intellectually stimulating and rewarding, the best way of appreciating the strengths and limitations of different

---

Box 10.8   Bradford Hill's criteria for causation

- Temporal sequence
- Dose–response relationship
- Strength of association
- Consistency
- Biological plausibility

---

approaches, and can even generate valuable new knowledge. An enquiring mind, careful planning and a determination to finish are enough for many research projects. Personal and financial assistance are not essential for descriptive and case-control studies, or systematic reviews, although they do help. On the other hand, sizeable grants and research teams are generally required for cohort studies, most clinical trials and technological investigations. We shall quickly run through the main stages in designing a research project (but see e.g. Lawrie et al 2000 for further details).

1. Have an idea   These may arise from clinical observations, discussion with other staff or reading the journals. Published articles often discuss what further studies are required. Simply attempting to replicate a particular study with minor alterations to clarify one issue can be an important contribution. Turning the idea into a question may help focus the idea, by clarifying the aims and hypotheses, and suggest a research design. It can be helpful to think in terms of the 'four part clinical question' (see Ch. 12): patient problem, exposure, outcome, and control subjects or interventions. Note that one aim and hypothesis is generally preferable, as it is more likely to be thoroughly addressed than when attempting to answer two or more.

2. Review the relevant literature   Truly original ideas are very rare. Getting up to speed with the available research is often the most time-consuming process in preparing a study, but is time well spent. It will identify what needs to be done, identify the strengths of weaknesses of particular research designs, what measures are potentially relevant, etc. If there is no recent good review article then you should write one or, preferably, do a systematic review. If you are thinking about a therapeutic question, look at the Cochrane Library. If you are prepared to do a systematic review, consider writing a Cochrane review, as you will get considerable methodological support and training to do it.

3. Consider the advantages and disadvantages of the various research designs   You must realistically evaluate what you are able to do. What sort of patients and controls, and how many of them, do you have access to? It is wise to study the sorts of patients you are likely to see anyway in your clinical work. How much time will you have? If, for example, you have one 4-hour session a week for research, and each subject's measures will take an hour, it will take you at least 6 months to recruit and assess 50 patients and 50 controls. Even this can only start once you have ethical approval (let alone grant funding) and have conducted a pilot study. Will you have any help? One assistant will halve the time required and will be able to ensure that any measures have 'inter-rater reliability' if that is required.

4. Write a research protocol (see Box 10.9).   At this stage it is worth consulting an experienced researcher and/or statistician if you have not already done so. Statistical and methodological support is very important at all stages of a study. Good research supervision will help to focus your idea, clarify the design and advise on sensible statistics. A protocol is essential for properly planning the study and will serve as a template for any ethical approval or grant applications you need to apply for.

A protocol starts with a title and *introduction*. This should discuss the issue you are addressing, briefly summarise the main findings and limitations of previous studies, and describe the aims of your study. If you are attempting to answer a particular question, as is preferable, you should predict what you expect to find and rephrase the prediction as a negative ('the null hypothesis'). You may find it helpful, in writing the introduction, to ask yourself

Box 10.9 A typical study protocol and suggestions on how to complete it

Box 10.9 A typical study protocol and suggestions on how to complete it

Title
- Keep it brief

Introduction
- Why do the study?
- Previous and pilot studies
- Aims and/or hypotheses

Methods
- Design (e.g. case-control)
- Subjects (who, where from and how defined); inclusion and exclusion criteria
- Measures (demographics, disease descriptors, exposures and outcomes)
- Power calculation and statistical tests

References
- Essential references only

Patient information and consent forms
- In lay language

why does this study need to be done, at this time and in this way?'.

The protocol should then describe the precise *methods* you intend to employ, particularly how you will identify and define *subjects*, the measurements you plan to make and the main statistical techniques you will use. Cases and controls should be as representative as possible of the entire populations from which they come. Controls are usually even more difficult to identify and recruit. Any psychiatric diagnoses must be verified, preferably by actually interviewing all the subjects — although this will take about an hour or more with most of the available structured psychiatric interviews (see the next section).

Inclusion and exclusion criteria are usually based on diagnosis and demographics, such as age. Do not make inclusion criteria too restrictive or exclusions too numerous, as your study will lose representativeness and the ability to examine any differences within your patient group, and may well suffer from the 'disappearing patient' phenomenon (sometimes called 'Lasagna's law'). Inclusions are best kept to the diagnosis of interest, and exclusions limited to important potentially confounding conditions such as, for example, neurological disease.

You must then describe the *measurements* you plan to make. Measures should ideally be reliable, valid, objective and standard. Only directly relevant data should be collected, to minimise the amount of time it takes you and the subjects to complete the study. Using at least some of the measures in some of the previous studies will aid comparison and clarification. Some of the more commonly used scales are described in the next section of this chapter. Basic demographics (age, sex, social class) can be obtained from simply asking the subjects, although some descriptors (e.g. intelligence) will require specific scales. Relevant disease parameters, such as duration, medication and number of admissions, can be easily and fairly reliably obtained from case notes. Symptom severity is generally worth measuring (see the next section) and may be the outcome of primary interest. These variables may modify any effects you discover, either in reality or as confounders. Important potential exposures and confounders need to be measured, as do outcomes. If you are interested in something for which there is no scale or questionnaire, it is probably better to devise one yourself than to forcefully adapt something else. Devised instruments

should be focused, brief and clear. If you need a simple measure of severity, for example, do not be afraid to ask subjects to mark a cross on a 10 cm line, as such visual analogue scales are often surprisingly useful.

You will also need to give some thought to how the data will be recorded, stored, checked and analysed. This and indeed all other aspects of your study can and should be examined in a pilot study.

5. Do a pilot study This may use up time and subjects, but is a crucial determinant of whether your aims, subject recruitment plans and methods are realistic. As important, a pilot study will give you the best available information for a power calculation to determine exactly how many subjects you will need to examine in the study. Further, many grant-giving bodies and ethical committees now require evidence from pilot studies to ensure that ideas are feasible before giving monies or subjecting participants to projects that are unlikely to give clear-cut results.

6. Plan the statistical analysis — before you start collecting data. The tests used will depend on the types and likely distribution of your data (i.e. parametric or non-parametric statistics), whether you are simply describing subjects or comparing them (i.e. descriptive or inferential statistics), the number of groups, and any planned analysis of potential confounders (e.g. by subgroups, analyses of covariance, regression) — see Chapter 11.

7. Write a patient information sheet and consent form Writing these will help you present your research idea in the sort of lay language that is required for ethical approval submissions (which always require information and consent sheets and often place the greatest emphasis on them) and may be required for some grant-giving bodies.

8. Keep your data safe and backed up Store your protocol, correspondence, any patient records and collected data in a locked, fireproof filing cabinet. Make regular copies or backups of your data and store this separately from your computer, preferably in a fireproof safe. All too often, computers are stolen, or floods and fire damage research offices, and data from important studies are irretrievably lost. Unfortunately, most researchers do not start to make regular backups until they have suffered some kind of major data loss.

9. Write your paper A good protocol will provide you with the bulk of the introduction and methods sections of any papers you write to get your research published. The purpose of a paper is to communicate the essence of a research project so that it can be appraised in the context of others. An introduction should briefly summarise what is known and what needs to be in a particular area. A detailed methods section should be written so as to allow your study to be exactly replicated (if anyone so desires). The results section should only give important positive and negative findings. The discussion should consider the results, strengths and limitations, and implications of your findings in the context of other studies. While you are waiting for the research to be published, you could always try to answer the new questions it will inevitably raise.

COMMONLY USED PSYCHIATRIC INTERVIEWS AND RATING SCALES

It is not possible here to describe all the properties of all the available interviews and rating scales used in psychiatric research, even if that were desirable. Rather, we shall describe the principal features of the main tools for general usage.

Structured psychiatric interviews

These are detailed, time-consuming and generally only recommended for use by trained personnel. However, they share the ability to improve the reliability of diagnosis of the major disorders, over standard clinical approaches, which is why they were first developed.

Present State Examination (PSE; Wing et al 1974)

The PSE is a semi-structured interview with probes for each symptom and a detailed list of signs to be evaluated. These are generally rated as absent, mild/possible and moderate/definite. It only covers the past 4 weeks, unless augmented by additional duration questions. There are 140 items in total, with particularly detailed coverage of different types of sensory distortion and delusion. This and the detailed appendix of how to score items are a great introduction to psychopathology for trainees. There is a computer program ('Catego') that can generate diagnoses for the major disorders but not for personality disorder, in children and adolescents, or the learning disabled.

Versions 7 and 8 were first used in two large international collaborations: the US UK Diagnostic Project and the International Pilot Study of Schizophrenia (see Ch. 19). The current version, PSE-10, was slightly adapted to generate most DSM-IIIR and then DSM-IV diagnoses as well as ICD-10. It is the central component of the *Schedules of Clinical Assessment for Neuropsychiatry (SCAN)*, which has become the standard instrument for clinical assessment worldwide (Wing et al 1990) and is complementary to the US-derived instruments for community screening (see below).

Schedule for Affective Disorders and Schizophrenia (SADS; Endicott & Spitzer 1978)

The SADS is entirely structured, with symptom rating criteria contained within the interview schedule. Symptom severity is assessed — on a 7-point scale where 3 or more is usually 'clinically significant' — for current episode, the previous week, the point of maximal severity and any previous episode. Not surprisingly, this can take up to 2 hours. There are now several versions available, including those for lifetime assessments, sensitivity to change and for children and adolescents. The SADS is not useful for organic disorders or anorexia, however. The same research group also developed a separate instrument, the Structured Clinical Interview for DSM (SCID), with the advantage that it is suitable for both clinical and research use, but the disadvantage that it is rarely used for either.

Diagnostic Interview Schedule (DIS; Robins et al 1981)

The DIS was specifically devised to be useful in all settings and for use by lay interviewers after 1–2 weeks training, so that the prevalence of DSM-III disorders (except organic and mental retardation) could be determined. The resulting Epidemiological Catchment Area (ECA) study of more than 18 000 urban residents in five US sites was extremely influential, although there are serious questions about the sensitivity of the tool (and particularly for schizophrenia). The DIS was revised to be suitable for DSM-IIIR but, rather embarrassingly, the subsequent National Co-morbidity Survey found rather different (usually higher) prevalences (see Narrow et al 2002 for an attempted resolution). Nonetheless, the DIS was then transformed, in line with ICD-10 and DSM-IV, into the *Composite International Diagnostic Interview (CIDI)*.

The development of the CIDI has been sponsored by WHO (Robins et al 1988), and is generally recommended for initial community screening to be followed by professional interviewing with the SCAN. Both are now available in several languages. These instruments are likely to become increasingly favoured over others, but will of course need amendment when DSM-V appears.

Symptom severity rating scales

The following are the most frequently used scales to assess symptoms, their severity and to monitor any change.

- *Brief Psychiatric Rating Scale* (BPRS; Overall & Gorham 1962). Originally composed of 16 general items (5 observational), rated 0–7, this was then revised to 18 (to include observations of excitement and disorientation), and some versions include up to 25 items. The semi-structured interview schedule is brief (18 minutes) and delivers reliable ratings, but the instrument is better for psychosis than depression or anxiety.
- *Krawiecka or Manchester scale* (Krawiecka et al 1977). Devised for rating chronic psychosis, with four symptoms and four signs (later revised to separate flat and incongruous affect) scored 0–4. No interview schedule is available, however.
- *Positive and Negative Symptoms Scale* (PANSS; Kay et al 1987). Measures general psychopathology (16 items), as well as positive and negative symptoms (7 items each) on a scale of 1–7 where 3 is mild. The PANSS takes longer than the BPRS but has been carefully validated against other instruments, especially for schizophrenia. Not to be confused with the Scale for the Assessment of Positive Symptoms (SAPS) and the equivalent for negative symptoms. The Scale for the Assessment of Negative Symptoms (SANS; Andreasen 1982) is by far the best option if negative symptoms are the focus of the study. It has 30 items, scored 0–5, in five domains (affective flattening, alogia, avolition-apathy, anhedonia-asociality, and attentional impairment).
- *Hamilton Rating Scale for Depression* (HRSD; Hamilton 1960). The original 21 items are commonly reduced to 17 (excluding the comparatively rare depersonalization, paranoia and obsessionality items, and missing out diurnal variation as this was thought to be related to the subtype of illness rather than severity). It is clinician rated, taking all available information into account. Although it is by far the most commonly used scale for depression, it is commonly misused as a diagnostic instrument, is biased towards biological symptoms over subjective distress, and has an unstable factor structure. Similar criticisms apply to the *Hamilton Rating Scale for Anxiety* (HRSA; Hamilton 1959) although this too has been extensively used for severity and change assessments.
- *Beck Depression Inventory* (BDI; Beck et al 1961). Self-completed 21-item inventory, which is sensitive to change, but biased to cognitive items.
- *Montgomery-Asberg Depression Rating Scale* (MADRS; Montgomery & Asberg 1979). Specifically designed as 10 items sensitive to change, it has good psychometric properties.
- *Hospital Anxiety and Depression Scale* (HADS; Zigmond & Snaith 1983). Specifically intended as a screening tool in medical patients, it contains seven items each on self-rated

depression and anxiety (scored 0–3) and is valid and sensitive to change.

- *State-Trait Anxiety Inventory* (STAI; Spielberger et al 1970). Two separate self-rated scales of 20 items each, which only take a few minutes to complete, and the state scale is sensitive to change.

The most widely used scale for obsessional symptoms is probably the Leyton Obsessional Inventory. There are few good scales for mania severity, which generally suffer from a difficulty capturing mixed states. Any of the various versions of the General Health Questionnaire (GHQ) are suitable for (postal) screening for psychiatric morbidity in the general population, although the follow-up interview is now rarely done with the Clinical Interview Schedule as was originally intended.

Outcome measurement in psychiatry

Diagnosis and symptom severity are obviously important determinants of functional ability and general well-being but by no means the only ones and sometimes not even the best. Doctors' realisation of this has accompanied an increased emphasis on patients' perceptions of their problems, together with the increasing drive to routine outcome monitoring in clinical practice. There is a bewildering array of scales and other potential outcome measures in medicine generally and psychiatry in particular. The Medical Outcomes Short Form — 36 items (SF36) has been most widely used, while the EuroQol or WHOQol seem to be emerging as the most likely alternatives for general use. The Health of the Nation Outcome Scales (HoNOS) have however been devised for such use in (UK) psychiatric settings specifically.

Outcome scales specific to psychiatry (and the UK) obviously cannot compare the outcomes of e.g. depression and heart failure (or internationally) in the way that the SF36 already has. The SF36 is a self-rated multidimensional measure of physical and emotional health, but the emotional symptom measures are very general. How it compares to the staff-rated HoNOS, and whether they are complementary, remain to be determined. The HoNOS covers a wider array of symptoms, behaviours and functions — and certainly appears preferable to the main alternatives such as the WHO's psychiatric Disability Assessment Schedule and the Global Assessment of Functioning in DSM. A Department of Health (Charlwood et al 1999) working group on outcome indicators in 'serious mental illness' recommended: the immediate implementation of mortality and homicide monitoring; the use (where locally possible) of both the HoNOS and a user-assessed 'quality of life' measure, augmented by measures of e.g. the numbers of patients discharged, defaulting from follow-up, in employment and suitable accommodation; with further indices to be considered subject to adequate information technology support.

One issue of particular note is that quality-of-life measures tend to be most useful if they help to plan clinical management. Although the SF36 and HoNOS can be used in this way and are sensitive to change, none of the above was specifically devised for 'needs assessment', although such instruments are available, e.g. the Camberwell Assessment of Need. There remains much work to be done in assessing the validity of generic and specific instruments in psychiatric populations, getting them into routine use, and evaluating them and clinical effectiveness generally (Gilbody et al 2002). Particular thought needs to be given to the reliability of ratings done by several staff. It is clear, however, that if routine outcome monitoring in psychiatry is to include functioning and well-being, clinicians will need to use at least some of the research methods already described in this chapter and the principles of measurement and statistics discussed in the next.

REFERENCES

Al-Shahi R, Warlow C 2000 Using patient-identifiable data for observational research and audit. British Medical Journal 321:1031–1032

Andreasen N C 1982 Negative symptoms in schizophrenia: definition and reliability. Archives of General Psychiatry 39:784–788

Assmann S F, Pocock S J, Enos L E, Kasten L E 2000 Subgroup analysis and other (mis)uses of baseline data in clinical trials. Lancet 355:1064–1069

Barker S, Lavender T, Morant N 2001 Client and family narratives on schizophrenia. Journal of Mental Health 10:199–212

Beck A T, Ward C H, Mendelson M et al 1961 An inventory for measuring depression. Archives of General Psychiatry 4:561–571

Bedi N, Chilvers C, Churchill R et al 2000 Assessing effectiveness of treatment of depression in primary care: Partially randomised preference trial. British Journal of Psychiatry 177:312–318

Carpenter W T Jr, Sadler J H, Light P D et al 1983 The therapeutic efficacy of hemodialysis in schizophrenia. New England Journal of Medicine 308:669–675

Carpenter W T Jr, Gold J M, Lahti A C et al 2000 Decisional capacity for informed consent in schizophrenia research. Archives of General Psychiatry 57:533–538

Chalmers T C, Celano P, Sacks H S, Smith H Jr 1983 Bias in treatment assignment in controlled clinical trials. New England Journal of Medicine 309:1358–1361

Charlwood P, Mason A, Goldacre M et al 1999 Health outcome indicators: Severe mental illness. Report of a working group to the Department of Health. National Centre for Health Outcomes Development, Oxford

CSBS 2001 Schizophrenia. Clinical Standards Board for Scotland, Edinburgh

Department of Health 2001 Treatment choice in psychological therapies and counselling. Evidence based clinical practical guideline. Department of Health, London

Dowrick C, Dunn G, Ayuso-Mateos J L et al 2000 Problem solving treatment and group psychoeducation for depression: multicentre randomised controlled trial. Outcomes of Depression International Network (ODIN) Group. British Medical Journal 321:1450–1454

Duffett R, Lelliott P 1998 Auditing electroconvulsive therapy: The third cycle. British Journal of Psychiatry 172:401–405

Edwards P, Roberts I, Clarke M et al 2002 Increasing response rates to postal questionnaires: systematic review. British Medical Journal 324:1183

Egger M, Smith G D, Altman D G 2001 Systematic reviews in health care. Meta-analysis in context. BMJ Books, London

Endicott J, Spitzer R L 1978 A diagnostic interview schedule for affective disorders and schizophrenia. Archives of General Psychiatry 35:837–844

Even C, Siobud-Dorocant E, Dardennes R M 2000 Critical approach to antidepressant trials. Blindness protection is necessary, feasible and measurable. British Journal of Psychiatry 177:47–51

Farmer A. The demise of the published case report — is resuscitation necessary? British Journal of Psychiatry 1999 174:93–94

Feinstein A R 1985 The architecture of clinical research. Saunders, Philadelphia

Geddes J, Freemantle N, Harrison P, Bebbington P 2000 Atypical antipsychotics in the treatment of schizophrenia: systematic overview and meta-regression analysis. British Medical Journal 321:1371–1376

Gilbody S, Whitty P 2002 Improving the delivery and organisation of mental health services: beyond the conventional randomised controlled trial. British Journal of Psychiatry 180:13–18

Gilbody S M, Song F 2000 Publication bias and the integrity of psychiatry research. Psychological Medicine 30:253–258

Gilbody S M, House A O, Sheldon T A. Outcomes research in mental health. British Journal of Psychiatry 2002 181:8–16

Grimes D A, Schulz K F 2002 Descriptive studies: what they can and cannot do. Lancet 359:145–149

Guyatt G, Sackett D, Taylor D W et al 1986 Determining optimal therapy — randomized trials in individual patients. New England Journal of Medicine 314:889–892

Hamilton M 1959 The assessment of anxiety states by rating. British Journal of Medical Psychology 32:50–55

Hamilton M 1960 A rating scale for depression. Journal of Neurology Neurosurgery & Psychiatry 23:56–62

Hennekens C H, Buring J E 1987 Epidemiology in medicine. Little, Brown, Boston

Hotopf M, Churchill R, Lewis G 1999 Pragmatic randomised controlled trials in psychiatry. British Journal of Psychiatry 175:217–223

Jones J, Hunter D 1995 Consensus methods for medical and health services research. British Medical Journal 311:376–380

Juni P, Altman D G, Egger M 2001 Systematic reviews in health care: Assessing the quality of controlled clinical trials. British Medical Journal 323:42–46

Kay S R, Fiszbein A, Opler L A 1987 The positive and negative syndrome scale (PANSS) for schizophrenia. Schizophrenia Bulletin 13:261–276

Kraemer H C, Stice E, Kazdin A et al 2001 How do risk factors work together? Mediators, moderators, and independent, overlapping, and proxy risk factors. American Journal of Psychiatry 158:848–856

Krawiecka M, Goldberg D, Vaughan M 1977 A standardized psychiatric assessment scale for rating chronic psychotic patients. Acta Psychiatrica Scandinavica 55:299–308

Last J M 1995 A dictionary of epidemiology. Oxford University Press, Oxford

Lawrie S M 2002 Clinical trial methodology. In: Reid I, Anderson I (eds) The fundamentals of psychopharmacology: The definitive guide, Martin Dunitz, London

Lawrie S M, McIntosh A M, Rao S 2000 Critical appraisal for psychiatry. Churchill Livingstone, Edinburgh

Lewis G, Pelosi A J 1990 The case-control study in psychiatry. British Journal of Psychiatry 157:197–207

Louis T A, Lavori P W, Bailar J C 3rd, Polansky M 1984 Crossover and self-controlled designs in clinical research. New England Journal of Medicine 310:24–31

Marshall M, Lockwood A, Bradley C et al 2000 Unpublished rating scales: a major source of bias in randomised controlled trials of treatments for schizophrenia. British Journal of Psychiatry 176:249–252

McMahon A D 2002 Study control, violators, inclusion criteria and defining explanatory and pragmatic trials. Statistical Medicine 21:1365–1376

Moher D, Cook D J, Eastwood S et al 1999 Improving the quality of reports of meta-analyses of randomised controlled trials: the QUOROM statement. Lancet 354:1896–1900

Moncrieff J, Wessely S, Hardy R 1998 Meta-analysis of trials comparing antidepressants with active placebos. British Journal of Psychiatry 172:227–231; discussion 232–234

Montgomery S A, Asberg M 1979 A new depression scale designed to be sensitive to change. British Journal of Psychiatry 134:382–389

Narrow W E, Rae D S, Robins L N, Regier D A 2002 Revised prevalence estimates of mental disorders in the United States: using a clinical significance criterion to reconcile 2 surveys' estimates. Archives of General Psychiatry 59:115–123

Naylor C D, Guyatt G H 1996 Users' guides to the medical literature. XI: How to use an article about a clinical utilization review. Evidence-Based Medicine Working Group. Journal of the American Medical Association 275:1435–1439

O'Brien T, Oxman A D, Davis D A et al 2002a Audit and feedback: effects on professional practice and health care outcomes (Cochrane review). In: The Cochrane Library, Issue 3. Update Software, Oxford

O'Brien T, Oxman A D, Davis D A et al 2002b Audit and feedback versus alternative strategies: effects on professional practice and health care outcomes (Cochrane review). In: The Cochrane Library, Issue 3. Update Software, Oxford

Offord D R, Kraemer H C 2000 Risk factors and prevention. Evidence-Based Mental Health 70:70–71

Overall J E, Gorham D R 1962 The Brief Psychiatric Rating Scale. Psychological Reports 10:799–812

Oxman A D, Guyatt G H 1988 Guidelines for reading literature reviews. Canadian Medical Association Journal 138:697–703

Peto R, Collins R, Gray R 1993 Large-scale randomized evidence: large, simple trials and overviews of trials. Annals of the New York Academy of Sciences 703:314–340

Pocock S J 1983 Clinical trials: a practical approach. John Wiley, Chichester

Pocock S J, Assmann S E, Enos L E, Kasten L E 2002 Subgroup analysis, covariate adjustment and baseline comparisons in clinical trial reporting: current practice and problems. Statistical Medicine 21:2917–2930

Roberts L W, Warner T D, Brody J L et al 2002 Patient and psychiatrist ratings of hypothetical schizophrenia research protocols: assessment of harm potential and factors influencing participation decisions. American Journal of Psychiatry 159:573–584

Robins L N, Helzer J E, Croughan J, Ratcliff K S 1981 National Institute of Mental Health Diagnostic Interview Schedule: its history, characteristics, and validity. Archives of General Psychiatry 38:381–389

Robins L N, Wing J, Wittchen H U et al 1988 The Composite International Diagnostic Interview: an epidemiologic instrument suitable for use in conjunction with different diagnostic systems and in different cultures. Archives of General Psychiatry 45:1069–1077

Sackett D L 1979 Bias in analytic research. Journal of Chronic Diseases 32:51–63

Sackett D L, Haynes R B, Guyatt G H, Tugwell P 1991 Clinical epidemiology: a basic science for clinical medicine. Little, Brown, Boston

Sackett D L, Straus S E, Richardson W S et al 2000 Evidence-based medicine: how to practice and teach EBM. Churchill Livinstone, Edinburgh

Savulescu J, Chalmers I, Blunt J 1996 Are research ethics committees behaving unethically? Some suggestions for improving performance and accountability. British Medical Journal 313:1390–1393

Schulz K F, Grimes D A 2002a Case-control studies: research in reverse. Lancet 359:431–434

Schulz K F, Grimes D A 2002b Unequal group sizes in randomised trials: guarding against guessing. Lancet 359:966–970

Schulz K F, Chalmers I, Hayes R J, Altman D G 1995 Empirical evidence of bias: dimensions of methodological quality associated with estimates of treatment effects in controlled trials. Journal of the American Medical Association 273:408–412

Spielberger C D, Gorusch R L, Lushene R 1970 STAI — Manual for the State-Trait Anxiety Inventory. Consulting Psychologists Press, Palo Alto

Stroup D F, Berlin J A, Morton S C et al 2000 Meta-analysis of observational studies in epidemiology. Journal of the American Medical Association 283:2008–2012

Thornley B, Adams C 1998 Content and quality of 2000 controlled trials in schizophrenia over 50 years. British Medical Journal 317:1181–1184

Vastag B 2000 Helsinki discord? A controversial declaration. Journal of the American Medical Association 284:2983–2985

Warlow C 2002 Advanced issues in the design and conduct of randomized clinical trials: the bigger the better? Statistical Medicine 21:2797–2805

Wing J 1981 Ethics and psychiatric research. In: Bloch S, Chodoff P (eds) Psychiatric ethics. Oxford University Press, Oxford, p 277–294

Wing J K, Cooper J E, Sartorius N 1974 The measurement and classification of psychiatric symptoms. Cambridge University Press, Cambridge

Wing J K, Babor T, Brugha T et al 1990 SCAN. Schedules for Clinical Assessment in Neuropsychiatry. Archives of General Psychiatry 47:589–593

Zigmond A S, Snaith R P 1983 The Hospital Anxiety and Depression Scale. Acta Psychiatrica Scandinavica 67:361–370

11 Research measurement and statistics

Andrew M McIntosh, Stephen M Lawrie

INTRODUCTION

The term statistics literally means 'numerical data', and statistics as a discipline is the science of assembling and interpreting numerical data (Bland 2000). Some form of numerical analysis is useful in most research, and all doctors should be able to understand and interpret the findings presented in medical journals that inform their clinical practice.

Almost all statistics are based on the premise that study of a sample of people with a condition allows the inference of something more general about the population from which they came. To do this, studies need to be valid (i.e. well designed and conducted) and present clear results using the appropriate tests. Statistics is concerned not merely with the results of an experiment or study, but also with its design. Badly designed studies are unlikely to yield reliable results, no matter how sophisticated the statistical analysis may be.

Most of the features determining the validity of a study have been covered in the previous chapter. This chapter will explain the most commonly used descriptive and inferential statistics relevant to data analysis and interpretation. By descriptive statistics we mean the summary, tabulation and graphical display of numerical information. By inferential statistics, we mean the inferences about the population that are drawn from the sample.

RESEARCH MEASUREMENT

Types of data

Data is conventionally classified as either discrete or continuous. Discrete data can only take a limited set of possible values (e.g. socio-economic status, sex) whereas continuous data have a potentially infinite series of values (e.g. height, temperature). In practice, the accuracy of data measurement usually means that continuous parameters such as height are measured to the nearest unit and are actually discrete variables. This qualification is not usually very important, however. Discrete data can be further subdivided into four types according to their properties:

- nominal or categorical;
- ordinal;
- interval;
- ratio.

Nominal or categorical data have values which are qualitatively different from one another but have no particular order (e.g. diagnosis). When there are only two possible values (e.g. gender), nominal data are sometimes also referred to as dichotomous. Ordinal data have a logical order in their values, but the differences between each of the values are not necessarily equal and the measurement has no true zero point (e.g. social class I–V, ward observation level). Interval and ratio data have very similar properties; in both, the differences between values are equal (e.g. the difference between a value of 1 and 2 is the same as the difference between 33 and 34). Ratio data have the additional property of having a true zero point (i.e. a complete absence of the quantity), though this distinction is rarely important. Distinguishing the various data types may seem like an irrelevant abstraction, but is essential in determining the correct method of data description and analysis. Discrete interval, discrete ratio and continuous data can be analysed using a group of related techniques called *parametric* statistics, subject to a limited number of additional considerations (see below). Data which are nominal or ordinal are analysed using *non-parametric* or distribution-free methods.

A further distinction in study data is made between variables that are *dependent* and those that are *independent*. Dependent variables are the characteristics we wish to investigate, whereas an independent variable refers to the data classification. For example, in a study where one compared the whole brain volume of patients with various psychiatric diagnoses, diagnosis would be the independent variable and brain volume the dependent variable.

Validity and reliability of measurement

- Validity is whether an instrument measures what it purports to measure.
- Reliability is whether repeated measurements of the same data give similar results.

There are several methods of determining the reliability and validity of a measure.

Validity

Validity of measurement can be assessed in many ways, but perhaps the simplest form of validity is when something 'looks right'. When a scale 'looks right' at brief inspection then it is said to have *face validity*. A related measure of validity is *content validity*. This refers to the individual items or content of a scale. For example an anxiety scale containing many items about psychosis is likely to have poor content validity.

With a new measurement technique there is often a *gold standard* against which it can be compared. If the new measurement gives consistently different results it cannot be valid. This form of validity is called *criterion validity* and should not be confused with reliability or repeatability, although the concepts are similar. If there is no clear gold standard then one has to compare the new measure with another measure of uncertain validity to see if it gives the results one could reasonably expect. For example, a scale measuring suicidal ideation might be found to predict deliberate self-harm. This property of having an appropriate relationship with other variables is known as *construct validity*. A final measure of the validity of a scale is whether the items on a scale are related to one another. This is known as *internal consistency* and can be measured using Cronbach's alpha. For more information about Cronbach's alpha the reader is referred to Bland & Altman (1997). For further information about the validity of scales the reader should consult Bland & Altman (2002).

Reliability

Researchers and clinicians often wish to obtain data from patients. Sometimes obtaining the information may be long and protracted (e.g. full clinical interview) or on other occasions it may entail the risk of harm to the patient (e.g. direct measurement of the CSF levels of drugs). In order to obtain the information more quickly, or with less risk to the patient, new methods may emerge whose level of agreement with the old techniques needs to be assessed. Measurements using a given technique should also be repeatable from researcher to researcher. For example: during a 10-year cohort study of people with schizophrenia it would be unlikely for the same researchers to be present throughout the whole study. We therefore need to be satisfied that, given the same material, the researchers would have a high level of agreement on its measurement. This form of reliability is sometimes known as *inter-rater reliability*.

The quantification of reliability between different raters (inter-rater) or between different methods in general can be accomplished by a number of means depending on the data type. For categorical data (e.g. whether someone has schizophrenia or not) the reliability of the results are usually measured using the kappa (κ) statistic. Kappa is calculated according to the following formula:

$$\kappa = \frac{P_o - P_e}{(1 - P_e)}$$

Where P_o is the proportion of observed agreement and P_e is the proportion of agreement expected by chance. Consider the example shown in Table 11.1, where two observers interview 100 patients and decide whether they have schizophrenia or not. In 50 cases, Observer 1 and Observer 2 agree that the person has schizophrenia, and in 20 that they do not, out of a total sample of 100. Therefore the observed agreement (P_o) is 0.7 or 70%. This is spuriously high, however, as the raters would agree by chance alone on a number of occasions. The expected chance agreement

Table 11.1 Example showing the level of agreement and disagreement between two observers

		Observer 1		
		Present	Absent	Total
Observer 2	Present	50	10	60
	Absent	20	20	40
	Total	70	30	100

can be calculated as follows: for each cell where there is observed agreement the row total is multiplied by the column total and divided by the total sample size. This comes to $60 \times 70/100$ (42) and $40 \times 30/100$ (12). Adding these together and dividing by the total sample size gives 56% expected agreement by chance alone. Therefore:

$$\kappa = \frac{(70/100) - (56/100)}{1 - 56/100} = 0.32$$

(a relatively unreliable result).

This method can be extended to situations where diagnoses or measurements are made in three or more ranked categories (e.g. no, borderline and definite diagnoses of mental illness), in which case kappa can be modified, or weighted, to account for partial agreement. The interested reader should consult Streiner & Norman (1996) for further details.

The reliability of interval, ratio or continuous measurements can be measured by a variety of other methods. The most *misused* method is to consider the association or correlation between the ratings of two or more observers using the Pearson or Spearman correlation coefficient. This approach is unsuitable because one investigator may consistently under-rate or over-rate compared with his colleague, and yet the degree of correlation between their scores could be very high. For example, one researcher may consistently over-rate the presence of positive symptoms compared with another at the same centre, but because the over-rating is consistent the correlations between scores may be perfect despite the fact that the raters never agree. A useful alternative to this approach is to use the *intra-class correlation coefficient (ICC)*. The ICC distinguishes the bias in the measurement from random variation of the instrument and produces a more accurate and representative value of reliability. It can also be adapted to situations where there are several observers and can be easily calculated from an analysis of variance (ANOVA) table (Streiner & Norman 1996).

No statistical test is however a substitute for clear graphical representation. The common error in representing agreement between two or more investigators is to plot the observations on a graph where the values given by each investigator are represented on each axis. This approach is similar to the method of correlation and can lead to misleading results. A more informative approach is to plot the difference between the investigators' measurements against the mean of the measurements (Fig. 11.1). Plotting the difference against the average will demonstrate whether the difference between the two methods is generally very small or very large. A mean difference between the methods can be calculated and, in situations where the mean difference is not zero, whether or not one method gives systematically higher or

Types of validity
• Face validity
• Content validity
• Criterion validity
• Construct validity
• Internal consistency

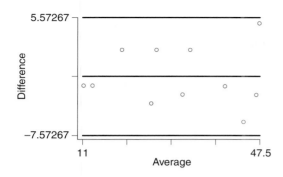

Fig. 11.1
Bland–Altman plot showing the differences between two measurements.

Reliability
• Can be between methods or raters (inter-rater) or within the same instrument or rater repeated on more than one occasion (intra-rater, test–retest) • Can be graphically represented on a Bland–Altman plot • Should not be measured by the simple correlation of different investigators' scores

lower scores than the other can be evaluated. Limits of agreement can be added around the average difference (as $d \pm 2s$) as a further refinement by calculating the mean difference (d) and its standard deviation (s). When these limits of agreement do not incorporate any clinically meaningful difference, the two methods may be used interchangeably. Further information about this approach is available from Bland & Altman (1986).

From the simulated example, illustrated in Figure 11.1, of two raters both using the same 60-point scale, the limits of agreement (reference range for difference) are –7.573 to 5.573, and the mean difference = –1.000. Since the reference range for the difference includes differences of up to 7 points on a 60-point scale, the inter-rater agreement may be too unsatisfactory for the results of one rater to be considered interchangeable with that of the other.

Similar techniques can be used to assess the reliability of a method repeated twice or more on the same material. As the variability between measurements is likely to be less, some of the sources of variation have been removed, and the methods above will need to be adapted for this purpose.

STATISTICS

Probability and risk

Probability and risk are interchangeable terms used to quantify uncertainty or the chance of an observation (or event) occurring. Probability always takes a value between 0, indicating that an event cannot occur, and 1 where it is a certainty. The probability of an event can be easily understood by referring to an unbiased six-sided die. If we ask ourselves the probability of throwing a 6, almost intuitively we come up with the solution 1 in 6, or 0.167. Without realising it we are undertaking the following calculation:

Probability = number of events / number of possible events

We know that each side of the die is equally likely (if the die is unbiased) and that there are six sides. Therefore the probability that any side will turn face up is 1 in 6. The probabilities of events in medicine are rarely quite as simple as this although the principles are the same. Consider a study of the probability of readmission following an acute episode of schizophrenia. In a study of 100 people over 1 year, let us say that 40 are readmitted. What is the probability of readmission over 1 year? From the above calculation we see that it is 40 (the number of events) divided by 100 (the number of possible events). Therefore the probability or risk of readmission is 0.4 or 40%.

There are alternative ways of stating the possibility that an event will occur. Those who are familiar with betting will recognise the term *odds*. This statistic is simply the ratio of events of interest to the non-events. To take the example of the die, the odds of throwing a 6 are 1 (the number of events) divided by (the number of non-events) 5. Taking the example of relapse in schizophrenia, we can see that the odds of relapse are 40 (the number of events) divided by 60 (the number of non-events) or 0.67. These examples illustrate several important points. The first is that we do not have to throw a die 100 times to calculate the probability of throwing a 6; we already have prior knowledge of its behaviour or probability distribution (i.e. it has a uniform distribution). In the second example, we do not know the probability distribution of readmission in schizophrenia so we determine it empirically. Secondly, note that the probability and odds are quite similar in the first example of the die, whereas in the second example they are quite different. This is because the event of interest in the first example is less frequent than in the second example. For very rare events the odds provide a good approximation to the probability and are preferred because of their mathematical properties, particularly for logistic regression (for further reading see the reference list). Thirdly, while probabilities range from 0 to 1, odds range from 0 to infinity and are often plotted on a logarithmic scale.

Where there is only one group of people and we wish to give an estimate of the chance with which an event will occur, the odds or probability will usually suffice. Odds and probability can be converted into one another using the following formulae:

$$\text{odds} = \frac{P}{1 - P} \quad \text{(probability of an event / probability of a non-event)}$$

$$p = \frac{0}{(1 + 0)} \quad (p, \text{ probability}; o, \text{ odds})$$

If we want to know the probability of two *independent* events (i.e. the outcome of one event will not influence the probability of the other), we multiply their probabilities together. Therefore, the probability of throwing two 6s in a row is 1/6 times 1/6, i.e. 1/36. If two events are mutually exclusive however (i.e. one event precludes the other) then the probabilities are added. For example the probability of throwing a six or a five is 1/6 plus 1/6, which equals 2/6 or 1/3. Similarly, in a study where 40 out of 100 people relapse and 60 do not, the probability of either relapse or non-relapse is 40/100 plus 60/100, i.e. 1.

In a clinical trial we generally compare the probability or odds of one or more outcomes in the two groups. If the treatment is efficacious, the probability of the adverse event (like relapse) will be less in the treated (or experimental group) than it is in the control group. These probabilities, or risks, are sometimes called the experimental event rate (EER) and control event rate respectively (CER). The experimental event rate is defined as the probability

Table 11.2 Contingency table showing relapse in haloperidol- and placebo-treated patients

	Relapse	Non-relapse	Total
Haloperidol	20	80	100
Placebo	50	50	100

of an event in the experimental group, and the control event rate is defined as the probability of an event in the control group. These terms are usually applied to undesirable events but are applicable to both undesirable and desirable events.

Consider, for example, a trial where patients are randomised to receive either haloperidol or placebo. One hundred people are treated in the haloperidol group and 100 are treated with placebo. Fifty people in the placebo group relapse over the course of the 6-week trial and 20 relapse in the haloperidol-treated group. We can represent the data in the form of a 2×2 (contingency) table, as shown in Table 11.2. The probability (or risk) of relapse in the haloperidol-treated group is 20/100 or 0.2. This is called the experimental event rate. Alternatively we could also say that the odds of relapse were 20/80 or 0.25.

The probability of relapse in the placebo-treated group is 50/100 or 0.5. This is called the control event rate. Alternatively, we could also say that the odds of relapse are 0.5/0.5 or 1.

These probabilities or odds can be combined to give a single measure of treatment effect. The simplest and most useful things to do are to divide probabilities or odds in the two groups, giving the *relative risk* and *odds ratio* respectively. Alternatively we could subtract the probabilities from each other giving an absolute risk or risk difference.

In the above example EER = 0.2 and CER = 0.5. Dividing these two risks we get 0.2/0.5 or 0.4 (40%). This is known as the *relative risk (RR)*.

$$\text{Relative risk} = \frac{\text{EER}}{\text{CER}}$$

Alternatively one could also say that the risk of relapse is reduced by 60% in the experimental group relative to the control group. This is known as the *relative risk reduction (RRR)*.

$$\text{RRR} = 1 - \text{RR}, \quad \text{or} \quad \text{RRR} = \frac{\text{CER} - \text{EER}}{\text{CER}}$$

Given the odds of relapse are 0.25 in the experimental group and 1 in the control group, their ratio (the *odds ratio*) is 0.25 divided by 1, or 0.25.

$$\text{Odds ratio} = \frac{\text{Odds of the event in the experimental group}}{\text{Odds of the event in the control group}}$$

Another way of summarising the difference between groups is to subtract the individual estimates of the probability of outcomes from one another. It makes no mathematical sense to subtract an odds from another odds so we will concentrate on the probabilities or risks. In the example above, the risk of relapse (EER) in the experimental group was 0.2 (or 20%) and the risk of relapse in the control group (CER) was 0.5. By subtracting these figures we can also say that the risk difference is 0.3 (30%). This is called the risk difference or *absolute risk reduction (ARR)*.

$$\text{Absolute risk reduction} = \text{CER} - \text{EER}$$

Absolute risk is a more clinically useful measure of treatment efficacy than the relative risk because the relative risk is relatively insensitive to the underlying or absolute risk in untreated individuals. If in our example, the EER were 0.02 instead of 0.2, and the CER were 0.05 instead of 0.5, the relative risk would remain the same and would suggest to the naïve reader that the treatment confers a considerable treatment benefit. However, because the risk to untreated individuals is comparatively low (0.05 or 5%) then the benefits of treatment in clinical practice would be less impressive. This is best illustrated by the ARR or risk difference, which in this case would be only 0.03 (3%) instead of 0.3 (30%). In other words, we would need to treat about 34 people to prevent one relapse instead of just 3.3. These figures are calculated by taking the reciprocal of the ARR to get the *number needed to treat (NNT)* (NNT = 1/ARR). These statistics and their applications are discussed in greater detail in the following chapter.

Incidence and prevalence

Epidemiology is the study of disease in populations. In many cases epidemiologists study populations by taking what they hope is a representative sample and inferring something about the population from which they were drawn. In order to do this, two numerical concepts must be introduced: *incidence* and *prevalence*. Incidence is the number of new cases arising in a given population in a defined time period. For instance, schizophrenia has an incidence of 2–3 cases per 10 000 population per year. Incidence is in fact an event rate, and the experimental and control event rates mentioned above are also incidence rates. Prevalence is the number of people within a population who have the disease of interest at any given time. The prevalence of schizophrenia is sometimes quoted as 0.5 per 100 (0.5%), meaning that at any time point, 5 in 1000 people fulfil diagnostic criteria for schizophrenia. Prevalence can be measured at a single point in time (point prevalence) or over a given time period (e.g. 1-month prevalence). Incidence and prevalence are related to each other though *chronicity*. When a disease is chronic, prevalence will be high relative to incidence. When a disease is acute and short-lived, the incidence may be high, but because few cases persist, prevalence will remain low.

Using data on incidence epidemiologists can investigate candidate risk factors. For example, when two populations exist, one of which is exposed to an agent (e.g. sheep dip) while the other is not, incidence of a disease (e.g. depression) can be measured in both groups. If the incidence of depression is greater in the exposed group, this suggests that sheep dip may cause depression. It would be unusual for the results of an epidemiological study to be as simple as this. Frequently two populations may differ on a number of other variables which may be associated with both the disease and exposure, in which case the study is said to be *confounded*. Quite often, the measurement of the disease frequency itself may be biased by a number of factors. Subject to these considerations, the ratio of the incidence in the exposed group to the incidence in the unexposed group is also referred to as the relative risk. Similarly, the subtraction of one risk from the other is referred to as the *absolute risk* (or risk difference) and has similar properties to the absolute risk reduction mentioned earlier.

The size of a relative risk or odds ratio is not however the only determinant of the importance of a putative risk factor or the incidence or prevalence of a disease. Analogously to the EER of 0.02/0.2 example above, a rare risk factor with a relative risk of 10 will be less important at a population level than a common risk factor with a relative risk of 2 (see, for example, family history and urban upbringing / season of birth in schizophrenia, Chapter 19). The concept of population *attributable risk* quantifies this relationship where, if an attributable risk is 10%, then removing that risk factor from the general population could avoid 10% of cases.

DESCRIPTIVE STATISTICS

It is difficult to make sense of a particular dataset without summarising its main characteristics in a meaningful way. In particular we often wish to know of what constitutes a typical value and the spread or distribution of other values around that number. There are several numerical and graphical methods of summarising datasets. We will consider the numerical methods first.

Measures of central tendency or location

The average (or *measure of central tendency or location*) is a general term for the typical value from a distribution and can be measured in a number of ways. First of all, let us consider that we have measured the height of 10 people in the street and we have obtained the following values (cm):

100, 120, 98, 132, 80, 140, 160, 138, 122, 108

Mean

The *mean* is simply the sum of all the values divided by the number of values. In our example this equals:

(100 + 120 + 98 + 132 + 80 + 140 + 160 + 138
+ 122 + 100) / 10 = 119 cm

Algebraically

$$\text{mean } (\bar{x}) = \frac{\Sigma x}{n}$$

(where Σx is used to denote the sum of all observations, and n is the total frequency or number of values)

Median

The median, or middle value, can be calculated by ranking the numbers from smallest to largest and taking the middle one. If there is an even number of values, the median is calculated by taking the arithmetic mean of the two middle values. Ranking our data:

80, 98, 100, 100, <u>120, 122</u>, 132, 138, 140, 160

the median is 121.

Mode

The mode is the easiest measure of central tendency to calculate as it is simply the most common value. As all of the numbers in our dataset occur once, with the exception of 100 which occurs twice, the mode is 100.

The relative benefits of the mean, median and mode are not apparent until one considers different datasets and the effect of extreme values on each estimate. For example, if socio-economic status were measured in 100 individuals on an ordinal scale of 1 to

6, the mean social class would be somewhat meaningless, as the differences between each point are not equal. The median would give a much more meaningful estimate of central tendency. The mean also gives a poor estimate of central tendency when there is skew in a distribution (i.e. when there are a disproportionately large amount of either small values or large values). These situations are illustrated graphically in Figures 11.2 to 11.4. In situations where the distribution is symmetrical (e.g. Normal

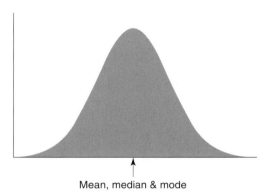

Mean, median & mode

Fig. 11.2
Symmetrical distribution.

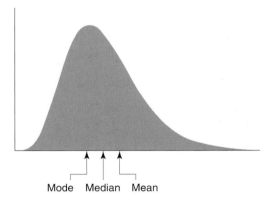

Mode Median Mean

Fig. 11.3
Positively skewed distribution.

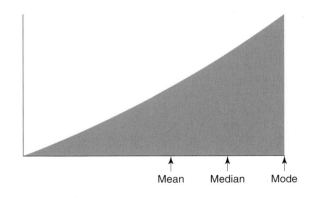

Mean   Median   Mode

Fig. 11.4
Negatively skewed distribution. (The differences between the mean, median and mode in this figure have been exaggerated for illustrative purposes.)

distribution, *t*-distribution), the mean, median and mode all take the same value and are equally good measures of central tendency. In skewed data, however, these statistics diverge.

Measures of dispersion

As well as describing the central location of a dataset, a statement of the data spread or dispersion is also helpful. There are several ways of doing this, and the best method often depends on the type of data and its distribution. The simplest method of describing dispersion is simply to give the range of values from smallest to largest. This measure is called the *range* and can be usefully represented on a 'box and whisker plot' (see Fig. 11.5). Another method, less influenced by extreme values, is to rank the distribution from smallest to largest value and divide the distribution into equal parts called *quantiles*. The most commonly used methods divide the distribution up into 4 quarters using 3 *quartiles*, or into 100 parts using 99 *percentiles*. By stating the difference from the first quartile (Q1) to the third quartile (Q3) we obtain the *interquartile range* (Q3–Q1) or IQR. Occasionally this range is further divided by 2 to obtain the semi-interquartile range. It is worth noting also that the second quartile and 50th percentile will always be equal to the median. This method is more robust to skewness but lacks the many useful mathematical properties of other methods.

A more popular method of determining spread is to measure how much each value differs from the mean and divide it by the number of values in the distribution. If we were to sum all of the differences we would however arrive at a value of 0 for every data set. Therefore the sign (+ or −) of each deviation is ignored. Each deviation is then added together for every value and then divided by the number of observations. This gives the *mean deviation*. Another method of overcoming the problem of differences summing to 0 is to square each deviation from the mean first. This value is always positive and is sometimes referred to the *sum of squares*. This figure is then divided by the total number of values minus 1 to give the *mean square* about the mean. This measure has the more familiar name of the *variance*. Algebraically,

$$\text{Variance} = \frac{\sum (x - \bar{x})^2}{n - 1}$$

The *standard deviation* (SD) is simply the square root of this value. The reason for dividing the squared deviations by *n* − 1 rather than *n* is that, given that you know the mean, the number of independent ways a data set can vary is always one less than the number of values. To illustrate, if a distribution of numbers had only one value, any measure of dispersion would be meaningless. Where a distribution has two values, it is possible to calculate how much each one varies around the mean, but dividing by *n* (2) would give a very misleadingly small estimate of the population variance from which the sample was drawn. *n* − 1 is sometimes called the *degrees of freedom*. When a distribution is skewed, the variance or standard deviation may mislead, as they are based on the deviations around the mean. When the mean is a poor estimate of central tendency, the variance and standard deviation will also be poor estimates of dispersion.

Table 11.3 summarises descriptive statistics appropriate for various types of data.

Descriptive statistics are usually quoted in published papers and can sometimes show that data are not normally distributed. This is particularly important if the investigators have gone on to use parametric statistics when they should have either transformed the

Table 11.3	Descriptive statistics for various types of data		
	Nominal	Ordinal (i.e. ranked)	Interval or ratio
Central tendency	Proportion	Median	Mean
Dispersion (spread)	NA	Interquartile range	Variance or SD

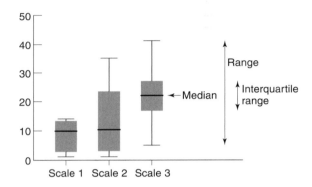

Fig. 11.5
Box-and-whisker plots of negatively skewed, positively skewed and normally distributed data.

data (e.g. by taking the log or square root of each value) or used a distribution-free (i.e. non-parametric) method. The simplest method is to look at the mean value and the range. If the range is asymmetrical about the mean, it is likely, although not certain, that the variable is skewed. For example if a variable has a mean of 5 and a range of 2–40 it is likely that the distribution is positively skewed, although the range represents the difference or interval between the largest and smallest values which are by definition somewhat atypical. An alternative method is to examine the first and third quartile, as these will also be symmetrical about the mean or median if the distribution is normal. A final quantitative method for detecting skewness is by examining the mean and standard deviation. Where a variable is normally distributed, the mean plus or minus two standard deviations will contain 95% (approximately) of the values. It follows therefore that if the mean is less than the value of the standard deviation then the data are likely to be skewed. These methods can be useful for showing that data *are* skewed, although if they do not suggest skewness, one cannot assume that they are normal distributed. Overall, perhaps the best method to detect skew is to examine the data visually (e.g. with a histogram or box-and-whisker plot; see Fig. 11.5). Other methods, such as normal probability plots can also be very useful, although they are beyond the scope of this chapter. Interested readers should consult Altman (1991) for further information.

INFERENTIAL STATISTICS — INTRODUCTION

In the previous section we considered the various ways in which data may be described. In many circumstances, however, one wishes to know whether two or more groups of measurements are different, or to be more precise, whether the difference is likely to be true or likely to have arisen by chance.

Table 11.4   Hypothesis testing and statistical power

Sample Study finding	Population	
	There is a difference	No difference
There is a difference (reject H_0)	Correct (true positive)	Incorrect (false positive) Type I error $p = \alpha$
There is no difference (accept H_0)	Incorrect (false negative) Insufficient power Type II error $p = (1 - \beta)$	Correct (true negative)

Conventionally, when we conduct a statistical test we are testing the statement, or null hypothesis (H_0), that there is no difference between two or more groups. When we conduct a test for association (correlation or regression analysis) we test for no association. Any p-value from a statistical test is simply the probability that the difference or association between variables is due to chance (i.e. a false positive). The arbitrary threshold for statistical significance is $p = 0.05$ (5/100 or 1 in 20), although the threshold can be set at any value, sometimes called *alpha*. When a statistical test is significant at $p \leq 0.05$ we reject the null hypothesis that there is no difference or association. If one finds no association or difference, then the null hypothesis cannot be rejected and there is no association or difference between two or more variables (true negative). Alternatively, we may find no difference when our study is not large enough or measurement is too imprecise (insufficient statistical power). This often happens when the spread of values is very large or when the effect one is trying to detect is very small. The probability that a study will not find a difference should one exist (false negative, or type II error) is sometimes called *beta*. $1 - \beta$ is the probability that we will find a significant difference should one exist and is sometimes referred to as the *power* of a study. The above concepts are demonstrated in Table 11.4.

The *power* of a study should always be considered in advance to ensure that a study is going to be large enough to reliably address a given research question. Underpowered studies are both unethical and a waste of effort. In order to calculate the power of a study and the number of people required to reject the null hypothesis, we need to set the level of statistical significance we require (usually $p = 0.05$) and the likely size of the treatment effect. If one requires a very high level of statistical significance (e.g. $p < 0.01$) one needs to recruit a far greater number of participants. Similarly, if comparatively small effects are envisaged, a much larger number of participants will be required than if the effect is very large. The relationship between sample size, significance and statistical power can be represented in the form of a graph (Fig. 11.6). Power is given on the right hand y-axis, and the p-values of 0.01 or 0.05 are represented by the two diagonal lines. The left hand y-axis is labelled 'standardised difference' and is a measure of the size of the anticipated effect. By setting a ruler on the expected effect and running it to the other side for the expected power, one can read off the number of study participants required to detect this result at $p = 0.05$ or 0.01.

There are a number of methods for calculating the *standardised difference*. When there are two groups of patients and the mean value and standard deviations in each group are known, then the standardised difference is given by:

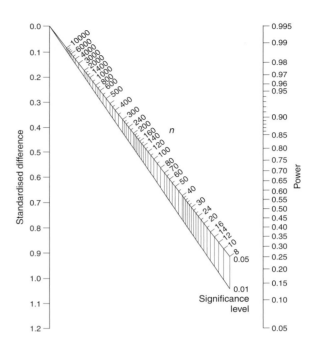

Fig. 11.6
Nomogram for the calculation of sample size. (Reproduced, with permission of D G Altman and BMJ Books, from Gore & Altman 1982.)

$$\text{Standardised difference} = \frac{\bar{X}_1 - \bar{X}_2}{\text{Pooled standard deviation}}$$

The means and standard deviations of each group will not be known with total accuracy (else there would usually be no point in doing the study), but they can often be estimated from existing data. Cohen's *d*, Hedge's *g* and Glass's Δ are related measures of standardised difference (or effect size) and are sometimes quoted in meta-analyses. For further information regarding the standardised difference, the interested reader should consult Egger et al (2001).

In addition to the nomogram given in Figure 11.6, there are a number of more accurate and reliable methods of determining sample size. Further details are available in Pocock (1983) and in the statistical software Epi-info, G-Power, STATA and SAS.

One-tailed and two-tailed tests of significance

In the above examples we have referred to the probability of rejecting the null hypothesis being alpha or the p-value. In rejecting the null hypothesis one is usually inferring that two or more groups are unequal in terms of a dependent variable (by dependent variable we mean the variable that is being compared between the groups), but that the difference might lie in either direction (e.g. group A > B or vice versa). Whichever group is bigger than the other is likely to be of some interest. For example, in a trial of olanzapine versus risperidone we would be interested to know whether olanzapine was better than risperidone, but we would be equally interested in the reverse. Occasionally, researchers have preconceptions about the direction of the difference and only test for a significant difference in one direction. Therefore the null hypothesis becomes H_0: 'olanzapine is not better than risperidone' instead of H_0: 'there is no difference'. In order to test whether there is a significant difference in one direction only, a *one-tailed test* (so called because only one tail of the distributions or differences is examined) is performed. If the investigator wishes to test for a difference in either direction, a *two-tailed test* will be conducted. However, one-tailed tests are almost never appropriate, as we are usually interested in a difference in either direction. The effect of using a one-tailed test is to increase the chance of finding a significant result, and this can lead to spurious positive findings (type I error). Further information on one-tailed and two-tailed tests is available in Altman (1991) and in a BMJ Statistics Note covering this issue (Bland & Altman 1994).

Multiple significance testing

Many published studies describe several significance tests which may generate conflicting results that are difficult to interpret. Part of this difficulty arises because, if many statistical tests are conducted, around one in twenty will show a significant result by chance alone. In an attempt to correct for the chance finding of a positive result, multiple significance tests are sometimes 'corrected'. The Bonferroni adjustment is perhaps the most commonly used of many methods for correcting significance tests.

False positive results occur (by definition) with a frequency of around 5% when the significance level is set to $p = 0.05$. When we conduct one significance test and find it to be significant, we are in fact saying that 'the probability of finding this result, or one that is more extreme, is less than one in twenty if the null hypothesis is true'. Therefore, if two independent tests are conducted simultaneously and the null hypothesis is true, the chance that one of them will be significant is 1 – (the probability that they are both non-significant) = $1 - (0.95)^2$ or 0.1 (approximately). The probability of a false positive increases with each independent test and approximates to the following relationship:

The probability that one or more significance tests will be positive when the null hypothesis is true	=	Significance level (α) (usually 0.05) $\times$ Number of individual significance tests

There are a number of approaches to this problem. The most conservative approach is the Bonferroni method which corrects for multiple significance testing by setting a higher threshold for statistical significance. The result of the correction is that the significance level for each individual test ($p_{corrected}$) when multiplied by the number of individual tests will be 0.05. By rearranging the above formula, we can see that if we conduct n independent tests and we want an overall significance level of 0.05, then the significance of individual findings will need to be (approximately):

$$p_{corrected} = \frac{0.05}{\text{Number of significance tests}}$$

Therefore, if we test two hypotheses, then the level of statistical significance required for each comparison will be approximately 0.025 or 2.5%.

Criticisms have been made of the Bonferroni method for several reasons (Perneger 1998). First, multiple hypothesis testing in a study is frequently done on variables which are not really independent. For example in a trial of chlorpromazine versus placebo which measured clinicians' global impression and patients' scores on the PANSS, it would be unreasonable to consider these two significance tests as independent from one another. Therefore, a

Bonferroni adjustment may be too stringent. Secondly, the Bonferroni adjustment is concerned with the null hypothesis that all null hypotheses are true simultaneously, a situation which is rarely of interest to researchers. Finally, using the Bonferroni adjustment to reduce the probability of false positives (type I error) will increase the probability of a false negative (type II error).

A similar problem arises in post hoc testing where researchers wish to look for significant findings when they did not set out to do this from the beginning (a priori). Such a *post hoc analysis* can often be very useful, previously unrecognised relationships can be explored and the need to conduct a further study can be determined. Secondly, if we conduct a significance test using three groups, we can test the hypothesis that the group means are different, but the significance test itself cannot tell us where the significant difference lies. However, the more statistical tests one conducts, the greater the chance of finding a false positive result, and this must be borne in mind when conducting any analysis. There are in fact many statistical approaches to this difficulty. The Scheffé and Tukey's Honestly Significant Difference are commonly used, but many others are available (SPSS lists more than 20). The details of each test are too complex to cover here but should be checked before their use as some tests make underlying assumptions about the nature of the underlying variables.

Confidence intervals

P-values tell the investigator how likely it is that the difference found in a study is due to chance. Studies often quote very small *p*-values in the hope that this demonstrates the certainty of their result. However, the *p*-value takes no account of the precision of the estimate and the likely range of plausible values that the value might take. For example, a treatment might be better than placebo at improving scores on the Hamilton Depression Rating Scale and be significant at $p = 0.01$ but have a wide range of possible effect sizes, some of which may not be *clinically significant*.

Confidence intervals are the range of plausible values that a variable may take in the 'real world' or population as a whole. For example, if a clinical trial showed that chlorpromazine was more effective than placebo for preventing relapse with a relative risk of 2.3 (with a 95% confidence interval of 1.2 to 3.5). We could be 95% certain that the true treatment effect lay between 1.2 and 3.5. The result is also statistically significant, as the confidence interval does not overlap 1 (the point of no effect or equal risk) though the range of possible risk ratios stretches from 3.5 (potentially very clinically important) to 1.2 (somewhat less clinically impressive). The result could also be said to be somewhat imprecise. By increasing the number of people in the study we could obtain a more precise estimate of the treatment effect. Alternatively we could combine several studies together in a *meta-analysis* producing a summary measure of treatment effect with an improved precision (and hence narrower confidence interval). This can be shown in the form of a *Forrest Plot* (Fig. 11.7). Each square represents the study size, its midpoint represents the effect size found in the individual study, and the horizontal bar represents the 95% confidence interval around the estimate. Studies which have larger sample sizes give rise to smaller confidence intervals. None of the trials shown in the Forrest Plot is significant in its own right but when combined give a more precise and statistically significant result. Further discussion of meta-analysis is given later in this chapter.

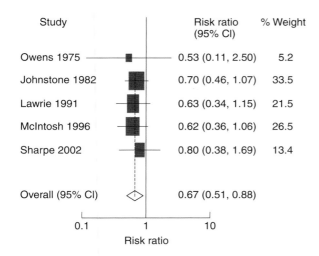

Study	Risk ratio (95% CI)	% Weight
Owens 1975	0.53 (0.11, 2.50)	5.2
Johnstone 1982	0.70 (0.46, 1.07)	33.5
Lawrie 1991	0.63 (0.34, 1.15)	21.5
McIntosh 1996	0.62 (0.36, 1.06)	26.5
Sharpe 2002	0.80 (0.38, 1.69)	13.4
Overall (95% CI)	0.67 (0.51, 0.88)	

Fig. 11.7
Forest plot of several simulated trials showing summary estimate and 95% confidence intervals.

Statistical distributions

Many variables in medicine follow a known distribution. For example, height and IQ follow an approximately normal distribution which is more or less symmetrical around a central mean. In a normal distribution it is also possible to say that 95% of possible values lie from the mean minus $1.96 \times$ the standard deviation to the mean plus $1.96 \times$ the standard deviation. Normally distributed variables also enable us to perform parametric statistical tests which have greater power than their non-parametric equivalents. Even if raw data in one study are not normally distributed, the sample means in several studies generally are (this is sometimes called the *central limit theorem*). For example, if we drew repeated samples of 40 people for a clinical study, the point estimates of each variable obtained from each sample would have a normal distribution with a mean equal to the true treatment effect in the population. The spread of the sample mean in this special case is also known as the *standard error*. The standard error is frequently misunderstood, as it is easy to confuse it with the standard deviation. In fact the standard error is the *standard deviation of the sample mean*. It may help to think of the sample error as a 'unit of uncertainty'. If we conduct a small study we can expect the standard error to be large. As we increase the sample size the standard error will reduce as the study provides a more precise estimate of effect. Confidence intervals are constructed from the standard error and are equal to the point estimate from the study plus or minus $1.96 \times$ standard error.

Sometimes other distributions are useful in medicine and psychiatry. Where events occur with a certain frequency over time or space (e.g. telephone calls to a switchboard or radioactive emissions) the variables frequently follow a *Poisson distribution*. When the result of a study is a proportion, the variables usually follow a *binomial distribution*. When a continuous variable is measured and its difference estimated between two groups (e.g. brain volume in schizophrenia vs controls) the mean difference follows a *t-distribution*. In most cases, however, as the sample size increases, the binomial, Poisson and *t*-distributions approximate to the normal distribution.

Parametric and non-parametric statistics

When we complete a study we usually want to do one of two things:

- test the hypothesis that some measurement is different between two or more groups of people;
- test the hypothesis that there is a relationship between two or more variables.

In order to test these hypotheses we have to re-frame each question as a null hypothesis (H_0: there is no difference or association), decide which *p*-value would lead us to reject this hypothesis and then conduct the appropriate statistical test. The correct choice of statistical test will depend on certain parametric assumptions:

- continuous data or at least interval discrete data;
- each unit of data collection should be independent of any other;
- data should be normally distributed;
- the variance of each group should be approximately equal

Where data meet these criteria we can use relatively powerful parametric statistical tests which use all of the data values, but where these criteria are not met we may need to use non-parametric statistics (distribution free tests) which require the conversion of raw values into ranks before analysis (Siegel 1988).

Parametric statistics are relatively robust to minor departures from a normal distribution, contrary to the common misperception that normality is the greatest underlying requirement. Where data are not normally distributed, it is often possible to transform them to normal distribution by taking the log or squaring each value. As a large number of transformations are possible, the interested reader should consult the suggestions for further reading at the end of this chapter for further information.

TESTING FOR DIFFERENCES

Chi-squared (χ^2) test

The χ^2 test is one of the most important statistical tests. It is one of the most commonly quoted tests in published papers, and other more complicated analyses can be derived from it.

The χ^2 test is a non-parametric test which is most commonly used to test whether the proportion of people with or without a certain characteristic differs between two or more independent groups. For example, the proportion of people improving on a certain drug, or the numbers of people of male gender in healthy controls compared with patients with schizophrenia. When conducting a χ^2 analysis, it can be helpful to represent the data in the form of a 2×2 table. Consider the data, shown in Table 11.5, from a study comparing the sexes of people with schizophrenia and healthy controls. The proportion of male subjects in both groups differs slightly; the null hypothesis is 'that there is no difference in the proportions in the population from which this sample was drawn'. In order to test the hypothesis we need to calculate the expected table values if there were no true difference between the groups. In order to do this, we multiply the row total by the column total for each cell and divide it by the total sample size, although in this case it seems perhaps intuitive that the expected values will each be 30. Once we have the observed and expected values from each cell, we can calculate the value of χ^2 using the formula:

Table 11.5 Example of subject group by gender

	Male	Female	Total
Schizophrenia	27	33	60
Healthy controls	33	27	60
Total	60	60	120

χ^2 test

- Is distribution free
- Compares expected with observed frequencies
- Should be modified when cell values are small
- The value of χ^2 and the degrees of freedom should always be stated

---

$$\chi^2_{1df} = \sum \frac{(O - E)^2}{E} = 1.2 \ (p = 0.27)$$

Because the probability of falsely rejecting the null hypothesis is 0.27, we cannot assume a difference in the population from which the sample was drawn. In practice χ^2, and the resulting p-value, are almost always calculated by computer.

Further refinements to the χ^2 test need to be made when the cell values are very small. When any expected frequency falls below 5, Yates's continuity correction or Fisher's exact test should be used. Usually these tests produce more conservative results and are less likely to lead to a false rejection of the null hypothesis when cell values are small. The χ^2 test (and its modifications) should be used where you want to test for a difference in the proportions between two or more groups. The values must take the form of absolute frequencies or counts and *not* percentages, which falsely inflate sample sizes.

The *t*-test

The *t*-test is one of the most common statistics quoted in medical research. There are two common uses of the *t* distribution. The two-sample *t*-test is used to examine differences in the means between two populations, provided there are independent samples from each, when the data are continuous or at least interval and approximately normally distributed with equal variances. Data from the same group measured on two separate occasions or from two different groups, where each individual member of one group is matched on key characteristics with an individual member of the other group, should be analysed by considering differences in scores between occasions, or between members of each pair. In such cases the paired *t*-test is applicable. You can also use a one-sample *t*-test to compare a sample mean with a known population mean; for example, you could compare the mean age of patients with dementia with the mean age of all elderly patients in a general hospital.

If your sample size is large, you can safely use the *t*-test even if some of the underlying assumptions are violated. The *t*-test is a parametric test which is relatively robust to departures from the usual assumptions underlying parametric statistics. However, there are modifications to the two-sample *t*-test that can be used if the assumption of equality of variance is violated.

The test statistic involves the calculation of the following:

---

t-test

- Is a parametric statistical test
- Compares the mean values of two independent groups
- Is relatively robust to departures from parametric assumptions
- The value of *t* and the degrees of freedom should always be stated

---

$$t = \frac{\text{Observed difference in means}}{\text{Standard error of the observed difference}}$$

with $n_1 + n_2 - 2$ degrees of freedom (where $n_1 + n_2$ is the total number of people in both samples combined). This tests the null hypothesis that there is no difference in the means of the two populations from which the samples were drawn. t becomes larger (and is more likely to be significant) as the difference in means increases, or when the standard error decreases (e.g. when the sample size increases). The significance of t can be obtained from tables, although it is usually calculated within the various statistical packages available.

Mann–Whitney U-test

The Mann–Whitney U-test is used when the aim is to show a difference between two groups in the value of an ordinal, interval or ratio variable. It is the non-parametric version of the *t*-test, which latter should be used for interval, ratio or continuous data unless there are large departures from the parametric assumptions. The process of calculating the test statistic is very simple but would use many lines of text to demonstrate here. The interested reader should refer to Bland (2000) for a clear and concise account of its derivation. It is worth noting that the test can detect differences in the spread as well as the location (median) of two variables, even when the medians are very similar (Hart 2001). Therefore, when presenting the results of Mann–Whitney tests, the median of each group should be presented along with a description of the skewness of each sample (e.g. a box plot). The Mann–Whitney test also assumes that the two groups are independent. Where the measurements are paired (i.e. are two measurements from the same individual), the Wilcoxon matched-pairs test should be used instead.

Analysis of variance (ANOVA)

All of the previous tests have concerned two groups of observations. When there are three or more groups, one tests the null hypothesis that there is no difference in the group means by examining the variances.

Consider the data, shown in Table 11.6, from three groups of 4 patients. There are several sources of variation in this sample.

Mann–Whitney U-test

- Is distribution free
- Is based on ranked values
- Is used to compare the medians of two independent groups
- The value of U and the degrees of freedom should always be stated

---

Table 11.6	Ages of three groups of 4 patients		
	Ages	Mean	Variance
Depressed	47, 52, 58, 66	55.75	66.9
Bipolar	25, 28, 32, 45	32.5	77.7
Schizophrenic	18, 27, 32, 28	28.75	71.6
Mean of whole sample = 39, variance = 214.5			

ANOVA

- Is a parametric statistical test
- Tests the null hypothesis that the mean values of three or more independent groups are equal
- The test statistic F is the ratio of the between-groups to within-groups variance
- The value of F and the two degrees of freedom should always be stated
- ANOVA has a non-parametric equivalent called the Kruskal–Wallis test (one-independent grouping only)

First, there is the total variation of the whole sample. To calculate this value one calculates the sample variance, ignoring the group to which each measurement belongs. This is sometimes called the total mean squares (MS_{total}) or total variance. Second, there is the variation of the group means about a grand mean of all observations. This is sometimes called the between-groups variance ($MS_{between}$) or sometimes MS_{treat}. Finally, there is the variation between the group measurements and their individual group means. This is sometimes called the within-groups mean squares or residual mean squares ($MS_{residual}$) or within-groups variance. The relationship between these sources of variation is:

$$SS_{total} = SS_{between} + SS_{residual} \left(MS = \frac{SS}{df} \right)$$

If each of the groups is drawn from the same population with equal population means, the between-groups variance will be comparable to the within-groups variation ($MS_{residual}$). Alternatively, if the three groups have different population means, the between-groups variation will be large compared with the within-groups variance. In order to test which one of these situations is more likely, we use the test statistic F.

$$F = \frac{\text{Variation between samples}}{\text{Variation within samples}} = \frac{MS_{between}}{MS_{residual}}$$

In the example above the total variance is calculated from the whole sample (as if they were not in groups). The between groups sum of squares is the sum of squared deviations between the group means and the overall mean multiplied by the number of observations in each group. The residual sum of squares is calculated usually by subtraction. Mean squares are the sum of squares divided by the appropriate degrees of freedom.

Most statistical packages when performing an ANOVA will produce an output similar to that shown in Table 11.7. The sum of squares is just the sum of the squared difference between each value and its corresponding mean. By dividing by the degrees of freedom, we can calculate the within-groups ($MS_{residual}$), between-groups ($MS_{between}$) and total variance.

In the above example, $F = 11.9$, which is significant, being less than 0.05. We can therefore reject the null hypothesis that there is no difference between the groups.

ANOVA can also be extended to the analysis of data which can be classified in a number of ways. For example, in an observational study measuring memory performance scores, patients may be classified by diagnosis, sex and treatment. If one wished to compare memory score by diagnosis, a one-way ANOVA (as above) could be conducted. However, if gender and treatment also affected memory score, the difference might not be due solely to the effect of diagnosis alone. To avoid this potential pitfall, a factorial ANOVA can include any number of the factors in a single experiment. The resulting analysis could give the effect of each factor independently, but can also provide information about interactions between factors. For example, a factorial ANOVA could detect that memory scores may be impaired in males with schizophrenia but not females, whereas a one-way ANOVA might fail to detect any differences.

An analysis of variance can be extended to include paired values from the same samples and is called repeated measures ANOVA. Where data can be classified in several ways (e.g. by group and gender) the appropriate statistical test is the factorial ANOVA. Other more complex models can also be used though their interpretation can be somewhat complex. We shall briefly consider one further extension of the ANOVA, the analysis of covariance (ANCOVA).

The analysis of covariance in used when we wish to see if the mean of a variable differs across three or more groups, while taking into account a possible confounder. If, for example, one examined cognition in the three groups of subjects above, their performance may be confounded by their premorbid general intellectual ability or their age. In order to take into account these factors we can either use a regression analysis (see later) or use ANCOVA, where IQ or age or both would be covariates.

Table 11.8 summarises tests for differences, for various data types.

TESTING FOR ASSOCIATION

Testing for an association between two variables is a common analysis in medical statistics and one that it sometimes misused. Often such analyses are undertaken in the hope that one variable causes a change in another, but the direction of effect cannot be

Table 11.7	Analysis of variance table				
	Sum of squares	Degrees of freedom	Mean square	F	Sig.
Between groups	1711.500	2	855.75	11.9	0.003
Within groups	648.500	9	72.1		
Total	2360.000	11	214.5		

Table 11.8 Summary of tests for differences

Two groups	Categorical	Ordinal (ranked)	Interval or continuous
Unpaired	Chi-squared test	Mann–Whitney U-test	Independent *t*-test
Paired	McNemar test	Wilcoxon matched pairs	Paired *t*-test
Three or more groups			
Unordered & unpaired	Chi-squared test	Kruskal–Wallis test	Analysis of variance (ANOVA)
Paired	Cochrane Q test	Freidman test	Repeated measures ANOVA

See Altman (1991) or Swinscow & Campbell (1996) for further details.

inferred solely from the results of the analysis (i.e. association is not causation). Two related techniques are available: correlation and regression. Correlating two variables is the simplest form of analysis and looks for a linear association between two variables (e.g. whole brain volume and IQ, or age and MMSE score) and can be conducted by a variety of parametric and distribution-free methods. Regression involves many of the underlying principles of correlation and is often extended to take account of several variables simultaneously.

Correlation

Consider the sample data, given in Table 11.9, from patients in an inpatient ward in whom performance IQ and duration of psychosis in months were measured. If we plot a graph of these values (Fig. 11.8) we can see that they appear to be related to one another.

In order to show a relationship we need to test the null hypothesis that there is no association between the two variables. If the parametric assumptions are met, we can calculate Pearson's product–moment correlation coefficient. If the assumptions are not met we can use Spearman's rank correlation coefficient, which is the corresponding distribution-free test. We will calculate both for the same data set.

Pearson's correlation coefficient (r) can take any value from -1 to $+1$. A correlation coefficient of 1 would indicate perfect positive correlation (both values rise together) whereas a correlation coefficient of -1 indicates perfect negative correlation. A correlation coefficient of 0 suggests that there is no relationship between two variables. Pearson's correlation coefficient is calculated using the method of least squares which tries to minimise the differences between each data point and a line of best fit. The line of best fit is shown on the graph above. For the dataset shown above, the correlation coefficient is -0.69 and the significance of the result is $p = 0.026$. This shows that duration of psychosis and performance IQ have a moderate to strong negative relationship with each other and that the relationship is significant at $p < 0.05$. In other words, as the duration of psychosis goes up, the performance IQ goes down, and the null hypothesis (that the correlation coefficient is zero and there is no relationship) can be rejected.

Spearman's rank correlation coefficient (ρ) can be calculated using the same dataset and is not dependent on a normal distribution of values. The value will lie between -1 and $+1$ and its interpretation is similar to that of Pearson's coefficient. In this case Spearman's correlation coefficient is -0.64, $p = 0.044$. The result is still significant, although slightly less so than before. This reflects the fact that distribution-free tests tend to have less power to detect associations or differences than parametric tests and yield

Table 11.9 Sample data on duration of psychosis and performance IQ

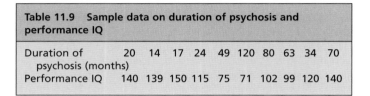

Duration of psychosis (months)	20	14	17	24	49	120	80	63	34	70
Performance IQ	140	139	150	115	75	71	102	99	120	140

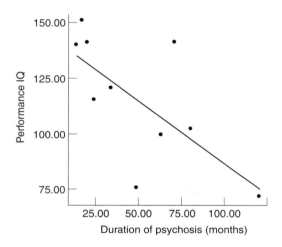

Fig. 11.8
Scatter plot of performance IQ against duration of psychosis, with line of best fit shown.

Pearson's correlation coefficient

- Is a parametric statistical test
- Measures the observed association between two variables
- Its significance or confidence interval should always be stated
- Is derived using the method of least squares

more conservative estimates if data is normally distributed. Spearman's coefficient however tends to exaggerate the association between variables when there are many tied values, in which case other measures may be more appropriate.

The simple correlation examples shown above can be extended to the situation where there is a third variable. In our example, this might be age or premorbid IQ. It is possible to calculate a partial correlation coefficient to take account of this confounder.

Table 11.10 summarises statistical tests for association.

Spearman's correlation coefficient

- Is a distribution-free test
- Converts raw values to ranks before measuring their association
- Tends to inflate the strength of the association when there are many tied values, in which case other tests may be more appropriate

Table 11.10   Statistical tests for association

Data	Test
Categorical data	Kappa
Ranked data	Spearman's rank correlation coefficient
Continuous or interval data	Pearson's correlation coefficient

Regression analysis

Regression analysis is the study of relationships between two or more variables and is usually conducted for the following reasons:

- when we want to know whether any relationship between two or more variables actually exists;
- when we are interested in understanding the relationship between two or more variables;
- when we want to predict a variable given the value of others.

In its simplest form regression analysis is very similar to correlation; in fact the underlying mathematical models are virtually identical. Regression analysis can however be used where there are many explanatory variables and where various data types are used together. The general regression model is:

$$Y = a + bX_1 + cX_2 + \ldots + \text{error}$$

Where a is a constant, X_1, X_2, etc. are the predictor variables, and the error term is the difference between the observed and predicted value of Y. A practical example of the above equation using the performance IQ data might take the following form:

$$\text{IQ} = 149 - 0.57 \times \text{duration of psychosis}$$

The error term is omitted here and is assumed to have a mean of 0. The distances between each data point and the line of best fit summarising their relationship are called the *residuals*. These are the differences between the observed and predicted values and are a measure of the unexplained variation. The model can be extended to more complicated examples, e.g. brain volume using the variables diagnosis, height and IQ. The equation might take the following form:

$$\text{Total brain volume} = 10 \times \text{diagnosis} + 0.03 \times \text{height} + \text{IQ}/20$$

Diagnosis is a categorical variable, and therefore it makes no sense to allocate a number to each diagnostic category as there is no order in the categories. Therefore we have to include a number of 'dummy variables' each one indicating the presence or absence of a diagnosis. The example above would be a suitable model when only one diagnosis is considered, as the variable diagnosis will only have to take values of 1 or 0.

Table 11.11   Analysis of variance table for a regression analysis in SPSS

	ANOVA				
Model	Sum of Squares	df	Mean Square	F	Sig.
1 Regression	6098.446	2	3049.223	22.744	0.001
Residual	938.454	7	134.065		
Total	7036.900	9			

Finally, if we expect an interaction between two terms (e.g. we might think that IQ is related to brain volume in healthy controls but not in people with schizophrenia, say) we can examine these interactions by including diagnosis × IQ as an explanatory variable in the regression equation. If we had further information about IQ we might want to include this in our regression analysis. The printout from our statistical software might look like: Table 11.11. The table is labelled ANOVA and it shows the mean squares about the regression model (similar to the between-groups variance) the residual mean squares (unexplained variance), their ratio F and its significance. What it does not tell us is whether there is an interaction between duration of psychosis and IQ or whether the addition of IQ to our model is better than having duration of psychosis as the only predictor variable. To test the first hypothesis, that there is an interaction between IQ and duration of psychosis, we would need to expand our model to include an interaction term. If we wanted to see which model is best (in terms of how much variance is explained overall) we need to either add or take away predictor terms to see which model fits the data best.

Most statistical packages have a variety of methods for doing this. The most common methods are called *forward entry*, *backward entry* and *stepwise*. Forward entry is a method of regression analysis whereby the predictor variable most significantly associated with the dependent variable is included in the model first, and if other predictor variables are also significantly associated with the dependent variable, they are entered into the model. Backward entry regression enters all of the terms into the regression equation first and removes successive terms if they do not predict the dependent variable. Stepwise regression is a combination of forward and backward entry methods.

The table in the regression analysis was titled ANOVA as regression and ANOVA use virtually identical underlying models. For instance, one could conduct a regression analysis where IQ was the dependent variable and duration of psychosis was the predictor. If we had done that we would have arrived at the same answer as an ANOVA.

There are however limitations to multiple regression. For example, as we enter more terms into our regression analysis, it becomes more and more difficult to interpret the results. In such cases clear descriptive statistics become invaluable. Further, in the above example we have only dealt with a situation in which the dependent variable is at least interval, ratio or continuous. When our dependent variable is an outcome (e.g. dead or alive) then we need to use a closely related technique called logistic regression. Other more complex models are available but are beyond the scope of this chapter (see Altman 1991 for more details).

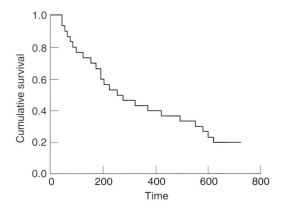

Fig. 11.9
Kaplan–Meier survival curve.

SURVIVAL ANALYSIS

Survival analysis, as its name implies, was originally related to the drawing of inferences from numerical data on length of life. However, the methods of survival analysis may be applied to the amount of time elapsing before any particular event, such as relapse, in the history of an individual. The quantity which is the subject of a survival analysis is the 'time to outcome', or survival time, of the individuals under study (Altman & Bland 2002). The survival time is the difference between two times or dates. The terminal event in psychiatric applications will not usually be death of the subject, but some other kind of event.

Perhaps the most important thing to appreciate about survival analysis is that by the end of any study the event will probably not have occurred in all patients. We will not know when or even whether they experience the event, only that they have not yet done so by the end of the study. Patients may also be lost to follow-up during the course of a study or may experience an event which is not the event of interest but means that their data is in effect 'censored'. An example of this might be the death of a patient from a lung tumour during the course of an antipsychotic trial to prevent relapse in schizophrenia. In survival analysis, it is assumed that those patients lost to follow-up have the same prognosis as those remaining in the study.

The aim of survival analysis is to model the survival experience of individuals and to estimate associated quantities of interest. Models may include explanatory variables of several types: such as group membership, a discrete variable which might indicate different treatment regimens, a continuous variable such as age which can be adjusted for in group comparisons, and other variables which may be of primary interest in themselves, or may be potential confounders of the relationships in question, and therefore need to be taken into account. Before conducting any of these analyses it is always helpful to graph the survival function against time, using the *Kaplan–Meier survival curve* (Bland & Altman 1998). This approach graphs the proportion of subjects surviving beyond any specified follow-up time (time p) as $S(t)$ and is estimated from the following equation:

$$S(t) = \frac{(r_1 - d_1)}{r_1} \times \frac{(r_2 - d_2)}{r_2} \times \ldots \times \frac{(r_p - d_p)}{r_p}$$

where r is the number of patients alive before a given time and d denotes the number who died at that time. This equation becomes much clearer when you consider the graph of $S(t)$ against time, as shown in Figure 11.9.

Significance tests applied to survival analysis

The purpose of undertaking a survival analysis and plotting a Kaplan–Meier curve is usually to demonstrate that the time to some event is greater in one group than in another. In such cases it is usual to perform a significance test to test the null hypothesis that the survival times are equal. The most common method of comparing two or more survival functions is the *log rank test*. This test is distribution-free and effectively yields a value which can be checked against statistical tables in order to give the significance level of the result. The log rank test assumes that survival times are at least ordinal and that the risk of one group relative to another does not change with time. This 'relative risk' is sometimes called the *hazard function* or ratio and the assumption that it is constant is called the *proportional hazards assumption*. The terms relative risk and hazard ratio, though they may be similar for specific time points, are not terms which should be used synonymously. For a more detailed consideration of this area the interested reader should consult Parmar & Machin (1995).

More complex methods of analysing survival data may be very useful, especially when two groups differ in the presence of one or more prognostic factor. Ideally, their effects should be corrected for in a type of multiple regression. The most common regression model applied to survival analysis is called *Cox's proportional hazards*.

MULTIVARIATE STATISTICS

Multivariate statistics refers to analyses in which there are multiple (more than one) *dependent* variables. This situation often arises in medicine when more than one outcome measurement is made (e.g. PANSS, BPRS, etc.) or sometimes when the same measurement is repeated on more than one occasion. A common mistake in the analysis of such data is to perform a series of one-way ANOVAs for each dependent variable separately. The problem with that approach is that every one-way ANOVA increases the chances of at least one type I error (false positive). In addition, the dependent variables are often correlated with one another, and including each variable in the same analysis can provide the researcher with more information (e.g. interactions between variables) than if several analyses are conducted separately. To overcome these problems, a series of multivariate techniques have been devised. For a more detailed account of them all, the reader should consult Norman & Streiner (1999).

Multivariate analysis of variance

In order to compare two or more group means we would conventionally conduct a one-way ANOVA. In more complicated situations, where there are several *independent* variables, a *factorial ANOVA* would be the appropriate technique. If one wishes to compare means between several groups while controlling for a confounder (e.g. when measuring current IQ in people with various diagnoses, one might with to control for premorbid IQ) the appropriate model is called an *analysis of covariance or ANCOVA*. Finally, when there are two or more *dependent* variables the amended ANOVA model is called a *multivariate analysis of variance* or *MANOVA* which can also be adapted to control for confounding variables (*MANCOVA*). The general mathematical model used in all of these approaches is very similar and often referred to as the *general linear model (GLM)*. For simplicity's sake the details have not been included in this chapter although further details can be found in Hand & Taylor (1987).

Factor analysis

Another method of dealing with large datasets is the technique of factor analysis. Factor analysis is a method of data reduction in which many variables are collapsed into a smaller number of different variables called *factors*. The variables can be reduced in this way when two or more variables are highly correlated and can effectively be replaced by a single factor without the loss of much information. Factors are effectively condensed statements of relationships between a set of variables and are sometimes referred to as *latent traits or variables* and also as *hypothetical constructs*.

> **Multivariate ANOVA**
>
> - Is a parametric statistical technique
> - Is based on the general linear model
> - Is a relatively computer intensive technique
> - A common test statistic is Hotteling's T^2, although others exist

One of the best known uses of factor analysis was in the field of intellectual ability. Spearman observed that the performances of people on a wide variety of tests of intellectual ability were highly correlated. Spearman, among others, thought that the reason for this finding was that performance on tests of intellectual ability could be explained by a single trait we now know as IQ. Evidence from factor analysis, and from other research, suggests that human abilities can indeed be explained partly by such a single factor. Research in the field of personality variation has also shown that human personality can be thought of as having five latent dimensions using the technique of factor analysis (see Chapter 6 for further details).

Taking a hypothetical example, if we measured the following list of variables on every admission to a hospital we might obtain the factors shown in Figure 11.10. This suggests that any patient's observed behaviour may be explained by three latent traits (arbitrarily) called hostility, mania and depression. It is worth noting that the names of the factors are descriptive and are not derived scientifically.

A frequent criticism of factor analysis is that it can be made to show almost anything you want. This criticism has some merit since the process of obtaining the factors involves several steps and, at each step, more than one technique is often available. The first step in factor analysis is to construct a correlation matrix. This is a table with all of the individual variables listed along the top and side of the table, with each individual cell showing the correlation coefficient between the two variables at the intersecting row and column. It may be obvious even at this stage that several variables are highly correlated with one another and might be explained by a single factor. The second step in the analysis is to extract the factors by using a linear combination of each variable. In the example shown in Figure 11.10, hostility might have been expressed by the following linear combination:

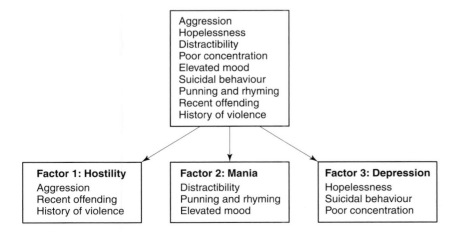

Aggression
Hopelessness
Distractibility
Poor concentration
Elevated mood
Suicidal behaviour
Punning and rhyming
Recent offending
History of violence

Factor 1: Hostility
Aggression
Recent offending
History of violence

Factor 2: Mania
Distractibility
Punning and rhyming
Elevated mood

Factor 3: Depression
Hopelessness
Suicidal behaviour
Poor concentration

Fig. 11.10
Factor analysis of patients' admission data.

Hostility =
0.75 × Aggression +
−0.1 × Hopelessness +
0.2 × Distractibility +
0.01 × Poor concentration +
0.6 × Elevated mood +
0.11 × Suicidal behaviour +
0.14 × Punning & rhyming +
0.9 × Recent offending +
0.82 × History of violence

The factors may be extracted in a way which maximises the amount of variance explained by the factor. You can see from the example above that aggression, a history of recent offending and a history of violence get the greatest weight and that hopelessness gets the least. These particular weights are the ones which explain the maximum amount of variance in the data set. The amount of variance accounted for by a factor is known as its *eigenvalue*. If a factor's eigenvalue is less than 1, it is worse than a single variable at explaining the overall variance. If however, the eigenvalue is equal to the number of variables, the factor explains all of the variance. In practice researchers often keep the factors with eigenvalues of 1 or more and discard the rest. Another approach is to take the first few factors which explain the largest amount of variance and when the amount of variance explained by successive factors diminishes, ignore subsequent factors. This second approach is usually performed with the aid of a *Scree Plot* (Kline 1994). The final step in factor analysis is to rotate the factors. This step is usually performed because some factor loadings will be negative and difficult to interpret and secondly because individual variables may 'load onto' two or more separate factors. Factor rotations are usually orthogonal (i.e. they minimise the correlation between factors) or oblique (they allow extracted factors to correlate with one another). One of the most common rotations used is the *Varimax rotation*. This technique is an orthogonal rotation which maximises the variance explained by each rotated factor (hence the name).

Factor analysis, as outlined above can be used for data reduction or data exploration. A further technique has evolved called *confirmatory factor analysis (CFA)* or *structural equation modelling* which can be used to test hypotheses about underlying factor structure. Further details are available in Kline (1994).

Cluster analysis

Cluster analysis is the name given to a set of techniques which ask whether people can be grouped into *categories* on the basis of their similarities or differences. It began when biologists began to classify plants on the basis of their various phyla and species and wanted to derive a less subjective technique. It has been applied to diagnostic classification in a similar way. To take a theoretical example, conventional categories of functional psychotic illness (depression, bipolar disorder and schizophrenia) are thought by many to be somewhat unsatisfactory concepts. They do not predict

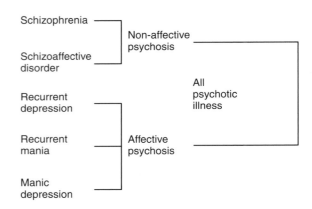

Fig. 11.11
Dendrogram of hypothetical cluster analysis of psychotic patients.

outcome particularly well and seem to share many risk factors. A researcher might attempt to collect data from people with psychosis and empirically derive their own categories using cluster analysis. The mathematical details are too complicated to explain here, but basically the researcher should first decide whether he wishes to use a hierarchical or partitioning method. Hierarchical methods involve the measurement of various variables on each subject. These variables are then compared between subjects and the clusters are derived in such a way as to minimise the differences ('*Euclidian distance*') between members within a category and to maximise the differences between people belonging to different categories. Each category can then be further subdivided into lower-order categories represented with a *dendrogram* (Fig. 11.11). Partitioning techniques assume each category is unique from all the others and are less commonly used.

To take the theoretical example of psychotic illness given above, a researcher might achieve the solution shown in Figure 11.11 to a cluster analysis.

META-ANALYSIS

A meta-analysis is the weighted average of the results from two or more studies. A meta-analysis is often conducted alongside a systematic review, but the terms are not synonymous (see Ch. 12). A meta-analysis of several studies may be misleading without a systematic review, since non-systematic reviews are more pone to bias, particularly in selectively citing studies which support a particular point of view. A meta-analysis of such studies will then provide a spuriously precise estimate of any overall effect failing to take into account other studies. Publication bias is also a threat to the validity of a meta-analysis, even when there has been a previous systematic review. Publication bias is the tendency for small, usually negative studies to remain unpublished. Finally, for studies to be meaningfully combined, the results must be broadly similar

Factor analysis
• May be obtained by several methods
• Can be used to simplify large data sets
• Produces latent variables or hypothetical constructs
• Rotations may be oblique or orthogonal

Common multivariate techniques in psychiatry
• Multivariate analysis of variance
• Factor analysis
• Cluster analysis

from study to study. When study results vary more than one would expect by chance, the results are said to demonstrate statistical *heterogeneity*. The finding of heterogeneity should prompt investigators to search for an explanation. Causes include differences in the characteristics of study participants and differences in methodology.

There are in fact a range of meta-analytic methods from which to choose. The choice of method will depend upon the measure of effect used in the individual studies and the presence or absence of heterogeneity. If the results of individual studies do not show heterogeneity, *fixed-effects* analyses should be used. These assume that there is a single underlying effect and that each individual study is an unbiased estimator of that effect. When heterogeneity is present, *random-effects* analyses should be used. These do not assume a single underlying treatment effect but estimate an average effect across all studies. Random-effect analyses produce a single overall estimate of treatment effect which is generally less precise than the corresponding fixed-effects analysis since the heterogeneity is also incorporated into the confidence interval of the overall effect estimate.

Fixed-effects analysis

Fixed-effects meta-analysis is a two-step process. The first step is to calculate a common unit of treatment effect, usually an odds ratio or relative risk of an event or a difference in two means for continuous data, for each individual study. The second stage is to calculate a summary statitic which is a weighted average of the results from individual studies. The weights used are usually the inverse of the variance (the square of the standard error) from the individual studies. Larger studies, which provide a more precise estimate of overall treatment effect, and have a relatively small variance, are given more weight than smaller trials with larger variances. This method can be expressed algebraically:

$$\theta_{IV} = \frac{\sum w_i \theta_i}{\sum w_i}$$

Where θ_{IV} is the pooled result using fixed-effects (inverse variance) analysis, θ_i is the result of individual studies, and w_i is the weight given to individual studies.

$$w_i = \frac{1}{SE(\theta_1)^2}$$

where $SE(\theta_i)$ is the standard error of the results of individual studies. The heterogeneity statistic Q is calculated as:

$$Q = \sum w_i (\theta_i - O_{iv})^2$$

Random-effects models

Random-effects analysis, sometimes referred to as DerSimonian and Laird random-effects models (DerSimonian & Laird 1986), do not assume one underlying treatment effect. The effect sizes from individual studies are assumed to be normally distributed with variance τ^2. The individual weights (w_i) for each included study are then:

$$w_i = \frac{1}{SE(\theta_i)^2 + \tau^2}$$

where $SE(\theta_i)$ is the standard error of the results of individual studies. And the pooled overall effect is:

$$\theta_{DL} = \frac{\sum w_i \theta_i}{\sum w_i}$$

Where θ_{DL} is the pooled result using random-effect (DL = DeLaird) analysis, θ_i is the result of individual studies, and w_i is the weight given to individual studies

As heterogeneity (and therefore τ^2) increase, the study weights given to individual studies will become more similar, and relatively more weight will be given to smaller studies compared with fixed-effects models. Random-effects models are more conservative than fixed-effects models, giving wider confidence intervals around the overall summary estimate.

Measuring publication bias

In order to assess whether the sample of studies you have obtained is likely to be biased because of selective publication or identification, a number of graphical and numerical methods are available. The simplest method of all is to construct a *funnel plot*. Essentially a funnel plot is a plot of the study effect size against its precision. The effect size is usually measured as a mean difference or standardised difference, for continuous data, or a relative risk or odds ratio for dichotomous or event-like data. Relative risks and odds ratios are usually plotted on a log scale so that effect sizes favouring an effect are plotted an equal distance away from the line of no effect as those showing an equal effect, but in the opposite direction.

Consider Figures 11.12 and 11.13. In Figure 11.12, we have 'found' 16 studies, some of which are large and have tight confidence intervals, some of which are small and have large confidence intervals. Overall the pooled estimate of treatment effect is non--significant, although its confidence intervals are quite narrow. In Figure 11.13 we present the same trials but leaving out those with small sample sizes ($n < 100$) that find a negative result. By removing the small negative findings we have changed the result of the whole meta-analysis to favour an overall effect. The funnel plot shows a corresponding gap or void in its lower right hand corner where one would expect to find small negative studies to be.

Further techniques have been developed to quantify funnel plot asymmetry. The interested reader should consult Egger et al (2001) for further details.

Qualitative data analysis

The aim of most medical research is to quantify differences or relationships between one or more groups of people according to an

---

Concerning meta-analysis

- Fixed-effects analysis — assume no or low heterogeneity and a single underlying effect
- Fixed-effects analysis — usually weight the results by the reciprocal of their variance
- Random-effects analysis — allow for heterogeneity, to give an average treatment effect across studies
- Random-effects analyses — incorporate heterogeneity as well as study variance into the weights given to individual studies
- Publication bias may be suggested by funnel plot asymmetry

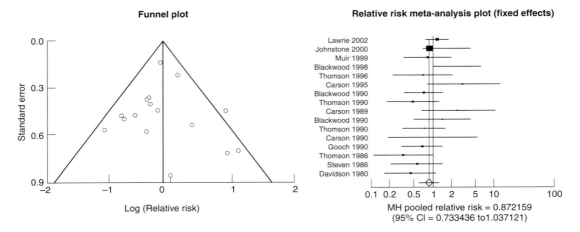

Fig. 11.12
Funnel and forest plot on all of 16 studies.

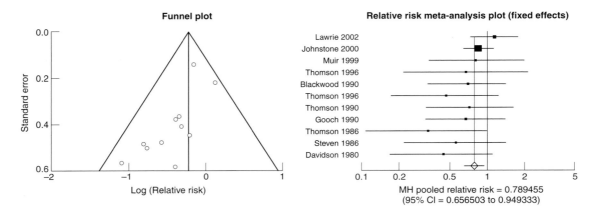

Fig. 11.13
Funnel and forest plot on studies where small negative findings have been removed.

exposure or experimental factor. However, sometimes researchers wish to interpret or explain something and may use qualitative rather than quantitative research methods in order to accomplish this. Qualitative research methods have been developed in order to provide reproducible and reliable methods of addressing questions usually about the beliefs or attitudes of a group of people.

Qualitative research methods are often inappropriate to the question being addressed and are more likely to be biased than quantitative methods. However, in situations where quantitative methods are impossible, or where they would reduce the apparent 'richness of information' obtained, qualitative methods may be appropriate. For example, a study examining the attitudes of patients with borderline personality disorder to their diagnosis may be less revealing if their attitudes are quantified along a series of Likert scales, than if the researcher attempts simply to describe what the patients *actually* said while studying them in their home environment.

Good qualitative research has several features. Firstly the perspective of the researcher must be considered in some detail. Secondly, the results should be confirmed using two or more methodologies (triangulation) and the theoretical framework to

the study should be described. Numerous papers on the subject of qualitative research have been published by the BMJ and are available by searching bmj.com using the search terms 'qualitative research'.

CONCLUDING REMARKS

This chapter has attempted to introduce the reader to the main statistical techniques used in medical and psychiatric research. (Figure 11.14 summarises basic statistical tests for various data types.) It is, however, difficult to fully appreciate some of the issues discussed without access to your own dataset and a suitable software package. We encourage readers to do this, once they have a grasp of the fundamentals, but also advise them to seek out sensible research design and statistical advice at an early stage. Statistical testing should be planned and should use research methods which are likely to yield a reliable and unbiased answer. No amount of analysis after the event can compensate for poor study design. Contrary to the cliché, statistics cannot be used to show anything one wants them to.

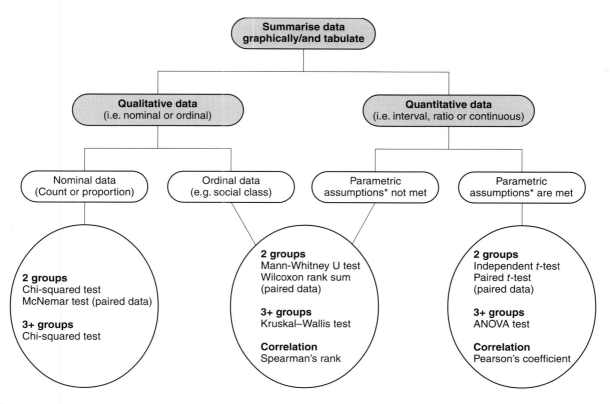

Fig. 11.14
Summary of basic statistical tests for various data types. *Assumptions underlying parametric statistics (approximately normal distribution, independence, equality of variance, at least interval data) are described in more detail on page 193.

FURTHER READING

Altman's *Practical Statistics for Medical Research* (see References) is a particularly useful text.

REFERENCES

Altman D G 1991 Practical statistics for medical research. CRC Press, Boca Raton, Florida

Altman D G, Bland J M 2002 Time to event (survival) data. British Medical Journal 317:468–469

Bland J M 2000 An introduction to medical statistics. Oxford University Press, Oxford

Bland J M, Altman D G 1986 statistical methods for assessing agreement between two methods of clinical measurement. Lancet i: 307–310

Bland J M, Altman D G 1994 Statistics notes: one and two sides tests of significance. British Medical Journal 309:248

Bland J M, Altman D G 1997 Statistics notes: Cronbach's alpha. British Medical Journal 314:572

Bland J M, Altman D G 1998 Survival probabilities (the Kaplan–Meier method). British Medical Journal 317:1572

Bland J M, Altman D G 2002 Validating scales and indexes. British Medical Journal 324:606–607

DerSimonian R, Laird N 1986 Meta-analysis in clinical trials. Controlled Clinical Trials 7:177–188

Egger M, Smith G D, Altman D G 2001 Systematic reviews in health care: Meta-analysis in context. BMJ Books, London

Gore S M, Altman D G 1982 Statistics in practice. BMJ Books, London

Hand D J, Taylor C C 1987 Multivariate analysis of variance and repeated measures. Chapman and Hall, London

Hart A 2001 Mann–Whitney test is not just a test of medians: differences in spread can be important. British Medical Journal 323:391–393

Kline P 1994 An easy guide to factor analysis. Routledge, London

Norman G R, Streiner D L 1999 PDQ statistics. BC Decker, Hamilton, Ontario

Parmar M K B, Machin D 1995 Survival analysis: a practical approach. Wiley, Chichester

Perneger T V 1998 What's wrong with Bonferroni adjustments. British Medical Journal 316:1236–1238

Pocock S J 1983 Clinical trials: a practical approach. Wiley, Chichester

Siegel S 1998 Nonparametric statistics. McGraw-Hill, Singapore

Streiner D L, Norman G R 1996 Health measurement scales: a practical guide to their development and use. Oxford University Press, Oxford

Swinscow T D V, Campbell M J 1996 Statistics at square one. BMJ Publishing Group, London

12 | Evidence-based medicine and psychiatry

Stephen M Lawrie, John R Geddes

Clinicians are under increasing pressure from a number of sources to keep up-to-date with the research literature and to ensure that their clinical practice is as effective as possible. The rapid expansion of the internet means that patients have increased access to knowledge about healthcare and understandably expect their doctors to be fully informed. Purchasers of healthcare expect maximum value for each pound spent. Clinicians, however, are faced with a substantial problem: the research literature is chaotic and rapidly expanding, and conventional approaches to keeping up-to-date are hopelessly inadequate. Evidence-based medicine (EBM), which consists of a coherent set of strategies based on developments in information technology and clinical epidemiology, has been proposed as a potential solution to this problem. EBM is a form of 'knowledge management' that has been developed to meet the needs of the practising clinician.

EBM involves several key steps:

1. the recognition of uncertainty and the formulation of an answerable question;
2. the reliable and efficient identification of the best available evidence;
3. the critical appraisal (in terms of validity and usefulness) of the evidence;
4. the integration of the appraised best available evidence with the clinician's own experience and the patient's own preferences, biology and social circumstances;
5. evaluation and improvement of the clinician's own performance at each stage of the process.

Together, the strategies of EBM facilitate a career-long, problem-based, self-directed process of learning with the fundamental aim of improving patient care. EBM was developed to assist the decision-making of the individual clinician helping a particular patient; however, the same process is also increasingly being used by policy-makers and purchasers of services.

In this chapter we will briefly describe the main historical developments leading to EBM and critically examine its potential clinical importance. We will then discuss in detail, with examples, how each of the components of EBM described above can be applied to the contemporary practice of psychiatry. Although EBM promises benefits for practitioners (and their patients) throughout their career, we appreciate that most readers of this textbook will be studying for postgraduate exams. We will therefore emphasise the processes of critical appraisal (Critical Review Paper Working Party 1997). This will be followed by an estimate of how much of current psychiatric practice is evidence based, and how it compares with other medical disciplines. Finally,

we will discuss the main problems facing EBM in general and evidence-based mental health (EBMH) in particular.

There has been a certain amount of misunderstanding about EBM (Sackett et al 1996). Some have suggested that there is nothing new in EBM; certainly, the principle of basing healthcare on good empirical evidence has been generally accepted for several decades, but the critical practical developments in information technology and epidemiology that make EBM feasible in the real world have only occurred recently. These same developments mean that EBM is not impossible, as some have suggested. EBM is not a purely academic pursuit — its whole theory and practice is targeted directly at the needs of busy clinicians and their patients. EBM does not ignore the results of research designs apart from randomised controlled trials (RCTs) or meta-analyses of RCTs; the most appropriate research design depends on the nature of the question being asked, e.g. whether the question is to do with diagnostic tests, making valid prognostic statements, or understanding patients' experiences. EBM has been confused with the guidelines 'industry', or managed care, which are often seen as attempts to restrict clinical practice inappropriately with a form of 'cook-book' medicine that ignores clinical expertise or patient preferences. However, this is a willful misunderstanding of EBM, because it has always been emphasised that the aim is to integrate research evidence with other forms of knowledge. Lastly, it does not play into the hands of those who wish to cut the costs of healthcare, as the best available treatment is often not the cheapest (although EBM may assist in the difficult process of balancing optimal practice against resource constraints).

HISTORICAL DEVELOPMENT

Sackett & colleagues (1996) have traced the philosophical origins of EBM to the spirit of enquiry and call for external evidence in 19th-century Paris. More specifically, the development of the RCT as the clinical equivalent of a scientific experiment — first described by Daniels & Hill (1952) — has probably done more than anything else to place medical practice on secure scientific foundations. The development and refinement of techniques of meta-analysis (Smith & Glass 1977, Egger et al 2001) has allowed the results of two or more studies to be summarised quantitatively.

EBM first became possible with developments in information technology which allowed rapid bibliographic searching and retrieval; coupled with the application of biostatistical principles, derived from population-based epidemiology, to the care of individual patients (Sackett et al 1991). At the same time, the increasing demand from consumers of healthcare and others for more explicit use of treatments of proven benefit increased the pressure on doctors to keep up to date and to ensure that their practice was based on the best available evidence (Cochrane 1972).

WHY EBM?

The central issue addressed by EBM is that keeping abreast of new medical developments is difficult. There are ever-increasing quantities of medical journals containing an ever-increasing literature to be sifted through. Relevant studies need to be read and assimilated and — when appropriate — new findings incorporated into clinical practice. Similarly, old practices need to be discarded as evidence emerges of lack of effectiveness or actual harm. For the average psychiatrist, as with most doctors, there are perhaps a handful of general medical journals and a similar number of specialist journals to be read, but time is limited and the journals are (clinically) disorganised. Moreover, there is evidence that the further physicians are from graduation, the more out of date they become (Ramsey et al 1991). Not only are we likely to need more time to study, but we are less likely to do so (and less able to assimilate new information, due to age-related cognitive decline).

This is not merely an academic issue. Studies suggest that the average physician, when asked, could usefully seek clinically relevant information in two out of every three patients seen, and that such information would change their clinical decisions in one of every four (Covell et al 1985, Smith 1996). It has long been recognised that the mass of potentially relevant information needs to be reliably reviewed and formatted for easy access in everyday clinical situations. The problem is that traditional updating methods — books, review articles and even continuing medical education — are unreliable and do not change clinical practice.

Textbooks are almost inevitably out of date by the time they are published. Most 'expert' review articles are unsystematic (in the selection and interpretation of studies for review) and often outdated. For example, conventional narrative review methods delayed the use of thrombolysis for myocardial infarction by about 10 years after a systematic review/meta-analysis would have shown convincing benefit (Antman et al 1992); while the dangerous, sometimes lethal, use of lignocaine prophylaxis for ventricular fibrillation was extended by about the same length of time after it had been shown to be counterproductive. By contrast, systematic reviews require a comprehensive search for relevant studies using an explicit strategy, bias-free citations, accurate judgement of scientifc quality of cited articles, and appropriate synthesis of the articles' conclusions. Unfortunately, but perhaps predictably, there is a strong inverse relationship ($r = -0.52$) between adherence to these standards and self-professed expertise of the reviewer (Oxman & Guyatt 1993).

Lastly, the processes of continuing medical education (CME) are often ineffective. As with reading, those motivated to attend CME courses are least likely to need to. It has been shown that many commonly used methods of CME do not change doctors' clinical behaviour and so are unlikely to bring about improvements in the quality of patient care (Davis et al 1995). The strategies of EBM offer a feasible alternative to haphazard reading and being at the mercy of pharmaceutical company representatives for keeping up to date. Although EBM itself is still in need of rigorous evaluation, there is some evidence that medical students at McMaster and Harvard universities, where the teaching has been problem- rather than knowledge-based for several years, find their undergraduate teaching more stimulating and satisfying and are better able to keep up to date with medical advances as postgraduates than students taught in more traditional curricula (Sackett et al 1997).

The Cochrane collaboration

The recognition of the need for systematic reviews of RCTs and the development of the scientific methodology of review articles has been one of the most important developments in health services research over the past decade. The Cochrane Collaboration was formed to 'prepare and maintain systematic reviews of randomised controlled trials of the effects of health care, and of other evidence when appropriate, and to make this information readily available to decision-makers at all levels of health care systems' (Cochrane Collaboration 1995). The first Cochrane Centre was established in Oxford, UK in 1992 as part of the NHS Research and Development (R&D) Programme, and centres have since been established in several other countries. The Cochrane Collaboration facilitates systematic reviews of RCTs of all aspects of healthcare, maintains a register of RCTs, organises training for reviewers, and establishes systems to update and efficiently disseminate the findings. Within this network, there are collaborative review groups, which co-ordinate reviews in a specific area of medical practice — for example, the Cochrane Depression Anxiety and Neurosis Group. Thus far, there are four other groups in psychiatry — covering dementia, schizophrenia, alcohol and drugs, and developmental disorders.

The Cochrane Library, containing all this information, is continually updated and published four times a year on compact disc and on the internet. As well as the Cochrane Database of Systematic Reviews (CDSR), the library contains the Database of Abstracts of Reviews of Effectiveness (DARE), the Cochrane Controlled Trials Register (of 160 000 controlled trials) and the Cochrane Review Methodology Database for those undertaking research synthesis (Cochrane Collaboration 2003).

By facilitating access to summaries of research evidence, the gradual evolution of the CDSR will greatly enhance the feasibility of evidence-based medical practice. The Cochrane Library is already the best available source of systematic reviews of the effectiveness of healthcare interventions. Its main strengths are in the continual updating of information and the dramatic advances in the methodology of systematic reviews that has accompanied the development of the Cochrane Collaboration (NHS Centre for Reviews and Dissemination (CRD) 1996). The Cochrane Collaboration builds upon contributors' existing interests, which improves the commitment to continual updating but means that reviews of very specialist interventions may be undertaken before reviews of more common and important treatments.

Improving access to high-quality evidence

Although these initiatives fulfil an essential role in producing regularly updated systematic reviews of evidence of clinical effectiveness, Cochrane reviews can be too unwieldy to be useful at the point of patient contact, and there is an inevitable delay between the publication of important evidence and its incorporation into a review. A further series of secondary publications are designed to provide more concise summaries and to alert clinicians to important new research findings. *Clinical Evidence* is a continuously updated compendium (published in both paper- and web-based versions: www.clinicalevidence.com) of the best available evidence of the effects of treatments: it includes a large mental health section. *Evidence-Based Mental Health* is a journal (with a full-text website: http://ebmh.bmjjournals.com/) that screens the mental health literature to locate the relatively small number of psychiatry research articles that are both valid and clinically important. These are then summarised into one-page structured abstracts with commentaries provided by experienced clinicians. Lastly, in the UK, the *National Electronic Library for Health* project aims to provide a common entry portal to all these new resources (http://www.nelh.nhs.uk/).

HOW TO PRACTISE EBM

EBM requires the acquisition of some new skills that many qualified clinicians will not possess. Learning the principles of EBM and beginning to employ them to improve patient care can be relatively quick, but acquiring detailed knowledge and experience demands regular and continuing reading and practice. What follows is enough to begin this hopefully lifelong process. Readers who want to further satisfy their curiosity and/or to take things further should consider: learning EBM by attending EBM and critical appraisal skills workshops, subscribing to the journals and discs described above, and/or setting up channels for regular communication with EBM teachers. (Indeed, a case can be made for at least one person in each service, perhaps the audit or R&D coordinator, doing all of these with a view to staff development and service evaluation.)

The five steps involved in EBM were outlined at the beginning of this chapter. Below we will illustrate the process of EBM as applied to a single treatment study, a diagnostic study, a prognostic study, a meta-analysis, and a clinical guideline. Critical appraisal criteria for audit and qualitative studies are briefly discussed in Chapter 10. It should be noted, however, that EBM also covers issues of aetiology, clinical decision analysis, economics, quality improvement, and others which are beyond the scope of this brief chapter. Those who are particularly interested or assiduous in preparing for exams are referred to Sackett et al (1997) and/or Lawrie et al (2000).

1. Framing questions

To be useful, such questions will be brief summaries of the clinical scenario and what information is required that are constructed in a way that makes searching for evidence likely to succeed. Specific questions will of course vary according to the situation, but productive questions tend to be composed of four parts, known as the PICO format: the **p**atient problem, the type of clinical issue or **i**ntervention being considered (e.g. diagnostic, prognostic or therapeutic), the **c**omparison intervention (if appropriate) and the clinical **o**utcome(s) of interest.

> Treatment example: *You are referred a 22-year-old female outpatient with a 5-year history of bulimia nervosa. She is not clinically depressed, but regularly abuses alcohol, and wishes some sort of talking rather than drug treatment. As a general adult psychiatrist, you are not sure what the best sort of treatment would be. You ask her to begin to record a diary of her eating*

and bingeing and arrange to do a literature search before you see her again in 2 weeks time.

Question: *In bulimia nervosa (problem), which psychotherapy (intervention) is most effective in securing recovery (outcome)?*

There are of course several questions that one could ask in this and any clinical situation — for example, how does drug treatment compare with psychotherapy? are there alternative treatments? The question will, of course, depend on what is most useful to you and your patient, what evidence you can actually find, and what might be of greatest benefit to know for similar common situations in the future. Of course, the number of possible questions will always be greater than the time available to answer them, but once one question is answered (and ideally recorded somewhere for easy access), others can be dealt with as and when the need and opportunity arises. Not only can several questions be asked within a domain (e.g. treatment) but several domains (such as clinical findings, aetiology, differential diagnosis, prognosis, therapy, prevention and even self-improvement) may be pertinent in any one consultation.

2. Searching for evidence

A really well-framed clinical question will make the literature search parameters obvious, but this may sometimes require further thought (and perhaps slight modification of the question). In obtaining evidence, one must next consider where and how to get it.

Electronic media for literature searching have several advantages, in terms of access time and completeness, over hand searching journals. The quickest and easiest way of identifying reliable information is to use evidence-based medical summaries generated by others, as mentioned above. However, if this does not answer the question, then a search of one of the computerised literature databases is often required.

MEDLINE, BIDS (Bath Information Database Service) and PsychLit are all useful resources, but have different databases stretching back to 1975, 1981 and 1990, respectively. It is important to appreciate that even a well-conducted search on one of these databases will probably only detect 30–50% of the relevant studies and that each will identify a different set of publications, but in practice MEDLINE has the advantage of being widely available, now with an improved user-friendly web interface (PubMed http://www.ncbi.nlm.nih.gov/entrez/query.fcgi).

A MEDLINE search demands search terms, as textwords or subject headings, to be typed in and allows certain operations to be performed to identify publications of a particular type. Ideally, when considering a treatment issue as in the brief example above, one would be able to identify one or more systematic reviews (indexed in MEDLINE under the heading 'meta-analysis') of RCTs which monitored and compared relapse rates on drug and placebo. However, it is more likely that no meta-analyses are available and one or more potentially relevant RCTs must be identified and then evaluated. *Evidence-Based Medicine* (EBM) suggests search terms to identify RCTs according to the year of publication — a 'high-quality yield search' with one item would use 'clinical trial (publication type [pt])' for 1990 and after, as well as 'random (textword [tw])' before 1990, although using more than one term will increase the number of studies identified (see inside back cover of EBM volume 1, part 7). PubMed now includes a 'clinical queries' service that automatically uses filters for the most reliable design to answer a clinical question (www.ncbi.nlm.nih.gov/entrez/query/static/clinical.html).

If you cannot find any relevant studies, a number of possible strategies are available. MESH (medical subject headings) search terms can be 'expanded' into a broader category, alternative words could be used, or another database may be worth consulting. However, it is more common to get too much rather than too little information from such a search. It is often useful to get help in searching, or learning how to search, from a trained librarian. Once the study or studies have been identified, they must be evaluated in terms of their validity and usefulness.

Literature search example: You remember seeing a structured review of a paper on psychotherapy for bulimia in a recent edition of Evidence-Based Medicine *(on disc or in print). Searching the disc/journal you find the one-page summary, although it was published longer ago than you thought (EBM Jan/Feb 1996). You note that the summary contains some of the EBM summary data you require.*

3. Appraising the evidence

The evidence needs to be critically appraised for its scientific validity and clinical importance. Validity criteria are essentially the same as the questions to be answered in critical appraisal (see Sackett et al 1997); while clinical importance can be determined by some of the summary measures EBM practitioners find useful (particularly for treatment studies).

Appraisal example: Although you know that Evidence-Based Medicine *only selects for inclusion treatment trials with random allocation, clinically important outcome measures and consistent data analysis, no system is infallible, and therefore you evaluate the paper for yourself (Fairburn et al 1995), following the checklist for treatment studies (see Box 12.1).*

The paper compares the outcome after cognitive-behavioral therapy (CBT), interpersonal therapy (IPT) and behaviour therapy. Treatment allocation was random (although the paper does not mention whether or not the randomisation list was concealed); 90% of the patients were interviewed at follow-up and the groups were analysed as randomised; the treatment was not blind (but outcome assessment was), the groups were treated equally other than with the interventions of interest and did not differ significantly at the start of the trial. You decide therefore that the study is valid.

At this point, it is worth briefly reviewing some of the measures of clinical effectiveness and how to calculate them for treatment studies. We are primarily interested in comparing the proportion of patients treated with a new treatment who get the outcome of interest — or the experimental event rate (EER) — with the proportion of patients treated with an alternative (standard) treatment who get the outcome of interest — or control event rate (CER). The difference between these two outcome rates is the absolute risk reduction (ARR), i.e. CER–EER (for an undesired outcome) expressed as a percentage. This tells us the difference in the number of patients with a specific outcome for every 100 patients treated in either way. The next term to introduce transforms this ARR into a more clinically useful number — the number needed to treat (NNT) — which is simply the reciprocal of the ARR and tells us how many such patients we would need to treat in a particular way so as to avoid one outcome event. As a

---

> **Box 12.1 Critical appraisal for single treatment studies**
>
> *Is the research valid?*
> - Was the assignment of patients to treatments randomised?
> - Was the randomisation list concealed?
> - Were all subjects who entered the trial accounted for at its conclusion?
> - Were they analysed in the groups to which they were randomised?
> - Were subjects and clinicians blind to which treatment was being received?
> - Apart from the experimental treatment, were the groups treated equally?
> - Were the groups similar at the start of the trial?
>
> *Is the research important?*
> - Absolute risk reduction (ARR, i.e. CER–EER) ARR =
> - Number need to treat (NNT, i.e. 1/ARR) NNT =
>
> *Can I apply it to my patient?*
> - Is this patient so different from those in the trial that the results do not apply?
> - How great would the benefit be for this particular patient?
> - What is the patient expected event rate (PEER) in my practice for patients like this one?
> - What is the (adjusted) NNT for this patient ? (PEER/CER = F, or estimate) NNT/F =
>
> *Is it consistent with my patient's values and preferences?*
> - Do I have a clear assessment of the patient's values and preferences?
> - Are they met by this intervention and its potential consequences?
>
> CER, control event rate; EER, experimental event rate.
> Source: Sackett et al (1997).

---

rough rule of thumb, NNTs of less than 10 usually denote a powerful and important treatment effect.

The results given in the paper are rates of still satisfying diagnostic criteria for bulimia at the end of the study: 37% for CBT, 28% for IPT and 86% for simple behavioural therapy. The ARR and NNT compared with simple behavioural therapy, are therefore 49% (86–37%) and 2 (95% confidence interval 1 to 4) for CBT, and 58% (86–28%) and 2 (1 to 3) for IPT. There seems little to choose between CBT and IPT, but the summary states that patients receiving CBT were less likely to have symptoms than those receiving either IPT or behavioural therapy, and that CBT complete remission rates were highest.

4. Implementation

We are here concerned with whether the results of valid, important studies can be applied to our particular patient or group of patients. In essence, this depends on the similarity and differences between the subjects in a paper and our own clinical population. Certain questions can be routinely asked for therapeutic studies, as shown in Box 12.1. In practice, it is often quickest to answer these applicability questions first, as this avoids the unnecessary evaluation of irrelevant papers, as long as the other stages of critical appraisal are not forgotten.

One further term needs to be introduced here. This is simply an estimate of your own patients' susceptibility to the outcome of interest as compared with the average patient in the trial — on the basis of age, sex, comorbidity, etc. This estimate is called F (for fraction), as many patients will be less susceptible than those in the RCT (e.g. F = $\frac{1}{2}$), although some patients may be more liable to benefit and the F will be greater than 1 in such cases. The NNT for any particular patient can be simply calculated by dividing the NNT by F.

> Implementation example: *Your patient is clearly similar in age and sex to those described in the study and would have been eligible for inclusion in the study. Interpersonal psychotherapy is not available locally — but cognitive-behaviour therapy is (and it produces the best remission rates). In your team, the clinical psychologist provides the CBT, and so you refer the patient. You tell him that there is a good chance of a successful outcome.*

5. Evaluation

The final stage of EBM is the continual evaluation and improvement of the specific skills involved at each stage of the process. It is useful to review periodically the clinical questions you have asked and your success in answering them. How well can you critically appraise the scientific literature, and is there any way that you can improve your skills (for example, by using critical appraisal checklists prepared by others)? Are you providing clinically useful summaries of the evidence — and keeping them up to date? It is useful to share any problems identified, by discussing with other local practitioners or clinical epidemiologists. You may benefit from attendance at an EBM or critical appraisal skills workshop.

One useful way of implementing EBM is to encourage a critical, but supportive, culture. Clinical colleagues should be asking each other for the evidence in support of some of their statements. Audit of how 'evidence-based' your practice is and what changes we should aim for, preferably with individualised feedback, will then be feasible. Similarly, it may be possible to begin to teach EBM principles to medical students or members of other disciplines. Existing structures, such as a journal club, can be reorganised along EBM lines (Sackett et al 1997).

> Evaluation example: *You ask the psychologist to inform you of the treatment outcome and decide to audit the treatments (and their outcome) you have offered to patients with bulimia you have seen over the past year. You discuss with your colleagues the possibility of a larger audit and ensuring that all such patients are treated with CBT in the future (for which resources will need to be identified).*

FURTHER EXAMPLES OF CRITICAL APPRAISAL AND IMPLEMENTATION

Diagnosis

Example: *With the advent of effective treatments for dementia, you and your primary care colleagues want to use a brief, but effective way of identifying dementia in elderly patients. The priority is to find an instrument that is quick and easy to use and reliably identifies patients who may be able to benefit from the new medicines. The test must have acceptable rates of both false positives and false negatives. Many colleagues are familiar with the Mini-Mental State Examination (MMSE) and have heard about a promising instrument: the modified MMSE.*

1. Question

How well does the modified MMSE screen for dementia in community living old people?

2. Literature search

You search PubMed clinical queries using the diagnosis filter with an emphasis on specificity. One article appears highly relevant: McDowell et al (1997).

3. Appraisal

McDowell et al conducted screening interviews with representative samples of people aged 65 or over in 36 communities in 10 Canadian provinces. The study was part of the Canadian Study of Health and Aging in which there were 8900 community participants; 1600 participants also underwent an extensive clinical and neuropsychological examination. Using the critical appraisal checklist (see Box 12.2) for diagnosis studies you decide that McDowell et al meets the validity criteria because there was an independent 'gold standard' for the diagnosis (DSM-IIIR criteria for dementia made by physician and neuropsychologist blind to the results of the screening instrument, with computerised verification and random reassessment), the sample of participants included an appropriate spectrum of those at risk, and the gold standard diagnosis was applied regardless of the diagnostic test result. The authors calculated the sensitivity and specificity at various cut-off points, and the results look as if they will be important and applicable to your question. There is, however, always a trade-off between sensitivity and specificity. If a cut-point with a high sensitivity is selected, then you can expect to pick up a high proportion of the cases. On the other hand, some of these will be false positives — in other words, they will screen positive, but not really have the disorder. To minimise the chances of false positives, a cut-point with a high specificity should be selected, but this will have the disadvantage of a high rate of missing cases (high false negative rate). Whether a particularly high specificity (or sensitivity) or a better balance is required depends on the disease and treatment available. In this example, where a possibly ameliorative treatment with few adverse effects could be prescribed for an incurable condition, we might wish to both maximise the number of people treated and minimise the number given an incorrect and distressing diagnosis. Sometimes, the aim is to maximise both the sensitivity and specificity, but this will invariably require a compromise of the optimal cut-point for either.

Any therapeutic decisions will, however, need to be taken after discussions with the patients (and any carers) who will want to know what their chances of developing dementia will be. This obviously depends on their score. In this example, if someone scores 61 their chance of developing dementia will be higher than if they scored 77, but how high will it be? This information comes from reading 'two by two tables' across rather than down (Table 12.1). Here, 151 of 188 people screening positive will actually have dementia – a 'positive predictive value' (PPV) of 80%; the study tells us that a cut-off of 61 would give a PPV of 80% (151 /{151 + 37}). These PPVs (and their negative counterparts, negative predictive values) are useful figures for clinicians and their patients, but they vary with the prevalence of the disorder. In this study of the over 65s in Canada the prevalence was 368/1600 or 23%. If the prevalence in your general practice was say 15% or 30% these PPVs would be

Box 12.2   Critical appraisal for diagnosis studies

Is the research valid?
- Was there an independent, blind comparison with a reference ('gold') standard of diagnosis?
- Was the diagnostic test evaluated in an appropriate spectrum of patients (like those in whom it would be used in practice)?
- Was the reference standard applied regardless of the diagnostic test result?

Is the research important?
The table below give the general formulae for the different test characteristics:

	Disorder present (according to gold standard)	Disorder absent (according to gold standard)	Row totals
Test positive	a	b	a+b
Test negative	c	d	c+d
Column totals	a+c	b+d	a+b+c+d

- Sensitivity = a/(a+c) = proportion of patients with the disorder who test positive
- Specificity = d/(b+d) = proportion of patients without the disorder who test negative
- Positive predictive value = a/(a+b) = proportion of patients with a positive test who have the disorder
- Negative predictive value = d/(c+d) = proportion of patients with a negative test who do not have the disorder
- Prevalence (= pre-test probability) = (a+c)/(a+b+c+d) = proportion of patients with the disorder in the whole sample
- Likelihood ratio = ratio of the probability that a positive test result came from someone *with* the disorder to the probability that a positive test result came from someone *without* the disorder = {a/(a+c)}/{b/(b+d)} = sensitivity/(1–specificity)

Can I apply it to my patient?
- Is the diagnostic test available, affordable, accurate and precise in your setting?
- Can you generate a clinically sensible estimate of your patient's pre-test probability (from practice data, from personal experience, from the report itself, or from clinical speculation)
- Will the resulting post-test probabilities affect your management and help your patient? (Could it move you across a test–treatment threshold? Would your patient be a willing partner in carrying it out?)
- Would the consequences of the test help your patient?

Source: Sackett et al (1997).

Table 12.1   Notional results of a test for dementia with a cut-off score of 61

Cut-off 61 results	Dementia	No dementia	Row totals
Test positive	151	37	188
Test negative	217	1195	1412
Column totals	368	1232	1600

unreliable (you might want to construct tables to prove this to your satisfaction). This is where likelihood ratios come in.

4.   Implementation

Likelihood ratios are calculated from the relatively prevalence-invariant measures of sensitivity and specificity to generate diagnostic test results of direct clinical relevance. In the current example, the likelihood ratio for a positive test (LR+, calculated as sensitivity /{1 – specificity}) using the 61 cut-off is 13.7 (0.41 / ({1–0.97}). This can be used to calculate the chance that a person scoring 61 on this test has dementia (more or less) regardless of the prevalence. First, as LRs are odds, the pre-test probability (P, which is also the prevalence or risk of having the disorder) must be converted into odds. Using the simple formula odds = P / (1 – P), the odds here are 0.29 (0.23 /{1–0.23}). Multiplying these pre-test odds by the LR+ gives the post-test odds of 3.97 (0.29 × 13.7). Converting back into a post-test probability (P = odds /{1 + odds}), for clinical use, someone scoring 61 or lower has a relatively high chance of being demented: 80% (3.97/4.97).

This is all a bit involved and can be done much more simply using the nomogram shown in Figure 12.1. Anchor a straight-edge along the left edge of the nomogram at the prevalence, or pre-test probability, of 23%. Pivot the straight-edge until it intersects the likelihood ratio for your patent's diagnostic test

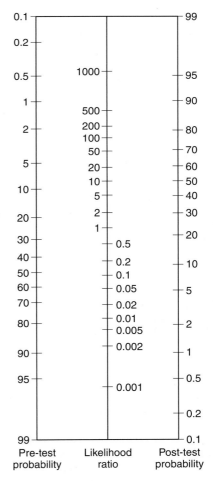

Fig. 12.1
Nomogram to calculate post-test probability.

result (about 14). It will intersect the right edge of the nomogram at your patient's post-test probability. Estimated this way the post-test probability is also about 80%.

Sixty-one is therefore a reasonably useful cut-off score for this test, since it makes the diagnosis very likely in those who screen positive. (Note, however, that it is not nearly so useful when it comes to ruling out the diagnosis and that a higher cut-off would do neither very well — you may wish to do the calculations for practice.) As a general rule, an LR+ of more than 10 is likely to be clinically useful.

5. Evaluation

You take your colleagues through these results and decide to use the test in routine practice (and to audit its use over 1 year).

Prognosis

Example: *A 25-year-old male patient currently hospitalised for his first episode of schizophrenia is nearing discharge. His ageing parents ask to see you to discuss the likely outcome for their son. At the meeting they are particularly interested in whether he will be able to live independently and obtain paid employment in the future. You tell them that the conventional wisdom is that about half of all patients with schizophrenia will return to their premorbid social situation but that the other half are likely to deteriorate progressively. They thank you for your time, but you are dissatisfied with the information you gave and sense that the parents were too. You resolve to search the literature for a recent prognosis study.*

1. Question

What percentage of patients in their first episode of schizophrenia will be living independently and in paid employment at 5–10 years?

2. Literature search

Using the MESH headings 'schizophrenia', 'cohort' and 'first episode' on MEDLINE you identify several studies. However, one catches your eye as it describes the results of a 13 year follow-up in Nottingham and mentions disability and residence in the structured abstract (Mason et al 1995).

3. Appraisal

Using the critical appraisal checklist for prognosis studies (Box 12.3), you decide that the Mason et al (1995) study meets the validity criteria because it studied all first-episode psychosis patients in a defined catchment area, obtained follow-up information in 94%, objective outcomes were determined with good reliability, and no subgroups with different prognoses were identified (making adjustment unnecessary), even though there was no independent 'test-set' group of patients. The results also look important — 57 of the 59 subjects (97%) had been living independently in the community for most of the past 2 years, 16 (28%) alone, and 22 (37%) had been employed for the past 2 years.

You then calculate *95% confidence intervals* for these outcomes to ensure that the results given in the paper are sufficiently precise to be useful in practice. The 95% confidence interval (CI) is the range of values in which you can be 95% sure that the true value

---

Box 12.3   **Critical appraisal for prognosis studies**
Is the research valid? • Was a defined, representative sample of patients assembled at a common (usually early) point in the course of their disease? • Was patient follow-up sufficiently long and complete? • Were objective outcome criteria applied in a 'blind' fashion? • If subgroups with different prognoses are identified, was there adjustment for important prognostic factors? • Was there validation in an independent group ('test-set') of patients? *Are the valid results of this prognosis study important?* • How likely are the outcomes over time? • How precise are the prognostic estimates? *Can you apply this valid, important evidence about prognosis in caring for your patient?* • Were the study patients similar to your own? • Will this evidence make a clinically important impact on your conclusions about what to offer or tell your patient?
Source: Sackett et al (1997)

lies. The approximate 95% CI for a proportion (expressed as a decimal) is the proportion plus or minus 1.96 times the square root of {[(the proportion) × (1-proportion)] / sample size}. For living independently, this is 0.97 ± 1.96 times the square root of $(0.97 \times 0.03)/59$, or 0.97 ± 0.04, or 93–100%. The other confidence intervals are 17–39% for living alone and 26–48% for employment (check them yourself for practice). The 95% CI gives an estimate of the uncertainty of the proportion.

4. Implementation

Again using the checklist (Box 12.3), you decide that the results can be applied to your patient because the study was of an unbiased inception (first-episode) cohort and your patient is just recovering from his first episode. The study was in a UK secondary-care setting similar to your own service. You also think that the information will be useful for you, your patient and his parents. You arrange to see them again briefly to discuss the results of your endeavours.

5. Evaluation

You note that the paper identified also gives information on symptoms and treatment outcomes and file your critically appraised summary of the paper under schizophrenia—prognosis. The summary will need to be updated as new evidence becomes available.

Systematic reviews and meta-analysis

Example: *You want to improve the local implementation of case management for the severely mentally ill. You are aware that there has been considerable uncertainty about the effectiveness of case management and for which patients it is most useful.*

1. Question

For patients with severe mental illness, what are the effects of case management on the clinical state and service utilisation?

2. Searching for evidence

You search for a relevant systematic review of RCTs in the CDSR (Cochrane Database of Systematic Reviews) on the Cochrane Library. You find a systematic review of case management for people with severe mental disorders which seems to address the issue (Marshall et al 2003).

3. Appraisal

Although the review has been conducted under the auspices of the Cochrane Collaboration, it is still important to critically appraise it for validity and usefulness (Box 12.4). The review includes eleven RCTs of case management versus standard care. The reviewers clearly describe the search strategy for identifying the primary studies, as well as the inclusion and exclusion criteria for including them in the review. All the studies investigated a form of case management which was broadly comparable; standard care was defined as the usual level of psychiatric care provided in the area where each study was conducted. The studies examined a range of clinical and health service utilisation outcomes. Although there was some variation between the studies, the reviewers investigated the reasons for this and concluded that it was mainly quantitative

---

Box 12.4   Critical appraisal for a systematic review

Is the research valid?
- Did the review address a clearly focused issue? (i.e. did the review describe: the population studied? the intervention given? the outcome considered?)
- Did the authors select the right sort of studies for review? (i.e. addressing the review question, with adequate study design)
- Were the important, relevant studies included? (Look for which bibliographic databases were used, personal contact with experts, search for unpublished as well as published studies, search for non-English language studies)
- Did the reviewers do enough to assess the quality of the included studies?
- Did they describe randomisation and/or use a rating scale?

What are the results?
- Were the results similar from study to study?
- Are the results of all studies clearly displayed?
- If the results are not similar, are the reasons for the variations discussed?
- What is the overall result of the review?
- Is there a clinical bottom line?
- What is the numerical result? (ARR = ?, NNT= ?)
- How precise are the results?
- Is there a confidence interval?

Can I apply the results to my patient(s)?
- Is my patient so different from those in the trial that the results may not apply?
- Should I apply the results to my patient(s)?
- How great would the benefit be?
- Is the intervention consistent with my patient's values and preferences?
- Were all the clinically important outcomes considered?
- Are the benefits worth the harm and costs?

Source: Sackett et al (1997).

---

rather than qualitative. You decide that the results of the overview are probably valid. As the primary studies were performed in the UK and USA, and included patients with severe mental illness (however defined), you also think that the review can be applied to your own clinical situation.

4. Implementation

The main findings of the review are that case management assists community psychiatric teams to maintain contact with patients. However, it also increases the rate of admission to hospital. There was no significant effect on other outcome variables (such as possible improvements in symptom severity or quality of life). Of 599 case managed subjects, 150 were lost to follow-up (EER = 25%), as compared with 195 of 611 standard care subjects (CER = 32%). The absolute benefit increase is 7% and the NNT is 15 (rounded up from 14.3). This means that 15 patients have to be treated with case management to prevent one less patient being lost to follow-up than would occur with standard care.

The ratio of the odds of being lost to follow-up in the case management group to the odds of the same in the standard care group was 0.70 (95% CI 0.50 to 0.98). You know from an audit of your own service, carried out before the implementation of the care programme approach, that only 10% of your own patients were lost to follow-up each year. This is the patient expected event rate (PEER) and is about 30% ($0.10/0.32 = 0.31$) of the CER in the review. Assuming that case management has a fairly constant effect in all patient groups, you can therefore adjust the NNT to apply to the loss of follow-up rate of your service by dividing it by this proportion, which is called the F value (Cook & Sackett 1995). This revised NNT is approximately 49 (15/0.31). However, among patients with a previous history of loss of contact, your drop-out rate was 80%. Adjustment in a similar way produces a second revised NNT of 6 for this 'high risk of drop-out' patient group.

5. Evaluation

You therefore decide not to use your scarce resources on routine case management (NNT 49), but to concentrate on those with whom you have previously lost contact (NNT 6). You audit the loss to follow-up in both groups over the next 6 months, both to ensure that your pre-case management audit figures are still applicable and to examine the effects of your decision to focus your care programming.

Clinical practice guidelines

Clinical practice guidelines have been defined as 'systematically developed statements to assist practitioner decisions about appropriate health care for specific clinical circumstances' (Field & Lohr 1990). Clinical practice guidelines are therefore a form of *policy statement*. The aim of guidelines, like that of EBM in general, is often misunderstood as an attempt to straightjacket clinical practice. To avoid this mistake, it is useful to consider a hierarchy of policy statements in which three levels can be distinguished that vary on two main dimensions: the degree of certainty about what will happen if the policy is followed (i.e. how convincing is the evidence on which it is based?) and the extent to which the patient's and clinician's preferences are both known and consistent with the likely outcomes (Eddy 1990). The three levels of statement are: options, clinical practice guidelines and clinical standards.

- *Options* are systematically derived statements, based on systematic reviews, that do not attempt to make general recommendations, recognising that implementation will depend on individual and local circumstances. The value of options is that they provide clinicians with a summary of up-to-date evidence and highlight current uncertainties.
- *Clinical practice guidelines* usually apply to the *average* patient and therefore need to be applied flexibly and tailored according to local circumstances and needs, including patient preference. To be valid for the average patient, clinical practice guidelines need to be based on a certain standard of evidence (see Box 12.5). Treatment recommendations are usually graded according to the strength of the evidence, and confident statements are usually only made about clinical issues that are reasonably supported by appropriate, randomised (in the case of treatment decisions) evidence. The key issue here is that, even with a reasonable level of evidence to make fairly general statements, there are likely to be occasions when adhering to a guidelines recommendation would do more harm than good.

Box 12.5   Classification of evidence and recommendations for a clinical practice guideline

Classification of evidence levels*

Ia   Evidence obtained from meta-analysis of randomised controlled trials

Ib   Evidence obtained from at least one randomised controlled trial

IIa Evidence obtained from at least one well-designed controlled study without randomisation

IIb Evidence obtained from at least one other type of well-designed quasi-experimental study[†]

III Evidence obtained from well-designed non-experimental descriptive studies, such as comparative studies, correlation studies and case studies

IV   Evidence obtained from expert committee reports or opinions and/or clinical experiences of respected authorities

Classification of grades of recommendations*

A   Requires at least one randomised controlled trial as part of a body of literature of overall good quality and consistency addressing specific recommendation (Evidence levels *Ia*, *Ib*)

B   Requires the availability of well-conducted clinical studies but no randomised clinical trials on the topic of recommendation (Evidence levels *IIa*, *IIb*, *III*)

C   Requires evidence obtained from expert committee reports or opinions and/or clinical experiences of respected authorities. Indicates an absence of directly applicable clinical studies of good quality. (Evidence level *IV*)

---

*Source: US Department of Health and Human Services, Agency for Health Care Policy and Research. Acute pain management: operative or medical procedures and trauma. The Agency, Rockville, MD, 1993. Clinical Practice Guideline No 1.

†Refers to a situation in which implementation of an intervention is outwith the control of the investigators, but an opportunity exists to evaluate its effect.

- *Standards*, on the other hand, need to be applied rigidly. Adherence to standards is one way of measuring the quality of a clinical service. To be valuable, there must be a high degree of certainty about the result of applying a standard, and patients and clinicians must agree about the desirability of the outcomes. The level of evidence must be very high. The construction of valid and useful standards is much more difficult when there is less certainty about the results of applying them. Most psychiatric treatments fall into this category. We are often reasonably sure that a treatment offers some overall benefit, on average. But we are less certain that the treatment should *always* be used for *all* patients.

Example: *You are trying to improve the quality of care for patients with bipolar disorder. You need a resource that has already summarised the best available evidence for several clinical decisions and, following due consideration of other factors relevant to the clinical situation, provides transparent recommendations for clinical practice. In this situation, a clinical practice guideline may be most helpful. Your initial aim is to see if there is a guideline that covers the area of bipolar disorder.*

1. Question

Usually, when a single clinical uncertainty arises, you formulate it into a structured and answerable clinical question and then systematically search for the best available evidence to answer that precise question. The evidence is then appraised and integrated with your clinical judgement and the patient's preferences. But in your current situation, you do not have time to search for all the evidence required to answer several clinical questions. The question therefore needs to be broad: For patients with bipolar disorder, what are the methods of assessment and therapy that lead to the best outcomes?

2. Literature search

It can be difficult to identify high-quality clinical practice guidelines. For example, within the UK, the National Institute for Clinical Excellence (www.nice.nhs.uk) is developing a series of clinical practice guidelines, but few have yet been completed. There is also a database of UK primary care guidelines (Prodigy: www.prodigy.nhs.uk) but these do not cover bipolar disorder. The respected guidelines of the Scottish Intercollegiate Guidelines Network (www.sign.ac.uk) do not include bipolar disorder (but one is planned). Therefore it is back onto PubMed with a simple text search for 'bipolar disorder', restricted to publication type (clinical guideline). You immediately find several, including the recent update of the American Psychiatric Association Guideline (2002).

3. Appraisal (see Box 12.6)

Guidelines involve making decisions, and therefore it is important that the developers have considered all the relevant treatment options and potential outcomes. In the APA bipolar guideline, basic interventions such as establishing a therapeutic alliance, providing education, enhancing compliance and monitoring clinical status are considered as well as specific interventions including medication for acute and maintenance treatment and specific psychotherapies. The outcomes of these interventions are described.

Are the recommendations in this guideline valid?
- Were all important decision options and outcomes clearly specified?
- Was the evidence relevant to each decision option identified, validated and combined in a sensible and explicit way?
- Are the relative preferences that key stakeholders attach to the outcomes of decisions (including benefits, risks and costs) identified and explicitly considered?
- Is the guideline resistant to clinically sensible variations in practice?

Is this valid guideline or strategy potentially useful?
- Does this guideline offer an opportunity for significant improvement in the quality of healthcare practice?
  — Is there a large variation in current practice?
  — Does the guideline contain new evidence (or old evidence not yet acted upon) that could have an important impact on management?
  — Would the guideline affect the management of so many people, or concern individuals at such high risk, or involve such high costs that even small changes in practice could have major impacts on health outcomes or resources (including opportunity costs)?

Should this guideline or strategy be applied in your practice?
- What barriers exist to its implementation? Can they be overcome?
- Can you enlist the collaboration of key colleagues?
- Can you meet the educational, administrative and economic conditions that are likely to determine the success or failure of implementing the strategy?
  — credible synthesis of the evidence by a respected body
  — respected, influential local exemplars already implementing the strategy
  — consistent information from all relevant sources
  — opportunity for individual discussions about the strategy with an authority
  — user-friendly format for guidelines
  — implementable within target group of clinicians (without the need for extensive outside collaboration)
  — freedom from conflict with economic incentives, administrative incentives, patient expectations and community expectations

As with other forms of research synthesis, such as systematic reviews, one of the fundamental requirements is that the identification of the primary studies was systematic, repeatable, unbiased and comprehensive. The APA guideline used a computerised search of the 'relevant' literature from MEDLINE and PsycINFO, and gives search terms and dates, but does not clarify how studies were assessed for inclusion or exclusion.

Guideline developers also need to explicitly rate the quality of the evidence used in the guideline, on a hierarchy of evidence (see Box 12.5). Randomised evidence is usually the most reliable form of evidence for treatment recommendations; in the APA bipolar guideline, *preference* was given to randomised controlled trials. However, the guideline statements were not directly linked to the level of available evidence, and no attempt was made to quantitatively review, or perform a meta-analysis, on the randomised controlled trials. The actual guideline recommendations should also

be directly linked to the evidence supporting them — this stage of the guideline development also has to take into account other factors, possibly from non-randomised sources, and guideline developers often use another hierarchy to describe the strength of the recommendation. The APA guideline does this fairly well.

Therefore the user of the guideline can be reasonably satisfied that the guideline was developed in an unbiased and appropriate manner — though a number of methodological approaches could have increased the user's confidence, and a quantitative review would have made the guideline more helpful. The limited amount of randomised evidence led the guideline developers to be appropriately cautious in their recommendations

4. Implementation

Of course, you want to be sure that any recommendations are fully evidence-based and realisable in your clinical environment. You decide that the guideline is valid enough, and useful enough, to help in your clinical service. One of the main reasons why you were searching for a guideline was that your clinical director had identified (with a little help from you) that there were substantial variations in clinical practice. This situation may present a good opportunity to introduce such recommendations, although the implementation of guidelines is more likely to be effective if they fully take into account local circumstances, are disseminated by an active educational intervention and implemented by patient specific reminders (NHS Centre for Reviews and Dissemination 1994).

5. Evaluation

You circulate the full guidelines and the executive summary to your colleagues. Some are keen to use them but others are not prepared to do so. You therefore agree that some consultants will use the guideline and others will stick to their standard practice, and to compare readmission rates and patient satisfaction with their care (measured on a simple 10-point Likert scale) over the next year.

HOW EVIDENCE-BASED ARE WE?

An obvious place to begin to evaluate our individual and collective practice is to ask how much of contemporary medical and specifically psychiatric treatment is evidence-based? We tend to assume that, because we are *trying* to do good, we *are* doing good. However, few of our treatments are evidence-based in the sense that they are supported by high-quality studies that would meet strict critical appraisal guidelines. Indeed, it has been estimated that perhaps 'only 15% of medical interventions are supported by solid scientific evidence' (Smith 1991).

This debate raises the question: how can we deem a treatment to be 'evidence-based'? One way of answering this is to identify how well the intervention is supported by evidence — using a hierarchy to rate the evidence according to the likelihood of its giving an unbiased estimate of the true effect. Most reliable are findings from systematic reviews of good-quality RCTs, followed by individual good-quality RCTs. However, there are certain clinical situations where benefits could be said to be obvious, or where RCTs would be difficult and, arguably, even unethical (e.g. admission and observation for suicidal ideation). Nonetheless, it might still be possible to conduct standard care versus alternative treatment RCTs in these areas. Alternatively, some useful information about treatments may be available from naturalistic follow-up studies, although the information gained from cohort studies and case-control studies is most reliable for prognosis and diagnosis, respectively. Lastly, uncontrolled studies, case series and individual case reports are too susceptible to bias to have general value, although they may sometimes identify a treatment effect or therapeutic hazard that would merit further study.

Using these criteria — where treatment is considered evidence-based if it is based on results from randomised evidence, either from systematic reviews or RCTs, or where benefit is obvious — how evidence-based is contemporary medicine and psychiatry? The answer crucially depends on whether we talk about treatments or diseases. Chalmers et al (1989) examined the evidence for 226 obstetric procedures: only 50% had been evaluated in RCTs, with only 20% of procedures having been shown to be beneficial; the other 30% were of dubious benefit or dangerous. On the other hand, taking patients as the denominator, Ellis et al (1995) reviewed the evidence for the main treatment of 121 consecutive admissions to a medical ward in Oxford over 1 month. One hundred and nine patients had an identified primary diagnosis, 58 (53%) of whom received evidence-based interventions (e.g. heparin and warfarin for deep venous thrombosis), a further 32 (29%) received treatments supported by convincing non-experimental evidence (e.g. antibiotics for infections, resuscitation for cardiac arrest), and the remaining 19 (18%) patients were given treatments without any substantial supporting evidence (e.g. support for stroke or overdoses, treatment of pain). Overall, therefore, 82% of the medical interventions were evidence-based, taking patients rather than procedures as the focus of interest. This apparent discrepancy between procedures or patients can be explained by the simple fact that there are many procedures which have never been evaluated, whereas patients tend to have common diseases which are easier to study and therefore more likely to have been subject to treatment trials. We can take issue with the Ellis and colleagues' approach, or some of the deficiencies of the study — such as potential problems with generalisability, the accuracy of diagnosis, the fact that few patients only have one problem in clinical practice, and that self-evident treatments are not necessarily effective — but the conclusion remains that most medical patients receive treatments backed up by evidence from RCTs. How does psychiatry compare?

Using a similar design, Geddes and colleagues (1996) evaluated the treatments received by 40 consecutive admissions to a general psychiatry ward in Oxford. Twenty-nine (65%) of these acute admissions received interventions supported by evidence from RCTs or meta-analysis. The main diagnoses and treatments they received are shown in Table 12.2. The other 14 (35%) acute admissions received treatments (usually combinations of medication) for which there was no good evidence of efficacy. This is a small study and subject to the same criticisms as apply to the study of Ellis et al (1995). Moreover, many of the primary trials were small, and the study only considered medical interventions: many other interventions are used in multidisciplinary inpatient (and particularly outpatient) settings.

Summers & Kehoe (1996) addressed some of these issues by examining 160 treatment decisions in 158 patients (56 inpatients, 29 daypatients and 75 outpatients). They reported that there was RCT evidence for 85 (53%) of the patient interventions (especially drug treatments), that 16 (10%) of the interventions could not be ethically subject to RCT evaluation (e.g. observation levels in

Table 12.2 Evidence-based treatments received by 29 out of 40 psychiatry patients	
Primary diagnosis (No. patients)	Primary treatment
Alcohol withdrawal (1)	Individualised chlordiazepoxide regimen
Acute schizophrenia (12)	Antipsychotic medication
Chronic schizophrenia (4)	Oral/i.m. antipsychotic medication
Acute mania (3)	Lithium
Bipolar affective disorder prophylaxis (2)	Lithium
Depressive disorder (4)	Antidepressants
Treatment-resistant depression (3)	Lithium augmentation
Source: Geddes et al (1996).	

suicide), and that the remaining 59 (37%) patients received supportive practical measures and psychotherapy. Thus, inpatient psychiatric treatment may be more evidence based than outpatient services, but, overall, psychiatry compares reasonably well with acute medicine. There is still a need, however, for further and more all-encompassing assessments of these questions in psychiatry as in other specialties.

PROBLEMS FOR EBM AND EVIDENCE-BASED MENTAL HEALTH

These studies highlight some of the problems facing EBM, although none is insurmountable. Most of the research done on treatments is conducted on patients with a particular diagnosis and no other comorbid or complicating conditions. This does not reflect the complexities of medical practice and raises questions about whether the results from RCTs apply to all patients. The adjustment of the results obtained from a trial, using PEER and F values (see above), are attempts to deal with this, but there is also an increasing recognition of the need for clinical trials which more closely resemble real-life clinical practice. These large-scale *pragmatic* trials aim to include a representative sample of patients rather than highly selected 'super-patients', the standards of interventions are similar to those achievable in (good) clinical practice, and outcomes are chosen which are meaningful to patients and clinicians. The science of research synthesis and statistical meta-analysis is complex and sometimes produces results which are inconsistent with subsequent large trials, but it is still in its infancy and methodological advances are occurring rapidly (Egger et al 2001).

Evidence-based mental health (EBMH), in particular, probably has a number of other problems to solve (Geddes & Harrison 1997). Clinical diagnoses in psychiatry are reliable if diagnostic criteria are followed, but this is probably rare in clinical practice. We need to continue to improve the quality of diagnostic decision making in clinical psychiatric practice (Zarin & Earls 1993). In psychiatry we have very few external validating criteria for diagnosis, so our diagnostic gold standard is the psychiatric interview — and yet symptom elicitation has low reliability unless a structured interview is employed (Mojtabai & Nicholson 1995). RCTs in psychiatry have tended to be small and from single centres. Treatment compliance is more of a problem in psychiatry than in other areas of medicine, which demands more studies of attempts to increase compliance. We are alone in medicine in facing the problems of trying to treat detained patients against their will and need to find ethically satisfactory ways of including such patients in treatment trials. The RCTs that have been done have used a host of incomparable outcome measures, usually of symptom severity rather than hard, practically relevant, dichotomous outcomes (e.g. recovered or not, employed or not). At the same time, we should not forget that hard end-points used in medical studies (usually death) ignore morbidity and quality of life. Finally, although various talking treatments are supported by RCT evidence, there are likely to be considerable variations in how these are practised clinically and this requires some form of clinical quality control.

THE FUTURE

What can be and needs to be done to promote EBM in general and EBMH in particular? The agenda could encompass virtually all aspects of medical care from research through to service provision and purchasing, but a few points merit particular mention.

Firstly, EBM itself still requires better evidence of its effectiveness. There are clear a-priori reasons to believe that EBM should lead to optimal patient outcomes, simply because it provides a coherent and consistent approach to helping clinicians ensure that patient care is based on the best available evidence. However, EBM itself has shown that such apparently convincing reasoning may be misguided, and that empirical, randomised evidence of efficacy is required. Moreover, is the time and effort required to practice EBM justified — that is, is EBM cost-effective?

There is some evidence for the effectiveness of specific components of EBM. Medical graduates of universities which offer courses in critical appraisal are more likely to keep up to date than their counterparts in traditional universities, but more work is required on the effects of evidence-based teaching on clinicians and any benefits for their patients.

Second, the numbers of people directly involved should, one hopes, steadily increase. EBM is most certainly not an elitist pursuit — it depends on the endeavours of too many and requires the help of still more. There is plenty of room, for example, for more contributors to the systematic reviews supervised by the Cochrane Collaboration, for ever-increasing numbers of EBM teachers, and local co-ordinators at a Trust or Directorate level.

Third, EBM readily identifies critical clinical areas that require further evaluation. As research becomes more responsive to the needs of patients and clinicians, and as clinicians become more skilled at basing their practice on high-quality evidence, it should become easier to co-ordinate the large-scale, pragmatic trials which are required. Equally as important, however, is the evaluation of the most effective methods of implementation — that is, changing clinical practice according to the evidence. Without this, even the highest-quality research becomes irrelevant. Each stage of the process need to be carefully linked — EBM is a form of information management in which high-quality knowledge is produced, disseminated and effectively implemented.

SUMMARY AND CONCLUSIONS

EBM attempts to help doctors to stay abreast of developments in medical research by integrating clinical epidemiology, biostatistics,

pathophysiological knowledge and clinical experience. Its underlying rationale is that healthcare decisions should be based on the best available evidence. For each kind of clinical question it is usually possible to identify the study design most likely to provide the most valid and useful information. Evidence is identified using the most efficient available methods, critically appraised using empirically derived criteria and integrated with clinical practice using meaningful measures and indices.

There are at least four specific advantages of EBM over previous attempts to keep doctors up to date, such as traditional methods of continuing medical education, audit and clinical guidelines:

- It facilitates the incorporation of the best available treatments into clinical practice as soon as there is sufficient evidence for their efficacy.
- It can identify which time- and resource-consuming medical procedures are required and which are not (and which require further evidence).
- It provides a common language and rules for communicating about effectiveness.
- It shows promise in improving undergraduate education and postgraduate training.

Archie Cochrane criticised psychiatry in 1972 for 'using a large number of therapies whose effectiveness has not been proven', stated 'it is basically inefficient', and suggested increasing 'grants for well-designed evaluatory research'. Some progress has been made in the past thirty years, and EBMH could deliver more. EBM offers a way of steadily improving patient care and job satisfaction throughout the average clinical career by replacing the tyranny of haphazard medical informatics with the rigour of a systematically gathered evidence base.

REFERENCES

American Psychiatric Association 2002 Practice guideline for the treatment of patients with bipolar disorder (revision). American Journal of Psychiatry 159(suppl 4): 1–50

Antman E M, Lau J, Kupelnick B et al 1992 A comparison of results of meta-analyses of randomized control trials and recommendations of clinical experts. Treatments for myocardial infarction. Journal of the American Medical Association 268:240–248

Chalmers I, Enkin M, Keirse M J N C 1989 Effective care in pregnancy and childbirth. Oxford University Press, Oxford

Cochrane A 1972 Effectiveness and efficiency: random reflections on health services. Cambridge University Press, Cambridge (reprinted 1989 by BMJ Publishing, London)

Cochrane Collaboration 1995 Cochrane collaboration handbook. Cochrane Collaboration, Oxford

Cochrane Collaboration 2003 The Cochrane Library. Update Software, Oxford

Cook R J, Sackett D L 1995 The number needed to treat: a clinically useful measure of treatment effect. British Medical Journal 310:452–454

Covell D G, Uman G C, Manning P R 1985 Information needs in office practice: are they being met? Annals of Internal Medicine 103:596–599

Critical Review Paper Working Party 1997 MRCPsych part II examination: proposed critical review paper. Psychiatric Bulletin 21:381–382

Daniels M, Hill A B 1952 Chemotherapy of pulmonary tuberculosis in young adults. An analysis of the combined results of three Medical Research Council trials. British Medical Journal 1:1162

Davis D A, Thomson M A, Oxman A D, Haynes R B 1995 Changing physician performance: a systematic review of the effect of continuing medical education strategies. Journal of the American Medical Association 274:700–705

Eddy D M 1990 Clinical decision making: from theory to practice. Designing a practice policy. Standards, guidelines, and options. Journal of the American Medical Association 263:3077,3081,3084

Egger M, Davey Smith G, Altman D 2001 Systematic reviews in health care. Meta-analysis in context. BMJ Publishing, London

Ellis J, Mulligan I, Rowe J, Sackett D L 1995 Inpatient general medicine is evidence-based. Lancet 346:407–410

Fairburn C G, Norman P A, Welch S L et al 1995 A prospective study of outcome in bulimia nervosa and the long-term effects of three psychological treatments. Archives of General Psychiatry 52:304–312 (summarised in Evidence-Based Medicine 1:48)

Field M J, Lohr K N 1990 *Clinical practice guidelines: direction of a new agency.* Institute of Medicine, Washington, DC

Geddes J R, Harrison P J 1997 Closing the gap between research and practice. British Journal of Psychiatry 171:220–225

Geddes J R, Game D, Jenkins N E et al 1996 What proportion of primary psychiatric interventions are based on randomised evidence. Quality in Health Care 5:215–217

Lawrie S M, McIntosh A M, Rao S 2000 Critical appraisal for psychiatry. Churchill-Livingstone, Edinburgh

McDowell I, Kristjansson B, Hill G B, Hebert R 1997 Community screening for dementia: the Mini Mental State Exam (MMSE) and Modified Mini-Mental State Exam (3MS) compared. *J Clin Epidemiol* 50(4):377–383

Marshall M, Gray A, Lockwood A, Green R 2003 Case management for people with severe mental disorders. Available in *The Cochrane Library.* Update Software, Oxford

Mason P, Harrison G, Glazebrook C et al 1995 Characteristics of outcome in schizophrenia at 13 years. British Journal of Psychiatry 167:596–603

Mojtabai R, Nicholson R A 1995 Interrater reliability of ratings of delusions and bizarre delusions. American Journal of Psychiatry 152:1804–1806

NHS Centre for Reviews and Dissemination 1994 Implementing clinical practice guidelines. Effective Health Care 8:

NHS Centre for Reviews and Dissemination 1996 Undertaking systematic reviews of research on effectiveness. Centre for Reviews and Dissemination, University of York

Oxman A, Guyatt G H 1993 The science of reviewing research. Annals of the New York Academy of Sciences 703:125–134

Ramsey P G, Carline J D, Inui T S et al 1991 Changes over time in the knowledge base of practicing internists. Journal of the American Medical Association 266:1103–1107

Sackett D L, Haynes R B, Guyatt G H, Tugwell P 1991 Clinical epidemiology: a basic science for clinical medicine. Little Brown, Boston

Sackett D L, Rosenberg W M, Gray J A et al 1996 Evidence-based medicine: what it is and what it isn't. British Medical Journal 312:71–72

Sackett D L, Richardson S, Rosenberg W, Haynes R B 1997 Evidence-based medicine: how to practise and teach EBM. Churchill Livingstone, London

Sheldon T A 1996 Research intelligence for policy and practice: the role of the National Health Service Centre for Reviews and Dissemination (EBM note). Evidence-Based Medicine 1:167–168

Smith M L, Glass G V 1977 Meta-analysis of psychotherapy outcome studies. American Psychologist (September): 752–760

Smith R 1991 Where is the wisdom. . . ? British Medical Journal 303:798–799

Smith R 1996 What clinical information do doctors need? British Medical Journal 313:1062–1068

Summers A, Kehoe R F 1996 Is psychiatric treatment evidence-based? Lancet 347:409–410

Zarin D A, Earls F 1993 Diagnostic decision making in psychiatry. American Journal of Psychiatry 150:197–206

13 | Clinical assessment: interviewing and examination

David G Cunningham Owens, Peter J McKenna, Richard Davenport

THE PSYCHIATRIC INTERVIEW

Medicine, it is often said, is as much art as science. There is, however, an additional dimension which is particularly pertinent to psychiatry — that of craft. Much of what comprises good psychiatric practice takes what is inherently 'good' about an individual's ability to relate to others and hones it, under the influence of a mentor of experience, into an effective set of professional skills. As a result, learning the tools of one's trade is, for most psychiatrists, an *apprenticeship*, best learned in the shadow of someone who does it well.

The present chapter cannot 'teach' interview skills. Its aim is more modest — to encourage an awareness of, first, the *process* elements of the psychiatric interview and, second, the importance of *structure* in organising clinical material. Its orientation is entirely pragmatic and does not emanate from any specific theoretical framework. Those interested in theoretical aspects are referred to the suggestions for further reading. Its target is predominantly trainees working in general adult services. Specialist practice will require new skills, though these will rest firmly on the principles relevant to general psychiatric practice.

PROCESS

There is no technology yet devised to replace the fundamental medical skill of interpersonal communication. For psychiatry, it is not just a core skill — it is *the* skill, competence in which forms the basis of any claim to professional expertise. Our ability to be effective in promoting a good clinical outcome can be clearly linked to the competence of our communication skills. It goes without saying therefore that being 'nice' and 'well-intentioned' is not enough. Psychiatric interviewing is not social chit-chat but a *professional* interaction geared towards engaging the patient in a therapeutic relationship. As such, there are certain factors which the interviewer must be aware of from his or her own, as well as the interviewee's, point of view — factors in the way the interaction is conducted, the circumstances in which it occurs, and external factors which act to promote or inhibit it.

Starting points: empathy and engagement

It has been shown that patients gauge a 'good' doctor on a simple measure: 'Is this someone I can trust?' Obtaining that trust is the doctor's most important goal, and while no-one will be able to achieve this with every patient, one will end up severely diminished therapeutically if one cannot go some way to achieving it with most.

The key to developing trust is the demonstration of *empathy*. Although this word has entered the vernacular, the concept itself is frequently misunderstood. Empathy refers to the ability to place oneself in the emotional perspective of another — *while maintaining one's own emotional perspective*. This latter point is crucial. Feeling your way into the patient's emotional environment — full stop — is *identification*, which, with all its biases and blinkered emotions, is the last thing a distressed patient requires of the doctor!

Recently, empathy has come to be seen not so much as a single process, but as a *cycle* of interaction between doctor and patient — one in which the doctor, via phrase, gesture, action, etc. plays the key initiating role. To maintain the cycle, the patient requires to register this initiating element for what it is and respond accordingly. This in turn must be picked up and responded to appropriately by the doctor, and so on. Empathy is therefore an *active* process, which should be ongoing throughout any interview. Work in the time-restricted settings of primary care has shown that the empathic cycle can be initiated simply — by expressions of personal concern or interest (e.g. about the patient's family), or raising matters of common interest other than those relating to the purpose of the visit (e.g. the weather!). Without an awareness of the central role and the dynamic of empathy, any interview may fail to start or is likely to derail or grind to a halt.

Empathy may be seen as one of the principal process mechanisms whereby one achieves *engagement* of the patient in the interview and its purposes, though it is not the only factor of relevance in this regard. Engagement is clearly helped by being 'engaging' — by projecting a warm, friendly and interested demeanour from the start — but there are risks in misjudging the means of doing this (see below). Some 'rules of engagement' are outlined in Box 13.1.

Barriers to engagement may emanate not only from the patient but also from factors inherent to the doctor or the circumstances of the interview. Some barriers are listed in Box 13.2. Those relating to the reasons why the consultation is taking place are obvious. However, other factors to do with the patient's personality, their lack of ease in a verbal medium, social or cultural alienation, past experiences of similar or other circumstances, or frank resentments at the whole exercise, are easily overlooked. Barriers presented by doctors may also relate to personality characteristics. Those in whom interest in the subject alone is the attraction to psychiatry are not immune from social awkwardness, lack of verbal fluency, aloofness or crass superficiality. Negative influences may also emerge from one's manner, be it disinterested, supercil-

---

Box 13.1 'Rules of engagment': some characteristics of a 'good' interviewer

- *Disposition* (encapsulated in the much-quoted words of Truax, as 'non-possessive warmth') — the natural qualities of character, or personality, one projects. There are two elements to this:
  - an open and friendly approach, which is not the same as trying to be seen as the patient's 'friend'. Friendship is a personal, intimate and possessive relationship, open to exploitation, and may represent an area of difficulty that brought the patient to psychiatric care in the first place.
  - respect for the patient as an individual, their beliefs and aspirations, often described under the general heading of 'autonomy'. This raises complex issues, especially when one's duty of care sets one against the patient's expressed wishes, but it is necessary for the effective psychiatrist to convey a respect for the patient as an individual and for the views they express, despite arriving at different perceptions.
- *Awareness* of the *process* elements of the interview. In busy clinical situations, it is easy to concentrate on the *content* of the interview — the factual material one is trying to acquire — to the exclusion of the methods one is employing. Psychiatric interviewing must always have a formality that separates it from social exchanges, and those who practice it must have a constant awareness of not just 'what' they are attempting, but 'how' they are attempting it. No question, comment or gesture should be without purpose and none should slip through unnoticed or without its place in the process clearly understood.
- A *demeanour* of confidence without dogmatism. Psychiatrists enjoy respect based on the understanding that they possess some particular expertise. Clinically it is helpful to project that expertise to patients — that one can be effective in addressing their concerns. However, expertise is as much about having the confidence to accept alternative opinion as it is about standing firm in splendid isolation. The 'good' psychiatrist will take on board not only alternative information, but alternative explanation, in constructing a picture that can be meaningfully viewed from many angles.
- A non-judgemental *attitude*. Many patients feel they have been judged and found wanting. This perception may extend beyond the obvious moral and ethical issues which may bring them into conflict with social norms. Those with psychotic symptomtatology may also feel that the validity of their experience is open to judgement and rejection. Maintaining a non-judgemental attitude is not the same as being complicit. Boundaries exist in all human relationships, and it is not helpful to create in the patient's mind the idea that this, for them, might not be so. It is, however, important that one is able to convey a sensitivity to their dilemma and to provide alternative models against which their situation may be appraised.
- A *sensitivity* to the subtleties of human interaction, both verbal and non-verbal. This is one aspect of psychiatric expertise that cannot be taught. You either have it or you have not! For those not gifted in this regard, the best that can be recommended is that they at least maintain awareness of their deficit — and that they read copiously from quality novels, for more will be found there about what they are missing than in the pages of any textbook.

Box 13.2 Some barriers to engagement

Patient	Doctor
• *Personality* insufficiently sophisticated, naturally diffident	• *Personality* aloof / socially awkward / diffident
• *Untrusting disposition* e.g. 'negative' past experience, rejection of authority	• *Disposition* condescending / paternalistic / patronising, 'rushed'
• *Insufficiently 'verbal' / articulate*, including first language not English	• *Verbal 'pitch'* too sophisticated / unsophisticated, says too much / too little, too much 'jargon'
• *Resentment*, e.g. 'negative' perceptions of psychiatry	• *Non-verbal communication* absent/inappropriate, open to misinterpretation
• *Circumstances*, e.g. 'forced' interview (e.g. prison)	• *Questions* — weak techniques (process/structure)
• *Mental state*, e.g. fear, perplexity, suspicion, preoccupation, retardation, cognitive impairment, intoxication	

---

ious, patronising or off-hand. One of the biggest problems for trainees in busy clinical contexts is to avoid the impression of being rushed — of seeing the patient as one more 'task' for the day. It can also be difficult for trainees to aim the 'pitch' of an exchange correctly, adopting a flexible presentational style appropriate to patients from 16 to 65 and all social and educational backgrounds. Undoubtedly the most important doctor-related barriers emerge from the style, structure and delivery of questions themselves.

Preliminaries

Before proceeding to aspects of questioning, it is worth raising some preliminary considerations.

The room

This is not something that doctors, especially trainees, may have a lot of say in, but arranging — or being seen to arrange — the most conducive environment can be taken as an empathic gesture, so a quick rearrangement of the seating as the patient enters, whether necessary or not, is to be commended. It is unhelpful to interview across a large and obstructing desk. In addition to creating a physical barrier, it creates a psychological one by reinforcing hierarchies. Seats should be high, comfortable and of comparable height for doctor and patient. The low, soft chairs so beloved of those who furnish outpatient departments should be avoided. They impose an uncomfortable posture and create a barrier to elegant exit for the elderly, the overweight and the even mildly parkinsonian. In arranging seating, it is best to avoid a direct face-to-face alignment, which can contribute to an inquisitorial atmosphere. Seating should be slightly off-centre, allowing the patient the opportunity to avoid the examiner, which may facilitate their comfort, without them having to turn away, which they might construe as rude. Seats should be sufficiently close to foster ease in the sharing of confidences, but not so close that legs and feet might touch.

Interview rooms should in general be spartan to avoid the temptation of transforming the attractive ornament into a missile. Telephone cables should be tightly fixed and as short as possible. Interviews should *never* be conducted with the patient seated between the doctor and the door. Alarms are a further necessity nowadays. Such simple safety points will seem trivial — until the day they are not!

While privacy is a basic expectation of anyone attending a psychiatric interview, psychiatrists must increasingly consider the value of a chaperone by appraising the risks of aggressive acts and the possibility of subsequent accusations of exploitation.

Introductions

First impressions count — especially to the anxious, the bewildered and those with negative preconceptions. Thus, it is essential that the 'obvious' — so easy to overlook — becomes an integral and formal part of every introduction.

The *attire* appropriate to a medical practitioner is a fraught topic and one on which, with increasing informality, there is unlikely to be a ready consensus. It furthermore may be one that is open to variability, depending on the doctor's 'target' population — those working with adolescents, for example, may find casual attire more conducive to engagement than a three-piece suit. Suffice to say that while 'casual' may have its place, untidy never does.

Informing the patient of *who* you are is common courtesy. No matter a doctor's eminence within his on her own institution or the wider profession, he or she is likely to be a stranger to the patient at first meeting. Furthermore, patients may have the notion that they are coming to see a specific individual, especially the consultant to whose clinic they have been referred. Sometimes patients may also have no awareness of *what* you are. It is not uncommon for patients to be referred by a colleague in another discipline who may, for whatever reason, have withheld the fact that you are a psychiatrist. The sudden realisation of your occupation may stimulate powerful emotions, including fear and anger, especially if you appear complicit in a deception. Secrets do not make for sound clinical relationships and, while there may be exceptions, it is generally better to be 'up front' and make it clear from the start in such situations not only who, but what, you are. One can, should there be concerns or objections, then work through them. Following on from that, it is also reasonable to inform the patient at the appropriate point what it is you are going to do, which might include an indication of the time the interview is likely to take.

A *hand-shake* is a widespread sign of introduction and welcome. However, there are limits to this. For example, a male doctor offering a hand to a traditional Muslim lady may create an uncomfortable dilemma for the patient. The same may pertain to patients who exude an obvious suspicion and anxiety. This raises the question of *touch*. A pat on the back, shoulder or forearm can be a potent and genuine signal of support or approbation, but because of its potency, touch can be all too easily misinterpreted as invasive or, worse, sexual in its connotations. In general, therefore, and especially with opposite-sex patients, it should be avoided.

When on 'your' territory — hospital or clinic — the patient occupies in effect the status of a guest. It should go without saying

therefore that, on entering the room, they should be *invited* to take a seat and not left to make awkward social assumptions. Some statement that they are *welcome* would also be appropriate, e.g.

> *'Good afternoon, Mrs X. My name is doctor Z. Do have a seat, and make yourself comfortable.'*

Mode of address is a further preliminary that is open to misinterpretation. We live in an increasingly informal society, in which the use of first names is taken as a sign of informality and friendliness, especially by the young. Equally, however, it may be seen as a reflection of superficiality and lack of respect. Doctors should make no presumptions in this regard and patients should always be addressed as 'Mr', 'Mrs' or 'Miss' until given leave by the patient to use a Christian name. It is usually best not to ask about use of first names immediately, but to wait until the formal exploratory part of the interview — i.e. after the 'presenting complaint' — before seeking leave. Even then, there is an argument that those considerably in advance of oneself in age deserve the respect of a formal mode of address throughout.

An additional common 'negative' on first contact is the impression of *lack of preparation*, which, in terms of the patient's expectations, is disrespectful and rude. It must be frustrating for a patient to have to sit in silence while an ill-prepared and discourteous doctor ignores him/her and instead reads a referral letter or familiarises himself/herself with past case note material. Any such preparation, no matter how brief, should be done in private and *before* first introductions.

To write or not to write

This is a question on which there can be little dogmatism. The rights and wrongs of taking a contemporaneous record will depend on the attributes of the interviewer (whether they can maintain engagement overall while intermittently disengaging to write), the interviewee (whether they feel diminished by, or suspicious of, slavish adherence to record keeping), and the nature of the interview (see below). There are, however, strong arguments that can be put forward to justify the recording of contemporaneous notes, especially of initial assessment/diagnostic interviews:

- First, no-one can remember *all* the information conveyed over a 45–50 minute exchange, not only factual material but, as importantly, how much structure had to be imposed, how much dissemblance was detectable, at what points particular emotions were shown, and so on.
- Second, there is no record so valuable as that liberally punctuated by verbatim quotations. This can be helpful in later consideration and evaluation of the issues; it can provide invaluable information for successors who may become involved in the case; and, crucially, it can provide unassailable evidence of what was actually said, should your opinions and recommendations come under subsequent challenge, be these legal or from patients who later deny their initial symptomatology.
- Third, it takes great skill to avoid an unbroken 50-minute interview from evolving into an interrogation or degenerating into chit-chat, and the breaks offered by a pause to write can provide useful oases of peace and reflection.

Engagement is facilitated by an initial period of overt attention to the patient's expressed concerns without the disengagement inherent to writing. Starting to write is something else best left till after one has clarified the 'presenting complaint'. A skilled interviewer will also cultivate the art of recording while maintaining the *flow* of the interview with simple social exchanges, facilitating comments (see below) or run-ins to the next question.

Types of interview

There are various ways of looking at psychiatric interviews, but two readily recognisable classifications relate to the *form* of the interview and its *purpose*. Three main *formal* types can be identified:

- *Structured interviews.* These have their origins in research and their form is determined by the requirements of the recording instrument, which may relate to just the areas that require to be covered or may in addition specify the precise questions. For example, the Present State Examination (Wing et al 1974), which comprises a mixed set of 140 symptom and behavioural items, bases its reliability largely on the fixed questioning presented in the manual and precise adherence to pre-defined anchor points. Such methods have not been widely applied in routine practice, but knowledge of them can provide a comprehensive mental state structure for routine use. They also provide a valuable insight into the levels of evidence necessary before the presence of psychopathology can be accepted with reliability.
- *Unstructured interviews.* These traditionally are associated with dynamically orientated practice, in which the way information emerges and its symbolic significance (i.e. the narrative) is considered as important as the factual information itself. The prolonged or open-ended contracts that usually go with such styles of interviewing are incompatible with routine practice.
- *Semi-structured interviews.* This is the usual format in routine practice. Such a format need not imply adherence to any particular school or specified set of questions, but merely suggests that the interviewer accepts a proactive role in establishing a core body of factual information and the structure within which such information can be sensitively acquired and evaluated.

Psychiatric interviews can also be considered in terms of the *purposes* they serve. *Initial interviews* are usually *diagnostic* assessments. They are likely to be the most structured, demanding as they do, the acquisition of a basic level of information. Diagnostic interviews are conventionally recommended as being 45–50 minutes in duration. This is not just tradition but reflects the difficulty that anyone — doctor or patient — has in maintaining active attention for longer.

Initial assessments however are not just about diagnosis. At a clinical level, diagnosis is the key to treatment planning and prognostication. In psychiatry, an initial interview may not provide sufficient information to formulate a diagnosis with the necessary probability of accuracy. Thus, in practice, diagnostic assessments are geared to provide a differential set of *possibilities*, ranked on a hierarchy of *probability*. Unlike in general medicine, psychiatry should not as a rule distinguish between 'the' diagnosis at the top and the group of 'differentials' which follow on. For us, first assessments should provide only 'differentials', albeit ranked by probability.

A modification of this type of interview is the *problem-orientated* interview, most effective in emergency and risk assessment situations, in which the evaluation of a specific presenting problem (usually a behaviour or set of behaviours) is of greater importance than a particular diagnosis.

Follow-up interviews are geared to *monitoring* the physical component of the treatment plan, which includes not only symptom remission and quality of life/psychosocial functioning, but issues relating to the treatment plan, including patient satisfaction. In addition, these interviews should incorporate a conscious element of *psychological* intervention, whether formal or informal, covering supportive issues, practical problem solving, adherence and so on. In general adult practice, such interviews are often conducted without structure in an *ad hoc* way, and can readily develop into chit-chat. It is important to keep in mind the *purpose* of the interview and to have at one's disposal a *structure* within which to address the key issues.

It is not uncommon, especially in specialist practice, that interviews must be geared towards a specific purpose which meets the needs of a third party, the most frequent examples of which are *legal reports*. In this situation, diagnostic issues may be of less import, having already been established, and interviewing may have to be modified to address the specific questions raised by those requesting the report.

Conduct of the interview

This is the most important component of professional interviewing and concerns the verbal and non-verbal interactions of both the interviewer and the interviewee. The 'patient' part will be the focus of the subsequent section on mental-state examination. Here, we will concentrate on the interviewer's contribution.

Open vs closed questions. Formal questions come in two main varieties. *Open* questions require some opinion or judgement from the respondent and allow for answers which are variable, open to debate or external response and interaction, e.g.

'How have you been sleeping recently?'
'How have you been feeling in your spirits recently?'

Both these would leave it open to the patient to provide a *qualitative* account of the area with which the question deals, and lend themselves to further probing with minimal intervention. *Closed* questions, on the other hand, are usually geared towards some factual response about which there is little room for debate, e.g.

'Have you been sleeping poorly recently?' — *'Yes'/'No'*
'Have you been feeling depressed recently?' — *'Yes'/'No'*

In general, 'open' questions open up an interview and allow a freer exchange of information, while 'closed' questions trim things down to basic, largely factual, exchanges. Over-reliance on either can result in major control problems: under-control in the former case, because of lack of constraint and inadequate direction; over-control in the latter from a failure to facilitate free expression. All interviews should start with an open question, e.g.

'What have been the difficulties that have brought you to see me?'

Thereafter, they should comprise a fluid mix of 'open' and 'closed' formats, with the balance *deliberately* chosen to facilitate the often competing requirements of (1) acquiring sufficient information, and (2) allowing the patient free expression of concerns. As a rule, 'open' questions will predominate in the earlier part of the interview, with 'closed' questions coming in later to fill in factual blanks. The important point is that, whereas in social contexts the interaction itself usually determines the balance, in formal settings the interviewer must *organise* the balance in order to maintain a reign on the interview. Thus, an interviewer must always be aware of where the interview is 'at', what type of question is being utilised and whether the best way to take it forward involves 'open' or 'closed' formats.

Brevity. Questions should be kept *short*. Verbose language has an enervating impact on the listener and lengthy questions bewilder. If possible, questions should be delivered in a single sentence. The only alternative is a succinct introductory (or 'lead') statement to preface a question that requires to be placed in some context, e.g.

'Depression is a word with many meanings. What does it mean to you?'

Simplicity. Questions should be *simple* (as opposed to 'compound') — that is, the interviewer should only be expecting the patient to address a single point with each answer, and that point should be clear. With compound questions it is not possible to be certain which part of the question the answer refers to, leaving it open for the interviewer to jump to false conclusions. Compound questions can come in remarkably straightforward guises, e.g.

'Do you feel sad and hopeless about the future?'

While depressed people often feel hopeless, hopelessness can have associations other than depression. A compound question can often be identified by the presence of a conjunction, though this is not always the case — an ill-chosen verb can produce a similar effect, e.g.

'Are you troubled by voices?'

The patient may indeed have voices but not be in the least 'troubled' by them — or may feel troubled in themselves without hallucinations as a feature of their mental state.

Leading questions. Avoid leading questions. This is perhaps the commonest mistake trainees make, particularly when they are losing control of an interview or, more commonly, are simply getting stuck. At best, leading questions place interviewees in a corner out of which they may not feel able to manoeuvre tactfully. At worst, they present the patient with a challenge to disagree, an offer most will feel unable to take up. Thus, they encourage the responses the patient thinks the doctor wants to hear. Leading questions come in two forms, positive and negative, of which the latter are the more powerful, e.g.

'You were depressed at that time (?)'
'You were not happy at that time (?)'

Trickiest of all, is to compound the error of a leading question by finishing it off with 'were you?', e.g.

'You were depressed at that time, were you?'

Leading questions are frequently prefaced by that sinister little word, 'So', e.g.

'So, you were depressed at that time, were you?'

This is a classic way of presenting the patient with a 'challenge'. Merely raising one's tone at the end of such sentences in an attempt to transform statements of opinion into 'questions' does not instil them with merit.

While as a general style, leading questions remain examples of unsophisticated interviewing, they can have a place in the psychiatric interview as part of a process of clarification where clarity remains elusive (see below).

Recapitulation and summarising. Utilise *recapitulation* and *summarising statements*. Direct statements used for recapitulation and summarising are an important part of the structure of psychiatric interviews. They allow for clarification while providing a natural break for 'air'. They also allow the examiner to facilitate the interview by offering approbation for the efforts so far (see below). And, they can very effectively begin with 'So'! — for example:

'So, am I correct in concluding . . .'
'So, is it the case that . . .'

Pitch Be aware of 'pitch'. This refers to the intellectual level at which you approach the patient (not one's voice register!). Even with intelligent individuals, vocabulary should be kept simple and devoid of technical jargon. This can be difficult in a specialty such as psychiatry, which shares an extensive technical language with lay usage.

Direct questions. Avoid asking direct questions, which are the key to interrogation. It is easy when conducting an interview to latch onto a particular piece of information that strikes one as important and, at the first opportunity, dive in with a frontal assault. One can still come across trainees enquiring along the lines of: 'Do you ever feel like killing yourself?'. Direct questioning should be resisted, largely because it will be interpreted as traumatising or quite simply, rude. Sensitive areas may indeed have to be explored, but ideally with a run in, in which the approach to sensitive issues can be 'softened', e.g.

'May I ask you, ...'

Even the addition of a couple of words that generalise a potentially embarrassing topic can improve its acceptability, e.g.

'Have you noticed any change in your interest in matters *of sex?'*

The imperative. Be prudent in the use of the imperative. The imperative is the case of command, something that is hard to avoid even with the most empathic delivery. For most, the distinction between 'Tell me what happened?' and 'Tell me what happened!' is easily blurred. One should similarly be wary of the word '*why*', which in splendid isolation, at best infers non-understanding, at worst censure or disapproval, e.g.

'Why did you do that?'

Both these styles suggest justification or accountability, neither of which should be expected of those participating in a psychiatric interview. A more empathic approach is to seek leave to explore the relevant issue, e.g.

'Would you tell me what happened?'
'Can you tell me why you did that?'

'Just'. Ban the word 'just' — as in, 'I would *just* like to ask you . . .'. It often seems that doctors are trained to view this word as a technical medical term, as it crops up so often: 'If I could *just* have a listen to your heart?'; or '*Just* a little prick in the skin'; and so on, ad infinitum. No doubt, those who come to rely on it do so in the belief that it is a 'softening' word, a way of making a request less like a command, or making something which is inherently unpleasant or embarrassing, less so. However, its effect on

the receiver is invariably negative, conveying hesitancy, uncertainty, or a general interpersonal awkwardness — or worst of all, an impression that the context in which it is used is actually not that important. In fact for most doctors it becomes a 'comfort' word, whose function is less to do with the patient than it is to relieve their own anxiety about communicating effectively.

Prompts and facilitators. Use prompts and facilitators judiciously. These are techniques, frequent in social interactions, which make it easier, by providing encouragement or approval, for the patient to continue. *Prompts* are usually pre-verbal — *Mmmm?*'s or *Uh-huh*'s — delivered with an empathic non-verbal gesture or expression, such as a raising of the eyebrows or a tilt or nod of the head. They convey curiosity, interest and understanding and act as a lubricant to promote the patient's participation. *Facilitators* are words, or more usually short phrases or sentences, which make it easier for the patient to respond, by conveying involvement or providing reinforcement of their efforts so far. They are demonstrations of concern and appreciation and are a key part of the examiner's 'returns' in maintaining the empathic cycle, e.g.

> *'I am sorry to hear that.'*
> *'You're doing very well.'*
> *'That must have been very difficult for you.'*

One eminent neurologist, after exploring the mysteries of the bizarre symptomatology that was his field, would conclude each section authoritatively with: 'Thank you, Mr X. That's clear to me' — whether it was or not!

It should also be remembered that statements of professional opinion can act as powerful facilitators. The classic way of putting this is: 'It seems to me . . .'. Although superficially presented as a statement of opinion — 'It seems to me you are very angry about this' — such comments can be similar in their effects to open questions, urging a reaction or opinion, and can act as powerful facilitators.

Intonation Remember the power of intonation. The natural rhythm, variability and inflection of the human voice is one of the most important elements in our communications, the subtleties of which can be powerful tools in the psychiatric interview. The 'way' a sentence is delivered can be as important as the words that are used. Written text can give little instruction on the 'goods' and 'bads' in this regard, and all that can be offered is further general encouragement to give as much attention to the 'how' of verbal exchange as to the 'what'.

Flow Be sensitive to the 'flow'. Human communication has a natural tempo, periods of intense exchange giving way to less emotive interactions when the 'static' is notably less evident; periods when interaction flows readily interspersed with spells when communication is less spontaneous. This natural 'ebb and flow' is to be encouraged, but always within a framework of control. Trainees often have difficulty with this aspect of the interview, reflecting their own insecurities in their professional role and lack of confidence in their process skills. As a result they can end up being either overwhelmed by a verbal deluge or excluded by a barrier of silence. In fostering the 'flow', it is important to be ready to intervene in the face of verbal onslaught, to recognise and respect natural pauses, and to provide lubrication to the points when the process seizes up.

Rambling verbosity is often a consequence of a timid, unconfident interviewer, unable to take hold of natural breaks (however short) to intervene effectively, and/or an interviewee who has little understanding of what is expected. Such interviews are best rescued by resolve — clear interventions on the part of the examiner, clear statements of the purpose of the questioning, and short, simple closed questions. Interviews which fail to get off the launch pad are usually influenced by barriers to engagement on the part of the patient, as noted above. Those which start, however tenuously, but come to an immovable halt, are usually inhibited by barriers from the interviewer. This can be evident in 'freezing' (silence from an interviewer unable to find a way forward) which especially arises during periods where the interviewer is emotionally overwhelmed or embarrassed, usually with overt or powerful displays of emotion, or when the interview takes on an unexpectedly disinhibited or inappropriately direct or aggressive quality.

A 'freeze' is different from a planned pause, which eases interpersonal tension and reinforces engagement. There are few more awkward atmospheres than those created by the psychiatrist who 'freezes' in mid-interview. 'Freezing' is the ultimate demonstration of loss of control and can readily turn one's best efforts at a therapeutic relationship into something distinctly counter-therapeutic. Such situations require a liberal use of empathic statements and gestures, carefully planted prompts and facilitators and an open questioning style.

Sometimes, 'freezes' can be helped by providing the patient with a statement to which they can respond that is 'one degree' removed from the painful emotional areas that may be silencing them. For example, rather than asking directly about fearfulness or anxiety per se, one might comment on their observed behaviour, e.g.

> *'You seem somewhat anxious at the moment.'*

Agreement on the presence of psychopathology may provide the necessary bridge to allow its further exploration.

Listening. Listen to what the patient says. How obvious this may seem, but the ability to convey a listening attitude is one of the most empathic, and engaging, of gestures. In the anxiety of trying to do everything else, however, it is not uncommon to find trainees paying greater attention to what the next question is going to be than to the answer they are getting to the one they have just asked. Most damaging of all is repeating a question already asked.

Non-verbal signals. While focusing on the verbal, do not ignore the non-verbal. Ethologists have suggested that non-verbal, behavioural elements constitute the major contribution to human communication. Be this as it may, evaluation of this will comprise an important part of your assessment of the patient — and a sizable component of their assessment of you! This element is crucial in setting the tone within which formal verbal elements are evaluated and is key in initiating and maintaining the empathic cycle that is such an important part of the 'work' of a psychiatric interview. It is a vast area whose insights and hypotheses are too numerous to be presented here. However, be wary of:

- *Facial expressions.* These can betray disinterest, disengagement, amusement, bewilderment, scepticism, and frank incredulity even in the presence of soothing and contrary words. While a controlled smile, judiciously used, can be a powerful signal of warmth, laughter — one of the most potent behaviours we share in social bonding — is as a rule too potent for the psychiatric interview, and hence too open to misinterpretation.

- *Interactive posture and gesture.* Engaging communication is fertilised by a general body posture that is open and gesture that is inviting. To lean slightly towards a speaker suggests confidentiality and interest; to slouch in one's chair, the opposite. For speakers, continuous direct eye contact is not essential — for listeners, it is (except when writing). Controlled use of hand movements can be a powerful sign of emphasis or encouragement; uncontrolled, they can be comedic, while 'professional bradykinesia' conveys a flatness interpretable as indifference.
- *Incidental, stereotyped movements.* To jiggle one's legs, or fiddle with pens etc. is to convey boredom, impatience or social anxiety. To sit with arms crossed over one's chest is to create barriers, while resting one's chin in a heavy hand wreaks of fatigue. 'Mirror' attitudes not infrequently develop in the course of therapeutic dyads, where patients come to adopt the postures, and possibly even the gestures, of their examiner. However, when it is the doctor who subconsciously comes to 'mirror' the patient, a serious control problem is evident!

STRUCTURE

Any separation of the process and structural elements of the psychiatric interview is somewhat artificial. However, in this section we shall refer briefly to the conventional way in which the material from a psychiatric interview is organised for presentational purposes (predominantly emphasising initial interviews). Psychiatric history taking is a complicated and extensive process, partly due to the need to obtain a considerable amount of information in order to place the patient's symptomatic material in its personal and social (including, on occasion, its hereditary) context. This makes for schemes with many headings and subheadings. A number of presentational schemes are in existence, and while the one illustrated here (and summarised in Box 13.3) is one of many, it contains the conventional core elements. Traditionally, the material comprising the patient's record has been referred to as the 'Case Notes' — which means it does not have to be written in perfect English. It is far more important that all relevant information is included than that the prose is perfect.

Preliminary and identifying statement

In writing up a case, and in presenting for examination purposes, it is useful to begin with a general introductory statement which 'sets the scene', e.g.

> Preliminary and identifying statement
> Mrs Margaret Smith, 51 years of age.
> Routine referral by General Practitioner (see letter).
> Interviewed in outpatient department.

Presenting complaint

This should be the starting point for every psychiatric interview and most commonly is taken from the patient's own words in response to a general enquiry. This should, where possible, be an 'open' question which is neither too pointed — 'Why are you here?' — nor too vague, allowing the patient to free associate. Examples might be:

> *'What have been the difficulties you've been experiencing recently?'*
> *'What are the major problems that have been troubling you recently?'*

A common introductory question — 'What brought you here today?' — should be avoided, in view of the common answer — 'An ambulance.'!

Standardised psychiatric assessments have different criteria for 'recently' (i.e. what 'present' means in relation to the *present* mental state). However, none restricts this to 'today', and in line with the Present State Examination (see below), we would recommend the previous 4 weeks to be a reasonable period for consideration.

Box 13.3 Summary of psychiatric assessment — history and mental-state examination

1. Reason for referral/contact
Presenting complaint
Patient and/or third-party sources
2. Symptomatic context
History of present episode/illness
Establishing boundaries — normal – syndromal
3. Social context
Family and personal
Family • Parents: — *alive*
  - ages/occupations
  - physical health
— *dead*
  - age at death
  - cause of death
  - occupation(s)
— *separated/divorced*
• Siblings: — number (incl patient's place)
  - alive/dead
  - ages
  - marital status
  - occupation(s)

- Relationships: past/present
- Medical histories
- psychiatric history — extended family (incl suicide/alcohol)
Personal • Date/place of birth
- Known obstetric problems
- Developmental milestones (if known)
- Early behavioural problems
- Schooling: elementary
  - special educational input
  - friendships
— secondary
  - special educational input
  - friendships
  - age of leaving
  - academic attainment
— higher (if relevant)
  - institution/course
  - attainments
- Employment record
  - attainments/failures

Continued

Box 13.3—Continued

— (e.g. promotion/
— demotion/dismissals)
- Psychosexual development
  — puberty
  — sexual orientation
  — relationships
    – cohabitation
    – marriage
    – separation/divorce
  — quality of adult relations
  — children
    – age(s)
    – difficulties
    – relationship
- Interests/hobbies/recreations
- Past psychiatric history*[†] (including treatments: satisfaction/dissatisfaction)
- Medical history*[†] (including known allergies)
- Substance use*
- Forensic history*
- Subjective appraisal of personality

4. Formal examination
   (a) *Mental state*
Appearance
Behaviour(/manner)
Speech
Thought: • Form
            • Content (including 'possession' – e.g. ruminations)
Perception: • Distortions
             • Deceptions
(Other abnormal mental contents)
Affect/mood**: • Subjective
                • Objective
Risk, e.g. suicide
Cognition: • Orientation
             • Concentration/attention
             • Memory: — short-term
                       — long-term (antero/retrograde)

- Executive function
- (Abstract thinking)
(Insight)
   (b) *Neurological assessment*
Observation — at rest: sitting/lying
- Abnormal postures: e.g. dystonia
- Restlessness: e.g. akathisia
- Additional movements: — Tremors
                        — Dyskinesias — choreoathetoid (sometimes mistaken for fidgetiness)
                        — tics
                        — jerks
- Lack (poverty) of movement: e.g. immobile facies/reduced blink rate
Examination: gross cognitive assessment (see above)
Observation
- Walking: *walk the patient 10 metres along a corridor, watch them turn and return*
- Gait: e.g. – 'waddling' in proximal muscle weakness
  — 'Marche à petit pas' (reduced length/height of step) in parkinsonism
  — Ataxia (broad-based, unsteady): e.g. cerebellar/ Huntington's
  — Stiff legged 'scissors' gait (spastic paraparesis)
  — 'Functional' gait disorder: e.g. dragging apparently useless limb behind one / exaggerated reliance on people or objects for support
  — Stooped posture, e.g. parkinsonism
  — Reduced/absent arm swing, e.g. parkinsonism
  — Instability on turning
Examination: *sit patient on edge of couch*
- Eye movements
- Arms above head
- Arms outstretched with eyes open and closed
- 'Piano-playing' / other fine repetitive movements with hands
Examination: *lie patient semi-recumbent*
- Tendon reflexes (brisk or normal)
- Plantar responses

*May be presented as separate headings.
[†]Often presented immediately after 2, 'History of presenting illness'.
** Often placed after 'Speech'.
( ) Optional.

Acutely disturbed patients may fail to acknowledge such enquiries with a simple statement — or any problem statement — so the 'presenting complaint' can be taken from third-party sources and can thus comprise either *subjective* or *objective* information.

In routine secondary-referral settings one will usually have a GP's letter, or some other referral information, and this can provide a smooth introduction, e.g.

'Your GP has given me an outline of your difficulties, but it would be helpful to me if you could summarise these in your own words.'

The 'presenting complaint' should be brief — it can literally be a single word, or short phrase. Only in exceptional circumstances, which usually relate to disturbed patients brought to medical attention by others, should it extend to more than a sentence. It can, where possible, be helpful to spend a few moments longer in introductory remarks, by explaining to the patient that to start with you would like to hear how he/she would summarise his/her difficulties — 'and by that I mean your main *symptoms*', — then explaining that you will go over the context in which these have developed subsequently.

Most of the rest of the interview is about placing the symptoms of the 'presenting complaint' in various contexts. In the example we develop, the 'presenting complaint' is as follows:

Presenting complaint
'I feel so miserable all the time.'

History of present illness

This covers, first, the *symptomatic* context (the way in which the lead symptomatology identified in the 'presenting complaint' blends with normality at one end and with the range of possible additional phenomena to form an identifiable syndrome at the other) and, second, the *temporal* context. For example, a patient complaining of anxiety would be asked about the nature of the symptomatology, whether it is associated with panic attacks, autonomic and other concomitant symptoms, whether it is free-floating or is confined to specific situations, the extent of any fluctuations, and how severe it gets, whether they have always been an anxious person, and how long the features they complain of have been present.

It is in establishing the symptomatic context that all those process elements noted above come into play — plus one not mentioned: curiosity. Curiosity is perhaps one of the surest qualities to guide a comprehensive psychiatric assessment — curiosity not only about the presence of mental state disorder, but about its unique and intricate detail, its boundaries and its impact. Demonstration of curiosity about the patient's experiences usually provides an invaluable fillip to the empathic cycle.

One of the most valuable pieces of information in mental state assessment is a history of *change* — to what extent does the patient's symptomatology represent a change from the norms, and in what way has it *evolved* over time? While many patients may chart their path to psychiatric care over many years, it is the identification of change in some aspect of mental state and/or psychosocial functioning, without spontaneous resolution, that is the strongest pointer to a diagnostic categorisation.

Whatever the initial complaint, it is always important to specifically explore *mood*. This is, first, because of the prevalence of disturbance in this area and its significance in differential diagnosis (major depression features as a possible primary diagnosis in patients presenting with everything from anxiety symptoms to psychosis) and, second, because of the key role it plays in risk assessment. It is also a useful domain to resort to at times when interviews are closing down or becoming difficult, as few people have reservations about discussing how they 'feel'.

While some presentational systems recommend that the so-called 'biological' or 'vegetative' features of affective disorders — affects on sleep, appetite, weight, etc. — should be presented in the mental-state examination, we would recommend that they are considered in this section, primarily because they are subjective phenomena, appropriately considered with other subjective symptomatologies. The wide range of other accessory depressive symptoms, such as anergia, poor concentration and memory, irritability, lack of interest, anhedonia and ideas of hopelessness, self-depreciation and self-blame should also be routinely explored and noted. By contrast, while questions about psychotic phenomena often come up in the course of history taking and are naturally explored here, such phenomena should be specifically commented on under the mental state.

Risk assessment is a further area that should be specifically addressed in this section, and is now of such potential importance as to justify a separate heading. This includes not only an assessment of suicide risk, but also of the possibility of harm to others. Planned, as opposed to impulsive, acts of self-harm tend to progress in significance along a continuum, and while establishing any patient's 'place' on the cascade does not allow for complacency, it does provide a measure of reassurance, or alarm, as the case may be. This 'pathway to suicide' is illustrated in Figure 13.1.

Diagnostic inferences. In forming diagnostic inferences, psychiatrists tend to operate somewhat differently from physicians. For the latter, presenting symptomatology tends to *open up* a range of possibilities, which are then explored by further questioning, examination, special investigations etc. In this process, *refutation* is as important as *confirmation* and the solution (i.e. the diagnosis) arises later. Psychiatrists on the other hand, have a tendency to take the presenting complaint as a pointer to *the* diagnosis, with subsequent questioning *closing down* the options to confirm an initial impression. Thus, diagnosis becomes largely a process of *construction*, in which refutation plays little part. Clearly, medicine in general tends to have wider diagnostic horizons to consider than psychiatry, but the danger of not 'testing' one's assumptions as the examination proceeds is that one merely ends up fulfilling one's own prophesy — which requires no expertise whatsoever!

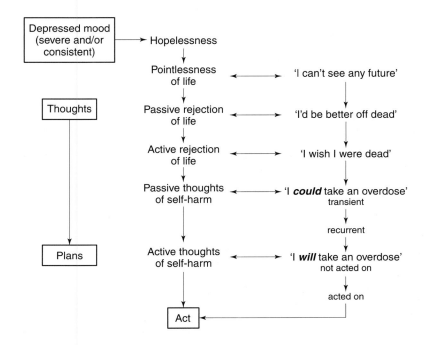

Fig. 13.1
Pathway to suicide

In assimilating the patient's history, it is important that neither deficient process elements in the interview nor initial bias limit a full and objective exploration of *all* potential symptomatology.

History of presenting illness

Lead symptom(s)
Feeling 'miserable' = 'depressed', 'sad all the time', 'awful'.

Elucidation of lead symptom(s)
Never felt like this before — 'I've had my moments, but this is different' — 'can't seem to shake myself out of it'. Feels depressed all the time — 'every day the same' — but worse in the mornings — 'that terrible feeing of dread' on waking. Eases as the day goes on but never feels her old self. No matter how much better she becomes in the evening, 'I can never carry that over to the next day'. Nothing can buck her up — 'I just can't see the joy in anything'. Doesn't know when she last enjoyed herself — 'last summer, probably' (i.e. 1 year ago).

Associated symptoms
Gets no pleasure from anything, even her grandson: 'He's become such a burden — that's terrible, isn't it'. Feels tearful sometimes but 'I can't cry' — 'Maybe I'd feel better if I did'. Feels guilty that she's letting everyone down — 'They all try so hard — but it's me'. Feels she's 'no good to anyone' — 'they (the family) would be better off without me'. Wonders if this is all a punishment for taking on too much — 'I tried to be superwoman — but I'm not'.
Has no energy — everything's 'an effort'. Even getting dressed some days is 'an uphill struggle'. Hasn't been out the house in some weeks — 'I get so anxious — it's ridiculous'. No appetite — 'The sight of food makes me feel sick'. Has lost about a stone or more in weight in the past couple of months. Sleep 'dreadful' — feels 'exhausted' in the evening and gets off to sleep without difficulty. Wakens at 4.00 a.m. — 'I could set my alarm by it'. Can't get over again. 'That's the worst time — that terrible churning in my stomach'. Getting about 5 hours sleep per night. Feels tired in the day but can't cat-nap. Concentration poor — 'I look at the television — but it goes right over my head'. Used to be an avid reader, but now 'can't be bothered'. Forgetful of everyday things, which she finds embarrassing.

Risk assessment (suicide/homicide)
Feels hopeless about the future — 'I can't see anything to look forward to — just more of the same'. Frequently wishes she was 'out of it'. Has thought of ending her life — 'It would be a release for everyone' — e.g. by taking an overdose or drowning herself, but says she would not do it — 'I'm too big a coward'. 'If only I could go to sleep and never wake up — I long for that'.

Evolution/associated factors
She relates the onset of her difficulties to being made redundant from her job 6 months ago. This was unexpected and came as 'a terrible blow'. 'I was told I wasn't up to it'. Admits that there had been 'problems' latterly in her job, but was 'shocked' when she was, as she sees it, 'fired'. Since then has brooded a lot on this and feels she was ill done by. Her problems have progressively worsened since then.

Personal and social history

Although the 'History' conventionally comprises a series of further headings, additional information is essentially about placing the symptomatic material in a *social* context. The order of presentation is not fixed. For example, some may see it as more logical to progress from details about the present episode to enquiry about the 'past psychiatric history', while for others this is part of the patient's wider personal life and would be more logically placed with 'personal history'.

Family history

After obtaining the symptomatic information, it is reasonable to explore the family relationships from which the patient has emerged and to which they may still belong.

It is traditional to begin with factual information: whether parents are alive and if so their ages and occupations, and whether they suffer from any physical illness; if they are deceased, their age at death and the cause. This is repeated for siblings. This is followed by enquiry about psychiatric disorder in all blood relatives, not just immediate family. If any positive responses are elicited, it is useful to supplement the enquiry with pointers to a likely diagnosis, if this is not known — e.g. 'he gets an injection every month' or 'she saw a counsellor for depression'. Frequently forgotten is the importance of enquiring about suicide within the extended family, and also alcoholism.

Having established a factual base, one may then explore *superficially* the patient's perception of the family's dynamics. In the 1960s and 1970s, social theory and family dynamics assumed a major role in paradigms of psychiatric disorder, for the most part in a far from positive way. Furthermore, in recent years the issue of childhood abuse has become prominent, as much with the lay public as professionals. Such areas, so dependent on inference and recollection in situations of charged emotions, must be explored not only sensitively, but with sophisticated, non-directive and ultimately non-collusive interview techniques which may be beyond the average trainee. The routine outpatient clinic is not, as a rule, the place for in-depth exploration of statements about early abuse or about family dynamics that the patient recalls as distorted.

Personal history

This should comprise a chronological account of the patient's personal experience, starting with their date of birth and birth details, and covering early development, schooling, early relationships, academic achievements, occupational history, adult relationships (psychosexual history, partner(s), children), present social circumstances.

While separate headings are often given to 'past medical history', 'forensic history', 'substance use' and so on, these are really subheadings of 'personal history', and it is reasonable to exercise judgement about whether to record any pertinent information separately or as part of 'personal history'.

Past psychiatric history

There is merit in specifically presenting details of past psychiatric disorder, as this may have a major bearing on the current presentation and on treatment options. Previous periods of identifiable illness should be summarised, which will often consist of episodes of diagnosed and treated illness. However, it is important to include any episode that comes to light on questioning, even if it did not come to formal medical attention at the time. For example, if a patient complaining of depression in the setting of considerable life stress describes a previous similar but milder episode some years previously which occurred without obvious precipitant, or if they give an account of a circumscribed period of apparent mild hypomania, this will have implications for the diagnosis.

It is important to record the patient's past treatment histories, though this can be a surprisingly difficult area in which to gain accurate information. The importance of past drug history extends beyond the obvious — such as avoiding re-use of preparations to which the patient may have developed bad reactions/ allergies in the past, being aware of possible interactions, etc. The patient will have expectations of the consultation which are likely to extend beyond merely a re-prescription of a previously failed regimen. If there are reasons to recommend a compound tried before, it is important to be able to justify this clearly, as a positive decision — in terms, for example, of its previous use being inadequate. This is not a position that can be adopted if prior regimens have not been elucidated in detail.

Personal and social history

Family history
Father died 5 years ago, aged 81. Had Alzheimer's disease. Retired engineer. Mother alive and well aged 78. Housewife. Lives independently. She sees her regularly.
Eldest of three siblings — Sister aged 49, married with three children. Housewife
Brother aged 44, married, one son. Lives in US. Advertising executive.
Describes a happy family life — remains close to her family and keeps in touch regularly.

Maternal uncle committed suicide in early adult life — 'alcohol problems, I think'. One cousin on mother's side treated for depression in the past — thinks she is still on antidepressants. No medical history of note in family.

Personal history
Born 14/10/53, Northern General Hospital. Normal full-term delivery. No early developmental or behavioural problems. Started school at 5 years old — enjoyed school and had many friends. High school from 12 — was popular and made friends easily. Academically successful. Left at 18 with 5 'Higher' grades (*2 'A's'/3 'B's*).

Went to Edinburgh University — honours course (MA) in politics/economics. Graduated 22 years. Joined Bank: 'fast-track' management programme. Achieved steady promotion until resignation with first pregnancy at 29. Worked from home as freelance financial advisor for 6 years before returning to work as financial analyst for an investment company. Promoted to team leader 4 years ago. Work 'stressful' but enjoyed and always felt capable. Achieved regular bonuses. Made redundant 6 months ago — was a reorganisation 18 months ago, though her role changed little. Told by senior colleague she was no longer able to do the job. Accepted a 'generous' settlement but felt 'devastated'.

Menarche aged 11 years. Regular periods. No problems. One steady boyfriend at school (not physical). Met husband at University. Lived together for 3 years before marriage.

Describes good relationship with husband, now partner in civil engineering firm. 'He's very understanding.' He travels extensively. She's always accepted this but recently 'I can't stand it when he's away'. Feels 'terrified' on her own, and stays with mother. Two children — son of 24 (married) works with airline, daughter of 19 (single), first year medical student in London. Children are 'wonderful'. One grandson (18 months old).

Owns own home. No money worries — 'life should be very comfortable'. Normally enjoys hill walking, country dancing and reading (lost interest in all in past few months).

Describes herself as diligent, 'slightly obsessive', gregarious. Has high expectations of others but feels she was 'a good manager' — was popular with staff.

Drinks moderately: 12–15 units per week. Mainly wine. Non-smoker. Denies illicit drug use.

No medical history of note.

Was on contraceptive pill for some years. Now takes HRT. Nil else.

No forensic history.

Sometimes, in patients with extensive histories and chronic symptomatology, separation of 'history of present illness' from 'past psychiatric history' can be difficult, and no hard and fast rules can be applied. On one occasion, where no clear breaks of well-being can be established, the best approach may be to chart the whole evolution of the patient's symptoms under 'History of present illness', even if this spans a number of years: on another, it may be sufficient merely to state that the patient has had 'N' previous admissions with similar symptomatology beginning at aged 'X', describing only those episodes which may not appear to fit the stereotype. For examination purposes, it is important to explain at the start of your presentation which approach you have opted for, and why.

Premorbid personality

Some schemes advocate specific assessment of 'Premorbid personality'. This is a complex area that requires expertise to make appraisals reliable, and the routine interview only allows for a 'stab' at this. One should begin with general enquiries, such as 'Would you say you were a shy person or an outgoing person?' and 'Is your mood generally stable?', though one must always remember to be diplomatic — no-one like to admit they have no friends, and it is better to approach this sort of area gently, e.g. 'Do you have lots of friends or just one or two close friends?'. One can then move on to more specific questions designed to elicit evidence of various different abnormal personality traits (Box 13.4). Questioning about premorbid personality provides little or no useful information about some personality traits, such as dissocial, histrionic or dependent.

MENTAL-STATE EXAMINATION

To some extent, examination of the mental state follows the conventions of general medicine, but with important differences. First, as Sims (1988) has pointed out, the distinction between symptoms (which the patient describes) and signs (the abnormalities the clinician elicits on examination) becomes blurred in psychiatry — many of the phenomena of interest to psychiatrists,

---

Box 13.4 Useful themes of enquiry for probing premorbid personality

Schizoid
- Does he* have solitary or eccentric hobbies?
- Does he have few friends?
- Is he shy?

Paranoid
- Has he ever had serious rows with people so that they have never spoken to him again.
- Has he ever taken anyone to court?
- Would other people regard him as a touchy person, i.e. quick to take offence
- Does he tend to take remarks the wrong way?
- Does he have any beliefs which he holds very strongly?

Anankastic (obsessional)
- Is he very tidy/fussy about the way things are arranged?
- Would other people regard her as being very houseproud?
- Is he the type of person who 'goes by the book' / believes in the motto 'a place for everything and everything in its place'?
- Does he find it difficult to make decisions about trivial things, such as what to wear, which restaurant to go to?
- Does he have to check things that he knows he has already done, such as doors being locked, appliances being switched off?

Hyperthymic
- Is he very extravert?
- Would people regard him as the life and soul of the party
- Does he need less sleep than most people.
- Does he suffer from brief spells of depression lasting a few days every so often?

Histrionic
- Is he the kind of person who likes to be the centre of attention at social gatherings?
- Can he be on top of the world one minute and then in the depths of despair the next?

Dissocial
- Does he lose his temper easily?

Dependent
- At what age did he leave home (for the first time)?

---

* Male personal pronouns are used to imply either male or female, unless a female form is more appropriate in the context.

---

in which some degree of cross-examination is inevitable. On the other hand, leading questions are often considered to be as inadmissible in the psychiatric interview as in the courtroom (see above). This issue has perhaps been best addressed in the preface to the Present State Examination (PSE), one of the most phenomenologically rigorous of the structured interview methods. Wing and colleagues note that 'some schools of psychiatric thought, particularly the psychoanalytic, regard diagnosis as a relatively unimportant part of their work and find cross-examination too "directive" a method of interviewing' but state their view that '. . . an interview designed to discover whether defined symptoms are present must be based to some extent upon the technique of "cross-examination". Patients find this completely acceptable and, to the extent that interviewer and patient are together successful in producing an exact description of the symptoms, it can be a rewarding and therapeutic experience in itself' (Wing et al 1974).

As with the history, categorising and recording the mental state has a fairly standard *structure*, covering the domains of appearance and behaviour, speech, mood and affect, thought content and perception, and concluding with cognition and insight. The exact ordering of the mental state examination is, however, determined largely by convention. While some will place 'mood/affect' immediately after the general descriptive components, others will consider it more logical to progress to 'thought' immediately after 'speech', as speech is the medium from which thought processes and contents are inferred.

Appearance

This initial category comprises a brief *descriptive* note of one's observations at first contact and through the interview. It refers not only to matters of dress and grooming, but would cover any physical characteristics worthy of note, such as posture, build, age-appropriateness of appearance, and so on. While facial expression is an evident part of one's 'appearance', this is best covered elsewhere.

Despite the wide range of dress currently acceptable in Western society, it is generally possible to judge, often 'at a glance', whether acceptable codes are being followed, and whether to an acceptable level. Thus a noteworthy comment may not only come from the 'codes' themselves but from whether they are presented tidily and neatly — i.e. whether the patient is *unkempt* or not. If a patient follows the fashion of some identifiable subculture — for example, new age travellers, punks, bikers, etc. — it is appropriate to record this, even although it is not in itself indicative of clinical abnormality.

Any degree of *self-neglect* may be seen in schizophrenia, and may be subtle or isolated — e.g. poor dental hygiene, odd socks, flies undone, etc. If a woman shows signs of letting her appearance go, as indicated by lack of make up or dishevelled hair, this can be a telling sign of depression. General decline in self-care may also be a marker of emerging dementia. While cognitive impairment may be evident in dress and grooming — e.g. buttons done up incorrectly — it is further worth remembering that some adverse treatment effects, especially parkinsonism, can impair dexterity, resulting in neglect which is more apparent than real.

Excessively *loud* (or, in females, *revealing*) clothes can be a sign of hypomania, as can garish or bizarre make-up, excessive jewellery, ornaments or inappropriate dress (e.g. evening clothes). Highly unfashionable and/or clashing garments may reflect long-standing schizoid personality traits or Asperger's syndrome, while an excessively neat appearance, sometimes disguised by a studied

whether described spontaneously or elicited by questioning, exist only as subjective descriptions of experience. Because of this, it is common practice to use the term 'symptom' to cover both types of phenomena. However, it is important for the clinician to keep an awareness of the distinction in mind.

Second, the identification and categorisation of mental symptoms depends on the discipline of *descriptive psychopathology*, or phenomenology. This attempts to recognise and categorise mental abnormalities *without embellishing them with explanation*, but at the same time trying to understand the nature of the experience as far as possible. This raises the question of the extent to which a patient should be pressed about his symptoms. On the one hand, diagnosis depends on determining whether a particular symptom is present, what its specific characteristics are, and how it can be differentiated from other similar symptoms, an exercise

casualness or even affectation, has been said to be a sign of obsessional personality (Enoch & Ball 2001). Judgement must however be exercised with such alleged 'signs'. The variation of those observed characteristics comprising 'appearance' in the normal population means they can never be strong indicators of disorder, far less of any specific disorder. While important to note, they can rarely provide more than adjunctive information.

Behaviour

Of necessity, the main focus of this part of the examination is on behaviour during the interview. However, it is perfectly acceptable to include accounts of noteworthy behaviour in prior contexts from reliable third-party sources (e.g. family, general practitioner, police, etc.).

Any *automatic* motor behaviours should be noted, such as restlessness, fidgetiness and nervousness, as well as *involuntary* movements such as orofacial dyskinesias. Any loss of expected motor activity in relation to, for example, facial expression, expressive posture and gesture, should also be noted. It is traditional to comment on the patient's eye contact when describing the mental state though, in fact, poor eye contact is of such low diagnostic significance as to be largely without value. It is more informative to note *gaze avoidance* if present, as this can be a sign of hostility.

The major abnormalities of movement and behaviour are those associated with schizophrenia and affective disorder. Acutely psychotic patients may act in response to delusions (searching for bombs in cupboards, etc.), or respond to abnormal perceptions ('behaving as if hallucinated'), or break social taboos without compunction (e.g. masturbate, make sexual advances or, in the tactful language of the PSE, 'pass loud flatus'!). They may be distractible by incidental noises, or so suspicious or bewildered as to be totally unforthcoming. *Catatonic* features are (or more properly, have become) uncommon in acute schizophrenic patients but remain surprisingly common in chronic patients (Rogers 1985, Lund et al 1991), and are also seen in both phases of affective psychosis, in learning disabilities, autism and some forms of organic brain disease (Rogers 1992, Wing & Shah 2000). Some of these wide-ranging phenomena are summarised in Box 13.5.

Lack of volition is one of the main negative features of schizophrenia (see below). As its name suggests, it refers to reduced motor behaviour which is based on a failure of motivation and interest. It is probably identical to, or at least shades into, *apathy*, although this term tends to be reserved for generally more severe states associated with marked emotional indifference seen in organic disorders, especially of the frontal lobe.

In affective disorders the main abnormalities are *retardation* and *agitation* in depression, plus a rather less well-defined set of inverse abnormalities (i.e. intuitively polar opposites) in mania. *Retardation* consists of delay in initiating and slowness in execution of motor acts, which sometimes gives the impression that the patient is attempting to overcome some inner inhibition. It may be subtle, where it is only noticeable as an *invariant facial expression* and *paucity of expressive gestures*, or more pronounced, manifesting itself in the classical bowed posture, slow hesitant actions and soft monotonous speech. The most extreme manifestation is *depressive stupor*, where the patient lies nearly motionless, struggles to whisper a few words and has, in the words of Kraepelin (1913a), a characteristic 'peculiar vacant, strained, disturbed, facial expression'.

Box 13.5   Catatonic symptoms

Disorders of movement
Stereotypies: purposeless motor acts which are carried out repetitively and with a high degree of uniformity, e.g. rocking, rubbing hands and tapping objects, more complicated, 'gymnastic' or 'contortionist' movements
Mannerisms: everyday goal-directed acts like washing, dressing and eating which are executed in idiosyncratic ways, e.g. keeping one arm tucked under armpit. (NB: In practice, it is difficult to separate stereotypies and mannerisms from one another; many patients show motor behaviour which is abnormal by virtue of varying degrees of repetitiveness, purposelessness, and stiltedness of execution.)
Manneristic gaits: e.g. over-precise or overelaborate, walking on the toes, with interpolated sidesteps and bowing
Posturing: hunched and constrained, hugging sides, sitting perched on edge of chair, adopting statuesque, 'pharaonic' poses (Sims 1988)
Other: grimacing, blocking/freezing, waxy flexibility (catalepsy), psychological pillow (where the patient lies with his head 2–3 inches off the bed)

Disorders of volition
Negativism: patients do the reverse of whatever is asked of them; e.g. hold their breath when asked to breathe deeply, resist attempts to get them to stand up, then refuse to lie down. Also gegenhalten (opposition): 'springy' resistance to passive movement which increases with the force exerted
Positivism (Lohr & Wisniewski 1987): includes echopraxia; mitgehen (passive movement overcomplied with, limbs elevate themselves at the slightest touch like an anglepoise lamp); and automatic obedience, where any suggestion (even one that is merely implied) is complied with in an exaggerated way
Other: ambitendence — the patient appears to simultaneously wish to and not wish to carry out some action, e.g. walking through a doorway

Disorders of behaviour
Catatonic stupor: the patient sits or lies motionless, mute, often in a contorted posture; waxy flexibility and gegenhalten may be evident. Although unresponsive, the patient is aware of his surroundings
Catatonic excitement: aimless overactivity, destructiveness and violence, often associatied with manneristic and stereotyped actions, e.g. moving around striking an endless series of quasi-symbolic poses
Catatonic impulsiveness: sudden, incomprehensible and often violent acts for which the patient is unable to give any more than a facile explanation. May interrupt stupor

Catatonic speech disorders
Aprosodic speech: speaks in monotone, peculiar scanning, automaton-like, telegrammatic sing-song, or affected intonations
Speech stereotypies and mannerisms: speaking in affected accents, adding -ism or -io to ever word
Other: mutism, echolalia and palilalia (repeating last word or last few words of a sentence over and over again)

From Lund et al (1991) and McKenna (1994).

Agitation is a much misused term which strictly describes patients who are in a state of severe motor unrest in the context of obvious distress. Agitated patients cannot remain seated, pace back and forth, wring their hands, pull their hair and clothes and make despairing gestures. Many psychiatrists also apply the term to lesser degrees of motor unrest accompanied by anxiety, but it should not be used merely to describe restlessness. Retardation and agitation can be present in the same patient.

Manic and hypomanic patients may appear infused with *energy*, drum their fingers impatiently, make emphatic and exaggerated gestures, smile broadly and display other emotions with animation. Restlessness, if present, usually reflects impatience and is without distress, and is indicated by fidgeting, walking around the room, leaving the room and coming back, etc. In more severe states patients may be continuously 'on the go', interfering and partaking in pointless acts which they are rapidly distracted from, sometimes referred to a *press of activity*.

A useful additional consideration at this point is the patient's *manner* towards you as the interviewer. What was their approach to you as an individual? Were they co-operative, forthcoming, engaged? Did they observe the social proprieties of politeness? — and so on.

Affect (mood)

The concepts of 'affect' and 'mood' are so confusing for psychiatry that a general consensus appears to have been reached that they should be considered to be interchangeable. This confusion was cemented with the designation of major *mood* disorders as 'affective disorders', attributed to Manfred Bleuler in the 1930s. In English-language psychiatry, many clinicians use the term 'affect' to refer to emotionality as judged objectively by the interviewer, and 'mood' to describe the patient's subjective account of their emotional state.

Strictly speaking, '*affect*' refers to that short-term component of emotionality which is responsive to circumstance and environment, and comprises a multitude of generally short-lasting feeling states, such as fear, anxiety, contentment, anger, jealousy, etc. (i.e. emotional 'waves'). '*Mood*', on the other hand, traditionally refers to one's longer-term emotional predisposition, as gauged along the dimension of elation–sadness (i.e. emotional 'currents'). While the theoretical niceties may indeed be of limited practical relevance (affective symptoms may be prominent elements of mood disorder, and happiness/despondency can be affects), an understanding of the distinction can nonetheless be helpful in interpreting complex emotional disorders.

Affective symptomatology, strictly defined, usually appears at different points in the presentation of mental-state material. Many affective features, for example, are best determined by questioning and hence will appear mainly in the 'history of the presenting complaint', while those which present overtly will usually be described under 'behaviour', as noted above. However, any affective symptomatology should be briefly brought together here — e.g. noting anxiety, anger, irritability, etc.

Subjective mood state should be explored and described in the history. However, it is important to bring together at this point in the MSE those elements of subjective mood previous elicited. This would include the patient's impression of severity and quality of mood change, the presence of *anhedonia* (inability to experience pleasure), and maintenance of *reactivity* (the patient can temporarily cheer up in the right circumstances).

The *objective* expression of mood should also be noted and can be considered along two axes — breadth and depth. Breadth refers to the variability of emotional display the patient is able to exhibit within the interview. Normal human interactions comprise a subtle array of changes in facial expression, interactive posture, gesture, intonation, flow of speech, etc., which vary in response to the emotional tone of the exchanges. Clinically significant depression usually imposes a limitation, or *restriction*, on the range of features appropriate to the interview. Such judgements are made on the basis of observation. Depth, on the other hand, is the one point in the MSE where empathy must be used to arrive at a judgement. This is gauged by the shear impact of the patient's presentation — their ability to convey a feeling state that is, literally, overpowering. In this regard, depressed patients often display a *heightened* depth of emotion, in which their presentation conveys to the examiner the full extent of their subjective distress.

It is clear that the above description might be seen to apply equally to *flattening of affect* associated with schizophrenia, but the two, which can be difficult to distinguish clinically, are not strictly the same. The latter is a limitation to the *display* of feeling states, in which not only the range is restricted, but so too is depth. However, an absence of emotional display does not allow the assumption that little subjective emotion is felt. Psychophysiological studies suggest that such individuals are often highly emotionally 'aroused'. It has been suggested that the key problem lies less with the absence of affect, than in its normal and fluid communication (Sims 1988), implicating a failure within the empathic cycle noted above.

Even experienced clinicians can disagree over the presence of milder degrees of affective flattening. Problems arise from the fact that there is wide variation in the display of emotion, both culturally and individually — some cultures value emotional reserve and some individuals always maintain an unemotive, 'dead-pan' demeanour. Many normal people will show (and feel) no grief when first bereaved and relatives of murder victims or other horrific crimes may show little emotion when the news is first broken to them. Some individuals with dissocial personality disorder react to appalling events with indifference (Hamilton 1984). Finally, the distinction between affective 'flattening' and drug-induced bradykinesia can be difficult, especially if no steps have been taken to examine for other parkinsonian features (Owens 1999).

Because of such variability and context, assessment of 'flattening' should never be a 'spot' diagnosis, and should come from observation of the *interaction* presented by an individual throughout the interview.

Blunting of affect is commonly used synonymously with affective 'flattening', but strictly speaking the two are separate phenomena. 'Blunting' refers to the coarsening of emotions and an insensitivity to social context — what Kraepelin referred to as a 'loss of the delicacy of emotion' (Kraepelin 1913b). For example, Sims (1988) described a schizophrenic woman who, with obvious relish for the sensational effect, took her visitors upstairs to view the corpse of her mother, deceased for 2 days.

Inappropriate or incongruous affect is the appearance of sudden emotional states which are out of keeping with events. In practice, this is invariably evidenced by patients laughing when describing distressing events. For example, when one patient was asked why there was a bandage on her wrist, she replied that she had been trying to kill herself that morning, and burst out laughing. It is important to remember, however, that inappropriate laughter may be a sign of social awkwardness or embarrassment, and assessment of affective incongruity should always be circumspect. Rightly or wrongly, sudden causeless laughter, essentially seen only in patients with severe, chronic schizophrenia, is considered by some to represent inappropriate affect, though clearly such an assumption must be based on the exclusion of private psychotic experience to which the response may be appropriate.

In mania, mood is most commonly one of *increased vitality*, gaiety and pleasure, with an infectious quality, rather than simple happiness, though *irritability* and adverse response to frustration may predominate. *Euphoria* — a heightened sense of happiness — may be seen, but is distinct from the typical mood change. Similarly, while in depression mood may be one of unexceptional sadness, patients not infrequently describe it as different from normal unhappiness, communicating a peculiarly painful quality.

Additional important affective abnormalities include *suspicion*, in which the palpebral fissures are narrowed, the mouth tightened and the eyes disproportionately alert and active in otherwise fixed facial contours; and *perplexity*, characterised by lowered brows, slowed gaze and partially open mouth. Perplexity is seen par excellence in puerperal psychosis, but can be present in any acute psychotic state, including organic ones. The so-called *omega sign*, in which the inner third of the eyebrows are depressed, the outer third elevated and vertical ridging is evident over the glabellar eminence, is said to be characteristic of major depression though is more likely to be a general expression of extreme worry. *Lability of mood*, where the emotional state shifts from cheerfulness to tears to irritability and back again over brief periods is common in mania, may be found in dementias or other organic states and is also a rare symptom of acute schizophrenia (Bleuler 1911). *Facile euphoria* is said to be characteristic of the frontal lobe syndrome and Korsakoff's syndrome. *Ecstasy* is a state of intense tranquil euphoria which usually has a religious colouring and often attracts descriptions like 'exalted' and 'transfigured' (Hamilton 1984, Sims 1988). Patients may become so absorbed in their inner state as to be unresponsive to the external world, and objectively appear to be in a state of so-called *euphoric stupor*. Other abnormalities said to be characteristic of particular disorders are the *catastrophic reaction* in early dementia, where a patient reacts excessively to realisation of failure on a cognitive task; the poor performance is abnormal but so is the response to it. So-called *obsessional affect*, described as 'warmth, with something held back', has been described as a feature of those with anankastic (obsessional) personality. *Histrionicity* is the exaggerated, melodramatic, but at the same time shallow, expression of emotions.

Speech and thought form

Strictly speaking, speech refers to the *motor component* of verbal expression — everything that happens from the central speech areas to the lips, and its abnormalities include dysarthria, dysphasias and disorders of articulation. However, there are other components to speech including pitch, power and intonation (or '*prosody*', the natural musicality of verbal expression), which are also the preserve of psychiatry, as are a number of so-called psychomotor qualities of speech, such as rate, quantity, flow and so on.

Many abnormalities of speech are fairly obvious counterparts of the disorders of behaviour described above, as applied to the particular motor act of speaking. Thus, speech may be soft, delayed and prone to tail off in depression and, conversely, may be loud and increased in quantity in mania. When speech is rapid and difficult to interrupt the term *pressure of speech* is applied. Although common in mania, 'pressured' speech can be a non-specific manifestation of social anxiety. Catatonia can also affect speech (see Box 13.5).

Speech latency refers to the time between a question being posed and an answer being given. Delays in providing response can be the result of an intense individual taking time to ensure the adequacy of his reply or can be found in the presence of anxiety intruding into the normal organisation of responses. Striking increases in speech latency are characteristic of profound depression but are also to be found in psychotically preoccupied patients. Strictly, this feature should be referred to as 'response latency', as it clearly reflects disorder of underlying thought rather than speech per se.

Poverty of speech is a characteristic negative symptom of schizophrenia, and can be regarded as the same disorder as lack of volition, affecting the domain of speech. Patients answer questions readily enough but use only the minimum necessary number of words. They do not elaborate on what they say, and make few spontaneous comments. Encouragement with open questions meets with little success. Despite its name, the presumption is that poverty of speech reflects a disorder of *thought*, specifically an inability to form and/or execute intentions to speak.

Speech is of course also the principal means by which we express thought. *Formal thought disorder* refers to abnormality in the coherence and logical structure of thought — the 'how' or 'mechanics' of thinking — which makes conversation difficult to follow or at times completely incomprehensible. Many different abnormalities have been proposed to account for the loss of coherence seen in schizophrenia, and in some cases the same phenomenon has acquired different terminologies — e.g. 'derailment' and 'knight's move thinking'. Current approaches, such as DSM-IV and structured interviews like the PSE, place emphasis on three or four types of disorder:

- *derailment* (loosening of associations, tangential thinking, 'knight's move' thinking): in which the 'train' of thought slips off the 'track'. Individual derailments may be slight, so the speaker only gradually, but progressively, digresses from the original point, though in some cases the links between ideas are clearly obscure and difficult to decipher.
- *incoherence* (word salad, schizophasia): where speech is completely incomprehensible. Typically, individual sentences themselves have no meaning, in contrast to derailment, where the meaning is lost over several sentences.
- *neologisms*: often found in conjunction with incoherence. This refers to the invention of new words (e.g. 'tarn-harn', 'bathroot'). The term has also been applied to the use of existing words in individualistic ways, though this is more precisely *idiosyncratic word usage* (e.g. the act of hallucinating as 'voicing'). A further variant is *word approximations*, where imprecise words or phrases are substituted for familiar ones — e.g. one patient spoke of having 'a menu three times a day' instead of three meals a day (Cameron 1938).
- *poverty of content of speech*: speech which is spontaneous and normal in quantity (i.e., as opposed to 'poverty of speech', the number of words used is normal/appropriate) but which fails to communicate any meaningful information. If 'incoherence' is the most severe expression of formal thought disorder, then poverty of content is the mild end of the spectrum. As has been pointed out, however: 'This symptom may appear to be readily recognisable in some of one's colleagues, therefore only rate it when it really is pathological' (Wing et al 1974)!

The two classical disorders of thought form in mania are: *flight of ideas* or *distractible speech*, in which the train of thought is distracted by irrelevant associations, either internal or external, which capture the patient's attention; and *clang associations*, composed of irrelevant connections made on the basis of assonance (similarity of sound), rhymes or puns.

In depression, thought may become narrowed and repetitive, in severe cases being reduced to a small circle of painful ruminations: in response to questioning on any topic, one patient would almost immediately revert to stereotyped repetitions of depressive delusions — 'my husband has been taken away . . . the house is boarded up . . . the children are on the street'.

Andreasen (1979) has developed a detailed classification of these and the many other abnormalities of thought form seen in psychiatry (Box 13.6). This is broad and includes abnormalities such as echolalia, a catatonic symptom, perseveration, the implication of which is most frequently an organic disorder, and circumstantiality which is not uncommon in normal individuals.

Trainees tend to absorb descriptively-based classifications of communication disorders in psychoses as if in clinical practice they have strong discriminative power, though in reality they often do not. When a patient is considered to show evidence of formal thought disorder it is *essential* to quote an example of the speech on which this conclusion is based. It is surprisingly easy to jot down a few consecutive sentences of speech while the patient is talking and this often appears considerably more disordered when it is read back outside the interview.

Thought content

Disorders of content relate to the 'what', as opposed to the 'how', of thinking — to the ideas and beliefs one holds. The prototypical abnormality is *delusions*. However, it is also appropriate to record here any other abnormal ideas and beliefs, including disorders of the possession of thought, overvalued ideas, obsessional ruminations, depressive ideas of self-depreciation, self-blame and guilt, simple ideas of reference, and so on.

Delusions are traditionally defined as *fixed, abnormal* beliefs which are out of keeping with the individual's *social* and *cultural* background, which are held with fixed *conviction* and are *impervious* to counter-argument (i.e. are 'incorrigible'). While this definition provides a useful yardstick for identifying most delusional beliefs, Jaspers (1963) has argued convincingly that it is superficial and there are exceptions to all its elements. For example, patients may experience *partial delusions*, which are beliefs expressed with doubt, as a possibility but not a certainty.

Delusional beliefs can be classified in many ways, perhaps the most comprehensive being that used in the PSE (Wing et al 1974), outlined in Box 13.7.

Patients will often refer to themselves as feeling 'paranoid' when experiencing probably the commonest type of delusion — *delusions of reference*. In this situation, the world becomes devoid of coincidence and, as the term implies, every incidental occurrence is referred directly to the patient, and has a personal significance for them, usually implying threat. The patient finds hints and double meanings in perfectly ordinary statements; things are done in a special way to convey a meaning; situations are specially arranged to test them out. There may be references to him in newspapers, magazines or on television — an extension the PSE calls *delusions of misinterpretation*.

Delusions of reference should be distinguished from *simple ideas of reference*, which are an exaggerated form of self-consciousness, usually driven by social anxiety. These comprise an

---

Box 13.6 Abnormalities of thought, language and communication

Poverty of speech. Restriction in the amount of spontaneous speech, so that replies to questions tend to be brief, concrete and unelaborated. Unprompted additional information is rarely provided

Poverty of content of speech. Although replies are long enough so that speech is adequate in amount, it conveys little information. Language tends to be vague, often over-abstract or over-concrete, repetitive and stereotyped. The interviewer may recognise this finding by observing that the patient has spoken at some length but has not given adequate information to answer the question. Sometimes characterised as 'empty philosophising'

Pressure of speech. An increase in the amount of spontaneous speech as compared with what is considered ordinary or socially customary. The patient talks rapidly and is difficult to interrupt. Some sentences may be left uncompleted because of eagerness to get on to a new idea. Even when interrupted, the speaker often continues to talk. Speech tends to be loud and emphatic

Distractible speech. During the course of a discussion or interview, the patient repeatedly stops talking in the middle of a sentence or idea and changes the subject in response to a nearby stimulus, such as an object on a desk, the interviewer's clothing or appearance, etc.

Tangentiality. Replying to a question in an oblique, tangential, or even irrelevant manner. The reply may be related to the question in some distant way. Or the reply may be unrelated and seem totally irrelevant

Derailment. A pattern of spontaneous speech in which the ideas slip off the track onto another one that is clearly but obliquely related, or onto one that is completely unrelated. Things may be said in juxtaposition that lack a meaningful relationship, or the patient may shift idiosyncratically from one frame of reference to another. At times, there may be a vague connection between the ideas; at others, none will be apparent

Incoherence. A pattern of speech that is essentially incomprehensible at times. The incoherence is due to several different mechanisms, which may sometimes all occur simultaneously. Sometimes the rules of grammar and syntax are ignored, and a series of words or phrases seem to be joined together arbitrarily and at random. Sometimes the disturbance appears to be at a semantic level, so that words are substituted in a phrase or sentence so that the meaning seems to be distorted or destroyed. Sometimes 'cementing words' (conjunctions such as 'and' and 'although' and articles such as 'the' 'a' and 'an') are deleted

Illogicality. A pattern of speech in which conclusions are reached that do not follow logically. This may take the form of non sequiturs, in which the patient makes a logical inference between two clauses that is unwarranted or illogical. It may take the form of faulty inductive inferences. It may also take the form of reaching conclusions based on faulty premises without any actual delusional thinking

Clanging. A pattern of speech in which sounds rather than meaningful relationships appear to govern word choice, so that the intelligibility of the speech is impaired and redundant words are introduced. In addition to rhyming relationships, this pattern of speech may also include punning associations, so that a word similar in sound brings in a new thought

continued

Box 13.6 Continued

Word approximations. Old words that are used in a new and unconventional way, or new words that are developed by conventional rules of word formation. Often the meaning will be evident even though the usage seems peculiar or bizarre

Circumstantiality. A pattern of speech that is very indirect and delayed in reaching its goal idea. In the process of explaining something, the speaker brings in many tedious details and sometimes makes parenthetical remarks. Circumstantial replies or statements may last for many minutes if the speaker is not interrupted and urged to get to the point. When not called circumstantial, these people are often referred to as 'long-winded'

Loss of goal. Failure to follow a chain of thought through to its natural conclusion. This is usually manifested in speech that begins with a particular subject, wanders away from the subject, and never returns to it. This often occurs in association with derailment

Perseveration. Persistent repetition of words, ideas, or subjects so that, once a patient begins a particular subject or uses a particular word, he continually returns to it in the process of speaking

Echolalia. A pattern of speech in which the patient echoes words or phrases of the interviewer. Typical echolalia tends to be repetitive and persistent. The echo is often uttered with a mocking, mumbling, or staccato intonation.

Stilted speech. Speech that has an excessively formal quality. It may seem rather quaint or outdated, or may appear pompous, distant, or overpolite. The stilted quality is usually achieved through use of particular word choices (multisyllabic when monosyllabic alternatives are available and equally appropriate), extremely polite phraseology ('Excuse me, madam, may I request a conference in your office at your convenience'), or stiff and formal syntax ('Whereas the attorney comported himself indecorously, the physician behaved as is customary for a born gentleman').

Self-reference. A disorder in which the patient repeatedly refers the subject under discussion back to himself when someone else is talking and also refers apparently neutral subjects to himself when he himself is talking.

From Andreasen (1979).

Box 13.7 The Present State Examination classification of delusions

Delusional mood. The subject feels that his familiar surroundings have changed in a puzzling way which he may be unable to describe, but which seems to be especially significant for him. The state often accompanies the development of full delusions

Delusions of reference and misinterpretation. What is said has a double meaning, someone makes a gesture which is construed as a deliberate message, the whole neighbourhood may be gossiping about the patient. He may see references to himself on the television, radio and in newspapers, or feel he is being followed, that his movements are observed, and that what he says is tape recorded. Circumstances appear to the patient to be arranged to test him out, objects are placed in particular positions to convey a meaning to him, whole armies of people are deployed to discover what he is doing or to convey some information to him

Delusions of persecution. The subject believes that someone, or some organisation, or some force or power, is trying to harm him in some way, to damage his reputation, to cause him bodily injury, to drive him mad or to bring about his death

Delusions of assistance. The subject believes that someone, or some organisation, or some force or power, is trying to help him

Delusions of grandiose ability. The subject thinks he is chosen by some power, or by destiny, because of his unusual talents. He thinks he is able to read people's thoughts, or that he is particularly good at helping them, that he is much cleverer than anyone else, that he has invented machines, composed music, solved mathematical problems, etc. beyond most people's comprehension

Delusions of grandiose identity. The subject believes he is famous, rich, titled or related to prominent people. He may believe that he is a changeling and that his real parents are royalty, etc.

Religious delusions. The patient believes he is a saint, an angel or even God, or has special spiritual powers, or a divine purpose

Delusional explanations. Explanation or elaboration of other abnormal experiences. This may be in terms of paranormal phenomena, including hypnotism, telepathy, magic, witchcraft, etc. Or it may be in terms of physical processes such as electricity, X-rays, television, radio or machines of various kinds. (This term largely replaces the older term 'secondary delusions'.)

Delusions of control. The subject experiences his will as replaced by that of some other force or agency. The basic, experience may be elaborated in various ways — the subject believes that someone else's words are coming out using his voice, or that what he writes is not his own, or that he is the victim of possession — a zombie or a robot controlled by someone else's will, even his bodily movements being willed by some other power. This is one form of passivity experience ('somatic passivity')

Sexual delusions. Delusions of having a fantasy lover, that one's sex is changing. Also delusions of pregnancy

Delusional memories and delusional confabulation. Experiences of past events which clearly did not occur but which the subject equally clearly remembers, e.g. 'I came to Earth on a silver star'. Delusional confabulations are beliefs which the subject either elaborates on or appears to make up on the spot

continued

uncomfortable feeling of undue attention from others. While the person cannot help thinking that others are taking notice of him, the feeling is recognised as originating from within himself. Many ordinary individuals experience this symptom at some time — e.g. on entering a room and noticing that the conversation seems to stop, though this would normally be followed immediately by insight into the nature and origins of the idea (or at least, by a decision to keep quiet about it!). Simple ideas of reference can however become pervasive and socially incapacitating in some conditions, such as anxiety and depressive states, or occasionally following some event perceived as embarrassing or shameful, or sometimes just in times of severe stress. The classification of beliefs as *delusions of persecution* should be reserved for situations in which the patient has a clear source for the adversity in their life, involving conspiracy and plot, often by an organisation such as the Freemasons, or the Government, which may result in dire consequences, including death. Occasionally, patients

---

Box 13.7   Continued

Fantastic delusions. Delusions which violate elementary common sense and logic, e.g. England's coast is melting, she has given birth to thousands of children

Simple delusions concerning appearance. The subject believes that something is wrong with his appearance. He looks ugly or old or dead, his skin is cracked, his teeth misshapen, his nose too large or his body crooked

Delusions of depersonalisation or nihilism. The subject has a conviction that he has no head, that he cannot see himself in the mirror, that he has a shadow but no body or that he does not exist at all

Hypochondriacal delusions. The subject feels that his body is unhealthy, rotten or diseased; he has incurable cancer, his bowels are stopped up or rotting away. (In schizophrenia there may be bizarre beliefs about bodily change or malfunction.)

From Wing et al (1974).

---

believe that the same individuals and organisations are working surreptitiously to help them, a phenomenon known as *delusions of assistance*.

Most delusional beliefs emerge over a period of time. However, they can emerge without detectable antecedents, in an 'autochthonous', or 'eureka' fashion (i.e. like a sudden brainwave). These sorts of beliefs have traditionally been referred to as '*primary delusions*', and while in practice there is some confusion surrounding this concept, there is merit in unequivocally identifying these on the rare occasions in which they are to be found because of the strong diagnostic inference of schizophrenia they allow. In the older literature, primary delusions were distinguished from 'secondary' delusions, where the abnormal belief seems to be based on, grow understandably out of, or represent an elaboration of some other element of psychopathology — as in depressed patients who develop beliefs that they have sinned greatly, have lost everything, have already died, etc. — though this term is less often used nowadays. Where a delusion seems obviously secondary to another *psychotic* symptom — e.g. a patient with auditory hallucinations who believes he has a radio transmitter in his head — the term *delusional explanation* is now preferred.

Subjective alterations in thought, or *disorders of the possession of thought*, include a heterogeneous group of phenomena covering core psychotic symptomatology, such as *thought insertion/withdrawal* and *thought broadcasting*, as well as obsessional patterns of thinking. Obsessional thoughts, or *ruminations*, have three characteristics: they are recognised by the patient as his own thoughts (i.e. despite having an imposed quality, they are 'non-alien'), their content is acknowledged as absurd, and there is an attempt to resist them, though the latter two qualities may be less evident in severe or chronic disorder. Other subjective alterations of thought include *slowness* in depression, and *crowding* or acceleration of thought in mania, in which ideas (and associated images) flash rapidly through the mind, each suggesting others.

Overvalued ideas are isolated beliefs which, though not obsessional in nature (i.e. they are not recognised as absurd or resisted), come to preoccupy an individual to the extent of dominating their life. Examples include querulous paranoid states, in which individuals pursue redress for some real or imagined wrong with extraordinary tenacity, and some forms of morbid jealousy and hypochondriasis. Another example of an overvalued idea, which also illustrates Jasper's argument that not all fixed, incorrigible beliefs are delusions, is the core belief of anorexia nervosa.

Abnormal perceptions

The most important type of misperception encountered in clinical practice is *hallucinations*, which are most simply defined as 'percepts without objects' (that is, they represent perceptual *deceptions*). There are however other definitions (Sims 1988), several of which emphasise the fact that, unlike tinnitus, the phantom limb syndrome and the like, patients with hallucinations usually consider their experiences to be real.

While hallucinatory experiences may occur in any sensory modality, in clinical practice hallucinations of hearing (*auditory hallucinations*) are the most frequent and important. 'Hearing voices' in the alert state can be found in individuals who do not demonstrate other features of illness (Dhossche et al 2002) and are not uncommon experiences in normal individuals in the phase of sleep induction (*hypnagogic* hallucinations), but the importance of these experiences is as a diagnostic pointer to psychotic illness, especially schizophrenia.

The range and variety of auditory hallucinations in schizophrenia is remarkable. They may be *elementary* (or rudimentary), comprising tapping, banging, music or pre-verbal whispers, mutterings and mumblings where individual words cannot be made out (but on to which the patient may still graft a content). They may comprise a single voice heard only sporadically, through conversations involving several parties, to thousands of voices babbling constantly (*mass hallucinations*). The voices(s) may be recognisable as family, friends, neighbours — even the patient's own voice — or may be total strangers. Their source may be localised in space to 'next door', 'the walls', 'behind my left shoulder', or they may seem to come from all around. They may arise from locations outside the normal perceptual sphere, e.g. 'from Italy' (*extracampine hallucinations*). They may occur spontaneously or occasionally require an additional stimulus of hearing to precipitate them (*functional* auditory hallucinations).

Traditional phenomenology makes a distinction between 'true' hallucinations and 'pseudohallucinations', though the basis of this is not well understood in English-language psychiatry (Taylor 1981). As a result, 'pseudohallucinations' has sometimes been erroneously applied to hallucinations which are recognised as being not 'real' by the patient or which are under some degree of voluntary control (Hare 1973). This probably accounts for the mistaken view that voices heard inside the head are not 'proper' hallucinations and therefore carry a lesser diagnostic implication. Many schizophrenic patients describe hearing voices inside their heads, which are typically as 'real' and compelling as those emerging from external space. In line with the PSE's convention, all hallucinatory experiences should be accorded equal diagnostic significance.

Visual hallucinations can be formless (shapeless images, lights, shadows) or formed objects (fiery crosses, faces, people). *Scenic* or *panoramic* hallucinations are visions of whole scenes such as battles, the crucifixion, etc. Visual hallucinations are perhaps most commonly seen in delirium, where they may take all these forms. In the elderly, they may take the characteristic form of 'silent boarders' — full-sized figures seen around the house who do not speak. Visual hallucinations are less common in schizophrenia than auditory hallucinations, but the view that they are so uncommon that their presence should point to an organic disorder (Hamilton 1984) is probably extreme. They are certainly seen in psychotic depression. Kraepelin (1913a) described patients as seeing evil spirits, corpses, crowds of monsters, and much else. As with hearing, visual deceptions can take the form of 'pseudohallucinations', where the images are seen 'in the mind's eye', or sometimes projected onto external space in an unreal way which the patient often finds difficult to describe clearly.

Somatic hallucinations can be classified on the basis of the specific sensation they replicate — e.g. *haptic* (touch, tickling, pricking), *thermic* (heat and cold), *hygric* (wetness), *kinaesthetic* (movement and joint position) (Sims 1988). Patients may complain of pain and sexual sensations, as well as more incomprehensible experiences of movement, vibrations, etc. inside the body. Somatic hallucinations are frequently inextricably bound up with delusional elaboration, to the extent that the relative contributions of hallucination and delusion are impossible to disentangle (Berrios 1982). One patient, for example, stated she had a Coca-Cola bottle in her stomach, while another felt semen travelling up his vertebral column to his brain, where it was laid out in sheets (Sims 1988).

Like somatic hallucinations, *olfactory* and *gustatory hallucinations* may be simple or elaborated in delusional ways.

Perception of real objects may also be changed (so-called perceptual *distortions*). The commonest distortions are the non-pathological *illusions*, such as *pareidolia* (elaboration of faces or human forms from complex backgrounds such as flames, carpets, wallpaper, etc.), and *affect illusions*, in which a heightened affective state leads to figures or forms being elaborated from poorly visualised, ambiguous stimuli (e.g. seeing a nocturnal stalker in wind-blown trees).

Analogous phenomena also occur in pathological states, but here the term 'illusion' tends to be avoided, with *perceptual misinterpretation* preferred, though the key elements of heightened affect and diminished attention are common to both. Perhaps the most familiar examples of this are seen in delirium, where, for example, patients may misperceive the window panes as bars in a cell (Lishman 1998).

Perception may in addition be 'heightened', 'dulled' or 'changed' (Wing et al 1974). In *heightened perception*, all sensation is experienced vividly — sounds seem unnaturally clear, loud or intense; colours appear more brilliant or beautiful; details of the environment seem to stand out in a particular way. In *dulled perception*, a rare symptom of depression, things seem dark, grey or colourless, with uniform, flat, uninteresting texture. Taste and appetite is blunted, colours may appear muddy or dirty, and sounds ugly or impure. Patients with *changed perception* experience objects changing in shape, size or colour, or complain that people appear different, ugly or facially distorted. One patient saw a chair take on a 'demonic' appearance.

Other abnormal mental contents

A number of other phenomena cannot readily be placed within the standard MSE headings and it is reasonable to keep a section for noting such features. This might include a précis of any descriptions of *depersonalisation/derealisation, obsessional images, déjà vu, out of body experiences, bodily experiences not obviously hallucinatory in nature*, including burning sensations, numbness, parasthesiae, and impulses, whether obsessional or otherwise.

Cognitive-state examination

The purpose of this is primarily to confirm the presence or absence of one of the two forms of global cognitive impairment — *delirium* (acute confusional state) or *dementia* — though it can also establish specific areas of neuropsychological deficit, such as *amnesia* or *frontal lobe syndrome*. In practice, however, such examination is only a crude 'broad brush' assessment to explore pointers that will already have become apparent and is not a substitute for formal neuropsychological evaluation.

Apart from the requirements of exams, there may in practice be little to be gained by a formal cognitive assessment in young individuals with an established non-organic psychiatric diagnosis, as it is only likely to confirm the obvious — diminished attention and impaired concentration. However, such screening should routinely be carried out in middle-aged and elderly patients, and in patients of any age in whom there is diagnostic uncertainty or physical illness that can affect brain function. In these contexts, cognitive evaluation should be combined with neurological examination and, often neglected, examination of the cardiovascular system.

A typical scheme for cognitive examination (after Hodges 1994) is shown in Box 13.8). Examination begins with general observations concerning behaviour and alertness, going on to cover orientation, attention and concentration, memory and executive function. This can be complemented by carrying out the Mini-Mental State Examination (Folstein et al 1975), a ubiquitous practice in psychogeriatrics, which provides a crude but useful measure of the severity of cognitive impairment. (See also the description of cognitive examination in chapter 17.)

Orientation

Orientation tends to be compromised progressively. Only 'time' is affected in mild disorder, followed by 'place', with 'person' only disrupted in severe cases. Most people are able to estimate the time to within half-an-hour, and any answer that is wrong by more

Box 13.8	Cognitive state examination
Alertness	Level of wakefulness and reactivity
Orientation	Time: day of week, time of day, month, year
	Place: Building, town, county, country
	Name, age, date of birth
Attention/concentration	Months of year backwards or serial 7s
Short-term memory	Digit span
	Immediate recall of name and address
Long-term memory	Delayed recall of name and address
	Recall of conversation, journey to hospital, recent news, famous events
Executive function	Proverbs, similarities, differences Verbal fluency
	Cognitive estimates

From Hodges (1994).

than this should be regarded as suspicious. Mildly disorientated patients often over- or under-estimate how long they have been in hospital, so as well as the standard questions, a question about this should be included. Also, it is surprising how often patients are unaware they are in hospital (Hodges 1994), and it is also worth asking 'What is the name of this place (building etc.)?'. In delirium, the degree of impairment characteristically fluctuates, and it is quite possible for orientation to be intact at the particular time the patient is being examined. When an organic condition is suspected, it is important to continue to check this aspect of mental state, for example by re-examining later in the day when fatigue may make subtle deficit more evident, or the next day, when recollection of the previous day's events is likely to be poor.

Attention and concentration

The suspicion of significant deficits in these areas is often raised by the patient's behaviour and responses during the preceding parts of the interview. For formal assessment, the 'serial-7's test' is conventional. However, normal elderly people may make errors on this, and even younger individuals require a certain level of numerical accomplishment to perform it accurately and with reasonable speed. Errors must therefore be interpreted. A simple alternative is asking the patient to recite the months of the year backwards. Because of the familiarity of the material, errors are more likely to reflect clinically significant disorder.

Memory

'Digit span' is a standard test of *short-term memory*, the store which holds a limited amount of information for periods of time up to 30 seconds. 'Immediate recall' of a name and address may also reflect partly or wholly the operation of short-term memory. Delayed recall of the same name and address tests *long-term memory*, the store of all information that needs to be held for more than 30 seconds.

A useful test of the ability to retain new information (*anterograde* memory) is to find a topic of interest, such as the patient's family or a recent holiday, and then tell the patient something about one's own family or recent holiday. The patient can then be asked about this later. *Retrograde* memory can be assessed by beginning with open-ended questions, such as 'What important events have been in the news recently?', and then asking about a standard list of famous events. Although there is no psychological support for the time-honoured clinical distinction between 'recent' and 'remote' long-term memory, patients with retrograde amnesia will usually show a temporal gradient of recall, with more impairment of recent and less impairment of remote events.

Executive function

Most of the commonly advocated 'bedside' tests of executive function are insensitive and will only pick up abnormality in gross cases. Furthermore, patients with frontal lobe lesions are notorious for performing normally on some, or even most, executive tests, while disastrously failing others.

One formal test that can be easily applied in the clinical setting is 'verbal fluency' — asking the patient to generate as many items as possible over a minute in a set category, such as animals, words beginning with 'S', or items that can be bought in a supermarket. Another is the Cognitive Estimates Test (Shallice & Evans 1978).

Box 13.9	The Cognitive Estimates Test

1. What is the height of the Post Office tower?

> 1500 ft	3	< 60 ft	3
= 1500 ft	2	= 60 ft	2
> 800 ft	1	< 100 ft	1

2. How fast do race horses gallop?

> 50 mph	3	< 9 mph	3
= 50 mph	2	< 15 mph	2
> 40 mph	1		

3. What is the best paid job or occupation in Britain today?

Manual workers	3
Car workers (or other special groups of well-paid blue-collar workers)	2
Professional (up to and including Prime Minister)	1

4. What is the age of the oldest person in Britain today?

> 115	3	< 103	3
= 115	2		
= 114	1	= 103	1

5. What is the length of an average man's spine?

> 5 ft	3	< 1 ft 6 in	3
> 4 ft	2		
= 4 ft	1	= 1 ft 6 in	1

6. How tall is the average English woman?

> 6 ft	3	< 5 ft 2 in	3
= 5 ft 11 in; 6 ft	2		
= 5 ft 9 in; 5 ft 10 in	1	= 5 ft 2 in	1

7. What is the population of Britain?

> 1000 million	3	< 2 million	3
> 500 million	2	< 3 million	2
= 500 million	1	< 10 million	1

8. How heavy is a full pint bottle of milk?

> 3 lb	3	< 1 lb	3
= 3 lb	1	= 1 lb	1

9. What is the largest object normally found in a house?

< Carpet	3
Carpet	2
Piano, sideboard, settee	1

10. How many camels are there in Holland?

Very large number	3	None	1

Responses are scored in terms of extremeness from 0 (normal) to 3 (very extreme). The signs < (less than) and > (greater) should be interpreted strictly, not as approximate values.
5th percentile cutoff for abnormality in 84 normal adults aged 17–68 with a wide range of estimated IQ = 12.75.
From Shallice & Evans (1978).

This requires the subject to give educated guesses to questions to which they are unlikely to know the exact answers — like, 'How fast do race horses gallop?' and 'What is the largest object normally found in a house?'. The full version of this is shown in Box 13.9. Sometimes the answers can be revealing: when asked what the population of Britain was, one patient with suspected frontal dementia replied 'About a thousand'. When the interviewer pointed out that there were probably a thousand people working in the hospital, she responded 'All right — two thousand' (R Dolan, personal communication).

Tests of abstract thinking — 'proverb interpretation' / 'similarities – differences' — are popular with psychiatrists and can provide useful clues to cognitive difficulty, such as early dementia, before orientation and memory impairment can be detected by routine bedside methods. However, it is important to remember that proverb interpretation is highly dependent on educational and cultural factors, and the choice should be restricted to simple, well-known examples. Many people (including some doctors!) do not know the meaning of: 'It's an ill wind that blows nobody any good'. Assessment should always be prefaced by: 'Have you heard the old saying . . .?', as ignorance is the surest way to 'fail' proverb interpretation!

Perseveration — the inappropriate repetition of words, ideas or themes — is a presumptive dysexecutive sign which has been considered to be a feature of schizophrenia, and was included by Andreasen (1979) as one of her abnormalities of thought, language and communication. Whether or not it is genuinely a symptom of schizophrenia or merely a reflection of the cognitive impairment found in this disorder, it is certainly a feature of organic disorders, particularly frontal lobe disease. Two striking examples of perseveration in patients with frontal dementia are shown in Figure 13.2.

Insight

Traditionally the mental state examination ends with a statement about insight, usually gauged simply on the patient's ability to accept that they are ill. Recent research has demonstrated that insight is a considerably more complex construct than this (David

et al 1995) and what meaningful information can be provided by rough bed-side appraisals must be open to question. Nonetheless, it is useful to explore at this point the patient's willingness to accept medical recommendations, response to which may in some circumstances have major implications for one's immediate decisions.

Formulation/summary

A traditional part of diagnostic assessments, especially in exams, has been the *formulation*. The '*exam formulation*' has been seen as a way of assessing a candidate's ability to focus thought on the essentials and to prioritise issues.

Unfortunately, 'formulation' means different things to different people and comes with heavy theoretical baggage. Its origins lie in psychoanalytical practice, where its functions are more explanatory than descriptive. This approach is illustrated, for example, in the views of the American analyst Karl Menninger, who considered individuals and their predicaments unique and incapable of classification. He, amongst others, rejected formal taxonomy in favour of *individualised formulations* that encompassed every facet of the patient's being and life experience that had brought them to a symptomatic state. Needless to say, this concept goes far beyond what is expected of the average examinee!

The concept of 'formulation' is too muddled for the examination room. If the skills of 'extraction' and 'prioritisation' are

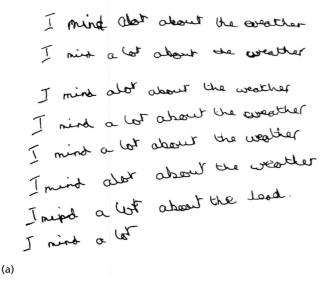

(a)

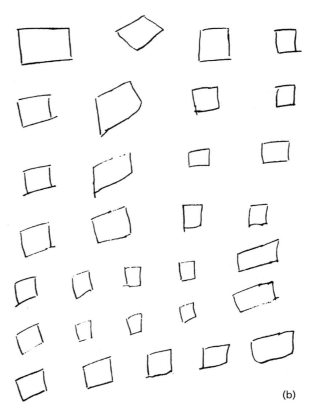

(b)

Fig. 13.2
Perseveration in fronto-temporal dementia. (a) The patient was asked to write a sentence about the weather, and then to write something about her stay in hospital. She continued to reproduce the original sentence despite repeated instructions to write something different. (b) The patient was asked to draw as many different designs as possible made up of four lines. (Reproduced with permission from Snowden et al (1996).)

deemed examinable, the same aim can be achieved by considering a 'summary' statement, which is entirely descriptive and has no theoretical implications. This should contain no more than three (occasionally four) brief sentences: the first, comprising basic demographic information, mode of referral and the presenting complaint, including its duration; the second, a précis of significant phenomenology elicited during the interview (only those features present, not those that were absent), its evolution and context; the third, key mental state disorders evident from formal examination. Differential diagnoses are too important to be 'summarised', and any proposed treatment plan deserves full exploration, so these should not be included. Unlike a 'formulation', a 'summary' should not encroach on speculative dynamics.

Proposals from some examination boards might now require trainees to present a 'psychodynamic formulation' or a 'behavioural formulation' of a case. This is to be regretted. Such skills are for those in specialist training to acquire and have as much relevance to the generalist as a formulation based on the patient's serotonergic receptor status.

Summary

A 51-year-old happily married professional lady with a family history of affective disorder, referred by GP with a 6-month + history of progressive, persistent depression of mood, associated with anhedonia, loss of emotional resonance, diurnal variation, early waking with daytime fatigue, poor appetite and weight loss and impaired concentration. She presents as mildly agitated and objectively depressed with ideas (but not delusions) of guilt, low self-esteem, and hopelessness associated with passive ideas of self-harm. (She relates the onset of her illness to enforced redundancy but admits to declining performance in the preceding months.)

CONCLUSIONS

A formal psychiatric interview should have a formal conclusion. This is not so much a statement or question — and is certainly not merely the passing on of a prescription! This is a section in itself, in which the doctor will, for initial contacts, provide some discussion of the problems as he or she sees them, including therapeutic recommendations, or for follow-up contacts, some assessment of progress and recommendations regarding on-going management. It is therefore important in busy outpatient settings that information gathering allows sufficient time for this crucial part of the exchange.

Ultimately, the examiner determines the structure and duration of most psychiatric interviews, but with skill and a competent exercise of control over process elements, he should nonetheless have allowed the patient ample opportunity to present issues of importance to them. This cannot however be guaranteed, and, especially if the patient has preconceptions that have not been fulfilled, they may still feel there are areas of significance that remain unaddressed. It is therefore often useful after concluding the above to give them the opportunity to note this. This might be done in the following way:

> *'We've covered a lot of issues during the interview. Are there any other issues we haven't covered that you feel it would be important for me to know about?'*

Alternatively, a useful signal to the patient that the information part of the exercise has been completed is to say:

> *'I've asked you a lot of questions. Are there any questions you would like to ask me?'*

Most individuals will not take this as an opportunity to ask about what is to come — i.e. treatment issues — but will relate it back to what has been before, to whether or not they are satisfied with what you have asked them about. Thus, it can act as a useful way of linking what has been established with what you will then be recommending.

A final and useful question at this juncture relates to the patient's expectations. One of the most powerful determinants of efficacy for any psychiatric intervention is the patient's belief in it. One will experience opposition, if not hostility, if one's recommendations are predominantly pharmacological when the patient's expectations were psychotherapeutic — and vice versa. Awareness of the patient's expectations is important in helping to frame recommendations sensitively, especially when they may not gel with what was anticipated. One might ask:

> *'In what way do you feel I might help you?'*

or

> *'What do you feel might be the best way forward?'*

In the concluding part of the interview, the psychiatrist's task is to provide an 'assessment' (not a 'formulation' which is too theoretically burdened; not a 'summary' which is too stark), a task relevant to both initial and follow-up interviews, though slightly different for each. The patient may wish a diagnosis, and if this is available with reasonable probability of accuracy, as with many non-psychotic disorders, it should be offered. However, many patients, especially those presenting with psychotic disorders, may not wish a diagnosis at an early stage — which is perhaps as well, because all that one may strictly be able to offer is a set of differential possibilities, which may be interpreted as lack of competence! Relatives may of course have profound interest in the outcome of the interview, and while every effort should be made to inform them — including the limitations imposed by cross-sectional evaluations — this must be within the bounds of patient confidentiality.

In considering the content and presentation of patient problems in interview contexts there are two 'rules' worth bearing in mind. The first, to paraphrase Kendell (1975), is what might be called the 'Rule of Intersubjective Certifiability'. While the central role of empathy in the conduct of the psychiatric interview has been emphasised, this must be rejected when it comes to evaluating the material comprising the MSE (with the possible exception of appraising depth of emotion, if one feels able to do this). As much of the MSE as possible must be submitted to *objective* appraisal, such that other examiners would reach similar conclusions to oneself. Not only must empathy be banned from the diagnostic process, so too should intuition, identification and any of the interminable dynamic 'insights' so beloved of experts with Sunday-supplement expertise. Possible roads to the disorder should be addressed *after* the disorder has been diagnosed, and that may include psychodynamic ones, but these principles should have no place in the diagnostic process itself.

The second rule might be called the 'Rule of Counter-Intuition'. It is everyday experience that, in all of us, difficult life circumstances produce unpleasant emotional consequences. However, what may be intuitive in relation to everyday life may not be so in relation to psychiatric disorder. It is well established that disordered mental states can themselves produce adverse life events — that is, that life events may bear a 'dependent' or an 'independent' relationship to psychiatric illness. The situation where psychiatrists have satisfied themselves that an event bears a causative relationship to the symptomatology they have elicited is one in which the principle of refutation should be invoked. The question 'Could it be the illness which created the event?' must be put forward for consideration. It is surprising how often 'intuitive' impressions fail to be sustained.

The reader will have noticed the recurrent use of 'recommendation' in this chapter and when it comes to proposing treatments, this word cannot be 'recommended' too strongly. While in psychiatric practice, 'recommendations' do sometimes have to be imposed, in the majority of instances the patient must be the willing recipient of professional advice. With its connotations of professional authority yet personal choice, it is the essence of what clinical practice is about.

BASIC NEUROLOGICAL EXAMINATION

Patients with neurological symptoms are often viewed with trepidation by doctors, with the neurological examination an impenetrable ritual understood only by neurologists, an aura of mystery they sometimes encourage. The nervous system is probably the most complex and poorly understood aspect of human function, producing symptoms that can be as vague as they are varied. Many neurological *diseases* are relentlessly disabling and untreatable, adding fear and anxiety to their presentations and worry in doctors that they may be missing something. Yet many neurological *symptoms* are benign and do not reflect organic pathology.

The division between neurology and psychiatry is in many ways artificial but likely to be maintained so long as training schemes are kept separate; and it remains the case that many psychiatrists, when confronted with potential neurological disease and the complexities of neurological examination, feel uneasy. The purpose of this section is not to turn psychiatrists into neurologists but simply to try and demystify the approach to neurological assessment and diagnosis. A secondary aim is to allow psychiatrists to feel comfortable about the limited expectations possible to them from a brief, standard neurological examination.

History taking

While diagnosis is the key aim of neurological assessment, neurologists — like psychiatrists — appreciate that many symptoms do not indicate disease and that some patients defy accurate diagnosis, certainly initially and perhaps indefinitely.

One should make no apology for emphasising an 'obvious' fact — in neurological assessment, there is no substitute for an accurate and well-interpreted *history*. Without an accurate history a neurological diagnosis is usually impossible, and many neurological diseases can be diagnosed on the history alone. This will be familiar to psychiatrists but, as in psychiatry, history-taking skills (as opposed to examination techniques) are rarely taught and published material is scarce (Thrush 2002).

There is no difference in taking a history from patients with neurological symptomatology than from those with any other types of presentation, though nervous system symptoms, 'psychiatric' or 'neurological', often require more patience to pursue. All history taking is an active process and while checklists or protocols

may be helpful for students or in diagnosing certain easily identified and specific disease processes, such as asthma attacks or stroke, they are hopelessly inadequate when pursuing less well-defined histories of the sort not uncommonly associated with neurological presentations. No two histories will be the same. One must be constantly listening, thinking and updating the potential differential diagnoses as one elicits the story, as this will open up new avenues of enquiry. In a further similarity with psychiatry, information from witnesses or third parties is often invaluable, though this is something that may be best obtained in private. With neurological presentations, family members or other witnesses may be embarrassed about discussing symptomatology in front of the patient, for example where cognitive problems predominate, or where relevant family histories have remained concealed or unspoken.

A neurological history can usefully begin with three standard question — *age, handedness* (a peculiar neurological obsession) and *occupation* (past and present) — and thereafter can be pursued within the same sort of traditional framework as noted above: the presenting complaint and its evolution; the past medical history; current and previous medications (prescribed and otherwise); and social and family history.

As many neurological and psychiatric disorders are chronic or relapsing/remitting in nature, *past histories* are crucial. This can be problematic, as patients often forget or dismiss previous symptoms, particularly if they have resolved and seemingly have little relevance to current complaints. Even if recalled, previous symptoms are often inaccurately placed in their timing or in the sequence of events. Sometimes they may be actively concealed. These pitfalls may be averted by reviewing contemporaneous medical records, and, although hospital practitioners rarely have easy access to primary-care records, obtaining these can at times be invaluable, even diagnostic. Simply knowing that the patient in front of you possesses a bulky set of primary-care records reflecting referral to several different departments and hospitals with a variety of ill-defined symptoms, can immediately alert one to the possibility of functional or factitious disorder. Alternatively, one may identify long-forgotten symptoms, such as a brief episode of reduced visual acuity in one eye in someone presenting years later with gait disturbance, indicating a probable diagnosis of multiple sclerosis.

By the end of the history taking, you should have a differential diagnostic list in your head. If you do not, the examination is unlikely to help.

The examination

Professional anxiety about the neurological examination can lead doctors to either omit it or, worse still, perform it incompetently, but a *basic* neurological examination should be within the grasp of all practising clinicians. There is, however, little point in nonneurologists attempting to learn a 'full' neurological examination — they are likely to get little opportunity to perform this regularly and, when they do, inexperience is likely to throw up false positive as well as false negative findings. Examination findings are subject to such variability that even experienced neurologists find themselves frequently disagreeing over 'hard' signs, like plantar responses.

Many practitioners place more faith in their abilities in undertaking an accurate neurological examination than in their history-taking skills, with the result that they are disproportionately influenced by isolated neurological 'signs', regardless of what the history is telling them. A reasonable neurological view would be that if you suspect neurological disease at the end of the history, you should refer the patient to a neurologist, regardless of what you may or may not have found on examination. Similarly, you can afford to ignore an isolated, potentially unreliable 'sign' if it makes no sense in the clinical setting. As a result, psychiatrists need only be competent in a very basic neurological examination (See Box 13.3).

A logical approach

A basic neurological examination does not require detailed neuro-anatomical knowledge. It is sufficient to consider the nervous system in three sections: cognitive apparatus, cranial nerve function, and limb function. Most neuropsychiatric syndromes, or neurological diseases presenting to psychiatrists will, with few exceptions, involve the central nervous system (i.e. brain and spinal cord), so one might particularly concentrate on cognitive disturbance and signs of upper motor neuron pathology.

1. Observation. Careful observation from the 'end of the bed' is the first stage of any examination, followed by observation of the patient *walking* an adequate distance down an uncluttered corridor. It is surprising how much information this can reveal (Box 13.3). Testing tandem gait (heel–toe walking) and for Romberg's sign (a test of proprioception) are common sources of false-positive errors and cannot be recommended for non-specialists. If the patient's standard gait appears normal, this can be accepted as a reasonable indication that legs and cerebellum are grossly intact. Finally, observing movements when undressing/dressing can also be instructive, though the importance of having a chaperone present cannot be over-emphasised.

2. Cognition. This has already been dealt with and only a couple of issues of importance in the neurological examination will be re-presented, especially from the perspective of 'bedside' testing as opposed to formal neuropsychological evaluation. Although clinicians enjoy eliciting the 'primitive' reflexes — e.g. the pout, snout, rooting and palmar-mental responses — in practice, these reflexes only infrequently add significantly to cognitive testing.

- *Consciousness.* This is a more complex issue than most clinicians appreciate or bedside testing allows for but, when required, the Glasgow Coma Scale is a widely utilised international standard. It should be remembered that it is a three-domain scale and findings should be presented as such, rather than as a composite score, which means little.
- *Orientation.* As noted above, page 235.
- *Attention.* As noted above, page 236.
- *Memory.* As noted above, page 236.
- *Executive function.* In addition to points noted above, testing motor sequences with the Luria 'three hand position' test can be useful.
- *Perception.* In a neurological context, this has a slightly different meaning than in psychiatry. Here, what is being tested is neurological substrate, not percepts themselves. This can be assessed with clock drawing tasks or line bisection.
- *Praxis.* This is difficult to assess unless marked, but can be roughly evaluated by testing the patient's ability to mime actions, such as lighting a cigarette, brushing his teeth or combing his hair.

3. Cranial nerves. Detailed assessment of all twelve pairs of cranial nerves is unnecessary in a psychiatric context, but certain signs are more common than others and worth looking for, particularly disorders of *eye movements*. Eye movement disorders occur in a number of neuropsychiatric disorders, and asking the patient to follow your finger in an 'H' pattern with the head fixed will identify gross abnormalities. The eye movements should be smooth and co-ordinated, without extra movements such as nystagmus. *Nystagmus* should be tested for in both the horizontal and the vertical planes of gaze. In interpreting eye signs, one must beware of *nystagmoid jerks* — which are common if the eyes are forced beyond their natural sweep, and indicate a faulty examiner, not a faulty patient! The interpretation of an eye movement disorder can be extremely difficult, even for specialists.

Simple observation of the face is likely to be more instructive than further detailed testing of facial sensation or movements — the immobile face of parkinsonism with reduced blinking and drooling; ptosis suggestive of myopathic or mitochondrial disorder; tics, blepharospasm or other dyskinesias. Lower cranial nerve dysfunction is most commonly manifest as dysarthria and may be accompanied by emotional lability. In general however, interpretation of cranial nerve deficits is best left to experts, and for the non-specialist it is sufficient to take observed abnormality as an indication for specialist referral.

4. The limbs. Gross motor power in the legs will already have been assessed by observing the patient walking. A common functional sign is the ability of the patient to walk (albeit oddly) yet to have virtually no power in the legs when examined on the bed — e.g. they appear unable to lift either leg off the bed despite having somehow got there in the first place!

The upper limbs may be grossly assessed in similar fashion by asking the patient to raise both arms above his head (gross motor power) then stretch them out in front with palms uppermost — initially with eyes open, then with eyes closed. One is looking for any 'drift' of the outstretched limb, often a subtle early sign of pyramidal disease. Lastly, with eyes open, the patient can be asked to wiggle his fingers in 'piano-playing' fashion, another subtle measure of pyramidal or extrapyramidal dysfunction, when fine finger movements are affected first. Interpretation of findings must bear in mind that the dominant hand will always be more dextrous than the non-dominant one. Other fine motor tasks that can be usefully observed include hand-writing and doing-up/undoing buttons.

Conventional teaching would dictate that the standard neurological examination should include a detailed assessment of resting *tone* and *power* in individual muscles. However it must be doubtful how useful these exercises actually are to the non-specialist. Assessing tone is difficult unless it is markedly increased, in which case there will be other, more obvious signs evident (such as exaggerated tendon reflexes and extensor plantars), and unless one possesses a working knowledge of the individual nerves and roots which supply individual muscles there would seem to be little point in testing them. It is far more important to decide whether or not the patient is *weak* (as opposed to stiff, apraxic, in pain, or subject to any of the other impairments which he may misinterpret as weakness), and if so, whether or not that weakness appears *consistent*. Simply observing gait, the ability to lift the arms above the head, and fine finger movements will usually identify significant weakness.

Testing upper (biceps, supinator, triceps) and lower (knee, ankle) limb *reflexes* should however be done, simply to see if they are exaggerated (which would *suggest* an upper motor neuron lesion) or not. But it should be remembered that absence of an isolated reflex in non-specialist hands is as often due to poor technique as to any underlying pathology. Interpretation should also be informed by the fact that deep tendon reflexes may appear brisk without indicating pathology, especially in anxious and tense patients. The *plantar response* should only be interpreted as abnormal (i.e. extensor) when it is *unmistakable* and *repeatable* and should not be confused with a *withdrawal response*, commonly found in people who dislike having their feet 'interfered with'.

As with any part of the examination, it is important not to fall into the trap of over-interpreting isolated signs. A patient with normal gait and otherwise entirely normal legs apart from an isolated extensor plantar probably has an intact motor system, while in the patient with a limp where it is suspected that the reflexes are brisk in the limping leg, a 'probable' extensor plantar on that side is altogether more suspicious of pathology within the central nervous system (which may or may not be relevant to the presenting complaint).

Summary

The concluding message is simple — dedicate your time to history and pursue all the witnesses available, including from medical records, especially in difficult cases. If you suspect a neurological disorder, refer the patient to a neurologist, indicating why you think this is the case. In making a referral, remember that the neurologist (a good one, at least) will be more interested in your history than your examination findings. Keep your own examination simple, for it is from simple observation and testing that the most reliable information will emerge; and be prepared to disregard signs which you find but which make no sense, as they are more than likely false positives. And remember that plenty of neurological disorders produce normal examinations.

EPILOGUE

Most of the aforegoing has been focused on the doctor–patient interaction. Like many things that 'go without saying', it is important to say that the quality of material relevant to any patient's case may be greatly enhanced by the addition of third-party information. Where possible — and where the patient is in agreement — third-party sources should be considered and where relevant sought, though the interview principles will be the same as those noted above.

Despite the many advances in psychiatric practice in the last half century, it remains the case that one of the most potent therapeutic tools available to the psychiatrist is the 'Dr' in front of his or her name. Despite increasing challenge, this still embodies powerful expectations on the part of most patients. Those who carry the title would do well to respect it.

FURTHER READING

Frith C D 1992 The cognitive neuropsychology of schizophrenia. Erlbaum, Hillsdale, NJ

Hawkes C H 1991 How to perform a rapid neurological examination. Hospital Update 17:125–131

Hawkes C H 1997 Diagnosis of functional neurological disease. British Journal of Hospital Medicine 57:373–377

Hersen M, Turner S M (eds) 1994 Diagnostic interviewing, 2nd edn. Plenum, New York

Kendell R E 1975 The role of diagnosis in psychiatry. Blackwell Science, Oxford

Memon A, Bull R (eds) 2000 Handbook of the psychology of interviewing. Wiley, Chichester

Myersough P R, Ford M J (eds) 1996 Talking with patients: keys to good communication, 3rd edn. Oxford University Press, Oxford

Shea S C 1998 Psychiatric interviewing, 2nd edn. Saunders, Philadelphia

Tasman A, Kay J, Lieberman J A (eds) 1997 Psychiatry. Saunders, Philadelphia

REFERENCES

Andreasen N C 1979 Thought, language and communication disorders, 1: Clinical assessment, definition of terms and evaluation of their reliability. Archives of General Psychiatry 36:1315–1321

Berrios G E 1982 Tactile hallucinations: conceptual and historical aspects. Journal of Neurology, Neurosurgery & Psychiatry 45:285–293

Bleuler E 1911 Dementia praecox or the group of schizophrenias (transl J Zinkin 1950). International Universities Press, New York

Cameron N 1938 Reasoning, regression and communication in schizophrenics. Psychological Monographs 50:1–34

David A, van Os J, Jones P et al 1995 Insight in psychotic illness: cross-sectional and longitudinal associations. British Journal of Psychiatry 167:621–628

Dhossche E, Ferdinand R, van der End J et al 2002 Diagnostic outcome of self-reported hallucinations in a community sample of adolescents. Psychological Medicine 32:619–627

Enoch M D, Ball H N 2001 Uncommon psychiatric syndromes. Arnold, London

Folstein M F, Folstein S E, McHugh P R 1975 'Mini-Mental State': a practical method for grading the cognitive state of patients for the clinician. Journal of Psychiatric Research 12:189–198

Hamilton M 1984 Fish's schizophrenia, 3rd edn. Wright, Bristol

Hare E H 1973 A short note on pseudohallucinations. British Journal of Psychiatry 122:469–476

Hodges J R 1994 Cognitive assessment for clinicians. Oxford University Press, Oxford

Jaspers K 1959 General psychopathology (transl J Hoenig, M W Hamilton 1963). Manchester University Press, Manchester

Kendell R E 1975 The role of diagnosis in psychiatry. Blackwell Science, Oxford

Kraepelin E 1913a Manic-depressive insanity and paranoia (transl R M Barclay 1921). Livingstone, Edinburgh

Kraepelin E 1913b Dementia praecox and paraphrenia (transl R M Barclay 1919). Livingstone, Edinburgh

Lishman W A 1998 Organic psychiatry: the psychological consequences of cerebral disorder. Blackwell Scientific, Oxford

Lohr J B, Wisniewski A A 1987 Movement disorders: a neuropsychiatric approach. Wiley, Chichester

Lund C E, Mortimer A M, Rogers D, McKenna P J 1991 Motor, volitional and behavioural disorders in schizophrenia, I: Assessment using the modified Rogers scale. British Journal of Psychiatry 158:323–327

McKenna P J 1984 Disorders with overvalued ideas. British Journal of Psychiatry 145:579–585

McKenna P J 1994 Schizophrenia and related syndromes. Oxford Medical Publications, Oxford

Owens D G C 1999 A guide to the extrapyramidal side-effects of antipsychotic drugs. Cambridge University Press, Cambridge

Rogers D 1985 The motor disorders of severe psychotic illness: a conflict of paradigms. British Journal of Psychiatry 147:221–232

Rogers D 1992 Motor disorders in psychiatry. Wiley, Chichester

Shallice T, Evans M E 1978 The involvement of frontal lobes in cognitive estimation. Cortex 14:294–303

Sims A 1988 Symptoms in the mind. Baillière Tindall, London

Snowden J S S 1996 Fronto-temporal lobar degeneration. Churchill Livingstone, New York

Taylor F K 1981 On pseudohallucinations. Psychological Medicine 11:265–271

Thrush D 2002 How to do it: take a good history. Practical Neurology 2:113–116

Wing L, Shah A 2000 Catatonia in autistic spectrum disorders. British Journal of Psychiatry 176:357–362

Wing J K, Cooper J E, Sartorius N 1974 The measurement and classification of psychiatric symptoms. Cambridge University Press, Cambridge

14 | Diagnosis and classification

Robert E Kendell, Stephen M Lawrie, Eve C Johnstone

INTRODUCTION

In psychiatry, as in the rest of medicine, the purpose of classification is to bring order to the wide range of complaints, behaviours and outcomes encountered in clinical practice. It allows us to identify groups of patients who have similar symptoms, responses to treatment and outcomes. In most branches of medicine the value of diagnosis is never questioned. Its importance is self-evident because treatment and prognosis depend upon it. In psychiatry the situation is rather different. With a few exceptions diagnoses continue to be based (largely) on the clinical syndrome and, although it is possible to achieve high reliability using structured interviews and operational definitions, everyday clinical diagnoses are still relatively unreliable. The therapeutic and prognostic implications of psychiatric diagnoses are also relatively weak. It is therefore not surprising that the value of psychiatric diagnoses has been questioned. Indeed, forty years ago American psychiatrists like Rogers and Menninger were arguing that psychiatry would be better off without any diagnostic categories at all. Although the current situation is very different and it is no longer necessary to defend the importance of diagnoses, it is, nonetheless, important to understand why classification is unavoidable, and to appreciate the ways in which it may be harmful as well as helpful to a patient to be given a diagnostic label.

THE INEVITABILITY OF CLASSIFICATION

Every patient possesses characteristics of three kinds:

1. those shared with all other patients
2. those shared with some other patients, but not all
3. those which are unique.

Insofar as the first of these three categories is dominant, classification or subdivision is pointless and unnecessary. All patients have fundamentally similar problems, and even if there are a few superficial differences between them they all require the same treatment. Insofar as the third category is dominant, classification is impossible. So too are learning from experience and useful communication with others. For if every patient is different from every other we can learn nothing useful from textbooks, from colleagues, or the accumulated wisdom of our predecessors. Indeed, we cannot even learn from our own personal experience if there are no significant similarities between our last patient and the next. Attention has, therefore, to be focused on the second category. What is more, as soon as one begins to recognise features that are common to some patients but not all, and to distinguish those which are important from those, like eye colour, which are not, one is classifying them, whether one realises it or not. And if we have more than one treatment available, as we have, and wish to use these different treatments with maximum efficacy, we must distinguish between one type of patient and another. Otherwise we are reduced to allocating successive patients to different treatment at random or on the basis of a whim. (Those who argued in the past that diagnostic categories should be abandoned did indeed believe that all patients required the same treatment — the 'moral regimen' of the asylum for Neumann and Prichard in the 19th century and psychotherapy for Rogers and Menninger in the 20th.)

A distinction between different kinds of mental disorder is therefore inevitable. The only open issues are what patient characteristics are going to be the basis of the classification, and whether this classification will be public or private, categorical or dimensional, reliable or unreliable, valid or invalid. Classifications of mental disorders may well be less useful than those of, say, cardiovascular disorders or gastrointestinal disorders, for they are still largely based on differences in symptomatology rather than on differences in aetiology, but the only viable option in this situation is to try to improve the classification we possess. It cannot simply be abandoned, and the idea that diagnosis can, or should, be replaced by a formulation is based on a fundamental misunderstanding of the nature of both. A formulation which takes account of the unique features of the patient and his environment, and the complex interaction between them, is often essential for any real understanding of his predicament, and for planning effective treatment, but it is unusable in any situation in which populations or groups of patients need to be considered. The essential feature of any population is that its members share at least one important characteristic in common. The essence of a diagnosis is that it embodies as many as possible of those characteristics which are common to several different patients (i.e. category 2 above), just as it is the essence of a formulation to embody those which are unique to the individual (category 3 above). Formulation and diagnosis are equally necessary, but for quite different purposes.

The shortcomings and disadvantages of diagnoses

If some form of categorisation or subdivision of mental disorders is inescapable, as it is, it is essential that we appreciate the limitations and potential ill-effects of allocating patients to diagnostic categories (Box 14.1). In the first place, psychiatric diagnoses are often an inadequate means of conveying what the clinician regards as the essence of his patient's predicament, and the better he

Box 14.1   Strengths and limitations of diagnoses

Strengths	Limitations
• Facilitate communication	• Convey limited information
• Can predict treatment and/ or prognosis	• Stereotypical
	• Can be pejorative

knows the patient the stronger this feeling becomes. To say that a woman has a depressive illness does not explain why she became depressed or how she came to medical attention, nor does it establish whether she is on the brink of suicide or merely despondent and dejected. She may have been ill for anything from a few weeks to several years and may require electroconvulsive therapy (ECT), antidepressant drugs or psychotherapy. Another important problem is that many patients do not conform to the tidy, stereotyped descriptions found in textbooks. They possess some, but not all, of the characteristic features of two or three different diagnostic categories and so have to be allocated more or less arbitrarily to whichever syndrome they seem to resemble most closely. As a result, disagreements about diagnosis are common-place, and hybrid terms like schizoaffective and borderline state have to be coined and pressed into service.

Many psychiatric diagnoses also have pejorative connotations. Terms like hysteric, neurotic, schizophrenic and psychopath are sometimes used as thinly disguised expressions of contempt, and even when this is not so the aura surrounding such terms can easily have harmful effects on the behaviour and attitudes of other people, and thus on the patient's own attitude to himself. Attaching a name to a condition may also create a spurious impression of under-standing. To say that a patient is suffering from schizophrenia actually means that he has some puzzling but familiar symptoms which have often been encountered before in other patients which are likely to reduce somewhat with treatment, but are also likely to denote a poor prognosis. To some psychiatrists, however, the impressive neologism 'schizophrenia' implies that the patient has a disease which was discovered by Kraepelin, or perhaps by Bleuler, which is fundamentally different from other diseases like bipolar disorder and whose cause will eventually be elucidated by medical science. Historically, of course, it has been very convenient for doctors to be able to conceal their ignorance from their patients by clothing it in Greek neologisms, but all too often they also deceive themselves. They 'reify' the diagnostic concept and treat the 'disease' instead of trying to relieve their patients' symptoms, anxieties and disabilities.

Diagnoses as concepts

It is important never to lose sight of the fact that all diseases and diagnostic categories are simply concepts. Schizophrenia and manic–depressive insanity were not discovered by either Kraepelin or Bleuler. It is closer to the truth to say that they were invented by them, and we continue to use the terms a century later only because the concepts they represent make it easier to make sense of the variegated phenomena of psychotic illness than it would otherwise be. The same is true, of course, of tuberculosis and migraine. To assert, as Szasz (1961) does, that 'there is no such thing as schizophrenia' is as trite an assertion as it would be to point out that there is no such thing as tuberculosis or poverty. None of these are objects; none has mass, velocity or position in

space. All of them are concepts which may in time lose their usefulness and pass out of use, as earlier concepts like phthisis and monomania have already done. But if this happens it will be because they have been replaced by other more useful concepts, not because of any sudden realisation that they do not exist. And, of course, to tell a bewildered patient who has been told he is suffering from schizophrenia that there is no such thing does not remove his disabilities, or prevent hallucinatory voices from tormenting him, any more than a man whose lungs have been destroyed by the tubercle bacillus would be prevented from dying by being told there was no such thing as tuberculosis.

Classification on the basis of symptoms

It is widely agreed that classifications of diseases should, wherever possible, be based on aetiology. This is simply because physicians have learnt by experience that aetiological classifications are almost invariably more useful than others. Classifications of infections based on the identity of the infecting organism are, for example, more useful than those based on purely clinical phenomena — the patient's fever, pulse rate, malaise and limb pains, the appearance of his tongue and the fetor on his breath — because they provide more information about the treatment required, the prognosis, and the risk to others. Unfortunately, apart from a few conditions like delirium tremens, Down syndrome and Wernicke's encephalopathy, the aetiology of most psychiatric disorders is still unknown, or all that is known for certain is that both genetic and environmental factors are involved. For this reason, most contemporary classifica-tions of psychiatric disorders are largely based on clinical symptoms, a term which includes the patients' complaints and abnormalities of subjective experience elicited by questioning, and clinical signs — a term referring to abnormalities of behaviour observed by the examiner (or described to him by others).

In all branches of medicine, diseases are usually defined initially by their clinical symptoms, largely because these are the overt manifestations of illness. They are the reasons why the patient seeks medical attention in the first place, or is identified as ill by other people. But in most other medical disciplines, apart perhaps from neurology and dermatology, this is no longer so. As their aetiology has slowly been elucidated, most diseases have come to be defined instead by the presence of some more fundamental characteristic — a distinctive morbid anatomy perhaps, or an infective agent or a biochemical defect. Phthisis, for example, which was originally defined by its symptoms and clinical course, became pulmonary tuberculosis, defined by a characteristic histology and the presence of *Mycobacterium tuberculosis*, when it became clear that this organism was ultimately responsible for the symptoms; and myxoedema, originally defined by the patient's complaints and appearance, became hypothyroidism, defined by an abnormally low serum thyroxine, when it was established that the syndrome was a consequence of thyroid deficiency. A few conditions, like migraine, trigeminal neuralgia and spasmodic torticollis, are still defined by their symptoms, but during the last hundred years these have dwindled to a small minority. We assume that the same transition will eventually take place for psychiatric disorders as their aetiology is slowly unravelled, but so far this has only occurred for a few conditions like Down syndrome and Creutzfeldt–Jakob disease. The majority are still defined, for the lack of something better, by their clinical features. In Scadding's terminology their defining characteristic is still their syndrome (Scadding 1967).

This has important consequences. Decisions about the presence or absence of symptoms are relatively unreliable: and, because few psychiatric illnesses have pathognomonic symptoms, most conditions have to be defined by the presence of some or most of a group of symptoms rather than by the presence of one key symptom. In the jargon of nosology they are *polythetic* rather than *monothetic*. This invites ambiguity and lowers reliability still further unless operational definitions are adopted (see below). Another important consequence is that most psychiatric diagnoses cannot be either confirmed or refuted, for there is no external criterion to appeal to. If two clinicians disagree about whether a patient is suffering from Creutzfeldt–Jakob Disease or Alzheimer's disease their disagreement can eventually be resolved by post-mortem examination of the brain, for the defining characteristic of both conditions is its histology. But if two clinicians disagree about whether a patient is suffering from a schizophrenic or an affective illness, no comparable criterion is available, for both schizophrenic and affective disorders are defined by their clinical syndromes. There is therefore no way of resolving the disagreement except by appeal to authority. One can only conclude either that the two clinicians have elicited different symptoms, or that they have different concepts (or are using different definitions) of schizophrenia and affective illness.

For these and other reasons it has often been suggested that symptoms should be ignored and a new classification developed on an entirely different basis. Psychoanalysts have frequently advocated a classification based on psychodynamic defence mechanisms and stages of libidinal development. In the 1950s, clinical psychologists extolled the advantages of a classification based on scores on batteries of cognitive and projective tests. More recently, learning theorists have argued that we should classify patients on the basis of a comprehensive analysis of their total behavioural repertoire. In principle all of these approaches are perfectly legitimate. In practice, however, none of them has ever progressed beyond the stage of advocacy. Although a series of different professional groups has, each in turn, proposed new classifications based on the mechanisms, scores, or behaviours they themselves were most interested in, none has ever made a serious attempt to develop, test and use the new classification they were advocating. It is likely that a classification based on psychodynamic defence mechanisms would be hamstrung by the low reliability common to all inferential judgements, that one based on cognitive and projective test results would yield even fewer useful therapeutic and prognostic distinctions than one based on symptoms, and that any classification aspiring to be based on an analysis of the patient's total behavioural repertoire would simply prove impracticable, but one can only suspect these things because such classifications have never been developed.

Two other alternatives are sometimes proposed: classification on the basis of treatment response and classification on the basis of the course or outcome of the illness. Unfortunately, neither is feasible. The fatal weakness of the treatment response proposal is that there are few, if any, specific treatments in psychiatry. Depressive, schizophrenic and manic illnesses may all respond to ECT; schizophrenic and manic illnesses or at least their 'positive' psychotic features both respond to antipsychotic drugs; depression and anxiety states both respond to antidepressants and cognitive psychotherapy; and so on. Worse still, these therapies are not mutually exclusive. The patient who responds to ECT often responds equally well to an antipsychotic. In any case, the fact that two disorders respond to the same treatment does not imply that they share the same aetiology.

Depression, panic attacks and nocturnal enuresis all respond to imipramine, and headaches, dysmenorrhoea, rheumatoid arthritis and rheumatic fever all respond to aspirin. Classification on the basis of outcome is equally impracticable, though for different reasons. One of the main functions of a diagnosis is to indicate the need for treatment, and the relative merits of different therapies. But if outcome were the defining characteristic, one would, logically, have to wait until the outcome was known before making the diagnosis and thus knowing which treatment to use. In any case most disorders, in psychiatry as in other branches of medicine, can have a wide range of outcomes. The fact that the patient recovered within a fortnight does not prove that he was suffering from chickenpox rather than smallpox; it merely makes it more likely. It is sometimes assumed that Kraepelin's classification, or at least his distinction between dementia praecox and manic–depressive insanity, was based on long-term outcome, but this is a misunderstanding. Kraepelin certainly emphasised the difference in the lifetime course of his two great rubrics, and perhaps subdivided the psychoses in the way that he did in order to maximise the difference in outcome between them. But he used outcome as a validating criterion (i.e. as evidence that his two rubries were fundamentally different disorders), not as a defining characteristic. Otherwise, when patients with dementia praecox recovered completely he would automatically have changed their diagnosis.

As things stand, therefore, we have no choice but to use a classification which is largely based on symptoms, despite its shortcomings and imperfections, because no practical alternative has yet been developed. Some psychologists have argued that we should identify, study and treat specific symptoms rather than diagnoses, but do not appear to appreciate the therapeutic implications of, for example, 'polypharmacy'.

THE DIAGNOSTIC INTERVIEW

So far, we have discussed why psychiatric disorders have to be classified and why that classification is based on symptoms. We have also noted that all diagnoses are arbitrary concepts, liable to be altered or discarded as circumstances change, and that psychiatric diagnoses are particularly likely to be misunderstood and misused. We must now consider the important practical implications of these decisions — in particular, how to elicit the patient's symptoms as completely and as reliably as possible, and how to make the appropriate diagnosis when this has been done. As the general principles of psychiatric interviewing are described in detail in Chapter 13, only matters bearing specifically on diagnostic interviews need be discussed here.

The conduct of the interview

Traditionally, psychiatrists, like other physicians, have usually detected symptoms by holding a free-ranging interview with the patient, and sometimes with his relatives also, and have assumed that the symptoms they elicited were present and that those they failed to elicit were absent. Unfortunately, these happy assumptions are unwarranted, as the reliability studies carried out in the 1950s quickly revealed. A well-known study of the reliability of clinical ratings made under ordinary National Health Service working conditions illustrates the scale of the problem. A series of 90 patients referred to an English mental hospital were re-interviewed by one of two research psychiatrists a few days after being seen as outpatients or on a domiciliary consultation by one of three consultants. All five of these interviewers recorded the presence or absence of 24 key symptoms in each patient. Despite having discussed their criteria beforehand, the average 'positive percentage agreement' between the first and second interviewers was only 46% (Kreitman et al 1961). In other words, when one psychiatrist recorded a symptom as present there was barely a 50:50 chance of his colleague agreeing with him. Diagnostic reliability has improved greatly since this time, at least for the major psychiatric disorders — probably due to the widespread use of diagnostic criteria — but remains little better than chance for some relatively 'minor' disorders, especially those of personality and for some key symptoms (see below).

Many factors contribute to this low reliability. There are behavioural differences between one interviewer and another. They ask different questions, show interest and probe further in different places, establish different sorts of relationship with their patients, and so on (see diagnostic/exposure suspicion bias in Chapter 11 on research methods). Their preconceptions are also important. If two interviewers are expecting to find different symptoms, both may succeed in fulfilling their expectations by means of subtle differences in the wording of their questions, and in the way in which they interpret ambiguous replies. Further, closed and forceful interviewing techniques can encourage patients to agree with doctors' perceptions (see 'obsequiousness bias'). Finally, important conceptual differences are often involved. Common terms like 'anxiety', 'delusion' and 'thought disorder' may be used in rather different ways by different psychiatrists without their being aware of the fact; and even when there is no disagreement over the meaning of a term, there is often disagreement over the extent to which graded characteristics, like depression or insomnia, have to be present to justify a positive rating. At worst, the diagnosis can influence the psychopathology detected. For example, a lack of emotional expression in schizophrenia may be called blunt or flat affect, but retardation in a patient with depression.

Because of these problems, unstructured interviewing methods are no longer used for research purposes. 'Structured' or 'standardised' interviews are employed instead. These specify not only, as rating scales do, the way in which symptoms are recorded, but also the manner in which they are elicited. Definitions, implicit or explicit, are provided for each item, and, subject to varying degrees of flexibility, the questions the patient is asked, and their order, are predetermined and ratings are made serially as the interview progresses rather than collectively at the end. The Present State Examination (Wing et al 1974) and the Diagnostic Interview Schedule (Robins et al 1981), now incorporated into the SCAN and CIDI respectively (see Chapter 11), are widely used examples; with such instruments, trained raters achieve considerably higher reliability than is possible under ordinary clinical conditions.

Structured interviews of this kind are generally unsuitable for ordinary clinical purposes, mainly because they are not sufficiently flexible. The need to cover a wide range of symptomatology makes them either too long or too sketchy, and they do not permit that rapid focusing on the patient's main difficulties that is the essence of a good assessment interview. Even so, much of the discipline involved in structured interviewing can be incorporated into any information-gathering interview. Most of the principles involved are simple enough, even self-evident, but this does not stop them being flouted, even by experienced clinicians who ought to know better. Knowing how to conduct a diagnostic interview — when to give the patient free rein and when to interrupt him, which

areas to concentrate on, and how to phrase one's questions so as to focus the patient's replies without putting words into his mouth — is a skill which is best learned by experience, although not necessarily acquired with it. Knowing how to interpret what the patient says and what information is necessary to establish the presence of particular symptoms is, or ought to be, a more simple matter. If the interviewer understands, and different interviewers agree, precisely what is meant by the technical terms like depersonalisation and delusion of control that are used to describe symptomatology, it will usually be clear to him what information he needs to establish the presence of the symptom in question. The problem is essentially one of definition. Adequate definitions are not provided in any systematic way in most textbooks, or even in psychiatric dictionaries or glossaries, and much of the low reliability of clinical ratings is attributable to this. A fairly comprehensive list can be found in the manual of the Present State Examination (Wing et al 1974).

Information from relatives

It is a sound principle always to obtain a collateral history from a relative, colleague or friend, if possible before making any decisions about management. Often 10 minutes will suffice to establish that the relative's perception of the situation is essentially the same as the patient's, but it is commonplace for his account to differ in important ways. He may describe a more alarming situation than the patient has admitted to, or make it clear that the symptoms the patient complains of are not a new development but have been present on and off for years. It is particularly important to get an independent history from someone else if there is any suspicion of alcohol or drug abuse. The capacity of people with alcohol problems to minimise or gloss over the ways in which their drinking has disrupted their lives is difficult to exaggerate, and the diagnosis will be missed time and again if the patient's account is accepted unchallenged.

THE RELATIONSHIP BETWEEN SYMPTOMS AND DIAGNOSIS

For the reasons discussed previously, diagnoses are mainly based on symptoms — the patient's complaints and descriptions of abnormal subjective experiences and the behavioural abnormalities evident on examination or reported by others. Other factors — like the patient's age, sex and personality and the previous course of the illness — are certainly taken into account, but the patient's symptoms, past and present, are the main determinants. Unfortunately, it is only comparatively recently that we have appreciated the need to specify the relationship between symptoms and diagnosis. Textbooks have always made it clear that the characteristic symptoms of schizophrenia, for example, were thought disorder, auditory hallucinations and delusions of control; that the characteristic symptoms of depression were anhedonia, retardation and early morning wakening; that the characteristic features of obsessional disorder were persistent, disabling compulsive acts or ruminations, and so on. They have not made it clear, however, which diagnosis should be attributed to someone with auditory hallucinations alone; or with obsessional ruminations in the presence of severe depression. As a result, psychiatrists frequently made different diagnoses when confronted with such situations, and diagnostic reliability was low.

What was needed were *rules of application* or *operational definitions* specifying the appropriate diagnosis for every possible combination of symptoms. Instead of simply listing the typical features of diagnosis X as A, B, C and sometimes D, as they had generally done in the past, textbooks and glossaries needed to say something like this: before diagnosis X can be made, A must be present, together with at least one of B, C and D, and E must be absent. As with symptoms themselves, the problem is primarily a matter of adequate definition. In the last 30 years, operational definitions of this kind have slowly come into widespread use. In 1972 Eli Robins and his colleagues in St Louis published operational criteria for 15 major diagnostic categories (Feighner et al 1972); since then, many alternative operational definitions have been published for most of the main syndromes, and their use has become the norm in clinical research. The most decisive change, however, was the American Psychiatric Association's decision to provide an operational definition for almost every diagnostic category in the third edition of its Diagnostic and Statistical Manual (DSM-III) (APA 1980). As a result, since 1980, American psychiatrists have been committed to using operational definitions for all their diagnostic terms, not just in research but in everyday clinical practice as well. (Incidentally, however, many senior American psychiatrists now lament their trainees' over-reliance on such criteria and their inability to conduct wider-ranging psychiatric interviews — see for example, Andreasen 2001).

The difference between these two types of definition, the descriptive and the operational, is best illustrated by an example. In the previous (ninth) revision of the International Classification of Disease (ICD-9), drug dependence was defined thus (WHO 1978):

A state, psychic and sometimes also physical, resulting from taking a drug, characterized by behavioural and other responses that always include a compulsion to take a drug on a continuous or periodic basis in order to experience its psychic effects, and sometimes to avoid the discomfort of its absence. Tolerance may or may not be present. A person may be dependent on more than one drug.

In contrast, the Dependence syndrome is defined by the research criteria of its successor, the tenth revision (ICD-10) as follows (WHO 1993):

Three or more of the following manifestations should have occurred together for at least 1 month or, if persisting for periods of less than 1 month, should have occurred together repeatedly within a 12-month period:
1. *a strong desire or sense of compulsion to take the substance;*
2. *impaired capacity to control substance-taking behaviour in terms of its onset, termination, or levels of use, as evidenced by: the substance being often taken in larger amounts or over a longer period than intended; or by a persistent desire or unsuccessful efforts to reduce or control substance use;*
3. *a physiological withdrawal state when substance use is reduced or ceased (sic), as evidenced by the characteristic withdrawal syndrome for the substance, or by use of the same (or closely related) substance with the intention of relieving or avoiding withdrawal symptoms;*
4. *evidence of tolerance to the effects of the substance, such that there is a need for significantly increased amounts of the substance to achieve intoxication or the desired effect, or a markedly diminished effect with continued use of the same amount of the substance;*
5. *preoccupation with substance use, as manifested by important alternative pleasures or interests being given up or reduced because of substance use; or a great deal of time being spent in activities necessary to obtain, take, or recover from the effects of the substance;*
6. *persistent substance use despite clear evidence of harmful consequences, as evidenced by continued use when the individual is actually aware, or may be expected to be aware, of the nature and extent of harm.*

Knowing that a patient was diagnosed as drug dependent using ICD-9 criteria was hardly more informative than knowing that he was so diagnosed 'by an experienced psychiatrist', or according to the description in a particular textbook, whereas to know that the ICD-10 research criteria were used gives a fairly precise indication of the behaviour he needed to display in order to qualify. This does, of course, require reliable interviewing, and leads to problems where, for example, only two rather than three or more features are present, but is surely an improvement on the former.

Diagnostic hierarchies

Insofar as there is a formal structure to the relationship between symptoms and diagnoses, it is hierarchical. At the top of this hierarchy come the so-called organic psychoses. If there is evidence of brain disease — perhaps clinical or EEG evidence of epilepsy or definite cognitive impairment — this overrides all other considerations, and whatever other symptoms the patient has, psychotic or neurotic, the diagnosis is organic. Schizophrenia has traditionally come next in the hierarchy. To many European psychiatrists, certain symptoms are regarded as diagnostic of schizophrenia, regardless of which other symptoms are also present, provided only that there is no question of cerebral disease. The 'symptoms of the first rank' which Schneider (1959) regarded as pathognomonic of schizophrenia 'except in the presence of coarse brain disease' constitute an explicit statement of this convention, and other clinicians have attached a similar significance to symptoms like thought disorder and incongruity of affect. For Schneider and his successors, third place in the hierarchy was occupied by the affective disorders. Even if the characteristic features of mania or melancholia were unmistakably present, organic or schizophrenic symptoms took precedence. As a result, patients with both schizophrenic and affective symptoms are regarded as suffering from schizophrenia, and were so classified in ICD-9. In ICD-10, however, schizophrenic and affective disorders are both at the same level. A diagnosis of schizophrenia cannot be made if the full depressive or manic syndrome is also present 'unless it is clear that schizophrenic symptoms antedated the affective disturbance'. Neurotic, stress-related and somatoform disorders come at the bottom of the hierarchy. In general, any given diagnosis *excludes* the presence of the symptoms of all higher members of the hierarchy and *embraces* the symptoms of all lower members.

It is no coincidence that the order in which diagnostic categories are arranged in the international and other classifications is the same as in this hierarchy, for both reflect the sequence of questions psychiatrists commonly ask themselves when arriving at a diagnosis. Indeed, a very similar sequence is involved in the decision pathways of computer programs for generating diagnoses, like Catego (Wing et al 1974). The psychologist Graham Foulds suggested that this structure was inherent in the nature of psychiatric illness, but it is more likely that it is a man-made convention.

It is a firm principle in medicine that every effort should be made to account for the patient's symptoms by a single diagnosis. In a situation in which most individual symptoms are liable to be encountered in the presence of a wide range of other symptoms, this is difficult to achieve unless the defining characteristics of different illnesses are in a hierarchical relationship to one another, with the least common symptoms at the top and the most common at the bottom. There is also some empirical justification for this arrangement. For example, when schizophrenic and depressive symptoms coexist, as they often do, the patient's prognosis and response to treatment are determined more by the former than by the latter, so if only one diagnosis is allowable it is more appropriate to regard the patient as suffering from schizophrenia than from depression. On the other hand, if patients do meet criteria for both, they are likely to benefit from both antipsychotics and antidepressants. This hierarchy was, however, largely abandoned by the American Psychiatric Association in 1987. In its revision of DSM-III (DSM-IIIR) the hierarchical relationship between depressive disorders and anxiety disorders was dropped, though that between organic and other disorders was retained. As a result, in both clinical and community studies, a high proportion of people fulfilling criteria for a depressive disorder were found to fulfil criteria for an anxiety disorder of some kind as well, a phenomenon which came to be known as comorbidity (Krueger 1999).

INTERNATIONAL DIFFERENCES IN DIAGNOSTIC CONCEPTS AND CRITERIA

As described above, until comparatively recently the relationship between symptoms and diagnoses was vague and ill defined. Many technical terms — like thought disorder, dependency and immaturity — were also poorly defined. As a result, trainees could only learn how to make diagnoses by modelling themselves on their teachers. In the absence of adequate rules the only way to learn which of their patients should be regarded as suffering, for example, from schizophrenia was to observe which patients their mentors gave this diagnosis to and do likewise. Diagnostic criteria were therefore at the mercy of the personal views and idiosyncrasies of influential teachers, and also liable to be affected by therapeutic fashions and innovations, and changing assumptions about aetiology. This led to the development of substantial differences in the way in which several key diagnostic terms were used in different centres. The less contact there was between two centres — and national boundaries and language differences were substantial impediments to such contact — the more likely it was that progressive differences in diagnostic usage would develop.

The best-documented of these differences in usage were those that developed between Britain and the USA in the 1940s and 1950s. The comparative studies carried out by the US/UK Diagnostic Project in the 1960s established that, in comparable series of patients, psychiatrists in New York diagnosed schizophrenia twice as frequently as their counterparts in London. Patients regarded in London as suffering from depressive illnesses or mania, or even from neurotic illnesses or personality disorders, were often diagnosed as schizophrenic in New York (Cooper et al 1972). The International Pilot Study of Schizophrenia confirmed that American psychiatrists had an unusually broad concept of schizophrenia, and also showed that the same was true, for quite different reasons, of Russian psychiatrists (WHO 1973). Of the nine centres involved, seven (London, Prague, Aarhus in Denmark,

Ibadan in Nigeria, Agra in India, Cali in Colombia and Taipei in Taiwan) shared a similar concept of schizophrenia, but Washington and Moscow both had a much broader concept. In Europe the situation was complicated by the fact that Norwegian and Danish psychiatrists made frequent use of a diagnosis of reactive or psychogenic psychosis which embraced many patients who would have been regarded as having schizophrenic or affective psychoses in Britain or Germany. And French psychiatrists used a number of categories like *délire chronique* and *bouffée délirante* which had no obvious counterpart in other nomenclatures. These differences are now disappearing, and for the younger generation of psychiatrists are already a thing of the past. The very broad American concept of schizophrenia was psychoanalytic in origin, and the decline of psychoanalytic influence in the 1970s, together with a renewed interest in descriptive psychopathology and classification, led to a rapid change. Indeed, the contemporary American concept of schizophrenia embodied in the operational criteria of DSM-IV is narrower than that of ICD-10. The adoption of the operational definitions of DSM-IV or ICD-10 in most parts of the world has also played a crucial role both in accustoming everyone to use the same diagnostic terms and in reducing international differences in usage.

It is important to realise that it is meaningless to ask who is right where any of these differences, past or present, are concerned. If two individual psychiatrists disagree about a diagnosis we are accustomed to assume that whichever of the two is more experienced, or whom we respect the more, is probably right. But if experienced psychiatrists in different centres consistently disagree with one another when presented with identical information, all one can say is that they have different concepts of that condition. The same is true of two psychiatrists using different operational definitions of the same syndrome. One can check that they are both using their respective definitions appropriately, but beyond that one can only conclude that the two definitions embrace different populations of patients. But although it is meaningless to ask who is *right*, it is perfectly legitimate, and necessary, to ask which concept or definition is more *useful*. Essentially, the choice between alternative definitions is, or should be, an issue of validity. If we knew more about the aetiology of psychiatric disorders we could decide which of the two alternative definitions of the syndrome correlated better with the underlying abnormality, just as we could easily decide which clinical definition of mitral stenosis was most reliably associated with narrowing of the mitral valve, or which clinical definition of Alzheimer's disease was most reliably associated with the characteristic histopathology of that condition. In the absence of this knowledge all we can do is ask which of the competing definitions most successfully meets some arbitrary criterion like homogeneity of outcome or treatment response. Unfortunately, different criteria may be best satisfied by different definitions, so the problem is not resolved. For example, the definition of schizophrenia which most successfully identifies patients who subsequently develop a defect state and become chronic invalids is different from the definition with the highest heritability (i.e. which gives the highest monozygotic: dizygotic concordance ratio in twin populations). We have to accept, therefore, that until we know more about the aetiology of the various syndromes we recognise and treat we cannot be sure how they should best be defined. As a result, we have to accept the coexistence of a number of rival operational definitions of syndromes like schizophrenia, and, in some areas like the personality disorders, of rival categories and classifications.

THE NATURE OF MENTAL DISORDER

If individual mental or psychiatric disorders are to be given operational definitions it would seem logical, even essential, for the parent concepts of disease (or disorder) and mental disorder to be provided with operational definitions themselves. To put the matter at its simplest, any organisation aspiring to produce a classification of diseases or mental disorders for general use ought to have a clear, public view of the nature of the diseases or disorders under consideration. In fact, medicine has never had an agreed definition of the term 'disease', or of illness, and most physicians naively assume that their meanings are self-evident. Significantly, the World Health Organization (WHO) has always avoided defining 'disease', or 'illness', or 'disorder' in the successive revisions of its International Classification of Disease (ICD); in its current (ICD-10) Classification of Mental and Behavioural Disorders it simply states that 'the term disorder is used throughout the classification, so as to avoid even greater problems inherent in the use of terms such as disease and illness. Disorder is not an exact term . . . it is used here to imply the existence of a clinically recognizable set of symptoms or behaviour associated in most cases with distress and with interference with personal functions' (WHO 1992). Recent editions of the Diagnostic and Statistical Manual (DSM) produced by the American Psychiatric Association (APA) have provided a detailed definition of the term 'mental disorder', but although this runs to 146 words in the current (DSM-IV) edition, it is preceded by a statement that 'no definition adequately specifies precise boundaries for the concept of mental disorder'. Although the APA's definition cannot be used as a criterion for determining what is and is not mental disorder, it does contain some important statements. It starts by observing that, unfortunately, the term 'mental disorder' implies a distinction between mental disorders and physical disorders 'that is a reductionistic anachronism of mind/body dualism'. It then makes it clear that the term 'mental disorder' — which it only continues to use for lack of any obviously more appropriate alternative — implies the presence 'of a dysfunction in the individual', and that this dysfunction may be 'behavioural, psychological or biological'. It is also emphasised that 'neither deviant behaviour nor conflicts between the individual and society' are mental disorders unless they are a symptom of 'dysfunction in the individual' (APA 1994).

Carefully chosen phrases such as these conceal the fact that several incompatible conceptions of disease or disorder are currently in competition, with little immediate prospect of a resolution. Because their underlying assumptions and implications are so different, all physicians, particularly psychiatrists, ought to be familiar with the main sources of disagreement. Four principal stances can be distinguished:

1. that disease is *a biological dysfunction* (an assumption made by most physicians). The most widely quoted purely biological definition is that of Scadding (1967), for whom disease was 'the sum of the abnormal phenomena displayed by a group of living organisms in association with a specified common characteristic or set of characteristics by which they differ from the norm for the species in such a way as to place them at a biological disadvantage'. Clearly, reduced life expectancy and impaired fertility are biological disadvantages, but many diseases, including many mental disorders, involve neither.

2. that disease is *a social concept* (an assumption made by most social scientists). The simplest plausible social definition is perhaps that a condition is regarded as a disease if it is agreed to be undesirable (an explicit value judgement) and it seems on balance that physicians (or health professionals in general) and their technologies are more likely to be able to deal with it effectively than any of the potential alternatives, such as the criminal justice system (treating it as crime), the church (treating it as sin) or social work (treating it as a social problem). This implies that, for example, the issue of whether restless, overactive children with short attention spans are best regarded as suffering from Attention Deficit Hyperactivity Disorder, or just as boisterous, difficult children, will depend simply on whether child psychiatrists are better at ameliorating the problem than parents and teachers. Worse, social desirability can change: for example, homosexuality was regarded as a disorder in the 1960s but is no longer.

3. that disease is *both a biological dysfunction and a social concept*. It may be argued that mental disorders are biological dysfunctions which are also harmful (again, a value judgement). Although this approach has the attraction of resolving the conflict between 1 and 2 above, it fails (as does the APA's definition of mental disorder) to provide an adequate means of recognising or defining the putative biological dysfunction underlying a clinical syndrome whose aetiology is largely unknown.

4. that disease is *an ostensive or Roschian concept*. This implies that disease is inherently indefinable. It is simply illustrated by its prototypes — which in the case of mental disorder might be schizophrenia or depressive disorder — and judgements about whether other similar conditions are also mental disorders can only be based on their degree of similarity to the agreed prototypes.

These rival conceptions of disease or disorder are not of merely theoretical interest. They have important implications for several controversial issues concerning mental disorders. For example, accepting that disease and mental disorder are ostensive concepts would explain why medicine seems to be incapable of defining these fundamental terms. The social concept of disease quoted above could provide a convincing answer to the accusation, often heard in North America, that psychiatrists are constantly inventing new and spurious mental disorders in order to increase their influence and their incomes. This social concept could also, unlike the other three definitions, enable 'relational disorders' (in which the complaint, and the focus of therapy, is on the relationship between two or more people rather than on an individual) to be regarded as mental disorders and included in psychiatric nosologies.

CONTEMPORARY CLASSIFICATIONS

The international classification

International classifications of mental disorders have existed for over one hundred years but had little influence before the late 1960s. In response to strenuous efforts by WHO, most countries were then persuaded to sacrifice their own traditions and aspirations in the interests of international communication and to use the nomenclature and definitions of the eighth revision of the *International Classification of Diseases, Injuries and Causes of*

Death (ICD-8), which came into use in 1969. This eighth revision was replaced by a ninth (ICD-9) a decade later (WHO 1978).

If one compares the successive revisions of the ICD from the sixth in 1948 to the ninth in 1978, each was an improvement on its predecessor. The mental disorders section of ICD-6 was primarily a classification of psychoses and mental deficiency. Its successors provided much more adequate coverage of commoner, less handicapping disorders, of the disorders of childhood, and of the wide range of conditions attributable to alcohol and drugs. Many new terms were introduced, a few obsolete ones like involutional melancholia were discarded, and every category was provided with a brief description. Despite these improvements the inherent problems associated with an international classification became more apparent with each revision. The brief descriptions provided in ICD-8 and ICD-9 were not operational definitions. They were simply 'thumbnail sketches' of the clinical concept in question. They described its essential features well enough but did not provide rules of application. A more fundamental problem was that radical change of any kind was very difficult to effect, because every country had to be willing to accept whatever innovations were introduced, and any attempt to force the pace risked damaging the fragile international consensus on which the whole enterprise was based. Another major problem was that, because national representatives were always prepared to argue more force-fully for the inclusion of their own favourite terms than they were to oppose the efforts of others to do likewise, there was a constant tendency for the classification to expand by incorporating alterna-tive and sometimes incompatible concepts. ICD-9 contained no less than 13 categories for patients with depressive symptoms, because in effect several different ways of classifying depressions were included alongside one another.

The tenth revision (ICD-10)

The text of ICD-10 was published in 1992 and came into use in the UK and most other countries in 1993. It had a new title — the *International Statistical Classification of Diseases and Related Health Problems* — and a new alphanumeric format (WHO 1992). The main purpose of the latter is to provide more categories (there are 26 letters in the alphabet, but only 10 digits) and so leave space for future expansion without the whole classification having to be changed. Each section has either 100, 1000, or 10 000 categories, depending on how many digits are used. The general format of the section entitled 'Mental, behavioural and developmental disorders' (F00–F99) is very similar to that of the APA's recent classifications because it incorporates many of the radical innovations introduced in DSM-III (see below). The traditional distinction between psychoses and neuroses has been laid aside, though the terms themselves are retained, and all mood (affective) disorders are brought together in a single grouping (F3). All disorders due to the use of psychoactive substances, including alcohol, have also been brought together under a common format (F1). Field trials of the 1986 draft text were held in 194 different centres in 55 different countries, and the final text benefited greatly from the comments of users in these very varied settings, and the evidence they provided of the acceptability, coverage and inter-rater reliability of the categories and definitions of that draft. Most categories in the final text are provided with both 'diagnostic guidelines' for everyday clinical use (WHO 1992) and separate 'diagnostic criteria for research' (WHO 1993). The classification will remain in use for considerably longer than the 10 years for

which ICD-6 to ICD-9 were each used, and may indeed be used by today's young psychiatrists for most of their careers.

The American Psychiatric Association's classifications

The first edition of the APA's *Diagnostic and Statistical Manual of Mental Disorders* (DSM-I) was published in 1952. Its format reflected the dominant Meyerian philosophy of the time and, although its influence was limited, it was the first official nomen-clature to provide a glossary of descriptions of the diagnostic cate-gories it listed. The second edition (DSM-II), published in 1968, was, like the corresponding WHO glossary, a national glossary to the nomenclature of ICD-8, the APA having been persuaded on this occasion to sacrifice its own diagnostic preferences in the interests of international conformity.

DSM-III

The third edition (DSM-III), published in 1980, was radically different from any previous classification (APA 1980). Its inno-vations were a response to the evidence that had accumulated over the previous 20 years that psychiatric diagnoses were generally unreliable, that there were systematic differences in the usage of key terms like schizophrenia between the USA and other parts of the world, and that major changes were needed to the overall format both of the international and of other existing classi-fications. It was also evidence of a sea change in the orientation of American psychiatry: the end of the psychodynamic era and the dawn of a new biological or 'neo-Kraepelinian' era. For the first time, almost every diagnostic category was given an operational definition to make it as clear as possible which patients were and were not covered by that rubric. Although this made the manual five times the size of its predecessors — and involved much discus-sion, argument and persuasion as well as extensive field trials in order to secure the necessary agreement — the result, as the field trials demonstrated, was that the reliability of most of its 200 categories was far higher than in any previous classification.

DSM-III was also a multiaxial classification with separate axes allowing the systematic recording of five different information sets: the clinical syndrome (Axis I); lifelong disorders or handicaps and specific developmental disorders (Axis II); associated physical conditions (Axis III); the severity of psychosocial stressors (Axis IV); and the highest level of social and occupational functioning in the past year (Axis V). The clinical syndromes coded on Axis I were also arranged in a novel sequence. In particular, the tradi-tional distinction between neuroses and psychoses was abandoned, mainly to allow all affective disorders to be brought together. A further important change was that most diagnostic terms were either explicitly divested of their aetiological implications or replaced by new terms devoid of such assumptions. As a result, many of the hallowed terms of psychiatry, like hysteria and manic–depressive illness, and even psychosis and neurosis, were discarded and replaced by stark, utilitarian terms like somatoform disorder, factitious disorder and paraphilia.

Classifications always tend to be controversial, if only because they involve fundamental concepts and important philosophical assumptions. Initially, DSM-III and its principal architect, Robert Spitzer, were bitterly criticised by many senior American psychiatrists for discarding the concept of neurosis and for introducing what they regarded as a crude 'Chinese menu' approach to diagnosis.

Such objections were elegantly expressed by Cancro (1983), who recommended that a few lines of Wordsworth could usefully be printed on every copy of DSM-III:

> *That false secondary Power*
> *By which we multiply distinctions, then*
> *Deem that our puny boundaries are things*
> *That we perceive and not that we have made.*

Clinical researchers and the younger generation of American psychiatrists, on the other hand, welcomed the new classification with enthusiasm (Jampala et al 1986) and it was soon clear the DSM-III was going to have a major influence on American psychiatry, particularly on clinical and biological research. Indeed, within a few years of its publication it had become an all-time psychiatric best-seller and made huge profits for the APA. It had also been translated into 13 other languages, and its operational definitions were being widely used in many countries. DSM-III also led to important changes in American usage of several diagnostic terms (Loranger 1990). Fewer patients were considered to have schizophrenia, and more were diagnosed as having unipolar or bipolar affective disorders. The creation of a separate axis and the provision of operational definitions also resulted in more extensive use of personality disorder diagnoses as well as a welcome increase in research into personality disorder.

DSM-IIIR

DSM-III was replaced by an extensive revision, DSM-IIIR, in 1987 (APA 1987). No fundamental changes were involved but a substantial number of minor alterations were introduced, including small changes to the wording of many of the 200 operational definitions. The classification of sleep disorders was expanded, mental retardation was moved from Axis I to Axis II, one or two categories were dropped (including homosexuality, even if egodystonic) and a few new ones introduced. DSM-III's hierarchical relationship between depressive and anxiety disorders was also abandoned, thus allowing several of these disorders to be present simultaneously. Individually, most of these changes were improvements. They involved either the correction of mistakes or misjudgements, or rational responses to new evidence, or to a change in the climate of opinion. Even so, it is doubtful whether it was wise to introduce a new classification after only 7 years, with all the disruption to newly established clinical concepts, to clinical and epidemiological research, and to clinical training programmes that new definitions inevitably involve.

DSM-IV

This further revision, published in 1994, was based on comprehensive literature reviews and analyses of several large data sets by 13 work groups (APA 1994). The most important change from DSM-III was that all decisions about the inclusion or exclusion of individual syndromes, and the detailed wording of their operational definitions, were based wherever possible on a systematic review of all relevant evidence rather than on expert opinion. A requirement that 'the disturbance causes clinically significant distress or impairment in social, occupational, or other important areas of functioning' was also added to the definitions of many syndromes. This was an attempt to restrict their application to people whose symptoms were genuinely clinically significant (i.e. handicapping and meriting treatment) made in response to criticisms of the unexpectedly high

prevalence of mental disorders in the American population as measured by surveys based on the definitions of DSM-III and -IIIR. DSM-IV has been even more successful than its predecessors, both financially and in the extent of its influence. It is widely used, at least for research purposes, throughout the world, has been translated into innumerable languages and had sold over one million six hundred thousand copies by the end of 2000.

Differences between ICD-10 and DSM-IV

The mental and behavioural disorders section of the ICD is one of 17 components of a comprehensive classification of all 'diseases and related health problems' and it has to meet the needs of, and formally secure the approval of, nearly two hundred countries throughout the world. The DSM, on the other hand, is produced by a national professional association to meet the needs of its own members, American psychiatrists. That fundamental difference virtually ensures that there will be differences between them. Even so, the APA and the staff of the WHO tried hard to minimise the differences between ICD-10 and DSM-IV. Unfortunately, because of the prior commitment to producing DSM-IIIR, the task force responsible for DSM-IV was not set up until 1988, by which time the main framework of ICD-10 had already been decided (Kendell 1991). As a result, the APA's task force was forced to choose between accepting the terminology and definitions of ICD-10 in order to harmonise the two nosologies as closely as possible, or accepting the recommendations of the work groups it had set up to produce draft proposals for the format and content of each individual section. Almost inevitably, it chose the latter. There are therefore many differences between the two nosologies, though none is sufficiently fundamental to make them incompatible, and in fact DSM-IV contains an appendix listing the ICD-10 codes corresponding to all its constituent categories of disorder. Some of the differences reflect important conceptual differences. Schizophrenia, for example, is required to have a minimum duration of 6 months by the DSM but of only 1 month by the ICD, chronicity being integral to the American concept of schizophrenia but not to the WHO concept. Most of the differences, however, are fairly trivial: minor differences in the number and names of subtypes of a major category (again, schizophrenia is an example) or, more commonly, seemingly trivial differences in the wording of operational definitions. Unfortunately, several of these definitional differences have important practical consequences. Andrews et al (1999) administered the Composite International Diagnostic Interview (CIDI) to 1500 Australians and compared the ICD-10 and DSM-IV diagnoses it generated. Overall, concordance between the two was only 68%. For some individual disorders like depressive episode and dysthymia it was over 80%, but for others, like substance abuse and post-traumatic stress disorder, it was as low as 33%.

The ICD is used by all countries, including the USA, for their annual statistical returns to WHO. It is also widely used by clinicians in Europe, Africa and Asia, but less so in the Americas. DSM-IV is used by all American psychiatrists and other healthcare professionals for routine clinical purposes, and used throughout the world for much clinical and epidemiological research. Neither is likely to replace the other in the foreseeable future.

Future classifications

Until more is known about the aetiology of the major syndromes like schizophrenia, bipolar disorder and obsessive–compulsive disorder it is unlikely that any future classification will be greatly superior to DSM-IV and ICD-10. Literature reviews, follow-up investigations, family studies, therapeutic trials and laborious analyses of sets of ratings derived from structured interviews with representative populations can only take us so far. Apart from one or two under-researched areas like the personality disorders, we may already be approaching the limits of what can be achieved by traditional clinical and epidemiological means. We should not be in a hurry, therefore, to develop new versions of comprehensive, formal classifications like the DSM and the ICD. It would be better to wait and see what novel concepts are introduced over the next decade by individual research groups, and what insights are gained from burgeoning developments in the neurosciences and human genetics. Other branches of medicine did not progress by a dogged pursuit of better and better classifications of their subject matter. They did so by acquiring new technologies, by developing radically new concepts and by elucidating fundamental mechanisms.

Although the APA is already committed to producing a DSM-V, its authors will face a fundamental dilemma. New classifications always have disadvantages as well as advantages because any change, however minor, is disruptive. A change in the wording of the operational definition of a disorder, for example, potentially changes almost everything that is known about that disorder — its incidence and prevalence, its response to therapeutic agents and its outcome. It will also involve changes in the questions asked by structured interviews like the CIDI and in computer programs. The disruption caused by major changes is often not much greater than that produced by minor ones, and the former are more likely to have real advantages to offset their disadvantages. For this reason, minor changes ought to be kept to a minimum, and restricted to the elimination of obvious anomalies.

There is another, more fundamental, reason for delay. It is becoming increasingly unlikely that any of the major syndromes of psychiatry is a 'disease entity'. Most attempts to demonstrate natural boundaries between related syndromes, or between a common syndrome like depression and normality, have ended in failure (Kendell & Jablensky 2003). It is increasingly probable that many different genes contribute to the aetiology of most of the major syndromes, and some of these genes appear to be risk factors for what have until now been regarded as unrelated syndromes, like schizophrenia and bipolar disorder. Environmental stress like abuse or neglect in childhood are likewise risk factors for several different disorders in adult life. The extent of comorbidity between depressive, anxiety and substance misuse disorders revealed by community surveys like the American National Comorbidity Survey also suggest that these disorders share major determinants and are not the independent conditions we often implicitly assume (Krueger 1999). Existing classifications do not reflect any of these complex relationships. But it is not yet clear what changes — possibly very fundamental changes — are required. As Allen Frances, chairman of the taskforce that produced DSM-IV, recently observed 'we are at the epicycle stage of psychiatry where astronomy was before Copernicus and biology before Darwin. Our inelegant and complex descriptive system will undoubtedly be replaced by ... simpler, more elegant models' (Frances & Egger 1999). It seems increasingly likely, in other words, that psychiatric nosology may be building up to a fundamental paradigm change. If that is so, it is not a good time to impose numerous minor changes on our existing classifications.

THE RELIABILITY AND VALIDITY OF PSYCHIATRIC DIAGNOSIS

Reliability

The reliability of psychiatric diagnoses is usually measured in one of two ways. Either a diagnostic interview is watched by a passive observer who makes his own independent diagnosis at the end (*observer method*), or else a second diagnostician conducts an independent interview with the patient a few hours or days after the first (*re-interview method*). The former overestimates reliability because all variation in the conduct of the interview is eliminated; the latter may underestimate it because the subject's clinical state may change in the interval between the two interviews, and he may react differently to the second interview simply because it is a repetition of the first.

Many reliability studies were carried out in the 1950s and 1960s and most of them found reliability to be depressingly low. The studies of Beck in Philadelphia and Kreitman in Chichester are often quoted because they were well designed and the participants were all experienced psychiatrists. Both used the re-interview method. Beck obtained 54% agreement for specific diagnosis, compared with the 15–19% agreement that could have arisen by chance alone. Kreitman, using a restricted range of 11 diagnostic categories, obtained 63% agreement.

There are three main ways of reducing disagreement: using structured or standardised interviews to minimise variation in the conduct of the interview; providing definitions for all the items of psychopathology covered by that interview (which together will help to minimise disagreements about which symptoms the subject exhibits); and using operational definitions to ensure that any given combination of symptoms always leads to the same diagnosis.

It has been shown repeatedly that research workers using standardised interviews can obtain considerably higher diagnostic reliability than is possible with unstructured interviews, and that further improvement can be obtained by adopting operational definitions for all diagnostic categories. For example, the field trials of DSM-III carried out in the USA in the late 1970s gave kappa values for the reliability of the major diagnostic categories varying from 0.65 to 0.83, compared with values ranging from 0.41 to 0.77 in comparable reliability studies carried out between 1956 and 1972. Organic and psychotic disorders generally have higher reliability than neuroses and personality disorders, and for this reason reliability studies based on inpatients tend to produce higher overall reliability than those based on outpatients. The comparatively low reliability of neuroses and personality disorders is probably due to the frequency of neurotic symptoms and maladaptive personality traits in the general population, and the fact that quantitative as well as merely qualitative judgements are involved.

There have been surprisingly few diagnostic reliability studies, whether in routine clinical situations or with the assistance of structured interviews, since the introduction of DSM-IV and ICD-10. Those that have been conducted, and published, do however suggest a dramatically better level of agreement than was evident fifty years ago. Most of the clinical reliability studies have been conducted in emergency services where, despite difficult circumstances, kappa values for the major diagnoses are generally between 0.4 and 0.8 ('moderate' to 'substantial'). There is, however, much less agreement on subsequent decisions, such as whether or not to admit and what treatment should be initiated (Way et al 1998). Similar levels of diagnostic agreement have been obtained in a number of studies by child and adolescent psychiatrists. Structured interviews increase agreement, to 'near perfect' values of 0.8 to 1.0, even if administered by allied professionals such as psychiatric nurses, particularly if supplemented by other information from medical records and/or informants (e.g. Basco et al 2000).

Although the 'minor' psychiatric diagnoses are less reliably made, we should not forget that diagnostic agreement (and specific symptom or sign reliability) can be similarly variable in the rest of clinical medicine and even in some 'objective' laboratory situations. Investigations, such as various body imaging techniques, require interpretation, and kappa values typically vary in the range 0.4–0.8 — with higher values for more readily identifiable abnormalities and diseases (McGee 2001). Even the assessment of malignancy from biopsy samples often has 10–20% disagreement or misdiagnosis (Fleming 2002). Tissue diagnosis is not necessarily a more reliable 'gold standard' than diagnostic criteria (although it probably has far greater validity).

In summary, although the studies conducted in the 1950s and 1960s demonstrated that the reliability of psychiatric diagnoses was often very low, the introduction of structured interviews and operational definitions has transformed the situation. In skilled hands, psychiatric diagnoses are now as reliable as the clinical judgements made in other branches of medicine, and sometimes more so. But reliability still does not, and probably never can, match the reliability of laboratory tests where the human eye is only required to judge the position of a needle on a scale or the timing of a colour change. Clinical judgements, whether they concern depersonalisation or bronchial breathing, are inevitably imprecise and imperfect, and the best we can do is to understand what the problems are and do our best to minimise them.

Validity

Reliability is a means to an end rather than an end in itself. Its importance lies in the fact that it sets a ceiling for validity; the lower it is the worse validity becomes. (Suppose, for example, that in reality syndrome A always responds to lithium whereas other superficially similar syndromes never do so. If diagnostic reliability is low and A is only correctly distinguished from B and C 50% of the time, this crucial difference will not be recognised. Instead, it will be believed that the chances of patients with syndrome A responding to lithium are about 50:50 and that B and C respond quite often as well.) The converse, however, is not true. Reliability can be high while validity remains trivial and, if so, high reliability is of limited value. One could, for example, increase the reliability of the diagnosis of schizophrenia by agreeing to apply the term to all those, and only those, with delusions of control. Nothing would be gained by doing this, though, because the response to treatment and long-term outcome of the population so defined would almost certainly be more variable than it is now.

Valid is defined in the Oxford dictionary as 'well founded and applicable; sound and to the point; against which no objection can fairly be brought'. Psychiatrists' assumptions about the concept of validity have always been strongly influenced by psychology texts, which generally adopt the American Psychological Association's distinction between face, content, criterion-related and construct validity. These terms, however, arose out of attempts to assess the validity of psychometric tests of various kinds, and they are not obviously relevant to the rather different issue of the validity of diagnostic concepts. This may explain why thinking and writing about diagnostic validity has remained so muddled, and why so few attempts have been made to measure the validity, or even to assess the comparative validity, of psychiatric diagnoses. It is difficult to measure something whose meaning is obscure.

Kendell & Jablensky (2003) have recently argued that when psychiatrists refer to the validity of diagnoses they are usually talking simply about their usefulness or utility. Sometimes this is explicit. Spitzer, for example, refers to 'clinical utility (validity)' and states that 'A diagnostic concept is assumed to have *validity* to the extent that the defining features of the disorder provide useful information not contained in the definition of the disorder. This may be about etiology, risk factors, usual course of the illness, whether it is more common among family members and whether it helps in decisions about management and treatment' (Spitzer 2001). More often, though, the virtual identity of the concepts of validity and utility is not appreciated by either writer or audience.

Discussions and concerns about the validity of diagnostic concepts are almost unknown in other branches of contemporary medicine. This is probably because nearly all their diagnoses are now defined at a more fundamental level than the clinical syndrome and there are usually clear, qualitative differences in aetiology even between disorders with similar syndromes. The clinical presentations of pulmonary tuberculosis and bronchial carcinoma, for example, may be very similar, but their histopathologies and aetiologies are quite distinct. Many infectious diseases present with fever, malaise, headache, abdominal symptoms and a skin rash, but their distinct identities are established by their different causative organisms. There are also some psychiatric disorders whose validity is never questioned: Down syndrome, fragile X syndrome, phenylketonuria, Huntington's disease and Creutzfeldt–Jakob disease, for example, and it is surely significant that all these conditions have a well-established aetiology which is distinct from that of other clinically similar disorders. The problem is posed, therefore, not by psychiatric disorders per se, but by disorders which are still defined by their clinical syndromes.

Against this background, Kendell & Jablensky have argued that disorders that are still defined by their syndromes should only be accepted as valid — as opposed to being useful — if it has been established that they are separated from other related syndromes, and from normality, by a natural boundary or 'zone of rarity' (i.e. that interforms, the 'greys' lying between the 'blacks' and the 'whites', are relatively uncommon). As things stand, most attempts to demonstrate such zones of rarity have been unsuccessful. Kendell & Brockington (1980), for example, failed to find any evidence of a natural boundary between schizophrenic and affective psychoses, and Kendler & Gardner (1998) failed to demonstrate a boundary between major depression and health or normality. This implies that the validity of most psychiatric disorders has yet to be established, even though in many cases their clinical utility is not in question. To some psychiatrists this is an alarming prospect. However, if many of psychiatry's familiar symdromes are not distinct disorders with demonstrable natural boundaries, but merely arbitrary loci in a multidimensional space (see below), they may well not survive exploration of their genetic and environmental determinants over the next few decades, and the accolade *valid* ought not to be accorded to a diagnostic concept which is not 'well founded . . . against which no objection can fairly be brought'.

CATEGORIES OR DIMENSIONS

Traditionally, psychiatry has always used a categorical classification or typology. That is, it has divided its subject matter, psychiatric illness, into a number of separate and mutually exclusive categories like schizophrenia, mania and Alzheimer's disease. The reasons it has done so are clear enough. Medicine is rooted in the biological sciences, and physicians were deeply impressed by the advantages botany and zoology derived from the development of detailed classifications of their subject matter into species, genera and orders in the 18th and 19th centuries. More compelling still, the structure of our language is based on classification. Every common noun — like 'tree', 'star' or 'fairy' — denotes the existence of a category or class of objects. There is, however, an alternative way of expressing the relationships between the members of a heterogeneous population, namely to assign each to a position on one or more axes or dimensions, that is to a locus in a uni- or multidimensional space.

There has been much debate about the relative merits of these two types of classification (see Box 14.2). In general, theoreticians like Eysenck have favoured a dimensional approach, while most practising clinicians — though not Kretschmer or Jung — have preferred a typology. It is important to appreciate that, in principle, both options — dimensions and categories — are available; there is no statistical technique or other criterion capable of deciding which is 'right'. The choice between the two is essentially a matter of deciding which is more useful, and the answer may well vary with the purposes for which the classification is required.

The main advantage of a dimensional classification is its flexibility. Consider, for example, the advantages of an Intelligence Quotient (IQ) — a dimensional representation of intelligence — over a typology with three categories (clever, average and stupid, say). Two individuals with IQs of 120 and 160 would both, presumably, be allocated to the 'clever' category, but this would involve losing sight of what in many situations would be an important difference between them. Conversely, two individuals with IQs of say 114 and 116 are in reality almost indistinguishable, yet one could be classified as normal and the other as clever. Moreover, a distribution of IQs can always be converted to any

---

Box 14.2 The relative merits of categories and dimensions

Advantages of categories
- They are familiar
- They are easy to understand, to remember, and to use
- Categorisation is a ready prelude to action, e.g. the diagnosis is X, and X is treated with drug D
- They are more acceptable to a somewhat conservative profession

Advantages of dimensions
- They convey more information because finer distinctions are possible
- They are more flexible, because they can easily be converted into any desired number of categories, and back again
- They do not imply the presence of unproven qualitative differences between members of different subpopulations
- They do not impose boundaries where none may exist in reality, and do not distort the observer's perception of individuals lying near the boundary between adjacent categories

---

number of categories as occasion demands, and the boundaries of these moved up or down the scale at will. But if the members of a population are all assigned to one of the three categories to begin with, this cannot subsequently be increased to four categories or reduced to two, except by splitting or combining some of the existing groups; nor is there any possibility of converting them to a dimension.

Another important advantage of dimensions is that they do not distract attention from the atypical in favour of the typical, or distort the observer's perception of individuals lying near the boundary between two adjacent categories. One of the most serious drawbacks of categorical classifications is the way in which they cause individuals who seem to lie halfway between two disorders, or between a disorder and health, to be overlooked or misrepresented. Patients exhibiting a combination of schizophrenic and affective symptoms illustrate this problem very clearly. Time and again in clinical research they have either been ignored, and the study confined to patients with typical schizophrenic or affective illnesses, or, if they were included, one or other component of their symptomatology was glossed over or ignored. In other words, using a typology leads us to expect, and so to perceive, our patients as fitting neatly into one or other of its categories, whether or not they actually do so.

The main disadvantage of dimensions is that any system involving more than one dimension can only be handled geometrically or algebraically, and, if there are more than three, only the latter is possible. This is why the only dimensional systems used in everyday life are those like height, weight and intelligence which only involve a single axis.

The most important advantage of a typology, apart from its familiarity, is the ease of description and conceptualisation it provides. A description of a typical member of a category provides a simple and easily remembered means of defining, and subsequently of recognising, the essence of that clinical concept, and of the essential differences between it and other categories. It is also difficult to ignore the fact that categorisation is the norm in most other areas of study and is inherent in the structure of our language. If we had good evidence that psychiatric illnesses were distributed in discrete clusters with natural boundaries (zones of rarity) between one disorder and the next, the arguments in favour of categorical classification would be very strong. Unfortunately, we still lack such evidence. As described above, attempts to demonstrate zones of rarity between related syndromes, or between disorder and health, by discriminant function analysis or other means have mostly been unsuccessful. The frequency with which psychiatrists are driven to employ such terms as schizoaffective, mixed anxiety depression, borderline syndrome and the like, and the difficulty they have in agreeing where to draw the boundary between one category and the next, is further evidence that in reality patterns of symptoms merge into one another and are not separated by zones of rarity. It is said that the art of classification lies in carving nature at the joints, but where psychiatric illness is concerned we cannot be sure that we have found the joints, or even that there are many to be found.

Despite the considerable theoretical attractions, it is unlikely that psychiatry will adopt a dimensional classification for ordinary clinical purposes in the foreseeable future. Old traditions die hard, other branches of medicine have always used a typology, and there is little immediate prospect of the advocates of dimensional systems agreeing how many dimensions are needed and what their identity should be, or of demonstrating how a dimensional representation would work in day-to-day clinical practice. After all, clinicians have to decide whom to treat and to follow-up and whom to detain under a Mental Health Act. In the long run, though, it is difficult to believe that personality disorder, and perhaps the symptoms associated with depression and anxiety as well, will not be more conveniently and usefully portrayed by a set of dimensions than by the numerous discrete categories we attempt to delineate at present. Indeed, it is quite possible that the classification of personality disorder in DSM-V will be dimensional. There is already broad agreement that the protean variations of normal personality are better portrayed by dimensions, and the continuity between normal personality and the clinical categories of personality disorder is increasingly difficult to ignore. Where psychotic illness is concerned, however, the balance of advantages and disadvantages is rather different, and it may well be that here a typology will continue to be preferable, even though the names of the disorders we recognise, and their defining characteristics, may change considerably as their aetiology is slowly elucidated.

REFERENCES

Andreasen N C 2001 Diversity in psychiatry: or, why did we become psychiatrists? American Journal of Psychiatry 158:673–675

Andrews G, Slade T, Peters L 1999 Classification in psychiatry: ICD-10 versus DSM-IV. British Journal of Psychiatry 174:3–5

APA 1980 Diagnostic and statistical manual of mental disorders, 3rd edn (DSM-III). American Psychiatric Association, Washington, DC

APA 1987 Diagnostic and statistical manual of mental disorders, 3rd edn, revised (DSM-IIIR). American Psychiatric Association, Washington, DC

APA 1994 Diagnostic and statistical manual of mental disorders, 4th edn (DSM-IV). American Psychiatric Association, Washington, DC

Basco M R, Bostic J Q, Davies D et al 2000 Methods to improve diagnostic accuracy in community mental health settings. American Journal of Psychiatry 157:1599–1605

Cancro R 1983 Towards a unified view of schizophrenic disorders. In: Zales M (ed) Affective and schizophrenic disorders. Brunner Mazel, New York

Cooper J E, Kendell R E, Gurland B J et al 1972 Psychiatric diagnosis in New York and London. Maudsley monograph 20. Oxford University Press, London

Feighner J P, Robins E, Guze S B et al 1972 Diagnostic criteria for use in psychiatric research. Archives of General Psychiatry 26:57–63

Fleming K A 2002 Evidence-based cellular pathology. Lancet 359:1149–1150

Frances A J, Egger H L 1999 Whither psychiatric diagnosis. Australian and New Zealand Journal of Psychiatry 33:161–165

Jampala V C, Sierles F S, Taylor M A 1986 Consumers' views of DSM-III: attitudes and practices of US psychiatrists and 1984 graduating psychiatric residents. American Journal of Psychiatry 143:148–153

Kendell R E 1991 Relationship between the DSM-IV and the ICD-10. Journal of Abnormal Psychology 100:297–301

Kendell R E, Brockington I F 1980 The identification of disease entities and the relationship between schizophrenic and affective psychoses. British Journal of Psychiatry 137:324–331

Kendell R E, Jablensky A 2003 Distinguishing between the validity and utility of psychiatric diagnoses. American Journal of Psychiatry 160: 4–12

Kendler K S, Gardner CO 1998 Boundaries of major depression: an evaluation of DSM-IV criteria. American Journal of Psychiatry 155:172–177

Kreitman N, Sainsbury P, Morrissey J et al 1961 The reliability of psychiatric assessment: an analysis. Journal of Mental Science 107:887–908

Krueger R F 1999 The structure of common mental disorders. Archives of General Psychiatry 56:921–926.

Loranger A W 1990 The impact of DSM-III on diagnostic practice in a university hospital. Archives of General Psychiatry 47:672–675

McGee S 2001 Evidence-based physical diagnosis. Saunders, Philadelphia

Robins L N, Helzer J E, Croughan J, Ratliff K S 1981 National Institute of Mental Health diagnostic interview schedule. Archives of General Psychiatry 38:381–389

Scadding J G 1967 Diagnosis: the clinician and the computer. Lancet ii: 877–882

Schneider K 1959 Klinische Psychopathologie, 5th edn. Hamilton M W (trans). Grune & Stratton, New York

Spitzer R L 2001 Values and assumptions in the development of DSM-III and DSM-IIIR. Journal of Nervous and Mental Disease 189:351–359

Szasz T 1961 The myth of mental illness. Hoeber-Harper, New York

WHO 1973 Report of the international pilot study of schizophrenia, vol 1. World Health Organization, Geneva

WHO 1978 Mental disorders: glossary and guide to their classification in accordance with the ninth revision of the international classification of diseases (ICD-10). World Health Organization, Geneva

WHO 1992 The ICD-10 classification of mental and behavioural disorders: clinical descriptions and diagnostic guidelines. World Health Organization, Geneva

WHO 1993 The ICD-10 classification of mental and behavioural disorders: diagnostic criteria for research. World Health Organization, Geneva

Wing J K, Cooper J E, Sartorius N 1974 Description and classification of psychiatric symptoms. Cambridge University Press, Cambridge

Way B B, Allen M H, Mumpower J L et al 1998 Interrater agreement among psychiatrists in psychiatric emergency assessments. American Journal of Psychiatry 155:1423–1428

15 | Clinical psychopharmacology

David G Cunningham Owens

The fact that human experience can be altered by drugs must rank, with fire, as one of man's earliest discoveries. References from the dawn of time bear witness to the use of plants, and plant extracts, for what might now be called 'recreational' purposes, with certain drugs coming to occupy central roles in religious and cultural mysteries still evident today. Even in medicine, the idea of medicaments having a 'tonic' or invigorating action, as much mental as physical, long antedated the emergence of psychiatry.

In this context, 'psychopharmacology' is a young specialty, the term being attributed to the American pharmacologist David Macht in 1920. Although it has now achieved professional acceptance, sections of the public remain wary. Humans may indeed use drugs to alter mental experience, but the idea of a professional, formalised 'psychopharmacology' holds potentially sinister overtones for many. The 'hard work' of modern psychiatric practice often seems equally spilt between promoting to a wary public the use of medically recommended drugs on the one hand while attempting to restrain the use of those not medically sanctioned on the other! What is rejected in the clinic is all too often accepted without question at the bus-stop outside!

The way by which the drugs considered in this section achieve their effects is by actions on *brain* substrates, and the term 'neuropharmacology' is more neutral. Nonetheless, the aim of drug treatments in psychiatric practice is to bring about beneficial changes in disorders affecting primarily the *mental state*, and, as such, the idea of 'clinical *psycho*pharmacology' is not misplaced.

Drugs which produce mental state changes within a therapeutic context have been referred to by a series of generic names, though nowadays the most commonly used is '*psychotropics*' (i.e. 'acting on the mind'). The term is not specific, however. A number of compounds used in medicine also affect mental state but are not given this generic classification, whereas some drugs used in psychiatric disorders have more peripheral than central actions. Also, an increasing number of illicit compounds are manufactured specifically to produce alterations in mental state, though without medical sanction these are not conventionally referred to as 'psychotropic'.

Despite the value of medications in the treatment of psychiatric disorders, they are rarely if ever 'insulin' to a psychiatric 'diabetes'. They can bring about undoubted clinical benefits, but these are almost invariably partial. The complex interplay of biological and social factors that contribute to the development of psychiatric disorders is poorly understood, and it remains the case that medication needs to be viewed as part of a treatment plan that incorporates a spectrum of approaches to management. Nonetheless, psychopharmacology can be justly credited with a major, and increasing, contribution to the well-being of those afflicted with psychiatric disorders and to an understanding of the neurochemical basis of these.

All the major classes of drugs used in psychiatry comprise compounds whose clinical characteristics were identified *empirically*. It is often said that the discovery and introduction of the first-generation drugs was 'serendipitous', but, while this may be credible for some, a prior scientific lineage can be identified for most.

The process began in 1949, when the Australian psychiatrist John Cade published the first account of the anti-manic and mood stabilising effects of lithium salts, though it was some years before this was brought to clinical realisation. The 'golden age', however, was the 1950s. In December 1950, Paul Charpentier synthesised chloropromazine, as the compound was initially called, and by 1952 its place was established as the foundation drug of the modern psychopharmacology era. In 1954 the rauwalfia alkaloid reserpine, long a tool of Indian Ayurvedic medicine, was introduced into western psychiatry by Nathan Kline, who was also instrumental in the development of monoamine oxidase inhibitors, introduced in 1957, following observations of the mood-elevating actions of certain anti-tuberculous agents. By the middle of the decade the first 'tranquilliser', meprobamate, became available and within 2 years rose to be the most widely prescribed drug in the USA. Also in 1955, the iminodibenzyl derivative of the renamed chlorpromazine was evaluated for antipsychotic efficacy with somewhat disastrous results, in that it seemed to promote manic-type symptoms in some patients. In 1957, however, its efficacy in 'vital depression' was demonstrated by Kuhn, and imipramine became the first tricyclic antidepressant, launched in 1958. In the same year, clozapine was synthesised, and around that time the behavioural properties of the 1,4 benzodiazepines were identified by Randall, culminating in 1960 with the launch of chlordiazepoxide.

Golden ages are by definition time limited, and so it was in psychopharmacology. For the next two decades what emerged was largely derivative, while clinicians developed an increasing awareness of the therapeutic limitations of these empirically derived classes and the mounting dilemmas their adverse effects could present.

From the 1960s, however, basic neuropharmacology started an exponential advance, aided by the new drugs, and in the past two decades psychotropic agents have started to emerge on the basis of specific hypotheses (though how accurate these hypotheses are remains to be seen!). This first impacted on antidepressant psychopharmacology in the 1980s and, since the early 1990s, has spread to the field of antipsychotics also. This process is set to continue, and, although it seems unlikely that this heralds a new 'golden age', these are exciting times in psychopharmacology.

The following provides an overview of the major drug treatments used in current psychiatric practice, with priority given to pharmacology. This is done in the belief that an awareness of the pharmacology of the drugs we use day and daily should form the *starting point* for clinical practice, not an optional extra. It is no longer an adequate practice standard for therapeutic recommendations to be predicated simply on a reading of the *British National Formulary* or, worse, on habit or expediency. It is furthermore important to ensure that the major sources of information are not the marketing literature for commercially available products.

Much pharmacokinetic work is undertaken in normal volunteers under ideal conditions. This ignores the influence of illness and lifestyle variables in determining kinetic parameters. For example, many psychiatric patients smoke, which alters a number of the pharmacokinetic parameters pertinent to most psychotropic drugs, something to which the literature has only recently paid attention. Furthermore, while diet is known to alter the kinetics of some drugs (e.g. valproate — see below) this aspect has been ignored in the literature on psychotropics. Thus, the following data on pharmacokinetics might be seen for the most part as representing a set of baselines derived from a more 'ideal' population than the target one.

In presenting therapeutic 'indications' for the use of various psychotropic drugs, it is important to realise that these may not necessarily correspond to 'licensed' indications. The licensing of pharmaceutical products is a process to ensure that marketing claims are justified on the basis of evidence (manufacturers are referred to as 'marketing authorisation holders' for licensing purposes). However, many uses of drugs, including in psychiatry, either antedate the introduction of modern licensing requirements or have evolved by 'practice and repute' and may not be supported by RCT or other higher levels of evidence. License recommendations are not legally binding on the prescriber but, with increasing introduction of therapeutic guidelines based on these, the distinction between 'clinical' and 'licensed' indications is becoming increasingly blurred.

One of the consequences of the times being psychopharmacologically 'exciting' is that advances are occurring rapidly, and some changes in the information presented here are almost inevitable prior to publication of the present volume.

ANTIPSYCHOTICS

Terminology

Soon after the introduction of chlorpromazine in 1952, its use was noted to be associated with the development of parkinsonism, as had been noted with reserpine. As this was largely a treatable and reversible phenomenon, it was for most psychiatrists not a matter of concern. Within a few years, however, these neurological effects came to be seen as pointing to an *essential* element of the pharmacology and to offer a window on the drug's mode of action. To reflect these views, Jean Delay coined, in 1955, the term by which this new class of drugs became universally known — 'neuroleptics' — i.e. compounds which forcibly 'grasp' or 'seize' neurons or the nervous system.

By the 1960s the idea that neurological effects were an essential herald of clinical efficacy had fallen into disrepute, though the term 'neuroleptics' has remained stubbornly entrenched. Nowhere else in pharmacology is a family of drugs classified on the basis of an adverse effect, and the durability of the term is to be regretted.

The ideal would be to classify on the basis of a unique pharmacological characteristic that corresponds in some way to clinical usage. This is not yet possible. While all currently available compounds share in common dopamine blockade, not all drugs which block dopamine are clinically effective in the management of major psychiatric disorders. In this situation, and again in line with convention, drugs which are clinically effective against psychotic disorders are best classified quite simply on the basis of this lead *clinical* function — that is, descriptively, as 'antipsychotics'. These compounds exert unique effects that are not mediated via sedation, and any reference to them being 'tranquillisers' — major or otherwise — is erroneous. These unique effects are, however, evident at the *symptom*, not the syndromal, level, so the class is diagnostically non-specific in its actions. It is therefore equally inaccurate to refer to them as 'anti-schizophrenics'.

Within the class of 'antipsychotics', it has in recent years become accepted practice to refer to older compounds as 'standard' (or 'conventional') antipsychotics and new drugs as 'atypical', the inference being that there are now 'two dichotomous groups' of antipsychotics (Kinon & Lieberman 1996). It is unclear, however, by what parameters 'atypicality' should (or can) be defined. If it could be demonstrated that on some *pharmacological* variable 'atypical' drugs clearly differ from 'standard' ones, this could form a basis of subclassification, especially if such a difference could be linked to a clinical variable also. Despite a number of proposals (e.g. $5HT:D_2$ ratios, balance of antagonism at dopamine receptor subtypes, $5HT_{1c}$ properties, etc.), no pharmacological proposal applies to new antipsychotics exclusively. While it has been suggested that 'atypical' clozapine-like effects may relate to weak (or 'loose') receptor binding characteristics, this only seems to be a property of quetiapine in addition to clozapine itself.

Essentially therefore, 'atypicality' is *clinically* defined, and clozapine remains the benchmark. Even here, however, there is no 'gold standard' of clinical characteristics. It is suggested that to be considered 'atypical', an antipsychotic should, like clozapine, at least:

- have an exceptionally low or absent liability to promote extrapyramidal neurological disturbances throughout the therapeutic dose range;
- not be associated with an elevation of serum prolactin or only produce transient, ill-sustained increases (Lieberman 1993).

Some suggest in addition that efficacy with negative features should be included.

By these criteria, not all that is new in antipsychotic psychopharmacology is 'atypical', and some 'old friends' start to look 'new'! There are two problems with criteria such as these. The first is that enhanced 'extrapyramidal' tolerability in practice refers to lower levels of parkinsonism on standard rating scales. As this is invariably assessed from an extremely limited rating perspective (using, for example, the Simpson–Angus Scale), it is difficult to say that benefits are genuine. More important, however, are the standards against which new antipsychotics are compared. These have predominantly been chosen to reflect 'routine' practice, especially in the USA, but raise questions about how appropriate they are. It would hardly be rocket science to show better tolerability for a new drug of broad spectrum used conservatively than for a high-potency, narrow-spectrum drug, such as haloperidol, used in higher clinical equivalent doses.

While this text may be swimming against the tide, we would recommend that the term 'atypical' be used with circumspection — not with the inference of defining a subgroup of antipsychotic drugs or dichotomising the class — but, for the present, merely as a marketing term — a synonym for 'new' (i.e. recently marketed).

Structures

Despite being appropriately classified for the purposes of clinical pharmacology by a single term, antipsychotics in fact represent a chemically diverse group of compounds (Fig. 15.1).

The phenothiazines constitute the largest group. The basic molecular structure was identified from methylene blue by August Bernthsen in 1883, and designated 'thiodiphenylamin'. Their modern name likewise reflects their essential composition — two benzene rings ('pheno'), linked by a central ring structure comprising a sulphur ('thio') and a nitrogen ('azo') atom, attached to which is a carbon side chain terminating in a tertiary amine or a cyclic structural analogue of a tertiary amine.

Two types of substitution are important in the clinical pharmacology of phenothiazines. The first are substitutions of electronegative moieties, such as Cl or S–CH_3, at the so-called R1 site (position 2) which greatly enhances antipsychotic efficacy, probably independent of positive effects on potency (Baldessarini 1985). The second is the nature of the R2 substituted side chains at position 10, which do affect potency but not efficacy and which form the basis of subclassification.

Dependent on the composition of these side chains, phenothiazines can be grouped as:

- *aliphatic* (or aminoalkyl), which have a straight chain of carbon atoms with methyl or alkyl substituents;
- *piperidine*, in which the amino nitrogen is incorporated into a cyclic structure;
- *piperazine*, in which the cyclic ring comprises two nitrogens and consequently is extended.

In all effective phenothiazines the side chain requires to comprise three carbon atoms.

As a rule, aliphatic compounds tend to be of low potency, with greater anti-autonomic and sedative actions. They are therefore overall possessed of higher profiles of *general* adverse effects but have a lower liability to promote *extrapyramidal* adverse effects (EPS). Piperazine compounds on the other hand tend to be of high potency, with a relatively greater propensity to neurological adverse effects, but better general tolerance. Those with piperidine side chains tend to adopt intermediate positions.

The thioxanthenes were synthesised in Denmark by Petersen and colleagues in 1958. Structurally they have been described as 'no more than a shift of emphasis' (Curry 1986) as they represent only a minor deviation from the phenothiazines, in which the nitrogen of the latter's central ring is substituted by a carbon atom. The consequence of this is that these compounds demonstrate *stereoisomerism* — that is, side-chain attachments can be in mirror image fashion. This translates into considerable differences in pharmacology, in that the affinity of different isomers for central dopamine (D_2) sites differs markedly. This group is represented by flupenthixol (flupentixol), the thioxanthene

analogue of fluphenazine, and zuclopenthixol (zuclopentixol), the analogue of perphenazine, as well as chlorprothixene and thiothixene.

The butyrophenones, which structurally can also be considered as *phenylbutylpiperidines*, represented an entirely new chemical group when haloperidol was synthesised by Paul Janssen in 1958. Janssen simply heated pethidine, creating norpethidine, which on further heating converted to haloperidol. Butyrophenones were subsequently shown to be amongst the most potent and selective D_2 antagonists and thus possess a high propensity for EPS induction, but have overall very good general tolerability. Since the withdrawal of droperidol for commercial reasons in 2000, haloperidol is the only significant representative of the group and was, in the 1980s, the world-wide market leader antipsychotic, mainly due to its enthusiastic adoption in the USA.

A modification to the side-chain structure of butyrophenones with the addition of an extra fluorinated benzene ring gives rise to the *diphenylbutylpiperidines*, which have some of the longest half-lives of any antipsychotics. Of this group, only pimozide has sustained a clinical profile, though some experimental compounds are also available, such as penfluridol.

Substituted benzamides. Multiple substitutions of the basic benzene ring have been of pharmacological interest for many years. In the 1960s, modifications to the metoclopramide molecule (itself a modification of the anti-arrhythmic procainamide) produced sulpiride, the first of the antipsychotic substituted benzamides. The basic pharmacology of sulpiride appeared somewhat different from that of the other subgroups of antipsychotics, possibly indicating a dose-dependent action at presynaptic dopamine sites. Clinically it was also felt that, especially at low doses, its use may be associated with lower rates of extrapyramidal dysfunction. For these reasons sulpiride was the first antipsychotic to be talked of as 'atypical' and 'novel'. The substituted benzamides represent one of the largest groups of psychotropic agents available worldwide, though only a few have effective antipsychotic properties. Remoxipride, a successful drug immediately following its launch, was withdrawn in most countries in 1993 after the identification of a cluster of aplastic anaemia cases associated with its use. Amisulpride, a broad-spectrum high-affinity compound is, despite these characteristics, included under the 'atypical' rubric, while the highly potent raclopride, to date confined to experimental receptor binding work, has been shown to be effective clinically (British Isles Raclopride Study Group 1992).

Piperazine derivatives of dibenzazepine. Interest in the piperazine derivatives of the dibenzazepine tricyclic molecule goes back to the early days of psychopharmacology, and modifications of this structure have proved a successful route to psychotropic drug development. With regard to compounds with antipsychotic properties, those with two nitrogen atoms in the central ring are termed *dibenzodiazepines*, the only currently available representative of which is clozapine. Substitution of one of the central ring nitrogens with an oxygen atom produces *dibenzoxazepines*, of which loxapine is the sole marketed representative, while substitution of the same nitrogen with a sulphur atom gives rise to *dibenzothiazepines*. This group has traditionally been represented by compounds such as metiapine and clothiapine (not available in the UK), though the new-generation antipsychotic, quetiapine, also belongs to this group. A slightly more radical modification of the basic dibenzazepine molecule involves substitution of one of the benzo rings with a thieno ring (*thienobenzodiazepine* structure), of which olanzapine is an example.

Phenothiazine

Thioxanthene

Butyrophenone

Diphenylbutylpiperidine

Benzamide

Dibenzazepine

Dibenzo**diaz**epine

Clozapine

Dibenzo**thi**azepine

Quetiapine

Compound	R$_1$ substitution	R$_2$ substitution
Aliphatic		
Chlorpromazine	Cl	—CH$_2$—CH$_2$—CH$_2$—N(CH$_3$)$_2$
Piperidine		
Thioridazine	S—CH$_3$	—CH$_2$—CH$_2$— (piperidine, N—CH$_3$)
Piperazine		
Trifluoperazine	CF$_3$	—CH$_2$—CH$_2$—CH$_2$—N(piperazine)N—CH$_3$
Flupenthixol	CF$_3$	—CH—CH$_2$—CH$_2$—N(piperazine)N—CH$_2$—CH$_2$—OH*

Compound	R
Haloperidol	
Pimozide	

Sulpiride

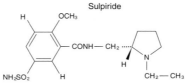

Dibenz**ox**azepine

Loxapine

Thienobenzodiazepine

Olanzapine

* Depot esterification site

Fig. 15.1
Structures of antipsychotics.

Other agents of more diverse chemical structure but with antipsychotic efficacy include the *benzisoxazole* derivative risperidone; the *benzisothiazoyl piperazine* ziprasidone (not licensed in the UK); and *indole* derivatives such as the long-available oxypertine and the more recent sertindole.

Pharmacokinetics

Oral formulations

Surprisingly little is known about the mechanisms mediating *absorption* of standard antipsychotics, but following oral ingestion most appear to be rapidly and completely absorbed from the proximal small bowel, which is also the case with all new-generation drugs. Times to peak blood levels (T_{max}) are in the range of 2–4 hours; though, for reasons that are unclear, wide discrepancies (0.5–6 hours) have been reported for haloperidol (Jorgensen 1986).

Orally administered antipsychotics are subject to *pre-systemic extraction* or *first-pass* effects with passage through the liver, the major clearing organ for these compounds. The extent of first-pass effects is dependent on a drug's *clearance* which, for almost all antipsychotics, is *flow*-limited and not capacity-limited (Greenblatt 1993). Thus the clearance depends only on the ability of the portal system to deliver drug to the liver and not on intermediate metabolism. The consequence of this is that the bulk of an orally administered antipsychotic dose does not reach the systemic circulation. Of that which does, only free drug is available for end receptor activity. However, all antipsychotics are highly membrane bound and protein bound, especially to albumen though also to other proteins such as α-1-glycoprotein. The bound fraction varies from around 90% to more than 99% (ziprasidone). Free drug is rapidly and widely *distributed* due to a particular physico-chemical property which is crucial to their effectiveness — lipophilicity. This not only means that unbound drug readily crosses the blood–brain barrier and is widely available to brain sites but also that uptake into peripheral organs is extensive. Antipsychotics therefore have a large *apparent volume of distribution*. Drug is reversibly and dynamically bound to peripheral sites, especially in lung and other organs with a rich blood supply, as well as in adipose tissue, from where it is readily released back into the systemic circulation as excretion progresses — a factor underlying the persistence of efficacy and adverse actions, and of active moieties in plasma long after cessation of treatment. As a result of these kinetic properties, standard antipsychotics have rather *low bioavailability*, which for chlorpromazine is in the region of 30%, though for haloperidol appears to be higher at around 60% (Dahl & Strandjord 1977). Generic preparations of clozapine, likely to become increasingly available, may not have the same bioavailability as Clozaril (Lam et al 2001), a point to note if preparations are changed.

The elimination half-lives ($t_{1/2}$) of antipsychotics, as with all drugs, bear a mathematical relationship to their hepatic clearance and volume of distribution. Despite their extensive clearance and wide distributions, the half-life of most antipsychotics is in the intermediate range at around 20 hours. Exceptions are sulpiride (see below), quetiapine and ziprasidone, all in the 6–8 hours range. On this parameter therefore, most antipsychotics are suitable for once daily dosing regimens, though half-life alone may bear only a tenuous relationship to receptor activity in drugs so widely distributed. However, wide distribution also means that, following cessation of treatment, drug can seep back into the systemic circulation over long periods. Thus, the *terminal phase* half-life of some of these compounds is very long (in the case of chlorpromazine up to 60 days), resulting in the persistence of detectable drug moieties for many months — if not years — after exposure has ceased (Curry 1986).

CSF levels have not been extensively studied but appear to represent only about 3–4% of plasma levels for chlorpromazine and haloperidol, which correspond approximately to free fractions in plasma, though they do seem to vary considerably in different individuals and with different preparations (Jorgensen 1986).

Metabolism is mainly in the liver, for the simple reason that lipophilic compounds must be transformed into water soluble ones in order to be excreted via the kidney. Antipsychotic metabolism is in general extensive, with little parent drug eliminated. The processes involved are for the most part unsophisticated, including oxidation, *N*-dealkylation and conjugation with glucuronic acid. Some metabolites are excreted in bile.

While some antipsychotics, such as flupenthixol and pimozide, do not appear to produce active metabolites, the majority do, and some produce several which have clinically significant antipsychotic actions. This has complicated the field of therapeutic blood monitoring, as the percentage of active metabolite varies considerably across individuals and these products have their own pharmacokinetic properties. Thus, although therapeutic monitoring has been a recurrent theme of mainly the American literature for over 20 years, it has not as yet lead to anything that is clinically useful.

An exception to the above general principles is sulpiride, which appears to have somewhat different — and less favourable — pharmacokinetic parameters than other antipsychotics. Considerable amounts of sulpiride can be recovered unchanged from faeces, implying that part of its low bioavailability (around 27%) is a consequence of relatively poor absorption. Poor absorption and difficulty in crossing the blood–brain barrier are undoubtedly both a result of the fact that, unusually for an antipsychotic, sulpiride is *water* soluble. The drug is subject to little in the way of first-pass effects and is substantially less protein bound than others of the class (approx. 40–50%). Estimated half-lives have been widely variable (Jorgensen 1986) but, with an average of approximately 8 hours, are in general shorter than those reported for most other drugs. On this basis, sulpiride is not suitable for once daily dosing, perhaps a more valid assumption for a drug of poor distribution than for ones with large distributions. Benzamides as a group are subject to a number of metabolic steps which produce inactive products. They are nonetheless excreted to a considerable extent unchanged in the urine.

The specific therapeutic actions of antipsychotics are invariably delayed. It is usually stated that antipsychotic efficacy does not become evident until about the third week of treatment, though this may to some extent reflect methodological issues in the relevant studies. Nonetheless it is clear that the desired effects emerge only after a week or two of regular exposure. This probably reflects partly receptor events that underlie the action of the drugs, though with antipsychotics, as with all drugs, it probably also reflects the time to steady state.

Steady state is achieved when the overall mean concentration of parent drug and active metabolites does not alter, so long as the daily does and factors influencing clearance do not undergo change. It is described by a constant relationship — namely, that four half-lives are required to achieve within 10% of the steady state condition (Greenblatt 1993). Clearly, drugs with very long half-lives, such as pimozide, will require much longer to achieve steady state than the likes of sulpiride, which has a much shorter half-life. The figure of four half-lives also applies to the time to achieve 90% elimination of a drug from plasma. Thus, in theory at least, drugs of short half-life may be associated with a more rapid onset of action but a swifter relapse rate on discontinuation. The trial evidence to support either of these assumptions is lacking, though at an anecdotal level the latter scenario might hold some truth.

Depot formulations

The kinetics of depot preparations are highly complex and markedly different from the above. Traditionally, depots are manufactured by esterification of a terminal side-chain hydroxyl group to a long-chain fatty acid, and the ester is dissolved in an inert oil base. The most common base is sesame oil, though the Lundbeck products (Depixol, Clopixol, Acuphase) use a synthetic triglyceride based on coconut oil, called Viscoleo. Following intramuscular injection, esters *slowly* diffuse from the oil base (though release may also be determined by partial metabolism of the oil) and are thereafter *rapidly* hydrolysed by plasma, and possibly muscle, esterases to release active drug.

Both the oily base and the fatty acid utilised in the esterification process are important in determining the kinetics of depot preparations. Viscoleo may be degraded more rapidly than sesame oil — one possible reason why the decanoate of flupenthixol is detectable for a less protracted period after last injection than that of fluphenazine. The role of the fatty acid in determining the rate of drug release can be seen with zuclopenthixol which, when esterified with acetic acid (Acuphase), gives plasma concentration curves closer to those of an aqueous solution than the characteristic depot curves found when the drug is esterified with decanoic acid (Clopixol).

These manufacturing principles radically alter the kinetics of depot preparations. This is because their pharmacokinetics are limited by the rate of drug *absorption*, not the rate of metabolism as is the case with other pharmaceuticals. Traditional pharmacokinetic models do not apply in such situations, and a so-called 'flip-flop' model, where the absorption rate constant is *less* than the elimination rate constant (Ereshefsky et al 1983, Jann et al 1985), has been proposed to describe the kinetics of depots. Interpreting plasma curves in this situation is difficult, as declines in blood levels reflect not only metabolism but also protracted absorption.

Most of the available long-acting depots (excluding zuclopenthixol acetate) share similar kinetic properties. Most achieve maximal plasma levels gradually over approximately 4–7 days followed by a gentle decline in the subsequent few weeks. The exception is fluphenazine decanoate which uniquely achieves peak levels rapidly within about 12–24 hours of administration, with an equally rapid decline to about one-third peak, followed by a more gradual reduction over the subsequent few weeks (Jann et al 1985). The reason for this rapid post-injection peak is not understood but may be related to the drug's vulnerability to muscle hydrolases. It probably underlies some difference in the pattern of early neurological adverse effects reported with depots (Owens 1999). Half-lives in the range 5–7 days following single doses of depots appear to increase with multiple dosing to something in the range 14–21 days (Jann et al 1985), though in a few individuals the half-life of flupenthixol decanoate has been found to be greatly extended (up to 112 days).

Like other new-generation antipsychotics, risperidone has no terminal hydroxyl group suitable for esterification, so Risperdal Consta, the first new antipsychotic 'depot', is differently formulated from standard depots and represents an innovation in the pharmaceutics of long-acting injectables.

The pharmacokinetics of depots have clear clinical implications. The first is, of course, that drugs in this formulation do not undergo first-pass effects, so the desired actions can be achieved with lower absolute doses. Of greater importance is the fact that depots take much longer than oral preparations to reach steady state and much longer to clear following discontinuation. Most achieve steady state after about 3 months, though again fluphenazine decanoate may be different, with a period of about 6 weeks reported (Jann et al 1985). This latter preparation can, however, be detected in plasma for up to 12 weeks, and occasionally longer, after cessation of treatment, while the decanoate of flupenthixol has, in general, been found to be present for only about half this time.

The clinical implications are that depots are not as a rule suitable for acute-phase management and that, after cessation, relapse may be substantially delayed by the actions of residual medication, a phenomenon perhaps more evident with Modecate than, for example, Depixol. Furthermore, dose regimens must be flexible and empirically derived in order to avoid detrimental cumulative effects in some patients.

Pharmacodynamics

Therapeutic (target) actions

From the chemical point of view, antipsychotics are a diverse class of compounds, and diversity is reflected in their clinical pharmacology. In general, those with more selective receptor binding actions tend to be possessed of less extensive general adverse effects, both peripherally and centrally mediated. A further general rule is that phenothiazines tend to be associated with higher levels of more varied adverse effects than other types of drugs (Edwards 1986), possibly a reflection of the known toxicity of the basic molecule that so hindered clinical development of the group for over half a century.

While peripheral actions of drugs are of practical importance in tolerability and safety, it is to the central pharmacology that we must look to understand efficacy. Again in line with their structural diversity, antipsychotics vary widely in their central pharmacology. Some examples are shown in Figure 15.2. In 1963, Carlsson and Lundquist suggested that antipsychotic drugs acted as postsynaptic dopamine antagonists, something that is now clearly established. In 1979, Calne and Kebabian classified central dopamine receptors into two types — D_1 and D_2—on the basis of the ability of the former to stimulate the synthesis of adenylate cyclase.

Whatever else these drugs may do in relation to other receptor systems, *all* currently known compounds of proven efficacy block central dopamine D_2 receptors at postsynaptic sites. While other targets have been explored and may ultimately hold potential, to date *no* strategies invoking other than postsynaptic D_2 antagonism have translated into effective antipsychotic treatments. However, it has become clear that the situation may be more complicated. With the introduction of molecular biological techniques, it has been established that the D_1/D_2 classification represents at least two 'families' of receptor subtypes: the D_1 'family' (comprising D_1 and D_5 isomorphs) and the D_2 'family' (comprising the so-called 'long' and 'short' varieties of D_2, plus the D_3 and D_4 isomorphs) (see Ch. 3). Antipsychotics differ considerably in their affinities for different isomorphs of the D_2 receptor, which is of some interest in exploring the detailed basis of the antipsychotic effect.

In addition, as Figure 15.2 shows, most antipsychotics are active at a range of other receptor types apart from dopaminergic ones. This was for many years felt to represent contamination contributing to adverse, rather than therapeutic, effects. The reason for this view springs from the inferences of the Dopamine Hypothesis of Schizophrenia (Box 15.1). Despite the fact that only the 'version' relating to the mode of action of antipsychotics has any substantive experimental support, the hypothesis has held a strong sway over perceptions about the pathogenesis of schizophrenia and the mechanisms underlying its treatment.

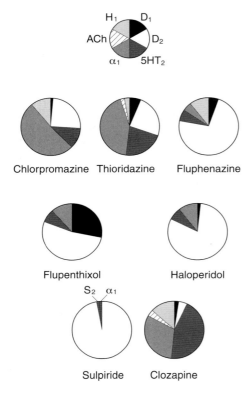

Fig. 15.2
Receptor-binding profiles of some commonly used antipsychotics. 5HT, serotonergic; α, alpha-adrenergic; ACh, cholinergic; D, dopaminergic; H, histaminic.

The thrust therefore was to produce increasingly selective D_2 antagonists that acted preferentially on the mesolimbic, as opposed to the nigrostriatal, dopamine system. The benzamides are to some extent the realisation of this. However, this approach was turned on its head by the demonstration that clozapine, a highly *un*selective transmitter antagonist (Fig. 15.2), was of superior efficacy to a standard drug (chlorpromazine) in, at least, treatment-resistant schizophrenia (Kane et al 1988). Drugs previously considered pharmacologically 'dirty' came to be seen as having 'rich and challenging' pharmacologies, and in the search for new treatments the highly selective approach has rapidly given way to the highly *un*selective approach.

Of the many possible models that could be extracted from the complex pharmacology of clozapine, the one which has been pursued most focuses on serotonergic mechanisms, and in particular the $5HT_{2a}$ receptor subtype. The new generation of antipsychotics all seek to combine D_2 antagonism with a powerful degree of $5HT_{2a}$ antagonism. However, it also seemed clear that if clozapine was our model, the 'ideal' drug should not be associated with the high affinity for D_2 receptors found with standard drugs. This view arose from in-vivo brain imaging, where it seemed that therapeutic doses of standard drugs were associated with 70–80% blockade of dopamine D_2 receptors whereas, with clozapine, efficacy was obtainable with occupancy levels in the range 50–60% (Farde et al 1992).

Thus the 'new' model of antipsychotic efficacy was predicated on a combination of relatively low affinity for D_2 receptors and relatively high affinity for $5HT_{2a}$ receptors. All the first wave of new-generation drugs have adopted this 'serotonin–dopamine' antagonist approach and have been marketed heavily on this basis. This interpretation of clozapine's benefits has resulted in a revivification of antipsychotic psychopharmacology by escaping from the confines of the classical Dopamine Hypothesis, but it is unlikely that this can form the basis of an antipsychotic revolution. While most of the new antipsychotics do have relatively high $5HT_{2a}$:D_2 affinity ratios (Box 15.2), some do not, and relatively high ratios can be found with a number of long-established compounds, including chlorpromazine. This is not the only model that can be proposed from clozapine's pharmacology, and it is to be hoped that in future years innovative explorations of alternatives will result in developments other than the repetitious production of further derivative compounds.

A further and potentially interesting approach to antipsychotic development is the use of drugs with partial agonist actions. A drug's biological effectiveness (technically referred to as 'intrinsic activity') is independent of its affinity for receptors. Partial agonists are compounds with *low* intrinsic activity but *high* affinity, as a result of which they can act to inhibit the actions of other agonist molecules with high intrinsic activity — i.e. they can antagonise

---

Box 15.1 The dopamine hypothesis

Mark 1:
Schizophrenia is the result of increased dopaminergic function in certain brain areas:
- from disruption at predominantly postsynaptic sites, e.g. increased postsynaptic receptor numbers (supersensitivity)
- from disruption at predominantly presynaptic sites, e.g. increased absolute levels/turnover (?mesolimbic system)

Mark 2:
Antipsychotic drug efficacy is mediated via postsynaptic dopamine (D_2) blockade (?mesolimbic system)

Box 15.2 $5HT_{2a}$:D_2 affinity ratios of some antipsychotic drugs

Olanzapine	50:1
Clozapine	30:1
Chlorpromazine	10:1
Risperidone	8:1
Loxapine	7:1
Thioridazine	5:1
Trifluoperazine	2:1
Quetiapine	1:1

them. They are called 'partial' agonists because they possess some limited intrinsic activity, but their net effect overall is to diminish the actions of the more powerful agonist. Partial agonism has been explored as a psychopharmacological tool; in relation to antipsychotics, aripiprazole, among other things a partial dopamine agonist, is likely to be the first to receive regulatory approval.

Adverse ('non-target') actions

General

Antipsychotics can be associated with the production of a wide range of general adverse effects (Table 15.1). Despite this, as a class, they are remarkably safe. With regard to adverse effects of major medical significance, therefore, antipsychotics have a *wide* therapeutic index. However, with regard to adverse effects that may not be medically significant but are nonetheless for the patient unpleasant and intrusive, their therapeutic index is far less favourable. It is important for doctors to acknowledge that what to them is minor, can be quite the opposite to the patient and may impact disproportionately on compliance.

Dry mouth, constipation, blurring of vision from impaired accommodation and, especially in males, *impaired urinary and sexual function* are not uncommon complaints from patients receiving antipsychotics, even those with little inherent anticholinergic activity. A 'background' level of such symptomatology is to be found in patients on placebo, and a proportion of these complaints undoubtedly reflect illness, rather than treatment, effects. Some are likely to have more complex origins than 'single transmitter' pharmacology would lead us to believe, and may be at least partially mediated by antiadrenergic as well as anticholinergic mechanisms. Problems of this sort are usually of little medical import, but they can be distressing or form the source of further medical problems. For example, a simple dry mouth can result in *stomatitis*, which may be present in the majority of patients, especially those with dentures, and can lay the seeds of oral *candidiasis* and long-term *dental caries* and *gum disease* (Lucas 1993), while paralysis of accommodation can precipitate *closed angle glaucoma* in those predisposed.

Clozapine may, in line with its potent anticholinergic actions, produce a dry mouth, but more commonly its use is associated with *increased salivation*. The pharmacological basis for this is unclear but may relate to cholinergic reuptake inhibition. As it is not extrapyramidal as such, it is best referred to descriptively as 'hypersalivation', rather than sialorrhoea which is more intimately associated with the bradykinesia of parkinsonism. Hypersalivation increases in frequency with continued exposure and can affect up to three-quarters of those on clozapine (Lieberman et al 1994). It can be obviated by small starting doses and very slow increments, or with hyoscine which can be applied by transdermal patches, but can remain an obstacle to continued treatment.

Weight gain can be a major problem with all antipsychotics but is particularly so with olanzapine, on which up to 30% of patients experience clinically significant increases (e.g. 3 kg over a 6-week acute exposure interval). This can be a major reason for non-compliance, as initially highlighted in women (Holden & Holden 1979, Silverstone et al 1988). Nowadays, however, neither gender is likely to accept significant weight gain with impunity. The mechanisms underlying this are unknown and may be multiple (e.g. hypothalamic H_1 antagonism / antiserotonergic actions).

Anti-autonomic actions result in an increase in resting *heart rate*, usually in the order of 10 beats per minute or less and not clinically significant. The more powerfully antiadrenergic drugs can also produce a significant fall in *blood pressure*, which is mainly *postural*. This is a potentially serious development that can precipitate myocardial ischaemia/infarction or cerebrovascular accident, especially in the elderly. It can occur with new-generation antipsychotics as well as with low-potency phenothiazines. For this reason, the latter should *never* be administered intravenously, and caution should *always* be exercised with intramuscular use.

Up to 25% of those receiving antipsychotics have ECG changes, including ST depression, T wave flattening and on occasion the emergence of U waves. Such changes seem to relate to the chemical structure of the drug and probably to potency. Hence, they are more associated with phenothiazines, and with chlorpromazine and thioridazine more than trifluoperazine (approximately 50% versus 16%, respectively) (Lipscomb 1980). However, the major ECG issue is delayed ventricular repolarisation, as evidenced in prolongation of the QT interval.

Since the last edition of this book, QT_c *prolongation* (i.e. duration of the QT interval corrected for heart rate) has gone from being of marginal to central concern in clinical pharmacology in general. The reason is increasing awareness of an association between QT_c prolongation and induction of serious tachyarrhythmias, such as the polymorphic ventricular tachycardia *torsade de pointes*, which can be fatal (see below). Epidemiological and other evidence suggests that certain psychotropic drugs can promote QT_c prolongation (Reilly et al 2000) and may also be associated with higher than expected rates of sudden death (Ray et al 2001). Risk also appears to increase in a dose-dependent manner, though there are inconsistencies here as QT prolongation has been reported with depot formulations, which are present in only nanomolar concentrations in blood. There are major problems in drawing clinical inferences from the QT_c measure, which is highly variable, with the boundaries of 'normal' arbitrarily defined (e.g. females < 450 ms, males < 430 ms). It varies in the same individual over time, and may show a diurnal pattern; it is longer in females, may be influenced by oestrogen and so change with the menstrual cycle; it may be dependent on autonomic (sympathetic) overactivity; and has variable determination depending on the method used to correct for heart rate (Bazett versus Fredericia methods). As a result, the dysrhythmogenic potential of any QT_c measure represents a *probability*, not an absolute. A QT_c > 500 ms would definitely increase the risk of dysrhythmias developing in any patient, and drugs 'lifting' patients to these levels could therefore be considered as having a *definite* risk associated with their use. Medications producing measures lower than this, but still raised from a pre-exposure 'baseline', are more open to doubt as to their potential for promoting serious dysrhythmias. Thus, while a QT_c between 450 and 500 ms *may* be of '*potential*' concern, this remains uncertain. Applying these sorts of criteria to antipsychotics, an *established* dysrhythmogenic risk can be attributed to thioridazine, haloperidol, pimozide, sertindole and ziprasidone (plus also lithium). Virtually all other antipsychotics licensed in the UK would be considered '*potential*' risk drugs — excluding half a dozen on which there are insufficient data (loxapine, oxypertine, perphenazine, pipothiazine, promazine and remoxipride).

Perhaps of greater importance than bald QT_c measures, is a heightened awareness of risk in those receiving antipsychotics who have other dysrhythmic risk factors, such as the elderly, those with pre-existing heart disease, those with electrolyte imbalance (e.g. hypokalaemia, hypomagnesaemia, hypocalcaemia), those receiving potassium-losing diuretics and other drugs which either interfere

Table 15.1   Non-neurological adverse (non-target) actions of antipsychotic drugs

Adverse reaction	Frequency	Comment
General		
Sedation	++	Esp. with low-potency standard and new-generation drugs
'Torpor' ('ataraxy')	+++	? Univeral action
Dry mouth, blurred vision, constipation, urinary difficulties	+	Conventionally viewed as anticholinergic, but ACh/NA imbalance also contributes
Priapism	Rare	
Weight gain	+++	Esp. clozapine and olanzapine
Stomatitis / oral candidiasis	Very common	Rarely clinically significant; may contribute to dental caries
Temperature change		Reduction, esp. with phenothiazines, usually not clinically significant; increase may result from impaired sweating ? NMS
Deep vein thrombosis	Rare	Relative risk increased substantially in those on low-potency standard drugs; ? immunopathic effect / ? secondary to weight gain, immobility, etc.
Cardiovascular		
Increased heart rate	+++	Vagal inhibition + reflex from hypotension; rarely clinically significant
Hypotension	++	Low-potency and new-generation drugs; can be serious, esp. in older patients
ECG changes	++	Quinidine-like effect; prolonged QT_c,? dose-related; caution when treating acute emergencies
Tachyarrhythmias	Rare	
Torsade de pointes	Very rare	? Sudden death; esp. thioridazine, pimozide, sertindole and? haloperidol
Myocarditis/cardiomyopathy	? Rare	Specifically clozapine; high mortality (~25%)
Endocrine		
Hyperprolactinaemia	+++	Universal effect with standard drugs, esp. sulpiride; variable–transient effect with new generation; relates to sexual side-effects
Galactorrhoea	Rare	Both sexes; rarely significant
Amenorrhoea	++	Multiple causes
Gynaecomastia	Rare	? Oestrogen:androgen imbalance
Altered glucose metabolism	++	Hypoglycaemia rare, usually with chlorpromazine; hyperglycaemia ? common, esp. with olanzapine
Dysmetabolic actions	?	Anti-insulin/dystriglyceridaemia, ? esp. with olanzapine
Inappropriate secretion of antidiuretic hormone	Rare	Thiazide-resistant oedema
Hepatic		
Impaired liver function	++	Transient changes common, esp. with olanzapine; jaundice esp. with chlorpromazine (1–2%)
Dermatological		
Skin rashes		
Erythematous	++	Chlorpromazine 5–10%
Urticarial	Rare	
Contact	Rare	
Photosensitivity	++	Esp. phenothiazines (Chlorpromazine); brightness more important than heat; can cause serious burning
Pigmentation	? Rare	? Associated with high doses
Alopecia	? Not uncommon	
Haematological		
Neutropenia	Rare	Higher risk with clozapine; reversible but can progress to agranulocytosis with continued exposure
Agranulcytosis	Very rare	Higher risk with clozapine (~ 1:1200)
Thrombocytopenia	Very rare	
Aplastic anaemia	Very rare	? Remoxipride
Haemolytic anaemia	Very rare	
Ophthalmic		
Lenticular deposits	Rare	Reversible with early detection
Pigmentary retinopathy	Rare	Higher risk with high-dose, long-term thioridazine; rarely with low dose
Immunological		
IgM isotype antiphospholipid antibodies	Very common (overall 40–50%)	Esp. with chlorpromazine; other drugs unclear; ? significance ? clotting diathesis
'Lupus anticoagulant' antinuclear antibody	? Common	? Significance
Rheumatoid factor	?	
Systemic lupus erythematosis	Very rare	With chlorpromazine

+, infrequent; ++, frequent; +++, very frequent.
Ach, acetylcholine; NA, noradrenaline; NMS, neuroleptic malignant syndrome
From Owens (1996).

| Box 15.3 | Factors predisposing to QT$_c$ prolongation |

Female gender
Elderly
- CHD
- Multiple medications
- Pharmacokinetic/dynamic changes
Electrolyte imbalance
- Hypokalaemia
  — Diuretic use
- Hypomagnesaemia
  — Vomiting/diarrhoea
Cardiac disease
- IHD — acute/chronic ischaemia
  — Predisposition to arrhythmia
- Cardiomyopathy
Drugs
- Dose-dependent action on ion channels which govern QT length
  — Therapeutic doses of drugs with known enhanced risk, or overdose of drugs with potential
- Pharmacokinetic
  — Raised blood level following especially inhibition of cytochrome P450 3A3/4 isozyme
Long QT syndrome
- Genetic
Sinus bradycardia
Psychological
- Sympathetic overarousal

CHD, coronary heart disease; IHD, ischaemic heart disease.

with antipsychotic metabolism (see below) or are themselves proarrhythmic (Box 15.3). Routine ECG monitoring is a 'good practice' principle in those with high atheromagenic and cardiovascular risk factors, as is the case with many of those for whom long-term antipsychotic medication is recommended.

Dysrhythmogenic potential may underlie the *sudden death syndrome*. Although a rare occurrence, usually involving apparently fit young males treated with high-dose regimens (Levinson & Simpson 1987), treatment with more than 100 mg thioridazine or its equivalent has been reported to increase the risk of sudden death approximately 2.5-fold (Ray et al 2001). A number of such sudden deaths occur in relation to the treatment of psychiatric emergencies. Extreme muscular overactivity can adversely alter the pharmacokinetics of certain agents (Jusic & Lader 1994) resulting in exceptionally high blood levels, possibly as a result of the loss of muscle storage sites. This emphasises the need to view psychiatric emergencies as potentially dangerous *medically*, requiring care and skill in their management. Although empirical, it may be worth considering their treatment as a 'two-step' process — where 'pre-treatment' with, for example, intravenous benzodiazepine may act against the kinetic effects of extreme muscular overactivity, making subsequently administered antipsychotic less risky, though the compound effects of sedation in complex strategies would require close monitoring.

Concern about the potential for sudden death and the promotion of prolonged QT$_c$ has led to restrictions in the use of certain antipsychotic drugs in recent years, or their voluntary removal from the market. Ceilings on recommended dose limits are set for pimozide (20 mg per day), while mandatory ECG monitoring is now required with pimozide, thioridazine and sertindole (recently relaunched in the UK under a very limited licence).

A further cardiological issue to emerge in recent years is the development of *myocarditis* and *cardiomyopathy* in patients receiving clozapine (Kilian et al 1999). Although the exact prevalence of this is unknown, it may be as high as 1 in 500 first exposures. The mechanism is unknown but may relate to direct binding of clozapine producing toxicity in myocardial tissue. Heart rate usually rises slightly in patients first exposed to clozapine, because of its anticholinergic (vagal) actions and as a reflex response to antiadrenergically mediated hypotension. However, a *persistent* increase in resting heart rate after initial dose titration and stabilisation, or the development of pain, exercise intolerance or palpitations, are indications for *full* cardiological investigation. Those starting on clozapine should, where practicable, have a pre-treatment ECG against which subsequent change may be measured. Because these problems may produce irreversible disability and may be associated with up to 25% mortality, clozapine *must* be stopped should the presence of myocarditis or cardiomyopathy be established.

Hyperprolactinaemia is inevitable with standard antipsychotics and results from blockade of tuberoinfundibular dopamine D$_2$ receptors. Rises in prolactin can be detected within a few hours of exposure, reaching a plateau within 4–7 days and remaining elevated for the duration of exposure (Meltzer & Fang 1976). Particularly high levels can be attained with sulpiride. The precise clinical consequences of antipsychotic-induced hyperprolactinaemia are unclear, though there is evidence that this plays a role in impaired sexual interest/performance (Smith et al 2002). It may also be associated with breast engorgement and *galactorrhoea* in both males and females and may contribute to *amenorrhoea*, though, in the emotionally disturbed, disorder of the menstrual cycle has complex origins. Clearly, these features can simulate pregnancy, a misattribution easily compounded by the tendency of phenothiazines to produce a false positive pregnancy test. Hyperprolactinaemia has also been related to a long-term loss of bone density, especially in females, though the *gynaecomastia* encountered rarely in males on long-term treatment is probably more the consequence of disturbances in oestrogen/androgen ratios (Edwards 1986).

In line with clozapine, most new antipsychotics produce either no increase in prolactin or only a transient, ill-sustained increase throughout the therapeutic range. Risperidone does produce a dose-related hyperprolactinaemia evident at the higher end of the therapeutic range (Ereshefsky & Lacombe, 1993).

Impaired glucose tolerance was described in schizophrenic patients before the introduction of phenothiazines, but there is evidence that the prevalence rose following their introduction. While hypoglycaemia may occur with chlorpromazine, *hypergly-caemia* from inhibition of insulin secretion is more common. Clozapine and olanzapine seem particularly likely to promote dysmetabolic effects, which may be independent of weight gain, and include both *anti-insulin actions* and *dyslipidaemia* (Haupt & Newcomer 2001). The detailed metabolic consequences of antipsychotic drug use have not been extensively investigated and the specificity of such changes remains to be established. However, they do raise questions about the appropriateness of long-term use of drugs with high liability to produce such effects in patients who already possess high atheromagenic and cardio-vascular risk factors.

Oedema, resulting from stimulation of antidiuretic hormone, may develop especially with phenothiazines, though is usually of little clinical significance. Other *endocrine changes* such as suppression of corticotrophin, growth hormone, thyroid stimulating hormone, folliclc-stimulating hormone and luteinising hormone are of uncertain and probably negligible clinical import (Edwards 1986).

Minor, transient *increases in hepatic enzymes* are not uncommon with antipsychotic treatment. Approximately 5–7% of those starting olanzapine will show transient, and probably clinically insignificant, rises in hepatic enzymes, but the biggest issue is again with standard antipsychotics, and especially chlorpromazine. About 1–2% of exposures to chlorpromazine will result in clinical *jaundice*, which represents a striking decline from the drug's early days (Regal et al 1987). The reason for this fall probably relates to better manufacturing resulting in removal of contaminants. It is widely believed that the hepatic damage underlying these changes is allergic, and this is undoubtedly part of the aetiology. However, histological examination shows not only allergically mediated cholestatic change but scattered hepatic necrosis. Hence direct toxicity is also part of the mechanism. Phenothiazine-induced jaundice is usually benign; although symptoms may resolve with continued exposure, this is not to be recommended. Cross-sensitivity among antipsychotics is rare, so a switch to another drug is usually all that is required for resolution, though this may take 6–8 weeks. A few cases of *primary biliary cirrhosis* have been reported, though this is very uncommon and the prognosis appears better than the idiopathic condition (Regal et al 1987).

About 5–10% of patients on chlorpromazine develop a typical erythematous hypersensitivity-type *skin rash* within 10–14 days of first exposure, though sooner if previously exposed. This can be treated with antihistamines, but again it is prudent to change the drug. Contact dermatitis has been described in medical and nursing staff handling chlorpromazine, though this again appears to be an infrequent observation nowadays. *Photosensitivity* is on the other hand far from infrequent, with dermatology derived prevalences of approximately 3% pertaining to severe cases. The pathology results from a mixture of phototoxicity and photoallergy, with an action in the UVA range. It is therefore less the heat that is important than the sun's 'brightness', so patients can receive considerable burns in conditions that subjectively feel cool. Similar problems may occur, less often, with other antipsychotics.

Pigmentation is again a problem largely associated with phenothiazines, and one rarely commented on nowadays. Earlier descriptions were of widespread deposition of a melanin-type pigment on mainly exposed areas, including eyes, though this *oculocutaneous melanosis* extends to pigmentary deposition in internal organs. Skin deposition imparts a silvery or bluish/purple hue to patients, most often females, who as a result used to be referred to as 'purple people'. It may be that this phenomenon results from chronic use of high-dose regimens, hence its decline. Deposition of pigment in the lens of the eye is still common, and although this infrequently impairs vision, the risk of *cataract* may be increased about 3–4-fold in those on long-term antipsychotics (Isaac et al 1991). Quetiapine has been reported to cause cataract formation in laboratory animals exposed in high dose, but this does not as yet appear to have translated into a clinical concern. Of much greater significance, though lesser prevalence, is retinal deposition of pigment. *Pigmentary retinopathy* has been most frequently associated with long-term use of high-dose thioridazine (Weekly et al 1960, Marmor 1990) and, as it is an important though probably reversible development, guidelines recommend, among other restrictions, that this drug should not be used in doses of more than 600 mg daily for longer than 4 weeks.

Hair loss is a not infrequent complaint of patients on psychotropics, especially women, and is a genuine observation, though is more likely to be associated with tricyclics and mood stabilisers than antipsychotics (Warnock 1991). Usually it represents merely a speeding up of normal shedding, and although the hair may thin, it does not as a rule result in patches of complete loss, though full *alopecia areata* has been described (Kubota et al 1994).

Antipsychotics can potently suppress marrow function. Although any type of drug can be implicated, the problems are individually greatest with clozapine, and collectively with phenothiazines. Clozapine-induced *neutropenia*, reversible on discontinuing the drug, has a cumulative incidence of 2.33% at 1 year, approximately 3% at 2 years, with a small (0.5–0.75%) but continuing risk thereafter (Owens 1996). *Agranulocytosis* with clozapine is also reversible following its early detection and discontinuation of the drug but can be fatal if allowed to persist. Data from long-term monitoring in the UK suggest an incidence of 0.73% at 1 year and 0.8% at 2 years (Atkin et al 1996). This probably represents an idiosyncratic allergic response in affected individuals but as yet no clear predictors have been identified. It occurs early in exposure, with over 80% of cases developing in the first 3 months, and the peak in the third month. No cases have emerged after 2 years. Clozapine may also produce an eosinophilia which appears benign.

Although other antipsychotics, especially phenothiazines, can produce similar effects on the granulocyte cell line, accurate comparative data are surprisingly not available. In the only systematic evaluation, undertaken in the 1970s, patients receiving various phenothiazines were monitored over 8 weeks. Transient leucopenia was noted in 10%, while agranulocytosis was estimated to occur in 1:1200 exposures (Pisciotta 1978). This is a higher risk than the 1:1400 exposures attributed to clozapine, but the data from which these calculations are derived are not comparable. It is generally agreed that agranulocytosis is an established but *rare* complication of phenothiazine treatment, the risk being less than with clozapine.

Suppression of other marrow lines, such as erythrocytes and platelets, has been associated with antipsychotic exposure, but as with haemolytic anaemia, these comprise only sporadic reports and the events must be very uncommon. However, a cluster of eight cases of *aplastic anaemia* occurring in patients receiving remoxipride (though none was on this alone) led to its withdrawal in most countries.

Clozapine (and remoxipride) requires regular haematological monitoring as a mandatory part of its administration.

Antipsychotics can mediate change in a number of *immunological* parameters. The development of IgM isotype antiphospholipid antibodies can be detected in up to 50% of patients, again particularly with chlorpromazine, though the significance of this is unknown, which is also the case for so-called 'lupus anticoagulant' (Canoso et al 1990, Zucker et al 1990). Recently, a high prevalence of venous thrombosis has been reported in patients receiving standard antipsychotics, especially low-potency drugs (Zornberg & Jick 2000). This may be the consequence of incidental factors, such as weight gain and immobility, but may be contributed to by immunopathic changes promoting a clotting diathesis. Very rarely, phenothiazines can cause drug-induced *systemic lupus erythematosis*. These immunological abnormalities are poorly understood but speak of pervasive drug effects that would justify more extensive investigation than has been undertaken to date.

Finally, depot formulations may on occasion cause *reactions* at their injection site. These have been reported with fluphenazine decanoate and haloperidol decanoate and comprise a firm, tender and sometimes pruritic mass which can remain for up to 3 months (Hamann et al 1990). These may not relate simply to flawed injection technique but are more likely to result from impaired vascularisation with consequent delayed absorption. For this reason, injection sites should be rotated.

Neurological — non-specific Antipsychotics are not, in classificatory terms, 'sedatives' — they do not bring about their desired effects in a barbiturate-like fashion. They can however produce *sedation* as a frequent adverse effect, especially the low-potency phenothiazines, early in exposure. This is probably a consequence of antihistamine (H_1) activity. Although an adverse effect, this is a property that can be therapeutically advantageous in the control of behavioural disturbance, particularly in acute management.

Almost all antipsychotics alter the EEG. With remoxipride, changes are minimal, though they are particularly evident (in a dose-related fashion) with clozapine, where up to one-third of patients may demonstrate striking changes. The effect is toward general slowing of waveforms, with a decrease in alpha waves and an increase in theta and delta waves. Chronic exposure results in increasing synchronisation, with increasing slow-wave activity and increasing amplitude. Spike and sharp waves can be superimposed, and paroxysmal discharges, similar to epileptiform activity, may be seen. As a result, a detailed drug history is essential for the interpretation of an EEG.

As a consequence of these electrophysiological actions, antipsychotics lower the seizure threshold. With standard drugs, there is approximately a 1% risk of precipitating *fits* (though this was not reported with remoxipride). The risk with low-dose clozapine (< 300 mg per day) does not appear to be increased, though with doses above 300 mg, prevalences as high as 14% has been reported. This results in an average risk for clozapine of about 4% (Baldessarini & Frankenburg 1991).

Antipsychotic-induced lowering of seizure threshold may result in fits in the context of some other predisposing factors, such as a past or family history of epilepsy, or pre-existing cerebral pathology. However, fits can be precipitated in the absence of such predisposition, and treatment variables such as polypharmacy, rapid increments and high-dose regimens may be relevant. In terms of a rank order of risk, after clozapine, chlorpromazine appears to top the list, with thioridazine, pimozide, haloperidol and fluphenazine at the bottom behind trifluoperazine, which appears intermediate (Cold et al 1990). Seizures in themselves are a potentially serious complication but, as they can usually be managed by a *gradual* switch to another preparation and/or the introduction of anticonvulsants, they do not represent a contraindication to antipsychotic use.

Antipsychotics can interfere with temperature control to produce two opposing clinical effects. Phenothiazines, and especially chlorpromazine, exert a *poikilothermic* action — i.e. they can lower core body temperature. This can result in clinical hypothermia, especially if the patient's alcohol intake is excessive and causes additional heat loss from peripheral vasodilatation.

Of greater interest in recent years has been the opposite action — namely, *hyper*thermia and the issue of *neuroleptic malignant syndrome*. This term has been applied to a syndrome of dramatic temperature rise (sometimes amounting to hyperthermia), extrapyramidal symptomatology (especially rigidity), confusion and autonomic lability. Creatine phosphokinase is usually strikingly elevated. The disorder has been reported most commonly in young males early in treatment. This is a rare development but published prevalences, which range from 0.02% to 2.4%, help us little in deciding how rare. The largest study to date, of almost 10 000 Chinese patients, suggested a figure of 0.12% (Deng et al 1990), which probably fits with clinical experience. There is however a problem with this concept, in that the diagnosis is often made in the presence of other medical conditions that could more readily explain the symptomatology (Levinson & Simpson 1986). Neuroleptic malignant syndrome has a reported mortality of around 20% (Shalev et al 1989) and can result in residual neurological deficits in survivors. However, it usually resolves on discontinuation of the implicated antipsychotic and the instigation of palliative measures, such as rehydration, correction of electrolyte imbalance, and if necessary the use of benzodiazepines. Anticholinergics may be tried in those with profound rigidity but must be used with care, as they may add to confusion and further impede heat loss by impairing sweating. Non-selective drugs (see below) should be avoided. The dopamine agonist, bromocriptine, may be helpful in a dose of up to 60 mg per day, but its use, and that of the peripheral muscle relaxant dantrolene (10 mg per kg) is empirical. Antipsychotics are not precluded in future by an episode of unequivocal neuroleptic malignant syndrome, but it is wise to change to an alternative compound and, most importantly, to introduce it *ultra-slowly*.

Neurological — extrapyramidal Neuroleptic malignant syndrome is sometimes classified as an 'extrapyramidal' adverse effect, though this heading usually refers to pure disorders of movement.

Extrapyramidally mediated movement disorders represent *the* major adverse effects associated with the use of standard antipsychotics. Up to three-quarters of all patients exposed may experience problems of this sort — and even that may be an underestimate! However, this does not mean that such a percentage of the patient population is inherently predisposed or that the use of antipsychotics (especially standard compounds) will inevitably result in this type of disorder. While antipsychotics differ in their inherent liabilities to promote extrapyramidal disturbance, the likelihood of any individual developing this is partly related to the way the drugs are used. Even high liability compounds like haloperidol, used in low but therapeutically, effective doses, may not produce extrapyramidal symptomatology (Rosebush & Mazurek 1999, Oosthuizen et al 2001). This is important to bear in mind when selecting an antipsychotic agent, be it a standard or new-generation drug.

Drug-induced extrapyramidal disorders remain poorly recognised, and their full impact is rarely acknowledged. There is no entirely satisfactory way of classifying them, but perhaps the simplest is the relationship that their onset bears to the duration of drug exposure. It is important to realise that, with the possible exception of tardive syndromes, these disorders comprise not only objective *signs*, but subjective *symptoms*.

The level of expertise in this area to which all psychiatrists should aspire cannot be provided by a general text. Only a brief overview is provided here (Box 15.4) in the hope that further *essential* information will be sought from dedicated works (e.g. Owens 1999).

Acute dystonias come on within 5 days of exposure or dose increment in 90% of instances. They affect up to one-third of patients on high-potency standard drugs but fewer on low-potency compounds. They may occur with some of the new

---

Box 15.4 Extrapyramidal non-target actions of antipsychotic drugs

Acute dystonias
- Prevalence: low-potency drugs 8–11%; high-potency 36%
- Gender: equal
- Risk factors: age (inverse relationship); potency/dose; rate of increment; cocaine use
- Distribution: inverse with age
- Onset: rapid (minutes–hours); 90% in first 5 days
- Treatment: anticholinergics
- Response: complete

Akathisia
- Prevalence/incidence: 30–40%
- Gender: equal
- Risk factors: potency/dose; rate of increment
- Onset: days–weeks, but can be after single dose (esp. high-potency/parenteral)
- Treatment: anticholinergics, beta-blockers, benzodiazepines
- Response: partial

Parkinsonism
- Prevalence: syndromal 15–30%; symptom? universal
- Gender: female predominance (? artefact)
- Risk factors: potency/dose; rate of increment; ? age; idiosyncratic (dopamine status)
- Onset: gradual — predominantly bradykinesia; signs and symptoms
- Course: signs tend to ease over first 3 months
- Treatment: anticholinergics
- Response: subjective good; objective? limited

Tardive dyskinesia
- Prevalence: 20–25% overall; up to 60% in selected samples
- Gender: equal (F > M is ? artefact)
- Risk factors: age; age at first exposure; potency/dose; drug-free intervals; prior akathisia; ? black race
- Onset: gradual, usually after years, but dystonia can be rapid (weeks)
- Course: variable — some tend to resolution
- Treatment: primary prevention; GABA agonists; ? free-radical scavengers; clozapine
- Response: unpredictable

Neuroleptic malignant syndrome

---

drugs, though liability is generally much reduced. No typical cases have been reported with clozapine. These disorders are heralded by increasing agitation and restlessness, and awareness of discomfort and impaired function in the affected part, followed by the sudden onset of, usually, static postural distortions that in adults tend to be localised to the head and neck (craniocervical dystonia), though in children may be generalised. The risk is inversely associated with age but relates positively to the potency/dosage and rates of increment. Acute dystonias respond readily to anticholinergics.

Parkinsonism comprises the same core triad of signs found in parkinsonism from all causes — bradykinesia, rigidity and tremor — though in drug-related disorder bradykinesia predominates. Motor slowing, loss of dexterity and postural instability emerge, with loss of pendular arm swing and postural tremor as early features. The flexed attitude of Parkinson's disease is uncommon except in upper limbs, a more frequent posture in the trunk being mild hyperextension. Sialorrhoea, probably a result of impaired swallowing, may emerge as may seborrhoea. Low-frequency, high-amplitude resting tremor, characteristic of idiopathic disease, is infrequent and a late sign, while rigidity is usually mild, requiring reinforcement to elicit.

Parkinsonism from whatever cause has a *subjective* component which may precede the onset of objective signs. Patients experience weakness or ready fatiguability, usually in axial trunk muscles or proximal limbs, apathy and social disengagement. In antipsychotic treated patients, other syndromes may present similarly.

The prevalence of drug-induced parkinsonism is difficult to assess but is usually quoted at between 15% and 40% in patients on standard antipsychotics. With careful examination over time the true prevalence is likely to be higher. Prevalences should, by definition, be lower with new-generation drugs, though comparative data are sparse.

Onset can begin within a few days of exposure or dose increment, with the majority evident within 2–3 months. Onset depends on drug potency, the dose regimen and the rate of dose increments. No age group is exempt, though the risk increases with age, when antipsychotics may release a tendency to Parkinson's disease.

The first step in management should be a reappraisal of the treatment plan, especially drug potency/dose and rate of dose increases. Specific interventions conventionally involve anticholinergics, and although patients may feel better, objective symptomatology often persists. Dopamine agonists have never found favour, though recent work with amantadine has shown equal efficacy compared with anticholinergics, but less impairment in memory and learning. Antiparkinsonian medication should not be started automatically with antipsychotics, the need being justified by emergence of symptomatology. Likewise, discontinuation should be attempted after 3–6 months, as there is a tendency towards resolution over time.

Akathisia comprises: an unpleasant (i.e. dysphoric) inner restlessness; and an urge to move, either individual body parts or the whole body (e.g. pacing). Incidence is up to 40% over 2 weeks in patients on standard drugs. Incidence rates with new drugs are unclear but seem to be lower. Even clozapine can produce a state of subjective restlessness phenomenologically similar to akathisia. Predisposing factors are again dependent on potency/dosage and rate of increment. Parenteral administration also increases the risk. Akathisia may have a very early onset — within hours of oral and 30 minutes of parenteral usage. Thus, akathisia may be readily confused with mental state disorder.

Some patients may show restless, non-goal-directed behaviour without feeling particularly agitated subjectively. This situation tends to emerge with chronic symptomatology and is best classified as *tardive* akathisia. The alternative term, *pseudoakathisia*, is more appropriately reserved for patients who look 'akathisic' but are victims of tardive dyskinesia, usually of dystonic type.

Acute akathisia responds disappointingly to specific interventions. After a review of treatment, the usual first choice is an anticholinergic. Results are variable, however, and these are perhaps most efficacious with the 50% of sufferers with coincidental parkinsonism. Benzodiazepines are popular, but their use is largely empirical. Advocacy for beta-blockers has waned as increasing trial evidence has failed to support initial enthusiasm.

Tardive dyskinesia refers to a *syndrome* of involuntary movements developing in the course of long-term exposure to antipsychotic (and other predominantly antidopaminergic) drugs. Any type of hyperkinetic movement disorder — tics, chorea, dystonia, etc. — may comprise the syndrome, except tremor, which is specifically excluded. Muscles of the lower third of the face comprise 80% of cases, giving rise to involuntary activity of the tongue, which may sweep the inner buccal surface ('bon-bon' sign) or irregularly protrude ('fly-catcher' sign). This can be combined with grinding/chewing lateral and/or anteroposterior jaw movements, and puckering/pursing movements of the lips. The combination of these signs is referred to as the 'bucco-linguo-masticatory' (BLM) triad. Symptomatology may, however, involve any or all body areas, including internal muscle groups (oropharynx, larynx, diaphragm).

Prevalence depends on a series of variables, especially the age of the sample. Overall, it has been estimated at 20–25%. In special populations, it is substantially higher. Incidence is 4–5% per year. Over time, however, some established cases resolve spontaneously. The risk appears greatest in the early years of exposure, but disorder can emerge without warning at any time. In patients first exposed in later life, incidence rates as high as 30% per year have been reported.

Predisposing factors from retrospective studies include age, drug-free intervals (> 1–3 months), alcohol abuse, metabolic disorders such as diabetes, plus cognitive impairment, affective symptomatology and negative schizophrenia. Reported associations with female gender probably reflect interposing influences, such as age. Prospectively, associations have been established with antipsychotic dosage, emphasising the need for cautious use of antipsychotics. In addition, intermittent exposure patterns (i.e. drug-free intervals) have again emerged, which should be considered with patients when recommending maintenance regimens. Associations with race (higher risk in Afro-Caribbeans; lower risk in Asians, especially Chinese) may represent genetic or treatment differences.

Tardive dyskinesia was for many years one of the major topics of psychiatric research, reflecting a perception of it as the most important extrapyramidal adverse effect of antipsychotics. It is doubtful if such a perception can be sustained in view of an increasing awareness of the intrusive nature of other neurological adverse experiences and the realisation that the course and outcome of tardive disorders is less relentlessly progressive than was once thought. The majority of cases of tardive dyskinesia remain mild and unobtrusive with a likelihood of resolving or declining in prominence over time. The importance of the issue is that in some cases (probably less than 10%), symptoms can be extremely severe and may be irreversible, especially in patients over 40 years of age. A further concern is cases in which *dystonia* dominates, for tardive dystonia is particularly incapacitating and resistant to intervention. The clinical dilemma is that at point of onset the ultimate extent of involuntary movements or the resultant incapacitation cannot be predicted.

Management of tardive dyskinesia remains predicated on primary prevention — strictly limiting indications for antipsychotic use, and utilising the lowest effective and simplest dose regimens during all phases of management. Incidental mental state disorder, such as depression or anxiety, should be adequately treated. Benzodiazepines may be helpful by virtue of their non-specific anxiolytic actions and because they are GABA-facilitatory. Further proposed, but unproven, interventions include the dopamine agonist bromocriptine and the presynaptic depleting agent tetrabenazine. The free-radical scavenger, alpha-tocopherol (vitamin E), has been reported as effective, and although the evidence is far from unanimous, this is a relatively safe intervention. The position of the new-generation antipsychotics remains to be established, but clozapine should always be considered, especially

> **Box 15.5 Indications for antipsychotics**
>
> - Treatment of acute schizophrenic episodes, including schizophreniform disorders, acute exacerbations of chronic schizophrenia, and schizoaffective disorders
> - Acute management of delusional (paranoid) disorders
> - Maintenance of remission in patients with recurrent psychotic disorders of schizophrenic type
> - Treatment of manic and hypomanic episodes with or without 'psychotic' symptomatology
> - Treatment of psychotic depression, characterised by the presence of 'psychotic' symptomatology
> - Maintenance of remission in patients with recurrent bipolar affective disorders in whom lithium or other mood-stabilising medication is ineffective or only partially effective
> - Management of psychotic symptomatology occurring in the context of acute or chronic organic syndromes (the tendency of antipsychotics to lower the seizure threshold reduces their value in withdrawal states)

in those whose disorder is predominantly dystonic. Clozapine may have antidystonic actions evident over a protracted time-scale (2–2½ years).

Therapeutics

Indications

In adult psychiatry it is possible to specify clinical indications for antipsychotics fairly clearly (Box 15.5), though in other areas of psychiatric practice indications may be less well defined. Clozapine is specifically indicated as a second- or third-line treatment in patients who are resistant to standard drugs given in adequate dose for an adequate time, and in those who demonstrate extrapyramidal intolerance. Clozapine is the first antipsychotic to which enhanced efficacy has been attributed, but it must be appreciated that, although its benefits can in some patients be striking, in objective terms advantages in *efficacy* are often slight. Its neurological *tolerability*, however, makes this an exceptional antipsychotic.

There has been great debate over the past twenty years as to whether antipsychotics 'treat' the negative features of schizophrenia. This has extended in recent years to encompass both standard and new-generation drugs. The problem is beset with conceptual problems as to what constitutes 'negative' symptomatology. There is also the additional issue of whether, having agreed what constitutes it, such features can be distinguished clinically with any confidence from other similar, but pathophysiologically distinct features, the most important of which are: anxiety and social withdrawal secondary to positive features; depressive retardation; and parkinsonian bradykinesia. The authentic deficits of the illness have been referred to as '*primary*' negative features, while those states that appear similar but are the result of other mechanisms have been designated '*secondary*' negative states (Carpenter et al 1985). Despite much written to the contrary, the view expressed in this volume is that there is *no* evidence that antipsychotic drugs have any therapeutic actions on *primary* negative symptomatology — and this conclusion applies to the new-generation compounds as much as to the standard ones (Moller 1993, Owens 1996).

Great care should be exercised in recommending the long-term use of antipsychotics solely as agents for non-specific behavioural control.

Strategies

There is *no* first-line antipsychotic for the treatment of acute psychotic states. Recent practice guidelines strongly favour the use of 'atypical' drugs (e.g. NICE 2002), but it would be a mistake to view this as inflexible dogma which renders clinical expertise redundant. The new-generation drugs are proving highly successful commercially, but the question of relative merits in relation to standard compounds remains unresolved, and a true understanding of the extent to which they may have shifted the cost:benefit ratio is not yet possible.

Rather than approaching antipsychotics as 'typical' or 'atypical', 'old' or 'new', attempts at rigid subclassifications, which are artificial, should be set aside. This volume would recommend a return to considering 'antipsychotics' as a *single* class of compounds comprising members of varied chemical and pharmacological characteristics, each of which has its own balance of risk:benefit, which the clinician should have the skills to utilise effectively in all the varied presentations of psychotic illness.

The two principles of antipsychotic use set out in Box 15.6 are designed to ensure that throughout the patient's illness the clinician brings to bear the medical expertise necessary to optimise the risk:benefit ratio.

Trial data do not confirm the intuitive belief that sedative, low-potency drugs have advantages in the management of agitated, behaviourally disturbed patients, though this may be one of those examples in which the unique circumstances of a clinical trial do not allow all findings to be carried over to routine treatment environments. Even allowing for this, there are two advantages of low potency drugs:

- they can impact immediately on non-specific symptomatology, such as agitation and insomnia, that patients find unpleasant and hence can produce some early signs of therapeutic advantage;
- they have an inherently lower liability to produce extrapyramidal adverse effects.

Their two major disadvantages are that their non-specific actions, such as sedation, may be intrusive to the patient, and as a rule they have a greater liability to produce a wider range of general adverse effects. However, while both doctors and patients are usually alert to general adverse effects, there is strong evidence that neither party is at all skilled in recognising extrapyramidal disorder, which means that the adverse experiences of patients on high-potency regimens may be persistently misattributed.

There is clear evidence that in routine practice unnecessarily high dose schedules for antipsychotics have become established. This is especially the case for the high-potency compounds. It has been shown in America that in terms of dose equivalence, haloperidol regimens were approximately four-fold greater than for patients treated with chlorpromazine itself, while for fluphenazine the figure was six-fold (Baldessarini et al 1984). This may illustrate a further possible advantage of low potency drugs — their general adverse effects may set a ceiling on over-generous and unnecessary dose regimens. It probably also illustrates the error of prescribing according to fixed schedules, as opposed to titrating schedules according to clinical need. The evidence is that the majority of schizophrenic patients in the throes of an acute episode of illness will respond to doses in the range 400–600 mg chlorpromazine per day or its equivalent (Kane 1987). The situation with their use in other clinical indications is less clear, but the same principles apply. While most antipsychotics may be suitable for single-dosing schedules, it can be useful to spread doses throughout the day to capitalise on any sedative effects that may ensue, at least during the acute phase. Some of the newer compounds (e.g. olanzapine, risperidone) now come in formulations which dissolve instantly on contact with saliva, allowing for rapid absorption from buccal mucosa and easier supervision of compliance.

Depots are widely used in the UK in maintenance plans, where they have been shown to enhance compliance (Davis et al 1994), though to a lesser degree than might be anticipated. There is, however, no evidence that they exert any preferential effects on outcome *independent* of compliance, and their pharmacokinetics can make 'fine tuning' of regimens difficult. Furthermore, by virtue of their administration by another individual, some patients feel the element of choice in their treatment is compromised. There is evidence that, for maintenance purposes, pimozide, a drug of exceptionally long half-life, may be effective in alternate-day or four times a week regimens (McCreadie et al 1980).

The question of antipsychotic dose equivalence is more craft than science. Equivalence tables, such as Table 15.2, are not based on data from objective scientific tests but are largely derived from clinical studies which adopted variable dose schedules. They do not take account of varied actions at other than dopamine receptors, the higher doses of high-potency drugs used to achieve containment in acute situations, nor, for the most part, pharmacokinetic factors. They are crude, poorly reliable (especially for the high-potency compounds) and should be considered as representing no more than the median points in *ranges* at which comparable efficacy can be reasonably expected. Conversion tables between oral and depot formulations are even less reliable, as most do not take into account pharmacokinetic factors which are particularly relevant to depot formulations. These 'calculations'

Box 15.6   Principles of antipsychotic drug use

- It is important to recognize that there is a temporal dissociation between the onset of adverse and therapeutic effects. Adverse effects may be evident after a single dose, and certainly within a few days, while the specific therapeutic action is inevitably delayed until at least the second week. The target actions cannot be accelerated by increasing doses rapidly; this will merely advance and escalate non-target actions, thereby seriously risking compliance. Over-rapid escalation is more likely when licensed dose indications are wide and loosely defined, as with older compounds, thereby contributing to the perception of a less favourable risk:benefit ratio
- A structure to the management of major psychiatric disorders should be maintained on the basis of the formulation of plans which:(a) prioritise problem areas; (b) identify clear goals; and (c) recognise, by regular monitoring, the evolution of these through different phases. With regard to the drug component of the treatment of schizophrenia, the primary aim of *acute phase* treatment is the control of acute, or 'positive', psychotic features and any behavioural disturbance that may be associated with them, using the minimum tolerable antipsychotic doses. In the *post-acute phase*, the aim is consolidation and rationalisation of administration schedules, doses and redundant medications. In *maintenance*, the primary role is maximising well-being on the minimum doses possible

Table 15.2 Antipsychotic dose equivalences	
Antipsychotic	Dose (mg)
Chlorpromazine	100/day
Orals	
Thioridazine	100/day
Pericyazine	24/day
Trifluoperazine	5/day
Fluphenazine	2/day
Perphenazine	8/day
Haloperidol	3/day
Pimozide	2/day
Flupenthixol	2/day
Sulpiride	200/day
Clozapine	50/day
Depots	
Fluphenazine decanoate	10–25/2 weeks
Flupenthixol decanoate	16–40/2 weeks
Zuclopenthixol decanoate	80–200/2 weeks
Haloperidol decanoate	40–100/4 weeks
Pipothiazine palmitate	20–50/4 weeks
From Atkins et al (1997).	

furthermore overlook the fact that depots are invariably used in maintenance management when overall dose requirements are less than during acute-phase treatment.

ANTIDEPRESSANTS

Introduction

In the late 1940s and early 1950s physicians caring for patients with tuberculosis noted that, when receiving treatment with certain antituberculous agents, most noticeably iproniazid, many seemed to experience an elevation of mood that was strikingly incongruent to their often parlous medical condition. These drugs were postulated, and subsequently shown, to non-selectively and irreversibly inhibit the action of monoamine oxidase, the major intracellular catabolic enzyme of biogenic amines, thereby resulting in an increase in the amount of transmitter available for recycling in neurotransmission. This laid the foundations for the first and most durable theory of the pathophysiology of affective disorders, though it is likely that the so-called Biogenic Amine Hypothesis is at best an oversimplification. Nonetheless with their launch in 1957 the monoamine oxidase inhibitors (MAOIs) became the first commercially available antidepressants.

Enthusiasm was soon tempered by concern. Although these new drugs were less hepatotoxic than the parent iproniazid, it was evident that they could produce serious and occasionally fatal side effects (see below). This, combined with the introduction of the tricyclics and the results of an influential trial sponsored by the Medical Research Council, showing no benefits over placebo, pushed these compounds into the therapeutic doldrums.

As was noted, imipramine was initially investigated as a potential rival to chlorpromazine, but it was its antidepressant properties that were identified by the Swiss psychiatrist Roland Kuhn, and for a quarter of a century the position of the tricyclics was unrivalled. In the 1980s, however, a series of new-generation antidepressants emerged for which a more selective pharmacology than that of

tricyclics was claimed, which translated into better tolerability and safety parameters. Furthermore, most of these new drugs could boast a theoretical foundation to support their efficacy, no matter that these foundations seem to tremble in proportion to the scrutiny imposed on the theory.

Unlike the antipsychotics, considerable differences exist within the class of antidepressants, which reflect in classification. Tricyclics continue to be classified on the basis of their *chemical structure*, whereas with the newer compounds — e.g. the selective serotonin reuptake inhibitors (SSRIs) — classification reflects their putative *mode of action*. This extends to moclobemide, which is considered an MAOI, although structurally it is in fact a substituted benzamide. Taking the tricyclics and MAOIs as the first-generation antidepressants, introduced empirically, those which have followed since the early 1980s might be considered together as 'new generation' because, although they may differ in their pharmacology, they share in common development on the back of at least some theoretical framework. It is accepted that the selective/reversible monoamine oxidase inhibitors sit uncomfortably within such a framework, but for convenience they will be considered with the traditional MAOIs, which they resemble more than other new-generation drugs.

Tricyclics

Structures

As their group name implies, tricyclics comprise two benzene rings joined by a central ring which in the classical compounds is seven membered (Fig. 15.3). Substitutions at position 5 can be either nitrogen, as with imipramine-type compounds, or carbon, as with amitriptyline. The former are therefore *dibenzazepine* analogues of phenothiazines whereas the latter, technically a *dibenzocycloheptene*, is closely related to the thioxanthenes. On the basis of their side-chain attachments at position 5 they may be classified as *tertiary* (e.g. imipramine, amitriptyline) or *secondary* (e.g. desipramine, nortriptyline) amines.

In general, most tricyclics vary only slightly in structure, based on modifications to their side chains, despite some differences (essentially of emphasis) in their pharmacology. A few deviate

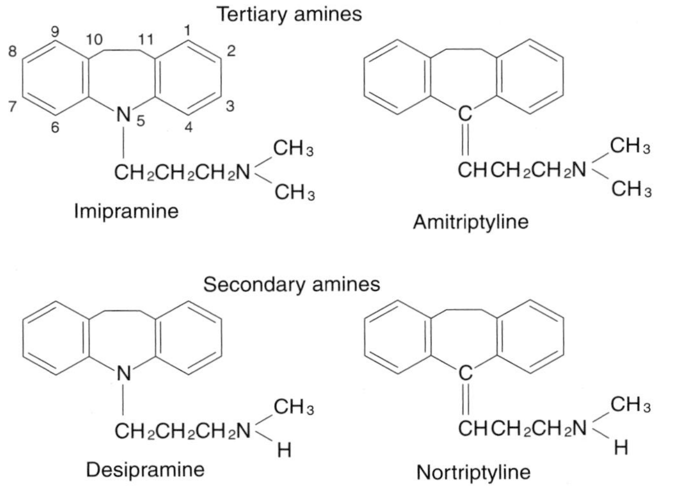

Fig. 15.3
Structures of tricyclic antidepressants.

somewhat more in their central ring structure. Amoxapine, for example, is a metabolite of the dibenzoxazepine antipsychotic loxapine (and might alternatively be referred to as norloxapine), while in maprotiline, a six-membered central ring is stabilised by an ethylene bridge. This compound has been considered by some as a 'tetracyclic' but is really a tricyclic variant.

Pharmacokinetics

Tricyclic antidepressants are all well absorbed from the gastrointestinal tract, a process not prone to interference by, for example, concomitant drug administration. The rate of absorption, and hence time to peak levels, is however more rapid for the tertiary amines (approximately 1–3 hours) than for the secondary amines (approximately 4–8 hours) (Preskorn 1993b). The speed of absorption (T_{max}) and the size of the post-absorption peak (C_{max}) may be related to the likelihood of certain adverse effects developing, such as sedation, agitation and membrane stabilisation which underlies the cardiac actions. Although this has been used as an argument in favour of the preferential use of secondary amine preparations, this is probably only of clinical significance in selected individuals, such as the elderly or those with a clear history of previous intolerance. Furthermore, divided-dose regimens may be used to attenuate C_{max} without altering steady-state levels.

All tricyclics are subjected to heavy first-pass effects, with only about 50–60% of an oral dose reaching the systemic circulation. The effect is particularly large with doxepin (average 70%). As with antipsychotics, at therapeutic levels clearance is flow-dependent and decreased by hepatic diseases or states which impede hepatic throughput. The major metabolic steps involve hydroxylation of the ring structures and demethylation of the terminal nitrogen (Baldessarini 1985). Hydroxylation appears to be the rate-limiting step and makes the largest contribution to breakdown, resulting in the formation of metabolites that in unconjugated form may be present in blood and brain in concentrations greater than those of the parent drug. Conjugated and unconjugated hydroxy metabolites account for up to 85% of an oral dose of imipramine and 55% for amitriptyline (Rudorfer & Potter 1987). The actions of hydroxylated tricyclic metabolites are, however, complex and difficult to study, especially for the tertiary amines. In vitro, and possibly in vivo, they do appear to share reuptake inhibition actions similar in type and degree to those of their parent drugs, and they make a contribution to efficacy and probably tolerability (Young 1991). There is a suggestion from animal studies that they may be more cardiotoxic than parent drugs, though it remains unclear if these data can be translated to humans. Demethylation of the side chain converts tertiary compounds to secondary amines, and these to primary amines. Secondary amines are of course active compounds, and a number are commercially marketed as such in their own right, whereas it appears that primary amines are inactive. Tricyclic metabolism may however not be unidirectional, as there is evidence that with administration of secondary amine compounds, some 15% of patients may develop detectable levels of tertiary drug in plasma — e.g. desipramine to imipramine (Rudorfer & Potter 1987).

A number of drugs interfere with hepatic metabolism of tricyclics (see below), but of particular note is alcohol, which has a triphasic effect. Acute ingestion to intoxication in a non-dependent individual impairs metabolism by competition, resulting in a two- to threefold increase in the amount of unaltered drug reaching the systemic circulation. This is one reason why combination overdoses can have such adverse medical consequences. A similar effect may be evident in chronically alcohol-dependent patients with coincidental hepatic cirrhosis and portocaval shunting. On the other hand, chronic alcohol ingestion without compromised hepatic blood flow increases the magnitude of first-pass metabolism via enzyme induction. A further reason why tricyclic effects can be so toxic in overdose relates to changes that occur in kinetic variables (see below).

Plasma protein binding for tricyclics is high (at around 90%), as is their lipophilicity. Elimination half-lives are on average in the region of 20–24 hours, with those for imipramine and desipramine somewhat less and for amitriptyline and nortriptyline rather longer. Protriptyline, with $t_{1/2}$ values in the region of 75–80 hours, is exceptional; with daily dosing regimens, accumulation is possible. Overall however, half-lives are compatible with once daily dosing and steady-state within 5–7 days. Amoxapine, with an average half-life in the region of 8 hours, may however be a doubtful candidate for single-dose regimens. Lofepramine also has a short half-life but, since this compound appears to function as a 'pro-drug' with rapid conversion to desipramine, the half-life figure is probably of less clinical importance.

The kidney is the major route for elimination of tricyclic antidepressants and is the most important source of alteration in pharmacokinetic parameters by age, illness or other incidental factors (Rudorfer & Potter 1987).

Pharmcodynamics

Mode of action Tricyclic antidepressants are typical of so-called pharmacologically 'dirty' drugs. This, and an absence for many years of specific screening tests for antidepressant activity, made it difficult to advance the pharmacotherapy of affective disorders by isolating the essential component(s) of efficacy.

The Amine Hypothesis of affective disorders was handed down from on-high on tablets of stone — or so it often seems observing the presentations of its protagonists. In its generic format it states that depression is associated with a functional deficit of neurotransmitter amines at critical CNS synapses and mania with a functional excess. This was refined into two subhypotheses when Schildkraut in 1965 postulated that the disturbance lay with catecholamine (predominantly noradrenergic) mechanisms, while Coppen pointed the finger at serotonin. The theory/theories arose from observations made of the effects on mood of various compounds used in humans, initially the presynaptic depleting agents and the monoamine oxidase inhibitors, and while there is much that supports it, there is much it does not explain. It would be miraculous indeed if the complexities of mood and its disorders could be reduced to a simple disturbance in a single neurochemical system that we just happened upon, and it would seem prudent from a clinical perspective to view the Amine Hypothesis as a set of working proposals that provide for the testing of certain essentially therapeutic models.

Tricyclics modify transmission by their receptor actions and by their effects on reuptake. As a group they have a strong affinity for histaminic (H_1), muscarinic cholinergic and α_1 adrenergic receptors (Table 15.3). They have only weak affinity for dopamine D_2 receptors, with amoxapine, trimipramine and clomipramine the most potent at these sites, though even these have only about one tenth or less of the affinity of chlorpromazine (Richelson 1996).

Presynaptic reuptake is an important mechanism in neurotransmission in order to prevent receptor overstimulation. As early as the 1960s, Axelrod and colleagues identified, from among their

Table 15.3 Binding affinities of various tricyclics for different receptor types (as percentage of reference compound)

| Tricyclic | Receptor type | | | |
	H_1*	$M^\dagger$	$\alpha_1{}^\ddagger$	D**
Imipramine	128	2.6	16.4	0.9
Amitriptyline	1282	13.3	55.2	1.9
Desipramine	12.8	1.2	11.5	0.6
Nortriptyline	141	1.6	25.4	1.6
Clomipramine	45	6.4	38.8	10
Trimipramine	5211	4	62.7	10.6
Doxepin	5915	2.9	62.7	0.8
Protriptyline	56.3	9.5	11.5	0.8
Amoxapine	56.3	0.2	29.9	11.7

* Histaminergic receptors: reference diphenhydramine.
† Muscarinic cholinergic receptors: reference atropine.
‡ α_1 Adrenoceptors: reference phentolamine.
** Dopamine D_2 receptors: reference chlorpromazine.
Data from Richelson (1996).

many actions, reuptake inhibition of amine transmitters as a possible mode of tricyclic action. These compounds are, however, relatively non-selective in this, blocking to varying degrees the reuptake of both noradrenaline and serotonin, though with only as a rule minimal effects on dopamine. In vitro, the secondary amines (e.g. desipramine, nortriptyline, protriptyline) are more potent and more selective inhibitors of noradrenaline reuptake than of serotonin, though there is doubt that such selectivity operates in vivo (Frazer 1997). Clomipramine is exceptional in having reuptake characteristics that are comparable to those of the SSRIs.

While reuptake blockade of amine neurotransmitter is accepted as the essential or necessary first step in tricyclic antidepressant action (Goodwin 1996), this rapid pharmacological process does not bear any relationship to the onset of clinical efficacy, and the nature of the secondary changes that seem likely to underlie the resolution of clinical symptomatology remains unclear. These undoubtedly reside in the complex modifications to receptor function that ensue from chronic exposure, including down-regulation of presynaptic α_2 adrenergic receptors and postsynaptic β_1 adrenergic and $5HT_{2a/2c}$ receptors, as well as up-regulation of postsynaptic α_1 adrenergic receptors, and the effect of these on cellular function.

Adverse effects A knowledge of the receptor antagonist properties of tricyclics can be helpful in understanding their adverse effect profiles (Table 15.4). There are, however, few hard and fast predictions that are possible for individual compounds because of the limitations of extrapolating in-vitro data to the clinical context, the interposing effects of pharmacokinetic variations and the fact that data on parent compounds does not allow for the effects of active metabolites. The generalities can however be clinically useful.

Tricyclics as a group are potent antagonists of histaminergic H_1 receptors. Some, such as doxepin and trimipramine, bind with some 50–60-fold greater affinity than reference antihistamines. Amitriptyline has approximately 10 times greater affinity than imipramine, which in its turn has approximately 2–3 times the affinity of protriptyline and clomipramine. Desipramine has on the other hand only very weak affinity for these receptors (Richelson 1996). Antihistaminic activity is thought to underlie the *sedative* side-effects of tricyclics, though it probably does not act alone in this regard. Nonetheless, in clinical situations where anxiety and

agitation are intrusive, capitalising on what is in effect an adverse action can be an aid to management.

Sedation diminishes *reaction time*. Absence of appropriate advice from doctors concerning driving, is one reason why patients taking tricyclics are disproportionately represented amongst those involved in road traffic accidents. As a consequence of sedative properties, tricyclics can increase sleep time. They are not as a rule sleep-inducers but rather act to *maintain* sleep in those with early wakening. They may however be associated with prominent and distressing *dreams* (perhaps a result of anticholinergic effects). Antihistaminic activity may also contribute to what is for patients one of the most unwanted of adverse effects, namely, *weight gain*. Increase in weight on these drugs can be considerable and a major reason for non-compliance. It is suggested that the likelihood is greatest with amitriptyline and least with the secondary amines (Fernstrom & Kupfer 1988). The mechanisms underlying it are complex and may involve factors such as carbohydrate craving.

Tricyclics have clinically relevant affinity for muscarinic cholinergic receptors, with amitriptyline and protriptyline the most potent antagonists and nortriptyline and desipramine the least. Indeed these latter drugs have less affinity for cholinergic sites than paroxetine (Richelson 1996). Anticholinergic actions, mostly peripheral, make a major contribution to the adverse effects patients complain of most. Impaired salivary flow, especially in the resting state, results in an uncomfortable *dryness in the mouth* which, as with antipsychotics, may promote low-grade but potentially significant oral infection and dental caries. A similar *reduction in lacrimation* may predispose to corneal infection and damage, especially in those who wear contact lenses. A relative paralysis of accommodation causes pupillary dilatation and *blurring of vision*, most marked with changes in focal length (e.g. in changing from distance sight to reading) and rarely, in predisposed individuals, may promote closed-angle *glaucoma*. Inhibition of the cardiac sphincter may result in *oesophageal reflux* and heartburn. *Constipation* is of course a constant concern for the general public though is rarely so for doctors. In the elderly, however, drug-induced bowel hypomotility may have major and sometimes catastrophic consequences, as for example when *paralytic ileus* ensues. Impaired elimination and frank *urinary retention* is usually, though not exclusively, a problem in males, especially those with underlying prostatic hypertrophy. Sexual dysfunction can undoubtedly be associated with the use of drugs with anticholinergic actions, especially *poorly sustained erections*, but contrary to popular medical belief these effects are probably a relatively minor contributor. A lack of cholinergic balance on particularly noradrenergic function may however underlie infrequent cases of *priapism*. Vagal blockade results in a mild *sinus tachycardia*, on average less than 10 beats per minute. This is rarely clinically significant but, especially when combined with a reflex tachycardia secondary to hypotension, may increase oxygen demand in those with ischaemic heart disease sufficiently to promote rate-related angina or so-called 'silent' ischaemia (Jefferson 1989). Central anticholinergic actions may produce *impairment of memory*, which is likewise usually not significant, though in the elderly this effect, exaggerated by pharmacokinetic changes, may promote learning and memory problems and frank *confusion* in those with a compromised brain substrate.

Separation of the tricyclics from the new-generation drugs is less clear on the basis of anti-α_1 noradrenergic actions than with actions at other receptor types. Doxepin, trimipramine and amitriptyline

Table 15.4 Adverse effects of antidepressant drugs

Mediated by receptor antagonism					Not mediated by receptor antagonism
H_1	ACh	NA	D_2	Na fast channels	
Sedation^T,Mz Lethargy^T ↓Reaction time^T ↑Weight^T ↑Sleep time^T	↑Dreams^T Dry mouth^T Impaired accommodation^T Oesophageal reflux^T Constipation^T Urinary difficulties^T Sexual difficulties^T,(Mz) Priapism^(T),Tz Impaired memory^T	Postural hypotension^T,Tz,(N),MP	Hyperprolactinaemia^T Movement disorders^T	Delayed AV conduction^T,(M) Delayed IV conduction^T AV block^T Cardiac dysrhythmias^T Hypomania^M Positive psychotic features^T,M	Sedation^M,Mo,Mi,S,Tz,N Agitation^M,Mo,S Akathisia^(T),S Insomnia^T,M,Mo,V,S Dry mouth^M,Mi,Tz Urinary difficulties^M Sexual difficulties^M,S,Ve Constipation^M Seizures^T,Mp Hyperhidrosis^T Nausea^V,S,Ve Vomiting^V,S,Ve Diarrhoea^S,Mo Headache^Mo,S Migraine^V Weight gain^M,Mz,Tz Weight loss^V,S Supine hypotension^Mp,M Hypertension^T,Ve Tremor^T,M,Mo,S Movement disorders^S Dizziness^Mo Bradycardia^S Rashes^(T),(S) Hepatic dysfunction^N,(T),(M),(S) Blood dyscrasias^(T),Mi

M, MAOIs; Mi, mianserin; Mo, moclobemide, Mp; maprotiline; Mz, mirtazapine; N, nafazodone; S, SSRIs; T, tricyclics; Tz, trazodone; V, viloxazine; Ve, Venlafazine.

all have strong affinity for α_1 receptors, with imipramine, clomipramine and nortriptyline intermediate and desipramine and protriptyline relatively weak. This compares with trazodone, which also has moderate affinity, and sertraline which has little (Richelson 1996). As a result of these actions, tricyclics can cause lightheadedness or a 'woozy' feeling on walking, especially when changing position, consequent upon *postural*, or orthostatic, *hypotension*. This occurs in about 5–10% of even young healthy individuals on tricyclics and up to 20% of older populations, 4% of whom may sustain injuries (Frazer 1997). The best predictor of orthostatic drop during treatment is simply a postural drop prior to exposure (Glassman et al 1979). Although often viewed as an inconvenience, postural hypotension deserves to be taken for the potentially serious adverse effect it is. It is a major cause of morbidity from falls, especially in the elderly, in whom hip fractures have been estimated to occur 2–3 times more often in those on tricyclics (Ray et al 1987), and on rare occasions can promote both cerebral and myocardial ischaemia. Noradrenergic antagonism at α_1 sites also mediates a reflex tachycardia and is probably the other major contributor to sexual dysfunction including impotence, impaired or premature ejaculation and anorgasmia.

Most tricyclics have little affinity for dopamine (D_2) receptors, the exceptions being amoxapine, trimipramine and clomipramine. In the case of amoxapine, this can cause the gamut of extrapyramidal movement disorders, and caution should be used in recommending long-term use of this drug or its use for any duration in the elderly. Clomipramine has been reported to produce the same clinical manifestations of hyperprolactinaemia as antipsychotics, but in practice the prevalence is lower and they only infrequently present a management problem. A higher risk of movement disorders has not been specifically attributed to either trimipramine or clomipramine.

Other important adverse effects of tricyclics do not relate directly to their properties of central receptor antagonism (Table 15.4). Increase in noradrenergic transmission is probably behind the development of *anxiety* and *agitation* in some patients, especially within a few days of exposure. This has been referred to as the 'jitteriness' or 'early tricyclic' syndrome, but to all intents and purposes appears phenomenologically similar to akathisia and might best be considered a variant of such. A similar mechanism is the likely explanation of the low-amplitude, high-frequency *tremor* that is not uncommon. Comparative studies suggest these symptoms are most frequent with desipramine and protriptyline (Cole & Bodkin 1990), which is in line with a pathophysiology based on the low affinity of these compounds for α_1 receptors in a climate of noradrenergic facilitation. In view of their reuptake inhibition properties, it is perhaps surprising that reports of *hypertension* are few. This may reflect an absence of routine monitoring, and it has been suggested that transient rises early in exposure are not uncommon, perhaps more with amoxapine and in those with pre-existing hypertension (Jefferson 1989). Sweating, sometimes amounting to *hyperhidrosis*, can affect up to 10% of patients, and probably also reflects a basic group action. Even in mild degrees, this can be subjectively distressing and is something worth asking about even if it is not volunteered spontaneously.

The most important actions not directly mediated via central receptor antagonism are the effects on *cardiac function*. For many years much of what was known about the cardiac effects of tricyclics was derived from studies of overdose, which no doubt contributed to the belief that these drugs were uniquely toxic. It is only in the past two decades that studies of the clinical pharmacology of these agents have been performed under therapeutic conditions, and a somewhat more favourable impression has emerged. The direct actions on the heart show mainly in the two crucial areas of rhythm and conduction.

Tricyclics have properties of Class I *antiarrhythmics*, promoting membrane stabilisation through inhibition of fast sodium channels. They share both Type IA effects, which are quinidine-like and result in decreased amplitude of Purkinje fibre action potentials and membrane responsiveness with slowed conduction, and Type IB (lidocaine-like) effects of decreased duration of action potentials and effective refractory period (Jefferson 1989). At therapeutic blood levels they are clinically effective in the treatment of supraventricular tachycardias and some dysrhythmias of ventricular origin. However, any drug with antiarrhythmic properties may be proarrhythmic in some patients, especially when blood levels are high or when two Type I drugs are combined. Thus, tricyclics should be avoided in patients already receiving a Type I antiarrhythmic.

On ECG, tricyclics can prolong the QT_c interval, both in therapeutic doses and in patients without pre-existing heart disease (Reilly et al 2000), and can produce T-wave changes. As noted above for antipsychotics, this is a potential concern, and the arguments about the extent to which this should translate into practical concern are as with antipsychotics. No reliable data as yet exist on relative risk, though the effect is probably a class one.

Tricyclics have little effect on AV nodal conduction but delay *intraventricular* conduction in the His–Purkinje system. In the most general terms the delay is related to blood levels. The major potential issue consequent upon this action is precipitating or advancing the level of *heart block*. In an important prospective study of this issue, however, only 0.7% of patients (1 of 150) with normal pretreatment ECGs developed a 2:1 block, and this was reversible on discontinuation of the drug (Roose et al 1987). In-situ electrophysiology subsequently showed this patient to have a conduction deficit. Thus, in patients with normal cardiac conduction, the risk of tricyclics precipitating abnormality is small. In those with confirmed pre-existing conduction disorder, no consequences of exposure to therapeutic levels of tricyclic were noted in this study in those with only first-degree block, but 2 (9%) of those taking imipramine who had pretreatment bundle branch block developed second-degree block during treatment, also reversible on discontinuation. In 2 others the QRS interval increased by more than 25%. Of 15 patients on nortriptyline, 1 developed sinus arrest requiring pacing and another, who had suffered a previous infarct, re-infarcted (Roose et al 1987). While the authors of this work acknowledged the increased risk of tricyclics exacerbating conduction disorders in those with pre-existing abnormality, they also pointed out that, from a cardiological perspective, tricyclics still represent relatively safe antiarrhythmic agents.

There remains debate about the effects of tricyclics on cardiac *contractility*, with animal studies suggesting an augmenting (positive inotropic) effect at low doses but a depressant effect at higher doses. The position in humans, especially those with heart disease, is unclear. Studies in this field are obviously difficult, but the evidence, which is only suggestive, does *not* support the view that tricyclics (nortriptyline, amitriptyline, imipramine and doxepin at least) adversely affect left ventricular performance (Glassman & Biggar 1981).

Therefore, the evidence to date is that at therapeutic levels tricyclics have few detrimental actions in the absence of pre-existing cardiac disease and in certain circumstances may have actions that are beneficial. With care, the evidence is that these drugs can be used with a relative margin of safety in most patients with signs of cardiac failure. Nonetheless, in view of increasing concern about the significance of prolonged QT_c, it is suggested that where tricyclics are recommended, ECG monitoring should be considered.

These drugs do, like most antipsychotics, alter the EEG and lower the seizure threshold. Hence they can precipitate seizures. The risk is low, however, with prevalence rates estimated to be in the region of 0.1–0.5% of patients (Skowron & Stimmel 1992). The risk does appear to be substantially higher with maprotiline, and this drug should be avoided in those in whom any family or personal predisposition can be elicited. The likelihood of an individual developing fits appears related to dose and the rate of dose increment.

For a number of years controversy existed about whether antidepressants in general, and tricyclics in particular, could precipitate *hypomania/mania* in non-bipolar depressed patients. The evidence is that this is unlikely and that those who do develop morbid elevation of mood while on treatment are predisposed to bipolar disorder or are experiencing withdrawal phenomena (Kupfer et al 1988). A disorder of speech, sometimes referred to as dysarthria but better described as *speech 'blocking'* or *hesitancy*, has been described with a rarity that probably does not reflect its true frequency. This adverse effect, resembling stammer, is easily confused with agitation associated with the depression itself.

Other rarely reported adverse effects include skin rashes, blood dyscrasias, cholestatic jaundice and hepatic necrosis (transient mild elevations in liver enzymes are not uncommon and usually of no clinical significance), oedema from inappropriate secretion of antidiuretic hormone, and non-vibratory tinnitus.

Although sometimes marketed as a new-generation drug, maprotiline is, as was noted, a modified tricyclic structure and in terms of its tolerability behaves, in general, similarly to amitripty-

line. Two additional problems are worthy of note, however. The first is an increased risk of skin rashes (approximately 3% in the first 2 weeks of treatment), and the second is a substantially increased likelihood of precipitating seizures, even in the absence of predisposing factors (Blackwell & Simon 1988).

The prevalence of adverse reactions to antidepressant drugs is difficult to estimate from published studies, which adopt differing methods and thresholds for recording. Their propensities would however seem to be less than clinical folklore indicates. The most systematic investigation reported a prevalence of 15.4% (Boston Collaborative Drug Surveillance Program 1972), which is comparable to the 18% found in comparative studies with newer antidepressants (see below).

Monoamine oxidase inhibitors

Structures

Although it is the antidepressant monoamine oxidase inhibitors that concern us, compounds acting by this mechanism have wide medicinal applications as antimicrobial, antineoplastic and antihypertensive agents.

Of the three traditional antidepressant monoamine oxidase inhibitors available in the UK, phenelzine and isocarboxazid are derivatives of *hydrazine* (NH_2NH_2), while tranylcypromine is a *cyclopropylamine*, formed by substituting the isopropyl side chain of amphetamine with a cyclopropyl side chain.

Advances in the pharmacology of drugs acting by monoamine oxidase inhibition have resulted in a number of new compounds with a selectivity and/or reversibility of action not seen with the traditional drugs. Moclobemide, originally developed as a potential lipid-lowering agent, is chemically a substituted benzamide and is the only one of these new MAOIs currently available in the UK as an antidepressant (Fig. 15.4). Selegiline (or –deprenyl), which

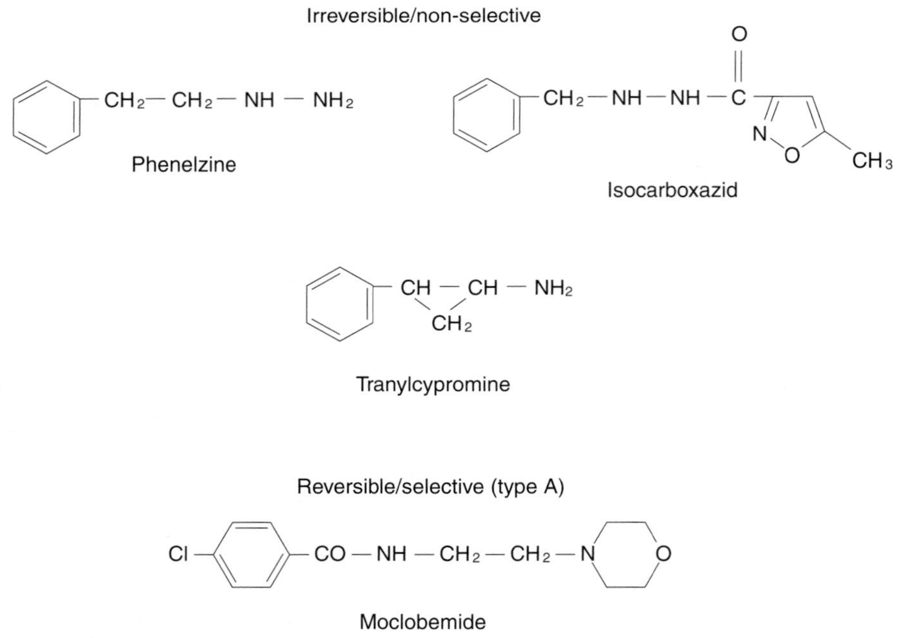

Fig. 15.4
Structures of monoamine oxidase inhibitors.

is a metamphetamine derivative, is pharmacologically within this group, however.

Pharmacokinetics

The pharmacokinetics of isocarboxazid have not been studied, but phenelzine and tranylcypromine appear to have fairly comparable properties (Mallinger & Smith 1991). They are readily absorbed and reach peak concentrations in 1–2 hours. Elimination of both drugs is also swift, with half-lives in the range of $1\frac{1}{2}$–4 hours (especially short for tranylcypromine). This is due to rapid and almost complete hepatic metabolism. Protein binding is high and bioavailability low. Even now, the steps underlying metabolism of these drugs are poorly understood. Acetylation was thought to be an important step in phenelzine metabolism, with 'acetylator status' (slow or fast) a major determinant of efficacy and especially tolerability. However, it is now unclear whether acetylation is the predominant metabolic route. Plasma steady-state levels of phenelzine appear to rise over the first 6–8 weeks of exposure, suggesting that either the drug (or a metabolite) may inhibit its own metabolism.

The traditional irreversible and non-selective MAOIs are unique psychopharmacological agents, in that their clinical effects bear little relationship to their pharmacokinetics. The reason for this is that these drugs mediate so-called *mechanism-based reactions*— that is, they are relatively inert compounds in themselves, but are converted by MAO into highly reactive intermediates which then inactivate the enzyme via a process of irreversible, covalent bonding (Amrein et al 1989). This results in what has been variously called a 'suicide' effect (in that the enzyme's affinity for the drug results in its irrevocable inactivation) and a 'hit-and-run' effect (because the action of the drug can be detected long after the drug itself has been completely eliminated).

The newer MAOIs also have 'breakneck' kinetics. Moclobemide is readily absorbed and reaches peak plasma concentrations in approximately 1 hour. Metabolism is rapid and complete, with elimination half-life in the range 1–3 hours. Some metabolites may be pharmacologically active but to a clinically insignificant degree. Protein binding, at around 50%, is relatively low but bioavailability appears to increase with regular dosing (Amrein et al 1989). A mechanism-based reaction has been postulated for moclobemide but, even if true, the consequences are fundamentally different than with the traditional drugs, as enzyme binding is reversible.

Pharmacodynamics

Mode of action

MAO is a flavin-containing enzyme situated mainly in the outer membranes of mitochondria. It has a wide and dense distribution. It is the major intracellular enzyme catalysing the oxidative deamination of biogenic amines, and in the CNS its function is intimately related to reuptake. By metabolising cytoplasmic amines and maintaining their concentration low, its action facilitates inward-directed transporter activity from the synapse. However, the precise relationship between these intracellular events and concentrations of monoamines in the extracellular space is more complex than was originally thought and remains unclear.

In 1968, Johnston identified two subtypes of MAO, referred to as 'type A' and 'type B'. These subtypes differ in their preferential substrates and inhibitors. The preferred substrates for type A include noradrenaline and serotonin, while phenethylamine, benzylamine and *N*-methylhistamine are preferential substrates for type B. Dopamine, tyramine and tryptamine have no preference for either subtype.

Some qualifications are necessary to the conventional wisdom about traditional MAOIs (Baldessarini 1985). The enzymatic 'hari-kari' that is the consequence of their mechanism-based action has allowed their effects to be viewed as irreversible, with inhibition only overcome by the manufacture of new enzyme. While this in general is true, a degree of reversibility is evident with tranylcypromine, and recovery of enzyme function is somewhat more rapid (7–10 days) following discontinuation of this than it is after cessation of treatment with hydrazine derivatives (2+ weeks). Secondly, although these drugs are considered non-selective, as is so often the case, this non-selectivity is relative. Phenelzine has an approximately 6:1 preference for type A, while tranylcypromine has a slight (2:1) predilection for type B. Only isocarboxazid has roughly equal affinity for both subtypes. It seems unlikely however that these differences translate into anything clinically meaningful. Finally, while mechanism-based reactions form the essential characteristic of the processes mediating efficacy, aspects of their adverse effect profile indicate that these drugs also partake in more conventional pharmacological interactions.

One of the problems in evaluating the place of traditional MAOIs in therapy relates to questions of dosing (see below). It has been suggested that in order to obtain therapeutic benefits, blockade of MAO must be in the region of 80–85%, levels only achieved by doses of phenelzine in the range 45–60 mg per day or above (Baldessarini 1985). However, these estimates may be flawed, as they refer to blockade performed on platelets, which contain only MAO-B. Nonetheless this does emphasise the obvious point — that even with drugs acting in the unique way that these do, adequacy of dosing is an essential prerequisite of therapeutic efficacy.

The identification of MAO subtypes led to the search for drugs with patterns of inhibition that were selective, particularly (in line with the Biogenic Amine Hypothesis) to type A (Rudorfer 1992). The first of these was still irreversible, so clorgyline, a selective inhibitor of MAO-A, has not found commercial sponsorship. The most prominent of the selective inhibitors of MAO-B, selegiline, is not useful in the treatment of depression because, in the higher doses necessary for antidepressant activity, selectivity is lost. Because of its dopaminergic actions, it has however become an important tool in the management of Parkinson's disease.

A number of selective inhibitors of MAO-A that are also reversible have been developed, including brofaromine, cimoxatone and toloxatone. Of these so-called RIMAs (**R**eversible **I**nhibitors of **M**AO type **A**), only moclobemide has thus far received a wide launch. Despite producing very similar plasma concentration time-course curves to tranylcypromine, the consequences of this with moclobemide are dramatically different, with maximum inhibition evident after the first dose (Mallinger & Smith 1991). Although moclobemide has a swift elimination half-life, it produces MAO-A blockade for 8–10 hours, though a decline in inhibition is evident towards the end of even a thrice daily dose schedule.

Traditional MAOIs and the RIMAs therefore produce very similar pharmacological effects but over strikingly different time scales — some 2 weeks with the former and almost immediate with the latter. Yet there is no evidence that the onset of clinical antidepressant action differs for the two types of drug. Once again the primary pharmacological action appears to represent only a necessary first step in the therapeutic process.

Adverse effects Studies of the pharmacology of the traditional MAOIs have focused on their enzyme-blocking action to the exclusion of other actions that may be more pertinent to some of their adverse effects (Table 15.4). Some adverse effects have been shown to relate to peak plasma concentrations, at least for tranylcypromine, the most studied of these drugs, and to be modifiable by alterations to methods of administration (Mallinger & Smith 1991). This is not compatible with exclusively mechanism-based activity.

The major adverse effect associated with the use of the traditional MAOIs is *hypotension*. Unlike tricyclics, where the effects are largely if not exclusively postural, with the traditional MAOIs, lowering of *supine* blood pressure is also evident. Hence, the overall clinical impact of any postural drop is more potentially disabling. The exact prevalence of reported postural hypotension varies considerably but may be in the region of 14% for tranylcypromine and slightly less for phenelzine (Rabkin et al 1985). The supine component of hypotension appears to develop relatively early (within the first week), but in a further difference with tricyclics, postural hypotension with traditional MAOIs may not be seen early in treatment but seems to build up, especially over the first 4 weeks or so of exposure. However, it may emerge at any point in the course of treatment, and it is important that this is appreciated by both physician and patient. This may be one of the adverse effects that relates to pharmacokinetic parameters, and therefore it may be useful to attempt to alter dose regimens as a first step in management.

The mechanism underlying the hypotensive actions of traditional MAOIs is unclear, though has been postulated to result from accumulation of biogenic amines (because of their slowed metabolism) with a consequent increase in the activity of precursors. This may result in the formation of amines with less direct sympathomimetic activity which, in effect, act as 'false transmitters' (Baldessarini 1985). This however remains a hypothesis.

Early in their use, it was reported that these drugs possessed antianginal properties, probably mediated via a diminution in sympathetically regulated arteriolar tone. However, although acting to alleviate pain, they do not modify ischaemic changes on ECG, so are in fact merely converting symptomatic to asymptomatic ischaemia (Jefferson 1989). Nonetheless, traditional MAOIs do not have any direct actions on cardiac rhythm, conduction or contractility, and a reduction in basal heart rate usually accompanies treatment, so they may be useful in treating depressed patients with cardiac disease who are receiving either no, or compatible, cardiac medication.

It is surprising that drugs with little antimuscarinic actions should in practice be associated with the development of adverse effects conventionally viewed as anticholinergic: *dry mouth*, *constipation* and *urinary difficulties*, including retention, and *sexual disturbance*, such as impotence and orgasmic dysfunction. Such symptoms, established mainly with phenelzine but also found with tranylcypromine, can be prominent, with urinary retention occasionally affecting females. Rather than reflecting a single receptor system (i.e. cholinergic) disorder, such adverse effects are probably manifestations of a peripheral cholinergic/noradrenergic imbalance, with an excess of adrenergic sympathetic function.

Traditional MAOIs can produce *elevation of mood* in those not predisposed to bipolar disorders, and hypomania/mania in those who are (Rudorfer 1992). They should also be avoided in schizophrenic patients, as they may precipitate or exacerbate '*positive*' psychotic symptomatology. Tranylcypromine is the sole first-generation antidepressant to which *abuse* and *dependency* can be attributed, a fact no doubt not unrelated to its close structural relationship to amphetamine, analogues of which are a product of its metabolism (Mallinger & Smith 1991).

As a result of their generally stimulant actions, traditional MAOIs may be associated with *insomnia* as well as agitation and general psychomotor 'arousal'. However, hydrazine compounds can be *sedative*, especially on first exposure. Prolonged phenelzine use has on occasion been reported to be associated with pyridoxine (vitamin B_6) deficiency, resulting in *peripheral neuropathy*. This appears to be reversible with B_6 supplements. Rare cases of diuretic-resistant oedema, probably associated with inappropriate antidiuretic hormone secretion, have been reported. The hepatotoxicity found with iproniazid does not appear to be an issue with the currently available drugs. However tranylcypromine should be avoided in those with pre-existing liver disease, as there appears to be a risk of precipitating an encephalopathic-type picture (Blackwell & Simon 1988).

The adverse-effect profile of moclobemide appears more favourable than those of tricyclics or the traditional MAOIs. In particular, autonomic side-effects seem less prevalent, especially dry mouth. Restlessness, disturbed sleep, daytime fatigue, and tremor can however occur, as can transient dizziness and headache (Baumhackl et al 1989). Confusion, reversible on discontinuation, has been reported rarely.

Hypertensive crises

The major source of concern with the traditional MAOIs is not strictly an adverse or toxic effect but rather a drug–drug (including food) interaction. This is the potential to precipitate a *hypertensive crisis*. These were described soon after their introduction and were crucial to the perception of risk that led to the side lining of the group from clinical practice. It was some years before the biochemistry of these potentially fatal reactions was understood (Blackwell 1963), and although this offers some reassurances, an element of unpredictability remains. Because of their early association with ingestion of strong cheeses, the syndrome is still sometimes referred to as the 'cheese reaction', but this is an unjustified narrowing of the concept.

Hypertensive crises have two causes. The first, and traditionally most common, results from the direct absorption of pressor amines formed as part of the bacterial decarboxylation of amino acid constituents of certain protein-containing foods. Normally these amines (e.g. tyramine, phenylethylamine and histamine) are neutralised by MAO in the gut wall, but the loss of this protective effect by the action of enzyme inhibition allows free passage of the amines into the systemic circulation. The second cause is the ingestion of sympathomimetic drugs, including ephedrine (and its derivatives) and phenylpropanolamine, which are common constituents of over-the-counter medicines, especially cold and cough remedies.

These types of compound stimulate inappropriate release of noradrenaline from sympathetic nerve terminals and/or adrenaline from the adrenal medulla, resulting in symptoms similar to phaeochromocytoma. Patients develop pallor, and feel anxious, nauseated and sweaty, with pounding occipital headaches and palpitations from both forceful and irregular heart beat. Associated with this is a dramatic paroxysmal rise in blood pressure. In severe cases, death can ensue from cerebrovascular accident or cardiac failure or arrest. The risk appears greatest with tranylcypromine.

When the mechanism of hypertensive crises was first delineated, an attempt was made to diminish the risk by defining the pressor amine content of foodstuffs, with the aim of removing from the diet those foods with the highest contents. In the USA, this led to listings of over 700 items (Frazer 1997) and a recommended diet not much more palatable than bread and water! Problems of estimation contaminated much of this work, and it is now clear that the dietary restrictions required of patients taking traditional MAOIs are in fact modest, with only gastronomes of a faddy disposition finding them in any way burdensome (Baldessarini 1985). Clear proscriptions apply to pickled herring, yeast extracts like 'Marmite' and fish and meat extracts, such as 'Bovril', and certain vegetable components such as broad bean pods and banana skins. It would also be prudent to go easy on the guacamole, and caviar should be kept for celebrating cessation of treatment. Most alcoholic drinks have low levels of pressor amines, and the problems with co-ingestion relate more to potentiation. Chianti wines, prohibited in the past, appear to have been somewhat unjustly singled out. Red wines have in general higher amounts of pressor amines than whites.

The position surrounding cheeses is less clear. Some, such as cottage or cream cheeses, are without risk, as are sour cream and yoghurt. However, the problem with other cheeses relates not so much to their absolute amine values — which, in reference lists, would indicate a limited source of concern — but to the fact that levels vary widely (up to 100-fold) and unpredictably in comparable samples. Manufacturing processes, especially of strong cheeses, lend themselves to wide variations in amine content across batches and to a lack of uniform distribution within samples produced from the same batch. Hence, caution should be exercised with all cheeses, especially matured ones. There is no particular proscription on 'blue' cheeses, as was once recommended, but the German 'Liederkranz', with its unusually high tyramine content, is verboten.

The risk of hypertensive crises with RIMAs is theoretically much reduced, though not completely eliminated. In practice, no specific dietary restrictions are necessary with moclobemide.

New-generation antidepressants

Structures

There is no unifying chemical structure to drugs considered under this heading. Among the survivors of the first wave are mianserin, a distant tetracyclic cousin of cyproheptadine, and trazodone, a triazolopyridine (or phenylpiperazine).

The selective serotonin reuptake inhibitors (SSRIs) can be conveniently seen as comprising the second wave. They are as a rule novel and complex molecules (Fig. 15.5) whose divergent structures help little towards understanding of their pharmacology. Bupropion, licensed in the USA as an antidepressant but in the UK only as an aid to smoking cessation, is an aminoketone whose efficacy appears predicated on reuptake inhibition — of dopamine!

A third wave of drugs has also emerged which inhibit the reuptake of both serotonin and noradrenaline (venlafaxine), selectively inhibit noradrenaline reuptake (reboxetine), or enhance serotoner-

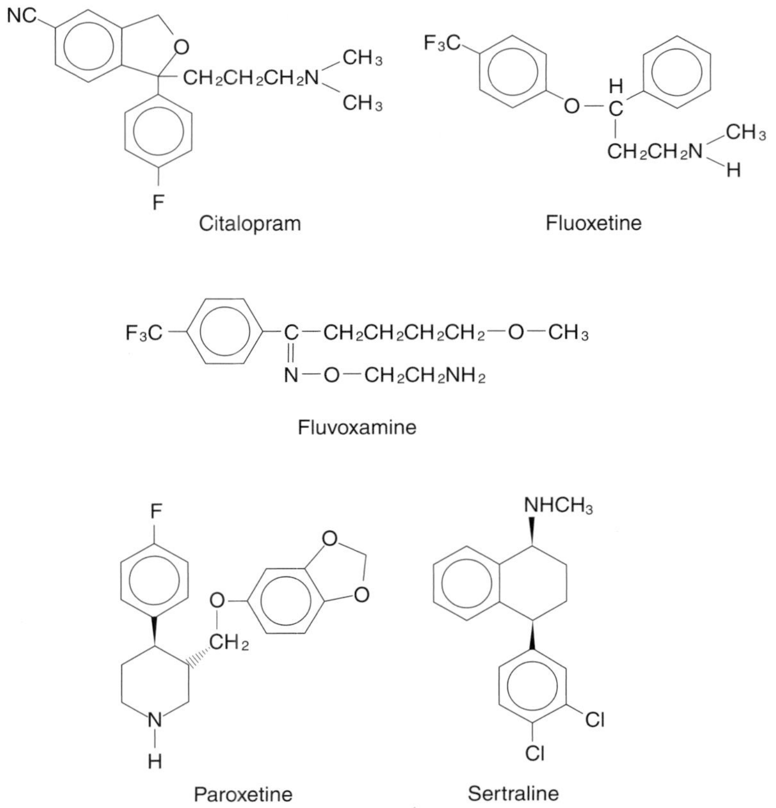

Fig. 15.5
Structures of selective serotonin reuptake inhibitors.

gic and noradrenergic transmission via antagonist actions at α_2 noradrenergic sites pre- and postsynaptically, such as mirtazapine, a close structural analogue of mianserin. Nefazodone, also a phenylpiperazine with complex receptor antagonist properties in addition to selective actions on serotonin reuptake, can be hepatotoxic and was withdrawn in Europe for commercial reasons in 2003. Escitalopram is a purified preparation of the active isomer of citalopram.

Pharmacokinetics

Mianserin is rapidly absorbed and subject to very extensive first-pass effects. Its bioavailability is less than 30%. Time to peak is in the region of 3 hours, and its half-life is between 10 and 20 hours but is much extended in the elderly. It is completely metabolised, and some products, such as desmethylmianserin, are weakly active.

Trazodone is rapidly absorbed (T_{max} = 1–2 hours) and prone to first-pass effects. Between 60% and 80% reaches the systemic circulation. First-pass metabolism may be saturable, and plasma levels may follow non-linear pharmacokinetics. The half-life is, for an antidepressant, relatively short at 5–9 hours, and excretion is mainly renal. A major metabolite of trazodone, *m*-chlorophenylpiperazine (*m*-CPP), has anxiogenic properties which counter the sedative properties of the parent. These may produce clinical effects in patients who attain high blood levels (Preskorn 1993b).

Pharmacokinetic variables are the main characteristics which distinguish the SSRIs from one another. The major parameters for currently available compounds are shown in Table 15.5. All are well, if slowly, absorbed; with fluoxetine, food may delay absorption further (Goodnick 1991). Likewise all are extensively metabolised. Both fluoxetine and paroxetine inhibit their own metabolism, and hence show *non-linear* pharmacokinetics, with increasing doses producing disproportionately large increases in blood levels (Preskorn 1993b). In the case of fluvoxamine and paroxetine, metabolism does not appear to result in active metabolites. The others do produce pharmacologically active breakdown products, though the contribution these make to efficacy is not uniform. Fluoxetine has as its major metabolite norfluoxetine, which is roughly equipotent in relation to serotonin reuptake inhibition as the parent drug. It also has an exceptionally long elimination half-life of 7–15 days. These variables may be extended in those with hepatic disease. In the case of fluoxetine therefore the metabolite has a major impact on the clinical action and on treatment decisions, especially following

discontinuation. The mono- and dimethylated metabolites of citalopram are likewise serotonin reuptake inhibitors, though they are respectively 4- and 13-fold less potent than the parent (Boyer & Feighner 1991). Desmethylcitalopram is, however, considerably more potent than its parent in inhibiting noradrenaline reuptake. The clinical impact of these in-vitro findings is likely to be modified by the fact that both metabolites penetrate the brain poorly and, although opinions at present differ, it appears they make little contribution to the therapeutic package. Citralopram's half-life is extended in the elderly. The primary metabolite of sertraline, desmethylsertraline, is a weak serotonin reuptake inhibitor, being about 5–10-fold less potent than the parent. Its elimination half-life however is, at over 60 hours, some two and a half times that of sertraline, and, whereas in the elderly this variable is unchanged for sertraline, the half-life of the metabolite is prolonged. For most clinical scenarios it seems unlikely that desmethylsertraline contributes to the therapeutic effect, though there may be some clinical effects in the elderly.

It can be appreciated that for some members of this group, steady state can take some time to achieve — for citalopram up to 2 weeks, for fluoxetine 2–3 weeks and for norfluoxetine anything from 4 to 8 weeks.

Venlafaxine is presented as a racemic mix of two active enantiomers. It is readily absorbed, with T_{max} values in the range 2–3 hours, and first-pass effects are substantial. Protein binding is low compared with other antidepressants (< 30%). Its half-life is also relatively short at approximately 5 hours, but that of its major metabolite — *o*-desmethylvenlafaxine, which is active — is about twice that of the parent. Excretion is almost exclusively renal.

Nefazodone is also rapidly and completely absorbed (T_{max} 1–3 hours) and is subject to substantial pre-systemic metabolism. It is uniquely highly protein bound (> 99%) and is also unusual in its rapid elimination half-life which, at 2–4 hours, is more like those of the MAOIs. The pharmacokinetics of nefazodone are non-linear, and *m*-CPP is a minor metabolic product (Malik 1996).

Reboxetine is structurally related to both fluoxetine and the now withdrawn viloxazine. It is presented, like a number of the new antidepressants, as a racemic mixture of two enantiomers which appear to have similar kinetics. Reboxetine is rapidly absorbed (T_{max} = approx. 2 hours), and its elimination half-life is in the region of 13 hours. It is highly protein bound, mainly to α_1 glycoprotein. Metabolism is extensive, with most excreted in the urine, though some may also be excreted in faeces in primates. Unlike most antidepressants, it appears to have little inhibitory effect on the cytochrome P450 system (Dostert et al 1997). This, together with its lack of action on serotonergic systems or against MAO, would indicate that its combined use with other drugs may be particularly uncomplicated, though this remains to be confirmed.

Mirtazapine is referred to as a NaSSA — a noradrenergic and specific serotonergic antidepressant. It is readily absorbed regardless of gastric contents, with a T_{max} value of around 2 hours, and the half-life, which varies from 20 to 40 hours, is sufficient for once daily dosing. It does not modify its own metabolism, which is mediated via several cytochrome isoenzymes.

Pharmacodynamics

Mode of action   Of these new-generation drugs, the SSRIs have putatively similar modes of action, and, although more diverse and intricate actions are claimed for the others considered here, the element of reuptake inhibition is common to most.

Table 15.5   Some pharmacokinetic parameters of SSRI antidepressants

	T_{max}(h)	Protein binding(%)	Half-life (h)	Active metabolites
Citalopram Escitaprolam	4–6	75 (or less)	30–36	+
Fluoxetine	6–8	94	24–72	+++
Fluvoxamine	2–8	77	15 (single dosing) 17–22 (multiple dosing)	–
Paroxetine	2–8	95	20	–
Sertraline	6–8	99	25	+

SSRIs selectively block the reuptake of serotonin relative to noradrenaline into the presynaptic bulb (Goodwin 1996, Frazer 1997). This selectivity is *relative*: all currently available drugs to some extent also block noradrenaline reuptake, though for the majority this action is weak and probably not relevant to their efficacy. Citalopram is the most serotonergically *selective* of the current drugs and paroxetine the most *potent* (Richelson 1996). Viewed by the criterion of *relative* selectivity, clomipramine could be viewed as an SSRI. In addition, however, those drugs classified as SSRIs are set apart by having little or no affinity for neurotransmitter receptors. Paroxetine has moderate affinity for muscarinic receptors, with which sertraline, fluoxetine and citalopram also interact detectably though very weakly. Sertraline also interacts with α_1 adrenoceptors, and fluvoxamine with dopamine D_2 receptors. This however represents overall a fairly inert receptor-binding profile.

Venlafaxine appears to be a pure reuptake inhibitor with no affinity for the commonly studied receptor subtypes (Richelson 1996), while trazodone (like its relative nefazodone) is a fairly potent α_1 antagonist. The efficacy of nefazodone, however, is postulated to lie in the combination of serotonin reuptake inhibition with potent $5HT_2$ antagonism. Reboxetine is a selective reuptake inhibitor of noradrenaline. Mirtazapine does not appear to inhibit monoamine reuptake but has a complex receptor-binding profile involving antagonism at especially presynaptic α_2 adrenoceptors and $5HT_{2a/2c/3}$ sites and is postulated to work by enhancing noradrenergic transmission, which is associated with a parallel increase in serotonergic function.

What essential components of action that can be extracted from the pharmacological melée that is antidepressant drugs in order to account for clinical efficacy is unknown — though there is no shortage of hypotheses. Antidepressant efficacy is associated with drugs which *selectively* block the presynaptic reuptake of noradrenaline *or* of serotonin, or are completely *non-selective* in inhibiting the reuptake of both. It may also be associated with the *facilitation* of serotonin reuptake, as with the atypical tricyclic tianeptine, or with inhibition of *dopamine* reuptake. It may occur in the context of direct receptor activity *or* no apparent receptor affinity. And of course one of our earliest lessons in antidepressant psychopharmacology was that it may occur in the *absence* of any direct effects on either reuptake or receptors. It may in future be more rational to classify *all* antidepressants in terms of their putative functional characteristics (Table 15.6), though as far as our attempts to *refine* the Biogenic Amine Hypothesis is concerned, the above does begin to look rather silly!

SSRIs, SNRIs, NaRIs or any other type of 'Is' are pharmacological tools for facilitating biogenic amine transmission in certain, probably specific, brain areas. This, it can be safely concluded, is the *necessary* first step. An advantage of the new drugs may lie in the precision with which they do this, as this may enhance tolerability and safety. This enhancement may be achieved solely by concentrating on serotonin or on noradrenaline separately or may be achieved by utilising the relationships between serotonin and noradrenaline, which may extend efficacy to more severe disorders. However, *no* antidepressant drug, new or old, has a pattern of clinical response that parallels its primary pharmacological action. Therefore it must be concluded that *other* changes mediate the desired clinical effect — and these certainly involve receptors and 'downline' changes in cellular metabolism.

A number of receptor changes have been associated with chronic antidepressant exposure (Baldessarini 1985). These include

Table 15.6 Classification of antidepressants by proposed modes of action	
Enzyme inhibitors	
Monoamine oxidase	
Irreversible/non-selective	e.g. phenelzine, tranylcypromine
Reversible/selective (type A)	e.g. moclobemide
Reuptake inhibitors	
Serotonin selective	e.g. fluoxetine, paroxetine
Noradrenaline selective	e.g. reboxetine
Serotonin and noradrenaline non-selective	e.g. venlafaxine
Dopamine and noradrenaline	e.g. bupropion
Reuptake inhibitors with specific receptor actions	
Serotonin reuptake inhibition +$5HT_{2A}$ antagonism	e.g. nefazodone
Reuptake inhibitors (non-selective) with multiple receptor interactions	
	e.g. imipramine, amitriptyline
Reuptake inhibitors (selective) with multiple receptor interactions	
	e.g. desipramine, clomipramine
Receptor interactions (selective) $5HT_{2A}/5HT_{2C}/5HT_3/\alpha_2$-NA	e.g. mirtazapine

desensitisation of cortical α_2 noradrenergic and presynaptic dopamine autoreceptors; up-regulation at α_1 and down-regulation at GABA-B sites; desensitisation and down-regulation of β-noradrenergic and $5HT_2$ receptors; and desensitisation and up-regulation of limbic $5HT_{1a}$ receptors.

Moulding these into a coherent hypothesis of universal applicability to the mode of action of antidepressant drugs is beyond the capabilities of the author to do and the needs of the reader to know!

Adverse effects   *Mianserin* is strongly sedative and, despite having no anticholinergic actions, can be associated with dry mouth and a non-significant increase in pulse rate. It can also promote fits but the risk is, if anything, lower than with tricyclics.

The major advantage of mianserin is that, apart from the above, it appears to have very little effect on cardiac function. Prolonged PR interval and decreased T-wave amplitude are inconsistent ECG findings with chronic treatment, and there is even the suggestion of enhanced cardiac function (non-significant) as shown by an increase in the ejection fraction (Kopera 1980).

There is, however, also a major potential problem. In 1979, blood dyscrasia associated with mianserin was described and in 1989 the Committee on Safety of Medicines issued a 'Current Problems' notice (No. 25) on a total of 239 cases received up to that time. Sixty-eight concerned agranulocytosis and 84 granulopenia or leukopenia, 17 of whom died. An excess of cases, and deaths, occurred in the over 65s. Reports from Australia and New Zealand put the overall rate of agranulocytosis at between 1:2000 and 1:4000 exposures (Blackwell & Simon 1988). These data remained controversial, and, in a unique move, the manufacturer went to Court to prevent withdrawal of the drug in the UK. Mianserin requires close *haematological monitoring* for at least the first 3 months of use, *particularly in the elderly*, something which limits its value in the population in whom, because of its lack of cardiotoxicity, it may otherwise be most useful.

Trazodone produces marked sedation and lethargy and, in some pharmacological models, has significant anti-anxiety effects. On the basis of this, it has achieved wide popularity in recent years. Once again it can be associated with dry mouth, blurred vision, etc. in the absence of cholinergic antagonist properties, probably relating to cholinergic–adrenergic imbalance promoted by its potent α_1 antagonist actions. This may also be the mechanism behind a uniquely high prevalence of *priapism* (Warner et al 1987), though this is not something that correlates with antiadrenergic actions in general. This is a potentially serious complication of trazodone, which may require surgical intervention, with impotence a not infrequent outcome. Male patients receiving trazodone should be advised to stop treatment at the first signs of any increase in the frequency and duration of erections. Trazodone appears to have minimal effects on cardiac function at therapeutic doses.

Contrary to developing lore, the *SSRIs* are not free from adverse effects (Table 15.4) but share a profile fairly characteristic of the group, though different from those of other antidepressants (Boyer & Feighner 1996). They all possess an increased liability to *gastrointestinal upset*, with *nausea* the commonest adverse effect (25–35%). Nausea of sufficient severity to force discontinuation affects 5–8% of patients. Abdominal discomfort/pain, frank vomiting and diarrhoea also occur with greater frequency than with other antidepressants. These effects develop early in exposure, before the establishment of steady state, and tend to ease as this is reached. Hence, they are likely to be mediated by local (GI) rather than central actions. Dry mouth and constipation may be more frequent with paroxetine, reflecting its weak receptor-binding profile. A further common group effects is *headache*, usually occipital in situation and pounding in quality. This tends to increase in frequency with continued exposure (Frazer 1997).

While these drugs cannot be conveniently considered as stimulant or non-stimulant, fluoxetine appears to be particularly associated with *nervousness, anxiety* and *agitation* which is likely to carry over into *insomnia* and reduced quality of sleep, even with the drug taken in the morning. The others, especially fluvoxamine and paroxetine, seem by contrast less likely to produce these effects and may indeed be associated with *sedation* and daytime fatigue.

It is not yet clear precisely where this restless state lies in relation to akathisia but, as with the tricyclics, it seems likely that it is phenomenologically very similar, if not identical. SSRIs do however possess the potential to cause *acute dystonic reactions*, and rarely *parkinsonism*, which are identical to those movement disorders caused by standard antipsychotics (Owens 1999). The prevalence of these is not as yet known but is likely to be considerably lower than with antipsychotics. SSRIs have also been reported to exacerbate *tardive* movement disorders. These adverse effects throw new light on the mechanisms underlying drug-related extrapyramidal dysfunction, and, although it is too early to say what might emerge with long-term exposure, this is a question that will require addressing.

The other major set of adverse effects associated with the SSRIs relate to *sexual dysfunction* (Lane 1997). The frequency of sexual side-effects is hard to specify, and figures differ between studies, but with widespread use it is becoming increasingly clear that problems such as abnormal ejaculation/orgasm, anorgasmia, impotence and decreased libido are common with this group, more

so than with tricyclics. One review suggested that 34% of patients on fluoxetine reported sexual difficulties — 10% with reduced libido, 13% decreased responsiveness and 11% both (Jacobsen 1992). There may be differences in prevalence with different compounds, though this cannot be concluded with certainty. Furthermore, the pattern may differ across drugs, with some, such as sertraline, causing more sexual dysfunction in males than females (Frazer 1997).

SSRIs have different effects on *weight* than traditional antidepressants (Boyer & Feighner 1996). Fluoxetine and sertraline have anorectic effects and are associated with a tendency to weight *loss*, especially in higher doses. Paroxetine appears unique in not possessing this property, and indeed patients on long-term treatment may gain somewhat. The others tend to be more neutral in this regard, at least in standard doses. It appears that absolute declines in weight during treatment depend on initial body weight, with greater loss being found in more obese patients, though there is also a suggestion (unconfirmed) that the elderly may be more liable to this action.

The SSRIs also exert virtually no effects on cardiac conduction and they are not dysrhythmogenic (Coupland et al 1997). However, they can produce *bradycardia* which may be clinically significant and symptomatic, especially in the elderly and those with certain forms of pre-existing heart disease.

A further uncommon adverse effect concerns the development of a *haemorrhagic diathesis* resulting in bruising and frank haematomata. This may be as a result of inhibition of platelet serotonin uptake and is more likely to be associated with laboratory abnormalities in platelet aggregation tests than in bleeding times. Intradermal bruising has been found in the offspring of laboratory animals exposed during pregnancy and is a strong reason for avoidance of this group of drugs during pregnancy until the position is clarified. Rarely, *skin rashes* and *hyponatraemia* with or without inappropriate ADH secretion have been reported, as have *seizures*, but the liability of the group in this regard is minimal and less than tricyclics.

One way of evaluating the impact of adverse experiences is from discontinuation rates in comparative clinical trials. In two large metanalyses of published studies (Montgomery et al 1994, Anderson & Tomenson 1995), fewer patients receiving SSRIs (14.9% and 14.4%, respectively) than tricyclics (19% and 18.8%, respectively) dropped out. In both these analyses the differences were *statistically* significant. However, they are far from dramatic and are unlikely to represent differences that are significant in *clinical* terms (Anderson & Tomenson 1995). A further metanalysis concluded that of every 100 patients treated with a tricyclic, 31 would be likely to drop out of treatment, while the comparable figure for those on an SSRI would be 28 (Hotopf et al 1997).

The other new-generation drugs appear to share the relatively favourable adverse-effect profile of the SSRIs. Little in the way of drowsiness or sedation has been reported with *venlafaxine*, which is in line with its minimal receptor binding, and any early nausea appears for the most part to resolve rapidly. However, it may cause a dose-related *increase in blood pressure* in 5–10% of patients, though this appears to be transient in about half (Frazer 1997). Effects on weight are inconsistent, with early tendency to lose being followed at 6–8 months by a slight increase, which may of course relate more to well-being than an adverse action. As with sertraline, sexual dysfunction may be more evident in males. *Trazodone* (like nefazodone) is sedative, and while both have potent anti α_1-noradrenergic actions, the latter seems to produce less postural hypotension than the former. One of the marketing points with nefazodone is its apparently low liability to produce disorders of sexual function, and interestingly this drug does not appear to share trazodone's priapismic proclivities. Nefazodone has however been associated with a worrying incidence of severe hepatic damage, sometimes requiring transplantation; in markets where it has not been withdrawn, monitoring of liver function would be important. Mirtazapine's receptor-binding profile would allow the assumption that it may be associated with less in the way of nausea ($5HT_3$ antagonism) but more in the way of day-time fatigue and impaired motor performance (H_1 antagonism) than the majority of the newer drugs.

As a scan of the web will show, there is considerable concern in some quarters about a putative association between SSRIs and suicidality, suicide acts and violent acts against others. The mechanism hypothesised relates to the liability to promote 'akathisia' and/or similar dysphoric mental state changes (see above). This remains a largely legal determination at present, as the data — which are predominantly based on individual case reports/experiences — can be interpreted variably. Some cases have been successfully prosecuted, others not. This association would at present be rejected by most clinicians in the UK but is a matter still under consideration, and one which those prescribing these compounds should be aware of. Currently in the UK, with the exception of fluoxetine, SSRIs (and Venlafaxine) are 'contraindicated' in major depression in those under 18 years.

Toxicity of antidepressants in overdose

For many years much of the little that was known about the clinical pharmacology of antidepressants was based on patients who had taken overdoses of tricyclics. In overdose, the clinical pharmacology of tricyclics is different from that of their therapeutic use, transforming these drugs into potentially lethal agents. Even today, the toxicity of antidepressants remains largely the toxicity of the tricyclics.

The pharmacokinetic parameters of tricyclics change following overdose, and this is the major factor underlying their toxicity in this situation (Jarvis 1991). First, *absorption* is substantially delayed, probably as a result of anticholinergic effects. It is common at postmortem to find drug residues in the stomachs of patients dying from tricyclic overdose. Furthermore, as was mentioned, considerable *enterohepatic recirculation* takes place, contributing to the maintenance of high blood levels.

At excessively high levels, tricyclics appear to shift from first-order to *zero-order kinetics* — that is, the amount metabolised is fixed rather than proportionate. This results from saturation of hepatic enzymes and in the case of tricyclics appears to relate to saturation of the rate-limiting hydroxylation pathways (Jarvis 1991). Thus, high blood levels in a way sustain themselves by delayed absorption, enterohepatic circulation and saturated metabolism, thereby prolonging the half-life by as much as twofold.

Furthermore, metabolism is dependent on cardiac output, and so any compromise in this will further impede metabolism. At high blood levels, tricyclics are profoundly *cardiotoxic*, mainly as a result of their potent actions in delaying ventricular conduction time, resulting in QT prolongation, QRS elongation and ventricular premature beats, which may progress to ventricular tachy-arrhythmias that can in turn be associated with strikingly inefficient pump action. In addition, a clinically unimportant positive inotropic action at therapeutic levels inverts to a negative action at high levels, which may further contribute to output failure.

Tricyclics at high blood levels can furthermore seriously impair gas exchange in the lungs. This is because of the central depressant effect common to the group, but also to increasingly recognised local alveolar damage (Roy et al 1989). The effect is *acidaemia*. Falls in pH are associated with reduction in the amount of drug that is protein bound and hence with an increase in the amount of pharmacodynamically active free drug. Because such a large proportion of tricyclic is protein bound, only very slight reductions in binding are necessary to greatly increase the percentage of free drug. For example, a reduction from binding levels of 95% to 93% could theoretically increase the free fraction by 50% (Jarvis 1991).

The major clinical manifestations of tricyclic toxicity are signs of *CNS and cardiovascular depression*. Patients may appear flushed and hot, with widely dilated pupils and peripheral tremulousness. Sedation and drowsiness, combined with motor signs of disco-ordination, progress to frank confusion as a prelude to coma. Breathing becomes rapid and shallow, and tachycardia of sinus or supraventricular type is usually evident. Cardiac irregularities may also be apparent. Around 4–8% of patients may fit or go into status, though the risk of fitting may be as high as 36% with overdose of maprotiline (Knudsen & Heath 1984). Of note are reports of acute renal failure in approximately 10% of amoxapine overdoses (Jennings et al 1983) and permanent neurological damage in 2% of maprotiline overdoses (Knudsen & Heath 1984), neither of which are features of uncomplicated overdoses of tricyclics in general.

For the reasons mentioned above, it is always important to attempt gastric lavage in tricyclic overdose patients, even if there has been a delay in discovering the individual. Otherwise treatment is essentially supportive. In view of the risks of antiarrhythmic drugs in overdose, and the fact that respiratory depression may require intubation, such supportive measures are for medical specialists. Even when the clinical situation appears stable, it is important for psychiatrists to be wary of over-zealous attempts by medical colleagues to return overdose patients to psychiatric units quickly. As a knowledge of the pharmacokinetics would suggest, half-lives — and risk periods — will extend for some days after a serious overdose.

The major advantage of the new-generation antidepressants is their safety profile in overdose (Boyer & Feighner 1996). Although isolated reports of fatality have appeared, especially with the earlier drugs, these have usually been in association with polydrug ingestion, in which the role of the antidepressant alone was unclear. The fundamental shift in the risk:benefit ratio for antidepressant treatment has allowed the potential benefits of therapy to be extended to those with relatively less severe disorders and to those in whom self-harm (both impulsive and planned) is a worrying reality, without the high levels of supervision and monitoring necessary with the older drugs. It could be argued that the introduction of antidepressants with a wide margin of safety has been one of the major advances in clinical psychiatric care over the past half century.

Antidepressant withdrawal ('discontinuation') syndromes

It has been known since 1959 that sudden cessation of treatment with tricyclics could be associated with the development of a withdrawal syndrome, though this was rarely commented on in the literature, and then only anecdotally. A similar phenomenon was noted with MAOIs. The issue has however received greater prominence in connection with SSRIs (Lejoyeux & Ades 1997).

In this context, the term 'discontinuation' has gained favour over the more usual 'withdrawal' for reasons that, although elegantly argued, are not always convincing. It is beyond the present chapter to review the meanings of 'dependency' and the implications of rebound symptomatology on cessation of regular drug ingestion, on which there is little expert consensus. From our point of view — and as far as the public understands the situation — the development of symptomatology on reduction or cessation of a drug is a reflection of a key role which that compound was playing in nervous system metabolism and, regardless of theoretical implications, represents *withdrawal* of that key function. Such symptomatology is therefore intuitively and, until proven otherwise, scientifically 'withdrawal' in nature. Attempts to term it something else are presently at best ill-founded, at worst deceptive.

Sudden cessation of protracted, and especially high dose, tricyclic regimens can be associated after a day or two with the development of symptomatology that can be considered in five categories (Dilsaver et al 1987):

- *somatic*, including nausea, vomiting, diarrhoea, sweating, malaise;
- *sleep*, including poor quality, decreased duration and vivid anxiety-laden dreams;
- *movement disorders*, especially akathisia and parkinsonian-type symptoms;
- '*activation*' symptoms, comprising mania/hypomania, anxiety, panic attacks and frank clouding;
- *cardiac arrhythmias*.

Despite reported prevalence figures ranging from 16% to 100%, these are probably uncommon in a degree that merits clinical attention. Prevalence may be greater with tertiary amine compounds than secondary ones, or alternatively the risk may relate more to the potency of the drug's cholinergic antagonist properties (as with antipsychotics), though neither of these possibilities has been established.

In line with conventional pharmacological actions in drugs of short half-life, withdrawal symptoms following MAOI treatment can be severe, especially with tranylcypromine (Halle & Dilsaver 1993), and include 'rebound' depression or manic/hypomanic symptomatology with agitation, irritability, insomnia, myoclonic jerks and frank confusion/delirium.

The renamed 'discontinuation syndrome' associated with stopping SSRIs is slightly different (Haddad 1997). It usually emerges within 24 hours of stopping and comprises anxiety and irritability, alteration in sleep and gastrointestinal symptoms with, in addition, flu-like symptoms of coryza, myalgia and shaking chills. Particular features include 'dizziness', consisting of both true movement-sensitive vertigo and a 'floating', 'spaced out' sensation akin to mild inebriation, ataxia and burning shock-like sensations (cf. benzodiazepine withdrawal), tingling or hypoaesthesias. It has also been suggested that aggressive and impulsive behaviour may represent a further novel SSRI 'discontinuation' phenomenon, but the few reports describing this may represent coincidental phenomenology (see above). These features can develop with all members of the group, though seem most likely to occur with compounds of shorter half-life. Thus, they appear relatively uncommon following cessation of

fluoxetine, but may affect up to one-third of those coming off paroxetine (Haddad 1997). A similar situation has been described after sudden discontinuation of venlafaxine.

Withdrawal syndromes can sometimes be dramatic, especially when patients stop medication without advice. This is particularly the case with the traditional MAOIs. Although in the vast majority of instances they are brief and self-limiting events lasting only 2 or 3 days, they may be more protracted especially with the older drugs. Most do not however require specific intervention. They do nonetheless emphasise the importance of gradual tapering of antidepressant regimens over days or preferably weeks, something which is made more problematic with the fixed dosing schedules of some of the newer drugs.

This is an issue much underestimated by doctors, both in its potential frequency and impact. In view of increasing patient awareness — and web-generated misunderstandings — it would be prudent for doctors to inform patients of the possibility of withdrawal symptomatology, even if, in practice, it will not be important for the great majority.

Therapeutics

Indications (Box 15.7)

There is still debate about the relative place of different antidepressant groups in clinical practice. As a rule, this is not about efficacy, as on the face of it the data indicate that all antidepressants are equivalent in this regard (Frazer 1997). The debate rests largely on the balance of tolerability and safety versus cost. There is however evidence that in severe depressions of the type most commonly seen in secondary care, especially those conforming to the traditional picture of 'melancholia', SSRIs at least are not as efficacious as tricyclics (Perry 1996). While this evidence remains soft, it is an impression based on clinical experience which the present volume would endorse. The position of other new-generation drugs remains to be seen.

Strategies

There has over the past few years been an effective — and *almost* convincing — campaign conducted against the use of tricyclics and in favour of new-generation antidepressants, an argument which has been presented in stark terms that serve to oversimplify a complex balance of choices.

It is often stated that all antidepressants are of equal efficacy, and that, by a modern reappraisal, that includes the MAOIs (Frazer 1997). But, as noted above, this does not mean that all are equally effective in all situations. Therapeutic choices must be balanced and include awareness of evidence that in some illnesses, especially the more severe 'melancholia' types, SSRIs may not be as effective as tricyclics (Perry 1996).

A second argument against tricyclics concerns tolerability. Meta-analyses of comparative studies consistently show better tolerability with SSRIs than with tricyclics, evaluated by patient withdrawals from trials. However, the differences are rarely marked, and, although on statistical analysis they reach significance, it is unlikely that they are significant clinically (Anderson & Tomenson 1995, Hotopf et al 1997). In routine practice, however, it may be that certain types of tricyclic-related adverse effects (e.g. anticholinergic) are simply more unpleasant in day to day terms and, although not leading directly to refusal, may impair quality of life.

Primary
- The treatment of acute episodes of major depression. Response is likely to be greater in depressions that are not secondary to other psychiatric disorders, but antidepressants, especially tricyclics, would also be indicated in secondary depressions, including post-psychotic (or schizophrenic) depressions
- The prevention of relapse in recurrent, non-bipolar depressions

Secondary
- Obsessive–compulsive disorder — both the tricyclic clomipramine and the SSRIs, especially fluoxetine and paroxetine, have proven efficacy in this condition
- Panic disorder — the work of Klein and colleagues established the efficacy of imipramine in the treatment of panic states, where this may be a preferable choice for long-term use than benzodiazepines. Recently, some SSRIs have been licensed for use in other manifestations of anxiety (e.g. social phobia)
- Eating disorders, especially bulimia nervosa — fluoxetine in high dose (e.g. up to 80 mg per day) has been reported as effective
- 'Atypical' depressions — Researchers in New York have refined this concept into what is sometimes referred to as 'Columbia atypical depression', after the authors' institution (Quitkin et al 1993). Theoretically, this is a somewhat uncomfortable concept for British audiences, combining as it does, analytically based concepts such as 'hysteroid dysphoria' (covering narcissism, romantic preoccupation and disappointment in relationships) with biological symptomatology, such as hyperphagia, hypersomnia, and profound fatigue associated with so-called 'leaden paralysis'. Nonetheless, the authors have presented data over the years to show that such patients respond preferentially to traditional MAOIs, especially phenelzine, compared with tricyclics
- Post-traumatic stress disorder, usually as an adjunct to psychological interventions
- Attention deficit disorder with hyperactivity in children. The strongest evidence relates to imipramine
- Pain syndromes — tricyclics have clear efficacy in the management of chronic pain syndromes. One meta-analysis concluded that of every 100 patients with pain from such diverse causes as diabetic neuropathy, post-herpetic neuralgia and atypical facial pain, 30 will experience a greater than 50% reduction of symptoms on a tricyclic, and that overall their efficacy is comparable to that of anticonvulsants (McQuay et al 1996)
- Enuresis in children (imipramine)
- Premature ejaculation (SSRIs)

Cost is an increasing consideration for prescribing, and a strong argument in favour of new drugs is that, although costing more in themselves, they are in fact, for a number of reasons, more cost effective in the long run. Considerable effort has gone into justifying this argument but it is clear that the outcome of such analyses depends on the information fed into the analytical models, i.e. one's assumptions. Thus far, such analyses have produced contrary conclusions (Hotopf et al 1996).

The one argument on which there is no contest is safety in overdose. All new-generation antidepressants have a more favourable toxicity profile than the tricyclics. Among the old drugs, amitriptyline, desipramine and dothiepin appear particularly associated with a fatal outcome after overdose (Cassidy & Henry 1987). The question then is the magnitude of the problem. Figures for the contribution made by the high-risk drugs to completed overdoses are variable. While some argue the contribution is substantial (Henry 1996), the data are open to different interpretations (Hotopf et al 1996).

Based on the figures of Montgomery and colleagues, derived from Coroners' returns for England and Wales for 1975–1985, the two worst offenders, dothiepin and amitriptyline, were each associated with between 45 and 50 deaths per million prescriptions (Montgomery et al 1989). In absolute numbers, this translates into approximately 170 deaths per year between them. Such data cannot reveal the extent to which these deaths represent the outcome of *inadequate treatment* — still a problem with tricyclic prescribing, especially in primary care (Beaumont et al 1996) — or *inadequate supervision*. It is furthermore not clear how many victims of tricyclic overdose might be saved by side-stepping these drugs, as the well-described phenomenon of 'substitution' might merely result in the determined resorting to other means.

Not all tricyclics are tarred with the same fatality risk in overdose as amitriptyline and dothiepin; clomipramine, protriptyline and lofepramine are apparently safer, though data on which these conclusions rest are open to greater criticism. The biggest problem with tricyclics is simply that a fatal overdose may be as little as 10–15 times the therapeutic dose, leaving the distressed patient little room for 'error'.

Although antidepressant prescribing choices remain more finely balanced than is sometimes made clear, there are situations in which new-generation antidepressants justify a first-line position:

- in patients in whom impulsive or planned misuse is an active or predictable issue;
- in primary-care situations where depressive disorders may be more amenable and where, by virtue of time constraints, high levels of support and close monitoring are not feasible;
- in cases of medical complexity such as severe heart disease, recent CVA, or coincidental complex drug regimens;
- in those in whom impaired motor performance may cause occupational restrictions;
- in those with previous intolerance of tricyclics;
- where there is a pressing need to cultivate clearly tenuous co-operation by the avoidance of unacceptable adverse effects — e.g. a fear of weight gain, etc.

The elderly present special considerations because, although for pharmacokinetic and other reasons they are undoubtedly more susceptible to the riskier adverse effects of tricyclics, they may also be more prone to depressions which respond less favourably to newer drugs.

It might be argued that poor compliance with tricyclics emanates from unsophisticated prescribing as well as from problems inherent to the group. By skilful application of some of the data presented above, tricyclics can be effectively and acceptably used, if indicated.

The traditional MAOIs remain third-line drugs, even in those with 'atypical' depressions, and their use is best reserved for specialist settings, while moclobemide can be prescribed more flexibly. Principles are outlined in Box 15.8.

Box 15.8	Principles of antidepressant drug use

- Assess the appropriateness of pharmacological intervention in the knowledge that this may not be the most suitable first-line recommendation
- Assess severity of the depression and the risk of self-harm independently. In general, the risk of overdose of prescribed medication is likely to parallel the severity of the depression; but attempts at self-harm may be impulsive and not necessarily related to severity of mood disorder as assessed at interview, especially in those with comorbidity (e.g. personality disorders)
- Allow levels of anxiety/agitation and sleep disturbance to influence prescribing decisions. Not all 'non-target' effects are 'adverse'
- Specific antidepressant efficacy is inevitably delayed, perhaps for longer than with antipsychotics. It is likely that about 10 days to 2 weeks will elapse before any benefits are evident, and these may take 4–6 weeks to maximise. Patients must be advised of this to avoid their giving up prematurely
- The possible adverse-effect profile of the chosen compound should also be discussed, as educating patients in this regard greatly enhances their willingness to tolerate any regimen and hence provides a boost to compliance
- Treatment must be adequate in terms of doses. The commonest cause of 'treatment resistant' depression is inadequate dosage. This contributes to unnecessary morbidity and increases the risk of self-harm while exposing patients to the likelihood of needless side-effects. This is less of an issue with the SSRIs, which tend to have narrower therapeutic dose ranges, but is pertinent to other new-generation drugs and especially to tricyclics, most of which have therapeutic doses in the range 150–225 mg per day
- Suboptimal or absent response after 6–8 weeks on an adequate dose regimen should indicate a change of drug (and probably of group)
- Treatment should also be adequate in terms of duration. Successful management should be extended for at least 6 months, and for up to 1 year in some cases, in order to minimise the risk of relapse

LITHIUM SALTS AND OTHER MOOD STABILISERS

Lithium

Introduction

Lithium was discovered in 1817 by the Swedes Arfwedson and Berzelius, who identified the sulphate from the mineral petalite. Elemental lithium was isolated by electrolysis in 1855. Lithium, a silvery-white alkali metal, is the lightest of all solids, occupying position 3 in the Periodic Table. As a highly reactive element, it has found wide commercial application in everything from processing rubber, to the manufacture of long-life batteries; from strengthening glass and ceramics, to the construction of nuclear bombs. Only about 1% of annual supplies is devoted to medicinal use.

The medical applications of lithium salts began in 1841 when Lipowitz recommended their use in gout. This followed the observation that in vitro they increased the solubility of urates. Despite half a century of use, this was not in fact an effective treatment, as very large and toxic doses would have been required to achieve the necessary concentrations. From 1864, however, lithium was listed in the British Pharmacopoeia, and the chloride, and especially bromide, salts were widely used as hypnotics throughout the latter part of the 19th and early 20th centuries. Lithium bromide was in addition one of the first compounds regularly employed as an antianxiety agent.

By the end of the 19th century, reports of toxicity with the medical use of lithium began to appear but despite this, unmonitored lithium chloride was enthusiastically endorsed in the 1940s as a salt substitute in the low-sodium diets then fashionable for the management of hypertension. In early 1949, considerable publicity surrounded fatalities from toxicity in the USA, which led to the FDA banning the use of lithium salts. This perception of hazard delayed the introduction of the present incarnation of lithium in America for over a decade.

In addition to their use in minor or non-specific psychiatric disorders, lithium salts were recommended early for the treatment of more severe forms of affective disorder. In the 1870s, the American physician William Hammond recommended massive oral doses of lithium bromide for the acute treatment of mania and melancholia, while in the 1880s the Danish neurologist Carl Lange favoured alkaline salts for the treatment of what he called 'periodic depression'. This was part of a belief, prevalent at the time, that some forms of mood disorder were one manifestation of the 'gouty diathesis', a concept on which James Parkinson, of 'shaking palsy' fame, wrote the monograph that first established his reputation. For a gouty diathesis, Lange recommended dietary restrictions, regular exercise — and prophylactic intake of alkaline salts!

The modern psychiatric use of lithium was begun by Dr John Cade, of the Victoria Department of Mental Hygiene in Australia. He hypothesised that mania might be the result of the build-up of some unidentified toxin, while depression might represent what he called 'a correspondingly deprivative condition'. Returning to purine metabolism, he noted that in guinea pigs urea produced a state of hyperexcitability, and he wished to see if uric acid enhanced the toxicity of urea. He therefore administered lithium urate, the most soluble of urate salts, and found that contrary to expectation, this protected the animals against the excitant properties of urea. On this flimsiest of bases, he gave lithium to excited patients in doses that he took from a 1927 text, Culbreth's *Manual of Materia Medica and Pharmacology*. In 1949, Cade published his results in a group of 10 patients, most of whom had been chronically symptomatic with mania. The findings were dramatic, with mood stabilisation in a week or so. By contrast, 6 schizophrenic patients did not improve significantly. The doses Cade chose, courtesy of Culbreth, were very high (one of the original group eventually died of toxicity), and it has been suggested that what was observed as improvement in the psychiatric illness may have been incipient toxicity. Cade's publication stimulated some interest in Australia but, it must be said, in few other places. One of these was Denmark, where Erik Stromgren suggested further exploration of the issue, thereby stimulating the work of the Aarhus group led by Mogens Schou, which was to be so influential in developing lithium as a safe and effective treatment.

Structure

The electrons orbiting the lithium nucleus comprise a pair at the lowest energy level plus a single outer electron. This outer electron is powerfully shielded from the attractive force of the nucleus, so the energy required to displace it from the atom is very low, whereas that required to displace one of the inner electrons is much higher. Thus, the chemistry of lithium is essentially that of the Li⁺ ion. Furthermore, as the therapeutic benefits of different salts in psychiatric applications are identical, the same applies to the pharmacology.

The major bulk lithium chemicals are the sulphate and carbonate salts and lithium hydroxide, though of these only lithium carbonate is now used in psychiatric practice. It is manufactured commercially from the reaction between lithium sulphate and sodium carbonate. Lithium citrate is also available and is particularly used in liquid form.

The lithium content of salts and of dosage formulations may vary; for accuracy, preparations should be compared on the basis of their lithium content in *milliequivalent* terms. In general, 37 mg of the carbonate salt is equal to 1 mEq of lithium (Baldessarini 1985). This has important implications for prescribing (see below).

Pharmacokinetics

Lithium has a narrow therapeutic index, and a knowledge of the pharmacokinetics of different formulations is important in maximising tolerability while minimising toxicity. There is however a difficulty with terminology, in that different preparations are marketed as having discrete absorption characteristics that may not in practice be quite so discrete.

Lithium is readily and almost completely absorbed. Some 20% of an orally administered dose is absorbed from the stomach, a process not apparently dependent on gastric acidity. Absorption is, however, predominantly (> 70%) from the small bowel and occurs by passive diffusion through the lateral intercellular spaces and the absorptive pores of the epithelial tight junctions (Diamond et al 1983). Absorption is hence fastest when concentrations in the bowel lumen are highest. The rise in plasma levels is rapid with standard preparations, peak levels being reached in 1–2 hours. Lithium is not protein bound, and its volume of distribution is approximately that of total body water. Oral bioavailability is 90% or above, though it varies with different formulations.

Unlike sodium and potassium, lithium shows no strong preferential distribution across cell membranes, but the rate of passage is not uniform across all body tissues, and at equilibrium there are some differences in a variety of tissue–plasma concentration gradients (Cooper 1987). Thus, in the liver the concentration of lithium tends to be lower than in extracellular fluid whereas in muscle, bone and thyroid it is two- to fourfold higher. The concentration in brain is roughly the same as that of extracellular fluid, which is approximately 50% of plasma concentration. This might indicate that in pharmacokinetic terms lithium is best represented by a two-compartment model (Poust 1987).

Half-life values vary considerably even after single dosing, something to which age may contribute. The shortest half-lives are generally found in young adults (e.g. 18–20 hours). Overall the half-life is regarded as being in the region of 22–24 hours and does not vary with different salts. Steady state is therefore achieved within 4–7 days. However, it seems clear that the half-life of lithium increases with long-term treatment by as much as 25–30% (Goodnick et al 1981). This has obvious clinical relevance in that accumulation may occur over time, with consequent increase in the risk of toxicity.

There are no metabolic steps in the body's handling of lithium, almost all of which is excreted via the kidneys, with less than 5%

accounted for by loss in faeces and from insensible sources. Lithium is secreted in most body fluids, including sweat, saliva, tears, ejaculate and breast milk and possibly also intestinal secretions. Being unbound, it is freely filtered by the renal glomerulus along with other cations, such as sodium and potassium. Also like sodium, some 70–80% of filtered lithium is reabsorbed in the proximal tubules by a mechanism which is competitive with sodium. However, while filtered sodium undergoes further reabsorption in the distal nephron (Loop of Henle, distal tubule and collecting ducts), lithium does not. The speed at which lithium is excreted — i.e. the lithium clearance — is therefore linked to proximal tubular fluid output, and as such is not constant. Clearance is increased with extracellular volume expansion, as for example during pregnancy but, more significantly, decreases with either water or sodium depletion. Thus, in terms of increasing the risk of toxicity, not only must disorders that impair glomerular filtration (such as renal disease and increasing age) need to be kept in mind, so too do states of decreased sodium intake or increased extrarenal loss (salt-depleting medications such as diuretics and dehydration). The adverse effects of water deficiency may be militated somewhat if dehydration is acquired via increased sweating, such as with inadequate fluid intake in hot climates or with fever, as increasing blood lithium levels will be associated with increased loss of lithium in sweat. However, this 'homeostatic' mechanism cannot be counted on to provide adequate protection, and patients must be given prudent advice.

The advantages of single dosing have long been evident. Single daily dosing of *standard* lithium is not as a rule possible in healthy individuals since, in order to maintain adequate levels over a 24-hour dosing interval, high average doses are required with peak levels well into the toxic range. Assuming a half-life of 24 hours, a single dose regimen of a standard preparation can be expected to produce 12-hour blood levels approximately 25% higher than those with the same daily dose given in a thrice daily schedule. Furthermore, giving a single dose of 900 mg standard lithium can result in peak levels almost four times those of trough levels, whereas on a thrice daily regimen the same daily dose results in a less than a twofold difference (Baldessarini 1985).

In order to minimise the size of the post-absorptive peak a number of formulations have been introduced which go by a number of names: 'slow release', 'controlled release', 'sustained release', etc. Various ingenious methods have been used to achieve the aim of a delayed rise to a lower peak level, including decreasing the solubility, embedding the drug in a non-digestible porous carrier or gel, and using ion exchange resins or controlled disintegration coatings, amongst others. After some unpromising starts, these appear to have resulted in preparations that have at least some of the desired characteristics which, unlike the early attempts, are attained at little, or sometimes no, cost to bioavailability (Goodnick & Schorr-Cain 1991). In general, peak levels with these formulations are achieved after 3–6 hours, with 'Liskonum' delayed somewhat more than others. 'Camcolit-400' and 'Priadel' appear to have similar characteristics, while lithium citrate achieves the lowest peak levels and also appears to have the lowest 12-hour plasma levels (Shelley & Silverstone 1987). Although data are contradictory, there is a suggestion that the area under the curve (AUC) is less with the citrate syrup than with carbonate in tablet form, suggesting lower bioavailability. Nonetheless, liquid citrate may be an option in those who find tablets difficult to swallow.

One complication in presenting the pharmacokinetic profile of lithium is that most studies have been done on normal volunteers, whereas there is evidence that the disorders for which the drug is being taken (i.e. affective disorders) may themselves alter pharmacokinetic data (Goodnick & Schorr-Cain 1991). This is something that has only been recognised in recent years and, while not altering the basic contention that an understanding of the drug's pharmacokinetics is an important aid to rational clinical practice, it does illustrate the need to utilise such information as a guide only.

Pharmacodynamics

Mode of action   The mode of action of lithium is unknown. As a widely distributed and highly reactive cation, lithium influences chemical processes at a series of physiological levels, yet clinically it seems to produce effects that are fairly focused. However, the lack of a tenable theory on the pathophysiology of affective disorders makes the task of unravelling the mode of action a 'needle in a haystack' task.

Lithium acts at three main neurochemical 'levels'. The *first* is on membrane electrophysiology. Lithium shares many of the physical properties of other physiologically active cations such as sodium, potassium and calcium, and can pass readily through ion channels associated with these. One of the earliest suggestions therefore was that it may stabilise electrolyte balances across neuronal membranes, something that may be disturbed in affective disorders. It may do this by stimulating Na/K-ATPase, the energy-dependent enzyme responsible for controlling the balance of sodium and potassium across cell membranes via the sodium pump mechanism. Lithium cannot however substitute for sodium in the pump arrangement, and so excessive replacement of sodium by lithium, as might happen in toxicity, could result in a failure of membranes to maintain polarisation and to conduct an action potential (Baldessarini 1985). This could underlie the catastrophic CNS collapse seen with severe and escalating toxicity.

The *second* level at which lithium acts is on neurotransmitters. It has been shown, as an acute effect, to increase neuronal uptake of catecholamines and, with chronic administration, to potentiate serotonergic and noradrenergic function, effects on the latter being less in degree though more consistent (Manji et al 1991). Lithium treatment may also prevent or modify the receptor supersensitivity response to chronic catecholamine antagonists, such as antipsychotics (Baldessarini 1985). However, this 'receptor stabilising' hypothesis, once promising, has been blighted by inconsistent data, especially at the clinical level. While it is likely that lithium's actions on catecholamine transmitter systems are regionally selective within the brain, there seems no doubt about this in relation to serotonin transmission. Short-term, lithium stimulates release of serotonin in especially the hippocampus and, longer term, may increase activity in presynaptic hippocampal neurons, resulting in receptor down-regulation. While some of these changes may be taken as consistent with the Biogenic Amine Hypothesis, they leave unexplained the compound's mode of action in these states.

The *third* and most complex level at which lithium may act is on so-called second messenger systems (Manji et al 1995). Neuronal membrane receptors mediate two sorts of events: those involving the propagation of electrical potentials on the membrane surface and those that result from the translation of receptor events into modifications in intracellular functioning (see Ch. 3). Agents mediating the first set of events — i.e. neurotransmitters themselves — might therefore be considered as the 'first' messengers in neurophysiological processes, while those mediating the transduction of electrical information at the receptor into changes at the level of intracellular effectors might then be thought of as 'second' messengers. These intracellular messengers, which include adenylyl cyclases, inositol 1,4,5-triphosphate, arachidonate, protein kinase C isoenzymes, guanine nucleotide binding- (or G-) proteins and calcium, act on specific target proteins to initiate signalling cascades. It is clear that lithium affects a number of signal transduction pathways.

Inositol phospholipids are relatively minor components of cell membranes but major participants in receptor-mediated signal transduction pathways. The activation of a number of receptor subtypes induces the hydrolysis of membrane phospholipids, a process involving the complex interaction of transmitters, including adrenaline and 5HT, with G-proteins which stimulate isoforms of the enzyme phospholipase C. These in their turn result in production of two intracellular second messengers: sn-1,2-diacylglycerol (DAG) and inositol 1,4,5-triphosphate. The brain is dependent on the recycling of inositol phosphates to maintain inositol levels, and lithium, which inhibits the intracellular enzyme inositol monophosphatase, results in a depletion of free inositol. While these appear to be robust findings, they seem unlikely in themselves to explain lithium's delayed and targeted actions.

A further receptor-coupled second messenger system on which lithium acts is the cAMP generation system. Lithium inhibits the accumulation of noradrenaline-induced cAMP. Indeed this attenuation of amine-induced coupling to adenylyl cyclase may also occur in peripheral cells and may underlie some of the drug's adverse effects, such as nephrogenic diabetes insipidus and possibly thyroid impairment. These effects may be mediated acutely via competition with magnesium for a binding site on the adenylyl cyclase molecule but, with chronic exposure, mediation seems to be via G-proteins (Manji et al 1995). G-proteins are a complex family of molecules that constitute an important signal transduction pathway. Long-term lithium exposure attenuates the actions of G-proteins by inhibiting their coupling to receptor proteins. It has further been suggested that by this mechanism (G-protein attenuation) lithium may prevent the development of receptor supersensitivity, though this is unproven.

The final intracellular system of interest with regard to the mode of action of lithium concerns a widely distributed and highly active set of enzymes collectively known as protein kinase C. These operate postsynaptically but are crucially important in presynaptic events also. Whereas acute administration of lithium activates this family of isoenzymes, chronic ingestion decreases the responses they mediate, including neurotransmitter release (Manji et al 1995).

Membrane events have been the traditional focus of neurophysiology but increasing understanding of *intra*cellular events has opened a new window on the complex systems that characterise cellular communication. It is not yet clear how the pervasive effects of lithium on the intracellular part of this communication highway relate to its therapeutic benefits (or for that matter to the pathophysiology of affective disorders) nor in what ways these may relate to other actions of the ion — e.g modifying early gene expression. Nonetheless, unravelling these complex events is likely to inform us more about the mechanisms underlying the modes of action of many psychotropics, including lithium, than approaches hitherto have done, as well as pointing the way to rational theories of pathophysiology at the molecular level.

Adverse effects   Lithium is a highly toxic ion and has the lowest margin of safety of any class of drugs used in clinical psychopharmacology. Although therapeutic monitoring has reduced the risk of toxicity dramatically, treatment can still be associated with a wide range of adverse effects (Table 15.7). Indeed, with close monitoring it has been suggested that only very few of those on standard lithium (around 10%) are likely to escape completely (Vacaflor 1975). The prevalence of most side-effects is lower with 'slow' or 'sustained' release formulations, now the most commonly used.

To some extent, many adverse effects of lithium and those of toxicity develop on a continuum and are matters of degree. Thus, while it is usually possible to distinguish between the major adverse effects that occur therapeutically and those indicative of toxicity, an overlap exists, and the distinction is, in the early stages of transition at least, largely a quantitative one. In fact, even with patients considered, on the basis of a standard 12-hour blood level, to be within the therapeutic range, adverse symptomatology can still be reported. This reflects both the rate of rise to, and the maximum height of, the post-absorptive peak, as well as rates of clearance. It is worth bearing in mind that over time patients can almost double their reference plasma levels but still remain within the defined 'therapeutic' level. Individuals running in the lower range and side-effect free, may start to develop adverse effects as, for example, age-related renal decline produces gradual rises in plasma levels. This may then start to produce adverse effects, even although plasma levels remain 'therapeutic'.

For purposes of emphasis, the features of toxicity are highlighted separately below, but it is important to appreciate that in practice they may not represent a discrete symptomatic break.

The most frequently reported adverse effects are gastrointestinal. The majority of patients will experience a degree of *nausea*, especially evident after starting lithium and prior to the establishment of steady state. For the reasons noted, some may continue to experience this for an hour or two after each dose. However, this usually abates with long-term treatment (> 1 year) (Schou et al 1970). Alternatively, patients may complain of bloated *epigastric discomfort*. Pain on the other hand is uncommon. Nausea seems to relate to the biochemical changes effected by lithium in the cells of the gut wall and as such is unlikely to be helped by taking the tablets with or after food.

Occasionally nausea may be associated with frank *vomiting* in the absence of toxicity, though this too usually settles rapidly. It appears that even small amounts of the lithium ion are irritant to the lower bowel, and *loose motions* are a common experience. Watery *diarrhoea* can be found at therapeutic levels, but in view of its potentially sinister implications, toxicity is usually a safer first assumption in this situation. Unlike most other adverse effects, lower intestinal symptomatology may be *more* frequently found with 'slow' or 'sustained' release products, as their mode of action, by significantly delaying absorption, delivers more ion to the lower bowel. It is important to take note of vomiting and diarrhoea that are sustained, if only for a few days, even in the presence of therapeutic blood levels, because of the consequences of fluid and sodium loss. Patients may complain of *constipation*, especially with chronic exposure.

Disturbed salivary flow, in the form of either an *increase in salivation* or *dryness* in the mouth, is also described. The former is frequent, something that with objective measurement is evident in over three-quarters of patients, and may be associated with salivary gland enlargement. The latter is, however, potentially more troublesome. For a number of years, concern was expressed about the high prevalence of dental caries in patients on lithium, which was

thought to reflect interference with enamel production. Lithium does not however appear to interfere with aspects of tooth development or maintenance (Curzon 1987), and it is now thought that decline in dental status is the consequence of a chronically dry mouth. Infrequently, patients may complain, sometimes bitterly, of a *metallic taste*, probably the result of salivary secretion of the ion.

The diuretic properties of lithium were noted by Garrod in the middle of the last century, and *polyuria* with compensatory *polydipsia* is commonly noted, affecting up to 50% of patients in some surveys (Walker & Kincaid-Smith 1987). The problem relates to a failure of concentration, and with laboratory evaluation it has been suggested that the majority of patients on lithium will show some increase in urine production on a normal fluid intake. Lithium appears to interfere with the action of vasopressin on the distal nephron, probably by inhibiting the adenylyl cyclase-mediated increase in the conversion of ATP to cyclic AMP. The effect can be a mild increase in urinary volume which is largely asymptomatic or that shows mainly as nocturia, through to full and profoundly incapacitating vasopressin-resistant nephrogenic *diabetes insipidus*. The natural assumption would be that this might be helped by spreading the administration of, particularly, slow release preparations over the day to attain lower peaks. There is however a suggestion that in the long-term, the lower *troughs* associated with once daily administration may be more protective to the kidney, and at a clinical level the most effective way of dealing with polyuria may be to utilise single-dosing regimens (Perry & Alexander 1987). An alternative strategy is the addition of the potassium-sparing diuretic amiloride, which decreases urinary output without reducing lithium clearance. Thiazide diuretics may also achieve a reduction in urine volume but at much greater risk of producing rises in lithium blood levels, which can be in the region of 20–25% and so require closer monitoring.

Impairment in urinary concentrating ability was for long thought to be reversible and of little consequence. This complacency was shattered in 1977 with the publication of the first of a series of reports suggesting a strong correlation between duration of exposure to lithium and impaired concentrating ability (Hestbech et al 1977). Of particular concern was the demonstration that the functional deficit correlated with histological abnormalities in the form of a chronic focal *interstitial nephropathy*. Long-term administration of lithium has been confirmed to be associated with structural changes, though the changes originally causing concern may in part be non-specific, as similar findings have also been reported in psychiatric patients not treated with lithium (Kincaid-Smith et al 1979). A common factor therefore may be long-term exposure to maintenance medications. However, it now seems clear that a potent predisposing factor to these 'non-specific' structural changes is *acute lithium toxicity*. In this situation, permanent renal damage may ensue that is associated with progressive impairment of concentrating ability. Lithium treatment does appear to be associated with a specific histological change in the form of *distal tubular dilatation*, following both acute and chronic exposure, though the long-term significance of this remains unclear.

Thus, with prolonged and stable exposure to lithium the likelihood of impairment of glomerular filtration rate and the risk of permanent or progressive renal damage is *slight*, though this risk is increased by episodes of *acute toxicity* (Hetmar et al 1991).

A low-amplitude/high-frequency *tremor* of predominantly postural type is a common complaint which may also be exceedingly inconvenient and embarrassing. This is one of the adverse experiences that most clearly relates to the rate and height of the post-absorptive peak and which may be helped by a change in preparation and/or schedule. It appears to be at least in part adrenergically mediated and may respond to a beta-blocker. Although tremor may be pronounced at therapeutic levels, moderately severe degrees of disorder or greater should arouse suspicion of toxicity. A further sign is that the quality of the tremor may change to one with coarser characteristics, although a coarsening with increase in amplitude may be simply a feature of ageing.

Lithium can affect *cardiac conduction*, and although this has not traditionally been considered a matter of concern (Martin et al 1987), there may be some cause for circumspection (Reilly et al 2000). The commonest ECG finding is a notched, flattened and occasionally inverted T-wave, which is not thought to be significant. However, conduction deficits at both the level of the sinoatrial and atrioventricular nodes have been reported. The former may result in *sick sinus syndrome* or *sinus node arrhythmias*, which may be asymptomatic or present with faintness or paroxysmal tachycardia, while the *AV block* associated with the latter is usually asymptomatic. Lithium can produce dispersion of cardiac repolarisation, as indicated by QT_c *dispersion*, which may be related to ventricular tachyarrhythmias (Reilly et al 2000).

Premature ventricular beats may occur from slowing of conduction in the Bundle of His. Those with pre-existing cardiac disease, especially conduction disorders, are at greater risk and require closer monitoring. Such changes appear to be reversible on stopping the drug.

Long-term ingestion of lithium can be associated with substantial *weight gain*. Reported prevalence rates vary widely from 20% to 75%, and the increases can in some cases be striking. This clearly can have major medical, as well as cosmetic, implications and is a further source of non-compliance. The mechanism is unknown.

Lithium interferes with a number of hormone functions, the most prominent of which involve the thyroid gland. Within a few months on treatment, slight falls in thyroxine (T_4) with compensatory rises in thyroid-stimulating hormone (TSH) are common. These do not usually take values beyond normal reference ranges and they usually stabilise within 12 months, though TSH may remain on the high side. Early in treatment, patients may develop signs of *hyperthyroidism*, though this is very uncommon. Of much greater frequency is the gradual development of *hypothyroidism*. Antithyroid antibodies are present in just under 10% of the general population and are more prevalent in females. Their presence rises sharply after

Table 15.7 Adverse and toxic effects of lithium

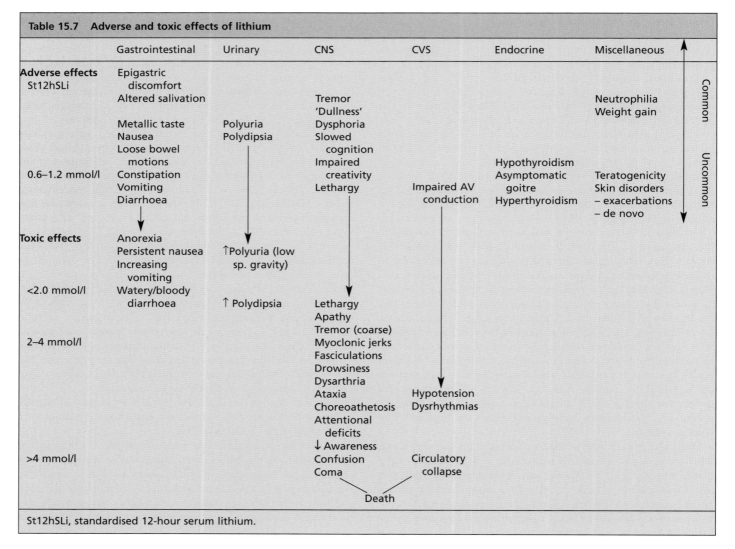

	Gastrointestinal	Urinary	CNS	CVS	Endocrine	Miscellaneous	
Adverse effects St12hSLi	Epigastric discomfort Altered salivation		Tremor 'Dullness'			Neutrophilia Weight gain	Common
	Metallic taste Nausea Loose bowel motions	Polyuria Polydipsia	Dysphoria Slowed cognition				
0.6–1.2 mmol/l	Constipation Vomiting Diarrhoea		Impaired creativity Lethargy	Impaired AV conduction	Hypothyroidism Asymptomatic goitre Hyperthyroidism	Teratogenicity Skin disorders – exacerbations – de novo	Uncommon
Toxic effects	Anorexia Persistent nausea Increasing vomiting	↑Polyuria (low sp. gravity)					
<2.0 mmol/l	Watery/bloody diarrhoea	↑ Polydipsia	Lethargy Apathy Tremor (coarse)				
2–4 mmol/l			Myoclonic jerks Fasciculations Drowsiness Dysarthria Ataxia Choreoathetosis Attentional deficits ↓ Awareness	Hypotension Dysrhythmias			
>4 mmol/l			Confusion Coma	Circulatory collapse			
			Death				

St12hSLi, standardised 12-hour serum lithium.

the middle of the fifth decade. Of those who demonstrate both autoantibodies and an elevated TSH, approximately 5% per year will develop hypothyroidism, with females about three times more represented than males (Myers & West 1987). Thus, it is likely that lithium is acting to promote disorder in predisposed individuals, rather than causing it de novo. The mechanism remains unclear but it is likely that there is no single pathway to lithium-induced hypothyroidism. One possibility is that in some patients with a predisposition to autoimmune thyroiditis, lithium may alter directly the rate of antibody formation. It may therefore be possible to identify the group most at risk as comprising females over 45, with circulating antithyroid antibodies, and a slight but sustained elevation of TSH. The risk of hypothyroidism necessitates regular (e.g. annual) monitoring of thyroid function, which should be extended to examination of the gland itself.

Lithium-induced *goitre* is rare and may not herald hypofunction, but it is better the physician discover it than the patient. Again, the mechanism is unknown but appears to reflect an impairment of iodine uptake and/or incorporation into thyroid hormone. The development of asymptomatic goitre or biochemical, or even clinical, hypothyroidism are not contraindications to continued use of lithium. Current recommendations are that sustained elevation of TSH, even in the presence of normal T_4, is sufficient indication for recommending thyroid supplement.

Lithium can alter a number of other endocrine functions, though not in ways that are clinically relevant. In a small number of patients, it can be associated with a rise in serum parathyroid hormone with associated hypercalcaemia, but the number of such cases is so low that they may merely reflect predisposing disorder of parathyroid function. Despite possessing some insulin-like properties, lithium probably does not alter glucose metabolism to any clinically significant degree, even in those with diabetes mellitus.

A series of skin disorders can develop in the coarse of lithium treatment, though the reported total prevalence of around 1% (Lambert & Dalac 1987) seems an underestimate. The commonest is *acne vulgaris*, which may present as a worsening of pre-existing disorder in the usual distribution or as a recrudescence of symptomatology long in abeyance. It may, however, also develop without prior abnormality, when the distribution may be eccentric and involve thighs or upper arms. It tends not to come in cycles as does idiopathic acne and may cause profound embarrassment which can lead to patients discontinuing treatment. It may improve slightly with dose reduction but this in itself is unlikely to be sufficient. Treatment should be conservative in view of a possible interaction between lithium and tetracyclines.

Of more serious import is *psoriasis*, which may also represent an exacerbation of prior disorder or, less commonly, the first manifestation of disorder. All types of psoriasis have been described, and the condition may be associated with characteristic nail changes. This does not usually respond well to conventional treatment, and may be a reason for cessation of treatment. Other skin disorders include seborrhoeic dermatitis, follicular keratosis and pruritic maculopapular erythematous eruptions. As with other psychotropic drugs, lithium treatment may be associated with *hair loss*, and frank alopecia may be a more frequent — though still rare — event than with previously discussed compounds.

While some patients with a relevant dermatological history may show increasing signs over the first 12 months of exposure, not all those with such histories experience exacerbations, so development of these problems is unpredictable. The pathophysiological mechanisms are unknown.

Increases in white blood counts of up to 40%, reflecting mainly a *neutrophilia*, are common in the first week of lithium exposure. A similar stimulatory effect may apply to *platelets*. Lithium has been suggested as a treatment of various marrow deficiency disorders but its action becomes less evident with prolonged use. It may be most apparent with lower doses. From a psychiatric perspective, this finding is an interesting curio, only worthy of note in order to prevent the enthusiastic going off down investigative blind alleys.

Controlled studies in normal volunteers have suggested that lithium produces a slight but detectable *impairment of cognition* and *subjective affective symptoms* of mental slowness, lethargy and dysphoria, sometimes with accompanying restlessness (Judd et al 1977a, 1977b). Some of this may be related to the increasingly appreciated tendency of lithium to promote or exacerbate mild pre-existing extrapyramidal dysfunction, and hence may represent the subjective manifestations of a subclinical parkinsonian-type disorder. In line with this is the descriptive language sometimes used to describe these types of features, such as feeling like 'a zombie'. Particular problems may be encountered by those whose occupation requires creativity.

Lithium does accumulate in bone, but earlier concerns about the possibility of prolonged treatment exacerbating osteoporosis seem unfounded. Caution should still be exercised with its long-term use in children and adolescents, in whom bone is still developing. There are rare reports of lithium worsening the symptoms of *myasthenia gravis*.

Although not strictly a side-effect, there has been concern in recent years about the risk of *rebound mania* occurring with greater than expected frequency following abrupt discontinuation of lithium (Faedda et al 1993). While this may relate to a possible 'withdrawal' type phenomenon, it may equally speak of the drug doing what is expected of it in holding off manic episodes which would have developed earlier in its absence. Certainly lithium, in line with all other psychotropics, should be discontinued *gradually* and never stopped suddenly.

There has been much discussion over the years about the *teratogenicity* of lithium; although the potential exists, the magnitude of the risk remains unclear. Lithium seems particularly prone to disrupt early morphogenesis, and especially development of the cardiovascular system. It therefore exerts its most serious effects during the *first trimester*. It was originally suggested that 11% of pregnancies exposed to lithium may result in congenital malformations, almost three-quarters of which involve the cardiovascular system, with a 2–3% risk of the particularly serious Ebstein's anomaly (Weinstein 1980). These data on the teratogenicity of lithium come from cases reported to the international lithium baby register, maintained for a number of years in the 1970s. The problems with this sort of methodology are legion and relate particularly to the preferential registration of abnormalities over pregnancies resulting in normal infants.

There is no doubt that lithium is potentially teratogenic, though the risks resulting from maternal ingestion are less than were at one time thought (see below). Although the overall risk of congenital malformations does not appear to be greatly increased, first-trimester fetal exposure increases the risk of major cardiac malformations, but no accurate figure can be placed on this at present. Nonetheless, patients need to be informed about this potential risk and strongly advised to avoid unplanned conception. Should the patient wish to become pregnant, lithium should be discontinued in the preconceptive period and for at least the first trimester. There is no specific information to guide the clinician thereafter, but common sense would suggest the merits of, wherever possible, maintaining the immature central nervous system free from exposure to such a pervasively active compound.

Toxicity

The upper limit of normal for the standard 12-hour blood level in most laboratories is 1.2 mmol/l. With modern methods of estimation, the test is readily standardised and the margin of error slight. Hence, this is now a fairly widely agreed figure. Accepting this as the upper limit does not of course mean that a value of 1.21 implies toxicity. There is no clear point of transition, and some patients may get substantially above this level before developing clinical features. Nonetheless patients showing an upward trend or a single reading above this level, which represents an uncharacteristically high value, and who develop a change in their pattern of tolerability should be suspected of moving to toxicity. Most patients will show an altered tolerance by the time blood levels are in the range 1.4–1.5 mmol/l, and clear signs of toxicity will be evident at levels over 2 mmol/l.

Most cases of lithium toxicity occur in the context of long-term administration and hence represent a relatively insidious departure from a stable situation. While symptomatology can emerge swiftly, their antecedents can usually be traced back over 24–48 hours.

Gastrointestinal features comprising *anorexia* and persistent or obtrusive *nausea*, culminating in *vomiting*, are usually the first signs of impending trouble (Table 15.7). At the same time patients may experience a dry mouth and insatiable *thirst* associated with production of voluminous amounts of dilute (i.e. low-specific-gravity) urine, which may contain glucose. *Diarrhoea* may then develop, which may be bloody. With this combination of disturbances, dehydration can rapidly ensue or progress. *Tremor* accentuates with a coarse, jerky quality emerging which may extend to all body parts. Patients feel increasingly *weak*. In addition, as levels rise, an appearance of restlessness is contributed to by *muscle fasciculations* and myoclonic-like *jerks* or typical *choreoathetoid* movements, associated with generalised *hypertonicity*. With progression, a general breakdown in neuromuscular co-ordination may show in *dysarthria* and *ataxia*. Disruption of higher mental functions is a sign of serious toxicity, with victims becoming increasingly *lethargic* and *drowsy*, with lack of interest and awareness, attention deficits and frank *confusion/delirium*. Incipient circulatory failure is signaled by *hypotension* and *irregularities of cardiac rhythm*. *Fits* are likely to emerge at this stage, which leads on to *stupor* and eventual preterminal *coma*.

It is important to bear in mind that because of delayed brain penetration and egression of lithium, clinical signs of CNS toxicity may not occur in unison with escalating blood levels, and may persist when levels are declining, and even after they are back to the therapeutic range.

It is essential to educate patients on the often simple measures that can be effective in avoiding lithium toxicity — such as maintaining hydration and salt intake, and being sensitive to any *change* in tolerability. In particular, the onset of gastrointestinal symptoms should always be emphasised as an important 'warning' where patients themselves can effectively intervene by simply stopping lithium for 1, or at most 2, days. Based on the half-life of lithium, blood levels can be expected to drop by about 50% in 24 hours, assuming maintenance of normal renal function, and

discontinuation is an effective, as well as necessary, strategy in the management of toxicity of any degree.

Where clinical symptomatology is in keeping with established toxicity, a so-called 'forced' diuresis is recommended (Thomsen & Schou 1975). This amounts to 1–2 litres of isotonic saline intravenously over a 6-hour period. The aim is volume repletion and a consequent increase in glomerular filtration, and hence lithium clearance. In patients with hyponatraemia, the use of saline is furthermore beneficial, by decreasing proximal reabsorption of lithium. Even with clinical improvement over the initial treatment cycle, i.v. fluids should be maintained to obviate the effects of delayed absorption, especially with slow-release preparations. A recommended aim is infusion at a rate sufficient to produce a 20% decline in lithium levels every 6 hours (Gomolin 1987). It must be borne in mind that a large urinary output in response to fluid replacement may reflect *renal damage*, in the form of impaired concentrating ability, and so electrolyte balance must be closely monitored. Some authors have recommended that the best results from diuresis are achieved when the urine is alkalinised ('forced alkaline diuresis'), but the increased hazard is not necessarily offset by an increased response, and a number of authorities now no longer recommend this.

Where toxicity is mild to moderately severe and unaccompanied by significant renal failure, such steps may be sufficient. However, with serum levels over 4 mmol/l or renal incompetence due either to pre-existing chronic failure or acute tubular necrosis related to the immediate problem, then such methods are unlikely to be adequate or fast enough. In this situation, dialysis is the recommended management. This can take the form of peritoneal dialysis, though haemodialysis is more efficient.

Lithium tends to be a drug patients treat with respect but, like all drugs, it can be a medium for overdose resulting in *acute toxicity*. In this situation, gastric lavage and induced emesis are widely utilised, especially when slow-release preparations have been ingested. One point in advocacy of these formulations has been that, because of their slow-release characteristics, such interventions are more likely to be worthwhile than with standard formulations. This is unlikely to be rational. As we have seen, little lithium is absorbed from the stomach, and the mechanism of slow release is to delay absorption from the small bowel. The only advantage of gastric lavage beyond 2–3 hours of any overdose is to remove excess lithium *secreted* in gastric fluid. The amounts that can be removed by this means are relatively small, and there is the very real risk of adding to any evolving electrolyte disturbance. Efforts at this stage are more profitably concentrated on measures to accelerate excretion, outlined above.

Other mood-stabilising agents

Anticonvulsants

It was noted in the 1960s that certain anticonvulsant drugs exerted effects on mood symptoms, when patients receiving carbamazepine for epilepsy reported feeling less anxious. The first report of their use in major affective disorders was by Takezaki and Hanoaka in 1971, though it was the report by Ballenger and Post 9 years later that stimulated widespread interest. To date, most work has concerned carbamazepine and sodium valproate, but with the introduction of a new generation of anticonvulsants, such as lamotrigine and gabapentin, interest is widening and anticonvulsants now occupy an important place in the treatment of major affective disorders. However, it is important for psychiatrists to realise that these compounds have complex kinetics and potentially serious adverse effects, making them different to handle compared with lithium.

Carbamazepine is a tricyclic compound, closely related structurally to imipramine (Fig. 15.6). It was synthesised in 1953 on the crest of the psychopharmacological excitement that followed the introduction of chlorpromazine. It was hoped that the new compound would emulate the actions of chlorpromazine, but it did not. It did however possess unique features of its own, and in the 1960s was introduced as a highly effective anticonvulsant.

Carbamazepine is rather slowly and erratically absorbed, with peak levels attained in 4–6 hours, though with Retard formulations T_{max} may be up to 24 hours. Bioavailability is in the range 80–90%. There are substantial first-pass effects. Its apparent volume of distribution is in the moderate range. At around 75%, it is relatively less protein bound than most psychotropics. Its half-life is dependent not only on its complex metabolism but also on the fact that for the first 2–3 months of chronic treatment it *induces* its own metabolism to a substantial degree. Thus, with single doses, half-life values are in the region of 25–45 hours, whereas with chronic administration these fall dramatically to 7–24 hours. After 1 month, the initial steady-state levels may have fallen by as much as 25% (Brodie 1987).

The major metabolic pathway in the liver is epoxidation by the enzyme arene oxidase to form carbamazepine-10,11-epoxide, which has a shorter half-life than the parent but is a pharmacologically active and toxic intermediate. This is, in turn, metabolised by epoxide hydroxylase to the inactive trans-carbamazepine-diol (or carbamazepine-10,11 dihydrodihydroxide), which is excreted in the urine. Fifteen to twenty percent of a carbamazepine dose is metabolised by direct conjugation with glucuronic acid. Epoxide hydroxylase is inhibited by a number of drugs, notably valproate, coadministration of which can result in a dramatic decrease in the ratio of carbamazepine to its epoxide metabolite (from 10:1 to 2:1). As a consequence, patients can experience signs of toxicity while still showing blood levels within the therapeutic range (Wilder 1992). Carbamazepine furthermore increases hormone clearance and can negate the actions of the contraceptive pill, especially low oestrogen formulations.

Sodium valproate is the soluble sodium salt of valproic acid, a poorly soluble branched chain carboxylic acid (Fig. 15.6). Absorption is rapid with unmodified formulations, peak levels being attained in 30–60 minutes. The drug is, however, a powerful gastric irritant, and a number of slow-release formulations, such as enteric coated tablets, are widely used which have T_{max} values in the region of 4–6 hours. Protein binding is up to 95% but is inversely dependent on the fat content of the diet. Binding

of valproate is saturable within the therapeutic range, thus rapid increases in dose can be associated with disproportionately large increases in free drug levels, which rapidly undergo metabolism, with consequently lower than expected blood levels. Valproate displaces carbamazepine from protein binding sites, and its introduction can result in transient toxicity of the latter. Half-life varies with preparation but is in the range 5–20 hours (Wilder 1992).

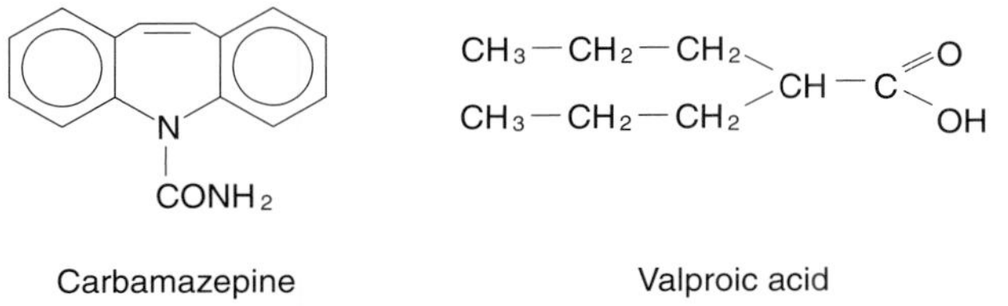

The metabolism of valproate is complex. One pathway is via the microsomal cytochrome P450 system, which produces two potentially toxic metabolites: 4-en- and 2,4-en-valproate. The more significant pathway — at least when the drug is administered alone — is via mitochondrial beta-oxidation, the pathway extensively utilised in the degradation of fatty acids in general. This produces 3-hydroxy- and 3-oxo- derivatives and 2-en-valproate, which has anticonvulsant properties and a long half-life. Therapeutic environments that stimulate P450 metabolism — for example coadministration of inducers, such as carbamazepine or phenobarbitone — can lead to excessive build-up of toxic metabolites, which may be the mechanism underlying the infrequently reported but potentially fatal *hepatic necrosis*. Another rare, but potentially serious scenario, is in those with *inherited* or *acquired metabolic diseases* who may be deficient in carnitine, an important constituent of fatty acid metabolism (Coulter 1991). Valproate decreases carnitine levels, and in this situation may precipitate *encephalopathy*.

Both these drugs can produce significant adverse effects. Both can cause gastrointestinal upset, and are sedative and can be associated with drowsiness. Carbamazepine can, like all tricyclic drugs, slow intracardiac conduction and produce arrhythmias. Hypocalcaemia can occur, and inappropriate ADH secretion may be associated with hyponatraemia and oedema. Idiosyncratic reactions include marrow suppression, hepatotoxicity, (morbiliform) skin rashes, photosensitivity and rarely Stevens–Johnson syndrome and a lupus-type syndrome.

Valproate can cause tremors, skin rashes and hair loss and may also be associated with oedema. Of greater importance are rare cases of acute pancreatitis, hepatotoxicity and hyperammonaemia, possibly progressing to coma, which may be related to the kinetic factors noted above. This drug can also affect ovarian function, and concern has been expressed about its chronic use and the possible development of polycystic ovaries and hyperandrogenism (Isojarvi et al 1993, 1996). Although apparently reversible, this is an important potential association in the context of the drug's increasing use as a mood stabiliser, which may restrict its future long-term use in women of child-bearing age.

Both carbamazepine and valproate are potentially *teratogenic* and should be *avoided in pregnancy*. Thus, use of anticonvulsants does not free psychiatrists from giving clear advice on avoidance of unplanned pregnancy any more than with those receiving lithium. Of the two, valproate probably presents the greater risk (Wilder 1992), including a 2% risk of hypospadias. Recently, concern has been expressed about a general developmental disorder, clinically not dissimilar to fetal alcohol syndrome, occurring in children exposed throughout pregnancy. This remains controversial but emphasises the new set of problems these drugs raise for psychiatric practice.

In recent years a new generation of largely 'add on' anticonvulsants has become available with novel modes of action. Their use as mood stabilisers has been expanding. *Lamotrigine* appears to inhibit the release of glutamate, and possibly other

Carbamazepine   Valproic acid

Fig. 15.6
Structures of mood stabilisers.

excitatory amino acids, from presynaptic terminals, while the evidence is that *gabapentin* attaches to high-affinity binding sites that, despite the drug's structural similarity to GABA, appear to be neither GABA recognition sites nor benzodiazepine receptors. Both these drugs have been recommended for mood-stabilisation purposes, though to date the trial evidence is stronger for lamotrigine.

Calcium channel antagonists

In 1981, Dubovsky and colleagues reported antimanic properties in a patient treated with the calcium channel antagonist *verapamil*. Since then a number of reports have appeared suggesting that this group of compounds may have clinical utility in bipolar affective disorders, though most of the evidence remains anecdotal or based on small or open studies (Dubovsky 1993). Much of the early interest remained with verapamil, whose value may be limited to patients with relatively mild disorder and/or patients who, for whatever reason, are unable to take lithium. More recent evidence has suggested that drugs of the dihydropyridine type, such as nifedipine and nimodipine, may be particularly useful in rapid-cycling bipolar disorders.

The calcium channel antagonists reduce calcium influx through potential-dependent calcium channels during cell stimulation. The actions of lithium on intracellular transduction pathways include desensitisation of the receptor-stimulated phophatidylinositol cycle that mobilises calcium, and inhibition of calmodulin, the calcium activation protein. Furthermore, both carbamazepine and at least some antipsychotics also antagonise calcium cellular influx. There is therefore good reason to explore the therapeutic application of these compounds, though the justification for their use at present remains largely empirical.

Therapeutics

Indications

The indications for lithium are more tightly circumscribed than those for other psychotropic agents (Box 15.9). The place of anticonvulsants remains under review. Both carbamazepine and valproate are increasingly used as alternatives to lithium, though the evidence base is strongest for the antimanic properties of valproate. Their place in the adjunctive treatment of resistant depressions and the prophylaxis of recurrent unipolar depressions have not as yet been established. Anticonvulsants are still usually reserved for second- or third-line, or combined, use in treatment-resistant situations.

Calcium channel antagonists have been insufficiently investigated for their relative place to be established clearly (a conclusion that might equally apply to antipsychotics!). They should therefore be reserved for empirical use in refractory bipolar disorders, especially rapid-cycling or ultradian (ultra-ultra rapid) types.

Box 15.9 Indications for lithium

- treatment of manic/hypomanic episodes
- prophylaxis of bipolar affective disorders
- prophylaxis of recurrent unipolar depressions
- as an adjunctive agent in the treatment of major depressive disorders unresponsive to antidepressants alone

---

Strategies

The role of lithium in the treatment of major affective disorders has been the subject of revision in recent years. Long-term follow-up studies suggest a less favourable impact on outcome than was thought, and although this is still the first-line approach in especially the prophylaxis of recurrent bipolar illnesses, some have even challenged its use in this situation (Moncrieff 1997). Where its use is decided upon, the major therapeutic principles are summarised in Box 15.10.

There is no hard and fast rule about how frequently serum lithium levels should be assessed but, in patients who are stable and compliant, three or four times per year is adequate. Thyroid function should be evaluated annually as routine, or 6-monthly in those at higher risk, such as middle-aged or elderly females with circulating autoantibodies. The advantages of routine monitoring of renal function are unclear, though this remains a conventional recommendation. It would certainly be indicated in the wake of an episode of frank toxicity. Following the decision to discontinue, lithium doses should be tapered downwards gradually over several weeks.

There are no such clear principles that apply to the other mood stablisers. Blood monitoring is often undertaken with carbamazepine, and increasingly with valproate, but its value is doubtful. There are as yet no clearly established therapeutic ranges for their use in affective disorders comparable to those for lithium. Blood levels may help identify poor or non-compliance; for carbamazepine, very high levels will increase the likelihood of toxicity. The most sensitive pointers to this are probably clinical, however, and regular symptomatic monitoring is a better practice principle than routine blood levels.

BENZODIAZEPINES AND OTHER SEDATIVES/HYPNOTICS

Introduction

There is, even today, no single antianxiety compound, but the search for medicaments which relieve anxiety and promote sleep is ancient and continuing. In the last century, alcohol and marijuana served this purpose, as did, if you could afford them, opium and laudanum (tincture of opium), the latter of which supported much of upper-class Victorian womanhood. Later, specific compounds structurally and pharmacologically similar to alcohol, such as chloral hydrate and paraldehyde, were introduced, while bromide salts found vogue well into the 20th century.

The first drugs to be termed 'sedatives' were the barbiturates, synthesised by Fischer and von Mering in 1903 from the condensation of malonic acid with urea (and called after 'a charming lady named Barbara'!). A large number of barbiturates were synthesised and, at their peak in the 1950s, accounted for 20% of all prescriptions in the UK. However, this group is blighted by a high dependency-producing potential and very narrow therapeutic index, problems which also afflict their various analogues, such as glutethamide and methaqualone, which temporarily found medical application in the 1960s and 1970s. Barbiturates are now obsolete, except in a very few cases of epilepsy, though even here their use is minimal. They and their kin have however held on with tenacity as the 'downers' of illicitly supplied, recreational usage; and, if anything, their availability is increasing with widespread access to 'on-line' pharmacies, usually

---

Box 15.10   Principles of lithium use

Major
- Because of its narrow therapeutic margin, it is important when starting lithium to establish a series of baseline parameters. These include routine haematological and biochemical screens, with particular attention to electrolytes, though baseline thyroid function is probably optional at this stage, except in high-risk patients. Routine ECG is also most pertinent to older age groups or those with pre-existing heart disease. It is furthermore important to be aware of the patient's renal status — or, more accurately, whether any significant pretreatment renal incompetence is present. Strictly speaking, this should be assessed by undertaking a lithium clearance but, in practice, creatinine clearance is the usual method. It is questionable, however, whether in the presence of a normal serum creatinine a full creatinine clearance actually provides meaningful additional information. Pregnancy should always be excluded in women of childbearing age
- Treatment plans must be geared around the maintenance of blood levels within a defined range, assessed by the standardised 12-hour serum lithium (Amdisen 1977). The assessment was originally validated in patients on multiple dosing regimens but is in fact equally applicable to once daily, 'nocte' regimens. The major requirement, apart from the patient being compliant, is that they must be in steady state. A plain blood sample is removed 12 hours after the last (nocte) dose and, if the patient is on a multiple dosing regimen, before the first dose of the morning. Therapeutic levels are now fairly standardised internationally within the range 0.6–1.2 mmol/l although in the context of maintenance, levels in the range of 0.45–0.5 may be adequate (Jerram & McDonald 1978)
- Lithium is the one drug in psychiatric practice that should never be prescribed generically. This is because, although bioavailability does not vary greatly with different formulations, it varies sufficiently to impact significantly on blood levels — e.g. for someone stabilised on 'Camcolit 400' who is then dispensed 'Priadel 400'. A further elementary error, especially in non-specialist pharmacies, is to dispense generic prescriptions on the basis of the most convenient tablet strength available. Thus, 'lithium, 1000 mg may be dispensed as 4×250 mg tablets, rather than 2.5×400 mg tablets. This may seem logical to an inexperienced pharmacist, but the tablet strength is the clue to the formulation — 400 mg tablets are slow/sustained release; 250 mg are not. Four tablets of standard lithium (250 mg) taken together will result in a very high C_{max}, which is likely to result in toxicity, something the author has encountered

Subsidiary
- Adverse effects may be obviated by flexibility both in the use of preparations and dosing schedules, with the aim of trying to reduce the rate and height of the post-absorptive peak
- Patients must be educated on an ongoing basis about the need to avoid dehydration and to maintain where possible relatively stable salt intakes

---

operating from developing countries. It is therefore possible that psychiatrists of the coming generation will encounter more problems with illicit use/misuse of these drugs than colleagues of the present one.

The first so-called 'tranquilliser' was meprobamate, a propanediol derivative synthesised in 1951. By the mid-1950s it was the most prescribed drug in America. However, although somewhat safer than barbiturates, it was still a drug with a relatively narrow therapeutic index and could also produce dependency.

Benzodiazepines

No class of psychotropic agent illustrates better the triumphs and failures of psychopharmacology than the benzodiazepines. By the end of the first decade of their use, they were the most prescribed group of drugs in the developed world; by the end of the second they were among the most vilified, an emblem of the public's perception that psychopharmacology was all about 'sorting' the ills of modern living with a pill. Neither of these two positions was, or is, justified. Benzodiazepines were undoubtedly excessively prescribed for problems better dealt with in other ways. But neither is psychopharmacology society's policeman. This class of drugs is highly effective as part of the management of specific *medical* conditions and, with the same levels of supervision demanded of any drug treatments, they remain valuable therapeutic agents.

The 1,4-benzodiazepine structure was discovered by the chemist Leo Sternbach who, in the mid-1950s, was searching for behavioural properties among a group of compounds thought to be benzheptoxdiazines, which he had investigated previously for their potential as dyes. In fact, the compounds being investigated were not benzheptoxdiazines, but a new analogue of quinazoline, a compound known since the 1890s. These investigations were not getting anywhere, and Sternbach was in the throes of what he later referred to as a 'house cleaning' operation, when in 1957 he submitted, without enthusiasm, one such compound for pharmacological screening (Sternbach 1983). This was later shown to have a different structure from what had been expected when it was created, and hence its production can indeed be seen as purely serendipitous. However, the pharmacologist Lowell Randell noted that in animals this derivative possessed a similar psychopharmacological profile to that of meprobamate. Confirmation of this in humans led in 1960 to the launch of the first commercial product, chlordiazepoxide, the vanguard of a pharmaceutical avalanche.

These were also the first drugs in which the influence of marketing strategies can be seen. Benzodiazepines have four main actions: antianxiety, hypnotic, anticonvulsant and muscle relaxant effects. There is, however, no evidence to support the view that different compounds have differential clinical profiles in these areas (Baldessarini 1985). Benzodiazepines differ in some pharmacological parameters, most notably potency and distribution, but not in terms of their differential effects. Even today, professional wisdom has it that different drugs in the class should be prescribed for different clinical indications, a perception no doubt encouraged by the somewhat irrational licensing conditions imposed by regulatory authorities.

Structures

The basic components of the majority of benzodiazepines comprise a benzene (or A) ring chlorinated at the R7 position, joined to a seven-membered diazepine (i.e. double nitrogen) ring (B ring), the two nitrogens of which are sited at the R1 and R4 positions (hence 1,4-benzodiazepines) and to which is attached a phenyl (or C) ring at position 5 (Fig. 15.7). The major variations in chemical substituents that characterise different drugs largely involve the B ring.

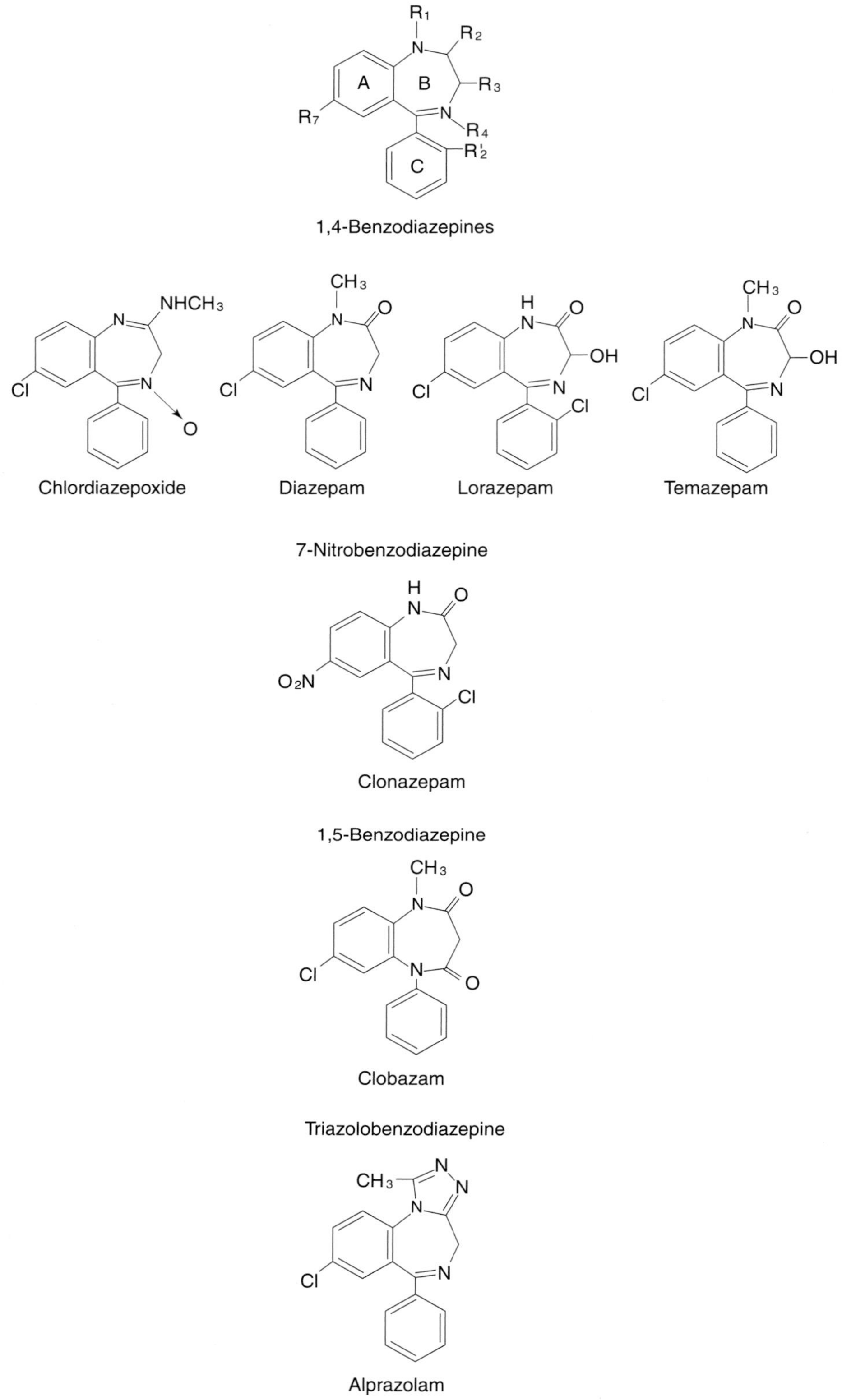

1,4-Benzodiazepines

Chlordiazepoxide

Diazepam

Lorazepam

Temazepam

7-Nitrobenzodiazepine

Clonazepam

1,5-Benzodiazepine

Clobazam

Triazolobenzodiazepine

Alprazolam

Fig. 15.7
Structures of the benzodiazepines.

This basic structure has been subject to modifications. The simplest is the transposition of one of the nitrogens from the R4 to the R5 position. The major representative of the 1,5-benzodiazepines is clobazam. Clonazepam is a 7-nitrobenzodiazepine. Other modifications produce compounds that, although originally described as 'non-benzodiazepines', are more appropriately considered benzodiazepine variants. These include the triazolobenzodiazepines, as exemplified by alprazolam and triazolam (withdrawn in the UK), and the thienodiazepines such as brotizolam, in which the benzene ring is replaced by a thiophene ring.

Pharmacokinetics

As with the SSRIs, benzodiazepines differ most from one another in their pharmacokinetic properties, which are not only varied but complex. Many of these variations relate to the differing physicochemical properties imparted by structural differences.

All benzodiazepines are weak organic bases which, when subjected to physiological buffering, become *lipid soluble* to varying degrees from moderate to high. This variability in lipid solubility is a major factor contributing to pharmacokinetic — and most importantly, clinical — distinctions between compounds. Of the drugs encountered in psychiatric practice, flurazepam is approximately 10% more lipid soluble than diazepam, whereas temazepam and lorazepam are only about 50% as lipid soluble. Midazolam, used in anaesthetics, is the most lipid soluble of all (50% more so than diazepam) (Greenblatt & Shader 1987).

Absorption from the GI tract is complete and followed by extensive first-pass metabolism for most compounds. For reasons not altogether clear, absorption is unpredictable from injection sites, especially in patients on continuous-dosing regimens. The exception may be lorazepam, which appears rapidly absorbed from intramuscular sites (Richens 1983). The rate of absorption, which is the rate-limiting step in the onset of action, varies but is overall rapid. Diazepam and flurazepam are among the most rapidly absorbed, while temazepam, despite its licensed indication, is among the slowest (Greenblatt & Shader 1987). In general, absorption can be slowed but not decreased by food, which delays gastric emptying and time to reach the proximal bowel. For some compounds, however, absorption may be impaired by aluminium-based antacids. Peak levels are usually achieved in 30–90 minutes with the rapidly absorbed compounds, and 2–4 hours for the slower ones. Rectal administration, in the UK mainly confined to children with epilepsy (though 'popular' in France), is a highly efficient administration route, especially if liquid formulations are used, with a T_{max} value of 15 minutes (Richens 1983).

The group as a whole are highly protein bound, mainly to albumen, with levels of up to 98% for diazepam and 94–97% for chlordiazepoxide. Lorazepam and nitrazepam are less protein bound at 85–90%, and alprazolam is the least, with a free fraction of about 30% (Moschitto & Greenblatt 1983).

Benzodiazepines are widely distributed, a function for each drug that is dependent on its lipophilicity. Thus, compounds such as diazepam, which are highly lipophilic, have large apparent volumes of distribution (V_d) and are widely and rapidly distributed, whereas drugs such as lorazepam have lower V_d values and are more slowly and less extensively distributed. The kinetics therefore technically conform to a two-compartment model, with the plasma concentration curve reflecting distribution as well as metabolism. Distribution characteristics have considerable clinical importance, especially with single parenteral dosing (see below). Half-lives also vary greatly across compounds and individuals, and are susceptible to the range of variables that influence both the delivery of drug to hepatocytes and the functional integrity of these, a point of particular note in predicting the susceptibility of neonates to these drugs. Flurazepam has a half-life that, at approximately 1–2 hours, is as short as any psychotropic agent, while that for clonazepam, at 50–70 hours, is as long as any. Figures for chlordiazepoxide, in the range 6–30 hours, are shorter than those for diazepam, which are in the region of 20 hours in most healthy adults, but may extend as high as 70 hours in some individuals.

Metabolism is hepatic, virtually total and, for most compounds, complex, though often incestuously inter-related (Fig. 15.8). For a few, such as lorazepam and temazepam, which share in common shorter half-lives, metabolism comprises simply conjugation with glucuronic acid, which produces the water solubility necessary for renal excretion (Richens 1983). These drugs therefore produce no active metabolites. For compounds undergoing more extensive metabolism, the fastest and hence first step involves dealkylation of alkyl substituents of the B ring, a process that strongly determines the half-life: where the alkyl group is large, or sited far from the ring itself, dealklyation is rapid and half-lives short (e.g. flurazepam); whereas with small alkyl substituents positioned close to the ring (e.g. chlordiazepoxide), dealkylation is slow and half-lives longer (Kaplan & Jack 1983). For drugs with methyl substituents at the N1 position, demethylation takes place, which is a relatively slow process. Perhaps the most important aspect of metabolism is hydroxylation at the R3 site which, for a number of drugs, produces desmethyldiazepam, a fully active metabolite which undergoes slow oxidation prior to excretion, and thus has a very long half-life (30–100 hours).

A knowledge of the pharmacokinetics of benzodiazepines illustrates the powerful impact that a drug's physicochemical properties and its intermediate metabolites can have on clinical expectations, and explains some apparent paradoxes. For example, knowledge of flurazepam's ultrashort half-life but the long half-life of its major and active metabolite, desalkylflurazepam (50–100

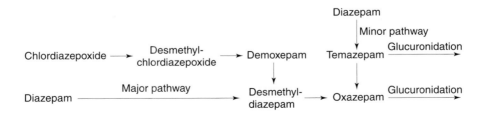

Fig. 15.8
Interconnected biotransformation pathways for some commonly prescribed benzodiazepines.

hours), allows one to predict the sometimes potent hangover, and even toxicity, effects that can be seen with this drug, especially in the elderly. Indeed, cumulative effects are to be anticipated with those drugs, such as diazepam, which have desmethyldiazepam as a metabolite, and advice on driving and contact with machinery is particularly important when recommending these.

The conflicting impact of distribution and half-life is evident with single intravenous use, a practice to which benzodiazepines lend themselves and that is widespread. Going by half-life values, it would be reasonable to expect that in the management of an acute situation intravenous diazepam would have a longer action than lorazepam, a drug with a much shorter half-life. This is not in fact the case, as diazepam is rapidly distributed, resulting in a swift decline in plasma levels to as low as one-fifth peak, and consequent loss of acute action. The less widely distributed lorazepam will maintain a longer action, despite its significantly shorter half-life (Greenblatt & Shader 1987).

Pharmacodynamics

Mode of action In 1977, excitement spread through the neuroscience community with the almost simultaneous discovery, by Braestrup and Squires in Denmark and Mohler and Okada in Switzerland, of specific benzodiazepine receptor sites in the mammalian brain that bound labelled diazepam with high affinity. Since then, these sites have been characterised in detail and are now known to represent part of a GABA-receptor–chloride ionophore complex (see Ch. 3).

Receptors for the major inhibitory amino acid neurotransmitter, γ-aminobutyric acid (GABA), come in two forms. These were delineated by Hill and Bowery in 1981 on the basis of sensitivity ($GABA_A$), or insensitivity ($GABA_B$), to bicuculline. These receptors have different distributions in the CNS and different patterns of agonist/antagonist interactions. Baclofen is the major agonist at $GABA_B$ sites, which may be predominantly presynaptic in location and are coupled to their signal transduction mechanisms by G-proteins. However, benzodiazepines do not interact with $GABA_B$ receptors.

The $GABA_A$ complex comprises a ring-shaped collection of transmembrane proteins which include representatives of at least 16 subunit proteins arranged in five groups (Fig. 15.9). These are given the Greek designations α, β, γ, δ and ρ. The α subunits are the sites at which benzodiazepines act as agonists, while the β subunits are the GABA sites. The α and β subunits interact insofar as each stimulates binding to the other, a relationship in which the γ subunits appear to be crucial. Co-assembly of an α, a β and a γ subunit is the minimum requirement for the production of a high-affinity benzodiazepine binding site, a motif sometimes referred to as the ω- (i.e. benzodiazepine-) 1 receptor.

These receptor components can be seen as the gatekeepers to the functional element of the complex, which comprises a gated ion channel for chloride. Despite the close functional relationship between subunits, it is solely the GABA-related subunits which control the channel. Stimulation of these opens the ion channel and produces an influx of chloride into the cell, resulting in a state of hyperpolarisation and hence a decreased firing rate of critical neurons. Benzodiazepines facilitate GABA inhibitory effects in the CNS by increasing the number of channels opened, rather than by prolonging the duration of opening of a few. The mechanism whereby GABA stimulation opens the chloride channels

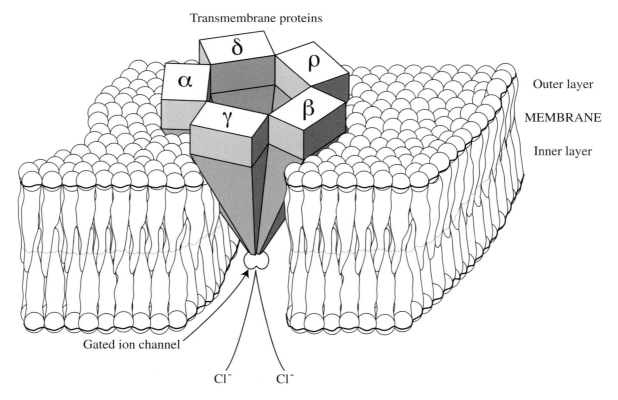

Transmembrane proteins

Outer layer

MEMBRANE

Inner layer

Gated ion channel

Cl⁻   Cl⁻

Fig. 15.9
$GABA_A$-benzodiazepine ionophore complex.

is thought to involve an element of physical distortion of the complex, a phenomenon known as *allosteric modulation*.

The elucidation of these intricate structural and functional relationships is one of the most impressive undertakings in modern psychopharmacology, but leaves unanswered two critical questions:

- How does this relate to the pathophysiology and alleviation of anxiety?
- What are the elusive endogenous ligand or ligands — so-called 'endozepines' — that, in the absence of man's intrusions, normally couple with benzodiazepine recognition sites?

Adverse effects Benzodiazepines have perhaps the highest therapeutic index of all psychotropic drugs, and are extremely effective. In view of their actions, it therefore becomes problematic as to whether patient complaints about 'side-effects' represent adverse effects as such, or merely the drug carrying out its intended function.

These drugs have little or no autonomic actions, though may promote mild *hypotension* with over-zealous intravenous administration. Some patients complain of *dry mouth* and *blurred vision*, though whether these are drug effects is unclear. Patients may however experience '*dizziness*' or 'wooziness' which lacks the rotational and impelled qualities of vertigo and is probably a form of lightheadedness, possibly related to mild blood pressure changes. Benzodiazepines do not alter the electrical or mechanical functioning of the heart. At therapeutic doses, they do not interfere with respiration but, when given rapidly by the intravenous route, they can produce significant respiratory depression and even arrest, especially those compounds which are distributed swiftly (e.g. diazepam). This can be reversed by the benzodiazepine antagonist *flumazenil*.

The commonest patient complaint is also the prime example of the efficacy versus tolerability question — namely, a feeling of *decreased mental acuity* or frank daytime drowsiness and sedation. This can be evident early in exposure, when it usually fades. It may however also emerge later in the course of chronic exposure as a result of the accumulation of drugs/metabolites of long half-life. Despite this, however, there seems to be a remarkable tolerance to such clinical consequences of accumulation (Baldessarini 1985).

Impaired psychomotor performance is an undoubted adverse effect, which results from a primary deficit in information processing and from sedation (Hindmarch 1980). As a group effect, benzodiazepines impair *reaction times* to a degree, which can lead to significant functional deficits. Some performance deficits can be demonstrated soon after exposure and, although some do appear to ease with the passage of time, deviations from the norm can also become evident as a consequence of accumulation. Even those drugs with the shortest half-lives and marketed as hypnotics are still associated with significant residual day-time blood levels, so one cannot take solace in the fact of the drug's ingestion the night before. It is imperative that doctors advise all patients taking a benzodiazepine of the impact this can have on daily tasks, such as driving or operating machinery. Those requiring high degrees of motor responsiveness, such as airline pilots, must be specifically apprised of the implications of residual blood levels on daytime performance.

Benzodiazepines also impair *short-term memory*. Although the traditional view is that this comprises a retrograde amnesia, controlled studies have in fact shown that the problem is almost exclusively an *anterograde* one, with impairments of recall relating solely to events after drug administration (King 1992). It further-

more appears to be secondary to sedation. Patients on routine treatment schedules are usually unaware of this effect, but after intravenous administration it can be striking. This is often used to therapeutic benefit in, for example, cardioversion and endoscopy, where patients given a benzodiazepine beforehand may afterwards not recall, or have only a hazy recollection of, basically unpleasant interventions. This action is being increasingly exploited in incidents of so-called 'date rape'.

In addition to the 'dizziness' noted above, patients occasionally develop *unsteadiness*, which more clearly relates to discoordination. In fact *ataxia*, *dysarthria* and a general breakdown of co-ordination are signs of the profound CNS depression that constitutes *intoxication*, and such features should be viewed in this light, even if the regimen recommended has been 'therapeutic'.

Rare reports have appeared over the years of skin rashes, blood dyscrasias, headache, gastrointestinal upset, weight gain, impaired sexual function and dyskinetic movement disorder associated with use of benzodiazepines, but in most instances these probably represented incidental disorder unrelated to the drug. Certainly, such problems, if genuine, are extremely rare.

Two other side-effects are important. Shortly after the introduction of chlordiazepoxide, a 'syndrome' of paradoxical behavioural disinhibition or '*dyscontrol*' was described (Ingram & Timbury 1960). The problem appears to be more frequent in women, and although reported most with chlordiazepoxide, is probably not unique to this preparation. The usual scenario is one of 'confinement', where the individual perceives herself as trapped, and is then challenged. Confrontation in this situation can be met with a rage response, associated with intemperate and assaultive behaviour. This is perhaps a better recognised phenomenon with other CNS depressants, especially alcohol, but it is important to bear in mind in psychiatric practice, as professional interventions, and especially inpatient environments, might be perceived by patients as confining and restrictive. By using benzodiazepines in an attempt to achieve behavioural containment, one might unwittingly produce the opposite.

Dependency and withdrawal. The final adverse effect is potentially the most serious, and was the one that forced a radical reappraisal of the risk–benefit ratio of benzodiazepines in the most public way. This is physiological dependency.

As early as the 1970s, it was clear that long-term use of benzodiazepines could be associated with tolerance effects. Patients frequently, if not usually, lost the sedation associated with early exposure, something known to happen rapidly over a few days. Also, the phenomenon of *REM rebound* was known from sleep EEGs of patients who had stopped long-term benzodiazepine hypnotics (Oswald & Priest 1965), and withdrawal type features, including fits, were well recognised after sudden cessation. However, full physiological dependency was thought to be a problem only in those who abused medication, and doubts continued as to whether these phenomena could occur with regimens used clinically. A further problem was that complaints from patients suddenly stopping these drugs had a familiar resonance with those of the conditions for which the drugs were used in the first place.

The issue was thrown into stark relief when Petursson & Lader (1981) showed conclusively that a *withdrawal syndrome*, and hence physical dependence, could develop with benzodiazepine regimens that were considered to be in the therapeutic range.

The symptoms of benzodiazepine withdrawal are unusual in that they are, as a rule, delayed in onset for longer than most withdrawal states. They are also unusual in that they combine *affective features* with unique *perceptual disturbances*. Some 5–7 days after stopping, patients start to feel increasingly unsettled, with anxious dysphoria. Sleep diminishes in both quality and duration, and daytime fatigue is prominent. Flu-like symptoms supervene, such as sweating, listlessness, anorexia, muscle aches and headache. Perceptual changes are evident in the form of heightened sensitivity to sounds, light and touch, and may develop a 'temporal lobe' quality of distorted environmental relationships — e.g. doors or fireplaces sloping to one side. Surroundings can seem alien, and frank depersonalisation may occur. In addition, bizarre paraesthesiae may be experienced (as with antidepressant withdrawal), such as numbness, tingling or a feeling of movement, or characteristically the sensation of walking on cotton wool. Fits are rare on withdrawal from therapeutic regimens.

There was a time when clinics were besieged by patients claiming persistence of such features months, or even years, after cessation of benzodiazepines, but this is untenable. Features of benzodiazepine withdrawal last for 1–2 weeks at most. Belief in the endurance of symptoms was, and is, a reflection of their impact, the patient's expectation and recurring anxiety.

The risk of dependency with chronic benzodiazepine use is even now not something that can be confidently quantified, as it depends on individual factors such as personality type, the duration of exposure, and pharmacokinetic parameters of the drug used. Overall, the best estimate is that after 6 months of continuous exposure, a risk in the region of 45% can be anticipated (Tyrer et al 1981). However, features such as withdrawal anxiety / sleep disturbance may be found in some patients after only 6 weeks of treatment (Power et al 1985). The risk must therefore be judged as substantial, though it appears to be greatest, as would be predicted, with drugs which have relatively short half-lives, such as lorazepam.

If the problem has resulted from use of a short-half-life compound, treatment should start by switching to diazepam which, with its relatively long half-life, should make the ultimate task of tapered reduction easier (Higgitt et al 1985). Beyond this, however, management rests essentially on the good practice principle of slow or ultra-slow reduction, preferably over weeks. Although a number of drugs have been recommended as useful in easing withdrawal symptomatology, propranolol is probably the only one with any merits, and even these are slight.

Benzodiazepines are very safe. Even in overdose, *fatality* is usually only associated with combined ingestion with other drugs, especially alcohol.

Other sedative / hypnotic agents

In recent years other compounds have been identified that structurally do not belong to the benzodiazepine group yet appear to act within the GABA$_A$–benzodiazepine–chloride ionophore complex.

The imidazopyridines bind selectively to the ω-1 motif, unlike benzodiazepines which bind non-selectively to each of the three types of ω receptor units (ω 1–3). This preferential and targeted binding is advocated as a substantive point of difference between the drug types. However, imidazopyridines can be displaced from their binding sites by the selective benzodiazepine antagonist flumazenil. At present this group is commercially represented by *zolpidem*, marketed as a hypnotic. There is some evidence that, notwithstanding zolpidem's marketed indication, this group may have more specifically targeted antianxiety actions.

The cyclopyrrolones likewise bind with high affinity to different elements of the same receptor complex and are postulated to mediate their response across the sedative/hypnotic range by producing a different pattern of allosteric modulation of chloride channels than other compounds. The only commercially available member of this group so far is *zopiclone*, also marketed as a hypnotic. Preliminary clinical evidence is that this drug (and hence probably the group) needs to be treated with the same care as standard benzodiazepines.

Much has been made of the focused mode of action of these non-benzodiazepine drugs, with the expectation that their use will not be associated with the same likelihood of physical dependency. It remains unclear however that, with long-term or unsupervised use, such optimism is justified.

An alternative approach to anxiety reduction is represented by *buspirone*, an azapirone (or azaspirodecanedione). This does not act on the GABA$_A$–benzodiazepine–chloride ionophore, though its complex actions are incompletely understood. It is a partial 5HT$_{1a}$ agonist and a relatively weak antagonist of dopamine, apparently at predominantly presynaptic sites. It is rapidly absorbed, undergoes extensive presystemic effects and has a very short half-life of only 2–4 hours. Buspirone's spectrum of action is restricted to anxiety management and it has no hypnotic, anticonvulsant or muscle relaxant properties. In a further departure from benzodiazepine pharmacology, its action is not instantaneous but requires some 10 days to become apparent and up to 3 weeks to develop fully. It should not be used to substitute for benzodiazepines or alcohol in withdrawal regimens and, in view of a pro-convulsant action, should be avoided in those at risk of fits. Its use may be associated with mild gastrointestinal upset and dizziness and, notwithstanding that its putative dopaminergic actions are on autoreceptors, it also elevates prolactin and can precipitate or exacerbate extrapyramidal disturbances. It must be avoided with traditional MAOIs. Because of its relative lack of interactions with other drugs, especially alcohol, and its apparent safety in overdose, buspirone may sometimes be useful in the management of chronic anxiety states, but its effectiveness remains a matter of debate, and it has as a rule found only limited clinical favour.

A disparate variety of other drugs are sometimes useful in the range of disorders covered by sedatives/hypnotics. The 'old standbys', *chloral hydrate* and *triclofos*, are still sometimes used in those rare situations in which hypnotics are indicated in children and can, in desperation, be tried in adults. Chloral, which added to alcohol comprised the original 'Mickey Finn', can be quite irritant to the stomach, and triclofos is in general better tolerated. The highly sedative antihistamines, such as *promethazine*, can sometimes be useful sleep inducers, but the thiamine analogue *chlormethiazole* is a potentially addictive and unpleasant compound whose use should be avoided.

Therapeutics

Indications

Indications for the use of sedatives/hypnotics must be strictly circumscribed (Box 15.11).

Strategies

The clinical use of sedatives/hypnotics, and especially benzodiazepines, is difficult, largely because it is at one level so easy. Because they are so effective and have a very high therapeutic index,

---

Box 15.11 Indications for sedatives hypnotics

Primary
- Short-term management of anxiety states, especially generalised anxiety disorder without depressive, hypochondriacal or other features
- Short-term management of panic disorder, especially without agoraphobia, the presence of which may necessitate inadvisably prolonged exposure before efficacy accrues. Nowadays, however, imipramine is often considered a preferential strategy for the drug treatment of panic states
- Short-term management of insomnia, especially when characterised by nocturnal anxiety and delayed initiation of sleep

For these indications, 'short-term' is usually defined as 2–4 weeks
- The emergency and prophylactic treatment of seizure disorders. The major value of benzodiazepines as a group is in the emergency treatment of status epilepticus, in which they are highly effective. They are also of great value in preventing seizure activity in states, such as withdrawal, where the seizure threshold is lowered. In the long-term prophylaxis of epilepsy, their ability to obstruct generalisation of a fit and to maintain an elevation of the seizure threshold tends to undergo tolerance, and they are of less value in this situation, although some, such as clonazepam which has an extremely long half-life, appear to be more effective in this regard
- Containment of psychiatric emergencies. In such situations their ease of administration, rapidity of onset and safety make them ideal for the management of severe behavioural disturbance associated with usually psychotic disorders, where they are safer than parenterally administered antipsychotics

Secondary
- It has been proposed that in high dose (e.g. diazepam up to 100 mg per day) benzodiazepines have a primary antipsychotic action (Lingjaerde 1991). The evidence for this remains unconvincing, but where these drugs may be helpful is as adjunctive treatments of acute psychotic states, particularly schizophrenia, In this situation their value may be in lessening the subjective anxious/dysphoria of 'akathisic-type' adverse effects, which have themselves been implicated in exacerbating the positive features of the illness (Owens 1999)
- In the treatment of non-extrapyramidally mediated rigidity/spasticity
- As pre-operative or inducing agents in relation to minor surgery

---

Box 15.12 Principles of sedative/hypnotic drug use

- Continuous treatment should be time-limited, as far as possible to 2–4 weeks
- An intermittent pattern of recommended use is preferable, where possible, particularly in relation to insomnia
- The risks of dependency should be explained to the patient prior to implementing treatment — but should be done in relation to the facts. One dose of temazepam on a long-haul flight is not the makings of a junky!
- Intramuscular use, as a rule, offers little advantage over the oral route in emergency situations, while application of some of the pharmacokinetic data can contribute to maximising their effects with emergency, 'stat' intravenous use

---

they appear to offer panaceas, in relation to their target disorders, which are in fact illusory. More than any other type of psychotropic agents, these drugs must be seen as part of a comprehensive package of management, with the drugs very much the junior partner. Principles of their use are summarised in Box 15.12.

While the new-generation drugs may offer some advantages, none of the compounds used for sedative/hypnotic purposes can at present be freed from the major risk of dependency.

MISCELLANEOUS DRUGS

Anticholinergics

Anticholinergics are among the most prescribed drugs in psychiatric practice yet are among the least studied. They are synthetic analogues of the belladonna alkaloids and have extensive applications in medicine in general, including cardiology, respiratory medicine and urology. These drugs act as antagonists at muscarinic cholinergic receptors. They have little action at nicotinic sites. They have been used in the treatment of Parkinson's disease since the 1920s, but have to a large extent been superseded by dopamine agonists. They are nonetheless effective in mild disorder and remain a cornerstone of the treatment of drug-related extrapyramidal disorders.

The pharmacokinetics of anticholinergics have been surprisingly little studied, and what is known has often been derived from patients with Parkinson's disease. Coincidental administration of antipsychotics has been reported to produce a kinetic interaction resulting in elevations of antipsychotic blood levels, or no effect. This may reflect different actions that attach to different combinations of drugs in each class.

Characteristics of subtypes In general, anticholinergics commonly used in psychiatry are of three main types.

Tertiary amines related to diphenhydramine. Orphenadrine combines antimuscarinic with antihistaminic properties. It has a variable therapeutic margin but can be fatal with overdoses as low as 10 times the therapeutic dose (Dutz 1992). Little is known about its pharmacokinetics, although with a reported half-life in the range 14–18 hours, it is suitable for twice daily dosing. It is doubtful if the combination of actions found in this drug offer any advantages for its indicated psychiatric use, and reports of its relative toxicity would suggest that it is best avoided.

Compounds combining atropine-like and diphenhydramine-like actions. The only widely used member of this group is benztropine, which is also the least selective, combining both atropinic and antihistaminic actions. Because of its wide spectrum of actions it is particularly likely to interact with other drugs sharing a similar broad spectrum, of which the low-potency antipsychotics are the most obvious examples. It is hard to see how such an unfocused compound could offer any clinical advantages. Furthermore, heat stroke has been described in association with benztropine use (Adams et al 1977), and it should be avoided in those living in hot climates or who have a prior history, or current suspicion, of neuroleptic malignant syndrome.

Trihexyphenidyl-related compounds. These include trihexyphenidyl itself (known in the UK as benzhexol), as well as biperiden and procyclidine. Several different types of muscarinic receptors have now been identified, of which the M_1 type is located in the CNS and is the desired target of anticholinergic drugs used to treat antipsychotic-related extrapyramidal disturbance.

Of the anticholinergics, biperiden is the most M_1 selective and benzhexol the least, with procyclidine only somewhat less selective than biperiden. The advantage of choosing a more selective drug is the lower likelihood of producing peripheral anticholinergic side-effects. A disadvantage of benzhexol is that it may be more prone to cause excitement (Dutz 1992).

Biperiden is rapidly absorbed, with a T_{max} of 1–2 hours. Its elimination half-life, in the region of 18 hours, might be compatible with once daily dosing. Procyclidine is also well absorbed but more slowly, with a T_{max} varying from 1 to 8 hours. It has a relatively short half-life ($t_{1/2}$ = 8–16 hours) suggesting that twice daily dosing is most appropriate. The routine practice of three times daily administration is probably unnecessary.

Therapeutics In general, anticholinergics should not be used in fixed-dose schedules but should be started in low doses (e.g. procyclidine 2.5 mg b.d.) and increased *flexibly* until resolution of target symptomatology (Owens 1999). Although they can sometimes produce sedation, the more usual response in low doses is excitement, and they should not be given after tea-time. Even on such schedules, they can significantly interfere with sleep (Johnstone et al 1983) though this action may undergo tolerance. They should furthermore be used *sparingly* — first, because even relatively selective drugs may produce their own pattern of side-effects, especially in combination with low potency antipsychotics; second, because they can produce an exacerbation of positive psychotic features; and third, because they are *euphorogenic* and have a well-established potential to be abused.

L-Tryptophan

L-tryptophan, an essential amino acid derived from dietary sources and the precursor of serotonin, has antidepressant properties, though it is not sufficiently efficacious to be used as first-line treatment. It has however an established adjunctive role, usually in combination with a tricyclic, in the management of treatment-resistant depression. It should be avoided in combination with an SSRI in view of the possibility of precipitating a serotonin syndrome.

In 1990, reports emerged of a serious multisystem allergic disorder called *eosinophilia myalgia syndrome* occurring in patients who had taken tryptophan from herbal sources, some of which proved fatal. No cases were reported with its medical use but, as a precaution, the purified preparation was also withdrawn. It was reintroduced in 1994, though its use remains strictly circumscribed to specialist settings. Patients and prescribers require to be registered, clozapine-like, with the Optimax Information and Clinical Support Unit (OPTICS) via the manufacturer.

Beta-noradrenergic antagonists

One of the oldest unresolved questions in psychology relates to the basis of anxiety symptoms — are they mediated by primarily central (Lange–James hypothesis) or peripheral (Cannon–Bard hypothesis) disturbances? Pharmacology has been of limited value in resolving the issue, as the most appropriate clinical tools tend to act both centrally and peripherally.

Beta-blockers, and particularly propranolol, have been widely used in psychiatry for the treatment of the somatic manifestations of anxiety though, in general, results are disappointing. Their major benefit may be in the management of symptomatology that is specifically environmentally triggered, such as performance anxiety in musicians or actors.

Propranolol was at one time advocated as an adjunctive treatment in severe or resistant schizophrenia, but this could be a risky undertaking in the high-dose regimens often advocated. It was subsequently shown that any benefits might well have resulted from a pharmacokinetic interaction of propranolol in increasing antipsychotic blood levels, and this approach has faded.

There has also been interest in propranolol as a treatment of akathisia. The greater the volume of trial literature on this topic the more sober the appraisal of efficacy, but in the low doses suggested (20–60 mg per day) propranolol is, in the absence of a history of asthma, safe and, if it is going to work, is likely to do so within a few days. This might however be seen as the first-line approach primarily in patients who develop akathisia in the absence of coincidental parkinsonism.

The $5HT_{1a}$ receptor antagonist pindolol has been advocated as an antidepressant augmentation strategy, but recent reviews highlight conflicting results (Olver et al 2000).

Drugs used in the treatment of dementia

The magnitude of the health problems presented by dementia, both now and in future, demands effective pharmacological strategies, which for many years seemed elusive. However, developments in the field of cognitive enhancement are arguably the most exciting in psychopharmacology since the last edition of this text.

Deficits in cholinergic transmission underlie the 'cholinergic hypothesis' of dementia (Bartus et al 1982), which formed the major starting point for drug development. The approach most pursued has been with compounds which inhibit the enzyme *acetylcholinesterase*, with the aim of extending the action of acetylcholine itself. The first widely studied acetylcholinesterase inhibitor was tacrine (or tetrahydroaminoacridine). Results were disappointing, especially in view of the drug's hepatotoxicity (approx. 28%), and, although licensed in the USA, tacrine remained an experimental drug in the UK.

In the last few years, several acetylcholinesterase antagonist drugs have been widely licensed. Donepezil and galantamine are reversible inhibitors of central acetylcholinesterase, with little effect on peripheral butyrylcholinesterase, while rivastigmine inhibits both enzymes. Galantamine further enhances acetylcholine synaptic activity by modulating nicotinic receptors. All are readily absorbed, rivastigmine and galantamine more rapidly so (T_{max} < 2 hours) than donepezil (T_{max} 3–5 hours). The former two compounds have low protein binding (< 40%), while binding is high for donepezil. Rivastigmine is predominantly metabolised by sulphate conjugation, whereas with donepezil and galantamine the main agents are CYP3A4 and 2D6 hepatic isoenzymes. Cholinesterase inhibitors demonstrate a non-linear relationship between dose and cholinesterase inhibition, with different drugs achieving their plateaux at different doses. Clinical improvement in cognition, functional abilities and behaviour are dose related and are suggested to result from 30–70% acetylcholinesterase inhibition (Jann et al 2002).

The introduction of acetylcholinesterase inhibitors may be the one example of the pharmaceutical industry underplaying its products. These drugs are indicated for early or mild dementia of Alzheimer's type, though empirically their use is being extended to other types of dementia, most notably arteriosclerotic. Furthermore, it seems that the initial impression of effects that were limited to a few months' duration may also be over-conservative, and benefits may be sustained for some years.

Although intuitively sound, acetylcholinesterase inhibitor strategies may be inherently limited, as the often profound decreases in the synthesis of M_1 receptor-linked phosphinositides found in the neurons of demented patients may not only reflect a reduction of M_1 receptor numbers, but point to a loss of functional competence in those which remain (Shvaloff et al 1996). A fascinating alternative strategy is inhibition of excitotoxic amino acid neurotransmitters. It has been postulated that excitatory amino acids play an important role in the pathophysiology of traumatically and degeneratively mediated brain pathologies, including dementias. Of those endogenous amino acids known to act in an excitatory transmitter role (e.g. glutamate, aspartate, homocysteine), receptors sensitive to glutamate are the best characterized. These comprise two groups: one *metabotropic*, activating the second messengers phospholipase C and adenylate cyclase (see Ch. 3); the other *ionotropic*, opening cation permeable channels mediating calcium and potassium influx. Of the latter type, *N*-methyl-D-aspartate (NMDA) receptors are the most studied. NMDA antagonism has been shown to promote a neuroprotective effect in a number of pathological states. The recently launched memantine is a voltage-dependent, uncompetitive NMDA receptor antagonist, licensed for more advanced dementia (moderate to severe) than the earlier compounds.

Other strategies involving *cholinergic agonism* with drugs such as arecoline, pilocarpine and carbachol, have been unsuccessful because of serious peripheral adverse effects, and the grandly named 'no-otropic' agents ('drugs which enhance cognitive performance'), such a piracetam, appear of little value in the context of a degenerate substrate. The uses of nerve growth factors and senile plaque inhibitors are interesting departures from conventional approaches but have yet to prove themselves. Patients with rheumatoid arthritis appear to have lower rates of Alzheimer's disease (Schneider 1996), and interest remains in the role of anti-inflammatory agents in the management of dementias. There is evidence that non-steroidal anti-inflammatories, such as indomethacin (and aspirin) might delay the onset and progression of dementia, though the relative place of such strategies, which might also include calcium channel antagonists, which increase cerebral perfusion, as well as lipid-lowering statins, remains to be determined.

From a protracted and shaky start, cognitive enhancement is now an extremely active area within psychopharmacology, with the possibility that such drugs may become 'lifestyle' agents, as well as therapies for defined illnesses.

Drugs used in the treatment of dependency states

In line with trends elsewhere in psychiatry, there is increasing interest in the use of pharmacological methods to manage disorders of dependency. The use of disulphiram is one of the more established techniques for attempting to maintain abstinence from alcohol. It is an inhibitor of hepatic aldehyde (including alcohol) dehydrogenases, resulting, with alcohol present, in the accumulation of acetaldehyde, which produces a garnut of unpleasant symptoms such as flushing, nausea, vomiting, lightheadedness and, in severe cases, collapse. Disulphiram has other complex actions that may underlie some of its effects. It can be a powerful spur to motivation but requires a deal of motivation to take in the first place. Reactions can be potentially dangerous, and patients must be advised of the need to avoid proprietary preparations containing alcohol (even over-liberal use of alcohol-based toiletries).

A different approach, which has some support from recent controlled trials, is the reduction of intake by controlling cravings for alcohol. Strategies for attempting this have included the use of the synthetic opiate antagonist naltrexone, and the GABA agonist acamprosate. Although increasingly used, such drugs only seem to exert benefits in the context of a comprehensive programme of management.

Buprenorphine, a synthetic opiate analogue, has been advocated in long-term management of opiate addiction as a safer alternative to methadone. It can be administered sublingually, which can facilitate administration and aid compliance.

DRUG INTERACTIONS

Polypharmacy is common across medical practice nowadays, including psychiatry, making drug interactions very likely. Most encountered in psychiatric practice do not, fortunately, have serious consequences, but even these may delay or obstruct the target effect or increase the likelihood of non-target effects. Some, however, can be fatal.

Interactions may be of two kinds.

- In *pharmacodynamic* interactions, a target action is magnified or diminished on the basis of the action of a second drug operating at the same target. These can produce responses that are strikingly different *qualitatively* from that of either drug alone. The *hypertensive crisis* with MAOIs is one example, where the second 'drug' can be food constituents. A further example is the serious interaction that can result from substituting fluoxetine with an MAOI or a tricyclic with serotonin reuptake inhibitory properties, such as clomipramine. The long half-life of fluoxetine, and especially norfluoxetine, results in an excess of serotonin in the synapse, which may result in a so-called *serotonin* or *serotonergic* syndrome. This is characterised by agitation, excitement, diaphoresis, hyperthermia, extrapyramidal signs especially rigidity, hyperreflexia, tachycardia, hypotension, confusion and coma. It may prove fatal. For this reason, a wash out of at least 5–6 weeks is recommended after stopping fluoxetine and prior to commencing these types of preparation.
- *Pharmacokinetic* interactions result when one drug produces an alteration, usually *quantitative*, in the target action of a second drug by altering its absorption, distribution, and especially its metabolism or elimination.

In psychiatric practice, pharmacokinetic interactions are not uncommon. The efficacy of most psychotropics correlates poorly or not at all with blood levels and the relationships with tolerability are only slightly more secure, so these have traditionally been seen as rarely producing problems of significance to routine practice. This may, however, be complacent. A more detailed understanding of the bases of such interactions may throw light on important clinical issues, such as differences in response rates and patterns of tolerability. Occasionally it may prevent potentially toxic elevations in blood levels.

The cytochrome P450 system This area has expanded dramatically following advances in understanding the cytochrome P450 system. These enzymes are of two types: *mitochondrial*, which mediate steroid synthesis; and *microsomal*, which mediate the oxidative metabolism of exogenous compounds. Although predominantly sited in the liver, P450 enzymes are widely distributed, including in gut wall and brain.

The cytochrome P (CYP) isoforms are characterised according to a genetic format, where the first number refers to the gene family, followed by the gene subfamily letter and finally the gene number itself: e.g. CYP-*2-D-6*. Over 30 CYP enzymes have been identified, with many still to be characterised (Ketter et al 1995, Ereshefsky et al 1996) but, in humans, four appear to be the most important: CYP1A2, CYP2C (comprising 2C9/10 and 2C19), CYP2D6 and CYP3A3/4. Most psychotropic drugs utilise the 2D6 system, while the importance of the CYP3A3/4 system lies in its being the most abundant, especially in intestinal mucosa. The activity of these enzymes is determined genetically, and striking interindividual differences in drug levels and tolerabilities of many psychotropic agents can to some extent be attributed to polymorphisms within these systems, especially the CYP2D6 genotype. These result from the combination of 'wild' alleles (which possess normal metabolic activity) and/or 'mutant' alleles, which may be characterised by decreased or absent metabolic capacity (Vandel 2003). The exact combination of polymorphisms in any individual determines their capacity to metabolise drugs which use that system — i.e. whether they are 'poor', 'intermediate', 'rapid' ('extensive'), or 'ultra-rapid' metabolisers — which has a bearing on dose–response relationships for both efficacy and tolerability. About 7% of Caucasians can be characterised as 'poor' (as opposed to 'extensive') metabolisers of drugs undergoing oxidative metabolism via 2D6, while the corresponding figure for Orientals is only 1% (Bertilsson 1995). On the other hand, 15–20% of Asians exhibit 2C19 polymorphisms, which are only evident in 3–5% of Caucasians.

An outline knowledge of those drugs which are metabolised by P450 enzymes and some of the commoner inhibitors and inducers can be helpful in predicting patterns of interaction that may have clinical relevance (Table 15.8). One might for example predict that fluoxetine, a potent inhibitor of the CYP2D6 isoenzyme and less so of the CYP3A3/4 group, would produce elevations in the blood levels of other psychotropics such as tricyclics, certain antipsychotics (e.g. haloperidol) and benzodiazepines such as alprazolam, which is the case. It may in addition increase carbamazepine levels. It can also be recommended that, for example, fluvoxamine, which inhibits the 3A3/4 group, should not be co-administered with alprazolam in view of the high levels of the latter that are likely to ensue. Of particular importance is the avoidance of combinations of tricyclics with potent inhibitors of CYP2D6, as tricyclics are dependent on this enzyme for their hydroxylation. It has been shown that the combination of a tricyclic (desipramine) with paroxetine or fluoxetine can result in a 3–4-fold increase in plasma desipramine levels, whereas co-administration with sertraline, a weaker inhibitor, produces only modest increases in desipramine levels.

A further non-psychiatric example is naringenin, a constituent of grapefruit juice, which inhibits the CYP3A3/4 system on which cyclosporin and a number of calcium channel antagonists, amongst others, depend for metabolism, resulting in significant elevations in blood levels and impaired tolerability. Although unidentified as being of clinical importance as yet, several similar examples pertinent to psychiatry could be postulated.

Most drugs have several potential metabolic pathways, and even now the necessary details of oxidative metabolism are still not known for the majority, so clinically it is not yet possible to apply information on the P450 system in a mathematical way. This is nonetheless an area of increasing importance.

PREGNANCY AND LACTATION

Most psychotropics can produce fetal maldevelopment when administered to pregnant laboratory animals, and the possible translation of such data to humans led at one time to considerable concern. This is reflected in the conservative recommendations usually offered by clinicians and the *British National Formulary*.

Systematic clinical evaluation of the question has however been sparse (Altshuler et al 1996). Meta-analysis of published data suggests that first-trimester exposure to low-potency phenothiazines imparts a small but significant increase in the risk of organ dysgenesis. The *additional* risk has been quantified at approximately 4 per 1000 live births. No specific increase in risk can be attributed to high-potency antipsychotics or tricyclics, and although SSRIs also appear safe, their limited use precludes definitive conclusions at present. Data from the lithium baby register have already been noted, which placed the rate of Ebstein's anomaly at 400 times that of the general population. However, more recent appraisal puts the risk at 10–20 times, which translates into an overall risk of approximately 0.1%. First-trimester exposure to carbamazepine is associated with a risk of spina bifida in the region of 0.5–1%, while the risk of this abnormality with valproate is around 2–5-fold greater. Valproate also imparts a 2% risk of hypospadias. Finally, although the data are somewhat contaminated, first-trimester exposure to benzodiazepines may be associated with a twofold increase in the risk of oral cleft abnormalities.

While these data would support caution in the use of most psychotropics during early pregnancy, they probably reflect *relative* rather than absolute risks, as the conditions for which these drugs are prescribed are themselves associated with an increased risk of fetal maldevelopment. Any drug with sedative properties should be avoided in the prenatal period, as this may complicate delivery.

The lipophilic properties of the great majority of psychotropic agents results in their being secreted in breast milk. However, the large apparent volume of distribution of such drugs means that the fraction of a maternal dose that is available for secretion in breast milk is small. The levels attained are also dependent on the lipid content of the milk sample. Thus, levels are as a rule higher in later-expressed (or hind-) milk, with its higher fat content, than in initial (or fore-milk) samples.

Formal study of the passage of maternal psychotropic drugs to breast-fed infants has also been slight, and differences in drug assay methodologies makes comparisons difficult. In view of immaturity of the liver, breast feeding by mothers receiving psychotropics should be *contraindicated* with babies born *prematurely* or who have *neonatal illness*. Otherwise the evidence to date suggests that, for mothers receiving most of the major classes of psychotropics, the decision to breast feed can, in terms of *safety*, be left to them (Yoshida & Kumar 1996).

There is a suggestion from a single case report that doxepin may cause toxicity (Matheson et al, 1985) but other tricyclics, although transferred, appear to be associated with very low or undetectable levels in infants. On the evidence to date, SSRI's also appear safe. Antipsychotics do attain measurable levels in breast fed infants and isolated reports of acute dystonic episodes and 'restlessness' with standard drugs have appeared. However, in general these too seem relatively safe. Despite its teratogenicity, there is no evidence that carbamazepine need be contraindicated post-natally (Yoshida & Kumar 1996). Care should be exercised

Table 15.8   Psychotropic drug Interactions: substrates and inhibitors for different isoforms of the cytochrome P450 system

Substrates	CYP1A2	CYP2D6	CYP2C9	CYP2C19	CYP3A3/4
Antidepressants	Tertiary amine tricyclics (*N*-demethylation)	Tertiary and secondary tricyclics (hydroxylation) Fluoxetine Paroxetine Nefazodone Venlafaxine (*O*-demethylation) m-CPP		Tertiary amine tricyclics (*N*-demethylation) Citalopram Moclobemide	Tertiary amine tricyclics (*N*-demethylation) Sertraline Nefazodone *O*-desmethylvenlafaxine
Antipsychotics	Clozapine	Haloperidol Thioridazine Perphenazine Risperidone			Clozapine
Sedative hypnotics				Diazepam (*N*-demethylation) Hexobarbital Mephobarbital S-mephenytoin	Diazepam (*N*-demethylation and hydroxylation) Alprazolam Clonazepam
Miscellaneous	Caffeine Propranolol Paracetamol Theophylline	Beta blockers Codeine Type Ic antiarrhythmics	Warfarin Phenytoin Tolbutamide	Propranolol Omeprazole	Carbamazepine Calcium channel antagonists Terfenadine Androgens/oestrogens Ethosuximide Cisipride Lidocaine Quinidine Erythromycin Cyclosporin
Inhibitors Strong ↓ ↓ ↓ ↓ Weak Inducers	Fluvoxamine	Quinidine Paroxetine Fluoxetine Norfluoxetine Sertraline Desmethylsertraline Fluvoxamine Nefazodone Venlafaxine Moclobemide Thioridazine	Fluoxetine Fluvoxamine	Ketoconazole Omeprazole Fluvoxamine	Ketoconazole Erythromycin Nefazodone Fluvoxamine Norfluoxetine Fluoxetine Sertraline Desmethylsertraline Paroxetine Venlafaxine Quinidine
	Fluoxetine Nefazodone Paroxetine Sertraline Cigarettes (?nicotine) Omeprazole	Haloperidol Perphenazine Erythromycin Ketoconazole		Fluoxetine Venlafaxine Rifampicin	Diltiazem Verapamil Dexamethasone Naringenin Carbamazepine Phenobarbital Phenytoin Rifampicin Dexamethasone

with benzodiazepines, as they may impair suckling from neonatal sedation and contribute to a 'floppy' baby.

The one possible proscription is on *lithium*, which is readily secreted and may attain plasma levels in the infant that are as high as one-third to one-half those of the mother. Because of immaturity of regulatory mechanisms, these may present a pharmacologically greater impact than comparable levels in adults, and cases of toxicity in breast-fed infants have been described. The consensus for avoiding breast feeding with lithium has been challenged (Linden & Rich, 1983) but, in the situation where a mood stabiliser is indicated, an alternative to lithium during the period of breast feeding would still seem the most prudent advice.

It is further reassuring that so far there is no evidence that exposure of the neonate to psychotropics produces any detectable early developmental delays (Altshuler et al 1996), though the question has only been systematically evaluated in relation to tricyclics (Yoshida et al 1997).

Thus, overall, the evidence is that the decision to breast feed can in most instances be left to individual mothers, without undue influence being brought to bear from psychopharmacological sources. The issue then becomes a 'gut' one — whether as a matter of principle the mother, or the clinician, has reservations about exposing the immature brain to centrally acting drugs of diverse and pervasive pharmacological actions. Placed in terms of such imponderables, it is likely most individuals would still opt for avoidance.

REFERENCES

Adams B E, Manoguerra A S, Lilja G P et al 1977 Heat stroke associated with medications having anticholinergic effects. Minnesota Medicine 60:103–106

Altshuler L L, Cohen L, Szuba M P et al 1996 Pharmacologic management of psychiatric illness during pregnancy: dilemmas and guidelines. American Journal of Psychiatry 153:592–606

Amdisen A 1977 Serum level monitoring and clinical pharmacokinetics of lithium. Clinical Pharmacokinetics 2:73–92

Amrein R, Allen S R, Guentert D et al 1989 The pharmacology of reversible monoamine oxidase inhibitors. British Journal of Psychiatry 155(suppl 6): 66–71

Anderson I M, Tomenson B M 1995 Treatment discontinuation with selective serotonin reuptake inhibitors compared with tricyclic antidepressants: a meta-analysis. British Medical Journal 310:1433–1438

Atkin K, Kendall F, Gould D et al 1996 Neutropenia and agranulocytosis in patients receiving clozapine in the UK and Ireland. British Journal of Psychiatry 169:483–488

Atkins M, Burgess A, Bottomley C et al 1997 Chlorpromazine equivalents: a consensus of opinion for both clinical and research applications. Psychiatric Bulletin 21:224–226

Baldessarini R J 1985 Chemotherapy in Psychiatry. Harvard University Press, Cambridge, Mass

Baldessarini R J, Katz B, Cotton P 1984 Dissimilar dosing with high-potency and low-potency neuroleptics. American Journal of Psychiatry 141:748–752

Baldessarini R J, Frankenburg F R 1991 Clozapine: a novel antipsychotic agent. New England Journal of Medicine 324:746–754

Bartus R T, Dean R L, Beer B et al 1982 The cholinergic hypothesis of geriatric memory dysfunction. Science 217:408–417

Baumhackl U, Biziere K, Fischbach F et al 1989 Efficacy and tolerability of moclobemide compared with imipramine in depressive disorder. British Journal of Psychiatry 155(suppl 6): 78–83

Beaumont G, Baldwin D, Lader M 1996 A criticism of the practice of prescribing subtherapeutic doses of antidepressants for the treatment of depression. Human Psychopharmacology 11:283–291

Bertilsson L 1995 Geographical/interracial differences in polymorphic drug oxidation. Clinical Pharmacokinetics 29:192–209

Blackwell B 1963 Hypertensive crisis due to monoamine oxidase inhibitors. Lancet ii: 849–851

Blackwell B, Simon J S 1988 Antidepressant drugs. In: Dukes M N G (ed) Meyler's side effects of drugs, 11th edn. Elsevier, Amsterdam, p 27–69

Boston Collaborative Drug Surveillance Program 1972 Adverse reactions to the tricyclic-antidepressant drugs. Lancet i: 529–531

Boyer W F, Feighner J P 1991 Pharmacokinetics and drug interactions. In: Feighner J P, Boyer W F (eds) Selective serotonin reuptake inhibitors. Wiley, Chichester, p 81–88

Boyer W F, Feighner J P 1996 Safety and tolerability of selective serotonin re-uptake inhibitors. In: Feighner J P, Boyer W F (eds) Selective serotonin re-uptake inhibitors, 2nd edn. Wiley, Chichester, p 291–314

British Isles Raclopride Study Group 1992 A double blind comparison of raclopride and haloperidol in the acute phase of schizophrenia. Acta Psychiatrica Scandinavica 86:391–398

Brodie M J 1987 Carbamazepine: pharmacokinetics and interactions. International Clinical Psychopharmacology 2(suppl 1): 73–81

Canoso R T, de Oliveira R M, Nixon R A 1990 Neuroleptic-associated autoantibodies: a prevalence study. Biological Psychiatry 27:863–870

Carpenter W T, Heindrichs D W, Alphs L D 1985 Treatment of negative symptoms. Schizophrenia Bulletin 11:440–452

Cassidy S, Henry J 1987 Fatal toxicity of antidepressant drugs in overdose. British Medical Journal 295:1021–1024

Cold J A, Wells B G, Froemming J H 1990 Seizure activity associated with antipsychotic therapy. DICP, Annals of Pharmacotherapy 24:601–606

Cole J O, Bodkin A 1990 Antidepressant drug side effects. Journal of Clinical Psychiatry 51 (suppl 1): 21–26

Cooper T B 1987 Pharmacokinetics of lithium. In: Meltzer H Y (ed) Psychopharmacology: the third generation of progress. Raven, New York, pp 1365–1375

Coulter D L 1991 Carnitine, valproate and toxicity. Journal of Child Neurology 6:7–14

Coupland N, Wilson S, Nutt D 1997 Antidepressant drugs and the cardiovascular system: a comparison of tricyclics and selective serotonin reuptake inhibitors and their relevance for the treatment of psychiatric patients with cardiovascular problems. Journal of Psychopharmacology 11:83–92

Curry S H 1986 Applied clinical pharmacology of schizophrenia. In: Bradley P B, Hirsch S R (ed) The psychopharmacology and treatment of schizophrenia. Oxford University Press, Oxford, p 103–131

Curzon M E J 1987 Teeth. In: Johnson F N (ed) Depression and mania — modern lithium therapy. IRL Press, Oxford, p 203–206

Dahl S G, Strandjord R E 1977 Pharmacokinetics of chlorpromazine after single and chronic dosage. Clinical Pharmacology and Therapeutics 21:437–448

Davis J M, Metalon L, Watanabe M D et al 1994 Depot anitpsychotic drugs: place in therapy. Drugs 741–773

Deng M Z, Chen G C, Phillips M R 1990 Neuroleptic malignant syndrome in 12 of 9,792 Chinese inpatients exposed to neuroleptics: a prospective study. American Journal of Psychiatry 147:1149–1155

Diamond J M, Ehrlich B E, Morawski S G et al 1983 Lithium absorption in tight and leaky segments of intestine. Journal of Membrane Biology 72:159–183

Dilsaver S C, Greden J F, Snider R M 1987 Antidepressant withdrawal syndromes: phenomenology and physiopathology. International Clinical Psychopharmacology 2:1–19

Dostert P, Benedetti M S, Poggesi I 1997 Review of the pharmacokinetics and metabolism of reboxetine, a selective noradrenaline reuptake inhibitor. European Neuropsychopharmacology 7(suppl 1): s23–s35

Dubovsky S L 1993 Calcium antagonists in manic-depressive illness. Neuropsychobiology 27:184–192

Dutz W. 1992 Drugs affecting autonomic functions or the extrapyramidal system. In: Duker M N G (ed) Meyler's side effects of drugs, 12th edn. Elsevier, Amsterdam, p 307–334

Edwards J G 1986 The untoward effects of antipsychotic drugs: pathogenesis and management. In: Bradley P B, Hirsch S R (ed) The psychopharmacology and treatment of schizophrenia. Oxford University Press, Oxford, p 403–441

Ereshefsky L, Lacombe S 1993 Pharmacological profile of risperidone. Canadian Journal of Psychiatry 38(suppl 3): s80–s88

Ereshefsky L, Saklad S R, Jann M W et al 1983 Pharmacokinetics of fluphenazine by high performance thin layer chromatography. Drug Intelligence and Clinical Pharmacy 17:436–437

Ereshefsky L, Riesenman C, Lam Y W F 1996 Serotonin selective reuptake inhibitor drug interactions and the cytochrome P450 system. Journal of Clinical Psychiatry 57(suppl 8): 17–25

Faedda G L, Tondo L, Baldessarini R J et al 1993 Outcome after rapid vs gradual discontinuation of lithium treatment in bipolar disorders. Archives of General Psychiatry 50:448–455

Farde L, Nordstrom A-L, Wiesel F-A et al 1992 Positron emission tomographic analysis of central D1 and D2 dopamine receptor occupancy in patients treated with classical neuroleptics and clozapine. Archives of General Psychiatry 49:538–544

Fernstrom M H, Kupfer D J 1988 Antidepressant-induced weight gain: a comparison study of four medications. Psychiatry Research 26:265–271

Frazer A 1997 Antidepressants. Journal of Clinical Psychiatry 58(suppl 6): 9–25

Glassman A H, Biggar J T 1981 Cardiovascular effects of therapeutic doses of tricyclic antidepressants. Archives of General Psychiatry 38:815–820

Glassman A H, Biggar J T, Giardina E V et al 1979 Clinical characteristics of imipramine-induced orthostatic hypotension. Lancet i: 468–472

Gomolin I H 1987 Coping with excessive doses. In: Johnson F N (ed) Depression and mania — modern lithium therapy. IRL Press, Oxford, p 154–157

Goodnick P J 1991 Pharmacokinetics of second generation antide-pressants: fluoxetine. Psychopharmacology Bulletin 27:503–512

Goodnick P J, Schorr-Cain C B 1991 Lithium pharmacokinetics. Psychopharmacology Bulletin 27:475–491

Goodnick P J, Fieve R R, Meltzer H L 1981 Lithium elimination and duration of therapy. Clinical Pharmacology and Therapeutics 29:47–50

Goodwin G M 1996 How do antidepressants affect serotonin receptors? The role of serotonin receptors in the therapeutic and side effect profile of the SSRIs. Journal of Clinical Psychiatry 57(suppl 4): 9–13

Gould G M, Murphy K M M, Reynolds I J et al 1983 Antischizophrenic drugs of the diphenylbutylpiperidine type act as calcium channels antagonists. Proceedings of the National Academy of Sciences of the USA 80:5122–5125

Gould R J, Murphy K M M, Reynolds I J et al 1984 Calcium channel blockade: possible explanation for thioridazine's peripheral side effects. American Journal of Psychiatry 141:352–357

Greenblatt D J 1993 Basic pharmacokinetic principles and their application to psychotropic drugs. Journal of Clinical Psychiatry 54(suppl 9): 8–13

Greenblatt D J, Shader R I 1987 Pharmacokinetics of antianxiety agents. In: Meltzer H Y (ed) Psychopharmacology: the third generation of progress. Raven, New York, p 1377–1386

Haddad P 1997 Newer antidepressants and the discontinuation syndrome. Journal of Clinical Psychiatry 58(suppl 7): 17–22

Halle M T, Dilsaver S C 1993 Tranylcypromine withdrawal phenomena. Journal of Psychiatry and Neuroscience 18:49–50

Hamann G L, Egan T M, Wells B G et al 1990 Injection site reactions after intramuscular administration of haloperidol decanoate 100 mg/mL. Journal of Clinical Psychiatry 51:502–504

Haupt D W, Newcomer J W 2001 Hyperglycaemia and antipsychotic medications. Journal of Clinical Psychiatry 62(suppl 27): 15–26

Henry J A 1996 Suicide risk and antidepressant treatment. Journal of Psychopharmacology 10(suppl 1): 39–40

Hestbech J, Hansen H E, Amdisen A et al 1977 Chronic renal lesions following long-term treatment with lithium. Kidney International 12:205–213

Hetmar O, Juul Povlsen U, Ladefoged J et al 1991 Lithium: long-term effects on the kidney. A prospective follow-up study ten years after kidney biopsy. British Journal of Psychiatry 158:53–58

Higgitt A C, Lader M H, Fonaghy P 1985 Clinical management of benzodiazepine dependence. British Medical Journal 291:688–690

Hindmarch I 1980 Psychomotor function and psychoactive drugs. British Journal of Clinical Pharmacology 10:189–210

Holden J M C and Holden U P 1979 Weight changes with schizophrenic psychosis and psychotropic drug therapy. Psychosomatics 11:551–651

Hotopf M, Lewis G, Norman C 1996 Are SSRIs a cost-effective alternative to tricyclics? British Journal of Psychiatry 168:404–409

Hotopf M, Hardy R, Lewis G 1997 Discontinuation rates of SSRIs and tricyclic antidepressants: a meta-analysis and investigation of heterogeneity. British Journal of Psychiatry 170:120–127

Ingram I M, Timbury G C 1960 Side effects of Librium. Lancet, ii: 766

Isaac N E, Walker A M, Jick H et al 1991 Exposure to phenothiazine drugs and risk of cataract. Archives of Ophthalmology 109:256–260

Isojarvi J I T, Laatikainen T J, Pakarinen A J et al 1993 Polycystic ovaries and hyperandrogenism in women taking valproate for epilepsy. New England Journal of Medicine 329:1383–1388

Isojarvi J I T, Laatikainen T J, Knip M et al 1996 Obesity and endocrine disorders in women taking valproate for epilepsy. Annals of Neurology 39:579–584

Jacobsen F M 1992 Fluoxetine-induced sexual dysfunction and an open trial of yohimbine. Journal of Clinical Psychiatry 53:199–122

Jann M W, Ereshefsky L, Saklad S R 1985 Clinical pharmacokinetics of the depot antipsychotics. Clinical Pharmacokinetics 10:315–333

Jann M W, Shirley K L, Small G W 2002 Clinical pharmacokinetics and pharmacodynamics of cholinesterase inhibitors Clinical Pharmacokinetics 41:719–739

Jarvis M R 1991 Clinical pharmacokinetics of tricyclic antidepressants overdose. Psychopharmacology Bulletin 27:541–550

Jefferson J W 1989 Cardiovascular effects and toxicity of anxiolytics and antidepressants. Journal of Clinical Psychiatry 50:368–378

Jennings A E, Levey A S, Harrington J T 1983 Amoxapine-associated acute renal failure. Archives of Internal Medicine 143:1525–1527

Jerram T C, McDonald R 1978 Plasma lithium control with particular reference to minimum effective levels. In: (Johnson F N, Johnson

S (eds) Lithium in medical practice. MTP Press, Lancaster, p 407–413

Johnstone E C, Crow T J, Ferrier I N et al 1983 Adverse effects of anticholinergic medication on positive symptoms. Psychological Medicine 13:513–527

Jorgensen A 1986 Metabolism and pharmacokinetics of antipsychotic drugs. In: Bridges J W, Chasseaud L F (ed) Progress in drug metabolism. Taylor & Francis, London, p 111–174

Judd L L, Hubbard B, Janowsky D S et al 1977a The effect of lithium carbonate on affect, mood, and personality of normal subjects. Archives of General Psychiatry 34:346–351

Judd L L, Hubbard B, Janowsky D S et al 1977b The effect of lithium carbonate on the cognitive functions of normal subjects. Archives of General Psychiatry 34:355–357

Jusic N, Lader M H 1994 Post-mortem antipsychotic drug concentrations and unexplained deaths. British Journal of Psychiatry 165:787–791

Kane J M 1987 Treatment of schizophrenia. Schizophrenia Bulletin 13:133–156

Kane J M, Honigfeld G, Singer J et al 1988 Clozapine for the treatment-resistant schizophrenic: a double-blind comparison with chlorpromazine. Archives of General Psychiatry 45:789–796

Kaplan S A, Jack M L 1983 Metabolism of the benzodiazepines: pharmacokinetic and pharmacodynamic considerations. In: Costa E (ed) The benzodiazepines: from molecular biology to clinical practice. Raven, New York, p 173–199

Ketter T A, Flockhart D A, Post R M et al 1995 The emerging role of cytochrome P450 3A in psychopharmacology. Journal of Clinical Psychopharmacology 15:387–398

Kilian J G, Kerr K, Lawrence C et al 1999 Myocarditis and cardiomyopathy associated with clozapine, Lancet 354:1841–1845

Kincaid-Smith P, Burrows G D, Davies B M et al 1979 Renal biopsy findings in lithium and prelithium patients. Lancet ii: 7001–7002

King D J (1992) Benzodiazepines, amnesia and sedation: theoretical and clinical issues and controversies. Human Psychopharmacology 7:79–87

Kinon B J, Lieberman J A 1996 Mechanism of action of atypical antipsychotic drugs: a critical analysis. Psychopharmacologica 124:2–34

Knudsen K, Heath A 1984 Effects of self-poinsoning with maprotiline. British Medical Journal 288:601–603

Kopera H 1980 Cardiac effects of mianserin: results of clinical pharmacological investigations. Current Medical Research and Opinion 6(suppl 7): 36–43

Kubota T, Ishikura T, Jubiki I 1994 Alopecia areata associated with haloperidol. Japanese Journal of Psychiatry and Neurology 48:579–581

Kupfer D J, Carpenter L L, Frank E 1988 Possible role of antidepressants in precipitating mania and hypomania in recurrent depression. American Journal of Psychiatry 145:804–808

Lam F, Y W, Ereshefsky L, Toney G B et al 2001 Branded versus generic clozapine: bioavailability comparison and interchangeability issues. Journal of Clinical Psychiatry 62(suppl 5): 18–22

Lambert D, Dalac S 1987 Skin, hair and nails. In: Johnson F N (ed) Depression and mania — modern lithium therapy. IRL Press, Oxford, p 232–234

Lane R M 1997 A critical review of selective serotonin reuptake inhibitor-related sexual dysfunction: incidence, possible aetiology and implications for management. Journal of Psychopharmacology 11:72–82

Lejoyeux M, Ades J 1997 Antidepressant discontinuation: a review of the literature. Journal of Clinical Psychiatry 58(suppl 7): 11–16

Levinson D F, Simpson G M 1986 Neuroleptic-induced extrapyramidal symptoms with fever: heterogeneity of the 'neuroleptic malignant syndrome'. Archives of General Psychiatry 43:839–848

Levinson D F, Simpson G M 1987 Serious nonextrapyramidal adverse effects of neuroleptics: sudden death, agranulocutosis and hepatotoxicity. In: Meltzer H Y (ed) Psychopharmacology: the third generation of progress Raven, New York, p 1431–1436

Lieberman J A 1993 Understanding the mechanism of action of atypical antipsychotic drugs: a review of compounds in use and development. British Journal of Psychiatry 163(suppl 22): 7–22

Lieberman J A, Safferman A Z, Pollack S et al 1994 Clinical effects of clozapine in chronic schizophrenia: response to treatment and predictors of outcome. American Journal of Psychiatry 151:1744–1752

Linden S, Rich C L 1983 The use of lithium during pregnancy and lactation. Clinical Psychiatry 44:358–361

Lingjaerde O 1991 Benzodiazepines in the treatment of schizophrenia: an updated survey. Acta Psychiatrica Scandinavica 84:453–459

Lipscomb P A 1980 Cardiovascular side effects of phenothiazines and tricyclic antidepressants: a review with precautionary measures. Postgraduate Medicine 67:189–196

Lucas V S 1993 Association of psychotropic drugs, prevalence of denture-related stomatitis and oral candidiasis. Community Dentistry and Oral Epidemiology 21:313–316

McCreadie R G, Dingwall J M, Wiles D H et al 1980 Intermittent pimozide versus fluphenazine decanoate as maintenance therapy in chronic schizophrenia. British Journal of Psychiatry 137:510–517

McQuay H J, Tramer M, Nye B A et al 1996 A systematic review of antidepressants in neuropathic pain. Pain 68:217–227

Malik K 1996 Nefazodone: structure, mode of action and pharmacokinetics. Journal of Psychopharmacology 10(suppl 1): 1–4

Mallinger A G, Smith E 1991 Pharmacokinetics of monoamine oxidase inhibitors. Psychopharmacology Bulletin 27:493–502

Manji H, Hsiao J K, Risby E D et al 1991 The mechanism of action of lithium, I: Effects on serotonergic and noradrenergic systems in normal subjects. Archives of General Psychiatry 48:505–512

Manji H, Potter W Z, Lenox R H 1995 Signal transduction pathways: molecular targets for lithium's actions. Archives of General Psychiatry 52:531–543

Marmor M F 1990 Is thioridazine retinopathy progressive? Relationship of pigmentary changes to visual function. British Journal of Ophthalmology 74:739–742

Martin C A, Dickson L R, Kuo C S 1987 Heart and blood vessels. In: Johnson F N (ed) Depression and mania — modern lithium therapy. IRL Press, Oxford, p 213–218

Matheson I, Pande H, Alertsen A P 1985 Respiratory depression caused by N-desmethyldoxepin in breast milk. Lancet 16:1124

Mehtonen O-P, Aranko K, Malkonen L et al 1991 A survey of sudden death associated with the use of antipsychotic or antidepressant drugs: 49 cases in Finland. Acta Psychiatrica Scandinavica 84:58–64

Meltzer H Y, Fang V S 1976 The effects of neuroleptics on serum prolactin in schizophrenic patients. Archives of General Psychiatry 33:279–284

Metzger E, Friedman R 1993 Prolougation of the corrected QT and torsades de pointes cardiac arrhythmia associated with intravenous haloperidol in the medically ill. Journal of Clinical Psychopharmacology 13:128–132

Moller H J 1993 Neuroleptic treatment of negative symptoms in schizophrenic patients: efficacy, problems and methodological difficulties. European Neuropsychopharmacology 3:1–11

Moncrieff J 1997 Lithium: evidence reconsidered. British Journal of Psychiatry 171:113–119

Montgomery S A, Baldwin D, Green M 1989 Why do amitriptyline and dothiepin appear to be so dangerous in overdose? Acta Psychiatrica Scandinavica 80(suppl 354): 47–53

Montgomery S A, Henry J, McDonald G et al (1994) Selective serotonin reuptake inhibitors: meta-analysis of discontinuation rates. International Clinical Psychopharmacology 9:47–53

Moschitto L J, Greenblatt D J 1983 Concentration-independent plasma protein binding of benzodiazepines. Journal of Pharmacy and Pharmacology 35:179–180

Myers D H, West T E T 1987 Hormone systems. In: Johnson F N (ed) Depression and mania — modern lithium therapy. IRL Press, Oxford, p 220–226

NICE 2002 Guidance of the use of newer (atypical) antipsychotic drugs for the treatment of schizophrenia: Technology appraisal guidance, No 43. National Institute for Clinical Excellence, London

Olver J S, Cryan J F, Burrows G D et al 2000 Pindolol angmentation of antidepressants: a review and rationale. Australian and New Zealand Journal of Psychiatry 34:71–79

Oosthuizen P, Emsley R A, Turner J et al 2001 Determining the optimal dose of haloperidol in first-episode psychosis. Journal of Psychopharmacology 15:251–255

Oswald I, Priest R G 1965 Five weeks to escape the sleeping pill habit. British Medical Journal ii: 1093–1095

Owens D G C (1996) Adverse effects of antipsychotic agents: do newer agents offer advantages? Drugs 51:895–930

Owens D G C 1999 A guide to the extrapyramidal side effects of antipsychotic drugs. Cambridge University Press, Cambridge

Perry P J 1996 Pharmacotherapy for major depression with melancholic features: relative efficacy of tricyclics versus selective serotonin reuptake inhibitor antidepressants. Journal of Affective Disorders 39:1–6

Perry P J, Alexander B 1987 Dosage and serum levels. In: Johnson F N (ed) Depression and mania — modern lithium therapy. IRL Press, Oxford, p 67–73

Petursson H, Lader M H 1981 Withdrawal from long term benzodiazepine treatment. British Medical Journal 283:643–645

Pisciotta V 1978 Drug-induced agranulcytosis. Drugs 15:132–143

Poust R I 1987 Kinetics and tissue distribution. In: Johnson F N (ed) Depression and mania — modern lithium therapy. IRL Press, Oxford, p 73–75

Power K G, Jerrom D W A, Simpsom R J et al 1985 Controlled study of withdrawal symptoms and rebound anxiety after six week course of diazepam for generalised anxiety. British Medical Journal 290:1246–1248

Preskorn S H 1993a Introduction — Pharmacokinetics of psychotropic agents: why and how they are relevant to treatment. Journal of Clinical Psychiatry 54(suppl 9): 3–7

Preskorn S H 1993b Pharmacokinetics of antidepressants: why and how they are relevant to treatment. Journal of Clinical Psychiatry 54(suppl 9): 14–34

Quitkin F M, Stewart J W, McGrath P J et al 1993 Columbia atypical depression. British Journal of Psychiatry 163(suppl 21): 30–34

Rabkin J G, Quitkin F M, McGrath P et al 1985 Adverse reactions to monoamine oxidase inhibitors, II: Treatment correlates and clinical management. Journal of Clinical Psychopharmacology 5:2–9

Ray W A, Griffin M R, Schaffner W et al 1987 Psychotropic drug use and the risk of hip fracture. New England Journal of Medicine 316:333–339

Ray W A, Meredith S, Thapa P B et al 2001 Antipsychotics and the risk of sudden cardiac death. Archives of General Psychiatry 58:1161–1167

Regal R E, Billi J E, Glazer H M 1987 Phenothiazine-induced cholestatic jaundice. Clinical Pharmacy 6:787–794

Reilly J G, Ayis S A, Ferrier I N et al 2000 QTc-interval abnormalities and psychotropic drug therapy in psychiatric patients. Lancet 355:1048–1052

Richelson E 1996 Synaptic effects of antidepressants. Journal of Clinical Psychopharmacology 16(suppl 2): 1s–9s

Richens A 1983 Clinical pharmacokinetics of benzodiazepines. In: Trimble M R (ed) Benzodiazepines divided. Wiley, Chichester, p 187–205

Roose S P, Glassman A H, Giardina E G V et al 1987 Tricyclic antidepressants in depressed patients with cardiac conduction disease. Archives of General Psychiatry 44:273–275

Rosebush P I, Mazurek M F 1999 Neurologic side-effects in neuroleptic-naïve patients treated with haloperidol or risperidone. Neurology 52:782–785

Roy T M, Ossorio M A, Cipolla L M et al 1989 Pulmonary complications after tricyclic antidepressant overdose. Chest 96:852–856

Rudorfer M V 1992 Monoamine oxidase inhibitors: reversible and irreversible. Psychopharmacology Bulletin 28:45–57

Rudorfer M V, Potter W Z 1987 Pharmacokinetics of antidepressants. In: Meltzer H Y (ed) Psychopharmacology — the third generation of progress. Raven, New York, p 1353–1363

Schneider L S 1996 New therapeutic approaches to Alzheimer's Disease. Journal of Clinical Psychiatry 57(suppl 14): 30–36

Schou M, Baastrup P C, Grof P et al 1970 Pharmacological and clinical problems of lithium prophylaxis. British Journal of Psychiatry 116:615–619

Shalev A, Hermesh H, Munitz H 1989 Mortality from neuroleptic malignant syndrome. Journal of Clinical Psychiatry 50:18–25

Shelley R, Silverstone T 1987 Lithium preparations. In: Johnson F N (ed) Depression and mania — modern lithium therapy. IRL Press, Oxford, p 94–98

Shvaloff A, Neuman E, Guez D 1996 Lines of therapeutic research in Alzheimer's Disease. Psychopharmacology Bulletin 32:343–352

Silverstone T, Smith G, Goodall E 1988 Prevalence of obesity in patients receiving depot antipsychotics. British Journal of Psychiatry 153:214–217

Skowron D M, Stimmel G L 1992 Antidepressants and the risk of seizures. Pharmacotherapy 12:18–22

Smith S M, O'Keane V, Murray R 2002 Sexual dysfunction in patients taking conventional antipsychotic medication. British Journal of Psychiatry 181:49–55

Smith W M, Gallagher J J 1980 "Les torsade de pointes" — an unusual ventricular arrhythmia. Annals of Internal Medicine 93:578–584

Sternbach L H 1983 The discovery of CNS active 1,4-benzodiazepines. In: Costa E (ed) The benzodiazepines: from molecular biology to clinical practice. Raven, New York, p 1–6

Thomsen K, Schou M 1975 The treatment of lithium poisoning. In: Johnson F N (ed) Lithium research and therapy. Academic Press, London, p 227–236

Tyrer P, Rutherford D, Huggett T 1981 Benzodiazepine withdrawal symptoms and propranolol. Lancet i: 520–522

Vacaflor L 1975 Lithium side effects and toxicity: the clinical picture. In: Johnson F N (ed) Lithium research and therapy. Academic Press, London, pp 211–225

Vandel P 2003 Antidepressant drugs in the elderly: role of cytochrome P450 2D6. World Journal of Biological Psychiatry 4:74–80

Walker R G, Kincaid-Smith P 1987 Kidneys and the fluid regulatory system. In: Johnson F N (ed) Depression and mania — modern lithium therapy. IRL Press, Oxford, pp 206–213

Warner M D, Peabody C A, Whiteford H A et al 1987 Trazodone and priapism. Journal of Clinical Psychiatry 48:244–245

Warnock J K 1991 Psychotropic medication and drug-related alopecia. Psychosomatics 32:149–152

Weekly R D, Potts A M, Reboton J et al 1960 Pigmentary retinopathy in patients receiving high doses of a new phenothiazine. Archives of Ophthalmology 64:95–106

Weinstein M R 1980 Lithium treatment of women during pregnancy and in the post-delivery period. In: Johnson F N (ed) Handbook of lithium therapy. MTP Press, Lancaster, p 421–429

Wilder B J 1992 Pharmacokinetics of valproate and carbamazepine. Journal of Clinical Psychopharmacology 12(suppl 1): 64s–68s

Wilt J L, Minnema A M, Johnson R F et al. 1993 Torsade de pointes associated with the use of intravenous haloperidol. Annals of Internal Medicine 119:391–394

Yoshida K, Kumar R 1996 Breast feeding and psychotropic drugs. International Review of Psychiatry 8:117–124

Yoshida K, Smith B, Craggs M et al 1997 Investigation of pharmacokinetics and of possible adverse effects in infants exposed to tricyclic antidepressants in breast-milk. Journal of Affective Disorders 43:225–237

Young R C 1991 Hydroxylated metabolites of antidepressants. Psychopharmacology Bulletin 27:521–531

Zornberg G L, Jick H 2000 Antipsychotic drug use and risk of first time idiopathic venous thromboembolism: a case-control study. Lancet 356:1219–1223

Zucker S, Zarrabi H M, Schubach W H et al 1990 Chlorpromazine-induced immunopathy: progressive increase in serum IgM. Medicine 69:92–100

16 | Psychological therapies

Chris Freeman, Else Guthrie

INTRODUCTION

Psychotherapies are 'talking' cures. Symptom relief is provided via the medium of a personal relationship, within the context of professional service or contract. Psychotherapy is not new and has been practised in some form or other for thousands of years. Every culture has devised ways of providing support, guidance and consolation for individuals at times of great stress. Often this has occurred via religious agencies, but in Western, secular society, it is increasingly being regarded as the state's role to protect the 'souls' of its people. Hence, following major disasters, or the disappearance of a child, it is expected that counsellors will automatically be supplied to comfort and help the stressed, shocked or bereaved. As Western cultures have become more technological and 'rational', psychological modes of healing have become more formalised and 'scientific'. Individuals have come to rely less on family and other social support systems, and much more upon formal organisations and healthcare.

All psychotherapies consist of two elements: professional service and personal attachment. There is a formal contractual arrangement between therapist and client, with the delivery of specific psychological technology and expertise. This takes place in the context of personal relationship, in which a bond develops between the two (or more) individuals engaged in the process.

The contribution of psychological therapies to the treatment of people suffering from mental illness is being increasingly recognised. In 1996, the Department of Health produced a strategic review of policy in relation to psychotherapy services in England. The importance of delivering evidence-based psychotherapies, to those individuals most in need of treatment, has been emphasised in the National Service Framework for Mental Health (for England) (Department of Health 2000). The government has also highlighted the importance of treatment choice in relation to psychological treatments and counselling (Department of Health 2001).

Common factors

Although, there are many different types of therapies and diverse approaches to the relief of psychological suffering, all psychotherapies have key common ingredients. These can be divided into three categories: support factors, learning factors and action factors (Lambert & Bergin 1994). Examples are listed in Box 16.1. The supportive factors include important aspects of therapy such as reassurance, and warmth and empathy from the therapist. Another supportive factor, the therapeutic alliance, has been

found consistently to correlate positively with therapeutic outcome (Horvath & Luborsky 1993, Gaston et al 1998, Martin et al 2000). In short-term therapy a strong early alliance has been found to be particularly important (Horvath & Symonds 1991). The therapeutic alliance has been conceptualised in a variety of different ways but includes the following:

- the ability of the patient to work purposefully in therapy;
- the capacity of the patient and therapist to form a strong affective bond between them;
- the therapist's skill at providing empathic understanding;
- an agreement between the client and therapist about goals and tasks;
- the ability of the therapist to identify and repair ruptures to the alliance.

Learning factors include giving advice, gaining insight, and the assimilation of problematic experiences. Action factors include modelling, testing of solutions, and mastery.

Types of psychotherapy

There are many different types of psychotherapy, but most can be grouped into four main categories: cognitive-behavioural therapies, psychodynamic–relational therapies, experiential–expressive therapies, and systemic therapies (Box 16.2). Cognitive-behavioural therapies have a shared emphasis upon the identification of maladaptive practices or thoughts produced by faulty learning or reasoning, and the correction of such problems in the context of a collaborative relationship. Modern psychodynamic therapies, which have been heavily influenced by interpersonal theory (Sullivan 1953) and object relations theory (Greenberg & Mitchell 1983) focus upon the correction of deeply ingrained and insecure patterns of attachment, or problematic ways of relating to others. The patient–therapist relationship is recognised as a powerful medium through which problematic patterns of relating can be elucidated and modified. Experiential–expressive therapies aim to restore well-being through the self-expression of distress. A supportive and safe framework is provided for the individual(s), within which to identify and find solutions to problems. Systemic therapies share a common approach in viewing an individual's behaviour as the product of a system. Emphasis is placed upon changing or altering the system rather than the individual.

The distinction between different therapeutic approaches is becoming gradually more blurred, and there is greater integration between different therapeutic approaches. Some therapies such as interpersonal therapy (Klerman & Weissman 1993) share elements of both cognitive-behavioural and relational approaches. Cognitive-analytic therapy (Ryle 1990) is another example of an integrative therapy which combines cognitive techniques within a framework of dynamic understanding. Psychodynamic–interpersonal therapy (Hobson 1985) combines elements of dynamic therapy, relational and experiential–expressive approaches. Key therapies, with either a strong evidence base, or a large practice base in the UK, will now be discussed.

PSYCHODYNAMIC THERAPY

Psychodynamic therapies developed from the work of Freud in the late 19th and early 20th century. Early theory (i.e. pre-1950s) focused upon the salience of motivational forces or innate drives (e.g. sexual drive or libido) of which individuals are unaware or partially unaware. Such drives resulted in unacceptable wishes or impulses which were kept out of conscious awareness, but resulted in the development of symptoms (either physical or emotional). Treatment was aimed at providing patients with awareness of (or insight into) these unacceptable wishes or conflicts, which could then be modified or resolved. Other key aspects of Freudian theory are summarised in Table 16.1. Many of Freud's original theories have been revised over the years. For example, in relation to development, other theorists such as Erikson (1950) and Mahler have focused on more social and interpersonal aspects of development, and extended the developmental period to include late life.

In the 1950s greater emphasis was placed on the role of attachment and on the important influence of early carer–infant/child relationships upon the stability and quality of relationships with significant others in adult life. This move, from a focus on the individual's internal conflicts, to an emphasis on the interactions he has with others, is represented by the development of object relations theory (Kernberg 1980). Writers such as Fairburn (1954) and Guntrip (1969) suggested that the primary innate drive in

hu-mans is to form a strong bond with a good object (i.e. person). This process begins during (some may argue even before) infancy and is characterised by complex two-way interactions between carer and infant. A stable, supportive, reciprocal relationship between carer and infant is regarded as the essential cornerstone for both emotional and cognitive development. Gradual separation of child from carer, with the eventual development of independent functioning by the child, is seen as a key developmental process. Disruption to the carer–infant relationship can occur at any stage, but early disruption produces long-term maladaptive patterns of behaviour in relation to others. Positive caring relationships are perceived as producing 'good objects' within people, whereas negative or abusive early relationships result in 'bad objects'. Objects are metaphors for the internalisation of emotional experiences. A preponderance of good over bad objects results in the individual being able to tolerate uncertainty, trust others and engage in warm and meaningful reciprocal relationships. A preponderance of bad objects over good objects produces difficulties in being able to care for and trust others, or tolerate disappointment. Thus, relationships are brittle and stormy. Object relations theory has much in common with the later ideas of schema-focused cognitive therapy, although initially the two approaches may seem very different.

Transference

Transference in its most basic form is the projection onto an individual of feelings and assumptions, which are derived from a previous important relationship (usually childhood). The feelings are experienced as real and there is no insight about their true derivation. A somewhat concrete, but real example of this involves a woman who was tortured and abused by her father when she was a child. He was a small man who wore round rimless glasses. As an adult, she regarded all men who wore such glasses as potential abusers. She described a hatred for her tutor at college, who she felt picked on her unfairly and humiliated her in class. This was not a view shared by her friends. It was only later on in therapy that she realised that, although her tutor did not wear glasses, he had certain facial characteristics which resembled those of her father. She realised that her perception of him had been clouded by her previous traumatic experiences.

Freud originally conceptualised transference as only occurring within psychotherapy, so that patients who had experienced such feelings as love, anger or a profound sense of gratitude towards their therapist may be expressing feelings which originated from relationships in early childhood, particularly with their parents. Freud broadened his view to accept that transference reactions occur throughout ordinary life and are part of most, if not all,

---

Box 16.1 Common ingredients of psychological treatment approaches

Support factors	Learning factors	Action factors
• Release of tension	• Advice	• Facing fears
• Trust	• Feedback	• Mastery
• Reassurance	• Insight	• Working through
• Structure	• Exploratory rationale	• Modelling
• Warmth	• Assimilation of problematic experiences	• Testing solutions
• Empathy		
• Therapeutic alliance		
• Acceptance		

Box 16.2 Different kinds of psychotherapy

Cognitive-behavioural therapies	Psychodynamic–relational therapies	Experiential–expressive therapies	Systemic therapies
• Behaviour therapy • Personal construct theory • Rational-emotive therapy • Dialectical behavioural therapy	• Psychodynamic therapy	• Client-centred psychotherapy • Gestalt therapy • Counselling • Supportive–expressive therapy	• Family therapy • Various group therapies • Therapeutic communities
• Interpersonal therapy • Cognitive-analytic therapy			
• Psychodynamic–interpersonal therapy			

Table 16.1   Key aspects of Freudian theory

Structural model of the mind

Component	Characteristics
Ego	• Part of the individual which mediates between the inner and outer world • Governed by the reality principle • No energy of its own
Id	• Respository of energy • Governed by the pleasure principle • Source of instinctual drives
Superego	• Conscience or moral agency of the mind • Develops through the successful resolution of the oedipal phase

Psychosexual development

Stages	Centre of erotic activity	Psychological objective	Disturbance produces
Oral (1–2 years)	Mouth	Establish trusting dependence upon a parent object	Excessive optimism, demandingness, dependency, rage when needs are not met
Anal (2–4 years)	Anal area	Develop greater self-control and separation from parent	Excessive rigidity, willfulness
Oedipal	Genital area	Gender identity, development of superego, tolerance of triangular relationships	Difficulty with authority, inability to take control, problems with competitiveness
Latency	Quiescence		
Genital stage	Other	Maturation of sexuality, separation from parents	Dependency problems with sexual partners

Dream terminology

• Manifest content — actual content of dream
• Latent content — masked meaning of dream
• Symbolism — visual expression of hidden ideas
• Condensation — single image represents several unconscious wishes
• Secondary revision — intellectual understanding of the dream by the dreamer

Depth psychology and the topographical model

• Unconscious — governed by primary process thinking; no sense of place, person, or time; ideas conveyed via images and symbols
• Preconscious
• Conscious — governed by rational thought processes

relationships. The most common example of transference is 'falling in love'.

In psychodynamic therapy, transference is used as an important (if not the most important) tool to understand an individual's difficulties or problems with relationships. Such problems come alive in therapy, and are re-enacted between the therapist and client. Analysis and interpretation of the transference is one of the most powerful therapeutic agents in psychodynamic psychoanalytic psychotherapy.

The core conflictual relationship theme method (CCRT), developed by Luborsky (Luborsky & Crits-Christoph 1990), can be used to objectively assess elements of the transference. Narratives from sessions of therapy are analysed according to three components: types of wishes, responses from other, and responses of the self. From this material, central relationship patterns, both adaptive and maladaptive, can be identified. The CCRT can be used to inform interpretations (see next subsection).

The term countertransference is used in a number of different ways by psychodynamic therapists. It most commonly refers to the therapist's emotional response to the client. The therapist's response will be made up of his own 'transference' feelings, which have a basis in the therapist's own prior experiences, and the therapist's reaction to the client's transference towards him. If a therapist can distinguish these two elements of the countertransference, he can gain valuable insight into the client's problems and ways of relating to others.

Interpretations

Interpretations are one of the main therapeutic tools used in dynamic therapies to aid conscious awareness of underlying conflicts or problems. They are attempts by the therapist to link conscious and unconscious determinants of an experience, feeling or symptom. An interpretation is not a dogmatic statement by the therapist, which is treated as being correct even if the patient disagrees with it. This, however, is how it is often portrayed. Interpretations are best understood as suggestions or tentative hypotheses which the patient is able to consider, and either agree with or reject.

There are a variety of measures which can be used to measure transference interpretations. Empirical research on the usefulness of interpretations has been reviewed by Piper et al (1993). Most studies of the effects of transference interpretations have been conducted on short-term therapies. Two aspects of transference interpretations have been studied: dosage (how many interpretations per session) and accuracy. The best outcome results are achieved from low frequency and high correspondence of transference interpretations (i.e. accuracy). For patients who score highly on object relations (see next subsection) transference interpretation variables can account for up to 40% of the outcome variance.

Object relations

Quality of object relations refers to a person's lifelong pattern of relationships, identified on a dimension ranging from primitive to mature. A measure has been developed by Azim and colleagues (1991) which enables patients' level of object relations to be rated on a nine-point scale. The measure is interview based and requires two 1-hour sessions to complete. Lifelong patterns of relation-ships are explored in reference to criteria that characterise five lev-els of object relations: primitive, searching, controlling, triangular, and mature. The criteria refer to behavioural manifestations, reg-ulation of affect, regulation of self-esteem, and historical an-tecedents. A tendency towards more mature object relations means the person enjoys equitable relationships characterised by love, tenderness and concern for objects of both sexes. There is a capacity to mourn and tolerate unobtainable relationships. A ten-dency towards primitive object relations means the person reacts to perceived separation or loss of the object, or disapproval or re-jection by the object, with intense anxiety and affect. There is in-ordinate dependence on the object who provides a sense of identity for the person.

Psychological mindedness

Psychological mindedness is the ability to identify dynamic or intrapsychic components and to relate them to one's difficulties. An individual is considered to be psychologically minded if the person is willing to talk about intrapsychic and interpersonal problems, has the capacity and motivation for behavioural change, and is interested in what motivates other people's behaviour.

McCallum & Piper (1997) have developed a procedure for assessing psychological mindedness: The Psychological Mindedness Assessment Procedure (PMAP). The subject is asked to watch two brief video clips of simulated patient–therapist scenarios. After viewing the videos, the person being assessed is asked for his general impressions of what is troubling the 'patient' on the tape. The person's responses are assessed by an individual assessor who grades the individual according to nine levels of psychological mindedness. They range from level 1, where a subject can recognise the patient's emotional state on the tape to level 9 where the subject is able to recognise that the 'patient' on the tape is behaving in a defensive way to protect herself from her true feelings. Patients who score low on psychological mindedness are more likely to drop out of therapy. There is also a strong positive correlation between psychological mindedness and work in therapy. There is also some, but not conclusive, evidence that psychological mindedness is also associated with outcome.

Defence mechanisms

Defence mechanisms are psychological strategies that are used to protect individuals from unbearable emotional distress. They are universal phenomena which all of us use at times to limit and con-strict awareness so that threatening cues, either from the inner or

outer environment, can be excluded. They appear to be invoked automatically and not under conscious control, and are psycho-logical measures which allow stressful situations to be coped with by distorting reality (Box 16.3). In a fascinating study, Valliant et al (1986) studied the defence mechanisms of 307 healthy middle-aged men followed up for 40 years and described the defence styles associated with coping and success. On the basis of this work the defence mechanisms measured in the study were grouped into hierarchical categories: mature, neurotic and immature defences. Individuals who tended to use mature defences had a better long-term outcome (both physical and mental) than those who used immature defences.

A small number of empirical studies of defensive mechanisms in relation to psychiatric disorder provide a degree of support for the validity of some aspects of psychodynamic theory. There is evi-dence that persecutory delusions reflect a defensive attributional style which protects the individual against feelings of low self-esteem (Lyon et al 1994). Panic disorder patients have a heightened use of reaction formation and undoing (Busch et al 1995). These findings are consistent with the psychodynamic formulation of panic that proposes that negative affects are threatening to panic patients because they represent a threat to the relationship to a sig-nificant other on whom the individual feels dependent. Patients with dysthymia score highly on immature defence mechanisms (Bloch et al 1993), and patients with a diagnosis of personality disorder use immature and primitive defensive mechanisms (Paris et al 1996).

The activation of mature mechanisms often result in a positive response from others (e.g. individuals who use humour or altruism are generally seen as likeable), whereas immature mechanisms may provoke a negative response from others. Thus mature defences are more adaptive and result in greater stability. Most individuals employ a repertoire of defence mechanisms, but when placed under stress or pressure, less mature defences tend to be deployed.

An analysis of an individual's repertoire of defence mechanisms can be a useful indicator of how that person may behave during psychotherapy. However, a finer grading system of categories of defensive control processes, which integrates both psychodynamic and schema-focused cognitive theory, may also be useful in under-standing maladaptive ways of coping with stress and anxiety (Horowitz et al 1997). The categories include:

- shifting attention;
- juggling concepts about a topic;
- sliding meanings and values;
- premature disengaging from topics;
- blocking apt modes of representation;
- shifting time span;
- using poor ideational linkage strategies;
- engaging inappropriate arousal levels;
- shifting self–other roles;
- rigidly stabilising compromise roles;
- altering valuation schemas (e.g. idealisation or denegration of others).

Evidence base

There are relatively few studies of psychodynamic therapies, in contrast with the large evidence base available for cognitive and behavioural interventions. In the last 15 years, there have been three systematic reviews. Svartberg & Stiles (1991) reviewed 19

Box 16.3   Common defence mechanisms

Mature
- Sublimation — partial expression of unacceptable desires in modified way which makes them acceptable or even desirable
- Suppression — partial prevention of unpleasant feelings at times when their expression would be socially unacceptable, but ability to acknowledge feelings at other times
- Anticipation — being able to anticipate and plan for distressing or difficult emotional events
- Altruism — meeting ones own emotional needs by helping others
- Humour — defusing difficult or conflictual situations by seeing the funny side

Intermediate/neurotic
- Displacement — transfer of negative feelings to a less threatening object
- Repression — anxiety-provoking thoughts are prevented from being made conscious
- Isolation — over-reliance upon self
- Reaction formation — opposite reaction to hide underlying true feelings

Immature
- Projection — internal anxiety/fear are attributed to an outside cause
- Schizoid fantasy — over-reliance upon fantasy to cope with life's disappointments
- Passive aggression — transformation of angry or aggressive impulses into passive resistance or refusal to comply with realistic goals
- Acting out — socially unacceptable behaviour prompted by underlying aggressive impulses (behaviour is usually self-injurious or directed at a key other person with whom the person is in conflict)
- Hypochondriasis — unacceptable feelings are converted into concerns about illness
- Dissociation — difficult feelings are split off from conscious awareness, and the individual becomes unconnected to reality (e.g. may develop fugue state or severe physical symptomatology)
- Splitting — People are perceived as being either all good or all bad

---

studies and found a negative outcome. Crits-Christoph (1992) focused on short-term interventions and included 11 studies, with favourable results for dynamic therapies. A more recent review by Anderson & Lambert (1995) included 26 studies and provided conclusions more similar to that of Crits-Christoph. Further evaluation of psychodynamic therapies is urgently required.

BEHAVIOURAL METHODS

In many early descriptions of behavioural approaches, emphasis was placed on the role of learning in the aetiology, maintenance and treatment of psychiatric problems. It was generally held that learning was a crucial concept in three main ways. First, some disorders were associated with a lack of learning, e.g. enuresis, or psychopathic behaviour. Second, some disorders were associated with overlearning, e.g. obsessional rituals and phobias. Third, some disorders were associated with loss of previous learning, by neurological dysfunction, e.g. aphasia, or through insufficient or inappropriate reinforcement as in institutionalisation. These notions provided the rationale for the application of learning theory to the amelioration of psychiatric problems. The links between behavioural approaches and learning theory have gradually become less direct, and methods of behaviour change have been sought from wider experimental psychology and other areas.

Systematic desensitisation (SD) (general exposure)

The original technique developed by Wolpe (1958) involved three stages:

1. training the patient to relax (see next subsection);
2. constructing with the patient a hierarchy of anxiety-arousing situations;
3. presenting phobic items for the hierarchy in a graded way, while the patient inhibits the anxiety by relaxation.

In this way, the patient, while never experiencing intolerable anxiety, proceeded from mildly frightening situations to previously terrifying ones.

Progress up the hierarchy can be made in imagination, in real life (in vivo) or by a combination of both, depending on such factors as the availability of the feared object or situation and how easily the graded steps can be reproduced in real life. Films, slides and recordings can also be used. The balance of evidence suggests that in-vivo SD is more effective, possibly because the treatment setting is more like the real-life situation, thus facilitating generalisation.

When SD is being conducted in imagination, the length of the session is generally about 40 minutes, depending on how long it takes to get the patient relaxed; moving up steps in the hierarchy rarely extends beyond 30 minutes. The number of sessions required varies (anything from 10 to 100 being possible), depending on the complexity of the problem and on the number of hierarchies to be worked through, for it is seldom that a patient presents with a single well-defined phobia. Patients are expected to practise at home what they have learned in the clinical session.

The following illustrates a section of a typical hierarchy for a patient with a phobia of shopping:

1. entering a quiet shop to purchase one article, e.g. a newspaper, with the exact purchase money in hand;
2. waiting behind one person, otherwise as (1);
3. purchasing more than one article, as (1);
4. as (3), but having to wait for change;
5. asking to see an article before purchasing;
6. as (4), but waiting in a queue of several people.

When SD is carried out in vivo, the patient is instructed how to relax and how and when to use relaxation in the clinic; but the actual desensitisation is done in the real situation. Often this 'homework' can be done while the patient is accompanied by a relative, and the presence of such a companion can act as an extra way of breaking down the hierarchy into smaller steps.

SD is one of the most intensively investigated of all kinds of psychological therapy, with over one hundred studies looking simply at the relative importance of the various elements involved. There is little doubt about its effectiveness, and it is extensively used as a treatment for phobic anxiety.

Relaxation

Behaviour therapists are not the only practitioners of relaxation, as other therapists have used it extensively. Nevertheless, since Wolpe (1958) advocated Jacobson's (1938) technique it has earned a firm place in the behavioural armamentarium. Its role has also gradually extended. Formerly, when used alone, it was regarded as a control procedure, lacking the essential conditioning elements of SD; but gradually evidence accumulated showing that it was often at least as effective as the treatment with which it was compared. This was particularly striking when it was being used as a control procedure with which to compare biofeedback (see below). It has now earned a place in its own right as an effective treatment for anxiety management, headaches, chronic pain, hypertension and other problems. A useful review of relaxation procedures has been provided by Lichstein (1988).

Flooding (rapid exposure)

Flooding involves exposing patients to a phobic object in a non-graded manner with no attempt to reduce anxiety beforehand. As with SD, flooding can be conducted in vivo or in imagination. In the latter case it is often referred to as implosive therapy, and as such was originally put forward as a psychoanalytic technique, with some similarity to abreaction. A recent application of imaginal flooding is to post-traumatic stress disorder (Cooper & Clum 1989).

Typically the patient is placed alone in a room with the phobic object, say a cat, and is required to stay there until the fear has diminished. It is argued that fear is maintained by the patient's avoidance of the phobic object or situation, and that if avoidance is not allowed the fear will diminish. The flooding session must be of long duration, normally an hour or more, to be effective. In general, the patient should stay in contact until there are clear indications of marked fear reduction; some reduction is normally seen after 15 minutes. Ending before this may represent another avoidance and could exacerbate the problem. This brings out a resemblance to SD which may not be obvious at first sight. In the initial stages of flooding, the anxiety is very high but, due to emotional exhaustion or habituation, after a time it starts to decline so that each recurrence of the frightening stimulus, e.g. a movement of the cat towards the patient, no longer leads to increased anxiety and the stimulus–response link between the cat and the fear has weakened. Another likely reason for success is the subject's 'reality testing' of the situation, whereby he discovers that he is less afraid of the phobic object than he had expected to be.

Several studies have compared flooding with SD in the treatment of phobias. Most have shown that there are no major differences in outcome. Flooding seems to be more effective with obsessive–compulsive patients when combined with response prevention (see below).

The decision whether to use flooding or not is by mutual agreement of patient and therapist. Most patients find it less frightening than they had imagined and it is usually much quicker acting than SD.

COGNITIVE THERAPY

Cognitive or cognitive-behavioural therapy refers to a method of therapy based on a theory of the emotional disorders (Ellis 1962, Beck 1967), a body of experimental and clinical studies (Blackburn 1988) and well-defined therapy techniques (Beck et al 1979, Beck & Emery 1985, Hawton et al 1989, Blackburn & Davidson 1990). Theoretically, the emphasis is on information processing; that is, individuals react, feel and behave according to how they process the information contained in their environment (Fig. 16.1).

Cognitive approaches to treatment were first developed for the management of depressive illness and labelled as cognitive therapy (Beck 1964) or as rational-emotive therapy (RET) (Ellis 1962). The theoretical underpinning and experimental studies were criticised (e.g. see Ledwidge 1978, Coyne & Gottlib 1983), but a more general positive reaction has led to a mushrooming of basic research and of therapeutic applications to disorders other than depression. The general principles of cognitive therapy will be described, followed by its specific applications. The main characteristics of cognitive therapy are described in Box 16.4.

General principles

Cognitive therapy, like behaviour therapy, is problem oriented. It is aimed at correcting psychological problems (emotional, cognitive and behavioural) and at improving coping skills (dealing with problem situations) to alleviate patients' distress. The main characteristics of cognitive therapy are that it is time limited, structured and problem oriented; it follows an explicit agenda, deals with the 'here-and-now', and adopts a learning rather than

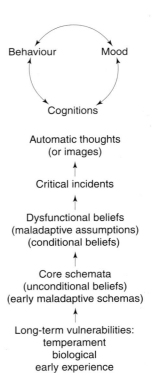

Fig. 16.1
The cognitive model.

Box 16.4 Main characteristics of standard cognitive therapy

- Time limited — 15–22 sessions over 3–4 months
- Structured — Each session lasts 1 hour and is structured by the use of an agenda to optimise the use of time
- Problem-oriented — Therapist and patient focus on defining and solving presenting problems
- A-historical — It deals with the here-and-now without recourse to the distant past history of the patient
- Learning — Does not use psychodynamic hypothetical constructs to explain the patient's behaviour. Rather, dysfunctional behaviour is attributed to maladaptive learning
- Scientific method — An experimental method is adopted: therapy involves collecting data (problems, thoughts, attitudes), formulating hypotheses, setting up experiments, and evaluating results
- Homework — The patient is given assignments for data collecting, verification of hypotheses, and practice of cognitive skills
- Collaboration — Patient and therapist work together to solve problems
- Active — The therapist adopts an active and directive role throughout treatment. He can be didactic sometimes but his main role is to facilitate the definition and resolution of problems
- Socratic questioning — The principal therapeutic method is socratic questioning, which is to ask a series of questions aimed at bringing the patient to identify his underlying thoughts, to perceive alternative solutions, or to modify his opinions
- Openness — The therapeutic process is not clouded in mystique; rather, it is explicit and open, therapist and patient sharing a common understanding of what is going on in therapy

---

psychodynamic model. It is a scientific method, involving the setting up and testing of hypotheses. Patients are given regular homework assignments, and a collaborative relationship between therapist and patient is developed.

Patients are provided with a rationale for understanding their problems, a vocabulary for expressing themselves, and a training in techniques for overcoming distressing affects and for solving problems. In addition to cognitive methods, cognitive therapy uses the whole gamut of behavioural techniques described earlier in the chapter. This is done not only to change behaviour but also to change interpretations, expectations and self-concept. These changes are not taken for granted, but put forward as hypotheses, and discussed after the behavioural experiments, which are repeated until both the therapist and patient are satisfied that cognitive changes have taken place. The main differences between cognitive-behavioural therapy and other therapies are listed in Box 16.5.

Cognitive therapy is more than the routine application of a series of techniques. In addition to mastering the basic therapeutic skills (Truax & Carkhuff 1967), the therapist must conceptualise each case within a cognitive therapy framework following a functional analysis which is similar to that described earlier in this chapter. The focus is on the cognitive factors which maintain emotional disturbance and maladaptive behaviour. Blackburn & Davidson (1990) described the main areas of enquiry to reach a formulation in cognitive therapy. These are:

- *Definition of the problem:* What are the major complaints? Which particular functions are affected?
- *Objective factors:* What are the current stresses, main past traumatic events and current living situation?
- *Internal vulnerability factors:* What are the main attitudes and beliefs which the patient holds about himself and his world? What types of events does he appear to be sensitive to?
- *Mediational cognitive factors:* What are the typical automatic thoughts which are expressed and which processing errors do they contain? (See next subsection.)
- *Current themes:* The recurring theme, for example, failure, loss of control, loss of love, or low self-image, will indicate particular vulnerabilities and help the therapist to hypothesise about basic schemata.
- *Coping skills:* What are the typical methods of dealing with problems? In what way are these helpful or unhelpful?

Box 16.5 How cognitive-behavioural therapy differs from other psychotherapies

- Open, explicit
- Structured, e.g. agenda
- Sets behavioural tasks
- Therapist more active
- Mainly uses here-and-now rather than past
- Does not use symbolism
- Uses specific cognitive techniques

- *Emotions:* What are the predominant emotions and what situations trigger them?

Specific techniques

The techniques first described for the treatment of depression (Beck et al 1979) are applicable, with some modifications and additions, to many different disorders (Hawton et al 1989): for example, anxiety, obsessional–compulsive and eating disorders, somatic problems, sexual dysfunction and chronic psychiatric handicaps. Beck (1987) has described the cognitive dysfunctions which maintain depression. These are seen at three levels of thinking, and cognitive therapy techniques are aimed at modifying each of these levels. An example is given in Figure 16.2.

The general aims of cognitive therapy are:

- to monitor negative automatic thoughts;
- to recognise connections between cognitions, affect and behaviour;
- to examine evidence for and against distorted automatic thoughts;
- to substitute more reality-oriented interpretations;
- to learn to identify and alter dysfunctional schemata.

The automatic thoughts (so called because they are the habitual and reflexive commentaries that we make to ourselves and of which we are not necessarily fully conscious) are the basic data of cognitive therapy. Several techniques have been described to help the therapist elicit and modify these thoughts, which maintain low or anxious or angry moods and dysfunctional behaviour (e.g. inactivity, ruminating, checking, bingeing, avoiding, etc.). The

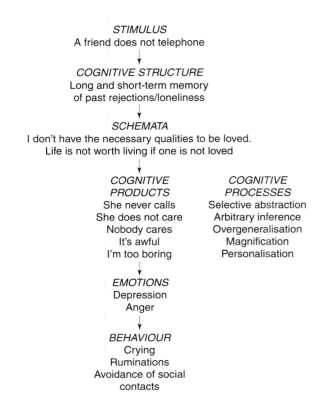

STIMULUS
A friend does not telephone

↓

COGNITIVE STRUCTURE
Long and short-term memory
of past rejections/loneliness

↓

SCHEMATA
I don't have the necessary qualities to be loved.
Life is not worth living if one is not loved

↓

COGNITIVE PRODUCTS	*COGNITIVE PROCESSES*
She never calls	Selective abstraction
She does not care	Arbitrary inference
Nobody cares	Overgeneralisation
It's awful	Magnification
I'm too boring	Personalisation

↓

EMOTIONS
Depression
Anger

↓

BEHAVIOUR
Crying
Ruminations
Avoidance of social
contacts

Fig. 16.2
Cognitive processes.

patient can be helped to access these thoughts through direct questioning, inductive questioning (a series of questions which guide the patient to discover the related automatic thought), using moments of strong emotion, re-enacting situations in role-plays, using mental imagery to recreate situations or using behavioural tasks to trigger the thoughts. The patient is asked to keep a diary (the 'daily record of dysfunctional thoughts'), using changes in emotions as cues to monitor thinking. These records are also used to practise challenging the automatic thoughts and substituting alternative interpretations which may lead to less distressing emotions. A variety of other techniques can also be used to modify automatic thoughts: for example, examining the evidence for and against, listing probabilities and collecting information which may invalidate the original interpretation. The basic principle in all these techniques is that the patient is taught to consider his thoughts not as facts but as interpretations which may be more or less accurate and which may be more or less functional in terms of the feelings and the behaviour that they trigger.

Identifying the basic schemata or beliefs which lead the patient to process information in idiosyncratic ways typically occurs later on in therapy and is generally more difficult and abstract than identifying automatic thoughts. It is also more difficult to modify the schemata, particularly in the personality disorders (Beck & Freeman 1990).

The schemata are inferred from the implicit or explicit rules which are exemplified in the automatic thoughts. The therapist and the patient, in collaboration, must look for common themes, for the 'shoulds' which are applied to the self and to others, and for the logical implications of automatic thoughts, by, for example, the 'downward arrow technique', of which an example (from Blackburn & Davidson 1990) is given in Figure 16.3.

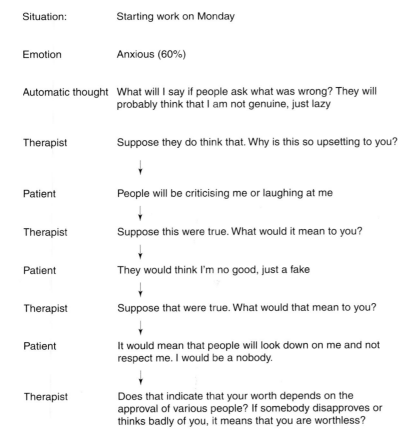

Situation:	Starting work on Monday
Emotion	Anxious (60%)
Automatic thought	What will I say if people ask what was wrong? They will probably think that I am not genuine, just lazy
Therapist	Suppose they do think that. Why is this so upsetting to you?
	↓
Patient	People will be criticising me or laughing at me
	↓
Therapist	Suppose this were true. What would it mean to you?
	↓
Patient	They would think I'm no good, just a fake
	↓
Therapist	Suppose that were true. What would that mean to you?
	↓
Patient	It would mean that people will look down on me and not respect me. I would be a nobody.
	↓
Therapist	Does that indicate that your worth depends on the approval of various people? If somebody disapproves or thinks badly of you, it means that you are worthless?

Fig. 16.3
Downward-arrow technique.

As with the automatic thoughts, modifying the schemata is done through collaborative discussion and the use of behavioural tasks. Thus, the patient may be asked to weigh up the advantages and disadvantages of holding the belief, to examine the evidence for and against the belief, to question the validity of the personal contract, to consider the short-term and long-term utility of the personal rule, to disobey the rule in a behavioural assignment and test the consequences. The latter technique is similar to response prevention in behaviour therapy.

Evidence base

There are numerous studies of cognitive-behavioural therapy which support its efficacy for a wide variety of disorders, including depressive disorders, anxiety states, somatisation and other neurotic conditions. The main evidence is reviewed at the end of this chapter.

INTERPERSONAL PSYCHOTHERAPY

Interpersonal psychotherapy (IPT) is a structured, individual, time-limited (12–16 sessions) psychotherapy which has been shown to be effective in clinical trials of major depressive disorder and bulimia nervosa.

There are many different types of interpersonal psychotherapy, but IPT refers specifically to the model of treatment proposed by Klerman and Weissman (Klerman et al 1984). It is of particular interest because it was devised by a biological psychiatrist and an epidemiologist.

IPT is based on the work of Harry Stack-Sullivan (1953). Sullivan taught that psychiatry includes the scientific study of people and the processes between people rather than focusing exclusively on the mind, society or the brain; hence the unit of clinical study is the patient's interpersonal relations at any one particular time.

IPT has two foci: to reduce depressive symptoms and to deal with the social and interpersonal problems associated with the onset of the symptoms. The initial sessions are devoted to establishing the treatment contract, dealing with the depressive symptoms, and identifying the problem areas. During the initial sessions, both the depression and the interpersonal problems are diagnosed and assessed. In these sessions, the therapist should accomplish six tasks:

- Begin dealing with the depression.
- Complete an interpersonal inventory and relate the depression to the interpersonal context.
- Identify the principal problem areas.
- Explain the rationale and intent of interpersonal therapy.
- Set a treatment contract with the patient.
- Explain the patient's expected role in the treatment.

Relating depression to the interpersonal context

Once the review of the depression has been completed, the therapist should direct the patient's attention to the onset of symptoms and to the reason for seeking treatment: what has been going on in the patient's social and interpersonal life that is associated with the onset of symptoms? The review of key persons and issues often follows easily. If not, it is useful to begin an inventory of current and past relationships to get a full picture of what the important current social interactions are in the patient's life.

The systematic review of current and past interpersonal relationships involves an exploration of the patient's important relationships with others, beginning with the present. This may all be done during the sessions or the psychotherapist may ask the patient to write an autobiographical statement containing interpersonal information.

In this inventory, the following should be gathered about each person who is important in the patient's life:

- interactions with the patient, including frequency of contact, activity shares, and so on;
- the expectations of each party in the relationship, including some assessment of whether these expectations were or are fulfilled;
- a review of the satisfactory and unsatisfactory aspects of the relationship, with specific, detailed examples of both kinds of interactions;
- the ways the patient would like to change the relationship, whether through changing his or her own behaviour or bringing about changes in the other person.

Although the inventory is constructed in the first two sessions, it may be added to less systematically as treatment progresses.

Problem areas

It is important to define the problem areas because they can help the psychotherapist formulate a treatment strategy with the patient. Since IPT is short-term, it is usually concentrated on one or two of the four problem areas that depressed patients commonly encounter. The main problem areas are usually:

- grief;
- interpersonal disputes with spouse, lover, children, or other family members, friends, or co-workers;
- role transitions — a new job, leaving one's family, going away to school, relocation in a new home or area, divorce, economic or other family changes;
- interpersonal deficits — loneliness and social isolation.

Diagnosis of interpersonal disputes

For the therapist to choose role disputes as the focus of IPT, the patient must give evidence of current overt or covert conflicts with a significant other. Such disputes are usually revealed in the patient's initial complaints or in the course of the interpersonal inventory. In some IPT research, role disputes with the spouse have been the most common problem area. In practice, however, recognition of important interpersonal disputes in the lives of depressed patients may be difficult

In developing a treatment plan, the therapist first determines the stage of the role dispute:

- *Renegotiation* implies that the patient and the significant other are openly aware of differences and are actively trying, even if unsuccessfully, to bring about changes.
- *Impasse* implies that discussion between the patient and the significant other has stopped and that the smouldering, low-level resentment typical of 'cold marriages' exists.
- *Dissolution* implies that the relationship is irretrievably disrupted.

Role transitions

Depression frequently results when a person recognises the need to make a normative role transition but has difficulty with the necessary changes required or when a person correctly recognises failure in a particular role but is unable to change the behaviour or to change roles. In depressions associated with role transitions, the patient feels helpless to cope with the change in role. The transition may be experienced as threatening to one's self-esteem and sense of identity, or as a challenge one is unable to meet.

In general, difficulties in coping with role transitions are associated with the following issues:

- loss of familiar social supports and attachments;
- management of accompanying emotions, such as anger or fear;
- demands for a new repertoire of social skills;
- diminished self-esteem.

Training

Didactic seminar   In a 2–5 day seminar, an attempt is made to help therapists identify what they are already doing that is like IPT, what they are doing that is not IPT, and the special skills needed for the IPT approach. This takes the form of an exegesis of the written material with extensive clinical illustration using videotaped case material.

Supervised casework   After the didactic seminar, therapists are assigned between two and four training cases each, on which they receive weekly supervision on a session-by-session basis. This is done on the telephone or in person after the supervisor has reviewed the videotape of the session. Both trainee and supervisor have videotape equipment and tapes available, so that they can watch specific segments as they discuss the session. The primary purpose of the supervision is boundary marking or helping the therapist learn which techniques are included and which are excluded in IPT. It is also helpful if the supervisor reviews the ratings made by the patient during the session as well as the observer ratings. The main areas of focus of IPT are listed in Box 16.6.

Evidence base

The main approach to IPT is described in a recent text (Weissman et al 2000). IPT is an efficacious treatment for the treatment of depression and was extensively evaluated in the large NIMH comparative study of CBT, IPT and antidepressants for major depressive disorder (Elkin et al 1989). It has also been used as a maintenance treatment for depression (Kupfer et al 1992, Reynolds et al 1992), to treat depression in HIV-positive individuals (Markowitz et al 1998), and is an effective treatment for bulimia nervosa (Fairburn et al 1986, 1995).

Box 16.6   Main areas of focus of IPT

- What has contributed to this patient's depression right now?
- What are the current stresses?
- Who are the key persons involved in the current stress?
- What are the current disputes and disappointments?
- Is the patient learning how to cope with the problem?
- What are the patient's assets?
- How can I help the patient ventilate painful emotions — talk about situations that evoke guilt, shame, resentment?
- How can I help the patient clarify his wishes and have more-satisfying relationships with others?
- How can I correct misinformation and suggest alternatives?

PSYCHODYNAMIC–INTERPERSONAL THERAPY

The model lies somewhere between traditional psychodynamic approaches and the interpersonal psychotherapy developed by Klerman and Weissman (Klerman et al 1984). Although, research into the model is at a relatively early stage, the findings to date suggest that this form of psychodynamic psychotherapy has clinical validity and is a valuable treatment for depression and somatisation.

Psychodynamic–interpersonal (PI) therapy was developed and refined over the course of thirty years by Hobson (1985). A training package and manual were first developed, and a subsequent brief manual and rating scale for the treatment of depression (Shapiro & Startup 1991) was published in 1991. A videotape teaching package was developed by Margison & Hobson (1983), which consists of three videotapes in which the main aspects of the model are described. The therapy is relatively easy to learn, and skills are maintained over at least a 2-year period (Moss et al 1991). A book which describes the development of the model, the manual and the research conducted upon it to date, is due to be published in 2004 (Barkham et al 2004). The model was originally called the 'conversational model' of psychotherapy, and it is theoretically derived from psychodynamic principles, but also draws upon humanistic and interpersonal concepts. The main task of the therapist in this model, is to develop, with the patient, what Hobson termed a 'mutual feeling language' and a relationship of 'aloneness-togetherness' (Hobson 1985).

Hobson developed the model as an attempt to move away from the traditional psychoanalytic approach of a one-sided asymmetrical relationship. He also wanted to convey to others a form of psychotherapy that was relatively 'jargon-free', yet had specified skills which could be learned, practised and tested. The model has been conceptualised as consisting of seven different but interlinking components. Some of these components are generic to all psychotherapies, but taken as a whole they constitute a specific definable model of therapy. They are listed in Box 16.7.

Box 16.7   Key components of psychodynamic–interpersonal therapy

- Rationale for exploratory therapy
- Developing a shared understanding
  - Negotiating style
  - Language of mutuality (I and we)
  - Metaphor (picking up metaphors used by client, or introduction of metaphors to deepen understanding)
  - Understanding hypotheses
- Focus on 'here and now'
  - Cue basis
  - Focusing
  - Staying with feelings
- Gaining better understanding of interpersonal problems
  - Patterns in relationships
  - Linking hypotheses
  - Explanatory hypotheses
- Structure
  - Sequencing of interventions
- Focus on change
  - Testing out solutions
  - Exploring barriers to change

Evidence base

Five randomised controlled trials have compared PI therapy with cognitive-behavioural therapy (CBT), for the treatment of depressive disorder (Shapiro & Firth 1987, Shapiro et al 1994, Shapiro et al 1995, Barkham et al 1996, 2000). All the studies showed broadly similar results and found little evidence for differences in outcome between PI therapy and CBT. There were slight advantages for CBT on the Beck Depression Inventory but no differences on any other major outcome measures of depression, psychological symptoms and social functioning. There were some advantages for PI for patients with more severe depression. Patients in all groups showed improvement, and confirmed that PI therapy is an effective treatment for depression and can be employed in a clinical NHS setting.

PI therapy also been evaluated as treatment for somatisation (Guthrie et al 1991, Hamilton et al 2000, Creed et al 2003), chronic, intractable depression and anxiety (Guthrie et al 1999) and deliberate self-harm (Guthrie et al 2001). Two of these trials have shown that significant healthcare cost reductions occur, in comparison with a control condition.

This model of therapy is relatively easy to learn, and can be practised by therapists from a wide range of different theoretical backgrounds, although it is preferable that therapists have a background training in either IPT or dynamic therapy. It may be a useful alternative to CBT, particularly if patients or clients have prominent interpersonal dilemmas or difficulties. The model requires further evaluation in a wider range of psychological disorders.

COGNITIVE-ANALYTIC THERAPY

This relatively new psychotherapy has a strong practitioner base in the UK. It has been developed by Anthony Ryle and the key text is his 1990 book *Cognitive-Analytic Therapy: Active Participation in Change*. Ryle describes how he recognises three essential patterns of what he calls neurotic repetition. These are:

- *traps* — negative assumptions generate acts which produce consequences which reinforce the assumptions;
- *dilemmas* — the person acts as though available action or possible roles were limited to polarised alternatives (false dichotomies), usually without being aware that this is the case;
- *snags* — appropriate goals or roles are abandoned either because the individual makes an assumption that others would oppose them or because they are perceived as forbidden or dangerous.

Several features differentiate cognitive-analytic therapy (CAT). The psychotherapy file (produced in full in Ryle's book) combines instructions for self-monitoring with descriptions of a range of traps, dilemmas and snags. It is normally given to patients at the end of their first interview. Ryle points out that the therapeutic relationship is clearly altered by a therapist who emphasises trying to work, offers concepts, prescribes reading, and suggests homework assignments, but these techniques do not make working with the transference impossible. One of the key theoretical concepts underlying the basis of CAT is the procedural sequence model (PSM). This gives an account of the sequence of mental and behavioural processes involved in carrying out an aimed directed activity. Ryle believes that these procedures are hierarchically structured. Describing them and helping alter them is one of the main features of the treatment.

Another central CAT principle is that, in social situations, the adoption of one pole of a reciprocal role exerts a pressure on others to reciprocate and adopt a congruent pole. In any situation, the role an individual adopts will be determined partly by his own state, and partly by the expectancies of others. The identification of characteristic or repeated reciprocal role relationships enables individuals to understand and modify their behaviour.

At the end of the assessment period, a reformulation is produced. This is given to the patient in written form at the end of treatment (usually after 10–12 sessions). A goodbye letter is written. Training is more comprehensive than for IPT or CBT and normally takes 2 years of individual or group supervision. A number of trials evaluating CAT are under way but as yet no randomised control trials have been published. Other forms of evaluative work have, however, shown promising results (Brockman et al 1987, Fosbury 1994).

SUPPORTIVE PSYCHOTHERAPY

This form of psychotherapy is as variously defined as it is widely used. Bloch (1979) describes it as a form of psychological treatment given to patients with chronic and disabling psychiatric conditions 'for whom basic change is not seen as a realistic goal'. This definition emphasises the notion of therapy as a prop or crutch and envisages the objectives of such an approach as the promotion of the patient's best possible psychological and social functioning, the bolstering of his self-esteem and self-confidence, the cultivation of his sense of and contact with reality, the prevention of relapse, and, in certain instances, the transfer of the source of support from professional to family or friends.

However, other definitions of supportive psychotherapy stress its role in enabling individuals to cope with and overcome psychological difficulties presenting more acutely. For example, a Royal College of General Practitioners' report (1981) on prevention of psychiatric disorders in general practice emphasised the importance of supportive intervention in enabling the individuals to negotiate 'psychosocial transitions' — particular life events and challenges which produce psychological reactions, symptoms and disorders commonly seen in patients presenting to general practitioners, health visitors and social workers. The objectives of such supportive psychotherapy include the minimising of the impact of the threatening event, the provision of protection and relief from responsibilities during the crisis or transition, the encouragement of the expression of emotions and talking through the difficulties, and support for the individual in his attempts to seek out new directions in life.

Supportive psychotherapy is also conceived of as the use of psychological means to build individuals up to a point where they can devote themselves to more profound, time-consuming and complex psychotherapeutic interventions and as a temporary expedient to contain individuals who are acutely ill and who are awaiting the therapeutic impact of other forms of psychiatric treatment, most notably pharmacological.

There is much more general agreement as to what constitutes the key elements of the supportive forms of psychotherapy (Box 16.8). It is now recognised that an interview itself can exercise a psychotherapeutic effect – that the mere act of a doctor listening carefully to what the patient is saying, and enabling the patient to give a full account of his situation and problems, can result in a significant improvement. This realisation has led in turn to

Box 16.8 Elements of supportive psychotherapy

- The interview
- Reassurance
- Explanation
- Guidance and suggestion
- Ventilation

attempts to dissect out those characteristics of the interview which may exercise particularly beneficial effect. To date, the bulk of the effort has been directed at identifying interview techniques which facilitate case detection but the implications for the facilitation of therapy seem clear. Among the interview techniques which appear important are the therapist's ability to note verbal and non-verbal cues, to ask questions in a sequence from open to closed, to avoid using too many direct questions and to emphasise the importance of understanding the here-and-now situation (Marks et al 1993).

Reassurance provided by a therapist equipped to use the therapeutic relationship constructively, able to be both detached and compassionate, and skilled in listening and providing information simply and comprehensively, is one of the basic elements of the supportive form of psychotherapy. Reassurance can be used to good effect to relieve fears, boost self-confidence and promote hope. But it is not without its problems. To promote a patient's hopes unreasonably by providing false reassurance, or to intervene prematurely before the patient has explained his situation fully, may be effective initially but eventually prove useless or worse. However, as Kessel (1979) has pointed out in a thoughtful essay on the subject, such a view at least partly reflects the perspective of the specialist psychotherapist concerned with the exploration rather than the alleviation of worry. The harmful effect of absolving a patient from his responsibilities and of getting between a patient and his recognition of underlying causes can be avoided once it is recognised.

Explanation is likewise an important element in psychotherapeutic support. Whereas reconstructive forms of psychotherapy emphasise non-directiveness, a degree of therapeutic passivity and active therapeutic interventions limited to the provision of interpretation, the supportive forms encourage the provision of explanations by the therapist of such diverse matters as the nature of the patient's symptoms, the choice of treatment, and the likely outcome. Explaining to a patient quite why certain symptoms are being experienced and the extent to which they are common can itself be reassuring and therapeutically effective. The goal is not so much to increase self-understanding as to enhance the patient's ability to cope by clarifying the nature of the problem faced, the symptoms experienced and/or the treatment recommended.

Guidance and suggestion involve the provision of direct and indirect advice. In general, therapists are encouraged to refrain from advising patients, yet in supportive therapy teaching a patient how and when to ask for help is often a crucial component. Advice may be necessary with regard to particular problems, such as optimal ways of relating to a particularly difficult relative or handling a job interview, or to general issues, such as making contact with members of the opposite sex. Occasionally, advice is ineffective, and persuasion, involving the therapist in a more direct, controlling role, is required. Suggestion involves the therapist using such techniques as the showing or withholding of approval in attempts to modify a patient's situation. Suggestion operates in all forms of psychotherapy, and it has even been postulated that the suitability of an individual for treatment is dependent on his potential openness to the suggestive influence (Strupp 1978). Variables which appear to regulate the forcefulness of suggestion include the significance of the therapist to the patient, the degree to which the patient is or can become dependent and the depth of the patient's anxiety or depression. Individuals whose coping strategies have been overwhelmed are believed to be particularly prone to cling with desperation to any potential helping resource and to respond dramatically to proffered advice, reassurance and guidance.

In recent years, the value of *ventilation* of feelings within the psychotherapeutic setting has received support, and interest has been stimulated in the old notion of catharsis by the rise of the so-called 'emotive release (body) therapies'. It does seem useful for patients to be able to express emotions such as anger, frustration and despair openly. Unfortunately, the amount and quality of emotional expression has rarely been assessed independently and related to outcome, so its value has received little direct experimental verification.

Supportive psychotherapy is widely used in psychiatric settings, in general practice and in settings in which patients with short-lived yet intense emotional crises are seen.

COUNSELLING

There has been an enormous expansion of counselling services in primary care in the UK over the last twenty years. The most commonly practised form is non-directive counselling. In this, the client is given opportunities to explore, discover and clarify ways of living more resourcefully. This occurs in the context of a therapeutic relationship, within which the counsellor uses a range of skills to facilitate the client's resolution of his problems. Counselling is based upon the general factors present in all kinds of psychotherapy (see Box 16.1). These include: developing a working relationship with the client, within a supportive framework; encouraging a frank and open discussion of the client's problems; adopting a non-judgemental attitude; the release of emotional distress and the facilitation of problem solution. Other forms of counselling, which involve specific tasks, are also used widely in the NHS setting. This can include information-giving (e.g. genetic counselling) or brief structured guidance (e.g. alcohol counselling).

The evidence base in support of counselling as an efficacious treatment is mixed. However, a recent, large, well-conducted study in primary care, has shown that there is no significant difference between counselling and cognitive therapy for the treatment of depression (Ward et al 2001).

GROUP THERAPY

There are many different forms of group therapy. They all, however, share certain characteristics. In addition to factors common to all therapies, groups enable people to share experiences and interact with each other, in a safe setting. Individuals within the group give and receive help from the other members. Yalom (1970) summarised the factors of group psychotherapy which can have beneficial (curative) effects:

- installation of hope;
- universality;

- imparting of information;
- altruism;
- corrective recapitulation;
- development of socialising techniques;
- imitative behaviour;
- interpersonal learning;
- catharsis;
- group cohesiveness.

Groups can be divided into the educational or therapeutic, fixed or open, and short or long term. Educational groups are common in the healthcare setting, and are usually time-limited and very structured. They usually have a clear leader and a timetable. Members of the group are invited to comment on the information they have been given and to discuss it.

Therapeutic groups are either fixed or open. Fixed implies that the membership of the group is determined before its start and does not change. 'Open' means that the membership of the group gradually changes over time; as one person leaves, another may join.

Most of the individual forms of therapy discussed above can be delivered in a group format, including CBT and psychodynamic therapy. Although the effects of group work are difficult to evaluate, over seven hundred studies have reported outcomes for various forms of group psychotherapy (Fuhriman & Burlingame 1994). Several meta-analytic studies have been carried out, some showing no difference between group therapy and individual therapy (Robinson et al 1990, Tillitski 1990) and some reporting an advantage for individual therapy over group (Dush et al, 1983; Hemmings & Gretter, 1987). Given the diversity of different treatment approaches, lengths of treatment, and conditions for which group therapy has been provided, the results are difficult to interpret.

Most analytic groups are 'slow, open' groups. This means they run for a lengthy period of time (several years) over which older members of the group may leave, and new members join. The group leaders may also change. Most members stay in the group for at least 2 years. Group members agree (before entry) to have no other contact with each other, outside the group setting. They are known to each other only by their first names. Most groups consist of 6–8 members, plus one or two therapists, and may meet either once or twice weekly. One group session usually lasts 90 minutes.

Groups of this nature are powerful mediators of change. Individuals within the group are faced with a variety of different interpersonal experiences. They may have to cope with an old member leaving the group, assimilate new people into the group, cope with peer relationships and also relationships with authority, as symbolised by the group leader. In addition, they have to interact with the other group members on a personal basis.

Transference and countertransference issues may become evident and played out within the group. As people get to know each other within the group, a cohesiveness develops, and the group becomes more than a set of individuals. This transpersonal network of communication is sometimes referred to as the group matrix.

As group work of this nature is quite intensive and expensive, it is usually only offered in the healthcare sector to individuals who have chronic psychological problems and a pattern of interpersonal disturbance.

Psychodrama

Psychodrama is a form of group therapy that was developed by Moreno. It usually occurs in a closed group setting. Each member of the group has an opportunity to become the focus of a particular enactment. Other members of the group role-play the person's family or friends. A particular problem will be re-enacted and discussed by the group, from which new understandings and solutions are generated. The enactments usually generate strong feelings in the person represented, but also resonate with other members of the group, who may share similar difficulties. Members can also swap roles, to help them appreciate the problem from a different perspective.

FAMILY THERAPY

Family therapy was developed in the 1950s. It involves working with the whole family or at least several family members. It is most widely practised in child and adolescent psychiatry, but is also used in a variety of other settings, including the treatment of schizophrenia in adults (Kuipers et al 1992) and the treatment of mental health problems in the elderly (Richardson et al 1994). There are many different forms of family therapy, but systemic family approaches are among the most commonly practised forms. In systemic family therapy, the whole family is seen as a system, in which the behaviour of one individual is understood as a reaction to other parts of the system. For example, the development of emotional symptoms in a child whose parents are experiencing marital difficulties, may be understood as a way of trying to keep the parents together. Alleviation of the symptoms will only occur if the fundamental problems with the system are addressed.

Another form of family therapy is attachment-based family therapy (ABFT) (Diamond & Siqueland 1995). The underlying assumption of ABFT is that poor attachment bonds, high conflict, harsh criticism, and low affective attunement can lead to physical or emotional neglect, abuse and abandonment. This kind of negative family environment inhibits children from developing the internal and interpersonal coping skills needed to buffer against the family, social and community stressors that can cause or exacerbate depression. An equally important assumption of ABFT is that attachment failures can be resolved, parents can become better caregivers, and adolescents can rebuild trust and communication with their parents.

Evidence base

There is a paucity of well-designed randomised controlled trials of systemic therapies with children and adolescents and those trials that do exist evaluate older therapies. Methodological limitations of existing research include the use of unrepresentative participants, small sample sizes and wide age ranges. There is a lack of credible no-treatment or alternative-treatment controls, tests of clinical as opposed to statistical significance, and conceptually relevant outcome measures that examine underlying interactional mechanisms. The term 'family therapy' encompasses a wide range of interventions, and it is not always clear what treatment intervention has been delivered. Nevertheless, there is good evidence for the effectiveness of systemic family therapies in the treatment of conduct disorders, substance misuse and eating disorders, and some support for their use as second-line treatments in depression and chronic illness (Cottrell & Boston 2002). Family and parenting interventions for juvenile delinquents and their families may have beneficial effects on reducing time spent in institutions and their criminal activity (Woolfenden et al 2002).

COUPLE THERAPY

Couple therapy involves the psychotherapeutic treatment of married or cohabiting partners. It is usually reserved for situations where there is clear marital or relationship conflict. Relatively little couple therapy is offered on the NHS, but it is widely available from non-statutory agencies such as RELATE.

There have been relatively few evaluations of couple therapy, and many of the problems highlighted above in relation to the evaluation of family therapy are equally relevant to couple therapy.

EMDR AND OTHER ULTRA-BRIEF THERAPIES

The late 1980s and the 1990s saw the emergence of a cluster of very brief therapies, sometimes labelled 'power' therapies. These include 'the five-minute phobia cure', TFT (Thought Field Therapy) and EMDR. Only EMDR (eye movement desensitisation and reprocessing) has an established evidence base (Foa et al 2000). EMDR was developed by Shapiro (1995) as a technique for mitigating the impact of traumatic memories. It was subsequently developed into a more comprehensive treatment for PTSD. The technique involves cognitive behavioural and emotional aspects. The patient is asked to hold in the mind a disturbing image, a negative cognition and the bodily sensations associated with that traumatic image. The clinician then moves his or her fingers back and forth approximately 25 cm in front of the patient's face while the patient tracks the moving fingers with his eyes. After approximately 20 back and forth eye movements (saccades) the clinician stops and asks the patient to let go of the memory, take a deep breath and provide feedback on any changes in the image, body sensations, emotions or thoughts about the self. This is repeated until the image begins to fade. The second stage is the installation of a positive cognition. The eye movements are the central stage in what is an eight-stage treatment process for which specific training and treatment manuals are available.

There is debate about whether the eye movements are necessary or sufficient for the treatment, and it seems likely that EMDR works because it is an accelerated form of behavioural exposure and cognitive reprocessing.

For such a new treatment, the evidence base is remarkably strong, with 12 good randomised, controlled trials comparing EMDR with wait list or other brief treatments, and there are four dismantling studies for PTSD. EMDR appears to be as effective as cognitive therapy or drug treatment and somewhat more efficient. The evidence base is, however, limited by the fact that most studies have treated single rather than multiple traumatic events.

The other ultra-brief therapy which has a robust evidence base is Richard Bryant's Four Session Cognitive Therapy for Acute Stress Disorder (Bryant et al 1998). This has been shown in several trials to be a highly effective treatment in reducing the symptoms of acute stress disorder and preventing the development of subsequent PTSD. Readers should be highly sceptical of claims made for other ultra-brief therapies.

The second cluster of brief treatments are those grouped under the rubric of psychological debriefing, including such packages as Critical Instant Stress Debriefing (CISD). These are psychological interventions delivered shortly after a major traumatic event, either individually or in groups. They aim to reduce or prevent the development of subsequent psychological disorders, such as PTSD, major depressive disorder and phobic disorders. The Cochrane Review (Rose et al 2002) has clearly demonstrated that a single episode of psychological debriefing delivered in the days after a traumatic event is ineffective. Some studies have shown higher rates of subsequent PTSD in those who were debriefed compared with those who were not. Ørner & Schnyder (2003) have recently comprehensively reviewed the whole area of 'early intervention after trauma'.

EFFICACY AND EFFECTIVENESS OF PSYCHOLOGICAL INTERVENTIONS

In this section, brief but structured evidence for efficacy of psychological treatment will be considered. Specific topics such as schizophrenia, alcohol and drug problems, sexual problems, deliberate self-harm and eating disorders are covered in other chapters in this book.

In any discussion of outcome, it is important to distinguish between efficacy and effectiveness. Efficacy refers to the performance of treatment in a (randomised) controlled trial, whereas effectiveness refers to its performance in a clinical setting. Randomised controlled trials of psychological treatment usually recruit highly selected patient populations, have strict exclusion criteria, and usually employ experienced or expert therapists to conduct the treatment, which is manual based and monitored closely. In clinical settings, patients have heterogeneous problems, therapy is not manual based, and is much less closely supervised or scrutinised than in a trial, and therapists have different degrees of expertise. It is perhaps not surprising that psychotherapies perform better in trial settings than in ordinary clinical settings (Weisz et al 1995).

Psychotherapy researchers were one of the first group of investigators to adopt meta-analytic methods, within the field of psychiatry, to evaluate outcome. The first meta-analytic reviews of psychotherapy were published in the 1970s. At the time of writing this chapter, meta-analyses and systematic reviews have become the gold standard in terms of evaluating the efficacy of a particular treatment approach.

Although meta-analyses have many positive aspects, some caution is required regarding their use in relation to psychotherapy outcome. Most meta-analyses of psychotherapy combine different patient groups, different treatments, evaluate change over different periods of time, and employ different outcome measures. These difficulties should, however, diminish somewhat with the passage of time as more trials are published. It is only in relation to cognitive-behavioural treatments that there are sufficient studies at present which meet the homogeneity that the meta-analytic method requires (for example, all studies using the same outcome measure in the treatment of the same condition).

Major depressive disorder (MDD)

Many of the large reviews of the efficacy of psychotherapy in major depression are now quite old and do not include many studies using modern psychotherapy techniques. Nevertheless, three reviews have focused on the efficacy of psychotherapy contrasted with pharmacotherapy: the Quality Assurance Project (1983), Steinbruek et al (1993) and Conte et al (1986). The most influential of these, the Quality Assurance Project, showed an effect size

Table 16.2   Meta-analyses of psychotherapy trials (Depression Guidelines Panel 1993)

Therapy	Overall efficacy (%)	No. trials analysed
Behaviour therapy alone	55.3	10
Brief dynamic therapy alone	34.8	6
Cognitive therapy alone	46.6	12
Interpersonal therapy alone	52.3	1
All therapies	50.0	29

for psychotherapy of 0.69, for tricyclic antidepressents of 0.55 and for monoamine oxidase inhibitors of 0.39. The Depression Guidelines Panel (1993) reported somewhat differently from most meta-analyses in that the effect size is not given but there is an expected response rate for each therapy. Details are given in Table 16.2. There are a relatively small number of studies on brief dynamic psychotherapy and only one on interpersonal psychotherapy in this review. Although cognitive therapy is undoubtedly efficacious in depression, whether it is more or less effective than other treatments is controversial (Wampold et al 2002). Two key studies are also worthy of attention: Hollon et al (1992), Elkin (1994).

Specific/simple phobia: key review

Emmelkamp (1994) reviews behaviour treatments for specific phobias. Overall improvement rates appear to be achieved in approximately 75% of cases. The general conclusion is that exposure is more effective than systematic desensitisation and that in-vivo exposure is the most effective. Treatments for circumscribed specific phobias can be brief, being carried out in a single prolonged session of 2 hours or over two to four sessions at weekly intervals. Key studies are Ost (1989), Liddell et al (1994).

Generalised anxiety disorder

Durham & Allan's review (1993) is important because they reviewed studies that had used the Hamilton Anxiety Scale and the State Trait Anxiety Inventory as outcome measures. Their results show that CBT produces best results, but there are some important qualifications. The rates of improvement varied markedly from study to study, CBT was not always the best treatment, and outcome and rates of improvement were modest, though significantly better than placebo drugs or anti-anxiety medication. Not all studies had reasonable follow-up periods. Approximately 55% of those who had received cognitive therapy were in the normal range on the two above measures at the end of treatment, and this compared with 22% who had received behaviour therapy without cognitive intervention. Key studies are Power et al (1990), Butler et al (1991), Durham et al (1994).

Panic disorder

Gould et al (1995) carried out a meta-analysis on 43 controlled studies for the treatment of panic disorder. Treatments included pharmacological treatment, cognitive-behavioural interventions, and combined pharmacological and CBT treatments. The long-term analysis favoured CBT above either CBT combined with pharmacotherapy or pharmacotherapy alone. However, there was

a paucity of trials in which CBT was directly compared with antidepressant medication. Key studies are Marks et al (1993), Clark et al (1994), Gould et al (1995).

Social phobia

There is one good meta-analysis of 10 trials of behavioural and cognitive therapy (Chambless & Gillis 1993). There were significant effects both on the positive symptoms of social phobia and on the fears of negative evaluation that social phobics have. Given the chronicity of this disorder, follow-ups were relatively brief at 1–6 months. A key study is Heimberg et al (1990).

Post-traumatic stress disorder

The most comprehensive review is that by Foa et al (2000). They point out that most studies have either been on Vietnam veterans or female rape victims. Effective techniques appear to be anxiety management, stress inoculation, training and cognitive restructuring. The role of exposure-based treatments remains controversial. The evidence-base for psychodynamic psychotherapy is unclear largely because of the poor quality of the studies. Although not part of Foa's review it is perhaps worth emphasising that as yet there is little evidence base for post-disaster counselling or post-disaster psychological debriefing. A recent review by Rose et al (2002) found no evidence for any benefits of post-disaster debriefing.

Psychological treatments in primary care

A systematic review by Churchill et al (2001) has been conducted on the effectiveness and cost-effectiveness of brief psychological treatments for depression in primary care. Low overall quality scores were recorded for many of the trials, and interpretation of the findings was limited by identification of probable bias in the funnel plots and heterogeneity and sensitivity analyses. Patients receiving variants of CBT were significantly more likely to improve than those receiving treatment as usual. There was very little available information concerning a comparison of CBT with other psychological treatments.

Seven trials of counselling in primary care have been evaluated in a recent systematic review (Bower et al 2002). Counselling produced significantly greater clinical effectiveness in comparison with usual care, and the levels of satisfaction with counselling were high. Long-term evaluation showed that the benefits were not sustained. Four trials reported that the total costs of counselling were similar to those for controls, so it may be delivered at no additional cost, but the economic analyses may be underpowered. Further high-quality trials of all types of psychological treatment (both brief and long-term) are required.

Conclusion

There is growing evidence that psychological treatment is efficacious for a wide variety of psychiatric disorders. However, in comparison to the evidence base for pharmacological treatment, there are still relatively few randomised controlled trials which have investigated the efficacy of psychological interventions. This partly reflects the lack of funding for psychotherapy research and the enormous resources available to the pharmaceutical industry for the development and evaluation of psychotropic treatments. The vast majority of randomised controlled trials of psychological treatment which have been published in the last 10 years involve evaluations of cognitive-behavioural therapy (or its derivatives). There is therefore a sound and robust evidence base for its use in clinical settings. Other psychological treatment approaches have not been evaluated to the same extent, and there is a clear need for further evaluation of these interventions.

FURTHER READING

Different types of psychotherapy

Forms of feelings: the heart of psychotherapy. R F Hobson. Tavistock, London, 1987

Introduction to psychotherapy: an outline of psychodynamic principles and practice, 3rd edn. Bateman A, Brown D, Pedder J. Routledge, London, 2000

Cognitive analytic therapy: active participation in change. Ryle A. Wiley, New York, 1995

Comprehensive guide to interpersonal therapy. Weissman M, Markowitz J C, Klerman G L. Basic Books, New York, 2000

Science and practice of cognitive behaviour therapy. Clark D M, Fairburn C G (eds) Oxford University Press, Oxford, 1997

Psychotherapy research

Handbook of psychotherapy and behaviour change. Bergin A E, Garfield S L (eds) Wiley, New York, 2003

The heart & soul of change: 'what works in therapy'. Hubble M A, Duncan B L, Miller S L (eds). American Psychological Association, Washington, DC, 2002

'What works for whom?' A critical review of treatments for children and adolescents. Fanagg P, Target M, Cottrell D, Phillips J, Kirtz Z (eds). Guilford Press, New York, 2002

The Society for Psychotherapy Research (SpR) is an international scientific organisation which is dedicated to the promotion of research into all aspects of psychotherapy. It emphasises the inclusiveness of professions, level of training, theoretical orientation, and treatment modality. Further information is available from http://www.psychotherapyresearch.org

For patient/client self-help and information

Know your own mind. Knowles J. Pandora, London, 1991

REFERENCES

Anderson E M, Lambert M J 1995 Short term dynamically oriented psychotherapy: a review and meta-analysis. Clinical Psychology Review 15:503–514

Andrews G, Singh M, Bond M 1993 The Defense Style Questionnaire. Journal of Nervous & Mental Disease 181:246–256

Azim H F A, Piper W E, Segal P M et al 1991 The Quality of Object Relations Scale. Bulletin of the Menniger Clinic 55:323–343

Barkham M, Rees A, Shapiro D A et al 1996 Outcome of time-limited psychotherapy in applied settings: replicating the Second Sheffield Psychotherapy Project. Journal of Consulting and Clinical Psychology 64:1079–1085

Barkham M, Guthrie E, Hardy G et al 2004 Psychodynamic–interpersonal therapy. Sage

Beck A T 1964 Thinking and depression, II: Theory and therapy. Archives of General Psychiatry 10:561–571

Beck A T 1967 Depression: clinical, experimental and theoretical aspects. Harper & Row, New York

Beck A T 1987 Cognitive models of depression. Journal of Cognitive Psychotherapy I:5–37

Beck A T, Emery G 1985 Anxiety disorders and phobias: a cognitive perspective. Basic Books, New York

Beck A T, Freeman A 1990 Cognitive therapy of personality disorders. Basic Books, New York

Beck A T, Rush A J, Shaw B F, Emery G 1979 Cognitive therapy of depression. Guilford Press, New York

Blackburn I M 1988 An appraisal of comparative trials of cognitive therapy. In: Peris G, Blackburn I M (eds) Cognitive psychotherapy: theory and practice. Springer-Verlag, Heidelberg

Blackburn I M, Davidson K M 1990 Cognitive therapy for depression and anxiety: a practitioner's guide. Blackwell Scientific, Oxford

Bloch S (ed) 1979 Supportive psychotherapy. In: An introduction to the psychotherapies. Oxford University Press, London

Bloch A L, Shear K, Markowitz J C et al 1993 An empirical study of defense mechanisms in dysthymia. American Journal of Psychiatry 150:1194–1198

Bower P, Rowland N, Mellor Clark J et al 2002 The Cochrane Library Issue 4. Oxford

Brockman B, Poynton A, Ryle A et al 1987 Effectiveness of time-limited therapy carried out by trainees: comparison of two methods. British Journal of Psychiatry 151:602–609

Bryant R A, Harvey A G, Sackville T et al 1998 Treatment of acute stress disorder: a comparison of cognitive behavioral therapy and supportive counseling. American Journal of Psychiatry 156:1780–1786

Busch F N, Shear K, Cooper A M et al 1995 An empirical study of defense mechanisms in panic disorder. Journal of Nervous and Mental Disease 183:299–303

Butler G, Fennell M, Robson P, Gelder M 1991 Comparison of behavior therapy and cognitive therapy in the treatment of generalised anxiety disorder. Journal of Consulting and Clinical Psychology 59:167–175

Chambless D L, Gillis M M 1993 Cognitive therapy of anxiety disorders. Journal of Consulting & Clinical Psychology 61:248–260

Churchill R, Hunot V, Corney R et al 2001 A systematic review of controlled trials of the effectiveness and cost-effectiveness of brief psychological treatments for depression. Health Technology Assessments 5:35 (Executive summary)

Clark D M, Salkovskis P M, Hackmann A et al 1994 A comparison of cognitive therapy, applied relaxation and imipramine in the treatment of panic disorder. British Journal of Psychiatry 164:759–769

Conte H R, Plutchik R, Wild K V, Karasu T B 1986 Combined psychotherapy and pharmacotherapy for depression. Archives of General Psychiatry 43:471–479

Cooper N A, Clum G A 1989 Imaginal flooding as a supplementary treatment for PTSD in combat veterans: a controlled study. Behavior Therapy 20:381–391

Cottrell D, Boston P 2002 Practitioner review: the effectiveness of systemic family therapy for children and adolescents. Journal of Child Psychology & Psychiatry & Allied Disciplines 43(5):573–586

Coyne J, Gottlib I 1983 The role of cognition in depression: a critical appraisal. Psychological Bulletin 94:472–505

Crits-Christoph 1992 The efficacy of brief dynamic psychotherapy: a meta-analysis. American Journal of Psychiatry 49:151–158

Department of Health 1996 NHS psychotherapy services in England: review of strategic policy. HMSO, London

Department of Health 2000 National service framework for mental health. HMSO, London

Department of Health 2001 Treatment choice in psychological therapies and counselling. HMSO, London

Depression Guidelines Panel 1993 Depression in primary care: detection, diagnosis and treatment: quick reference guide for clinicians. Clinical Practice Guideline No 5, AHCPR publication No 93-0552. US Department of Health and Human Services, Public Health Service, Agency for Health Care Policy and Research, Rockville, MD

Diamond G S, Siqueland L 1995 Family therapy for the treatment of depressed adolescents. Psychotherapy 32:77–90 (special issue: Adolescent Treatment: New Frontiers and New Dimension)

Durham R C, Allan T 1993 Psychological treatment of generalized anxiety disorder: a review of the clinical significance of outcome studies since 1980. British Journal of Psychiatry 163:19–23

Durham R C, Murphy T, Allan T 1994 Cognitive therapy, analytic psychotherapy and anxiety management training for generalised anxiety disorder. British Journal of Psychiatry 115:315–323

Elkin I 1994 The NIMH treatment of depression collaboration research program: where we began and where we are. In: Bergin A E, Garfield S L (eds) Handbook of psychotherapy and behaviour change, 4th edn. Wiley, New York

Elkin I, Shea M T, Watkins J T et al 1989 National Institute for Mental Health Treatment of Depression Collaborative Research Program: general effectiveness of treatment. Archives of General Psychiatry 46:971–982

Ellis A 1962 Reason and emotion in psychotherapy. Citadel Press, Secaucus, NJ

Emmelkamp P M G 1994 Behavior therapy with adults. In: Bergin A E, Garfield S L (eds) Handbook of psychotherapy and behavior change, 4th edn. Wiley, New York

Erikson E H 1950 Identity and the life cycle. International Universities Press, New York

Fairbairn W R D 1954 An object-relations theory of personality: psychoanalytic studies of the personality. Basic Books, New York

Fairburn C G, Kirk J, O'Connor M 1986 A comparison of two psychological treatments for bulimia nervosa. Behaviour Research & Therapy 24:629–643

Fosbury J A 1994 Cognitive analytic therapy with poorly controlled type I diabetic patients. Paper presented at the European Association for the study of diabetes 27 September to 1 October, Dusseldorf, Germany

Gaston L, Gallagher D, Cournoyer L, Gagnon R 1998 Alliance, technique and their interactions in predicting outcome of behavioural, cognitive and brief dynamic therapy. Psychotherapy Research 8:190–209

Gould R A, Otto M W, Pollack M H 1995 A meta-analysis of treatment outcome for panic disorder. Clinical Psychology Review 15(8):819–844

Guntrip H 1969 Schizoid phenomena, object relations, and the self. International Universities Press, New York

Guthrie E, Creed F, Dawson D, Tomenson B 1991 A controlled trial of psychological treatment for the irritable bowel syndrome. Gastroenterology 100:450–457

Guthrie E, Moorey J, Margison F et al 1999 Cost-effectiveness of brief psychodynamic-interpersonal therapy in high utilizers of psychiatric services. Archives of General Psychiatry 56:519–526

Guthrie E, Kapur N, Mackway-Jones K et al 2001 Randomised controlled trial of brief psychological intervention after deliberate self poisoning. British Medical Journal 323:135–138

Hamilton J, Guthrie E, Creed F et al 2000 A randomized controlled trial of psychotherapy in patients with chronic functional dyspepsia. Gastroenterology 119:661–669

Hawton K, Salkovskis P M, Kirk J, Clark D M 1989 Cognitive behaviour therapy for psychiatric problems: a practical guide. Oxford University Press, Oxford

Heimberg R G, Dodge C S, Hope D A 1990 Cognitive behavioral treatment of social phobia: comparative to a credible placebo control. Cognitive Therapy & Research 14:1–23

Hobson R F 1985 Forms of feeling. Tavistock, London

Hollon S D, Du Rubeis R J, Evans M D et al 1992 Cognitive therapy and pharmacotherapy for depression: singly or in combination. Archives of General Psychiatry 49:774–781

Horowitz M J, Mibrath C, Stinson C H 1997 Assessing personality disorders. In: Strupp H H, Horowitz L M, Lambert M J (eds) Measuring patient changes. APA, Washington, DC, p 401–432

Horvath A O, Luborsky L 1993 The role of the therapeutic alliance in psychotherapy. Journal of Consulting & Clinical Psychology 61:561–573

Horvath A O, Symonds D B 1991 Relationship between working alliance and outcome in psychotherapy: a meta-analysis. Journal of Counselling Psychology 38:139–149

Jacobson E 1938 Progressive relaxation. University of Chicago Press, Chicago

Kernberg O 1980 Internal world and external reality: object relations theory applied. Aronson, New York

Kessel N 1979 Reassurance. Lancet i:1128

Klerman G L, Weissman M M 1993 New applications of interpersonal psychotherapy. American Psychiatric Press, Washington, DC

Klerman G L, Weissman M M, Rounsaville B J, Chevron E S 1984 Interpersonal psychotherapy of depression. Basic Books, New York

Kuipers L, Leff J, Lam D 1992 Family work for schizophrenia: a practical guide. Gaskell, London

Kupfer D J, Frank E, Perel J M et al 1992 Five year outcome for maintenance therapies in recurrent depression. Archives of General Psychiatry 49:769–773

Lambert M J, Bergin A E 1994 The effectiveness of psychotherapy. In: Bergin A E, Garfield S L (eds) Handbook of psychotherapy and behaviour change, 4th edn. Wiley, New York

Ledwidge B 1978 Cognitive behaviour modification: a step in the wrong direction. Psychological Bulletin 85:353–375

Lichstein K L 1988 Clinical relaxation strategies. Wiley, New York

Liddell A, di Fazio L, Blackwood J, Ackerman C 1994 Long-term follow-up of treated dental phobics. Behaviour Research Therapy 32:604–610

Luborsky L, Crits-Christoph P 1990 Understanding transference: the CCRT (The Core Conflictual Relationship Theme) method. Basic Books, New York

Lyon H M, Kaney S, Bentall R P 1994 The defensive function of persecutory delusions: evidence from attribution tasks. British Journal of Psychiatry 164:637–646

McCallum M, Piper W E 1997 The psychological mindedness assessment procedure. In: McCallum M, Piper W E (eds) Psychological mindedness. Lawrence Erlbaum, Hillsdale, NJ, p 27–58

Margison F, Hobson R F 1983 A conversational model of psychotherapy. (Videotapes) Tavistock, London

Markowitz J C, Kocsis B, Fishman L A et al 1998 Treatment of HIV-positive patients with depressive symptoms. Archives of General Psychiatry 55:452–457

Marks I M, Swinson R P, Basoglu M et al 1993 Alprazolam and exposure alone and combined in panic disorder with agoraphobia. Journal of Psychiatry 162:776–787

Martin D J, Garske J P, Davis M K 2000 Relation of the therapeutic alliance with outcome and other variables: a meta-analytic review. Journal of Consulting & Clinical Psychology 68:438–540

Moss S, Margison F, Godbert K 1991 The maintenance of psychotherapy skill acquisition: a 2 year follow-up. British Journal of Medical Psychology 64:233–236

Ørner R, Schnyder U 2003 Reconstruction early intervention after trauma. Oxford University Press, Oxford

Ost L G 1989 One session treatment for specific phobias. Behaviour Research & Therapy 25:397–409

Paris J, Zweig-Frank H, Bond M, Guzder J 1996 Defense styles, hostility and psychological risk factors in male patients with personality disorders. 184:153–158

Piper E R, Joyce A S, McCallum M, Hassan F A 1993 Concentration and correspondence of transference interpretations in short-term psychotherapy. Journal of Consulting & Clinical Psychology 61:586–595

Power K G, Simpson R J, Swanson V, Wallace C A 1990 A controlled comparison of cognitive behaviour therapy, diazepam, and placebo alone and in combination, for the treatment of generalised anxiety disorder. Journal of Anxiety Disorders 4:267–292

Quality Assurance Project 1983 A treatment outline for depressive disorders. Australian & New Zealand Journal of Psychiatry 17:129–146

Reynolds C F, Frank E, Perel J M et al 1992 Combined pharmacotherapy and psychotherapy in the acute and continuation treatment of elderly patients with recurrent major depression: a preliminary report. American Journal of Psychiatry 149:1687–1692

Richardson C A, Gilleard C J, Lieberman S, Peeler R 1994 Working with older adults and their families: a review. Journal of Family Therapy 16(3):225–240

Rose S, Bisson J, Wessely S 2002 Psychological debriefing for preventing post traumatic stress disorder (PTSD). The Cochrane Library, Issue 4, Oxford

Royal College of General Practitioners 1981 Prevention of psychiatric disorders in general practice. RCGP, London

Ryle A 1990 Cognitive-analytic therapy: active participation in change. Wiley, Chichester

Schnyder U, Orner R 2003 Reconstructing early intervention

Shapiro D, Firth J 1987 Prescriptive v exploratory psychotherapy: outcomes of the Sheffield Psychotherapy project. British Journal of Psychiatry 151:790–799

Shapiro D A, Barkham M, Rees A et al 1994 Effects of treatment duration and severity of depression on the effectiveness of cognitive-behavioural and psychodynamic-interpersonal psychotherapy. Journal of Consulting & Clinical Psychology 62:522–534

Shapiro D A, Rees A, Barkham M et al 1995 Effects of treatment duration and severity of depression on the maintenance of gains following cognitive-behavioural and psychodynamic-interpersonal psychotherapy. Journal of Consulting & Clinical Psychology 63:378–387

Shapiro F 1995 Eye movement desensitisation and reprocessing: basic principles, protocols and procedures. Guilford Press, New York

Steinbruek S M, Maxwell S E, Howard G S 1983 A meta-analysis of psychotherapy and drug therapy in the treatment of unipolar depression with adults. Journal of Consulting and Clinical Psychology 51:856–863

Strupp H M 1978 Psychotherapy research and practice – an overview. In: Bergin A E, Garfield S L (eds) Handbook of psychotherapy and behaviour change, 2nd edn. Wiley, New York

Svartberg M, Stiles T C 1991 Comparative effects of short-term psychotherapy: a meta-analysis. Journal of Consulting and Clinical Psychology, 59:704–714

Sullivan H S 1953 Interpersonal theory of psychiatry. Norton, New York

Truax C B, Carkhuff R R 1967 Toward effective counselling and psychotherapy: training and practice. Aldine, Chicago

Valliant G E, Bond M, Valliant O 1986 An empirically validated hierarchy of defense mechanisms. Archives of General Psychiatry 43:786

Wampold B E, Minami T, Baskin T W, Callen T S 2002 A meta (re)analysis of the effects of cognitive therapy versus 'other therapies' for depression. Journal of Affective Disorders 68(2–3): 159–165

Weissman M M, Markowitz J C, Klerman G L 2000 Comprehensive guide to interpersonal psychotherapy. Basic Behavioural Science. Basic Books, New York

Weisz J R, Donenberg E R, Man S S, Weiss B 1995 Bridging the gap between laboratories and clinic in child and adolescent psychotherapy. Journal of Consulting & Clinical Psychology 63:688–701

Wolpe J 1958 Psychotherapy by reciprocal inhibition. Stanford University Press, Stanford, CA

Woolfenden S R, Williams K, Peat J K 2002 Family and parenting interventions for conduct disorder and delinquency: a meta-analysis of randomised controlled trials. Journal of Pediatrics 141(5):738

17 | Organic disorders

Alan Carson, Adam Zeman, Tom Brown, Michael Sharpe

INTRODUCTION

At the interface between psychiatry and neurology lies a range of disorders that have been traditionally termed 'organic' in order to differentiate them from functional psychiatric disorders such as schizophrenia. Scientific advances have rendered this distinction an anachronism (Lipkin 1969) as few would dispute that organic changes in the brain underpin the psychopathology of traditional 'functional' disorders such as schizophrenia. And ironically, much less is understood about the neuropathology of many of the traditional 'organic' disorders, such as Gilles de la Tourette's syndrome, than about those disorders previously regarded as 'functional'. Although discarded in DSM-IV the category of 'organic disorders' has been retained in ICD-10 (F00–F09) and consequently we use it here. This chapter broadly follows the ICD-10 classification (Box 17.1). The pathology of the dementias is covered in detail in Chapter 4 and their management in Chapter 26. In relation to 'Other mental disorders due to brain damage and dysfunction and to physical disease (F06.0–9)', we have described the cognitive and psychological consequences of common neurological disorders that the psychiatrist is likely to encounter.

Clinical practice at this interface between psychiatry and neurology is often called neuropsychiatry. Neuropsychiatry is based on: (a) a systematic clinical approach to patient assessment, based on the known psychological and behavioural correlates of damage to different parts of the brain (Fig. 17.1) and (b) a clinical assessment not only of this impairment but also of the psychological and social factors associated with the subsequent disability and handicap (see Box 17.2)

This two-pronged assessment will generate both a diagnosis and a problem list. Together they form the essential prerequisite for the drawing up of individually tailored management plans. Because in many cases our ability to reverse the neuropathology giving rise to the impairment is limited, management focuses on addressing the psychological and social factors driving disability and handicap. Hence psychological, environmental and social interventions are as important in the management of the organic disorders as pharmacology. The principles behind psychological and behavioural interventions are described in Chapter 16. In this chapter we concentrate on pharmacological interventions but hope the reader will understand that both assessment and management require an appropriate multidisciplinary contribution.

CLINICAL ASSESSMENT

A systematic approach to clinical assessment is the basis of safe and effective practice. See also Chapter 13.

Cognitive examination

The cognitive examination is described briefly in Chapter 13. A somewhat more detailed description is given here as it is central to the assessment of organic disorders. It is organised according to the capacities it aims to assess, as follows.

Wakefulness

Wakefulness depends on normal cerebral arousal by the brainstem and thalamic ascending activating system. A subject whose conscious level is impaired will inevitably perform poorly on cognitive testing. The Glasgow Coma Scale (GCS) provides a widely used assessment tool which uses three parameters: eye opening, verbal responses and motor behaviour (Table 17.1).

Orientation

Orientation in place and time depends on multiple psychological functions, and a finding of disorientation therefore implies cognitive failure in one or several domains. It is helpful to test orientation near the start of the cognitive examination.

Attention

Attention can be 'sustained', 'selective', 'divided' or 'preparatory' or classified in terms of its object, for example 'spatial' and 'non-spatial'. The form most relevant to the cognitive examination is the sustained attention that allows us to concentrate, which depends on the concerted functioning of a number of brain regions, including subcortical arousal centres, frontal 'executive' regions and posterior sensory or language areas. Disruption of attention — often by factors that disturb brain function in a diffuse way, such as drugs, infection or organ failure — is the hallmark of a confusional state or 'delirium'. Sustained attention is best tested using moderately demanding, non-automatic tasks like reciting the months backwards or, as described in the Mini Mental State Examination (MMSE)

Box 17.1 ICD-10 organic disorders

F00–F09
Organic, including symptomatic, mental disorders
F00	Dementia in Alzheimer's disease
F01	Vascular dementia
F02	Dementia in other diseases classified elsewhere (Includes dementia in Pick's disease, Creutzfeldt–Jakob disease, Huntington's disease, Parkinson's disease, and human immunodeficiency virus [HIV] disease)
F03	Unspecified dementia
F04	Organic amnesic syndrome, not induced by alcohol and other psychoactive substances
F05	Delirium, not induced by alcohol and other psychoactive substances
F06	Other mental disorders due to brain damage and dysfunction and to physical disease (Includes organic psychoses and organic mood disorder)
F07	Personality and behavioural disorders due to brain disease, damage and dysfunction (Includes Organic personality disorder, Postencephalitic syndrome, and Postconcussional syndrome)
F09	Unspecified organic or symptomatic mental disorder

Box 17.2 WHO definitions of impairment, disability and handicap

Impairment:	The loss or abnormality of structure or function
Disability:	The restriction or lack of ability to perform an activity in the manner or within the range considered normal for a human being
Handicap:	The disadvantage for an individual that prevents or limits the performance of a role that is normal for that individual

Table 17.1 The Glasgow Coma Scale

Feature	Scale responses	Score
Eye opening	Spontaneous	4
	To speech	3
	To pain	2
	None	1
Best verbal response	Orientated	5
	Confused conversation	4
	Words (inappropriate)	3
	Sounds (incomprehensible)	2
	None	1
Best motor response	Obey commands	5
	Localise pain	4
	Flexion to pain	3
	Abnormal flexion	2
	Extension to pain	2
	None	1
Total coma 'score'		**3–15**

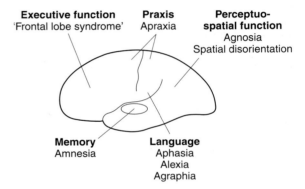

Fig. 17.1
Functional topography of the cerebral cortex, and the various syndromes that arise from impairment in particular areas.

(Folstein et al 1975), spelling *WORLD* backwards or subtracting 7 serially from 100.

Memory

Figure 17.2 depicts a widely accepted taxonomy of memory. There is an important distinction between explicit or declarative memory and implicit or procedural memory. Declarative memories can be articulated whereas procedural memories are enacted, as when, for example you ride a bicycle. Working (or 'short-term') declarative memory allows you to keep information in mind while you use it, for example remembering a telephone number from looking it up in the directory to dialling it. Long-term declarative memory is divided into episodic, the memory for unique events like your last holiday, and semantic, the database of knowledge about language and the world which we constantly use to interpret what we perceive. These distinctions have a neurobiological basis. Working memory depends on frontal executive structures which direct attention, and posterior areas relevant to the material being rehearsed. The acquisition of new long-term declarative memories requires the integrity of limbic regions connected in the 'circuit of Papez' (Fig. 17.3), particularly the hippocampus and adjacent structures in the medial temporal lobes, the fornix and the anteromedial thalamus. Damage to these structures underlies the classical 'amnestic syndrome'. Procedural memory is

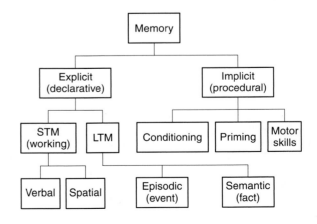

Fig. 17.2
A taxonomy of memory. LTM, long-term memory; STM, short-term memory.

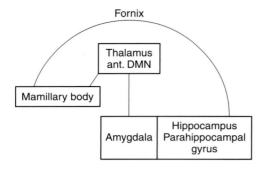

Fig. 17.3
Schematic diagram of the 'circuit of Papez' linking limbic structures essential to the formation of new long-term declarative memories. ant. DMN, anterior and dorsomedial nuclei.

substantially independent of declarative memory and is based in different brain structures — including the cerebellum, which mediates classical conditioning, and the basal ganglia.

Memory is usually tested clinically by asking the patient to register information, such as a name and address or three words (working memory), and to recall the same information after an interval of at least one minute, while performing other mental tasks to prevent rehearsal. General knowledge questions are often asked to tap semantic memory (which is also probed by questions requiring visual recognition and naming).

Executive function

'Executive function' refers to the complex of abilities which allow us to plan, initiate, organise and monitor our thoughts and behaviour. These abilities, which are located mainly in the frontal lobes, are essential for normal social performance. Functional subdivisions are recognised within the frontal lobes. Motor and premotor areas in and adjacent to Brodmann Area 4 more or less directly govern movement. Dorsolateral prefrontal cortex, lying anterior to motor and premotor cortex is particularly involved in attention, working memory and organisation of thought and behaviour; orbitofrontal cortex is concerned with regulation of social behaviour; medial frontal cortex, including the anterior cingulate gyrus, is closely connected to the limbic system and mediates motivation and arousal.

Frontal lobe disorders are notoriously difficult to test but often make themselves apparent in social interaction with the patient. Specific tasks which can be used to clarify deficits in frontal lobe function include:

- verbal fluency, for example listing as many animals as possible in one minute;
- motor sequencing, for example asking a patient to copy a sequence of three hand positions;
- the go–no-go task, requiring the patient to tap the desk once if the examiner taps once, but not to tap if the examiner taps twice;
- tests of abstraction ('what do a tree and a snail have in common?').

Language

The left hemisphere is dominant for language in almost all right-handed persons and also in most left-handers. The brain areas critical for language cluster around the Sylvian fissure ('perisylvian area'), and include three main components:

- Broca's area in the inferior frontal lobe, required for fluent language production;
- Wernicke's area, in the posterior superior temporal lobe, required for language comprehension;
- the arcuate fasciculus, the white matter tract which connects them.

Damage to Broca's area causes dysphasia characterised by effortful, dysfluent speech with reduced use of 'function words' (prepositions, articles, etc.) and 'phonemic paraphasias' (incorrect words approximating to the correct one in sound), with well-preserved comprehension. Damage to Wernicke's area produces a dysphasia characterised by fluent speech with both phonemic and semantic paraphasias (incorrect words approximating to the correct one in meaning) and poor comprehension. The stream of incoherent speech and lack of insight in patients with Wernicke's dysphasia sometimes leads to misdiagnosis of a primary thought disorder and consequently to a general psychiatric referral: the clue to the diagnosis of a language disorder in such cases is the severity of the comprehension deficit. Global dysphasia combines features of Broca's and Wernicke's dysphasias. Damage to the arcuate fasciculus leads to a conduction aphasia in which speech is normal but repetition markedly defective. The non-dominant hemisphere also plays a part in speech by enabling the appreciation of the emotional overtones of language.

When assessing dysphasia, first listen to the characteristics of the patient's speech (is it dysfluent or paraphasic?), then assess their comprehension. Naming is impaired in both major varieties of dysphasia, and 'anomia' can be the clue to mild dysphasia. Selective impairment of repetition characterises 'conduction aphasia'. In 'transcortical' dysphasia, repetition is spared, but damage closely adjacent to Broca's or Wernicke's area causes patterns of deficit otherwise typical of Broca's or Wernicke's dysphasia. It can also be helpful to assess reading and writing ability. The main dysphasic syndromes are described in Table 17.2.

Arithmetic

Arithmetical skills are located in the dominant hemisphere, particularly in the region of the angular gyrus, in the inferior parietal lobe. Damage to the angular gyrus gives rise to Gerstmann's syndrome of dyscalculia, dysgraphia (difficulty with writing), confusion of left and right, and 'finger agnosia' (difficulty in identifying individual fingers).

Praxis

'Praxis' refers to the ability to perform skilled actions. Dyspraxia is the inability to perform skilled actions despite intact basic motor and sensory abilities. Knowledge of how to do such things as use a screwdriver or brush teeth depends on areas in the frontal and parietal lobes of the dominant hemisphere. Dysphasia and dyspraxia often occur together. These abilities can be tested by asking a subject to mime actions, and by asking him to copy unfamiliar hand positions.

'Gait apraxia' is difficulty in initiating and maintaining gait despite intact basic motor function of the legs, and is associated with bilateral medial frontal pathology, caused, for example, by hydrocephalus.

Table 17.2 Classification of dysphasic syndromes

Aphasia type	Fluency	Comprehension	Repetition	Naming
Global	+	+	+	+
Broca's	+	–	+	+
Wernicke's	–	+	+	+
Conduction	–	–	+	+
Transcortical sensory	–	+	–	+
Transcortical motor	+	–	–	+
Anomic	–	–	–	+

+, affected; –, relatively spared.
After Hodges (1994).

'Dressing apraxia' describes a difficulty in dressing caused by inability to puzzle out the spatial arrangement of clothes in relation to the body and is a perceptual rather than a motor dysfunction.

Perception

The right hemisphere is 'dominant' in tasks requiring an appreciation of spatial relationships. The syndrome of 'neglect' involves a failure to attend to or act towards the side of space contralateral to a brain lesion; as this is usually in the right hemisphere, it is usually the left side of space that is neglected. The right hemisphere is also dominant in other perceptual tasks. 'Prosopagnosia', for example, a selective difficulty in recognising familiar faces, is more common after right than left hemisphere damage. Agnosia is difficulty in recognising objects where basic sensory functions are intact. Agnosia can be 'apperceptive', if relatively 'early' processes of percept formation are involved, or 'associative' if the failure lies in perceptual memory. Associative agnosias merge into deficits of semantic memory. Perception is tested using naming tasks, which depend on both recognition and name finding, and by testing copying, which taps perceptual as well as motor processes.

Standard assessment instruments

The Mini-Mental State Examination (MMSE) (Folstein et al 1975) is the most widely used brief instrument, The Addenbrooke's Cognitive Examination is a more extensive 'bedside' battery (Mathuranath et al 2000). Both are described in detail in Chapter 26.

Neurological examination

Psychiatrists should be able to perform a competent basic neurological examination, as this often provides the crucial clues to a neuropsychiatric diagnosis. A neurological examination for psychiatrists is described in Chapter 13. Here we highlight some findings of particular relevance to the assessment of organic psychiatric disorders.

Dyskinesias

Involuntary — or semi-voluntary — movements of face, trunk or limbs are known as 'dyskinesias'. The family of dyskinesias includes several types:

- *Tics* are habitual, usually jerky, movements which can be voluntarily suppressed for a time.
- *Myoclonus* describes rapid, 'shock-like', muscle contractions which can be focal or generalised (we all experience generalised myoclonus from time to time as we drop off to sleep).
- *Tremor* is rhythmic alternating contraction of agonist and antagonist muscles, occurring with the arms outstretched in 'postural tremor', often due to benign familial tremor, or at rest in the pill-rolling tremor of Parkinson's disease, or when nearing a target in the 'intention tremor' of cerebellar disease.
- *Chorea* describes the fidgety, changeful, distal movements which accompany some disorders of the basal ganglia such as Huntington's disease (*athetosis* is the proximal equivalent of chorea, *hemiballismus* its pathological extreme).
- *Dystonia*, relatively sustained abnormalities of posture, occurring focally in writer's cramp or torticollis, globally in generalised dystonia, is also thought to reflect basal ganglia dysfunction.
- *Tardive* orofacial dyskinesia sometimes induced by antipsychotics is particularly familiar to psychiatrists.

Abnormalities of gait

Characteristic patterns include:

- the flexed, unsteady, small-stepping gait of Parkinson's disease with diminished arm swing;
- the broad based, unsteady gait of cerebellar disease;
- the lurching, chaotic gait of Huntington's chorea;
- the stiff-legged, scissoring gait of upper motor neuron dysfunction ('spasticity');
- the failure of 'gait ignition' in gait apraxia, due for example to hydrocephalus;
- the high-stepping gait accompanying foot drop.

Abnormalities of visual fields and eye movements

Markedly reduced acuity of recent onset should raise suspicion of a central scotoma linked to optic nerve disease, for example in multiple sclerosis. A hemianopia to left or to right present in both eyes' fields ('homonymous') points to pathology behind the optic chiasm, probably within the hemispheres. A hemianopia affecting the temporal field in each eye (bitemporal) suggests pathology at the chiasm, most often due to compression by a pituitary tumour.

Palsies of gaze, for example inability to direct either eye to one side, indicate pathology in the brainstem or in tracts descending to the brainstem from the hemispheres. Inability to trigger rapid voluntary vertical eye movements ('saccadic' movements) is an early feature of progressive supranuclear palsy.

Pyramidal signs

Dysfunction of the 'pyramidal tracts', the direct descending pathway from the motor cortex to the brainstem and spinal cord, gives rise to 'upper motor neuron signs'. These are increased tone in the limbs with a 'clasp-knife' or 'catch-and-give' quality, weakness particularly affecting extensor muscles in the arms and flexors in the legs, excessively brisk reflexes and extensor (upgoing) plantar reflexes. Such signs are commonly seen after stroke and in multiple sclerosis. Pyramidal signs in the limbs may be associated with 'pyramidal' dysfunction of bulbar muscles (a 'pseudo-bulbar palsy', giving rise to dysphagia and dysarthria), and with lability of emotional expression or 'pseudo-bulbar affect' (easily provoked 'pathological' crying).

Frontal 'release' signs

Certain 'primitive' reflexes can be released by impairment of frontal lobe function. These include the pout reflex (a pouting movement stimulated by stroking the upper lip or tapping the lips), the grasp reflex (flexion of the patient's hand around the examiner's finger despite a request 'not to grip'), and the palmomental reflex (puckering of the ipsilateral chin in response to drawing an orange stick briskly across the thenar eminence). These reflexes should be regarded as abnormal in young adult patients, but can return with advancing age. They may accompany the behavioural abnormalities associated with the frontal lobes or their connections.

Extrapyramidal signs

Dysfunction of the basal ganglia (caudate, putamen, globus pallidus and linked subcortical regions) can cause either a 'negative' or a 'positive' neurological syndrome. The negative syndrome is typified by Parkinson's disease, with difficulty in initiating and slowness in performing movements (bradykinesia), reduction of automatic movements such as facial expression and arm swing, increased limb tone with a 'lead-pipe' or cogwheeling quality (rigidity), rest tremor and postural instability. The positive syndrome, typified by Huntington's disease, or over-treated Parkinson's disease, involves an excess of movement with choreo-athetosis. The neurological signs of basal ganglia disease are often accompanied by psychological symptoms such as slowing of cognition in Parkinson's disease and impulsivity in Huntington's chorea.

Cerebellar signs

Cerebellar dysfunction impairs the coordination of movement. Signs include nystagmus, dysarthria, gait ataxia, inco-ordination of limb movements (e.g. 'finger–nose') and impairment of rapid alternating movements (e.g. tapping with one hand on the upper and lower surface of the other hand alternately). The role of the cerebellum in co-ordinating thought and emotion as well as movement is a focus of current research.

Lower motor neuron signs

These result from disorders affecting the brainstem, spinal cord or peripheral nerves, for example in patients with peripheral neuropathies. The signs are muscle wasting and fasciculation, muscle weakness which is often generalised, and loss of reflexes. Disorders causing lower motor neuron signs can also be associated with impairment of brain function, for example in dementia associated with motor neuron disease, leucodystrophies and HIV infection.

Sensory signs

Sensory signs are generally the least reliable or helpful neurological findings. They can, however, occasionally give useful clues — as, for example, loss of joint position and vibration sense in a patient with dementia due to vitamin B_{12} deficiency.

General medical examination

Like the neurological examination, a careful general medical examination should be a routine part of the assessment of organic psychiatric disorders. The cause of dementia, for example, may come to light when pallor (due to the anaemia of vitamin B_{12} deficiency), lymphadenopathy (associated with HIV infection), slow pulse (of hypothyroidism), hypertension (causing subcortical ischaemia), or a testicular tumour (associated with paraneoplastic limbic encephalitis) is detected.

THE DEMENTIAS

Definition

Dementia is defined as a syndrome due to disease of the brain, usually of chronic or progressive nature, in which there is disturbance of multiple higher cortical functions but no clouding of consciousness. The nature and management of the senile dementias of Alzheimer's, vascular, and Lewy body types are described in detail in Chapter 26.

A clinical approach to the diagnosis of dementia

Careful clinical assessment will reveal the diagnosis in the majority of patients with complaints which raise a suspicion of dementia and should include:

- a history-taking from the patient, which both supplies relevant factual information and provides an opportunity to appraise cognitive function;
- a history from an informant, which is essential in the assessment of all patients with cognitive complaints;
- a general medical, neurological and mental-state assessment including a cognitive examination.

In our own memory clinic this assessment is performed jointly by a neurologist and a psychiatrist who see patients consecutively; the total assessment takes around 90 minutes.

Three key questions need to be answered by the clinical assessment:

- Is there a significant cognitive problem? A proportion of the patients referred will be 'worried well'; if so, clinical assessment and reassurance may be all that is needed.

- Is there a psychiatric diagnosis other than dementia, in particular does the patient have a depressive or anxiety disorder? The presence of these does not rule out concomitant dementia, but early recognition of psychiatric disorder is helpful, as it may be treated. Sometimes the mood disorder will turn out lie at the root of the cognitive symptoms.
- If dementia is present, what is its cause? Will clinical assessment and 'standard' investigations (see below) suffice to establish a specific diagnosis, or is a more intensive approach required?

History-taking

As well as documenting the details of the cognitive disorder, it is important to obtain a good background medical and psychiatric history, including previous episodes of affective illness, a history of vascular disease, or the consumption of prescribed or recreational drugs. Each of these could point to the cause of a patient's cognitive impairment. Both patient and informant should be interviewed alone. We generally find it convenient to take the initial history with both present, then to interview the informant alone, and finally to perform the examination with the patient alone. The aspects of the history to be covered are listed in Box 17.3.

Examination

The approach to clinical examination is outlined above and in Chapter 13. However, it should be remembered that both a gen-

eral medical and neurological examination is required. The medical examination may contribute important diagnostic information. The mental-state examination should always include a cognitive assessment. While the MMSE is the minimum required, it should be remembered that it is insensitive to early cognitive decline in people with high IQ, and also insensitive to impairment in some cognitive domains, for example praxis and executive function. We have described supplements to the MMSE above.

Investigations

Where the clinical assessment suggests that a dementia is likely, most patients will be suffering from one of the three most common causes: Alzheimer's disease, vascular dementia, or Lewy body disease. If the clinical features are in keeping with one of these diagnoses, a set of 'standard' investigations (Box 17.4) will generally suffice to support the diagnosis and exclude several of the more readily reversible causes of dementia (Box 17.5). These relatively inexpensive tests should be performed unless there is a good reason not to. It is a moot point whether formal neuropsychological testing should always be requested; careful 'bedside' cognitive assessment is often sufficient in straightforward cases.

More intensive investigation will generally be required if an unusual cause is suspected. The clinical features which should excite suspicion of an unusual cause include:

- early onset (under the age of 65);
- rapid progression (beyond the approximate 3 point annual decrement on the MMSE which is expected in Alzheimer's disease);

Box 17.3   History-taking in dementia

Enquire (from patient, informant, or both) about:
- Course and duration of symptoms
- Cognitive symptoms:
  — Concentration: ?absent mindedness and slips of attention
  — Memory: episodic, semantic
  — Executive function: planning and organisation of activities
  — Language: word-finding, comprehension, reading, writing
  — Calculation: finances
  — Spatial/perceptual function: route finding, face recognition
  — Praxis: ?preserved motor skills
- Psychological and behavioural symptoms:
  — Personality change
  — Mood disturbance
  — Psychotic phenomena
  — Altered eating habits
  — Sleep disturbance
  — Altered sexual behaviour
- Activities of daily living:
  — Washing
  — Dressing
  — Shopping
  — Cooking
  — Housework
  — Work
  — Driving
  — Hobbies
  — Social activities

Box 17.4   'Standard' investigations in dementia

- Neuroimaging:
  — CT or MRI
- Blood screen:
  — FBC, ESR
  — U+E, LFT, Ca
  — Glucose, cholesterol
  — B_{12} and folate
  — Thyroid function
  — Syphilis serology

Box 17.5   Reversible causes of dementia

- Wilson's disease
- Whipple's disease
- Hashimoto's encephalopathy
- Vasculitis
- Hydrocephalus, chronic subdurals, benign CNS tumours
- Hypothyroidism
- Vitamin deficiencies, e.g. B_{12} deficiency
- Prescribed and recreational drugs
- Obstructive sleep apnoea
- Depression

NB: This list highlights causes which can sometimes be *reversed*; several other causes of dementia can be *treated* medically with some success, e.g. Alzheimer's disease, Lewy body disease and HIV-related dementia.

Table 17.3   Delirium versus dementia

Feature	Delirium	Dementia
Onset	Acute or subacute	Insidious
Course	Fluctuating	Slowly progressive
Duration	Hours–weeks	Months–years
Alertness	Abnormally low or high	Typically normal
Sleep–wake cycle	Disrupted	Typically normal
Attention	Impaired	Relatively normal
Orientation	Impaired	Intact in early dementia
Working (ST) memory	Impaired	Intact in early dementia
Episodic (LT) memory	Impaired	Impaired
Thinking	Disorganised, delusional	Impoverished
Speech	Slow or rapid, incoherent	Word-finding difficulty
Perception	Illusions, hallucinations common	Typically unimpaired in early dementia (LBD is an exception)
Behaviour	Withdrawn or agitated	Varies with type of dementia but often intact in early stages

LBD, Lewy body disease; LT, long-term; ST, short-term.
After Hodges (1994).

Box 17.6   Additional investigations which may be helpful in atypical dementia

- Formal psychometric assessment
- Neuroimaging: MRI, SPECT
- Other imaging: e.g. CXR
- Specialised blood tests, e.g.
  — Genetic testing, e.g. Huntington's, CADASIL, mitochondrial disorders, familial AD, familial prion dementia
  — White-cell enzyme studies in leucodystrophy
  — HIV test
  — Connective tissue serology in suspected CNS inflammation, e.g. ESR, antinuclear factor (ANF), anticardiolipin antibodies, antineutrophil cytoplasmic antibodies (ANCA), antibodies to extractable nuclear antigens (ENA), rheumatoid factors, complement fractions
  — Antithyroid antibodies in suspected Hashimoto's encephalopathy
  — Caeruloplasmin in suspected Wilson's disease
- EEG
- CSF examination
- Brain biopsy

CADASIL, cerebral autosomal-dominant arteriopathy with subcortical infarcts and leucoencephalopathy.

- a family history of the presence of systemic or neurological features other than those associated with the three common dementias;
- the presence of certain distinctive combinations of features: for example, limb apraxia, myoclonus and alien limb phenomena in corticobasal degeneration; or dysarthria, dysphagia and personality change in the frontal lobe dementia linked with motor neuron disease.

Where an atypical cause is suspected, but its nature is unclear, a range of further tests is worth considering (Box 17.6).

Diagnosis

It is helpful to bear in mind two major distinctions during the clinical assessment of patients with possible dementia. The first is the distinction between delirium (or 'confusion') and dementia (Table 17.3). The presence of dementia is a risk factor for delirium, and some dementing illnesses, notably Lewy body disease, incorporate elements of delirium. However, the causes and management of delirium and dementia are largely distinct, and the separation is therefore useful.

The second distinction is between cortical and subcortical dementias (Table 17.4). Cortical dementias, such as Alzheimer's disease, and some cases of cerebrovascular dementia, disrupt the 'modules' of cognitive function identified in the first section of this chapter — language, praxis, perception, etc. The classical syndromes of 'dysphasia', 'dyspraxia', 'agnosia' ensue. In subcortical dementias these cortical functions remain more or less intact, but their subcortical activation and interaction are impaired: the cardinal feature of the resulting cognitive impairment is *slowness*, often accompanied by behavioural change reminiscent of the apathy and inertia which can follow damage to the frontal lobes. Subcortical cognitive impairment of this kind is seen in disorders as varied as 'small vessel' cerebrovascular disease, multiple sclerosis, HIV infection, Huntington's disease and progressive supranuclear palsy. The distinction between 'cortical' and 'subcortical' dementias can be helpfully refined by recognising that some 'cortico-subcortical' disorders combine features of both (for example Lewy body dementia and prion dementia). Box 17.7 lists causes of dementia.

Inherited dementias

Huntington's disease

Definition   Huntington's disease (HD), also known as Huntington's chorea, was first described in Long Island in 1872 by George Huntington. This dominantly inherited disorder, which causes a combination of progressive motor, cognitive, psychiatric

Table 17.4 Cortical and subcortical dementia

Function	Cortical dementia, e.g. Alzheimer's disease	Subcortical dementia, e.g. Huntington's disease
Alertness	Normal	'Slowed up'
Attention	Normal in early stages	Impaired
Executive function	Normal in early stages	Impaired
Episodic (LT) memory	Amnesia	Forgetfulness (improves with cueing)
Language	Aphasic features	Normal except for reduced output
Praxis	Apraxia	Normal
Perception, visuospatial abilities	Impaired	Impaired
Personality	Preserved (unless frontal type)	Apathetic, inert

After Hodges (1994).

Box 17.7 Causes of dementia

Inherited
- Huntington's disease
- Wilson's disease
- Leucodystrophies

Acquired
- Primary degenerative dementias
  - Alzheimer's disease
  - Dementia with Lewy bodies
  - Frontotemporal lobar degeneration (including Pick's disease)
  - Progressive supranuclear palsy
  - Corticobasal degeneration
- Vascular dementia
  - Multi-infarct
  - Subcortical
  - Strategic infarction
- Infective
  - HIV
  - Transmissible spongiform encephalopathies (prion dementias)
  - Herpes simplex encephalitis
  - Whipple's disease
  - SSPE

- Inflammatory
  - Multiple sclerosis
  - Vasculitis
  - Hashimoto's encephalopathy
- Neoplastic
  - Primary and metastatic CNS tumours
  - Paraneoplastic: limbic encephalitis
- Traumatic
  - Post head-injury
- Structural
  - Hydrocephalus
  - Chronic subdurals
- Metabolic/endocrine
  - Hypothyroidism
- Deficiency disorders
  - Vitamin B_{12}/folate deficiency
- Sleep-related
  - Obstructive sleep apnoea
- Substance-induced
  - Alcohol
  - Anticholinergics, antiepileptics, neuroleptics, hypnotics, etc.
- Psychiatric
  - Depression ('pseudodementia)

SSPE, subacute sclerosing panencephalitis.
NB: This simple classification of the causes of dementia is for dementia defined as significant cognitive impairment affecting more than one cognitive domain, which is not primarily due to delirium. The list is not comprehensive, but the great majority of the causes of dementia fall under the categories listed. All dementias can be palliated; this list also includes causes which are potentially reversible, for example hydrocephalus, Wilson's disease and sleep apnoea. Rarely, some of the 'acquired' dementias listed here can be inherited (e.g. dominantly inherited Alzheimer's disease, inherited frontotemporal dementia, and some prionopathies; see text).

---

and behavioural dysfunction results from an abnormality in the *IT-15* gene on chromosome 4 encoding the protein Huntingtin.

Epidemiology Huntington's disease occurs with a prevalence of approximately 6 per 100 000, with wide regional variation. The sexes are affected equally. Onset can occur at any age, but most commonly in young or middle adulthood. The disorder exhibits 'anticipation', that is the age of onset tends to decrease through the generations, especially with paternal transmission (see below).

Clinical features Chorea, involuntary fidgety movements of the face and limbs, is the characteristic motor disorder. As the disease progresses, other extrapyramidal features, including rigidity, dystonia and bradykinesia, can develop, with associated dysphagia,

dysarthria and pyramidal signs. Epilepsy can occur. Cognitive dysfunction goes hand in hand with the motor disorder. The dementia is predominantly 'subcortical', with impairment of attention, executive function, speed of processing, and memory. Psychiatric symptoms and behavioural change are common: depression, apathy and aggressivity occur very commonly, with psychosis, obsessional behaviour and suicide in a significant minority. Progression to a state of immobility and dementia typically occurs over 15–20 years. Cognitive and behavioural change may predate the clear-cut emergence of more obvious symptoms.

Pathology and aetiology The epicentre of the pathology lies in the striatum, the caudate and putamen. The loss of small neurons in the striatum is accompanied by loss of neurons in the cerebral cortex, cerebral atrophy, ventricular dilatation and, eventually, neuronal depletion throughout the basal ganglia. The underlying genetic abnormality is expansion of a 'base triplet repeat' within the *Huntingtin* gene. The function of Huntingtin remains uncertain.

Investigation and differential diagnosis A number of disorders can cause a combination of chorea and cognitive change, including other inherited disorders such as neuroacanthocytosis and dentato-rubro-pallido-luysian atrophy (DRPLA), and acquired disorders such as SLE. The diagnosis can now be made with confidence by DNA analysis. Counselling by a clinical geneticist is mandatory before pre-symptomatic testing and should also be considered in other circumstances.

Management Patients may seek treatment for the chorea but this is usually best avoided, given the psychological and extrapyramidal side-effects of the agents required — antipsychotics, dopamine-depletors such as tetrabenazine, or benzodiazepines. Other psychological and behavioural symptoms should be treated in the usual way.

Wilson's disease (hepatolenticular degeneration)

Definition First described by Wilson in 1912, Wilson's disease is a rare, autosomal-recessive, progressive but eminently treatable disorder of copper metabolism, causing personality change, cognitive decline, an extrapyramidal disorder and cirrhosis of the liver.

Epidemiology Wilson's disease is rare, with a prevalence of 1 in 30 000 live births, and is distributed worldwide. Because there is a high mortality associated with failure to diagnose the disease the point prevalence is lower than frequency at birth.

Clinical features The onset of Wilson's disease is most common in childhood or adolescence but can be as late as the fifth decade. It can present to psychiatrists with personality change, behavioural disturbance, including psychosis, or dementia, and to neurologists with a variety of extrapyramidal features, including tremor, dysarthria and drooling, rigidity, bradykinesia and dystonia. In virtually all symptomatic cases, there are 'Kayser–Fleischer rings', rings of greenish-brown copper pigment at the edge of the cornea (in suspected cases an ophthalmologist should be asked to look for this with a slit lamp). Liver failure and the psychiatric symptoms can occur together or independently.

Pathology and aetiology The causative mutation is in the copper-transporting P-type ATPase coded on chromosome 13. The result is excessive copper deposition in brain, cornea, liver and kidneys and increased copper excretion in urine. The globus pallidus and putamen (together known as the lenticular nucleus) are most severely affected, but the other basal ganglia and the cerebral cortex are also involved.

Investigation and differential diagnosis Almost all patients have low levels of the copper-binding protein, caeruloplasmin, in the serum. A normal caeruloplasmin and the absence of Kayser–Fleischer rings render the diagnosis very unlikely. Difficult cases may require measurement of urinary copper excretion, and liver biopsy for measurement of copper content. The differential diagnosis varies with the type of presentation. The combination of psychological disturbance and unusual neurological features has led to misdiagnosis as conversion disorder.

Management Copper-chelating agents are effective but carry a risk of significant side-effects. Penicillamine is currently the most widely used agent; alternatives include tetraethylene tetramine (trientine) and zinc acetate.

Leucodystrophies

Leucodystrophies, recessively inherited or X-linked disorders of myelination, can present with psychiatric symptoms, usually with associated neurological symptoms.

Degenerative dementias

Frontotemporal lobar degeneration (including Pick's disease)

Definition This group of disorders is of importance to psychiatrists, as personality change and behavioural disturbance may be the presenting features. The frontotemporal dementias (FTDs) are a clinically and pathologically diverse group of focal dementias presenting with either features of frontal lobe dysfunction or features of temporal lobe dysfunction or both.

Epidemiology Although a rare cause of dementia overall, frontotemporal dementia (FTD) accounts for approximately 10–15% of cases occurring before the age of 65. Some cases are familial.

Clinical features

Dementia of 'frontal type', or 'frontal variant FTD', is characterised by the features listed in Box 17.8. The temporal lobe variant presents most commonly with 'semantic dementia', a syndrome of progressive word-finding difficulty, loss of language comprehension, depletion of conceptual knowledge (apparent on non-verbal as well as verbal tests), and impairment of object recognition. These features reflect left temporal lobe dysfunction. If the right temporal lobe is more severely affected, prosopagnosia (impaired face recognition) and loss of knowledge about people may be especially prominent.

Pathology and aetiology Several types of pathology can underlie the symptoms of FTD. The five principal types are:

Box 17.8   Criteria for a diagnosis of dementia of frontal type

- Presentation with an insidious disorder of personality and behaviour
- The presence of two or more of the following features: loss of insight, disinhibition, restlessness, distractibility, emotional lability, reduced empathy or unconcern for others, lack of foresight, poor planning or judgement, impulsivity, social withdrawal, apathy or lack of spontaneity, poor self-care, reduced verbal output, verbal stereotypes or echolalia, perseveration, features of Kluver–Bucy syndrome (gluttony, pica, sexual hyperactivity)
- Relative preservation of day-to-day (episodic) memory
- Psychiatric phenomena may be present (mood disorder, paranoia)
- Absence of past history of head injury, stroke, alcohol abuse or major psychiatric illness

After Gregory & Hodges 1993.

- classical Pick's disease pathology, with tau- and ubiquitin-positive cortical inclusions (Pick bodies) and ballooned neurons;
- neuronal loss with microvacuolation of outer cortical layers and astrocytosis;
- tau-positive inclusions in neuronal and glial cells in familial FTD with parkinsonism, linked to mutations in the *tau* gene on chromosome 17;
- motor neuron disease type pathology;
- corticobasal degeneration (CBD) type pathology (see below).

The role of tau protein accumulation in Pick's disease, inherited FTD linked to chromosome 17, and CBD, is a focus of current research.

Investigation and differential diagnosis Neuropsychological examination is particularly helpful in identifying these clinical syndromes. Imaging should reveal corresponding focal atrophy. A younger person presenting with an atypical dementia requires a full neuropsychiatric assessment.

Management There is no proven specific treatment for these conditions (with the possible exception of riluzole for motor neuron disease).

Progressive supranuclear palsy

Progressive supranuclear palsy (PSP) is characterised by: a supranuclear gaze palsy (inability to direct eye movements voluntarily, especially vertical eye movements, in the presence of normal reflex eye movements); truncal rigidity, akinesia, postural instability and early falls; bulbar features, with dysarthria and dysphagia; subcortical dementia and changes in mood, personality and behaviour. Neurofibrillary tangles, consisting of tau protein, are found in neurons of the basal ganglia and brainstem. Midbrain atrophy may be apparent on MRI.

Corticobasal degeneration

Corticobasal degeneration typically presents with a combination of limb apraxia, usually asymmetric at onset, alien limb phenomena, limb myoclonus, parkinsonism and cognitive decline. The pathology involves neuronal loss in both the basal ganglia and the frontal and parietal cortex, with intraneuronal accumulations of tau protein resembling those seen in PSP. MRI usually reveals frontoparietal atrophy.

Infective dementias

Human immunodeficiency virus-1 (HIV-1) infection

Definition Human immunodeficiency virus-1 which causes the acquired immunodeficiency syndrome, or AIDS, can cause a dementing illness or HIV-1-associated dementia. This is the AIDS-defining illness in approximately 5% of patients with AIDS.

Epidemiology About one quarter of patients with AIDS will present with or develop HIV-1-associated dementia. Dementia develops within 2 years of the AIDS-defining illness in about half these patients. Given the global prevalence of HIV-1 infection, it is a major cause of dementia in young people worldwide.

Clinical features The dementia is usually subcortical and presents insidiously. Difficulty with concentration, forgetfulness, cognitive slowing, apathy and social withdrawal are early features.

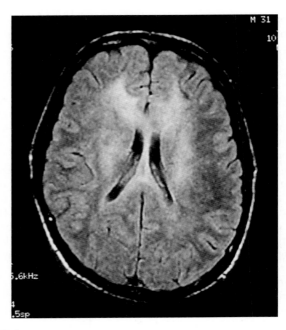

Fig. 17.4
MRI scans in HIV-1 dementia typically reveal cerebral atrophy with regions of increased signal in the white matter and basal ganglia.

Global dementia eventually ensues. Neurological features, including pyramidal and cerebellar signs, appear as the dementia progresses. A milder disorder, HIV-1-associated minor cognitive/motor disorder, which is not an AIDS-defining illness, is also recognised.

Pathology and aetiology HIV-1 virus crosses the blood–brain barrier early in the course of infection, often at the time of the initial viraemia, and persists within the CNS. The cells infected with HIV in the CNS are predominantly macrophages and microglia; these give rise to the microscopic hallmark of HIV dementia, the presence of multinucleated giant cells (MGCs).

Investigation and differential diagnosis HIV testing, following appropriate counselling, should be considered in patients with unexplained dementia, particularly where the patient has risk factors for HIV infection (homosexuality, unprotected sex with multiple partners, intravenous drug abuse, blood or blood product transfusions, etc.). MRI scanning typically reveals cerebral atrophy with regions of increased T2 signal in the white matter and basal ganglia (Fig. 17.4). The CSF usually shows an increased cell count, elevated protein and the presence of oligoclonal bands of immunoglobulin.

There are causes of cognitive decline in patients with known HIV infection besides HIV associated dementia. These include the effects of depression, drugs and substance abuse, systemic illness, opportunistic infections and HIV-related tumours of the CNS, particularly lymphoma. Causes of CNS infection to consider in this context include toxoplasmosis, tuberculosis, cryptococcosis, cytomegalovirus (CMV), syphilis and progressive multifocal leucoencephalopathy (PML).

Management HIV is now a treatable, if not curable, cause of dementia. Combined therapy with antiviral agents reduces the risk of progressing from HIV-infection to AIDS and HIV-associated dementia.

Transmissible spongiform encephalopathies (prion dementias)

Definition The transmissible spongiform encephalopathies (TSEs) are a group of rare dementias caused by an accumulation of abnormal prion protein within the brain. Related illnesses occur in animals; indeed, one recently described disorder, variant Creutzfeldt–Jakob disease (vCJD), is thought to result from infection of humans by consumption of beef products from cattle with bovine spongiform encephalopathy (BSE) . The term 'prion' stands for 'proteinaceous infectious pathogen'.

Epidemiology All the TSEs are rare. Sporadic Creutzfeldt–Jakob disease (spCJD), the most common human TSE, occurs with an annual incidence of one per million population, usually affecting people between the ages of 55 and 70. Variant CJD has been diagnosed in approximately only 150 individuals at the time of writing, almost all resident in the UK. It usually develops in younger subjects than spCJD, and most cases have presented in the second to fourth decades of life.

Clinical features Sporadic CJD typically causes a rapidly progressive dementia, with early changes in behaviour, visual symptoms and cerebellar signs. Within weeks to months, marked cognitive impairment develops, often progressing to mutism, with pyramidal, extrapyramidal and cerebellar signs and myoclonus. The median duration of symptoms to death is only 4 months. Iatrogenic cases of CJD (iatCJD) have occurred when CNS tissue from patients with spCJD has unwittingly been transferred from patient to patient by surgical instruments, or used in medical procedures as a source of growth hormone, gonadotrophins, dura mater or corneal grafts.

Variant CJD differs markedly from spCJD. The initial symptoms are usually psychiatric — in particular anxiety or depression — often sufficiently severe to lead to psychiatric referral (Spencer et al 2002). Limb pain or tingling is common early in the course of the illness. After some months cognitive symptoms typically develop, causing difficulty at school or work, together with varied neurological features including pyramidal, extrapyramidal and cerebellar signs and myoclonus. The disorder evolves more slowly than spCJD, with an average duration to death of 14 months.

Pathology and aetiology The light microscope reveals 'spongiform change' in the brain associated with neuronal loss, gliosis and deposition of 'amyloid'. Immunocytochemistry and direct biochemical analysis indicate that the amyloid is composed of a protease-resistant form of prion protein (PrP). PrP is a membrane-associated neuronal protein coded on the short arm of chromosome 20. In TSEs, PrP is thought to undergo a conformational change to a disease associated form, PrP^{sc}, which both renders PrP resistant to normal degradation, and confers upon it the capacity to convert other molecules of PrP to PrP^{sc}. This process of catalysis gradually results in the toxic accumulation of PrP^{sc}. In spCJD the initial conformational change occurs 'spontaneously'; in transmitted cases it is catalysed by exogenous PrP^{sc}; and in inherited cases, a mutation in the *PrP* gene renders the molecule more than usually vulnerable to spontaneous transformation to PrP^{sc}. This radical 'prion hypothesis' explains how one and the same disorder can occur in sporadic, infective and inherited forms (Aguzzi et al 2000).

Investigation and differential diagnosis In spCJD the EEG shows 1–2/second triphasic waves in 80% of cases at some time during the course of the illness. Detection of 14-3-3 protein in CSF has a sensitivity and specificity of 90% for spCJD. Brain

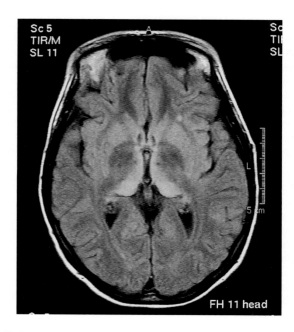

Fig. 17.5
MRI scans in vCJD are characterised by high signal intensity in the pulvinar nucleus.

biopsy is usually diagnostic but rarely performed. In vCJD the EEG and CSF examination are less useful, but characteristic MRI abnormalities (especially high signal in the pulvinar nucleus; see Fig. 17.5) are found in a high proportion of cases, giving a sensitivity of 78% and specificity of 100% in one study. Tonsillar biopsy has also been used as a confirmatory test PrP^{sc} is found in lymphoid tissue in vCJD. In suspected cases of familial TSE, sequencing of the *PrP* gene will identify the causative mutation.

Management At present, there is no proven remedy for prion-associated disease. In the UK the CJD Surveillance Unit, based in Edinburgh, can mobilise the substantial package of support which is now available for patients with CJD, and, in the interests of accurate disease surveillance, it is vital that all cases should be reported to the Unit.

Other rare infective causes of dementia

Whipple's disease Whipple's disease is rare but important because it is treatable. Infection with *Tropheryma whippelii* typically causes a multisystem disorder with prominent steatorrhoea, weight loss and abdominal pain. CNS involvement is common, and neurological symptoms and signs, psychiatric symptoms and dementia can occur in the absence of systemic features. Antibiotic treatment can be effective.

Subacute sclerosing panencephalitis Subacute sclerosing panencephalitis (SSPE) is a rare complication of childhood measles, due to intraneuronal persistence of a defective form of the virus in the CNS causing a continuing immune response with high levels of measles antibody in the CSF. Neurological signs, including myoclonus, accompany the dementia. Average life expectancy from onset is 1–2 years.

Progressive multifocal leucoencephalopathy Progressive multifocal leucoencephalopathy (PML) is caused by activation of JC Papova virus within the CNS in an immunocompromised patient. The resulting demyelination gives rise to pyramidal signs, visual impairment and a subcortical dementia usually progressing to death over months.

Herpes encephalitis Herpes encephalitis, which spreads through limbic pathways, can leave dementia in its wake if treatment of the acute encephalitis is unsuccessful or delayed.

Inflammatory dementias

A number of inflammatory conditions affecting the CNS can cause dementia. The diagnosis will generally be suggested by the presence of features that are atypical for other common causes. These may be systemic, such as the butterfly rash, arthralgia and renal impairment often associated with systemic lupus erythematosus, or the oral and genital ulcers and iritis of Behçet's syndrome, or neurological, such as the headache and fluctuating confusion of cerebral vasculitis, or the upper motor neuron signs which usually occur in multiple sclerosis. Features likes these — or unexplained dementia in a younger person — call for 'additional investigations' listed in Box 17.6, in particular serological tests for inflammatory disorders, neuroimaging with MRI, and CSF examination.

Multiple sclerosis

A demyelinating disorder of the central nervous system, MS causes some degree of cognitive impairment in almost half of cases and can present with unexplained subcortical dementia. The disorder can also cause and occasionally present with affective disorders. The presence of high signal abnormalities on T2-weighted MRI, and of oligoclonal bands of immunoglobulin in the CSF, help to confirm the diagnosis.

Systemic lupus erythematosus

Systemic lupus erythematosus (SLE) is a multisystem inflammatory disorder which can be accompanied by CNS involvement. The mechanisms are vascular and immunological, with psychiatric and cognitive symptoms sometimes amounting to delirium or dementia. Serological tests for antibodies including antinuclear factor, DNA-binding and anticardiolipin are helpful. Immunosuppression is indicated in 'cerebral lupus'.

Cerebral vasculitis

Inflammation of blood vessels within the CNS (cerebral vasculitis), can occur in association with several systemic vasculitic disorders, such as polyarteritis nodosa, Wegener's polyarteritis, and Churg–Strauss syndrome, or as an isolated process ('isolated angiitis of the CNS'). It can present with headache and confusion, often accompanied by neurological signs and sometimes seizures. If untreated, dementia may result. Immunosuppression can be effective, but brain biopsy is usually required for a confident diagnosis.

Hashimoto's encephalopathy

This is a recently recognised disorder associated with high titres of antithyroid antibodies causing either a progressive dementia, often with psychotic features, or a more acute illness with stroke-like episodes, confusion and seizures. The diagnosis should be suspected in patients with known autoimmune thyroid disease and unexplained cognitive impairment, and in patients with unexplained atypical dementia.

Neoplastic dementias

CNS tumours

While primary and metastatic CNS tumours typically present with headache, focal neurological signs or seizures, they can also cause cognitive impairment and occasionally mimic a dementing illness. CT scanning should reveal their presence, although diffusely infiltrating tumours are occasionally missed in the early stages. The diagnosis of paraneoplastic 'limbic encephalitis' is more challenging. This disorder results from immunological cross reaction between tumour antigens and antigens present within the CNS. It can give rise to a range of presentations, including confusional states, a pure amnesic syndrome and affective symptoms. Small-cell lung cancer is the most common cause, but breast cancer, gynaecological tumours, renal carcinoma, testicular tumours and lymphoma can also be responsible. The tumour may be small and sometimes undetectable by imaging initially. The diagnosis is supported by the detection of antineuronal antibodies in serum or CSF, most commonly 'anti-Hu'; the CSF often contains oligoclonal bands of immunoglobulin.

Traumatic dementias

Trauma is one of the few causes of abrupt-onset dementia and is discussed further under traumatic brain injury

Structural dementias

Hydrocephalus

Definition Hydrocephalus (HC) is dilatation of the ventricles within the brain caused by elevation of the pressure of the CSF synthesised within them. It is 'communicating' when the block to CSF flow occurs outside the ventricular system and non-communicating when the block is within the ventricles (for example in the narrow acqueduct of Sylvius, a common site of obstruction to CSF flow). In 'compensated' hydrocephalus, the clinical signs and CSF dynamics stabilise at an elevated level of CSF pressure. In 'normal pressure hydrocephalus', the ventricles enlarge despite apparently normal CSF pressure, possibly as a result of intermittent surges of high pressure.

Clinical features Hydrocephalus can cause a wide range of neurological and psychiatric symptoms and signs. Manifestations include enlargement of the head (if present in infancy), headache, sudden death due to 'hydrocephalic attacks' with acute elevation of intracranial pressure, progressive visual failure, gait disturbance (often 'gait apraxia'), incontinence and subcortical cognitive impairment progressing to dementia. 'Normal pressure hydrocephalus' in older people is classically associated with the triad of gait apraxia, incontinence and cognitive decline.

Investigation and differential diagnosis In a younger person the radiological signs of hydrocephalus are usually clear-cut on CT scanning. This is sometimes true in the elderly, but in other older patients an apparent hydrocephalus is sometimes due to atrophy of the brain rather than to dilatation of the ventricles. When enlargement of the ventricles raises a suspicion of communicating hydrocephalus in an older person, specialised studies are required to determine whether the scan appearance is relevant to the clinical problem (usually either serial lumbar punctures with observation of the clinical effects, or neurosurgical CSF pressure studies).

Management The insertion of a 'shunt' that allows the diversion of CSF from the CSF space to venous system or peritoneum, can be beneficial or even life-saving. However, it is prone to complications, including subdural haematomas and infection and should not be undertaken lightly.

Subdural haematoma

Definition Subdural haematomas are accumulations of blood and blood products in the space between the fibrous dura mater and the more delicate arachnoid membrane which encloses the brain. Acute subdural haematomas accumulate rapidly following head injury; chronic subdural haematomas can sometimes, but not always, be traced back to a head injury.

Clinical features Acute subdural haematomas are, by definition, diagnosed close to the time of trauma, as a result either of symptoms present at the time — headache, depressed level of consciousness, focal neurological signs — or from a CT scan. Chronic subdurals give rise to more gradually evolving symptoms and signs. While they, also, can cause headache, depressed consciousness and focal signs, they sometimes result in predominantly cognitive features, including confusion and dementia. Marked variability of the mental state, and sometimes also of the neurological features, is often a clue to the diagnosis. Seizures can occur.

Pathology The variability of the clinical features is explained by the tendency of the size of chronic subdurals to wax and wane as a result of alternating phases of bleeding and of breakdown of the contents of the chronic haematoma.

Investigation and differential diagnosis Subdural haematomas can generally be diagnosed on CT scanning (Fig. 17.6). They are occasionally 'isodense' with brain and therefore easily missed, especially if bilateral. It is important to recognise that a small subdural can be an incidental finding: cerebral atrophy occurring in the course of a dementing illness, for example, predisposes to subdural haematoma as vulnerable bridging veins are

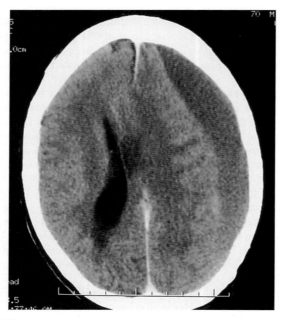

Fig. 17.6
CT scan of large subdural haematoma showing compression of the ventricles and midline shift.

stretched between the dura and the arachnoid. In these circumstances treatment of the subdural is unlikely to be helpful.

Management This requires liaison with a neurosurgical team. Small subdural haematomas often resorb spontaneously. If a subdural is considered to be relevant to a patient's problems, and drainage is required, several surgical approaches are available.

Metabolic and endocrine dementias

Hypothyroidism

Thyroid function tests should always be performed in patients with cognitive decline, as hypothyroidism can present with cognitive symptoms, progressing to dementia, and is readily treated. The early cognitive symptoms are usually mental lethargy and slowing of cognition. A wide range of physical symptoms, apathy, depression, confusion or psychosis ('myxoedema madness') may also occur.

Deficiency disorders

Vitamin deficiency

Deficiency of B vitamins, especially B_1 (thiamine) and B_{12} (cobalamin compounds), and of folic acid are important organic causes of organic psychiatric disorders. B_1 (thiamine) deficiency, causing Wernicke's encephalopathy in the acute phase, and Korsakoff's psychosis if untreated, is discussed under amnestic syndromes. Vitamin B_{12} and folate deficiency are relatively rare but highly treatable causes of dementia, and the concentration of these vitamins in the blood should be checked in patients with cognitive decline.

Sleep-related dementias

Obstructive sleep apnoea

Obstructive sleep apnoea typically presents with excessive daytime sleepiness (EDS) on a background of snoring and intermittent apnoea due to upper airways obstruction in sleep, most often in obese middle aged men. The patient is often unaware of the extent of his sleep disturbance, and present with non-specific symptoms such as fatigue, forgetfulness or impaired concentration.

Substance-induced dementias

Alcohol and recreational drugs

The question of whether excessive alcohol intake alone damages the brain — as opposed to the associated thiamine deficiency, head injury, secondary hypoglycaemia and other consequences — has been much debated. The balance of evidence suggests that alcohol itself can cause cognitive impairment and cerebral atrophy, although its effects are often compounded by additional factors. Chronic misuse of other substances and its complications can cause or contribute to cognitive decline. It is important therefore to take a history of recreational drug use, including alcohol, in patients with cognitive symptoms.

Medication-induced dementias

Occasionally, prescribed medication causes or contributes to cognitive impairment. Drugs which can be responsible include anticholinergics, anticonvulsants (especially barbiturates), hypnotics and neuroleptics.

FUNCTIONAL PSYCHIATRIC DISORDERS THAT CAN MIMIC DEMENTIA

Depressive, hysterical and simulated 'pseudodementia' and the Ganser syndrome

Definition

In 'pseudodementia', which is a functional psychiatric disorder or rarely a deliberate simulation, the clinical picture is similar to that of an organic dementia. However, there are differences which aid in differential diagnosis:

- *Depressive pseudodementia* is cognitive impairment on the background of a depressive illness, sometimes in the absence of typical symptoms of depression.
- *Hysterical pseudodementia* is cognitive impairment mimicking organic dementia which proves not to be due to organic pathology. 'Functional dementia' might be a more appropriate term for both depressive and hysterical pseudodementia.
- *Simulated dementia* is cognitive impairment that has been feigned deliberately in the pursuit of some form of gain.

Clinical features

Depression is the most common potentially reversible cause of cognitive impairment encountered in memory clinics. Where cognitive impairment occurs in someone who is overtly depressed, the diagnosis will be immediately suspected. But when loss of interest in the environment is coupled with slowing of thought and behaviour, in the absence of overt sadness, an organic cause, such as a subcortical dementia, might well be considered. On cognitive examination, depressive pseudodementia is likely to produce slowed responses, paucity of speech and impaired concentration in the absence of 'cortical' deficits such as dysphasia or agnosia.

Hysterical pseudodementia is suggested by unexpectedly severe and inconsistent impairment of cognitive function, especially in the context of other 'functional' symptoms and signs. Some cases occur on a background of dramatic psychological precipitants.

Aetiology

A number of cognitive mechanisms, including a tendency to retrieve distressing memories, and an over-general retrieval style, help to explain the cognitive deficits associated with depression. There is also recent evidence, from a combination of animal and human studies, that both depression and stress affect structure and function in the hippocampus by modulation of circulating glucocorticoids, mineralocorticoids and monoaminergic inputs.

Investigation and differential diagnosis

The most commonly encountered clinical dilemma is the distinction between a primary depressive illness causing cognitive impairment and an organic dementia with associated mood disturbance. The diagnoses of dementia and depression are not, of course, mutually exclusive. Features which may point towards depression being the primary process include the recent occurrence of negative life events, a relatively abrupt onset, and variability of cognitive dysfunction. Psychometric testing can be helpful but sometimes it is only possible to reach a definite conclusion in retrospect, after conducting an adequate trial of treatment for depression and allowing the passage of time.

Management

Depression should be treated in the usual way. There is little evidence to guide our management of 'hysterical pseudodementia', but the generally agreed approach is strong reassurance that the disorder will improve, followed by rehabilitation. 'Abreaction' (interviewing under light sedation with diazepam or sodium amytal) has sometimes been used to good effect as a diagnostic and therapeutic tool, as it may alleviate functional impairment, but is likely to exacerbate most types of organic cognitive impairment.

DELIRIUM

Delirium occurs most commonly but not exclusively in the elderly and is described in Chapter 26.

Definition

Delirium has a number of synonyms, including 'acute confusional state', 'acute brain syndrome', 'acute organic reaction' and 'acute brain failure'. It is defined as an aetiologically non-specific syndrome characterised by concurrent disturbances of consciousness and attention, perception, cognition, behaviour, emotion and the sleep–wake cycle. It is transient and fluctuating.

Epidemiology

Most prevalence studies of delirium have been carried out in hospitalised, medically ill patients, in whom the prevalence is about 25%. This rises with age, and is greater in the terminally ill and in certain groups of post-operative patients (Table 17.5).

Clinical features

Delirium is characterised by marked abnormalities of attention accompanied by generalised cognitive impairment affecting orien-

Table 17.5	Prevalence of delirium
Setting	Percentage with delirium
Hospitalised medically ill patients*	10–30
Hospitalised elderly patients	10–40
Hospitalised cancer patients	25
Hospitalised AIDS patients	30–40
Terminally ill patients	80

* High risk conditions and procedures include cardiotomy, hip surgery, transplant surgery, burns, renal dialysis, and lesions of the central nervous system.
Prevalence figures from *Practice guideline for the treatment of patients with delirium*, American Psychiatric Association, 1999.

tation, memory and planning skills. Variability in alertness and awareness of the environment are almost invariably present. Disturbances of the sleep–wake cycle, affect, perception and psychomotor performance are also clinically important for diagnosis and management. 'Clouding' of consciousness is no longer included within current definitions, as it is hard to define. The onset is usually acute and develops over hours to days. The symptoms fluctuate, and are usually worse at night. The fluctuations often delay diagnosis, but should alert clinicians to the presence of delirium (Brown & Boyle 2002).

Three clinical variants of delirium have been described (Lipowski 1989):

- a hyperalert-hyperactive type;
- a hypoalert-hypoactive type;
- a mixed type.

Identification is usually straightforward in the hyperalert/hyperactive patient. The hypoalert/hypoactive variant causes more problems and is under-recognised and occasionally misdiagnosed, for example, as depression. The hyperalert-hyperactive form of delirium is more often accompanied by psychotic symptoms (hallucinations and delusions), and agitation and disorientation, whereas the hypoalert-hypoactive form is characterised by confusion and sedation and fewer psychotic symptoms.

Patients with delirium have a reduced ability to focus and sustain attention. This is clinically important, not only in the assessment of delirium but also in its management. Even simple procedures, such as blood tests and physical examinations, may need to be explained on more than one occasion if they are not to be misperceived as an assault. Such misperception may precipitate aggressive behaviour. The memory impairment in delirium reflects lack of attention, and, if attention can be sustained, retrograde memory will often be intact. However, more often there is a dense amnesia with islands of memory during periods of lucidity.

Disorientation for time and place is almost universal, with difficulties in identifying the day of the week, the month or the year, or even the approximate time of day. Hospitalised patients may believe that they are still in their own homes or at their place of work. Perceptual disturbances include hallucinations and misinterpretations and delusions. Visual hallucinations are typical and can be particularly vivid and frightening. Illusions are common, and perceptual distortions, including micropsia and macropsia, also occur. Fleeting transitory delusions may result from these misinterpretations — for example, patients may see a nurse add sugar to their cup of tea and develop the belief that they are being poisoned. The patient's ability to think coherently is usually impaired, with marked disorganisation and poor direction of thought. This contributes to difficulties with the planning of the simplest of actions.

Disturbance of the sleep–wake cycle is invariable, with reversal of the normal cycle being usual. Patients may be drowsy during the day and agitated during the night. Such sleep as the patient does get is often accompanied by frightening nightmares which can merge imperceptibly with the hallucinations the patient has on wakening.

Abnormalities of mood are common and can range from apathy to anxiety, agitation and fear. As with other features of this disorder, mood may rapidly fluctuate rapidly from one emotional state to another.

Pathogenesis and aetiology

A reduction in cerebral-oxidative metabolism and an imbalance of neurotransmitter synthesis is presumed to be the final common pathway, but the mechanism is not established. Cholinergic deficits appear to particularly important. The cholinergic system is widely distributed through the brain and is involved in vision, attention, memory and sleep, all of which can be disturbed in delirium. The underlying causes include a lack of oxygen, glucose and amino acids, vitamin deficiency, deficient synthesis and blockade of neurotransmitters, accumulations of toxins and false transmitters, impaired cerebral blood flow, increased permeability of the blood–brain barrier, and damage to cell membranes. These cellular mechanisms are reflected in the risk factors for delirium — age, impaired cognitive functioning, severe physical illness, use of alcohol and drugs, dehydration and infection, electrolyte disturbance and low albumin (Box 17.9).

Delirium is often due to multiple aetiologies. The most common single cause of delirium, particularly in the elderly, is intoxication due to prescribed drugs. Drugs with anticholinergic activity (such as tricyclic antidepressants) are particularly likely to cause delirium. Theophylline, digoxin, benzodiazepines and narcotic analgesics are also common culprits. However, any drug should be considered a potential cause of delirium. The medical conditions that most commonly cause delirium are listed in Box 17.10.

Withdrawal from alcohol or sedative hypnotic drugs is also a common cause and should be considered in patients who have recently been hospitalised and separated from their supply. Delirium tremens, the form of delirium associated with alcohol withdrawal, is worthy of special attention as it is so common. In delirium tremens, anxiety and autonomic hyperactivity are particularly prominent. There are often associated metabolic disturbances and withdrawal seizures.

Box 17.9   Risk factors for delirium

Patient factors
Individual:
- Age
- Pre-existing cognitive deficit
- Severe comorbidity
- Previous episode of delirium
- Personality before illness

Perioperative:
- Course of postoperative period
- Type of operation (for example, hip replacement)
- Emergency operation
- Duration of operation

Specific conditions: burns; AIDS; fracture; hypoxaemia; organ insufficiency; infection; metabolic disturbances (for example, dehydration, low serum albumin concentration)

Pharmacological factors
- Treatment with many drugs
- Dependence on drugs or alcohol
- Use of psychoactive drugs or alcohol

Environmental factors
- Extremes in sensory experience (for example, hypothermia)
- Deficits in vision or hearing
- Immobility or decreased activity
- Social isolation
- Novel environment
- Stress

> **Box 17.10   Common medical causes of delirium**
>
> - Intoxication with drugs — many drugs implicated especially anticholinergic agents, anticonvulsants, anti-parkinsonism agents, steroids, cimetidine, opiates, sedative hypnotics, also alcohol and illicit drugs
> - Withdrawal syndromes — Alcohol, sedative hypnotics, barbiturates
> - Metabolic causes:
>   — hypoxia, hypoglycaemia, hepatic, renal or pulmonary insufficiency
>   — endocrinopathies (such as hypothyroidism, hyperthyroidism, hypopituitarism, hypoparathyroidism or hyperparathyroidism)
>   — disorders of fluid and electrolyte balance
>   — rare causes (such as porphyria, carcinoid syndrome)
> - Infections
> - Head trauma
> - Epilepsy — ictal, interictal, or postictal
> - Neoplastic disease
> - Vascular disorders:
>   — Cerebrovascular (such as transient ischaemic attacks, thrombosis, embolism, migraine)
>   — Cardiovascular (such as myocardial infarction, cardiac failure)

Infections are common precipitants, and even innocuous, non-life-threatening infections, particularly in the elderly, can precipitate delirium. Post-operative delirium occurs in 10–15% of elderly surgical patients and is particularly common in those taking anticholinergic drugs or misusing alcohol.

Detection of delirium

Systematic surveys show that half the cases of delirium in hospital go unrecognised (Meagher 2001). Failure to diagnose delirium is important because it has been associated with a poorer outcome; although most patients with delirium do recover, a significant proportion progress to stupor, coma, seizures or death. Death occurs because of failure to recognise and treat the underlying medical disorder, or from the sequelae of delirium associated behavioural disturbance. Inactivity may cause pneumonia and decubital ulcers, and wandering may lead to fractures from falls.

Differential diagnosis

The most important distinctions are (1) between delirium and dementia, (2) between delirium (hypoalert/hypoactive type) and depression and (3) between delirium and a functional psychotic illness (schizophrenia or mania). The history provides the most important diagnostic clues and usually requires good third-party information from nurses or relatives.

In differentiating delirium and dementia, delirium should be suspected when the onset is acute or subacute and the course fluctuates markedly. Hallucinations and delusions can occur in dementia but are more common in delirium, where they are more vivid and detailed. Delirium is not uncommonly superimposed on a pre-existing dementia. There can be particular difficulty in distinguishing Lewy body dementia from delirium, because of its fluctuant course, although the presence of parkinsonian symptoms in Lewy body dementia may help to discriminate.

Delirium of hypoalert and hypoactive type differs from depression in that sustained low mood and/or anhedonia is absent and fluctuating disorientation is present. Antidepressant agents are likely to make delirium worse.

The hyperalert/hyperactive variant of delirium is differentiated from functional disorders by the presence of markedly fluctuating mental state and impairment of attention and memory.

Occasionally delirium is confused with dissociative disorder. Both disorders are often sudden in onset. In dissociative disorders loss of personalised identity commonly occurs where it does not in delirium. The memory loss in dissociative disorders tends to be circumscribed (for example to past personal memories) and does not correspond with accepted patterns.

Investigations

Investigation should be guided by the history and as careful a physical examination as the patient will permit. Urgent blood sugar and blood gas analysis may be required. Additional investigations to consider are full blood count, C-reactive protein, urea and electrolytes, liver function tests, thyroid function, blood glucose, urine analysis and culture of midstream urine and chest radiography. Where the diagnosis is genuinely in doubt, an electroencephalogram may be helpful and shows diffuse background slow-wave activity in delirium.

If these initial investigations reveal no underlying causes for delirium, it may be necessary to carry out further investigations. Occasionally, even rarer disorders have to be considered (see Boxes 17.9 and 17.10).

Management

There are four key aspects to the management of delirium:

- identifying and treating the cause;
- paying attention to environmental and general supportive measures;
- drug management and pharmacological interventions;
- review and follow-up.

Identifying and treating the cause

Identifying causes can be difficult, especially when patients are unable to give a coherent history or to co-operate with physical examination. Occasionally it may even be justifiable to judiciously sedate a patient to enable an adequate physical examination to be conducted (see below). When a cause is identified, appropriate treatment of the underlying cause should be started without delay.

Environmental and supportive measures in delirium

The provision of adequate trained nursing staff is critical. The patient should be nursed by as few nurses as is feasible. Particular attention should be paid to clear, repeated and concise communication with the patient. The need for constant and repeated orientation, particularly to time, place and identity of important individuals, should also be highlighted. Involving family and friends in assisting with orientating the patient and helping the patient comply with management can be invaluable.

Attention should also be paid to the environment in which the patient is nursed, ensuring adequate lighting and a limited

---

> **Box 17.11   General management of delirium**
>
> - Education of all who interact with patient (doctors, nurses, ancillary and portering staff, friends, family)
> - Reality orientation techniques:
>   — firm clear communication, preferably by same member of staff
>   — use of clocks and calendars
> - Creating an environment that optimises stimulation (adequate lighting, reducing unnecessary noise, mobilising patient whenever possible)
> - Correcting sensory impairments (providing hearing aids, glasses, etc.)
> - Ensuring adequate warmth and nutrition
> - Making environment safe (removing objects with which patient could harm self or others)

---

number of attendants. Clocks, calendars and objects familiar to the patient can assist orientation. The safety of the environment should also be considered, and objects that the patient might use to harm himself or others should be removed. Simple matters, such as correcting sensory impairments, e.g. by ensuring the patient has a hearing aid or spectacles, are sometimes overlooked, and attending to nutrition, hydration and toileting needs should not be forgotten (Box 17.11).

Pharmacological management

Drug treatment should be used only when essential and then only with care. It requires consideration of the risks of such management as well as the potential benefits. Drugs often make delirium worse by exacerbating underlying causes, precipitating falls and worsening cognitive impairment. Doctors are often pressurised by other medical colleagues, nurses and relatives to sedate people inappropriately, and caution is required.

Antipsychotic drugs   For delirium other than that caused by withdrawal from alcohol or benzodiazepines, antipsychotic drugs are the most appropriate. A randomised, double-blind controlled trial (Breitbart et al 1996) has demonstrated their superiority over benzodiazepines. Doses of haloperidol between 1 mg and 10 mg per day are adequate for most patients, and can be administered intramuscularly if required. The dose in the elderly should be low, and starting doses of 0.5 mg b.d. are often adequate. It is preferable to use a fixed dosing regimen. Patients should be monitored regularly for both response and emergence of side-effects. Particularly troublesome side-effects include sedation, anticholinergic effects and α-adrenergic effects, in particular hypotension, and these should be specifically monitored. Some authorities recommend a baseline electrocardiogram because of the risk of prolonged QT_C interval leading to torsades de pointes, ventricular fibrillation and sudden death. New-generation antipsychotics, e.g. olanzapine, have the advantage of having fewer extrapyramidal side-effects.

Benzodiazepines   These are the preferred drugs when delirium is associated with withdrawal from alcohol or sedatives. They are also sometimes used as alternatives or additives to antipsychotics when these are ineffective or causing unacceptable side-effects. They can of course be rapidly reversed with flumazenil. Lorazepam is the drug of choice as it has a relatively short duration of action, has no active metabolites and can be given intra-

muscularly. No more than 2 mg of lorazepam every 4 hours should be required. Much lower starting doses are recommended, especially in the elderly.

Regular review

A common shortcoming in the management of delirium is a failure to review the patient on a regular basis. Patients are often seen with acute symptoms out of hours by on-call junior staff or on-call psychiatrists, and not reviewed the following day when these doctors are no longer in the hospital. The management of delirium, and its underlying causes, should be reviewed daily, for the duration of the hospital stay, and drugs used to treat it stopped as soon as possible.

Treatment of delirium in patients with dementia

Patients with dementia (particularly Lewy body dementia) are particularly vulnerable to treatment with antipsychotics. They are also particularly vulnerable to delirium. Doctors involved in the management of elderly patients with delirium need to be aware of this and to use them only when the benefits to the patient outweigh the risks. In patients with known Lewy body dementia, antipsychotic drugs should be avoided.

AMNESTIC SYNDROMES

The amnestic or amnesic syndrome describes a condition in which learning and memory are affected out of all proportion to other cognitive functions, in an otherwise alert and responsive patient. The most common cause is Wernicke–Korsakoff syndrome as a result of nutritional depletion and in particular thiamine deficiency. Other causes include carbon monoxide poisoning, herpes simplex encephalitis and other infections (see the section on dementia), hypoxic and other acquired brain injuries (see the section on acquired brain injury), vascular disorders (stroke), deep midline cerebral tumours and surgical resections. In the vast majority of cases the pathology lies in midline or medial temporal structures, but there are a number of case reports of amnestic disorder following frontal lobe lesions.

Wernicke–Korsakoff syndrome

Wernicke–Korsakoff syndrome is the result of thiamine depletion, and any cause of this can lead to the syndrome (Zubaran et al 1997). The overwhelming majority of cases arise secondary to alcohol abuse as a result of decreased intake and absorption of thiamaine. A genetic defect for thiamine metabolism has been described in a proportion of patients. The chronic amnestic or Korsakoff syndrome (or psychosis) usually follows an acute Wernicke's encephalopathy, hence Wernicke–Korsakoff syndrome. Wernicke's encephalopathy is characterised by confusion, ataxia, nystagmus and ophthalmoplegia. There can also be peripheral neuropathy. Wernicke's encephalopathy is a medical emergency, and parenteral administration of high-dose vitamins to prevent the development of the chronic amnestic syndrome is indicated.

Patients with the chronic Korsakoff syndrome may perform well on standard tasks of attention and working memory (serial sevens and reverse digit span), but may struggle on more complex tasks involving shifting and dividing attention. Memory impairments

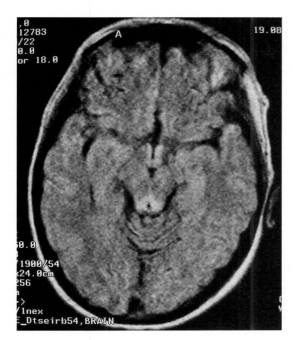

Fig. 17.7
MRI scans in Wernicke–Korsakoff syndrome frequently show atrophy in the diencephalon.

involve both anterograde and retrograde deficits. Defective encoding of new information has been implicated as a core to the memory disorder. Some learning may be possible particularly if patients are given a strategy to follow. Confabulation commonly occurs, particularly early in the disorder. Procedural memory remains relatively intact.

The pathology consists of neuronal loss, microhaemorrhages and gliosis in the periventricular and periqueductal grey matter. The mamillary bodies, the mamillothalamic tract and the anterior thalamus appear to be the key structures involved. There is also likely to be a degree of generalised cortical atrophy, more marked in the frontal lobes. This may be non-specific, secondary to the years of alcohol abuse. MRI indicates specific atrophy in diencephalic structures (Fig. 17.7).

The prognosis is variable. For the acute episode, one quarter of patients recover, half improve but have some persistent impairment, and the remaining quarter remain severely impaired. Some die. High-dose vitamins should be given to all patients acutely and may also have some efficacy even after the acute phase has passed.

Transient amnesic syndromes

Transient amnesia can occur with several disorders: Transient global amnesia (TGA) is a distinctive benign disorder affecting middle-aged or elderly subjects who become amnesic for recent events, and unable to lay down new memories, for a period of about 4 hours. Repetitive questioning by the patients of their companions is a characteristic feature. Episodes can be provoked by physical or emotional stress and are usually isolated. There is evidence that the disorder results from reversible medial temporal lobe dysfunction, but the aetiology is uncertain. Temporal lobe epilepsy occasionally mimics TGA ('transient epileptic amnesia'), but episodes are typically briefer, lasting less than an hour, recurrent (several/year), and often occur on waking. Other causes of transient amnesia include transient cerebral ischaemia (usually

accompanied by other neurological symptoms and signs), migraine, drug ingestion and head injury.

ACQUIRED BRAIN INJURY

In industrialised countries advanced trauma and life support techniques have led to dramatic reduction in mortality rates from acquired brain injury (ABI), but an increasing number of survivors — the majority young adult males who have suffered head injuries — although physically fit, have severely damaged brains and multiple cognitive and emotional disabilities.

Epidemiology

The incidence in Scotland is 330/100 000 per year. Of these, approximately 80% are mild, 10% moderate and 10% severe. Post-injury life expectancy, although reduced, is measured in decades, and as a result the prevalence of ABI-associated disability is increasing annually. The disability will depend on both the severity and the nature of the injury, as well as on the premorbid state of the patient. This latter issue is of considerable importance as people who have problems with substance or alcohol abuse, violent tendencies or risk-taking traits in their personalities are more likely to suffer brain injury.

Severity of injury

There is no single definitive marker of severity of brain injury. The Glasgow Coma Scale has been a major advance in documenting the severity of coma (Table 17.6). It is highly predictive of both mortality and need for surgical intervention. However, it is less useful in predicting long-term outcomes, particularly when coma duration has been brief. The length of post-traumatic amnesia (PTA) is the other main predictor of severity of injury (Table 17.7). Studies in which both methods have been used find good agreement but with a substantial number of discrepant cases.

Table 17.6 Assessment of outcome after acute brain injury — Glasgow coma scale	
Scale score	Injury
13–15	Mild
9–12	Moderate
3–8	Severe

Table 17.7 Assessment of outcome after acute brain injury — duration of post-traumatic amnesia	
Duration of PTA	Injury
< 10 min	Very mild
10–60 min	Mild
1–24 h	Moderate
1–7 days	Severe
> 7 days	Very severe

Post-traumatic amnesia

The duration of post-traumatic amnesia is defined as the time from the moment of injury to the time of resumption of normal continuous memory. The termination of PTA is often abrupt except in cases where enduring memory difficulties supervene. Brief islands of memory can punctuate the period of PTA. Behaviour within the period of PTA can be normal but more commonly there is defective memory and mental confusion that is obvious to others. Studies of cognitive function during PTA are rare but illustrate that some procedural memory functions remain intact, while episodic memory is impaired.

Retrograde amnesia

Retrograde amnesia is defined as the time between the moment of injury and the last clear memory from before the injury that the patient can recall. It can usually be indicated with reasonable precision. It is usually dense and much shorter than PTA. It is of less predictive value.

Mechanism of injury

Penetrating injuries

In general, cognitive symptoms after a penetrating injury will correspond to the area of the brain that is damaged. They are also generally accompanied by impairment in memory and attention and general cognitive slowing reflecting associated diffuse damage.

Closed head injury

Both primary and secondary injuries can occur. The primary injury is the damage that occurs at the time of impact. There are three main mechanisms:

- the *coup*, which corresponds to damage to the cortex under the site of a direct blow, and the *contrecoup*, in which the brain sustains a bruise in the area opposite the injury;
- bruising which occurs as a result of rapid deceleration leading to the brain hitting the bony structures of the floor of the skull;
- shearing injury which occurs when a moving head comes to a rapid stop. This leads to a generalised shearing injury of the axons known as *diffuse axonal damage*.

The secondary injury consists of the effects of the physiological processes set in motion by the primary injury, and can often be the more destructive. Of major importance is an increase in intracranial pressure (ICP) which results either from oedema in injured cerebral tissue or from secondary haematomas. The control of intracranial pressure is consequently the most important consideration in acute care of the head-injured patient.

Clinical features

The immediate effect of a brain injury is concussion. This can be mild, without total loss of consciousness, and characterised by symptoms such as 'seeing stars' and disorientation, with or without amnesia. Or, it can be more severe with reversible coma at the instant of trauma, accompanied by neurological, cardiovascular and pulmonary changes.

Cognitive effects of ABI

Coup and contrecoup lesions result in direct impairment of cortical function at the site of the lesion. Bruising tends to affect the frontal and temporal lobes and leads to problems in control of behaviour, in conceptual thinking and problem solving and with various memory and learning tasks. Diffuse damage from shearing reduces speed of processing, attentional functions, cognitive efficiency and high-level concept formation and complex reasoning. This can be seen directly or as irritability, fatigue and a general inability to do things as well as before the accident. Tasks requiring selective or divided attention tend to be particularly sensitive to diffuse effects, and patients will perform poorly on tests of oral or sequential arithmetic. Few patients with moderate or severe injury demonstrate only one pattern of impairment, and generally there is a combination of all three.

Sensory impairment

This is a common complication of ABI and often underlies difficult or disturbed behaviour. A loss of the sense of smell is frequently the result of damage to the olfactory nerve during a bruising injury to the frontal pole of the brain, although it can indicate damage to limbic structures in the temporal lobe. Visual disturbance is common, and its nature will be dependent on the nature of the damage to optic pathways. Hearing and balance defects are common and may be associated with tinnitus.

Mild head injury

This will involve short duration of loss of consciousness (< 30 min) and PTA measured in hours not days. Around 80% of injuries are mild. Patients generally describe a triad of attention deficits, impaired verbal retrieval and emotional distress. Headache, dizziness and photophobia are also common accompaniments. This usually appears within a few days of the injury, but can be delayed for days or weeks. Although communication deficits and perceptual disturbance are commonplace in the acute phase of injury, after they have settled down most head injury patients show few deficits in overlearned verbal material (excepting when language centres have been directly damaged) but will still display some dysnomias and occasional paraphrasias.

Emotional distress is often accompanied by marked fatigue and concern over perceived cognitive deficits. The effort needed to overcome attentional deficits is particularly distressing. Frank depressive illness itself, however, tends to be a later complication of injury, not occurring until some 3–6 months after the event.

The effects of mild brain injury are synonymous with post-concussional syndrome, although the latter term is generally reserved for situations where dramatic disability occurs following a mild brain injury. The physical symptoms are usually marked, and fatigue in particular can be highly disabling. Noise sensitivity and intolerance are commonplace, and symptoms more typical of a somatoform disorder frequently appear after a latent period of several months. Most accept that a multidimensional model of aetiology underlies the presentation and involves not only the direct effects and secondary consequences of brain injury but also those factors more commonly described in somatoform disorders. However, studies have noted microscopic lesions observable at postmortem, abnormalities on functional imaging and delayed brainstem evoked potentials.

Moderate head injury

A patient with a Glasgow Coma Scale score of 9–12 and post-traumatic amnesia of less than 24 hours is likely to be classed as moderate. Headaches, memory problems and difficulties with everyday life are the most common complaints. Two-thirds of patients will not return to work. Most patients exhibit some evidence of frontal or temporal bruising. Impulsivity, diminished initiative, affective muting and temper outbursts are all common. Temporal lobe damage is displayed as a true learning disorder with lateralisation for verbal and non-verbal material.

Severe head injury

Although accounting for less than 10% of ABI cases, the complex rehabilitation and long-term care required make severe head injury a major problem for health services. The associated impairments are generally categorised as occurring in three main areas: cognitive, emotional and executive.

Cognitive deficits are usually multiple, with individual patterns being unique — some neural functions being severely impaired and others functioning at near normal levels. Attentional deficits are particularly common and when very severe can place barriers to any form of retraining. Memory impairment usually affects acquisition and retrieval of semantic and episodic memory, and procedural and working memories are relatively spared. Frontal lobe injuries can be particularly handicapping and interfere with patients' abilities to use knowledge and skills appropriately.

Emotional disorders generally involve the exaggeration or muting of affective responses but, as well as reflecting the nature of the organic damage, will also be influenced by premorbid personality and mental state. Frontal lobe damage is associated with both excitability, impulsivity, and lability, and with apathetic, flat, uninterested and non-initiating responses. Damage to temporal limbic structures tends to result in emotionalism with sudden temper outbursts or pathological crying.

Executive dysfunction involves impairment of self-determination, self-direction and self-control and regulation. This involves not just the cognitive ability itself but also the ability to express it. Such patients frequently need external cues for activity, and perseveration (repetition) of behaviours is common.

Both psychotic symptoms and major depressive disorders occur. Early psychosis usually involves delusions of misidentification, and reduplicative paramnesias are particularly associated with brain injury. In this striking disorder, the patient believes himself to be in a different place despite all evidence to the contrary. The majority remit spontaneously. Late presentations of psychotic illness also occur, with an increased risk of a schizophreniform psychosis. Paranoid states, frequently related to memory impairment, also occur and can be hidden by communication difficulties. These psychiatric syndromes should be treated in the usual way but with increased caution about unwanted drug effects. The presentation and management of depressive disorders is discussed under stroke.

Agitation and aggression

Agitation and aggression cause clinically significant problems in around 10% of brain injured patients acutely. In the chronic phase,

Table 17.8	Disability 1 year after head injury		
Initial injury	Severe disability	Moderate disability	Good outcome
Mild	20%	28%	45%
Moderate	22%	24%	38%
Severe	29%	19%	14%
From Thornhill et al (2000).			

such behaviours can be a major cause of disability and are one of the most frequent complaints of relatives and carers. Cognitive impairments, and in particular communications disorders, are more likely to be the cause than psychotic disorders or depression. Drug treatment is complicated and almost always needs to be supplemented with behavioural interventions. The evidence is best for high-dose propranolol. Carbamazepine, valproate, trazodone and atypical antipsychotic drugs have all been advocated.

Prognosis

This varies according to the severity of injury (Table 17.8). Recent outcome studies have highlighted a high rate of chronic disability and failure to return to work (Thornhill et al 2000). Although there is general agreement on the cause of the acute impairments, the reason for long-term complaints is still a matter of debate. Clinical experience suggests that psychological and social factors become increasingly important the more distant from the injury, but it is seldom possible to tease out the exact contribution of each in any individual patient (Lishman 1988).

In more severe injuries, following return to consciousness, patients are generally delirious for a period of days to weeks. In such states they usually display restlessness, agitation and incomprehension and are unco-operative. Over the first 6 months many aspects of physical and cognitive function improve dramatically and then plateau — particularly those relating to attention. Activities relating to new learning tend to improve over a far longer period of time but seldom return to premorbid levels. Improvements after the first year tend to be more related to the development of compensatory strategies than to resolution of the underlying impairment.

Litigation

Compensation claims are frequently made after accidental head injury and often involve considerable sums of money reflecting long-term loss of earnings and a need for long-term care. Specialist assessments are required. Studies have found little difference between those patients who seek compensation and those who do not, with the possible exception that the former may complain more of their impairments.

STROKE

Definition

A cerebrovascular accident or stroke is 'a rapidly developed clinical sign of a focal disturbance of cerebral function of presumed vascular origin and of more than 24 hours duration'. One of two pathological processes can be responsible: cerebral infarction or cerebral haemorrhage. Infarction may result from thrombosis of vessels or emboli lodged within them. Haemorrhage can be into either brain tissue directly or into the subarachnoid space. Infarctions are four times more common than haemorrhages and, as a result of a lower immediate fatality rate, are a much greater source of enduring disability.

Epidemiology

Strokes are the third commonest cause of death in the Western world. The Oxford community stroke project reported an annual incidence of 2 per 1000 (Bamford et al 1988) for first ever stroke. Stroke is more common in men, and a quarter of those affected are under 65 years of age. Psychiatrists are not usually involved in the diagnosis of acute stroke but occasionally can be in several of the less typical cerebral syndromes where altered mental state and cognitive function dominate the clinical picture.

Clinical features

The clinical features depend largely on which area of the brain is damaged, which in turn depends on which artery is affected (Fig. 17.8).

Middle cerebral artery occlusion produces a contralateral hemiparesis and sensory loss of a cortical type. This is often accompanied by a hemianopia if the optic radiation is affected. If the lesion is in the dominant hemisphere then dysphasia may be expected whereas a non-dominant lesion will be accompanied by neglect or perceptual disturbance.

Anterior cerebral artery occlusion leads to contralateral hemiparesis affecting the leg more severely than the arm. A grasp reflex and motor dysphasia may be present. Cognitive changes resembling a global dementia may occur and be accompanied by incontinence. Residual personality changes of a frontal type can occur.

Posterior cerebral artery occlusion presents with a contralateral hemianopia sometimes accompanied by visual hallucinations, visual agnosias or spatial disorientation. Cognitive disturbance can again predominate, with transient confusion serving to obscure the detection of hemianopia. The vital memory structures are supplied from the posterior cerebral artery, and in a proportion of normal subjects both medial thalamic areas are supplied by a single penetrating artery. Dense amnestic symptoms occur if the hippocampus and other limbic structures are involved bilaterally. Such disorders can be a particular diagnostic dilemma as early CT scan investigations are often negative, although subsequent MRI scans will show the bilateral lesions.

Internal carotid artery occlusion may be entirely asymptomatic but much depends on the efficiency of collateral circulation and the Circle of Willis in particular. The clinical picture is often that of middle cerebral artery occlusion. However, in some situations cognitive and behavioural symptoms are predominant, with general slowing, decreased spontaneous activity and dyspraxia. In these situations it is important to pay attention to the abruptness of onset of the symptoms.

Vertebrobasilar strokes can be extremely diverse in their manifestations. Total occlusion of the basilar artery is usually rapidly fatal. Partial occlusions can be very diverse but the hallmark is brainstem involvement with a combination of unilateral or bilat-

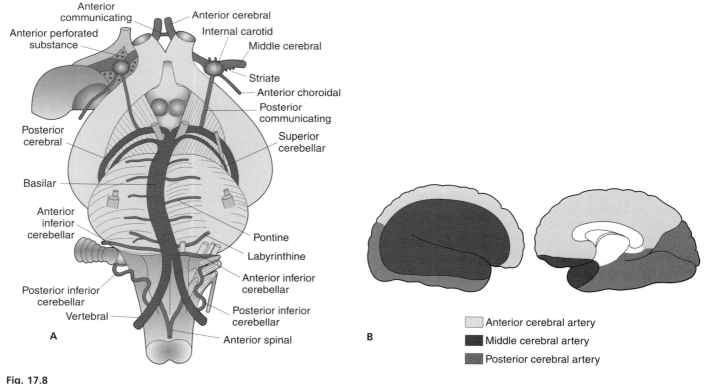

Fig. 17.8
(A) The Circle of Willis and the arteries of the brainstem. It should be noted that the arterial 'circle' lies in a horizontal plane and the basilar artery is vertical. (B) The lateral areas (left) and the medial areas (right) supplied by the cerebral arteries.

eral pyramidal signs and ipsilateral cranial nerve palsies. One, thankfully rare, variant is the 'locked in' syndrome where total paralysis is accompanied by full wakefulness and alertness. Occlusions of the rostral branches of the basilar artery can result in infarction of the midbrain, thalamus and portions of the temporal and occipital lobes.

Psychiatric manifestations and their management

Delirium and cognitive impairment

Delirium affects 30–40% of patients in the first week after stroke. It is important to distinguish delirium from focal cognitive deficits affecting declarative memory. Although this can often be complicated by the presence of an agitation, the disturbance of attention and fluctuating pattern of impairment that accompany delirium are often absent in the latter. The presence of delirium after stroke is associated with poorer prognosis, longer duration of hospitalisation and increased risk of subsequent dementia. Dementia following stoke is common, and approximately one quarter of patients are found to be demented at 3 months after a stroke. This figure rises significantly if focal cognitive impairments are also counted.

Behavioural changes

Global aphasia leads to the abolition of all linguistic faculties, and recording of mood and emotion is speculative. Some accounts associate Broca's aphasia with intense emotional frustration that may be secondary to problems in social interaction, and Wernicke's aphasia may be associated with lack of insight, irritability and rage, with recovered patients reporting that they thought their examiner was being deliberately incomprehensible.

Anosognosia refers to partial or complete unawareness of a deficit. It may coexist with depression, suggesting two separate systems for emotional assessment. Anosognosia for hemiplegia is perhaps most described, but it can affect any function and is commonly associated with visual and language function. It occurs more frequently with right-sided lesions, particularly in middle cerebral artery territory.

Affective dysprosodia is the impairment of the production and comprehension of language components which allow the communication of inner emotional states in speech, such as stresses, pauses, cadences, accent, melody and intonation. Its presence is not associated with an actual deficit in the ability to experience emotions, just in the ability to communicate or recognise them in the speech of others. It is particularly associated with right-sided lesions.

Apathy manifests as reduced spontaneous actions or speech, and delayed, short, slow or absent responses. Apathy is frequently associated with hypophonia, perseverations, grasp reflex, compulsive manipulations, cognitive and functional impairment and older age. Hypoactivity of frontal and anterior temporal regions have been observed.

Depression after stroke is also common, occurring in about a quarter in the first year. Depressive disorder is usually defined according to standard DSM-IV or ICD-10 criteria. However, these criteria may be hard to apply because of communication problems and difficulties in deciding whether to attribute symptoms such as sleep disturbance to the stroke or to the depression. Possible solutions are to use the accounts of informants and to place more weight on mood change and loss of interest that on somatic symptoms (see also Chapter 28). Most clinicians take a pragmatic approach and will treat depression in patients who have suggestive symptoms, although this is not without the risk of causing complications such as delirium. There has been much controversy over the cause of depression after stroke. Much emphasis has been placed on the site of the stroke lesion, and in particular on the hypothesis that damage to the left frontal area causes depression. However, a recent meta-analysis found no support for this hypothesis (Carson et al 2000). The disability caused by the stroke is clearly a likely cause of depression in many cases but the association of depression and anasagnosial states indicates that this is not the sole cause. There are disappointingly few RCTs of treatments for depression after stroke. Both SSRI and tricyclic antidepressants have been shown to be effective, and although SSRI drugs are probably better tolerated (Andersen et al 1994), nortriptyline was superior to fluoxetine in the only head to head trial. Certainly stroke patients who are prescribed antidepressants should be closely monitored for both treatment effectiveness and for adverse drug effects. The use of psychological treatments, in particular cognitive-behavioural therapies, potentially offers a solution to this problem but has not been adequately evaluated and trials so far have been negative (Lincoln & Flannaghan 2003).

Anxiety disorders are also common after stroke. They probably share the same risk factors as depression. Stroke is a sudden and unpredictable life-threatening stressor, and post-stroke anxiety states may be associated with fear of recurrence. This can lead to agoraphobia and to the patient's misinterpretation of somatic symptoms of anxiety as frightening evidence of recurrent stroke. Although there is a paucity of evidence from RCTs the standard drug and psychological therapies are probably effective.

Emotionalism or emotional lability, with an increase in laughing or crying with little or no warning signals, is frequent in acute stroke. There is an association with depression but the two can exist independently (House et al 1989). It has been suggested that the abnormality is serotonergic and that there is a specific response to SSRIs.

Catastrophic reactions manifest as disruptive emotional behaviour when a patient finds a task unsolvable. They are often associated with aphasia and it has been suggested that damage to language areas is a critical part of the aetiology. They generally exist independent of depression in acute strokes, but many patients showing catastrophic reactions will over time develop depression.

Psychosis and in particular mania are occasionally reported following acute stroke. Old age and pre-existing degenerative disease seem to increase the risk. Treatment is assumed to follow that of psychosis generally. Reduplicative paramnesias can occur and are usually short lived, although a small number of chronic cases have been reported.

PARKINSON'S DISEASE

Definition

Parkinson's disease is a degenerative condition characterised by the triad of tremor, rigidity and bradykinesia.

Epidemiology

The prevalence of Parkinson's disease is 200–300 per 100 000. The prevalence rises with age and increases with distance from the equator.

Aetiology

The cause of Parkinson's disease remains unknown. Genetic forms have been described, but account for a minority of cases. Similarly, environmental causes such as viral infection have been suggested, but no single exposure has been consistently replicated, with the exception of cases associated with the recreational drug MPTP. Cigarette smoking decreases risk.

Clinical features

Rest tremor is the most characteristic feature of Parkinson's disease and is found in most patients. In the early stages of disease it is described as 'pill-rolling'. The rigidity manifests as fixed abnormalities of posture and resistance to passive movement throughout the range of the joint. Concurrent tremor can give this a 'cogwheel' sensation. Bradykinesia is usually of insidious onset and the most disabling feature. Postural instability is a common additional feature, giving rise to an increasing liability to falls as the disorder progresses. Abnormal involuntary movements are common, both as a result of the disease process and of dopaminergic replacement therapy. Freezing of gait is one of the most poorly understood features of the disease but is one of the most disturbing to patients. Freezing to visual cues may be misinterpreted as voluntary behaviour. Non-motor manifestations are common and include autonomic (particularly orthostatic hypotension, bladder and gastrointestinal disturbances), sensory (pain), cognitive and emotional symptoms.

Cognitive symptoms

Approximately one-third of patients with Parkinson's disease have symptoms of dementia. Impairment of 'frontal' functions is detectable from very early in the disease process. Hallucinations and delusions are a common feature of dementia in Parkinson's disease. Clinically it is important to distinguish between a delirium of acute onset with disorientation, impaired attention, perceptive and cognitive disturbance and alteration to the sleep–wake cycle, on the one hand, and an iatrogenic dopaminomimetic psychosis, which is a subacute, gradually progressive psychotic state without a primary deficit of attention. The former state is often induced by dopamine agonists (such as selegiline) or anticholinergic medication. Appropriate examination and laboratory tests should be performed to detect underlying aetiological factors. For the latter a reduction in the dose of dopaminomimetic drugs can be considered, but is seldom successful, and antipsychotic drugs are often required but may worsen motor function. Clozapine and Quietapine are favourite agents.

Emotional symptoms

Depression is common in Parkinson's disease, with a prevalence of around 50% (Burn 2002). There is a bimodal distribution with peaks at early and late stages of disease. Large-scale studies have demonstrated that depression is one of the major determinants of quality of life in Parkinson's disease. The degree to which it is neurogenic remains uncertain. Mood changes can accompany the late-stage fluctuations to levodopa, known as on–off phenomena. Bipolar mood changes reflecting the on–off phases have been described.

Anxiety is also common in Parkinson's disease. It tends to occur with depression and is associated with the severity of motor symptoms. In particular, marked anticipatory anxiety concerning freezing of gait is a common phenomenon. Treatment with antidepressant drugs and cognitive behavioural therapy, particularly if delivered in conjunction with an active physiotherapy programme, can be helpful. Benzodiazepines may be required.

EPILEPSY

Definition

Epilepsy is an episodic condition associated with cerebral seizure activity. A seizure is a transient cerebral dysfunction resulting from an excessive abnormal electrical discharge of neurons (Fig. 17.9). The clinical manifestations are numerous. As a result the psychiatrist commonly encounters epilepsy both when considering whether epilepsy is the primary cause of paroxysmal psychiatric symptomatology and when treating its significant psychiatric complications.

Epidemiology

The prevalence of active epilepsy is around 7 per 1000 in the developed world. There is a higher incidence in developing nations, probably as a result of increased rates of birth trauma and head injury. Most studies show a bimodal distribution of the incidence with increased rates below 10 years and above 60 years old. It is twice as common in men.

Aetiology

In less than one third of cases is a specific cause identified. These include perinatal disorders, learning disabilities, cerebral palsy, head trauma, CNS infection, cerebrovascular disease, brain tumours, Alzheimer's disease and substance misuse. Many idiopathic seizures are likely to have a genetic basis.

Clinical features

Epilepsy refers to a heterogeneous group of disorders with multiple causes and manifestations, and its clinical features reflect this diversity. The key clinical distinction is between seizures with a focal or a generalised cerebral origin. The former are more likely to be associated with a detectable and potentially remediable cerebral lesion; the latter more likely to start in childhood or adolescence and to be familial. Despite the wide variety of possible seizure manifestations, an individual patient's seizures are usually stereotyped. Their clinical features result from a recurrent pattern of cortical hyperactivity during the ictal event followed by hypoactivity in the same area post-ictally (Fig. 17.10). This gives rise to predictable set of symptoms dependent upon the brain region affected (Fig. 17.11).

Tonic-clonic seizures are the most dramatic manifestation of epilepsy and are characterised by motor activity and sudden loss of consciousness. In a typical seizure a patient has no warning with the possible exception of a couple of myoclonic jerks. The seizure begins with sudden loss of consciousness and a tonic phase during which there is sustained muscle contraction lasting 10–20 seconds. This is followed by a clonic phase, of repetitive muscle contraction that lasts approximately 30 seconds. A number of autonomic changes may also occur including an increase in blood pressure and pulse rate, apnoea, mydriaisis, incontinence, piloerection, cyanosis

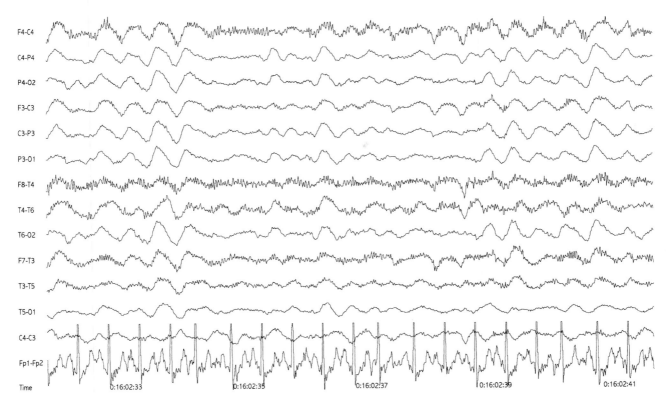

Fig. 17.9
This EEG shows bursts of bilateral anteriorly dominant 2–3 Hz delta rhythmical EEG activity which corresponded with the patient reporting a sense of 'impending doom'. The focus of the seizures was deep in the frontal cortex.

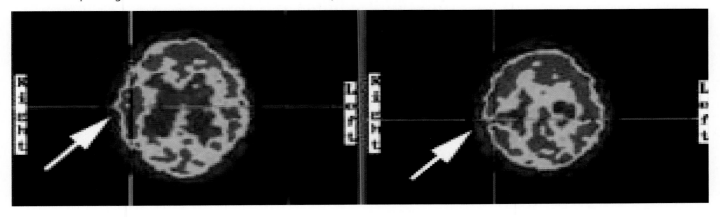

Fig. 17.10
SPET scans during epileptic seizures show hyperactivity in the region of onset at the time of the seizure, then hypoactivity postictally in the same area. The symptoms seen during a fit will correspond to the brain regions affected.

and perspiration. In the post-ictal period the patient is drowsy and confused. Abnormal neurological signs are often elicited.

Partial seizures are categorised according to whether they are simple (without impairment in consciousness) or complex (with impairment of consciousness). This classification is problematic in clinical practice and it may be abandoned.

Simple partial seizures have features that depend on the brain region activated. Although the initial area is relatively localised, it is common for the abnormal activity to spread to adjacent areas, producing progression of the seizure pattern. If the activity originates in the motor cortex, there will be jerking movements in the contralateral body part. This will cause progressive jerking in contiguous regions, known as Jacksonian march. Activity in the supplementary motor cortex causes head turning with arm extension on the same side — the classic 'fencer's posture'. Seizures originating in the parietal lobe can cause tingling or numbness in a bodily region or more complex sensory experiences such as a sense of absence on one side of the body, asomatognosia. Seizures in the inferior regions of the parietal lobe can cause severe vertigo and disorientation in space. Dominant hemisphere parietal lobe seizures can cause language disturbance. Seizures of the occipital lobe are associated with visual symptoms which are usually elementary, such

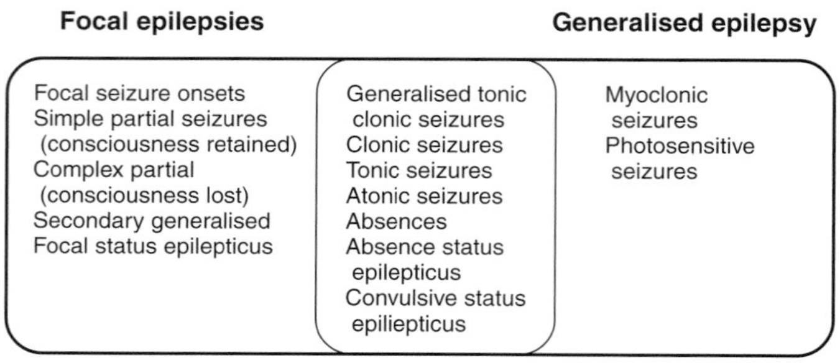

Focal epilepsies   **Generalised epilepsy**

Focal seizure onsets	Generalised tonic	Myoclonic
Simple partial seizures	clonic seizures	seizures
(consciousness retained)	Clonic seizures	Photosensitive
Complex partial	Tonic seizures	seizures
(consciousness lost)	Atonic seizures	
Secondary generalised	Absences	
Focal status epilepticus	Absence status	
	epilepticus	
	Convulsive status	
	epiliepticus	

Fig. 17.11
A simplified version of the ILA classification of epilepsy.

as simple flashing lights. However, if the seizure occurs at the border with the temporal lobe more complex experiences can occur, including micropsia, macropsia and metamorphosia as well as visual hallucinations of previously experienced imagery. Seizures affecting the temporal lobe can be the most difficult to diagnose, but it is also the most common site of onset accounting for 80% of partial seizures. Symptoms include auditory hallucinations ranging from simple sounds to complex language. Olfactory hallucinations, usually involving unpleasant odours, follow discharge in the mesial temporal lobe. Seizures in the sylvian fissure or operculum will cause gustatory sensations, and epigsatric sensations such as nausea or emptiness are generally secondary to a temporal lobe origin. The well-known emotional and psychic phenomena of temporal lobe seizure activity can occur in simple seizures but are more common in complex partial seizures

Complex partial seizures are commonly associated with an aura at the onset of the seizure. The aura is a simple partial seizure lasting seconds to minutes. It should be distinguished from a prodrome, which is not an ictal event, and can last for hours or even days before a seizure. Prodromes usually consist of a sense of nervousness or irritability. The content of the aura will depend on the location of the abnormal discharge within the brain. Thus it may consist of motor, sensory, visceral or psychic elements. This can include hallucinations, intense affective symptoms such as fear or depression or panic, and cognitive symptoms such as aphasia or depersonalisation. Distortions of memory can include dreamy states, flashbacks and distortions of familiarity with events (déjà vu or jamais vu). Occasionally, rapid recollection of episodes from past life experiences occurs (panoramic vision). Rage is rare, but when it does occur it is associated with lack of provocation and abrupt abatement. This is then followed by impairment of consciousness and a seizure usually lasting 60–90 seconds. It may generalise into a tonic-clonic seizure. Automatisms may be present and can involve an extension of the patient's actions prior to seizure onset. They commonly include chewing or swallowing, lip smacking, grimacing, or automatisms on the extremities including fumbling with objects, walking or trying to stand up. Post-ictal confusion is usually significant and would be expected to last for 10 minutes or longer. Complex partial seizures of a frontal lobe origin tend to begin and end abruptly, with minimal post-ictal confusion, and often occur in clusters. The attacks are usually bizarre, with motor automatisms such as bicycling, or sexual automatisms and vocalisations.

Absence seizures are well-defined clinical and EEG events. The essential feature is an abrupt, brief episode of decreased awareness without any warning, aura or post-ictal symptoms. At the onset

there is a disruption of activity, and a simple absence seizure is characterised by only an alteration in consciousness. The patient remains mobile, breathing is unaffected, there is no cyanosis or pallor and no loss of postural tone or motor activity. The ending is abrupt and the patient resumes his previous activity immediately, often unaware that a seizure has taken place. An attack usually lasts around 15 seconds. A complex absence seizure displays additional symptoms such as loss or increase of postural tone, minor clonic movements of face or extremities, minor face or extremities automatisms or autonomic symptoms such as pallor, flushing, tachycardia, piloerection, mydriasis or urinary incontinence.

Violent behaviour of an undirected nature can occasionally arise from the emotional changes associated with temporal lobe seizures. However, in the overwhelming majority of cases violence is in response to being restrained during a seizure. We suggest that psychiatrists are very cautious indeed before attributing other violent assaults to a seizure. The following criteria should be considered before making such a link.

- Has known epilepsy.
- Clear evidence of a seizure at the time of the offence.
- The offender's usual seizure phenomena might explain behaviour at time of offence.
- Behaviour at time of offence within range of known ictal/post-ictal behaviours — in particular, no evidence of structured thought such as going to a specific drawer in a different room to find a knife then returning to commit an assault.
- No external motive for the offence.

Differential diagnosis

Documentation of the clinical features of the seizure is usually the key to diagnosis. As first-hand observation is seldom possible, unless seizures are very frequent, the history of the episode, including an eye-witness account (or a home video), is of paramount importance. The chief differential diagnosis of epilepsy is from non-epileptic attack disorder and syncope. It also needs to be distinguished from other paroxysmal disorders, including transient ischaemic attacks, panic attacks, hyperventilation attacks, hypoglycaemia, migraine, transient global amnesia, cataplexy, paroxysmal movement disorders and paroxysmal symptoms in multiple sclerosis. Attacks during sleep can pose particular difficulties as informant reports are often less reliable.

Non-epileptic attack disorder (NEAD) previously referred to as 'pseudo-epilepsy' or 'psychogenic epilepsy' is an important differential diagnosis. It accounts for around 30% of patients attending clinics with suspected epilepsy. Some patients have both epilepsy and non-epileptic attacks, but probably only around 10% of those with NEAD fall into this category. Many of these patients are learning disabled and at increased risk of both epilepsy and psychiatric disorders. The diagnosis of NEAD can often be made on the basis of a careful history and examination. Clinical clues include:

- the presence of prior or current psychiatric disorders, including somatoform disorders;
- atypical varieties of seizure, especially the occurrence of frequent and prolonged seizures in the face of normal interictal intellectual function and EEG;
- a preponderance of seizures in public places, especially in surgeries and hospitals;

Box 17.12   Distinguishing NEAD from epilepsy

More likely in NEAD
- Resistance to eye opening
- Eyes shut during attack
- Responsive during generalised shaking attack (or can interrupt seizure)
- Memory of seizure
- Weeping during or after a seizure
- Generalised attack lasting longer than 2–3 minutes

Unhelpful in distinguishing NEAD from epilepsy
- Aura or post-ictal confusion
- Tongue biting
- Injury (carpet burns may indicate pseudoseizure)
- Incontinence
- Pelvic thrusting
- Attack during sleep
- 'Status epilepticus'
- Patient alone during a seizure
- Elevation of post-ictal prolactin — may be elevated in syncope

---

- behaviour during an apparently generalised seizure which suggests preservation of awareness, for example resistance to attempted eye opening and persistent aversion of gaze from the examiner.

A history of childhood abuse is common but by no means universal. Where doubt remains after careful clinical assessment and standard investigations, the gold standard for diagnosis is the observation of attacks during videotelemetry. A normal EEG during or immediately after an apparently generalised seizure provides strong evidence against epilepsy (Box 17.12).

Syncope is due to temporary interruption of the blood supply to the brain. It should be noted that it is often accompanied by myoclonic jerks which may be misinterpreted as epileptic by both lay and medical onlookers. The occurrence of more complex movements, eye deviation, eyelid flicker or vocalisations can confuse the diagnosis further. Similarly, the majority of subjects recall aura symptoms including epigastric, vertiginous, visual and somatosensory experiences.

Sleep disorders, including sleepwalking, night terrors and confusional arousals, all of which occur from slow-wave sleep, REM sleep behaviour disorder, and a variety of other parasomnias including bruxism, rhythmic movement disorder and periodic limb movements, must all be distinguished from epilepsy.

Investigation of seizures

Epilepsy is a clinical diagnosis, and the use and interpretation of investigations must reflect this. Routine blood tests should include full blood count, urea and electrolytes, liver function tests, glucose, and calcium. An ECG should always be performed. An EEG is helpful if there is doubt about the diagnosis, or a need to clarify the type of epilepsy (generalised or focal). However, the EEG is insensitive: a single interictal EEG will detect clearly epileptiform abnormalities in only about 30% of patients with epilepsy. Therefore a normal EEG does not exclude epilepsy, just as minor non-specific abnormalities do not confirm it. Serial recordings, including sleep-deprived recordings, increase the diagnostic yield to about 80%. EEG can be supplemented with video recording to allow the correlation between clinical symptoms and EEG abnormality to be examined (videotelemetry). Twenty-four-hour ambulatory monitoring is sometimes helpful. Some form of neuroimaging should be performed to exclude tumours and major structural abnormalities. Measurement of serum prolactin is of limited value as false positives and negatives occur. Additional cardiac investigations which may be helpful in selected cases include 24-hour ambulatory ECG to identify cardiac dysrhythmias, echocardiography to identify structural cardiac abnormalities, and tilt table testing to help confirm the diagnosis of syncope.

Treatment of seizures

The mainstay of management is with anti-epileptic drugs. A large number are available. The principles of drug treatment are:

- Use a single drug whenever possible.
- Increase the dose slowly until either the seizures are controlled or toxicity occurs.
- If a single drug does not control seizures without toxicity then switch initially to another drug used alone.
- Drug level monitoring is generally unnecessary except in the case of phenytoin, and is sometimes misleading: some patients do well with drug levels below or above the 'therapeutic range'.
- Consider using two drugs only when monotherapy is unsuccessful.
- Be aware that the ability to metabolise anticonvulsant medication is different in the young, the elderly, pregnant women and patients with chronic disease, particularly hepatic and renal, and be on the lookout for drug interactions.

Approximately 20–30% of patients do not achieve seizure control with drug treatment. In carefully selected cases surgery can be effective. It is noteworthy that poor psychological outcomes occasionally accompany good post-operative seizure control and some patients need considerable psychological help in adjusting to life without seizures.

Vagal nerve stimulation has been shown to reduce seizure frequency in some patients with refractory epilepsy, but probably no more so than the addition of the newer anticonvulsants to established therapy.

Psychiatric manifestations of seizures and their management

Studies have found greatly increased rates of psychiatric disorder in both men and women with epilepsy when compared with healthy controls, but not when compared with controls with a chronic medical condition.

Psychoses

In describing the psychiatry of epilepsy, symptoms are usually related temporally to seizure events. Hence psychotic symptoms generally divide into transient post-ictal psychoses and chronic interictal psychoses. The former often present with manic grandiosity, religious and mystical features. A number of small studies have suggested that such patients are more likely to have psychic auras, bilateral interictal spikes and nocturnal secondarily generalised seizures than other epilepsy patients. In general, psychotic episodes do not start immediately after a seizure but follow a lucid interval of 2–72 hours. In contrast, patients with chronic interictal psychoses had a higher frequency of perceptual delusions and auditory hallucinations than patients with post-ictal psychoses.

Anti-epileptic drugs may also contribute to the development of psychotic symptoms, especially newer agents. Vigabatrin, an irreversible inhibitor of GABA transaminase, has been shown to precipitate psychotic and affective symptoms in 3–10% of patients. This is more likely in patients with significant past psychiatric histories.

Depression and anxiety

Depressive and anxiety disorders affect approximately one-third of patients with epilepsy. Neurobiological, psychological, social and iatrogenic factors have all been suggested and probably all are relevant. Notably the drugs used to treat epilepsy can also be a cause of depression. Anxiety probably has a similarly complex aetiology. Anticipatory anxiety about having a seizure, in the absence of a warning, can lead to considerable secondary disability in the form of agoraphobic-like symptoms and behavioural response. The treatment of depressive and anxiety disorders follows the normal principles of treatment of anxiety and depression in the medically unwell. Care needs to be taken, however, not to exacerbate the epilepsy, as antidepressant agents tend to lower seizure threshold.

TIC DISORDERS

These are a type of movement disorder. Tics are sudden, rapid, repetitive, twitch-like movements

Gilles de la Tourette's syndrome

Definition

This is an idiopathic condition in which multiple tics are associated with forced involuntary vocalisations which may take the form of obscenities (coprolalia).

Clinical features

The condition is characterised by a combination of multiple, waxing and waning motor and vocal tics. These vary from simple twitches and grunts to complex stereotypies. Premonitory sensations in body parts that 'need to tic' are a common feature and complicate the picture, as their temporary suppressibility lends them a voluntary component. Other features are echolalia and coprophasia, particularly in severe cases. The syndrome is strongly associated with obsessive–compulsive disorder, but many claim that it is qualitatively different — with concern with symmetry, aggressive thoughts, forced touching, and fear of harming self being prominent compared with typical symptom clusters of hygiene and cleanliness. Depressive symptoms are commonplace, and attention deficit hyperactivity disorder has been described, but the issue of appropriate comparison groups has led to debate over its relevance.

Epidemiology

The prevalence is around 5 per 10 000 with a 4:1 ratio of males.

Aetiology

Genetic studies have suggested a strong hereditary component but without a specific pattern of inheritance. Similarly the neuro-

biology remains elusive, with dysfunctional dopaminergic basal ganglia circuitry receiving most attention. Structural imaging is usually normal and functional imaging data are contradictory at the current time.

Management

Management must address the educational, social and family consequences of the disorder. Dopamine antagonists remain the mainstay of pharmacological management, with haloperidol the most widely used. Pimozide has been shown superior in one of the few RCTs conducted, but the potential cardiac side-effects limit its use.

DYSTONIAS

Definition

The dystonias are a group of movement disorders characterised clinically by involuntary twisting movements and abnormal postures.

Clinical features

The traditional clinical categorisation is based on age at onset, distribution of symptoms and site of onset. Early-onset dystonia often starts in a limb, tends to generalise and frequently has a genetic origin. By contrast adult-onset dystonias usually spare the lower limbs and frequently involve the cervical or cranial muscles, with a tendency to remain focal. They appear sporadic in most cases. Dystonias tend to improve with relaxation, hypnosis and sleep. With the exception of cervical dystonia, pain is uncommon. The fluctuant nature of the symptoms, the ability to use 'tricks' to suppress them, and their association with task-specific symptoms (e.g. writer's cramp) can often lead to the erroneous assertion of a functional disorder.

Aetiology

Primary torsion dystonias are commonly associated with the *DYT1* gene on chromosome 9. The inheritance is autosomal dominant with reduced penetrance. It usually begins in childhood, in a limb, then generalises to other body parts.

Focal dystonia is the most prevalent form of the disorder, starting in adulthood and remaining focal such as an isolated torticollis. The majority of cases appear sporadic, although some family pedigree studies have shown an increased risk of autosomal-dominant focal dystonias in other family members.

Dopa responsive dystonia (DRD) is characterised by childhood onset, diurnal fluctuation of symptoms and a dramatic response to levodopa therapy. It generally has autosomal-dominant inheritance although recessive forms associated with mutations in the tyrosine hydroxylase gene have been described.

Management

Medical treatment involves oral drugs and botulinum injections. Botulinum therapy is the most effective treatment for focal dystonias such as torticollis. In generalised dystonia, a trial of levodopa should be considered in all early onset cases. Thereafter the first-line treatment is usually anticholinergics, followed by baclofen and possibly benzodiazepines and dopamine depletors such as tetrabenazine. Surgical treatment is by selective peripheral denervation or functional brain surgery.

SUMMARY

There is increasing recognition of the overlap between neurological and psychiatric practice. Many of the patients traditionally seen by psychiatrists are increasingly recognised to have structural brain abnormalities, and many neurological patients have none (Martin 2002). It will be increasingly important both for neurologists to be able to perform mental-state assessments and for psychiatrists to be competent to perform basic neurological assessments and to interpret neurological investigations. This is especially important for those psychiatric disorders traditionally regarded as organic.

ACKNOWLEDGEMENTS

The authors would like to thank Dr Rod Duncan, Consultant Neurologist, Glasgow, for providing information on violence and epilepsy, and Dr Don Collie, Consultant Neuroradiologist, Edinburgh, for providing the MRI scans.

FURTHER READING

Bogousslavsky J, Cummings J L 2000 Behaviour and mood disorders in focal brain lesions. Cambridge University Press, Cambridge

Hodges J R 2001 Early-onset dementia: a multidisciplinary approach. Oxford University Press, Oxford

Lance J W, Goadsby P J 1998 Mechanism and management of headache, 6th edn. Butterworth-Heinemann, Oxford

Lishman A W 1998 Organic psychiatry: the psychological consequences of cerebral disorder, 3rd edn. Blackwell Science, London

Mayou R, Sharpe M, Carson A J 2002 ABC of psychological medicine. BMJ Press/Tavistock, London

O'Brien J, Ames D, Burns A 2000 Dementia, 2nd edn. Arnold, London

REFERENCES

Aguzzi A, Klein M A, Montrasio F et al 2000 Prions: pathogenesis and reverse genetics. Annals of the New York Academy of Sciences 920:140–157

Andersen G, Vestergaard K, Lauritzen L 1994 Effective treatment of poststroke depression with the selective serotonin reuptake inhibitor citalopram. Stroke 25:1099–1104

Bamford J, Sandercock P, Dennis M et al 1988 A prospective study of acute-cerebrovascular disease in the community: the Oxfordshire Community Stroke Project 1981–86, 1: Methodology, demography and incident cases of first-ever stroke. Journal of Neurology, Neurosurgery & Psychiatry 51:1373–1380

Breitbart W, Marotta R, Platt M M et al 1996 A double-blind trial of haloperidol, chlorpromazine, and lorazepam in the treatment of delirium in hospitalized AIDS patients. American Journal of Psychiatry 153:231–237

Brown T M, Boyle M F 2002 Delirium. British Medical Journal 325:644–647

Burn D J 2002 Depression in Parkinson's disease. European Journal of Neurology 9(suppl 3): 44–54

Carson A J, Machale S M, Allen K et al 2000 Depression after stroke and lesion location: a systematic review. Lancet 356:122–126

Folstein M F, Folstein S E, McHugh P R 1975 Mini-Mental State. Journal of Psychiatric Research 12:189–198

Gregory C A, Hodges J R 1993 Dementia of frontal type and the focal lobar atrophies. International Review of Psychiatry 5:397–406

Hodges J R 1994 Cognitive assessment for clinicians. Oxford University Press, Oxford

House A O, Dennis M, Molyneux A et al 1989 Emotionalism after stroke. British Medical Journal 298:991–994

Lincoln N B, Flannaghan T 2003 Cognitive behavioral psychotherapy for depression following stroke: a randomized controlled trial. Stroke 34:111–115

Lipkin M J 1969 Functional or organic? a pointless question. Annals of Internal Medicine 5:1013–1017

Lipowski Z J 1989 Delirium in the elderly patient. New England Journal of Medicine 320:578–582

Lishman W A 1988 Physiogenesis and psychogenesis in the postconcussional syndrome. British Journal of Psychiatry 153:460–469

Martin J B 2002 The integration of neurology, psychiatry, and neuroscience in the 21st century. American Journal of Psychiatry 159:695–704

Mathuranath P S, Nestor P J, Berrios G E et al 2000 A brief cognitive test battery to differentiate Alzheimer's disease and frontotemporal dementia. Neurology 55:1613–1620

Meagher D J 2001 Delirium: optimising management. British Medical Journal 322:144–149

Spencer M D, Knight R S G, Will R G 2002 First hundred cases of variant Creutzfeldt–Jakob disease: retrospective case note review of early psychiatric and menrological features. British Medical Journal 324:1479–1482

Thornhill S, Teasdale G M, Murray G D et al 2000 Disability in young people and adults one year after head injury: prospective cohort study. British Medical Journal 320:1631–1635

Zubaran C, Fernandes J G, Rodnight R 1997 Wernicke–Korsakoff syndrome. Postgraduate Medical Journal 73:27–31

18 | Misuse of, and dependence on, alcohol and other drugs

Malcolm Bruce, Bruce Ritson

INTRODUCTION

It is hard to think of any country which does not rely on some drug or other to facilitate social relations, mark festivals or enhance religious rituals. In Britain, alcohol is the most widely used and misused drug, but other forms of drug misuse are not new (Geikie 1904).

In considering the consequences of drug use, it is helpful to differentiate between the pharmacology of the drug, the hazards inherent in the route of administration, the dose and frequency of use and the health and personality of the user. Finally, and perhaps more crucial, is consideration of the setting in which the drug is taken, the immediate surroundings, the presence of friends, their attitudes and expectations, the culture and folklore surrounding the drug as well as the legal sanctions on its use. Drugs regarded as hazardous and illegal in one culture or time in history have been condoned or even promoted in another.

Historical and cultural aspects of alcohol consumption

Ethyl alcohol is a natural product of the breakdown of carbohydrates in plants, Its euphoriant and intoxicating properties have been known from prehistoric times, and almost all cultures have had some experience of its use. Early Egyptian and Greek writings make several references to alcohol and distinguish between its beneficial effects in moderation and the problem of drunkenness. Throughout the 17th century in Britain drunkenness was widespread. In an effort to promote agriculture and obstruct competition from French brandies, positive incentives were given to produce cheap gin. This policy succeeded so completely that by 1736 consumption of spirits was approximately one gallon a head per annum (Dillon 2002). Gradually, by means of licensing and taxation, consumption was reduced, only to rise again during the 19th century. The chief opponent of drunkenness at that time was the Temperance Movement. Initially it advocated moderate consumption but later moved to champion total abstinence. Some physicians such as Benjamin Rush, in the USA and Thomas Trotter in Scotland pointed out both medical and psychological consequences of alcohol misuse, and moved toward the contemporary concept of alcohol addiction.

The Temperance Movement scored its greatest victory in the 18th Amendment of the US Constitution, which prohibited the manufacture and sale of alcohol except for therapeutic or sacramental purposes. The Amendment was difficult to enforce and led to gangsterism. Because of these social consequences and lack of public support, it was repealed in 1933. (It is noteworthy that cirrhosis mortality declined during the years of prohibition.) The Temperance Movement never attained the political strength in Britain which it enjoyed in the USA or some Scandinavian countries. Nonetheless, it was a considerable force by the end of the 19th century and it facilitated the introduction of control measures which Lloyd George imposed during the First World War

There is nothing fixed or unchanging about a nation's drug or alcohol usage. Habits have changed dramatically in Britain during the past century, most often in response to economic and social influences. 'Dry' generations are often followed by those that are relatively 'wet'. The consequences of excess give rise to the reinstatement of controls, and the cycle repeats itself. These cycles, which are evident in many countries, should be an encouragement to preventive strategies which we might hope to influence the tide of change and fashion in the direction of harm reduction.

PREVENTION OF MISUSE

General issues

In the past, primary prevention of both drug and alcohol misuse has focused principally on controlling availability, or strengthening the resistance of the individual by education and persuasion. The health and social costs of a substance are not necessarily reflected in the effort invested in education or control. Tobacco, which is a more damaging drug in health terms, is legally available and advertised in many countries. This chapter will not be concerned with tobacco but it is important to recognise its addictive properties, damaging health consequences and the difficulty experienced by individuals in changing this habit once they have become addicted.

Prevention of alcohol misuse

For alcohol-related problems, prevention should be better than cure because the efficacy of treatment is uncertain and the problem is endemic in most industrialised countries. The mean per caput level of alcohol consumption in a population and the prevalence of heavy drinking are closely correlated ($r = 0.97$) (Rose & Day 1990). Thus a 10% decline in consumption would reduce the number of heavy drinkers by a similar percentage. While excessive drinkers experience many more alcohol-related problems than other drinkers, their contribution to the level of alcohol-related harm in a community is lower than that arising from the much larger population of moderate and light drinkers. Focusing a preventive strategy only on those at 'high risk' would have less impact on the overall level of harm than would a population-based approach. This is termed *the preventive paradox* (Kreitman 1986).

Prevention is most visibly effective when a specified effect can be traced to a cause which is readily amenable to influence. For example, the association between drink-driving and road accidents is clear-cut, and the 1967 legislation imposing penalties on those driving in the UK with a raised blood alcohol level had an immediate effect in reducing the number of road fatalities by 15%, although the effect diminished as drivers began to realise that the risk of detection was low. There is evidence that the introduction of random breath testing would lead to a further decline in alcohol-related accidents.

Primary prevention

Primary prevention is aimed at reducing the prevalence of hazardous drinking, or in some cases the hazards of drinking (for example by separating drinking from driving) in the population. It relies on three strategies: control of availability, education about sensible use, and providing alternative pursuits (Table 18.1). These approaches are not mutually exclusive alternatives but are interdependent. For instance, it would be politically unwise to introduce controls which did not enjoy a measure of public acceptance, an aim which would have to be pursued first by an active public education programme. There is considerable scope for local action aimed for instance at licensing practices, road safety or providers of alternative leisure pursuits (Ritson 1995). In some cases the task is to separate drinking from certain contexts such as drinking and work, sport such as swimming, or driving.

Controls of availability Prohibition is an extreme form of control. It proved effective in reducing mortality from liver cirrhosis in the USA in the 1920s, but these gains were outweighed by other social problems which arose. The limitations of prohibition and similar restrictive endeavours include the public resentment which they may generate, difficulties with enforcement, loss of tax revenue (currently over £10 000 million per annum in the UK), and the growth of smuggling and illicit production of what may prove to be lethal brews. Most countries now endeavour to control rather than prohibit availability. (An exception is within Islam where cultural tradition sustains prohibition.)

Major restrictions on permitted hours of sale of alcohol in Britain were introduced by the Prime Minister Lloyd George in 1915 in an effort to ensure that the workforce was sufficiently sober to meet the demands required by the war effort. Consumption dropped at that time and remained low for more than a decade. In the UK the control, and particularly enforcement, of licensing laws and permitted hours of opening is amenable to considerable local influence and can be seen as one example of the importance of local action in influencing the level of alcohol-related harm in a community. Other examples are the designation of zones where public drinking is banned and restrictions on alcohol at sporting events; both have been shown to lead to an improvement in public order in the target areas.

Most countries impose a minimum age at which young people are allowed to drink in public. In the USA and Canada experience has shown that states or provinces which lowered the permitted age experienced a rise in motor accidents and drink-driving offences amongst the young.

Advertisers argue that they are simply concerned with promoting or sustaining brand loyalties among drinkers, but research suggests that they also stimulate overall consumption. The effects of advertising on the young are a particular concern, and most counties have controls on advertising that specifically seeks to attract youngsters or is placed near schools. In some communities there has been a total ban.

Price Over the past three hundred years, alcohol consumption in Britain has shown marked fluctuations. Every time the price of alcohol relative to disposable income has fallen, as it has done almost continuously since 1945, consumption has risen. In 1981 an increase in the excise duty on beer and spirits caused their price to rise faster than the retail price index and average disposable incomes. These economic changes were associated in Edinburgh with a decline in alcohol consumption of 18% and a reduction in alcohol-related harm of 16%. Contrary to predictions, heavy drinkers and even dependent drinkers reported a disproportionate reduction in their consumption (Kendell et al 1983).

The health lobby is but one competing interest group in the debate about controlling the availability and consumption of alcohol. Other groups argue in favour of continuing growth in the alcohol market. There is, for instance, the employment argument and the needs of the tourism and advertising industries.

Education Education needs to take into account the medium, the audience and the message. Target groups include the general public or specific segments of the population such as schoolchildren, the elderly or ethnic minorities, or particular high-risk groups such as pregnant women, drivers, or those in hazardous occupations. In the past, education for young people has often been woolly in focus and content, but even with

Table 18.1 Primary prevention strategies		
Strategy	Method/target	Aim
Controls	Fiscal Legislative	To reduce availability
Education	The general public Young people and at-risk groups Key professionals; politicians	To foster moderate informed drinking and promote awareness of hazards
Provision of alternatives	Promoting alternative leisure activities, facilitating sensible drinking, for instance with meals, ensuring that inexpensive non- or low-alcohol beverages are readily available	To promote sensible drinking

carefully designed and evaluated campaigns the lasting impact may be disappointingly small (Foxcroft et al 1997).

Education in schools should recognise that in the UK there is evidence that children know about alcohol from the age of 6 onwards and that their attitudes towards drinking change markedly and become more positive between 11 and 14, as the peer group begins to exert more influence than parents or teachers. Information about the alcohol content of various alcoholic beverages, sensible drinking practices and safe limits for consumption are facts which should be part of every young person's knowledge of the world. Evidence shows that it is easier to improve knowledge than to influence attitudes or particularly behaviour.

Public education can be concerned with informing the public about alcohol problems along with specific advice about where to seek help. Campaigns of this kind have not influenced drinking habits but have often produced an increase in utilisation of treatment and counselling facilities. Wallack et al (1993) has pointed to the importance of influencing the media to ensure that health issues are given a fair hearing and presentation in public debate.

Provision of alternatives Many communities are heavily dependent on drinking places as a principal source of entertainment. Clearly the pub has a significant social role in its neighbourhood, but those concerned with planning should ensure that other leisure pursuits are encouraged and that other non-alcoholic beverages are readily available. The promotion of low-alcohol beers and wine has proved helpful.

Secondary prevention

Secondary prevention aims to prevent the further progression of a condition by identifying and treating cases at an early stage. Symptom-free excessive drinkers see little reason to change their habits. However, a primary-care worker, consulted perhaps for some other reason, can take the opportunity to educate and persuade an excessive drinker to cut down.

There are a number of questionnaires available which facilitate early recognition of hazardous drinking. For general screening purposes AUDIT (Alcohol Use Disorders Test) is most effective at detecting hazardous or harmful drinking. Primary-healthcare physicians can also use the mean corpuscular volume (MCV) and gamma-glutamyl transpeptidase (gamma GT) in screening, since about 60% of heavy drinkers will show an elevation on one or other test. Carbohydrate deficient transferring (CDT) is another useful measure but less widely available in the UK. Blood tests are probably more useful in monitoring progress or augmenting the findings of screening questionnaires than for initial screening (Fiellin et al 2000).

A sensible policy which would enhance recognition would be to follow the Royal College of Physicians (1987) recommendation that every person seen in general practice or in hospital should be asked about his or her alcohol intake as a matter of routine, along with questions about smoking and medication, and the answers recorded.

A number of studies have shown that simple advice given by a suitably trained doctor or nurse can produce a significant decline in hazardous drinking with demonstrable benefit to health. For example, Wallace et al (1988) randomly allocated heavy drinkers to a treatment or control group. Treatment involved simple advice from the general practitioner about reducing consumption, and follow-up at 3-monthly intervals. After 1 year, 44% fewer men were drinking excessively in the treatment group than at baseline, compared with 26% fewer amongst controls, and 48% fewer women were drinking heavily in treatment than at baseline, compared with 29% in controls. Meta-analysis shows the health benefits of brief intervention for hazardous drinking (Waller et al 2002).

Prevention of drug misuse

Reducing supply through customs and enforcement agencies is outwith the scope of this chapter. However, reducing demand through health promotion does justify elaboration. Current strategies in drug education can be divided into a number of categories (Box 18.1). The first strategy, information type programmes, may slow transitions to heavier or hazardous use but do not stop experimentations. As for the second strategy, there is no support from outcome studies in adopting a moral-value or living-skills approach to drug prevention. The third, resistance strategies, may reduce experimentation but it promotes a polarised community, and drug use in those that use tends to be more hazardous. Providing alternatives, the fourth strategy, appears ineffective, but if linked to broader community initiatives, may prove useful. The fifth strategy, secondary prevention in the form of harm minimisation for those already using, has shown substantial benefits elaborated further on page 379. The final strategy requires further research, but studies suggest a positive response (Dorn & Murji 1992).

Prevention is not only limited to stopping initial drug use but may also be related to detecting use at an earlier stage, and this involves targeting, among others, parents to educate them about drugs and solvents so that the thresholds for detection in their children are lowered (Health Publications Unit 1993). Hair analysis for drugs has also produced a technological breakthrough along with an ethical quagmire, depending on your point of view (Strang et al 1993). Special circumstances are found in prison, and the introduction of mandatory drug testing in British prisons in February 1995 to detect, deter and prevent drug use may be having unexpected results, such as the switching from cannabis to injectable shorter-acting drugs to avoid detection (Gore et al 1996). Attempts at lowering the threshold of detection, and early intervention, to prevent serious drug problems, have also been attempted in the workplace. Training staff has been evaluated and shown to improve the confidence and the ability of staff to deal with drug and alcohol problems and hence their willingness to intervene (Gossop & Birkin 1994).

Box 18.1   Current strategies in drug education
• Providing information (whether 'scare' or 'balanced')
• Seeking to remedy supposed deficits of moral values or living skills
• Promoting decision-making skills in the context of anti-drug norms
• Providing alternatives to drug use through youth and community participation
• Secondary prevention by harm minimisation
• Peer-lead approaches involving youth groups with facilitators

EPIDEMIOLOGY

Epidemiology of drinking and alcohol-related harm

Epidemiology is concerned with the prevalence and incidence of illness in a population. When considering alcohol-related problems, the problem of 'caseness' is a significant barrier. The harm experienced with alcohol depends on age, gender, setting, culture, genetic make-up and pattern of consumption. Nonetheless, guidelines for risk and alcohol consumption have been agreed in the UK based on the unit system (note that the definition of a unit of alcohol varies between countries, and care should be taken in extrapolating from one country to another unless the units are defined). In the UK a unit of alcohol is equal to 8 g alcohol, which is 10 ml of 100% alcohol (roughly equivalent to half a pint of normal-strength beer, a small glass of wine or single measure of spirits). The levels of risk associated with consumption are shown in Table 18.2.

One in four adults in the UK is drinking in a hazardous way, and one in 25 adults is dependent on alcohol. Among 16–24-year-olds, 38% of men and 5% of women regularly drink twice the recommended safe levels of alcohol (Alcohol Concern 2000).

The prevalence of alcohol-related problems in a population is linked to the alcohol consumption per person in that population. There is a close correlation between national consumption and cirrhosis mortality. Within countries, fluctuations in consumption over time are positively correlated with fluctuations in cirrhosis mortality (Skog 1980). Changes which increase consumption, such as price, enhanced availability, more advertising or sales outlets or greater social permissiveness, also contribute to rising problem rates. Of course, overall consumption is not the only influence: different styles of drinking are linked to different problems. In cultures where a bout pattern of drinking predominates, there is a higher level of social harm than in areas where consumption is less episodic.

Influences on consumption

Government revenue statistics are the usual source of information about overall national alcohol consumption. The lowest point in per caput consumption of all forms of alcohol for three centuries occurred in the 1930s. In common with many other countries, consumption of alcohol in the UK rose steadily from 1945 to 1980.

Since then consumption has increased only slightly in many countries. While consumption among adults in UK has remained steady, drinking among young teenagers and young women has increased rapidly in recent years. In southern Europe wine consumption has declined by 42% in the past 30 years. This has been partially offset by an increased popularity of beer. Death rates from cirrhosis of the liver have fallen significantly in France and Italy over the same period of time (Gual & Colom 1997). In 1988 there were severe restrictions of official production and sales in Russia, and consumption declined, but with the advent of free-market competition the 1990s have seen a dramatic growth in alcohol use and alcohol-related problems. In the UK, and particularly Scotland, cirrhosis mortality has risen steeply in recent years.

In the UK beer and spirit consumption peaked in 1980, but wine consumption has almost quadrupled in the past 25 years. Increased advertising and marketing, increasing numbers of

Table 18.2 Alcohol consumption and risk

Risk	Consumption
Low risk — intake unlikely to be associated with the development of alcohol-related harm if taken over the 7 days	< 21 units/week for men < 14 units/week for women
Hazardous drinking — intake likely to increase the risk of developing alcohol-related harm (physical and/or psychological)	22–50 units/week for men 15–35 units/week for women
Harmful drinking — a pattern of drinking associated with the development of alcohol-related harm	> 50 units/week for men > 35 units/week for women

In 1995 the Department of Health revised the previous low-risk drinking limits of 21 units for men and 14 for women per week to daily benchmarks of 3–4 units for men and 2–3 units for women and placed greater emphasis on pattern of drinking than previously

outlets, extension of licensing hours and falling relative price have been shown in Britain and in other countries to contribute to rises in consumption. It has become unusual for alcohol not to be served at both private and public functions. 'Going out for a drink' is England's most popular leisure activity.

Drinking by women This has increased greatly, particularly when the second half of the 20th century is compared with the first. Changes in the woman's role, with the result that she enters more male environments and has more income, have contributed. Advertising directed specifically at women has possibly played a part too. In 1998 24% of young women were drinking over recommended limits, a rise from 18% in 1995. Although all age groups for women have shown a rise in excess drinking, younger age groups have shown the largest (Scottish Executive 2002).

Regional differences within the united kingdom Surveys show that, although the mean consumption and the proportion of drinkers who are heavy drinkers is similar in all parts of the UK, in Scotland drinking seems to be concentrated into fewer days of the week. Among males the highest weekly consumption is found in the North of England. In Northern Ireland the proportion of abstainers is much higher than elsewhere in the UK. In all parts of the UK there is a close relationship between alcohol-related harm and social deprivation.

Ethnic and religious minorities Islam, Hinduism, Sikhism, Seventh Day Adventism and the Baptist Church oppose or prohibit consumption of alcohol. The percentage drinking over 36 units/week among Afro-Caribbean men is about half the national average for men of comparable age and social status. Some heavy drinkers are to be found among people from India and Pakistan (Cochrane & Bal 1990).

Occupation There are various reasons for the association of heavy drinking and certain occupations: availability of alcohol at work (e.g. the licensed trade); social expectations (e.g. the business lunch); separation from normal social and sexual relationships (e.g. seamen, servicemen). Men in the drinks industry have the highest average per person consumption, while the construction industry has the highest proportion of men who drink 'heavily' (over 50 units per week). Freedom from supervision may contribute to why doctors, lawyers and senior executives have an increased risk of being heavy consumers.

The prevalence of alcohol-related disorders

Attempts to estimate the prevalence of 'alcoholism' are misleading, and epidemiologists now study the elements of this conglomerate concept, for example breaking it down into identifiable components such as alcohol dependence and the adverse health and social consequences of drinking. Data on the prevalence of physical damage from alcohol are available in mortality records and hospital admissions statistics. Mortality from cirrhosis is greatest in the grape-growing countries of central and southern Europe, where consumption is higher. The increase in cirrhosis deaths in the UK which has occurred since 1945 is accounted for by an increase in alcoholic cirrhosis (Saunders et al 1981). By 1980 a peak had been passed in the USA, Canada and Sweden and a decrease noticed, the reasons for which remain to be clarified (Smart & Mann 1991). The majority of studies show a dose–response relationship between alcohol consumption and hepatic cirrhosis. In 1990, alcohol-related deaths accounted for 1 in 100 deaths in Scotland; by 1999 this had risen to 1 in 40. The majority of these deaths were from alcohol-related liver disease (Scottish Executive 2002). In general hospitals 20–30% of all male admissions and 5–10% of female admissions are deemed to be 'problem drinkers'.

Alcohol disorders account for approximately one-fifth of psychiatric first admissions, but admission figures are influenced by availability of beds, and fashions in day- and outpatient care versus inpatient care.

The general population survey permits a prevalence estimate that is not subject to the vagaries of hospital admission and referral policies or the defining processes of social agencies. However, the door-to-door interviewer has difficulty in finding the heavy drinker at home, and when found at home he or she tends to under-report consumption and problems. Estimates are very sensitive to alterations in the definition of a case: for example, the number and severity of alcohol-related symptoms required to reach the criterion for inclusion, and whether or not past as well as present symptoms are counted. A survey of the prevalence of psychiatric morbidity in adults (age 16–64) living in private households in the UK was conducted in 1993. The annual prevalence rate of symptoms of alcohol dependence was 4.7%, compared with illicit drug dependence at 2.2%. Men were three times more likely to be alcohol dependent than women. The prevalence was particularly high among young men (Mason & Wilkinson 1996).

In North America DSM-III criteria have been applied in general population surveys. The St Louis sample revealed a lifetime prevalence of alcohol dependence of 16.1% for men and 3% for women. The same instrument, DIS (Diagnostic Interview Schedule), was translated for use in Korea and Taiwan, where rates among men were 20% and 3%, respectively, perhaps reflecting the less severe oriental flushing reaction in Koreans than Taiwanese as well as the high tolerance, indeed encouragement, of drinking in males in South Korean society (Helzer et al 1990).

Level of consumption and adverse consequences
Community samples must be studied if estimates are to be made of the risk to health of drinking at particular levels. It has been shown for a particular district in France, by comparing what cirrhotics drink and what a sample from the rest of the population drinks, that the risk of cirrhosis increases logarithmically with increasing consumption, starting at 6 units per day in women and 8 units per day in men. At 12 units per day the risk in men is increased 14-fold. The risk for delirium tremens begins at 12 units per day. This research is based on what people admit to drinking. The risk of being admitted to a medical ward for a variety of diagnoses (gastrointestinal, liver, cardiovascular disorders, myocardial infarction) was shown in a sample of Scottish men to rise at 21 units per week (Chick et al 1986). Stroke death in Chicago was found to begin to be linked with alcohol when consumption reached 42 units per week (Dyer et al 1980).

Estimates have been made of the contribution of alcohol to the death rate, using data from follow-up studies where self-reports of alcohol consumption were obtained at entry to the study. Anderson (1988) arrived at a figure for England and Wales, for ages 15–74, of 28 000 excess deaths per year. Those who drink 1–3 units of alcohol per day have a lower death rate than abstainers, but it is likely that this is due partly to the light drinkers being over represented in those whose lifestyle is healthy in other ways. Mortality risk rises in men taking more than 3 units per day and women more than 2 units per day. Current evidence suggests that low to moderate consumption of alcohol may protect middle-aged men and post-menopausal women from developing coronary heart disease. In younger people, of course, any benefits are more than countered by the relationship between alcohol use and accidents and suicide.

It is clear that the risk of psychosocial harm also rises with increased consumption. Many of the social costs associated with drinking impinge principally or even exclusively on third parties such as the drinker's partner, pedestrians, bystanders or workmates. Room et al (1995) have shown that the frequency of having five drinks or more per occasion is at least as important as the overall intake in predicting alcohol-related personal and social problems.

Patterns of illegal drug use and their related problems

The majority of drug users are not known, and, as the behaviour is illegal, they wish it to remain that way. Therefore, anonymity and confidentiality are essential in trying to access this hidden population. Assessing the pattern of drug use in Britain is like putting together a jigsaw with most of the pieces missing. The British Crime Survey (BCS) now provides the best national longitudinal estimate of drug misuse. It has been carried out every 2 years since 1992 and will be undertaken annually from 2000 (Ramsay & Partridge 2001). It is estimated that of the adult population, 6% (2.8 million people) have ever tried, and in any one year at least 3% will take, an illegal drug (Drugscope 2002). Most take cannabis, and most use it only occasionally. Data from the BCS are shown in Table 18.3. The essential current trends over time in adults above 15 years old are that in those under 19 years old the prevalence of any drug use may be dropping from a peak in 1996. At the extremes of use, cannabis, heroin and MDMA ('Ecstasy') are unchanged. Amphetamine and LSD use is falling, and cocaine use is rising. Other figures show a female:male sex ratio of 1:1.4 for lifetime use of any drug, increasing to 1:2.3 for use within the last month. Drug use does not vary by education, social class, employment or income, except for one drug, namely heroin. Heroin is six times more prevalent in the more excluded groups within society.

Table 18.3   population averages of drug use

(a) Prevalence for 16–59-year-olds, 1994–2000 (%)

	1994	1996	1998	2000
Lifetime	28	29	32	34
Within the last year	10	10	11	11
Within the last month	6	6	6	6

(b) Proportion of young adults who have used drugs in their lifetime, in the last year or in the last month, for the years 1996, 1998 and 2000 (%)

Age range	16–19 years			20–24 years			25–29 years		
Year of survey	1996	1998	2000	1996	1998	2000	1996	1998	2000
Lifetime	45	49	42	49	55	58	41	45	50
Last year	31	31	27	27	28	30	17	19	20
Last month	19	22	15	18	17	20	10	11	12

(c) Proportion of young adults who have used various drugs in the last year, for the years 1996, 1998 and 2000 (%)

Age range	16–19 years			20–24 years			25–29 years		
Year of survey	1996	1998	2000	1996	1998	2000	1996	1998	2000
Cannabis	27	28	25	24	26	27	15	16	17
Amphetamines	11	9	6	11	10	6	3	4	4
MDMA	6	4	5	6	5	6	2	2	4
LSD	5	2	2	3	3	2	1	1	1
Cocaine	1	1	4	2	5	6	1	3	5
Heroin	–	–	1	–	–	1	1	–	1

Source: British Crime Survey 2000 (Ramsay & Partridge 2001).

The longest-running longitudinal study of knowledge and experience of young people (aged 14 and 15 years old) regarding drug misuse has been monitored every 5 years since 1969 in one English town. Over this period, the proportion of people who knew someone taking drugs increased from 15% to 58% (peak 65% in 1994), and the proportion who had been offered drugs increased from 5% to 48%. The major change occurred primarily between 1989 and 1994. Stimulants were more commonly mentioned than opiates (Wright & Pearl 2000). Cross-sectional studies across the United Kingdom have shown that, in pupils aged 15 to 16, at least 40% had used illicit drugs at some time, mainly cannabis. Geographical variations also occur, for example levels of drug use are higher in Scotland (Miller & Plant 1996). In a cross-sectional study in Scotland, many of the findings by Miller & Plant (1996) were confirmed. Typically, cannabis was reported most commonly — in at least 40% of the group of 14–15-year-olds — and then, in descending order, pain killers, solvents, amphetamine, magic mushrooms, LSD, tranquillisers, MDMA, cocaine and heroin. Only 1.2% have tried heroin. In the 14–15-year-old group, 14% used drugs once a week or more, 15% once a month and 10% once a year (Fast Forward Positive Lifestyles 1996, National Centre for Social Research 2001). The evidence is for increasing use of 'soft' drugs, but the use of heroin seems to be fairly stable across Europe, with a typical lifetime risk of around 2% and a male to female ratio of 2 to 1 (Hartnoll 1994).

Regular users of drugs may subsequently develop problems related to their drug use and may then present to the Criminal Justice System, the Health Service, or other caring agencies outside the Health Service.

Criminal statistics include a variety of data on drugs, including the quantities, number of seizures by customs and by police as well as a record of the number of offences against the 1971 Misuse of Drugs Act. Cannabis remains the most common drug seized: 73% of cases in 2000. Whereas overall drug seizures have fallen since a peak in 1998, seizures of class A drugs (heroin, cocaine etc.) have continued to increase. The purity of some drugs remains stable, with amphetamines at around 5%, but heroin and cocaine purity seems to be increasing above 50%, and crack cocaine above 70%. Typical retail prices of drugs on the illicit market have tended to be stable since the early 1990s, suggesting that the supply and demand match is relatively constant. Most police forces in Scotland have seizures above the UK average per head of population (Home Office Statistical Bulletin 2002).

Prior to May 1997 there used to be a statutory obligation for doctors to provide information to the Home Office Addicts Index on people presenting to the Health Service who were dependent on opiates or cocaine (details in the *British National Formulary* prior to June 1997). There was undoubtedly under-reporting, however, and the Index's prime value was as an indicator of trends; the number of notifications to the Home Office in the last few years up to 1997 increased year on year by 15% (Home Office Statistical Bulletin 1995). Prevalence tends to be higher in major cities: typically two to three times the national average. The highest published population rates are for Glasgow: 700–1200 per 100 000 in 1989 (Frischer 1992). The methodological and practical issues in accessing this hidden population of drug users not in contact with services has been explored by Griffiths and colleagues (1993). The Capture, Re-capture Technique is explained and promoted by others as being the method for prevalence estimation when direct methods are not feasible (Domingo-Salvany et al 1995). The National Addiction Centre in London has also used a ratio estimation method for determining prevalence of cocaine in the UK; they suggest there may be a multiple of 1.6 on the number of heroin users, i.e. 116 000 cocaine users. (Gossop et al 1994). There is a strong association between social deprivation and rates of drug dependence, with the most deprived areas having the highest rates.

Drug-related deaths continued to rise across the UK in 2000. Opiates were one of the most common groups associated with drug-related deaths. In Scotland more than 23 heroin users were killed by necrotising fasciitis in 2001. For the UK, among intravenous drug users (IVDU) as a whole, HIV infection has remained low and stable (at between 1% and 2%), but the transmission of hepatitis C and B has become a major problem, with respective prevalence rates of approximately 30% and 5%, with wide ranges depending on population subgroup selected. In 2000 in England, Scotland and Wales combined, 40 430 drug users sought treatment for their drug use in the 6-month period ending 30 September. This was an increase of 7% in relation to the same period in 1999 and a 45% increase on the same period in 1995. Heroin was the main drug of use in over half of the reported cases in 2000, a slight increase from 1999, but the proportion said to be injecting heroin as their main drug has remained stable from 1995 to 2000 (Drugscope 2002).

Natural history of problem drinking

The problem drinker is not an individual irredeemably condemned to addiction; many people move into and out of problem drinking. Surveys record low rates of drinking problems after age 50. One-half to one-third of respondents in several large US surveys who reported a given 'problem' no longer reported that problem when re-interviewed four years later. Though some of these had developed a different alcohol-related problem instead, others had stopped or reduced their drinking. Positive changes in social circumstances such as job and personal relationships are important in the history of these recovered individuals (see p. 376). In a Swedish general population cohort, re-interviewed after a 15-year interval, 41% of the 71 alcoholics identified originally and still alive were completely free of drinking problems (Ojesjo 1981). A similar proportion (45%) of 120 problem drinkers from the Boston inner-city sample (Vaillant 1995) followed during 20 years on average were no longer in difficulties. However, 10% had died and 40% continued to have drinking problems. At conscription to the Swedish armed forces, men who are drinking over 30 units per week had three and a half times the expected death rate in the following 15 years (Andreasson et al 1988), which is similar to the excess rate shown by those who are discharged from hospital diagnosed as alcoholics.

Natural history of drug taking

The vast majority of non-regular drug users do not become regular users. Non-regular users tend to use to keep-in with their friends and to 'act hard'. It is only when they begin to use drugs to forget about problems, or to avoid boredom, or primarily to get a good feeling, that they risk becoming regular users (Fast Forward Positive Lifestyles 1996). Natural history tends to vary with culture, social setting, drug and route of use. For heroin, in

a community sample of London users, there was a move from smoking to injection, but this was not inevitable. The majority of smokers never moved to regular injecting, despite often using high doses for many years. Women were less likely to move to injecting — 16% of the sample smokers had previously been regular injectors, and this is a less well-known natural progression (Griffiths et al 1994). In a 22-year follow-up study of heroin addicts from a London clinic, the mortality rate was assessed at 2% annually, an excess mortality ratio of 12. No sex differences in mortality rates were demonstrated, but the excess mortality was concentrated at younger ages. No prediction of survival could be made on the length of heroin use or age at intake into the study (Oppenheimer et al 1994). In those that survived, two-thirds were not using opiates and had not transferred their dependence onto other substances, such as alcohol, but there was a high incidence of smoking.

The natural history of cocaine remains uncertain. A longitudinal study in Canada on 100 adult users in the community in 1990, with 54 re-interviewed at 1 year, showed that the fear of adverse health, social and financial consequences, cautioned users. Most had quit or reduced their use without professional help, suggesting that the natural history of cocaine use is of a self-limiting phenomenon of relatively short duration (P G Erickson, unpublished work 1993).

DEFINITIONS OF DEPENDENCE ON PSYCHOACTIVE SUBSTANCES

'Alcoholism' still has currency amongst many clinicians and therapists in the field and is still used at times in this chapter. Though imprecise, the term carries the implication that the drinker is dependent and has incurred harm to himself or others. The ICD-10 categorises the mental and behavioural disorders due to psychoactive substance use by drug types. Within each drug category, there is then the possibility of a number of clinical conditions (where 'X' refers to the drug type). The clinical condition F1X.2, Dependence syndrome, has diagnostic guidelines based on the Edwards & Gross paper on the alcohol dependence syndrome (1976); see Box 18.2.

Narrowing of the personal repertoire of patterns of psychoactive substance use has also been described as a characteristic feature of the dependence syndrome. There was a move to have tolerance and withdrawal as a mandatory requirement for the diagnosis of the dependence syndrome. This would be in keeping with the prominence that was historically given to 'dependence' and 'physical dependence'. However, studies have shown that

---

Box 18.2 ICD-10 diagnostic guidelines for dependence syndrome

- A strong desire or sense of compulsion to take the substance
- Difficulties in controlling substance-taking behaviour in terms of its onset, termination or level of use
- A physiological withdrawal state when the substance use has ceased or been reduced
- Evidence of tolerance
- Progressive neglect of alternative pleasures or interests
- Persistence with substance use despite clear evidence of overtly harmful consequences

tolerance and withdrawal do not emerge as superior to other dependence criteria on several indicators of concurrent and predicted validity, including severity (Carroll et al 1994a). The original dependence syndrome developed on studies of alcohol dependence, and there is only limited support for other individual drug classes — in the case of hallucinogens, none at all (Morgenstern et al 1994). In contrast to the ICD10, the American diagnostic system DSM-IV has a measure of severity. The measure of severity correlates reasonably well with measures of quantity and frequency of drug use and associated problems. It may be useful in the future to incorporate this within the ICD-11, as severity is one of many factors that can influence outcome (Woody et al 1993). The ICD-10 diagnosis of harmful use has poor agreement with the DSM-IV category of abuse, and future revisions may see changes in these definitions (Rounsaville et al 1993).

COMORBIDITY

Comorbidity has implications for aetiology, diagnosis, management and prognosis. For the purposes of this chapter, the term comorbidity (rather than dual diagnosis) will be used throughout and one diagnosis will be a mental and behavioural disorder coexisting with psychoactive substance use. Some research does not distinguish clearly between alcohol and other drugs of misuse or between abuse and dependence, so extrapolation to individual groups needs to be done with care. The second diagnosis will not be confined to severe mental illness but will include other psychiatric disorders including personality disorder.

Which condition occurs first? In the case of an initial substance misuse problem, intoxication, withdrawal, or chronic effects with or without continued drug use, can lead to psychiatric complications and long term 'comorbidity' issues. However, drug-induced psychiatric states are not true comorbidity and should be seen as secondary phenomena. In the case of an initial psychiatric condition, this may be precipitated in a vulnerable individual by drug misuse, but in addition there is increased drug use within this group for a variety of reasons such as common risk factors between psychiatric illness and substance misuse. Some suggest a preferential use of particular drugs for 'symptomatic relief', others that a sense of control is exerted by the use of drugs in some people who have psychotic phenomena.

The importance of this issue is underlined by three editorials in the *British Journal of Psychiatry* in 1997, dedicated to: comorbidity of mental disorders and substance misuse (Hall & Farrell 1997); service provision for this group of patients (Johnson 1997); and suicide and substance misuse (Neeleman & Farrell 1997).

Comorbid mental disorders

Schizophrenia In schizophrenia, complications arising from comorbidity include increased rates of violence, suicide, non-compliance with treatment, earlier psychotic breakdown, exacerbation of psychotic symptoms, relative neuroleptic refractoriness, increased rates of hospitalisation, tardive dyskinesia, homelessness, and overall poor prognosis (Smith & Hucker 1994). However, they also point out that, should the substance misuse problem be dealt with, then the overall prognosis is better

than for poor-prognosis schizophrenia. Substance misuse is the most prevalent comorbid condition associated with schizophrenia, and recent prevalence studies suggest that substance misuse amongst patients with schizophrenia is increasing.

In at least 80–90% of cases, substance misuse occurs before the symptoms of schizophrenia. When the first psychotic episode occurs, there is a suggestion that it may have an earlier onset, be more abrupt, and with less negative symptoms of schizophrenia than in those who do not misuse substances. Typical drugs of abuse are cannabis and amphetamines, but many of the American studies report extremely high rates for cocaine use, which is currently less available and more expensive in Europe. In an Australian study looking at self-report of substance misuse in patients with schizophrenia, 40% of patients used cannabis and 8% used amphetamines, with 20% using more than one substance. Patients associated their substance misuse with the initiation or exacerbation of their schizophrenic illness. Despite this, their substance misuse continued. Initial reasons for starting drugs were either peer pressure or in 30% of cases to relieve dysphoria and anxiety, less frequently just for experimentation. Continued use in 80% of cases was because the drugs were perceived as relieving dysphoria or anxiety or to enhance social interaction within their cultural subgroup. This may also contribute to the association between the denial of the diagnosis of schizophrenia among substance-misusing patients and resistance to follow-up attempts. Patients preferred activating drugs in the form of amphetamine, cannabis, hallucinogens or cocaine as they were felt to relieve the depression or dysphoria and the negative symptoms of schizophrenia, even at the price of exacerbating some positive symptoms (Baigent et al 1995). Generally, patients with comorbidity were found to be young males with depressive symptoms or possibly negative symptoms, and these symptoms were identifiable triggers for substance misuse in this condition and could be amenable to treatment; therefore clinical efforts should be made towards this end.

Relapse with positive schizophrenic symptoms is also associated with substance misuse. In one study looking at compulsory admissions for 'dangerousness' in a mixed diagnostic group, patients with a positive urine result for drugs recovered more quickly over a 5-day period than those with no drugs in their urine. The exception was when patients had a history of personality disorder in addition to their severe mental illness (Sanguineti & Samuel 1993). Others have reported higher readmission rates for abuse rather than for dependence syndrome. The 'natural history' of comorbidity in schizophrenia shows that, over a 7-year follow-up period in 29 subjects, of those that abused substances, 46% still continued to abuse substances at follow-up. In those that had a dependence syndrome, 69% continued to abuse substances at follow-up. This suggests a chronic relapsing condition (Bartels et al 1995).

A study of the effects of substance misuse on treatment response in chronic schizophrenic patients showed that young substance misusers had higher rates of visual and olfactory hallucinations and decreased treatment responsiveness of auditory and tactile hallucinations as a result of their continued substance misuse (Sokolski et al 1994).

The problem of service delivery to patients with comorbidity has been reviewed extensively by Drake and colleagues (1996). In their paper they reviewed 13 projects in addition to their review of the literature and identified nine key principles of treatment for this group. The principles are: assertiveness, close monitoring, integration, comprehensiveness, stable living environment, flexibility in specialisation, stages of treatment, longitudinal perspective, and optimism.

Johnson (1997) in her review of the case for specialist services outlines the need for integration. Psychiatric staff often lack training, expertise and confidence in the treatment of substance misuse disorder, and only experience these patients in crisis, i.e. when intoxicated or in withdrawal states. This often results in the patients being confronted with a punitive response. This is perpetuated by the specific exclusion of substance misuse disorder from these units. As a result, staff do not gain experience in the overall management of substance misusers who are not in crisis. Substance misuse staff have the converse problem in that their experience of general psychiatric conditions is not as up-to-date as that of their colleagues. Many may also work in a highly confrontational, high-arousal environment with a low tolerance of relapse, which would be likely to exacerbate schizophrenia. Parallel treatments can lead to miscommunications, contradictory recommendations and non-compliance, and are not seen as in the best interests of the patient. In the USA, dedicated teams for comorbidity providing 24-hour care with caseloads of 12 patients per keyworker, have been shown to decrease hospitalisation, increase functioning and show 50% abstention from substance misuse at 3-year follow-up. However, Johnson argues that with the difference in training of staff in substance misuse in the UK, such units may not be necessary. Options put forward are for increased training of respective staff within the separate units.

Mood disorders   Mood disorders are also associated with a four-fold increased risk of subsequent substance misuse if a mood disorder has developed before the age of 20 (Burke et al 1994). The largest study in patients with bipolar affective disorder comorbidity looked at 188 cases, with a comorbidity rate of 35% (Feirnnan & Dunner 1996). They analysed the data comparing three groups: bipolar affective disorder only; bipolar affective disorder with late onset substance misuse; initial substance misuse disorder with later onset of bipolar affective disorder. The most common drugs abused by this group, in more than 50% of cases, were stimulants, typically cocaine or amphetamine. Across the groups, findings were: an increased family history of substance misuse in those with a diagnosis of substance misuse; a female preponderance in those with an exclusive affective disorder; a male preponderance in early-onset substance misuse with subsequent affective disorder; and fewer suicide attempts and panic attacks within the exclusively affective disorder patients. Those who demonstrated mood changes rapidly over a period of days or hours were patients with an initial diagnosis of substance misuse.

Neurotic and stress-related disorders   Alcohol disorders are associated with an increased prevalence of neurotic and stress-related disorders. There are fewer data on the illicit substances. However, one American study compared initial-onset anxiety disorder with initial-onset substance misuse disorder and looked for substance-specific and diagnosis-specific interactions. They found little support for the self-medication hypothesis but did find an increased risk of opiate misuse in those with an initial diagnosis of post-traumatic stress disorder. However, their strongest finding was for an avoidance of stimulant drugs in those with a primary diagnosis of anxiety disorder. This was not found in those with a primary diagnosis of substance misuse disorder (Goldenberg et al 1995).

Obsessive–compulsive disorder   In a study selecting its patients from a substance misuse setting, comorbidity of obsessive–compulsive disorder (OCD) was found to be 11%, at least four times the incidence of that found in the general population (Fals-Stewart & Angarano 1994.) Accurate diagnosis of OCD within substance misuse patients has been shown to be important as regards outcome (Fals-Stewart & Schafer 1992). An outcome study at 12-month follow-up, showed that patients with comorbidity who received treatment for their OCD and substance misuse, stayed in treatment longer, showed greater reduction in OCD symptom severity and higher overall abstinence.

Post-traumatic stress disorder   The course of symptoms in post-traumatic stress disorder (PTSD) has been shown to begin with hyper-arousal, progress onto avoidance behaviour and peak with intrusive re-experiencing of the trauma. The time course for this can be a period of years, and when substance misuse has been observed in this group, it has been found to parallel the development of the PTSD. This supports the hypothesis that substance misuse in PTSD is a form of self-medication. In addition, there seems to be a selective use of sedatives, primarily alcohol, cannabis, heroin and benzodiazepines, which would depress hyper-arousal and induce 'numbing' on exposure to stimuli specific for the PTSD and also suppress or 'forget' re-experiences. It has also been found that these patients avoid stimulants such as cocaine and amphetamines (Bremner et al 1996).

Eating disorders   An extensive review of the literature regarding eating disorders and substance misuse has being carried out by Holderness and colleagues (1994). In this they present the three main theories of the association between substance misuse and eating disorders: eating disorders are a form of addiction; substance misuse is a form of self-medication; or the two disorders have a common aetiology such as dysfunctional families. In all studies, bulimia is found to be more strongly associated with substance misuse than is anorexia. Typical prevalence of substance misuse in bulimic patients is 20%. The drugs misused were, in descending order, cannabis, amphetamine, benzodiazepines and then other drugs. In clinical samples, subgroups of bulimics have been postulated with a 'multi-impulsive' disorder. There have been no studies of treatment for comorbid conditions or of outcome following different treatments. The clinical implications of the comorbidity of eating disorders and substance misuse therefore remain unexplored.

Personality disorder   The research in this area comes exclusively from the USA and deals primarily with the antisocial personality disorder (ASPD) subtype. The typical prevalence of ASPD is 5% of males and just less than 1% of females. When there is a comorbid diagnosis of substance misuse disorder, ASPD rates rise to 18%. Higher prevalence rates are found in different subpopulations; for example, in intravenous drug users, prevalence is as high as 44%. When the diagnostic criteria 'onset prior to the age of 15 with conduct disorder' is removed (this results in a diagnosis similar to antisocial personality disorder used in the ICD-10) then prevalence rises to near 70% (Cottler et al 1995).

ADHD   Attention deficit hyperactivity disorder (ADHD) (in ICD-10 these patients would be classified as having hyperkinetic disorders) is a condition which is becoming increasingly diagnosed. The research into ADHD and substance misuse is exclusively from the USA. The hypothesis put forward by researchers is that ADHD in childhood progresses into adulthood in at least 50% of cases. In adults, ADHD leads to self-medication and comorbid substance misuse. Drugs used are typically stimulants. Therapeutic trials in adults have been shown to be effective with this group (Schubiner et al 1995).

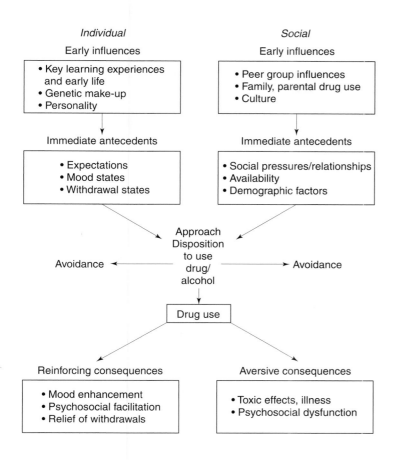

Fig. 18.1
Factors influencing an individual's drug/alcohol use.

Detection and management

There continues to be a need for doctors to have a low threshold for the detection of substance misuse in the assessment of their patients. Typical figures for inpatient psychiatric units are between 20% prior to drug screening and 35% following drug screening; depending on the catchment area and the specific type of institution, higher rates of comorbidity can be found, typically among young, male, urban, lower-income groups. Instances can be as high as 65%. Failure to recognise substance misuse results in incorrect diagnosis, poor management and a worse prognosis. There is no conclusive evidence as to whether sequential treatment, initially of the substance misuse and then of the comorbid psychiatric disorder is indicated, or a simultaneous approach is more effective. However, case studies support a simultaneous approach.

AETIOLOGY

Aetiology of alcohol dependence and misuse

Availability of alcohol is a powerful determinant of level of consumption, and culture and tradition are potent influences on the pattern and context, but many other factors play a part in determining the individual development of harmful drinking and dependence. For some problem drinkers the causes are to be found principally in their environment, for others there is a major genetic contribution (dealt with in Ch. 9). On present evidence it seems likely that alcohol dependence is a phenomenon that has many forms which, though phenotypically similar, are genotypically

different, and to which the degree of environmental contribution varies. There is good epidemiological evidence that heavy drinking runs in families. (Marshall & Murray 1991). A summary of factors influencing an individual's disposition to use a drug or drink alcohol is shown in Figure 18.1.

Personality

Sufferers from alcohol-related problems who attend clinics are more likely to have personality deviations and early family disturbance than are the general population. This is partly to be expected since clinics in the UK tend to be based in psychiatric services and thus attract psychiatrically disturbed cases. In the general population, follow-up studies of young men show that the impulsive, rebellious, more extrovert individual is somewhat more at risk of developing alcoholism, particularly alcohol-related social problems. Childhood conduct disorder also predicts alcohol-related problems, typically of early onset and linked to criminality. A debate developed in the 1980s about whether there is a type of male alcoholism, with early onset, severe problems, especially social problems, a manner that is socially detached, distractible and confident, and also linked to a similar pattern in the biological father ('Type 2' — Cloninger 1987), which contrasts with a more dependent, anxious, rigid, less aggressive, more guilty alcoholic ('Type 1') with either biological mother or father an alcoholic. Some have felt that Type 2 is best seen as alcoholism secondary to antisocial personality (ASP) (Schuckit & Irwin 1989). ASP greatly increases the risk that a man or a woman will have an alcohol problem in longitudinal and cross-sectional community studies. ASP and/or family history of alcoholism was found in 48% of male alcoholics and 63% of female alcoholics in a large community study (Lewis & Bucholz 1991).

Drake & Vaillant (1988), in a 33-year longitudinal study of 456 inner-city adolescent boys chosen as non-delinquent at that age, found that in this sample adolescent indicators of personality disorder were good predictors of adult personality disorder, but not alcoholism. Having an alcoholic father was the best predictor: 28% of sons developed alcoholism compared with 12% of sons of non-alcoholic fathers. Apart from the severe disturbance associated with childhood conduct disorders and parental drinking habits, community studies do not usually, especially in middle-class subjects, find evidence linking parenting styles to subsequent alcoholism (Vaillant 1995). As well as antisocial personality disorder in the community, alcohol dependence is found to be associated with phobic disorder, anxiety disorder, other psychotropic substance misuse (notably tranquilliser dependence) and (especially in women) depression (e.g. Lewis & Bucholz 1991).

Alcohol may be used to anaesthetise grief by the bereaved and may complicate pathological grief. Phobias, especially agoraphobia, are common in alcoholics attending psychiatric hospitals (Kushner 1996). Alcohol, because it is a short-acting sedative causing rebound arousal, may exacerbate or even precipitate anxiety states. However the phobia in some instances clearly predates the alcohol dependence. Bipolar disorder, including the manic phase, may result in drinking to the point of physical dependence.

Psychological aspects of alcohol dependence in women

Women make up a third of alcoholics seen in psychiatric practice. There is often a male heavy drinker either in the family history or the marriage. Women more often than men attribute the onset of problem drinking to a particular life-stress. However, community surveys have not shown either in Scotland or in North America that adverse life events predict whose drinking will increase during a follow-up period (Romelsjo et al 1991). Depression in middle life following the departure of the children ('the empty nest'), or in the lonely spinster or widow, can lead to excessive drinking. Typically this is at home and in secret, and associated with considerable shame and denial. Traditionally, women have been much more abstemious than men, but this has changed significantly, particularly amongst younger economically independent women who now pursue more male patterns of socialising and excessive drinking

Childhood experience of sexual abuse, when asked for in a research interview, is more commonly reported in women alcoholics than in the general population. It is not yet known if it is more common than in other psychiatric disorders (Hurley 1991).

Female patients, whether presenting with dependence, psychiatric or medical complaints, often give a shorter history of excessive drinking than men and tend to report a lower intake of ethanol, even after correction for body weight. This may partly be explained by the greater stigma attached to women's drinking, which might lead to their minimising their consumption. However, a given dose per kilogram body weight of ethanol produces a higher peak blood level in a woman than in a man. This may be due in part to the female body having a lower ratio of water to fat than the male body (alcohol dissolves more readily in water than in fat), and to lower activity of alcohol dehydrogenase in the gastric mucosa.

Role of marital relationships

In an alcoholic's marriage, hostility, mistrust and attempts by one partner to control the other are common. Women problem drinkers sometimes have husbands whose energies are all directed toward their work or their hobbies, or husbands who make them feel worthless. It is difficult to disentangle cause from effect, and adequate research which would need to be longitudinal has not yet been conducted. However, many marital problems undoubtedly improve when the drinking ceases.

Aetiology of drug use

Factors vary, depending on what stage of drug use one is examining (Table 18.3). Factors determining initiation of drug use may differ from those influencing continuation of drug use, the move into dependent use, and from the causes of relapse. The aetiology of relapse is discussed later in the chapter.

Initiation of drug use

Whether an individual will take a particular drug will depend on its availability, cost, legal status, alleged effects and risks and, in some case, the form of the drug. Why one particular individual will chose to use a drug whereas another will not, given the same situation, is more complex. Personality traits, such as rebelliousness and curiosity, are thought to contribute to drug experimentation, as is a wish to express independence or hostility. The wish to seek peer group approval may also contribute. Individuals are also influenced by families and society, and here role models and group pressure may result in some individuals taking drugs, whereas others do not. In some instances, initiation to drug use is iatrogenic: for example, treatment of severe pain.

Continued use

The factors involved in the initiation of use may play greater or lesser importance in subsequent drug behaviour; however, additional factors come into play when people continue to take drugs. For an individual drug to be continued, it must give positive effects and minimal negative effects. These positive effects will be the beginning of the development of 'positive outcome expectancy', which later with continued reinforcement develops into craving. With use, classical and other conditioned responses become more apparent. The pharmacology of the drug determines much of what users then chose to do. On the individual level, continued use is associated with general non-conformity. Understanding of genetic contributions to individual differences in sensitivity to drugs and their influence on behaviour is not fully developed, but will play a part in a future account of why some people move from experimental to recreational and then dependent use (Morse et al 1995). Individual distress or unrecognised psychiatric illness can lead on to self-medication and the short-term alleviation of symptoms by continued use.

Dependent use

Once the dependence syndrome has developed, tolerance and withdrawal symptoms are frequently a feature of the condition, and the substance type primarily determines the quality and severity of withdrawals. Avoidance of withdrawal then becomes a major factor in continued drug use. At the individual level, personality traits in people dependent on drugs, particularly heroin addicts, are certainly different from those of normal controls. There is an increased incidence of: low self-esteem; submissiveness; dependence on others and a craving of approval; lack of self-confidence; a learned helplessness; low expectations for the future; and a tendency to give up easily. However, is this a cause or an effect of the dependence syndrome? This has not been resolved by prospective studies. Much is said about individual denial of problems related to drug use, or at least a lack of awareness. Dependent drug users may chose to continue using because the benefits of giving up are outweighed by the advantages of continued use. An alternative theory of continued drug use in dependent users is that they have not developed alternative coping mechanisms for dealing with problems, and that their use of drugs is their main coping mechanism.

THE PSYCHOBIOLOGY OF ALCOHOL DEPENDENCE

Initiation and reinforcement

Initiation into drinking and other forms of drug taking is influenced by the setting, the company and expectancies about the likely effects. All of these contribute as much or more than its pharmacological action to whether alcohol has a relaxing or euphoriant impact (Young et al 1990).

The consequences of drinking for the novice drinker may well have an effect on his subsequent drinking career. Individuals with high levels of anxiety will be conscious of alcohol's relaxing properties. At low doses alcohol has an euphoriant effect for some individuals in some settings, and this is a potent reinforcer of continued drinking. Genetic factors may make some individuals experience euphoria or tension reduction more intensely at this stage (Marshall & Murray 1991). It is also interesting that there is a greater concordance in drinking style in monozygotic than in dizygotic twins, even allowing for the greater social closeness of the former (Heath & Martin 1988).

The main approaches of genetic studies have been by linkage and association methods. The principal consistently reproduced finding has been the genetic transmission of alcohol-metabolising genes in oriental populations. Orientals have varying degrees of acetaldehyde dehydrogenase deficiency, and the consequent 'flushing' reaction to alcohol is a deterrent to drinking for some (though alcohol dependence does develop in some Orientals despite flushing).

Sons of alcoholics, identified both from among sons of clinic attenders in a general population cohort and by questionnaire survey, for example in college students, have been compared with controls on numerous measures (Pihl et al 1990). In sons of alcoholics, alcohol has a greater dampening effect on the physiological correlates of stress than is seen in controls. Children of alcoholics, of school age, tend to be distractible, quick to resort to aggression and often in trouble with authority. A twin study did not find cognitive impairment (nor cortical atrophy) in the non-alcoholic MZ twins in discordant pairs, which also provides some evidence against the hypothesis that an inherited predisposing trait in alcoholism might be cognitive impairment. It points to aspects, at least, of cognitive impairment being a result rather than a precursor of the drinking (Gurling et al 1991).

Trait markers

A number of biological markers have been identified which may predict a vulnerability to developing alcohol-related problems. Mostly they have been observed in the detoxified alcoholic and in greater frequency in the offspring of alcoholics. They include reduced EEG alpha activity and reduced P300 wave amptitude. Autonomic responsiveness to stress also has been shown to be greater in the sons of alcoholics.

A search is being made for biochemical abnormalities which occur in alcoholics and can also be demonstrated in their pre-drinking children. After drinking, alcohol levels of prolactin are lower in offspring with a family history of alcoholism than in controls. The rise in cortisol and adrenocorticotrophin (ACTH) following a drink of alcohol is less among those men with a family history than those without. This is one of a number of illustrations of the way in which genetic predisposition may in a variety of subtle ways make individuals more at risk of drinking in a harmful way.

Tolerance and withdrawal

As drinking becomes a regular habit, many drinkers find that they have to take more to obtain the desired effect; this is evidence that tolerance is increasing, and this may make reduction in intake seem more difficult.

A behavioural explanation of tolerance and withdrawal is that an organism 'expects' the drug because it is confronted with signals that previously heralded the drug. 'Drug compensatory conditional responses' act to cancel the effect of the drug, producing tolerance if the drug is administered, or a 'withdrawal' state if the drug is withheld. Thus animals may only display tolerance to alcohol in an environment where the alcohol was initially administered and not in a novel setting. Nonetheless, it seems probable that the development of neurophysiological tolerance is a key step along the way to establishing dependence. The understanding of the neurochemical basis of the actions of alcohol is developing rapidly. This has occurred because new neuroimaging techniques, positron emission tomography (PET) and single photon emission computed tomography (SPECT), have enhanced the capacity to study and understand the biological basis of dependence. Prior to these developments much of the research was reliant on animal studies (Nutt 1999).

Alcohol, in common with other neuroactive drugs, alters brain transmitter function. It has several actions on different brain sites, including dopamine release in the nucleus acumbens. When alcohol is stopped, dopamine release drops below normal, which may account for the depressed mood associated with early withdrawal. It is thought that overactivity of dopamine contributes to the excitability observed in delirium tremens. Alcohol also appears to act through gamma-aminobutyric acid (GABA) and excitatory amino acid receptors; genetic influences on these systems and their response to alcohol may prove of critical importance in understanding different propensities to develop tolerance and responsiveness to pharmacotherapy.

There is evidence that endogenous opioid transmitters also play a part in the effects of alcohol. It has also been shown that relapse in dependent alcoholics can be mitigated by opiate antagonists (e.g. naltrexone). The activity of noradrenaline (norepinephrine) is decreased by opioids, and withdrawal symptoms are in part thought to be an expression of a rebound of noradrenaline activity.

Ion channels in the cell membrane are a particular target for alcohol. Calcium homeostasis is critical to all cells, and several different calcium channels control the passage of this ion across cell membranes. Alcohol reduces entry through the channels. As a result they increase in number. One consequence of this is that during withdrawal, calcium flux becomes excessive. Some speculate that this intense calcium flux contributes to neuronal death (Nutt 1996). The varied actions may account for the euphoriant and anxiety-reducing properties of the alcohol.

The original demonstration that 'rum fits' and delirium tremens were withdrawal symptoms of alcohol dependence was made by Isbell et al (1955). In this experiment, recovered opiate addicts consumed between 1 and $1\frac{1}{2}$ bottles of spirits (250–370 g ethanol) per day for 7 weeks. On cessation all had withdrawal symptoms, and some had fits or delirium. Such a short history is unusual in clinical practice. Usually the tendency to drink such large amounts over successive days takes years to develop. Nevertheless, traces of withdrawal phenomena (insomnia, restlessness, increased REM sleep) occur even after single large doses of a sedative such as alcohol. Hangover is in part a mild withdrawal state.

Relapse and reinstatement

Some clinicians believe that there is a protracted physiological withdrawal state which outlasts the visible tremor, tachycardia, sweating and anxiety of the initial 3–10 days. Cognitive deficits are still improving several months after abstinence; cerebral atrophy also resolves in some patients, and cerebral blood flow improves. During this time, abnormalities in EEG evoked response and sleep architecture, and complaints of insomnia persist; patients complain of anxiety and depressive symptoms, diminishing proportionally with the length of abstinence; and there appears to be reduced suppression in the dexamethasone-suppression test and blunted thyrotrophin response to thyrotrophin-releasing hormone (Garbutt et al 1991). The indications are that GABA receptors, their chloride channels, and perhaps up-regulation of NMDA receptors continue to be abnormal. (For further discussion see Nutt 1996.)

During this time, some patients feel an urge to drink and they struggle with craving. There are of course psychological and social processes during this period, as well as neurochemical ones. These include a range of cues to drinking that have been learnt over the years. Such cues may be environmental: social situations, the pub or club. Cues may also be internal; for example, drinking may have become associated with feeling happy, sad, angry, tired, hungry, or all of these.

During these initial months some contend that further, even slight, use of alcohol may erode resolve about further consumption, and lead to relapse. Many alcoholism recovery programmes recommend absolute abstinence. After tolerance has been lost, five or six drinks may be sufficient to dissolve one's intention not to take a seventh. However, there seems no obvious reason why that should lead to a return in the next day or so to heavy harmful drinking, reinstatement of craving and withdrawal symptoms. There is no evidence that one drink sets off a neurophysiological tripwire, but disposition to drink in alcoholics (measured objectively as work done to obtain alcohol or speed of drinking under standard conditions) has been shown in laboratory settings to increase after as little as three large measures of spirits. It seems as if relapse occurs after a certain level of priming dose has been reached. Increased disposition to drink in abstinent alcoholics has also been demonstrated on the morning after a dose of alcohol.

Thus, in alcohol-dependent individuals who have been abstinent for some time, the pattern of response to renewed drinking is 'carried over' from their previous drinking period. Carry-over has been demonstrated in monkeys and in rats: physical dependence (tendency to withdrawal phenomena) is more easily evoked in animals who have been previously made physically dependent, even after 37 days' abstinence. 'Reinstatement' is also used to describe the carry-over phenomenon.

As well as a learning theory/neurophysiological view of reinstatement a cognitive explanation has also been put forward. It is said that abstinent alcoholics who relapse on recommencing drinking do so because they believe, as a result of treatment or attendance at Alcoholics Anonymous, that one or two drinks necessarily leads to harmful drinking — 'the self-fulfilling prophecy'. Of course, having a drink can also be seen as a stimulus with a long-ingrained conditional response — taking another drink. This view has led some to advocate cue-exposure, including exposure to drinking environments, as a way of reducing severity of relapse. This approach is not yet proven as a treatment method (Drummond et al 1990).

PSYCHIATRIC COMPLICATIONS OF ALCOHOL MISUSE

Withdrawal states with delirium (ICD-10 F10.4)

The condition commonly known as delirium tremens (DTs) is often taken as a hallmark of alcoholism but it is relatively rare, being reported by only about 5% of patients attending alcoholic clinics. It occurs when an individual who is severely dependent on alcohol stops or reduces drinking.

The full syndrome is characterised by marked tremor of the limbs, body and tongue, restlessness, loss of contact with reality, clouding of consciousness, disorientation and illusions progressing to terrifying hallucinations which are most commonly visual, but may be auditory or tactile. Delusions often of a paranoid kind may also occur, often associated with the hallucinations. Sweating and tachycardia are pronounced. The disturbance usually develops out of milder withdrawal symptoms 1 day after cessation of drinking and rarely persists for more than 4 days. Symptoms are often worse at night. There is a significant mortality (approximately 10%), partly because it often complicates other medical emergencies such as infections or injuries. The development of fever, dehydration and signs of shock are ominous prognostic signs. It is important to remember that concomitant infection, Wernicke's encephalopathy, metabolic disturbance, hypoglycaemia or head injury may complicate the clinical features and prognosis. Withdrawal fits may occur at any time from the first to the 14th day (Isbell et al 1955). The development of DTs can often be aborted by prompt and adequate sedation with benzodiazepine.

Admission to hospital will usually be necessary. The patient's environment should be safe, uncluttered and uniformly lit to avoid ambiguities. Parenteral multivitamin preparations (Parentrovite) may be given provided resuscitation equipment is available. Electrolytes and plasma glucose should be checked. An oral benzodiazepine, such as chlordiazepoxide, commencing at 100–150 mg/day and reducing after the second or third day, will usually be sufficient to contain the patient's agitation and can be stopped after a week. It is important that the dosage should be progressively reduced, and should not be continued after, at most, 14 days.

Psychotic disorder — alcoholic hallucinosis (F10.5)

In this condition hallucinations occur in clear consciousness. Sometimes these are a continuation of hallucinations first experienced during withdrawal from alcohol. However, hallucinations may also commence de novo in a patient who is still drinking. Usually these experiences are auditory and begin as fragmentary sounds. The sounds gradually become formed and voices are heard, often making unpleasant remarks: 'She ought to be ashamed of herself, 'He's a lush', etc. The voices may give commands to do things against the subject's will, and persecutory delusions may develop. The experiences may be very compelling and distressing, occasionally resulting in violence or suicide.

In one series it was observed that men who developed hallucinosis were significantly younger at the onset of alcohol problems, consumed more alcohol per occasion, developed more alcohol-related life problems and had higher rates of drug experimentation (Tsuang et al 1994). In two large series of cases studied by Bendetti (1952) and Victor & Hope (1958) only a few cases (5–10%) continued to have symptoms for 6 months or more if abstinence was maintained. Renewed drinking, however, tended to bring about a return of hallucinations.

Despite the close resemblance of the hallucinations to those of acute schizophrenia, only a few go on to show typical schizophrenic deterioration: 4 out of 76 in Victor & Hope's series and 13 out of 113 in Bendetti's series; but Cutting in a more recent series (1978) observed 19%. In distinguishing this condition from schizophrenia, it is noteworthy that premorbid adjustment in the social and sexual spheres tends to be normal. A family history of schizophrenia is usually absent except in the cases where hallucinations persist and schizophrenic personality deterioration occurs. There is no close relationship with gross cognitive impairment. The basis of alcohol hallucinosis is presumably subtle alcohol-induced damage or dysfunction, perhaps of the temporal lobes, though this has not been proven.

Management commonly requires admission to hospital, withdrawal from alcohol and, if the hallucinations still continue, antipsychotics. It is usually possible to stop the antipsychotics after 2 or 3 months. Thereafter the patient usually has full insight into the illness.

Pathological jealousy (Othello syndrome) (F10.5)

Firmly held delusions of infidelity are not uncommon in patients who misuse alcohol. They may be precipitated by the patient's feeling of inadequacy stemming from alcohol-induced impotence and further aggravated by the spouse's growing indifference towards a drunken partner. The patient's accusations become repetitive, and aggressive demands for proof may be reinforced by violence. No amount of contrary evidence will dispel the delusion, and cases sometimes end tragically in assault or murder. Alcohol abuse is not the only cause of this syndrome (see Ch. 19, on schizophrenia). Treatment is of the underlying condition. Sometimes the only feasible and safe solution is for the couple to separate permanently.

Depression and anxiety

Symptoms of depression are common among excessive drinkers. This is understandable considering the lifestyle of dependent drinkers, who frequently wake with a hangover facing a day overshadowed by the problems caused by their drinking. Biological changes induced by excessive drinking may also contribute to depressed mood.

Excessive drinking may mask the symptoms of depressive illness, an association more common in females. Alcohol also releases inhibitions, which makes it easier to express feelings of sadness and to give way to self-destructive impulses. It is therefore hardly surprising that alcohol figures so prominently in studies of parasuicide and successful suicide. Factors increasing risk are previous attempts, a history of depression, and evident physical and social problems. If secondary diagnoses of alcoholism are included the proportion of suicides affected ranges from 20% to 40% or to 55% if only males are included (Duffy & Kreitman 1993).

Depression is a primary factor in a relatively small number of alcohol-dependent individuals. This is more commonly the case in women. At presentation to an alcohol treatment service 42% of men had significant depressive symptoms but only 5% were depressed after 4 weeks of abstinence (Brown & Schuckit 1998) The clinician should discriminate between those patients whose alcohol misuse is symptomatic of depression and the much larger number who have become depressed because of their drinking. In the latter, improvement usually follows cessation of drinking and appropriate therapy, whereas the former may require antidepressant medication, combined with a period of abstinence.

Alcohol is often used as a means of lowering anxiety, particularly in stressful social situations. While this may relieve anxiety at low doses, greater quantities and chronic use generates anxiety symptoms, and of course the characterstics of a mild withdrawal state often mimic those of acute anxiety. It is important to avoid making a diagnosis of anxiety state until an alcohol-dependent patient has been abstinent for 3–6 weeks. In the majority of cases anxiety and phobic symptoms will resolve, leaving about 10% of patients who have a primary anxiety disorder which will require treatment in its own right. Great care should be taken in prescribing anxiolytics to such patients because of the hazards of substituting one dependence for another; behavioural approaches are preferrable.

Cognitive impairment and brain damage

Some 50–60% of alcoholics attending psychiatrists perform worse on cognitive testing than would be predicted from their verbal intelligence educational level and age. They commonly show:

- impairment of memory, visual more than verbal;
- narrowing and rigidity of thought processes, i.e. difficulty changing from one way of construing and categorising to another;
- difficulty learning new material;
- impairment of visuospatial and visuoperceptive skills.

Patients often find it very difficult to judge objects in space. A variety of factors may contribute to cognitive impairment among excessive drinkers: the neurotoxic effect of alcohol; thiamine deficiency; repeated head injury; and the consequences of alcohol withdrawal fits. A spectrum of cognitive disabilities has been observed extending from mild impairment to end-stage alcoholic dementia. That some of these deficits might predate the heavy drinking has been discussed earlier.

Imaging techniques show cortical atrophy and ventricular enlargement in 50–70% of patients admitted with alcohol dependence. There are modest correlations between atrophy and cognitive impairment. Magnetic resonance imaging (MRI) relaxation time and brain density measured during computerised tomography (CT) are altered in proportion to lifetime consumption. The shrinkage is mainly in white matter. In liver cirrhosis hepatic encephalopathy is an additional factor.

Cognitive deficits often improve with long-term abstinence. Social functioning is of paramount importance, and good outcome has been observed in abstinent alcoholics despite significant impairment on formal testing (Lennane 1988). It is prudent to give thiamine-containing vitamin supplements for at least 4 months. Small bowel malabsorption, in addition to poor intake and excessive utilisation, contributes to vitamin deficiency in alcoholics. Since this may take some weeks to recover, parenteral vitamins are necessary initially, despite their small risk of anaphylactic reaction. In many cases impaired memory and attention improve following withdrawal. Cognitive assessment is inappropriate during the first 3 weeks after withdrawal. A great deal of improvement can be observed during the first 3 weeks, and this continues gradually up to a year after stopping.

Formal cognitive testing should be postponed until the patient has been abstinent for at least 3 weeks, and then the patient should be monitored thereafter at 3 monthly intervals. The uses of testing include:

- providing a more formal judgement where there is clinical evidence of impairment; this is particularly helpful in assessing whether the patient is likely to be able to utilise certain cognitive behavioural techniques and make changes in his way of life;
- providing a basis for feedback to the patient, who may need to know that drinking has affected his memory or intellectual powers; this often proves a powerful motivating influence;
- monitoring progress, both for the clinician and patient;
- providing a guide to employability and any hazards which may be experienced in particular occupations or driving.

Testing will often reveal a decline in intellectual ability and poor performance on visuospatial tasks, impaired planning and reduced co-ordination ability. In common with all tests, the patient's attention and mood are confounding factors. More ecologically based tests are currently being explored which will provide a better measure of the patient's capabilities in tackling real-life situations.

MEDICAL COMPLICATIONS OF EXCESSIVE DRINKING

Cancer (oesophageal and oropharyngeal), cardiovascular disease, cirrhosis, pancreatic and gastrointestinal disease, accidental death, suicide and greater vulnerability to infection such as TB, all contribute to the raised mortality amongst excessive drinkers.

Neurological complications

Wernicke's encephalopathy. The triad of confusion, ataxia and ocular palsy was described by Wernicke in 1881. Patients dying of this condition show haemorrhages in the brainstem and hypothalamus. Identical lesions have been produced in thiamine-deficient animals. The condition responds to urgent treatment with intravenous thiamine and withdrawal of alcohol, but even with such measures there is often a residual dementia or Korsakoff psychosis

(Victor 1962). This condition is often overlooked, and it is essential not to wait for the classical triad of symptoms before commencing therapy. Mental changes of confusion, drowsiness, and precoma or coma are common and sometimes the only clinical findings.

Treatment of Wernicke's encephalopathy should be in hospital and the patient given intravenous thiamine, for instance as Pabrinex 2 ampoules pair three times daily for 2–3 days followed by Pabrinex IVHP 1 ampoule pair daily for 3–5 days. Each ampoule should be diluted in 50–100 ml N saline or 5% N/V glucose and infused over 30 minutes. Because of a small risk of anaphylaxis, facilities for treating anaphylactic shock should be available. General and psychiatric hospitals should have agreed protocols for the management of alcohol withdrawal including delirium tremens and Wernicke's encephalopathy (Thomson 2000). The merits of continuing longer-term oral thiamine supplements are less clear, but in a poorly nourished and/or impaired patient it seems a sensible preventative strategy

Disturbance of consciousness in the alcoholic must also raise the suspicion of traumatic subdural haematoma, though unilateral signs will then probably be present. Hepatic encephalopathy and hypoglycaemia should also be considered. Occasionally, dementia is marked and accompanied initially by incontinence, generalised weakness, tremor persisting long after withdrawal from alcohol, slurred speech and ataxia. Alcoholic cerebellar degeneration presents as ataxia of stance and gait.

Korsakoff's psychosis This late consequence of alcohol misuse is characterised by impairment of short-term memory with a tendency to confabulate. In most cases it will have been preceded by Wernicke's encephalopathy. The defects are less clear cut than at one time thought, and a wide range of other memory and cognitive defects may be also present. Total recovery, even after abstinence and treatment with thiamine, is rare, but significant functional improvement is often observed over many months. Observed pathological changes are chiefly necrosis and gliosis in the mamillary bodies.

Polyneuropathy contributed to by vitamin deficiency, is common in alcoholics in at least a mild form, with asymptomatic absence of the ankle jerks, and calf tenderness. In the established condition the patient complains of muscular cramps and unpleasant paraesthesiae in the feet and calves and unsteadiness of gait. All forms of sensation are impaired in a stocking distribution. Flaccid weakness in the limbs may progress to wrist drop. The cranial nerves are spared.

Alcoholic myopathy presents as chronic weakness with wasting, punctuated by exacerbation during bouts of drinking.

Gastrointestinal complications

Gastritis, presenting as upper abdominal pain and haematemesis, perhaps accompanied by acute gastric erosions, is common in those who drink excessively. Peptic ulcer, though it occurs in 10% of alcoholics, is as common in the general population, so it is unlikely that alcohol is a cause. Alcohol nevertheless provokes the symptoms of an ulcer and probably delays healing. Severe diarrhoea sometimes occurs in excessive drinkers, and small bowel damage leading to malabsorption exacerbates dietary vitamin deficiency. Chronic relapsing pancreatitis is characterised by recurring acute abdominal pain with inflammation, fibrosis and eventually calcification of the pancreas. It is usually associated with an alcohol intake of over 20 units per day. A protein-deficient diet and hyperlipidaemia are believed to contribute.

Deaths from cancer of the mouth, pharynx, oesophagus and liver are elevated in heavy drinkers. The risk is augmented further in those who also smoke. Some, but not all, studies have also found a relationship between alcohol and cancer of the pancreas, breast and rectum.

Alcohol and liver disease

Over 90% of ingested alcohol is converted by an obligatory oxidative process in the hepatocytes to acetaldehyde, thence to acetate and finally to carbon dioxide and water. Fat deposition in liver cells (steatosis) almost invariably accompanies heavy drinking and may be present even though liver function tests are normal. Less fortunate drinkers go on to develop hepatitis or cirrhosis. Cirrhosis of the liver is nowadays among the five commonest causes of death in those under 60 in most industrial countries.

Liver injury is related to volume and duration of alcohol consumption and not to type of beverage. It is now thought that obesity alone can also cause fatty liver and produce a picture indistinguishable from alcohol-related damage. Cirrhosis can be induced in the individual who has drunk moderately for years and then rapidly escalates consumption for 1 or 2 years. Women may be more vulnerable than men, and there are indications that progression to cirrhosis depends on immune responses and also, from studies of the human leucocyte antigen system, that heredity contributes.

Modern treatments, despite being expensive, do not appear to have been very successful in reversing the complications of cirrhosis (hepatic failure, variceal bleeding, ascites and primary liver cancer), and there have not been improvements in recent years in the survival of patients with alcoholic cirrhosis. About one-third of patients will still be alive after 5 years, though with abstinence the survival rate doubles, so that those with compensated cirrhosis at presentation have a 90% 5-year survival (Saunders et al 1981). Death from variceal haemorrhage or hepatic or renal failure may also result from alcoholic hepatitis in the absence of cirrhosis.

Alcoholics who are candidates for liver transplantation are usually expected to demonstrate an ability to abstain and a commitment to maintaining this after surgery. Despite this, many will drink again, particularly after the period of intensive follow-up ends (Howard et al 1994). Nonetheless, patients transplanted for alcoholic liver disease appear to have a better survival than those with viral hepatitis. Liver transplant units should have the assistance of a liaison psychiatrist and alcohol specialist nurse to ensure detailed assessment of the patient's drinking history and long-term follow-up with relapse prevention therapy.

Metabolic complications

Life-threatening hypoglycaemia occasionally follows 6 to 8 hours after heavy alcohol consumption in previously fasting individuals. It may follow imperceptibly from alcoholic stupor. Treatment is by urgent intravenous administration of glucose. Insulin-dependent diabetics who ingest moderate to large amounts of alcohol with little carbohydrate may become hypoglycaemic, as may well-fed normal subjects who undertake vigorous exercise in the cold. Chronic alcoholics are prone to reactive hypoglycaemia following a carbohydrate-rich meal, perhaps related to their known accelerated gastric emptying.

Acute renal failure after a beer-drinking binge has been reported in Britain and several other countries.

Cardiovascular disease

There is evidence that drinking 1 to 3 units per day diminishes the risk of coronary disease, but heavier consumption is related to increased morbidity and mortality from this cause. These benefits are only evident in men over 40 and post-menopausal women. Drinking more than 6 units per day is associated with rising blood pressure and an increased risk of cerebrovascular accidents.

Alcohol is a cause of supraventricular arrhythmias, and of cardiomyopathy leading to congestive cardiac failure. Arrhythmias are particularly prone to occur after bouts of excessive drinking.

Sexual impairment

High blood alcohol level impairs penile erection by a direct pharmacological effect. Heavy drinkers who repeatedly fail to maintain an erection become anxious about their sexual performance, which itself leads to further failure. Alcohol also has direct toxic effects on the Leydig cells of the testis, resulting in reduced testosterone production, impaired spermatogenesis, infertility and testicular atrophy. A significant improvement in sperm count and fertility was noted in a sample of men attending an infertility clinic when they reduced their alcohol intake.

Fetal alcohol syndrome

Heavy drinking during pregnancy is associated with spontaneous abortion, intra-uterine growth retardation and the fetal alcohol syndrome. This syndrome has been observed in children born to mothers who have severe alcohol problems. It is characterised by developmental and growth retardation and facial and neurological abnormalities. These children often show continuing developmental difficulties. It may be that there are critical developmental stages when alcohol is most likely to do damage. It is also likely that other drugs used, particularly smoking (Plant 1987), are confounding factors.

Forrest et al 1991 could not detect any effect of moderate maternal consumption on the development of offspring at 18 months and concluded that pregnant mothers could safely consume 70–85 g of alcohol per week. Health authorities now advise women either to abstain or confine their drinking during pregnancy to one or two drinks once or twice a week. Antenatal clinics should screen for hazardous drinking and alcohol-related problems.

Alcohol and accidents

Alcohol is a factor in as many as one-third of all accidents. They are particularly likely to occur amongst young men; road traffic accidents, drownings, pedestrian deaths and accidents in the home are all common during intoxication. This relationship between alcohol accidents and violence points to the importance of identifying alcohol-related problems in accident and emergency departments and carefully screening all adults who have suffered injury.

ALCOHOL-RELATED SOCIAL HARM

As alcohol comes to play an increasingly salient part in the drinker's life, he or she often experiences a number of distressing social consequences. Frequently these have their first impact on family and work. Most of the social disabilities which arise are easier to list than quantify. They include the following:

Disruption of family relationships

Alcohol misuse contributes to as many as one-third of divorces, and domestic suffering and violence are commonplace. Disappointments may lead to depression in the parent, child or spouse, or to a numbed state in which the drinker is disowned. The children of problem drinkers are specifically at risk of developing behaviour problems and alcohol problems later in life. They often show a facade of premature adult responsibility, losing the experiences of childhood in consequence. A fellowship of support groups formed for adult-children of alcoholics has been prominent in the USA in recent years.

Economic factors

Alcohol is expensive, and the family budget suffers accordingly. Earning power is usually reduced, which compounds the disability. The quality of accommodation which the heavy drinker can sustain may decline, leading to homelessness.

Employment problems

Alcoholic employees usually develop a poor work record with frequent absences due to sickness, erratic time-keeping, low productivity and a greatly increased risk of accidents involving themselves and others. The cost of all this to the employer has prompted many companies to set up programmes to encourage employees with drinking problems to seek early treatment (see below).

Crime

As many as 60% of prisoners report significant alcohol problems. A quarter of young prisoners had been drinking when they committed their crime. Over 50% of male prisoners in the UK were drinking hazardously in the year before coming in to prison. Young offenders whose crimes are alcohol related have been shown to benefit from attendance at alcohol education courses designed to promote sensible drinking practices (Baldwin 1991).

Drink-driving offences are common among dependent drinkers. One in three of all drivers killed have more than the legal limit of alcohol in their blood. Offenders whose blood alcohol is found to be exceptionally high (over 150 mg%), or who have previous drink-driving convictions, are particularly likely to be alcohol-dependent. Many drink-driving offenders have an elevated serum gamma glutamyl transpeptidase, indicating that they are regular heavy drinkers. Drink-driving offences are also common in patients with other alcohol-related problems.

Drunkenness offences

The majority of men and women charged by the police with drunkenness offences have been shown to be alcohol-dependent, and 60% are homeless or living in hostels. The *Report on the habitual drunken offender* (Home Office 1974) recognised that processing these unfortunate people through the courts was wasteful, and even dangerous as alcoholics sometimes died in police custody. Concern about the revolving door for these habitual offenders passing in and out of the penal system gave rise

to a number of alternative approaches. In some countries, such as Finland, parts of Canada and the USA, public drunkenness was decriminalised, while in Britain the approach has been to divert the habitual drunken offender out of the courts into a medicosocial system. The Criminal Justice Acts in both England & Wales and Scotland now allow the police to take an individual charged with simple drunkenness to a 'designated place' for detoxification and rehabilitation. Very few of these places exist in Britain, and policy has moved away from detoxification toward police cautioning which takes no account of rehabilitation. It has been shown in this population that severe withdrawal symptoms are surprisingly rare and that non-medical detoxification is often sufficient, providing nursing and medical help is available for the 5% who become seriously disturbed. An effective detoxification service can be used as an entrée to a more stable lifestyle.

RECOGNITION AND CLINICAL MANAGEMENT OF ALCOHOL RELATED PROBLEMS

This section deals with specific treatment approaches; the organisation of services within which these are located, is discussed later in the chapter.

Identification and assessment

The clinical manifestations of alcohol misuse are many and varied. The sickness certificates of people eventually diagnosed as alcohol-dependent reveal, for example, anxiety states, depression, injuries, 'gastritis', 'debility'. The general practitioner may have been aware of frequent absences from work for minor symptoms, or stress symptoms in other members of the family, but the contribution which alcohol makes to these symptoms has been overlooked or ignored. Patients rarely acknowledge alcohol as a problem at a first interview. They may be evasive because they are sensitised to criticism about their behaviour. Sometimes it is better to avoid focusing the whole interview on the drinking, taking instead a problem-orientated approach starting with questions about the reason for seeking help. With respect to the drinking, enquire about a recent period (e.g. the past 7 days) by asking in detail about work, leisure activities, the company kept, and the amount and type of beverage consumed. Spirits, wines and beers should be enquired into separately. Reconstruct the cues which have been important triggers to drinking.

The first principle for the clinician, whether psychiatrist, physician, surgeon or general practitioner is always to bear alcohol in mind as a possible cause of presenting symptoms and to ask some questions about alcohol use as part of routine case taking. There is good evidence that this simple step is often overlooked in both hospital, psychiatric and general practice. Basic questions should include:

- How often do you take a drink? (= x)
- On a day when you drink, how many drinks would you typically take? (= y) (Multiplying x and y together gives a very rough estimate of number of units per week.)
- Have there been any days in the past month when you have had more than 10 units?
- Have you had any problems from drinking in the past year?

These simple questions should be asked of all newly admitted and referred patients.

Box 18.3 CAGE questionnaire

- Have you ever felt you should cut down on your drinking?
- Have people annoyed you by criticising your drinking?
- Have you ever felt bad or guilty about your drinking?
- Have you ever had a drink first thing in the morning to steady your nerves and get rid of a hangover (eye-opener)?

There are standard brief questionnaires which can be used in screening, such as AUDIT (Babor et al 1989) or the very brief four-question FAST derived from AUDIT for use in A & E departments (Hodgson et al 2002), and CAGE (Ewing 1984). The latter is more useful in identifying established serious drinking problems, the four questions being as shown in Box 18.3.

Severity of dependence is assessed as follows. Mildly dependent patients will regularly notice restlessness at certain times of the day or in certain situations and at these times wish to have alcohol or seek out their drinking companions. If they occasionally have very heavy sessions, they may relieve the next morning's hangover with a drink, but this will not be more than once or twice a week at most. More severely dependent patients report that the restlessness they feel without a drink is noticeable at times to colleagues or family, or prevents them from getting on with other activities. They organise their day to ensure that they are able to have a drink at times when they predict they will need one. There may be times when they feel unable to think of anything but getting a drink. Morning nausea, sweating and relief drinking may be reported for periods of many days consecutively. Insomnia becomes frequent unless late evening intake relative to daytime drinking is very heavy. Wakefulness in the small hours of the night, like daytime tenseness and anxiety in the dependent drinker, can be, of course, an effect of a falling blood alcohol level. A widely used rating scale is the Severity of Alcohol Dependence Questionnaire (Stockwell et al 1979).

Adverse consequences in the areas of health, work, family, friends and the law should be explored. An epileptic fit for the first time in an adult should raise the suspicion of alcohol dependence. A withdrawal fit may occur without other gross signs. Tremor of the outstretched fingers or tongue, injected conjunctivae and sclerae, stigmata of liver disease, excessive facial skin capillarisation, and alcohol on the breath are valuable clues.

The mean cell volume is raised (without anaemia) in 30–50% of patients, probably due to a direct toxic action of alcohol on the marrow. The gamma glutamyl transpeptidase and/or other liver enzymes are elevated in 60–70% of patients, due to enzyme induction and/or liver damage. They are markers of heavy drinking in the preceding weeks. Other conditions such as liver disease or some medications can cause similar elevations. Carbohydrate deficient transferrin is also used as a marker, but the test although valuable is less widely available in the UK. A specimen for blood alcohol or a reading on a portable breathalyser may help. In a 70 kg man one unit of alcohol produces a peak blood alcohol concentration of 15 mg% after about half an hour, and takes an hour to be metabolised. Assessment of brain damage, important in planning future treatment, should be left until the patient has been free of alcohol for 3 weeks.

If possible the spouse or partner or other relatives should be interviewed, to add objectivity and to assess the quality of their relationship with the drinker. The spouse often feels angry and guilty and is reassured when these feelings are acknowledged and understood. At this stage avoid reaching premature conclusions about 'motivation'. A moment's introspection shows that our own motivation to change familiar habits varies greatly from day to day. Problem drinkers are no exception. Clinicians have to work with fluctuating levels of motivation. Probably the psychiatrist's most important first step is to acquire the trust of the patient and to establish an atmosphere in which frankness prevails and confrontation is seen as caring. Patients will then be able to start making decisions about themselves and plan to change their way of life.

Early intervention

There is good evidence showing the benefits of intervention including advice about 'sensible drinking' given at an early stage in the patient's drinking career when they are drinking in a hazardous way (i.e. drinking in a way which if sustained is likely to risk physical or psychological harm) or have first experienced evidence of alcohol problems. It is much better to help the patient at this stage before they have developed more serious and intractable problems related to their drinking. In these circumstances, simple focused advice given in a primary healthcare or general hospital setting, can be very effective. There have been many controlled studies of the efficacy of brief interventions in a variety of healthcare settings, and most produced significant reductions in alcohol use (Moyer et al 2002).

Helping patients change their drinking habits

Helping patients change their habits often requires a considered and phased approach. At first a patient's decision to seek help is often fleeting and characterised by ambivalence about change. The clinician can help by clarifying reasons for changing: for example, by asking the patient to draw up a balance sheet of the benefits versus the harms of continuing to drink in this way. It is often helpful to explain the physiology of symptoms that may be due to physical dependence, and the role of alcohol in other presenting symptoms, be it sleep disturbance, tension, depression or family disharmony. The status and role of a physician is a powerful persuasive force. Often patients respond to an interview style which results in the patient arguing their own case for a change in drinking habits (Miller & Rollnick 2002). This approach is known as motivational interviewing.

Motivational interviewing

While a significant number of patients seen in primary healthcare and in hospital settings will respond to simple advice about changing their drinking habits, others will require considerable help in making a commitment to change. Motivational interviewing is a technique which helps the patient reach his own decision about changing his habits. The majority of early intervention strategies are focused on returning to problem-free drinking rather than total abstinence. Bien et al (1993) summarised the essential components of brief intervention in the acronym FRAMES (Box 18.4).

Motivational interviewing arises from the concepts of Prochaska & Di Clemente (1992). They observed that patients came to see clinicians at different stages of readiness to make changes and that motivation was not a fixed and unchanging entity, but fluctuated from day to day and in different circumstances. They divided

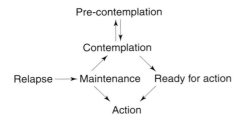

Fig. 18.2
Stages of change. (After Prochaska & Di Clemente 1992.)

patients into those who came at a pre-contemplative stage before they had even recognised that alcohol was contributing to their problems, and others at a contemplative stage where they were beginning to recognise that drinking was a problem but were ambivalent about making change. They also recognised a 'readiness for action' stage when they would be willing to accept positive advice for change. The circle was completed by a period of relapse or faltering of resolutions, requiring maintenance. The stages of change are summarised in Figure 18.2.

Other strategies for helping to achieve change

Set goals Goals should be specific, attainable, short-term, immediately rewarding and ones which the patient defines. For example: no alcohol for 4 weeks; rewards: better physical health, better family atmosphere. Abstinence is often immediately rewarding and is an easier target for many than partial reduction of drinking. However, some see abstinence as totally inappropriate. For them a goal might be: reduce intake by half; or, reduce gamma glutamyl transpeptidase to below 50 units when the reward is the satisfaction of watching this measure of liver function improve over the next 2–3 months.

Involve the family Family distress is common, and advice on being firm with the drinker, not entering into fruitless struggles, but remaining caring and positive, is often beneficial. Without information from those near at hand, the clinician may not get the full picture from the patient.

Enhance self-esteem Often patients feel powerless to change their lives. The doctor should convey hope and encourage patients to believe in their own ability to change things.

Review impediments to change such as former cues and triggers to drinking. Such cues may be subjective, for instance the feelings of anxiety or depression which experience suggests will be relieved by a drink; or external, like the atmosphere among friends in the pub. The barriers to change are varied (Box 18.5). Encourage substitute activities: alternatives to drinking. For some, physical dependence and the experience of withdrawal symptoms

will be a significant impediment necessitating detoxification as the initial step.

Identify associated conditions such as depressive illness or phobias that might respond to specific treatment, but bear in mind that many will be secondary to the drinking.

Consider other agencies such as voluntary councils on alcohol which may provide a counselling service or a social programme, such as Alcoholics Anonymous (see below), or hostels for recovering alcoholics.

Follow-up Active follow-up is one of the ingredients of successful treatment. Relapse is common in the first 6–12 months after treatment. Brief but regular appointments help to remind the patient of goals and to provide an opportunity perhaps to repeat mean corpuscular volume or serum gamma glutamyl transpeptidase or breath alcohol measure. It is important to be prepared to confront patients when necessary and risk anger. The spouse or partner should usually be encouraged to attend follow-up sessions. Relapse, if and when it occurs, should be viewed as an opportunity for further learning, not as an irrevocable catastrophe.

Close study of the precipitants of relapse shows that they have a lot in common across a range of addictions. Marlatt & Gordon (1984) analysed 311 relapses among patients with a variety of addictive behaviours (problem drinking, smoking, heroin addiction, gambling and overeating). They identified three high-risk situations which accounted for three-quarters of all relapses: negative emotional states, interpersonal conflicts and environmental triggers. In therapy, the patient should learn to identify cues to relapse and develop strategies for handling them.

Faith and hope Faith in the therapist, faith in the treatment, and the warmth, empathy and authenticity displayed by the therapist have often been termed non-specific ingredients of therapy, but they have a major influence on efficacy. In a two-year follow-up study of outpatient treatment of problem drinkers, low-empathy therapists were associated with the same or even a worse outcome compared with giving patients a booklet only, while high-empathy therapists significantly improved on the booklet-only outcome (Miller & Baca 1983). Non-specific factors in therapy need to be transformed into clearly defined specifics.

Pharmacotherapy and alcohol dependency

Detoxification

Medication to minimise withdrawal symptoms makes stopping drinking easier. Hospital admission is only essential when delirium threatens or there is a history of fits or current medical or psychiatric illness. A long-acting benzodiazepine such as chlordiazepoxide (starting at 60–80 mg/day and reducing to nil over 5–7 days) is usually adequate for community detoxification. Larger doses may be needed in hospital to control agitation and offset the likelihood of confusional states. The final dose should be determined by regular clinical monitoring, but the maximum dose should not exceed 400 mg chlordiazepoxide in 24 hours (CRAG/SCOT-MEG 1994). It should not be continued for more than 10 days. If there is a history of fits, greater initial doses of the benzodiazepine should be given. In any circumstance the final dose should be determined by regular monitoring. Chlormethiazole is probably even more addictive than long-term benzodiazepines. Alcohol/chlormethiazole interactions causing respiratory depression and even death have occurred. Chlorpromazine is less effective and may increase the risk of withdrawal fits (Mayo-Smith 1997)

When the patient is reasonably well-intentioned and there is someone at home, or a nurse or family doctor who can call, where there is no history of fits and no confusion, withdrawal can be undertaken at home (Stockwell 1987). The patient should be advised to take time off work, to rest and to drink fruit juices and other soft drinks, but avoid large quantities of caffeine-containing tea and coffee. In more severe withdrawal it is sensible to check serum urea and electrolytes and aim to maintain an oral fluid intake of 2–2½ litres daily.

In view of the frequency of cognitive impairment in heavy drinkers and its probable relation to vitamin depletion, vitamin supplements should be given to most patients, particularly those who are poorly nourished, and if there is any evidence of cognitive impairment or neuropathy, they should be given orally for several months.

Alcohol-sensitising agents

Disulfiram (Antabuse) is an alcohol-sensitising deterrent drug which interferes with the breakdown of alcohol and floods the system with acetaldehyde. Disulfiram is a useful adjunct in the follow-up phase of treatment until a new lifestyle has developed. The disulfiram effect lasts for several days. Acetaldehyde is a toxic substance and produces an unpleasant reaction with flushing, headache, nausea, tachycardia, laboured breathing and hypertension. On rare occasions the reaction may be life threatening, particularly in those who have cardiovascular disease.

Disulfiram should not be taken until the breath alcohol has returned to zero. The patient and partner should be fully informed about the mode of action of the drug and its hazards. With the recommended dose of 200 mg daily, side-effects of disulfiram are uncommon, although tiredness and halitosis is sometimes noted. For these reasons some patients prefer to take the drug at night. Reversible neuropathies and confusional states have also been reported. It should not be given to patients with recent heart disease, suicidal impulses or who take hypertensive drugs. It should also be avoided when there is very active liver disease. To ensure success, the patient will often agree to the nomination of a supervisor, for example, the spouse, general practice, the clinic, or an occupational health nurse in cases with employment problems. The supervisor ensures that the compound is dispersed in water and swallowed. These measures improve compliance which greatly improves efficacy. Disulfiram, when dispensed by a spouse as part of a contract, or by a clinic as part of an arrangement with the patient's employer, is of proven efficacy in maintaining abstinence for substantial periods (Chick et al 1992), in reducing absenteeism at work (Robichaud et al 1979) and is also of proven value with socially deteriorated clients (Bourne et al 1966).

Other drug treatments

There has been understandable resistance to the use of psychotropic drugs in the treatment of alcohol problems because of the risk of precipitating a further addiction. Drugs which have specific effects on neurotransmitters have been shown to reduce alcohol consumption in animal experiments. Several studies have suggested that the frequency and severity of relapse can be reduced by use of the opiate antagonist naltrexone, particularly when combined with coping skills therapy (O'Malley et al 1992); others have shown benefits from acamprosate, which is a GABA agonist and glutamate antagonist (Whitworth et al 1996). The use of acamprosate is well established in the UK and the rest of Europe whereas at present naltrexone is more available in the USA and not currently licensed in the UK. Both have demonstrable effectiveness when combined with psychosocial interventions and improve drinking outcomes in one-third of dependent patients compared with one-quarter in controls. At present most follow-up periods have been less than 2 years.

Antidepressant and other antipsychotic medications are of benefit to those problem drinkers who have associated psychiatric disorders, but it is important to keep in mind that most symptoms of anxiety and depression will clear after 2–3 weeks of abstinence without further drug therapy.

Non-drug treatments

Social skills training

Many excessive drinkers are influenced by social cues, and many report that they feel deficient in social skills. Refusing drinks, buying non-alcoholic drinks, applying for jobs, being firm with subordinates, expressing affection to loved ones and expressing annoyance without being insulting are some of the items of interpersonal behaviour that alcoholics find it useful to role-play in social skills training groups. In one of the best-known methodological analyses of controlled trials for treatments for alcohol disorders, social skills therapy was one of the most consistently highly rated of the psychological treatments (Miller & Wilbourne 2002).

Group therapy

Participating in treatment in a group facilitates identification and enhances self-esteem. Fellow problem drinkers are quick to expose the rationalisations and self-deception of their peers, but often do so sympathetically and with great tolerance. The importance of Alcoholics Anonymous in the recovery of many alcoholics is one indication of the value of the group process and the fellowship this provides.

Conjoint and family therapy

Cohesiveness of marriage and family life is a predictor of recovery. Family interviews enable members to have their views heard, without the discussion spiralling into denials, accusations and counter accusation. The patient can be helped to see that family members are bound to feel hesitant at first but that this need not imply that they do not care or appreciate the efforts that are being made. The man who has opted out of married and family life, or who has gradually been extruded because of his drinking, may suddenly want to resume his roles of husband and father, ignoring the fact that others in the family now have their own way of doing things (Chick & Chick 1992).

Other members of the family sometimes fear that the therapist is going to blame them for the patient's drinking. The psychiatrist's invitation to them might be 'to hear their views of how things have been, and to have their opinions on how X can best be helped'. Involving a partner or relative in therapy improves outcome and should be part of both assessment and treatment whenever possible (Edwards & Steinglass 1995). Family therapy improves outcome over the first 18 months of rehabilitation in dependent alcoholics (O'Farrel 2001).

Social behaviour and network therapy

One of the strongest predictors of improvement is a beneficial change in the patient's social network. Recently a variety of treatments have extended the concept of social skills acquisition to engage family and friends of the patient as part of the recovery process. Thus key members of the patient's social network are involved to help reward positive changes in behaviour (sometimes known as community reinforcement therapy) and develop strategies for dealing with crises. In contrast with family therapy, in this approach network members are part of the therapist's working team, not subjects of treatment (Galanter 1999).

To drink or not to drink

Abstinence is the safest goal, particularly for those who have sustained physical damage from alcohol or who have been physically dependent, and for patients aged 40 and over. However, in young people, particularly those who have not been severely physically dependent, return to limited drinking after a few month's abstinence is sometimes appropriate. Therapist and patient can work out appropriate strategies together (Fig. 18.3):

- stick to drinks that are low in alcohol (e.g. low-strength beers rather than those that are extra strong);
- avoid buying rounds;
- intersperse drinks with non-alcoholic drinks;
- go to the pub at 9.30 p.m. instead of 7.00 p.m.;
- sip rather than gulp;
- no lunch-time drinking;
- eat while drinking;
- completely avoid situations or company where heavy drinking is likely;
- set a limit (e.g. never more than 6 units per day).

Keeping a daily record of consumption can help monitor progress and review goals. Controlled studies on clinic attenders aimed at demonstrating the efficacy of controlled drinking remain few and need replication (Heather & Robertson 1997).

Specialist services

Units for the treatment of alcohol problems

These units offer a specialised service in most regions of Britain. They have a responsibility for treatment, training and research,

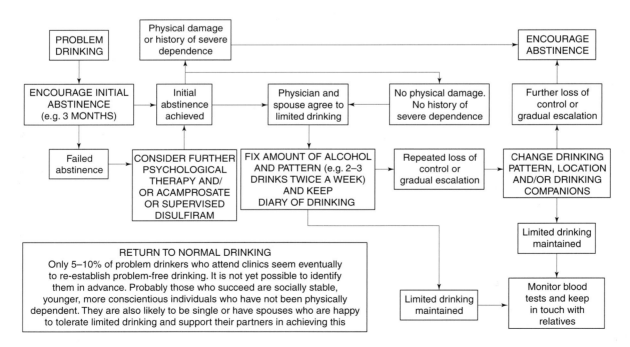

Fig. 18.3
Advice to patients who have found total abstinence difficult.

and facilities of a similar kind are to be found in many parts of the industrial world. Traditionally they offered inpatient treatment of 6 to 8 weeks' duration with an emphasis on group therapies. In recent years there has been a shift away from this devotion to inpatient treatment toward outpatient therapy combined with brief inpatient or day-patient treatment. In response to evaluation studies which have cast doubts on the importance of very intensive forms of therapy, these units have become more flexible, offering a range of approaches, including behaviour therapy, marital and family therapy as well as more familiar but unproven group and individual psychotherapy.

Glaser (1980) has criticised the tendency for specialist services to act as if the alcoholic population were homogeneous and to offer a single form of treatment for all. This is clearly inappropriate, and a careful assessment of each patient's needs and matching of these to a range of treatment options is required (US Department of Health and Human Services 1990).

Councils on alcohol and alcohol advice centres

Many countries now have counselling services separate from psychiatric or medical clinics. Problem drinkers or their families may initiate the contact, and referrals will be accepted from doctors.

Alcohol-related offences are commonplace, and some courts now have access to programmes which help offenders learn to drink sensibly and break the link between crime and alcohol. Similar strategies have been used in rehabilitating persistent drink driving offenders.

Employment policies

Employers who are prepared to face the issue of drinking problems among their workforce may negotiate an *alcohol in employment* policy and arrange with their employees and trade union for those whose drinking is impairing performance to seek help at an early stage. When drinking has led to a breach of work regulations, the employee may be offered the opportunity of attending a treatment service rather than facing disciplinary proceedings. The outcome of problem drinkers identified and treated in the work context tends to be good.

Alcohol misuse among doctors and other health professions has been a particular concern because of the impaired performance which can result. The majority of cases coming to the attention of the General Medical Council in the UK concern alcohol misuse. With appropriate help, doctors can make good recoveries and return to practice, but it is important that problems are identified at an early stage.

Alcoholics Anonymous

Since the meeting of its two founder members, Dr Bob and Bill W in Akron, Ohio, in 1935, Alcoholics Anonymous (AA) has spread to most countries of the world. It grew particularly in the 1960s and 1970s in the USA and the UK, and is currently growing at a rate of 15% per annum. Members meet regularly and share a common faith that as alcoholics they are powerless where alcohol is concerned and that total abstinence is the only route to recovery.

The principles on which AA was founded are open self-scrutiny, the giving of aid to others, and fellowship. The AA programme offers hope and clear, simple advice (e.g. avoid the first drink; attend meetings; take life one day at a time; stay sober for yourself). A prayer is said at every meeting. Potential affiliates need not be put off by AA's spiritual language.

AA groups usually offer to meet a new affiliate personally and introduce him or her, though they will also make the new member welcome simply by attending the local meeting. Records are not kept and all members are anonymous, but observation shows that AA helps large numbers of regular attenders (Robinson 1979). Those most likely to adhere to AA tend to have suffered much harm from their drinking, but this is by no means always the case.

Al-Anon is a parallel organisation for the spouses of alcoholics, to whom it offers an opportunity for mutual support and understanding. Affiliated to their organisation is Al-ateen for the teenage children of alcoholics. This offers them a chance to share some of the tensions and problems which they commonly experience.

Services for the homeless alcoholic

The homeless alcoholic usually finds abstinence unattainable unless he can be helped out of the 'skid row' environment of lodging houses or sleeping in the open. Engaging such individuals in treatment is often difficult, and outreach services have been developed working with rough sleepers and the homeless, to maintain contact and encourage them to utilise services.

Hostels are an important part of rehabilitation. Most hostels for alcoholics require abstinence as a condition of residence, and they usually provide a therapeutic programme in which the residents help each other to find a new lifestyle. After a residence of up to 1 year, many find the transition to independent life extremely difficult, and some areas provide half-way houses and supported accommodation as the next stage. In some cities there is accommodation for alcoholics who continue to drink. These so called 'damp houses' provide some shelter and support, on the way, one hopes, to longer-term rehabilitation.

Most hostels are managed by church or other voluntary organisations. In some cities they are also provided by the social work department.

MANAGEMENT OF DRUG MISUSE

Assessment and management of clinical conditions associated with drug use

Every doctor is now likely to see patients who misuse drugs, be it a member of staff in the accident and emergency department dealing with an acutely intoxicated patient, the general practitioner confronted with concerns around the harmful use of various substances, the obstetrician faced with a pregnant patient whose drug use has been disclosed because of concerns about the child, the police surgeon attending a patient in the cells with a drug-induced psychosis, the house officer in the general hospital confronted with a patient undergoing withdrawal from drugs, the psychiatrist having to differentiate drug-induced psychopathology from other causes, or the specialist drug service trying to help patients with a dependence syndrome who have already failed to give up the substance by themselves. Prior to assessment, a low index of suspicion of drug misuse is required; early detection is preferable to the subsequent management of the dependence syndrome. Assessment is based on standard clinical skills of history, examination and investigation. However, emphasis is given to:

- drug use and previous treatment;
- objective signs of withdrawal;
- needle marks;
- urine toxicology;
- mental state;
- comorbid, physical and mental conditions, e.g. HIV;
- areas of conflict: relationships, jobs, debt, the law;
- support structure;

During the late 1980s and early 1990s, much of the funding and impetus for the setting up of services for drug use and its associated problems was motivated and driven by concerns around HIV. This is now less of an issue among drug users as injecting declines and knowledge exists within the drug-using subculture about the risks of spread of HIV and hepatitis B and C. That said, knowledge in itself does not change behaviour, and the incidence of sharing among those that inject continues to be high. As a result, detailed questioning may be required if injecting is practised.

For each clinical condition induced by drug use, there are general principles of management. Specific drug and treatment options are discussed later in the chapter.

Acute intoxication (ICD-10 F1X.0)

This may require the medical or surgical management of injuries occurring secondary to the intoxication. It may also require observation of any head injuries. Life support may be required in the event of coma, and in some instances (e.g. opiates) antagonists may be available and given to reverse drug effects. Offensive or dangerous disinhibited behaviour may require containment until drug effects decline. Acute intoxication is a transient phenomenon, and recovery is therefore complete.

Harmful use (F1X.1)

A patient may be recovered from intoxication or be presenting with some other medical condition and has raised drug use as a personal concern. Education is required around the dangers of drug use and the options explained about how to change that behaviour. Some patients may not see their drug use as a problem, and the theory proposed by Prochaska & Di Clemente (1992) is a useful working model when helping patients (see Fig. 18.2). If patients are experiencing harmful use but are in a pre-contemplative phase (i.e. do not recognise their drug problem), then efforts to encourage abstinence will fail. In this case, the process of motivational interviewing (see p. 373) can be used to effect change in the direction of awareness and a wish to move away from harmful drug use (Miller & Rollnick 1991).

Dependence syndrome (F1X.2)

Once this is developed, management will depend on the patient, drug and the patient's environment (Department of Health 1999). If the patient is continuing to use (F1X.24), management is as outlined above for harmful use. Alternatively, if abstinent and in the community (F1X.20), then the focus should be on relapse prevention techniques which are discussed later in the chapter (p. 381). Other alternative categories within the dependence syndrome include the patient being abstinent but in a protected environment (F1X.21). These treatment settings may be divided into four groups: rehabilitation houses; religious units; community crisis rehabilitation units; and residential 12-step programmes. The essential elements of management within these units are to provide a safe drug-free environment, to address pre-existing causes, solve current problems, and equip patients with greater personal resources for their discharge back to the community. Another category concerns the patient who is abstinent but receiving treatment with antagonist drugs (F1X.23) (e.g. opiate dependence, receiving naltrexone). Management in this instance usually involves a partner supervising daily consumption at the start of a period of abstinence, and the provision of some chemical support while relapse prevention techniques are acquired. The final category is that of the patient in a clinically supervised maintenance or replacement regimen (controlled dependence) (F1X.22). In maintenance programmes, chaotic illegal dependence is replaced with controlled legal dependence. Once established, then management is similar to that of those who are in protected environments.

Withdrawal state, with (F1X.3) or without delirium (F1X.4)

Withdrawal states may be managed by acute abstinence and symptomatic supportive measures or, more commonly, the initiation of substitute medication and then a graduated, more humane withdrawal over a period of time. The types of withdrawal and the drugs that may be used are discussed later under the individual drug types.

Psychotic disorder (F1X.5)

This requires management as any other psychotic disorder, but the aetiology is drug induced. The disorder typically resolves at least partially within 1 month and fully within 6 months and, as long as the patient remains drug-free, is unlikely to reoccur.

Residual and late-onset psychotic disorders (F1X.7)

Here a variety of conditions may be present which have been caused by drug use but are now persisting despite termination of drug use. These conditions include flashback phenomena (F1X.70), personality or behavioural disorder (F1X.71), residual affective disorder (F1X.72), dementia (F1X.73), other persisting problems of impairment (F1X.74) and late-onset psychotic disorders (F1X.75). The management of these conditions is symptomatic.

Goals of treatment

The rationale for this heading may seem obscure, because the goal of treatment is cure. However, cure has been associated with abstinence. An expectation on the part of many in the medical profession that their goal is abstinence in drug users with a dependence syndrome, has led to a sense of therapeutic nihilism. To avoid this, it is important to elaborate on the goals of treatment. Most clinical conditions are self-limiting and only require supportive management. A few residual states exist where the management is no longer directed at drug use but at helping people live with their changed state. The difficulty comes when confronted with people who continue to use drugs, or are dependent on drugs, and require help in gaining awareness of the

---

Box 18.6   Hierarchy of therapeutic goals for intravenous drug users

1. Reduction of sharing of injecting equipment
2. Reduction in injecting
3. Reduction in street drug use
4. Stabilisation on substitute prescribing
5. Management of features associated with dependence syndrome
6. Reduction in substitute prescribing
7. Maintenance of abstinence from psychoactive drugs

---

problems that their drug use is causing them. The hierarchy of goals and harm reduction for intravenous drug users and others is given in Box 18.6.

Health professionals are primarily focused on health issues. However, it needs to be accepted that in cost–benefit terms a motivating factor, as HIV becomes less of a driving force in establishing and maintaining services for drug users, will become drug-related crime and its prevention. It is estimated that the costs sustained by victims of drug-related crime by dependent heroin users alone, is between £58 million and £864 million annually (1997 costs). The cost to the criminal justice system of dealing with drug users is similarly substantial, in excess of £500 million per year. Similar papers by UK political parties also support this view. So far the rehabilitation of dependent drug users by the criminal justice system has been less successful than that achieved by the health system. Diversion from the criminal justice system into healthcare will become more important in this decade.

Specific drugs and treatment options

Opiates

Acute intoxication with opiates can result in respiratory depression and sometimes death. This is not an uncommon event. A recent Australian study of heroin users indicated that two-thirds had had a drug overdose, and a third had had one within the past year (Darke et al 1995); others have reported lower incidents (Gossop et al 1996). One reason for this may be that the purity of heroin varies such that, when injecting, the exact dose being taken is unpredictable. Alternatively, a dose of drug that takes the user near to the edge of death may maximise the euphoric effect. An increasing presentation of opiate intoxication is methadone overdose. The reasons for this are complex, but undoubtedly more users are presenting to services with methadone as their route into opiate dependence rather than heroin. Methadone overdose can be difficult to control and follows an unpredictable course in non-tolerant patients, who are at risk of sudden death (Cairns et al 1996). Clinical management of opiate overdose follows general guidelines. The opiate antagonist naloxone may be used in a dose of 0.4 mg i.v. to reverse respiratory depression, but as it is short-acting, and the overdose may be of a long-acting drug such as methadone, subsequent infusion may be required. Concern about the mortality of accidental opiate overdose has made some advocate the 'take-home' of naloxone by opiate addicts (Strang et al 1996b).

Patients with an opiate dependence syndrome traditionally constitute the bulk of specialist drug services work. Their management depends on their current drug use. If still using, and not prepared to move towards abstinence from street drugs, then harm reduction strategies should be employed as mentioned above. Some may be abstinent and concentrating their therapy on relapse prevention techniques. Some may be abstinent and supplementing their relapse prevention techniques with a trial of naltrexone at a dose of 50 mg a day. This is an opiate antagonist similar to naloxone but can be administered orally and lasts for over 24 hours. A comprehensive review has been carried out by Kirchmayer and colleagues (2002). However, most abstinent drug users chose not to carry on with naltrexone. There has been some promising work using naltrexone as a condition of treatment for people who repeatedly offend to finance their drug habit. The best results with naltrexone treatment have been reported in studies with certain target groups (particularly people who are highly motivated, e.g. doctors) who have developed a drug dependence syndrome on opiates (Washton et al 1984). A select group of patients may elect to go into drug-free rehabilitation programmes. Inpatient detoxification prior to transfer to a rehabilitation programme may improve retention rates, as there is often a high dropout if patients go direct to drug-free rehabs while still using.

However, the majority of patients with opiate drug dependence syndrome tend to be managed at least at some point in a maintenance programme. This is probably the most extensively evaluated treatment within this field, and repeated reviews of the literature have confirmed that compliance with the treatment is good and that it reduces illicit drug use (Mattick et al 2002a). There is less-robust evidence that methadone reduces criminal activity, lowers risk of seroconversion for HIV, hepatitis B and hepatitis C, and improves re-socialisation (Farrell et al 1994). It needs to be remembered, however, that methadone itself is not the treatment, and needs to be given in conjunction with a full package of care (Hagman 1994). The research on maintenance prescribing is primarily with oral methadone. Doses in the UK were primarily aimed at the minimum dose to avoid withdrawal symptoms, but if the goal is the reduction of illicit drug use then a higher dose is usually needed. A typical dose may be in the region of 60–120 mg methadone mixture, 1 mg/ml, per day. Doses of 50 mg and above have been associated with death in naive drug users. In addition, approximately 10% of substitute methadone prescribing in Britain is in an injectable form, a practice which used to be exclusive to the UK and has some research support for its use (Strang et al 2000), but the case for injectable substitute prescribing is by no means made (Zador 2001). The remaining 10% of methadone prescriptions are for the tablet form, which is readily acknowledged as being easy to reconstitute for injection and therefore is specifically now contraindicated in dependent opiate users (Department of Health 1999). In the UK there is greater provision of 'take-home' medication than in the USA or Australia, where the majority of medication is dispensed on a daily basis and often with supervised consumption at the point of collection. In the UK, nearly a third of all methadone is dispensed by weekly or fortnightly pick-up and a further third by daily pick-up (Strang et al 1996a). Buprenorphine is also an effective intervention for use in the maintenance treatment of opiate dependence, but it is not more effective than methadone at adequate dosages (Mattick et al 2002b). What buprenorphine may offer is an increased dispensing interval (up to once every four days) compared with methadone (Petry et al 2001).

The opiate withdrawal syndrome can be characterised by nausea, vomiting, muscle aches, lacrimation, rhinorrhoea, pupillary dilatation, pilo-erection, sweating, diarrhoea, yawning, fever and insomnia. The severity and length of withdrawal is dependent on the drug of abuse, shorter-acting drugs tending to have more severe withdrawal over shorter periods than do longer-acting drugs. Some describe withdrawal as a 'flu-like illness' but others demonstratively have a severe reaction. This may in part be due to expectation, but the level of tolerance and dependence on the drug also contribute. The withdrawal is managed with substitution of the opiate, usually methadone, and a gradual reduction is then carried out over a period of time. The shortest period advocated is 24 hours (Carreno et al 2002) — this needs to be carried out in an intensive care unit and involves naltrexone-induced withdrawal, with heavy sedation. More typical withdrawal periods are of 10–21 days on an inpatient basis (Gowing et al 2002a). Symptomatic treatment may be given with, for example, α_2 adrenergic agonists such as clonidine or lofexidine, but these drugs have no effect on the insomnia, craving and muscle aches associated with withdrawal. Longer out patient maintenance to abstinence programmes are also used (Farrell 1994).

Recently introduced for the treatment of opiate withdrawal, buprenorphine has potential to ameliorate the signs and symptoms of withdrawal from heroin, and possibly methadone, but many aspects of the treatment protocols and the relative effectiveness need to be investigated further (Gowing et al 2002b).

The medical management of opiate withdrawal is not complicated other than in the very short procedures. The difficulty is in achieving continued abstinence, and this is discussed further under relapse prevention (p. 381). However, approaches that might increase compliance with subsequent naltrexone maintenance treatment, such as antagonist-induced regimens, require further research to confirm their relative effectiveness, as well as variables influencing the severity of withdrawal and adverse effects (Gowing et al 2002c).

Stimulants

Intoxication with stimulants appears to be less common, possibly because there is a loss of pleasurable effect at high doses, the mental state becomes associated with paranoia and psychosis, and convulsions may result. Treatment is symptomatic along general guidelines. Patients with a stimulant dependence syndrome in the UK usually abuse amphetamines, but increasingly cases of dependence on cocaine, and in some areas 'crack' cocaine, are occasionally seen. If patients continue to use, then harm reduction advice is essential as with any other substance. However, treatment options based on the literature are limited in that they are exclusively abstinence orientated, with the majority involving residential settings (Schuckit 1994). Therefore the main focus is in relapse prevention. Various drugs have been suggested as being useful in the stimulant dependence syndrome, including bromocriptine, which theoretically should alleviate the hypothesised dopamine depletion of chronic stimulant abuse. Other drugs which boost dopamine activity include mazindol, flupenthixol and amantadine. Unfortunately, research results do not justify their use as part of a standard therapy for stimulant-dependent individuals. Antidepressant medication has been used in view of the mood swings experienced following stimulant abstinence. Again, while theoretically sound, the research does not provide support for antidepressant use in day-to-day practice (Lima et al 2002). There are no randomized controlled trials published to support maintenance prescribing or maintenance to

abstinence prescribing for stimulant dependence syndrome, although a pilot feasibility study has now been carried out (Shearer et al 2001). However, within specialist drug units in the UK, some prescribing along these lines does occur (Bradbeer et al 1998). More research needs to be done in this area before it can be advocated as a treatment. Stimulant withdrawal has been suggested by some to be a triphasic state with a 'crash', 'withdrawal' and 'extinction' phase. The crash typically occurs within 30 minutes and may last up to 40 hours. The withdrawal phase tends to peak at 2–4 days, and various depressive symptoms last for several weeks after that, including hypersomnia, fatigue, anhedonia, sadness, suicidal ideation and general malaise (Lago & Kosten 1994). However, this description of stimulant withdrawal has not been repeated by others, who find a persistent, gradual improvement throughout the withdrawal period. There is no specific symptomatic treatment, and the majority of stimulant users end their dependence without resorting to medical support.

Sedatives and hypnotics

Illicit use of drugs in this group is now almost exclusively of benzodiazepines, although historically barbiturates have been important. The management of benzodiazepine acute intoxication follows general principles, and the benzodiazepine antagonist flumazenil may be used to reverse the onset of respiratory depression and coma. Sedatives and hypnotics are also commonly used in conjunction with other drugs, particularly stimulants and alcohol. There is extensive harmful use of this class of drugs, the harm including increased risk behaviour by intravenous drug users (Strang et al 1994), an increased association with accidents (Currie et al 1995), aggression (Bond et al 1995), deterioration in performance (Kerr et al 1992), and amnestic effects which can be used medically to good purpose in surgical premedication (Hindmarch et al 1993). Iatrogenic initiation of benzodiazepines, with subsequent dependence, remains a concern (Surendrakumar et al 1992), despite the recommendations from the Committee on Safety of Medicines (1998) to limit treatment to short courses only. Medical negligence maybe claimed in these cases, and long-term use requires careful consideration (Hallstrom 1990). Iatrogenic benzodiazepine drug dependence is more common than high-dose illicit benzodiazepine drug dependence (usually in the context of multiple drug use). The latter group poses a significant clinical challenge, but has been studied the least. As to the former, the clinical management has been reviewed (Higgitt et al 1985) and guidelines have been issued (Substance Abuse Committee of the Mental Health Foundation 1992). The best outcome in this group is associated with younger patients, fewer withdrawal symptoms and at 6 months post-withdrawal less personality disturbance and longer duration of use prior to withdrawal (Holton et al 1992). In high-dose illicit use, management of a dependence syndrome may be different. One finding is that drug users prefer high-dose short-acting compounds and are more likely to seek these out (Griffiths & Wolff 1990). There is no research support for maintenance prescribing.

The withdrawal state has features which are clinically similar and sometimes indistinguishable from anxiety states. Additional features include hypersensitivity in all senses, de-realisation and de-personalisation. Late presentations of withdrawal include psychotic states and convulsions. The management of withdrawal involves substitute prescribing of a long-acting benzodiazepine (e.g. diazepam). Then gradual controlled withdrawal with the co-operation of the patient can take place over a period of months. Rapid inpatient detoxification may be unsafe (Robertson & Bell 1993). Associated features of withdrawal are managed symptomatically as they arise, as outlined above in the treatment of iatrogenic dependence.

Hallucinogens

There is a large variety of hallucinogens that may be used and could produce clinical conditions. These include psilocybin and mescaline (primarily found in fungicides), lysergic acid diethylamide (LSD), and 3,4-methylenedioxymethamphetamine (MDMA) and many other compounds with botanical origin (DeSmet 1996). The main drugs which sometimes present with clinical conditions are LSD and MDMA and will be discussed further. Hallucinogenic intoxication usually only presents when there is a 'bad trip'. This is primarily dependent on the mental set and environmental setting of the user. If the user is not relaxed, or is feeling under pressure of time, or had a recent argument, or holding major resentments, this may lead to a bad trip. In addition, solitary experimentation in an over-stimulated environment can also precipitate bad experiences. These experiences usually wear off before medical intervention is sought. However, treatment should be directed at preventing the patient from physically harming themselves, or others. Reducing external stimulation and focusing on a single individual, preferably a friend, may be used to help the user calm down. The somatic (dizziness, paraesthesiae, weakness and tremor), perceptual (altered reality) and psychic (labile mood, dreams, altered time sense and de-personalisation) symptoms may be so severe as to require antipsychotic medication, such as chlorpromazine. Some of the adverse reactions that occur after LSD are not due to the drug but to contaminants, such as phencyclidine (PCP). There appears to be no significant dependence syndrome or withdrawal state for the hallucinogenic group. There is some concern over the hallucinogenic residual state of flash-backs, which occurs in a small proportion. Over time, their intensity, frequency and duration diminish (Frankel 1994). There is no evidence of any neurotoxic effect of LSD, but this is not the case for MDMA.

Acute intoxication with MDMA can produce a syndrome similar to the serotinergic syndrome and neuroleptic malignant syndrome (Demirkiran et al 1996). This condition is managed as for the neuroleptic malignant syndrome. Harmful use of MDMA occurs as a result of tolerance, where users may increase the dose to achieve the original effect, and this may result in neurotoxicity. Subjects may take large doses (Green & Goodwin 1996), but the significance of this in practical terms for users has been challenged (Merrill 1996). The use of hallucinogenic drugs to explore neurochemistry and in psychotherapy research disappeared during the 1970s and 1980s but has re-emerged (Strassman 1995).

Cannabis

As with hallucinogens, the premorbid state and setting are influential in determining reactions to acute ingestion. In a dose–response manner, acute intoxication with cannabis can result in disturbances of perception and, in severe cases, psychotic states (Ghodse 1986, Thomas 1993, Johns 2001). Treatment for these conditions follows general guidelines. A dependence syndrome for cannabis occurs in a small minority of users; treatment tends to be aimed at reduced consumption and abstinence. Withdrawal from cannabis is also reported for high-dose chronic users, but the literature is poor and unclear as to what the withdrawal features are (Smith 2002). Little evidence has been found (Ashton 2001) of long-term negative consequences for chronic users, but marijuana smoke contains the same carcinogens as tobacco smoke, usually in somewhat higher concentration, and therefore long-term physical health may well be damaged. Cannabis has been made available on prescription in two American states. This is for symptomatic treatment of various conditions, including cancer, chronic pain and spasticity. Randomised controlled trials are underway in the UK and, if positive, are likely to lead to cannabis prescribing for specific medical conditions.

Solvents

Acute intoxication with solvents can produce coma and death. In addition, there are quite specific problems of sudden death with solvents, usually related to cardiac arrhythmia, or vasovagal inhibition resulting in cardiac arrest. There is no place for harm reduction in solvent misuse, and the sole goal is one of abstinence. There is limited evidence that a dependence syndrome with specific withdrawal occurs. Residual states due to long-term use can occur, as there is extensive multiple organ damage with protracted use. Treatment is symptomatic. The main focus for solvents is prevention, early detection and abstinence (Advisory Council on the Misuse of Drugs 1995).

RELAPSE PREVENTION

Once a former user is abstinent from the substance, the process of keeping him drug-free can be described as relapse prevention. The psychological and psycho-biological models of this process are well developed (Connors et al 1996). However, there has been limited outcome research to support the models with regard to addictions other than alcohol. Substance misuse needs to be seen as a chronic relapsing disorder. Progress in the area is hampered by variation in the definition of relapse itself. Reported outcomes can vary between studies depending on whether they report on a continuous basis along a dimension, or just for short periods repeatedly throughout that dimension. Also, is relapse focused just on the substance misused or is there a more comprehensive assessment, including other areas of physical psychological and social functioning? In addition, the threshold at which a drug is being used, and what constitutes a relapse needs to be defined. Does any use constitute a relapse or may it just be seen as a lapse which is rapidly followed by reinstatement of abstinence? The inclusion of assessments of whether there is transfer to another substance or behaviour of dependence, and issues around verification and the importance placed on this, are also undecided and make analysis across studies difficult (Miller 1996). The continued development and harmonisation of accepted standards of outcome measures makes it more likely that, in the future, studies of individual groups can be generalised beyond the setting of the research. Miller and colleagues in 1996 conducted an analysis of alcohol relapse that could be extended to other substances. In addition to pre-treatment characteristics, they identified five factors mediating tendency to relapse (Box 18.7).

The practical process of applying relapse prevention involves various key themes outlined by Daley & Marlatt (1992) (Box 18.8).

Box 18.7   Factors mediating tendency to relapse

- Negative life events
- Cognitive appraisal, including self-efficacy, expectancy and motivation for change
- Client coping resources
- Craving experiences
- Affective/mood status

From Miller et al (1996).

Box 18.8   Themes important in relapse prevention

- Help patients identify their high-risk relapse factors and develop strategies to deal with them
- Help patients understand relapse as a process and as an event
- Help patients understand and deal with substance cues as well as actual cravings
- Help patients understand and deal with social pressures to use drugs
- Help patients to develop a supportive relapse prevention network
- Help patients develop methods of coping with negative emotional states
- Help patients learn methods to cope with cognitive distortions
- Help patients work towards a balanced lifestyle
- Help patients develop a plan to interrupt a lapse or relapse

---

Some specific work has been done with opiate addicts to assess whether they can predict their own relapse (Powell et al 1993). In this study, 43 opiate addicts who had undergone inpatient detoxification were followed-up at 6 months. Those with lower self-esteem and higher positive expectancies were using less often. Latency to first lapse was longer in subjects with higher anxiety and neuroticism score. It is suggested that greater awareness of personal vulnerability may promote effective coping strategies. Experimental models have also been used with this population to examine mood effects (euphoria, depression, anxiety and anger). This showed that induced depression increased drug craving, and tended to increase opiate withdrawal symptoms. Other trends were also outlined and a suggestion was made that these may become a conditioned stimulus to trigger a relapse (Childress et al 1994). The role of attribution in abstinence, lapse and relapse has also been explored (Walton et al 1994).

A well-designed study was carried out by Carroll and colleagues (1994b). This study was a 1-year follow-up of 121 cocaine abusers who underwent two forms of psychotherapy — either relapse prevention or clinical management — and also were treated with either desipramine or placebo. Their analysis suggested a delayed improved response during follow-up in patients who received relapse prevention compared with supportive clinical management alone.

EVALUATION OF TREATMENTS

Evaluation of treatments for drug misuse

Of the various treatments discussed in this chapter, methadone maintenance has been evaluated to a greater extent than any other.

There is an extensive review of the literature by Ward and colleagues (1998). In the USA in 1992, there were about 120 000 patients in treatment. In the UK and the rest of Europe, numbers are increasing. Research shows increased compliance with treatment, reduction in crime by 50% year on year, reductions in illicit drug use, reductions in sharing and improvements in psychosocial functioning. Inpatient detoxification is also advocated within the UK, and outcome studies do show abstinence rates near 50% at 6-month follow-up (Johns 1994). As for other treatments in substance misuse, not all treatments work on all patients. The attempts in alcohol research to match patients to particular treatments will no doubt be duplicated in other drugs.

An evaluation of treatments in the opiate dependence syndrome is being carried out by The National Treatment Outcome Research Study (NTORS). This involves 1110 people who entered treatment in 1995, who were in either residential programmes, inpatient units, methadone maintenance or methadone reduction programmes. The findings after 5 years have been published (National Treatment Outcome Research Study 2001). These show reductions in:

- heroin and other drug use (at 5 years abstinence rates for opiates were 47% in the residential settings and 35% for those previously taking methadone; continued daily opiate use was about 20% for both groups, and 40% were still using heroin at least once a week);
- injecting (60% falling to 37% in both groups);
- sharing injecting equipment (falling from 14% to 5% in the 5 years);
- physical and psychological ill health (improved but still with an annual mortality rate of 1.2% — much higher than age-matched peers);
- criminal activity (reduced by 50% at 1 year and then largely dependent on whether heroin use continued).

An economic evaluation of treatment showed that for every £1 spent on treatment £3 was saved in the criminal justice system. However, the more important results addressing questions such as the relationship between client characteristics and treatment outcome, or the relationship between treatment structure, process and outcome, will follow in the coming years.

Evaluation of treatment for alcohol misuse

There have been a large number of studies evaluating the effectiveness of treatment for alcoholism, alcohol dependence and alcohol-related problems. Patient characteristics, particularly social and marital stability and, to a lesser extent, severity of dependence, often prove better predictors of outcome than specific features of therapy. During the past 20 years there have been an increasing number of good quality controlled trials for the treatment of alcohol use disorders. Miller and his colleagues have periodically reviewed the evidence derived from these studies. The most recent report in this series is based on 361 clinical trials and shows that brief intervention is the most consistently effective approach, although only a minority of the reported studies concerned a clinical population. Other effective treatment approaches included were motivational enhancement (again less so with clinical populations), social skills training, community reinforcement, behaviour contracting and behavioural marital therapy. Drug treatments with acamprosate or naltrexone were also effective. Most of the psychosocial approaches favoured are based on cognitive-behavioural principles, while more traditional approaches such as psychotherapy and 'general alcoholism counselling' were not shown to be effective (Miller & Wilbourne 2002).

Another major study that has proved very influential is project MATCH which aimed to demonstrate the merits of matching clients to three different and carefully defined treatments: Twelve Step Facilitation (a 12 week guided introduction to the principles of AA); motivational enhancement therapy (four sessions); coping skills therapy (twelve sessions). The study involved a total of 1726 clients treated in various centres in the USA. Relatively few matching effects were observed at 3-year follow-up. All proved very effective. It is noteworthy that motivational enhancement therapy was just as effective in most cases as the more intensive therapies and emerged as the most cost-effective approach. Another aspect of this study is the way in which the therapists employed were carefully trained, worked to a manual and had their practice reviewed by regular video recording. This overcame uncertainties about the quality and character of the treatments offered and may have contributed to the excellence of the overall outcome (Project MATCH Research Group 1998).

Controlled studies of AA have not been conducted, but follow-up studies in the USA indicate strongly its efficacy. For example, Vaillant (1995) followed 100 patients at regular intervals for 8 years. Of the 39 men attaining stable abstinence, two-thirds did so through AA. In the same city, 120 problem drinkers identified in the community and not at clinics, and who were followed for between 10 and 30 years, yielded 34% who became stable abstainers. Of those, a third were regular AA attenders and many had commenced abstinence through that route.

There is considerable instability in the drinking status of samples of patients followed up in the first 2–4 years after commencing treatment (Polich et al 1981). Ten studies are published where follow-up was at least 8 years and objective as well as subjective data are available on outcome. A fifth of subjects died (a mortality two to three times greater than expected). Of the survivors, half to two-thirds were still in some difficulty with their drinking. Of those who were well, most were abstainers. Some 5–10% had been drinking without problems for a year or more. It is clear, however, from following problem drinkers identified in the community that many change their habits without professional help (Vaillant 1995).

Most of the studies reported by Miller & Wilbourne (2002) concerned specific therapies rather than treatment programmes. In large samples of patients, inpatient treatment has not shown clear advantages over outpatient treatment. Oxford & Edwards (1977) randomly allocated 100 married male alcoholics to two treatment groups: one was offered intensive therapy, including admission to hospital when indicated; the other was assessed and given carefully chosen advice in a single session. The two groups were followed closely for 1 year. A total of 60% improved but no difference was found between the two groups, although 2-year follow-up suggested that severely dependent patients did better if given intensive treatment.

Many controlled studies have examined the influence of duration and intensity of treatment on prognosis. With remarkable consistency these studies have failed to demonstrate any relationship (Institute of Medicine 1990). Chick et al (1988) compared very minimal treatment with a broad package of treatments, including some inpatient and group therapy, using a systematic follow-up for those patients who accepted it. This research showed that the stable abstinence rate was no higher after 2 years in the more intensively treated group; however, the intensive group had experienced fewer total problems related to their drinking than the advice-only group. Before concluding that there are no advantages inherent in more intensive treatment it is worth recording that relatively few studies have adequately characterised the total treatment package, and there are indications that more severely dependent patients do have a better outcome if offered somewhat more intensive treatment.

The overall picture is that approximately two-thirds of individuals receiving treatment show improvement and that treatment is significantly better than no treatment. Considering the costs to society of alcohol problems, there is good evidence of the cost benefits of providing treatment to individuals with alcohol problems (Holder & Blose 2000).

ORGANISATION OF SERVICES

Alcohol

Alcohol-related problems are extremely common and protean in their clinical manifestations. It is estimated that about one in twenty patients seen by a general practitioner will have an alcohol problem, and a further 10–20% will be drinking amounts which increase their risk of future problems. In general medical and general psychiatric wards approximately 20% of men and 12% of women will be found to be drinking at levels that are damaging to their health.

The manifestations of alcohol-related problems are diverse and extend from hazardous drinking patterns which may prove harmful in time or in certain contexts to complex and severe problems including dependency and physical and psychological harm. It is therefore unrealistic to expect one single therapeutic strategy to meet all these needs.

A framework of health and social services is required which takes into account this range of problems. This should extend from services that provide identification and assessment often coupled with brief intervention, commonly provided by generalists, and extend to more specialist services that cater for patients who have complex needs including comorbidity or have proved unresponsive to simpler approaches. Any framework of services should ensure that help is readily accessible, non-stigmatising and equitably available. This 'stepped care approach' ensures that patients receive the least intrusive and most cost-effective intervention and only draws specialist services into direct service provision when necessary (Raistrick et al 1999).

There is an opportunity for change inherent in each crisis, provided the problem is recognised and the primary-level agency has received adequate training and feels competent in coping with the problem and giving advice. The different layers of increasingly specialised intervention are illustrated in Box 18.9.

Front-line services will require support from agencies, such as councils on alcohol, Alcoholics Anonymous and specialised treatment units. The majority of alcohol problems can be managed in the community, while a smaller number require some initial inpatient treatment and/or residential hostel care. Community alcohol teams have evolved as a means of providing support to the primary level and linkage with specialist resources. Their joint plan for each district should be concerned with both prevention and treatment and will involve multi-agency co-operation often enhanced by the formation of an alcohol action team to take forward the local plan (Ritson 1995, Scottish Executive 2002).

Box 18.9 Levels of intervention relevant to an effective response to alcohol problems	
Level 1	The drinker, the family and friends
Level 2	Employers, work colleagues, police, bartenders, social welfare
Level 3	Primary healthcare, accident and emergency services, hospitals, social work, probation, counsellors
Level 4	Alcoholics Anonymous, councils on alcohol, specialist alcohol treatment services

Level 1: Awareness of hazardous drinking can lead to 'spontaneous' improvement, influenced by health promotion and the attitude of the family. Level 2: Although care is not their primary responsibility, these agencies are well placed to initiate an effective intervention. Level 3: Primary-level caring agencies can be effective with sufficient training and support. Level 4: Specialist services (responsible for direct care as well as giving consultation and support to levels 2 and 3).

In an early report which remains relevant, the Department of Health and Social Security (1978) recommended that 'treatment and care should be provided at a primary level' and identified that the main tasks of the primary-level workers were to:

1. recognise hazardous and harmful drinking, its causes and effects;
2. have adequate knowledge of the help required by the problem drinker and the family;
3. give appropriate advice and help where necessary;
4. know where and when to seek more specialist help;
5. provide continuing care, support and follow-up.

Primary-level workers are often ill-equipped to provide this kind of service unless they receive adequate training and continuing support from a specialist team. The role of the specialist in alcohol problems increasingly involves providing this kind of support. Within hospital settings there is good evidence that the presence of a specialist alcohol nurse can enhance the likelihood of detecting alcohol problems at an early stage. These nurses should work closely with liaison psychiatrists or with outreach from the alcohol treatment services.

Drugs

With specific reference to drugs, there have been three recent documents dedicated, at least in part, to the organisation of services: one produced by The Advisory Council on the Misuse of Drugs (1993), the second the result of the establishment by the Secretary of State for Scotland of a ministerial drugs task force (1994), and thirdly the English Task Force to Review Services for Drug Misusers (1996). This last task force made 12 recommendations that would greatly improve the effectiveness of drug services (Box 18.10). The report by the Advisory Council on the Misuse of Drugs made 33 similar recommendations but, in addition, included a recommendation to expand outreach to try and contact hidden populations of drug users. The Scottish ministerial drugs task force examined drug misuse and made recommendations including some in the area of services. It acknowledged the lack of expert advice on the effectiveness of provision, types or combination of types of service required to meet the needs of different drug users. It recommended the establishment of such expert advice.

Box 18.10 Recommendations suggested to improve the effectiveness of drug services
• A shared-care model between specialist services and general practice. (However, the General Medical Services Committee has defined shared-care arrangements with regard to treatment in drug dependence as non-core services. It seems that unless funding is available to support GPs in this extra work, resistance may occur regarding GP involvement.)
• Opportunities should be taken when drug misusers present to the criminal justice system. Treatment within the prison service and on release should be continuous with treatments in the community
• Maintenance of syringe exchange facilities
• Basic health checks at first point of contact with drug users
• Hepatitis B vaccination being made available to injectors
• Counselling and support services as co-components of treatment
• Availability of: methadone reduction programmes; oral methadone maintenance programmes; residential rehabilitation programmes; specialist inpatient drug dependency units
• An end to the prescribing of methadone tablets to drug users
• A limitation to the licence to prescribe injectable drugs to drug misusers
• Maximum waiting times
• Flexible opening times reflecting needs of drug users
• Monitoring of key indicators of treatment organisations and outcomes

From Task Force to Review Services for Drug Misusers (1996).

It is clear that there are many similarities in the problems experienced by those who misuse alcohol or other drugs, and multiple drug misuse is commonplace. Nonetheless, difference of age, life-style and the legal status of the drugs involved results in many agencies retaining some separation in the treatment systems for individuals who misuse alcohol or other drugs while working closely together when this is advantageous.

Services for young people

Among young people alcohol and drug misuse is often associated with increased dropout from school, poor scholastic attainment, delinquency, early pregnancy, family difficulties and mental health problems. The evidence on optimal organisation of services for young people is limited and principally from the USA. The Health Advisory Service (Gilvarry 2001) in England recently reviewed the available evidence and proposed a tiered approach to services, emphasising the need to integrate drugs, alcohol and other child care services (Box 18.11).

As with all services, emphasis should be placed on early recognition with particular attention to screening among vulnerable groups such as: young offenders; runaway homeless children; all those in the 'looked-after' system or in contact with social services; children with behavioural or learning problems at school; those subject to family disturbance; attenders at accident and emergency departments with trauma or self harm. While many young people mature out of alcohol or drug misuse, a significant minority progress to greater harm.

Box 18.11 Health Advisory Service (2001) suggested approach to services

- Tier 1: Universal-generic primary services
- Tier 2: Youth-orientated services offered by practitioners with some drug and alcohol experience and youth specialist knowledge
- Tier 3: Services provided by specialist teams. Such teams would entail collaboration between mental health, paediatrics and addiction workers, alongside education and social services
- Tier 4: Very specialised services — these would work in continuity with Tier 3, often providing short periods of residential care including detoxification at times of crisis. They would be concerned with adolescents with very complex needs

Any framework for services needs to recognise that some groups find it difficult to access or utilize mainstream adult services. These groups include women (see p. 366), ethnic minorities, the homeless, the elderly (in whom alcohol problems are commonly overlooked or misdiagnosed) and young people. Despite widespread concern about drug and alcohol misuse and smoking among teenagers, particularly in the UK (Hibell et al 1999), there is a dearth of appropriate services for their needs.

WEBSITES

The following websites give up-to-date information.

- National guidelines for the management of drug misuse — full text
  www.doh.gov.uk./pub/does/doh/dmfull.pdf
- Drug misuse in Scotland
  www.drugmisuse.isdsscotland.org
- UK government policy and research on drug misuse
  www.drugs.gov.uk
- European Monitoring Center for Drugs and Drug Addiction (EMCDDA)
  www.emcdda.org
- American drug information & research
  www.nida.nih.gov
- Systematic reviews
  www.cochrane.org
- UK drug resource centre
  www.drugscope.org.uk
- Society for the Study of Addiction with excellent links page to many countries' drug databases
  www.addiction-ssa.org
- Alcohol use and misuse in Scotland: National Plan
  alcoholaction@scotland.gsi.gov.uk
- UK alcohol resource centre
  www.alcoholconcern.org.uk
- Alcohol review of relapse prevention
  www.htbs.co.uk
- Medical information about alcohol
  www.medicouncilalcol.demon.co.uk
- American alcohol information and research
  www.niaaa.nih.gov

REFERENCES

Advisory Council on the Misuse of Drugs 1993 Aids and drug misuse update. Department of Health, HMSO, London

Advisory Council on The Misuse of Drugs 1995 Volatile substance abuse. Home Office, HMSO, London

Alcohol Concern 2000 Straight Talk 15. Alcohol Concern, London

Anderson P 1988 Excess mortality associated with alcohol consumption. British Medical Journal 297:824–826

Andreasson S, Alleback P, Romelsjo A 1988 Alcohol and mortality among young men: longitudinal study of Swedish conscripts. British Medical Journal 296:1021–1025

Ashton C H 2001 Pharmacology and effects of cannabis: a brief review. British Journal of Psychiatry 178:101–106

Babor T 1994 Demography, epidemiology and psychopharmacology — making sense of the connections. Addiction 89:1391–1396

Babor T F, Ritson E B, Hodgson R J 1986 Alcohol related problems in the primary health care setting: a review of early intervention strategies. British Journal of Addiction 81:23–46

Babor T F, de la Fuente J R, Saunders J 1989 AUDIT: The Alcohol Use Disorder Identification Test: guidelines for use in primary care. World Health Organisation, Geneva

Baigent M, Holme G, Hafner R J 1995 Self reports of the interaction between substance abuse and schizophrenia. Australian & New Zealand Journal of Psychiatry 29(1):69–74

Baldwin S 1991 Alcohol education and young offenders. Springer-Verlag, Berlin

Bartels S J, Drake R E, Wallach M A 1995 Long-term course of substance use disorders among patients with severe mental illness. Psychiatric Services 46(3):248–251

Bendetti G 1952 Die Alkoholhalluzinosen. Thieme, Stuttgart

Bien T H, Miller R W, Tonigan J S 1993 Brief intervention for alcohol problems: a review. Addiction 88:315–336

Bond A J, Curran H V, Bruce M S et al 1995 Behavioural aggression in panic disorder after 8 weeks' treatment with alprazolam. Journal of Affective Disorders 35(3):117–123

Bourne P G, Alford J A, Bowcock J Z 1966 Treatment of skid row alcoholics with Disulfiram. Quarterly Journal of Studies on Alcohol 27:42

Bradbeer T M, Fleming P M, Charlton P, Crichton J S 1998 Survey of amphetamine prescribing in England and Wales. Drug and Alcohol Review 17:299–304

Bremner J D, Southwick S M, Darnell A, Charney D S 1996 Chronic PTSD in Vietnam combat veterans: course of illness and substance abuse. American Journal of Psychiatry 153(3):369–375

British Medical Association 1998 The misuse of alcohol and other drugs by doctors. BMA, London

Brown S A, Schuckit M A 1998 Changes in depression among abstinent alcoholics. Journal of Studies on Alcohol 49:412–417

Burke J D Jr, Burke K C, Rae D S 1994 Increased rates of drug abuse and dependence after onset of mood or anxiety disorders in adolescence. Hospital & Community Psychiatry 45(5):451–455

Cairns A, Roberts I, Benbow E 1996 Characteristics of fatal methadone overdose in Manchester, 1985–1994. British Medical Journal 313:264–265

Carreno J E, Bobes J, Brewer C et al 2002 24-hour opiate detoxification and antagonist induction at home — the 'Asturian method': a report on 1368 procedures. Addiction Biology 7(2):243–250

Carroll K M, Rounsaville B J, Bryant K J 1994a Should tolerance and withdrawal be required for substance dependence disorders? Drug & Alcohol Dependence 36(1):15–22

Carroll K M, Rounsaville B J, Nich C et al 1994b One-year follow-up of psychotherapy and pharmacotherapy for cocaine dependence: delayed emergence of psychotherapy effects. Archives of General Psychiatry 51(12):989–997

Chambers R A, Krystal J H, Self D W 2001 A neurobiological basis for substance abuse comorbidity in schizophrenia. Biological Psychiatry 50(2):71–83

Chick J 1992 Doctors with emotional problems: how can they be helped? In: Hawton K, Cowen P (eds) Dilemmas in the management of psychiatric patients, vol 2. Oxford University Press, Oxford

Chick J, Chick J 1992 Drinking problems: information and advice for the individual, family and friends, 2nd edn. MacDonald Optima Press, London

Chick J, Duffy J C, Lloyd G G, Ritson B 1986 Medical admissions in men: the risk among drinkers. Lancet ii: 1380–1383

Chick J, Ritson B, Connaughton J et al 1988 Advice versus extended treatment for alcoholism; a controlled study. British Journal of Addiction 83:159–170

Chick J, Gough K, Falkowski W et al 1992 Treatment of alcoholism. British Journal of Psychiatry 162:84–89

Childress A R, Ehrman R, McLellan A T et al 1994 Can induced moods trigger drug-related responses in opiate abuse patients? Journal of Substance Abuse Treatment 11(1):17–23

Cloninger C R 1987 Neurogenetic adaptive mechanisms in alcoholism. Science 23:410–415

Cochrane R, Bal S 1990 The drinking habits of Sikh, Hindu, Muslim and white men in the West Midlands: a community survey. British Journal of Addiction 85:759–769

Committee on Safety of Medicines 1988 Benzodiazepine dependence and withdrawal symptoms. Current Problems 21

Connors G, Maisto S, Donovan D 1996 Conceptualisation of relapse: a summary of psychological and psychobiological models. Addiction 91 (suppl): S5–S14

Cottler L B, Price R K, Compton W M, Mager D E 1995 Subtypes of adult antisocial behavior among drug abusers. Journal of Nervous & Mental Disease 183(3):154–161

CRAG/SCOTMEG 1994 The management of alcohol withdrawal and delirium tremens. Scottish Office, Edinburgh

Currie D, Hashemi K, Fothergill J et al 1995 The use of anti-depressants and benzodiazepines in the perpetrators and victims of accidents. Occupational Medicine 45(6):323–325

Cutting J 1978 A reappraisal of alcoholic psychosis. Psychological Medicine 8:285–296

Daley D, Marlatt G 1992 Relapse prevention: cognitive and behavioural intervention. In: Lowinson J, Ruiz P, Millman R (eds) Substance abuse: a comprehensive textbook, 2nd edn. Williams & Wilkins, Baltimore, p 533–542

Darke S, Ross J, Hall W 1995 Overdose among heroin users in Sydney, Australia, 1: Prevalence and correlates of non-fatal overdose. Addiction 91:405–411

Demirkiran M, Jankovic J, Dean J M 1996 Ecstasy intoxication: an overlap between serotonin syndrome and neuroleptic malignant syndrome. Clinical Neuropharmacology 19(2):157–164

Department of Health 1995 Sensible drinking: The report of an interdepartmental working group. Department of Health, London

Department of Health 1999 Drug misuse and dependence — guidelines on clinical management. TSO, London

Department of Health and Social Security 1978 The pattern and range of services for problem drinkers. HMSO, London

De Smet P A 1996 Some ethnopharmacological notes on African hallucinogens. Journal of Ethnopharmacology 50(3):141–146

Dillon P 2002 The much lamented death of Madam Geneva — the eighteenth century gin craze. Review, London

Domingo-Salvany A, Hartnoll R L, Maguire A et al 1995 Use of capture–recapture to estimate the prevalence of opiate addiction in Barcelona, Spain, 1989. American Journal of Epidemiology 141(6):567–574

Dorn N, Murji K 1992 ISDD Research Monograph 5 — Drug prevention: a review of the English language literature. ISDD, London

Drake R E, Vaillant G E 1988 Predicting alcoholism and personality disorder in a 33-year longitudinal study of children of alcoholics. British Journal of Addiction 83:799–807

Drake R, Mueser K, Clark R et al 1996 The course, treatment and outcome of substance disorders in persons with severe mental illness. American Journal of Orthopsychiatry 66:42–51

Drugscope 2002 National Audit of Drug Misuse in Britain 2001 College Hill Press, London

Drummond D C, Cooper T, Glautier S P 1990 Conditioned learning in alcohol dependence: implications for cue exposure treatment. British Journal of Addiction 85:725–743

Duffy J Kreitman N 1993 Risk factors for suicide and undetermined death among in-patient alcoholics in Scotland. Addiction 88:757–766

Dyer A R, Stamler J, Oglesby P et al 1980 Alcohol consumption and 17-year mortality in the Chicago Western Electric Company study. Preventive Medicine 9:78–90

Edwards G, Gross M 1976 Alcohol dependence: provisional description, of a clinical syndrome. British Medical Journal i: 1058

Edwards M E, Steinglass P 1995 Family therapy treatment outcomes for alcoholism. Journal of Marital and Family Therapy 21(4):475–509

Ewing J A 1984 Detecting alcoholism: the CAGE questionnaire. Journal of the American Medical Association 252:1905–1907

Fals-Stewart W, Angarano K 1994 Obsessive–compulsive disorder among patients entering substance abuse treatment: prevalence and accuracy of diagnosis. Journal of Nervous & Mental Disease 82(12):715–719

Fals-Stewart W, Schafer J 1992 The treatment of substance abusers diagnosed with obsessive–compulsive disorder: an outcome study. Journal of Substance Abuse Treatment 9(4):365–370

Farrell M 1994 Opiate withdrawal. Addiction 89(11):1471–1475

Farrell M, Ward J, Mattick R et al 1994 Methadone maintenance treatment in opiate dependence: a review. British Medical Journal 309:997–1001

Farrell M, Howes S, Bebbington P et al 2001 Nicotine, alcohol and drug dependence and psychiatric comorbidity: results of a national household survey. British Journal of Psychiatry 179:432–437

Fast Forward Positive Lifestyles Limited 1996 Scottish Schools Drug Survey 1996. Scotland Against Drugs, Readpath, Edinburgh

Feirnnan J A Dunner D L 1996 The effect of alcohol and substance abuse on the course of bipolar affective disorder. Journal of Affective Disorders 37(1):43–49

Fiellin D A, Reid M C, O'Connor P G 2000 Screening for alcohol problems in primary care: a systematic review. Archives of Internal Medicine 160(13):1977–1989

Forrest F, Floray C du V, Taylor D et al 1991 Reported social alcohol consumption during pregnancy and infant development at 18 months. British Medical Journal 303:22–25

Foxcroft D R, Lister-Sharp D, Lowe G 1997 Alcohol misuse prevention for young people. Addiction 92(5):531–537

Frankel F H 1994 The concept of flashbacks in historical perspective. International Journal of Clinical & Experimental Hypnosis 42(4):321–336

Frischer M 1992 Estimated prevalence of injecting drug use in Glasgow. British Journal of Addiction 87:235–243

Galanter M 1999 Network therapy for alcohol and drug abuse. Guilford Press, New York

Galanter M, Egelko S, Edwards H, Vergaray M 1994 A treatment system for combined psychiatric and addictive illness. Addiction 89:1227–1235

Garbutt J C, Mayo J P, Gillette G M et al 1991 Dose-response studies with thyrotropin-releasing hormone (TRH) in abstinent male alcoholics: evidence for selective thyrotropin dysfunction. Journal of Studies on Alcohol 52:275–280

Geikie Sir A 1904 Scottish reminiscences. Maclehose, Glasgow

Ghodse H 1986 Cannabis psychosis. British Journal of Addiction 81:473–478

Gilvarry E 2001 The substance of young needs: review 2001. Health Advisory Service, London

Glaser F B 1980 Anybody got a match? Treatment research and the matching hypothesis. In: Edwards G, Grant M (eds) Alcoholism treatment in transition. Croom Helm, London

Goldenberg I M, Mueller T, Fierman E et al 1995 Specificity of substance use in anxiety-disordered subjects. Comprehensive Psychiatry 36(5):319–328

Goldstein D B 1979 Some promising fields of inquiry in biomedical alcohol research. Journal of Studies on Alcohol Supplement 8:204–247

Gore S, Bird A, Ross A 1996 Prison rights: mandatory drug tests and performance indicators for prisons. British Medical Journal 312:1411–1413

Gossop M, Birkin R 1994 Training employment service staff to recognise and respond to clients with drug and alcohol problems. Addictive Behaviors 19(2):127–134

Gossop M, Strang J, Griffiths P et al 1994 A ratio estimation method for determining the prevalence of cocaine use. British Journal of Psychiatry 164(5):676–679

Gossop M, Griffiths P, Powis B et al 1996 Frequency of non fatal heroin overdose: survey of heroin users recruited in non-clinical settings. British Medical Journal 313:402

Gowing L, Farrell M, Ali R, White J 2002a Alpha2 adrenergic agonists for the management of opioid withdrawal (Cochrane Review). In: The Cochrane Library, Issue 4, Oxford

Gowing L, Ali R, White J 2002b Buprenorphine for the management of opioid withdrawal (Cochrane Review). In: The Cochrane Library, Issue 4, Oxford

Gowing L, Ali R, White J 2002c Opioid antagonists with minimal sedation for opioid withdrawal (Cochrane Review). In: The Cochrane Library, Issue 4, Oxford

Green A, Goodwin G 1996 Ecstasy in neurodegeneration. British Medical Journal 312:1493

Griffiths R, Wolff B 1990 Relative abuse liability of different benzodiazepines in drug abusers. Journal of Clinical Psychopharmacology 10:237–243

Griffiths P, Gossop M, Powis B, Strang J 1993 Reaching hidden populations of drug users by privileged access interviewers: methodological and practical issues. Addiction 88(12):1617–1626

Griffiths P, Gossop M, Powis B, Strang J 1994 Transitions in patterns of heroin administration: a study of heroin chasers and heroin injectors. Addiction 89(3):301–309

Gual A, Colom J 1997 Why has alcohol consumption declined in countries of Southern Europe. Addiction 92 (suppl 1): S21–S31

Gurling H M D, Curtis D, Murray R 1991 Psychological deficit from a co-twin study. British Journal of Addiction 86:51–155

Hagman G 1994 Methadone maintenance counselling: definition, principles, components. Journal of Substance Abuse Treatment 11(5):405–413

Hall W, Farrell M 1997 Co-morbidity of mental disorders with substance misuse. British Journal of Psychiatry 171:425

Hallstrom C 1990 Benzodiazepines and medical negligence. Hospital Update 1990:569–571

Hartnoll R 1994 Opiates: prevalence and demographic factors. Addiction 89:1377–1383

Health Publications Unit 1993 Drugs and solvents, you and your child. DSS Distribution Centre, London

Heath A C, Martin N G 1988 Teenage alcohol use in the Australian Twin Register: genetic and social determinants of starting to drink. Alcoholism (NY) 12:735–741

Heather N, Robertson I 1997 Problem drinking. Oxford University Press, Oxford

Helzer J, Canino G, Yeh E-K et al 1990 Alcoholism — N America and Asia. Archives of General Psychiatry 47:313–319

Hibell B, Andersson B, Ahlstrom S et al 2000 The 1999 ESPAD report: Alcohol and drug use in 30 European countries. Swedish Council for Information on Alcohol and other Drugs and Council of Europe (Pompidon Group), Stockholm

Higgitt A, Lader M, Fonagy P 1985 Clinical management of benzodiazepine dependence. British Medical Journal 291:688–690

Hindmarch I, Sherwood N, Kerr J S 1993 Amnestic effects of triazolam and other hypnotics. Progress in Neuro-Psychopharmacology & Biological Psychiatry 17(3):407–413

Hodgson R, Alwyn T, John B et al 2002 The FAST Alcohol screening test. Alcohol & Alcoholism 37:61–66

Holder H, Blose J O 2000 The reduction of health care costs associated with alcoholism treatment: a 14 year long standing study. Journal of Studies on Alcohol 53:293–302

Holdemess C C, Brooks-Gunn J, Warren M P 1994 Co-morbidity of eating disorders and substance abuse: review of the literature. International Journal of Eating Disorders 16(1):1–34

Holton A, Riley P, Tyrer P 1992 Factors predicting long-term outcome after chronic benzodiazepine therapy. Journal of Affective Disorders 24(4):245–252

Home Office 1974 Report on the habitual drunken offender. HMSO, London

Home Office Statistical Bulletin 1995 Statistics of drug addicts notified to the Home Office, United Kingdom, 1994. Research and Statistics Department, Home Office, Croydon

Home Office Statistical Bulletin 2002 Statistics of drugs seizures and offenders dealt with, United Kingdom, 2000. Research and Statistics Department, Home Office, Croydon

Hough M 1996 Drug misuse and the criminal justice system: a review of the literature. Drug Prevention Initiative Paper 15. Home Office, HMSO, London

Howard L, Fahy T, Wong P et al 1994 Psychiatric outcome in alcoholic liver transplant patients. Quarterly Journal of Medicine 87:731–736

Humphries T, Bennet M, Ray C 1991 Alcohol can damage your health. Alcohol Concern, London

Hurley D L 1991 Women, alcohol and incest: an analytical review. Journal of Studies on Alcohol 52:253–268

Institute for the Study of Drug Dependence (ISDD) 1995 National audit of drug misuse in Britain 1994. College Hill Press, London

Institute of Medicine 1990 Prevention and treatment of alcohol problems — research opportunities. National Academy Press, Washington

Isbell H, Fraser H F, Wikler D W et al 1955 An experimental study of the etiology of 'rum fits' and delirium tremens. Quarterly Journal of Studies on Alcohol 16:1–23

Isometsa E T 2001 Psychological autopsy studies — a review. European Psychiatry 16(7):379–385

Johns A 1994 Opiate treatments. Addiction 89:1551–1558

Johns A 2001 Psychiatric effects of cannabis. British Journal of Psychiatry 178:116–122

Johnson S 1997 Dual diagnosis of severe mental illness and substance misuse: a case for specialist services? British Journal of Psychiatry 171:205–208

Kendell R E, de Roumanie M, Ritson E B 1983 Effect of economic changes on Scottish drinking habits 1978–1982. British Journal of Addiction 78:365–372

Kerr J S, Hindmarch I, Sherwood N 1992 Correlation between doses of oxazepam and their effects on performance of a standardised test battery. European Journal of Clinical Pharmacology 42(5):507–510

Kirchmayer U, Davoli M, Verster A 2002 Naltrexone maintenance treatment for opioid dependence (Cochrane Review). In: The Cochrane Library, Issue 4, Oxford

Klein-Schwartz W 2002 Abuse and toxicity of methylphenidate. Current Opinion in Pediatrics 14(2):219–223

Kreitman N 1986 Alcohol consumption and the preventive paradox. British Journal of Addiction 81:353–363

Kushner M G 1996 The relation between alcohol problems and anxiety disorders. American Journal of Psychiatry 153:139–140

Lago J A, Kosten T R 1994 Stimulant withdrawal. Addiction 89(11):1477–1481

Lennane K J 1988 Patients with alcohol related brain damage: therapy and outcome. Australian Drug and Alcohol Review 7:89–92

Lewis C E, Bucholz K K 1991 Alcoholism, antisocial behaviour and family history. British Journal of Addiction 86:177–194

Lima M S, Reisser A A P, Soares B G O, Farrell M 2002 Antidepressants for cocaine dependence (Cochrane Review). In: The Cochrane Library, Issue 4, Oxford

Lynskey M T, Hall W 2001 Attention deficit hyperactivity disorder and substance use disorders: Is there a causal link? Addiction 96(6):815–822

Marlatt G A, Gordon J R 1984 Relapse prevention: maintenance strategies in addictive behaviour. Guilford, New York

Marshall E J, Murray R M 1991 Familial alcoholism: inheritance and initiation. British Medical Journal 303:72–73

Mason P, Wilkinson G 1996 The prevalence of psychiatric morbidity. British Journal of Psychiatry 168:1–3

Mattick R P, Breen C, Kimber J, Davoli M 2002a Methadone maintenance therapy versus no opioid replacement therapy for opioid dependence (Cochrane Review). In: The Cochrane Library, Issue 4, Oxford

Mattick R P, Kimber J, Breen C, Davoli M 2002b Buprenorphine maintenance versus placebo or methadone maintenance for opioid dependence (Cochrane Review). In: The Cochrane Library, Issue 4, Oxford

Mayo-Smith M F 1997 Pharmacological management of alcohol withdrawal: a meta-analysis and evidence based practice guideline. American Society of Addiction. Journal of American Medical Association 278(2):144–151

Merrill J 1996 Advice is that "less is more". British Medical Journal 313:423

Miller P, Plant M 1996 Drinking, smoking, and illicit drug use among 15 and 16 year olds in the United Kingdom. British Medical Journal 313:394–397

Miller W 1996 What is a relapse? 50 ways to leave the wagon. Addiction 91(suppl.): S15–S27

Miller W R, Baca L 1983 Two year follow-up of bibliotherapy and therapist-directed controlled drinking training for problem drinkers. Behaviour Therapy 14:441

Miller W R, Hester R K 1986 The effectiveness of alcoholism treatment methods, what research reveals. In: Miller W R, Heather N (eds) Treating addictive behaviors: processes of change. Plenum, New York

Miller W, Rollnick S 1991 Motivational interviewing: preparing people to change addictive behaviour. Guilford Press, London

Miller W R , Rollnick S 2002 Motivational interviewing: preparing people for change, 2nd edn. Guilford Press, New York

Miller W R Taylor C A 1980 Relative effectiveness of bibliotherapy, individual and group self-control training in the treatment of problem drinkers. Addictive Behaviours 5:13

Miller W, Westerberg V, Harris R, Tonigan J 1996 What predicts relapse? Prospective testing of antecedent models. Addiction 91(suppl): S155–S172

Miller W R, Wilbourne P L 2002 Mesa Grande: a methodological analysis of clinical trials for alcohol use disorders. Addiction 97:265–277

Ministerial Drugs Task Force 1994 Drugs in Scotland: meeting the challenge. HMSO, London

Mitchison M, Hartnoll R 1980 Evaluation of heroin in a maintenance controlled trial. Archives of General Psychiatry 37:877

Morgenstern J, Langenbucher J, Labouvie E W 1994 The generalizability of the dependence syndrome across substances: an examination of some properties of the proposed DSM-IV dependence criteria. Addiction 89(9):1105–1113

Morse A C, Erwin V G, Jones B C 1995 Pharmacogenetics of cocaine: a critical review. Pharmacogenetics 5(4):183–192

Moyer A, Finney J W, Swearingen C E, Vergun P 2002 Brief interventions for alcohol problems: a meta-analytic review of controlled investigations in treatment-seeking and non-treatment seeking populations. Addiction 97:279–292

Nakamura H, Overall J, Hollister L, Radcliffe E 1983 Factors affecting outcome of depressive symptoms in alcoholics. Alcoholism: Clinical and Experimental Research 7:188–193

National Centre for Social Research 2001 Smoking, drinking & drug use among young people in Scotland in 2000. Department of Health, TSO, London

National Treatment Outcome Research Study 1996 Summary of the project, the clients and preliminary findings. Department of Health, HMSO, London

National Treatment Outcome Research Study 2001 NTORS after 5 years. Department of Health, TSO, London

Neeleman J, Farrell M 1997 Suicide and substance misuse. British Journal of Psychiatry 171:303–304

Nigam R, Schottenfeld R, Kosten T R 1992 Treatment of dual diagnosis patients: a relapse prevention group approach. Journal of Substance Abuse Treatment 9(4):305–309

Nutt D J 1996 Addiction: brain mechanisms and their implications for treatment. Lancet 347:31–36

Nutt D J 1999 Alcohol and the brain. Pharmacological insights for psychiatrists. British Journal of Psychiatry 175:114–119

O'Farrell T F 2001 Family-involved alcoholism treatment: an update. Recent Developments in Alcoholism 15:329–356

Ojesjo 1981 Long-term outcome in alcohol abuse and alcoholism among males in the Lundby general population British Journal of Addiction 76:391–400

O'Malley S S, Jaffe A J, Chang G 1992 Naltrexone and coping skills therapy for alcohol dependence. Archives of General Psychiatry 49:881–887

Oppenheimer E, Tobutt C, Taylor C, Andrew T 1994 Death and survival in a cohort of heroin addicts from London clinics : a 22 year follow-up study. Addiction 89:1299–1308

Oxford J, Edwards G 1977 Alcoholism. Oxford University Press, Oxford

Petry N M Bickel W K Badger G J 2001 Examining the limits of the buprenorphine interdosing interval: daily, every-third-day, and every-fifth-day dosing regimens. Addiction 96(6):823–834

Pihl R, Paterson J, Finn P 1990 Inherited pre-disposition to alcoholism: characteristics of the sons of male alcoholics. Journal of Abnormal Psychology 99:271–301

Plant M 1987 Women drinking and pregnancy. Tavistock, London

Plant M A, Peck D F, Samuel E 1985 Alcohol, drugs and school leavers. Tavistock, London

Plant M A, Pirie F, Kreitman N 1979 Evaluation of the Scottish Health Education Unit's 1976 campaign on alcoholism. Social Psychiatry 14:11

Poikalainen K 1999 Effectiveness of brief interventions to reduce alcohol intake in primary health care populations: a meta analysis. Preventative Medicine 28:503–509

Polich J M, Armor D J, Braiker H 1981 The course of alcoholism four years after the treatment. Wiley, New York

Powell J, Dawe S, Richards D 1993 Can opiate addicts tell us about their relapse risk? Subjective predictors of clinical prognosis. Addictive Behaviors 18(4):473–490

Prochaska J Di Clemente C 1992 Stages of change in the modification of problem behaviours. In: Hersen M, Eisler R, Miller P (eds) Progress in behaviour modification, vol 28 Sycamore Publications, Sycamore, Illinois

Project MATCH research group 1998 Matching alcoholism treatments to client heterogeneity: three year outcomes. Alcoholism Clinical and Experimental Research 22:1300–1311

Raistrick D, Hodgson R, Ritson B 1999 Tackling alcohol together. Free Association Books, London

Ramsay M, Partridge S 2001 Drug misuse declared in 2000: results from the British Crime Survey. Home Office Research Development & Statistics Directorate, London

Ritson B 1995 Community and municipal action on alcohol. WHO Euro No 63 Copenhagen

Roberts L J, Shaner A, Eckman T A et al 1992 Effectively treating stimulant-abusing schizophrenics: mission impossible? New Directions for Mental Health Services 53:55–65

Robertson M, Bell J 1993 Are rapid inpatient benzodiazepine detoxifications unsafe? Medical Journal of Australia 158(8):578–579

Robichaud C, Strickler D, Bigelow G, Liebson I 1979 Disulfiram maintenance alcoholism treatment: a 3-phase evaluation. Behaviour Research and Therapy 17:618–621

Robinson D 1979 Talking out of alcoholism: the self help process of Alcoholics Anonymous. Croom Helm, London

Romelsjo A, Lazarus N B, Kaplan G A, Cohen R D 1991 The relationship between stressful life situations and changes in alcohol consumption. British Journal of Addiction 86:157–169

Room R, Bondy A, Ferris J 1995 The risk of harm to oneself from drinking, Canada 1989. Addiction 90:499–513

Rose G, Day S 1990 The population mean predicts the number of deviant individuals. British Medical Journal 301:1031–1034

Rounsaville B J, Bryant K, Babor T et al 1993 Cross system agreement for substance use disorders: DSM-III-R, DSM-IV and ICD-10. Addiction 88(3):337–348

Royal College of Physicians 1987 A great and growing evil. Tavistock, London

Royal College of Physicians, Royal College of Psychiatrists, Royal College of General Practitioners 1995 Alcohol and the heart in perspective, London

Royal College of Psychiatrists 1986 Alcohol our favourite drug. Tavistock, London

Russell M A H, Wilson C, Taylor C, Baker C D 1979 Effect of general practitioners' advice against smoking. British Medical Journal 2:231

Sanguineti V R Samuel S E 1993 Comorbid substance abuse and recovery from acute psychiatric relapse. Hospital & Community Psychiatry 44(11):1073–1076

Saunders J B, Walters J R F, Davies P, Paton A 1981 A 20-year prospective study of cirrhosis. British Medical Journal 282:263–266

Schubiner H, Tzelepis A, Isaacson J H et al 1995 The dual diagnosis of attention-deficit/hyperactivity disorder and substance abuse: case reports and literature review. Journal of Clinical Psychiatry 56(4):146–150

Schuckit M A 1986 The genetic and clinical implication of alcoholism and affective disorder. American Journal of Psychiatry 143:140–146

Schuckit M A 1994 The treatment of stimulant dependence. Addiction 89(11):1559–1563

Schuckit M A, Irwin M 1989 An analysis of the clinical relevance of type 1 and type 2 alcoholics. British Journal of Addiction 84:869–876

Scottish Executive 2002 Plan for action on alcohol problems. Scottish Executive Health Department, Edinburgh w.w.w.scotland.gov.uk/health/alcohol problems

Shaper A G, Wannamethee G, Walker M 1988 Alcohol and mortality in British men: explaining the U-shaped curve. Lancet ii: 1267–1273

Shearer J, Wodak A, Mattick R P et al 2001 Pilot randomized controlled study of dexamphetamine substitution for amphetamine dependence. Addiction 96:1289–1296

Skog O J 1980 Liver cirrhosis epidemiology: some methodological problems. British Journal of Addiction 74:282–283

Smart R G, Mann R E 1991 Factors in recent reductions in liver cirrhosis deaths. Journal of Studies on Alcohol 52:232–240

Smith J, Hucker S 1994 Schizophrenia and substance abuse. British Journal of Psychiatry 165(1):13–21

Smith N T, 2002 A review of the published literature into cannabis withdrawal symptoms in human users. Addiction 97:621–632

Sokolski K N, Cummings J L, Abrams B I et al 1994 Effects of substance abuse on hallucination rates and treatment responses in chronic psychiatric patients. Journal of Clinical Psychiatry 55(9):380–387

Stevenson R 1994 Winning the war on drugs — to legalise or not. Paper 124, Institute of Economic Affairs, London

Stewart S H, Kushner M G 2001 Introduction to the Special Issue on "Anxiety Sensitivity and Addictive Behaviors". Addictive Behaviors 26(6):775–785

Stockwell T 1987 The Exeter home detoxification projects. In: Stockwell T, Cleriene S (eds) Helping the problem drinker. Croom Helm, London

Stockwell T, Hodgson R, Edwards G et al 1979 The development of a questionnaire to measure severity of alcohol dependence. British Journal of Addiction 73:79–87

Strang J, Griffiths P, Powis B, Gossop M 1992 First use of heroin: changes in route of administration over time. British Medical Journal 304:1222–1223

Strang J, Black J, Marsh A, Smith B 1993 Hair analysis for drugs: technological breakthrough or ethical quagmire. Addiction 88:163–166. Comments in Addiction 1994 89:295–300

Strang J, Griffiths P, Abbey J, Gossop M 1994 Survey of use of injected benzodiazepines among drug users in Britain. British Medical Journal 308:1082

Strang J, Sheridan J, Barber N 1996a Prescribing injectable and oral methadone to opiate addicts: results from the 1995 national postal survey of community pharmacies in England and Wales. British Medical Journal 313:270–272

Strang J, Darke S, Hall W, Ali R 1996b Heroin overdose: the case for take-home naloxone. British Medical Journal 313:1435

Strang J, Marsden J, Cummins M et al 2000 Randomized trial of supervised injectable versus oral methadone maintenance: report on feasibility and six-month outcome. Addiction 95:1631–1646

Strassman R J 1995 Hallucinogenic drugs in psychiatric research and treatment: perspectives and prospects. Journal of Nervous & Mental Disease 183(3):127–138

Straw J 1996 Breaking the vicious cycle: Labour's proposals to tackling drug-related crime. Labour Party, London

Substance Abuse Committee of the Mental Health Foundation 1992 Guidelines for the prevention or treatment of benzodiazepine dependence. The Mental Health Foundation, London

Surendrakumar D, Dunn M, Roberts C 1992 Hospital admission and the start of benzodiazepine use. British Medical Journal. 304:881

Tarter R E, Hegedus A M, Goldstein G et al 1984 Adolescent sons of alcoholics: neuropsychological and personality characteristics. Alcoholism: Clinical and Experimental Research 8:216

Task Force to Review Services for Drug Misusers 1996 Report of an independent review of drug treatment services in England. Department of Health, HMSO, London

Thomas H 1993 Psychiatric symptoms in cannabis users. British Journal of Psychiatry 163:141–149

Thomson A D 2000 Mechanisms of vitamin deficiency in chronic alcohol misuers and the development of the Wernicke-Korsakoff syndrome. Alcohol & Alcoholism supplement 35 (suppl 1): 2–7

Tsuang J W, Irwin M R, Smith T L, Schukit M A 1994 Characterstics of men with alcoholic hallucinosis. Addiction 89:73–78

U S Department of Health and Human Services 1990 Alcohol and health. DHHS, Rockville, Md

Vaillant G E 1995 The natural history of alcoholism revisited. Harvard University Press, Cambridge, Mass

Victor M 1962 Alcoholism. In: Baker A B (ed) Clinical neurology, vol 2. Hoeber-Harper, New York

Victor M, Hope J M 1958 The phenomenon of auditory hallucinations in chronic alcoholism. Journal of Nervous & Mental Disease 126:451–481

Wallace P, Cutler S, Haines A 1988 Randomised controlled trial of general practitioners in patients with excessive alcohol consumption. British Medical Journal 297:663–668

Wallack L, Dorfman L, Jernigan D, Themba M 1993 Media advocacy and public health: power for prevention. Newbury Park, Sage

Waller S, Naidoo B, Thom B 2002 Prevention and reduction of alcohol misuse: evidence briefing. Health Development Agency, London

Walton M A, Castro F G, Barrington E H 1994 The role of attributions in abstinence, lapse, and relapse following substance abuse treatment. Addictive Behaviors 19(3):319–331

Ward J, Mattrick R, Hall W 1992 Key issues in methadone maintenance treatment. New South Wales University Press, New South Wales, Australia

Ward J, Mattrick R, Hall W 1998 Methadone maintenance treatment and other opioid replacement therapies. Harwood, Australia

Washton A M, Potash A, Gold M 1984 Naltrexone in addictive business executives and physicians. Journal of Clinical Psychiatry 45:39–41

Weaver T, Renton A, Stimson G, Tyrer P 1999 Severe mental illness and substance misuse. British Medical Journal 318:137–138

West R 2001 Theories of addiction. Addiction 96 (1): 3–14

Whitworth A B, Fischer F, Lesch O et al 1996 Comparison of Acamprosate and placebo in long-term treatment of alcohol dependence. Lancet 347:1438–1442

Williams R, Cohen J 2000 Substance use and misuse in psychiatric wards. Psychiatric Bulletin 24:43–46

Wolfe W L, Maisto S A 2000 The relationship between eating disorders and substance use: moving beyond co-prevalence research. Clinical Psychology Review 20(5):617–631

Woody G E, Cottler L B, Cacciola J 1993 Severity of dependence: data from the DSM-IV field trials. Addiction 88(11):1573–1579

Wright J D, Pearl L 2000 Knowledge and experience of young people regarding illicit drug use 1969–1999 Addiction 95(8):1225–1235

Young R M, Oei T P S, Knight R G 1990 The tension reduction hypothesis revisited: an alcohol expectancy perspective. British Journal of Addiction 85:31

Zador D 2001 Injectable opiate maintenance in the UK: is it good clinical practice? Addiction 96:547–553

19 | Schizophrenia and related disorders

Stephen M Lawrie, Eve C Johnstone

Schizophrenia is the heartland of psychiatry and the core of its clinical practice. Every layman knows that the term means 'split mind', and his concept of madness is largely based on the oddities and abnormalities of those who suffer from this enigmatic illness. Because it is a relatively common condition, which often cripples people in adolescence or early adult life, without greatly reducing their life expectancy, it has been described as the worst disease affecting mankind. It probably causes more suffering and distress and blights more lives than any cancer, and certainly represents a major burden for carers, health services and society as a whole. About 25 years ago, when most patients were hospitalised for most of their lives, schizophrenia was the single most expensive illness for the UK National Health Service to manage, and in the USA all costs were estimated as 2% of the gross national product. Recent figures suggest the total societal costs are in excess of £2.6 billion per year for England alone.

HISTORICAL INTRODUCTION

Although brief descriptions of an illness with some resemblance to schizophrenia are to be found in the Hindu Ayurveda as long ago as 1400 BC, and in the writings of the Cappadocian physician Aretaeus in the 2nd century AD, recognisable descriptions of schizophrenia are considerably less common, in historical medical texts or literature generally, than those of melancholia or mania. The earliest unambiguous descriptions date only from the end of the 18th century, and it was a further hundred years before the syndrome was defined with any clarity.

That crucial step was achieved by Emil Kraepelin, professor of psychiatry at the University of Munich, in the fifth (1896) edition of his *Psychiatrie, ein Lehrbuch für Studierende und Ärzte*. Throughout the 19th century, psychiatrists had struggled, with scant success, to develop a satisfactory classification of insanity. In 1856 Morel had coined the term *démence précoce* to describe an adolescent patient, once bright and active, who had slowly lapsed into a state of silent withdrawal. In 1868 Kahlbaum had described the syndrome of *Katatonie*, and 3 years later Hecker had described *Hebephrenie*. But it was Kraepelin who first succeeded in going beyond straightforward clinical description, by his division of the myriad and shifting forms of insanity into two main groupings on the basis of their symptoms and long-term course. The first, which he called manic–depressive insanity, pursued a fluctuating course with frequent relapses but full recovery after each. The second, for which he used Morel's term dementia praecox, embraced Kahlbaum's catatonia, Hecker's hebephrenia and his own dementia paranoides, was a progressive disease which either pursued a steady downhill course to chronic invalidism or, if improvement did occur, resulted only in partial recovery. Initially, Kraepelin was criticised for introducing yet another classification without any aetiological or pathological basis, but it was not long before the force and utility of his unifying concepts impressed themselves on his contemporaries and they started to come into general use.

In 1911, however, while acceptance of this new classification was still incomplete, the Swiss psychiatrist Eugen Bleuler published his *Dementia Praecox or the Group of Schizophrenias*, which was to be at least as influential as Kraepelin's *Lehrbuch*. Although Bleuler regarded himself as confirming and developing Kraepelin's concept of dementia praecox, in fact he changed it fundamentally, and it was his term *schizophrenia* which eventually won universal adoption. Kraepelin had assumed, in the tradition of Griesinger and other German academic psychiatrists, that dementia praecox was a disease of the brain. Bleuler, influenced by the writings of Sigmund Freud and the infant school of psychoanalysis, coined the term schizophrenia, meaning 'split mind', because he believed that the disorder was due to a 'loosening of associations' between different psychic functions, affecting both the transition from one idea to the next in thought and speech and the co-ordination between emotional, volitional (conative) and intellectual (cognitive) processes in general. He also drew a distinction between his 'four As' (see Box 19.1), which he regarded as the 'fundamental symptoms', and the more obvious hallucinations, delusions and catatonic phenomena which for him were accessory phenomena of less importance. This led him to conclude that schizophrenia could develop and be diagnosed in the absence of hallucinations and delusions, and so to add a fourth type, simple schizophrenia, to the hebephrenic, catatonic and paranoid forms recognised by Kraepelin.

Although Bleuler's term 'schizophrenia' eventually displaced Kraepelin's 'dementia praecox', and his assumptions about the nature of the disorder became very influential, particularly in the USA, Kraepelin's original concept remained dominant in many European centres. This failure to resolve the incompatibility of the Kraepelinian and Bleulerian approaches, together with the inherent ambiguities of each, resulted in considerable confusion and seriously hindered fruitful research for the next half century.

The crucial characteristic of Kraepelin's dementia praecox — what distinguished it from manic–depressive insanity — was its prognosis. The illness progressed to a state of permanent impairment, and any recovery was either temporary or incomplete. However, it was soon recognised that some patients with the typical clinical characteristics of the condition did recover, and remained well indefinitely without any detectable defect.

Kraepelin himself eventually accepted that this occurred in 13% of his own cases. Unfortunately, the implications of this were never properly faced. Kraepelin and most of his contemporaries had assumed that dementia praecox was a 'disease entity' with its own characteristic symptomatology, aetiology, pathology and course. But the aetiology and neuropathology remained a mystery, and here was evidence that the course was variable and inconstant. Understandably, the predominant reaction to this quandary was to assume that this variable prognosis was an artefact, occurring because patients with a superficially similar psychosis of good prognosis were being confused with those suffering from real dementia praecox/schizophrenia. Determined efforts were therefore made to distinguish the two.

In Europe, the Norwegian psychiatrist Langfeldt sought to distinguish between schizophrenia and what he called 'schizophreniform psychosis' on the basis of a detailed study of the symptomatology of the illness. He presented evidence to suggest that the two had quite different outcomes, and that electroconvulsive therapy (ECT) and insulin coma therapy were ineffective in schizophrenia itself (Langfeldt 1960). Although his methodology had clear limitations, his claim was initially widely accepted because it was so welcome. In the USA, similar efforts were made by clinical psychologists, and a series of rating scales — the Elgin, Phillips and Kantor Scales — were developed to discriminate between what they called *process* and *non-process* schizophrenia, mainly on the basis of the premorbid personality and psychosexual adjustment. Both Langfeldt and these American workers assumed that true process schizophrenia was endogenous and hereditary, and that schizophreniform or non-process ('reactive') psychoses were psychogenic, but neither succeeded in demonstrating a clear demarcation between the two.

The principal problem with Bleuler's concept of schizophrenia was its lack of clear boundaries. Although he provided little empirical evidence to justify his belief that his 'fundamental symptoms' were indeed fundamental, his assumptions were widely accepted, particularly in the USA, and as a result the diagnosis of schizophrenia came to be based on the presence of one or more of the so-called 'four As' (Box 19.1), whether or not the patient was psychotic. Unfortunately, all four of these phenomena are intangible qualities which can be detected in most psychiatric patients and in some healthy people, particularly when under stress. Their use as diagnostic criteria therefore led to a marked expansion of the concept of schizophrenia, to the point at which it was degenerating into a vague synonym for severe (and sometimes not so severe) mental illness. Indeed, in the 1950s USA, patients were diagnosed as having schizophrenia without having any characteristic features at all. An example of this diagnostic practice is the concept of 'pseudoneurotic schizophrenia' (Hoch & Polatin 1949), where patients had a wide range of neurotic symptoms, such as phobias, obsessions and depersonalisation, often associated with severe anxiety and attacks of psychotic disturbance lasting days, hours or perhaps only minutes.

Between 1920 and 1960 the confusion increased steadily. With the partial exception of French psychiatry, which pursed its own traditions untroubled by outside influences, the term 'schizophrenia' was used throughout the world, but in a bewildering variety of different ways which were rarely made explicit. Some authorities, like Kleist and Leonhard in Germany and Langfeldt in Norway, insisted that the term should be restricted to illnesses resulting in permanent damage to the personality; others were prepared to use it freely regardless of outcome. Some psychiatrists would only make the diagnosis in adolescents or young adults; others were willing to do so at any age. Some insisted on the presence of certain key symptoms; others were prepared to make a confident diagnosis on the basis of indefinable subjective impressions, the so-called 'praecox feeling'. In the USA Bleuler's views predominated, largely because his concept of schizophrenia as a psychological, and possibly psychogenic, disorder was readily compatible with the prevailing psychoanalytic orientation. The overuse of the term was therefore most marked in that country. In most of Europe, on the other hand, Kraepelin's concepts still held sway. In most of the German-speaking world schizophrenia was regarded as an endogenous and hereditary psychosis and the diagnosis was restricted to patients exhibiting certain cardinal symptoms, mainly hallucinations and delusions of particular kinds. Kleist and Leonhard developed very detailed classifications of different forms of schizophrenia, mainly on the basis of a meticulous study of the chronic stage of the illness.

Of greater influence, however, were the teachings of Kurt Schneider, who focused attention on the earlier acute stage of the illness and described a number of 'symptoms of the first rank' (Box 19.2) which he considered to be diagnostic of schizophrenia in the absence of overt brain disease (Schneider 1959). Many of these hallucinations and delusions can be interpreted as the result

---

Box 19.1   Bleuler's fundamental symptoms ('the four As')

- Loosening of Associations (thought disorder)
- Blunt or incongruous Affect
- Autism (social withdrawal)
- Ambivalence (apathy)

Box 19.2   Kurt Schneider's 'symptoms of the first rank'

1. Auditory hallucinations taking any one of three specific forms:
   a. Voices repeating the subject's thoughts out loud (Gedankenlautwerden or écho de la pensée), or anticipating his thoughts
   b. Two or more hallucinatory voices discussing the subject, or arguing about him, referring to him in the third person
   c. Voices commenting on the subject's thoughts or behaviour, often as a running commentary
2. The sensation of alien thoughts being put into the subject's mind by some external agency, or of his own thoughts being taken away (thought insertion or withdrawal)
3. The sensation that the subject's thinking is no longer confined within his own mind, but is instead shared by, or accessible to, others (thought broadcasting)
4. The sensation of feelings, impulses or acts being experienced or carried out under external control, so that the patient feels as if he were being hypnotised, or had become a robot (passivity)
5. The experience of being a passive and reluctant recipient of bodily sensation imposed by some external agency (somatic passivity)
6. Delusional perception — a delusion arising fully-fledged on the basis of a genuine perception which others would regard as commonplace and unrelated

of a failure to distinguish between ideas and impulses arising in the patient's own mind and perceptions arising in the external world, a so-called 'loss of ego boundaries'. Schneider was less interested in the theoretical significance of these symptoms than in their practical utility, regarding them as convenient diagnostic aids that were pathognomonic of schizophrenia in the absence of brain disease. He accepted that some patients with otherwise typical schizophrenic illnesses never exhibited any of these symptoms, and that all of them could occur at times in epileptic and other organic psychoses, but he regarded them nonetheless as sufficiently characteristic to be worth distinguishing from what he called 'second rank' symptoms like perplexity, emotional blunting, and hallucinations and delusions of other kinds.

DEFINITIONS

The confusion caused by the unresolved differences between Kraepelin's and Bleuler's concepts of schizophrenia was at its worst in the 1950s, and the best known and most extensively studied differences were Anglo-American. Spurred by the observation that the first-admission rate for schizophrenia was considerably higher in the USA than in England and Wales, and that for manic–depressive illnesses the difference was the other way about, detailed studies were mounted of series of consecutive admissions to mental hospitals in the two countries, using identical interviewing methods and diagnostic criteria (Cooper et al 1972). These comparisons showed that the symptoms of patients admitted to public mental hospitals in New York and London were virtually identical, but the proportion of patients given a diagnosis of schizophrenia was nearly twice as high in New York as in London because the New York psychiatrists' concept of schizophrenia embraced many patients who in London would have been regarded as suffering from depressive or manic psychoses, or even from neurotic illnesses or personality disorders. Shortly after this the International Pilot Study of Schizophrenia confirmed that psychiatrists in Washington — and also, for rather different reasons, in Moscow — had a considerably broader concept of schizophrenia than their counterparts in the other seven countries involved, namely Colombia, Czechoslovakia, Denmark, India, Nigeria, Taiwan and the UK (WHO 1973).

Increasing awareness in the 1970s of the scale and consequences of international differences of this kind, and of the low reliability of psychiatric diagnoses generally, led to a widespread realisation that key terms like schizophrenia must be operationally defined in order to make it quite clear what criteria had to be satisfied to establish the diagnosis (see Ch. 14). Because schizophrenia, like most other psychiatric disorders, is still recognised by its syndrome and its aetiology is still obscure, it must be defined by the presence of particular symptoms or combinations of symptoms, or by its course, or by some combination of the two. In the last twenty years many different operational definitions of schizophrenia have been proposed, and this has inevitably led to comparisons of their relative merits. High reliability and a reasonable concordance with traditional usage are obviously important qualities, but not sufficient by themselves. What we are really trying to do when faced with a choice between alternative definitions is to decide which is likely to be more useful in predicting response to treatment or long-term course, or which is likely to correspond most closely with the putative biological abnormality underlying the disorder. Because the syndrome of schizophrenia appears to

merge into related syndromes, because we have not yet identified the underlying biological abnormality, and because political considerations are also involved, there is not yet any single agreed definition, nor any immediate prospect of a global consensus.

Areas of agreement are however increasing. Bleuler's fundamental symptoms, and thought disorder in particular, have lost their former influence, mainly because they are too intangible, and therefore incapable of being reliably identified. Schneider's first-rank symptoms are still influential in Britain and Germany, partly because their presence can be reliably rated, but several studies have demonstrated that they have little significance for long-term prognosis. The presence of first-rank symptoms in the acute illness does not predict either incomplete recovery or the development of a schizophrenic defect state (Kendell et al 1979), and it is not uncommon for these symptoms to develop in the course of what are in other respects typical, manic illnesses (Brockington et al 1980). In fact, none of the symptoms of the acute illness is as good a predictor of the long-term course as the duration and mode of onset. If the initial illness starts insidiously and lasts for several months, a poor long-term prognosis is much more likely than if it starts acutely in association with obvious stress and lasts only a few weeks, regardless of the detailed symptomatology.

There are now only two widely used definitions of schizophrenia — the American Psychiatric Association's DSM-IV (APA 1994) criteria and ICD-10 (WHO 1992) — and they are much more similar than previous versions (Table 19.1). They both require clear evidence of psychosis, currently or in the recent past, and specify particular kinds of hallucinatory experience or delusional ideation (among other possible symptoms). Both stipulate that affective symptoms must not be prominent. Indeed, the principal difference is in the minimum duration of illness, being 1 month for ICD-10 and 6 months for DSM-IV. DSM-IV is used for both clinical and research purposes in the USA. ICD-10 has both clinical and research criteria but the latter are rarely used, and DSM-IV is preferred by researchers worldwide. The more restrictive DSM-IV criteria have the merit of defining a group of patients with a poor long-term prognosis akin to Kraepelin's original dementia praecox, but diagnostic criteria for schizophrenia of less than 6 months duration are then required — even though such a 'schizophreniform disorder' may have limited validity.

It is, of course, very confusing for everyone, not least for students, to have alternative definitions of a single disorder, particularly when it is commonplace for a patient to fulfil one set of criteria but not another. Under present circumstances, however, this is inevitable; and it is better for differences of this kind to be overt than to be concealed and unsuspected. The existence of a number of definitions also helps to emphasise that all definitions are arbitrary, justified only by their usefulness, and liable to be altered or supplanted.

CLINICAL PRESENTATION AND SYMPTOMATOLOGY

It follows from what has been said above about the definition of schizophrenia that the symptoms and other characteristics of the condition will vary somewhat, according to the way in which the syndrome is defined. There is nonetheless a core group of patients who fulfil most definitions, and international comparisons using films or videotapes of diagnostic interviews confirm that

Table 19.1   A comparison of DSM-IV and ICD-10 diagnostic criteria

	DSM-IV	ICD-10
Symptoms	1 of: Bizarre delusions / Scheiderian hallucinations or 2 of: Delusions 　　　Hallucinations 　　　Disorganised speech/behaviour 　　　Negative features	1 of: Scheiderian delusions/hallucinations or 2 of: Catatonic behaviour 　　　Hallucinations 　　　Disorganised speech 　　　Negative features
Dysfunction	Social/occupational	Not specified
Duration	At least 6 months	One month
Exclusions	Mood disorder Substance abuse Pervasive developmental disorder	Mood disorder Substance abuse Organic brain disease

psychiatrists throughout the world will consistently identify these as people suffering from schizophrenia.

Premorbid characteristics

Personality

Schizophrenia can develop in personalities of all kinds, but some adults with schizophrenia were 'odd' as children. Observations in support of this view have been made since the time of Kraepelin, and the premorbid personality traits most often described are those of solitariness and coldness of affect. Some are noted to have been inclined to suspiciousness or to have abnormal speech patterns. These are often called schizoid/schizotypal traits. The relationship of such premorbid traits to the development of schizophrenia has not been easy to determine. In a review of early German studies of premorbid personality in schizophrenia, Cutting (1985) concluded that the schizoid trait complex was described in 25% of schizophrenic patients and other personality variants (e.g. paranoid) in a further 15%. Such retrospective data suggest the existence of unusual personality characteristics prior to the onset of schizophrenic illness but offer no information as to whether such traits occur more often in those destined to develop schizophrenia than in their peers who will remain well, and they do not allow us to determine whether the schizoid/schizotypal trait complex is a risk factor which contributes independently to the disease or is in fact a preclinical manifestation of the disorder itself.

Development

A number of prospective studies have addressed these issues in the past ten years. Done et al (1994) used data from the 1958 UK National Child Development Survey as this had included assessments of social behaviour at the ages of 7 and 11 years. Those who went on to develop schizophrenia in adult life were compared with those who developed other psychiatric disorders and those who remained well. At 7 and 11 years pre-schizophrenic boys showed significantly more anxiety, hostility and inconsequential behaviour than those who would remain well, and at 11 years pre-schizophrenic girls were significantly more withdrawn than those who did not become mentally ill. Those destined to develop affective psychosis in later life differed little from normal controls. Jones et al (1994) conducted a similar study using the 1946 British

National Survey of Health and Development and found delayed motor development, especially walking, as well as speech problems and preference for solitary play as early as the age of 4. Both studies found evidence of relatively low IQ, and all these findings have since been replicated in other countries. Clearly, therefore, many years before illness develops, there are significant excesses of abnormal neurodevelopment and social behaviour in children destined to develop schizophrenia in adult life. Nonetheless, by no means all who go on to develop schizophrenia have been considered to be abnormal in any way, and some have shown very high levels of social, academic and occupational functioning.

Prodromal symptoms

Quite what marks the transition from such abnormalities to psychotic symptoms and frank psychosis is largely unknown, but a number of prospective studies of individuals at high risk of developing schizophrenia have given us an insight into the timing of these events. McGhie & Chapman (1961) revisited the psychotherapy notes of 26 patients who were subsequently diagnosed with 'schizophrenia'. Subjective difficulties were recorded in focusing attention on pertinent rather than irrelevant stimuli (e.g. in someone else's speech) and thinking clearly, accompanied by relatively minor perceptual disturbances, anxiety and perplexity, and a reduced sense of control. Individual delusions or hallucinations may be evident several years before someone would meet diagnostic criteria for schizophrenia, but the bulk of the available evidence suggests that it is more common for anxiety, depression and negative symptoms to precede psychosis by 5 or even 10 years (see e.g. Miller et al 2001). These may gradually give way to delusional mood — the experience that something non-specific about the external world is unusual or even disturbing, and thence to frank hallucinations and delusions. Klosterkotter et al (2001) examined 160 outpatients with 'diagnostic problems' from 1987 to 1998, over which time 79 developed DSM-IV schizophrenia. Prodromal symptoms were sensitive predictors of psychosis, while individual delusions and hallucinations were more specific, but neither effect was sufficiently strong to be useful clinically. This is because, as an increasing number of studies demonstrate, 10–20% of the general population may experience individual psychotic symptoms at some point in their lives, especially as adolescents, but do not develop a psychotic illness (Verdoux & van Os 2002).

The acute illness

Onset

Schizophrenia can occur at any age from 7 to 70, but the onset is usually in adolescence or early adult life. Often it develops insidiously. A youth, whose previous behaviour has been unremarkable, slowly becomes more withdrawn and introverted. He may acquire a new interest in religion, psychology or the occult and drift away from his friends. He also loses his drive and determination and may fail to complete a university degree or an apprenticeship that had previously seemed well within his grasp. His parents may be worried by his failures, his apparent lack of interest in achievement and his progressive estrangement from them but they do not suspect that he is ill until one day, months or even years later, it suddenly becomes apparent that he is entertaining delusional ideas, or hearing voices. In other cases the onset is acute. Sometimes in the aftermath of some obvious stress, perhaps being spurned by a girlfriend or failing an exam, or while in the unfamiliar environment of a foreign country and possibly dabbling with drugs, the subject becomes obviously and sometimes floridly ill over the course of a few days. He becomes convinced that he is being watched or followed, may attach great significance to the colours of clothes or postage stamps, talk of Martians, laser beams or hypnosis, or suddenly be found, mute and inaccessible, kneeling on a floor.

Delusions

The delusions of the acute illness are very variable in type and even more so in their detailed content. Table 19.2 shows the frequency of the most common delusions and hallucinations, elicited by one of the authors using the Present State Examination (PSE), in large samples of first-episode and chronic patients. Delusions of reference and persecutory, grandiose, religious and hypochondriacal ideas of various kinds are all common but the most specifically characteristic of schizophrenia are a variety of *passivity phenomena*. The subject feels that he is no longer in control of his own thoughts, feelings or will and that he is being influenced or controlled by some mysterious, alien force. Thoughts which are not recognised as his own are put into his mind (*thought insertion*), or his own thoughts are taken away (*thought withdrawal*) or somehow have become accessible to other people (*thought broadcasting*). Or he may be convinced that someone is trying to hypnotise him or impose their will on his. The subject's interpretation of these phenomena, which lie beyond the bounds of normal experience, depends on his cultural background. Our forefathers attributed them to God or the Devil; some people from other cultures attribute them to spirits or witchcraft; and the inhabitants of modern industrial countries tend to attribute them to electricity, X-rays, television, laser beams and satellites. In short, the subject endeavours to make an unintelligible (primary) experience intelligible by (secondarily) attributing it to some powerful, invisible force with which he is conversant but does not fully understand.

Hallucinations

The hallucinations are equally varied and may involve any of the five senses (see Table 19.2). Auditory hallucinations in the form of voices are the most common, however, and the visual, olfactory, gustatory and tactile hallucinations are all uncommon in the absence of hallucinatory voices. Although Schneider and others have drawn attention to particular types of hallucinatory voices that are characteristic of schizophrenia (see Box 19.2), it is commonplace for schizophrenics to hear voices talking to them as well as about them, and the content is very variable. Indeed, from a diagnostic point of view the duration is probably more important than the detailed perceptual characteristics or the content, because hallucinatory voices rarely continue all day long, week after week, in other psychoses. Schizophrenic hallucinations frequently have a quality intermediate between that of a genuine auditory perception and a thought. Although the subject speaks spontaneously of a 'voice' he will often admit on questioning that he does not really hear it out loud or with his ears. It is in the mind, a 'silent voice', which is nonetheless insistent, troublesome and sometimes fright-

Table 19.2	Frequency of specific psychotic symptoms by stage of illness	
	First episodes (*n* = 242)	Chronic patients (*n* = 354)
Delusions		
Delusional mood	86%	25%
Delusions of reference	77%	60%
Delusions of misinterpretation	74%	52%
Delusions of persecution	70%	50%
Alien penetration	52%	–
Thoughts read	48%	–
Delusions of grandiose ability	40%	31%
Delusions of catastrophe	–	24%
Thought insertion	–	22%
Hallucinations		
2nd person hallucinations	48%	28%
Non-verbal auditory hallucinations	34%	15%
Other (tactile, gustatory)	36%	16%
3rd person hallucinations	32%	16%
Olfactory hallucinations	27%	13%
Visual hallucinations	23%	11%
From Johnstone et al (1986, 1991).		

ening. Often, too, the subject has difficulty describing what it says. Doubtless this is often due to embarrassment, or a reluctance to divulge what the subject suspects his questioner will regard as evidence of insanity, but it does sometimes seem that the patient has genuine difficulty in describing the content of the hallucination, perhaps because the normal link between perception and memory is only partly established.

Affect

The patient's affect during the acute illness is as variable as his thought content but is nearly always disturbed in some way. Perplexity is a common and characteristic feature of acute schizophrenic illnesses. The subject suspects that something strange is going on around him but is not sure what, and ideas may come and go in rapid succession as he seeks to integrate his changing perceptions and affective state with his premorbid experience (*delusional mood*). At other times the subject may be depressed, elated or angry, and it is sometimes difficult to tell whether the content of the delusions and hallucinatory voices is derived from the prevailing mood or vice versa. In more established cases a general flattening or blunting of affective responses often occurs. This term refers to a loss of the ability to feel, or at least to express, any deep or profound emotion, and a matching inability to evoke a sympathetic response in other people. (Technically, flattening refers to a reduced range of emotional expression and blunting to a reduced sensitivity to others, but the distinction is unclear and probably of little clinical relevance.) Incongruity of affect — that is a mismatch between the subject's emotional responses and the setting or the topic of conversation — silly giggling while important or distressing events are taking place being the most common example, may occur in both acute and more chronic states. Sometimes the patient knows that this is happening and may be able to explain that the emotion he expresses is quite different from that which he feels.

Behaviour

Finally, the patient's general behaviour is affected. Again, the nature of the change is variable but characteristically involves withdrawal from contact with and interest in other people, and actions which seem bizarre or inexplicable to the onlooker. Occasionally, the patient displays the particular behavioural abnormalities of Kahlbaum's catatonia, becoming mute, or stuporose, or adopting strange postures, sometimes for hours on end. Catatonic phenomena of this kind used to be common and figured prominently in Kraepelin's original descriptions of dementia praecox. These included: *automatic obedience* (a wooden, robotic response to all requests or commands, however silly or pointless); *negativism* (a similarly wooden response, but the opposite of that required by the request); and *waxy flexibility* (a curious disturbance of muscle tone in which the patient's limbs could be moved only slowly into new positions, but would then remain exactly as placed for minutes on end). Catatonic phenomena of this kind are rarely seen nowadays in acute states but continue to occur to some degree in chronic patients (Lund et al 1991). The reason why this should be so is a mystery, but it serves to emphasise that the clinical features of the illness are not inherent and predetermined but are partly the result of the subject's background and expectations. The behavioural abnormalities prior to first admission for schizophrenia were studied in over 250 cases (Johnstone et al 1986). In addition to

bizarre non-understandable behaviour such as that described, property damage or potentially threatening behaviour to the life of the patient, or indeed to that of others, occurred in at least 25% of patients.

The chronic stage

Sooner or later the hallucinations and delusions of the acute illness become less intense (see Table 19.2). Often they disappear completely, and if they do persist for months or years on end their influence on the patient's behaviour usually wanes. Unfortunately, this rarely indicates a recovery, even temporarily. Recovery is often complete after one or two short-lived episodes of illness, but the more episodes a patient has had, and the more insidiously developing and longer lasting these have been, the more likely it is that some residual damage will remain. This 'defect state' is much less conspicuous than the florid symptoms of the acute illness and may not be apparent at all to those who did not know the patient well before his illness. But in the long run it is a far more serious handicap. In its mildest form it involves nothing more than a subtle loss of vivacity, enthusiasm and emotional responsiveness. More commonly, however, the patient's drive and determination are affected. He becomes apathetic, no longer strives, and no longer cares. At the same time, and perhaps fundamentally for the same reason, he loses interest in other people. He talks much less ('poverty of speech'), and his capacity to form enduring emotional relationships is greatly reduced. He is no longer capable of falling in love or even developing new friendships, and if unmarried is likely to remain so. It is this apathy and emotional loss which make schizophrenia the terrible illness it is, because there are permanent changes in the personality which handicap the subject in every sphere — his ability to get and keep a job, to be an effective husband, wife or parent, to achieve anything, and even to fully enjoy anything.

Most patients with chronic schizophrenia have recurrent psychotic episodes with hallucinations and delusions, usually taking much the same form on each occasion, or faded remnants of earlier delusional systems, as well as this characteristic apathy and emotional blunting. Depression is also a common and important feature of chronic schizophrenia. Indeed, ICD-10 recognises post-schizophrenic depression as a distinct subtype of schizophrenia. Some patients become depressed in the immediate aftermath of their original psychotic episode, others make an apparently full recovery only to return weeks or months later with widespread depressive symptoms. It is sometimes suggested that this lowering of mood is induced by antipsychotics, but there is no convincing evidence from controlled trials that this is so. More likely, it is partly inherent to schizophrenia and partly an understandable psychological reaction to its dire effects and implications. Although the depression of chronic schizophrenia is rarely as severe, or accompanied by such a widespread disturbance of sleep, appetite and concentration as primary depressive disorders often are, it is nonetheless an important cause of suffering and disability. Furthermore it is often treatable (see below).

Suicide and homicide

Many schizophrenics, at least in the early stages of their illness, are well able to appreciate that it has deprived them of their capacity to enjoy or feel deeply about anything. Self-harm is common — 32% of a sample of 532 individuals with recurrent schizophrenia had harmed themselves at least once (Johnstone et al 1991), and some 10% die by suicide, usually in the early years of the illness and often around the time of admission or discharge. Homicide, despite all the media attention it generates, is rare. Patients with schizophrenia do have an increased rate of violent and non-violent crime, but any member of the public is far more likely to be attacked by a member of their own family, and if one is assaulted by a stranger he is more likely to be well than mentally ill (Walsh et al 2001).

Symptoms or syndromes?

Hughlings Jackson, a 19th-century neurologist, used to distinguish between positive and negative symptoms in neurological diseases — the former being based on some active disturbance of cerebral function, the latter reflecting a reduction or loss of normal function. Crow (1980) developed these concepts in relation to schizophrenia by proposing that there are two pathological processes in the disorder that can occur separately or together in an individual case. Crow's type I syndrome was characterised by positive symptoms (delusions, hallucinations and thought disorder) and thought to be acute, while the type II syndrome was characterised by negative symptoms (affective flattening, apathy and poverty of speech) and chronic. Problems with this formulation included the question of whether the important factor was the type of symptomatology or the chronicity, and the issue of whether thought disorder should be considered as a positive or a negative symptom. Liddle (1987) then developed these issues further by examining the pattern of correlation between schizophrenic symptoms in a group of patients with illnesses of similar chronicity and found that the symptoms segregated into not two but three distinguishable syndromes:

- *psychomotor poverty* (poverty of speech, flat affect, decreased spontaneous movement);
- *disorganisation* (disorder of form of thought and inappropriate affect);
- *reality distortion* (delusions and hallucinations).

This pattern of segregation into three syndromes has been replicated in many other studies employing factor analysis of schizophrenic symptoms, including patients with illnesses of variable chronicity, although a lot of the variance in symptom aggregations is not explained in such studies and additional, possibly developmental, factors need to be considered (Smith et al 1998). This work has, however, been developed by neuropsychological studies, which show that each syndrome is characterised by a specific pattern of test performance (see Frith 1992 and below), and by studies of regional cerebral blood flow using position emission tomography (Liddle et al 1992) which show that the different syndromes are associated with altered perfusion in different sites in the brain.

A note on thought disorder

Thought disorder is a characteristic feature of schizophrenia. It is, however, an unsatisfactory term that has traditionally been applied to a variety of ill-defined abnormalities of the subject's speech and writing which are assumed — and it is an assumption — to be secondary to a more fundamental disturbance of thinking. (The term 'formal thought disorder' is sometimes used to emphasise that it is an abnormality of the form rather than of the content of speech, i.e. thought disorder does not embrace delusional ideation.) These abnormalities were first noted by Hecker in 1871 ('a peculiar departure from normal logical sentence structure, with frequent changes in direction that may or may not lose the train of thought'), and then by Kraepelin, but they were studied and described in much more detail by Bleuler who regarded them as a direct consequence of the 'loosening of associations' which he thought was the fundamental deficit of schizophrenia. It is therefore to Bleuler that we owe the long-lived assumption that thought disorder was of cardinal importance, aetiologically and diagnostically, being exhibited by all schizophrenics and by no one else. These were unfortunate assumptions for several reasons. No one has ever succeeded in producing a satisfactory definition of the term thought disorder, or in identifying any fundamental psychological or linguistic deficit capable of accounting for the various observable abnormalities of schizophrenic speech. Worse still, few of the abnormalities Bleuler and his successors identified have proved to be specific to schizophrenia, and none to be manifested by more than a proportion of patients with what in other respects are typical schizophrenic illnesses. Indeed, large studies of the symptomatology of schizophrenia (for example, Johnstone et al 1991) show them to be rare in comparison to delusions and hallucinations.

The most obvious abnormality in the early stages of the illness is the subject's inability to give a straight answer to any but the simplest of questions, so that the interviewer suddenly realises, after talking to his patient for 5 or 10 minutes, that he has not yet learned anything useful. Usually none of the patient's statements or replies has been obviously nonsensical or bizarre, but almost every one has been vague or irrelevant, and as a result little useful information has been transmitted. This abnormality is sometimes referred to as 'poverty of thought content'.

It is sometimes said that thought disorder involves the semantic content rather than the syntactic structure of speech and that the latter remains intact until a very late stage. This is not so. It has been demonstrated by detailed linguistic analysis that the syntactic structure of schizophrenics' speech is quite different from both that of manic and of normal controls (Morice & Ingram 1982), and also that these abnormalities progress with the passage of time. Schizophrenic speech may be harder to comprehend in the acute illness, partly because the patient is often excited and preoccupied with delusional ideas, but its structure is more abnormal in the chronic stage. Sentence structure becomes more primitive, with fewer and less deeply embedded subordinate clauses, and grammatical errors of varied kinds become more frequent. Above all, the total quantity of speech is reduced ('poverty of speech').

Bleuler and Kretschmer regarded thought disorder as a result of a generalised 'dissociation' of psychic functions. Subsequently, Babcock suggested that it was simply due to a slowing of all intellectual processes, but later work showed that, although schizophrenics were indeed slower than normals, so too were depressives and psychotics in general. In the 1940s Cameron suggested that 'over-inclusiveness' was the fundamental disability, by which he meant an inability to maintain conceptual boundaries because of a failure to exclude irrelevant associations. This has some empirical support from object sorting tests, and has interesting parallels with the psychophysiological evidence (and subjective accounts) that schizophrenics have difficulty discriminating between relevant and irrelevant sensory information. Both, in other words, might be due to the breakdown of some hypothetical filtering or attentional focusing mechanism. In the 1960s it was claimed, though never confirmed, that schizophrenic speech tended to be less 'redundant' (more 'condensed') than normal speech, so that, if every fourth or fifth word was deleted (the Cloze technique), naive readers were less successful at guessing the identity of the missing words. It is established, however, that schizophrenics tend to use a more restricted range of words, and hence to have a lower 'type:token ratio' than normal people, and that this tendency to repetition applies to syllables as well as to words and phrases, indicating that the cause is something more fundamental than simply having a limited vocabulary. It has also been shown that, in terms of Kelly's personal construct theory, schizophrenics' constructs are less stable and more idiosyncratic than those of other people.

Unfortunately, none of these observations has yet proved to be of much practical use, and none of these various hypotheses has illuminated the fundamental nature of thought disorder. Andreasen (1979) attempted to define 20 of the terms most widely used to describe different facets of thought disorder, including derailment, tangentiality, clanging and illogicality (see Box 19.3). She succeeded in demonstrating that most of these terms can be defined and rated with reasonable reliability, and showed which were relatively specific to schizophrenia and which equally or more common in mania. She also suggested replacing the term thought disorder with the less ambiguous but more cumbersome phrase 'disorders of thought, language and communication'. These are valuable achievements, but a more radical approach is needed. Seventy years of research into thought disorder has achieved little, not because Bleuler was wrong in believing that there was something very odd about the speech of many schizophrenics, but because that research was conducted, often without adequate controls, by psychiatrists and psychologists who knew nothing of linguistics. It remains to be seen whether modern linguistic analysis will be any more successful, but future research is more likely to illuminate the fundamental nature of thought disorder if it is based on linguistic concepts like cohesion, lexical density and dysfluency rather than on ancient clinical metaphors like derailment.

Varieties of schizophrenia

Kraepelin recognised three varieties of schizophrenia — hebephrenic, catatonic and paranoid — and Bleuler added a fourth — simple schizophrenia. Bleuler also said that, although he assumed schizophrenia to be a group of allied conditions rather than a single disease, he regarded these subdivisions as purely provisional, like a classification of tuberculosis into cases with and without haemoptysis, or with and without amyloidosis. It is ironical, therefore, that his four varieties have figured in most classifications of schizophrenia ever since. Although several additional varieties have often been added, no schema which attempted to supplant them has ever won more than local acceptance. The expansion of the concept of schizophrenia which took place in the 1940s and 1950s was partly due to the emergence of a series of new concepts, like residual schizophrenia, latent schizophrenia, schizoaffective psychosis (Kasanin 1933), which were added to the original four and had the effect of bringing new types of patients under the schizophrenic rubric.

The new (10th) revision of the ICD (WHO 1992) recognises seven varieties: Bleuler's original four (paranoid, hebephrenic, catatonic and simple) plus undifferentiated schizophrenia, residual schizophrenia and post-schizophrenic depression. Schizoaffective states are classified separately from both schizophrenic and affective disorders. Schizotypal disorder, 'a disorder characterised by eccentric behaviour and anomalies of thinking and affect which resemble those seen in schizophrenia, though no definite and characteristic schizophrenic anomalies have occurred at any stage', is now included. Although schizotypal disorder does sometimes evolve into overt schizophrenia, it is usually a stable and enduring personality disorder which is relatively common in the close relatives of schizophrenics and assumed to be part of the genetic 'spectrum' of schizophrenia (Kendler et al 1991).

In day-to-day clinical practice most psychiatrists content themselves with a plain diagnosis of schizophrenia and only use the subcategories for the minority of patients whose symptomatology corresponds closely to one of the subcategory stereotypes (see Box 19.4). Although the hebephrenic and catatonic forms tend to have the worst prognosis and the paranoid form the best, there are no consistent differences in response to treatment or prognosis between the various categories, and patients may show the characteristic symptoms of different varieties at different stages in their careers. Nor is there convincing evidence from family studies that the different varieties 'breed true'. Partly for these reasons, contemporary interest is focused primarily on how schizophrenia should best be defined rather than on how it should be subdivided. The current American classification, DSM-IV (APA 1994), for example, recognises only five varieties — disorganised (hebephrenic), catatonic, paranoid, undifferentiated and residual — and emphasises that the distinction between them is based only on 'the predominant clinical picture that occasioned the most recent evaluation or admission to clinical care' and may therefore change over time.

Box 19.3   **Examples of types of thought disorder**
• Derailment — spontaneous speech in which ideas slip off track (cf. flight of ideas in pressured speech)
• Tangentiality — replying to a question in an oblique or irrelevant manner
• Incoherence — incomprehensible speech ('word salad') due to misuse of grammar or syntax and/or missing or substituted words
• Illogicality — false conclusions based on faulty premises or inductive inferences
• Clanging — word sounds rather than meaning appear to govern use
From Andreasen (1979).

Box 19.4   **Subtypes of schizophrenia**
• Hebephrenic — the illness starts early and insidiously and is dominated by thought disorder and disturbance of affect
• Catatonic — motor abnormalities like posturing or stupor are present
• Paranoid — hallucinations and delusions are prominent and the personality relatively well preserved
• Simple — progressive deterioration and increasing eccentricity develop in the absence of overt psychotic symptoms
• Residual — the original psychotic symptoms have died away, leaving only the apathy, emotional blunting and eccentricity of the defect state

EPIDEMIOLOGY

Frequency

In most of the industrial countries in which population surveys have been carried out the lifetime risk of schizophrenia is about 1%, with an incidence of approximately 15 new cases per 100 000 population per annum and a prevalence of 2–4 per 1000. In the American Epidemiologic Catchment Area (ECA) survey, for example, which was based on over 18 000 interviews with random population samples, the lifetime risk for schizophrenia using DSM-III criteria was 1.3% (Regier et al 1988). Studies in Africa and Asia are less numerous and have tended to produce somewhat lower estimates. The International Pilot Study of Schizophrenia established that substantial numbers of schizophrenics were admitted to psychiatric hospitals in all the countries involved (Colombia, Czechoslovakia, Denmark, India, Nigeria, Russia, Taiwan, the UK and the USA) and that their symptoms were remarkably similar in all nine, despite major differences in language, religion, culture and degree of urbanisation (WHO 1973).

The main findings of an even larger cross-cultural comparison by the World Health Organization, based on nearly 1400 patients from 12 centres in 10 countries, have also been reported (Sartorius et al 1986). This study attempted to identify all schizophrenics making a first contact with any treatment agency, including religious institutions and traditional healers, within a defined geographical area, and so was able to generate incidence or inception rates. Although affective symptoms (mainly depressive) were more common in the industrial countries, and visual and auditory hallucinations and catatonic symptoms more common in the developing countries, the core symptoms of schizophrenia were again remarkably similar in all centres. So too were the inception rates, and also the reasons for admission or referral. When the same operational definition (PSE Catego class S+, which effectively identifies patients with Schneiderian first-rank symptoms) was applied in all centres the inception rate ranged only from 7 per 100 000 population per year in Aarhus (Denmark) to 14 in Nottingham, with both the urban and rural areas in Chandigarh (India), Dublin, Honolulu, Moscow and Nagasaki in between. This strongly suggests that the incidence of schizophrenia is fairly stable across a wide range of cultures, climates and ethnic groupings. There appears to be far less variation in the incidence of schizophrenia than for most other common diseases, apart from mental handicap and epilepsy.

Changing incidence? It used to be thought, mainly on the strength of historical studies, that the incidence of schizophrenia had not changed since the first decades of the 19th century despite the profound social and cultural changes that have taken place since that time. Hare (1988) marshalled a mass of historical data to suggest that schizophrenia either arose de novo, or at least became much more common, towards the end of the 18th century, and that its prevalence increased steadily for the next 100 years. This view has however not found widespread support, although it is generally accepted that the presentation of the illness has changed, at least in Europe and North America, since the beginning of the 20th century. The hebephrenic and catatonic forms seem to have become much less common and the paranoid form considerably more common since Kraepelin and Bleuler wrote their classical descriptions. These changes were accompanied by a rise in the average age of onset and a gradual improvement in prognosis, at least prior to the introduction of more restrictive diagnostic criteria (Hegarty et al 1994). There have also been several reports of declining hospital first-admission rates for schizophrenia in industrial countries in the last 25 years. Eagles & Whalley (1985) drew attention to a 40% fall in the first-admission rate in Scotland between 1969 and 1978, and similar declines have since been reported in other European countries, North America and New Zealand (Cannon & Jones, 1996). Although the consistency of these reports is impressive it seems likely that the observed decline is due either to changing diagnostic criteria or to an increasing reluctance to admit schizophrenics to hospital, or some combination of the two.

Onset

The onset of the disease is characteristically between the ages of 15 and 45 years, but it may be before puberty, or delayed until the seventh or eighth decades. Although schizophrenia is equally common in men and women, male schizophrenics are consistently admitted to hospital 4 or 5 years earlier than females, and this appears to reflect a genuine and unexplained difference in the age of onset between the two sexes (Häfner et al 1989). The incidence is considerably higher in the unmarried than the married in both sexes and both also have a considerably reduced fertility.

Fertility

The fertility of schizophrenics has been studied many times, and there is general agreement that they marry less often than other people, remain childless more often even when they do marry, and have fewer children than other people in or out of wedlock. In the past this was usually attributed to their confinement in sexually segregated asylums. However, it is now apparent that their fertility is low even before admission to hospital, and studies carried out in the 1960s and 1970s after the introduction of 'open door' policies confirm that, despite the increased opportunities for marrying and conceiving thus provided, schizophrenics still have far fewer children than other people. It remains uncertain as to whether social or biological factors are responsible.

Mortality

Schizophrenics also have a substantially raised early mortality. Studies in Europe and North America suggest that their relative risk of early death is increased two- or three-fold. This increased risk is largely attributable to suicide, and is shared by other forms of mental illness, but there are also increased rates of death by homicide, accidents and physical illnesses (Joukamaa et al 2001). There have been repeated claims of associations, both positive and negative, between schizophrenia and various physical illnesses. The best-established of these relationships is a negative, and as yet unexplained, association between schizophrenia and rheumatoid arthritis. Despite many conflicting claims, it is not established that schizophrenics are either more or less likely to develop cancers in general, or any particular form of cancer, than other people. Nor is the claimed association between schizophrenia and coeliac disease supported by convincing evidence. There are, however, a number of reports of an increased risk of death from respiratory disease, presumably related to smoking.

Table 19.3 Risk factors for schizophrenia and their estimated relative risks/odds ratios	
Risk Factor	RR/OR
Family history	RR 5–50×
Immigrant/ethic minority status	OR = 5
Developmental delay/abnormality	OR = 3
Chronic cannabis/stimulant use	OR = 3
Childhood solitariness	OR = 2
Urban birth/residence	OR = 2
Obstetric complications	OR = 2
Ventriculomegaly/cerebral 'atrophy'	OR = 2
Maternal flu/malnutrition	OR = 2
Others, e.g. winter birth	OR < 2
After Cannon & Jones (1996)	

Risk factors

Risk factor epidemiological investigation in schizophrenia has, with the main exception of genetic studies, followed rather than preceded studies of biological disruptions. Table 19.3 summarises the epidemiological evidence and gives best-estimates of the likely strength (as risk or odds ratios) of these effects (adapted from Cannon & Jones 1996). The relative risk of developing schizophrenia if one has an affected first degree relative ranges from about five (for parents of an affected child), to ten (for children or sibs), to fifteen (two or more first degree relatives) and onto about fifty times if one has an affected identical twin. The other effects are comparatively weak, and in many cases it is still unclear whether they are true risk factors rather than early expressions of the disease (or a genetic or environmental liability to it). We will discuss those with known or likely biological effects in the next section and those of unknown pathophysiological significance here.

Urban residence

The first-admission rate for schizophrenia is generally higher in urban than in rural areas, and much higher from the central areas of large cities than from the surrounding suburbs. Faris & Dunham (1939) first drew attention to this striking phenomenon in Chicago, and it has since been confirmed in several other American and European cities. The highest admission rates are consistently from the poor working-class areas and the lowest rates from the middle-class suburbs. This geographical gradient is accompanied by an equally impressive social class gradient — the admission rate of social classes IV and V (unskilled and semiskilled manual workers) being consistently higher than that of other occupational groupings. These findings were originally regarded as evidence that being brought up in a working-class family, or in the central slum areas of a big city, created a predisposition to develop schizophrenia. Goldberg & Morrison (1963) were able to show, however, by examining the birth certificates of a series of 672 young male schizophrenics, that although they themselves were predominantly from social classes IV and V, their fathers' social class had not differed from that of the general population, and that the disparity between the two was due to a 'downward drift' of the sons a few months or years before their admission to hospital. This normal distribution of social class at birth and decline prior to onset has been well replicated (Cannon & Jones

1996), but there are an increasing number of studies which also suggest an effect of urban as opposed to rural birth. Most notably, Mortensen et al (1999) linked the Danish birth and psychiatric registers and found a relative risk of 2.4 for those with an urban birth after controlling for any (first degree) family history of schizophrenia. This effect could, however, be attributable to any number of factors, including selective migration.

Ethnicity and migration

Pockets of high prevalence have been reported in isolated parts of Scandinavia, Ireland and the Balkans, but these are probably artefactual. In the ECA study, black people had a slightly higher prevalence than whites. Migration, on the other hand, has long been associated with a substantially increased risk of schizophrenia. Odegaard (1932) found the Norwegians who had emigrated to Minnesota had a higher risk of schizophrenic breakdown than those who had remained in Norway, and Malzberg & Lee (1956) showed that immigrants to New York had a much higher hospital admission rate than native born Americans, with their children half-way between. More recently, Cochrane (1977) has shown that most immigrant groups to England and Wales, particularly West Indians, Asians and Poles, have higher hospital admission rates for schizophrenia than the English and the Scots. Similar findings have been reported from other countries, but the relationship is not invariable. At times the cause of this increased risk has had considerable political as well as scientific significance, with the host country or community being tempted to attribute the phenomenon to a selective migration of unstable undesirables, and the immigrants themselves and their fellow-countrymen back home attributing it to the stresses of living in a foreign and sometimes hostile land. In reality, it is not yet firmly established that the incidence of schizophrenia is increased in immigrants. Most studies have been based on hospital admissions, and psychiatrically disturbed immigrants are more likely to be admitted to mental hospitals than other people. Once admitted they are also at greater risk of being labelled as schizophrenic, particularly if their behaviour is unusual and the examining doctor has difficulty communicating with them. Moreover, most comparisons between immigrant and native populations have not matched the two for age, a crucial omission because most immigrants are young adults and schizophrenia is a disease of young adults.

It has however been reported that the Afro-Caribbean populations of several English cities have extremely high hospital admission rates for schizophrenia, perhaps 10 times as high as that of their white neighbours, with possibly even higher rates in their offspring (McGovern & Cope 1987). It seems unlikely that differences of this magnitude could be generated by racial biasing of diagnostic criteria, inaccurate demographic assumptions or ethnic differences in contact rates with psychiatric services. The offspring effect and the fact that the incidence of schizophrenia is not elevated among Afro-Caribbeans in the Caribbean argue against selective migration and for post-migration factors. Recent studies suggest that these are more likely to be social (such as discrimination or isolation) than biological (such as cannabis abuse or obstetric complications). Boydell et al (2001), for example, found that the incidence of schizophrenia increased in non-white people in Camberwell, South London, as the proportion of such ethnic minorities in the local population fell. This issue will however remain controversial and politically sensitive until rigorously designed epidemiological comparisons have been carried out and adequate explanations for the very high hospital admission rates offered at an individual level.

Other factors

One of the most important reasons for studying the epidemiology of a disease is to obtain clues to its aetiology. At one time the striking relationships found between schizophrenia and the central areas of big cities, low social class, being unmarried and being a migrant all seemed capable of providing that vital clue. But the relationships with urban birth/upbringing and migration are still unclear, and the other two have turned out to be consequences rather than causes of the disorder. There are, however, other important associations that cannot be consequences: e.g. season of birth and maternal nutrition/influenza. The relationship between schizophrenia and season of birth has been found in virtually every country in the temperate latitudes of the northern hemisphere. First admissions are more likely to have been born in the early months of the year than the rest of the population, and correspondingly less likely to have been born in July to September. This relationship is not shared by other diagnostic categories and, although the excess of births in January to March is only about 8%, it is consistent and highly significant statistically (Bradbury & Miller 1985). The odds ratio may only be about 1.1, but the population attributable risk for such a relatively common event may be as high as 10% (Mortensen et al 1999). In Australia and South Africa the excess of births is in July to September (i.e. the winter months, as in Europe), although the data are less conclusive. Preliminary evidence also indicates that the siblings of schizophrenics show the same distribution of birth dates as the general population and that the excess of winter births of schizophrenics is greater the colder the winter. This suggests that the incidence of schizophrenia is influenced by some widely distributed seasonal variable, probably infective or dietary, acting either in utero or in the early months of life.

Intrauterine viral infection is one such possibility, for many viral infections have a well-defined seasonal variation, and rubella demonstrates that an inconspicuous infection in a young woman may cause permanent damage to the fetal nervous system if she is pregnant at the time. There are indeed intriguing but unreplicated reports of associations between rubella and toxoplasmosis, and schizophrenia. There have been several reports in recent years, from Finland, Denmark, England and Scotland, that fluctuations in the birth dates of schizophrenics can be related to fluctuations in the incidence of influenza in the preceding few months (for example, see Sham et al 1992). This is particularly notable in a relationship between the 1957 influenza epidemic and the fact of mothers of people who later developed schizophrenia being in the second trimester of pregnancy. This suggests (but does not prove) that possible damage to the fetus may be aetiologically important.

Another related issue of interest is severe maternal food deprivation during pregnancy. This is of course by no means rare but is often associated with civil disorganisation and a lack of organised records such as registration of births. In northern Holland, at the end of the Second World War, the entire population was severely deprived of food during the winter of 1944–1945. The deprivation was relatively circumscribed in time, and organised record keeping was maintained. An increased rate of schizophrenia was found in the daughters of women who suffered severe food deprivation during the first trimester of pregnancy (Susser & Lin 1992). These and other suggestions of severe maternal 'stress'

being associated with schizophrenia require independent replication. Further, until the mechanism involved is established, the meaning of these potentially important findings will remain unclear.

AETIOLOGY AND PATHOPHYSIOLOGY

It should be clear that the causes of schizophrenia are far from fully understood but that a number of aetiological factors are now known to be relevant. We have moved a very long way from the position outlined by Kraepelin in 1919: 'the causes of dementia praecox are at the present time still mapped in impenetrable darkness'. Indeed, Weinberger (1995) recently commented that 'Twenty years ago, the principal challenge for schizophrenia research was to gather objective scientific evidence that would implicate the brain. This challenge no longer exists'. Efforts must now be directed to exploring the mechanisms by which the factors known to be relevant to the aetiology interact and produce the clinical features of schizophrenia.

Neurobiological factors

The biological factors known to be relevant to the aetiology of schizophrenia may conveniently be considered under the headings listed in Box 19.5.

Familiality

It has long been known that schizophrenia aggregates in families. This suggests that genetic factors are likely to be important, but disorders can of course be familial because family members share the same disadvantaged environment. As far as schizophrenia is concerned the matter of whether the relevant factor was shared genetic material or shared environment was elegantly clarified by the adoption studies of Kety et al (1975), who found high rates of schizophrenia in the biological relatives of schizophrenics who had been adopted away at birth and high rates of the later development of schizophrenia in the children of schizophrenic mothers who had been adopted away at birth. Further details of such genetic studies in schizophrenia are described in Chapter 9.

It is, however, less clear which specific genes are involved. Linkage studies have implicated several promising regions of several chromosomes; replications have been inconsistent but pooled analyses strongly suggest that there are susceptibility loci on chromosomes 6p, 8p, 13q and 22q, although the latter two in particular may also be associated with bipolar disorder. More

---

Box 19.5 Biological factors relevant to the aetiology of schizophrenia

- Familiality of the disorder
- Occurrence of 'schizophrenia-like' psychoses
- Pharmacological mechanisms of antipsychotic drugs
- Substance use
- Pregnancy and birth complications
- Deficits in intellectual function
- Structural brain changes
- Changes in regional cerebral blood flow on functional imaging

---

specifically, systematic reviews and meta-analyses have found homogenous and publication-bias-free evidence to implicate polymorphisms of the dopamine D_3 and $5HT_{2a}$ genes (or genes in linkage disequilibrium with them). This is in keeping with what is known about the effects of antipsychotic drugs, although the odds ratios are only in the region of 1.2 (Williams et al 1997, 1998) and other genes with possibly stronger effects await discovery.

'Schizophrenia-like' psychoses

This term refers to primary cerebral disease or to systemic disease affecting the brain and causing 'secondary' schizophrenia — not to the subtle abnormalities which modern techniques, such as imaging, can show to be present in schizophrenia. In the great majority of patients the illness develops in the absence of demonstrable organic disease; but certain 'organic' diseases, which could not result from any of the social and environmental disadvantages secondary to the disorder, occur in association with schizophrenia more often than would be expected by chance. Davison & Bagley (1969) reviewed the early literature on CNS disorders and concluded that certain tumours and head injuries, temporal lobe epilepsy, Huntington's disease, Sydenham's chorea and Wilson's disease, as well as some infections (general paresis and rheumatic encephalitis) were reported in association with schizophrenia to a greater extent than would be expected by chance. Notwithstanding the effects of reporting bias, the conditions are so varied that it is difficult to see any common path by which they could all come to produce the same clinical picture, although there is a tendency for them to affect the temporal lobes and diencephalon. When the occurrence of these conditions was studied in relation to a large defined cohort of first schizophrenic episodes (Johnstone et al 1987), underlying organic disease of at least possible aetiological significance was found in 15 of 268 cases (6%) and some overlap was apparent (Table 19.4). The worrying possibility that other organic cases are missed is obvious, but this cohort was followed up for a further 5 years and no additional relevant illnesses were known to develop. A small number of subsequent reports continue to hint at but not confirm an association with head injury and cerebral infections, particularly in children and adolescents. Clarification of these effects and any mechanism by which those conditions produce 'secondary schizophrenia' could illuminate our understanding of the pathogenesis of the illness in general.

The effects of antipsychotic drugs

Chlorpromazine was introduced into psychiatric practice by Delay & Deniker in 1952, and by the early 1960s it was clear that phenothiazines relieved schizophrenic symptoms and were not simply supersedatives. A large number of other antipsychotic agents were introduced, and it became evident that they all shared the property of blockade of D_2 dopamine receptors and that their antipsychotic efficacy was proportional to their ability to block these receptors. By the early 1970s a number of pieces of evidence led to the conclusion that antipsychotic drugs acted by blocking D_2 receptors. Although there was no evidence of an excess of dopaminergic transmission, the fact that reduction in such transmission by antipsychotic drugs was consistently effective in controlling the disorder made it likely that dopaminergic transmission had a central role in the underlying mechanisms of schizophrenia (see Ch. 15).

The evidence for this position was made much less clear by the demonstration that clozapine (a weak D_2 antagonist with a wide range of other pharmacological effects) is generally of greater efficacy against psychotic symptoms than traditional antipsychotics which are much more effective D_2 blockers. The conclusion is that D_2 blockade and some other pharmacological mechanism is more effective in antipsychotic terms than D_2 blockade alone. It used to be thought that $5HT_{2a}$ blockade, and the ratio of this to D_2 blockade in particular, was an important determinant of 'atypicality' — and indeed may of the newer drugs were developed with this in mind — but $5HT_{2a}$ blockade is evident at subtherapeutic doses. An alternative view is that clozapine and the newer 'atypicals' have a faster dissociation off the dopamine receptor, making them more accommodating of physiological dopamine transmission (see e.g. Seeman 2002). This theory can account for the reduced extrapyramidal side-effects and hyperprolactinaemia observed on the atypicals.

In the meantime, however, several studies have reinforced the 'dopamine hypothesis' (Jones & Pilowsky 2002). It is now clear that dopamine receptors are elevated in number and the dopaminergic system is overactivated in schizophrenia, and this is not entirely attributable to therapeutic blockade. We have in effect moved from an over-simplistic view about *the* disturbance of neurotransmission involved — such that various other transmitter systems are implicated (e.g. serotonin, glutamate) — but dopamine almost certainly has *a* role. More generally, these neuropharmacological studies provide important evidence for disturbances at the synaptic level in schizophrenia.

Substance use

An association between various illicit drugs and psychotic symptoms has been commonly observed. Psychotic 'reactions' to cannabis, LSD, amphetamines and more recently to Ecstasy and ketamine ingestion occur, but it can be difficult to distinguish them from delirious states or drug taking as a reaction to psychosis. There is certainly no convincing evidence for *specific* cannabis or amphetamine psychoses. While drug challenge with methylphenidate and ketamine can provoke psychotic symptoms in schizophrenics, it can also do so in controls and only has transient effects in both groups. The mechanisms of such effects remain unclear, although cannabis and stimulants increase dopamine release and LSD is a $5HT_{2a}$ agonist.

The prospective Swedish conscript study of cannabis use and psychosis did provide good evidence that cannabis use can precede

Table 19.4 Organic diagnoses in Northwick Park study of 268 first episodes	
Organic diagnosis	No. of cases
Alcohol excess/withdrawal	3
Drug abuse/withdrawal	2
Syphilis	3
Carcinoma of the lung	1
Autoimmune multisystem disease (systemic lupus erythematosus)	1
Thyrotoxicosis	1
Cerebrovascular accident	1
Sarcoidosis	2
Cerebral cysticercosis with secondary epilepsy	1
From Johnstone et al (1987)	

the onset of psychosis. Andreasson et al (1987) linked information about drug use, in approximately 50 000 young men conscripted in 1969/70, to a national register of psychiatric admissions up to 1983. They found that cannabis use was associated with a 2.4-fold increased risk of a subsequent admission for schizophrenia, and that the relative risk was 6 in more frequent users, but could not exclude the possibility that other drugs were responsible or that the 'pre-psychotic' turned to cannabis after the development of early symptoms but before the onset of psychosis. Zammit et al (2002) recently updated the study, with linkage to admission data up until 1996, and were able to control for these and other potential confounders. They demonstrated that stimulant use was not responsible, and that the elevated risk of admission for schizophrenia in cannabis users held in those who were admitted more than 5 years after conscription. A number of case-control studies also support the association between cannabis and schizophrenia, as do some more recent cohort studies (see e.g. Miller et al 2001). Further, this observational evidence that cannabis is psychotomimetic is strongly supported by a recent meta-analysis of randomised controlled trials (RCTs) of cannabinoid anti-emetics or placebo in cancer patients, which found a relative risk of approximately 6 for hallucinations and 9 for delusions.

Pregnancy and birth complications

This evidence includes the well-documented tendency for individuals who later develop schizophrenia to have been born in the winter months of the year, and the possible effects of maternal influenza or food deprivation in pregnancy described above. More specifically, a large number of studies have examined the frequency of obstetric complications in individuals with schizophrenia as compared with controls. Individual studies have produced variable findings, as one would expect, but a number of systematic reviews provide evidence that such complications are associated with the later development of schizophrenia.

Cannon et al (2002) have summarised this literature and conducted a meta-analysis on recent prospective studies. There is good evidence that low birth weight (especially below 2 kg) increases the risk of schizophrenia. It is unclear whether this is attributable to genetic or environmental factors, but the increased rates of congenital malformations and 'minor physical anomalies' in schizophrenia implicate the genetic control of fetal growth and development. On the other hand, perinatal problems like pre-eclampsia, uterine atony and emergency sections suggest possible hypoxic brain damage. Direct evidence of birth asphyxia in neonates who go on to develop schizophrenia is limited, but the hippocampus is very sensitive to such effects and a number of structural brain imaging studies suggest that the hippocampus is small in schizophrenia and that this may be related to obstetric complications.

Changes in brain structure

Pneumoencephalographic studies conducted from the 1920s indicated that there is a degree of ventricular enlargement and a reduction of brain tissue in schizophrenia, but they were difficult to interpret because of the problems of conducting this investigation in control subjects. The introduction of non-invasive imaging allowed controlled studies to be carried out, and the finding of enlarged ventricular spaces in schizophrenia (Johnstone et al 1976) has been widely replicated. A host of structural MRI

Table 19.5 Evidence for cortical dysconnectivity in schizophrenia	
Investigation	Finding
Structural MRI	Inter-regional volume correlations reduced
Diffusion tensor imaging	White matter tract integrity reduced
Postmortem neurochemistry	Reduced synaptophysin mRNA expression
Postmortem microscopy	Reduced dendritic spines
Cognitive	Organisation of encoding and retrieval may be responsible for impaired memory
Functional imaging	Altered relationships between frontal and temporal lobe activity on certain tasks

studies suggest that schizophrenics have reduced volumes of the whole brain, the prefrontal lobe and the thalamus, and parts of the temporal lobes in particular (see Ch. 5). These findings are evident in first-episode patients and even in relatives and subjects at high risk (Lawrie et al 2001), suggesting a developmental cause. There are specific indications of apparent genetic effects in the prefrontal lobes and environmental (obstetric) effects in the medial temporal lobe, but there may be additional changes around the time of onset.

Neuroimaging studies stimulated a resurgence of interest in neuropathological work in schizophrenia that was first conducted in the early part of this century. The whole brains, temporal lobes and the thalamus of patients with schizophrenia are consistently smaller and lighter than in controls. This appears to be due to smaller neurons and less neuropil rather than a loss of neurons (Harrison 1999). Reductions in the numbers of dendritic spines and the expression of synaptophysin mRNA (a marker of synaptic activity) support imaging findings that suggest subtle differences in inter-regional connectivity may underlie schizophrenia (see Table 19.5). There is also an absence of gliosis, interpreted as indicative of a disorder of neurodevelopment (Weinberger 1995). A variety of subtle cytoarchitectural abnormalities in the hippocampus and in the cerebral cortex have been reported but none has been convincingly replicated (Harrison 1999). Indeed, neuropathology studies do not consistently find reductions in the size of medial temporal lobe structures — although it is difficult to get large numbers of well-preserved brains, and most MRI studies therefore have much more power to detect such differences. The postmortem and MRI studies do however agree that these macroscopic structural changes are associated with cognitive disturbances.

Cognitive dysfunction

In his original monograph Bleuler had maintained that intelligence, and cognitive function in general, was unimpaired in schizophrenia, and this view was generally accepted until recently. It was well known, of course, that many schizophrenics performed poorly on formal tests of intelligence, but it was assumed that this could usually be explained as a secondary consequence of apathy, or of the subject's preoccupation with hallucinatory experiences or delusional ideas. There was no doubt too that chronic schizophrenia was compatible, at least in some people, with high intellectual achievement, and that some of the patients who scored badly on an intelligence test on one occasion performed far better on re-testing. This view was challenged by the demonstration of ventriculomegaly on computerised tomography (Johnstone et al 1976), and members of the same research group at Northwick Park soon showed that many chronic schizophrenics were disoriented in time and some did not even know how old they were (Crow & Stevens 1978). When the cognitive abilities of chronic schizophrenics were examined in detail, evidence of widespread impairments was found.

General intelligence is reduced in patients with schizophrenia and to a lesser extent in their healthy sibs. This appears to largely predate the illness, but there may also be further reductions around the time of onset. There does not appear to be any progressive dementia as such, even though some patients with longstanding illnesses appear to be impaired to such a level. Performance IQ is lower than verbal IQ, and there are notable deficits in reaction time and motor skill (Heinrichs & Zakzanis 1998).

There are also clear impairments on tests of attention, executive function and memory, although it is difficult to reliably demonstrate that these are greater than the global problems already described. Frith (1992) deals with this by providing evidence for relationships between particular cognitive disturbances and specific types of symptoms (see below), each of which can be mapped onto regional abnormalities on functional imaging. Several studies do however suggest that there may be particular problems with memory (Heinrichs & Zakzanis 1998). Implicit memory and the ability to learn new information are relatively preserved, but working, episodic and semantic memory are impaired — deficits that are if anything improved by antipsychotic medication but exacerbated by anticholinergics (see Ch. 8). There are, in particular, strong suggestions that hallucinations are related to difficulties in remembering the source of episodic memories (cf. monitoring whether stimuli are internally or externally generated) and that schizophrenics have difficulty organising the encoding and retrieval of memories. The latter is another pointer to the importance of dysconnectivity in schizophrenia, as functional imaging in healthy volunteers reliably activates frontal and temporal lobes during such activity and these activation patterns are disturbed in schizophrenia.

Changes in regional cerebral blood flow

In 1974, Ingvar & Franzen demonstrated that patients with schizophrenia had relatively reduced cerebral blood flow in the frontal lobes. This 'hypofrontality' was confirmed in some subsequent studies but not in all, and some even found 'hyperfrontality'. Other studies compared activity during performance of certain neuropsychological tests and that in a reference condition ('cognitive challenge' studies), with if anything even more variable results. The key issue seems to be whether or not the patients can or will actually do the test in the scanner.

Greater success has been evident in establishing the neuroanatomical correlates of specific symptoms — such as mapping auditory hallucinations to language areas of the brain (see e.g. Frith 1992, 1996). There is also a remarkably consistent body of evidence from various ligand studies that presynaptic dopamine activity is increased (see Ch. 5). The current focus of much functional imaging research in schizophrenia is on dysconnectivity and reduced frontotemporal connectivity in particular (Friston & Frith 1995). A variety of studies have been carried out and, taken together, they suggest imbalances between neuronal activity at diverse interconnected brain sites rather than abnormal function at a single location (see e.g. Lawrie et al 2002).

Social factors

Although the twin and adoption studies prove beyond reasonable doubt that schizophrenia is genetically transmitted, this evidence has also established that environmental influences must play a major role as well, for estimates of the concordance rate in monozygotic twins are consistently 50% or lower. If someone whose genetically identical twin develops schizophrenia has less than a 50:50 chance of doing the same, whether or not he does must depend on his past or present environment.

Abnormal family relations?

In the last forty years the possibility that pathological relationships or patterns of communication within the nuclear family may lead, at least in genetically vulnerable children, to the eventual development of schizophrenia has received a great deal of attention, particularly in the USA. In the 1940s Fromm-Reichmann coined the phrase 'schizophrenogenic mother' and later workers supported the concept, with claims that the mothers of schizophrenics were both overprotective and hostile to their children. A few years later Gregory Bateson suggested that schizophrenia was produced by the constant reception of incongruent messages from a key relative — to take a trite example, the verbal message 'You know that Mummy loves you' accompanied by non-verbal behaviour implying something quite different — and this 'double-bind hypothesis' remained in vogue for a decade or more. Shortly afterwards, Lidz and his colleagues at Yale carried out a series of intensive studies of 17 upper middle-class families with what they regarded as schizophrenic children. They described several highly abnormal relationships within these families which differed with the sex of the schizophrenic child and which they suggested were associated with the development of schizophrenia in this son or daughter. Their work aroused great interest and their terms 'marital schism' and 'marital skew' obtained the same wide currency as Bateson's 'double-bind'. Around the same time, and with a similarly dramatic impact, R D Laing published his influential book *The Divided Self*. Unfortunately, these studies all had serious methodological defects and owed their influence more to their catch phrases and the prevailing climate of opinion than to objective evidence. They were not conducted blind, had no adequate control groups, involved a very diffuse concept of schizophrenia and were retrospective, so that it was difficult to tell which of the observed abnormalities had preceded the onset of schizophrenia in the child, and might therefore have some aetiological significance, and which were merely reactions to the child's illness.

Alongside these global studies of parental personalities and family interactions a series of more limited and better designed studies of communication patterns in schizophrenic and non-schizophrenic families was carried out. The most influential of these were by Singer & Wynne (1965) who gave Rorschach tests to the parents of schizophrenics and claimed that they consistently produced more deviant responses (i.e. that they were more 'thought disordered') than control parents. However, when

Hirsch & Leff (1975) repeated this work they were unable to replicate the finding. Although there was a significant difference between the average deviance scores of the parents of schizophrenics and the parents of neurotic controls, the overlap was considerable and the higher deviance scores of the former were entirely due to the fact that they spoke at greater length, i.e. there was no difference in the *rate* at which the two groups made deviant responses. The results of other studies have been similarly mixed.

What then survives from all this? There is some evidence that the parents of schizophrenics are emotionally disturbed more often than the parents of normal children and that more of the mothers have schizoid personality traits. Moreover, it is claimed that the parents of schizophrenics seem to be in conflict with one another more often than the parents of other psychiatric patients, and that the mothers are more concerned about and protective towards their children. These unfortunate people do of course have a very great deal to worry them. It could be claimed that there was scope in all this for baneful influence on the pre-schizophrenic child, but as yet there is no convincing evidence that any of these influences do in fact precede the development of schizophrenia. Furthermore, any well-substantiated parental abnormalities are easily explicable in genetic terms, and none is invariably present. Indeed, genetic studies suggest that environmental factors contributing to aetiology of schizophrenia are much more likely to be unique or 'non-shared' rather than familial.

Life events

Events in the weeks or months immediately prior to the onset of illness have received less attention than the events during childhood, but there is some evidence that they may be important. Steinberg & Durrell (1968) showed that the schizophrenic breakdown rate of recruits to the US army was much higher in their first month of military service than at any time in the next 2 years, suggesting that the transition from civilian life to recruiting barracks was a contributing factor. The effect was the same in volunteers as in enlisted men, and they were able to produce fairly convincing evidence that the illnesses presenting in the first month of service were indeed new and not merely newly detected. Further evidence was provided by Brown & Birley (1968), who obtained detailed information about the events of the previous 12 weeks from 50 patients with schizophrenic illnesses of recent onset and 400 controls from the same neighbourhood. They found that the schizophrenics had experienced significantly more life events than the controls in the 3 weeks immediately prior to the onset of illness, but only in those 3 weeks. The difference between schizophrenics and controls remained, even when all events that might have been a consequence of incipient illness (e.g. losing a job by being sacked rather than by closure of the firm) were eliminated. It has to be borne in mind, however, that the concept of schizophrenia employed in both these studies was a broad one. In Brown & Birley's study, 24 patients were only 'probably schizophrenic' and, furthermore, only 24 of the 50 were first admissions.

Subsequent work has been scanty and largely unable to overcome the major methodological problems of identifying enough independent events in people with reliably diagnosed first-episode psychosis. This is not surprising given the findings already described that prodromal symptoms may precede psychosis by years. There is, however, a general consensus that major life events

can precipitate symptoms in the predisposed (see e.g. Miller et al 2001).

Expressed emotion

More attention has been paid to the determinants of relapse in those who have already had one episode of schizophrenia, mainly because the comparatively high probability of a further episode makes it feasible to mount prospective studies. Brown et al (1972) showed that the relapse rate over the next 12 months in young men who had just recovered from a first episode of schizophrenia was far higher (58% versus 16%) in those who returned to live with a relative, usually a parent or wife, who was prone to make critical comments about them than in those who lived with a relative who was more tolerant and accepting. Moreover, the ill-effects of what the authors called 'high expressed emotion', or high EE, were mitigated to some extent if the patient was receiving antipsychotic drugs, and also if patient and relative were in contact with one another for less than 35 hours a week, i.e. social withdrawal seemed to be protective. These findings have since been widely although not invariably replicated; a systematic review of 27 studies demonstrated a robust effect, especially in chronic patients, albeit less than in affective and eating disorders (Butzlaff & Hooley 1998).

The origins of the behaviour measured by EE are, however, uncertain. It is possible that the EE measure is predictive at least in part because relatives respond in a particular way to sufferers whose illness in any case has a poor prognosis. There is evidence that at least some components of high EE are associated with a variety of abnormalities in the patient, and Birchwood & Smith (1987) argue that high EE develops over time as part of the coping style of relatives in response to the difficulty of living with someone with schizophrenia. The fact that high EE is less evident in relatives of first-episode patients than in those with subsequent admissions is used in support of this argument.

Psychological factors

Innumerable psychological theories of both the aetiology and the pathogenesis of schizophrenia have been proposed in the past. Many were derived from psychoanalysis, others from behavioural psychology. Apart from the defective filter theory of sensory overload, few were backed by any substantial empirical data and most are now of only historical interest. Recently, however, some new and more promising models have been propounded from a cognitive neuropsychological perspective.

A number of studies have examined psychotic symptoms, especially delusions, in terms of what is known about the determinants of social interaction, sensory experience and belief formation. Delusional content, for example, may reflect everyday concerns about being attacked or excluded, or people's preoccupations with spiritual matters. People tend to have 'attributional styles', such as tendencies to egocentricity, externalising (attributing events to outside forces) or intentionalising (attributing intentions to others' behaviour). There is some evidence that those with delusions are disposed to jump to conclusions and stick to them ('reasoning biases'), despite limited information, especially if the material is emotionally salient. Thus, persecutory delusions could be related to some combination of personality factors, focusing on a specific stimulus (perceptual/attentional bias), misinterpreting it and ignoring information that goes against that interpretation

(Blackwood et al 2001). These concepts are rather vague and overlapping, and sound a little like simple reformulations of descriptive psychopathology, but do perhaps offer the prospect of a scientific study of these experiences. This kind of approach has certainly been successful in understanding the Capgras delusion — as the exact opposite of prosopagnosia. Facial processing in Capgras subjects is normal, but the emotional concomitants of familiar face perception appear to be somehow disconnected from it, leading to an anomalous affectless experience that can be explained in the delusion (Halligan & David 2001).

Frith (1992) suggested that it is possible to explain the symptoms and signs of schizophrenia in terms of abnormalities of three main cognitive processes:

- Negative symptoms and some inappropriate behaviours (e.g. perseverations) may be considered as the result of inability to generate spontaneous (willed) actions.
- Some positive symptoms, e.g. passivity experiences, auditory and somatic hallucinations, may be considered the result of a lack of awareness of the prior intention that accompanies a deliberate act. Being unaware of their own intentions, patients will experience their own actions, thoughts and subvocal (and perhaps vocal) speech as resulting from some source other than themselves.
- Delusions of persecution and reference may be understood as the result of an inability to correctly infer the intentions of other people. Similarly the patient's inferences about what other people are thinking may be incorrectly perceived as information coming from an external source. This could provide an explanation for third person auditory hallucinations.

In terms of this theory, schizophrenia may be explained as a defect of the mechanism (referred to as 'meta-representation' or 'theory of mind') which enables us to be aware of our goals and our intentions and to infer the beliefs and intentions of others (see Table 19.6).

Frith developed this work in relation to changes in regional cerebral blood flow in response to provocative neuropsychological tests (see above). This led him to suggest that the failure of some schizophrenic patients to distinguish between their own actions and intentions and internal events may be due to a functional disconnection between frontal brain areas concerned with action and more posterior areas concerned with perception (Frith 1996). Much of this model has since been independently replicated, particularly regarding some auditory hallucinations and negative symptoms. It has the additional appeal of being compatible with much of what is known about the biology of the disorder.

Animal and computer models

Animal models of serious mental disorders have obvious problems and are less fashionable than they were at one time. Latent inhibition has however continued to be studied. It is a phenomenon, readily demonstrable in animals and man, whereby repeated exposure to a stimulus without consequence retards subsequent conditioning to that stimulus. (For example, a rat repeatedly exposed to a particular odour will take longer to learn the significance of that odour if it is subsequently paired with a rewarding or punishing stimulus.) An early study found that although schizophrenics in remission displayed latent inhibition in the same way as normal controls, acutely ill schizophrenics did not (Baruch et al 1988). Quite apart from the intrinsic interest of a simple and widely applicable paradigm in which schizophrenics perform 'better' (respond more) than normals, latent inhibition is known to be abolished in rats by amphetamine, and to be strengthened by antipsychotics. It has the makings, therefore, of a possible animal model of schizophrenia. Work also continues on pre-pulse inhibition, as an index of 'sensorimotor gating', as do efforts to breed strains of animals and to knock-out particular genes with specific performance patterns on these tests (Kilts 2001).

The advent of artificial intelligence as a tool to understand information processing in the human brain has also led to new approaches to psychosis, and hallucinations in particular. Through computational modelling of neural networks that have been trained on empirical data, putative pathologies can be introduced into the system and the effects monitored. For example, it has been shown that 'pruning' modelled synaptic connections in a speech system results in initial improvements in word detection but that, after about 40% pruning, hallucinations are simulated, as speech percepts with no input (McGlashan & Hoffman 2000). This approach offers great potential for integrating what is known about schizophrenia and developing it by modelling various insults that could in turn refine empirical research in patients.

Summary

The most plausible synthesis of the genetic, neuropathological and epidemiological evidence described above is that schizophrenia is a neurodevelopmental disorder, as Weinberger (1987, 1995) has suggested. The structure of the hippocampus and other parts of the temporal lobe, and the connections between these and the frontal lobes, are abnormal in at least a substantial proportion of schizophrenics. These abnormalities may either be genetically determined or produced by injury to the developing brain (mediated perhaps by disruption of the normal sequence of neuronal migrations), either in utero or at the time of birth. This would account for the changes in the brains of schizophrenics, found on structural imaging and at postmortem examination, and the subtle intellectual and social disabilities of schizophrenic children before the overt onset of their illness. The 20–30 year delay before the onset of the psychosis could be explained in maturational terms.

Table 19.6 Three principal abnormalities of cognitive process that underlie schizophrenia	
Process	**Associated symptoms**
Inability to generate willed action	Poverty of action Perseveration Inappropriate action (distractibility, disorganised behaviour)
Inability to monitor willed action	Delusions of passivity Certain auditory hallucinations Thought insertion
Inability to monitor the beliefs and intentions of others	Delusions of reference Paranoid delusions Third-person hallucinations Certain kinds of incoherence
From Frith (1992).	

Myelination and synaptic pruning are not complete in the frontal lobes until puberty, or later, and it has been shown that the behaviour of infant monkeys with surgical lesions of their dorsolateral prefrontal cortex does not become overtly abnormal until they are adult (Weinberger 1987, 1995, McGlashan & Hoffman 2000). A model of this kind could explain many of the established facts about schizophrenia. There are, of course, speculative elements in the model, and the role of psychosocial factors remains poorly specified, but it does at least provide a plausible conceptual framework to guide future research.

COURSE AND PROGNOSIS

Kraepelin's original concept of dementia praecox was founded on the belief that such illnesses all progressed to a state of global deterioration, or at least resulted in permanent damage to the personality. The outcome of schizophrenic illnesses, as Kraepelin himself eventually came to realise, is however very variable, regardless of how the syndrome is defined. Some resolve completely, with or without treatment, and never recur. Some recur repeatedly with full recovery every time. Others recur repeatedly but recovery is incomplete; that is, there is a persistent defect state that does not improve or tends indeed to deteriorate with successive relapses. Finally, some illnesses pursue a progressive downhill course from the beginning. The relative frequency of these different outcomes depends a great deal on how schizophrenia is defined. If it is defined in such a way as to exclude those with prominent affective symptoms, the proportion of patients making a full recovery is reduced; and if the diagnosis is also restricted, as it is by e.g. the DSM-IV criteria, to patients with a 6-month history, the proportion recovering without permanent defect is reduced still further (Hegarty et al 1994).

Outcome predictors

The matter of predicting the type of course that the illness of individual patients will take is naturally an issue of clinical importance. In the days before operational definitions for schizophrenia were used, Vaillant (1964) and others identified factors predictive of outcome. To some extent these were of features less than central to the disorder (see Box 19.6).

The development of more closely defined criteria for schizophrenia might have been expected to improve the prediction of outcome, but this hope has not really been realised. Studies have been conducted in which more and less restrictive criteria for the diagnoses have been applied to groups of patients who were then followed up for several years (e.g. Hawk et al 1975, Kendell et al 1979). On the whole the criteria were not very successful in identifying groups of patients with a poor outcome,

and in general what success there was lay in defining symptomatic rather than social outcome.

Outcome seems to be determined more by the circumstances under which the illness develops and the premorbid personality than by the symptomatology of the illness itself. Illnesses that develop acutely in response to stress have a much better prognosis than those that develop insidiously for no apparent reason. And if patients have prominent schizoid personality traits, particularly if they are also young, of low intelligence and have a poor work record, the outlook is much bleaker than if they are married, more mature and have a more 'normal' personality. Several studies have also reported a worse prognosis, at least where hospital discharge rates are concerned, in men than in women. Social considerations may be partly responsible for this difference. In most societies women are more likely to possess the basic housekeeping skills needed for survival outside hospital, and also pose less threat of violence to others. But the fact that women also have a later age of onset than men suggests that there are intrinsic differences in the nature of the illness between the sexes.

Outcome frequencies

Numerous studies of outcome have been published over the years. Many of these studies class patients in simple categories of outcome such as 'recovered', 'improved' and 'not improved'. Interpretation of even such simple terms can vary: some classing patients as recovered when their delusions, although present, are not readily revealed, and others classing such individuals as having continuing symptoms. Notwithstanding these limitations, most studies report that about 50% of people with schizophrenia will improve and 20% or so will recover (Hegarty et al 1994). A particularly large study of 532 patients discharged from inpatient care in a London borough between 1975 and 1985 and followed up between 1987 and 1990 was conducted by Johnstone et al (1991) and provides detailed information about various outcomes. The heterogeneity of outcome in schizophrenia was very evident in this study and, while there were some striking successes, unemployment, social difficulties and a restricted lifestyle were common and many patients had continuing symptoms. Of particular concern are the findings that the mean number of admissions required during the follow-up period was 5.4, and on average patients spent 14 months out of 10 years as inpatients. A slightly more encouraging picture emerged from a 13-year follow-up of a representative cohort of 67 first-episode patients, of whom approximately 40% had been employed over the previous 2 years and 20% were living independently (Mason et al 1995). Table 19.7 gives summary estimates of the frequency of outcomes based on these studies.

Influences on outcome

Illnesses, of course, do not have an outcome in vacuo, or even a pure 'natural history'. Outcome is always affected for good or ill by treatment and other environmental influences, and there is little doubt that the outcome of schizophrenia has improved considerably in the last fifty years. Hegarty et al (1994) have systematically reviewed this literature. Follow-up studies conducted in the 1920s and 1930s, before any effective treatments were available, only reported full recovery in about 10% of patients, and at least 60% were either unimproved or dead at the time of assessment. Since the 1950s all comparable follow-up studies have shown much better results. To what extent this improvement was

---

Box 19.6	Vaillant's predictors of a good prognosis

- Acute onset
- A stressful precipitating event
- Family history of depressive illness
- No family history of schizophrenia
- Absence of schizoid traits in the premorbid personality
- Confusion or perplexity
- Prominent affective symptoms

Table 19.7 Frequency of desirable outcomes in first episode schizophrenia (estimates)

Outcome	Frequency
Improvement	50%
No further episodes	20%
Employment / higher education	40%
Live independently	20%

due to the phenothiazine drugs introduced in 1952 and to what extent it was due to the changes in the milieu of mental hospitals and in public attitudes to mental illness taking place simultaneously is difficult to determine, but the combination certainly produced a substantial change. In most industrial countries the number of mental hospital beds fell by at least 50% between 1950 and 1990, and although financial and political considerations played an important role in many places, the major cause of this massive reduction was the changed outlook and management of schizophrenia. There is little doubt, though, that the effects of antipsychotics on the long-term prognosis of schizophrenia are less impressive than the short-term effects. Although contemporary patients spend less time in hospital than their predecessors, and are far less likely to end their days as permanent hospital invalids, a disturbingly high proportion still remain chronically handicapped by defect states or recurring hallucinations and delusions and still require repeated admissions to hospital despite longterm drug therapy.

Cultural influences

The vast majority of these follow-up studies were carried out in the industrialised countries of Western Europe and North America. There is, however, fairly substantial evidence that the prognosis of schizophrenia is considerably better in so-called 'underdeveloped' countries, despite their meagre psychiatric services. The most important evidence to this effect comes from the International Pilot Study of Schizophrenia. In that study a large series of psychotic patients, the majority of whom were schizophrenics, were studied in nine different centres in different parts of the world. The same structured interviewing methods were used in all nine centres and the patients were re-interviewed at 2 years and 5 years, again using the same methods and criteria throughout. Quite unexpectedly, the average outcome was considerably better in the underdeveloped countries (Colombia, India and Nigeria) than in the industrialised countries (Czechoslovakia, Denmark, the UK, the USA and Russia) (Sartorius et al 1977). The difference did not lie in the proportion of patients pursuing a steady downhill course; this was much the same throughout. Rather, it lay in the proportion suffering recurrent relapses. Despite the much more extensive follow-up treatment available in the industrial countries, a high proportion of their patients had further psychotic episodes, whereas Colombian, Nigerian and Indian patients did not. The same finding had emerged from an earlier comparison of the outcome of schizophrenia in London and Mauritius. Although careful comparisons of the initial symptomatology and other characteristics of the patients from the nine study centres did not reveal any important differences between them, the possibility that these differences in outcome were due to unrecognised differences in the types of patients admitted to

hospital in the nine centres can obviously not be excluded. Certainly, people with acute behavioural disturbances are more likely to come to medical attention in settings where psychiatric services are novel and thinly spread than are those with insidiously developing disorders that do not cause the same alarm; and the former are, of course, likely to have a better prognosis than the latter.

Partly to elucidate these intriguing differences in outcome the WHO mounted a further international comparison, involving 12 centres in 10 countries, known as the Determinants of Outcome of Severe Mental Disorders Programme. The preliminary results of this major study confirm that, at follow-up 2 years after their initial inception into treatment, schizophrenic illnesses have a better prognosis in developing than in developed countries (Sartorius et al 1986). Part, but only part, of this difference is attributable to a higher proportion of illnesses in the developed countries having a relatively insidious onset. It seems likely, therefore, that there is something about the social organisation of contemporary industrial societies, or their family structure or attitude to mental illness, which has a deleterious effect on the course of schizophrenic disorders. Not only is the outcome worse in industrial than in developing countries, it is probably worse in urban than in rural areas within industrial countries. A recent comparison has shown that the functioning of schizophrenic patients in the rural district of Nithsdale in south-west Scotland was higher than that of similar patients from south London (McCreadie et al 1997). To what extent this is due to the much higher use of the psychiatric services by the Nithsdale population is a matter for speculation.

To summarise, schizophrenia used to be regarded as a steadily progressive disease with a poor prognosis. It is now clear that this is not so, or perhaps no longer so. The long-term prognosis is rather better than we used to believe, and the course of the illness is very variable. On the whole, patients do not deteriorate further after the first 5–10 years, but even chronic patients may show surprising changes, either improvement or deterioration, after many years of apparent stability. These facts are difficult to reconcile with the idea that schizophrenia is a steadily progressive brain disease; they force us to consider aetiological hypotheses of quite different kinds. Schizophrenia also seems to have a better prognosis now than it had at the beginning of the 20th century and, at least in industrial countries, its clinical presentation has changed. The catatonic and hebephrenic forms have become much less frequent, and paranoid forms more frequent. These changes and differences are usually attributed to advances in treatment and to the pathoplastic effects of cultural differences and social changes. It is possible, however, that they are actually due to a slowly progressive change in the nature of the disease, as occurred with general paresis during the 19th century and with scarlet fever in the 20th. If such a change has indeed taken place, it is likely to be due to some change in the environmental factors contributing to the aetiology of the condition; if so, identifying these could inform therapeutic and even preventative approaches.

TREATMENT

Before the 1930s there was no effective treatment for any of the so-called functional psychoses, and the prime function of mental hospitals was to keep their patients in tolerable comfort and physical health in the hope that spontaneous remission would take place. Regimens were essentially custodial, with whatever occupational, recreational and spiritual accompaniments local custom and resources allowed. The introduction of Sakel's insulin therapy in 1933, Moniz's prefrontal leucotomy and von Meduna's convulsive therapy in 1935 and Cerletti's ECT in 1938, and the possibilities of cure which these dramatic new therapies seemed to offer, had a profound effect on the atmosphere and morale of mental hospitals throughout the world. ECT and insulin coma therapy were both widely used throughout the 1940s, and thousands of patients were enthusiastically subjected to prefrontal leucotomy. The discovery of the calming effects of chlorpromazine by Henri Laborit in the early 1950s had an even more profound effect, and within a few years of the introduction of these new phenothiazine drugs the insulin coma regimen and leucotomy both passed into a rapid decline. ECT remained in widespread use much longer, mainly in combination with phenothiazines or as a second-line treatment for patients who had failed to respond to these drugs, but is now very rarely used.

Antipsychotic drugs

The various types and preparations of antipsychotic drugs are now the mainstay of schizophrenia management. Most have been evaluated in RCTs and shown to be of benefit. It is beyond doubt that they ameliorate acute episodes, such that placebo-controlled trials in this situation would be unethical. The RCTs are, however, generally small and short-lived, so that potentially important benefits of antipsychotics or differences between them are quite likely to be missed (Thornley & Adams 1998). The Cochrane collaboration (see Ch. 12) has a schizophrenia section and already includes more than 100 systematic reviews and meta-analyses of pharmacological (and psychosocial) treatments. Space precludes them being individually cited here, but many are summarised in *Clinical Evidence* (Lawrie & McIntosh 2002). Even this secondary research and reporting does not however provide particularly good evidence on the harmful effects of treatment, which is probably most reliably determined from large observational studies. In what follows we therefore refer to key individual studies and systematic reviews where possible.

Treating acute symptoms

The phenothiazines, butyrophenones and thioxanthenes were initially used in schizophrenia for the purpose of treating the positive symptoms of acute episodes. In the 1960s several large-scale trials demonstrated that these drugs were highly effective in combating such symptoms and were not merely supersedatives (Hollister et al 1960, National Institute of Mental Health 1964). Nonetheless, about 30% of patients show only limited effects in such trials (Davis 1976) and about 10% of cases do not appear to show any response at all, even to prolonged treatment (Johnstone et al 1986). The Cochrane review of chlorpromazine, for example, found that an average of 55% of patients had a 50% or greater improvement in general over 6–8 weeks, but that many suffered from sedation and/or movement disorders. Haloperidol is less sedative but also more likely to cause dystonia, akathisia and parkinsonism. Pimozide and sulpiride were greeted with much enthusiasm in the 1980s, but have relatively slight advantages and disadvantages (Cochrane Library 2002, Lawrie & McIntosh 2002).

Partly because of individual differences in absorption and metabolism, the dose required to bring psychotic symptoms under control varies considerably from one patient to another, from 150 mg/day in chlorpromazine equivalents to as much as 1000 mg/day. Baldessarini et al (1988) comprehensively reviewed the published controlled trials of different antipsychotic dosages in the treatment of schizophrenia. They concluded that, in the acute illness, moderate doses (chlorpromazine 300–600 mg/day, or equivalent doses of other antipsychotics) are most effective. They also found evidence of a biphasic or inverted-U dose–response relationship, suggesting that if a patient does not respond to moderate doses of antipsychotics it is as logical to decrease the dose as to increase it.

The 'atypical' antipsychotics

Until the early 1980s the psychopharmacology of acute schizophrenia was dominated by the idea of the relevance of dopamine receptor blockade. This situation changed with the comeback of the 'atypical' antipsychotic clozapine. The concept of atypical antipsychotic drugs was originally derived from the idea that the antipsychotic and extrapyramidal effects of such drugs are linked, so that in order for a drug to be an effective antipsychotic it must necessarily produce extrapyramidal side-effects (EPSE) in patients. Clozapine produces minimal extrapyramidal effects. It was introduced in the 1970s but withdrawn from use in the USA, Great Britain and much of continental Europe after it was shown to be associated with agranulocytosis in a small percentage of cases. However, Kane et al (1988) reported a large multicentre trial in the USA concerning 268 patients with chronic schizophrenia who had failed to respond to at least three different antipsychotics and also to a 6-week trial of haloperidol 60 mg/day. In this situation clozapine (in doses of up to 900 mg/day) was found to be more effective than chlorpromazine in doses up to 1800 mg/day; in a 6-week double-blind comparison, 30% of clozapine versus 4% chlorpromazine patients achieved preset standards of improvement. Clozapine has a wider ranging pharmacological profile than most traditional antipychotics. It has a relatively modest affinity for D_1 and D_2 receptors and effects upon many other neurotransmitter receptors, including other dopamine receptor subtypes, serotonin and adrenergic receptors. Which, if any, of these effects is relevant is not established at the present time (see Seeman 2002). The disadvantages of clozapine are its very high cost, a tendency to cause hypersalivation, and that frequent neutrophil counts are necessary in order to detect incipient marrow depression and to prevent deaths from agranulocytosis.

Other 'atypical' antipsychotics have been introduced. Individual trials suggest they may have benefits compared with 'typical' drugs on overall efficacy, side-effects, compliance and various aspects of functioning. The vast majority of these trials have however been sponsored by the pharmaceutical industry, and Cochrane reviews show much less dramatic benefits (Cochrane Library 2002, Lawrie & McIntosh 2002). Further details are given in Chapter 15.

The adverse effects of the newer 'atypicals' are different from those of traditional antipsychotics, the main problems being obesity and undesirable cardiac effects. In short, the newer atypicals have a different profile of adverse effects. Allied to this, there is virtually no evidence that these drugs are effective in first-episode patients and relatively few studies demonstrating benefits in the medium to long-term. Nonetheless, the recent NICE guidelines (2002) advocated their use as first-line treatments in newly diagnosed patients. The management of the positive symptoms of acute episodes is however only one aspect of the management of schizophrenia, and it is not difficult to make the case that the reduction of relapse rates and the treatment of the negative symptoms of the defect state are at least as important.

Relapse reduction

Many studies have focused upon the role of antipsychotic drugs in reducing schizophrenic relapse. The benefits of both oral (Leff & Wing 1971) and depot medication (Hirsch et al 1973) have been clearly demonstrated. Reviewing 24 controlled studies, Davis (1976) concluded that the evidence for the efficacy of maintenance antipsychotic treatment was overwhelming. The drugs do not, however, abolish the tendency to relapse. In a 2-year follow-up study of oral antipsychotics versus placebo, the rate of schizophrenic relapse in placebo-treated patients was 80%, whereas that of patients on active antipsychotics was 48% (Hogarty et al 1974). Gilbert et al (1995) systematically reviewed studies comparing medication maintenance and withdrawal, and found an overall 37% reduction in relapses over an average of about 8 months in the continuation groups.

Although individual trials suggest that oral haloperidol and chlorpromazine continue to reduce relapses at 3 years (Cochrane Library 2002), there is no good reason to select one drug over another. Compliance is however a major problem. Patients with schizophrenia are often unreliable at taking tablets once their acute symptoms have subsided and they have left hospital. There are several reasons for this. They may not accept that they have been ill in the first place, and, even if they do, may not accept that there is any risk of the illness recurring. The drugs often cause akathisia and other unpleasant side-effects which are more obvious than their antipsychotic effect. For these reasons 'depot' preparations capable of producing adequate serum levels when administered at intervals of 2 weeks or more have been developed. The introduction of these injectable depot preparations over thirty years ago was hailed as a great advance, and they are now widely used, often with special clinics and elaborate follow-up arrangements to ensure that patients do not miss their regular injection every 2, 3 or 4 weeks. They are probably a significant advance, but it is important not to forget that no trial comparing long-term relapse rates on daily tablets and fortnightly injections has demonstrated any clear advantage for the latter. For example, Hogarty et al (1979) conducted a further study comparing maintenance prophylaxis with oral and with depot antipsychotics. There was no difference between the two groups, and the 2-year relapse rate remained substantial. These trials have, however, generally been so small that one cannot rule out a clinically significant advantage (Cochrane Library 2002).

There is, however, consistent evidence that reducing or stopping medication, even after a prolonged period of maintenance and well-being, is a risk for relapse. Concern about the extrapyramidal side-effects of antipsychotics led to several attempts to maintain chronic patients on very small doses of antipsychotics, or to give these drugs only at the first sign of impending relapse. The results have been disappointing. Johnson et al (1987), for example, found that if chronic schizophrenics who were well controlled on relatively low doses of Flupentixol (up to 40 mg i.m. fortnightly) were transferred double-blind to half that dose, their relapse rate over the next 3 years was significantly increased. Although Baldessarini et al (1988) found that quite low doses (chlorpromazine 50–100 mg/day or equivalent) provide adequate maintenance therapy in about 50% of patients, subsequent systematic reviews of

RCTs have shown that relapse rates are lower on doses of 200–500 mg (Barbui et al 1996) or 166–375 mg (Bollini et al 1994). Higher doses than this merely increase the side-effect burden.

Managing EPSE

Because they also affect the dopamine receptors of the nigrostriatal system, all conventional antipsychotics tend to produce troublesome extrapyramidal side-effects (EPSE). For this reason some clinicians prescribe antiparkinsonian drugs routinely whenever they want to use more than a small dose of an antipsychotic. This is not good practice, for a variety of reasons. Akathisia and parkinsonism are the most common and troublesome EPSE, and there is little evidence that the routine prescribing of antiparkinsonian drugs reduces them to any worthwhile extent. There is also some evidence that the use of these drugs may impair the efficacy of antipsychotics, particularly in controlling positive symptoms, and increase the incidence of tardive dyskinesia; and because they have mild stimulant properties some patients abuse them or become dependent. What trial evidence there is suggests that benzodiazepines may be the best treatment for akathisia (Cochrane Library 2002). In general, therefore, antiparkinsonian drugs should only be used if the patient actually develops an acute dystonia or troublesome parkinsonism and it is not feasible to reduce the dose of antipsychotic. And even if this is necessary, and successful, an attempt should be made to withdraw the antiparkinsonian agent after a couple of months because it will often be possible to do so without the extrapyramidal symptoms returning.

The case for giving antipsychotic drugs to chronic schizophrenics year in, year out is less compelling than the case for using them during acute episodes or exacerbations — about 20% of patients will not have further episodes, and a similar percentage will relapse regardless. The disadvantages of chronic medication are also substantial. Many patients are seriously distressed by akathisia or rigidity, and others who are fortunate enough not to suffer in this way are understandably reluctant to continue 'taking drugs' indefinitely. There is also the long-term risk of tardive dyskinesia (TD) to consider; which, even though the patient may be unaware of it, is often all too obvious to the general public. The incidence of TD may be as high as 5% per year on medication, but such figures can give a distorted idea of the frequency as some cases remit spontaneously. TD at least partially reflects the underlying brain disruption in schizophrenia. Certainly, it is well established that indistinguishable involuntary movements are not uncommon in elderly schizophrenics who have never received antipsychotics of any kind (for example, see Owens et al 1982) and that persistent chewing movements and other dyskinesias were observed in chronic schizophrenics long before antipsychotics existed (Farran-Ridge 1926). This interaction may explain why TD is so difficult to treat — despite several trials of several different interventions, the only (possibly) effective approach is to reduce the dose of antipsychotic (Cochrane Library 2002).

On the other hand, it is also important to realise that stopping patients' maintenance medication may, paradoxically, result in their receiving an increased rather than a decreased total dose over the next year or two, because they may relapse and then require a substantially larger dose to bring their hallucinations or other symptoms back under control (Johnson et al 1983). Only rarely is it appropriate to give patients two or more different antipsychotics simultaneously. Sometimes there are good reasons for temporarily increasing the effective dose in a patient on an injectable depot preparation by giving a second drug orally as well; and some patients cannot tolerate an adequate dose of one drug because of its hypotensive or sedative effects, or an adequate dose of another because of its extrapyramidal effects, but can tolerate a mixture of the two in lower doses. Most polypharmacy however, simply a public display of pharmacological ignorance.

Negative symptoms

Clear benefits of antipsychotic medication have been demonstrated in the treatment of acute episodes and in the reduction of relapse rates, but there is no drug treatment that can reliably be recommended as relieving negative symptoms in the same way that antipsychotic agents relieve positive symptoms. The effect of these drugs on negative symptoms is uncertain. Controlled trials have yielded conflicting evidence; traditional antipsychotics have been found to improve, to have no effect upon, or to exacerbate negative symptoms. The same is true of both dopamine agonists and antidepressants.

There may be, however, slightly more encouraging results from RCTs of the 'atypicals', in particular clozapine and amisulpiride. Clozapine reduced negative symptoms in the original treatment resistance study (Kane et al 1988), and both drugs appear to do so in general (Cochrane Library 2002). It is important to note however that the four small clozapine trials included in the Cochrane review found greater benefits than typical drugs; the improvements may therefore have been attributable to reductions in negative symptoms secondary to positive symptoms or EPSE, rather than primary negative symptoms. Similarly, the four amisulpiride trials were only placebo controlled, such that the apparent benefits may have been due to reductions in positive or depressive symptoms. Storosum et al (2002) have however reviewed these trials from this perspective and found that these explanations are unlikely, although they noted a relatively high placebo response rate and suggest that there may be both enduring and non-enduring primary negative symptoms.

Depressive symptoms

Tricyclic and other antidepressants are frequently given to schizophrenics in an attempt to relieve their associated depressive symptoms. The apathy and flattening of affect of the schizophrenic defect state can resemble depression but, in addition to this, the occurrence of depressive symptoms in schizophrenic patients when they are not actively psychotic (in what is sometimes called secondary or post-psychotic depression) has increasingly been recognised (McGlashan & Carpenter 1976). The value of adjunctive antidepressant treatment both on an acute (Siris et al 1987) and on a maintenance basis (Siris et al 1994) has been demonstrated, although the trials may have overestimated the therapeutic benefits (Cochrane Library 2002).

Evidence-based prescribing

The results of these clinical trials provide the basis of a rational prescribing policy (see Box 19.7). Acute schizophrenic illnesses should almost invariably be treated with antipsychotic agents, and it is probably wise to try to keep most patients on a maintenance dose for at least a year or two thereafter, even if their recovery is complete and rapid. With so many similar preparations to choose

> **Box 19.7 An evidence-based prescribing policy for schizophrenia**
>
> *Acute episode*
> Chlorpromazine equivalents 300–600 mg per day orally
> — If acute dystonia, administer i.v. anticholinergic
> — If akathisia, reduce antipsychotic dose / prescribe concurrent oral benzodiazepine
> — If parkinsonism, reduce antipsychotic dose / prescribe concurrent oral anticholinergic
> If intolerant of side-effects, change to 'newer' (atypical) drug
>
> *Maintenance*
> Oral / i.m. antipsychotic 150–500 mg chlorpromazine equivalents per day for up to 2 years
>
> *Treatment resistance*
> Change to clozapine
>
> *Comorbid depression*
> Concurrent antidepressants

from, the choice of drug is largely a matter of personal preference and relative costs. Many psychiatrists will use chlorpromazine in the acute phase, and, if the patient is overactive or frightened, its sedative effects are valuable. However, the hypotensive effects of chlorpromazine (and of thioridazine) may be dangerous in the elderly or in patients with a history of heart disease, and in them a drug like trifluoperazine may be preferable (see Ch. 15). Usually the drug can be given orally, but intramuscular injection (or liquid medication) may be necessary initially if the patient is aggressive, refusing to take tablets, or if there are doubts about compliance.

If EPSE are a particular problem, and not improved by reducing antipsychotic dosage, it probably makes sense to switch to a new 'atypical' drug. Some of these drugs may yet prove to have a role in managing treatment-resistant patients, but most of the trials to date have included both resistant and intolerant patients. Clozapine remains the only proven drug treatment in resistant cases, but there are suggestions that both ECT and certain psychological approaches may be valuable.

ECT

Although antipsychotics have been central to treatment of acute schizophrenia for the past 40 years, ECT has been extensively used in some centres, though less so now than in the past. In May's (1968) pivotal trial, patients treated with ECT fared significantly better than those who only received psychotherapy, though less well than those receiving phenothiazines. Subsequent trials, including those comparing both real and dummy ECT under double-blind conditions, found it to have genuinely beneficial effects in acute schizophrenia, though these are no longer detectable 3–6 months later (Cochrane Library 2002). For this reason the principal indication for using ECT in the treatment of schizophrenia nowadays is for severe schizoaffective illnesses (see below). The statement that ECT has value in the treatment of cases of catatonic stupor tends to be passed down in editions of textbooks over the decades. The condition is so vanishingly rare that there is little evidence one way or another, but a placebo-controlled trial in the 1950s showed no advantage of active treatment. However, a recent large trial of 114 patients with treatment-resistant schizophrenia, defined in the same way as by Kane et al (1988), found that ECT and flupentixol led to remission in 58 cases, and that the combination of weekly and then fortnightly continuation ECT with flupentixol kept the vast majority well (Chanpattana et al 1999). The study requires replication, and the treatment may not be acceptable to many patients, but it does at least suggest a therapeutic option in patients who do not respond to or cannot tolerate clozapine.

Social and psychological measures

Although, in the short run, antipsychotics have a much more dramatic effect on the symptoms of schizophrenia than any other therapeutic measure, there is a great deal more to the treatment of the disorder than prescribing antipsychotic agents. There is abundant evidence that the course of schizophrenic illnesses and the resulting social handicaps can be affected, for good or ill, by the patient's social environment, and it has been known for thirty years that many of the most obvious behavioural abnormalities of chronic schizophrenics, like posturing and talking to themselves, are not intrinsic or inevitable, but are to a considerable extent the product of a monotonous, unstimulating environment. This was well illustrated by Wing & Brown's (1961) comparison of three mental hospitals in southern England. In their hospital C, patients had few if any personal possessions, little liberty, spent much of the time unoccupied in the wards, and were generally treated as 'inmates'; whereas in hospital A they had their own clothes and other personal possessions, spent most of the day actively employed and generally lived as free and normal a life as possible. A third hospital, B, was intermediate. The incidence of social withdrawal (underactivity, lack of conversation, neglect of hygiene and personal appearance) and socially embarrassing behaviour (incontinence, mannerisms, purposeless overactivity, threats of violence, talking to self) was higher in hospital C than it was in A (B was intermediate in all respects) — despite the fact that these patients' initial type and severity of illness appeared to have been the same, and there were no important differences in the prescribing and discharge policies of the two hospitals.

Too much stimulation, or stimulation of the wrong kind, can also be harmful. There is, for example, the evidence that schizophrenic illnesses may be precipitated by events in the previous few weeks, pleasant and unpleasant, which disrupt the subject's normal lifestyle (Brown & Birley 1968). There is also the evidence that returning to live with a critical or hostile relative after a schizophrenic illness greatly increases the relapse rate over the next 12 months (Brown et al 1972). The overall management of schizophrenia is based, therefore, on an attempt to avoid both extremes. To this end, attempts are made to get the patient out of hospital and into an occupation and a domestic setting in which they have some real but limited responsibilities, in which they have a daily routine which is ordered and predictable without being too monotonous, and in which they are protected from emotional demands they cannot meet. This is often easier said than done.

Service organisation

For the last forty years, partly because of the realisation that mental hospitals themselves could have detrimental effects on their patients if their stay was prolonged, and partly for straightforward financial reasons, intensive efforts have been made to discharge schizophrenics as soon as their psychotic symptoms have resolved and to keep them 'in the community' as much as possible thereafter. To be successful, or for the patient to be better off, such a policy requires the provision of a range of hostels, day centres, 'half-way houses' and occupational placements in the community. Unfortunately, these facilities have not yet materialised in anything like adequate numbers. For this reason many psychiatrists (though not hospital managers) are increasingly questioning whether early discharge is always in the patient's interests, and whether mental hospitals have not been too eager to discard their traditional 'asylum' role. A back bedroom can be just as deprived and harmful an environment as a back ward, and a park bench even more so. There is in fact some evidence that these 'innovations' were associated with an overall worsening of outcome, between 1981 and 1996, in a representative sample of patients in Nithsdale, Scotland (Kelly et al 1998), although wider socio-economic changes are an alternative explanation.

Various approaches to organizing community services have been implemented and examined over that time. The principal two — case management or the care programme approach (CPA) and assertive community treatment (ACT) — seem to have surprisingly different effects (at least as evaluated in RCTs). CPA mainly involves planning community management prior to discharge, with the involvement of patients and all their carers, so that each professional involved has a specific remit. One of the key goals of CPA is to maintain service contact with patients, which it certainly does, but at the price of prolonging hospital stays and increasing readmissions without any obvious gains in clinical outcome (Cochrane Library 2002). CPA was politically enforced in England & Wales in the 1990s and probably just put further pressure on already stretched services. ACT, on the other hand, involves identifying the most appropriate keyworker to co-ordinate a therapeutic package, with specific treatments being provided by particular staff. ACT certainly maintains patient contact better than standard care, and probably also reduces readmissions and their duration, and homelessness, while increasing employment and independent living (Cochrane Library 2002). The vast majority of the trials were however conducted in the USA, and studies which found the most impressive results were conducted on the first trenche of patients to be de-institutionalised — who presumably had the best prognoses. These studies also usually have ACT teams with relatively high staff:patient ratios, although it appears that this is less important than the frequency and aims of the patient contact. Both of these models of service delivery are compatible with the community mental health teams (CMHTs) commonly employed in the UK and elsewhere, which in themselves do little more than improve patient and carer satisfaction (Cochrane Library 2002). The obvious danger is that CMHTs attempting to provide ACT 'on the cheap' can end up providing something more akin to the CPA. On the other hand, Ziguras et al (2002) systematically reviewed both RCTs and non-randomised controlled trials and found positive effects of the CPA on many aspects of patient functioning, although the improvements were still better for ACT. It is a moot point as to whether the RCTs' higher internal validity or the controlled trials' possibly greater external validity should guide service planners. However, no study has as yet randomised or otherwise allocated treatment providers (rather than patients) to different approaches, in an attempt to control for the likely 'therapeutic zeal' in a new or experimental service that would be less likely to be maintained in long-term routine clinical practice.

Rehabilitation

Some patients have a home and a job to return to, or succeed in obtaining accommodation and employment without the aid of any formal rehabilitative measures. Most are too badly handicapped by the effects of illness on their drive, initiative and demeanour, by the social stigma of having been mentally ill, and often too by their previous lack of education and marketable skills, to be capable of obtaining a job without assistance. In the past it was one of the primary functions of rehabilitation programmes to help people who had schizophrenia to obtain suitable paid employment. However, this has become increasingly difficult, mainly because fundamental industrial changes have resulted in a substantial reduction in the need for unskilled or semiskilled workers. As a result, rehabilitation programmes are increasingly geared to help patients with defect states or recurring psychotic episodes to cook and shop for themselves, to obtain temporary or unpaid employment and to use their leisure time productively.

It remains possible, however, to train some patients for full-time paid employment, but it is clear that supported employment is superior to pre-vocational training (Crowther et al 2001). Sheltered workshops and work skills training have at most temporary benefits and do not increase the likelihood of gaining competitive employment. Supported employment places patients directly into competitive jobs, with support from trained 'job coaches', and five American RCTs have shown that it leads to paid employment in about a third of trial participants. There is clearly a need to develop and evaluate such programmes outside the USA. Social skills and cognitive abilities tend to predict successful vocational rehabilitation, and adding these elements into these treatments may enhance their efficacy.

Some people with schizophrenia have become homeless by the time they are first admitted to hospital; others become so after a series of further relapses and readmissions. Accommodation has to be found for most such patients if they are ever to leave hospital, and many of them are unable to cope in ordinary rented accommodation even if landlords can be persuaded to take them. Other types of accommodation geared to their needs have to be provided. In the past, hostels were often provided by psychiatric hospitals themselves, either on the hospital site or elsewhere, and supervised to varying extents by nurses. Now hostels, group homes, flats and bed-sitters reserved for former psychiatric patients tend to be provided by local authority social work departments and voluntary organisations. The amount and quality of supervision provided is very variable, and not all of it is supportive of the proven elements of psychiatric management, but the greater quantity and variety of protected housing available increases the likelihood that individual patients will eventually find a suitable niche. It is, however, deeply regrettable that the provision of suitable supported accommodation remains insufficient.

Family treatments

Discharging patients from hospital when adequate community facilities are not available may also place a heavy burden on relatives, a burden which service providers may do little to relieve. A particular difficulty sometimes arises when the patient is living with a relative, usually a spouse or parent, who is willing to have him back, but it becomes clear while the patient is in hospital that this relative cannot accept and adapt to the change that has come over the patient and remains angry, frightened and critical. There are various ways of trying to deal with this potentially hazardous situation. It may be possible to arrange for the patient to move into a hostel instead of returning home; but suitable accommodation is not always available, and even if it is it may be impossible

to persuade either the patient or the relative that this is preferable to returning home. Indeed, it is often the mothers who are most critical of their schizophrenic son's or daughter's behaviour who are least willing to be parted from them. An alternative strategy in such circumstance is to mitigate the ill-effects of the relative's emotional involvement by reducing the time the two spend in one another's company. A full-time job is, of course, the best way of doing this, but, if this is impossible, regular attendance at a day hospital or day centre of some kind may achieve the same ends.

A further preventive strategy is to try to alter the attitudes and behaviour of the relatives, and various forms of family therapy to this end have been developed in the last two decades. Several small-scale but important clinical trials have now been reported. In the first, 24 schizophrenics who were all living in a 'high expressed emotion' environment, and therefore at high risk of relapse, were randomly allocated either to routine outpatient care or to receive a special package of social interventions consisting of factual talks to their relatives about schizophrenia, fortnightly group meetings for the relatives designed to help them share experience, and regular family therapy sessions in the patient's home designed to lower expressed emotion and face-to-face contact (Leff et al 1982). All 24 patients received depot antipsychotics throughout. After 9 months the relapse rate was 50% in the controls but only 9% in the treatment group, and the only patients in the treatment group to relapse were the two in whom no reduction in expressed emotion (EE) or face-to-face contact was achieved. This trial therefore adds to the evidence that high expressed emotion can provoke relapse and that reduced face-to-face contact is protective. It does not, of course, reveal which elements of the treatment package were most important.

There are now at least 25 trials of various family interventions (and several systematic reviews of them). Each has included education about the illness, but usually combined with one or more approaches described as crisis management, problem solving or family therapy. There is no doubt that these all tend to reduce relapse rates, and there is good agreement that longer treatment is more likely to be successful (Cochrane Library 2002, Pitschel-Walz et al 2001). The mode of action remains unclear however. There is no good evidence that any one therapeutic model is better than another, and thus education may be the key component. Medication compliance may be improved, and the general support given may be reassuring, but the ability of a family to 'cope' with patients does not seem to be affected (Cochrane Library 2002). Reducing EE does not appear to be crucial; indeed, provided the patient intervention is comprehensive, the family need not necessarily be involved (Pitschel-Walz et al 2001).

These uncertainties, and the time-consuming nature of the treatment, may explain why such a successful intervention is rarely implemented in clinical practice. Family interventions can however be successfully delivered in a group setting, which may provide an additional source of information and reassurance. What effectiveness studies there are suggest that relatives feel they benefit most from education and support. Nonetheless, these approaches are by definition not of any value to the many patients who no longer have contact with their families or do not wish them to be involved in their treatment.

Education

Information about the illness and its management can of course be provided to patients themselves. The early trials, of what has sometimes been called psycho-education (sic), tended to provide other interventions as well, such that the specific effects of education were difficult to determine. More recent studies have focused on education, usually given didactically to groups of both patients and families. Even relatively brief programmes, of ten sessions or less, seem to reduce relapse rates over the subsequent 9–18 months, with an effect (number needed to treat, NNT 12) comparable to that of lengthier treatment (NNT 9) and that of family interventions (NNT 7, Cochrane Library 2002). The 95% confidence intervals of these NNTs overlap, meaning that there may be no substantial difference in their effects on relapse. Education also appears to improve global functioning and, perhaps surprisingly, to reduce relatives' expressed emotion, but these results are derived from two or three small studies. Medication compliance may be improved, but behavioural techniques appear to be more successful in this regard (see below and Lawrie & McIntosh 2002).

The clinical 'bottom-line' is that a relatively brief series of educational sessions may be as good as any psychosocial intervention in terms of reducing relapse rates. Patients and their families may however wish a more flexible system that they can use at times of particular difficulty. Regardless, it should be borne in mind that education could potentially have undesirable effects, perhaps particularly in newly diagnosed patients hearing about the likelihood of poor outcomes, just as family interventions can actually increase EE in low EE families.

Psychotherapy

Some of the benefits of these interventions may be attributable to 'supportive psychotherapy', but it is clear that anything resembling psychoanalysis is at best worthless and at worst positively harmful in schizophrenia. The results of May's (1968) trial in California indicated quite unequivocally that psychodynamic psychotherapy was valueless in the active phase of the illness. The only detectable effects, whether psychotherapy was given alone or in combination with a phenothiazine, were on the duration and cost of hospital treatment, both of which were substantially *increased*.

The effect of psychoanalytically oriented social casework on patients in their postpsychotic, posthospital phase of the illness were explored in a large American trial (Goldberg et al 1977). Four hundred newly discharged schizophrenics were randomly allocated to one of four groups and followed up for 2 years. The first group received maintenance chlorpromazine plus what the authors called 'major role therapy' (a combination of intensive psychoanalytically oriented social casework and vocational rehabilitation); a second group received maintenance chlorpromazine but only minimal contacts with a social worker; a third group received placebo tablets and 'major role therapy'; and a fourth group received placebo tablets and minimal social contacts. As expected, the relapse rate was much lower in patients on maintenance chlorpromazine than in those on placebo (48% versus 80%). Overall, 'major role therapy' had no effect on the relapse rate. But more detailed analysis showed that in patients who might have been expected to have a good prognosis the relapse rate was reduced by this treatment, and in those who might have been expected to have a relatively poor prognosis the relapse rate was increased. In other words, some patients benefited but others were harmed, and the two tended to cancel each other out. What the mechanism of harm is we can only speculate, but it is easy to imagine how an intensive relationship with a keen social worker

might create something akin to a 'high expressed emotion' situation. The moral is clear. Emotional pressures, including those from well-meaning psychotherapeutic interventions, may be positively harmful to those who have recently had a schizophrenic illness, and so should only be offered if it is quite clear that the patients are capable of responding. Emotional withdrawal may be a valuable self-protective strategy as well as a symptom.

Behavioural and cognitive interventions

As trials of the efficacy of psychotherapy have demonstrated in other settings, behavioural and cognitive approaches to psychosis tend to be much more valuable in general. Probably the first technique to be used and evaluated was the *token economy*, in which a desired behavioural change was fostered by giving tokens as rewards for designated desirable behaviours. The tokens could be exchanged for cigarettes, food etc. Token economy programmes were widespread in the 1970s but became restricted to long-stay wards, where socially appropriate behaviours were rewarded in long-stay patients who were preparing to be transferred to the community. They were regarded as effective in reducing some psychotic behaviours, and improving personal care and work capabilities in hospital, but early controlled trials did not adequately control for medication effects and lacked community follow-up data. Despite this, it is not clear why the treatment fell out of favour, particularly as a small number of RCTs do suggest the token economy may be one of the few effective treatments of negative symptoms (Cochrane Library 2002).

As enthusiasm for psychotherapy and the token economy as treatments for schizophrenia waned, interest developed in *social skills training*. This involves various combinations of instruction, modelling, rehearsal, feedback and homework, usually with the main aim of improving communication skills to enhance access to resources and reduce stresses. Early controlled studies suggested benefits in reducing relapse rates, but often included other therapeutic elements. A recent systematic review and meta-analysis of ten RCTs between 1983 and 1998 found no such benefit at 1 year, but some effect at 2 years into treatment (Pilling et al 2002).

Other active therapies, in particular *cognitive behavioural therapy* (CBT), seem to offer greater benefits with less input. CBT involves challenging key beliefs, problem solving and coping enhancement, and has been enthusiastically advocated for patients with schizophrenia for almost a decade. Early RCTs suggested relapse rates were reduced but suffered from the perennial problems of not controlling for therapist time, non-blind outcome raters and not being able to identify which elements of the treatment were effective (see Cochrane Library 2002). Two recent studies merit particular mention. Sensky et al (2000) randomised 90 patients, who had at most partially responded to chlorpromazine, to an equal amount of manualised CBT or 'empathic, non-directive' befriending. Blind raters assessed positive and negative symptom severity at baseline, treatment termination and after 9 months follow-up. Both treatments appeared effective on both measures at the end of treatment, but the group treated with CBT showed further improvements at follow-up whereas the befriended group lost some of their earlier gains. This well-conducted trial demonstrates that CBT may be effective for treatment resistance and negative symptoms, but used experienced therapists to provide lengthy and intensive treatment. It is not likely that this could be made available for anything more than a fraction of the patients with schizophrenia in most health services. Turkington et al (2002) therefore conducted a pragmatic trial of brief CBT given by newly trained psychiatric nurses to a representative sample of patients in secondary care. The intervention led to a greater improvement in overall symptoms, insight and depression, and fewer treatment drop-outs, than standard care. It remains to be seen whether this would hold true in treatment-resistant patients, who may require more skilled treatment. CBT may prove to be the single most useful psychosocial intervention for schizophrenia, but further evaluation of its essential components and practicality is required before it should be advocated for routine use.

CBT techniques have been adapted and integrated with motivational interviewing principles for patients with poor medication compliance or substance abuse comorbidity. These are both very common clinical problems which worsen overall outcome. Psychiatrists tend to underestimate their prevalence, which may be as high as 50%, and have almost no treatments of proven efficacy to deal with them. There are suggestions from systematic reviews that ACT, family interventions and education may increase the amount of medication patients say they take (Cochrane Library 2002). This is however an obviously unreliable outcome measure (albeit perhaps the most practical one), and as a rule complex interventions including reminders and rewards are more effective than education alone in general medical patients (Cochrane Library 2002). A few preliminary trials suggest this holds true in schizophrenia, although focused treatments, such as *compliance therapy*, show promise (Lawrie & McIntosh 2002). Similarly, integrated mental health and substance abuse therapeutic programmes or what might be called 'comorbid substance abuse therapy' may reduce substance abuse — although there is a notable discrepancy between open and controlled versus randomised trials (Cochrane Library 2002). It is also far from clear that improving compliance or reducing abuse necessarily leads to improved outcomes. Clearly, much more work on these neglected aspects of clinical care is required.

Cognitive remediation is a relatively new and developing treatment for the increasingly recognised cognitive deficits in patients with schizophrenia. Typically, patients receive guided practice on tests of attention, memory and/or higher functions such as planning. A number of controlled studies suggest, not surprisingly given patients' preserved ability to learn, that performance improves with practice. However, these studies and systematic reviews of the few available RCTs (Cochrane Library 2002, Pilling et al 2002) suggest this does not generalise to other tasks, let alone to more clinically relevant measures. Future studies might more profitably address the value of compensatory strategies such as simple diary keeping and other memory aids.

Evidence-based principles of psychosocial management

In summary, the best available evidence suggests that the management of schizophrenia after discharge from hospital is best accomplished through assertive community treatment (ACT) in general and using additional therapies as indicated (see Box 19.8). Illness education and family treatments appear to be more or less equally effective at reducing relapse rates and can be initiated during periods of inpatient care. Education provided routinely to patients, and their carers when requested, may be the most cost-effective general approach. Given financial constraints, CBT may be best reserved for treatment-resistant patients who can use it. If patients

---

> **Box 19.8 Evidence-based principles of psychosocial interventions for schizophrenia**
>
> 1. ACT is preferable to CPA
> 2. Supported employment is better than pre-vocational training
> 3. Education may be as effective as other PSI for reducing relapse rates
> 4. Psychodynamic psychotherapy is of no general value
> 5. Token economy may reduce negative symptoms (in restricted ward settings)
> 6. Social skills training improves communication abilities after 2 years
> 7. CBT may reduce positive and negative symptoms and may be effective in treatment resistance
> 8. Cognitive remediation by guided task practice is ineffective
>
> ACT, assertive community treatment; CBT, cognitive behavioural therapy; CPA, care programme approach; PSI, psychosocial interventions

have a realistic wish to obtain paid employment, sheltered employment schemes are clearly preferable to pre-vocational training. Dynamic psychotherapies appear to have no demonstrable place in the management of schizophrenia, although some patients still want them and some practitioners (generally in the private sector) are prepared to provide them.

As the number and quality of RCTs evaluating these interventions increases, it is more difficult to sustain the view that their benefits are simply attributable to enhanced medication compliance and non-specific support. More importantly, we need to know whether, for example, optimised antipsychotic regimens and psychosocial therapies are complementary, if clozapine and CBT have additive effects in resistant patients or on negative symptoms, etc. A particularly comprehensive systematic review and meta-analysis has suggested that generic drug and non-drug treatments do indeed have additive effects, particularly in chronic patients (Mojtabai et al 1998). The methods and results of that review can be criticised on several grounds — as it was based on controlled trials, did not find any specific effects of different treatments, and there was some evidence of publication bias — but clinicians and patients are probably right to want to use both approaches. Whatever else, we must now pay far more attention to the views and wishes of patients and their families than in the past, and they clearly want and appreciate time being spent with them. That time should be used to provide treatments in line with the best available evidence. Indeed, the careful implementation and evaluation of this is likely to be the best way of refining the delivery of the most effective therapies in an integrated clinical service.

Prevention

We have already discussed many aspects of secondary and tertiary prevention, but not what is sometimes called 'early intervention'. In one of the first studies of 'relapse prevention', Jolley et al (1990) attempted to maintain schizophrenic outpatients in stable remission off all medication, but to ensure that they received oral haloperidol at the first signs of relapse by warning both patients and their relatives what those signs were likely to be and providing both monthly follow-up appointments and a 24-hour telephone contact. Unfortunately, the experiment failed, partly because only 50% of the relapses were preceded by any prodromal symptoms at all; and, although the drug-free patients had fewer extrapyramidal symptoms than their controls, this was not accompanied by any improvement in social functioning. Subsequent studies have rarely taken such an ambitious approach, usually comparing the effects of various doses or frequencies of medication with or without psychosocial approaches. It does appear to be possible to reduce relapse rates on low dose or intermittent medication with sufficiently frequent relapse education and monitoring, perhaps particularly in first-episode rather than chronic patients, but much more evaluation of such interventions is required.

Given the obvious limitations of our currently available treatments for schizophrenia, primary prevention or early intervention in the first episode (if successful) are extremely desirable goals. This has been reinforced by several recent studies suggesting that the duration of untreated psychosis (DUP) prior to initiating treatment is associated with a variety of markers of a poor outcome. Ironically, however, the first demonstration of such an effect does not stand up to close examination. Johnstone et al (1986) randomised 120 first-episode patients, about to be discharged, to maintenance antipsychotics or placebo. Although the treatment reduced relapse rates at 2 years, the most important determinant was a year or more of untreated psychosis prior to admission — but this did not hold if the DUP was set at 3 months or 6 months. None of the subsequent studies suggesting the importance of DUP have been conducted in the context of a trial, and the association of a long DUP with a poor outcome may simply reflect confounding due to the well-recognised tendency for illnesses with a gradual rather than acute onset to be more severe. Indeed, the only study to directly control for premorbid characteristics and illness severity found no significant DUP effect (Verdoux et al 2001), although it remains possible that these are all on the same causal chain.

True prevention remains the ultimate goal. The literature thus far is, however, enthusiastic and descriptive rather than experimental, with one exception. Building upon their innovative service for young adults presenting with psychotic symptoms in Melbourne, McGorry et al (2002) randomised 59 patients to 'needs-based' supportive psychotherapy and case management with or without low-dose risperidone and CBT for 6 months. At the end of treatment, 3 (10%) of those receiving risperidone and CBT had developed psychosis as compared with 10/28 (i.e. c. 30%) who did not. However, a further 3 people in the experimental treatment arm went on to develop psychosis in the following 6 months, rendering the difference non-significant.

Whether this represents incidence reduction or delayed onset remains to be seen and requires replication. Similar trials are ongoing in England and The Netherlands, and results are awaited. It has to be said however that the conversion rate to psychosis in Australia is substantially higher than preliminary results suggest elsewhere and has been recorded in Germany (Klosterkotter et al 2001) and Scotland (Miller et al 2001). Why this may be is uncertain, but it is important that we do not let our enthusiasm for prevention of this most disabling disorder lead us to instigate incompletely evaluated new treatments. Patients with schizophrenia have all too often been let down by overenthusiastic advocates of experimental treatments in the past. After all, in any financially constrained service, every resource consumed on exciting innovations is one that could have been spent on interventions with a more rigorous evidence-base.

RELATED DISORDERS

Disorders 'related' to schizophrenia include a variety of conditions, described by a wide range of terms, which share some of the features of schizophrenia, but not all. In general they tend to be characterised by psychotic symptoms but they do not have the chronicity, the lack of a mood-related component, or perhaps the poor prognosis. As noted above, the range of disorders given the diagnosis of schizophrenia has at times been very wide, and whether or not a psychotic episode will fulfil criteria for schizophrenia depends very much upon the operational definition used. Definitions like that in DSM-IV, in which a 6-month duration is obligatory, exclude many first-episode cases, and cases with a duration of at least 1 month and less than 6 months would be classed as 'schizophreniform' disorder (APA 1994). This is the most obviously arbitrary and probably invalid by-product of operational definitions in this area (and not to be confused with the term 'schizophrenia-like' disorder in ICD-10 (WHO 1992) to refer to conditions with features of schizophrenia but which are due to brain damage and dysfunction or to systemic physical disease). The other schizophrenia-related disorders in these classifications which are discussed below have a much longer pedigree and stronger evidence of distinctive characteristics.

Persistent delusional disorder

Persistent delusional disorder (PDD) is characterised by one or more non-bizarre delusions or a delusional system. Formerly known as 'paranoia' or 'paranoid psychosis', Kahlbaum and Kraepelin distinguished it from schizophrenia, as do contemporary classifications, although Bleuler and Schneider appear to have viewed them as subtypes of schizophrenia with a good prognosis. Both ICD-10 (WHO 1992) and DSM-IV (APA 1994) stress the importance of excluding subcultural beliefs and features of schizophrenia, depression or organic brain disease. However, the duration criterion for ICD-10 is 3 months, while that for DSM-IV is only 1 month, and ICD-10 recommends delusions of less than 3 months duration should be coded as an 'acute and transient psychotic disorder' (see below). Paraphrenia is included as a persistent delusional disorder in ICD-10, but as schizophrenia in DSM-IV (in which patients over the age of 40 are regarded as having paraphrenia and those over 60 as having late paraphrenia). However, most patients in these age groups who have delusions usually also have hallucinations and therefore a diagnosis of schizophrenia (see Ch. 26).

Subtypes

Five subtypes of delusional disorder are described in DSM-IV, according to the predominant delusional theme (see Table 19.8). ICD-10 also includes the categories of self-referential and litigious, which are incorporated into the persecutory subtype in DSM-IV. The latter is the classical and probably the most common form of PDD. It, and the jealous variant, are often said to be most likely to be associated with dangerous behaviour. This is however a recognised risk of other types if patients become angry or frustrated with the attention or lack of it that they are receiving.

The hypochondriacal or somatic subtype merits particular consideration, both because of its number and variety of synonyms

Table 19.8	Subtypes of delusional disorder	
Subtype	Related terms	Relative frequency*
Persecutory	Self-referential	39/71
	Litigious (querulous paranoia)	
Grandiose	Monosymptomatic	2/71
Hypochondrial (somatic)	hypochondriacal psychosis	4/71
	Delusional dysmorphophobia	16/71
Jealous	Morbid jealousy	
	Othello 'syndrome'	
	Delusional jealousy	
Erotomanic	De Clerambault's 'syndrome'	2/71
* From Opjordsmoen (1988)		

and because it has been said in the past (probably incorrectly) to specifically respond to pimozide (Munro 1988). Munro popularised the term monosymptomatic hypochondriacal psychosis and in a case series of 50 patients described three main types of delusion:

- olfactory (in which the patient complained of extreme halitosis or body odour);
- infestation (insect, worms or foreign bodies under the skin);
- dysmorphic delusions (of ugliness or mis-shapenness).

Patients with these disorders typically present to physicians, requesting cosmetic surgery or treatment which is rarely beneficial. Munro's patients were in a wide age range, but Trabert (1995) described a generally older age of onset in a review of 1223 case reports of delusional infestation. Rather confusingly, monosymptomatic hypochondriacal psychosis of the dysmorphic type is sometimes referred to as delusional dysmorphophobia, whereas non-delusional dysmorphophobia or body dysmorphic disorder is essentially a variant of hypochondriasis. The borderline between overvalued ideas and delusions in these areas is discussed in Chapter 13.

It is likely that dysmorphic ideas are on a continuum with dysmorphic delusions, as is increasingly recognised for most psychotic phenomena. These difficulties are worsened when psychiatrists loosely use terminology such as 'Othello syndrome' and de Clerambault's syndrome (see Table 19.8) when they are actually referring to abnormal ideas of specific content. It should not be forgotten that most such ideas when seen in clinical practice do indeed present as part of a syndrome — but that syndrome is schizophrenia, depression, or indeed an organic disorder. The same is equally true of the 'delusional misidentification syndromes' such as Capgras and Fregole.

Epidemiology and aetiology

There are no population surveys of the prevalence of delusional disorder. The best available evidence is therefore from reviews of hospital admission data (Kendler 1982) or large case series (Opjordsmoen 1988). The prevalence of PDD in the general population is estimated to be about 0.03%, with no apparent sex difference. Delusional jealousy (where it is in fact the ideas of infidelity that are delusional) is probably more common in men

and erotomania in women. The age at onset is typically later than in schizophrenia, and delusional jealousy tends to present at an older age than other subtypes. Hypochondriacal delusions can however occur in young people, and may represent the prodrome to schizophrenia in up to 20% of cases. The course is quite variable — outcome is generally better than in schizophrenia (Opjordsmoen 1988), but is often chronic, especially in the persecutory type (APA 1994).

The aetiology and pathophysiology of delusional disorder remain obscure, not least because of the difficulties in assembling a large enough cohort for meaningful studies. There is no clear evidence that it is genetically inherited, and most studies suggest that the prevalence of schizophrenia is not raised in the relatives of people with delusional disorder. There may however be a tendency for 'feelings of inferiority', paranoid personality traits and delusional disorder itself to run in families (Kendler et al 1985). Although a number of organic brain conditions can lead to secondary delusions, there is no clear pattern in their lesions or location. Immigrants may be at elevated risk. Hearing loss is, however, clearly associated with an increased risk of paranoid psychosis in the elderly (Cooper et al 1974).

The associations with immigrant status and hearing loss hint at the relevance of psychosocial factors. A lack of sensory information and/or an unfamiliar environment may precipitate psychosis in those predisposed through personal cognitive biases, leading to the formation of persecutory delusions. These mechanisms are, of course, likely to be the same as in the formation of delusions in schizophrenia (see psychological theories above), but there is, in addition, some specific evidence that patients with delusional disorder may have a liability to make external attributions for negative events, a particular sensitivity to threatening stimuli, a tendency to 'jump to conclusions' and to be more likely to remember negative feelings than specific events (Kaney et al 1999).

Management

Paranoid delusions have little diagnostic value, and the diagnosis of a delusional disorder requires excluding organic, schizophrenic, affective and sometimes neurotic features. In the latter situation, as in paranoid personality disorder, the beliefs are not of delusional intensity nor held with absolute conviction, i.e. patients may acknowledge alternative interpretations of their complaints. In induced delusional disorder ('folie à deux') the symptoms are usually paranoid or grandiose and arise within the confines of a close relationship in two (or more) people who are otherwise socially isolated (Silveira & Seeman 1995) — the treatment being separation or perhaps psychotherapy for the recipient and treatment of the underlying condition in the dominant partner.

Separation of the patient from the focus of the delusions, where possible, and supportive psychotherapy are the principles of psychosocial management. It is often quite difficult to establish a therapeutic relationship — these people do not usually view themselves as ill, often continue to function relatively well, and may wish to see a different type of doctor, if any. Suicidal and homicidal thoughts in delusional disorder may be particularly likely and need to be taken seriously.

Antipsychotic drugs are the mainstay of treatment. There are no trial data to back up claims that pimozide is particularly effective. Antidepressants, particularly those with serotoninergic effects, appear to be effective in treating obsessive and depressive symptomatology — and indeed the delusions (Phillips et al 2002).

Acute and transient psychotic disorders (ATPD) / brief psychotic disorder (BPD)

If persistent delusional disorder is a rag-bag of historical 'syndromes', then acute and transient psychotic disorders are more so. Several early European psychiatrists described syndromes with symptoms like those in schizophrenia but with an acute onset and usually a favourable outcome — including Legrain's bouffée délirante, Wimmer's reactive psychosis, Leonard's cycloid psychoses, etc. Many of these survived into ICD-9, as did 'hysterical psychosis'. ICD-10 has improved matters slightly by subdividing the diagnostic categories into acute polymorphic (i.e. changeable) psychotic disorder with or without symptoms of schizophrenia and an acute schizophrenia-like psychotic disorder. The DSM-IV criteria for 'brief psychotic disorder' are much clearer, although not necessarily any more valid, in essentially defining it as schizophrenia of less than 1 month's duration and with a full return to premorbid functioning. ICD-10 demands an acute onset and a duration of less than 3 months, but does not make any outcome restrictions. Pillmann et al (2002) examined 1036 patients admitted to a German hospital over a 5-year period with psychosis and found that 4% met criteria for ATPD, of whom 62% fulfilled criteria for BPD, the remainder mainly having schizophreniform disorder.

The essential clinical features are perplexity, confusion, rapid shifts in intense affect, and disorganised behaviour. Epidemiological information is extremely limited, but there appears to be an association with pre-existing personality disorder, female sex and a relatively young age of onset (APA 1994). There may also be strong cultural influences on presentation and duration. It has been suggested that ATPDs may be particularly common in African Caribbeans living in London — which may partly explain the increased rates of psychosis and use of the Mental Health Act to detain them in hospital. In the Northwick Park functional psychosis study, researchers followed-up patients with illnesses which did not fulfil operational criteria for schizophrenia after 2 years and compared them with those who did. 'Partial' illnesses, where delusions were not held with full conviction, had a similar prognosis to that of schizophrenia; whereas 'transient' psychoses (with short-lived symptoms) had good symptom and social outcomes, although they tended to recur (Johnstone et al 1996).

The differential diagnosis includes delirium and substance intoxication, as well as factitious disorder and malingering. There is obviously some phenomenological overlap with the 'Ganser syndrome' (see Ch. 29). Management is as for an acute schizophrenic episode, although particular care may need to be taken to ensure adequate hydration and nutrition, and there may be a particularly high risk of suicide.

Schizoaffective disorder

Following Kraepelin's separation of dementia praecox and manic–depressive disorder, it was soon recognised that a considerable proportion of patients with functional psychotic illnesses did not fit neatly into either category, having features typical of both. The term schizoaffective psychosis was introduced by Kasanin (1933) and is still to be found in ICD-10 and DSM-IV. Both classification systems stress that there must be a period of 2 weeks with at least one typical symptom of schizophrenia and of affective disorder to be able to make the diagnosis, but DSM-IV demands that full criteria for the two disorders be met. Both have manic/bipolar and depressive subtypes, while ICD-10 has an additional mixed type subcategory. It is likely that these criteria have improved the reliability of the diagnosis and possibly even increased the notoriously low levels of agreement between various definitions of schizoaffective psychosis (Brockington & Leff 1979), but it is difficult to know because the condition is so infrequently studied. When it is, it is usually as an indistinguishable subgroup of people with schizophrenia.

Psychiatrists are still reluctant to make the diagnosis clinically, as it smacks of 'fence-sitting', which may account for the impression that the disorder is relatively rare. What evidence there is suggests that it is uncommon (Johnstone et al 1992), but this may be an artefact of psychiatric classification. This is an important point, as it strongly argues against the view that there may be a 'continuum of psychosis' and for the Kraepelinian distinction between the functional psychoses.

The family studies that have been conducted suggest that there is an increased risk of both schizophrenia and mood disorders in the relatives of patients with schizoaffective disorder, and that the outcome is typically somewhere between that of affective disorder and schizophrenia. Management, similarly, usually consists of treating psychotic symptoms with antipsychotics and mood disturbance with antidepressants and/or mood stabilisers. However, a recent systematic review of controlled treatment studies of schizoaffective disorder suggests that antipsychotics alone may be just as effective, or even more so, for schizoaffective disorder currently depressed; with little evidence that lithium or anticonvulsants were better than antipsychotics alone in the manic subtype (Levinson et al 1999). Atypical antipsychotics, such as clozapine, may prove advantageous, but this is not yet clear. The evidence, such as it is, suggests a clear difference in the therapeutic response of schizoaffective disorder and post-psychotic depression, and demonstrates the importance of distinguishing between them.

Concluding remarks

It is clear that there are several disorders that are related to schizophrenia and share some features but are sufficiently different to merit the distinction. Ideally, however, future studies need to examine the full range of these diagnoses to accurately define their similarities and differences. In particular, if we exclude milder variants, a poor prognosis in schizophrenia becomes a self-fulfilling tautology and aetiological research runs the risk of telling us more about the influences on the severity of psychosis rather than schizophrenia per se. It is the case, nonetheless, that the use of diagnostic criteria has facilitated an exponential rise in our understanding of these disorders and indeed an increase in the array of effective treatments we have at our disposal. If one compares what we have learned in the past 100 years, 50 years, 25 years and even the last 10 years, ever increasing progress is clearly being made. It is therefore entirely reasonable to suggest that some important genes and pathophysiological mechanisms will be identified, newer and more effective treatments will be developed, and outcomes generally improved over the next 10–20 years. The ultimate goals of an aetiological classification, valid diagnostic tests and prevention are further off, but perhaps not too far behind.

REFERENCES

Allison D B, Mentore J L, Heo M et al 1999 Antipsychotic-induced weight gain: a comprehensive research synthesis. American Journal of Psychiatry 156:1686–1696

Andreasen N C 1979a Thought, language, and communication disorders, I: Clinical assessment, definition of terms, and evaluation of their reliability. Archives of General Psychiatry 36:1315–1321

Andreasen N C 1979b Thought, language, and communication disorders, II: Diagnostic significance. Archives of General Psychiatry 36:1325–1330

Andreasson S, Allebeck P, Engstrom A, Rydberg U 1987 Cannabis and schizophrenia: a longitudinal study of Swedish conscripts. Lancet ii: 1483–1486

APA 1994 Diagnostic and statistical manual of mental disorders, 4th edn. American Psychiatric Association, Washington, DC

Baldessarini R J, Cohen B M, Teicher M H 1988 Significance of neuroleptic dose and plasma level in the pharmacological treatment of psychoses. Archives of General Psychiatry 45:79–91

Barbui C, Saraceno B, Liberati A, Garattini S 1996 Low-dose neuroleptic therapy and relapse in schizophrenia: meta-analysis of randomized controlled trials. European Psychiatry 11:306–313

Baruch I, Hemsley D R, Gray J A 1988 Differential performance of acute and chronic schizophrenics in a latent inhibition task. Journal of Nervous and Mental Disease 176:598–606

Birchwood M, Smith J 1987 Schizophrenia in the family. In: Oxford J (ed) Coping with disorder in the family. Croom Helm: London

Blackwood N J, Howard R J, Bentall R P, Murray R M 2001 Cognitive neuropsychiatric models of persecutory delusions. American Journal of Psychiatry 158:527–539

Bleuler E 1911 Dementia praecox, or the group of schizophrenias (translated 1950 by J. Zinkin). International University: New York

Bollini P, Pampallona S, Orza M J et al 1994 Antipsychotic drugs: is more worse? A meta-analysis of the published randomized control trials. Psychological Medicine 24:307–316

Boydell J, van Os J, McKenzie K et al 2001 Incidence of schizophrenia in ethnic minorities in London: ecological study into interactions with environment. British Medical Journal 323:1336–1338

Bradbury T N, Miller G A 1985 Season of birth in schizophrenia: a review of evidence, methodology, and etiology. Psychological Bulletin 98:569–594

Brockington I F, Leff J P 1979 Schizo-affective psychosis: definitions and incidence. Psychological Medicine 9:91–99

Brockington I F, Wainwright S, Kendell R E 1980 Manic patients with schizophrenic or paranoid symptoms. Psychological Medicine 10:73–83

Brown G W, Birley J L 1968 Crises and life changes and the onset of schizophrenia. Journal of Health and Social Behaviour 9:203–214

Brown G W, Birley J L, Wing J K 1972 Influence of family life on the course of schizophrenic disorders: a replication. British Journal of Psychiatry 121:241–258

Butzlaff R L, Hooley J M 1998 Expressed emotion and psychiatric relapse: a meta-analysis. Archives of General Psychiatry 55:547–552

Cannon M, Jones P 1996 Schizophrenia. Journal of Neurology, Neurosurgery and Psychiatry 61:604–613

Cannon M, Jones P B, Murray R M 2002 Obstetric complications and schizophrenia: Historical and meta-analytic review. American Journal of Psychiatry 159:1080–1092

Chanpattana W, Chakrabhand M L, Sackeim H A et al 1999 Continuation ECT in treatment-resistant schizophrenia: a controlled study. Journal of ECT 15:178–192

Cochrane Library 2002 Issue 4. Update Software, Oxford

Cochrane R 1977 Mental illness in immigrants to England and Wales: an analysis of mental hospital admissions, 1971. Social Psychiatry 12:25–35

Cooper J E, Kendell R E, Gurland B J et al 1972 Psychiatric diagnosis in New York and London. Maudsley Monograph 20. Oxford University Press: Oxford

Cooper A F, Curry A R, Kay D W K et al 1974 Hearing loss in paranoid and affective psychoses of the elderly. Lancet ii: 851–857

Crow T J 1980 Molecular pathology of schizophrenia: more than one disease process? British Medical Journal 280:66–68

Crow T J, Stevens M 1978 Age disorientation in chronic schizophrenia: the nature of the cognitive deficit. British Journal of Psychiatry 133:137–142

Crowther R E, Marshall M, Bond G R, Huxley P 2001 Helping people with severe mental illness to obtain work: systematic review. British Medical Journal 322:204–208

Cutting J 1985 The psychology of schizophrenia. Churchill Livingstone: Edinburgh

Davis J M 1976 Recent developments in the drug treatment of schizophrenia. American Journal of Psychiatry 133:208–214

Davison K, Bagley C R 1969 Schizophrenia-like psychoses associated with organic disorders of the central nervous system: a review of the literature. In Harrington R N (ed) Current problems in neuropsychiatry. Headley Brothers: Kent

Done D J, Crow T J, Johnstone E C, Sacker A 1994 Childhood antecedents of schizophrenia and affective illness: social adjustment at ages 7 and 11. British Medical Journal 309:699–703

Eagles J M, Whalley L J 1985 Decline in the diagnosis of schizophrenia among first admissions to Scottish mental hospitals from 1969–78. British Journal of Psychiatry 146:151–154

Faris R, Dunham W 1939 (reprinted 1960). Mental disorders in urban areas. Hafner: New York

Farran-Ridge C 1926 Dementia praecox and epidemic encephalitis. Journal of Mental Science 72:513–523

Friston K J, Frith C D 1995 Schizophrenia: a disconnection syndrome? Clinical Neuroscience 3:89–97

Frith C D 1992 The cognitive neuropsychology of schizophrenia. Erlbaum, Hove

Frith C D 1996 Neuropsychology of schizophrenia. In: Biological psychiatry. British Medical Bulletin 52:618–626

Geddes J, Freemantle N, Harrison P, Bebbington P 2000 Atypical antipsychotics in the treatment of schizophrenia: systematic overview and meta-regression analysis. British Medical Journal 321:1371–1376

Gilbert P L, Harris M J, McAdams L A, Jeste D V 1995 Neuroleptic withdrawal in schizophrenic patients: a review of the literature. Archives of General Psychiatry 52:173–188

Goldberg E M, Morrison S L 1963 Schizophrenia and social class. British Journal of Psychiatry 109:785–802

Goldberg S C, Schooler N R, Hogarty G E, Roper M 1977 Prediction of relapse in schizophrenic outpatients treated by drug and sociotherapy. Archives of General Psychiatry 34:171–184

Häfner H, Riecher A, Maurer K et al 1989 How does gender influence age at first hospitalization for schizophrenia? A transnational case register study. Psychological Medicine 19:903–918

Halligan P W, David A S 2001 Cognitive neuropsychiatry: towards a scientific psychopathology. Nature Review Neuroscience 2:209–215

Hare E H 1988 Schizophrenia as a recent disease. British Journal of Psychiatry 153:521–531

Harrison P J 1999 The neuropathology of schizophrenia: a critical review of the data and their interpretation. Brain 122:593–624

Hawk, A B, Carpenter W T, Jr, Strauss J S 1975 Diagnostic criteria and five-year outcome in schizophrenia: a report from the International Pilot Study of schizophrenia. Archives of General Psychiatry 32:343–347

Hegarty J D, Baldessarini R J, Tohen M et al 1994 One hundred years of schizophrenia: a meta-analysis of the outcome literature. American Journal of Psychiatry 151:1409–1416

Heinrichs R W, Zakzanis K K 1998 Neurocognitive deficit in schizophrenia: a quantitative review of the evidence. Neuropsychology 12:426–445

Hirsch S R, Leff J P 1975 Abnormalities in parents of schizophrenics. Maudsley monograph 22. Oxford Universisty Press: London

Hirsch S R, Gaind R, Rohde P D et al 1973 Outpatient maintenance of chronic schizophrenic patients with long-acting fluphenazine: double-blind placebo trial. Report to the Medical Research Council Committee on Clinical Trials in Psychiatry. British Medical Journal 1:633–637

Hoch P, Polatin P 1949 Pseudoneurotic forms of schizophrenia. Psychiatric Quarterly 23:248–256

Hogarty G E, Goldberg S C, Schooler N R, Ulrich R F 1974 Drug and sociotherapy in the aftercare of schizophrenic patients, II: Two-year relapse rates. Archives of General Psychiatry 31:603–608

Hogarty G E, Schooler N R, Ulrich R et al 1979 Fluphenazine and social therapy in the aftercare of schizophrenic patients: relapse analyses of a two-year controlled study of fluphenazine decanoate and fluphenazine hydrochloride. Archives of General Psychiatry 36:1283–1294

Hollister L E, Trauts L, Prusmack J T 1960 Use of thioridazine for intensive treatment of schizophrenia refractory to other tranquillizing drugs. Journal of Neuropsychiatry 1:200–204

Ingvar D H, Franzén G 1974 Abnormalities of cerebral blood flow distribution in patients with chronic schizophrenia. Acta Psychiatrica Scandinavica 50:425–462

Johnson D A W, Pasterski G, Ludlow J M, Street K 1983 The discontinuance of maintenance neuroleptic therapy in chronic schizophrenic patients: drug and social consequences. Acta Psychiatrica Scandinavica 67:339–352

Johnson D A, Ludlow J M, Street K, Taylor R D 1987 Double-blind comparison of half-dose and standard-dose flupenthixol decanoate in the maintenance treatment of stabilised out-patients with schizophrenia. British Journal of Psychiatry 151:634–638

Johnstone E C, Crow T J, Frith C D et al 1976 Cerebral ventricular size and cognitive impairment in chronic schizophrenia. Lancet ii: 924–926

Johnstone E C, Crow T J, Johnson A L, MacMillan J F 1986 The Northwick Park Study of first episodes of schizophrenia, I: Presentation of the illness and problems relating to admission. British Journal of Psychiatry 148:115–120

Johnstone E C, Macmillan J F, Crow T J 1987 The occurrence of organic disease of possible or probable aetiological significance in a population of 268 cases of first episode schizophrenia. Psychological Medicine 17:371–379

Johnstone E C, Leary J, Frith C D, Owens D G 1991 Disabilities and circumstances of schizophrenic patients — a follow-up study. Police contact. British Journal of Psychiatry (Suppl) 159:37–39, 44–46

Johnstone E C, Frith C D, Crow T J et al 1992 The Northwick Park 'Functional' Psychosis Study: diagnosis and outcome. Psychological Medicine 22:331–346

Johnstone E C, Connelly J, Frith C D et al 1996 The nature of 'transient' and 'partial' psychoses: findings from the Northwick Park 'Functional' Psychosis Study. Psychological Medicine 26:361–369

Jolley A G, Hirsch S R, Morrison E et al 1990 Trial of brief intermittent neuroleptic prophylaxis for selected schizophrenic outpatients: clinical and social outcome at two years. British Medical Journal 301:837–842

Jones H M, Pilowsky L S 2002 Dopamine and antipsychotic drug action revisited. British Journal of Psychiatry 181:271–275

Jones P, Rodgers B, Murray R, Marmot M 1994 Child development risk factors for adult schizophrenia in the British 1946 birth cohort. Lancet 344:1398–1402

Joukamaa M, Heliovaara M, Knekt P et al 2001 Mental disorders and cause-specific mortality. British Journal of Psychiatry 179:498–502

Kane J, Honigfeld G, Singer J, Meltzer H 1988 Clozapine for the treatment-resistant schizophrenic: a double-blind comparison with chlorpromazine. Archives of General Psychiatry 45:789–796

Kaney S, Bowen-Jones K, Bentall R P 1999 Persecutory delusions and autobiographical memory. British Journal of Clinical Psychology 38:97–102

Kasanin J 1933 The acute schizoaffective psychoses. American Journal of Psychiatry 90:97–126

Kelly C, McCreadie R G, MacEwan T, Carey S 1998 Nithsdale schizophrenia surveys 17: fifteen year review. British Journal of Psychiatry 172:513–517

Kendell R E, Brockington I F, Leff J P 1979 Prognostic implications of six alternative definitions of schizophrenia. Archives of General Psychiatry 36:25–31

Kendler K S 1982 Demography of paranoid psychosis (delusional disorder): a review and comparison with schizophrenia and affective illness. Archives of General Psychiatry 39:890–902

Kendler K S, Masterson C C, Davis K L 1985 Psychiatric illness in first-degree relatives of patients with paranoid psychosis, schizophrenia and medical illness. British Journal of Psychiatry 147:524–531

Kendler K S, Ochs A L, Gorman A M et al 1991 The structure of schizotypy — a pilot multitrait twin study. Psychiatry Research 36:19–36

Kety S S, Rosenthal D, Wender P H 1975 Mental illness in the biological and adoptive families of adopted individuals who have become schizophrenic: a preliminary report based on psychiatric interviews. Proceedings of the Annual Meeting of the American Psychopathology Association 63:147–165

Kilts C D 2001 The changing roles and targets for animal models of schizophrenia. Biological Psychiatry 50:845–855

Klosterkotter J, Hellmich J, Steinmeyer E M, Schultze-Lutter F 2001 Diagnosing schizopohrenia in the initial prodromal phase. Archives of General Psychiatry 58:158–164

Kraepelin E 1896 Lehrbuch der Psychiatrie. Barth: Leipzig

Kraepelin E 1919 Dementia praecox and paraphrenia (translated by RM Barclay). Livingstone: Edinburgh

Langfeldt G 1960 Diagnosis and prognosis of schizophrenia. Proceedings of the Royal Society of Medicine 53:1047–1052

Lawrie S, McIntosh A 2002 Schizophrenia. In: Clinical Evidence (7th issue). BMJ Publishing, London, p 920–944

Lawrie S M, Whalley H C, Abukmeil S S et al 2001 Brain structure, genetic liability and psychotic symptoms in subjects at high risk of developing schizophrenia. Biological Psychiatry 49:811–823

Lawrie S M, Buechel C, Whalley H C et al 2002 Reduced frontotemporal functional connectivity in schizophrenia associated with auditory hallucinations. Biological Psychiatry 51:1008–1011

Leff J P, Wing J K 1971 Trial of maintenance therapy in schizophrenia. British Medical Journal 3:599–604

Leff J, Kuipers L, Berkowitz R et al 1982 A controlled trial of social intervention in the families of schizophrenic patients. British Journal of Psychiatry 141:121–134

Levinson D F, Umapathy C, Musthaq M 1999 Treatment of schizoaffective disorder and schizophrenia with mood symptoms. American Journal of Psychiatry 156:1138–1148

Liddle P F 1987 The symptoms of chronic schizophrenia: a re-examination of the positive-negative dichotomy. British Journal of Psychiatry 151:145–151

Liddle P F, Friston K J, Frith C D et al 1992 Patterns of cerebral blood flow in schizophrenia. British Journal of Psychiatry 160:179–186

Lund C E, Mortimer A M, Rogers D, McKenna P J 1991 Motor, volitional and behavioural disorders in schizophrenia, I: Assessment using the modified Rogers Scale. British Journal of Psychiatry 158:323–327

McCreadie R G, Leese M, Tilak-Singh D et al 1997 Nithsdale, Nunhead and Norwood: similarities and differences in prevalence of schizophrenias and utilisation of services in urban and rural areas. British Journal of Psychiatry 170:31–36

McGhie A, Chapman J 1961 Disorders of attention and perception in early schizophrenia. British Journal of Medical Psychology 343:103–116

McGlashan T H, Carpenter W T, Jr 1976 Postpsychotic depression in schizophrenia. Archives of General Psychiatry 33:231–239

McGlashan T H, Hoffman R E 2000 Schizophrenia as a disorder of developmentally reduced synaptic connectivity. Archives of General Psychiatry 57:637–648

McGorry P D, Yung A R, Phillips L J et al 2002 Randomized controlled trial of interventions designed to reduce the risk of progression to first-episode psychosis in a clinical sample with subthreshold symptoms. Archives of General Psychiatry 59:921–928

McGovern D, Cope R V 1987 First psychiatric admission rates of first and second generation Afro-Caribbeans. Social Psychiatry 22:139–149

Malzberg B, Lee E S 1956 Migration and mental disease: a study of first admission to hospitals for mental disease, New York, 1939–1941. Social Science Research Council: New York

Mason P, Harrison G, Glazebrook C et al 1995 Characteristics of outcome in schizophrenia at 13 years. British Journal of Psychiatry 167:596–603

May P R A 1968 Treatment of schizophrenia. Science House: New York

Miller P, Lawrie S M, Hodges A et al 2001 Genetic liability, illicit drug use, life stress and psychotic symptoms: preliminary findings from the Edinburgh study of people at high risk for schizophrenia. Social Psychiatry & Psychiatric Epidemiology 36:338–342

Mojtabai R, Nicholson R A, Carpenter B N 1998 Role of psychosocial treatments in management of schizophrenia: a meta-analytic review of controlled outcome studies. Schizophrenia Bulletin 24:569–587

Morice R D, Ingram J C L 1982 Language analysis in schizophrenia: diagnostic implications. Australian and New Zealand Journal of Psychiatry 27:11–21

Mortensen P B, Pedersen C B, Westergaard T et al 1999 Effects of family history and place and season of birth on the risk of schizophrenia. New England Journal of Medicine 340:603–608

Munro A 1988 Monosymptomatic hypochondriacal psychosis. British Journal of Psychiatry (suppl 2) 37–40

National Institute of Mental Health 1964 Psychopharmacology Service Center Collaborative Study Group. Phenothiazine treatment of acute schizophrenia. Archives of General Psychiatry 10:246–261

NICE 2002 Technology Appraisal Guidance No. 43 — Guidance on the use of newer (atypical) antipsychotic drugs for the treatment of schizophrenia. National Institute for Clinical Excellence, London

Odegaard O 1932 Emigration and insanity: a study of mental disease among Norwegian-born population of Minnesota. Acta Psychiatrica et Neurologica Scandinavica (suppl 4)

Opjordsmoen S 1988 Long-term course and outcome in delusional disorder. Acta Psychiatrica Scandinavica 78:576–586

Owens D G, Johnstone E C, Frith C D 1982 Spontaneous involuntary disorders of movement: their prevalence, severity, and distribution in chronic schizophrenics with and without treatment with neuroleptics. Archives of General Psychiatry 39:452–461

Phillips K A, Albertini R S, Rasmussen S A 2002 A randomized placebo-controlled trial of fluoxetine in body dysmorphic disorder. Archives of General Psychiatry 59:381–388

Pilling S, Bebbington P, Kuipers E et al 2002 Psychological treatments in schizophrenia, II: Meta-analyses of randomized controlled trials of social skills training and cognitive remediation. Psychological Medicine 32:783–791

Pillmann F, Haring A, Balzuweit S et al 2002 The concordance of ICD-10 acute and transient psychosis and DSM-IV brief psychotic disorder. Psychological Medicine 32:525–533

Pitschel-Walz G, Leucht S, Bauml J et al 2001 The effect of family interventions on relapse and rehospitalization in schizophrenia — a meta-analysis. Schizophrenia Bulletin 27:73–92

Regier D A, Boyd J H, Burke J D et al 1988 One-month prevalence of mental disorders in the United States. Archives of General Psychiatry 45:977–986

Sartorius N, Jablensky A, Shapiro R 1977 Two-year follow-up of the patients included in the WHO international pilot study of schizophrenia. Psychological Medicine 7:529–541

Sartorius N, Jablensky A, Korten A 1986 Early manifestations and first-contact incidence of schizophrenia in different cultures. A preliminary report on the initial evaluation phase of the WHO Collaborative Study on determinants of outcome of severe mental disorders. Psychological Medicine 16:909–928

Schneider K 1959 Clinical Psychopathology. Grune and Stratton: New York

Seeman P 2002 Atypical antipsychotics: mechanism of action. Canadian Journal of Psychiatry 47:27–37

Sensky T, Turkington D, Kingdon D et al 2000 A randomized controlled trial of cognitive-behavioral therapy for persistent symptoms in schizophrenia resistant to medication. Archives of General Psychiatry 57:165–172

Sham P C, O'Callaghan E, Takei N et al 1992 Schizophrenia following pre-natal exposure to influenza epidemics between 1939 and 1960. British Journal of Psychiatry 160:461–466

Silveira J M, Seeman M V 1995 Shared psychotic disorder: a critical review of the literature. Canadian Journal of Psychiatry 40:389–395

Singer M T, Wynne L D 1965 Thought disorder and family relations of schizophrenics. Archives of General Psychiatry 12:187–212

Siris S G, Morgan V, Fagerstrom R et al 1987 Adjunctive imipramine in the treatment of postpsychotic depression: A controlled trial. Archives of General Psychiatry 44:533–539

Siris S G, Bermanzohn P C, Mason S E, Shuwall M A 1994 Maintenance imipramine therapy for secondary depression in schizophrenia. A controlled trial. Archives of General Psychiatry 51:109–115

Smith D A, Mar C M, Turoff B K 1998 The structure of schizophrenic symptoms: a meta-analytic confirmatory factor analysis. Schizophrenia Research 31:57–70

Steinberg H R, Durrell J 1968 A stressful social situation as a precipitant of schizophrenic symptoms: an epidemiological study. British Journal of Psychiatry 114:1097–1105

Storosum J G, Elferink A J A, van Zwieten B J 2002 Amisulpride: Is there a treatment for negative symptoms in schizophrenia patients? Schizophrenia Bulletin 28:193–201

Susser E S, Lin S P 1992 Schizophrenia after prenatal exposure to the Dutch Hunger Winter of 1944–1945. Archives of General Psychiatry 49:983–988

Thornley B, Adams C 1998 Content and quality of 2000 controlled trials in schizophrenia over 50 years. British Medical Journal 317:1181–1184

Trabert W 1995 100 years of delusional parasitosis: meta-analysis of 1,223 case reports. Psychopathology 28:238–246

Turkington D, Kingdon D, Turner T 2002 Effectiveness of a brief cognitive-behavioural therapy intervention in the treatment of schizophrenia. British Journal of Psychiatry 180:523–527

Vaillant G E 1964 Prospective prediction of schizophrenic remission. Archives of General Psychiatry 11:509–518

Verdoux H, van Os J 2002 Psychotic symptoms in non-clinical populations and the continuum of psychosis. Schizophrenia Research 54:59–65

Verdoux H, Liraud F, Bergey C et al 2001 Is the association between duration of untreated psychosis and outcome confounded? A two year follow-up study of first-admitted patients. Schizophrenia Research 49:231–341

Walsh E, Buchanan A, Fahy T 2001 Violence and schizophrenia: examining the evidence. British Journal of Psychiatry 180:490–495

Weinberger D R 1987 Implications of normal brain development for the pathogenesis of schizophrenia. Archives of General Psychiatry 44:660–669

Weinberger D R 1995 From neuropathology to neurodevelopment. Lancet 346:552–557

WHO 1973 Report of the International Pilot Study of Schizophrenia. World Health Organization: Geneva

WHO 1992 ICD-10. The ICD-10 classification of mental and behavioural disorders: clinical descriptions and diagnostic guidelines. World Health Organization: Geneva

Williams J, McGuffin P, Nothen M, Owen M J 1997 Meta-analysis of association between the 5-HT2a receptor T102C polymorphism and schizophrenia. EMASS Collaborative Group. European Multicentre Association Study of Schizophrenia. Lancet 349:1221

Williams J, Spurlock G, Holmans P et al 1998 A meta-analysis and transmission disequilibrium study of association between the dopamine D3 receptor gene and schizophrenia. Molecular Psychiatry 3:141–149

Wing J K, Brown G W 1961 Social treatment of chronic schizophrenia: a comparative survey of three mental hospitals. Journal of Mental Science 107:847–861

Zammit S, Allebeck P, Andreasson S et al 2002 Self reported cannabis use as a risk factor for schizophrenia in Swedish conscripts of 1969: historical cohort study. British Medical Journal 325:1199

Ziguras S J, Stuart G W, Jackson A C 2002 Assessing the evidence on case management. British Journal of Psychiatry 181:17–21

20 | Mood disorder

Guy Goodwin

INTRODUCTION

Mood disorder is the term now widely applied to a range of conditions in which the most prominent symptom is elevation or depression of mood. It is used synonymously with affective disorder. The most extreme forms of elation (mania) or depression (melancholia) have been recognised since the writings of Hippocrates or before. There is continuing uncertainty about how to subclassify the less severe syndromes of mood disorder. Understanding is also coloured by the experience and perception of normal mood both by patients and healthcare workers. Normal mood necessarily has an uncertain boundary with minor illnesses.

NORMAL MOOD

A moment's introspection will tell us that we use the word mood to describe pervasive feelings that are in part purely psychical but also have a powerfully physical component. When we feel happy we tend to have positive thoughts, feel more energetic, physically comfortable and lighter in limb. In the opposite state we are more prone to pessimistic and negative ideas, may feel literal physical discomfort and find action more effortful. What is perhaps most characteristic about mood is that it captures the character of any transient state of consciousness. Since it can dramatically change, what has the most power to change it? This can obviously be answered easily, if anecdotally: events, relationships, music, alcohol. There is no shortage of ordinary experience, therefore, that informs both our prejudices and our expectations of theories of mood.

The most influential contemporary psychological approach to mood has been cognitive. It supposes that a critical part of what determines mood tone is thinking and reflection. Beliefs and assumptions will clearly influence how we think. Abnormal beliefs or habits of thought could then provide an explanation for why optimistic or depressive interpretations might be made of events or experience. The extension of this view, usually attributed to Beck (1976), would place 'cognitive distortions' at the heart of mood disorder. Efforts to treat depression have been devised that are intended to change the beliefs of individuals with depressive illness. Notice that this view of mood disorder lends itself to an exclusively mentalistic view of mood. The Cartesian split between mind and body tends to make us think of 'mental illness' as not physical. The simplest cognitive account of mood perpetuates this. The prominence given to beliefs allows little credible room for biological mechanisms because, while we know that beliefs must be a product of brain function, they are so high level as to make the point academic.

Nevertheless, the broad alternative to a cognitive formulation of mood is a more biological one. Where cognitive psychology correctly emphasises the potential for thoughts to influence mood, more biological theories highlight the potential for mood to induce particular patterns of thought. Biochemical tone may determine unconscious biases at various levels of neuropsychological function in attention, encoding, stimulus evaluation and recall. The widespread use of alcohol and stimulant drugs is informal testimony to the power of brain chemistry over human experience and behaviour through broadly mood-related mechanisms. In addition, the idea that 'stress' can modify body and brain states is also an old one. The relevance of this to our understanding of clinical states and their treatment will emerge below. However, it is also now accepted that essentially automatic mechanisms have the potential to change emotional experience and memory. In part this is based on a growing understanding of the neural basis of emotional learning in animals and the development of parallel observations in man (LeDoux 2000)

Importantly, the parallel strands provided by cognitive mechanisms on the one hand, and biological on the other, do not offer mutually exclusive alternatives: they demand some form of unification. William James famously proposed that emotion rested on the perception of the peripheral autonomic/somatic response to any emotion-provoking stimulus, although he also allowed that the efferent outflow might itself contribute feedback to the percept. This essentially placed peripheral bodily structures in series with brain regions mediating emotional experience. It predicted the abolition or at least modification of normal emotion by, for example, spinal transection, and the induction of strong emotion by peripheral autonomic agents such as adrenaline. The idea appears to have been widely discounted after an influential critique by Cannon (1927). However, that the balance of autonomic and motor input/output may modify emotional experience still seems likely in view of the prominence of adverse visceral and muscular sensation in mood disorder. The evaluation of afferent information probably requires a particular central set or context which may easily be thought of as having either or both a cognitive and a neurochemical component. A direct experimental confirmation of the interaction between cognitive input and drug-induced autonomic changes was provided by Schachter (1966). Hence a strong interoceptive stimulus must be interpreted in an emotional context derived from other mainly cognitive clues. This seemed best to reflect anxious or angry responding and is close to or identical with contemporary ideas about the evolution of panic anxiety from the misinterpretation of bodily cues (see Ch. 21).

Emotion emerges from such analyses as something of a subjective by product. However, the history of human folly, and human triumph, suggests that it may influence our reason in most potent ways. Damasio has re-established this precedence experimentally rather than experientially by showing that somatic and autonomic factors are critical to normal *cognitive* performance in the domains of planning and judgement, not just in domains that are conventionally emotion laden. He has developed his arguments from the observation that brain lesions in critical areas produce impairments of online decision making and processing of emotion. These areas are the ventromedial prefrontal cortex, the amygdala and the somatosensory cortex in the right hemisphere. The relevance of these arguments to the neurobiology of mood disorder will be developed below. The ideas are extremely important for psychiatry generally in embracing a unitary approach to the mind–body problem, and Damasio's book *Descartes' Error* should be required reading for all disciplines working with mentally ill patients (Damasio 1994).

MOOD DISORDER: AN ILLNESS OR A WEAKNESS?

It is a powerful idea that we give meaning to our experiences in part by interpreting the mood states that they provoke or recall. It means that subjective psychology and philosophy can accommodate disorders of mood into normalising views of human experience. It can give rise to the view that depressive illness does not in some sense exist at all. The argument behind this is usually that the concept of depressive illness is 'not scientific' because it is based on arbitrary diagnostic criteria, or cannot be shown to be an illness in the way that, say, bacterial endocarditis can. Instead, the argument tends to go, it should be viewed as an existential struggle against despair. This point of view is put most uncompromisingly in books for popular consumption. The manner in which authors such as Dorothy Rowe or Peter Breggin set out to convince is to demand premature certainties of psychiatry. The scientific need to embrace hypotheses provisionally and cautiously can then be taken as proof of the discipline's failure and, further, as licence for an author's personal agenda to be imposed instead. It is one of the more curious aspects of human psychology that unfounded intuitive certainty, like fundamentalism in its many forms, exercises a greater attraction for a significant section of the population than the reliable methods of scientific inquiry. Perhaps emotion intrudes into its own interpretation.

This chapter is written from the point of view that mood can show extreme manifestations, like other natural biological phenomena such as the level of blood pressure or blood sugar. It would be nonsense to dismiss descriptions of hypertension or diabetes by referring to the normality of having a blood pressure or a blood sugar level. By the same token, extremes of mood cause 'disease' in the people who suffer from them. The burden that mood disorder imposes on patients is actually much greater than that associated with hypertension and diabetes (Murray & Lopez 1997). Psychiatry aspires to bring the methods of science to bear on the problem: there have been some successes. However, in clinical circumstances psychiatrists and psychologists have to make what can be an arbitrary distinction between the two domains of

normal experience and mood disorder. They have a boundary, and at this boundary distinctions are difficult. Clinically the best guide to where one lies is in the realm of the phenomena we call symptoms, and it is to these that we will turn first in outlining a disease-orientated understanding of mood disorder.

SYMPTOMS AND DIAGNOSIS OF MOOD DISORDER

Operational diagnosis of psychiatric disorder has been the major advance in psychiatry within the last 40 years. It seeks simply to identify the pattern of symptoms that most reliably characterises a given illness. It makes no claims about aetiology but, instead, makes possible the fundamental scientific activity of classification and, thereby, communication about similar patients. Clinicians can share experience and base their observations of treatment interventions on a sound footing. The identification of symptoms is, however, an arbitrary process and is based upon a judgement of severity, duration and, in some cases, quality of experience. Case identification can be made by self-rating or observer-rating methods. Observer-rating relies upon the interview of the patient by another person, usually a psychiatrist, and tends to be regarded as more reliable than self-rating. The use of operational criteria strengthens the reliability of a conventional clinical interview. The symptoms that comprise a diagnosis of major depression are shown in Box 20.1. Notice that the symptoms have to be present for at least 2 weeks, although in practice they may often have been present for longer before a patient consults the doctor. The subjective experience of patients commonly leads them to describe their mood as depressed or negative and/or to describe a loss of interest and pleasure in life. Suicidal thoughts and in some cases specific plans are quite common. While these symptoms may often be seen as the core of depressive illness, such experience is described by a range of people in unhappy situations, with unhappy backgrounds or with abnormal personalities. For that reason the additional symptoms necessary for a diagnosis of depressive illness are critical and must always be sought and identified with confidence. In clinical practice, diagnosis may rely particularly on evidence of impaired social, occupational or other function together with additional symptoms. If operational criteria are used, five symptoms from Table 20.1 are necessary for a diagnosis of major depression according to DSM-IV (APA 1994); comparable rules apply for a depressive episode (F32) in ICD-10 (WHO 1992). This is a relatively undemanding threshold and, as will be obvious on a moment's reflection, could include patients with a range and diversity of symptoms. Indeed two patients may score their five symptoms in a way that barely overlaps given the alternatives shown in Box 20.1. This remains an unsatisfactory but unresolved paradox at the heart of diagnosis and classification of mood disorder.

Specimen cases

Cases 1 and 2 (see Boxes 20.2 and 20.3) illustrate contrasting types of clinical syndrome. They were chosen both to be males although either could have been female. The emphasis is on presentation and symptoms. The features that contribute to diagnosis are emboldened.

What is striking about Case 1 is the extreme contrast between the patient when well and the state of depression. This man has

---

Box 20.1 Criteria for major depressive episode (DSM-IV)

Five (or more) of the following symptoms have been present during the same 2-week period and represent a change from previous functioning; at least one of the symptoms is either (1) depressed mood or (2) loss of interest or pleasure.
Note: Do not include symptoms that are clearly due to a general medical condition, or mood-incongruent delusions or hallucinations.

1. Depressed mood most of the day, nearly every day, as indicated by either subjective report (e.g. feels sad or empty) or observation made by others (e.g. appears tearful). Note: In children and adolescents, can be irritable mood
2. Markedly diminished interest or pleasure in all, or almost all, activities most of the day, nearly every day (as indicated by either subjective account or observation made by others)
3. Significant weight loss when not dieting or weight gain (e.g. a change of more than 5% of body weight in a month), or decrease or increase in appetite nearly every day. In children, consider failure to make expected weight gains
4. Insomnia or hypersomnia nearly every day
5. Psychomotor agitation or retardation nearly every day (observable by others, not merely subjective feelings of restlessness or being slowed down)
6. Fatigue or loss of energy nearly every day
7. Feelings of worthlessness or excessive or inappropriate guilt (which may be delusional) nearly every day (not merely self-reproach or guilt about being sick)
8. Diminished ability to think or concentrate, or indecisiveness, nearly every day (either by subjective account or as observed by others)
9. Recurrent thoughts of death (not just fear of dying), recurrent suicidal ideation without a specific plan, or a suicide attempt or a specific plan for committing suicide

---

Box 20.2 Case 1

A 48-year-old self-employed businessman presented with a **5-week** history of increasing **loss of interest** and **impairment of concentration**. In the preceding 4 months he had experienced problems following the death of a close friend who was also a business colleague. This had resulted in unexpected company debts, increased pressures of work and concerns about the security of his colleague's family.

In the last 2 weeks he was **unable to work at all** and spent much of the time at home **pacing up and down** and **unable to make decisions**. He became increasingly convinced that **his business was going to fail and that he was probably already bankrupt. His sleep was grossly disturbed** and he had **impaired appetite** and **no sexual interest**. There was **some diurnal variation** of mood such that he tended to be more withdrawn and quiet in the early part of the day. He frequently expressed concern that the problems were of **his own making** and his life was a failure. On direct questioning he volunteered that he had had thoughts of **ending his life by jumping** from a bridge close to his house.

---

markedly endogenous features (see below) despite an obvious precipitant, and he poses a suicide risk. His beliefs about being bankrupt were almost delusional. Note that he did not complain specifically of being depressed but of his loss of interest and the capacity to solve problems. Paradoxically, therefore, he has a severe

---

Box 20.3 Case 2

A 20-year-old male university student presented complaining of **increasing worries** about work. He dated these difficulties to a change in tutor who had been appreciably more aggressive in handling his written work. This had also activated resentments about coming to this particular university to please his parents. He described **crying virtually every day** for the last **3 weeks** and that his head felt 'about to burst'. He had **withdrawn from social activity** and was avoiding lectures. His anxiety was greatest in relation to work-related situations but he could **no longer concentrate** at all on reading. He was **low in spirits** and often **ruminated about the probability of his failure** and his lack of any subsequent prospects. He could see no future for himself and had **thoughts of impulsively taking an overdose** of paracetamol. He found such thoughts frightening but was concerned that he might nevertheless act on them. He described **sleeping for longer than usual** with occasional wakenings and bad dreams. His sleep, however, was unsatisfying and he felt **tired all the time**. Food consumption was normal but he had **no interest in sex**.

---

illness but the diagnosis could be missed if one has an approach to depressive mood disorder based on 'understandability' and experience of our everyday manageable misery. As William Styron (1990) pinpointed, 'Depression . . . used to be termed melancholia. . . . "Melancholia" would still appear to be a far more apt and evocative word for the blacker forms of the disorder, but it was usurped by a noun with a bland tonality and lacking any magisterial presence, used indifferently to describe an economic decline or a rut in the ground, a true wimp of a word'.

The patient in Case 2 is a man with prominent subjective distress who will be much more easily identified and may be more likely to seek help. The irony here is that, while he has a diagnosis of major depression (see the marked symptoms), the prominence of his anxiety symptoms may result in an explanation based on his 'personality' or the 'stress' of his academic schedule. The essence of an operational approach is that it identifies the relevant pattern of symptoms. This discipline is essential to clinical assessment before one addresses the more obvious psychosocial issues that seem to have precipitated illnesses of the sort described here. Nevertheless, the description of both these cases as major depression clearly misses something else, which is that they may represent different types of illness.

Subclassification of major depression

Subclassification of major depression is primarily to identify the more severe sort of disorder (as in Case 1 above) which is known as melancholia (DSM-IV) or somatic syndrome (ICD-10). The important additional symptoms include complete loss of pleasure in virtually all activities, lack of reactivity, a distinct almost painful quality to the depressed mood, motor slowing, agitation, marked disturbance of sleep and appetite and diurnal variations of symptoms. Guilt may be excessive or even psychotic. The patient is more likely to require inpatient admission. Melancholia is often diagnosed when there is a previous history of similar episodes responsive to treatment and showing full recovery (recurrent mood disorder). There is commonly a family history of mood disorder. An understanding of where the pressure for this sort of division of mood disorder originates can best be appreciated by a brief survey of the history of diagnosis in this area; a fuller account is given by Parker and colleagues (Parker & Hadzi-Pavlovic 1996).

Severe depression has always been seen as the preserve of psychiatrists. Psychotic depression may result in a patient becoming virtually immobile, mute, indifferent or negative towards food and fluids, and incontinent. The severity of these illnesses was well recognised in the 19th century, as was their tendency to show recovery. It is worth remembering, however, that patients might in some cases require 2 or 3 years in hospital, during much of which time they might require tube feeding to support their normal physiology (in depressive stupor). There was an associated acute mortality. When a classification of psychiatric disorder was being developed, these patients were placed in the general framework of manic–depressive psychosis; this of course was Kraepelin's contribution to the subdivision of psychosis in general.

Patients with severe depression may show both delusions and hallucinations, although they are usually mood congruent. In other words, the delusions will have a deeply depressive colouring: the patient is bankrupt, he has a malignancy, infection or infestation, he is evil, can harm others, etc. Hallucinations will be accusing and derogatory. This territory of mood disorder was (and remains) very different from that inhabited by relatively minor cases of mood disorder seen in the community. Minor cases were initially seen as the preserve of doctors offering supportive psychological treatment. The extension of psychiatric boundaries from the gates of the lunatic asylum to the greener pastures of primary care resulted in broadening of the umbrella under which mood states could be encompassed. It was helped along by the discovery of effective medicines; Healy (1997) gives an exceptional account of this phenomenon. However, the historical dichotomy between very severe illnesses (endogenous, psychotic) and less severe illnesses (reactive, neurotic) became controversial.

There was a seminal debate between the Newcastle School (Carney et al 1965), which claimed that suitable statistical treatment of symptom profiles resulted in a bimodal distribution of cases, and the Maudsley School, which denied that such operations were effective or that, when they were, they were influenced by the preconceptions of the doctors making the ratings (Lewis 1934, Kendell 1968). Broadly speaking, the Maudsley view prevailed and major depression came to be seen as displaying a continuum of symptoms from psychotic to neurotic.

It is probably correct that many individual patients cannot be readily dichotomised on the basis of interviews that seek subjective phenomena as the criteria for diagnosis. However, an interesting alternative approach has been developed within the last few years by Parker and colleagues. This has sought to base classification upon what they describe as a sign- rather than a symptom-based typology. In other words, they suggest that to observe particular signs in patients is more discriminating than eliciting the common subjective clinical symptoms. The reason for this is made obvious in Table 20.1, which shows the relative frequency of signs and symptoms in psychotic, endogenous and neurotic cases with major depression. A symptom such as suicidal ideation is common in all groups. Thus it is a good identifier for major depression but a poor discriminator between the putative subtypes. By contrast, a sign such as slowing of speech rate is very unusual in neurotic depression but occurs in almost 30% of endogenous cases. Accordingly, it would be a poor item for diagnosis of major depression but a good discriminator between endogenous/psychotic and neurotic cases. Identification of a group of signs contributing this pattern of difference made possible the construction of an endogenicity measure (the CORE). It shows a bimodal distribution across the patient population where symptom scores (and the Hamilton rating scale) do not (Fig. 20.1). The existence of such bimodality is what much of the preceding debate had been about. A re-analysis of Lewis's own data (Parker & Hadzi-Pavlovic 1993) gave the same result! In addition, entirely

Table 20.1 Percentage of patients with particular selected signs and symptoms rated as present in each of three diagnostic subgroups of major depression

Clinical feature	Percentage affirming feature			
	Psychotic ($n = 73$)	Endogenous ($n = 140$)	Neurotic ($n = 200$)	Odds ratio
Signs				
Non-reactivity	96	84	33	14.6***
Delay in responding verbally	64	39	4	22.1***
Poverty of associations	84	61	10	20.8***
Delay in motor activity	44	29	1	103.8***
Slowing of speech rate	36	27	2	28.2***
Symptoms				
Appetite loss	83	82	57	3.4***
Weight loss	78	69	45	3.1***
Indecisive	82	93	83	1.6
Unpleasant thoughts	94	82	84	1.2
Suicidal thoughts	71	62	76	0.6
Loss of interest in pleasurable activities	96	96	88	2.1
Energy worse in morning	42	60	43	1.5

Odds ratio comparing psychotic + endogenous depressed with neurotic depressed *** p < 0.001.
Data from Parker & Hadzi-Pavlovic 1996.

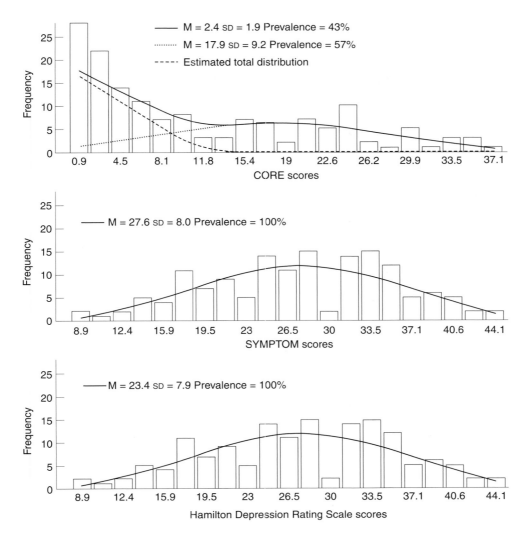

Fig. 20.1
Normal distributions fitted by mixture analysis to CORE scores (top), SYMPTOM scores (middle) and Hamilton scores (bottom). Number of distributions plotted determined by significance test.

objective tests of psychomotor speed give a bimodal result (Parker & Hadzi-Pavlovic 1996). This is the revised basis for thinking of mood disorder as having two somewhat separate incarnations as melancholic or non-melancholic illnesses. That the separation may nevertheless be largely an effect of severity of illness is suggested by analysis of the genetics of melancholic depression, albeit defined primarily by symptoms rather than signs (Kendler 1997). Only a molecular genetic account is likely eventually to clarify the true relationship between the phenotypes.

Although there is a general belief that DSM-IV and ICD-10, in their slightly different ways, are no better than provisional classifications, there is no consensus on how they could be improved. Indeed, they are the only consensus. The terminology is outlined in Table 20.2. Alternative classifications are of limited interest. For example, the distinction between primary and secondary depression is one that has found some favour in the USA (Winokur 1990). Secondary depressions are defined as being preceded by another psychiatric illness (alcohol dependence, eating disorder, anxiety disorder) or accompanying a serious physical illness.

Primary depressions may only be preceded chronologically by mania. Like other diagnostic schema this is an attempt to isolate a core depressive syndrome and separate it from the many other cases where the diagnosis of depression is complicated by a variety of other features. The primary advantage of this classification has been assumed to be that it will identify a subgroup of patients with a specific (genetic) aetiology; in fact, it performed poorly in a twin study to estimate heritability for different definitions of illness (Kendler et al 1992). The classification seems unlikely to be adopted for clinical purposes as it has little to contribute to prognosis and treatment.

Atypical depression

The use of this term has varied over the years but has increasingly converged on a presentation where there are reversed biological symptoms (increased eating and sleeping) and unusual reactivity of mood. There may also be a characterological sensitivity to personal rejection. Indeed the apparent prominence of personality

Table 20.2 Classification of depressive disorders	
DSM-IV	ICD-10
Major depressive episode	*Depressive episode*
Mild	Mild
Moderate	Moderate
Severe	Severe
Severe with psychosis	Severe with psychosis
	Other depressive episodes
	Atypical depression
Major depressive disorder	*Recurrent depressive disorders*
recurrent	Currently mild
	Currently moderate
	Currently severe
	Currently severe with
	psychosis
	In remission
Dysthymic disorder	*Persistent mood disorders*
	Cyclothymia
	Dysthymia
Depressive disorders not	*Other mood disorders*
otherwise specified	Recurrent brief depression
Recurrent brief depression	
Hypomanic episode	*Manic episode*
Manic episode	Hypomania
Mild	Mania
Moderate	Mania with psychosis
Severe	
Severe with psychosis	
Bipolar I and bipolar II	*Bipolar affective disorder*
disorder	Currently hypomanic
Current (or most recent	Currently manic
episode)	Currently depressed
Hypomanic	Currently mixed
Manic*	In remission
Depressed	
Mixed*	
Cyclothymia	
* Excludes bipolar II.	

difficulties may serve to distract the clinician from identifying the major depressive episode. It is claimed that the response to monoamine oxidase inhibitors (MAOIs) is better than to tricyclic antidepressants (Quitkin et al 1988, 1989). A subclassification of depressive syndromes on the basis of likely therapeutic response retains an important potential value for clinical practice. The differential effect of phenelzine relative to imipramine is also seen at withdrawal after 6 months. Phenelzine-treated atypicals were much more likely to relapse if it was discontinued compared with those treated with imipramine (Stewart et al 1997). Any illness defined by what it is not (melancholic or 'typical' depression) risks including a rag bag of different conditions or, more likely, cases drawn from the ends of a set of orthogonal symptom dimensions. Parker et al (2002) suggest that atypical depression may best be thought of as a spectrum disorder in which rejection sensitivity (a personality style) occurs alongside prominent anxiety symptoms; they de-emphasise mood reactivity. However, the larger point is that these are patients in whom a depression diagnosis (and the potential for treatment) may be missed in favour of a diagnosis of personality disorder.

Brief recurrent depression

The existence of short episodes of severe but transient depression of mood lasting 2–7 days and recurring frequently is not a new finding (Paskind 1929). However, recurrent brief depression was first formally described for community samples by Angst and colleagues (Angst et al 1990). There may be an important relationship with similarly short periods of anxiety (Angst & Wicki 1992) and with the risk of deliberate self-harm (Angst & Hochstrasser 1994). The comorbidity with major depression (and dysthymia) is striking, and patients may serially show conversion from major depression to recurrent brief depression and vice versa (Angst 1996). Recurrent brief depression is a category in ICD-10 (F38. 10) but the concept has been slow to be adopted in the USA (Keller et al 1995). Treatment trials have been disappointing (Montgomery et al 1994). The area is likely to remain important because, together with the problem of residual symptoms, a shift to longer-term treatment in mood disorder will raise the importance of longer-term outcomes, both in the domains of symptoms and of personal or social function.

Minor depression, dysthymia and depressive personality

Minor depressive states still present a diagnostic muddle. Efforts to wring meaningful classifications out of minor symptoms, present to a greater or lesser degree either with more obvious temperamental abnormality or with more prominent anxiety symptoms, remain of dubious clinical value. Symptoms that are both milder and are present for longer periods of time have attracted attention recently. DSM-IV includes a category of mood disorder described as dysthymia, where fewer depressive symptoms are present for over 2 years. As well as the symptoms contributing to a diagnosis of major depression, this category is characterised by symptoms such as feelings of pessimism, low self-esteem, low energy, irritability and decreased productivity. In the past these clinical cases would have been largely subsumed under the notion of neurasthenia or depressive personality (Hirschfeld 1994), but interest in them has been provoked by the reports of responsiveness to pharmacological treatment (Baldwin et al 1995, Thase et al 1996). This is of particular relevance given the availability of agents of greater specificity and therefore of lower side-effect profile than tricyclic antidepressants and old-style MAOIs. The diagnosis is sometimes made in patients with superimposed major depression.

The status of depressive personality disorder is uncertain. Personality disorder must be present from adolescence, invariant, more or less, throughout life. Akiskal has argued that temperament is critical to understanding the spectrum of chronic affective disorder (Akiskal 1983), and this has echoes of the emphasis of an earlier generation of clinicians on illnesses as reactions by personality types (Slater & Roth 1969). Certainly, the stability of measures of personality such as neuroticism (N) is well established across the lifespan by very large studies (Costa & McCrae 1994), and the disposition in high-N subjects to react negatively appears to have validity in acute experimental studies (Larsen & Ketelaar 1989). What makes the notion of depressive personality disorder difficult is the addition of yet another arbitrary threshold for 'diagnosis'. Personality dimensions par excellence seem to require continua not categories. It seems quite likely that diagnosis of discrete syndromes would in general be enriched by systematic measures of personality. This is no less true in states where euphoria may alternate with depression, as will be described below.

Mania

The development of manic states is a feature of those mood disorders described as bipolar or manic–depressive. Association of manic states with depressive states serially in the same individuals was a key observation of Kraepelin. The symptoms of mania are characterized by disinhibition of psychomotor function. Patients are more active, experience pressure of thought and may show flight of ideas as thoughts crowd in faster than the patient can speak. Projects get started and not finished. They frequently attribute an increased importance and meaning to their thoughts and plans. The emotional rapport is often infectiously euphoric, but opposition may be met with irritability and even violence. The presentation may be frankly psychotic, and delusions are typically grandiose in content. In the most severe illnesses, patients may also experience hallucinations of the sort usually associated with schizophrenia. Distinction between psychotic and non-psychotic mania is an arbitrary one. However, patients generally show impaired judgement in manic states. In their expansive state of mind they may spend large amounts of money, indulge in risky or undesirable sexual activity which they subsequently regret and may be extremely difficult with the people around them. Dangerous driving is a particular hazard, and patients with a history of severe mania are required to notify the licensing authorities and are disqualified from driving for 6 months after a severe episode. Since patients may have a good deal to lose by exposing people in the family, and particularly at work, to their behaviour when manic, it would be wrong to see the boundary between psychotic and non-psychotic mania as a particularly critical one in terms of management. Patients also show prominent sleep disturbance, commonly going for days without feeling the need for sleep, the sleep deprivation probably thereby contributing to their irritability and erratic behaviour. The diagnostic criteria for mania are shown in Box 20.4. Unipolar recurrent mania is unusual but has been described. However, more common is a lifetime history of mood disorder characterised by episodes of mania and depression.

Hypomania is the term that describes states of euphoria and overactivity short of mania. DSM-IV defines hypomania to be a milder condition (literally below mania) whereas in ICD-10 hypomania is an almost superfluous term that describes mild mania. In UK psychiatry and possibly elsewhere, hypomania is used as an unhelpful diminutive for patients who clearly have mania (e.g. inpatients). DSM-IV offers us something different and more useful, and the term should be employed in that sense (Goodwin 2002).

Subjectively, hypomanic patients tend to feel unusually well and energetic. Their capacity to work and be creative may be genuinely increased, but the limits over which they may slip to become judgement impaired are always uncertain. Subjective accounts capture the experience very graphically. It is a particular problem that hypomania is usually, perhaps understandably, viewed very positively by patients (Jamison 1995). Poor compliance with pharmacological treatment and the denial of more severe disturbance is often related to the wish to experience hypomania in its least troubled forms. Unfortunately, hypomania, like mania, is also associated with depressive swings.

The depressive states of bipolar disorder are indistinguishable from those of severe unipolar depression. The only difference

---

Box 20.4   Criteria for manic episode (DSM-IV)

A. A distinct period of abnormally and persistently elevated, expansive, or irritable mood, lasting at least 1 week (or any duration if hospitalisation is necessary)
B. During the period of mood disturbance, three (or more) of the following symptoms have persisted (four if the mood is only irritable) and have been present to a significant degree:
   1. Inflated self-esteem or grandiosity
   2. Decreased need for sleep (e.g. feels rested after only 3 hours of sleep)
   3. More talkative than usual or pressure to keep talking
   4. Flight of ideas or subjective experience that thoughts are racing
   5. Distractibility (i.e. attention too easily drawn to unimportant or irrelevant external stimuli)
   6. Increase in goal-directed activity (either socially, at work or school, or sexually) or psychomotor agitation
   7. Excessive involvement in pleasurable activities that have a high potential for painful consequences (e.g. engaging in unrestrained buying sprees, sexual indiscretions or foolish business investments)
C. The symptoms do not meet criteria for a Mixed Episode.
D. The mood disturbance is sufficiently severe to cause marked impairment in occupational functioning or in usual social activities or relationships with others, or to necessitate hospitalisation to prevent harm to self or others, or there are psychotic features
E. The symptoms are not due to the direct physiological effects of a substance (e.g. a drug of abuse, a medication, or other treatment) or a general medical condition (e.g. hyperthyroidism)

---

emerging from modern comparisons has been shorter episodes and more agitation in the melancholic forms of bipolar depression (Mitchell et al 1992). This may reflect the underlying neurobiology that underpins the manic upswing. In addition, mixed states may be seen where symptoms of mania and depression may be co-mingled or alternate over short periods of time.

In recent years, there has been increasing interest in the occurrence of hypomania in association with recurrent major depression (bipolar II disorder in DSM-IV). This may, in over 10% of cases, be succeeded by the development of a frank manic episode. However, more important conceptually is the idea that, since hypomania is defined in an arbitrary way, bipolarity in its minor or temperamental forms is much more common than is currently appreciated. Thus a relaxation of the DSM-IV criteria for hypomania identifies increasing numbers of patients with major depression who meet soft definitions of bipolarity (Angst et al 2003). The iceberg of bipolar spectrum disorder that emerges from unipolar disorder is illustrated in Figure 20.2.

Cyclothymia also identifies a subsyndromal predisposition to cyclical mood change. The most persuasive proponent of the importance of subsyndromal mood disorder is, again, Akiskal (Akiskal & Akiskal 1988). The dilemma, as ever with DSM-type classification, is where to draw the line around a syndrome of a particular severity and finite duration and where we should be seeking to capture the quantitative and qualitative range of individual temperament. However, there is the further problem that while premorbid personality measures of subjects with a subsequent unipolar course show high neuroticism, bipolars appear to

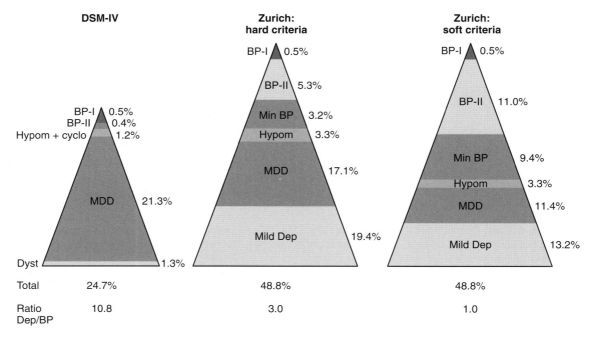

Fig. 20.2
Prevalence rates of bipolar and depressive spectra in the Zurich community study. On the left, diagnosis by DSM-IV criteria; to the right by increasingly relaxed criteria for hypomania (hard, middle, and soft, right). Note the change in the ratio of unipolar to bipolar cases (Dep/BP). For further details, see Angst et al (2003). BP, bipolar disorder; cyclo, cyclothymia; dyst, dysthymia; hypom, hypomania; MDD, major depressive disorder.

be normal (Clayton et al 1994). Retrospective measures of temperament may be influenced by a recent illness: the so-called scar effect on personality. The issue awaits resolution and is not simply academic if mood-stabilising agents are a better choice in patients with minor bipolar disorders than antidepressants alone.

CLASSIFICATION OF MOOD DISORDER BY CLINICAL COURSE

Mood disorders tend to recover but to recur. Kraepelin placed a central emphasis on recovery between episodes in his great division between schizophrenia and manic–depressive psychosis. Unipolar depression describes patients having recurrent depressive episodes, and the term bipolar disorder is reserved for patients with a history of mania. Unipolar mania is sufficiently unusual to be ignored. The bipolar/unipolar distinction was proposed by Leonhard and popularised in the English language literature by Perris and others. However, it was intended to apply to recurrent endogenous illness, so the extension of the term unipolar to all cases of major depression is arbitrary. The unipolar/bipolar division is clinically useful because it appears to have implications for treatment. Patients with bipolar illness show a constant higher risk of recurrence over time than unipolars (Angst et al 2003). The contemporary classification of mood disorders in DSM-IV and ICD-10 is shown in Table 20.2.

Seasonal affective disorder

Mood has a seasonal variation within the normal population. Seasonal affective disorder (SAD) was a term introduced to describe patients who answered newspaper advertisements designed to recruit people who thought they had a seasonal mood disorder. It turned out that they tended to describe rather consistent atypical symptoms: hypersomnia, hyperphagia, tiredness and low mood in winter (but the syndrome does not include rejection sensitivity) (Rosenthal et al 1984). It was initially claimed that the condition was responsive to bright-light therapy in the early morning and this was attributed to a physiological resetting of the photoperiod (perhaps involving melatonin). This turns out to have been a beautiful hypothesis rather spoiled by the facts. It has proved difficult to show any benefit in SAD of bright light over dim light (Levitt et al 1994, Wileman et al 2001) or of early morning exposure compared with midday (Jacobsen et al 1987, Lafer et al 1994) or increased sensitivity to light in the suppression of melatonin (Murphy et al 1993). Furthermore, community studies do not support the notion of a specific syndrome, although there is some seasonality of mood disorder in general, as long recognised (Wicki et al 1992). The status of SAD and light therapy accordingly remains unclear. There continue to be positive reports of the benefits of light therapy, but the sizes of the trials have been disappointing and the specificity of the light effects difficult to disentangle from placebo. Patients with winter episodes of major depression are best treated conventionally.

EPIDEMIOLOGY OF THE DEPRESSIVE DISORDERS

Our knowledge of the incidence and prevalence of mood disorders comes from detailed structured interviews of representative population samples. This is a relatively recent innovation (see Ch. 10) so that our understanding of the extent of mood disorder is better now than it has ever been. However, there are difficulties. Population studies immediately throw up a boundary problem. There appears to be a more or less continuous variation between the well and the ill with regard to subjective distress, identification of particular symptoms or groups of symptoms, and duration and degree of impairment. Where one sets the threshold for defining a case of depression therefore determines what actual percentage value one obtains for incidence and prevalence. In the epidemiological catchment area (ECA) programme in the USA, representative samples of more than 18 000 adults aged 18 years or over were interviewed in five representative centres (Regier et al 1988). The lifetime prevalence for all DSM-III affective disorders was between 6.1% and 9.5%. Major depression was the most common diagnosis, showing a lifetime prevalence in women between 4.9% and 8.7% and for men of 2.3% to 4.4%. These studies have now been extended multinationally (Weissman et al 1996). The lifetime rates for major depression varied across countries, ranging from 1.5 cases per 100 adults in Taiwan to 19.0 cases per 100 adults in Beirut. The annual rates ranged from 0.8% in Taiwan to 5.8% in New Zealand. The mean age at onset showed less variation (range 24.8–34.8 years). There was an increased risk of comorbidity with substance abuse and anxiety disorders. Individuals who were separated or divorced had significantly higher rates of major depression in most of the countries, and the risk was somewhat greater for divorced or separated men than women in most countries. The rates of major depression are usually higher for women than men. As a rule the multiplier is approximately 2–3 and appears at puberty (Angold & Worthman 1993). The cause of this female excess is a source of controversy. At least in part, it could be an artefact. Men may be less likely to admit to having depressive symptoms and more likely to forget previous symptoms that they have experienced (Angst & Dobler-Mikola 1984). However, a genuinely higher prevalence of depressive disorder in women is still widely accepted. The relative contribution of psychological, social and biological influences to the sex difference is not understood. The potential explanatory factors include psychological attributes (temperament, personality and attributional/coping styles) and the experience of psychosocial adversity — the need for social support seems stronger in women. Menstruation, childbirth and child-rearing may also increase the risk of depression. The possible biological underpinnings of such differential mechanisms will be considered with other aspects of the neurobiology. Whatever the mechanism, the consequences of mood disorder may be worse in men even when symptoms are mild, with increased premature mortality described in the Stirling County cohort (see below). Recent studies of male/female twins largely controlled for genetic and early environmental differences: on average, women reported more fatigue, hypersomnia and psychomotor retardation, men reported more insomnia and irritability (Khan et al 2002).

Major depression overlaps critically with dysthymia. A survey of five American communities showed that dysthymia affected approximately 3% of the adult population (Weissman et al 1988). It had a high comorbidity with other psychiatric disorders, particularly major depression; only about 25–30% of cases occur over a lifetime in the absence of other psychiatric disorders. Although the onset and highest risk for more severe mood disorder was young adulthood, a residual state of dysthymia occurs typically in middle and old age.

All cross-sectional epidemiological studies risk confounding incidence with recurrence. A longitudinal investigation of psychiatric epidemiology in a general population — the Stirling County study (Murphy et al 1989) — has suggested that the incidence of depression and anxiety disorders is low relative to prevalence because these disorders have long durations. In an average year approximately 9 adults among 1000 experienced a first-ever episode of one of these disorders. This work highlights the difficulty of interpreting retrospective accounts of symptoms. Recovery to some criterion may distort a true picture of long-term symptoms and difficulties, the severity of which waxes and wanes. This affects the vexed question of whether the incidence of mood disorder is rising.

Are we in an age of melancholia?

Recent epidemiological studies have suggested that the risk of major depression has been increasing in recent decades. In 1985, the results of interviews with 2289 relatives of 523 probands with affective disorder in the USA were published (Klerman et al 1985). It was observed that the lifetime occurrence of depression was higher in younger relatives than older relatives: the opposite of what would be expected if risk had remained constant. When the relationship between decade of birth and risk of illness by age was analysed, the effect was even more striking. For women born after 1950, the risk of major depression appears to be almost 70% by age 30! This appears to represent a major shift forward in the age of onset and the lifetime risk. All these relatives necessarily had an increased risk of mood disorder compared with the general population but the same pattern has been observed in the ECA population study (Klerman 1988, Klerman & Weissman 1989). Indeed there is also prospective longitudinal evidence favouring a trend to earlier onset of depression from the Stirling County study (Murphy 1994). Simple memory artefacts in older subjects, while they must occur along with other biases, appear not to be a full explanation for the cross-sectional findings (Warshaw et al 1991). Interpretation should remain cautious because the same pattern of increasing risk in recent birth cohorts is seen for mania (Lasch et al 1990), which appears much more epidemiologically stable (see below). What such findings actually imply, if correct, can only be guessed at. Social changes could be exercising strong and changing influences on the risk for depression of Western populations but, specifying how, for example, family relationships or the frequency of life events has changed over the last century will not be feasible. It also seems improbable that the social change should have been so consistently for the worse. For the moment, we have no way of knowing whether these findings represent an accurate basis for predicting further growth in the burden of disability imposed on societies by mood disorder in the coming decades. It is safe to predict a growth on the basis of improved detection of cases.

EPIDEMIOLOGY OF BIPOLAR DISORDER

The lifetime rates for bipolar I disorder are much lower and more consistent across countries (0.3/100 in Taiwan to 1.5/100 in New Zealand), the sex ratio is more equal and the onset age is earlier than for major depression. It is of particular interest that female sufferers have proportionately fewer manic episodes. It is increasingly claimed that the onset of bipolar disorder may often be in the teenage years, when the diagnosis may be missed. Systematic epidemiological studies are limited and diagnostic criteria remain controversial. Kessler et al (2001) suggest that as many as 25% of adolescents will have an episode of major depression and 2% of mania. The figures for mania appear too high and must be set besides an increasing vogue in North America for diagnosing bipolar disorder in children under 10 years of age. European clinicians are skeptical about the meaning of these diagnoses, which may be confused by prevailing ideas about attention deficit hyperactivity disorder (ADHD) and the surprisingly widespread use of stimulants as treatment in such patients in North America. The children (aged 12–21 years) of bipolar parents studied in the Netherlands did not show elevated rates of psychopathology (Wals et al 2001).

The unipolar–bipolar conversion rate is of the order of 5%. New onsets may increase in the elderly (Eagles & Whalley 1985). The very stability of its demographic characteristics favours a primarily biological explanation for the causes of bipolar I illness. As already indicated, bipolar II disorder is of emerging interest. It appears likely to be more common than bipolar I disorder (Simpson et al 1993) and clinically must often be misclassified as unipolar depression. Uncertainty over how to diagnose hypomania contributes to this problem (Goodwin 2002). The existence of minor elated states means that the classification of the major depressive states in the community as bipolar spectrum depression is likely to increase.

AETIOLOGY OF MOOD DISORDER

Our understanding of the aetiology of mood disorder is developing rapidly on the basis of critical scientific inquiry. It is important not least for the emphasis properly placed on alternative modes of treatment. More biologically determined conditions appear more likely to require medicines. More psychosocial causes of mood disorder may more plausibly prompt psychological interventions.

Individual cases of unipolar depression often appear to have understandable antecedents (life events or difficulties) which precipitate an illness. The extent to which such events independently and literally *cause* a depressive illness is always more questionable. The majority of individuals appear to negotiate the same losses and disappointments without decompensating and becoming ill: they cope. The failure to cope appears to be strongly determined by vulnerability factors which may in some cases be largely genetic, and in others the consequences of adverse early environmental experience. Recovery may be spontaneous or promoted by pharmacological or psychological intervention. The aetiology of individual cases is always more speculative than that of experimental cohorts but it is worthy of formulation both as an exercise for the clinician but also as a help for the patient. Interpersonal psychotherapy (IPT) (Klerman et al 1984) has as its central ingredients clear identification of symptoms, diagnosis and formulation of causal factors. Improved objective understanding of aetiology can be used constructively by patients in managing their illnesses. Self-management of mood disorder is likely to assume increasing importance as patients become better informed about what is known of their conditions.

Studies of the inheritance of mood disorder

Family studies

As has been noticed in the preceding section, affective disorder is more common in the relatives of identified probands with affective

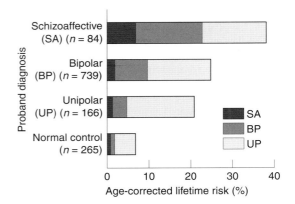

Fig. 20.3
Affective disorders in patients, siblings and adult offspring of probands in Bethesda, USA (Gershon et al 1982).

disorder than in the general population. The highest risks are seen with the most severe illnesses. This is illustrated in Figure 20.3, which shows the relative risks of different sorts of affective disorder for the first-degree relatives of normal controls and of patients with unipolar disorder, bipolar disorder or schizoaffective disorder. The striking conclusion is that, across these three illnesses, the risk of unipolar illness is about constant (around 20%) in the relatives of patients with each illness. However, there is an increased risk of bipolar and schizoaffective disorder, respectively, in the relatives of patients with these illnesses. These findings are compatible with the view that the more severe the illness in an index case, the greater the risk of a severe illness in first-degree relatives.

Twin studies Clearly, average risks of the sort described above may underestimate or overestimate the risks in a single family. For example, the family of Vincent van Gogh, who had a severe mood disorder and, of course, committed suicide, had above-average rates of severe psychiatric disorder (Jamison & Wyatt 1992). Such observations do not of course prove a genetic cause: families might influence the risks of mood disorder by their interactions and behaviour. Proof requires twin studies, where a discrepancy is sought between the concordance for monozygotic or genetically identical twins and dizygotic twins who should show simply the first-degree risks shown by other siblings. Such studies have been conducted classically on twin series from hospital registers but more recently also upon large community samples of twins. We now know a great deal about the relationship between genetic risk, environmental or familial influences and mood disorder.

The genetic basis is strongest for bipolar disorder, where almost 60% of identical twins will develop the same bipolar illness as cotwins in monozygotic samples, compared with something of the order of 14% in dizygotic pairs. Severe unipolar illness shows similarly high concordance for hospital samples. For example, probands with major depressive disorder ascertained via the Maudsley Hospital Twin Register showed proband-wise concordance of 46% in monozygotic ($n = 68$) and 20% in dizygotic ($n = 109$) twins. There was no evidence of a sex difference in heritability or of shared environmental effects. A duration of longest episode of less than 13 months, multiple episodes, and an endogenous rather than neurotic pattern of symptoms tended to predict a higher monozygotic:dizygotic concordance ratio (McGuffin et al 1996). Heritability was between 48% and 75%.

The links between genetic, temperamental and other risk factors and major depression have been forged most significantly by the ground-breaking work of Kendler's group at the Medical College of Virginia. They originally interviewed a large sample of female–female twin pairs and used nine definitions of major depression, producing lifetime prevalence rates from 12% to 33% (Kendler et al 1992). For seven of the definitions, the estimated heritability of liability ranged from 33% to 45%. For the two definitions that included only primary cases of depression, the heritability was lower (21% to 24%). The critical conclusions were that the tendency for depression to aggregate in families results largely from shared genetic and not from shared environmental factors, and the magnitude of genetic influence was similar in broadly and narrowly defined forms of major depression. Most environmental experiences of causative importance for depression are those not shared by members of an adult twin pair (i.e. more likely to be individual events rather than shared environmental factors) (Kendler et al 1992). Genetic factors are apparently shared between major depression and generalized anxiety disorder. Whether a vulnerable woman develops major depression or generalized anxiety disorder is a result of her individual environmental experiences (Kendler 1996).

Synthesis of the findings from different twin studies shows striking consistency (Sullivan et al 2000). The essential conclusion is that major depression in community samples is a markedly, but by no means overwhelmingly, genetic condition. Genetic explanations that ignore environment are likely to be partial. However, environmental explanations that ignore genetics will, equally, be misleading.

Of the genetic liability to major depression, 55% appeared to be shared with the personality trait neuroticism or N. A value for N 1 SD above the mean increased the risk of major depression within the next year by 100–130%. In fact, Kendler's group developed an exploratory but comprehensive model that accounted for 50% of the variance in the liability to major depression in a 1-year follow-up. Stressful life events, genetic factors, a previous depressive episode and N emerged as the best predictors of a subsequent depressive episode. The best-fitting model to an updated version of the same data from female twins again explained half the variance in liability to episodes of major depression. The three strongest risk factors were dependent and independent stressful life events in the last year and N. The development of risk for major depression in women may result from three broad pathways reflecting internalizing symptoms, externalizing symptoms, and psychosocial adversity (Kendler et al 2002).

The heritability of neurotic traits has also emerged from smaller studies. A genetic analysis was conducted on trait neuroticism and symptoms of anxiety and depression in 462 mixed-sex twin pairs from the Australian Twin Registry interviewed five times at regular intervals (Andrews et al 1990). When the lifetime history of these subjects was determined, rates of diagnosable disorder were low, and the study lacked the power to detect a genetic pattern. However, there was substantial genetic involvement in the average level of neuroticism and current symptoms. Neither genes nor the shared environment of the twins was a significant cause of lability in these measures, which was primarily affected by adverse life events.

The co-occurrence of mood disorder with alcohol and illicit substance abuse/dependence

The association between alcohol misuse and mood disorder is both clinically and theoretically important. There were significant genetic correlations (from +0.4 to +0.6) between major depression and alcoholism in women, which were higher using narrower criteria for alcoholism (Kendler et al 1993a). Thus, comorbidity in women appears to result largely from genetic factors that influence the risk of both disorders. Other genetic factors exist that independently influence the liability to mood disorder without influencing the risk of alcoholism, and vice versa. Cigarette smoking is also weakly related to the risk of mood disorder: twin analysis suggests that it results solely from genes that predispose to both conditions (Kendler et al 1993c). It is tempting to speculate that abnormal function in reward mechanisms may underpin these associations.

Molecular genetic findings in mood disorder

Genome scans The molecular genetic approach promises to give us clues to the underlying biochemistry of mood disorder (see Ch. 9). The inheritance of mood disorder is unlikely to be due to the gene mutations that underlie the best known (but much rarer) genetic diseases such as Huntington's chorea or the larger deletions of genetic material that underlie many severe congenital diseases, in most cases leading to mental handicap. These are genetic mistakes which can express their consequences independent of environmental influence. More common diseases are likely to be related to the presence of what are called polymorphisms. These are different forms (or alleles) of normal genes, present at different rates in the population, whose variation may be benign under most circumstances but still increases the risk of a disorder via dysfunction of the physiology that they control.

The role of putative loci can be established by linkage or allelic association studies. The best known linkage study was of a large Old Order Amish pedigree which was originally believed to show linkage of bipolar affective disorder to markers on chromosome 11 (Egeland et al 1987). Unfortunately this proved to be the first of several (false) positive studies announcing the linkage of the major psychiatric disorders to loci that could not subsequently be confirmed (Kelsoe et al 1989, Pauls et al 1991). The effort has, however, continued with renewed caution in accepting initial positives. The pooling of findings from individual studies offers an obvious way of increasing power for comparable populations. This has been performed recently for all the published genome scans for bipolar disorder and schizophrenia (Badner & Gershon 2002). The strongest evidence for susceptibility loci was on 13q and 22q for bipolar disorder, and on 8p, 13q and 22q for schizophrenia. There have been other putative reports of linkage of bipolar disorder to chromosome 4 (Blackwood et al. 1996), chromosome 18 (Berrettini et al 1994, Freimer et al 1996) and chromosomes 6 and 15 (Ginns et al 1996). Single studies of this sort need to be adequately powered because, where they are not confirmed, it is impossible to decide between the possibility of a type 1 error or a population specific (potentially important) positive. These effects appear worryingly small, and it remains to be seen how many of these findings will prove to be sufficiently localising to identify the relevant gene involved. If the function of the gene is known, the progress is likely to be straightforward. If it is not, then efforts to determine the function of individual genes are extremely complicated, and a long time is likely to elapse between the identification of the site and an understanding of why it is important.

An alternative approach to the illness phenotype is via quantitative traits known to be associated with the risk of, for example, major depression. Neuroticism is the most obvious candidate relevant to mood disorder as the Kendler group's work has shown. In addition, large samples of randomly screened siblings can be used to focus on phenotypically extreme individuals to increase power to detect genetic linkage in complex traits. Recently, a genome-wide linkage scan was completed using 87 extreme discordant and 190 extreme concordant sibling pairs, selected from 34 000 sibships who completed a personality questionnaire. Neuroticism was linked to loci on chromosomes 1p, 7p, 11q, 12q and 13q (Fullerton et al 2003). The locus on chromosome 1 is syntenic with that reported for QTL mapping of rodent emotionality, an animal model of neuroticism (Fernandez-Teruel et al 2002). This is the first report of the successful application of extreme selection strategies to identify QTL and suggests that animal and human QTL may be homologous for a behavioural trait relevant to depression and anxiety disorder. If this heralds the development of valid animal model of mood disorder it will have been a landmark discovery.

Allelic association studies It is now quite easy to genotype large numbers of patients and controls and to determine whether or not particular alleles are present in excess in patient populations. In consequence, allelic association studies of so-called 'candidate' genes are proliferating. In the original work of this sort, findings from the gene coding for the serotonin transporter protein (SERT) attracted particular attention because of the importance of the serotonin transporter as a singular site of action for antidepressants such as fluoxetine and the other selective serotonin reuptake inhibitors (SSRIs) (see below). An association between the rare allele of a variable number tandem repeat (VNTR) sequence in an intron of the SERT and mood disorder (both unipolar and bipolar patients) was described (Battersby et al 1996, Ogilvie et al 1996). This association could have represented a type 1 error, a direct effect of the allele on the function of the gene or linkage disequilibrium with a site close by of more direct relevance to the actual effect. That we remain unsure offers some understanding of the subsequent history of this field. Thus, in the first meta-analysis of findings for this original polymorphism and for a second SERT polymorphism in the promoter region of the same gene (Furlong et al 1998), there was no demonstrable allelic association of the VNTR polymorphism with affective disorder for a large combined bipolar and unipolar group, whereas promoter allele 2, which has previously been shown to result in lower levels of serotonin transporter transcription, did appear to be associated with affective disorder risk (estimated odds ratio 1.21; 95% confidence interval 1.00–1.45). While it was undeniably interesting to implicate a gene that is coding for a protein critical to the action of antidepressants, the effects were small and remained at the edge of statistical significance even with a total pooled sample of over 1000. Indeed a subsequent larger single sample failed to confirm the positive effect (Serretti et al 2002). The contribution of these genes to the risk of mood disorder may be too low to be important. It is possible that particular medicines may be differentially effective in individuals carrying particular

polymorphisms, but this and the literature surrounding innumerable other largely unsuccessful allelic association studies is beyond the scope of this chapter.

The significance of advances in this area will be to confirm the role of particular neurotransmitters and their receptors for mood disorder. There is also the potential to identify entirely new receptor mechanisms or pathways which may become a target of yet more effective and more focused treatments. At present the total risk seems to be contributed by many factors of small effect. Whether genetics makes any impact at all in shaping our approach to treatment of mood disorder will depend on whether subsidiary mechanisms (not the phenotype itself) can be more potently linked to individual gene function. If all the genes discovered are in fact of small effect, it is possible that genetics will offer no logical way to increase the effectiveness of our existing pharmacological treatments.

Environmental risk factors for affective disorder

While genetic factors determine the major risk of bipolar and severe unipolar disorder, there is an appreciable environmental contribution to the timing of severe illnesses and the incidence of less severe depressive illness. We have already noticed the variation in incidence of major depression between different societies and apparent increases in its frequency over time which seem to imply a major cultural effect on its expression. Kendler's exploratory attempt to weight the contributions of multiple factors to the onset of depression in the community is an important framework for starting to understand the role of 'social' factors as independent variables (Kendler et al 1993b). The studies that have hitherto attracted most attention in 'social psychiatry' have not controlled for the effects of genes. Surveys of inner-city populations of working-class and single mothers have indicated that adverse experiences in childhood and adolescence (involving parental indifference, and sexual and physical abuse) considerably raise the risk of both depression and anxiety conditions (with the exception of mild agoraphobia and simple phobia) in adult life (Brown & Harris 1993, Brown et al 1993). Given a strong prevailing bias to construe minor psychiatric disorder in these terms, the idea that vulnerability to depression is a socially determined risk has enjoyed easy acceptance. However, there is a quantitative balance between what is genetic and what is purely social. An early exposure to inadequate parenting may well be a consequence of the genetic endowment of the parent, as well as environmental misfortune. Only what is left after the appropriate control for genetic factors should be regarded as the 'environmental variance', and this must also contain error and chance. Conventional observational studies of the social origins of depression must have overstated the contribution of early environment. The problem is an intriguing one and even intrudes in the case of 'independent life events'.

Life events emerged strongly from Kendler's studies as predictors of the onset of major depression. In the best-known social studies, the impact of specific life events has been estimated with a strong emphasis on their context (Brown 1993). This means that life events are not judged as simple objective setbacks, such as the loss of a spouse or parent, but instead are given a weighting which relates to the closeness of the lost relative and the impact upon the individual patient. While this clearly has clinical meaning, it risks incorporating factors that are equally to do with personality and, potentially, genetic endowment. It confounds these factors, while attributing to them an independent status. Despite this, the differential effects of threat and loss events (to produce anxiety or depression) have been strengthened by genetically controlled studies.

The less rigorous methodology has also suggested a useful difference between first episodes and recurrences in more endogenous cases, with life events playing a part in the former, but not to the same extent in the latter conditions (Brown et al 1994). Such 'kindling' effects of recurrent illness are also seen in the female twins (Kendler et al 2001). The association between stressful life events and major depression declined as the number of previous depressive episodes increased. This decline was strongest in those at low genetic risk and was weak to absent in those at high genetic risk. Thus genetic risk factors for depression produce a 'pre-kindling' effect rather than an increase in the speed of kindling. The vulnerable state, in which depressive episodes occur with little provocation, may be reached by two pathways: many previous depressive episodes and perhaps multiple adversities, or high genetic risk.

However, the new genetic findings suggest that genes also contribute significantly to the vulnerability that is sometimes regarded as entirely social in origin (Kendler et al 1993b) and even to the exposure to life events. The 'heritability of life events' had been highlighted in other studies (McGuffin et al 1988, Thaper & McGuffin 1996). In Kendler's community sample, genetic liability to major depression was associated with a significantly increased risk of assault, serious marital problems, divorce/breakup, job loss, serious illness, major financial problems and trouble getting along with relatives/friends. The effect was not due to events occurring during depressive episodes (Kendler & Karkowski-Shuman 1997). About 10% of the total genetic liability to major depression may be mediated by genetically determined life events. In other words, certain traits appear to predispose individuals to select high-risk environments.

The significance of genes for social activity remains controversial. However, if we concede that socialisation has been a critical evolutionary development for the human species, it is difficult to argue that genes will have had no impact on behaviour and predispositions within it. The interaction of genes with early experience of loss and adversity that can predispose to depression is uncertain. Kendler's model has limited power to distinguish between various pathways to vulnerability (Kendler et al 2002). Nevertheless, these largely conform with clinical experience and highlight separate broadly internalising, externalising and deprivation-based routes to depression in women.

The relationship between lack of adequate parental care in early life and an increased risk of depression is convincing. Abuse and neglect are, however, highly non-specific factors which increase the risk of psychiatric disorder generally, and reflect gross disruption of the nurturing process. It is more difficult to decide whether more subtle disturbance of the parent–child relationship contributes as much as is popularly believed to the development of adult psychopathology. Adult reports of childhood difficulties can be systematised with the Parental Bonding Instrument (Parker 1983, Parker 1986, Parker & Barnett 1988). It identifies two dimensions: caring/non-caring and protective/overprotective. Non-caring and overprotective parental styles are associated with mood disorder in later life, but most strikingly with non-melancholic disorder (Parker et al 1987, 1995). There are non-causal explanations of this association: current depression might influence judgement of parental characteristics, reported parental characteristics may simply be wrong and those with a depressive predisposition might elicit less parental care and greater overprotection. The first two explanations appear to be excluded by appropriate experiments (Parker 1981). However, the determinants of parenting are obviously complicated, and a recent examination of the same measures in twins suggested that parental warmth was influenced by personality factors in both parents and children, while authoritarianism was related to educational and religious background (Kendler et al 1997a).

Recovery and improvement, when compared with conditions not changing, has been claimed to be associated with a prior positive event (Brown et al 1992). Such events were characterised by one or more of three dimensions:

- the 'anchoring' dimension involved increased security;
- 'fresh-start' involved increased hope arising from a lessening of a difficulty or deprivation;
- 'relief' involved the amelioration of a difficulty not involving any sense of a fresh start.

Events characterised by anchoring were more often associated with recovery or improvement in anxiety, and those characterised as fresh-start were associated with recovery or improvement in depression. Recovery or improvement in both disorders was more likely to be associated with both anchoring and fresh-start events. The effects of improved mood per se on the social measures could not be clearly differentiated, and these ideas remain highly provisional. Again, genes play a part. In a twin design, the four variables that influenced the time to recovery from depressive episodes were financial difficulties, obsessive–compulsive symptoms, severe life events and genetic risk (Kendler et al 1997b). All depressive episodes meeting symptomatic DSM-IIIR criteria were divided into early (5–28 days) and late (> 28 days) phases. Cases with more chronic depression showed an effect of personality, financial problems and genetic risk as predictors of slow time to recovery, suggesting different processes in recovery from brief versus prolonged depressions.

Bipolar disorder

The effects of life events on the recurrence or onset of bipolar disorder have received much less attention than for non-endogenous major depression. There appears to be a small excess of life events in advance of manic recurrence in bipolar illness (Hunt et al 1992a). The best known example of a life event precipitating mania is childbirth, where 1 in 500 mothers may develop a psychosis within 3 weeks of delivery, which is usually manic in form (Kendell et al 1987). Manic illness appears not to occur in any particular season, but bipolar depression may be more common in the autumn (Silverstone et al 1995). Perhaps 10% of patients appear to manifest an individual seasonality (Hunt et al 1992b): this can be clinically useful in advising patients on self-management.

Drugs and hormones

Depressive symptoms are strongly associated with the withdrawal of alcohol or stimulants like amphetamine or MDMA (ecstasy) (Peroutka et al 1988). Ecstasy has relatively selective effects on the serotonergic system, and it is tempting to suppose that these effects are generally related to serotonergic projections, because specific depletion of these neurons produces depressive symptoms (see below). Certainly, compared with other drug use, ecstasy appears to affect mood and aggressivity in particular. Women are more susceptible than men to mid-week low mood following weekend use of MDMA; however, both men and women show increased self-rated aggression (Verheyden et al 2002). It remains to be seen whether the predicted long-term adverse effects are seen on a population basis (Green & Goodwin 1996). The current widespread availability and use of ecstasy by young people could result in a later epidemic of mid-life depression attributable to neurotoxic effects on serotonergic neurons.

A more specific problem is posed by corticosteroids, which appear to increase the risk of affective disturbance and, in particular, of mania or hypomania, in relation to dose. Almost 3% of patients treated with a high dose of steroid may develop a clinically significant disorder of mood, and this is by far the highest sort of risk known for an exogenous stimulus (Boston Collaborative Drug Surveillance Program 1972). Recent controlled studies have confirmed high rates of subclinical mood elevation after 1 week of steroid administration (Naber et al 1996). Chronic exposure to corticosteroids, as in Cushing's syndrome, tends to be associated with depression of mood (see below). There are many anecdotal claims associating specific drug classes with effects on mood, but only calcium channel blockers and digoxin have been associated with depression by replicated, well-conducted studies (Patten & Love 1997). β-Adrenoceptor blockers and thiazide diuretics probably do not have important effects on mood.

Physical illness

Physical illness increases the risk of developing depressive illness (see also Ch. 28). While this may be understandable in the sense that the threat of a severe illness to an individual may provide a very powerful and pervasive negative context to his life, the depressive episode nevertheless merits treatment. There are some specific associations which may turn out to be of particular aetiological interest and will be described here.

Depressive illness and stroke

It has been suggested that depression is common after stroke and that the particular site of the brain insult may influence the risk of subsequent mood disorder. Thus, as well as a non-specific risk from the severe illness there may be a specific neuropsychiatric impact, depending on the localisation of the lesion. The original studies concentrated on selected groups of patients requiring hospital admission and longer-term care. They suggested an association between depression and left frontal pole regions, and euphoria and right hemisphere lesions (Robinson et al 1983). This is of some interest given the neuroimaging findings implicating left frontal cortex in mood disorder (see Ch. 5). Even in an unselected series of patients recruited from the community, in the 12 months after the stroke emotionalism was 10–20% and there was again an association with left-sided anterior lesions (House et al 1989), but there was a smaller number of cases of major depression. However, subsequently, the same study was summarised much more negatively as showing low rates of mood disorder and no evidence for localising lesions (House et al 1990). A comparably negative study has been reported using a similar patient sample (Burvill et al 1996). Clearly rates of depression vary between series (Andersen et al 1994) and are likely to be influenced by a range of general risk factors for depression that may often swamp the effects of the site of lesion (Burvill et al 1997). The question of whether, in an appropriate case-control series, there are nested associations between lesion location and risk of depression remains of neurobiological interest. For example, lesions in the region of the left basal ganglia have been suggested to be more specifically associated with depression (Herrmann et al 1995). Larger community studies of cardiovascular disease (not stroke per se) have also suggested an association between depressive symptoms and lesions of the basal ganglia (Steffens et al 1999).

Whatever the aetiology, depression is also of appreciable practical importance for the management of stroke patients (Robinson 1997). Depressive symptoms shortly after stroke (not major depression itself) predict increased mortality in unselected stroke patients (House et al 2001). Pharmacological treatment of post-stroke depression has been subjected to a number of small controlled trials. The evidence is that antidepressants are effective, although some tricyclics may be prone to produce confusion (Robinson et al 1995).

Heart disease

Findings in patients with myocardial infarction (MI) with depressive symptoms are surprising and interesting. Several studies have now described an association between short-term mortality following MI and the presence of significant depressive symptoms. For example, 222 patients were interviewed between 5 and 15 days following the MI and were followed up for 6 months (Frasure-Smith et al 1993). Depression was a significant and independent predictor of mortality from cardiac causes (95% CI 4.61 to 6.87). The effect was confirmed at 18 months (Frasure-Smith et al 1995). Traditionally, it might be supposed that depressive symptoms after MI would be reactive. In fact, there is evolving evidence that depressive symptoms can predict an elevated risk of MI many years before it occurs (Barefoot & Schroll 1996) and/or in the few weeks before an acute admission (Carney et al 1990). A follow-up of the Baltimore cohort of the ECA study showed that, compared with respondents with no history of dysphoria, the odds ratio for MI associated with a history of dysphoria was 2.07 (95% CI 1.16 to 3.71), and with a history of major depressive episode was 4.54 (95% CI 1.65 to 12.44), independent of coronary risk factors (Pratt et al 1996). A recurrence detectable in the coronary care unit may carry a particularly poor prognosis (Lesperance et al 1996). Patients with severe affective disorder have long been known to have an increased mortality from cardiovascular causes, and the association between the two is of considerable evolving interest. The most common cause of death is probably cardiac arrhythmia (Frasure-Smith et al 1995). It is interesting that depressed patients with stable heart disease have higher resting heart rates and lower variability during ordinary activity (Stein et al 2000). Autonomic dysfunction may be the cause of subsequent fatal arrhythmia.

If patients with heart disease are depressed, will they respond to antidepressants, and will antidepressants improve cardiovascular outcomes? A recent treatment study (SADHEART) comparing sertraline with placebo in patients with recent MI or unstable angina was able to demonstrate reduced depressive symptoms after sertraline, especially in more depressed patients. However, cardiovascular effects were not discriminable. A cardiovascular benefit may be present, because the trial was underpowered to detect worthwhile differences in rates of severe events (Glassman et al 2002).

NEUROBIOLOGY

There are no even partly satisfactory animal models of mood disorder but there is a highly relevant emerging literature on the understanding of emotion in animals. Behaviour theory was erected on the idea of primary reinforcing stimuli, positive ones such as taste and smell increasing associated responses, negative ones such as pain producing avoidant responses. Secondary associations are postulated to grow out of the pairing of primary reinforcers with a particular context. The complex emotional associations we experience with social situations, specific people and events could clearly be elaborated upon a basic theory of this sort. Intriguingly we are beginning to understand where the neural processing must be occurring. The key areas appear to be the amygdala and inferior frontal cortex. Primary reinforcing stimuli such as taste and smell are modalities whose representation in secondary sensory areas is directly within the inferior frontal region (Rolls 1990). Visual input is from much more highly elaborated representations that have already been processed through a number of cortical association areas. Are we in a position to say whether a lesion in inferior frontal areas renders people incapable of experiencing emotion? The answer is, probably, yes: the experience of emotion is different in such individuals (Rolls et al 1994), and the failure of their online monitoring of interoceptive bodily feelings seems to deprive them of 'gut feelings' that are essential for normal cognition (Damasio et al 1990, Bechara et al 1996). The question of pathological depression or elation of mood is more difficult since 'normal emotion' usually refers to anxiety. However, imaging studies have tended to localise the critical areas for mood change in mesial frontal cortex (Goodwin 1996).

The understanding of mood *disorder* in terms of neurobiology remains tentative while we have limited animal models. The identification of trait neuroticism as a risk factor with a significant heritability should be understandable in biological terms. Gray (1982) explicitly proposed that it might reflect an enhanced sensitivity of a 'behavioural inhibitory system' to negative experiences, which echoes Eysenck's own approach to understanding neuroticism in man. Experimentally, high-N individuals show a greater sensitivity to negative mood induction, while high E (extraversion) is associated independently with a greater sensitivity to positive mood induction (Larsen & Ketelaar 1989, 1991, Watson et al 1994). Why some depressive states persist and seem to become metastable is not understood. How cognitive information is processed may be important (Carr et al 1991, Dritschel & Teasdale 1991). The differences in cognitive function between individuals may be manifestations of different neuronal connectivity. Alternatively, there may be local properties of the brain areas directly involved in subserving mood that decide mood stability. For example, it has been claimed that a lobule of inferior frontal cortex, thought to be a critical node for the integration of mood, is atrophic in major depressive illness (Drevets et al 1997). Other abnormalities in brain structure might influence inferior frontal cortex through diffuse failures in afferent input. Severe mood disorder tends to be associated with ventricular enlargement and sulcal prominence (Elkis et al 1995). First episodes of severe depression occur more frequently with increasing age and tend to be more refractory to treatment (See Ch. 26). Such illnesses are associated with evidence of structural abnormality in the brain (Soares & Mann 1997) and cognitive impairment (Abas et al 1990, Beats et al 1996). Therefore, imaging suggests that something is permanently wrong in the brains of patients with particularly intractable mood disorder. Indeed this finding may be linked to poor outcome (Hickie et al 1995). This emphasises the need to ground explanations of illness in a unitary appreciation of psychological and biological variables. Structural brain abnormality is not of course an explanation for the more familiar illnesses that do show recovery.

The role of monoamines

Most of what we know, or think we know, about the neurobiology of mood disorder is based on the modulation of mood by pharmacological treatments. In other words the reversibility of mood disorder has seemed to require a neurochemical rather than a structural basis. It has given rise to what is generally called the monoamine hypothesis of affective disorders. Reserpine, which depletes monoamines, can induce a depressed mood, whereas amphetamine and, particularly, ecstasy, which releases monoamines, can induce euphoria, overactivity and excitement. Because these drugs modulate the levels and release of monoamines in the brain, this provides prima facie evidence of monoamines' relevance to the normal regulation of mood and possibly to the mechanisms of mood disorder. The monoamines concerned are noradrenaline (norepinephrine), dopamine, 5-hydroxytryptamine (5HT, serotonin) and acetylcholine. Cells containing these chemicals are present in neurons whose cell bodies are in the brainstem and midbrain. They project diffusely into forebrain areas where they appear to regulate global behavioural states or functions such as the sleep–wake cycle, appetite, motivation, motor activity, aggressiveness, sexual responsiveness and aspects of learning and memory. The evidence for involvement in these integrated behavioural responses is derived from animal experimentation, but it will be immediately obvious that these functions echo elements of psychiatric symptomatology described in depression. The first generation of agents discovered to treat mood disorder also have their primary actions on monoamines. Monoamine oxidase inhibitors (MAOIs) inhibit the breakdown of monoamines via the enzyme monoamine oxidase which exists in two forms: the A form catalyses the breakdown of noradrenaline and 5HT and the B form that of dopamine (and 5HT). The original MAOIs were non-selective between the A and B form and irreversible in their action. Subsequently, agents more selective for monoamine oxidase A and showing reversibility (e.g. brofaromine, moclobemide) have been shown to be effective antidepressants.

The other mechanism for antidepressant action is via the inhibition of monoamine reuptake. The tricyclic antidepressants appear primarily to act in this way, inhibiting the reuptake of both noradrenaline and 5HT (but not dopamine at clinical doses). Their antidepressant actions were discovered initially by accident through the clinical investigation of imipramine (Kuhn 1958). This led to the discovery that imipramine and the other tricyclics inhibit the reuptake of monoamines. Reuptake was recognised as a novel means of terminating neurotransmitter action both in the periphery and in the brain. Blockade of these receptors prolongs transmitter availability.

The most important development since then has been that of genuinely selective inhibitors of the reuptake of 5HT. The SSRIs have been shown to be effective antidepressants at doses where their action must be essentially on a single receptor. This is an exceedingly important theoretical and practical observation. It means that a highly complex disease can be treated by a medicine acting at a single receptor in the brain. This is in itself a powerful argument that reduced serotonergic function is a central abnormality in mood disorder and that its correction leads to clinical response. Other evidence supports the proposition that 5HT is unusually and specifically involved in mood disorder. The evidence for this is based on a number of different lines of enquiry. It will serve as the introduction to a neuroscience literature which is too large to survey here comprehensively. However, the fundamental weakness of the monoamine theory is its failure to take account of what is most puzzling and important about mood disorder: its poor outcome in a significant number of severe cases.

CSF metabolites

The monoamines are metabolised by relatively simple pathways that give rise to a small range of metabolites. These can readily be measured in cerebrospinal fluid (CSF) and allow rough estimates of transmitter turnover. In general these have revealed small and not always consistent differences in neurotransmitter metabolism in patients compared with controls. The National Institute of Mental Health (NIMH) study showed a tendency for increased levels of metabolites of noradrenaline and dopamine in the manic state compared with controls, and a relative depression of levels in the depressed state, particularly in dopamine turnover (Koslow et al 1983). The findings for 5HT suggest increases in the manic state, particularly in women, and did not show significant decreases in depression. Reduced 5HT metabolite level (and, hence, turnover) has been described in a variety of other studies. Most consistently this has implicated violent acts either towards the patients themselves (Traskman et al 1981) or others (Virkkunen et al 1994). The association between violent and impulsive behaviour and reduced 5HT function also emerges from studies of non-human primates (Mehlman et al 1994). A series of patients undergoing neurosurgery for depression also had depressed 5HT metabolites in CSF (Francis et al 1993). Even if the results had been entirely consistent it would have been difficult to distinguish between different possible causes because the physiology of people who are significantly sleep disturbed or who have lost weight may be different from that of normal controls but be only indirectly related to disturbance of mood.

It has already been noticed that the relationship between genetic findings and abnormalities of the phenotype is uncertain. CSF monoamine levels appear to be related to polymorphism in relevant genes. Polymorphisms in the dopamine transporter (DAT), serotonin transporter (SERT) and norepinephrine transporter (NET) genes have been examined. For both of the two SERT polymorphisms and the NET polymorphism, significant relationships were found with CSF 3-methoxy-4-hydroxyphenylglycol (MHPG) levels. No relationship was found with CSF homovanillic acid (HVA) and 5-hydroxyindoleacetic acid (5HIAA) levels (Jonsson et al 1998).

Tryptophan depletion

Perhaps the most convincing evidence that 5HT is involved in mood disorder comes from depletion of its amino acid precursor tryptophan. Tryptophan, both in peripheral blood and in brain, can be driven to very low levels by loading with large neutral amino acids which both compete with it for access to the brain amino acid transporter and increase the metabolism of all large neutral amino acids peripherally. The consequence is reduced synthesis and release of 5HT. Tryptophan depletion might be expected to uncover vulnerability to depressive symptoms normally gated by 5HT neurotransmission. That it does so is very important confirmation of the 5HT hypothesis. Tryptophan depletion produces reductions in mood in females, not males (Ellenbogen et al 1996), which may parallel both the vulnerability of women in general to mood disorder and the greater vulnerability of the serotonergic system to dietary perturbation (Goodwin et al 1987). There is a similar effect in males with a family history of mood disorder (Benkelfat et al 1994). However, much more striking is that, in patients who have recovered from a depressive episode during treatment with a 5HT selective reuptake inhibitor, tryptophan depletion produces a transient but clear-cut return of severe symptoms (Delgado et al 1990, 1991). Patients treated with an inhibitor of noradrenaline reuptake, such as desipramine, do not appear to show the effect. This finding has now been extended to patients with a history of recurrent major depression who are euthymic but off all medication (Smith et al 1997). These findings directly implicate 5HT specifically in the mechanism involved in the development of mood disorder. What is particularly intriguing is that prominent objective symptoms of retardation and cognitive distortion return in both a stereotyped and severe way, reflecting symptoms when previously ill. The apparent immediacy of the link between neurotransmitter function and symptoms may be the reason why the most vulnerable groups need long-term treatment with antidepressants to remain well.

Hypercortisolaemia

It is well established that patients with major depression have a raised cortisol output and that this tends to normalise on recovery. The most significant effect appears to be an elevation of the usual nadir in the evening, although cortisol levels are increased generally. The meaning of this phenomenon is still highly uncertain. An attempt was made to develop a test for severe depression based on the suppression of endogenous cortisol secretion by dexamethasone (the dexamethasone suppression test or DST). Suppression occurs when the sensitivity of the normal glucocorticoid receptor-mediated inhibitory feedback to the hypothalamus is present: non-suppression of endogenous cortisol occurs, for example, in Cushing's disease. It implies either reduced feedback and/or enhanced central drive to release cortisol. The initial findings were that the 1 mg DST showed high specificity (96%) and sensitivity (67%) for melancholia (Carroll et al 1981). This result has proved difficult to replicate. The high specificity was only established against normal controls and is clearly much less when other patient groups are included (Berger et al 1984). Non-suppression reflects hypercortisolaemia and there is quite a strong association between hypercortisolaemia and psychotic illness in general, particularly psychotic mania (Christie et al 1986). It is also possible that some patients show DST non-suppression as a result of weight loss (Mullen et al 1986), or because of altered metabolism of dexamethasone (Holsboer et al 1986).

In some respects the cortisol story has been too quickly devalued because of its failure to tie in with conventional ideas about how mood disorder should be diagnosed. Instead it should perhaps have been regarded as a phenomenon to be explained rather in the way that we may regard retardation, itself not specific to depression. Hypercortisolaemia certainly occurs and is both easy and objective to measure. This is of course less true of other symptoms that we identify as part of the depressive syndrome. In addition, relatively impaired glucocorticoid feedback has been described in the relatives of patients with mood disorder (Holsboer et al 1995). It appears that increased cortisol production is associated both with an increased release of hypothalamic β-endorphin (Goodwin et al 1993) and probably a pulsatile increase in adrenocorticotrophin (ACTH). However, in addition there appears to be peripheral hypertrophy of the adrenal glands which results in a measurable increase in size on magnetic resonance imaging (MRI) and an enhanced response to a given dose of corticotrophin (Gerken & Holsboer 1986). Like the hypercortisolaemia itself, the MRI change is reversible on recovery (Rubin et al 1995).

What remains unclear is whether cortisol actually contributes to the clinical picture by a direct action on the brain. This is of interest because of the association between exogenous cortisol administration and affective symptoms. It has led to efforts to treat mood disorder by inhibition of cortisol synthesis with metyrapone: preliminary results suggest this may be effective (O' Dwyer et al 1995, Thakore & Dinan 1995). This has led to the speculation that excessive cortisol secretion can produce depressive symptoms, as, indeed, seems to occur in Cushing's disease (Loosen 1994). Cortisol could of course be a plausible mediator between a variety of stresses and the biological components of mood disorder (Stokes 1995). Thus, the onset of depressive symptoms and their diurnal change could be accounted for by altered diurnal modulation of cortisol secretion. This concept of 'cortisol toxicity' remains to be convincingly tested. If this were indeed the explanation for mood disorders, in general, antagonists of cortisol's action should be extremely effective antidepressants. Evidence is awaited.

There are other contradictory aspects of these findings. For example when depressed patients are given large doses of cortisol, they tend to show acute mood enhancement (Goodwin et al 1992). This could lead to a mirror image hypothesis that actually cortisol is a euphoriant (or antidepressant) and therefore the hypercortisolaemia is an effort to mount an antidepressant action via the stress regulating mechanisms of the brain.

Although we measure steroids in the extracellular compartment, the primary actions are likely to be intracellular. Transport of steroids across the plasma membrane may be one of the mechanisms disturbed in mood disorder. Depression could be associated primarily with low intracellular cortisol. It is an interesting new idea that antidepressants may actually modulate this mechanism and serve to increase intracellular levels of cortisol (Pariante & Miller 2001).

An additional complication is that cortisol is believed to act on two receptors in the brain (the glucocorticoid and mineralocorticoid receptors) which may have opposed actions (DeKloet et al 1997). There is accordingly scope for opposing hypotheses of glucocorticoid action. Furthermore there is some emerging evidence that patients with early experience of abuse and neglect and individuals with post-traumatic stress disorder may show hypocortisolaemia. The future development of this field requires the elucidation of the psychotropic effects of cortisol itself upon the brains of patients who are potential hyper- or hyposecretors. The lumping together of depressions with different aetiology may explain our failure to find consistency hitherto. Given that hypercortisolaemia remains one of the more robust biological findings in mood dis-

order, we will have to return to it eventually for our understanding of the neurobiology to be complete.

Other endocrine abnormalities

There is also persistent interest in the role of the thyroid axis in mood disorder. There are abnormalities of the thyrotrophin (TSH) response to thyrotrophin-releasing hormone (TRH). The TSH secretion that results is impaired in some patients with depressive illness, but this effect is poorly understood and has few accepted clinical associations. The use of thyroid hormones in treatment is sufficiently interesting to suggest that there is more to be learned than we know currently about this endocrine axis. There is certainly evidence that thyrotrophin has important interactions with transmitter systems within the brain, and whether these are abnormally regulated in mood disorder remains unknown.

Sleep disturbance

Sleep is disturbed in depression in a variety of ways. The most typical, early morning waking, is by no means the only pattern that is seen, and trouble getting to sleep, frequent wakings and unsatisfactorily prolonged sleep are also common. Like other biological manifestations of the disorder, the extent to which sleep is simply a consequence of depression or contributes to its biology is tantalisingly uncertain. In favour of the latter view, patients even with severe depression may respond to sleep deprivation with a transient increase in mood. This occurs in patients refractory to other forms of treatment but has a limited value because the effect is rarely sustained and the consequences of chronic sleep deprivation are too difficult to make it a practical alternative. The fundamental involvement of the sleep–wake cycle in mood disorder is, however, interesting in view of the rhythmicity seen in bipolar disorder in particular and the possibility that some of the mechanisms that are involved may overlap and have a common biology. EEG recording either in a sleep laboratory or using ambulant methods has allowed the characterisation of the sleep disturbances in mood disorder (Berger & Riemann 1993). In melancholia the most characteristic effects are a reduction in the total length of slow-wave sleep and a shortened latency to the appearance of rapid eye movement or REM (dreaming) sleep. REM induction has been claimed to represent a cholinergic mechanism that may be abnormal in depression (Giles et al 1988, Berger & Riemann 1993), although its fundamental involvement in mood disorder is made less likely by the observation that REM changes can be mimicked by sleep restriction (Mullen et al 1986).

General problems with biological investigations of mood disorder

There are rather few measures of physiological, neuropharmacological, neuroanatomical or biochemical abnormality in the brain or blood or urine of subjects that could not be made the subject of a study that contrasts patients with mood disorder with normal controls. Attention has been focused here on those areas that have been most interesting. However, the acute disturbances of physiology and behaviour that are seen in severe depression are such that almost no aspect of the performance of an organism is likely to be entirely untouched by the state of depression. This implies that any of the changes that have been seen may be epiphenomena of the physiology that is so obviously disturbed in depression and mania (Mullen et al 1986, Goodwin et al 1987). What would be much more interesting is an abnormality that is demonstrably present in the euthymic condition. There is likely to be particular value in studying patients who are at high risk of mood disorder but are well. Such studies must also recognise our improved understanding of aetiology. Abnormalities in vulnerable subjects when compared with low-risk individuals are much more potentially interesting and much more potentially relevant to the development of new interventions.

EFFECT OF BRAIN AGEING

Age is an important risk factor for the development of severe mood disorder. This is true of both mania and depression (Eagles & Whalley 1985, Young & Klerman 1992) and may provide additional clues to the pathophysiology of mood disorder at the level of regional connectivity and in relation to specific markers. Normal ageing is accompanied by a decline in a variety of indices of monoamine function, including presynaptic markers of 5HT innervation. There is some evidence for reduced binding at these sites postmortem in depression (Perry et al 1983) and suicide (Mann et al 1996). Whether a reduced serotonergic innervation is the critical change that increases the vulnerability to mood disorder of patients with advancing years is not yet established. Postmortem studies in elderly depressed patients appear likely to have more potential validity than the (much more numerous) reports on schizophrenia: a definitive study is awaited.

TREATMENT OF DEPRESSION — PRIMARY CARE

If patients are reluctant to seek treatment and the detection of less severe depressive illness in primary care is relatively low, then many, perhaps the majority of episodes of depression receive no treatment at all. Where depression is detected and endures, there is a range of effective treatments. The most widely available are antidepressants. Antidepressants are not, as is widely believed, addictive. Unlike drugs that are, they do not have primary rewarding properties, do not display tolerance and produce, at worst, mild physical symptoms on withdrawal. The choice of effective medicines that we now have available is quite large. In addition we have at least two classes of psychological treatment which also have efficacy relevant to treatment in primary care: cognitive behaviour therapy (CBT) and interpersonal psychotherapy (IPT) and the related method of problem solving. At present we really have no way of deciding which should be regarded as best practice. There are a number of issues, which include relative efficacy, adverse effects, subsequent risk of recurrence, costs both direct and indirect, and last, but not least, acceptability to patients. Readers can find useful guidelines for the use of antidepressants at http://www.bap.domainwarehouse. com/ (Anderson et al 2000).

Reuptake inhibitors

Tricyclic antidepressants and the newer, more selective compounds (selective serotonin reuptake inhibitors or SSRIs) act primarily to block active transport of neurotransmitters back into neurons (see Ch. 15). The older compounds (amitriptyline, imipramine, chlomipramine) are still widely used and, if anything, are more effective than the newer antidepressants in patients with severe

illness (Anderson & Tomenson 1994). Quantitative reviews comparing the actions of the tricyclic antidepressants with the newer compounds suggest equality of efficacy in less severe illness (Song et al 1993). The major problem with the tricyclics is the need to employ doses of at least 150 mg at night (correspondingly lower in older patients). At such therapeutic levels there are commonly important side-effects. These are due to actions at cholinergic receptors (dry mouth, sweating, mild tachycardia), histamine receptors (sedation, weight gain), serotonergic receptors (weight gain, disturbed sexual function). Amitriptyline tends to have more actions of this sort, imipramine (and especially desipramine) rather less. However, the sedative action is sometimes valued by patients who are having difficulty sleeping or who have marked anxiety symptoms. These side-effects are usually, however, a disadvantage and a reason why patients may discontinue treatment (Anderson et al 1994, Maddox et al 1994). Taken with the greater danger of tricyclics in overdose, there is an argument that newer compounds should be employed because of their greater acceptability. In principle, more patients will be treated effectively with an antidepressant that they will take than with one that they will not. The alternative newer compounds are as follows.

SSRIs (selective serotonin reuptake inhibitors)

These agents work at a single receptor, and their adverse effects are accordingly related to their central therapeutic action. These effects include nausea and even vomiting (tending to diminish with time), orgasmic impotence which is a major problem in long-term use for some patients (albeit a possible advantage for male patients with premature ejaculation), and sleep disturbance. All these effects can be related to the physiology of 5HT. The SSRIs available in the UK are fluoxetine, paroxetine, sertraline and citalopram. While pharmacologically similar they are not identical. Sertraline and fluoxetine appear to be more activating. Also, some patients experience idiosyncratic reactions to one of the agents that they do not experience on others (for example, marked agitation). Paroxetine appears to be associated with, usually mild, physical withdrawal effects more often than other SSRIs. The use of the SSRIs has increased dramatically since their introduction. What is interesting is that most of this increase in prescribing appears to be additional to, not just instead of, tricyclic prescribing. This may reflect the greater acceptability of SSRIs. They are also easier to prescribe because of their simple dosing requirements. In Scandinavian countries the introduction of SSRIs has been associated with a reduction in suicide rates.

There have been regular efforts in the courts to obtain compensation from parent companies after patients taking SSRIs have committed suicide or even homicide. The relationship between these mercifully rare events and any prescription is obscured by the confound of the depressed state itself. There is no signal from existing databases or population frequencies to suggest that SSRIs cause patients to commit suicide. Indeed, the evidence noticed above suggests the opposite.

Receptor antagonists

Other antidepressants increase the availability of monoamines (specifically 5HT and noradrenaline) by mechanisms other than reuptake inhibition (Davis & Wilde 1996). The most widely prescribed include mianserin and its successor mirtazapine. Compounds such as trazodone may also fall into this category.

Reversible inhibitors of monoamine oxidase

The conventional MAOIs (see below) would rarely be considered first-line treatments in primary care but their successors are reversible compounds which require fewer dietary precautions, are safer in overdose and carry a lower risk of interactions with tyramine-containing foodstuffs. Moclobemide may, accordingly, be an adequate antidepressant for use in primary care. Its relative advantages are not yet established. Particular caution is required if patients are prescribed moclobemide and an SSRI sequentially. There is then the risk of a combined overdose which can produce a very dangerous toxic serotonin behavioural syndrome with hyperthermia (Neuvonen et al 1993). The MAOIs and SSRIs (and clomipramine) should never be used together because they can produce related toxic effects at therapeutic doses.

TREATMENT OF DEPRESSION — SECONDARY CARE

Tricyclic antidepressants

Tricyclic antidepressants remain an important and useful class of medicines for treatment of severe depression in secondary care. As already indicated, the main problem is the need to treat with doses which almost inevitably incur adverse effects, although many patients are prepared to persevere with treatment because of the severity of their mood disturbance. The apparent advantages of tricyclic antidepressants over newer compounds are most clearly seen in older inpatients, where clomipramine has been shown to be superior to citalopram and paroxetine (Gram 1986, Anderson et al 1990, Anderson & Tomenson 1994). This is a theoretically important finding if it reflects the action of clomipramine on both noradrenergic and serotonergic reuptake sites to facilitate transmission in both pathways. A drug that had these tricyclic-like actions without the toxicity inherent in the chemistry of the tricyclics would be a major advance. Venlafaxine is a compound which inhibits reuptake in vitro at both sites but has few other actions. It shows the predicted superiority to SSRIs but not tricyclics in a meta-analysis (Smith et al 2002). Milnacipram has the same sort of profile, but is not widely available. The selectivity of these antidepressants with a double action (including mirtazapine) confers advantages compared with tricyclics in the treatment of patients in secondary and tertiary care because they induce fewer side-effects and are safer in overdose.

Monoamine oxidase inhibitors

Patients who fail to respond to tricyclic antidepressants may respond to monoamine oxidase inhibitors. The previous reputation of these compounds for lack of efficacy resulted from the use of too small a dose in influential trials (Medical Research Council 1965). Phenelzine, for example, should be given at doses above 45 mg daily. The major disadvantage with the MAOIs is the requirement for strict dietary avoidance of fermentation products to prevent the so-called cheese reaction (the ingestion of tyramine-containing foods that are toxic in the presence of complete and irreversible monoamine oxidase inhibition). They may also produce postural hypertension at relatively low doses. Severe cases of mood disorder merit a trial of an MAOI where tricyclics have failed.

Electroconvulsive therapy

ECT is an important treatment for severe depression. The indications are usually psychotic or endogenous features and, commonly, the failure of pharmacological treatment. In addition, ECT is indicated in emergencies where depressed patients are refusing food and drink, on the basis of extreme retardation or nihilism. ECT is now always administered under general anaesthesia with a neuromuscular blocking agent 2 or 3 times per week. Its unpleasantness is about the same as going to the dentist. The effectiveness of ECT is well supported by clinical trials and there are no established long-term adverse sequelae. Despite this, the rate of administration clearly varies a good deal from region to region and consultant to consultant, probably reflecting the ebb and flow of opinion about its use, which has long been controversial. The Royal College of Psychiatrists produces regular guidelines to regulate practice and maintain standards. The 'dose' of ECT will always require clinical judgement because efficacy and adverse cognitive effects both increase along with stimulus intensity. Bilateral ECT is moderately more effective than unilateral ECT, and higher-dose ECT is more effective than lower-dose. Seizure duration should be monitored as greater than 20 s to ensure optimal efficacy. The number of administrations required varies a good deal but is usually between 4 and 6 treatments. The earliest changes occur in feeding and locomotion, and the response rate under naturalistic conditions should be about 80%. The problem is sometimes to maintain improvement in patients who may be relatively refractory to pharmacological treatments.

Combination treatments

Patients seen by psychiatrists are much more likely to have a poor outcome or fail to respond at all to first-line treatments than those seen in primary care. Their management is therefore empirically based upon the use of logical pharmacological combinations. The discussion of the pharmacology of this approach is beyond the scope of this chapter, and experience and considerable care are probably required to avoid problems. That said, the most important options are the following.

- *Augmentation with lithium*. The addition of lithium to either tricyclic antidepressants, SSRIs or MAOIs appears to be associated with an acute antidepressant effect in up to 50% of patients otherwise refractory to monotherapy. This is a relatively simple combination but there is uncertainty about its longer-term benefits. Use of lithium increases the complexity and difficulty for the patient because of the need for continuing plasma monitoring.
- *Addition of tryptophan*. It was probably the first application of rational psychopharmacology to add tryptophan in the treatment of patients refractory to MAOIs (Coppen et al 1963). It may also be a useful adjunct to treatment with clomipramine, and there are advocates for the addition of both tryptophan and lithium to either an MAOI or clomipramine in the treatment of the most severely refractory patients. The withdrawal of tryptophan (because of fears about impurities) produced relapse in the patients treated long term with these combinations (Ferrier et al 1990). With appropriate monitoring for an eosinophilia syndrome, use of tryptophan is still a safe and convenient augmentation strategy. Successful addition of tryptophan implies that patients may be depleted of substrate. Another possibility is

that they may use substrate less effectively because of cofactor deficiency. Plasma homocysteine is a sensitive measure of functional folate deficiency, and a biological subgroup of depression with folate deficiency, impaired methylation, and monoamine neurotransmitter metabolism has been described (Bottiglieri et al 2000). There is growing interest in folate as a relevant supplement in such cases. A controlled trial has suggested efficacy for folate, specifically in women (Coppen & Bailey 2000).

- *Thyroid augmentation*. There is evidence to support the augmentation of antidepressant treatment with tri-iodothyronine (T_3) (Joffe et al 1993, Aronson et al 1996).

In general this is an area of considerable uncertainty, and efforts to trial different combination treatments, preferably combined with newer compounds of dual action, would be welcome.

STRATEGIES OF MANAGEMENT IN MAINTENANCE AND CONTINUATION TREATMENT

In primary care, the primary objective is to treat, be it with pharmacological or psychological methods, to a good short-term outcome over about 6 months. At that point (in fact, often sooner) treatment is usually withdrawn; many patients will have only a single episode of mood disorder. We are very unsure whether active treatment affects the long-term outcome of mood disorder in individual patients. Since many patients must be untreated, the natural course of illness in younger patients may be spontaneous recovery. It seems reasonable to assume that more decisive treatment is necessary with later onset or with chronic or repeated illnesses. The evidence for this remains circumstantial, however. Recurrent depressive episodes may be a potent reason for long-term treatment with antidepressants even in primary care (Geddes et al 2003 and see below)

Patients referred to psychiatrists tend by definition to have more severe illnesses either in relation to the severity of symptoms, their duration or their tendency to recur. The strategy for treating most patients with mood disorder seen in secondary and tertiary care should be, first, to get effective acute treatment using the necessary strategies outlined above, and then to continue with an acceptable maintenance treatment indefinitely. At present this is a difficult conclusion for many doctors and patients themselves to accept. The evidence is, however, that with each recurrence the risk of a further subsequent illness is increased and the time at which it will occur tends to advance.

There is evidence that long-term treatment with lithium is effective in unipolar disorder (Souza & Goodwin 1991). This is a logical continuation treatment for patients who have required lithium augmentation in the acute phase of their illness but seems not to be very commonly considered because there is no particular evidence of an advantage over the use of long-term reuptake inhibitors. There have been good long-term studies demonstrating the efficacy of imipramine up to 5 years in patients showing recurrent unipolar depression (Kupfer et al 1992). Treatment for up to 2 years has been examined for the SSRIs and for the other new antidepressants. As already noticed, the results of relapse prevention studies are remarkably consistent in showing continuing and substantial relative reductions in risk of relapse independent of the duration of preceding treatment (Geddes et al

2003). This is important and poorly appreciated by doctors and patients alike When the risk of recurrence is high, treatment may be highly effective.

Compliance, adherence, concordance

Patients may show compliance with doctors' orders (unfashionable), adherence to prescribed medicines (neutral) or concordance (new speak) with a shared treatment plan. The bottom line is that medicines will not work if patients do not take them. While short-term compliance may be dominated by issues relating to side-effects, in the long term it is likely to be much more to do with a patient's beliefs and perceptions (Horne & Weinman 1999). Interventions to enhance adherence should increase the effectiveness of prescribing. This is a neglected area in psychiatry, highly relevant to long-term treatment in mood disorder.

THE PLACE OF PSYCHOLOGICAL TREATMENTS

The idea that a psychological treatment might be as effective as a pharmacological treatment in acute illness and offer greater protection from recurrence is an attractive one (Andrews 1996). Maintaining recovery is an important objective of effective psychological treatments for panic disorder or eating disorders. Trials in primary care have tended to suggest a particular benefit from CBT in depression (Blackburn et al 1981, 1986), although most such patients recover, however treated (Scott & Freeman 1992).

For more severe depressive illness, however, there is reasonable evidence from a large NIMH multicentre trial (Elkin et al 1995) that cognitive therapy is not particularly effective in the acute treatment phase. Indeed IPT was probably superior. Although the original analysis of this study was probably inadequate, re-analysis has not changed the conclusions, much as it has served to sharpen the debate. The tentative finding that patients failing CBT respond to imipramine (Stewart et al 1993) underlines the conclusion that severe depressive illness is best treated with an effective antidepressant. The issue, which remains uncertain, is whether, nevertheless, CBT may improve the long-term outcome. This can only be answered by a trial of cognitive therapy specifically directed at the prevention of relapse or recurrence. Modest benefits have been reported when a complex CBT package was compared with treatment as usual in patients with residual depressive symptoms (Paykel 2001). How much is specific in such interventions and how much is a result of enhancing the structure of care in quite a non-specific way is uncertain. This is of interest because the difficulty with cognitive therapy is that it is complicated and requires extensive training. Interpersonal psychotherapy (Klerman et al 1984) and its close relation, problem-solving psychotherapy, is easier to teach and, because it focuses almost exclusively on relationship, is a more generic approach to the problems of patients of all sorts. In relative terms it remains neglected compared with CBT but merits much more attention that it has so far received.

TREATMENT OF MANIA

Mania is often an indication for admission to a specialised psychiatric unit. Detention under the appropriate section of the Mental Health Act may also be necessary because of the loss of judgement and insight associated with severe upswings in mood. In the past, severe manic states were associated with increased mortality as a result of exhaustion, dehydration and hyperthermia. Although modern practice has reduced this particular risk considerably, it needs to be remembered, together with the potential for suicide, although this is rarely an important risk in uncomplicated mania. Admission allows the supervision and titration of adequate pharmacological treatment, and a well-run ward is an important component of treatment.

Pharmacological treatment

The objectives are to control behaviour, to terminate the episode and to prevent early recurrence. Dopamine receptor antagonists (major tranquillisers or antipsychotics) are the first-line agents in acute severe mania. The dose must be established empirically by giving repeated small doses of the chosen compound until an adequate effect is established. The urgency of this titration clearly depends upon the patient. Where there is a fear of violence or conflict it is easy to get drawn into using high doses of antipsychotics. However, it is probably wrong to think too readily of antipsychotics as achieving 'tranquillisation'. The most beneficial effects of antipsychotics may relate to psychomotor slowing and antipsychotic effects. Sedation by antipsychotics may require very high doses, and this is increasingly realised to be undesirable and potentially dangerous. The difficulty with antipsychotics resides in their actions on myocardial transmission and the risk of sudden death. There is therefore contemporary interest in developing alternative regimens which depend upon an antipsychotic in low to moderate doses combined with more-explicitly sedative compounds such as lorazepam or clonazepam. The advantage of benzodiazepines is their remarkable safety at high doses.

The number of trials in mania has been nothing like the number in schizophrenia. Indeed, the classical antipsychotics have scarcely been examined in mania against placebo. There is increasing interest in atypical antipsychotics in the treatment of acute mania. A better therapeutic ratio for extrapyramidal effects is an important advantage of such medicines. Olanzapine, quetiapine, risperidone, aripiprazole and ziprasidone have been shown to be anti-manic in placebo-controlled randomised clinical trials.

The usual duration of treatment is dictated by the time of remission of symptoms. Depressive symptoms may develop and require treatment in their own right. In fact the resolving phase of an acute manic disturbance is often difficult to treat, and patients are frequently discharged from hospital before they are completely well. Recovery usually takes approximately 6 months.

Lithium is itself effective in acute mania and is advocated especially in the USA (see below). It is not very sedative and does not reach adequate intracellular concentrations quickly when given in conventional doses of 800–1600 mg daily. It should be chosen only after careful medical screening. A plasma concentration of about 1 mmol/l, i.e. the upper end of the therapeutic range (or higher), is said to be superior in acute illness. Careful monitoring of plasma concentrations is essential. Concurrent use of a dopamine blocker is often necessary but must be cautious (see description of neurotoxic effects below).

Valproate (as semisodium valproate) has been shown to be as effective as lithium in acute mania (Bowden et al 1994). Valproate is used in the USA for most severities of mania and may be the preferred choice when rapid cyclical mood changes or mixed mania (combining manic and depressive features during the course of the day) are prominent.

Any sedative agent may be useful in refractory mania, and there is anecdotal experience to support the use of barbiturates, high-potency benzodiazepines as described and even paraldehyde. Whether any of these medicines influence the course of the underlying disorder is uncertain, and they are often used together with antipsychotics. ECT can be very useful in refractory mania, and there is also evidence for a paradoxical tranquillising effect of amphetamine. Finally, verapamil and other calcium antagonists may have anti-manic actions, the pharmacological basis for which is poorly understood. It is important to understand that alternatives to antipsychotics remain in the absence of a therapeutic response to conventional management.

Treatment of mania is regarded by American authorities as revolving round the choice of a mood stabiliser as primary treatment (lithium or an anticonvulsant) and necessary 'adjunctive' treatments (antipsychotic and benzodiazepines). To describe an antipsychotic as a first-line medicine (as above) would then be to fail to treat the disorder. Caution appears necessary in accepting the distinction between mood stabilisers and adjunctive treatments. This may be more a linguistic convention than an empirical difference.

Prevention of recurrence

Lithium

The usual indications for starting treatment with lithium in otherwise uncomplicated cases are two illnesses within 2 years or three illnesses in 5 years. This is both arbitrary and conservative. It is also of limited average effectiveness. Although its use can transform the occasional individual's life, disappointingly few patients with an established recurrent illness achieve long-term mood stability on lithium monotherapy (Markar & Mander 1989). Given an early onset, a strong family history, and severe disorder, the destructive potential of bipolar illness justifies prophylactic treatment after the first episode. In practice, however, the resistance of the patient or the family to an indefinite course of pharmacological treatment before the illness has shown evidence of recurrence may limit the clinician's actions. In any case, on average, recurrence with subsequent illnesses is the rule rather than the exception.

There have been adequate numbers of patients randomised into placebo-controlled long-term or maintenance trials of lithium treatment (Burgess et al 2001). Relapse rates on lithium over a year or so were 40% compared with 61% on placebo. That means in general one would need to treat about 4 patients for a year with lithium to avoid 1 relapse. The patients who do well on lithium continue to do well on it. There is a 40% relative reduction in risk of manic relapses compared with 23% for depressive relapses. In fact lithium is only just effective on current evidence at protecting against depressive relapses. Thus, the use of the term mood stabiliser, implying that a medicine will be equally effective against both the manic and the depressive poles of bipolar illness may be overoptimistic. In the case of lamotrigine (see below) the effects are in the opposite direction — it is a 'mood stabiliser' more effective against depression than mania. We are uncertain of the true magnitude of relevant efficacy against recurrent mania and depression for other medicines used long term in bipolar disorder, simply because there have been insufficient numbers of patients entered into randomised clinical studies.

If we remain significantly uncertain as to the extent that most medicines used for long-term treatment in bipolar disorder actually do 'stabilise' mood, then the term 'mood stabiliser' may best be discarded in favour of the more neutral 'long-term treatment'

Baseline investigation of renal and thyroid function and an electrocardiograph are advised before starting lithium. It can usually be prescribed as a single does at night. The unusually low therapeutic index requires monitoring of plasma concentration. Blood should be regularly sampled 12 hours after the last dose; a concentration of 0.5–1.0 mmol/l is usually effective. Plasma concentrations over 1.1 mmol/l or certainly 1.5 mmol/l are predictive of toxicity. Recommendations about how frequently levels should be checked vary enormously; once the level is stable, every 3 months is probably prudent. Concentrations at the lower end of the range are usually adequate for prophylaxis. Efforts to raise lithium levels to 0.8 mmol/l will increase side-effects and non-adherence.

The most common side-effects are tremor, polyuria and weight gain. It is worth lowering the does to try to reduce these symptoms, as all may affect compliance. If necessary, tremor can be treated with a beta blocker and polyuria with amiloride. The introduction of any diuretic requires careful monitoring of the plasma lithium concentration. Neurotoxicity is an important but rare complication. It can develop insidiously, sometimes after a dose increase, sometimes at notionally 'therapeutic' levels, sometimes in conjunction with other medicines, especially antipsychotics, sometimes in association with intercurrent illness or other brain pathology (Kemperman & Tulner 1990, Bell et al 1993). The resulting encephalopathy has no defining features and may be reversible. However, the most characteristic bad neurological outcome is a cerebellar syndrome.

Manic illness following discontinuation of lithium in bipolar patients is a particular problem. Suppes and colleagues reviewed 14 studies involving 25 patients with bipolar disorder, and found that more than 50% of new episodes of illness occurred within 10 weeks of stopping treatment (Suppes et al 1991). The length of treatment preceding discontinuation varied widely, but averaged about 30 months. This risk means that prophylactic treatment with lithium must continue for longer than 2 years because premature withdrawal may bring forward the time of the next recurrence of mania (Goodwin 1994). A long period of mood stability while taking lithium is not a guarantee of stability on its withdrawal. In addition, anecdotal evidence suggests that symptoms after withdrawal may be refractory to subsequent treatment (Post et al 1992). For these reasons, indefinite maintenance treatment with lithium is often recommended.

Alternatives to lithium prophylaxis

Valproate is regarded as an alternative to lithium in North America. It has been studied in a single statistically inconclusive RCT, showing rates for all relapses of 24%, against placebo at 38%. This suggests a relative risk reduction of about 37%, numerically comparable with that for lithium. Target dose for maintenance is around 1000 mg. It may show superior acceptability, especially if lithium is used at relatively high plasma levels.

Carbamazepine was the first medicine after lithium to be advocated for long-term treatment of bipolar disorder (Okuma &

Kishimoto 1998). It has been re-examined in two recent trials, which showed a substantial benefit to lithium compared with carbamazepine in preventing relapse. It may be useful in patients with atypical (i.e. non-euphoric) cases. Lamotrigine maintenance trials individually support an effect against depression, as against mania.

Long-term treatment with antipsychotics

Antipsychotics are used in as many as 50% of bipolar outpatients for long-term treatment. The evidence supporting such a strategy is mainly by extension from schizophrenia and clinical audit (e.g. Littlejohn et al 1994). Depot antipsychotics have the advantage of ensuring adherence. The disadvantages of classical antipsychotics relate primarily to their extrapyramidal effects, which may be more likely to occur in patients with affective illness. Some patients taking lithium have regular (e.g. seasonal) manic upswings that can be managed by giving an oral antipsychotic for a few weeks as an outpatient. It is advisable to provide an advance supply of the medicine for this purpose to responsible patients. Antipsychotics are commonly used in combination with other agents.

Olanzapine has been shown to be effective in long-term relapse prevention studies. Other atypical antipsychotics are also under active investigation. Given the reduced risk of adverse motor effects, atypical antipsychotic agents may be appropriate for the long-term management of bipolar patients, especially where the illness is driven by recurrent episodes of mania.

Long-term treatment with antidepressants

Long-term treatment of bipolar I patients with antidepressants is also common in clinical practice. Given the significant burden of disease imposed by chronic depressive symptoms and recurrent depressive episodes, this may not be surprising. The evidence supporting the use of antidepressants in the long-term prophylaxis of unipolar depression is unusually strong. The equivalent evidence for bipolar patients is almost completely absent. Antidepressants may precipitate and even exacerbate mania. There is non-random evidence for successful long-term prophylaxis with antidepressants in bipolar patients also receiving an anti-manic agent to avoid provoking mood instability and manic relapse.

Bipolar II patients and, in particular, patients with bipolar spectrum depression have not been sufficiently investigated. Anecdotally, some authorities believe that effective treatment with antidepressants is possible without an additional anti-manic medicine. This is an area that merits further investigation as the diagnostic issues become more widely understood.

Antidepressant-induced mania or hypomania merits co-administration of an anti-manic medicine such as valproate or lithium.

Lamotrigine is recommended for the treatment of bipolar depression in North America. This is because the few placebo-controlled data which bear on the use of conventional antidepressants are thought to compare unfavourably with the evidence for lamotrigine.

Long-term treatment — winning combinations

It follows that if no single medicine is maximally effective against both poles of the illness then in future efforts must be directed to identifying the best combination of agents for individual patients or groups of patients. We would not treat cancer with a single compound until it was shown to be ineffective. The study of combinations of the currently available medicines with anti-manic and antidepressant properties to determine the optimal choice for patients under all conditions appears increasingly necessary. Effective prevention of disease progression may require combination treatment from as early in the illness course as possible. At present we are uncertain as to what combination if any to recommend from a first episode. The solution will be pragmatic clinical trials which are large, simple and conducted in partnership with, but independent of, the pharmaceutical industry, an approach that has paid off in other branches of medicine concerned with long-term treatment strategies (Geddes & Goodwin 2001).

COURSE AND OUTCOME OF MOOD DISORDERS

It is appropriate, and necessarily humbling, to return to a consideration of the course and outcome of mood disorder after reviewing our current treatment options. The seriousness of mood disorder is still something that needs formally to be reaffirmed for the medical profession and public alike, and there remain many problems in the delivery of the treatments we have, before we achieve their known limitations (Hirschfeld et al 1997). It is an irony of the mood disorders that the most severe episodes of mania and psychotic depression have in some senses the best short-term outcome. Patients have a high probability of short-term recovery but the near certainty of subsequent recurrence with or without treatment. How the outcome should be represented for the whole spectrum of mood disorder remains uncertain.

Approximately half of all incident cases of major depression in the community will not have a subsequent episode. The mean time to recurrence with the second episode is about 15 years, and to the third episode about 10 years. However, this sort of retrospective reporting is subject to obvious biases. The longer-term prospective studies are only now becoming available (Murphy 1994).

The best-known follow-up studies have been based on inpatient cohorts. For example, a 40-year follow-up of a cohort of patients admitted to the Iowa Psychopathic Hospital between 1934 and 1945 allowed the contrast to be drawn between the mood disorders and schizophrenia. Depressive disorders generally had a better outcome than schizophrenia but that is not to say very much. The general conclusion from studies of this sort is that the outcome is poor. This is perhaps underlined by detailed follow-up studies of more recent cohorts. Lee & Murray (1988) showed that only 11 of 89 patients first seen in the 1960s after admission to the Maudsley Hospital had a good outcome. Twenty-five had an extremely poor outcome. This finding was echoed by a very similar study from Australia (Kiloh et al 1988). The Maudsley depressives showed the worst outcome for those who had the most psychotic or endogenous symptoms at the index admission.

The outcome in severe mood disorder is similar in bipolar and unipolar samples. For example, in a recent 27-year prospective study of 186 unipolar depressives and 220 bipolars, there was a progression from unipolar depression, schizodepression, pure affective bipolar disorder to schizobipolar disorder showing a systematic decrease in age of onset and length of episode. When compared with unipolar disorders, the bipolars showed more-frequent but shorter episodes. The only difference in course between schizoaffective subjects and those with pure affective disorder was a greater frequency in episodes requiring hospitalization among schizoaffectives (Angst & Preisig 1995a). Eleven percent of the sample had committed suicide, and the risk was associated with clinical severity and onset prior to the age of 60. Late onset of affective illness was associated with chronicity (10–19% of cases), and recovery was more frequent among unipolar than among bipolar patients. The 5-year remission rates (26% in unipolars, 16% in bipolars) were independent of the number of episodes (Angst & Preisig 1995b).

Mortality

Patients with mood disorder have a reduced life expectancy (Black et al 1987). This is true for all severities of illness. The primary causes in younger age groups are cardiovascular disease and suicide. A recent naturalistic retrospective 17-year follow-up of 472 bipolar patients showed greater mortality from suicide and cardiovascular and respiratory causes compared with the general population (Sharma & Markar 1994). The deceased were more likely to have been unmarried, showed greater frequency and duration of admissions, a shorter follow-up period and were less likely to have received lithium treatment. Patients with mood disorder tend to smoke more than the average for the population. The suicides were significantly younger at onset and death than the index and control groups, and suicide was uncommon where follow-up extended over 10 years. The increased risk of suicide in bipolar and unipolar patients previously admitted to hospital is confirmed by Angst's major longitudinal survey (Angst et al 2002).

Suicide

Depressive illness is often characterised by bleak and persistent thoughts of suicide. Only rarely are such thoughts the logical conclusion of an autonomous person performing some existential calculus. On recovery they usually disappear completely. It is not surprising, therefore, that depressive illness is the most common single antecedent to suicide, and suicide is the most common cause of death in affective disorder. Social 'explanations' for suicide rates can seem blind to the concept of depressive illness even though the social factors that are invoked to account for changes in suicide rates may operate in large part through the agency of affective disorder. The association is also poorly understood by the public and the media, who almost invariably report celebrity suicides as unaccountable and mysterious. Improved public understanding of the relationship between the risks of suicide and the prevalence of mental illness is desirable simply to reduce the reluctance of some individuals to seek help. In the UK, voluntary organisations have tended to take the lead in popularising a psychosocial interpretation of suicide and parasuicide. While appropriate to the latter phenomenon, it may simultaneously do disservice to the former.

The broad issue of suicide is covered in Chapter 27, in which it is emphasised that there are no psychological or biological measures that can be used to estimate the risk of subsequent suicide in an individual being treated for depression. However, since psychiatric referrals with depression collectively represent an identified group at relatively high risk of suicide, general improvement in their care would be as appropriately targeted as any. That could mean clearer adherence to the principles of treatment outlined above. It is reasonable to ask whether prophylactic treatment reduces mortality. At present the most positive findings come from specialised lithium clinics where suicide rates may actually appear lower than expected (Coppen et al 1991, Ahrens et al 1995, Muller-Oerlinghausen et al 1996). The obvious difficulty is that such clinics will tend to select patients with the best compliance, best insight, and, one might suggest, the best likely outcome. Detailed clinical audit of case series also supports the finding that lithium treatment is associated with lower rates of suicidal acts (Tondo et al 1998).

EVIDENCE-BASED MENTAL HEALTH

The challenge in devising treatments in future will be to improve the basis on which we currently make clinical decisions. This involves the collation of the trials that already exist to form meta-analyses that can better inform choices between different pharmacological treatments. It also means providing up-to-date guidelines and quantitative reviews to all clinicians via advanced communication links. If you have a problem deciding what to do in a clinical setting you should be able to click onto an appropriate body of evidence immediately from the computer at your elbow.

While the use of evidence, rather than authority and opinion, is a traditional strength of medical practice, the explosion of information taking place in recent decades requires novel solutions to avoid information overload. Evidence-based medicine is an approach to teaching and learning designed to allow continuous updating of a clinician's knowledge and understanding. It grew out of the teaching innovations at McMaster University in Canada (Sackett et al 1997). It places a premium upon understanding the statistical meaning of evidence and its critical appraisal. The explicit introduction of this way of thinking into psychiatry is an important contemporary development which should have an impact in all treatment modalities (see Ch. 12). It encourages clinicians to ask critical questions about their practice. The development of this approach can best be appreciated by looking at the work of the Evidence Based Mental Health Unit and the Cochrane Collaboration in Oxford. Interested readers may access materials via appropriate web sites (for links, contact http://www.psychiatry.ox.ac.uk/).

CONCLUSION

The challenge of the mood disorders lies in their apparently rising incidence and prevalence, the realisation that long-term disability and even mortality is likely to be increasingly evident, and the need for better delivery of more effective treatments. Against these challenges can be set our improving understanding of aetiology and the likely development of novel treatments. Long-term treatments must be informed by independent large-scale clinical trials. That we have a capacity, albeit finite, to treat mood disorder is one of its recurring clinical rewards.

REFERENCES

Abas M A, Sahakian B J, Levy R 1990 Neuropsychological deficits and CT scan changes in elderly depressives. Psychological Medicine 20:507–520

Ahrens B, Muller-Oerlinghausen B, Schou M et al 1995 Excess cardiovascular and suicide mortality of affective-disorders may be reduced by lithium prophylaxis. Journal of Affective Disorders 33:67–75

Akiskal H 1983 Dysthymic disorder: psychopathology of proposed chronic depressive sub-types. American Journal of Psychiatry 140:11–20

Akiskal H S, Akiskal K 1988 Reassessing the prevalence of bipolar disorders: clinical significance and artistic creativity. Psychiatrie et Psychobiologie 3:29s–36s

Andersen G, Vestergaard K, Riis J O, Lauritzen L 1994 Incidence of post-stroke depression during the first year in a large unselected stroke population determined using a valid standardized rating scale. Acta Psychiatrica Scandinavica 90:190–195

Anderson B, Brosen K, Christensen P et al 1990 Paroxetine: a selective scrotonin reuptake inhibitor showing better tolerance, but weaker antidepressant effect than clomipramine in a controlled multicenter study. Journal of Affective Disorders 18:289–299

Anderson I M, Tomenson B M 1994 The efficacy of selective serotonin re-uptake inhibitors in depression: a meta-analysis of studies against tricyclic antidepressants. Journal of Psychopharmacology 8:238–249

Anderson I M, Nutt D J, Deakin J F W 2000 Evidence-based guidelines for treating depressive disorders with antidepressants: a revision of the 1993 British Association for Psychopharmacology guidelines. Journal of Psychopharmacology 14:3–20

Andrews G 1996 Talk that works: the rise of cognitive behaviour therapy. British Medical Journal 313:1501–1502

Andrews G, Stewart G, Allen R, Henderson A S 1990 The genetics of six neurotic disorders: a twin study. Journal of Affective Disorders 19:23–29

Angold A, Worthman C W 1993 Puberty onset of gender differences in rates of depression: a developmental, epidemiologic and neuroendocrine perspective. Journal of Affective Disorders 29:145–158

Angst J 1996 Comorbidity of mood disorders: a longitudinal prospective study. British Journal of Psychiatry 168:31–37

Angst J, Dobler-Mikola A 1984 The Zurich study III. Diagnosis of depression. European Archives of Psychiatry and Neurological Sciences 234:30–37

Angst J, Hochstrasser B 1994 Recurrent brief depression: the Zurich study. Journal of Clinical Psychiatry 55:3–9

Angst J, Preisig M 1995a Course of a clinical cohort of unipolar, bipolar and schizoaffective patients. Results of a prospective study from 1959 to 1985. Schweizer Archiv für Neurologie und Psychiatrie 146:5–16

Angst J, Preisig M 1995b Outcome of a clinical cohort of unipolar, bipolar and schizoaffective patients. Results of a prospective study from 1959 to 1985. Schweizer Archiv für Neurologie und Psychiatrie 146:17–23

Angst J, Wicki W 1992 The Zurich study XIII. Recurrent brief anxiety. European Archives of Psychiatry and Clinical Neuroscience 241:296–300

Angst J, Merikangas K, Scheidegger P, Wicki W 1990 Recurrent brief depression: a new subtype of affective disorder. Journal of Affective Disorders 19:87–98

Angst F, Stassen H H, Clayton P J, Angst J 2002 Mortality of patients with mood disorders: follow-up over 34–38 years. Journal of Affective Disorders 68:167–181

Angst J, Gamma A, Benazzi F et al 2003 Toward a re-definition of subthreshold bipolarity: diagnosis and epidemiology of bipolar-II, minor bipolar disorders and hypomania. Journal of Affective Disorders 73:133–146

APA 1994 Diagnostic and statistical manual of mental disorders, 4th edn. American Psychiatric Association, Washington, DC

Aronson R, Offman H J, Joffe R T, Naylor C D 1996 Tri-iodothyronine augmentation in the treatment of refractory depression: a meta-analysis. Archives of General Psychiatry 53:842–848

Badner J A, Gershon E S 2002 Meta-analysis of whole-genome linkage scans of bipolar disorder and schizophrenia. Molecular Psychiatry 7:405–411

Baldwin D, Rudge S, Thomas S 1995 Dysthymia: Options in pharmacotherapy. CNS Drugs 4:422–431

Barefoot J C, Schroll M 1996 Symptoms of depression, acute myocardial infarction, and total mortality in a community sample. Circulation 93:1976–1980

Battersby S, Ogilvie A D, Smith C A D et al 1996 Structure of a variable number tandem repeat of the serotonin transporter gene and association with affective disorder. Psychiatric Genetics 6:177–181

Beats B C, Sahakian B J, Levy R 1996 Cognitive performance in tests sensitive to frontal lobe dysfunction in the elderly depressed. Psychological Medicine 26:591–603

Bechara A, Tranel D, Damasio H, Damasio A R 1996 Failure to respond autonomically to anticipated future outcomes following damage to prefrontal cortex. Cerebral Cortex 6:215–225

Beck A T 1976 Cognitive therapy and the emotional disorders. New American Library, New York

Bell A J, Cole A, Eccleston D, Ferrier I N 1993 Lithium neurotoxicity at normal therapeutic levels. British Journal of Psychiatry 162:689–692

Benkelfat C, Ellenbogen M A, Dean P et al 1994 Mood-lowering effect of tryptophan depletion: enhanced susceptibility in young men at genetic risk for major affective disorders. Archives of General Psychiatry 51:687–697

Berger M, Riemann D 1993 REM sleep in depression – an overview. Journal of Sleep Research 2:211–223

Berger M, Pirke K M, Doerr P et al 1984 The limited utility of the dexamethasone suppression test for the diagnostic process in psychiatry. British Journal of Psychiatry 145:372–382

Berrettini W H, Ferraro T N, Goldin L R et al 1994 Chromosome 18 DNA markers and manic-depressive illness: evidence for a susceptibility gene. Proceedings of the National Academy of Sciences of the USA 91:5918–5921

Black D W, Winokur G, Nasrallah A 1987 Is death from natural causes still excessive in psychiatric patients? A follow-up of 1593 patients with major affective disorder. Journal of Nervous and Mental Disease 175:674–680

Blackburn I M, Bishop S, Glen A I M et al 1981 The efficacy of cognitive therapy in depression: a treatment trial using cognitive therapy and pharmacotherapy, each alone and in combination. British Journal of Psychiatry 139:181–189

Blackburn I M, Eunson K M, Bishop S 1986 A two-year naturalistic follow-up of depressed patients treated with cognitive therapy, pharmacotherapy and a combination of both. Journal of Affective Disorders 10:67–75

Blackwood D H R, He L, Morris S W et al 1996 A locus for bipolar affective disorder on chromosome 4p. Nature Genetics 12:427–430

Boston Collaborative Drug Surveillance Program 1972 Acute adverse reactions to prednisone in relation to dosage. Clinical Pharmacology and Therapy 13:694–698

Bottiglieri T, Laundy M, Crellin R 2000 Homocysteine, folate, methylation, and monoamine metabolism in depression. Journal of neurology, neurosurgery and psychiatry 69:228–232

Bowden C L Brugger A M, Swann A C et al 1994 Efficacy of divalproex vs lithium and placebo in the treatment of mania. Journal of the American Medical Association 271:918–924

Brown G W 1993 Life events and affective disorder: replications and limitations. Psychosomatic Medicine 55:248–259

Brown G W, Harris T O 1993 Aetiology of anxiety and depressive disorders in an inner-city population: 1. Early adversity. Psychological Medicine 23:143–154

Brown G W, Lemyre L, Bifulco A 1992 Social factors and recovery from anxiety and depressive disorders. A test of specificity. British Journal of Psychiatry 161:44–54

Brown G W, Harris T O, Eales M J 1993 Aetiology of anxiety and depressive disorders in an inner-city population: 2. Comorbidity and adversity. Psychological Medicine 23:155–165

Brown G W, Harris T O, Hepworth C 1994 Life events and endogenous depression: a puzzle reexamined. Archives of General Psychiatry 51:525–534

Burgess S, Geddes J, Hawton K et al 2001 Lithium for maintenance treatment of mood disorders. Cochrane Database Syst Review 2001; 3:CD003013

Burvill P W, Johnson G A, Chakera T M H et al 1996 The place of site of lesion in the aetiology of post-stroke depression. Cerebrovascular Diseases 6:208–215

Burvill P, Johnson G, Jamrozik K et al 1997 Risk factors for post-stroke depression. International Journal of Geriatric Psychiatry 12:219–226

Cannon W J 1927 The James–Lange theory of emotions. American Journal of Psychology 39:115–124

Carney M W P, Roth M, Garside R F 1965 The diagnosis of depressive syndromes and the prediction of ECT response. British Journal of Psychiatry 111:659–674

Carney R M, Freedland K E, Jaffe A S 1990 Insomnia and depression prior to myocardial infarction. Psychosomatic Medicine 52:603–609

Carr S J, Toasdalo J D, Broadbent D 1991 Effects of induced elated and depressed mood on self-focused attention. British Journal of Clinical Psychology 30:273–275

Carroll B J, Feinberg M, Greden J F 1981 A specific laboratory test for the diagnosis of melancholia. Archives of General Psychiatry 38:15–22

Christie J E, Whalley L J, Dick H et al 1986 Raised plasma cortisol concentrations a feature of drug-free psychotics and not specific for depression. British Journal of Psychiatry 148:58–65

Clayton P J, Ernst C, Angst J 1994 Premorbid personality traits of men who develop unipolar or bipolar disorders. European Archives of Psychiatry and Clinical Neuroscience 243:340–346

Clerc G E, Ruimy P, Verdeau Pailles J 1994 A double-blind comparison of venlafaxine and fluoxetine in patients hospitalized for major depression and melancholia. International Clinical Psychopharmacology 9:139–143

Collier D A, Arranz M J, Sham P et al 1996 The serotonin transporter is a potential susceptibility factor for bipolar affective disorder. NeuroReport 7:1675–1679

Coppen A, Bailey J 2000 Enhancement of the antidepressant action of fluoxetine by folic acid: a randomised, placebo controlled trial. Journal of Affective Disorders 60:121–130

Coppen A, Shaw D M, Farrell J P 1963 The potentiation of the antidepressive action of a monoamine-oxidase inhibitor by tryptophan. Lancet i: 79–81

Coppen A, Standish-Barry H, Bailey J et al 1991 Does lithium reduce the mortality of recurrent mood disorders? Journal of Affective Disorders 23:1–7

Costa P T J, McCrae R R 1994 Stability and change in personality from adolescence through adulthood. In: Halverson C F Jr, Kohnstamm G, Martin R P (eds) The developing structure of temperament and personality from infancy to adulthood. Lawrence Erlbaum, Hillsdale, NJ, Ch 7, p 139–150

Damasio A R 1994 Descartes' error: Emotion, reason and the human brain. Picador, London

Damasio A R, Tranel D, Damasio H 1990 Individuals with sociopathic behavior caused by frontal damage fail to respond autonomically to social stimuli. Behavioural Brain Research 41:81–94

Davis R, Wilde M I 1996 Mirtazapine: A review of its pharmacology and therapeutic potential in the management of major depression. CNS Drugs 5:389–402

DeKloet E R, Vreugdenhil E, Oitzl M S, Joels M 1997 Glucocorticoid feedback resistance. Trends in Endocrinology and Metabolism 8:26–33

Delgado P L, Charney D S, Price L H et al 1990 Serotonin function and the mechanism of antidepressant action: reversal of antidepressant-induced remission by rapid depletion of plasma tryptophan. Archives of General Psychiatry 47:411–418

Delgado P L, Price L H, Miller H L et al 1991 Rapid serotonin depletion as a provocative challenge test for patients with major depression: relevance to antidepressant action and the neurobiology of depression. Psychopharmacology Bulletin 27:321–330

Drevets W C, Price J L, Simpson Jr J R et al 1997 Subgenual prefrontal cortex abnormalities in mood disorders. Nature 386:824–827

Dritschel B H, Teasdale J D 1991 Individual differences in affect-related cognitive operations elicited by experimental stimuli. British Journal of Clinical Psychology 30:151–160

Eagles J M, Whalley L J 1985 Ageing and affective disorders: the age at first onset of affective disorders in Scotland, 1969–1978. British Journal of Psychiatry 147:180–187

Egeland J A, Gerhard D S, Pauls D L et al 1987 Bipolar affective disorders linked to DNA markers on chromosome 11. Nature 325:783–787

Elkin I, Gibbons R D, Shea M T et al 1995 Initial severity and differential treatment outcome in the National Institute of Mental Health treatment of depression collaborative research program. Journal of Consulting and Clinical Psychology 63:841–847

Elkis H, Friedman L, Wise A, Meltzer H Y 1995 Meta-analysis of studies of ventricular enlargement and cortical sulcal prominence in mood disorders. Archives of General Psychiatry 52:735–746

Ellenbogen M A, Young S N, Dean P et al 1996 Mood response to acute tryptophan depletion in healthy volunteers: Sex differences and temporal stability. Neuropsychopharmacology 15:465–474

Fernandez-Teruel A, Cubin M, Tiwari H et al 2002 A quantitative trait locus influencing emotionality in the laboratory rat. Genome Research 12:618–626

Ferrier I N, Eccleston D, Moore P B, Wood K A 1990 Relapse in chronic depressives on withdrawal of L-tryptophan. Lancet 336:380–381

Francis P T, Pangalos M N, Stephens P H et al 1993 Antemortem measurements of neurotransmission – possible implications for pharmacotherapy of Alzheimer's disease and depression. Journal of Neurology, Neurosurgery and Psychiatry 56:80–84

Frasure-Smith N, Lesperance F, Talajic M 1993 Depression following myocardial infarction: impact on 6-month survival. Journal of the American Medical Association 270:1819–1825

Frasure-Smith N, Lesperance F, Talajic M 1995 Depression and 18-month prognosis after myocardial infarction. Circulation 91:999–1005

Freimer N B, Reus V I, Escamilla M A et al 1996 Genetic mapping using haplotype, association and linkage methods suggests a locus for severe bipolar disorder (BPI) at 18q22–q23. Nature Genetics 12:436–441

Fullerton J, Cubin M, Tiwari H et al 2003 Linkage analysis of extremely discordant and concordant sibling pairs identifies QTL that influence variation in the human personality trait neuroticism. American Journal of Human Genetics 72:879–890

Furlong R A, Ho L, Walsh C et al 1998 Analysis and meta-analysis of two serotonin transporter gene polymorphisms in bipolar and unipolar affective disorders. American Journal of Medical Genetics 81:58–63

Geddes J G, Goodwin G M 2001 Bipolar disorder: clinical uncertainty, evidence-based medicine and large scale randomised trials. British Journal of Psychiatry 178(suppl 41): s191–s194

Geddes J R, Carney S M, Davies C et al 2003 Relapse prevention with antidepressant drug treatment in depressive disorders: a systematic review. Lancet 361:653–661

Gerken A, Holsboer F 1986 Cortisol and corticosterone response after syn-corticotropin in relationship to dexamethasone suppressibility of cortisol. Psychoneuroendocrinology 11:185–194

Gershon E S, Hamovit J, Guroff J J et al 1982 A family study of schizoaffective, bipolar I, bipolar II, unipolar, and normal control probands. Archives of General Psychiatry 39:1157–1167

Giles D E, Biggs M M, Rush A J, Roffwarg H P 1988 Risk factors in families of unipolar depression. I: Psychiatric illness and reduced REM latency. Journal of Affective Disorders 14:51–59

Ginns E I, Ott J, Egeland J A et al 1996 A genome-wide search for chromosomal loci linked to bipolar affective disorder in the Old Order Amish. Nature Genetics 12:431–435

Glassman A H, O'Connor C M, Califf R M et al, Sertraline Antidepressant Heart Attack Randomized Trial Group 2002 Sertraline treatment of major depression in patients with acute MI or unstable angina. Journal of the American Medical Association 288:701–709

Goodwin G M 1994 Recurrence of mania after lithium withdrawal. British Journal of Psychiatry 164:149–152

Goodwin G M 1996 Functional imaging, affective disorder and dementia. British Medical Bulletin 52:495–512

Goodwin G M 2002 Hypomania – what's in a name? British Journal of Psychiatry 181:94–95

Goodwin G M, Fairburn C G, Cowen P J 1987 The effects of dieting and weight loss on neuroendocrine responses to tryptophan, clonidine, and apomorphine in volunteers: Important implications for neuroendocrine investigations in depression. Archives of General Psychiatry 44:952–957

Goodwin G M, Muir W J, Seckl J R et al 1992 The effects of cortisol infusion upon hormone secretion from the anterior pituitary and subjective mood in depressive illness and in controls. Journal of Affective Disorders 26:73–83

Goodwin G M, Austin M P, Curran S M et al 1993 The elevation of plasma beta-endorphin levels in major depression. Journal of Affective Disorders 29:281–289

Gram L F 1986 Citalopram: clinical effect profile in comparison with clomipramine. A controlled multicenter study. Psychopharmacology 90:131–138

Gray J A 1982 The neuropsychology of anxiety. Oxford University Press, Oxford

Green A R, Goodwin G M 1996 Ecstasy and neurodegeneration. British Medical Journal 312(7045):1493–1494

Healy D 1997 The antidepressant era. Harvard University Press, Cambridge, Mass

Herrmann M, Bartels C, Schumacher M, Wallesch C W 1995 Poststroke depression: is there a pathoanatomic correlate for depression in the postacute stage of stroke? Stroke 26:850–856

Hickie I, Scott E, Mitchell P 1995 Subcortical hyperintensities on magnetic-resonance-imaging – clinical correlates and prognostic significance in patients with severe depression. Biological Psychiatry 37:151–160

Hirschfeld R M A 1994 Major depression, dysthymia and depressive personality disorder. British Journal of Psychiatry 165:23–30

Hirschfeld R M A, Keller M B, Panico S et al 1997 The National Depressive and Manic-Depressive Association consensus statement on the undertreatment of depression. Journal of the American Medical Association 277:333–340

Holsboer F, Wiedemann K, Boll E 1986 Shortened dexamethasone half-life in depressed dexamethasone nonsuppressors. Archives of General Psychiatry 43:813–815

Holsboer F, Lauer C J, Schreiber W, Krieg J C 1995 Altered hypothalamic-pituitary-adrenocortical regulation in healthy-subjects at high familial risk for affective-disorders. Neuroendocrinology 62:340–347

Horne R, Weinman J 1999 Patients' beliefs about prescribed medicines and their role in adherence to treatment in chronic physical illness. Journal of Psychosomatic Research 47:555–567

House A, Dennis M, Molyneux A 1989 Emotionalism after stroke. British Medical Journal 298:991–994

House A, Dennis M, Warlow C et al 1990 Mood disorders after stroke and their relation to lesion location: a CT scan study. Brain 113:1113–1129

House A, Knapp P, Bamford J, Vail A 2001 Mortality at 12 and 24 months after stroke may be associated with depressive symptoms at 1 month. Stroke 32:696–701

Hunt N, Bruce Jones W, Silverstone T 1992a Life events and relapse in bipolar affective disorder. Journal of Affective Disorders 25:13–20

Hunt N, Sayer H, Silverstone T 1992b Season and manic relapse. Acta Psychiatrica Scandinavica 85:123–126

Jacobsen F M, Wehr T A, Skwerer R A et al 1987 Morning versus midday phototherapy of seasonal affective disorder. American Journal of Psychiatry 144:1301–1305

Jamison K R 1995 Manic-depressive illness and creativity. Scientific American 272:62–67

Jamison K R, Wyatt R J 1992 van Gogh, Vincent: illness. British Medical Journal 304:577–577

Joffe R T, Singer W, Levitt A J, MacDonald C 1993 A placebo-controlled comparison of lithium and tri-iodothyronine augmentation of tricyclic antidepressants in unipolar refractory depression. Archives of General Psychiatry 50:387–393

Jonsson E G, Nothen M M, Gustavsson J P 1998 Polymorphisms in the dopamine, serotonin, and norepinephrine transporter genes and their relationships to monoamine metabolite concentrations in CSF of healthy volunteers. Psychiatry Research 79:1–9

Keller M B, Klein D N, Hirschfeld R M A et al 1995 Results of the DSM-IV mood disorders field trial. American Journal of Psychiatry 152:843–849

Kelsoe J R, Ginns E I, Egeland J A et al 1989 Re-evaluation of the linkage relationship between chromosome-11p loci and the gene for bipolar affective-disorder in the Old Order Amish. Nature 342:238–243

Kemperman C J F, Tulner D M 1990 Neurotoxicity of lithium. Lithium 1:195–202

Kendell R E 1968 The classification of depressive illness. Maudsley monograph. Oxford University Press, Oxford

Kendell R E, Chalmers J C, Platz C 1987 Epidemiology of puerperal psychoses. British Journal of Psychiatry 150:662–673

Kendler K S 1996 Major depression and generalised anxiety disorder. Same genes, (partly) different environments – revisited. British Journal of Psychiatry 168:68–75

Kendler K S 1997 The diagnostic validity of melancholic major depression in a population-based sample of female twins. Archives of General Psychiatry 54:299–304

Kendler K S, Karkowski-Shuman L 1997 Stressful life events and genetic liability to major depression: genetic control of exposure to the environment? Psychological Medicine 27:539–547

Kendler K S, Neale M C, Kessler R C 1992 A population-based twin study of major depression in women: the impact of varying definitions of illness. Archives of General Psychiatry 49:257–266

Kendler K S, Heath A C, Neale M C 1993a Alcoholism and major depression in women: a twin study of the causes of comorbidity. Archives of General Psychiatry 50:690–698

Kendler K S, Neale M, Kessler R 1993b A twin study of recent life events and difficulties. Archives of General Psychiatry 50:789–796

Kendler K S, Neale M C, MacLean C J et al 1993c Smoking and major depression: a causal analysis. Archives of General Psychiatry 50:36–43

Kendler K S, Sham P C, MacLean C J 1997a The determinants of parenting: an epidemiological, multi-informant, retrospective study. Psychological Medicine 27:549–563

Kendler K S, Walters E E, Kessler R C 1997b The prediction of length of major depressive episodes: results from an epidemiological sample of female twins. Psychological Medicine 27:107–117

Kendler K S, Thornton L M, Gardner C O 2001 Genetic risk, number of previous depressive episodes, and stressful life events in predicting onset of major depression. American Journal of Psychiatry 158:582–586

Kendler K S, Gardner C O, Prescott C A 2002 Toward a comprehensive developmental model for major depression in women. American Journal of Psychiatry 159:1133–1145

Kessler R C, Avenevoli S, Ries-Merikangas K 2001 Mood disorders in children and adolescents: an epidemiologic perspective. Biological Psychiatry 49:1002–1014

Khan A A, Gardner C O, Prescott C A, Kendler K S 2002 Gender differences in the symptoms of major depression in opposite-sex dizygotic twin pairs. American Journal of Psychiatry 159:1427–1429

Kiloh L G, Andrews G, Neilson M 1988 The long-term outcome of depressive illness. British Journal of Psychiatry 153:752–757

Klerman G L 1988 The current age of youthful melancholia – evidence for increase in depression among adolescents and young adults. British Journal of Psychiatry 152:4–14

Klerman G L, Weissman M M 1989 Increasing rates of depression. Journal of the American Medical Association 261:2229–2235

Klerman G L, Weissman M M, Rounsaville B J, Chevron E S 1984 Interpersonal psychotherapy of depression. Aronson, London

Klerman G L, Lavori P W, Rice J et al 1985 Birth-cohort trends in rates of major depressive disorder among relatives of patients with affective-disorder. Archives of General Psychiatry 42:689–693

Koslow S H, Maas J W, Bowden C L et al 1983 CSF and urinary biogenic amines and metabolites in depression and mania. A controlled, univariate analysis. Archives of General Psychiatry 40:999–1010

Kuhn R 1958 The treatment of depressive states with G22355 (imipramine hydrochloride). American Journal of Psychiatry 115:459–464

Kupfer D J, Frank E, Perel J M et al 1992 Five-year outcome for maintenance therapies in recurrent depression. Archives of General Psychiatry 49:769–773

Lafer B, Sachs G S, Labbate L A 1994 Phototherapy for seasonal affective disorder: a blind comparison of three different schedules. American Journal of Psychiatry 151:1081–1083

Larsen R J, Ketelaar T 1989 Extraversion, neuroticism and susceptibility to positive and negative mood induction procedures. Personality and Individual Differences 10:1221–1228

Larsen R J, Ketelaar T 1991 Personality and susceptibility to positive and negative emotional states. Journal of Personality and Social Psychology 61:132–140

Lasch K, Weissman M, Wickramaratne P, Livingston-Bruce M 1990 Birth-cohort changes in the rates of mania. Psychiatry Research 33:31–37

LeDoux J E 2000 Emotion circuits in the brain. Annual Review of Neuroscience 23:155–184

Lee A S, Murray R M 1988 The long-term outcome of Maudsley depressives. British Journal of Psychiatry 153:741–751

Lesperance F, Frasure-Smith N, Talajic M, Cameron O 1996 Major depression before and after myocardial infarction: its nature and consequences. Psychosomatic Medicine 58:99–112

Levitt A J, Joffe R T, King E 1994 Dim versus bright red (light-emitting diode) light in the treatment of seasonal affective disorder. Acta Psychiatrica Scandinavica 89:341–345

Lewis A J 1934 Melancholia: a clinical survey of depressive states. Journal of Mental Science 80:277–378

Littlejohn R, Leslie F, Cookson J 1994 Depot antipsychotics in the prophylaxis of bipolar affective disorder. British Journal of Psychiatry 165:827–829

Loosen P T 1994 Cushing's syndrome and depression. Endocrinologist 4:373–382

Maddox J C, Levi M, Thompson C 1994 The compliance with antidepressants in general practice. Journal of Psychopharmacology 8:48–53

Markar H R, Mander A J 1989 Efficacy of lithium prophylaxis in clinical practice. British Journal of Psychiatry 155:496–500

McGuffin P, Katz R, Bebbington P 1988 The Camberwell Collaborative Depression Study. III: Depression and adversity in the relatives of depressed probands. British Journal of Psychiatry 152:775–782

McGuffin P, Katz R, Watkins S, Rutherford J 1996 A hospital-based twin register of the heritability of DSM-IV unipolar depression. Archives of General Psychiatry 53:129–136

Mann J J, Henteleff R A, Lagattuta T F et al 1996 Lower ^{3}H-paroxetine binding in cerebral cortex of suicide victims is partly due to fewer high affinity, non-transporter sites. Journal of Neural Transmission 103:1337–1350

Medical Research Council 1965 Clinical trial of the treatment of depressive illness. British Medical Journal 1:881–886

Mehlman P T, Higley J D, Faucher I et al 1994 Low CSF 5-HIAA concentrations and severe aggression and impaired impulse control in nonhuman primates. American Journal of Psychiatry 151:1485–1491

Mitchell P, Parker G, Jamieson K et al 1992 Are there any differences between bipolar and unipolar melancholia? Journal of Affective Disorders 25:97–105

Montgomery D B, Roberts A, Green M et al 1994 Lack of efficacy of fluoxetine in recurrent brief depression and suicidal attempts. European Archives of Psychiatry and Clinical Neuroscience 244:211–215

Mullen P E, Linsell C R, Parker D 1986 Influence of sleep disruption and calorie restriction on biological markers for depression. Lancet ii:1051–1054

Muller-Oerlinghausen B, Wolf T, Ahrens B et al 1996 Mortality of patients who dropped out from regular lithium prophylaxis – a collaborative study by the international group for the study of lithium-treated patients (IGSLI). Acta Psychiatrica Scandinavica 94:344–347

Murphy D G M, Murphy D M, Abbas M et al 1993 Seasonal affective disorder: response to light as measured by electroencephalogram, melatonin suppression, and cerebral blood flow. British Journal of Psychiatry 163:327–331

Murphy J M 1994 The Stirling County study: then and now. International Review of Psychiatry 6:329–348

Murphy J M, Sobol A M, Olivier D C 1989 Prodromes of depression and anxiety. The Stirling County study. British Journal of Psychiatry 155:490–495

Murray C J, Lopez A D 1997 Global mortality, disability, and the contribution of risk factors: Global Burden of Disease Study. Lancet 349:1436–1442

Naber D, Sand P, Heigl B 1996 Psychopathological and neuropsychological effects of 8-days' corticosteroid treatment: A prospective study. Psychoneuroendocrinology 21:25–31

Neuvonen P J, Pohjola Sintonen S, Tacke U, Vuori E 1993 Five fatal cases of serotonin syndrome after moclobemide–citalopram or moclobemide–clomipramine overdoses. Lancet 342:1419

O'Dwyer A M, Lightman S L, Marks M N, Checkley S A 1995 Treatment of major depression with metyrapone and hydrocortisone. Journal of Affective Disorders 33:123–128

Ogilvie A D, Battersby S, Bubb V J et al 1996 Polymorphism in serotonin transporter gene associated with susceptibility to major depression. Lancet 347:731–733

Okuma T, Kishimoto A 1998 A history of investigation on the mood stabilizing effect of carbamazepine in Japan. Psychiatry and Clinical Neurosciences 52:3–12

Pariante C M, Miller A H 2001 Glucocorticoid receptors in major depression: relevance to pathophysiology and treatment. Biological Psychiatry 49:391–404

Parker G 1981 Parental reports of depressives: An investigation of several explanations. Journal of Affective Disorders 3:131–140

Parker G 1983 Parental 'affectionless control' as an antecedent to adult depression: A risk factor delineated. Archives of General Psychiatry 40:956–960

Parker G 1986 Validating an experiential measure of parental style: the use of a twin sample. Acta Psychiatrica Scandinavica 73:22–27

Parker G, Barnett B 1988 Perceptions of parenting in childhood and social support in adulthood. American Journal of Psychiatry 145:479–482

Parker G, Hadzi-Pavlovic D 1993 Old data, new interpretation: a reanalysis of Sir Aubrey Lewis' MD thesis. Psychological Medicine 23:859–870

Parker G, Hadzi-Pavlovic D 1996 Melancholia: a disorder of movement and mood. Cambridge University Press, Cambridge

Parker G, Kiloh L, Hayward L 1987 Parental representations of neurotic and endogenous depressives. Journal of Affective Disorders 13:75–82

Parker G, Hadzi-Pavlovic D, Greenwald S, Weissman M 1995 Low parental care as a risk factor to lifetime depression in a community sample. Journal of Affective Disorders 33:173–180

Parker G, Roy K, Mitchell P et al 2002 Atypical depression: a reappraisal. American Journal of Psychiatry 159:1470–1479

Paskind H A 1929 Brief attacks of manic-depressive depressions. Archives of Neurology 22:123–134

Patten S B, Love E J 1997 Drug-induced depression. Psychotherapy and Psychosomatics 66:63–73

Pauls D L, Gerhard D S, Lacy L G et al 1991 Linkage of bipolar affective disorders to markers on chromosome 11p is excluded in a second lateral extension of Amish pedigree 110. Genomics 11:730–736

Paykel E S 2001 Continuation and maintenance therapy in depression. British Medical Bulletin 57:145–159

Peroutka S J, Newman H, Harris H 1988 Subjective effects of 3,4-methylenedioxymethamphetamine in recreational users. Neuropsychopharmacology 1:273–277

Perry E K, Marshall E F, Blessed G et al 1983 Decreased imipramine binding in the brains of patients with depressive illness. British Journal of Psychiatry 142:188–192

Post R M, Leverich G S, Altshuler L, Mikalauskas K 1992 Lithium-discontinuation-induced refractoriness: preliminary observations. American Journal of Psychiatry 149:1727–1729

Pratt L A, Ford D E, Crum R M et al 1996 Depression, psychotropic medication, and risk of myocardial infarction – prospective data from the Baltimore ECA follow-up. Circulation 94:3123–3129

Quitkin F M, Stewart J W, McGrath P J et al 1988 Phenelzine versus imipramine in the treatment of probable atypical depression: defining syndrome boundaries of selective MAOI responders. American Journal of Psychiatry 145:306–311

Quitkin F M, McGrath P J, Stewart J W et al 1989 Phenelzine and imipramine in mood reactive depressives. Further delineation of the syndrome of atypical depression. Archives of General Psychiatry 46:787–793

Regier D A, Boyd J H, Burke Jr J D et al 1988 One-month prevalence of mental disorders in the United States, based on five epidemiologic catchment area sites. Archives of General Psychiatry 45:977–986

Robinson R G 1997 Neuropsychiatric consequences of stroke. Annual Review of Medicine 48:217–229

Robinson R G, Starr L B, Kubos K L, Price T R 1983 A two-year longitudinal study of post-stroke mood disorders: findings during the initial evaluation. Stroke 14:736–741

Robinson R G, De Carvalho M L, Paradiso S 1995 Post-stroke psychiatric problems. Diagnosis, pathophysiology and drug treatment options. CNS Drugs 3:436–447

Rolls E T 1990 A theory of emotion and its application to understanding the neural basis of emotion. Cognition and Emotion 4:161–190

Rolls E T, Hornak J, Wade D, McGrath J 1994 Emotion-related learning in patients with social and emotional changes associated with frontal lobe damage. Journal of Neurology, Neurosurgery, and Psychiatry 57:1518–1524

Rosenthal N E, Sack D A, Gillin J C et al 1984 Seasonal affective disorder. A description of the syndrome and preliminary findings with light therapy. Archives of General Psychiatry 41:72–80

Rubin R T, Phillips J J, Sadow T F, McCracken J T 1995 Adrenal-gland volume in major depression – increase during the depressive episode and decrease with successful treatment. Archives of General Psychiatry 52:213–218

Sackett D L, Richardson W S, Rosenberg W, Haynes R B 1997 Evidence based medicine. Churchill Livingstone, Edinburgh

Schachter S 1966 The interaction of cognitive and physiological determinants of emotional state. In: Spielberger C D (ed) Anxiety and behaviour. Academic Press, London, p 193

Scott A I F, Freeman C P L 1992 Edinburgh primary care depression study: treatment outcome, patient satisfaction, and cost after 16 weeks. British Medical Journal 304:883–887

Serretti A, Lilli R, Lorenzi C et al 2002 Serotonin transporter gene (5-HTTLPR) and major psychoses. Molecular Psychiatry 7:95–99

Sharma R, Markar H R 1994 Mortality in affective-disorder. Journal of Affective Disorders 31:91–96

Silverstone T, Romans S, Hunt N, McPherson H 1995 Is there a seasonal pattern of relapse in bipolar affective disorders? A dual northern and southern hemisphere cohort study. British Journal of Psychiatry 167:58–60

Simpson S G, Folstein S E, Meyers D A et al 1993 Bipolar II: The most common bipolar phenotype? American Journal of Psychiatry 150:901–903

Slater E, Roth M 1969 Mayer–Gross, Slater and Roth's clinical psychiatry, 3rd edn. Baillière Tindall, London

Smith D, Dempster C, Glanville J et al 2002 Efficacy and tolerability of venlafaxine compared with selective serotonin reuptake inhibitors and other antidepressants: a meta-analysis. British Journal of Psychiatry 180:396–404

Smith K A, Fairburn C G, Cowen P J 1997 Relapse of depression after rapid depletion of tryptophan. Lancet 349:915–919

Soares J C, Mann J J 1997 The anatomy of mood disorders – review of structural neuroimaging studies. Biological Psychiatry 41:86–106

Song F, Freemantle N, Sheldon T A et al 1993 Selective serotonin reuptake inhibitors: meta-analysis of efficacy and acceptability. British Medical Journal 306:683–687

Souza F G M, Goodwin G M 1991 Lithium treatment and prophylaxis in unipolar depression: a meta-analysis. British Journal of Psychiatry 158:666–675

Steffens D C, Helms M J, Krishnan K R, Burke G L 1999 Cerebrovascular disease and depression symptoms in the cardiovascular health study. Stroke 30:2159–2166

Stein P K, Carney R M, Freedland K E et al 2000 Severe depression is associated with markedly reduced heart rate variability in patients with stable coronary heart disease. Psychosomatic Research 48:493–500

Stewart J W, Mercier M A, Agosti V et al 1993 Imipramine is effective after unsuccessful cognitive therapy: sequential use of cognitive therapy and imipramine in depressed outpatients. Journal of Clinical Psychopharmacology 13:114–119

Stewart J W, Tricamo E, McGrath P J, Quitkin F M 1997 Prophylactic efficacy of phenelzine and imipramine in chronic atypical depression: likelihood of recurrence on discontinuation after 6 months' remission. American Journal of Psychiatry 154:31–36

Stokes P E 1995 The potential role of excessive cortisol induced by HPA hyperfunction in the pathogenesis of depression. European Neuropsychopharmacology 5:77–82

Styron W 1990 Darkness visible. Cape, London

Sullivan P F, Neale M C, Kendler K S 2000 Genetic epidemiology of major depression: review and meta-analysis. American Journal of Psychiatry 157:1552–1562

Suppes T, Baldessarini R J, Faedda G L, Tohen M 1991 Risk of recurrence following discontinuation of lithium treatment in bipolar disorder. Archives of General Psychiatry 48:1082–1088

Thakore J H, Dinan T G 1995 Cortisol synthesis inhibition: a new treatment strategy for the clinical and endocrine manifestations of depression. Biological Psychiatry 37:364–368

Thapar A, McGuffin P 1996 Genetic influences on life events in childhood. Psychological Medicine 26:813–820

Thase M E, Fava M, Halbreich U et al 1996 A placebo-controlled, randomized clinical trial comparing sertraline and imipramine for the treatment of dysthymia. Archives of General Psychiatry 53:777–784

Tondo L, Baldessarini R J, Hennen J et al 1998 Lithium treatment and risk of suicidal behavior in bipolar disorder patients. Journal of Clinical Psychiatry 59:405–414

Traskman L, Asberg M, Bertilsson L, Sjostrand L 1981 Monoamine metabolites in CSF and suicidal behavior. Archives of General Psychiatry 38:631–636

Verheyden S L, Hadfield J, Calin T, Curran H V 2002 Sub-acute effects of MDMA (+/− 3, 4-methylenedioxymethamphetamine, "ecstasy") on mood: evidence of gender differences. Psychopharmacology 161:23–31

Virkkunen M, Rawlings R, Tokola R et al 1994 CSF biochemistries, glucose metabolism, and diurnal activity rhythms in alcoholic, violent offenders, fire setters, and healthy volunteers. Archives of General Psychiatry 51:20–27

Wals M, Hillegers M H, Reichart C G et al 2001 Prevalence of psychopathology in children of a bipolar parent. Journal of the American Academy of Child and Adolescent Psychiatry 40:1094–1102

Warshaw M G, Klerman G L, Lavori P W 1991 Are secular trends in major depression an artifact of recall. Journal of Psychiatric Research 25:141–151

Watson D, Clark L A, Harkness A R 1994 Structures of personality and their relevance to psychopathology. Journal of Abnormal Psychology 103:18–31

Weissman M M, Leaf P J, Livingston Bruce M, Florio L 1988 The epidemiology of dysthymia in five communities: rates, risks, comorbidity, and treatment. American Journal of Psychiatry 145:815–819

Weissman M M, Bland R C, Canino G J et al 1996 Cross-national epidemiology of major depression and bipolar disorder. Journal of the American Medical Association 276:293–299

WHO 1992 International statistical classification of diseases and related health problems, 10th revision. World Health Organization, Geneva

Wicki W, Angst J, Merikangas K R 1992 The Zurich Study. XIV: Epidemiology of seasonal depression. European Archives of Psychiatry and Clinical Neuroscience 241:301–306

Wileman S M, Eagles J M, Andrew J E et al 2001 Light therapy for seasonal affective disorder in primary care: randomised controlled trial. British Journal of Psychiatry 178:311–316

Winokur G 1990 The concept of secondary depression and its relationship to comorbidity. Psychiatric Clinics of North America 13:567–583

Young R C, Klerman G L 1992 Mania in late life – focus on age at onset. American Journal of Psychiatry 149:867–876

21 | Neurotic, stress-related and somatoform disorders

Phil Harrison-Read, Peter Tyrer, Michael Sharpe

INTRODUCTION AND DEFINITION

The term neurosis is used to refer to a group of conditions that have been traditionally grouped together in psychiatric classifications. These conditions describe a range of psychological and somatic symptoms, which are neither psychoses nor organic disorders and which lack the lifelong duration of personality disorders. The previously well-established concept of neurosis was abandoned as a term and classificatory principle in DSM-III as being both too general and too associated with psychoanalysis (Editorial 1982). It was counter argued that it still served a useful function of grouping together a number of conditions that share common features and which are not easily defined or classified in any other way (Gelder 1986). Subsequently it has remained absent from DSM but has been retained as a term and organising principle, although not as a diagnosis, in ICD-10 as 'neurotic, stress-related and somatoform disorders (F40 to F48)'; these conditions are listed in Box 21.1

A short history of neurosis

In order to understand the concept of neurosis it is helpful to briefly consider its history. This will arbitrarily be divided into three phases.

Phase 1: the early years, 1700–1890

The term neurosis was coined in 1772 by the Edinburgh physician William Cullen (1710–1790) to mean any disorder of the nervous system without obvious symptoms or signs of physical disease such as fever. A later term for the same concept was 'functional nervous disorder', which persists to this day mainly to describe medically unexplained somatic symptoms. During the following 150 years or so, this rather vague concept of neurosis was modified and refined by advances in the understanding of physical diseases affecting the nervous system, and to a lesser extent by interest in the mental disorders that might result. Originally the 'psychoses' (a term introduced in 1845) were regarded as severe forms of neurosis, i.e. functional mental disorders. Later, functional psychoses were classified as separate conditions and the term neurosis came to mean less severe or 'minor' forms of mental illness.

Phase 2: the psychoanalytic concept of neurosis, 1890–1950

In the latter part of the 19th century, the importance of psychological factors in neuroses was increasingly recognised. This was exemplified by the French neurologist Jean-Martin Charcot who was particularly interested in hysteria. In the early part of his career he regarded this as a brain disease but in his later years was increasingly convinced of the role of psychological factors. A major change in the theoretical views of neurosis was brought about by Sigmund Freud (1856–1939) and his colleagues. Freud began his career as a neuroanatomist and neurologist, and his early writings were heavily influenced by the mechanistic neuroscience of his day. Also important however was the influence on Freud's ideas of the social milieu of 19th century Vienna where he lived and worked, which was rigidly hierarchical and sexually repressed. Initially Freud focused on one aspect of neurosis (conversion hysteria), which particularly affected his mainly wealthy female patients, but it was not long before the phenomenon of anxiety assumed a central role in his thinking.

Freud's early views (1895) of the neuroses in general and of anxiety neurosis in particular were that they resulted from the *discharge* of thwarted or 'damned-up' instinctual drives, e.g. sexual energy or libido. These so-called 'actual neuroses' (neurasthenia and anxiety neurosis) were conceived of in physiological or physical terms. They were contrasted with the 'psycho-neuroses' (hysteria and phobic and obsessional states) which were explained initially as resulting from *suppression* of sexual drives and later as maladaptive attempts of the adult individual to deal with childhood trauma, specifically premature sexual awareness and experience. Freud developed the concept of self-protective psychic defence mechanisms, analogous to the behavioural defences of fight, flight or submission observed in animals. When exaggerated or operating excessively these defence mechanisms were considered to produce particular types of neurotic symptoms (obsessional, phobic, hysterical and depressive).

In Freud's later writings, which incorporated his theories about the organisation of the mind, anxiety neurosis was conceptualised in a similar way to the other psychoneuroses, with 'signal anxiety' (roughly analogous to 'free-floating' or general anxiety) representing the subjective experience of failing defence mechanisms unsuccessfully attempting to exclude from consciousness unacceptable impulses and desires (i.e. anxiety about a danger that has yet to be discovered). However, unlike other neurotic symptoms, which represented excessive or maladaptive psychic defences, anxiety was viewed as a symptom of a more fundamental problem, i.e. conflict between what is acceptable to the 'ego' and what is imposed or demanded by the 'id' and 'superego' respectively. 'Primary anxiety', in Freud's later view, represented the overwhelming subjective experience resulting when psychic defence mechanisms actually fail, and therefore was analogous to the extreme form of emotion (terror, panic) originally included in the earlier concept of 'actual neurosis'. Freud's theoretical work established the 'talking cure' of psychoanalysis as the mainstay of treatment for neurotic disorders during the first part of the 20th century.

Psychoanalytic ideas had a major influence on the conceptualisation and management of other types of traumatic neurotic conditions, which have both historical and contemporary significance: combat or war neuroses and post-traumatic stress disorder. All these conditions have in common an element of 'dissociation'. Dissociation was a concept developed by Pierre Janet (1859–1947), a pupil of Charcot. These ideas, as well as those of his collaborator Joseph Breuer, had a major influence on Freud's psychoanalytic conceptualisation of neuroses. Janet's concept of dissociation as a psychological reaction to severe trauma or stress included a loss of normal integration between various components of cognitive functioning, resulting in altered states of awareness and altered responsiveness to surroundings and suggestions. Freud's development of Janet's ideas and the related concept of 'conversion' by which psychological conflicts and traumas are expressed as physical symptoms did not attract widespread interest until the First World War (1914–18) when there was a dramatic increase in the incidence of 'hysterical' and other psychological disorders in the form of combat neuroses or 'shell shock'.

This gave a new impetus to psychotherapeutic techniques of managing neurotic disorders using Freudian principles, which reached its peak during and shortly after the Second World War (1939–45) when an even greater number of neurotic casualties arose. It was also during this period that group psychoanalysis and 'therapeutic communities' became established. In devising and delivering eclectic psychiatric treatment to large numbers of war combatants suffering from neurotic disorders, much of the philosophy and framework for the new specialty of psychological medicine in the post-war National Health Service was established. In the aftermath of the American Vietnam War during the 1970s, and later wars and local disasters, dissociative disorders took on a new mantle in the form of post-traumatic stress disorder.

Phase 3: The subdivision of neurosis on the basis of response to treatment 1950–80

The next phase in the history of the neuroses is concerned with two interconnected themes: first, the extent to which neurotic conditions are psychologically as opposed to neurobiologically

determined and second, whether they are best considered as made up of a number of different conditions, more-or-less distinct from one another with characteristic aetiological and clinical features and responsiveness to different forms of treatment.

An early sceptic of Freud's theoretical explanations for and distinctions between different types of neurotic disorders was Karl Jaspers (1923) who pointed out that 'there is no sharp line to be drawn between types (of neurosis), nor between what is healthy and what is not' and that 'it is difficult to bring any diagnostic order of practical value into shifting phenomena which continually keep merging into one another'. Jaspers's views were echoed by Freud's follower Carl Jung (1875–1961). Writing in 1945, Jung scathingly argued that there is little to be gained by subdividing neurotic disorders and 'fixing a more or less lucky label' to each, because this does not improve prediction of prognosis or response to different forms of therapy.

This state of affairs is exactly what changed in the 1950s, when there began a gradual process of subdividing neurosis into various more-or-less distinct disorders based on an apparently differential response to treatment. Firstly, there was the demonstration by early behaviour therapists that situational anxiety states (phobic disorders) responded to the technique of 'reciprocal inhibition' or graded exposure and desensitisation to the feared situation, whereas other forms of anxiety responded less well or not at all. Furthermore, when present in the same phobic patients, 'free-floating' or anticipatory general anxiety tended to interfere with the therapeutic response to behaviour therapy. Later studies of behaviour therapy in phobic disorders demonstrated that isolated phobias responded more readily to desensitisation and exposure than social phobias or agoraphobia, especially when the latter were accompanied by, or maintained and even initiated by, the occurrence of panic attacks. It was argued that these findings justified different diagnostic categories of anxiety disorder, phobic disorders having a predominantly psychological basis, in contrast to general anxiety and panic disorder, which might have a greater neurobiological component.

In keeping with this idea, Donald Klein claimed in the 1960s that prolonged treatment with the tricyclic antidepressant drug imipramine was slowly effective in helping (Klein used the term 'blocking') spontaneous (non-situational, unexpected) panic attacks which he believed were often the cause of agoraphobia. This finding was used to support the case for a separate condition called panic disorder characterised by spontaneous panic attacks with or without secondary agoraphobia and with a predominantly neurobiological causation. Conversely, generalised anxiety responded well to benzodiazepine drugs, which were much less effective against panic attacks. Although the blocking action of imipramine on panic attacks could not be regarded as a specific effect of the drug (because imipramine is also an effective antidepressant), it is an example of treatment selectivity, in that imipramine appeared to be ineffective against generalised anxiety.

These initial findings of treatment specificity have not gone unchallenged, however. For example Johnstone reported a trial in which a wide range of mostly chronic neurotic disorders, including 'neurotic depression', mixed anxiety and depression and various other anxiety disorders, responded similarly well to a 4-week trial of a tricyclic antidepressant drug, amitriptyline, but rather poorly to a benzodiazepine drug, diazepam (Johnstone et al 1980). However, patients with panic disorder were not separately identified in this study. Other later studies have confirmed that generalised anxiety disorder is as responsive as panic disorder to a range of antidepressant drugs independent of the presence of depressive symptoms, and that benzodiazepines when given in sufficiently high doses have anti-panic properties after all. Furthermore, these and more recent studies have shown that behavioural and cognitive therapies are helpful in all types of anxiety disorder including those with panic attacks, particularly if longer-term outcomes are considered.

Despite the limited evidence for specificity of treatment response, it led to a splitting of the neurosis entity into literally dozens of different diagnoses. This is illustrated by the changes in the classification systems: In ICD-8, neurotic disorders were grouped together as manifestations of a common condition 'without any demonstrable organic basis in which the patient may have considerable insight ... The principal manifestations include excessive anxiety, hysterical symptoms, phobias, obsessional and compulsive symptoms and depression'. In ICD-10 although the term 'neurotic' is retained as a heading, the concept of neurosis is abandoned 'as a major organising principle' and instead, 'disorders are arranged in groups according to major common themes or descriptive likeness'. Similarly in DSM, beginning with DSM-III, successive revisions have also introduced increasing numbers of diagnostic categories with fewer exclusion criteria, opening up the possibility of multiple diagnoses to many patients who would previously have received a single diagnosis of neurosis. This vexed subject of 'comorbidity', in particular the boundaries between neurosis, depressive disorders and personality disorders, is the subject of substantial on-going investigation and debate.

A modern conception of neurosis

Given the controversy over whether neuroses are best regarded together (as proposed by the 'lumpers') or as separate conditions (as advocated by the 'splitters') we will consider neurosis from both perspectives. First we will consider these disorders together around the concept of anxiety. Anxiety, is at the heart of much of human experience and a large part of mental pathology, but it is only in this group of conditions that, peacock-like, it displays its many features in all their magnificent colours. Second, we will consider them each briefly as separate syndromes as classified in ICD-10 and DSM-IV.

COMMON FEATURES OF NEUROSES

What do the neuroses have in common?
The common characteristics of the neuroses are:

1. An emotional disturbance that is disproportionately severe or prolonged considering the person's experiences and external circumstances. By implication, it reflects a disorder of psychological functioning, which has a more or less discrete onset, and cannot be entirely accounted for by the patient's usual personality. The presence of an external focus or trigger helps to provide the basis for a classification of these disorders.
2. The accompaniment of the emotional disturbance by:
   (a) distressing alterations in bodily sensations reflecting the physiological changes underlying heightened arousal (autonomic and somatic) and defensive reactions ('fight and flight', avoidance and response suppression). They include psychiatric disorders presenting with predominantly somatic or other medically unexplained

symptoms. The somatic symptoms common in neuroses are listed in Box 21.2;
   (b) altered cognition by which everyday situations provoke apprehensive expectation, and perturbing events (e.g. novelty, uncertainty) are processed as though aversive; threatening or noxious events may produce extreme or catastrophic responses (e.g. panic, terror);
   (c) changes in self-image and self-awareness which are not ascribed to alterations in external reality.
3. The accompaniment of emotional disorder associated with thoughts (e.g. self-reassurance, obsessions) and behaviours (e.g. avoidance, rituals) which may be regarded as attempts to reduce anxiety, but which are in fact maladaptive in that they exacerbate or perpetuate the problem. Thoughts may be judged as unacceptable or absurd by the patient but are recognised as their own. Behaviour may be highly disruptive and disabling for the individual, but usually remains within socially acceptable limits.
4. The disorder cannot entirely be explained by the presence of medical conditions including organic brain disease, psychosis, depressive mood states or personality disorders as defined elsewhere in this book, although one or more of these conditions may coexist with a neurotic disorder in the same patient.

The boundaries of the concept of neurosis

Problems of living or psychiatric illness?

Since neurotic disorders can be viewed as quantitatively rather than qualitatively different from normal experience, the suggestion that they represent an overmedicalisation of problems of

---

Box 21.2 Somatic or bodily symptoms commonly found in neurotic disorders

Motor symptoms
- Keyed up, 'on edge'
- Restlessness, fidgetiness
- Exaggerated startle response

Neuromuscular symptoms
- General muscle aches and pains (especially in neck, shoulder and back)
- Muscle tension, 'tension headaches'
- Trembling, shaking, action or intention tremor
- Numbness, 'tingling sensations' in the face, hands and feet

Autonomic arousal symptoms
- Excessive sweating
- Dry mouth
- Sensation of difficulty swallowing ('lump in the throat')
- Epigastric discomfort, dyspepsia
- Nausea
- Stomach churning ('butterflies in the stomach')
- Abdominal pain, bloating and flatulence
- Frequent loose motions
- Urinary frequency
- Tachycardia
- Palpitations, pounding heart
- Chest pain or discomfort
- Difficulty in breathing (sense of 'incomplete' inspiration)
- Tachypnoea, hyperventilation
- Feeling dizzy, light-headed, unsteady

living rather than 'psychological illness' is a common one. The mental and physical accompaniments of challenging situations can therefore hardly be called 'symptoms' of an illness. These experiences become symptoms when they cause distress and disability to the individual that exceeds generally agreed thresholds. These thresholds are as much determined by cultural norms as by medical criteria, although in Western societies they are usually the prerogative of doctors.

Neurosis or personality disorders: the general neurotic syndrome

Neurosis is differentiated from personality disorder by having a definite onset and meeting symptom defined criteria. However, it has long been known that there is an association between neurosis and personality disorder. First chronic neurosis with onset in early life may merge into personality disorder, and second certain neurosis may appear as exaggeration of personality traits. The general neurotic syndrome is a name suggested for a condition in which various neurotic symptoms are present simultaneously or successively and which is associated with certain kinds of personality disorder (Tyrer 1985) (see Table 21.1). The characteristic features of personality disorder associated with the general neurotic syndrome include excessive timidity, poor self-esteem, avoidance of anxiety-provoking situations and dependence on others. In terms of the current classification of personality disorders used by ICD-10, these features are covered by Anxious (Avoidant) (F60.6) and Dependent Personality Disorders (F60.7), although there are also features of Obsessive–Compulsive (Anankastic) Personality Disorder (F60.5) (indecision and excessive caution).

The general neurotic syndrome allows the possibility of a common heritable component to both neurosis and personality disorder, and accounts for the different mood states and possible diagnostic change that follow from different life experiences. It is postulated to have a chronic course, a high incidence of relapse and change to other diagnoses within the neurotic spectrum, and poor response to treatment with the possible exception of long-term antidepressants. In practice, the syndrome often coexists with personality disorder and both should be coded.

Neurosis and depression

Neurosis commonly coexists with depressive disorder. One way of differentiating them is to focus on the symptom of anhedonia. Anhedonia is defined as a reduction in the capacity to experience pleasure or interest, and is regarded by some as a core feature of

Table 21.1 Cothymic disorders: neurotic, mood and other conditions in which symptoms of anxiety and depression occur together with non-specific symptoms such as fatigue and irritability

ICD-10 code/category name	Onset/duration criteria	Clinical/diagnostic features
F48.9 Neurotic disorder, residual category	Duration: ≥1 week	NS > A = D
F43.22 Mixed anxiety–depressive reaction	Onset within 1 month of stressful life event; duration: ≥ 1 week, ≤ 6 months	NS = A = D (highly variable)
F41.2 Mixed anxiety–depressive disorder	Duration: ≥ 1 month (DSM-IV), ≥ 6 months (ICD-10), ≤ 2 years (?)	NS = A = D* ICD-10 emphasises autonomic symptoms of anxiety
F41.3 Other mixed anxiety disorders	Duration: ≥ 6 months	A > NS > D General anxiety disorder (F41.1) plus prominent, transient 'other' neurotic disorders (F40–49) which fail to meet full diagnostic criteria
F48.0 Neurasthenia	Duration: ≥ 6 months (ICD-10 Primary Care version)	NS >> A = D* Mental &/or physical fatigue after minimal effort, autonomic and musculoskeletal somatic complaints, irritability, etc. predominate over anxious, depressed mood
F34.1 Dysthymia	Duration: ≥ 2 years	D† > NS ≥ A Depressive symptoms are similar to those in (major) depressive episode (F32–F33) but are less numerous and severe and predominate over non-specific and anxiety symptoms
No code General neurotic syndrome	Duration: > 2 months (usually chronic)	D† > A > NS Requires current or recent depressive episode (F32–F33) or dysthymia (F34.1) plus current or recent, transient anxiety disorder(s) (F40–F42; F44–F45) excluding adjustment disorders (F43), dependent (F60.6), avoidant (F60.6), or anankastic (F60.7) personality disorder

A, anxiety symptoms;	≥, equal to or more than;
D, depressive symptoms;	>>, much more than;
NS, non-specific neurotic symptoms.	≤, equal to or less than;
* Anhedonia only included by ICD-10.	?, uncertain or unclear.
† Includes anhedonia.	

major depressive illness. Anhedonia is a characteristic feature even of mild depressive mood states which are placed outside the neurotic spectrum by DSM and ICD (Mild Depressive Episode, F32.0; Dysthymia F34.1). By contrast, in the conditions which feature low dysphoric mood typically of mild degree but *without anhedonia*, neurotic symptoms (e.g. anxiety, worry, fatigue, irritability and difficulty falling asleep) are found in abundance. This type of mood disorder has been referred to as 'neurotic depression'. However the term neurotic depression is no longer used in formal classificatory systems, although confusingly it is sometimes used as a synonym for Dysthymia, and its classification code (300.4) in DSM-IV is the same as depressive neurosis in the old ICD classifications. In ICD-10, the category Mixed Anxiety–Depressive Disorder (F41.2) describes most of the features previously associated with the concept of neurotic depression, although of course the co-occurrence of anxiety with depression in approximately equal proportions is given even greater emphasis. In summary, DSM-IV regards anhedonia as a hallmark of major depressive disorders, and dysthymia as a milder, chronic variant of these conditions which are outside the spectrum of neurotic disorders. By contrast, ICD-10, which unlike DSM-IV includes mixed anxiety–depressive disorder as a category in its own right under the heading of neurotic disorder, fails to make a clear distinction between mixed anxiety–depressive disorder and dysthymia.

Neurosis and general medical conditions

For each of the diagnoses listed in this section, and particularly those that present with loss of function, the occurrence of a pathologically defined general medical condition that could cause similar symptoms is regarded as an exclusion. Hence a person who has symptoms of chronic severe anxiety would be regarded as suffering from a generalised anxiety disorder but, if those symptoms were found to be associated with clear evidence of thyrotoxicosis, the appropriate diagnosis is that of thyrotoxicosis. Underlying this distinction is the theoretical concept of 'mental' as compared with 'physical' conditions. The mental conditions are generally assumed to have a psychological aetiology whereas physical conditions have an aetiology based in malfunction of the body. This is a useful working distinction and one that the psychiatric clinician must be vigilant to.

However, our greater understanding of neurosis makes this theoretical distinction increasingly dubious. The greater understanding of the biology of neurosis as exemplified by the account in this chapter, and the increasing understanding of the role of psychological factors in the aetiology of so called medical conditions, questions this simple dichotomy. Rather than regarding 'mental' and 'physical' disorders as having clearly separate natures and aetiologies it is probably more helpful to simply acknowledge that the psychiatric disorders are diagnosed on the basis purely of symptom criteria whereas the medical disorders are diagnosed on the basis of identifiable bodily pathology. There is no theoretical reason why an agitated state accompanied by a high level of thyroxin should be regarded as fundamentally different from an agitated state associated with altered neurotransmission. The differentiation between psychiatric and medical disorders can consequently be regarded as ultimately arbitrary but indicating which medical specialty is best equipped to manage them. Furthermore this boundary is potentially changeable, as certain conditions previously diagnosed as hysteria have been found to be associated with neurological pathology, and other conditions previously regarded to have specific

medical cause are no longer regarded as having such. In summary, while in practice the psychiatric versus medical distinction is important for patient management, care should be taken in assuming that it represents a fundamental distinction of illness and in any sense 'carves nature of the joints'. For a further discussion of the issue see Chapter 28.

Summary

In summary, the concept of neurosis may be defined by both the commonalities of the neurotic conditions which centre on the concept of anxiety and associated psychological, behavioural and physiological abnormalities. It is also differentiated by its boundaries, which are with normality, mood disorder, personality disorder, and symptoms more usefully attributed to general medical conditions.

THE CLASSIFICATION OF NEUROTIC DISORDERS

The current classification of neurotic disorders in ICD-10 is shown in Box 21.1. In considering classification it is helpful to address some basic assumptions of how this is achieved.

Categories or dimensions?

Past and present versions of the ICD and DSM systems of classification and diagnosis of neurotic and mood disorders are essentially categorical ones, despite the fact that features of depression, anxiety and other neurotic symptoms do not behave in an all or nothing way. That is, they coexist in the same patients in proportions that vary over time and with the severity of illness. In order to achieve a workable categorical system the variable mixture of clinical features and the overlap between states of anxiety and depression were dealt with in DSM-III by imposing strict hierarchical rules. These allowed only one principal diagnosis, with major depression taking precedence over all anxiety disorders, and general anxiety disorder only being diagnosed in the absence of any other disorder. In DSM-III therefore generalised anxiety disorder was at the bottom of the hierarchy of mood and anxiety disorders. The assumptions underlying a hierarchy of this sort are that conditions at a higher level of the hierarchy are less prevalent, more disabling and more likely to coexist with conditions lower down the hierarchy. In other words, the most 'serious' conditions such as major depression are likely to incorporate the symptoms of less serious ones. However, since the severity and seriousness of a condition are partly defined and determined by the number of symptoms present, explanations for this involving a hierarchy of disorders may be unnecessary.

After the introduction of DSM-III it was recognised that some of the assumptions underlying the strict diagnostic hierarchy used may not be valid. Furthermore, in applying the hierarchy in epidemiological surveys and research studies, information about conditions lower down the hierarchy was being concealed or lost. Finally, as the diagnostic thresholds for the conditions lower down the hierarchy were relatively high, a large proportion of subjects with clinically relevant, disabling and distressing symptoms, were not given a diagnosis at all, or fell into a residual category, 'not otherwise specified'.

With so many diagnostic categories, it can be argued that DSM-IV and ICD-10 are in effect 'pseudo-categorised dimensional systems'. Furthermore, for many categories of disorder, hierarchical rules still apply. For example in ICD-10, when a depressive episode occurs in the same patient at the same time as an anxiety disorder which fulfils all criteria of symptom type, severity and duration, etc., the anxiety disorder is not diagnosed separately if the depressive episode dominates the clinical picture and/or preceded the anxiety disorder. In the case of Generalised Anxiety Disorder (F41.1), Mixed Anxiety–Depressive Disorder (F41.2), and Adjustment Disorders (F43.2), the presence of a depressive episode or any other anxiety disorder invalidates the diagnosis. In DSM-IV, if criteria for generalised anxiety disorder are met exclusively during a major depressive episode, the diagnosis of generalised anxiety disorder is not allowed. Panic attacks occurring only during a depressive episode cannot be classified as Panic Disorder (F41.0) in ICD-10 although this is allowed in DSM-IV, with more than half the cases of panic disorder being comorbid with major depressive episode. ICD-10 has higher diagnostic thresholds and more hierarchical rules and exclusion factors than DSM. The relationships between anxiety and depressive symptoms are illustrated in Figure 21.1.

Levels of categorical diagnosis

Neurotic disorders as defined in categorical terms can be considered at various levels, which comprise:

- *individual symptoms:* isolated or small numbers of individual symptoms without any one predominating and which may or may not be persistent;
- *sub-syndromal disorders:* mixtures of several (typically three or more) symptoms which are relatively consistent, severe and enduring or recurring, but which fail to meet diagnostic criteria for full-blown anxiety states or other related disorders;
- *specific syndromes:* categories of mental disorder which fulfil diagnostic criteria in terms of content, severity and duration of one or two characteristic symptoms, but which still show a wide range of clinical features and other symptoms, many of which are common to a number of different syndromes.

Symptoms

Diverse psychological and somatic complaints which cannot be explained by identifiable physical disease and which appear to be accompaniments or expressions of emotional distress are common in the general population. Transient symptoms are common but we are not good at detecting which will persist and which will recur. A few symptoms lasting less than 2 weeks are unlikely to cause significant disability, and there appears to be an approximate correlation between the number of symptoms causing distress and the likelihood of spontaneous remission, particularly if the symptoms are an understandable reaction to stressful life events. Nonetheless, the common assumption that neurotic symptoms are trivial and transient is not always justified. In milder neurotic disorders, features of anxiety and depression, as well as common non-specific features such as fatigue and insomnia, are likely to occur together in the same individuals so that it may be difficult to decide which if any particular category of neurotic disorder the patient has. For this reason, it has often been proposed that neurotic disorders are better described clinically and conceptualised theoretically by their position on one or more dimensions or continua, rather than by placing them into discrete categories (Kendell 1975). Study of the links between personality traits and

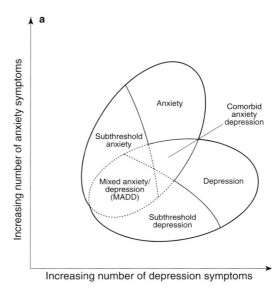

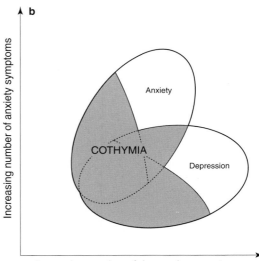

Fig. 21.1

Neurotic disorders as mixed states: the concept of cothymia. (a) Distribution of hypothetical individual scores for symptoms of anxiety and depression in patients suffering from neurotic disorders. All subjects will score for both anxiety and depression, and therefore in one sense all conditions are mixed states. Anxious and depressive subjects with higher levels of the alternate mood states will reach the criterion or threshold for a 'diagnosable' disorder at a lower level of the predominant mood state. A relatively large number of subjects fail to reach the diagnostic thresholds for discrete anxiety or depressive syndromes or disorders. Of these subsyndromal mixed states, a minority (10–20%) have approximately equal numbers of anxiety and depressive symptoms ('mixed anxiety and depressive disorders'). Of the subjects that can be diagnosed with a clear-cut anxiety or depressive disorder, about a quarter will meet diagnostic criteria for the other condition (comorbid anxiety and depression). (b) Cothymia is the term given to neurotic conditions featuring various combinations of anxiety and depressive symptom which fail to met formal diagnostic criteria for either an anxiety disorder or a depressive disorder. Syndromal anxiety disorders and depressive conditions occurring in the same individual (comorbid anxiety and depression) may also sometimes be included in the concept of cothymia.

attributes and susceptibility to neurotic disorders also supports a dimensional view of both personality and neurosis. The fact that in psychiatric practice there is still a dogged perseverance with a categorical view of neurotic and other mental illnesses may both illustrate and explain the lack of impact of the theories of Alexander, Eysenck, Gray and others on clinical practice.

'Sub-syndromal' disorders

Because syndromes are defined by arbitrary cut-offs on a dimension of severity, there will be many patients who have significant symptoms but who do not quite meet criteria for a syndromal diagnosis. These patients may be considered as 'sub-threshold' for anxiety and depressive disorders. They usually have varying mixtures of milder anxiety and depressive symptoms, as well as non-specific symptoms such as fatigue. In ICD-10, these 'sub-syndromal' conditions include Mixed Anxiety and Depressive Disorder (F41.2) and Neurasthenia (F48.0), which will be considered here, as well as three categories of Adjustment Disorder: Brief Depressive Reaction (F43.20), Prolonged Depressive Reaction (F43.21) and Mixed Anxiety and Depressive Reaction (F43.22). As illustrated in Figure 21.1b and Figure 21.2, the term 'cothymia' has been used to describe conditions characterised by a mixture of neurotic symptoms which do not clearly and consistently qualify for a diagnosis of a depressive or anxiety disorder (Tyrer et al 2003).

Syndromal disorders

There is a widespread basic assumption that, despite qualitative differences, most if not all neurotic disorders share common characteristics and possible causal mechanisms. These operate together with increasing intensity in a single or several closely related dimensions to give multiple symptoms causing increasing distress and disability in a diminishing number of subjects (Goldberg et al 1987). This dimensional view of neurotic disorders justifies the concept of a case threshold, i.e. a level of severity of symptoms which defines the boundary of clinically

significant impairment. For example, a score of 12 or more on the Revised Clinical Interview Schedule (CIS-R) used in the UK National Psychiatric Morbidity (NPM) Household Survey (Meltzer et al 1995) defined 'caseness' in terms of neurotic and related mood disorder. The case threshold in the NPM Household Survey was reached or exceeded by 16% of the population (Fig. 21.3). The syndromal neurotic disorders are considered individually later in this chapter.

EPIDEMIOLOGY

Neurotic illnesses are common. They affect at least 15% of the adult population of Great Britain at any time. In the UK and Europe, a high proportion (at least half) of people suffering from neurotic symptoms approach their doctors for help and make up a quarter to a third of all consultations in general practice. However, according to epidemiological surveys the large majority of neurotic patients are not appropriately diagnosed or treated.

Community surveys

This section summarises the results from four epidemiological studies in which the prevalence rates of neurotic and mood disorders have been assessed in very large populations. The US Epidemiologic Catchment Area (ECA) study (Regier et al 1984), the US National Comorbidity Study (NCS) (Kessler et al. 1994a) and the UK NPM Household Study (Meltzer et al. 1995) (see Table 21.2) are community surveys which sampled subjects in several areas or in the general population who had not necessarily been previously identified as ill.

By contrast, the worldwide WHO–Psychological Problems in General Health Care Study (World Health Organization 1995) screened a large number (25 916) of adults who were consulting primary-healthcare services. Of these, 5438 (21%) were identified by the 12-item GHQ as suffering from some form of psychiatric disorder and were subjected to further investigation using standardised interviews. These in turn generated ICD-10

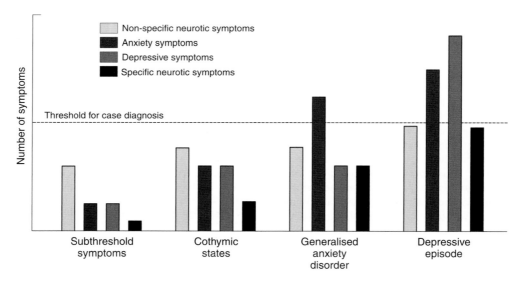

Fig. 21.2
Hypothetical scores for four types of neurotic/mood symptoms in four syndromes of increasing overall severity. Note that in the depressive episode, all symptom types are more numerous (severe) than in the other three syndromes.

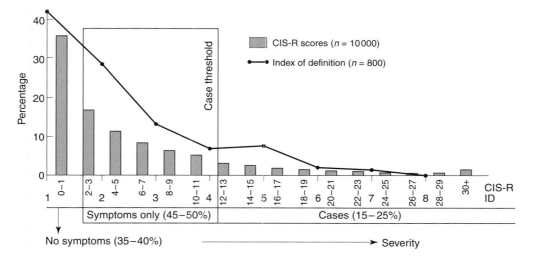

Fig. 21.3
Distribution of scores derived from clinical interview indicating severity of psychiatric disorder in the general adult population. Data are derived from two large community surveys carried out in the UK. The histogram plots data from Meltzer et al (1995). Revised Clinical Interview Schedule (CIS-R) scores of 12 or above attained by 16% of the sample indicate clinically significantly neurotic or mood disorder in the previous week. The graph plots data from Bebbington et al (1981). Scores from the Present State Examination (PSE) were used to derive an index of definition (ID) which measures the degree of certainty with which a mental disorder is deemed to be present in the last month. ID scores of 4 or above indicate a probable or definite mental disorder (predominantly anxiety, depression and related conditions). Approximately 18% of the sample exceeded this criterion (11% had definite mental disorder).

Table 21.2 Prevalence (%) of neurotic disorders in the UK from the National Psychiatric Morbidity (NPM) Household Survey (Meltzer et al 1995)

Diagnostic category	Women	Men	All	All*
Non-specific neurotic disorder (NSND)	9.9	5.4	7.7	7.7
Generalised anxiety disorder (GAD)	3.4	2.8	3.1	4.5
Depressive episodes	2.5	1.7	2.1	2.3
All phobias	1.4	0.7	1.1	1.8
Obsessive–compulsive disorder (OCD)	1.5	0.9	1.2	1.6
Panic disorder	0.9	0.8	0.8	1.0
Any neurotic or mood disorder	19.5	12.3	16.0	16.0
Alcohol abuse/dependence[†]	2.1	7.5	4.8	–
Drug abuse/dependence[†]	1.5	2.9	2.2	–

Prevalence figures for mutually exclusive diagnostic categories obtained after ascertaining the duration of symptoms present during the past week and applying the following hierarchy to ICD-10 diagnoses: psychotic disorder > depressive episode (severe and moderate) > agoraphobia > panic disorder > OCD > depressive episode (mild) > social phobia > GAD > specific phobia > NSND. Non-specific neurotic disorder mainly corresponds to ICD-10 Mixed Anxiety–Depressive Disorder but would also include Adjustment Disorders and Neurasthenia.
* Prevalence rates with hierarchical rules abandoned, so that categories are no longer mutually exclusive and the total exceeds that for 'any disorder'.
[†] Annual prevalence rates.

diagnoses and 1-month and lifetime prevalence rates calculated using the total sample as a denominator.

The results of these epidemiological surveys are summarised in Table 21.3. It is not possible to compare in detail the prevalence data generated by the various surveys for several reasons. For example no survey used the same interview schedule and diagnostic system, and whereas the American studies (which used DSM-III or DSM-IIIR) calculated annual prevalence rates, the WHO–PPGHC study and the NPM Household Survey (which both used ICD-10) calculated 1-month and 1-week prevalence rates, respectively. Despite these discrepancies between the surveys, they show a fair degree of concordance. There are however two major exceptions. First, the prevalence rates for depressive episode are extremely low in the NPM Household Survey, even allowing for the fact that only disorders present during the previous week were considered. Prevalence rates of depressive episodes in the ECA study are also low in comparison with the NCS and WHO–PPGHC study; it is likely that, owing to various methodological limitations of the ECA study, the higher estimates of prevalence of depressive illness (approximately 10%) are more likely to be valid. The second discrepancy concerns the prevalence of phobic disorder. The two American studies, particularly the NCS, examined the prevalence of phobic states in some detail, distinguishing between simple phobias, social phobias and agoraphobia. The 1-year rate for social phobia was particularly high in the NCS (7.9% versus 4.2% in the ECA). This partly explains the somewhat higher overall prevalence rate for any phobic disorder reported in the NCS compared with the ECA study. However, both these figures are an order of magnitude higher than the figure obtained for all phobic disorders in the NPM Household Survey, which is likely to be an underestimate. This may partly reflect the higher diagnostic threshold for phobic

Table 21.3 Summary of results of population surveys giving prevalence rates (%) of neurotic, depressive and substance misuse disorders

| Survey (reference) | GAD | Phobic disorders | | Panic disorder | OCD | Any anxiety disorder | Depressive episode | Alcohol misuse dependence | Drug misuse/ dependence |
		All	Agor. only						
ECA (Regier et al 1990)	3.7[c,d]	10.9[c]	5.8[c,f]	1.3[c]	2.1[c]	**12.6**[c]	5.7[c]	7.0[c]	2.8[b]
NCS (Kessler et al 1994)	3.1[c]	11.9[c,d]	2.8[c,f]	2.3[c]	NA	**17.2**[c]	10.3[c]	9.7[c]	3.6[c]
NPM HS (Meltzer et al 1995)	4.5[a,e]	1.8[a,e]	NA	1.0[a,e]	1.6[a,e]	**13.9**[a,d]	2.3[a,e]	4.8[c]	2.2[c]
WHO–PPGHC (Sartorius et al 1996)	7.9[b]	NA	1.5[b,f]	1.1[b]	NA	**10.2**[b]	10.4[b]	NA	NA
Mean	4.8	8.2	3.4[f]	1.4	1.8	**13.5**	7.2	7.2	2.9

GAD, generalised anxiety disorder; NA, not assessed or result not available; OCD, obsessive–compulsive disorder.
[a] 1-week prevalence.   [d] Residual or estimated value.
[b] 1-month prevalence.   [e] Diagnostic hierarchy suspended.
[c] 1-year prevalence.   [f] Agoraphobia only.

disorders in ICD-10 compared with DSM-III and DSM-IIIR. In the WHO–PPGHC study the only phobic disorder considered was agoraphobia, which limits comparison with the other surveys.

From the overall pattern of results shown in Table 21.3, the prevalence of any anxiety disorder (10–17%) consistently matches or exceeds the rates for depressive episodes (7–10%). Earlier studies had shown that depressive disorders are somewhat more prevalent than anxiety disorders. These findings therefore suggest either that anxiety disorders are becoming more common or that they are being better recognised. Within the group of anxiety disorders, generalised anxiety disorder and phobic disorders tend to occur at more than double the rate of panic disorder and obsessive–compulsive disorder.

The summary scores in the table indicate that phobic disorders are the most prevalent anxiety disorders of all, although the prevalence of the 'sub-syndromal' residual category of mixed anxiety–depressive disorder, reported as 7.7% in the NPM Household Survey, would probably have been comparable to that of phobic disorder had it been considered in the other surveys.

Social and demographic correlates of neurosis

Gender

Neurotic symptoms are more prevalent in females than in males in a ratio of approximately 3:2. Similarly all neurotic disorders and depressive episodes tend to be more prevalent in women than in men, although the sex difference is most marked for milder conditions such as mixed anxiety–depressive disorder and generalised anxiety disorder, and least for panic disorder. This supports the view that neuroses seem to be more common in women partly because milder symptoms are reported more frequently and reliably by women than by men. In more severe disorders (e.g. panic disorder), this difference in communication of distress between women and men would have a smaller impact on whether a disorder is recognised and diagnosed.

Age

The overall prevalence of neurotic disorders increases slightly with age until about the age of 40, after which neurotic disorders are diagnosed less often, particularly in men. However, the age at which neurotic disorders and especially mood disorders peak may show a cohort effect: a younger age of maximum prevalence and a general increase in the prevalence of all conditions is apparent in more recent surveys. In other words these conditions may be getting more common especially in younger people. Phobic disorder, especially social phobia, is particularly common in younger people and seems to predispose to the later development of depressive disorders and substance misuse.

Social and family relationships

Neurotic disorders in both marital partners occur more often than predicted by chance. Neurotic individuals may be more likely to marry other neurotics (assortative mating), or neurotic disorder in one partner may create problems and stress which make it more likely that the other partner will develop a neurotic disorder later. This is a more likely explanation than assortative mating because concordance for neuroses increases with the length of time that people are married. Single people, especially those who are divorced, separated or widowed, and lone parents are more likely to have neurotic disorders (especially mixed anxiety–depressive disorder) than married or cohabiting couples.

Socio-economic status, employment, housing and urban living

The prevalence of anxiety disorders varies inversely with people's income and educational attainments. The latter finding may suggest that stress due to social hardship and disadvantage tends to cause more threats and losses, and more anxiety and depression. In the NPM Household Survey, unemployed men and women showed particularly high rates of neurotic and mood disorders independent of other factors such as poverty. The increased prevalence of anxiety and mood disorders in people living in urban versus rural areas reported in the NPM Household Survey appeared to be independent of other explanatory variables.

Mortality

Neurotic disorders appear to be linked with increased mortality due to suicide, accidental death and alcohol and drug dependence or misuse. In severe anxiety disorders, the risk of suicide may be as high as in depressive illness, although it is unclear what effect treatment of the anxiety disorders has on the risk of suicide.

Recognition and treatment

Extrapolating from the UK NPM Household Survey, the average GP with a list of 1800 patients (63% aged 16–64) will have care of about 160 adults suffering from anxiety disorders or other neurotic conditions, which also amounts to about 9% of the GP's list. The international WHO–PPGCH study found that about 30% of all patients consulting GPs had a neurotic or mood disorder, although, of these, nearly half just failed to meet diagnostic criteria according to ICD-10. About 16% of patients were suffering from a clinically significant anxiety disorder, compared with 20% with a depressive condition such as depressive episode, sub-threshold depressive episode or dysthymia. Six percent suffered from both anxiety and depression at the same time.

The commonest anxiety disorder identified in the WHO–PPGHC study was generalised anxiety disorder, which affected nearly 8% of the sample. However, nearly as many subjects (6.3%) qualified for sub-threshold anxiety disorder, with 1.3% having an equal mixture of anxiety and depressive symptoms (mixed anxiety–depressive disorder). As in the much earlier study (Johnstone & Goldberg 1976), GPs in the WHO–PPGHC study failed to detect nearly half of the patients who met diagnostic criteria for anxiety disorders. These findings suggest that, as well as GPs missing many cases, nearly as many other patients were incorrectly identified as having psychiatric disturbance, because this could not be confirmed after standardised interview. Most (80%) patients with anxiety disorders identified by GPs were offered some form of treatment, usually counselling. The co-occurrence of anxiety states and depression greatly increased the likelihood that GPs would recognise the disorder and offer appropriate treatment, probably because GPs are better informed about depressive disorders. Only about half of the cases of anxiety disorders recognised by GPs were offered any drug treatment. Antidepressant drugs were prescribed for both depressed and anxious patients, but only about 10% of anxious patients who would have benefited from these drugs received any drug treatment. On average, an even smaller number (about 5%) of anxious patients received rapidly acting anxiolytic drugs (e.g. benzodiazepines), but there were very wide geographical differences in rates of prescribing anxiolytics.

Taken overall, these findings are quite discouraging. There seems to have been little improvement over 20 years or so in the accurate detection of anxiety and other neurotic disorders in primary care, and less than 10% of patients received effective treatment from their GPs. The importance of striving to improve the detection and treatment of neurotic disorders in general practice is illustrated by a study carried out by Mann et al (1981), who followed up non-psychotic patients presenting to their GPs. After 1 year, although a quarter of patients had improved, 50% showed intermittent illness and 25% were chronically adversely affected by their symptoms.

Summary

In summary, neurotic symptoms and neurotic disorders are highly prevalent in the general population and in persons attending general practitioners. The most common neurotic disorders are anxiety disorders, and anxiety and depression frequently coexist.

Neurotic symptoms are more prevalent in females and in those of low socio-economic status. The prognosis for neuroses seen in general practice is poor for a quarter of cases, and the relatively low rates of recognition and treatment could probably be improved. A strong case can be made for psychiatry devoting more attention to neuroses as highly prevalent, treatable but neglected psychiatric disorders.

AETIOLOGY

The aetiology of neuroses is best understood by considering the combined effect of biological, psychological and social influences.

Biology

Genetics

Although neurotic disorders tend to run in families, this can partly be explained by findings that adverse early experiences and high rates of stressful life events are also common to members of the same family. Whereas environmental factors can fairly specifically determine whether anxiety, depression or a mixture of neurotic symptoms dominates the clinical picture, it seems that genetic factors determine only non-specific general vulnerability to neurotic and mood disorders. The vulnerability which is inherited may be roughly analogous to constitutional emotional reactivity as reflected by Eysenck's concept of 'neuroticism' or by personality traits resembling anxious (avoidant) personality disorder. Twin studies show that similar or identical genes are responsible for generalised anxiety disorder and major depression (Kendler 1996). Other anxiety disorders may be heterogeneous in terms of genetic influence, as there is some evidence that phobic disorders and especially panic disorder are inherited in a different way from generalised anxiety disorder and major depression. However, the evidence is not clear, and a partially inherited general susceptibility to all types of neurotic disorder seems most likely (Andrews 1996).

Neurotransmitters and neural circuits

Current neurobiological theories of neurotic disorders are dominated by three brain neurotransmitter receptor systems: (1) the $GABA_A$–benzodiazepine receptor complex (Nutt & Malizia 2001); (2) the serotonin ($5HT_{1A}/5HT_{2C}$) receptor group (Deakin 1998) and (3) the noradrenergic system (Nutt 1992). These brain receptor systems mediate the effects of benzodiazepines, selective serotonin reuptake inhibitors (SSRIs) and tricyclic antidepressants (TCAs), the three main classes of drugs currently used for treating neurotic disorders.

GABA Gamma-aminobutyric acid (GABA) is the most important inhibitory neurotransmitter in the central nervous system (see Ch. 3). GABAergic interneurons and afferent fibres inhibit brain neurons and are in balance with excitatory inputs (mostly glutamatergic) which cause neuronal excitation. Enhancement of GABAergic-induced neuronal inhibition is associated with reduced behavioural arousal (sedation), amnesia and ataxia, whereas attenuation of the effects of GABA causes increased arousal, enhanced memory, anxiety, restlessness, insomnia, exaggerated reactivity (startle) and convulsions. Many of the behavioural inhibitory effects of GABA are believed to be mediated by suppression of neuronal activity in the serotonergic and noradrenergic systems described later.

Serotonin (5HT) Catecholamine neurotransmitters (noradrenaline [norepinephrine] and dopamine) are known to be important in mediating psychological processes such as arousal, reward, punishment, attention and memory which are all disrupted in neurotic and mood disorders. However, the indolamine neurotransmitter serotonin (5-hydroxytryptamine, 5HT) may serve an equally important role in these processes, and in particular may explain many of the mechanisms of therapeutic drug action in neurotic and mood disorders.

There are two important serotonergic systems in the brain which mediate different types of defensive or coping responses to aversive and threatening events. The central projections of the brainstem dorsal raphé nucleus (DRN) are activated by aversive stimulation and cause release of 5HT onto neurons in the amygdala, frontal cortex and basal ganglia. The same structures also receive a dopaminergic innervation which acts in functional opposition to the serotonergic inputs at low levels of neuronal and behavioural activity. By contrast, at high levels of functional activity, serotonin and dopamine appear to interact co-operatively. The DRN 5HT signal is mediated by postsynaptic $5HT_{2C}$ receptors and results in fear and anxiety and acute adaptive responses such as inhibition of ongoing behaviour followed by avoidance of the perceived source of danger or threat.

Psychosocial stress causing neurotic symptoms such as anxiety and mild depression is associated with activation of $5HT_{2C}$ receptors. Drugs which block or downregulate $5HT_{2C}$ receptors (all antidepressants when given for several weeks or more), or which reduce serotonergic activity and 5HT release onto $5HT_{2C}$ receptors (benzodiazepines and buspirone) are therefore effective in reducing states of anticipatory (generalised) anxiety. Buspirone exerts its main effect by stimulating $5HT_{1A}$ autoreceptors which inhibit 5HT cell firing and 5HT release, thereby switching off the $5HT_{2C}$ anxiety signal. This effect persists because the autoreceptors in the DRN-$5HT_{2C}$ system appear relatively resistant to compensatory desensitisation or down-regulation. Despite the reduction in synaptic 5HT, $5HT_{2C}$ receptors gradually downregulate or decrease in number in response to prolonged administration of buspirone. The net effect of prolonged administration of antidepressants and particularly of buspirone is likely to be a marked reduction in $5HT_{2C}$ neurotransmission.

As well as mediating fear and anxiety by $5HT_{2C}$ receptor activation in the amygdala and associated limbic structures, serotonergic projections from the DRN onto $5HT_{2C}$ receptor sites in other parts of the amygdala, and in the hypothalamus and periaqueductal grey matter (PAG system), inhibit the escape (flight) response which is activated during panic attacks. Thus $5HT_{2C}$ systems have different effects on generalised anxiety and panic depending on the site of action in the brain. High levels of anxiety associated with a high $5HT_{2C}$ signal are therefore linked to a lower probability of panic attacks occurring. Although this seems counterintuitive, it does agree with clinical observations. Drug treatments which enhance $5HT_{2C}$ receptor functioning in the PAG system (e.g. high doses of SSRIs given chronically) exert an anti-panic effect, whereas $5HT_{2C}$ receptor-blocking drugs can aggravate panic attacks.

The DRN-$5HT_{2C}$ fear system may also exert an inhibitory effect on the repetitive defensive thoughts and behaviours associated with obsessive–compulsive disorder (OCD). Underactivity in the system, which seems to occur in OCD, may therefore exacerbate if not necessarily cause symptoms of OCD. This probably explains why treatments which selectively increase serotonergic activity at $5HT_{2C}$ receptors (e.g. certain hallucinogenic drugs and SSRIs administered chronically in high dosage) exert an appreciable anti-obsessional effect, whereas $5HT_{2C}$ receptor blockers may make the condition worse.

The median raphé nucleus (MRN) sends serotonergic projections to areas of the frontal cortex and hippocampus which are also richly innervated by noradrenergic neurons and in which there is a high density of postsynaptic $5HT_{1A}$ receptors. Enhancement of $5HT_{1A}$ functioning occurs with chronic psychosocial stress and adversity, and results in re-emergence of previously suppressed behaviours, and disengagement from maladaptive cognitive-behavioural sequences. Thus the $5HT_{1A}$ receptor system is involved in longer-term adaptive responses to aversive stimuli which encourage coping mechanisms and resilience. In predisposed individuals, continued stress may result in underactivity and failure of the MRN-$5HT_{1A}$ system as demonstrated by reduced neuroendocrine responses to administration of the 5HT precursor tryptophan. Breakdown in the MRN-$5HT_{1A}$ resilience system appears to result in learned helplessness and depressive illness, and may also encourage maladaptive behavioural coping strategies such as compulsive rituals and addictive behaviour.

Several factors may determine whether and to what extent the MRN-$5HT_{1A}$ system breaks down. For example, there is evidence that the DRN-$5HT_{2C}$ fear system, which is activated by acute and chronic stress and mediates the effects of anticipatory anxiety, has an inhibitory influence on the MRN-$5HT_{1A}$ system, and may contribute to its failure if stress is severe and prolonged. This fits with the evidence mentioned earlier that anxiety states often precede and may predispose to depressive episodes. Another mechanism which may contribute to the breakdown of the MRN-$5HT_{1A}$ resilience system involves increased secretion of cortisol caused by chronic psychosocial stress and social isolation. Raised levels of cortisol may compromise the effectiveness of the MRN-$5HT_{1A}$ system by reducing the availability in the brain of the serotonin precursor tryptophan and also by directly or indirectly interfering with the functioning of $5HT_{1A}$ receptors in the hippocampus.

Restoration of normal functioning in the MRN-$5HT_{1A}$ resilience system may explain some of the therapeutic effects of antidepressant drugs in anxiety and depression and perhaps, to a lesser extent, their anti-obsessional effects as well. All effective antidepressants, including tricyclic antidepressant drugs and SSRIs, share the ability by one mechanism or another to enhance $5HT_{1A}$ neurotransmission, although this effect typically requires several weeks to develop fully. In most cases this delay is probably due to the need for inhibitory 'autoreceptors' located on the serotonergic neurons and presynaptic nerve endings to become gradually desensitised, so allowing antidepressant drugs to bring about increased neuronal release of serotonin onto postsynaptic $5HT_{1A}$ receptors.

Noradrenaline (norepinephrine) Animal studies indicate that acute stress and aversive stimulation increase the release of noradrenaline in the brain, as well as that of 5HT. Noradrenaline causes heightened arousal and focuses attention on the source of threat, whereas, as discussed earlier, the DRN-$5HT_{2C}$ system inhibits ongoing behaviour and flight responses. Patients suffering from chronic anxiety states show abnormal neuroendocrine and physiological responsiveness to drugs which stimulate or block α_2-adrenoceptors. This implies abnormal regulation or lability of noradrenergic systems in anxiety disorders.

Summary

Because the neuroses have, at least in recent history, been regarded as psychological conditions, there may be a tendency to ignore the fact that they have associated neurochemical changes. Our knowledge of these is such as to not only identify that such changes occur but to start to identify with some degree of specificity what these changes are. Increasing sophistication of understanding of the biological basis of neurosis is likely to lead to more rational design of pharmacotherapy.

Psychological factors

Behavioural factors

Behaviourists use learning theory to explain the development of anxiety disorders and to provide a basis for treatment. The best known example of this approach is the two-stage model of Mowrer proposed in 1939. In this, phobias are believed to result from the association of neutral stimuli or situations with fear-evoking or traumatic events. Some stimuli are less neutral and more likely to promote phobias than others. This may partly reflect people's inherent fearfulness of particular stimulus properties, objects or situations, and also the effect of observing other people's responses to these (modelling). As a result of classical conditioning, previously more-or-less neutral situations come to evoke fear and avoidance behaviour. Avoidance, which is an integral part of phobic disorders, reduces anxiety and is therefore reinforced and maintained by operant conditioning. This formulation gives a clear indication and justification for behavioural treatment since exposure to the feared situation will allow extinction or habituation of conditioned fear by removal of the source of the reinforcement (relief after avoidance). When exposure to feared situations is difficult in real life, as in the case of performance anxiety or certain specific phobias (e.g. phobia of vomiting), exposure in fantasy or imagination can be effective. A very similar argument applies to anticipatory anxiety in panic disorder and to anxiety occurring as part of an obsessional state which may be temporarily relieved by performing a compulsive ritual. The latter is thereby positively reinforced (increased probability of behaviour occurring), and will persist and be repeated unless the patient is exposed to the feared situation by response prevention, i.e. banning or physically preventing rituals from being carried out. Other behavioural techniques used in treating neurotic disorders include response modelling, relaxation therapy and social skills training. Some of these techniques are described in more detail elsewhere in this book.

Cognitive factors

Cognitive factors refer to how information is interpreted, stored and recalled. Cognitive factors are important in the aetiology of neurosis and are central to many psychological theories. They are also an important focus of treatment in cognitive therapy or cognitive-behaviour therapy. Given that neuroses are largely exaggerated forms of normal emotional and behavioural reactions to stressors, the interpretation of stressors is considered to be one of the factors in the aetiology of such marked reactions. The role of cognition in mediating the interpretation of experience is particularly clear in the anxiety disorders. Prominent in driving the symptoms of generalised anxiety is ongoing worry, in phobic anxiety a negative prediction of what would happen if the person exposed himself to the feared stimulus, and in panic a catastrophic interpretation of the physical symptoms of autonomic arousal associated with anxiety. Cognitive factors in the form of memory of trauma are core to post-traumatic stress disorder. The potential role of cognitive factors is well illustrated with the example of panic disorder.

In panic disorder, it seems likely that a combination of biological and psychological predisposing factors and unexpected situational anxiety trigger an initial 'spontaneous' panic attack. This in turn initiates a cascade of catastrophic thoughts and beliefs which establish a high level of anticipatory anxiety and phobic avoidance of situations associated with panic attacks or from which escape is judged to be difficult or impossible. Consequently, agoraphobia is commonly comorbid with panic attacks, although it is by no means always certain that panic attacks precede the avoidance behaviour. Panic attacks may subsequently decrease in frequency as a result of phobic avoidance, but spontaneous panic attacks may still occur unexpectedly, often when the patient is relatively relaxed and anxiety-free.

Psychodynamic theory

Psychoanalytical theory explains anxiety disorders as a result of unconscious internal conflicts, particularly those involving sexual and aggressive impulses. From this perspective, anxiety and other neurotic disorders occur when defence mechanisms are over-used, and particularly when they begin to fail or actually break down. General anxiety disorder is seen as the result of unacceptable impulses that the conscious mind blocks out of awareness. These repressed or inhibited impulses produce a constant state of anxious apprehension and tension, but since they are unconscious, the patient is unaware of the source or cause of their anxiety. It can be argued that phobias occur if an individual displaces anxiety onto a relatively neutral stimulus, situation or social function which can easily be avoided in contrast to the unconscious impulses or conflict from which the anxiety originates. Furthermore, it is believed that this 'virtual avoidance' is capable of relieving the conscious experience of anxiety. According to psychoanalytical theory, panic disorder and agoraphobia both have their origin in childhood experiences of separation anxiety. When adults who have had this experience perceive threat of separation or actually experience separation and loss of a loved one, panic will be evoked.

Summary

There has been considerable theoretical and empirical exploration of the neuroses from a psychological point of view. This has been associated with the development of effective cognitive and behavioural treatments for many neuroses. One should be cautious about regarding neuroses as purely psychological phenomena, however, as they are also associated with physiological disturbance and with interpersonal predicaments. Although unfashionable, psychodynamic theory may still offer useful hypotheses for empirical testing.

Social factors

Social situation

We have already referred to the importance of various socio-demographic variables in determining the prevalence of a range of neurotic disorders. The nature and degree of life events can determine the type and severity of neurotic disorders with which they are associated, but more enduring risk factors include social isolation and lack of support, unemployment and poverty. Urban life appears to represent an independent risk factor for neurosis, at least in the UK.

Life events

It seems likely that whereas major adverse life events can provoke neurotic disorders in previously stable individuals, less serious adversity will only cause illness in predisposed subjects. Major life events involving loss or bereavement are more likely to trigger depression, whereas events involving danger and threats are more often associated with anxiety disorders. Serious life events involving both loss and danger tend to be associated with mixed anxiety and depressive disorders (Finlay-Jones & Brown 1981). Adversities in childhood, for example due to parental neglect and physical and sexual abuse, are common antecedents of both anxiety and depressive disorders, but current adverse psychosocial factors such as lack of family supports are more strongly linked to depressive disorders than to anxiety states. Some chronic stressors and life events may be the result rather than the cause of personality traits which independently predispose to neurotic disorders. Current adversity arising in this way will tend to amplify the extent to which certain personality traits and temperament increase the risk of developing neurosis. The therapeutic implications of these epidemiological findings are obvious, but equally obviously, improvement in people's social and economic circumstances is often beyond the scope of psychiatric treatment.

Summary

Regarding the neuroses as disorders of the individual may lead to a neglect of social factors in their aetiology. There is good evidence that life stresses, childhood adversity, and lack of social support are relevant to the aetiology and perpetuation of neurotic disorders.

Multifactorial aetiology

The aetiology of neuroses is best addressed by considering the interaction of multiple factors which may be arbitrarily divided into biological, psychological and social realms. Furthermore the action of these factors may usefully be conceptualised as having their main impact at different times. Some may predispose, some may precipitate and some may perpetuate neurotic disorder. Hence for example a person may be predisposed to anxiety by genetics and early upbringing, the anxiety may be triggered by a life event occurring in a certain social situation, and the anxiety may then be perpetuated by brain changes, catastrophic cognitions and continuing social difficulties. The implication of this complex model of aetiology is that in many cases single targeted interventions may be ineffective to fully resolve a neurotic condition and that multifaceted management may be necessary, particularly where neurosis is chronic. Multifactorial aetiology is illustrated in Table 21.4.

DIAGNOSIS AND ASSESSMENT

Principles of psychiatric assessment of neurosis

Much of general psychiatry now is concerned with the diagnosis and assessment of the psychotic patient and associated assessment

Table 21.4 Multiple factors in the aetiology of neuroses

	Predisposing cause	Precipitating cause	Perpetuating cause
Biological	Genetic Biological vulnerability	Illness or injury	CNS changes Autonomic arousal
Psychological & behavioural	Childhood factors Vulnerable personality (neuroticism)	Psychological stress	Depressed mood Fears and beliefs Avoidance
Social	Lack of support	Life	Reinforcement of unhelpful cognitions & behaviour
		Social stress	Social stress

of risk. When assessing the patient with neurosis the approach has to be somewhat different. The main difference is that much more emphasis has to be placed on the patient's own history rather than on observation of the patient and on the differentiation of the phenomena they report from normality. Neuroses are not generally associated with violent or disturbed behaviour. Risk assessment is relevant only insofar as neurosis may be a manifestation of another condition, particularly mood disorders.

Differential diagnosis

The main differential diagnoses of neurosis are from other psychiatric conditions, from general medical conditions, particularly neurological and organic brain diseases, from lifelong problems, especially personality disorders, and from variations of normality.

Other psychiatric diagnoses

Psychosis can present with neurotic phenomena, particularly with anxiety. This is a common catch in psychiatric practice. For example a patient presented with severe paroxysmal anxiety and was treated with a benzodiazepine. Further enquiry revealed that the anxiety reflected delusional beliefs that the patient was being watched by others. It is generally believed that treatment of psychosis will produce resolution of the neurotic symptoms and, while this is often the case, it is not always. For example a patient who has developed agoraphobia in the context of a psychotic disorder may need specific exposure treatment for agoraphobia even after the psychosis has resolved.

General medical conditions and organic brain disorders

The differentiation of neurosis from general medical conditions is important. Some specific neurotic phenomena such as derealisation may result from organic brain disease such as temporal lobe epilepsy. There is also a range of general medical conditions which may mimic neurotic phenomena. For example the agitation and tremulousness associated with thyrotoxicosis is a differential diagnosis for generalised anxiety disorder, and the episodic physical symptoms associated with phaeochromocytoma constitute a rare differential for a diagnosis of panic disorder. The differentiation from medical conditions is particularly important in those with somatic symptoms highly suggestive of disease, as in the somatoform disorders. Care has to be taken however to balance the risk of missing a medical diagnosis with the psychological harm that may result from excessive investigation and inappropriate medical treatment.

Personality disorders

The differentiation of neurosis from lifelong problems or personality disorder is important for prognosis and predicting response to treatment. An inadequate history may identify apparently neurotic phenomena without ascertaining that these are in fact lifelong. Useful questions to include in the history are 'When did these symptoms begin?' and 'When were you last well?'. When a person is unable to answer this question it should lead to concern that the symptoms are better regarded as manifestations of personality. Some personality disorders, such as avoidant personality disorder, merge into neurotic conditions such as social phobia.

Differentiation from normality

Most neurotic phenomena are exaggerations of normal human experience and behaviour. In this sense the diagnosis of illness is arbitrary and the cutoff is based on convention. While it can be reassuring to tell patients that their symptoms are simply an extreme variant of something that everyone experiences, it is important not to convey the impression that one is minimising their suffering. For example a patient who presents with severe fatigue and is told that 'we all get tired' is likely to think that you have failed to understand the severity of his suffering. The differentiation of neurotic from normal phenomena is usually based on the criteria of duration and severity. The duration criteria vary between diagnoses but some degree of persistence is usually required. Severity is usually defined in terms of the person being distressed, suffering impairment of the usual functioning, or both.

Diagnosis and formulation

Diagnosis

Often in cases of neurotic disorder a single diagnosis does not adequately describe the range of problems. Rather than struggle to force all the phenomena into a single condition, it is often helpful to list the disorders for which the patient meets criteria and then to prioritise these in a hierarchy (see above). For example if a patient has both a major depressive disorder and a panic disorder, simply characterising the disorder as a major depression does not do justice to the panic phenomena, and it is now usually considered best to list both.

Formulation

For many neurotic conditions diagnosis alone provides an inadequate understanding of the illness, and a formulation is often used to convey a fuller account. This formulation usually consists of the following:

- a brief statement about the patient and the presenting symptoms;
- the principal diagnoses and subsidiary diagnoses;

> **Box 21.3   Sample formulation**
>
> Mrs Smith is a 29-year-old married woman who is currently unemployed and presents with a 6-month history of fatigue, low mood and episodic dizziness.
>
> The principal diagnoses are that of major depressive disorder, as evidenced by pervasive low mood and other physical symptoms, and panic disorder as evidenced by episodes of acute paroxysmal anxiety accompanied by multiple physical symptoms. The differential diagnosis is principally from a medical condition which has been excluded and a personality disorder which is also excluded by the evidence of good premorbid functioning up to the onset of the illness. There was no evidence of psychotic phenomena, and the symptoms she describes are causing significant impairment and distress and should clearly be regarded as illness.
>
> She was predisposed to developing depression by strong family history and probably by the death of her parents in childhood. Her current illness seems to have been precipitated by the loss of her job and perpetuated by continuing financial difficulties, loss of social contact and inactivity.

- an outline of likely relevant aetiological factors categorised into predisposing, precipitating and perpetuating.

An example is show in Box 21.3.

PRINCIPLES OF TREATMENT

General considerations

There are two standard ways of describing treatments for a range of disorders: the treatments can be listed and their applications to various disorders discussed, or the disorders described separately together with their individual treatments. As might be predicted from the earlier part of this chapter, we choose the first of these, mainly because the overlap of treatment effects across disorders is so great.

There are many merits in viewing the range of conditions as a spectrum, called affective spectrum disorders (Hudson & Pope 1990). The proposed range of disorders are those that respond to antidepressant drug therapy and include depression, anxiety, phobias, obsessions, panic and eating disorders, which it is proposed could all be grouped together as having the same biological basis. We prefer to delimit three groups with regard to treatment: *adjustment reactions* (which includes, but also includes more than, adjustment disorders in the current classification), *anxiety–depressive disorders* (including cothymia, the mixed group), and *complex neurotic disorders* in which anxiety and/or depression are normally present but there are also behavioural accompaniments that dominate the clinical presentation (phobic, obsessional and eating disorders). See Table 21.5.

The three-way classification of neurotic disorders is based on the principles of clinical validity (Kendell 1989) and of clinical utility defined as 'of use to those involved in managing and treating the patient'. The three groups are different in that they have different natural histories, clinical presentations and associated personality features, and tend to be seen in different settings. The arguments against the conventional classifications of DSM and ICD are primarily that they are too heterogeneous and often include all three of the groups. Response to treatment is therefore equally heterogeneous.

Table 21.5   Suggested three-category classification of the main neurotic disorders

Clinical feature	Adjustment reactions	Anxiety–depressive disorders	Complex neurotic disorders
Course	Self-limiting with spontaneous improvement	Episodic, except in some instances of pure disorders, with worse outcome in mixed group (cothymia)	Persistent, so that treatments, when successful, often have to be given long-term or with frequent recourse to brief treatment
Recommended treatment	Correction or avoidance of stressor	Anxiolytic or antidepressant drug therapy in short term with cognitive and related therapies in longer term	Specific treatments for the main behavioural component of the syndrome together with treatment for the anxiety–depressive component
Abnormal personality features	Prominent in recurrent disorders, absent in single reactions	Common, most often in association with cothymia	Generally common except with encapsulated single disorders, particularly with cluster C personality disorders
Most common treatment setting	Primary care	Primary and secondary care equally	Secondary specialist care for specific treatment, primary care for general treatment

The therapeutic relationship

Explanation

The explanation of the illness given to the patient, and his agreement with this, are essential to management. Patients may be concerned that they are developing a psychotic illness or be subject to compulsory treatment, particularly when the phenomena they are experiencing are alarming such as those of obsessive–compulsive disorder. They may also be reluctant to accept a psychiatric label because of stigma. An explanation which both validates the reality of their experience and indicates that it is closer to variations of normality than to madness is often necessary. Many patients feel that it is blameworthy to develop a neurosis and require an explanation that neuroses are understandable conditions with genetic vulnerability factors and a real but usually reversible substrate in altered brain functioning.

Collaboration

The management of neurosis almost always involves the voluntary co-operation of the patient. It is therefore essential that the patient understands and agrees with the need for and the nature of the treatment. This applies both to pharmacological treatment and to psychological and behavioural therapies. It is important to explain that antidepressant drugs, although marketed under this label, actually have a wide range of action and affect sleep, energy and anxiety among other things. The second major concern patients have about drugs is that they might in some way be harmful or addictive. This issue is clearly a complex one and may require some detailed discussion with the patient. Psychological treatments will only be effective if the patient is a willing and active collaborator. Some patients may feel that a psychological treatment implies that their symptoms are not real or are in some way imaginary, and it can be helpful in such cases to emphasise that psychological treatment is to help the patient cope positively with the illness she has and it does not imply that the illness is a purely psychological phenomenon. Advice about general behaviour and lifestyle can also be an important part of the treatment of neurosis. Advice, for example on employment, stress, relationships and physical activity, can not only be helpful but also gives the patient some active role in management.

Box 21.4   Categories of treatments for neuroses

Biological
- Drug therapy
- (Neurosurgery and transcranial magnetic stimulation)

Psychological & behavioural
- Behaviour therapy
- Cognitive-behaviour therapy
- Other psychotherapies

Social
- Lifestyle, relationship and occupational changes

It is quite common for the management of neurosis, particularly when chronic, to require a multifaceted approach. That is, it may be necessary to combine drug therapy with psychological treatment and with general life changes and advice. The broad categories of treatment for neurosis are listed in Box 21.4.

Because management is often complicated, it is helpful to write out a detailed management plan and not just name a single therapy. Given the necessity to obtain the patient's collaboration, providing a copy of this written plan to the patient, perhaps in the form of a letter to a general practitioner, is good practice that may improve the patient's adherence to the prescribed regimen.

Services

Delivering effective treatments to patients with neurosis can be difficult. Specialist psychiatric services have in recent years increasingly concentrated on psychosis and risk management. Inpatient psychiatric wards are rarely suitable places to which to admit the neurotic patient, and specialist services such as those providing cognitive-behavioural therapy are usually in short supply. Increasingly the management of neurosis appears to be delegated to primary care. It is important therefore when planning management that the psychiatrist remembers that he or she is in a position of advising the general practitioner and being mindful of the limitations of resources in primary care for the management of such patients. For more severe cases of neurosis, ongoing support and advice to the patient and/or general practitioner can be important, and management can often be greatly enhanced by

Table 21.6 Classification of drugs in the treatment of neurotic disorders		
Drug group	Common members of group	Main mechanism of action
Sedative/hypnotic	Main group: benzodiazepines Subsidiary groups: barbiturates cyclopyrrolones propanediols miscellaneous	Facilitation of GABA transmission
Azospirodecanediones	Buspirone	Partial agonists of 5HT$_{1A}$ receptors
Beta-blocking drugs	Propranolol Atenolol	Peripheral beta-blockade
Antihistamines	Promethazine Chlorpheniramine	Histamine-receptor blockade
Antipsychotic drugs	Chlorpromazine Flupentixol (flupenthixol)	
Tricyclic antidepressants	Amitriptyline Dothiepin Clomipramine Lofepramine	See text
Monoamine oxidase inhibitors (MAOIs)	Phenelzine Moclobemide	Increase in central monoamine levels
Selective serotonin reuptake inhibitors (SSRIs)	Citalopram* Fluoxetine[†] Paroxetine* Sertraline	Probably linked to changes (down-regulation) in noradrenergic and 5HT receptors after regular treatment for 3 or more weeks. Short-term relief of anxiety may be immediate with the more sedative tricyclic antidepressants
Selective noradrenaline and serotonin reuptake inhibitors	Venlafaxine**	

* Licensed for treatment of depression, panic disorder and generalised anxiety disorder.
[†] Licensed for treatment of depression and bulimia nervosa.
** Licensed for treatment of generalised anxiety disorder and depression.

the provision of joint consultations between general practitioner, psychiatrist and patient.

Drug treatments

Apart from benzodiazepines and buspirone, tricyclic, SSRI and other antidepressant drugs (e.g. monoamine oxidase inhibitors) are the main drug treatments for neuroses (see Table 21.6).

Benzodiazepines

Whereas buspirone, tricyclic antidepressants and SSRIs need to be taken for several weeks before an appreciable anxiolytic or antidepressant effect is obtained, benzodiazepines act rapidly and effectively to reduce symptoms of anxiety but not of depression. Given their safety and freedom from serious adverse effects with acute administration, benzodiazepines are uniquely useful anxiolytic drugs for short-term use. Benzodiazepines are particularly effective in reducing somatic symptoms of anxiety, but their therapeutic effect on psychic anxiety and on panic attacks is less marked and may require higher doses causing excessive sedation. Obsessive–compulsive disorder may not be helped at all by these drugs, and benzodiazepines do not have antidepressant properties. With longer-term administration, benzodiazepines are relatively ineffective as treatments for neurotic disorders compared with tricyclics. Benzodiazepines are no longer the most commonly prescribed psychotropic drugs in the world but are still prominent in the treatment of anxiety.

Benzodiazepine dependence   The main reason for their loss of popularity is the fear of addiction, an understandable concern, but one that has been variously interpreted, ranging from the view that it is a minor handicap that has been greatly overstated to the assertion that these drugs should be regarded as treatments of last resort because of their short- and long-term dangers. Benzodiazepine dependence has been recognised as a significant issue in the prescription of tranquillising drugs for twenty-five years.

The common symptoms of the benzodiazepine withdrawal syndrome are those of anxiety (palpitations, tingling, sweating, difficulty in concentration, irritability, tremor), hypersensitivity to sensory stimuli of all kinds (tinnitus, blurring of vision), formication (feeling of things crawling on the skin), and (much less common) neurological symptoms such as epilepsy, paranoid psychotic symptoms and muscular twitching (Tyrer et al 1990). These can almost be predicted from knowledge of the actions of benzodiazepines. They are all rebound effects that are the opposite of anxiety reduction, sedation and anticonvulsant effects. These can be predicted from the effects of benzodiazepines on GABA transmission, and exactly the same symptoms can be created by giving a GABA antagonist (e.g. picrotoxin), suggesting that dependence problems can be described in terms of GABA stimulation.

The 'withdrawal symptoms' of *low-dose dependence* are not always what they seem. First, they overlap considerably with ordinary symptoms of anxiety and none is pathognomonic in itself; second, they are not confined to low-dose use and are fundamentally no different in high-dose use; third, only about one in three patients prescribed benzodiazepines long-term develops withdrawal symptoms when they reduce their tablets — and this applies in both sudden and tapered withdrawal. A significant proportion of patients develop 'pseudo-withdrawal symptoms' (Tyrer et al 1983) even in the absence of genuine medication reduction. People with dependent and anxious personalities are more likely to develop withdrawal symptoms when they stop taking benzodiazepines.

To make the diagnosis of the benzodiazepine withdrawal syndrome the following are necessary:

- Symptoms must always follow drug reduction or withdrawal (usually within 5 days).
- There may be an increase in the previous symptoms of anxiety and/or emergence of new symptoms that have not been experienced before.
- Some improvement should occur after the first 14 days of reduction.

There is no real consensus of the recommended usage of benzodiazepines and their related compounds. There is a significant problem of dependence with these drugs but it has been overstated. Although long-term treatment of anxiety states with benzodiazepines may be effective and justified for many patients not responding well to other treatments, concerns centring on the minority of patients at risk of experiencing long-term problems such as drug abuse and withdrawal effects, as well as the sedation and cognitive impairments that may be troublesome especially in elderly people, have led most licensing authorities to recommend a restricting of the use of benzo-diazepines for treating anxiety to periods of less than 4 weeks. In practice, however, many chronically anxious patients are still successfully maintained on benzodiazepines with more benefit than harm and no significant waning of therapeutic effect. By exploiting the rapid-onset anxiolytic action of these drugs, the strategy of intermittent benzodiazepine use may be particularly helpful in treating people with chronic anxiety disorders, which typically show short-term exacerbations.

The benzodiazepines are remarkably safe, although there can be additive effects with alcohol and other depressant drugs, particularly other drugs of the sedative–hypnotic type. A major indication of excessive dosage is drowsiness. Anterograde amnesia (i.e. amnesia from the time of onset of drug action) may also be a problem in higher dosage, although it may be a beneficial effect in some conditions (e.g. pre-medication for dental phobia). All benzodiazepines (and all other sedative drugs) have a risk of psychomotor impairment. This is of special relevance when carrying out tasks that need co-ordination and vigilance (e.g. driving, monitoring machinery). Because anxiety fluctuates considerably from hour to hour, unwanted effects such as psychomotor impairment may be noted after acute anxiety has passed but the effects of the drug persist.

Buspirone

This drug is a member of the azospirodecanediones. Buspirone, a $5HT_{1A}$ partial agonist drug which enhances $5HT_{1A}$ activity and indirectly reduces $5HT_{2C}$ neurotransmission, appears to be particularly useful in treating generalised anxiety disorder, in which after several weeks of administration it is highly effective.

Buspirone has one major advantage over the benzodiazepines: it does not produce dependence, and so there is no reason in principle why it should not be continued for several months or even longer (although its main indication is for treatment of short- and medium-term anxiety). Despite this obvious advantage it has not proved to be a particularly popular drug, and this appears to be a

consequence of its major disadvantage: it is dysphoric, or more simply, it makes people feel bad. When this is combined with a short delay before its full effects are shown it is easy to see why it has not become well established.

Beta-blocking drugs, antihistamines and other anti-anxiety drugs

Beta blockers Beta-blockers are of limited value in anxiety disorders. Their central actions do not contribute significantly to reducing generalised anxiety or blocking panic attacks, and they are most useful for reducing autonomic and somatic arousal symptoms by an action on peripheral beta-adrenoceptors. It is likely that their major effects on the emotions are indirect due to their peripheral effects, hence somatic symptoms mediated through beta-receptors are most likely to be helped. These include awareness of fast heart beat, flushing, palpitations and tremor. The most obvious use of beta-blockers is in the treatment of performance anxiety in acute stress situations, such as speaking in public or playing a musical instrument. If avoidance of tremor is particularly important (e.g. playing the violin) beta-blocking drugs may be of particular help. The main advantage of beta-blockers is that they cause no sedative effects or sensori-motor impairment and no risk of dependence.

Antihistamines Antihistamines are well-established drugs with a long history of successful use in the treatment of mild anxiety and insomnia from childhood onwards. The sedative effects are rapid in onset but these overlap with drowsiness which can become a severe problem in daytime use. Although the dependence risk of these drugs is low, there is still some potential for abuse, with both cyclizine and diphenhydramine being reported as addictive. However, problems of withdrawal following long-term low-dose treatment have not been reported.

Antipsychotic drugs These drugs, ranging from the prototype chlorpromazine introduced in 1950 to the newer 'atypical' drugs such as risperidone, clozapine and olanzapine, are all effective in treating anxiety. They have not been subjected to rigorous comparison with other established drugs, but older studies show them to be of roughly equivalent efficacy. However, the main reason for caution is the danger that the irreversible syndrome of tardive dyskinesia might develop, especially with the older drugs; this confines their use to the short-term only, unless they are given for the treatment of anxiety in conjunction with psychotic disorders.

Antidepressants

It has become increasingly clear that antidepressants are the first-line drug treatment for all persistent neurotic disorders, including mixed anxiety–depressive disorder, generalised anxiety disorder, obsessive–compulsive disorder and panic disorder. The effectiveness of these drugs in treating anxiety states is not dependent on the presence of comorbid depressive disorder, although when anxiety and depressive symptoms are present together, antidepressants reduce both type of symptoms equally well. This multiple action of antidepressants has sometimes been used as an argument against attempting to distinguish between different types of neurotic disorder, or even in support of the hypothesis that anxiety states and depressive disorders are different manifestations of the same underlying condition.

However, whereas both noradrenergic and serotonergic actions of these drugs may be equally important in mediating their antidepressant effects, their therapeutic actions in anxiety and neurotic disorders in the main appear to result directly or indirectly from drug-induced alterations in serotonergic (5HT-dependent) brain activity. Brain 5HT systems, especially the MRN-5HT$_{1A}$ pathway, are closely functionally related to the noradrenergic system, usually in a co-operative fashion. Drugs principally affecting the noradrenergic system may therefore indirectly exert therapeutic effects through serotonergic mechanisms. Whereas in depression and possibly in generalised anxiety disorder, drugs with a dual action on serotonergic and noradrenergic functioning (e.g. amitriptyline, venlafaxine) may have a therapeutic advantage, antidepressant drugs which act primarily on the serotonergic systems (SSRIs) appear to be most effective in treating panic disorder and especially obsessive–compulsive disorder. SSRIs may even benefit phobic disorders, especially social phobia, conditions which previously were not considered to be drug-responsive.

Although most antidepressants are not licensed for the treatment of anxiety (citalopram and paroxetine are exceptions) they have been used increasingly for this purpose since concerns over benzodiazepine dependence first began in the 1980s. This is not surprising, since, from the mid 1960s, evidence had emerged that antidepressants were effective in the treatment of anxiety, even though, unlike the benzodiazepines, which helped immediately, their effects took 2–4 weeks to develop adequately. Because antidepressants were not considered to produce dependence it was natural to change from sedative drugs with increasing problems associated with their use to well-tried 'clean' antidepressants without such problems. This pressure became even stronger when the new class of antidepressants, the SSRIs, were introduced to a market saturated with antidepressants. These new antidepressants were of similar efficacy to the old ones in the treatment of depression but were less likely to lead to suicide in overdose, because they were less toxic. When additional evidence came along that the SSRIs were possibly more effective in treating anxiety associated with depression than standard tricyclic antidepressants, an additional reason for choosing these drugs was found. The position now is that anxiety is now regularly treated with antidepressants in all forms of clinical practice, and the only variation is in the diagnostic choice for each compound or group.

In general the SSRIs are more effective in obsessional disorders, in which clomipramine, despite being a tricyclic antidepressant, is also included as it has partial serotonin selection. Imipramine and other tricyclic antidepressants still vie with SSRIs in the treatment of panic and generalised anxiety, and SSRIs are now being investigated more in the treatment of phobias. The monoamine oxidase inhibitors, particularly the new reversible compounds that do not have the dietary restrictions associated with the old agents such as phenelzine and tranylcypromine, are now being targeted on social phobia. Preliminary evidence suggests that moclobemide, the main exemplar of the new compounds, is not as effective as phenelzine in treating social phobia. The problems of dependence are not just confined to the benzodiazepines; they occur to some extent with the antidepressants also.

Choice of drug treatment in anxiety

In choosing a drug treatment for anxiety there are several issues which need to be addressed. The main one is the likely duration of treatment. If it is likely that the drug will only be needed for a short time (e.g. for an adjustment disorder) then it is likely that a mild sedative (including among the possibilities an antihistamine) will be chosen unless the patient has characteristics predisposing to dependence. If, however, the event leading to the anxiety is of particular emotional significance for the patient it would be wise not to give a benzodiazepine in high dosage in case anterograde amnesia (amnesia during the period of major drug action) developed and prevented subsequent adjustment to the event.

If the anxiety is likely to need longer-term treatment an antidepressant might be considered but, as there is a delay in the onset of therapeutic effects, a benzodiazepine might be given for a short time (e.g. 2 weeks) simultaneously, on the clear understanding that this will not be repeated. Although the tricyclic antidepressants are now generally considered to be 'dirty old drugs' in many quarters because of their many side-effects, it is important to note that one of these side-effects, sedation, can be very helpful to the anxious patient. The sedation, unlike the main anti-anxiety effects, begins immediately after administration of the drug, and so could take the place of a sedative–hypnotic drug during the first 20 days of therapy. Trimipramine (100–200 mg), dothiepin (75–150 mg) and amitriptyline (75–175 mg) are the main sedative antidepressants available and, if a benzodiazepine is being given simultaneously for the first few weeks, it may be more successfully withdrawn under cover of the antidepressant.

If dependence is considered to be a major risk (e.g. in the treatment of alcohol withdrawal) then buspirone could be used in the longer term while the risks of epilepsy and other acute problems could be offset by prescribing a benzodiazepine such as chlor-diazepoxide (20–100 mg daily) in steadily reducing dosage. Low-dose antipsychotic drugs such as trifluoperazine (2–4 mg daily) and flupentixol (flupenthixol)(0.5–1.5 mg daily) could also be considered if dependence is considered a long-term risk. However, antipsychotic drugs should not be used for long-term treatment of anxiety because of the significant risk of tardive dyskinesia even with low doses.

The choice of an SSRI or an MAOI such as moclobemide, in place of a tricyclic antidepressant, may also be made. Clomipramine is a cheap compromise in this task; no studies have shown clomipramine (50–200 mg/day) to be less effective than a more respectable SSRI in the treatment of anxiety. The main problem will be when the treatment is considered to be over and 'discontinuation problems' may arise. The additional provision of brief psychotherapy during the treatment may help to maintain progress after the antidepressant is withdrawn.

The full choice is shown in Table 21.7. It is not always an easy one, and it helps to consider all aspects of drug treatment, initial therapy, maintenance treatment, and effects of withdrawal, before the choice is made.

Summary

Drugs are effective in anxiety but their correct use involves judicious selection of the right compound, using it for the most appropriate time and anticipating, not merely reacting to, problems. Combining drug and psychological treatments is also an excellent way of getting the best out of both of them. The exact diagnosis of the patient being treated is of lesser importance; do not let it get in the way of answering the other questions.

Psychological treatments

The main psychological treatments available for anxiety are based on the notion that pathological anxiety in its many forms consists of maladaptive and inappropriate responses to stimuli which have been generated as much from past experience as constitution. These

Table 21.7   Comparison of the issues determining the choice of an anti-anxiety drug

Drug group	Speed of action	Sedation and sensorimotor impairment	Risk of dependence	Efficacy	Main indications
Sedative/hypnotics	Fast (< 2 h)	Significant but dose-related	Relatively great in long-term treatment	Excellent	Time-limited treatment (e.g. alcohol withdrawal)
Azospirodecanediones	Fairly slow (2–5 days)	Very little	Very low	Good	Anxiety in abuse-prone situations (e.g. chronic alcohol abuse)
Antipsychotic drugs	Fairly slow	Little in low dosage	Very low	Fair	Anxiety in presence of psychotic symptoms
Antihistamines	Fast	Present to some degree	Slight	Fair	Mild anxiety and insomnia
Antidepressants — tricyclic	Slow (2–5 wks)	Variable, depending on dose and drug	Very low	Good	Persistent anxiety/panic associated with chronic insomnia
Antidepressants — SSRIs and reversible MAOIs	Slow (2–5 wks)	Very little	Low	Very good	Complex — see text
Beta-blocking drugs	Fast	None	None	Good in some instances	Performance anxiety

treatments are behaviour therapy, cognitive therapy and related techniques such as anxiety management training. There is also a range of alternative therapies which are less well researched but are worthy of mention, not least because anxiety disorders are extremely prone to the placebo effect.

Behaviour therapy

Behavioural therapies are based on learning theory. This is described in Chapter 6.

Exposure therapy   Exposure therapy is used to treat phobias. In learning terms exposure therapy regards the phobia (unreasonable fear) and subsequent avoidance of the phobic stimulus as maladaptive conditioned behaviour that needs to be extinguished. This is best achieved by deconditioning the maladaptive behaviour patterns and counter conditioning them with better adaptive ones. The principles of exposure therapy are extremely straightforward; indeed they were presented in almost their current therapeutic form by Charles Darwin in 1872. Despite this, the application of this approach in psychiatry has not been a particularly smooth one. The original form of exposure was desensitisation, and originally this was presented as desensitisation in imagination. The sufferer had to think about the phobic stimulus when in a relaxed state, and the intention was for the relaxation feeding to be paired with the phobic thinking so that it no longer evoked fear. The theory came from the work of a South African Psychiatrist, Joseph Wolpe, who introduced a theory of reciprocal inhibition derived from neurology, which postulated that it was necessary to present both the agonist (fearful) and antagonist (relaxation) stimuli together in order to get a learned association and thereby therapeutic improvement. In fact, many studies have shown that desensitisation in imagination is not as effective as exposure in vivo, and has limited application in behaviour therapy nowadays. The evidence that exposure therapy is effective in phobic disorders has now been shown in over one hundred studies. The type of phobia has relatively little impact on the success of treatment, although there is good evidence that phobias that are more specific, such as most of

the simple phobias (like fears of lightning, thunder, dogs, etc.) are more successfully treated than the more diffuse phobias of agoraphobia and social phobia. Unfortunately the simple phobias are also the least handicapping, and so the introduction of behaviour therapy has not had the effect predicted by the late Hans Eysenck, who predicted in 1975 'that within a generation psychologists in mobile treatment trucks will travel round the country and eliminate phobias and other neurotic disorders entirely'.

Cognitive therapy

Cognitive therapy originally was developed in the treatment of depression and involved the novel concept that the symptoms of this disorder might be a consequence of cognitive dysfunction rather than the cause of such dysfunction (Kovacs & Beck 1978). It soon became apparent that with relatively few changes this treatment could easily be transferred to the treatment of panic, anxiety and phobias. The main difference was that it was not the negative cognitive triad of depression that was being generated by cognitive dysfunction but a threatening triad of catastrophic thinking, alarm and insecurity that constituted anxiety generation.

The main principles of cognitive therapy are described in reference texts (e.g. Clark & Fairburn 1997). See also Chapter 6. Cognitive therapy is usually combined with behavioural treatment strategies such as exposure to constitute cognitive-behaviour therapy (CBT). Comparisons of cognitive therapy and behaviour therapy in generalised anxiety disorder have shown cognitive therapy to be generally superior, with fewer dropouts from treatment (Butler et al 1991). Cognitive therapy is also effective in GAD (Gale & Oakley-Browne 2002), PTSD (Bisson 2002) and panic disorder (Kumar & Oakley-Browne 2002).

Anxiety management and relaxation training

Anxiety management training is a form of combined relaxation and behavioural training. It was developed primarily as a treatment of generalised anxiety disorder and is undoubtedly effective in the condition (Butler et al 1987) but has no special advantages over cognitive and behavioural therapy.

Relaxation training, particularly progressive relaxation, first developed by Wolpe in the 1950s with some derivation from Jacobson's instructions to aid muscular relaxation, is a useful, if basic, treatment for anxiety. A variant of this treatment, applied relaxation, which involves control of breathing and the induction of positive mental imagery has been claimed to be superior to progressive relaxation and is possibly as effective as exposure and cognitive therapy (Ost et al 1993).

Hypnotherapy

Hypnotherapy is one of the oldest treatments in psychiatry. It was developed by Mesmer, a Viennese physician, who developed dramatic cures in patients by talking to them in a commanding voice, inducing sleep in some cases, and laying his hands over the body to redistribute 'magnetic fluid' within the body. He called this phenomenon 'animal magnetism'; others called it Mesmerism (a word that has persisted in the language). Hypnosis has fallen from grace in the past fifty years. The small number of randomised trials has yielded mixed results. For example it was found to be of no benefit in the treatment of phobias (Marks et al 1968) but recently to have some effectiveness in conversion disorder (Moene et al 2003).

Self-help

When one considers the large number of people with neurosis in the population at any one time it is clear that there will never be sufficient therapists to treat it by psychological means, nor sufficient physicians to treat with pharmacological ones (even if this approach were considered desirable). Self-help has been shown in a number of studies to be effective. With newer forms of technology it is now possible to develop sophisticated self-help packages which include all the elements of instruction involved in live therapy. In its simplest form, self-help is given as bibliotherapy, self-teaching reading material, and this has been shown to be effective in treating panic (Lidren et al 1994). However, some degree of therapist contact seems to improve the effectiveness of self-help (Newman et al 2003).

The place of psychological therapies in the treatment of neurotic disorders

For the motivated patient the brief cognitive therapies are at least as good as any other treatments for anxiety. The research data, taken together, look more impressive than is probably the case, as they refer to treatment given by enthusiastic therapists who are optimally trained, but these are not the norm in a clinical service. However, there is some evidence that when trained, psychiatrists, nurse practitioners and psychologists who normally work with pharmacological treatments can be effective in administering such therapies (Welkowitz et al 1991).

Combined psychological and pharmacological therapy

In general the data support the combination of pharmacological and psychological treatments in anxiety with few if any negative interactions. Thus the combination of buspirone and CBT is more effective than either (Cottraux et al 1995), and CBT combined with diazepam is superior to either diazepam or CBT alone in the treatment of generalised anxiety disorder (Power et al 1990). In a meta-analysis (the combination of results from several trials) of controlled studies of the treatment of agoraphobia and panic conditions, the combination of antide-pressants with exposure in vivo was the most effective treatment out of seven types of intervention (van Balkom et al 1997). Advantageous effects of combined treatment modalities depend on either treatment alone being suboptimal, which is not always the case.

Summary

The treatment of the patient with neurosis must start with development of a collaborative therapeutic relationship. Treatments for neurosis require the patient's active co-operation and cannot succeed without this. There is good evidence for the effectiveness of both pharmacological and psychological therapies and some evidence that they may be more effective when used together. Psychological treatments arguably have a better long-term outcome but are difficult to provide for the large number of patients with neurosis. It is likely that the future will see an increasing role for self-help treatments, at least for those patients who are able to use them.

PROGNOSIS

The classical outcome data apply to all neurotic conditions — one-third recover completely, one-third show improvement but not resolution, and one-third fare poorly. For example one large follow-up study found that 40% of patients with a variety of neurotic diagnoses continued to be handicapped either intermittently or continuously throughout the 5-year period. Specific disgnosis is not a strong predictor of outcome, which is better predicted by age, personality and recency of onset than by other clinical variables with the exception of initial response to treatment (Seivewright et al 1998).

In the future we should have better guidelines on how to treat the neurotic disorders. At present we have an à la carte menu rather than a clear set course. Our suggestions (p. 463, Table 21.5) about a tripartite diagnosis of:

- specific (complex) neurotic disorders (focused drug or psychological treatment);
- adjustment disorders (little in the way of specific treatment as self-resolving);
- mixed disorders (including cothymia and the general neurotic syndrome — no specific effective treatment yet demonstrated)

have face validity and overcome the problems of comorbidity described earlier in this chapter, but they do not yet have a firm evidence base.

SPECIFIC NEUROTIC SYNDROMES

PHOBIC ANXIETY DISORDERS

Phobic anxiety disorders have as their core anxiety evoked by specific situations or objects which are perceived as more dangerous than they actually are and lead to avoidance.

There is a potentially large range of specific or isolated phobias defined by the stimulus giving rise to anxiety. Previously all phobias were grouped together but differences, including age of onset (Marks & Gelder 1966), were noted and separate categories made in DSM-III. The common types of phobia include fear of the sight of blood or injury, animals, flying, small spaces and heights. Two other types of phobias are specifically listed in ICD-10: social phobia (social anxiety disorder) and agoraphobia (which is strongly associated with panic).

The essence of the treatment of all phobias is by exposure to the feared stimulus. This allows extinction of the anxiety response when the feared consequences do not occur and removal of the reinforcing effect of anxiety-relief on avoidance. Treatment with exposure may be amplified by examination of the fear catastrophe using cognitive techniques. For example the person who is fearful that he will collapse in public may be asked if this has ever actually occurred. Treatment may also involve dealing with comorbid problems such as anxiety and alcohol dependence.

Specific phobia

Definition

Specific phobias are characterised by a marked and persistent fear that is excessively unreasonable and is associated with the presence or anticipation of a specific object or situation.

Clinical features

The most commonly feared objects and situations are animals, aspects of nature, and blood. For phobia to be an illness there needs to be not just a degree of fear but interference with the person's life caused by the avoidance. Panic attacks may be precipitated by exposure to the feared stimulus.

Epidemiology

The National Comorbidity Study (NCS) (Kessler et al 1994b) reported a 12-month prevalence rate of 8.8% for simple phobia. Simple phobia tends to begin early in life and is more common in women.

Aetiology

There is evidence for a familial pattern of phobias with a probable genetic contribution. Freud's classic case of little Hans provides a model for the psychoanalytic approach. Freud's hypothesis was that phobias reflected internal psychological conflict. This hypothesis was illustrated by the case of a boy called little Hans who developed a fear of horses. Freud proposed that it resulted from unconscious oedipal fears which were denied and projected onto the horses, thereby keeping the real source of anxiety from consciousness.

Classical conditioning theory puts forward the alternative hypothesis that phobias arise more directly as a result of a negative experience with the objective situation — in this case being frightened by horses. The two-factor learning theory that purports to explain the perpetuation of the phobia is described above. It has also been argued that phobias do not occur randomly but that humans have an inherited tendency to fear specific stimuli such as snakes.

Treatment

Exposure is the core of most successful treatments. This may be combined with a cognitive approach. Drug treatments alone are relatively ineffective.

Social phobia

Definition

The essence of social phobia is a persistent fear of social situations in which embarrassment occurs, and this fear leads to avoidance of such situations.

Clinical features

The embarrassment often focuses on an exaggerated perception of some minor defect in social performance, such as shaking, stammering or blushing. A vicious circle may then arise in which the anxiety associated with the perceived criticism leads to autonomic arousal, then to exaggeration of the defect (such as shaking or blushing), greater anxiety and so on. Social phobia may be associated with depression and understandably can lead to excess alcohol intake and alcohol dependence. The precise focus of social anxiety may vary between cultures. For example in Japan social anxiety often centres on the concern that one's body odour will be offensive to others, a form much less common in Europe.

Epidemiology

Social phobia often begins early in life. It is more common in women. The 12-month prevalence in the NCS was 8%.

Aetiology

There is some tendency for social phobia to be familial, probably reflecting both genetic and environmental factors.

Diagnosis

Social phobia may occur in the presence of other depressive and anxiety disorders. It may also be more likely in those with lifelong sensitivity to social criticism and in this sense may coexist with or even shade into avoidant personality disorder.

Treatment

The treatments of choice are cognitive-behavioural therapy (CBT) based on exposure, and antidepressant medication (Fedoroff & Taylor 2001). There is evidence of the effectiveness of both SSRIs and monoamine oxidase inhibitors. Beta-blockers and benzo-diazepines may be helpful, though the risk of dependence with the latter should be noted. Comorbid conditions such as associated alcohol misuse may also require attention.

Agoraphobia

Definition

Agoraphobia is anxiety associated with places or situations from which either escape may be difficult or in which help may not be available in the event of having a panic attack or panic-like symptoms. Agoraphobia means literally fear of the market place. It is strongly associated with panic. This association is underlined by the DSM-IV classification of agoraphobia which divides agoraphobia into panic with agoraphobia (which is considered the most common form) and agoraphobia without panic. Confusingly ICD-10 emphasises phobia and consequently classifies agoraphobia as agoraphobia with and without panic (see also the section on panic).

Clinical features

Persons with agoraphobia typically find it difficult to shop in busy supermarkets and to go to crowded places such as the theatre or cinema. Avoidance of these situations is a prominent feature. They may however feel better if accompanied by someone else. As with other phobias, those with the condition may have relatively low levels of baseline anxiety if they are able successfully to avoid the phobic situations. Clearly however, agoraphobia is severely disabling. Approximately half of people diagnosed with panic disorder in community samples also have agoraphobia.

Epidemiology

Agoraphobia is more prominent in females, and agoraphobia with very extensive avoidance is much more common in females. Epidemiological surveys have found large numbers of people seen in the community who have agoraphobia without panic disorder and who seldom come to medical attention (Regier et al 1990).

Aetiology

Family and twin studies suggest that genetic factors are relevant. However, the onset of agoraphobia often follows a precipitating event, which may be a panic attack or may be other potentially frightening incident which leads to subsequent avoidance.

Treatment

As with other phobias, treatment requires exposure, and this is effective. If there is coexisting panic, this also needs to be treated by either cognitive-behavioural or pharmacological means (see below).

PANIC DISORDER

The central component in panic disorder is a panic attack. The notion of the panic attack is an ancient one; the word 'panic' derives from experience suffered by travellers through the woods in ancient Greece who experienced acute attacks of anxiety when the mischievous god, Pan, jumped out in front of them or teased them in other frightening ways. The description of the panic attack as a central symptom of anxiety is also not new, and is well summarised in one of Sigmund Freud's earlier papers.

Definition

Panic attacks only become panic disorder when they are recurrent and are associated with worry about further panic attacks. The diagnosis 'agoraphobia with panic attacks' was allowed as a joint diagnosis in DSM-III. This reflected the views of Donald Klein, who maintained that a natural consequence of panic disorder was agoraphobia.

The criteria for diagnosing agoraphobia with or without panic disorder are dependent on the absence or presence of panic attacks provided that these cannot be accounted for better as part of another diagnosis such as social anxiety. The accompanying symptoms of panic (see below) are mostly those of the bodily manifestations of sympathetic nervous activity. To qualify for a panic attack these symptoms have to be generated within a short time (an outer limit of 10 minutes) and also not be persistent, as physiological overdrive at this level is unlikely to be maintained for more than around 30 minutes at any one time.

Clinical features

Panic attacks present with a sudden onset of multiple somatic symptoms including those listed in Box 21.2. They are of sudden onset and usually last for several minutes but sometimes much longer. They are usually accompanied by a subjective experience of extreme anxiety often with the thought that a catastrophic consequence is imminent such as death, collapse or loss of control. In some cases the anxiety may not be reported, a picture that has been described as 'non-anxious panic'. Panic may also occur from sleep. A substantial number of people who suffer from panic attacks go on to avoid situations associated with the panic, leading to the picture of panic with agoraphobia. Panic disorder may be complicated by alcohol abuse.

Diagnosis

The main differentiation is from generalised anxiety, phobic anxiety and from medical conditions. In GAD, concern with factors other than panic, such as finances and work, is predominant as well. Panic attacks may also occur in phobias but only on exposure to the feared situation. Panic attacks may also occur in the context of PTSD and OCD, but the other features of those syndromes predominate.

Given the large number of somatic symptoms of panic, it is not surprising that it often results in a presentation to medical services and that panic has to be differentiated from medical causes of similar symptoms. The differential diagnosis will depend somewhat on the predominant picture of panic symptoms but includes cardiac problems, seizures, asthma, and metabolic disturbance (classically including phaeochromocytoma) as well as the effects of substance misuse.

Epidemiology

The large population surveys have found that clearly defined panic attacks occur in approximately 10% of the population, with similar fearful spells occurring much more frequently. Panic disorder as defined in ICD-10 and DSM-IV has a much lower prevalence, however, of approximately 2%. Panic disorder is twice as common in females as males.

Aetiology

Available evidence suggests that there is a genetic contribution to vulnerability to panic and that early childhood trauma is also associated. There are also commonly precipitating events in the form of medical illness or life stress.

Biological models Noradrenergic brain symptoms appear to be involved in the production of panic attacks, as noradrenergic agents such yohimbine and isoproterenol will trigger panic attacks, in patients with panic disorder. It is further suggested that this is associated with increased activity in the locus ceruleus, which has been described as the brain's 'alarm system'. GABA systems also appear to be involved, as evidenced by the effectiveness of benzodiazepines in treatment. The evidence for disturbance in serotonergic brain systems is less clear, although the effectiveness of SSRI antidepressants in reducing panic attacks indicates that an increase in serotonergic transmission decreases panic. Pentagastrin can produce panic attacks in humans with panic disorder. See Bourin et al (1998) for a review.

Psychological models The psychological model of panic emphasises the critical importance of the catastrophic misinterpretation of bodily symptoms. The model proposed by Clark (1986) is that of a vicious circle in which somatic symptoms are misinterpreted as evidence of a feared catastrophe such as impending collapse, which leads to increased apprehension, to further autonomically mediated symptoms of anxiety, and to apparent confirmation of the initial catastrophic misinterpretation, and so on. Certainly, cognitive therapy which focuses on addressing these misinterpretations is highly effective (see below).

Treatment

There is evidence for the effectiveness of antidepressant drugs, particularly SSRIs, in the treatment of panic. In the practical treatment of panic with SSRIs it is necessary to address the temporary exacerbation that many patients experience when starting medication. If this is not done as many as half the patients treated may drop out from treatment. It should be stressed to the patient that this temporary exacerbation is transitory and, once overcome, increasing doses of medication will lead to abolition of panic. Benzodiazepines are also effective but their use is hampered by the risks of dependence as described. CBT based on addressing misinterpretations is a highly effective treatment — of equivalent effectiveness to imipramine but probably with greater long-term efficacy (Barlow 1997). In uncomplicated cases of panic, CBT can be effective in only a few sessions of treatment (Clark et al 1999). Coexisting agoraphobia required exposure therapy (van Balkom et al 1997).

GENERALISED ANXIETY DISORDER

DSM-III split anxiety neurosis, leaving generalised anxiety disorder (GAD) as a residual category. As discussed above, there are questions about its validity as a condition distinct from other anxiety and mood disorders.

Definition

The core feature of generalised anxiety is persistent anxiety and worry that is disproportionate to circumstances. The worry may shift in its focus from one topic to another and is perceived as difficult to control. Somatic symptoms including muscular tension, fatigue, and bowel symptoms are common. Both DSM-IV and ICD-10 require a period of 6 months generalised anxiety and worry associated with somatic symptoms.

Clinical features

The clinical features are feelings of tension often with associated muscle discomfort and fatigue, autonomic symptoms such as sweating, tachycardia and bowel disturbance, uncontrollable worry which may shift in its focus from one topic to another, and disturbed and unrefreshing sleep. The patient with GAD may look tense with an anxious expression and be restless. Because of its somatic manifestations GAD may present to medical services. Aches and pains with fatigue and bowel and bladder symptoms are common and may lead to a diagnosis of a functional syndrome such as fibromyalgia or irritable bowel syndrome (see Ch. 28).

Epidemiology

The exact prevalence depends on the duration criteria applied, but the community surveys described above place the prevalence at about 3%. It commonly coexists with other anxiety and mood disorders, and nearly two-thirds of persons with GAD have an additional diagnosis, most commonly of phobias, panic, or depression.

Aetiology

GAD is more common among family members of those with the condition. It appears that genetic factors do play some role in the aetiology but the association may be mediated by the vulnerability to depressive disorders rather than to GAD. However, GAD and other anxiety disorders may precede and predispose to depressive disorders. There is evidence for abnormalities in neurotransmitters, particularly the noradrenergic system (see above), and in the hypothalamic–pituitary axis. From a cognitive perspective the main problem is inability to control worry. Stressful life events have been associated with onset of GAD, as has a style of parenting characterised by excessive control (overprotection) and lack of warmth and responsiveness (emotional deprivation).

Diagnosis

Because generalised anxiety can be present in all other anxiety and related diagnoses, there have to be a number of exclusion clauses to make sure that the condition is not over-diagnosed.

Treatment

Benzodiazepines are effective, although their use is complicated by the risk of dependency (see above); there is also a potential role for buspirone, but probably the most widely used drugs are the antidepressants. Psychological therapy, particularly anxiety management training (which emphasises relaxation), are widely used and probably effective, although not for everybody (Butler et al 1987).

More-specific cognitive therapies that target worry have been developed and also appear to be of some therapeutic value. The strongest evidence for efficacy is for cognitive therapy using a combination of behavioural intervention such as exposure, relaxation, and cognitive techniques. Relaxation on its own is probably less effective. There is no good evidence that beta-blockers are helpful. However, there have been no controlled trials of beta-blockers in generalised anxiety disorder. For a review of the evidence for the various treatments see Gale & Oakley-Browne (2002).

MIXED ANXIETY – DEPRESSION

We have discussed the potentially artificial separation of depression and anxiety disorders. It is conventional to either choose to make a diagnosis of depressive disorder or anxiety disorder when one set of symptoms predominate and in other cases to make both diagnoses. The category of mixed anxiety and depressive disorder in ICD-10 is used when symptoms of both anxiety and depression are present but neither set of symptoms considered separately is sufficiently severe to justify a diagnosis. Mixed anxiety and depressive disorder is not listed as a diagnosis in DSM-IV but is contained in Appendix A1 for further study.

OBSESSIVE–COMPULSIVE DISORDER

Definition

Obsessive–compulsive disorder (OCD) is a relatively common and chronic neurotic disorder which can cause severe distress and disability. The diagnostic criteria for OCD in ICD-10 and DSM – IV are quite similar and require the presence on most days for 2 weeks or more of either obsessions or compulsions or both. Obsessions and compulsions share the following common features, all of which must be present:

- They must be acknowledged as originating in the patient's mind and not from outside the patient.
- They are persistent, repetitive, intrusive and repugnant. At least one obsession must be acknowledged as excessive, senseless or unreasonable.
- At least one obsession or compulsion must be unsuccessfully resisted, suppressed or neutralised in some way, although when symptoms are long-standing, resistance may be minimal.
- The obsessions or compulsions are not intrinsically pleasurable and usually cause anxiety and distress and/or interfere with social functioning or lifestyle, usually by taking up excessive amounts of time (DSM-IV defines this as more than an hour per day).
- The obsessions and compulsions cannot be entirely accounted for by the presence of another mental illness such as schizophrenia or mood disorder.

Clinical features

The key and defining feature of OCD is the presence of recurrent, unpleasant and intrusive thoughts, mental images or impulses (obsessions) which have a compulsive quality and cause anxiety, disgust or disavowal and evoke attempts to avoid, suppress or resist them. Many patients with OCD also perform repetitive mental routines and behaviours which sometimes occur as a response to obsessions or may have no obvious connection with them and may occur on their own. These mental and behavioural routines (rituals) also have a compulsive quality and may be resisted. However, in many situations rituals appear to represent maladaptive attempts to cope with and relieve the anxiety produced by obsessional thoughts or fears, and are entered into and pursued with determination. Rather confusingly, ritualistic behaviours occurring in OCD are now simply called 'compulsions', whereas the cognitive and mental phenomena are grouped together as 'obsessions', despite the fact that all the behaviours and cognitive phenomena occurring in OCD have both obsessive (persistent and preoccupying) and compulsive qualities (demanding attention or action).

Most patients with OCD have multiple obsessions and compulsions which persist over long periods, although the nature, quality and severity of symptoms may vary considerably over time. There are several well-recognised patterns of obsessional symptoms. The most common pattern is a preoccupation with contamination, dirt or infection, which are perceived as being difficult to avoid and which evoke washing or cleansing rituals. Another common pattern involves excessive questioning or uncertainty about previous behaviour and routines, mostly centring on issues of safety or security. These obsessional doubts result in compulsive checking behaviour, which, like cleansing rituals, only temporarily relieves the anxiety associated with the obsessional thoughts. Instead, checking subsequently creates further worry and doubt, so establishing a vicious cycle. The third pattern involves intrusive abhorrent thoughts or impulses of a sexual, aggressive or violent nature with a fear of acting upon them. So-called obsessional phobias typically apply to potentially harmful objects such as knives or to situations where giving in to the obsessional impulses would be most embarrassing or damaging (e.g. shouting obscenities in public). Finally some people suffering from OCD show an excessive insistence on order, tidiness, symmetry or precision, frequently associated with pedantic speech and extreme slowness in carrying out everyday tasks. This is distinct from the time-wasting associated with carrying out repetitive rituals. The fact that all of these abnormal thoughts and behaviours associated with OCD are perceived by the patient as unreasonable, absurd or even 'crazy', leads to secondary self-doubt, guilt or shame. These in turn may reinforce some of the obsessional fears, and so establish another vicious cycle.

Epidemiology

Obsessions and compulsions as isolated symptoms may occur in up to a tenth of the general population at any one time (Meltzer et al 1995). In most cases these are mild, transient phenomena which do not meet the diagnostic criteria for OCD. Patients with anankastic (obsessional) personality traits may be more likely to show transient obsessional symptoms, but these subjects are no more predisposed to OCD than to other types of neurotic disorder. About a quarter of subjects with OCD have premorbid anankastic traits. Unlike other neuroses, OCD is only slightly more common in women than men (ratio 1.5:1). The mean age of onset is at about age 20.

Diagnosis

The main differential diagnosis is from phobia, depression or psychosis. Although the fears associated with phobic disorder are irrational, they are only evoked by the anticipation of or actual encounter with the phobic situation. Avoidance is the hallmark of phobic disorder, whereas OCD patients typically seek out and engage with the objects of their obsessions. These tend to be difficult to avoid, such as dirt or 'germs', as opposed to the usual objects of phobic anxiety which are readily avoided, albeit at the cost of limiting or impairing social functioning. Another feature distinguishing OCD from phobic disorder is that the fears in OCD often concern harm to other people, whereas in phobic disorder the fears are for the subject's own safety or wellbeing.

Depressive episodes are often accompanied by obsessional symptoms which resolve as the depression improves and do not necessarily qualify for a separate diagnosis of OCD. However about 15% of people reporting a lifetime history of major depression have also suffered from OCD. Conversely, patients suffering from OCD often experience depressive mood swings which constitute depressive episodes in about a third of cases, with up to two-thirds experiencing a depressive episode at some stage. The occasionally bizarre quality of obsessions and compulsions in OCD may resemble features of schizophrenia. In particular it may be difficult to decide whether the patient perceives and believes that obsessive–compulsive symptoms originate from his own mind rather than from external sources. This distinction may be difficult if the obsessions and compulsions are no longer ego-dystonic and fail to evoke marked anxiety and resistance. Although it is unlikely that OCD represents a significant risk factor for schizophrenia, many schizophrenic patients experience typical obsessive–compulsive symptoms, particularly in the early, prodromal stages of psychosis when the diagnosis may still be in doubt. About 15% of schizophrenic patients qualify for an additional diagnosis of OCD which tends to be associated with a relatively poor prognosis of both conditions (Berman et al 1995). Finally, obsessional-like symptoms may occur in various organic brain syndromes such as Sydenham's chorea, temporal lobe epilepsy and cases of encephalitis lethargica. A high percentage of patients suffering from Tourette's syndrome complain of obsessional symptoms, and a minority of patients with OCD suffer from tics.

Aetiology

The rate of OCD in first-degree relatives of OCD patients is about three times higher than predicted by chance, and is more markedly increased when considering patients with childhood-onset OCD. Although, it does seem likely that there is a genetic component to OCD, investigation of a possible candidate, the 5HT-transporter gene, has failed to identify any differences between OCD patients and controls. Three brain diseases which are known to affect the extrapyramidal system of the brain, particularly the caudate nucleus, typically include descriptions of obsessive–compulsive symptoms. These three conditions are encephalitis lethargica, Tourette's syndrome and Sydenham's chorea. The clinical manifestations of these brain disorders, including the obsessive–compulsive components, are believed to involve abnormalities in the basal ganglia (comprising the caudate nucleus and putamen, together known as the striatum). The basal ganglia have connections with the orbitofrontal cortex and are believed to modulate cortical circuitry involved in the expression of over-learnt cognitive and behavioural sequences. Abnormalities in this modulatory function may underlie obsessive–compulsive symptoms.

Brain structure and function Early computerised tomography (CT) studies found that caudate nucleus volume was bilaterally decreased in male adults with childhood-onset OCD, although subsequent CT and magnetic resonance imaging (MRI) studies have not always shown consistent structural brain abnormalities in OCD. Functional neuroimaging techniques such as single photon emission computed tomography (SPECT), positron emission tomography (PET) and functional magnetic resonance imaging (fMRI) have provided more consistent data indicating increased metabolic activity in the orbitofrontal cortex, the anterior cingulate gyrus and related subcortical structures such as the caudate nucleus and thalamus. Taken together, these findings suggest that there is abnormal connectivity between brain areas which modulate and control repetitive behavioural and cognitive routines which may be abnormal in OCD. A causal link is suggested by findings that some of these functional abnormalities normalise when symptoms improve with successful pharmacological or psychological treatment (Saxena et al 1998). Furthermore neurosurgical procedures which interrupt pathways from the orbitofrontal cortex and the anterior cingulate gyrus (cingulotomy) can help patients with otherwise intractable OCD symptoms.

Neurotransmitters There is now good evidence that drug-induced enhancement of serotonergic (5HT) activity in the brain has a marked impact in reducing symptoms of OCD. However, the precise nature of the serotonergic enhancement remains elusive, and it now seems rather unlikely that abnormal 5HT function provides a pathophysiological basis for OCD. Serotonin is not the only neurotransmitter to be implicated in OCD. Dopamine, noradrenaline (norepinephrine) and various neuropeptides may also be involved (Baumgarten & Grozdanovic 1998).

Psychological factors According to learning theory, compulsive rituals in OCD reduce anxiety and are therefore positively reinforced, just as avoidance responses in phobic disorders are reinforced by the relief of anxiety that they afford. This formulation logically leads to one of the most effective treatments for OCD: exposure and response prevention. However, in reality, the situation is more complex as anxiety reduction only occurs during the early stages of ritualistic behaviour, with increases in anxiety shortly afterwards. Cognitive theories focus on the OCD subject's dysfunctional reactions to intrusive thoughts which themselves are regarded as infrequent features of normal experience. The subject with OCD shows excessive fear and concern for the negative consequences, particularly for others, of their obsessional ideation. In particular, they fear acting on their impulses, and this triggers a cascade of cognitive and behavioural strategies to reduce their anxiety, but which usually only serve to perpetuate their dysfunctional thought processes.

According to psychoanalytical theory, OCD results from fixation at and regression to the anal phase of childhood development which is characterised by ambivalence toward the parent or caregiver, and particularly involves unconscious aggressive or sexual impulses. According to Freud, the anxiety generated by these impulses is contained by three major psychological defence mechanisms which are important in OCD: isolation, undoing and reaction formation. Isolation resembles the concept of dissociation in that affect is removed from anxiety-provoking ideas. Undoing similarly deals with disconnecting affect from otherwise anxiety-evoking impulses and materialises as a compulsive act which is performed in order to prevent or undo the anticipated consequences of obsessional thoughts or impulses. Reaction formation manifests as a reversal of negative emotions into their positive counterparts e.g. angry impulses translating into excessive care and concern.

Treatment

Given the fact that OCD is usually a chronic disorder which runs a fluctuating course, symptoms may sometimes improve without or in spite of treatment. The negative impact of OCD on social functioning and quality of life may persist despite short-term improvements in symptomatology, and this needs to be borne in mind in planning and assessing the outcome of different treatment strategies. Given the likelihood that the majority (up to two-thirds) of patients with OCD will suffer from a depressive illness at some time during the course of their disorder, a careful check for characteristic depressive symptoms should be made when patients are reviewed.

Drug therapy

The effectiveness of clomipramine in OCD was first reported in 1967, and has since been confirmed in numerous randomised placebo-controlled trials. Following the introduction of selective serotonin reuptake inhibitors (SSRIs) in the mid-1980s, many controlled studies have been conducted in OCD patients. Most of the studies carried out in the 1990s obtained a somewhat smaller reduction in baseline OCD scores compared with the earlier clomipramine studies (about 30% versus 40–50%). Furthermore, the placebo response in these later studies was higher (20% versus less than 10% in the earlier studies). This suggests that the later OCD trials using SSRIs studied milder, often previously treated cases of OCD which showed smaller specific drug responses.

In addition to tricyclic antidepressants other than clomipramine, monoamine oxidase inhibitors, lithium, antipsychotic drugs, benzodiazepines and electroconvulsive therapy have all proved ineffective as monotherapy for OCD. Adding a typical or atypical antipsychotic drug to partially effective clomipramine or SSRI treatment may bring about an additional improvement in OCD symptoms, particularly in patients with comorbid tics and schizotypal disorder who may otherwise not respond well to serotonergic drugs.

It is likely that anxiolytic drugs can be helpful in the short term, especially when starting behaviour therapy which can be very daunting to some OCD patients. However since OCD is a long-term problem, benzodiazepines are generally not recommended for treating this condition.

Summary In summary, SSRIs or clomipramine are the first-line treatment for OCD. Dosage of SSRIs should be built up gradually to values higher than those usual for treating depression (e.g. 60 mg per day of fluoxetine), allowing at least 12 weeks for the anti-obsessional effect to become noticeable. In contrast to the use of SSRIs in other anxiety disorders (especially panic disorder), there is not usually an exacerbation of symptoms in the early stages of drug treatment of OCD. In the case of clomipramine, the dose should be built up to 200 mg or even 300 mg a day over a 2–3 week period, and once again 12 weeks should be allowed for the treatment effect to develop. If clomipramine is ineffective or cannot be tolerated owing to side-effects, the patient should be tried on an SSRI. Similarly if after an adequate trial of an SSRI at the full dosage the patient does not respond satisfactorily, clomipramine should be tried. If after switching medications in this way, the patient still fails to respond adequately, it is worth trying different SSRIs, and/or adding an antipsychotic drug.

Psychological treatment

Behaviour therapy Behaviour therapy for OCD comprises exposure to situations or stimuli which evoke obsessive–compulsive symptoms combined with response (ritual) prevention. There are no randomised control trials of behaviour therapy versus no treatment, but in comparison with relaxation therapy or general anxiety management, behaviour therapy has convincingly been shown to be effective in OCD (Abramowitz 1997). Because behaviour therapy concentrates on compulsive behaviour, patients who show clear cut rituals tend to respond best. Obsessional thoughts which are closely associated with the rituals usually greatly improve at the same time. When obsessional thoughts occur in relative isolation without associated compulsive behaviour, behaviour therapy is less feasible and effective. In these situations, the technique of 'thought stopping' is used. In practice this may do little more than distract the subject from their obsessions. Although double-blind controlled comparisons are not possible, it seems that behaviour therapy is as effective as SSRIs and clomipramine in OCD. As with drug treatment, up to half of OCD patients may show an unsatisfactory response to behavioural treatment, with at least 10% not responding at all. However, in contrast to drug treatment, the benefits of behaviour therapy are likely to persist beyond the period of treatment. In one study (Marks et al 1975) 20 OCD patients who had successfully received behaviour therapy in a randomised controlled trial were followed up over 2 years, with nearly 80% sustaining their improvement.

Cognitive therapy Cognitive therapy focuses on obsessional thoughts, but rather than emphasising 'thought stopping', patients are encouraged to expose themselves to repetition of their obsessional ruminations (sometimes using a tape recording of their own voice) in order to focus attention on the content of the obsessions and to draw out their inherent absurdity or implausibility. This is essentially an extension of behaviour therapy in imagination but can be combined with more specific cognitive techniques which challenge the convictions and fears which patients have about their obsessional thoughts and impulses. Although cognitive therapy sounds very plausible, particularly when obsessions are the main clinical feature, there is no good evidence that it is more effective than behaviour therapy. However, patients may be less resistant to a cognitive approach than to exposure with response prevention in the first instance, although the difficulties associated with the shortage of therapists remain the same.

Combining pharmacological and psychological treatments

Patients may be unwilling to embark upon long-term SSRI treatment for OCD because of concerns about drug-related side effects and drug dependency. A significant minority (25%) of OCD patients may be reluctant to start exposure therapy because of the initial high levels of anxiety that it engenders. Starting treatment with SSRIs and then introducing behaviour therapy later when OCD symptoms have improved may be a useful strategy in these patients, with the option of phasing out medication once behaviour therapy is well underway.

The anti-obsessional effects of clomipramine and SSRIs probably last only as long as the medication is continued, suggesting that, to obtain maximum benefit, patients should remain on drug treatment for as long as they can tolerate it. For those patients who will accept long-term treatment with clomipramine or SSRIs, combining this with behaviour therapy appears to be a logical and helpful strategy in order to exploit the advantages of both treatments. The evidence in favour of this approach is actually rather limited, but there is no suggestion that drug and psychological therapy negatively interact in OCD.

Neurosurgery and repetitive transcranial magnetic stimulation

In the 5–10% of patients with very severe, treatment-refractory OCD, neurosurgery may be considered. The most frequently used neurosurgical procedures are cingulotomy, capsulotomy, limbic leucotomy and subcaudate tractotomy. Evaluation of outcome is difficult because the patients referred for neurosurgery are already at the extreme end of symptom severity and disability. Not surprisingly, there have been no prospective controlled trials carried out in this field, and the long-term results are particularly uncertain. Given the risks of short-term post-operative complications, epilepsy and personality change, it is obvious that neurosurgery should only be considered for the most difficult cases in which other treatments have been exhaustively evaluated and have failed. For a review of this interesting area see Jenike (1998). Transcranial magnetic stimulation is an established technique to non-invasively stimulate the cerebral cortex, which has been used in the treatment of depression. No anaesthetic is required and the procedure appears safe, with a low risk of inducing seizures over periods of 2–3 weeks of daily treatments. Preliminary evidence suggests that repetitive transcranial magnetic stimulation may have benefits in OCD (Greenberg et al 1997) but further studies are needed.

REACTIONS TO SEVERE STRESS (PTSD) AND ADJUSTMENT DISORDERS

Until relatively recently, the nature and limit of people's responses to everyday adverse life events and catastrophes were not considered to be the concern of psychiatrists. During the First World War these notions and conventions were seriously challenged when large numbers of apparently normal people showed psychological reactions to war and combat which were reminiscent of the most extreme cases of neurosis. Nonetheless, the focus remained on the physical and mental vulnerabilities of the affected individuals who at best were assumed to have been harbouring covert personality disorder, pre-existing neurotic conflicts or mental illness, and at worst were accused of malingering and cowardice. Despite the Second World War, the Holocaust and numerous later wars and conflicts, the position did not change significantly until the 1970s in the aftermath of the American War in Vietnam. The new generation of war veterans appeared to suffer much the same as their predecessors, but for complex reasons, as much social and political as psychiatric, the emphasis shifted so that exposure to extreme stress or traumatic events was now regarded as *both necessary and sufficient* to explain the occurrence and form of much of the psychiatric morbidity shown by war veterans. The diagnostic category *post-traumatic stress disorder* (PTSD) evolved during the 1970s and was formally first introduced in 1980 with the publication of DSM-III. PTSD and the closely related category acute stress disorder, as well as adjustment disorders, were and remain unique in being the only psychiatric disorders currently defined as much by their aetiology as by their clinical features.

In ICD-10 and subsequent revisions of DSM, the defining features of traumatic stressors necessary for the diagnosis of PTSD were modified and broadened to accommodate the experiences of non-combatant civilian populations. In DSM-IIIR it was no longer necessary for the criterion traumatic events to be 'outside the range of usual human experience' and in ICD-10 only that they are of 'an exceptionally threatening or catastrophic nature, which is likely to cause pervasive distress in almost anyone'.

Another less obvious aspect of the focus on triggering events, rather than on individual vulnerability in defining PTSD, is that unique amongst psychiatric diagnosis, PTSD has causes which are viewed as relatively independent of and largely outside the control and responsibility of the affected individual. Not only does this exculpate them for many of the long-term adverse consequences associated with the disorder, but it may also shift blame onto others, either individuals or institutions, and lead to claims for compensation which no other psychiatric diagnosis can justify so well. This section will deal with acute stress reactions, and the closely related categories of acute stress disorder and post-traumatic stress disorder. Adjustment disorders will be covered in a later section. In ICD-10 these disorders are placed in a separate category (F43) distinct from anxiety and other neurotic disorders, whereas in DSM-IV acute stress disorders and PTSD are considered along with other anxiety disorders, only adjustment disorders being assigned a category of its own.

Acute stress reaction

Definition

ICD-10 specifies a condition called *Acute Stress Reaction* (F43.0) which is very similar to one of the two essential criteria for both acute stress disorder and PTSD, as defined in DSM-IV. The triggering traumatic events for an acute stress reaction as described in ICD-10 are quite similar to those for ICD-10 PTSD and for DSM-IV acute stress disorder as well as for PTSD, and will be described in more detail later. An acute stress reaction as defined in ICD-10 usually occurs within minutes of the triggering event and resolves rapidly, for example within a few hours if the stressor is removed, and within 1–3 days even if it is not.

Clinical features

Typical clinical features include marked symptoms of anxiety and increased arousal along with 'dissociative' symptoms such as reduced awareness of and responsiveness to other people and surroundings, disorientation, agitation, inappropriate or purposeless activity, irritability or aggression, and panic attacks. The acute stress reaction specified as a necessary precursor of acute stress disorder and PTSD in DSM-IV requires that the individual experiences intense fear, helplessness, or horror, and in children the response must involve disorganised or agitated behaviour.

Management

Three time-honoured strategies for reducing the adverse impact of extremely stressful experiences are: (1) the acute or short-term use of sedative drugs such as alcohol or benzodiazepines; (2) general support, reassurance and assistance with coping responses; and (3) psychological 'debriefing' which involves encouraging detailed recollection of traumatic events shortly after they have occurred.

Drug treatment There is little evidence to justify the use of sedative and hypnotic drugs in people who have recently suffered extreme traumatic stressors as a means of preventing PTSD.

Psychological debriefing Providing debriefing, that is having the person talk about the trauma in detail, has high face validity and is usually readily acceptable to trauma victims. However, systematic review of the evidence suggests that early debriefing is ineffective in preventing PTSD and may even increase it (Bisson 2002)

Acute stress disorder

Definition

Whereas the acute stress *reaction* defined in ICD-10 typically lasts considerably less than 48 hours, the category acute stress *disorder* described in DSM-IV begins during or shortly after experiencing the precipitating traumatic and distressing event and must last *at least 48 hours* to meet diagnostic criteria. Except for the different defining time frame, the clinical features of acute stress disorder are similar to those of PTSD, including the criteria for the triggering traumatic stressors.

Clinical features

A striking characteristic feature of acute stress disorder is the presence of prominent dissociative symptoms, including 'being in a daze', derealisation, depersonalisation, and amnesia for key aspects of the traumatic experience (dissociative amnesia). Reduced emotional responsiveness, detachment or numbing of feeling are also regarded as dissociative symptoms. If an acute stress disorder as defined by DSM-IV lasts longer than 1 month, the diagnosis is automatically regraded to PTSD.

Management

Pharmacological and psychological treatments given at this early stage after stress exposure are similar to those used for established PTSD (see later), and may be beneficial in reducing the development of PTSD (Bisson 2002). Patients with marked dissociative symptoms have in the past sometimes been managed by 'abreaction reaction' techniques involving acute administration of potent sedative drugs such as barbiturates or benzodiazepines. Reducing the hyperarousal that accompanies dissociative states may allow the patient to access and verbalise traumatic memories. However there is no evidence that these techniques assist in reducing intrusive re-experiencing or flashbacks, probably because memories accessed in drug-induced states do not readily transfer to normal states of consciousness.

Post-traumatic stress disorder

Definition

PTSD is a delayed and/or protracted response to exceptionally threatening or catastrophic events or situations (traumatic stressors). DSM-IV specifies these stressors in detail as well as requiring that the individual shows an acute stress response to them involving fear, helplessness or horror. DSM-IV defines an extreme traumatic stressor as the experiencing or witnessing of an event or series of events that involve actual or threatened death or serious injury, or threat to the physical integrity of the self or to other people. For example, learning about the unexpected death of a family member or loved one might represent a traumatic stressor, just as would direct personal experience of a life-threatening situation. To meet the diagnostic criteria for PTSD in DSM-IV, at least one feature from each of the re-experiencing, avoidance and hyperarousal symptom clusters must have occurred following a specified traumatic stressor which also evoked an acute stress reaction. In addition, the condition must have been present for *1 month* or more and caused significant distress and social dysfunction. The criterion duration of 1 month for DSM-IV PTSD ensures that the condition cannot be diagnosed until at least 1 month after the traumatic event and, in this sense, is by definition a delayed reaction. The diagnostic criteria for PTSD in ICD-10 are similar to those in DSM-IV except that the 1 month delay/duration criterion is not specified and resulting significant distress and social dysfunction are not essential.

Clinical features

The most specific group of symptoms involve intrusive and uncontrollable *re-experiencing* of aspects of the provoking stressor or trauma in the form of fragmented images, memories, 'flashbacks' (in which the individual feels or even acts as if the event were still happening) and distressing dreams and nightmares of the traumatic events. Despite involuntary re-experiencing or remembering, intentional recall of the trauma is frequently incomplete and disorganised, and there may even be complete amnesia for salient aspects of the event. Disturbing memories of the trauma may be triggered by situations or sensory experiences. This is associated with the second main group of symptoms which involves the individual's deliberate attempts to avoid remembering or re-living the traumatic experience. Related to these avoidance responses is a diminished interest in activities in general, and a sense of detachment and difficulty in feeling ordinary emotions ('numbness'). The third cluster of symptoms typical of PTSD and acute stress disorder are those of hyperarousal, including increased vigilance, exaggerated startle response, irritability, poor concentration and insomnia.

Diagnosis

Adjustment disorders are distinguished from acute stress disorder and PTSD by the fact that the latter has characteristic symptoms that are triggered by extremely threatening stressful events which evoke fear and horror, whereas in adjustment disorders, the precipitating stress is typically less catastrophic, and the psychological reaction less specific. Some of the symptoms of an acute stress reaction or disorder such as reduced awareness and responsiveness, 'confusion' and irritability resemble those associated with brain injury which must be ruled out in cases involving actual or probable physical trauma. A brief psychotic reaction to an extreme stressor (Acute Polymorphic Psychotic Disorder, F23.0) may also mimic an acute stress disorder with an abrupt onset, 'confusion' and emotional turmoil. However hallucinations and delusions are usually obvious. Dissociative Disorders (F44) and Depersonalisation–Derealisation Syndrome (F48.1) also share some of the clinical features of an acute stress disorder, but if diagnostic criteria for the latter are met, this takes precedence.

With the virtual abandonment of a diagnostic hierarchy in respect of PTSD, comorbidity with other psychiatric diagnoses can be expected. PTSD is associated with very high rates of depression, anxiety disorders, and especially alcohol and substance misuse/dependency. Overall about 80% of people with PTSD have other psychiatric diagnoses, the majority of which follow the onset of PTSD. Depression and dependence on drugs and alcohol are very common in subjects with PTSD.

Epidemiology

Most people living in developed western countries will experience during their lifetime a traumatic event meeting criteria for traumatic stressors preceding PTSD. At a conservative estimate, on average about 10% of people experiencing a significant traumatic event actually go on to develop PTSD (Kessler et al 1995). Estimates of prevalence of PTSD will clearly depend on which population is being considered. The US National Comorbidity Survey estimated lifetime prevalence for PTSD in the general population of 5% for men and 10% for women using DSM-IIIR criteria. More recent US studies using DSM-IV criteria have reported a 1-month prevalence of PTSD of 1.2% for men and 2.7% for women (Stein et al 1997). Much higher rates of PTSD have been reported in groups of individuals exposed to frequent traumatic stressors such as volunteer fire fighters.

Risk factors The risk of developing PTSD following a traumatic stressor depends on a number of variables. Women are twice as likely as men to develop PTSD, despite experiencing fewer stressors overall. Women are more likely to experience 'high impact' stressors such as rape, and also appear to have a greater susceptibility to PTSD. A personal and family history of psychiatric disorder and a previous history of traumatic experiences in childhood (sexual and physical abuse and parental separation) are also associated with an increased risk of developing PTSD after acute traumatic stressors in adult life. Low intelligence and certain personality traits ('neuroticism') and disorders may also predispose to PTSD by increasing vulnerability to traumatic stress. However, the same or related personality variables may be also associated with attitudes and lifestyles which put the individual at greater risk of encountering traumatic events. It has long been suspected that patients who have lost consciousness due to injury or other factors whilst undergoing an acute traumatic stressful event are less likely to develop PTSD subsequently. However it does appear that PTAD can develop in those who have lost consciousness in car accidents (Mayou 2002).

The trauma The severity of physical injury is a weaker predictor of the likelihood of developing PTSD than the severity of psychological distress. Examples of stressors with their relative impact are listed in Box 21.5.

Aetiology

Genetics Susceptibility to PTSD seems to be partly genetically determined. In a study of 2224 monozygotic and 1818 dizygotic twins who were all Vietnam War combat veterans there was a higher concordance of PTSD among monozygotic than dizygotic twins. It was calculated that genetic factors explained approximately one-third of the variance in susceptibility to PTSD (True et al 1993).

HPA axis Patients with PTSD have reduced basal concentrations of cortisol in the blood, with exaggerated suppression of cortisol when given low doses of dexamethasone (Yehuda et al 1990). Subjects exposed to traumatic stressors who fail to develop PTSD do not show these changes. This suggests that in PTSD there is exaggerated negative feedback inhibition of the hypothalamic–pituitary–adrenal (HPA) axis by glucocorticoids. There may be a link between this dysregulation of the HPA axis and reduced hippocampal volume in PTSD since glucocorticoid receptors are found in the hippocampus, which is sensitive to damage by raised level of glucocorticoids. The dysregulation of the

---

> **Box 21.5 Common and less common traumatic stressors with moderate or high 'impact' in producing PTSD**
>
> **Common traumatic stressors of moderate impact (precede PTSD in 5–20%)**
> - Diagnosis of life-threatening illness in self or loved one
> - Sudden death of a loved one (witnessed or reported)
> - Witnessing death or serious injury of another person in an accident or crime
> - Direct involvement in a serious accident (not necessarily related to severity of injury)
> - Involvement in fire, flood or small-scale natural disaster
>
> **Common high-impact traumatic stressors (precede PTSD in > 20%)**
> - Being mugged or threatened with weapon (less impact in men than in women)
> - Serious domestic violence to women
> - Rape (more impact in men than in women)
> - Sexual and/or physical abuse in childhood
>
> **Uncommon high-impact traumatic stressors**
> - Participation in war and combat
> - Being kidnapped, held hostage or tortured
> - Prisoner of war; survivor of Holocaust (may be associated with enduring personality change)
> - Witnessing or participating in torture, war atrocities
> - Direct involvement in large-scale natural or man-made disasters (earthquake, terrorist bombing, etc.)

HPA axis in PTSD is unlike that found in depressive disorders, in which increased secretion of CRF is associated with hypercortisolaemia and normal or impaired dexamethasone suppression of blood cortisol.

Brain structure and function A number of studies using magnetic resonance imaging have demonstrated decreased hippocampal volume in combat veterans and other subjects with chronic PTSD, sometimes with a negative correlation between hippocampal volume and severity of symptoms or amount of exposure to traumatic stressors. It is unclear whether decreased hippocampal volume represents a risk factor for or a consequence of PTSD. Positron emission tomography studies suggest that in PTSD there is increased functional activity in the amygdala relative to areas in the hippocampus and prefrontal cortex which both have connections from the amygdala. Amygdala activation is most pronounced in PTSD subjects re-experiencing memories of trauma. Taken together, neuroimaging studies suggest that PTSD symptoms are associated with exaggerated activity in the amygdala and with structural and functional deficits in the hippocampus and related cortical areas including the left inferior cortex (Broca's area). It has been suggested that these findings are compatible with increased encoding of emotionally charged 'sense memories' at the expense of memories which can be consciously recalled and expressed in language. Although these findings may not be specific to PTSD, there is limited evidence that they normalise after successful treatment. For a review see Hull (2002).

Neurotransmitters Glutamatergic neural pathways mediating excitatory neuronal responses through NMDA receptors in hippocampus and amygdala appear to be crucial in encoding normal and aberrant long-term memories. GABAergic neurons mediating inhibitory neuronal effects in the same brain areas via $GABA_A$–benzodiazepine receptors induce forgetting and amnesia. In PTSD there may be an imbalance between these two brain systems, which are affected by a number of other neuro-transmitters. A role for altered opioid functioning in the brains of subjects with PTSD has been suggested, since it can be argued that PTSD symptoms resemble both the direct actions of opioids (e.g. emotional numbing and raised pain thresholds) as well as opioid withdrawal (agitation and fear responses). There is some evidence that endogenous opioids are secreted by PTSD patients re-experiencing traumatic stressors. For review see Nutt (2000).

Psychological factors Under normal circumstances, experiences are mainly processed as autobiographical explicit memories which are recalled in a verbal form without vivid emotional overlay. Memories of highly emotionally charged traumatic situations are probably encoded differently as implicit memories, principally as sensations as opposed to personal narratives. However, with time, these 'trauma memories' 'get put into words' and become linked to autobiographical context and explicit memory. If this process of 'cognitive restructuring' is impeded, memories of traumatic experiences continue to be easily triggered by stimuli similar to the original stressor. The trauma memory therefore remains encoded in implicit memory and retains its powerful emotional impact and ability to make the PTSD patient feel as though he were vividly reliving the past. In PTSD, it is hypothesised that there is an imbalance between implicit and explicit memory processes dependent on the amygdala and hippocampus, respectively. This results in impairment in the processing of trauma memories. Although trauma memories are not easily accessed voluntarily or readily processed using language, this is what may need to be achieved in order to restore an appropriate balance between implicit and explicit memory processes and to reduce PTSD symptoms. Traumatic memories must be evoked or activated, discussed and 'worked through', in order to reduce their persistent intrusive power. Viewed in this way, the involuntary re-experiencing phenomena characteristic of PTSD may represent an exaggerated or aberrant mechanism for integrating trauma memories with episodic memory. If so, PTSD should be self-limiting. This does appear to be the case in many subjects with PTSD, although it does not account for the 25% or more of subjects who experience PTSD symptoms for many years. For a review see Brewin & Holmes (2003).

Management

Recovery from PTSD is facilitated by good social support, and by minimising the negative personal and social consequences of the traumatic life event (especially survivor guilt), and of course reducing the likelihood of further traumatic life events occurring.

Psychological treatment Behaviour therapy for PTSD usually involves exposing the subject to re-evoked memories of past trauma. This may be achieved individually or in groups by watching films or hearing audio tapes of similar experiences to their own, or making an audio tape of their own verbal account and replaying this. A recent variant of behaviour therapy for PTSD involves the technique of eye movement desensitisation and reprocessing (EMDR). In this technique, the patient recalls traumatic events while in a state of induced relaxation resulting from focusing their attention on the therapist's voice and following the therapist's rapid finger movements. However, it appears that the resulting saccadic eye movements are not essential for the effectiveness of EMDR. In general, exposure treatment is effective in many cases of PTSD, particularly if the traumatic stressor is a discreet event rather than chronic, repeated traumas. Cognitive therapy for PTSD involves identifying and challenging dysfunctional thoughts surrounding the traumatic incident and is often combined with exposure therapy as in CBT. For a summary of systematic reviews and randomised controlled trials of psychological treatments in PTSD see Bisson (2002).

Drug treatment

Most randomised-controlled studies of drug therapy have been of short duration (12 weeks or less). A wide range of drugs has been studied, with the largest and best quality studies being devoted to SSRIs. Treatment with all these drugs is capable of reducing all core features of PTSD. Although tricyclic antidepressants may be effective in PTSD, the evidence is not strong, and tricyclic noradrenergic reuptake inhibitors appear to be ineffective. Monoamine oxidase inhibitors such as phenelzine have been shown to be effective in PTSD in randomised controlled trials, but the results with these drugs seem to be less consistent than with SSRIs (Bisson 2002).

Adjustment disorders

Definition

An adjustment disorder is any distressing and disabling response to a stressful life event or series of events which fails to meet diagnostic criteria for another psychiatric syndrome. Adjustment disorders may manifest as emotional and/or behavioural symptoms. Since adjustment disorders are the only psychiatric diagnoses without any characteristic clinical features, they are essentially sub-syndromal conditions at the very bottom of the diagnostic hierarchy referred to earlier in this chapter. By convention, if following exposure to a stressful event, a subject's psychological or behavioural reactions meet diagnostic criteria for any other psychiatric disorder; the label adjustment disorder is abandoned, even if the stressful circumstances persist. Although adjustment disorders are by definition triggered by life events, crises or adversity, and would not otherwise have occurred without these events, in contrast to the situation with acute stress reactions/disorder and PTSD, these external stressors are not defined or characterised in detail. Instead, the emphasis is on the individual's predisposition and vulnerability in determining and shaping her abnormal reaction to a particular set of stressful circumstances. Broadly similar adverse life events may produce a diverse range of reactions in different people, depending on their personality, past and present social circumstances, and their cultural and religious background. In making a diagnosis of adjustment disorder, a clinical judgement has to be made that the individual's response to a particular stressor is disproportionate or maladaptive, since some degree of distress and disability would form part of a normal reaction to stress. In the past, such normal reactions which might come to the attention of psychiatrists were called 'transient situational disturbances', a term which is no longer current in diagnostic systems. Both DSM-IV and ICD-10 subdivide adjustment disorders (F43.2 in ICD-10) into those in which disturbance of mood or other emotions occur and coexist in various combinations. Inevitably, more than with any other psychiatric condition, the diagnosis of adjustment disorder requires a cross-cultural perspective if it is to have any validity.

DSM-IV requires that the psychological disturbance constituting an adjustment disorder must begin *within 3 months* of the onset of the stressor, and last no longer than 6 months after the stressor or its consequences have ceased. However, if the stressful circumstances persist or are recurrent, the adjustment disorder diagnosis continues to apply unless the disorder, considered in its entirety, subsequently meets the diagnostic criteria for another psychiatric condition, e.g. dysthymia. In ICD-10, the timing criteria for adjustment disorders are less clearly defined — 'the onset is usually within one month of the occurrence of the stressful event or life changes and the duration of symptoms does not usually exceeds six months'. If symptoms do persist beyond 6 months (2 years in the case of a prolonged depressive adjustment reaction, F43.21), or if symptoms subsequently meet criteria for another ICD-10 diagnosis, the adjustment disorder diagnosis is dropped. In the former case the individual will now no longer qualify for an ICD-10 diagnosis, even though they may still be significantly distressed and disabled. Clearly DSM-IV has an advantage over ICD-10 in this respect.

Clinical features

Adjustment disorders may manifest with a wide variety of emotional and behavioural symptoms. Subtypes have been distinguished on the bases of these and include depressed mood, anxious mood, mixed anxiety and depressed mood, disturbance of behaviour, and mixed disturbance of emotion and behaviour. The behavioural disturbances may take the form of withdrawal or of disturbed and aggressive behaviour including violence. They are often complicated by substance misuse.

Epidemiology

Adjustment disorders have been excluded from consideration in all the major epidemiological surveys of recent times. It has been estimated that 2–20% of patients attending a psychiatric outpatient service could be diagnosed with an adjustment disorder. However, given that adjustment disorders with appropriate depressive clinical features would only need to be present for 2 weeks or more to qualify for a diagnosis of major depression or depressive episode, many examples of depressive adjustment disorders are not officially recognised as such. In other words, it is likely that many cases of major depression are adjustment disorders in all but name. This is not merely a semantic nicety, since depressed patients who are adjusting to life events may benefit more from problem-solving and coping strategies than depressed patients in whom stressful events are less clearly linked to symptomatology. Essentially this is revisiting the supposedly obsolete reactive–endogenous distinction with respect to diagnosis of mood disorder. However, it may be that combining and incorporating the concept of adjustment disorder with major depression may prove more fruitful than is acknowledged by ICD-10 and DSM-IV.

Diagnosis

Other psychiatric disorders which occur in response to stressful events and circumstances (acute stress disorder, PTSD) require external triggers which are exceptionally threatening and have a characteristic constellation of clinical features. By contrast, adjustment disorders involve diverse, unspecified reactions to a wide range of possible stressors. DSM-IV states that in adjustment disorders, symptoms should 'not represent bereavement', that is 'an expected (normal) response to the death of a loved one'. However, DSM-IV does allow that a diagnosis of adjustment disorder may be appropriate when the bereavement reaction is inappropriately excessive or prolonged. This same distinction between normal and abnormal grief reactions is attempted in ICD-10, but with even less clarity.

Treatment

Helping patients adjust to bereavement, physical illness and other specific life situations, is covered elsewhere in this book. In general, treatment is aimed at helping the patient cope with current difficulties and to address the precipitating problems. If adverse external circumstances cannot be improved, at least the individual may be helped to adapt to them. The main techniques used are confronting and reducing patients' denial and avoidance of their difficulties, whilst helping them develop workable solutions to their psychological and practical difficulties. Sometimes, underlying personality difficulties or disorder may be brought to the fore by the subject's experience of challenging life events and stressors.

Prognosis

Approximately 80% of individuals identified as suffering an adjustment disorder will be well 5 years later, and in most, symptoms will have resolved rapidly. However, given the ambiguous nature of the adjustment disorder diagnosis and the ease with which it may convert to major depression or depressive episode, there is a danger that many subjects undergoing adjustment reactions will receive unnecessary psychiatric interventions. On the other hand, the minority of adjustment disorders which are sub-syndromal for other psychiatric diagnoses and yet represent prolonged and disabling reactions to chronic adversity may well benefit from more intensive psychiatric intervention. On the whole, the concept of adjustment disorder as elaborated in ICD-10 and DSM-IV does not help make this distinction.

DISSOCIATIVE (CONVERSION) DISORDERS

The dissociative (conversion) disorders are modern terms for disorders previously referred to as hysteria. The essential characteristic is a loss of a normal mental or physical function. Although hysteria was abandoned, in part because of its inappropriate anatomical implications, the term dissociation is itself hardly atheoretical. Indeed it stems from psychoanalytic theory which aimed to explain how such loss of function could occur without any evidence of structural disease. The theory is that the normally integrated functions of consciousness, memory, identity and perception become disrupted or disintegrated. Specific functions that may be affected in this way are memory (dissociative amnesia), memory associated with sudden unexpected travel (fugue), consciousness (trance), identity and personality (multiple personality disorder), and other states.

Definition

The main features of dissociative (conversion) disorder are: symptoms of loss of function regarded as indicating a loss of normal integration between psychological systems; the absence of a medical disorder to explain them, and evidence of psychological causation in the form of association in time with stressful events, problems or disturbed relationships

ICD-10 and DSM-IV differ principally over how they classify loss of physical function. In DSM it is called conversion disorder. The term conversion disorder also reflects a psychoanalytic theory that aimed to explain how the proposed psychological conflicts that caused the loss of function were converted into physical symptoms. In DSM-IV conversion disorder is placed within the somatoform disorders. In ICD-10 conversion disorders are named dissociative motor disorder, dissociative convulsions, and dissociative anaesthesia. In both classifications it is presumed that psychological factors are involved but that these are unconscious.

Conversion disorder Conversion disorder can present with sensory, motor or mixed symptoms. Consequently cases are more likely to be found in neurological and medical departments than in psychiatric clinics. Motor symptoms may be of weakness or paralysis, tremor, seizures, loss of speech or other movements. Atasia-abasia refers to difficulty in standing and walking. Sensory symptoms include numbness, blindness or deafness. Typically the symptoms are discrepant with the anatomical deficit expected with a pathological lesion; for example the loss of sensation does not follow known nerve distribution but may be of a limb with a line where the limb meets the body. 'Belle-indifference', the apparent lack of emotional concern about the deficit is not a reliable sign. See Stone et al (2002b) for a practical review of assessment and diagnosis.

Dissociative amnesia Dissociative (psychogenic) amnesia is occasionally seen by those working in psychiatric services. The patient typically complains of a sudden onset of loss of memory of important personal information such as name and address. Care should be taken to ensure that acute neurological conditions such as stroke are excluded. However, the presentation of total loss of memory for personal information but preservation of other mental functions is characteristic of dissociative amnesia. The diagnosis is supported if the onset of amnesia arose in the context of severe psychological stress.

Dissociative fugue Fugue refers to travelling away from home, usually during an amnesiac episode. This often purposive travelling away from home may be in the context of the person taking up a new identity and disclaiming knowledge of their previous identity.

Dissociative trance or stupor This is part of a differential diagnosis of stupors or trance states. The patient may sit or lie motionless for long periods but maintains normal muscle tone, posture and eye movements.

Dissociative personality disorder (multiple personality disorder) This refers to a phenomenon described in the literature where people present themselves as having more than one independent personality to another person, usually a therapist. The syndrome is certainly rare and there has been controversy about whether is exists as a dissociative phenomenon rather than the shaped behaviour of vulnerable, suggestible persons.

Hysterical psychosis Occasionally a patient presents as apparently psychotic, although the implausibility of the presentation, and suddenness of onset in relation to trauma, suggests that this is a dissociative rather than a truly psychotic phenomenon. Furthermore the form of psychosis may reflect that of the person's belief of what psychosis is like rather than that more familiar to the psychiatrist. An example might be an individual who says that he had an hallucination of his friend's head turning through 360 degrees 'like in the film The Exorcist'. The rapid onset and offset of a condition would be suggestive, although differentiation from true brief psychotic states may clearly be difficult. Dissociative psychosis is almost certainly rare.

Dissociation in special circumstances Dissociative and conversion reactions occurring in group situations have received particular attention and special labels. Epidemic hysteria or mass hysteria refers to apparently contagious dissociative phenomena which take place in large groups of people or institutions under conditions of anxiety. Typically, they are described as taking place in schools where episodes of illness or fainting appear to spread through the school with rapidity. Clearly the differential diagnosis is from an epidemic of illness such as viral illness. A classic and controversial example is an episode of acute illness which took place mainly in nurses of the Royal Free Hospital in 1955 during an epidemic of polio. Their symptoms were regarded by some as being evidence of 'atypical' polio infection but by others as evidence of mass hysteria (McEverdy & Beard 1970). The controversy remains unresolved to the present day.

Combat hysteria, shell shock and battle neurosis During wartime, soldiers are subject to a very great degree of stress and may develop dissociative conversion disorders of acute onset. These disorders are often interpreted has having the function of preventing the person from having to continue fighting. For example they may become blind or unable to use their right arm. Clearly, in such circumstances differentiation from malingering is both difficult and fraught.

Epidemiology

There are limited data on the epidemiology of dissociative disorders. For conversion disorder (as defined in DSM-IV) a wide range of prevalence has been described, but these are almost certainly underestimates because patients with disorders suggestive of neurological deficit are much more likely to present to neurological clinics than to mental health services. Indeed a recent survey in Edinburgh suggested that conversion disorder with loss of motor function may be as common in neurological services as multiple sclerosis.

Conversion disorder appears to be more frequent in women than in men. Assessment of the validity of possible differences in prevalence between cultures has been made difficult by the fact that altered mental and physical states may not be regarded as medical problems (that is in some cultures they may be regarded as manifestation of religious rather than medical phenomena). It has commonly been suggested that conversion symptoms are more common on the left side of the body, although a recent systematic review has suggested that this is not borne out by the literature and may reflect bias in previous reporting (Stone et al 2002a).

Aetiology

Old ideas about hysteria refer to migration of the uterus around the body. With increasing anatomical sophistication the cause was later thought to be disease of the brain, and in the late 1800s when the brains of people with hysteria who died were found to be of normal structure, these gave way to ideas of altered brain functioning.

In the early 20th century Freud and the psychoanalysts developed the idea that hysterical phenomena were psychogenic. That is that they were manifestations of unconscious mental phenomena with the physical symptoms being a way of resolving a mental conflict and indeed often symbolising it. Thus for example someone who was conflicted about leaving home might find that they were unable to walk. Associated theoretical notions were the concept of primary gain and secondary gain. Primary gain was defined as the internal psychological benefit the person would obtain by resolving the conflict. Secondary gain has been used to refer to the practical advantages that may follow from being sick (for example receiving care and attention). Janet, also writing in the early 20th century, emphasised the splitting of mental functions (dissociation) and the importance of the person's idea of disease shaping the form of the symptom. Modern ideas of the aetiology of dissociation continue to emphasise the role of psychological factors. Previous experience (such as childhood abuse) is a predisposing factor, psychological or physical trauma a precipitating factor, and special rewards for disability a perpetuating factor. There has also been increased interest in the neurobiology of dissociation, with preliminary work on functional brain imaging suggesting identifiable changes which are different from those of people feigning illness (Halligan et al 2000).

Diagnosis

In practice the diagnosis of these conditions can be difficult. First one has to be sure by appropriate medical assessment and investigation that the loss of function is not a result of identifiable neurological disease. Although not entirely straightforward the difficulty of this has previously been overestimated (Stone et al 2002b). More controversial is the diagnostic requirement that psychological factors, usually in the form of a psychological trauma or conflict, are deemed relevant to the aetiology. This requirement is both theoretically based and potentially unreliable. Most difficult is the requirement to differentiate dissociative and conversion states from those which are malingered. This is because there is no reliable way of differentiating conscious from unconscious processes. In practice the test that is often used is that of consistency. If someone presents with a clear deficit and then is seen in another circumstance to not have that deficit (for example a patient who attends in a wheelchair and then is seen to be walking briskly down the road outside the clinic) this would sway a diagnostic judgement towards intentional production of symptoms. In summary the definition of these syndromes is unsatisfactory and would benefit from revision that provided simpler operational definitions less influenced by theory.

Treatment

There are few trials to guide our treatment of dissociative and conversion states. Treatments that have been suggested include simple encouragement, hypnosis, abreaction (in which the person is encouraged to talk about the traumatic event, often under sedation) and a variety of other means. Most but not all patients improve, and an approach which involves support, encouragement to treatment of associated disorder, and the resolution as far as possible of current stressors, is generally felt to be appropriate. The role of abreaction remains controversial.

OTHER NEUROTIC DISORDERS

Neurasthenia

The term neurasthenia has a long history and before Freud was essentially an amorphous concept covering all neurotic disorders. The terms was particularly prevalent during the First World War as applied to soldiers suffering from combat neurosis but without signs of dissociative/conversion disorders (hysteria). The new emphasis on physical and mental 'weakness' as defining clinical features also carried pejorative connotations of failings of character and cowardice when applied to soldiers who were unable to cope psychologically with active service. Subsequently, neurasthenia was used much more narrowly to describe neurotic conditions (including depression) in which chronic fatigue was the main feature, and this is how the term is still used in ICD-10.

Definition

Neurasthenia (F48.0) is included in ICD-10 as a category distinct from the Somatoform Disorders (F45), whereas in DSM-IV it is subsumed under the heading 'undifferentiated somatoform disorder'. Neurasthenia as defined in ICD-10 is characterised by a persistent and distressing complaint of increased fatigue after mental effort or persistent and distressing complaints of bodily weakness and exhaustion after minimal effort. Neurasthenia is broadly equivalent to the medical functional syndrome of chronic fatigue syndrome (CFS). Whether these conditions are identical to myalgic encephalomyelitis (ME), regarded by some as a specific neurological disease, is highly controversial. However, in the absence of any definitive evidence of specific brain disease the existence of ME as a specific subgroup of neurasthenia must remain speculative. For a review see Sharpe (1996).

Clinical features

Patients with neurasthenia present with the predominant compliant of physical and mental fatigue that is exacerbated by exertion. They commonly have symptoms of depression and anxiety but the fatigue is predominant. These patients are more commonly seen in medical than psychiatric settings and often receive diagnosis such as post-viral fatigue or sometimes ME. They may develop strong beliefs about a medical aetiology for their condition which reduces the acceptability of psychiatric management.

Aetiology

Current understanding of aetiology is that it is probably multifactorial. There is some evidence for a genetic predisposition. There is also some evidence for precipitating life events and possibly a triggering role for medical conditions such as viral infection. Neurasthenia can certainly develop after acute Epstein–Barr virus infection (glandular fever). Neurasthenia is not necessarily a stable diagnosis, and cases of neurasthenia may change to cases of depression or anxiety. It has been proposed that there are subgroups of neurasthenia which have different and specific organic aetiologies, although this remains to be established.

Epidemiology

Fatigue is common in the general population but the diagnosis of neurasthenia less so. One study found that although 13% of the population complain of prolonged and excessive fatigue, less than 2% met ICD-10 criteria for neurasthenia and less than 0.5% neurasthenia without comorbid anxiety and depression (Hickie et al 2002). Neurasthenia (and CFS) is more common in women.

Treatment

The available evidence suggests that antidepressant treatments are of limited value, but there is good evidence for rehabilitative psychological treatments including CBT and simple graded exercise therapy (Whiting et al 2001).

Prognosis

Mild cases of fatigue tend to fluctuate, although established cases of neurasthenia tend to persist and to follow a chronic course.

Depersonalisation–derealisation syndrome

Depersonalisation and derealisation refer to a fairly common symptom in which the person reports that their perceptions are changed in quality in a way that makes them unreal or distant.

Definition

The definition in ICD-10 is of a syndrome in which the person experiences depersonalisation and/or derealisation, the condition is accepted by the person as a subjective and spontaneous change, and there is no organic cause such as delirium or epilepsy.

Clinical features

When the description is applied to the patient's body this is usually termed depersonalisation. Such individuals may feel that they are somehow separate from all of their body and looking down upon themselves or that parts of their body such as a limb feel different and no longer belong to them. When referring to the outside world it is called derealisation. In derealisation the quality of the external world is changed so that surroundings no longer seem substantial or solid looking, sometimes being described as being 'like a film set'.

Aetiology

Depersonalisation and derealisation commonly occur under stress, with drug intoxication and sleep deprivation. They may also be a symptom of depressive or anxiety disorders. The phenomena must be differentiated from psychotic phenomena and from brain disease, including dementia and temporary epilepsy.

Treatment

When they occur on their own the conditions are reified as depersonalisation–derealisation syndrome. Reassurance and explanation, antidepressant drugs, exercise and relaxation have all been tried. There is, however, little in the way of clinical trial evidence to guide treatment.

Prognosis

The condition is usually transient but may become chronic.

SOMATOFORM DISORDERS

Somatoform disorders became a necessary category in DSM-III following the abolition of the general category of neurosis. They continue to exist in ICD-10 (F45) under the general heading 'Neurotic Stress Related and Somatoform Disorders'. The earlier concept of neurosis encompassed a range of psychological and somatic symptoms that were not attributable to a medical condition. The differentiation of neurosis into specific subcategories, particularly into the mood disorders and the anxiety disorders, left those who presented with predominant somatic symptoms and few if any psychological phenomena, homeless in the classification. Hence the creation of the category of somatoform disorders. Somatoform simply means in physical form and it is historically closely related to the idea of somatisation (which in turn is related to conversion). This is a theoretical mechanism to explain how somatic symptoms which are not due to organic disease could be produced by psychological phenomena. That is, a psychological problem or conflict is made physical or 'somatised'.

Definition

The common feature of somatoform disorders is a repeated presentation of somatic symptoms, often with requests for medical investigation despite repeated negative findings and reassurance, where the symptoms are not explained by a medical condition.

Clinical features

Somatoform disorder category contains a wide range of phenomena which are unified only by the factor that they tend to present with physical symptoms to non-psychiatric physicians. This appears to be a poor basis for classification.

Specific syndromes included under this heading vary somewhat between DSM-IV and ICD-10 but both include a chronic condition with multiple symptoms including conversion symptoms termed somatisation disorder (previously Briquet's syndrome), a condition characterised by somatic symptoms accompanied by anxiety that the symptoms represent a serious disease (hypochondriasis). The other conditions refer to a variety of presentations which have as a common feature a concern about physical symptoms. These include dysmorphophobia or body dysmorphic disorder where the concern is about bodily or facial appearance, pain disorder where the concern is over bodily pain of psychogenic origin, and undifferentiated somatoform disorder which describes medically unexplained or functional somatic symptoms. These conditions mostly present to non-psychiatric physicians and are all considered in more detail in Chapter 28.

REFERENCES

Abramowitz J S 1997 Effectiveness of psychological and pharmacological treatments for obsessive–compulsive disorder: a quantitative review. Journal of Consulting & Clinical Psychology 65:44–52

Andrews G 1996 Comorbidity and the general neurotic syndrome. British Journal of Psychiatry 168(suppl 30): 76–84

Barlow D-H 1997 Cognitive-behavioral therapy for panic disorder: current status. Journal of Clinical Psychiatry 58(suppl 2): 32–36

Baumgarten H G, Grozdanovic Z 1998 Role of serotonin in obsessive–compulsive disorder. British Journal of Psychiatry Supplement 13–20

Bebbington P, Hurry J, Tennant C et al 1981 Epidemiology of mental disorders in Camberwell. Psychological Medicine 11:561–579

Berman I, Kalinowski A, Berman S M et al 1995 Obsessive and compulsive symptoms in chronic schizophrenia. Comprehensive Psychiatry 36:6–10

Bisson J 2002 Post-traumatic stress disorder. Clinical Evidence 7:913–919

Bourin M, Baker G B, Bradwejn J 1998 Neurobiology of panic disorder. Journal of Psychosomatic Research 44:163–180

Brewin C R, Holmes E A 2003 Psychological theories of posttraumatic stress disorder. Clinical Psychology Review 23:339–376

Butler G, Cullington A, Hibbert G et al 1987 Anxiety management for persistent generalised anxiety. British Journal of Psychiatry 151:535–542

Butler G, Fennell M, Robson P, Gelder M G 1991 Comparison of behavior therapy and cognitive behavior therapy in the treatment of generalized anxiety disorder. Journal of Consulting & Clinical Psychology 59:167–175

Clark D M 1986 A cognitive approach to panic. Behaviour Research & Therapy 24:461–470

Clark D M, Fairburn C G 1997, Science and practice of cognitive behaviour therapy. Oxford University Press, Oxford

Clark D M, Salkovskis P M, Hackmann A et al 1999 Brief cognitive therapy for panic disorder: a randomized controlled trial. Journal of Consulting & Clinical Psychology 67:583–589

Cottranux J, Note I D, Cungi C et al 1995 A controlled study of cognitive behaviour therapy with busbirone or placebo in panic disorder with agoraphobia. British Journal of Psychiatry 167:635–641

Deakin J F 1998 The role of serotonin in panic, anxiety and depression. International Clinical Pharmacology 13 (suppl 4): S1–S5

Editorial 1982 Goodbye neurosis? Lancet i: 29

Fedoroff I C, Taylor S 2001 Psychological and pharmacological treatments of social phobia: a meta-analysis. Journal of Clinical Psychopharmacology 21:311–324

Finlay-Jones R, Brown G W 1981 Types of stressful life event and the onset of anxiety and depressive disorders. Psychological Medicine 11:803–815

Gale C, Oakley-Browne M 2002 Generalised anxiety disorder. Clinical Evidence 883–895

Gelder M G 1986 Neurosis: another tough old word. British Medical Journal 292:972–973

Goldberg D P, Bridges K, Duncan Jones P, Grayson D 1987 Dimensions of neuroses seen in primary-care settings. Psychological Medicine 17:461–470

Greenberg B D, George M S, Martin J D et al 1997 Effect of prefrontal repetitive transcranial magnetic stimulation in obsessive–compulsive disorder: a preliminary study. American Journal of Psychiatry 154:867–869

Halligan P W, Athwal B S, Oakley D A, Frackowiak R S 2000 Imaging hypnotic paralysis: implications for conversion hysteria. Lancet 355:986–987

Hickie I, Davenport T, Issakidis C, Andrews G 2002 Neurasthenia: prevalence, disability and health care characteristics in the Australian community. British Journal of Psychiatry 181:56–61

Hudson J I, Pope H G 1990 Affective spectrum disorder: Does antidepressant response identify a family of disorders with a common pathophysiology? American Journal of Psychiatry 147:552–564

Hull A M 2002 Neuroimaging findings in post-traumatic stress disorder: systematic review. British Journal of Psychiatry 181:102–110

Jenike M A 1998 Neurosurgical treatment of obsessive–compulsive disorder. British Journal of Psychiatry 173 (suppl 35): 79–90

Johnstone A, Goldberg D 1976 Psychiatric screening in general practice: a controlled trial. Lancet i: 605–608

Johnstone E C, Owens D G, Frith C D et al 1980 Neurotic illness and its response to anxiolytic and antidepressant treatment. Psychological Medicine 10:321–328

Kendell R E 1975 The role of diagnosis in psychiatry. Blackwell Scientific, Oxford

Kendell R E 1989 Clinical validity. Psychological Medicine 19:45–55

Kendler K S 1996 Major depression and generalised anxiety disorder: same genes, (partly) different environments – revisited. British Journal of Psychiatry 168 (suppl 30): 68–75

Kessler R C, McGonagle K A, Zhao S et al 1994a Lifetime and 12-month prevalence of DSM-III-R psychiatric disorders in the United States. Results from the National Comorbidity Survey. Archives of General Psychiatry 51:8–19

Kessler R C, McGonagle K A, Zhao S et al 1994b Lifetime and 12-month prevalence of DSM-III-R psychiatric disorders in the United States. Results from the National Comorbidity Survey. Archives of General Psychiatry 51:8–19

Kessler R C, Sonnega A, Bromet E et al 1995 Posttraumatic stress disorder in the National Comorbidity Survey. Archives of General Psychiatry 52:1048–1060

Kovacs M, Beck A T 1978 Maladaptive cognitive structures in depression. American Journal of Psychiatry 135:525–533

Kumar S, Oakley-Browne M 2002 Panic disorder. Clinical Evidence 906–912

Lidren D M, Watkins P L, Gould R A et al 1994 A comparison of bibliotherapy and group therapy in the treatment of panic disorder. Journal of Consulting & Clinical Psychology 62:865–869

McEvedy C, Beard A 1970 Royal Free Epidemic of 1955: a reconsideration. British Medical Journal 1:7–11

Mann A H, Jenkins R, Belsey E 1981 The twelve-month outcome of patients with neurotic illness in general practice. Psychological Medicine 11:535–550

Marks I M, Gelder M G 1966 Different ages of onset in varieties of phobia. American Journal of Psychiatry 123:218–221

Marks I M, Gelder M G, Edwards G 1968 Hypnosis and desensitization for phobias: a controlled prospective trial. British Journal of Psychiatry 114:1263–1274

Marks I M, Hodgson R, Rachman S 1975 Treatment of chronic obsessive–compulsive neurosis by in-vivo exposure. A two-year follow-up and issues in treatment. British Journal of Psychiatry 127:349–364

Mayou R A 2002 Psychiatric consequences of motor vehicle accidents. Psychiatric Clinics of North America 25:27–41, vi

Meltzer H, Gill B, Pettigrew M, Hinds K 1995 The prevalence of psychiatric morbidity among adults living in private households. HMSO, London

Moene F C, Spinhoven P, Hoogduin K A, van Dyck R 2003 A randomized controlled clinical trial of a hypnosis-based treatment for patients with conversion disorder, motor type. International Journal of Clinical & Experimental Hypnosis 51:29–50

Newman M G, Erickson T, Przeworski A, Dzus E 2003 Self-help and minimal-contact therapies for anxiety disorders: Is human contact necessary for therapeutic efficacy? Journal of Clinical Psychology 59:251–274

Nutt D J 1992 Pharmacoendocrine studies in anxiety. Clinical Neuropharmacology 15 (suppl 1, Pt A): 214A–215A

Nutt D J 2000 The psychobiology of posttraumatic stress disorder. Journal of Clinical Psychiatry 61 (suppl 5): 24–29

Nutt D J, Malizia A L 2001 New insights into the role of the $GABA_A$–benzodiazepine receptor in psychiatric disorder. British Journal of Psychiatry 179:390–396

Ost L G, Westling B E, Hellstrom K 1993 Applied relaxation, exposure in vivo and cognitive methods in the treatment of panic disorder with agoraphobia. Behaviour Research & Therapy 31:383–394

Power K G, Simpson R J, Swanson V, Wallace L A 1990 Controlled comparison of pharmacological and psychological treatment of generalized anxiety disorder in primary care. British Journal of General Practice 40:289–294

Regier D A, Myers J K, Kramer M et al 1984 The NIMH Epidemiologic Catchment Area program. Historical context, major objectives, and study population characteristics. Archives of General Psychiatry 41:934–941

Regier D A, Narrow W E, Rae D S 1990 The epidemiology of anxiety disorders: the Epidemiologic Catchment Area (ECA) experience. Journal of Psychiatric Research 24 (suppl 2): 3–14

Sartorius N, Ustun T B, Lecrubier Y, Wittchenh H U 1996 Depression comorbid with anxiety: results from the WHO study on psychological disorders in primary health care. British Journal of Psychiatry 168 (suppl 30) 38–43

Saxena S, Brody A L, Schwartz J M, Baxter L R 1998 Neuroimaging and frontal-subcortical circuitry in obsessive–compulsive disorder. British Journal of Psychiatry 173 (suppl 35):26–37

Seivewright H, Tyrer P, Johnson T 1998 Prediction of outcome in neurotic disorder: a 5-year prospective study. Psychological Medicine 28:1149–1157

Sharpe M 1996 Chronic fatigue syndrome. Psychiatric Clinics of North America 19:549–574

Stein M B, Walker J R, Hazen A L, Forde D R 1997 Full and partial posttraumatic stress disorder: findings from a community survey. American Journal of Psychiatry 154:1114–1119

Stone J, Sharpe M, Carson A et al 2002a Are functional motor and sensory symptoms really more frequent on the left? A systematic review. Journal of Neurology, Neurosurgery & Psychiatry 73:578–581

Stone J, Zeman A, Sharpe M 2002b Functional weakness and sensory disturbance. Journal of Neurology, Neurosurgery & Psychiatry 73:241–245

True W R, Rice J, Eisen S A et al 1993 A twin study of genetic and environmental contributions to liability for posttraumatic stress symptoms. Archives of General Psychiatry 50:257–264

Tyrer P 1985 Neurosis divisible? Lancet i: 685–688

Tyrer P, Owen R, Dowling S 1983 Gradual withdrawal of diazepam after long-term therapy. Lancet i: 1402–1406

Tyrer P, Murphy S, Riley P 1990 The Benzodiazepine Withdrawal Symptom Questionnaire. Journal of Affective Disorders 19:53–61

Tyrer P, Seivewright H, Johnson T 2003 The core elements of neurosis: mixed anxiety–depression (cothymia) and personality disorder. Journal of Personality Disorders 17:129–138

van Balkom A J, Bakker A, Spinhoven P et al 1997 A meta-analysis of the treatment of panic disorder with or without agoraphobia: a comparison of psychopharmacological, cognitive-behavioral, and combination treatments. Journal of Nervous & Mental Diseases 185:510–516

Welkowitz L A, Papp L A, Cloitre M et al 1991 Cognitive-behavior therapy for panic disorder delivered by psychopharmacologically oriented clinicians. Journal of Nervous & Mental Diseases 179:473–477

Whiting P, Bagnall A, Sowden A et al 2001 Interventions for the treatment and management of chronic fatigue syndrome: a systematic review. Journal of the American Medical Association 286:1360–1368

World Health Organization 1995 Mental illness in general health care: an international study. Wiley, Chichester

Yehuda R, Southwick S M, Nussbaum G et al 1990 Low urinary cortisol excretion in patients with posttraumatic stress disorder. Journal of Nervous & Mental Diseases 178:366–369

22 | Eating disorders

Chris Freeman

INTRODUCTION

This chapter describes the characteristic psychopathology, clinical course and treatment of the two eating disorders that present most commonly to psychiatrists and psychologists: anorexia nervosa (AN) and bulimia nervosa (BN). It also reviews binge eating disorder (BED). It does not cover obesity despite the many common areas of interest and overlap.

The research and clinical fields of obesity and eating disorders have developed quite separately. Obesity research has largely had its roots in physiology and the health risks of obesity, whereas eating disorders have been based in the disciplines of psychiatry and psychology. This split is unfortunate.

HISTORICAL PERSPECTIVE

Eating disorders are widely thought to be a 20th-century Western phenomenon. Several detailed reviews have shown this not to be the case (Parry-Jones & Parry-Jones 1995, Silverman 1995, Russell 1997).

In his book *Treatise on Consumption*, published in 1689, Richard Morton describes cases of anorexia nervosa in an 18-year-old woman and a 16-year-old man. The young woman died, though we do not know if this was because of the treatment or the disorder. The outcome of the young man is unknown. He was advised to abandon his studies, move to the country, take up riding and drink an ass's milk diet. In 1767 Robert Whytt, Professor of Medicine at Edinburgh University, described a case in a young woman which appears to have started with a medically prescribed diet. This patient survived and made a complete recovery. There is a description of slow and gradual re-feeding to avoid undue gastric dilatation.

The French physician Louis-Victor Marcé, most renowned for his descriptions of postpartum disorders, clearly described the syndrome of anorexia nervosa though he did not name it (Marcé 1860). He recommended that such patients could not be treated without removal from the family and entrusting the patient's care to strangers so as to circumvent the habitual circle of obstinate resistance that such patients and their families present. He recommended that if food refusal continued, intimidation and force should be employed and that, if necessary, an oesophageal sound should be used.

The two physicians whose names are most associated with the description of AN are Charles Lasegue and William Gull. Lasegue, from La Pitié in Paris, who described 'de l'anorexie hystérique', warned against giving friendly advice, medicines and, most impor-

tantly, intimidation: 'with hysterical subjects a first medical fault is never repairable'. He advised watchful waiting and described in detail the physical symptoms that would develop and the gradual increase in distress in the family and relatives. A point would be reached where the patient herself would receive a shock to her self-satisfied indifference, and at this point the physician should carefully move in and resume authority. William Gull's papers appeared a year later (Gull 1874). He described three starving teenage patients, Misses A, B and C. Gull too, described gradual re-feeding and thought that the main psychopathology in AN was 'perversions of the ego'.

Pierre Janet divided AN into an obsessional and a hysterical type. He clearly described the loathing that such women felt for their bodies and their refusal to eat in spite of ravenous hunger. This clearly raises the issue that anorexia is not the correct description for all such disorders.

Hilda Bruch was the first modern author to describe anorexia nervosa, and her views still have clear validity and appropriate influence today (Bruch 1965). She described the three core psychological features of the disorder as being

- body image disturbance;
- interoceptive disturbance;
- pervasive feelings of ineffectiveness.

Interoceptive disturbance refers to the inability of such individuals to accurately identify and respond to internal sensations, e.g. hunger, fullness, mood states and sexual arousal. Other important modern influences have been Gerald Russell and Arthur Crisp, whose work will be referred to later in the chapter.

Earlier descriptions of AN do exist, mainly in early religious literature. Such individuals were often starving to purify themselves or to attain closeness to God, and the descriptions lack the characteristic psychopathology described above.

Turning to bulimia nervosa, there is a clear starting point when Russell (1979) described his 'ominous' variant of AN. Since that date, BN has emerged as a common disorder affecting nearly 2% of the female population. In a scholarly text Parry-Jones & Parry-Jones (1991) review the history prior to 1979. Literally translated, bulimia means ox-hunger. They found historical reference to a number of cases occurring in the middle ages and up to the beginning of the 19th century, where there were clear descriptions of rapid ingestion of food, secret eating, night bingeing, self-induced vomiting and all accompanied by normal weight. St Catherine of Siena (died 1380) may have been the first case description of BN. She certainly self-induced vomiting by passing straws into her throat. William Cullen in 1780 described three types of bulimia, one of which (bulimia emetica) is very similar to the modern concept of BN. Other types of bulimia may have been related to head injury and infestation with worms.

Russell (1997), gives three detailed descriptions of these early cases: the case of Nadia (Janet 1903); the case of patient D (Wulff 1932); and the case of Ellen West (Binswanger 1994), all of whom may have met modern diagnostic criteria for BN. These cases clearly describe the bodily loathing, the cravings for food, a history of sexual abuse, a family history of depression, and the use of other methods of purging such as laxatives.

DIAGNOSTIC ISSUES

The clinical syndromes of anorexia nervosa and bulimia nervosa are described separately below, but it is important to realise that there is much overlap (Fig. 22.1) and that, during their eating disorders career, individuals may move from one disorder to the other, not just on one, but on several occasions.

Current diagnostic criteria dictate that anorexia nervosa 'trumps' bulimia nervosa. In other words if an individual meets the diagnostic criteria for AN, then this is the primary diagnosis whether or not they binge or purge. Table 22.1 and Figure 22.2 show diagnostic criteria and a flow chart, respectively, as aids to differentiating AN, BN and BED.

The most common direction of movement is from anorexia to bulimia, with some 50% of those who initially meet the diagnostic criteria for AN graduating to bulimia. Movement in the opposite direction — that is, an individual starting with normal weight bulimia and then developing AN — does occur but is less common. Boxes 22.1 and 22.2 give the diagnostic criteria for the two main disorders according to ICD-10. The criteria according to DSM-IV are similar but less detailed for AN. ICD-10 requires a body mass index of 17.5 or less whereas DSM-IV only requires a body weight of 85% or less of that which would be expected. ICD-10 gives more detailed criteria for the symptoms to be expected in pre-pubertal AN. DSM-IV subdivides AN into a restricting and a binge eating/purging type.

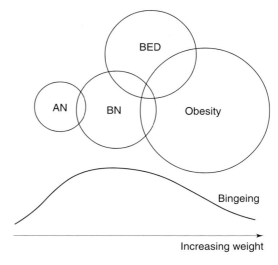

	AN	BN	BED
Annual prevalence	1% or less	2–4% depending on population	4–5% depending on definition
Dietary restraint (all 3 groups dieting)	↓↓↓	↓↓	↓
Bingeing	+	+++	++
Purging	++	+++	−

Fig. 22.1
Relationship of eating disorders to each other. AN, anorexia nervosa; BED, binge eating disorder; BN, bulimia nervosa.

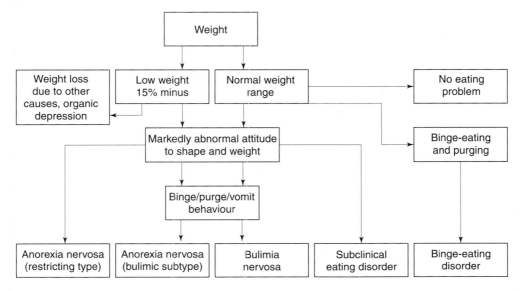

Fig. 22.2
Diagnostic flow chart for anorexia nervosa, bulimia nervosa and binge eating disorder.

Table 22.1   Diagnostic criteria for anorexia nervosa, bulimia nervosa and binge eating disorder

	Anorexia nervosa (restricting subtype)	Anorexia nervosa (bulimic subtype)	Bulimia nervosa	Binge eating disorder
Characteristic extreme concerns about shape and weight	Yes	Yes	Yes	Maybe
Behaviour designed to control shape and weight	Yes	Yes	Yes	No
Bulimic episodes	No	Yes	Yes	Yes
Low weight according to population norms	Yes	Yes	No	No
Amenorrhoea	Yes	Yes	Maybe	No

The ruling that anorexia nervosa 'trumps' bulimia nervosa is adopted.

Box 22.1   ICD-10 diagnostic criteria for anorexia nervosa

For a definite diagnosis all of the following are required:

1. Body weight is maintained at least 15% below that expected (either lost or never achieved), or Quetelet's body mass index is 17.5 or less. Body weight is maintained at least 15% below that expected (either lost or never achieved), or Quetelet's body mass index is 17.5 or less. Prepubertal patients may show failure to make the expected weight gain during the period of growth
2. The weight loss is self-induced by avoidance of 'fattening foods'. One or more of the following may also be present: self-induced vomiting; self-induced purging; excessive exercise; use of appetite suppressants and/or diuretics
3. There is body image distortion in the form of a specific psychopathology whereby a dread of fatness persists as an intrusive, overvalued idea and the patient imposes a low weight threshold on himself or herself
4. A widespread endocrine disorder involving the hypothalamic-pituitary-gonadal axis is manifest in women as amenorrhea and in men as a loss of sexual interest and potency. (An apparent exception is the persistence of vaginal bleeds in anorexic women who are receiving replacement hormonal therapy, most commonly taken as a contraceptive pill.) There may also be elevated levels of growth hormone, raised levels of cortisol, changes in the peripheral metabolism of the thyroid hormone, and abnormalities of insulin secretion
5. If onset is prepubertal, the sequence of pubertal events is delayed or even arrested (growth ceases; in girls the breasts do not develop and there is a primary amenorrhoea; and in boys the genitals remain juvenile). With recovery, puberty is often completed normally, but the menarche is late

Atypical anorexia nervosa. This term should be used for those individuals in whom one or more of the key features of anorexia nervosa, such as amenorrhoea or significant weight loss, is absent, but who otherwise present a fairly typical clinical picture. Such people are usually encountered in psychiatric liaison services in general hospitals or in primary care. Patients who have all the key symptoms but to only a mild degree may also be best described by this term. This term should not be used for eating disorders that resemble anorexia nervosa but that are due to known physical illness

---

Box 22.2   ICD-10 diagnostic criteria for bulimia nervosa

For a definite diagnosis all of the following are required:

1. There is a persistent preoccupation with eating, and an irresistible craving for food: the patient succumbs to episodes of overeating in which large amounts of food are consumed in short periods of time
2. The patients attempts to counteract the 'fattening' effects of food by one or more of the following: self-induced vomiting; purgative abuse; alternating periods of starvation; use of drugs such as appetite suppressants, thyroid preparations, or diuretics. When bulimia occurs in diabetic patients they may choose to neglect their insulin treatment
3. The psychopathology consists of a morbid dread of fatness, and the patient sets herself or himself a sharply defined weight threshold, well below the premorbid weight that constitutes the optimum or healthy weight in the opinion of the physician. There is often, but not always, a history of an earlier episode of anorexia nervosa, the interval between the two disorders ranging from a few months to several years. This earlier episode may have been fully expressed, or may have assumed a minor cryptic form with a moderate loss of weight and/or a transient phase of amenorrhoea

Atypical bulimia nervosa This terms should be used for those individuals in whom one or more of the key features for bulimia nervosa is absent but who otherwise present a fairly typical clinical picture. Most commonly this applies to people with normal or even excessive weight but with typical periods of overeating followed by vomiting or purging. Partial syndromes together with depressive symptoms are also not uncommon, but if the depressive symptoms justify a separate diagnosis of a depressive disorder, two diagnoses should be made

---

For BN, DSM-IV has stricter criteria for a binge in that it has to occur in a discrete period of time (within 2 hours). ICD-10 describes more fully the common earlier history of AN, which may have been fully expressed or cryptic. DSM-IV divides BN into a purging type where there is self-induced vomiting or the misuse of laxatives, diuretics or enemas, and a non-purging type where binge eating alternates with other compensatory behaviours such as fasting or excessive exercise.

Binge eating disorder does not yet have separate diagnostic criteria in either DSM-IV or ICD-10, though papers are now regularly appearing on the aetiology, epidemiology and treatment of this disorder. There are research criteria for BED DSM-IV, and these are given in Box 22.3. It can be seen that the main differences are concerned with the lack of inappropriate compensatory behaviours such as purging, fasting and excessive exercise.

As far as other atypical eating disorders are concerned, DSM-IV has only one category — eating disorder not otherwise specified (EONOS) — whereas ICD-10 has five: atypical anorexia nervosa; atypical bulimia nervosa; overeating without other psychological disturbances; vomiting associated with other psychological disturbances; and other eating disorders. There is very little research on this group, and the term 'atypical' includes a number of cases who have partial syndromes of either AN or BN, sometimes referred to as subthreshold disorders. Other disorders classified here would be overeating that leads to obesity, vomiting that may occur in hypochondriacal or dissociative disorders, and other types of psychogenic vomiting. Pica of non-organic origin occurring in adults, and psychogenic loss of appetite which is not caused by major depression, would also be classified here.

The diagnostic criteria for all these disorders are continually under review, and it will be interesting to see what emerges in DSM-V. Simple changes can make major differences to the size of different diagnostic groups. It was only a few years ago that the diagnostic criteria for AN were altered. The threshold for the amount of weight loss required used to be 25% or greater and is now 15%. This is clearly one way to make a disorder much more common overnight. We still do not know what the optimal weight threshold is and whether amenorrhea is essential. Conversely there are moves to tighten the criteria for bulimia nervosa and to only include the group currently described under DSM-IV's binge/purge type. If this were to happen, the non-purging type of BN would probably be included with BED. Details of the incidence of anorexia nervosa given in Table 22.2.

Box 22.3 DSM-IV research criteria for binge eating disorder

A. Recurrent episodes of binge eating. An episode of binge eating is characterised by both of the following:
 (1) Eating, in a discrete period of time (e.g. within any 2 hour period), an amount of food that is definitely larger than most people would eat in a similar period of time under similar circumstances; and
 (2) A sense of lack of control over eating during the episode (e.g. a feeling that one cannot stop eating or control what or how much one is eating)
B. The binge-eating episodes are associated with three (or more) of the following:
 (1) Eating more rapidly than normal
 (2) Eating until feeling uncomfortably full
 (3) Eating large amounts of food when not feeling physically hungry
 (4) Eating alone because of being embarrassed by how much one is eating
 (5) Feeling disgusted with oneself, depressed or very guilty after overeating
C. Marked distress regarding binge eating is present.
D. The binge eating occurs, on average at least 2 days a week for 6 months.
 Note: The method of determining frequency differs from that used for bulimia nervosa: future research should address whether the preferred method of setting a frequency threshold is counting the number of days on which binges occur or counting the number of episodes of binge eating.
E. The binge eating is not associated with the regular use of inappropriate compensatory behaviours (e.g. purging, fasting, excessive exercise) and does not occur exclusively during the course of anorexia nervosa or bulimia nervosa.

ANOREXIA NERVOSA

Clinical presentation

The core feature of AN is a profound psychological disturbance which centres on an overwhelming concern about body size, shape and weight. Sufferers feel fat even when emaciated, are terrified of any weight gain and preoccupied with elaborate plans to reduce weight further. Such psychopathology has variously been described as hysterical, a phobia of weight gain, an obsessional symptom and clearly delusional. To some extent it simply represents a marked exaggeration of ideas that are widespread in our society, and it is perhaps best conceptualised as a set of overvalued ideas. Multiple theories exist as to why these beliefs should be so firmly held. They include fear of maturation, fear of secondary sexual characteristics, fear of separation usually from a maternal figure, fear of oral impregnation, through to addictive and

Table 22.2 Incidence of anorexia nervosa

Area	Authors	Period	Annual incidence per million population
Southern Sweden	Theander (1970)	1931–1940	0.08
		1941–1950	0.19
		1951–1960	0.45
North-east Scotland	Kendell et al (1973)	1966–1969	1.60
	Szmukler et al (1986)	1978–1982	4.06
Zurich canton	Willi & Grossman (1983)	1963–1965	0.55
		1973–1975	1.12
	Willi et al (1990)	1983–1985	1.43
Monroe County	Kendell et al (1973)	1960–1969	0.37
New York State, USA	Jones et al (1980)	1970–1976	0.64
Rochester, Minnesota, USA	Lucas et al* (1991)	1950–1954	4.63
		1980–1984	14.20

* Increase in incidence occurred principally in females 10–19 years old.

biological models. (See the section on aetiology, below.) What patients themselves nearly always say, is that the central feature for them is that they fear loss of control and that this is countered by the increased sense of self-control, from strict dieting and from being able to determine one's size and shape. This of course is one of the many paradoxes of AN — while trying to achieve that sense of autonomy and self-control sufferers end up trapped in a disorder which profoundly controls them. Patients rarely say that their starvation was designed to make them more attractive to others, though they do feel that gaining even a small amount of weight would make them even less attractive. Weight gain and 'fat' in particular come to symbolise laziness, self-indulgence, lack of control, and self-loathing.

As well as self-induced starvation, there are a whole range of other behaviours designed to reduce weight. These are summarised in Box 22.4. Many of these behaviours develop into very obsessional or ritualistic patterns, so that exercise has to be for a prescribed number of minutes every day and can never be less than that carried out the day before.

The intense dietary restraint is characterised by a narrowing of the range of foods eaten, a complete avoidance of certain foods which are seen as 'fattening', and usually some method of calorie counting with a predetermined daily calorie limit of well under 1000 calories.

The body image disturbance is an unusual and not very well understood symptom. There are at least two components: first, a perceptual distortion of body size and shape so that either the whole body or specific parts of the body appear larger or fatter to the sufferer. Anorexia nervosa sufferers can accurately gauge the size of other people's bodies and of inanimate objects but not of their own. There is some evidence that they distort meal size as well. They will often report that when caught unaware by a mirror image, they did not recognise themselves and truly saw a thin, emaciated figure. The second component is of body disparagement. This can be generalised or again focused on specific parts. There is an intense dislike amounting to hatred of the patient's own body. (For a detailed review, see Smeets 1997.)

General psychopathology

Depressed mood and lability of mood are common features, and in more chronic cases hopelessness and thoughts of suicide may be present. Anxiety symptoms, usually related to situations which

Mr A B had been a junior cross-country champion. Even at 14-years he had prided himself in keeping his body fat below 10%. This was measured regularly by his coach using skin callipers. He did not have to restrict his intake, as he ran a half marathon 5 days per week and swam for 2 hours on the other 2 days. At 15-years, while studying for his 'O' Grade exams, he had to exercise less and compensated by reducing his intake. By 16½ years he had the full blown syndrome of anorexia nervosa with a BMI of 13 and a weight of 35 kg. He achieved straight 'A's in 'O' Grades and 'A' levels and entrance to medical school. He presented for treatment towards the end of his first year at medical school having not been picked up at university entrance and with the headmaster's reference from his school mentioning nothing of his problems. His presenting complaint was because of pain in his ankles. Examination showed that he had bilateral stress fractures of both ankles, moderately severe osteoporosis and marked lack of secondary sexual characteristics. By this time he was existing on a diet of vitamin pills and white boiled fish. His parents would deliver a crate of fish weekly to his hall of residence. He would eat only one meal per day would boil the fish for 2 hours, standing with a whole roll of paper towel dabbing the globules of oil and fat that rose to the surface as the fish was being boiled. He could no longer run but he walked at least 5 miles a day in extreme pain. He had kept up his pattern of severely restricted eating for over 4 years, never losing control.

Repeated inpatient treatment programmes in various specialists units around the country produced only modest and short-term improvement, with weight gains of 6–7 kg being lost within 6 months of discharge.

Fifteen years later, Mr A B has chronic but stable AN with a weight which fluctuates between 37 and 40 kg, a very restricted and stereotyped eating pattern, a rigid plan of exercise, and severe osteoporosis despite several years of testosterone replacement. He did complete a degree though not in medicine and leads a lonely, isolated life dominated by routine and ritual. He would clearly meet the diagnostic criteria for obsessive–compulsive disorder.

involve eating, are also encountered and many sufferers develop marked socially phobic symptoms, not being able to eat in public at all. Outside interests are often reduced, and there is usually marked social withdrawal. Obsessional features may be present and frequently cause food preparation and eating to become slow and ritualistic. Work or school performances are often maintained despite increasing impairments of concentration and marked emaciation.

The contribution of starvation — the Minnesota experiments

All those working with patients suffering from eating disorders should be familiar with a key set of studies carried out towards the end of the Second World War and published over 50 years ago by Ancel Keys (Keys et al 1950). Thirty-six men who were the youngest, healthiest and most psychologically normal from 100 volunteers were selected to take part in this study of starvation. By volunteering, the men avoided military service. During the first 3 months they ate normally while their behaviour, personality and eating patterns were monitored. During the next 6 months, the

Case History 2: Ms C D

Ms C D presented at the age of 16 years with severe anorexia nervosa but with only a 9-month history. She had gone on a diet when her first relationship had ended just after her 15th birthday. Other triggering factors appeared to be the loss of a close girlfriend at her female boarding school who had become jealous of her relationship with her boyfriend, and her parents deciding to move to Spain leaving her and her youngest sister at boarding school in the UK. She had lost just under 17 kg in 9 months and had amenorrhoea for 6 months.

Physical examination showed she was emaciated, covered in fine downy hair (lanugo) and with bright orange palms and soles (carotenaemia). Her blood pressure was low, with a bradycardia of under 50 bpm, and she was markedly depressed. She had not been compulsively exercising or using any other weight control measures.

For the previous 3 months she had been existing on cups of tea and coffee with skimmed milk, oxo cubes and plates of boiled vegetables. She would chew the vegetables for long periods but not swallow them, spitting each mouthful out after approximately 10 minutes of mastication.

Her Dexa bone density scan showed no osteoporosis. She had been a very fit and active adolescent with an early puberty and menarche and had fully mineralised her bones by the age of 16 years.

Her initial weight loss had been profoundly rewarding. Two other boys in the local village had shown interest in her and she had been able to brush them aside. Her status with her peers at school increased and she moved from just being able to get into size 12 clothes to easily being able to fit into a size 10. She could even wear her younger sisters' clothes. Her more severe weight loss caused her mother to return from Spain and to rent a house close to the school.

Treatment consisted of 10 weekly outpatient sessions followed by monthly follow-ups for the next 9 months. Elements of treatment were the institution of a regular meal plan, self-monitoring with diaries, and two extended family interviews, for one of which her father came back from Spain. She also had repeated medical investigations, the results which were fed back to her in detail. The individual sessions used both cognitive, behavioural and interpersonal techniques, examining each significant relationship in detail and using cognitive therapy to help her identify her dysfunctional attitudes and beliefs and to challenge them.

Weight gain occurred slowly over the next year and levelled out at about 4 kg less than her pre-disorder weight, giving her a BMI of just under 20.

Follow-up over the next 9 years has shown no recurrence of her eating disorder apart from a brief 3-month period of binge eating towards the end of first year at university, again associated with the break-up of a relationship. Menstruation returned within 9 months and fertility has not been impaired. Ms C D, now aged 24 years, has been in a stable and sexually active relationship for the past 2 years.

Interestingly the first annual bone scan showed a marked drop in bone density into the osteoporotic range, even though weight had been largely restored by that time. Follow-up showed it was 7 years before she regained the bone density she had had at age 16 years. This occurred without specific treatment.

loss, there was a further 3 months of rehabilitation/re-feeding with a 9-month post-starvation monitoring occurring in some subjects. The importance of this study is that many of the symptoms thought to be characteristic of AN occurred in these men. When treating sufferers it is important to appreciate just how much of the psychological and behavioural symptoms are a *result* of starvation state and not a cause of it.

The men became increasingly preoccupied by food, they found it difficult to carry out their usual daily activities because they were plagued by incessant thoughts of food and eating. Food became the principal topic of conversation or reading and of daydreams. The men began to smuggle bits of food out of the dining room, hid food and ate food in secret in long rituals. Men who had no previous interest in food or cooking became intensely interested in menus, cookbooks, dietetics and even food production. The men reported getting vicarious pleasure from watching other subjects eat. Hoarding was not just confined to food but included cooking utensils, recipes and even non-food-related items. The men spent much of the day planning how they would eat their daily allotment of food. They made unusual concoctions of food, often ate in silence and ate in a quite ritualistic way, dawdling over food so that even small meals would take several hours.

Other behaviours such as rummaging through garbage cans, binge eating and marked increase in coffee intake were reported in some subjects. Mood swings were common, and about a quarter of the men had significant depression. Irritability and frequent outbursts of anger were common. Two subjects developed more serious psychiatric symptoms requiring hospital admission.

During the re-feeding phase the behavioural changes did not immediately reverse. In some men they persisted throughout the follow-up period. Some men became more depressed when re-feeding. One man chopped three fingers off his hand in a fit of severe depression.

Marked social and sexual changes also occurred, so that the men became progressively more withdrawn and isolated with little sense of humour or comradeship. Most men responded to increasing starvation with a decrease in physical activity, but a few exercised deliberately, feeling that they would be able to eat a little more if they did so.

Physical complications

Details of these are given in Table 22.3. For a comprehensive review, see Sharp & Freeman (1993). The main laboratory abnormalities are also shown in the table.

Most of the many complications associated with AN are found in uncomplicated starvation, and are reversed by return to a normal healthy diet, but there are important differences between anorexia and starvation. In anorexia, protein intake is usually adequate, but carbohydrates, fats and therefore calories are lacking. Vitamin deficiencies are uncommon. The complications are numerous. For a detailed review, see Sharp & Freeman (1993).

Cardiac abnormalities may occur at some stage, in over 80% of anorexic patients. These include bradycardia, tachycardia, hypotension, ventricular arrhythmias, cardiac failure and a variety of ECG changes. Congestive cardiac failure may occur as a terminal event in the disorder but is also a well-recognised complication of re-feeding, first described in survivors of the concentration and prisoner of war camps in the Second World War.

Most of the gastrointestinal complications, such as oesophagitis, erosions and ulcers, are a result of frequent exposure to gastric

men were restricted to approximately half their former food intake and lost on average a quarter of their former weight. They were thus starved down into the AN range. After 6 months of weight

System	Starvation	Bingeing/purging/vomiting
Cardiovascular	Bradycardia	Arrhythmias
	Hypotension	Cardiac failure
	Sudden death	Sudden death
	Mitral valve dysfunction	
Renal	Mild pitting oedema	Severe oedema
	Electrolyte abnormalities: hypophosphataemia, hypomagnesaemia, hypocalcaemia	Electrolyte abnormalities: hypokalaemia, hyponatraemia, hypochloraemia, metabolic alkalosis (vomitors), metabolic acidosis (with laxative abuse) hypomagnesaemia, hypophosphataemia, hypocalcaemia
	Renal calculi	Renal calculi
	Hypokalaemic nephropathy	Hypokalaemic nephropathy
	Proteinuria	
	Reduced glomerular filtration	
Gastrointestinal	Parotid swelling	Parotid swelling
		Oesophageal erosion
		Oesophageal/gastric perforation
	Delayed gastric emptying	Gastric/duodenal ulcers
	Re-feeding pancreatitis	Pancreatitis
	Nutritional hepatitis	
	Constipation	Constipation, steatorrhoea
Skeletal	Osteoporosis	Osteoporosis
	Pathological fractures	Pathological fractures
	Short stature	
Endocrine	Amenorrhoea	
	Low LHRH, LH and FSH	
	Low oestrogen and progesterone	
	Low tri-iodothyronine (T_3)	
	High cortisol	
	High fasting growth hormone	
	Erratic vasopressin release	
Haematological	Anaemia	
	Leukopenia	Leukopenia, lymphocytosis
	Thrombocytopenia	
	Bone marrow hypoplasia	
	Reduced serum complement levels	
	Low ESR	
Neurological	Generalised seizures	Generalised seizures
	Confusional states	Confusional states
	EEG abnormalities	EEG abnormalities
	Peripheral neuropathies	Peripheral neuropathies
	Ventricular enlargement	
Metabolic	Impaired temperature regulation	Impaired temperature regulation
	Hypercholesterolaemia	Hypercholesterolaemia
	Hypercarotenaemia	Hypercarotenaemia
	Hypoproteinaemia	Hypoproteinaemia
	Impaired glucose tolerance	Fasting hypoglycaemia
	High β-hydroxybutyrate	High β-hydroxybutyrate
	High free fatty acids	High free fatty acids
	Impaired calcium metabolism	
Dermatological	Lanugo, brittle hair and nails	Calluses on dorsum of hands

acid. In clinical practice delayed gastric emptying is responsible for the feelings of fullness and bloating reported by patients after eating which are often wrongly interpreted as the deposition of fat. Pancreatic disease is uncommon but occasional cases of acute pancreatitis have been reported in the re-feeding phase.

Liver changes are common in protein-calorie malnutrition. Nutritional hepatitis, manifested by low serum protein and raised serum bilirubin levels along with raised lactate dehydrogenase and alkaline phosphatase occur in about one-third of subjects.

Pancytopenia is common in severe anorexia, with mild anaemia and thrombocytopenia reported in about one-third of patients and leucopenia in up to two-thirds.

Patients with early-onset AN tend to be shorter than their peers, and bone mineralisation can be markedly impaired during adolescence. Osteoporosis and pathological fractures are common, and demonstrable osteoporosis can occur within 2 years of the onset of AN.

Anorexia nervosa is one of the most lethal of all psychiatric disorders. The mortality rate is over 20% at 30-year follow-up (Theander 1985). More recent follow-up studies show mortality rates of 5–10% at 10 years. Two-thirds of fatalities result from the direct effects of the disorder, one-third from suicide.

Outcome of course of anorexia nervosa and bulimia nervosa

Sullivan (2002) has produced a useful review of outcome which is summarised in Table 22.4. He estimated the risk of death from AN to be 6% per decade. Recovery rates in those who survive were similar for AN and BN, with little evidence of excess mortality for BN.

Aetiology of anorexia nervosa

Most women who suffer from this order will talk about control as being the central issue. They will describe the sense of power and achievement they get from self-induced starvation and denial, particularly when they feel that the rest of their life is out of control. Nevertheless it is clear that AN does not develop from a single cause. When thinking about the aetiology a number of factors have to be considered (Fig. 22.3). The disorder is overwhelmingly one of women; the majority of cases start in adolescence, with the average age of onset being 16 years, but it can start at any time from childhood to late middle age. Strict self-starvation is a key feature, but most women do not have a history of obesity. No biological or organic cause has been found, and at present we have to conclude that the disorder is mainly psychological in origin.

Genetic factors are probably involved, as both AN and BN run in families. The evidence from twin studies suggests that specific genetic factors are more important in AN — and particularly in restricting AN, where the concordance rate from monozygotic twins is approximately 65% and for dizygotic is 32%. The vulnera-

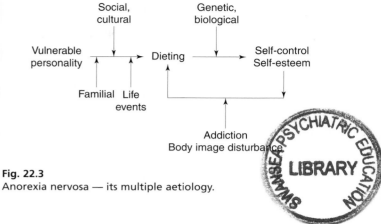

Fig. 22.3
Anorexia nervosa — its multiple aetiology.

bility to AN appears to be a specific one and not a general predisposition to 'neuroticism' or psychiatric disorder. The non-affected twins of monozygotic pairs appear remarkably normal in contrast to those with BN, where there seems to be an inheritance of a more general predisposition with links with substance abuse, affective disorder and obesity. The finding of high rates of perfectionism in the non-affected dizygotic twins has led to the view that this could be the vulnerability trait.

Sociodemographic factors, social class, parental age, family composition and family size have all been suggested as contributing factors to the development of this disorder. However, none of these has been found consistently across studies. An examination of social class distribution by Gard & Freeman (1996) found that it is only in clinic samples that there is an excess of social classes 1–3 and that, in community samples, eating disorders are spread evenly across the social classes. Of the other factors mentioned above, only parental age has some support, with several studies consistently finding that AN sufferers have older parents.

Adverse events

Although childhood sexual and physical abuse are common, they do not appear to be more common than in other psychiatric disorders, nor is there an excess of parental loss due to death or break up of a family.

Individual and family pathology

One way of viewing the psychology of AN is to see it as an adaptive process. Self-induced starvation serves many positive roles for a young woman, providing an increased sense of control and autonomy relating to her own body while at the same time developing increased dependence on her nuclear family. Basic beliefs relating to perfectionism, high achievement and ascetisim are all enhanced, while maturational tasks such as individuation and separation are avoided. Secondary sexual characteristics do not develop, and a peri-pubertal state of development is ensured. It may well be that these psychological factors initiate the disorder and then biological and addictive processes take over, ensuring the clinicity and resistance to treatment.

Family studies, particularly those reported by Minuchin and Selvini-Palazoli were very influential in the 1970s and 1980s. Certain characteristic family styles and patterns of interaction were said to increase the likelihood of producing an anorexic daughter. The concept of the anorexogenic mother probably has as much

Table 22.4	Outcomes of anorexia nervosa and bulimia nervosa	
Domain	Intermediate to long-term outcome of index disorder (10 years) after clinical referral	
	Anorexia nervosa	Bulimia nervosa
Death	10%	–1%
Persisting index eating disorder	10%	10%
Subthreshold eating disorder	15%	20%
'Crossover' (i.e. anorexia nervosa to bulimia nervosa or vice versa)	15%*	–1%
No clinical eating disorder at follow-up	50%	70%

Estimates are qualitative approximations from the accumulated literature, from Sullivan (2002).
* About half would have met criteria for bulimia nervosa at some point.

validity as the schizophrenogenic mother and has probably done as much harm. Mothers of anorexic girls already feel profoundly guilty and responsible, and theories that blame them are hardly useful therapeutically. Our own studies (Blair & Freeman 1995) comparing normal families, families with a cystic fibrosis child and families with an anorexic daughter showed little difference between the three groups. The most important finding was that family disturbance increased with the chronicity of the disorder, suggesting it was the disorder which largely caused the family disturbance rather than vice versa. We did not find that concepts such as rigidity, enmeshment or weak generational boundaries differentiated the groups. It seems much more likely that these were features of upper middle-class families whether or not they have an ill child.

Biological factors

Hypothalamic disturbance has been most frequently cited as the most likely biological factor contributing to aetiology. However, the hypothalamic dysfunction found is similar to that found in starvation due to other causes and it tends to return to normal when the patient regains weight. Several studies have found neuropsychological deficits such as reduced vigilance and attention span, impairment of visuospatial processing, and impaired associate learning. Again, most of these seem to return to normal limits with weight gain. Brain scans have found significant sulcal widening and/or ventricular enlargement which again appears reversible with renutrition. In a minority of cases these abnormalities do not reverse, even though the degree of abnormality was related to the rapidity of the original weight loss. The most interesting findings are those recently reported by Gordon et al (1997). In a small sample of children and adolescents with AN, 13 of 15 patients had unilateral temporal lobe hypoperfusion as demonstrated by regional cerebral blood flow radio-isotope scans. These findings are of particular interest because the changes are unilateral and therefore unlikely to be due directly to starvation. Attempts to link these abnormalities with specific psychopathology such as impairment of visuospatial processing, leading to vulnerability to body image distortion, are at present complete speculation but nevertheless interesting. The potential role of leptin, a protein produced by fat, has excited much interest in the genetics and development of obesity, but so far its role in AN and BN is unclear.

Treatment of anorexia nervosa

There is surprisingly little research evidence to guide us in treatment. There have been very few controlled trials, and most of the published work consists of lengthy descriptions of treatment programmes with a striking lack of detail about their effectiveness. One exception to this is the series of trials from the Maudsley Hospital comparing family with individual therapy and different types of family intervention. We therefore have to be guided by what is seen as current best clinical practice. There is general agreement that no one treatment modality is sufficient and that, for most moderately severe and severe cases, combined treatment approaches are required and that it is a matter of skill to introduce these elements in sequence so as to provide a coherent treatment programme.

Perhaps the single most skilled task is to engage the patient in treatment in the first place. Many anorexia sufferers feel very strongly that they do not want or need treatment. The following general principles represent the consensus of most specialists.

- The initial interview/assessment and subsequent engagement and treatment is of vital importance and requires both time and skill.
- Psychological treatment/psychotherapy is the treatment of choice. Experience in treating such patients is probably much more important than the type of psychotherapy used.
- Inpatient treatment may be required for some patients, and a small number will require compulsory treatment to stop them dying.
- Psychological treatment is of little benefit and difficult to administer in severely starving patients who need a degree of weight restoration.
- The treatment must first involve significant others (family of origin and/or partner), though this does not need to be in the form of systematised family therapy.
- Treatment needs to be flexible and adapted to suit the patient's needs. Treatment approaches in the past have probably been too rigid.
- Treatment will not be brief, and treatment services need to be organised so as to provide continuity of care.

Inpatient treatment

Weight restoration is the primary goal for emaciated and medically compromised anorexic patients. However, Hsu (1988) has demonstrated that weight restoration to normal or near normal weight alone is a weak predictor of long-term outcome.

It is difficult to tease out the active components of treatment from comprehensive treatment regimens which often include supervised eating, medication, nutritional education, individual and/or family psychotherapy, operant conditioning methods and coercion. Agras & Kraemer (1984) described 21 published treatment studies which they classified into drug therapy, behaviour therapy and medical therapy. They found that medication did not add benefit to hospitalisation and that behavioural therapy produced more rapid weight gain. Touyz et al (1984) compared the effects of strict versus lenient operant conditioning programmes on weight gain in a sample of 65 anorexic inpatients. The lenient programme produced just as much weight gain and was far more acceptable than the strict programme. It was also associated with higher motivation to participate in other aspects of treatment and required less nursing time.

Indications for inpatient treatments include serious physical complications or suicidal risk. When weight loss is extreme, with a BMI below 13, or rapid then admission should be considered. Patients can survive at extremely low weights providing the weight is stable and providing there is careful monitoring of white cell count, haemoglobin, electrolytes and creatinine kinase. However, patients whose weight loss has been rapid, especially after previous re-feeding can be medically compromised at much higher weights. Sometimes hospitalisation is needed to separate the patient from the family or partner where there is a high degree of negative expressed emotion, or where the family feels overwhelmed or helpless. Coercive procedures should be reserved for the very small group of non-compliant patients whose situation is truly life threatening; if possible they should be avoided altogether.

Involuntary treatment

The legal system in most countries allows the committal of severely emaciated anorexic patients to hospital against their will, and patients should not be allowed to die. There is, however, currently an active debate as to whether there could be occasions when it might be appropriate to let severely ill chronic patients who have had unsuccessful treatment die with dignity rather than be subjected to yet another episode of what would almost certainly be coercive re-feeding.

Drug treatment

Nearly all studies in which the efficacy of different types of psychotropic medication have been assessed have shown very disappointing results. Antipsychotics, antidepressants, lithium, and minor tranquillisers have all been shown to have little or no value. There has been some recent work using fluoxetine showing that this may aid re-feeding in hospitalised anorexics. This may appear a paradoxical result given that fluoxetine tends to cause weight loss and increase satiety. If it is effective it may work because it decreases obsessional preoccupation with food and therefore anxiety around eating.

Individual and family therapy

There have been no satisfactory studies comparing different models of individual psychotherapy either for weight-restored anorexics or for anorexics treated from the start with psychotherapy. Psychotherapy should not be used as a sole treatment but should be combined with appropriate medical care.

Russell et al (1987) showed that one group of patients, those with early-onset anorexia (before the age of 19 years) and with a short history (less than 3 years) were very much better 1 year after discharge from hospital if they had received family therapy as opposed to individual supportive psychotherapy during that year. However, another group in this study, those with late onset, did slightly better with individual supportive therapy rather than family therapy. The most important finding overall of this study is that at 5 year follow-up those young patients who had received family therapy were doing better both at 1 year and at 5 years. A subsequent study compared conjoint with separated family therapy and found that patients in high expressed emotion families did better with separated family therapy in terms of both engagement and outcome (Eisler et al 2000).

Although cognitive therapy has been widely proposed as part of a multidimensional treatment approach to anorexia, there is only limited evidence for its efficacy (Channon et al 1989), with no difference between behaviour therapy and cognitive therapy. Two studies have compared cognitive-behaviour therapy (CBT) with nutritional counselling: Serfaty et al (1999) and Pike (unpublished). In Serfaty's study 100% of those allocated to nutritional counselling dropped out and refused further contact, where as 92% of CBT patients persisted. Pike found similar findings on engagement, and 44% of CBT patients had good outcome compared with 6% of those receiving nutritional counselling. A large multicentre study is now under way in the USA. Currently, there is a move towards day patient or partial hospitalisation rather than inpatient treatment. This is led partly by cost considerations and partly because of the disappointing results of inpatient treatment, the high relapse rate and repeated need for readmission. There is no doubt that some patients respond to inpatient re-feeding by 'eating their way out of hospital'. Although such treatment may seem to be partially successful because weight has been restored, the patient feels even more guilt and self-loathing and feels a failure not just as an individual but as an anorexic, often resolving to starve even more vehemently as soon as discharge is achieved.

EATING DISORDERS IN MALES

Community-based studies have shown ratios of 1 male case to 6 female cases, of both AN and BN, compared with ratios of 1:10 in clinical samples. In the pre-adolescent age group, the ratio is about 1:4.

A diagnosis of AN is probably more often missed in males. There is no obvious marker such as cessation of menstruation, and loss of sex drive occurs gradually with weight loss as testosterone falls.

So called 'reverse anorexia nervosa' or 'muscle dysmorphia' occurs almost exclusively in males. These men subjectively perceive themselves as thin even when highly muscular. Anabolic steroid use is common.

Differences from female sufferers include more rapid and severe development of osteoporosis (Andersen et al 2000), a history of gender identity conflicts, a higher rate of homosexuality and a higher rate of premorbid obesity (50%). Carlat et al (1997) provides a good review.

Treatment outcomes in men are similar to those in women but men often feel isolated in all-female programmes.

BULIMIA NERVOSA

As previously described, Russell (1979) proposed the term bulimia nervosa to describe a disorder, first recognised in the mid 1970s, in which young women present with bouts of uncontrolled overeating. Many other names were at first used, including bulimarexia, dietary chaos syndrome, bulimia, and binge eating syndrome. The term bulimia nervosa is now the accepted and preferred one. It emphasises the close links between this disorder and anorexia nervosa and it specifies the 'nervosa' part of the syndrome characterised by drive for thinness, distorted body image, and body disparagement. The ICD-10 diagnostic criteria are given in Table 22.1.

Clinical features

Like AN, this is predominantly a female disorder, and in most clinics male cases of BN are rarer than those of AN. It is a disorder of young people, tending to start most commonly in mid-adolescence. Cases present for treatment somewhat later: typically in the early 20s. Between a third and a half of cases have previously been through a clear cut episode of AN or a subclinical episode. The term cryptic anorexia nervosa has been used to describe these latter cases. These are women who would have been at the upper end of the normal weight range for height or mildly obese, who diet so that when they present they are in the middle of the normal weight range. They are classified as normal-weight BN but in fact have engaged in marked dietary restraint which has triggered off their binge episodes.

Specific psychopathology

The clinical picture is very similar to that found in AN, with overvalued ideas concerning shape and weight, and numerous methods of weight control including intense dieting, self-induced vomiting, laxative and diuretic use. There are the same preoccupations with food, eating, shape and weight. There is, however, often less of a preoccupation with intensive exercising compared with AN.

The two main distinguishing features from AN are normal weight and the bulimic episodes themselves. These binges can be massive, involving many thousands of calories and in severe cases will occur 10–15 times per day.

Bulimic episodes are often planned, the food being bought specifically to binge on. Binges are arranged at a time when they will not be interrupted. Binge foods are usually high-energy, high-fat, sweet foods and may be selected because they are 'easy' to binge on. Binge eating is usually rapid, with food being vomited very shortly after it has been consumed. In more severe cases, binge-vomit cycles will go on for many hours. In large case series, the average number of binge episodes is 5–6 per week. Vomiting is usually induced by activating the gag reflex by inserting fingers into the throat. Many women soon learn to vomit simply by contracting thoracic and abdominal muscles and can then vomit at will and with ease. Some patients find great difficulty in triggering vomiting. Calluses may develop on the knuckles of the index and middle fingers where they are abraded by the palate during repeated efforts to trigger vomiting (Russell's sign). I have had patients who had to use balls of cling film inserted into the throat (a highly dangerous practice) or rolled up copies of the *Radio Times* because of its rough texture. Gastric lavage is sometimes used instead of vomiting. A patient of mine graduated from aquarium hose to a garden hose and finally to her washing machine waste hose with a diameter of some $3\frac{1}{2}$ cm. This finally resulted in the rupture of thoracic oesophagus. The use of Ipecac to induce vomiting is not common in the UK, but is more frequent in the USA.

Figure 22.4 shows a typical binge of over 20 000 calories and shows a number of features. A patient was out with her husband for a social meal. At the point at which she ate the potato salad she crossed her own threshold for her calorie intake for the day of 1000 calories. She deliberately ate the beetroot, thinking this might mark the onset of her bingeing. Everything she ate from

this point on was labelled by her as a binge and therefore if she could vomit the beetroot back she would have got rid of all the binge food. She managed to stay in the restaurant for a further half hour, getting increasingly distressed, and then ran out leaving her husband. The baked potatoes bought on the way home and much of the rest of the food was consumed over the 45 minutes she had at home before her husband arrived. Much of it was straight from the freezer and semi-frozen. She managed to make herself sick just before her husband returned.

Figure 22.5 shows typical diary pages for two days from a patient with severe BN.

Patients are very secretive about their behaviour and may go on for several years before they seek help. Although initially the binges may be exciting or at least provide some relief from anxiety or depression, as the binge progresses there is profound dysphoria, depression, guilt and self-loathing, only partially relieved by self-induced vomiting. Once established, BN becomes self-sustaining, with a number of feedback loops maintaining the disorder (Fig. 22.6).

A minority of patients start with self-induced vomiting, progressing subsequently to bingeing. For the majority the vomiting occurs immediately after the first binge or is discovered 'after some months of bingeing'. Initially, vomiting produces a great sense of relief in that control over bingeing is now less required, but progressively the binges get more and more out of control.

General psychopathology

The commonest comorbid symptoms are those of anxiety and mood disorders. Laessle et al (1987) found that 46% of BN subjects had a history of major depression. At presentation, depressive symptoms are certainly common, but these are often secondary to the eating disorder and disappear when the eating disorder is treated without the use of antidepressant medication. Clinically the presence of major depressive disorder in patients with BN does not imply a poor prognosis. Clinical trials of both psychological and drug treatments have found that current or past depressive disorder is not related to outcome. There is an excess family history of both major depression and obesity in the families of BN subjects, but no corresponding excess of eating disorders in the families of those with major depression. This indicates that there is not a common pathogenesis between BN and major depression.

A minority of BN sufferers have multiple dyscontrol behaviours indicative of marked personality disturbance. These include cutting, burning, multiple taking of overdoses, alcohol and drug misuse, promiscuity, shop-lifting and other self-damaging behaviours. This subgroup have been given the term multi-impulsive BN by Lacey (1993). Lacey's criteria require at least three of the following behaviours:

- drinking at least 36 units of alcohol per week;
- taking heroin, LSD or amphetamines or purchasing street tranquillisers on at least four occasions in the previous year;
- stealing at least ten times in the previous year;
- at least one overdose in the previous year; and severe regular self-cutting or self-burning.

These patients also show marked affective dysregulation with mood swings of depression, anger and elation. This group are older when they first seek help and are more likely to have been sexually abused.

A BINGE	
1 gin and bitter lemon	2 profiteroles & cream
prawn cocktail	& choc. sauce
roll and butter	1 can diet coke
2 glasses wine	1 can 7-up
1 slice roast beef	large gin and bitter lemon
1 slice roast pork	5 sandwiches & meat filling
1 slice ham	6 pancakes & butter
portion potato salad	7 scones & butter & jam
portion beetroot	bowl ice cream (1 litre)
portion sweetcorn	2 slices date & walnut cake
portion coleslaw	1 litre fresh orange
lettuce, cucumber & tomato	3 glasses lemonade
portion curried rice	packet crisps
large baked potato & dressing	cup of tea
1/2 large bakewell tart	2 slices fruit cake
4 oz. Black Magic	4 biscuits
1 lb tablet	packet Polos

Fig. 22.4
A typical binge.

	Monday 11th June		Vom	Lax	Other
A	**Breakfast** 2 slices brown toast Primula cheese and marmite 1 medium apple				
A	½lb Muesli/bran type biscuits 1 tin Vienna biscuits (17½oz) 2 slices bread + slices cold butter + 2 tsps. apricot jam 2 mugs milky tea + cup fresh orange juice		1 vomit + 26 Vomit Rinsing Cycles		
A	**Lunch** Scrambled eggs (2 large) on 1 slice (brown) toast + outline marg. 1 tomato. 1 lg. orange ¼lb seedless grapes. Mug milky tea				
A	1 loaf large, brown bread ¼lb butter, 6 heaped tsps golden syrup, 3 oz pate, 8 oz pork pie, tin Heinz coleslaw ½ tube Smarties, mug milky Ovaltine, 2 Farley's rusks 1 large glass orange juice, fresh		1 vomit + 30 cycles		
	1 cold large potato, 4 cold sausages, 1 glass diluted Ribena, 4 Opal Fruit sweets, 2 slices cold ham		Rinsing + Vomiting		
A	14 oatcakes + 3 oz chedder cheese 4 boiled potatoes in melted butter, 1 apple, 2 pkts crisps, 2 mugs milky coffee, 4 choc ices, 1 small Aero, mug milky coffee, 1 medium apple		1+ 5 cycles		
a		Totals			

Monday June 11th Continued

1 bowl veg soup (Heinz)
3 slices toast and butter
6 pkts crisps, 1 tablet jelly
1 large pkt chocolate digestives
12oz uncooked biscuit mixture:
(Comprising – 12oz margarine
– 12oz flour
– 6oz icing sugar
– 6oz custard powder)
2 cans Fresca drink
} A — 1 Vomit + 30 Rinsing and Vomiting cycles

Evening meal
Lettuce, cucumber, tomato
2oz chicken, 2 boiled pots (med)
1oz veg salad (Heinz), 1 beetroot,
2 spring onions, 1 orange (large)
2 slices toast + outline + Marmite
1 5oz flavoured yoghurt.
2 cups tea with milk
mug Ovaltine ½ milk ½ water — 1 Vomit

1.30 A.M.
1 loaf bread (toasted) + 6oz butter
½ pot jam + ¼ pot marmalade
6 mugs milk + Ovaltine
1 mug milky tea
} A — 2 Vomits

TOTAL CALORIES: 26 000

TOTAL 7 VOMITS + 91 RINSING AND VOMITING CYCLES

Fig. 22.5
Diary pages of a patient with bulimia nervosa: (a) binge/purge day. Bracket indicates binge; A indicates eating alone.

Physical complications

Many patients have no physical complaints at all, though BN can be associated with significant adverse medical sequelae. Compared with AN, however, medical complications are relatively benign, and the mortality seen appears to be very low. Enlarged submandibular and parotid salivary glands resulting in a puffy face occur commonly after bingeing. In the majority of patients these swellings go down after a day or two but in a small number there appears to be permanent hypertrophy. Dental enamel erosion of the palatal surface of the upper teeth can be severe, and dentists can easily identify cases of BN by mouth inspection. Dental amalgam is more resistant to gastric acid than the surrounding tooth enamel, so fillings tend to protrude above the teeth. The majority of patients who have been vomiting for several years will have obvious evidence of dental enamel erosion. Vigorous toothbrushing is understandable following self-induced vomiting, and may increase dental enamel wear.

The other major complication is hypokalemia. About 50% of bulimia patients have electrolyte abnormalities, which can be detected on routine screening. Frank metabolic acidosis is less common but can occur because of the dehydration and the loss of large amounts of potassium in the urine, and chloride in the emesis, leading to a picture of raised serum bicarbonate, hypochloraemia and/or hypokalaemia. Metabolic acidosis can also occur in patients abusing large amounts of laxatives. This is caused by the loss of carbonate-rich fluid in the faeces. The hypokalaemia can lead to chest pain and cardiac arrhythmias, and I have had one case of cardiac arrest.

Less frequent complications include oesophagitis, oesophageal perforation, Mallory–Weiss tears in association with vomiting, gastric diliatation and gastric rupture. ECG changes are usually secondary to low potassium.

Menstruation is absent or irregular in about half of severe cases and many demonstrate low oestradiol and progesterone levels. Lacey (1993) has reported an association with polycystic ovarian disease. See Table 22.3 for a comprehensive list of physical consequences.

Epidemiology

The point prevalence of BN among young females, using strict diagnostic criteria, is approximately 1%. A further 1% have significant symptoms of eating disorder pathology, and less than half of these are known to their GPs (Fairburn & Beglin 1990). Hoek (1991) found the incidence in primary care in the

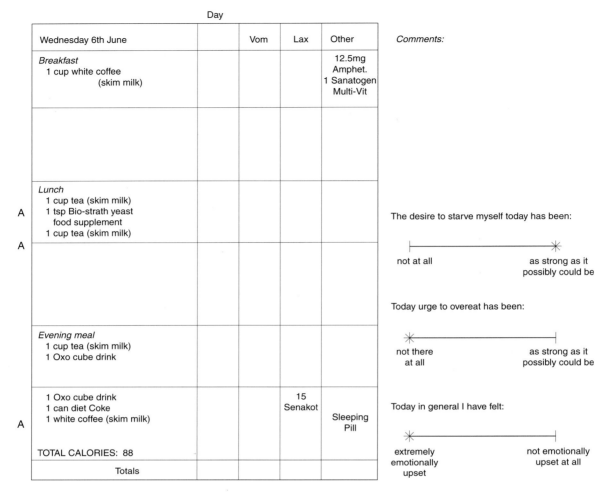

Day					
Wednesday 6th June		Vom	Lax	Other	*Comments:*
Breakfast 1 cup white coffee (skim milk)				12.5mg Amphet. 1 Sanatogen Multi-Vit	
Lunch 1 cup tea (skim milk) 1 tsp Bio-strath yeast food supplement 1 cup tea (skim milk)					
Evening meal 1 cup tea (skim milk) 1 Oxo cube drink					
1 Oxo cube drink 1 can diet Coke 1 white coffee (skim milk)			15 Senakot	Sleeping Pill	
TOTAL CALORIES: 88					
Totals					

The desire to starve myself today has been:

not at all ——————————————✳ as strong as it
                                possibly could be

Today urge to overeat has been:

✳——————————————————
not there   as strong as it
at all   possibly could be

Today in general I have felt:

✳——————————————————
extremely   not emotionally
emotionally   upset at all
upset

Fig. 22.5
Continued (b) Restricting day. A indicates eating alone.

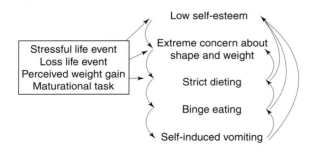

Fig. 22.6
Triggering and maintenance of bulimia nervosa.

Netherlands to be 11.4 per 100 000 of the population per year during the period 1985–1989. In the same population he found the 1-year community prevalence rate to be 1.5%. Only 11% of these community cases were detected by GPs, and half of those were referred on to mental health facilities. It seems that for BN the interface between community and primary care is fairly impermeable. Fairburn's studies indicate community cases are no less severe than those detected by GPs. This low detection rate appears to arise from a combination of the secretive and private behaviour of those who suffer from the disorder and low awareness by GPs.

The apparent sudden appearance of patients with BN in the late 1970s may be because the diagnosis was missed by clinicians prior to that date or because there has been a large increase in frequency over the past 20 years. Kendler et al (1991) interviewed over 2000 female subjects from a twin register in Virginia, USA. He examined the lifetime cumulative risk for definite and probable BN in three cohorts: (1) patients born before 1950; (2) those born between 1950 and 1959; (3) those born after 1959 (Fig. 22.7). The three curves obtained were quite different and show that the lifetime prevalence increased progressively according to recency of birth. Kendler calculated that for cohort (1) the prevalence of the disorder by the time they were 25 was 0.8%, for cohort (2) it was 1.1%, and for the most recent cohort (3) it was 3.7%. However, Fombonne (1996), reviewing all studies, concluded that rates have not increased since 1980.

Aetiology of bulimia nervosa

Given that 50% of patients with BN have a past history of AN, it is clear that the aetiology of the two conditions must have a great deal in common. Nevertheless, there are some factors which may

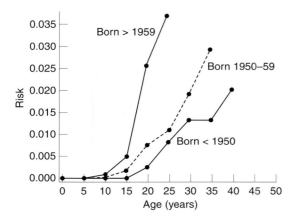

Fig. 22.7
Lifetime prevalence of bulimia nervosa (Kendler et al 1991).

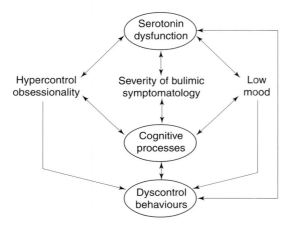

Fig. 22.8
Proposed relationship between bulimia symptoms and dyscontrol behaviours.

be specific to BN These include a personal and family history of obesity, a family history of affective disorders and a family history of substance misuse.

If we accept that the prevalence of AN has stayed relatively constant over time but that of BN has risen, then it may be that cultural and social factors play a more important role in the aetiology of BN and that the increased preoccupation with dieting and slimness is one reason why this disorder has become more common.

Cowen et al (1996) studied the effect of moderate dieting in healthy women on the prolactin response to the serotonin receptor agonist m-chlorophenylpiperazine (MCCP). This is a measure of the sensitivity of postsynaptic $5HT_{2C}$ receptors. They proposed that dieting in women is associated with the development of a functional supersensitivity of $5HT_{2C}$ receptors, probably in response to lower levels of 5HT, and that this might be a vulnerability factor aiding the dysregulation of eating that occurs in some women following dieting. Figure 22.8 gives a suggested method of how serotonin dysregulation and cognitive factors can combine to produce both over-control and dyscontrol.

Although frequently cited, there is little evidence that childhood sexual abuse is a specific risk factor for BN. Pope et al (1994) compared young American, Austrian and Brazilian women who suffered from DSM-IIIR bulimia. Childhood sexual abuse was reported by 24–36% of the women in the three countries, though only 15–32% reported abuse before the onset of their bulimia. These rates are no higher than those that occur in general psychiatric populations. It may well be that sexual abuse is a risk factor for psychiatric disorders in general but not specifically for BN. Their study did not find that bulimic women had endured more severe sexual abuse or that sexual abuse was associated with the severity of bulimic symptoms.

Treatment of bulimia nervosa

Despite its relatively recent appearance, there have now been over 50 good randomised trials of treatment for BN. Four main types of treatment have been investigated: self-help (usually guided self-help), cognitive-behavioural therapy (CBT), interpersonal psychotherapy (IPT), and drug treatment using SSRIs. Nearly all patients with BN can be managed on an outpatient basis. Inpatient treatment is only indicated if the patient is suicidal or there is concern about her physical health because of very high-frequency vomiting. Very occasionally, patients who have proved refractory to all other methods of treatment may require admission. However, this is often extremely difficult to manage on general psychiatric wards because of the type and structure of treatment that is required. The only other indication for inpatient treatment is early pregnancy, as high rates of spontaneous abortions have been reported. Figure 22.9 gives a sequential tiered model for treatment, modifications of which are now in place in most eating disorders specialist treatment centres.

Pharmacological treatment studies

Earlier drug studies evaluated tricyclic antidepressants or phenelzine. Modest efficacy has been demonstrated in the short term for imipramine (Pope et al 1983, Mitchell et al 1990); desipramine (Hughes et al 1986) and phenelzine (Walsh et al

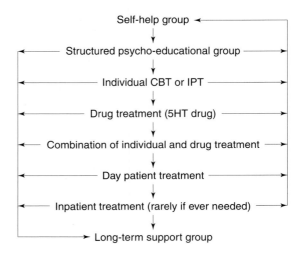

Fig. 22.9
Tiered approach to the treatment of bulimia nervosa.

1988). These were all short-term studies with the drug being given usually for 8–12 weeks. However, there seemed little evidence of any continued gain once the drug has been discontinued. Where attempts have been made to assess long-term efficacy (Walsh et al 1991) drop-out and relapse rates have been so high that no conclusions could be drawn. Several of the above authors have commented that there are major problems with compliance if antidepressants are the main mode of treatment. Many bulimic patients are reluctant to take medication, and complaints of side-effects produce a high discontinuation rate.

The largest antidepressant study has been with fluoxetine (Fluoxetine Bulimia Nervosa Collaborative Study Group 1992). 387 women received either 20 or 60 mg of fluoxetine daily or a placebo. Fluoxetine at 60 mg a day was found to be significantly superior to placebo. After 8 weeks of treatment results with the standard antidepressant dose of fluoxetine 20 mg did not differ from those with placebo. On the 60 mg dose, however, 63% of women had a reduction of 50% or greater in their binge frequency.

Clinical experience shows that if drugs are used, they have to be used for periods of up to a year and that, unless combined with non-pharmacological treatments, relapse is high when the drug is discontinued. It was clear that fluoxetine works as an anti-bulimic and not just as an antidepressant agent, as baseline depression is not associated with response.

Psychotherapeutic treatments

CBT has been the best-evaluated treatment. Several research groups working in different centres have found similar results, with an average reduction in binge and purge frequency of approximately 70% and between one-third and one-half of patients stopping bingeing altogether at the end of a 10–16 week course of outpatient individual CBT (Fairburn et al 1993, Freeman et al 1988, Garner et al 1993). Unlike drug treatments, several studies have had follow-up periods of 1 year and one of 6 years. Follow-up shows that treatment gains are largely maintained. Patients with markedly low self-esteem and with severe personality disorder do less well and are more likely to drop out.

Interpersonal psychotherapy (IPT) was developed as a treatment for depression and used in the NIMH study on the treatment of depressive illness. It has been less evaluated than CBT but, in one group of studies (Fairburn et al 1993), it has been shown to be as effective as CBT. CBT acted more quickly, with symptom improvement in IPT occurring for up to a year after the end of treatment.

Guided self-help

In this treatment approach, patients are given a comprehensive self-help treatment manual and have a limited number of brief sessions with a therapist who introduces them to the manual and who is available to check on progress and encourage compliance over subsequent weeks. Several studies have shown modest benefits from this approach, and it may form a useful first step in treatment.

Drug treatment versus psychotherapy

There are no studies that have compared fluoxetine and psychotherapy directly. Mitchell et al (1990) randomised 254 patients to: imipramine 300 mg per day maximum; placebo treatment; imipramine plus intensive group CBT; and placebo plus intensive group CBT. The main treatment effect was for group CBT. The addition of imipramine did not give additional benefit when compared with group therapy alone, though it did help relieve depressive symptoms. Forty percent of the patients on imipramine dropped out, mainly because of side-effects.

Agras et al (1992) compared desipramine with CBT. Again, psychotherapy alone or psychotherapy in combination with drugs were superior to drugs alone.

REFERENCES

Agras W S, Kraemer H C 1984 The treatment of anorexia nervosa: do different treatments have different outcomes? In: Stunkard A J, Stellar E (eds) Eating and its disorders. Raven Press, New York, pp 193–207

Agras W S, Rossiter E M, Arnow B et al 1992 Pharmacologic and cognitive-behavioural treatment for bulimia nervosa: a controlled comparison. American Journal of Psychiatry 149:82–87

Andersen A E, Watson T, Schlechte J 2000 Osteoporosis and osteopenia in men with eating disorders. Lancet 355:1967–1968

APA 1994 Diagnostic and statistical manual of mental disorders, 4th edn. American Psychiatric Association, Washington, DC, p 731

Binswanger L 1958 The case of Ellen West. In: May R, Angel E, Ellenberger U F (eds) Existence: a new dimension in psychiatry and psychology. Simon & Schuster, New York, pp 237–364

Blair C, Freeman C P L, Cull A 1995 The families of anorexia nervosa and cystic fibrosis patients. Psychological Medicine 25:985–993

Bruch H 1965 Anorexia nervosa and its differential diagnosis. Journal of Nervous and Mental Disease 141:556–566

Carlat D, Camargo C A, Herzog D 1997 Eating disorders in males: a report on 135 patients. American Journal of Psychiatry 154:1127–1132

Channon S, DeSilva P, Hemsley D, Perkins R 1989 A controlled trial of cognitive-behavioural and behavioural treatment of anorexia nervosa. Behaviour Research and Therapy 27:529–535

Cowen P J, Clifford E M, Walsh A E S et al 1996 Moderate dieting causes 5-HT$_{2C}$ receptor supersensitivity. Psychological Medicine 26:1155–1159

Cullen W 1780 Synopsis methodicae exhibens . . . systema nosologica. Creech, Edinburgh

Eisler I, Dare C, Hodes M et al 2000 Family therapy for adolescent anorexia nervosa: the results of a controlled comparison of two family interventions. Journal of Child Psychology & Psychiatry 41:727–736

Fairburn C G, Beglin S J 1990 Studies of the epidemiology of bulimia nervosa. American Journal of Psychiatry 147:401–408

Fairburn C G, Jones R, Peveler R C et al 1993 Psychotherapy and bulimia nervosa: longer-term effects of interpersonal psychotherapy, behavior therapy and cognitive behavior therapy. Archives of General Psychiatry 50:419–428

Fluoxetine Bulimia Nervosa Collaborative Study Group 1992 Fluoxetine in the treatment of bulimia nervosa: a multicentre, placebo-controlled, double-blind trial. Archives of General Psychiatry 49:139–147

Fombonne E 1996 Is bulimia nervosa increasing in frequency? International Journal of Eating Disorders 19:287–296

Freeman C P L, Barry F, Dunkeld-Turnbull J, Henderson A 1988 A controlled trial of psychotherapy for bulimia nervosa. British Medical Journal 296:521–525

Gard M C E, Freeman C P 1996 The dismantling of a myth: a review of eating disorders and socio-economic status. International Journal of Eating Disorders 20:1–12

Garner D M, Rockert W, Garner M V et al 1993 Comparison of cognitive-behavioural and supportive-expressive therapy for bulimia nervosa. American Journal of Psychiatry 150:37–46

Gordon I, Lask B, Bryant-Waugh R et al 1997 Childhood-onset anorexia nervosa: towards identifying a biological substrate. International Journal of Eating Disorders 22:159–165

Gull W W 1874 Anorexia nervosa (apepsia hysterica, anorexia hysterica). Transactions of the Clinical Society of London 7:22–28

Hoek H W 1991 The incidence and prevalence of anorexia nervosa and bulimia nervosa in primary care. Psychological Medicine 21:455–460

Hsu L K G 1988 The outcome of anorexia nervosa: a reappraisal. Psychological Medicine 18:797–812

Hughes P L, Wells L A, Cunningham C J, Ilstrup D M 1986 Treating bulimia with desipramine: a double-blind placebo controlled study. Archives of General Psychiatry 3:182–186

Janet P 1903 Les obsessions et la psychasthénic. Vol 1, sect 5: L'obsession de la honte du corps. Germer Baillière, Paris

Jones D J, Fox M M, Babigian H M, Hutton H E 1980 Epidemiology of anorexia nervosa in Monroe County, New York: 1960–1976. Psychosomatic Medicine 42:551–558

Kendell R E, Hall D J, Hailey A, Babigian H M 1973 The epidemiology of anorexia nervosa. Psychological Medicine 3:200–203

Kendler K S, Maclean C, Neale M et al 1991 The genetic epidemiology of bulimia nervosa. American Journal of Psychiatry 148:1627–1637

Keys A, Brozek J, Henschel A et al 1950 The biology of human starvation (2 vols). University of Minnesota Press, Minneapolis

Lacey J H 1993 Self-damaging and addictive behaviour in bulimia nervosa: a catchment area study. British Journal of Psychiatry 163:190–194

Leassle R G, Kittl S, Fichter M M et al 1987 Major affective disorder in anorexia nervosa and bulimia: a descriptive study. British Journal of Psychiatry 151:785–789

Lucas A R, Beard C M, O'Fallon W M, Kurland L T 1991 50-year trends in the incidence of anorexia nervosa in Rochester, Minn.: a population-based study. American Journal of Psychiatry, 148:917–922

McCluskey S, Evans C, Lacey J H et al 1991 Polycystic ovary syndrome and bulimia. Fertility & Sterility 55:287–291

Marcé L V 1860 Note sur une forme de délire hypochondriaque consécutive aux dyspepsies et caractérisé principalement par le refus d'aliments. Annales Medico-Psychologiques 6:15–28

Mitchell J E, Pyle R L, Eckert E D et al 1990 A comparison study of antidepressants and structured intensive group psychotherapy in the treatment of bulimia nervosa. Archives of General Psychiatry 47:149–157

Morton R 1689 Phthisiologia, seu exercitationes de phthisi. Smith, London

Parry-Jones B, Parry-Jones W L 1991 Bulimia: an archival review of its history in psychosomatic medicine. International Journal of Eating Disorders 10:129–143

Parry-Jones B, Parry-Jones W 1995 The history of bulimia and bulimia nervosa. In: Brownell K D, Fairburn C G (eds) Eating disorders and obesity. Guilford Press, New York, ch 26

Pope H G, Hudson J I, Jonas J M, Yurgelun-Todd D 1983 Treatment of bulimia with imipramine: a double-blind placebo controlled study. American Journal of Psychiatry 14:554–558

Pope Jr H G, Mangweth B, Brooking N A et al 1994 American Journal of Psychiatry 151:732–737

Russell G F M 1979 Bulimia nervosa: an ominous variant of anorexia nervosa. Psychological Medicine 9:429

Russell G F M 1997 The history of bulimia nervosa. In: Garner D M, Garfinkel P E (eds) Handbook of treatment for eating disorders, 2nd edn. Guilford Press, New York, p 11–12

Russell G F M, Szmukler G, Dare C, Eisler I 1987 An evaluation of family therapy in anorexia nervosa and bulimia nervosa. Archives of General Psychiatry 44:1047–1056

Serfaty M A, Turkington D, Heap M et al 1999 Cognitive therapy versus dietary counseling in the outpatient treatment of anorexia nervosa: effects of the treatment phase. European Eating Disorders Review 7:334–350

Sharp C W, Freeman C P L 1993 The medical complications of anorexia nervosa. British Journal of Psychiatry 162:452–462

Silverman J A 1995 The history of anorexia nervosa. In: Brownell K D, Fairburn C G (eds) Eating disorders and obesity. Guilford Press, New York, p 141–144

Smeets M A 1997 The rise and fall of body size estimation research. In: Anorexia nervosa: a review and reconceptualization. Eating Disorders Review 5(2):75–79

Sullivan P F 2002 Course and outcome of anorexia and bulimia nervosa. In: Fairburn C, Brownell K D (eds) Eating disorders and obesity. Guilford Press, New York, p 226–230

Szmukler G I, McCance C, McCrone L, Hunter D 1986 Anorexia nervosa: a psychiatric case register study from Aberdeen. Psychological Medicine 16:49–58

Theander S 1970 Anorexia nervosa: a psychiatric investigation of 94 female patients. Acta Psychiatrica Scandinavica Suppl 214

Theander S 1985 Outcome and prognosis in anorexia nervosa and bulimia. Some results of previous investigations compared with those of a Swedish long-term study. Journal of Psychiatric Research 19:493–508

Touyz S W, Beaumont P J V, Glaun D et al 1984 A comparison of lenient and strict operant conditioning programmes in refeeding patients with anorexia nervosa. British Journal of Psychiatry 144:517–520

Walsh B T, Gladis M, Roose S P et al 1988 Phenelzine versus placebo in 50 patients with bulimia. Archives of General Psychiatry 45:471–475

Walsh B T, Hadigan C M, Devlin M J et al 1991 Long-term outcome of antidepressant treatment for bulimia nervosa. American Journal of Psychiatry 148:1206–1212

WHO 1992 The ICD-10 classification of mental and behavioural disorders: clinical descriptions and diagnostic guidelines. World Health Organization, Geneva, p 176–181

Wulff M 1932 Ueber einen interessanten oralen Symptomen-komplex und seine Beziehung zur Sucht. Internationale Zeitschrift für Psychoanalyse 18:281–302

Willi J, Grossman S 1983 Epidemiology of anorexia nervosa in a defined region of Switzerland. American Journal of Psychiatry 140:564–567

Willi J, Giacometti G, Limacher B 1990 Update on the epidemiology of anorexia nervosa in a defined region of Switzerland. American Journal of Psychiatry 147:1514–1517

23 Personality disorders

David J Cooke, Stephen D Hart

PERSONALITY DISORDER: A SOURCE OF CLINICAL CONCERN

Personality disorders, although long recognised, are oft disregarded by clinicians. Many factors militate against personality disorders being of central concern: they appear elusive in that the boundaries between the pathological and non-pathological are not distinct; reliable diagnostic tools are only now becoming available; and pessimism abounds regarding therapy. Personality disorders are given limited consideration in most clinical training. Yet, they are prevalent disorders; estimates suggest that 10–14% of the general population meet diagnostic criteria for at least one personality disorder (Widiger & Rogers 1989, Weissman 1993, Pilkonis et al 1997).

A personality disorder is a chronic disturbance in one's relations with self, others and the environment that results in distress or failure to fulfil social roles and obligations (e.g. WHO 1992b, APA 2000). There is growing awareness that personality disorders are important clinical conditions that have significance for the individual sufferer, their family and society at large. Personality disorders impact through their links with child abuse, spousal assault, suicide, school drop-out, employment problems, homelessness, raised mortality in early adulthood and relationship disruption — this is a worldwide phenomenon (Desjarlais et al 1995). Costs to society through the burden that the personality disordered places on the health, social welfare and criminal-justice systems are considerable (Coid 2003). Further, those suffering from severe mental illness, and who have a comorbid personality disorder, have poorer outcomes in community treatment compared with those with a singleton diagnosis (Tyrer & Simmonds 2003). Awareness of these disorders is important for all clinicians; unfortunately, many mental health clinicians pay comparatively little attention to the diagnosis and treatment of these disorders.

In this chapter we examine the history of the concept of personality disorder; we then examine current diagnostic systems, aetiological theories and risk factors. Discussion of the assessment and treatment of personality disorders is followed by an account of forensic issues in relation to them. We start by considering the concept of personality and related constructs.

WHAT IS PERSONALITY?

Personality is a term oft used but rarely defined adequately in mental-health texts (Livesley 2001). There are many definitions of personality, but there are two common and key features of all mainstream definitions (Hogan et al 1997). First, personality is concerned with consistency and regularity of thoughts, feelings and behaviour across time and across settings. The focus is thus on characteristic — rather than rare or episodic — thoughts and behaviours. Second, personality is more than the sum of traits, thoughts and behaviours, it encompasses the fundamental psychophysiological systems that organise and lend coherence to these aspects of the individual.

The term personality should be distinguished from two common related terms, namely, temperament and character. Traditionally, temperament has been used to encompass the simple features of personality, thought to be essentially biological in origin, that are evident in infancy, rather than the more complex mesh of thoughts, feelings and behaviour that are identifiable in adulthood (Rutter 1987). Character, by way of contrast, traditionally refers to enduring traits and behaviour patterns; however, more recent usage implies that while temperament may be fundamentally biological in origin, character should be viewed as the consequence of the interplay between temperament and experience. Unfortunately, this simple dichotomy is not consistent with the behavioural-genetic data that suggest that all personality traits are heritable (Livesley 2001). Thus, the distinction between temperament and character may be more apparent than real.

THE HISTORY OF THE CONCEPT OF PERSONALITY DISORDER

The concept of personality *disorder* is as old as the concept of personality, being evident in the writings of classical times (Morey 1997). Modern conceptions of personality disorder can be traced back to Pinel's concept of *manie sans délire* (madness without confusion of mind) (Pinel 1801/1962). Pinel was among the first to recognise that that psychological disturbance could occur even when powers to reason were intact, and without a loss of contact with reality (Pinel 1801/1962, Millon & Davis 1996). Pritchard expanded and refined these notions and indicated that the impairments of 'feelings, temper, or habits' could underpin certain forms of insanity and that these impairments could be viewed as exaggerations of 'natural' behaviours: that is, they could be regarded as qualitatively rather than as quantitatively distinct variations. Pritchard's contribution went further. He clarified the distinction between elements of psychopathology that are linked to transient symptomatic states and those that are linked to more enduring characteristics (Berrios 1996); by doing so, Pritchard laid the foundations for the disorders of personality to be regarded as a new diagnostic grouping (Livesley 2001).

These foundations were built upon by Kurt Schneider in his seminal volume *Psychopathic Personalities* (Schneider 1923/1958). In this volume Schneider clarified the distinction between personality disorders and other forms of mental disorder. He distinguished between two important concepts: *abnormal personality* and *psychopathic personality*. He defined abnormal personality as: 'a variation upon an accepted yet broadly conceived range of average personality. The variation may be expressed as an excess or deficiency of certain personal qualities and whether this is judged good or bad is immaterial to the issue. The saint and the poet are equally abnormal as the criminal. All three of them fall outside the range of average personality as we conceive it so that all persons of note may be classed as abnormal personalities' (Schneider 1923/1958 pp. 2–3).

This definition of abnormal — essentially, deviation from the average — could not provide a useful definition of pathology; indeed, certain abnormality could be viewed as indicative of health rather than pathology. Schneider proposed that psychopathic personalities were: 'abnormal personalities who either suffer personally because of their abnormality or make a community suffer because of it' (Schneider 1923/1958 p. 3)

In his volume Schneider focused on psychopathic personality rather than abnormal personality. He described ten variants of psychopathic personality: fanatical, depressive, hyperthymic, insecure (sensitives and anankasts), labile explosive, affectionless, weak-willed, asthenic and attention-seeking. It should be self-evident that the Schneiderian concept of psychopathic personality is much broader than the Anglo-American construct of psychopathy, a construct that has most in common with Schneider's 'affectionless' psychopath. This classification provided the first taxonomy of personality disorders to be used generally in psychiatry and provided the basis for much of the taxonomy used in both the DSM-IV (APA 2000) and the ICD-10 (WHO 1992b) systems.

The publication of DSM-III (APA 1980) was critical in promoting both clinical and research interest in the personality disorders and lead to an exponential rise in the number of research papers on the topic (Blashfield & McElroy 1987). This first attempt to describe personality disorders within the DSM system was found to be unsatisfactory in terms of diagnostic reliability; as a consequence more behavioural criteria were introduced in the next revision (APA 1987). These criteria, despite promoting the study of personality disorders, highlighted some of the major problems in achieving adequate descriptions. From a clinical perspective, it was found that the distinct disorders have limited clinical utility because comorbidity among disorders is very common and, therefore, specific diagnoses have limited value in predicting treatment outcome. From the research perspective, the diagnoses are so heterogeneous that attempts to link specific categories with basic psychological or biological processes are fraught with difficulties.

CLINICAL CLASSIFICATIONS OF PERSONALITY DISORDERS

Currently there are two main systems that are used to classify personality disorders: the DSM-IV system and the ICD-10 system. We will focus on the former because, not only does it have wider acceptance, but also it is underpinned by a larger corpus of research evidence. There is naturally a considerable overlap between the two systems, as illustrated in Table 23.1. It is noteworthy that there is

no equivalent in the ICD-10 system to the diagnoses of *Schizotypal* or *Narcissistic* Personality Disorders found in DSM-IV. The degree of concordance between the two systems depends on both the personality disorder being considered and the approach to description: that is, whether a categorical or dimensional approach is being applied (Ottoson et al 2002). These authors found that when a categorical approach was adopted concordance between the two systems ranged from 26% (Schizoid) to 88% (Histrionic); whereas when a dimensional approach was adopted the lowest concordance was 79% (Antisocial [DSM]/Dissocial [ICD-10]).

A general definition of a personality disorder is provided in the DSM-IV (APA 2000 p. 685):

> *A personality disorder is an enduring pattern of inner experience and behavior that deviates markedly from the expectations of the individual's culture, is pervasive and inflexible, has an onset in adolescence or early adulthood, is stable over time, and leads to distress or impairment.*

In essence this definition encapsulates the 'three Ps' of personality disorder: the symptoms must be pathological, pervasive and persistent. The *pathological* aspect of the disorder is manifest in the domains of cognition, affect, interpersonal functioning or impulse control, resulting in problems that lead to either distress or impairment in the individual's functioning. While the majority of personality disorders lead to the individual's feeling distress, this is not always the case; the traits may be ego-syntonic. The *pervasive* aspect of the disorder is manifest by the fact that impairment is not limited to a particular aspect of the person's life but is widespread across roles, including intimate, social and occupational roles. The *persistent* aspect of the disorder is manifest by the fact that the individual's difficulties can be traced back to adolescence or early adulthood and they often persist throughout adulthood.

In coming to a diagnosis of a personality disorder it is essential to rule out other possible explanations of why the symptoms are manifest, including other mental disorders, the effects of substances and general medical conditions, including head trauma.

We now examine the essential features of the DSM-IV definitions of personality disorders, reviewing the key diagnostic features, the prevalence of the disorders, familial pattern and comorbidity. It should be noted that we only provide a summary of the criteria and that diagnosis should only be made after full consultation with the diagnostic manual.

Within DSM-IV, Personality Disorders are grouped into three clusters: the 'Odd–eccentric', the 'Dramatic-emotional or erratic' and the 'Anxious-fearful'. Within the odd–eccentric cluster, disorders are characterised by asociality and unusual thoughts and behaviour. Cluster B disorders, labelled dramatic–erratic–emotional, are characterised by impulsive behaviour and affect. Finally, Cluster C, the anxious–fearful disorders are characterised by negative affectivity.

Cluster A: 'Odd–eccentric' Personality Disorders

This cluster is composed of three disorders: Paranoid Personality Disorder, Schizoid Personality Disorder and Schizotypal Personality Disorder.

Paranoid Personality Disorder

The key defining feature of Paranoid Personality Disorder is the distrust of others and suspiciousness about their motives; others

Table 23.1 Relationship between ICD-10 and DSM-IV descriptions of personality disorders

ICD-10 description	DSM-IV description
Paranoid Suspiciousness, excessive sensitivity to setbacks, bears grudges, believes conspiratorial explanations, self important, combative in regard to personal rights	*Paranoid* Distrust and suspiciousness of others, interprets others as having malicious intent
Schizoid Emotionally cold, flat affect, does not derive pleasure from activities, solitary, lacks close friends, eccentric and prone to excessive fantasy and introspection	*Schizoid* Detachment from social relationships, restricted emotional expression in interpersonal settings
No equivalent	*Schizotypal* Social and interpersonal deficits leading to inability to maintain, and acute discomfort in, close relationships. Cognitive and perceptual distortions and eccentricities of behaviour
Histrionic Overly dramatic, exaggerated expression of emotion, shallow and labile affect, suggestible, desires to be centre of attention, inappropriately seductive, overly concerned with appearance	*Histrionic* Excessive emotionality and attention-seeking behaviour
Dissocial Gross disparity between behaviour and prevailing social norms, callous, irresponsible behaviour, unstable intimate relationships, low frustration tolerance, blames others, does not learn from experience	*Antisocial* Disregard for the rights of others, violation of these rights
No equivalent	*Narcissistic* Grandiosity, need for admiration and a lack of empathy for others
Emotionally Unstable Acts impulsively without considering consequences, affective instability, fails to plan, unstable relationships, suicidal threats or acts of self-harm	*Borderline* Unstable interpersonal relationships, self-image and affects. Marked impulsiveness
Anakastic Excessive doubt and caution, preoccupied with rules and organisation, perfectionism that leads to failure in task completion, pedantic, rigid and stubborn	*Obsessive–Compulsive* Preoccupied with orderliness, perfectionism that results in inadequate flexibility, openness and efficiency
Dependent Subordinates own needs to needs of others, uncomfortable or helpless when alone, fear of abandonment, cannot make decisions without reassurance, needs others to make decisions for him/her	*Dependent* Excessive need to be taken care of. Fear of separation leads to submissive and clinging behaviour
Anxious/Avoidant Feelings of tension and apprehension, believes inferior to others, hypersensitive to criticism, avoids social activities	*Avoidant* Feelings of inadequacy, social inhibition, hypersensitive to negative evaluation

are regarded as having malevolent intent. To meet the diagnostic criteria individuals must meet four or more of the following criteria:

- considers, without adequate evidence, that others aim to harm, deceive or exploit him/her;
- preoccupied by doubts regarding the loyalty or trustworthiness of friends and associates;
- scared to confide in case information is used against him/her;
- misinterprets remarks as designed to threaten or demean;
- bears grudges, does not forgive insults, injuries or slights;
- misperceives attacks on his/her character and is quick to respond angrily;
- recurrent unjustified suspicions about the fidelity of intimate partner

As a consequence of these traits, those suffering from Paranoid Personality Disorder may have difficulty in close relationships; they may be guarded and secretive, hostile and sarcastic. They frequently demand control of those around them and are unable to collaborate or accept even mild criticism. Criticism may lead to anger and threats of litigation. They may hold grandiose views and are concerned with power and rank. In coming to this diagnosis it is important to establish that the symptoms do not only occur during the course of schizophrenia, a mood disorder with psychotic features or other psychotic disorder.

Paranoid Personality Disorder — basic facts Paranoid Personality Disorder is more common among males. The prevalence of the disorder is estimated to be between 0.5% and 2.5% in the general population and can be around 10% in outpatient settings and as high as 30% in inpatient settings (Table 23.2; APA 2000, Mattia & Zimmerman 2001, Bernstein et al 2001, Coid 2003). Onset may be evident from childhood difficulties, including idiosyncratic fantasies, withdrawal, hypersensitivity and social anxiety; these may result in bullying. Relatives of probands with schizophrenia have a higher risk of this disorder. It is frequently comorbid with other personality

Table 23.2 Prevalence of and gender differences in personality disorders

Personality disorder	Prevalence in general population	Prevalence in outpatient clinics	Prevalence in inpatient settings	Gender difference
Paranoid*	0.5–2.5%	2–10%	10–30%	More common in males
Schizoid*	0.4–1.7%	***	***	Slightly more common in males
Schizotypal*	0.1–5.6%	***	***	Slightly more common in males
Antisocial[†]	0.6–2%	***	***	3:1 M:F in general population
Borderline[†]	0.7–2%	10%	20%	1:3 M:F in general population
Histrionic[†]	2–3%	10–15%	10–15%	Slightly more common in females
Narcissistic[†]	> 1%	2–16%	2–16%	More common in males
Avoidant[‡]	0.5–5.0%	10%	NA	Equally common in males and females
Dependent[‡]	1.0–1.7%	NA	NA	Equally common in males and females
Obsessive–Compulsive[‡]	1.7–2.2%	3–10%	NA	2:1 M:F in general population

* Cluster A Personality Disorders, 'Odd or eccentric'
[†] Cluster B Personality Disorders, 'Dramatic, emotional, or erratic'.
[‡] Cluster C Personality Disorders: 'Aanxious or fearful'.
NA No adequate estimates available.
Sources: APA 2000, Mattia & Zimmerman 2001, Coid 2003.

disorders, including Borderline, Avoidant, Schizotypal, Schizoid, Antisocial and Narcissistic. Paranoid traits may be adaptive, for example, within the criminal subculture or within minority groups. Paranoid Personality Disorder comorbid with Antisocial Personality Disorder is frequently a risk factor for violent crime (Coid 2003). Paranoid traits, including suspiciousness, have been found to have a heritability of around 40% (Kendler & Hewitt 1992, Livesley 1998).

Schizoid Personality Disorder

The key defining features of Schizoid Personality Disorder are detachment from social relationships, together with limited emotional expression in interpersonal interactions. To meet the diagnostic criteria individuals must meet four or more of the following:

- does not seek or enjoy close relationships;
- generally chooses solitary activities;
- no interest in sexual experiences with others;
- does not experience pleasure in many activities;
- lacks close friends or confidants outwith family;
- indifferent to praise or criticism;
- emotionally cold, detached or affectively flattened.

As a consequence of these traits, those suffering from Schizoid Personality Disorder may have difficulty expressing anger and may act passively when under stress. Their lives frequently lack direction, and their lack of social skills and lack of desire for close relationships results in few friendships or intimate partnerships. Their occupational functioning is frequently impaired if it requires significant interpersonal interaction.

Schizoid Personality Disorder — basic facts Schizoid Personality Disorder is slightly more common among males. Studies indicate that the prevalence of the disorder is between 0.4% and 1.7% in the general population; no adequate prevalence

estimates for inpatient or outpatient settings are available (Kalus et al 1995, APA 2000, Mattia & Zimmerman 2001, Coid 2003; see Table 23.2). Those suffering from this condition rarely present in clinical contexts, because of their aloofness.

Onset may be evident from childhood difficulties, including school underachievement, solitariness and poor relationships with peers. Being a victim of teasing is not uncommon. Schizoid Personality Disorder has increased prevalence among relatives of those suffering from schizophrenia or Schizotypal Personality Disorder. It is frequently comorbid with other personality disorders, including Avoidant, Schizotypal and Paranoid. Little empirical evidence is available about the course of the disorder. Wolff & Chick (1980) followed-up 20 schizoid children over 10 years, and the vast majority retained their symptoms despite intensive psychotherapy.

In coming to this diagnosis it is important to establish that the symptoms do not only occur during the course of schizophrenia, a mood disorder with psychotic features, or other psychotic disorder.

Schizotypal Personality Disorder

The key defining features of Schizotypal Personality Disorder are acute discomfort with close relationships, eccentricities of behaviour and a range of cognitive or perceptual distortions. To meet the diagnostic criteria individuals must meet five or more of the following:

- ideas of reference;
- odd beliefs or unusual thinking, including magical thinking, that influence behaviour;
- unusual perceptual experiences;
- odd thinking and speech, e.g. vague, metaphorical, circumstantial or stereotyped;
- paranoid ideation or suspiciousness;
- inappropriate or constricted affect;

- odd, peculiar or eccentric behaviour or appearance;
- lack of confidants or close friends outwith family;
- high levels of social anxiety linked to paranoid thinking rather than low self-esteem.

As a consequence of these traits, those suffering from Schizotypal Personality Disorder may seek treatment for symptoms of dysphoria. They may experience transient psychotic episodes often in response to stress.

In coming to this diagnosis it is important to establish that the symptoms do not only occur during the course of schizophrenia, a mood disorder with psychotic features, other psychotic disorder, or a pervasive developmental disorder.

Schizotypal Personality Disorder — basic facts Schizotypal Personality Disorder is slightly more common among males. The prevalence of the disorder is estimated to be between 0.1% and 5.6% in the general population; no adequate prevalence estimates for inpatient or outpatient settings are available (see Table 23.2). Onset may be evident from childhood difficulties, including idiosyncratic thoughts and language, withdrawal, hypersensitivity, social anxiety and underachievement at schools; these features may result in the individual being a victim of bullying. Schizotypal Personality Disorder has a higher frequency amongst first-degree relatives of those suffering from schizophrenia. It is frequently comorbid with other personality disorders, including Borderline, Avoidant, Paranoid and Schizoid. There is evidence to suggest that the diagnosis is underpinned by a taxon or discrete diagnostic entity (Lenzenweger 1999, Blanchard et al 2000). This is the only personality disorder for which such evidence is available.

Cluster B: 'Dramatic–emotional–erratic' Personality Disorders

This cluster is composed of four disorders: Antisocial Personality Disorder, Borderline Personality Disorder, Histrionic Personality Disorder and Narcissistic Personality Disorder.

Antisocial Personality Disorder

The key defining feature of Antisocial Personality Disorder is a pervasive disregard for the rights of others, including the violation of these rights. To meet the diagnostic criteria individuals must be over 18 years of age and have met three or more of the following since the age of 15:

- lack of conformity with social norms, behaviour being grounds for arrest;
- deceitfulness; lies and cons others both for profit and pleasure;
- impulsivity and failure to plan;
- irritability and aggression that leads to fights and assaults;
- reckless with regard to the safety of self and others;
- irresponsible, fails to honour obligations;
- lack of remorse, indifferent to the mistreatment of others.

In addition to the above criteria, there must also be evidence of, although not necessarily a full diagnosis of, Conduct Disorder (APA 2000) with onset prior to 15 years of age. In coming to this diagnosis it is important to establish that the antisocial behaviour does not occur only during the course of a schizophrenic or manic episode.

As a consequence of these traits, those suffering from Antisocial Personality Disorder have a high risk of offending. They may have a history of multiple sexual partners and an inability to sustain close confiding relationships, they may neglect and mistreat their children, and they have an elevated risk of premature demise through suicide, homicide or accidents. They are likely to be involved in substance abuse and may have problems with gambling.

A noteworthy difficulty with the DSM-IV definition of Antisocial Personality Disorder is that, while suggesting that this disorder can be considered to be the same as psychopathy, sociopathy or dissocial personality disorder, it relegates, to the category of associated features, characteristics thought by many commentators to be the key features (e.g. Cleckley 1976, Hart & Hare 1996, Cooke & Michie 2001). These characteristics include arrogant self-appraisal, lack of concern for the future, superficial charm and lack of empathy; rather unusually these are regarded as being particularly diagnostic in forensic settings; thus, diagnostic category is a function not merely of the patient's characteristics but also of their setting.

Antisocial Personality Disorder — basic facts Antisocial Personality Disorder is three times more common among males than among females. The prevalence of the disorder is estimated to be between 0.6% and 2% in the general population; no adequate prevalence estimates for inpatient or outpatient settings are available (see Table 23.2). The prevalence of Antisocial Personality Disorder, and the related construct psychopathy, varies across cultures (Compton et al 1991, Robins et al 1991, Cooke 1998, Cooke & Michie 1999). In prison populations its prevalence may range from 50% to 75%; this has led some commentators to suggest that the diagnosis merely medicalises criminality. By definition evidence of Antisocial Personality Disorder is present in childhood. Comorbidity of Conduct Disorder and Attention Deficit/Hyperactivity Disorder is a particular risk factor for the development of the disorder in adulthood. Antisocial Personality Disorder has a higher frequency among first degree relatives of those suffering from the disorder compared with the general population. It is frequently comorbid with other personality disorders, including Borderline, Histrionic and Narcissistic.

Borderline Personality Disorder

The key defining features of Borderline Personality Disorder are impulsivity together with instability of affect, self-image and interpersonal relationships. To meet the diagnostic criteria individuals must meet five or more of the following:

- frantically avoids real or imagined abandonment;
- unstable and intense interpersonal relationships; alternates between idealisation and devaluation of others;
- unstable sense of self or self-image;
- impulsivity in more than one area, e.g. spending, substance abuse, reckless driving, sexual behaviour;
- recurrent self harm or parasuicidal behaviour;
- unstable affect and marked reactivity of mood;
- chronic feelings of emptiness;
- inappropriate intense anger or failure to control anger;
- brief dissociative experiences or paranoid thoughts linked to stress.

As a consequence of these traits, those suffering from Borderline Personality Disorder may undermine themselves just at the point of success (e.g. getting a new job, developing an intimate relationship); a proportion may develop psychotic-like symptoms under stress, e.g. ideas of reference, body image distortions and hallucinations. Broken relationships, disrupted education and disrupted employment are common.

Borderline Personality Disorder — basic facts Borderline Personality Disorder is three times more common among females than among males. Studies indicate that the prevalence of the disorder is between 0.7% and 2.0% in the general population, can reach 10% in outpatient settings and be as high as 20% in inpatient settings; as a group they are typically treatment seeking (see Table 23.2). During adolescence, problems of impulsivity and discontrol may lead to frequent contact with physical and mental health services; deliberate self-harm is common. Stability may emerge in the third and fourth decade of life.

In coming to this diagnosis it is important to establish that the symptoms do not only occur during the course of schizophrenia, a mood disorder with psychotic features, or other psychotic disorder. Borderline Personality Disorder has a higher frequency amongst first-degree relatives of those suffering from the disorder compared with the general population. It is frequently comorbid with other personality disorders, including, Antisocial, Histrionic and Avoidant.

Histrionic Personality Disorder

The key defining features of Histrionic Personality Disorder are emotionality and attention-seeking behaviour. To meet the diagnostic criteria individuals must meet five or more of the following:

- uncomfortable when not the centre of attention;
- interacts in a provocative or sexually seductive manner;
- displays of emotions are shallow and change rapidly;
- uses physical appearance to draw attention to self;
- speech lacks detail and is impressionistic;
- emotion is displayed in a theatrical, exaggerated or self-dramatic manner;
- suggestible;
- thinks relationships are more intimate than they are.

As a consequence of these traits, those suffering from Histrionic Personality Disorder may have difficulty in forming and maintaining intimate relationships; they control their relationships by manipulation and flirtation, while remaining overly dependent. Their flirtatiousness may threaten their relationships with same-gender friends. They are sensation seeking and prone to boredom; they can become frustrated when instant gratification is denied.

Histrionic Personality Disorder — basic facts Histrionic Personality Disorder is slightly more common among females. The prevalence of the disorder is estimatd to be between 2% and 3% in the general population and can be as high as 10–15% in outpatient and inpatient settings (see Table 23.2). It is frequently comorbid with other personality disorders, including Borderline, Antisocial, Dependent and Narcissistic. It is associated with unexplained physical complaints among women and substance abuse among men (Coid 2003).

Narcissistic Personality Disorder

The key defining features of Narcissistic Personality Disorder are grandiosity, lack of empathy and a need for admiration. To meet the diagnostic criteria individuals must meet five or more of the following:

- grandiose sense of self importance;
- fantasises about success, power, brilliance, beauty or ideal love;
- believes him/herself to be special and only to be understood by high-status people;
- needs excessive admiration;
- sense of entitlement; demands automatic compliance with his/her expectations;
- exploits others to achieve his/her own ends;
- lacks empathy;
- envious of others or believes others are envious of him/her;
- arrogant and haughty.

Those suffering from Narcissistic Personality Disorder frequently have vulnerable self-esteem; criticism results in feelings of humiliation or emptiness that they do not display outwardly. They may counterattack with rage, disdain or sarcasm. Within their relationships they demand recognition and admiration, and have a profound sense of entitlement.

Narcissistic Personality Disorder — basic facts Narcissistic Personality Disorder is more common among males. The prevalence of the disorder is estimated to be under 1% in the general population and 2–16% in outpatient and inpatient settings (see Table 23.2). It is common in forensic samples (Coid 2003). Narcissistic traits may be evident from early adolescence; however, their presence does not mean that the individual will progress to the full disorder (Ronningsham 1999). It is frequently comorbid with other personality disorders, including Borderline, Histrionic, Paranoid and Antisocial.

Cluster C: 'Anxious–fearful' Personality Disorders

This cluster is composed of three disorders: Avoidant Personality Disorder, Dependent Personality Disorder and Obsessive–Compulsive Personality Disorder.

Avoidant Personality Disorder

The key defining features of Avoidant Personality Disorder are inhibition in social situations, a sense of inadequacy, and hypersensitivity to negative evaluation. To meet the diagnostic criteria individuals must meet four or more of the following:

- avoids occupational activities that entail interpersonal contact that may result in disapproval, criticism or rejection;
- avoids relationships unless sure that they will be liked;
- restrained within intimate relationships because of fear of ridicule or being shamed;
- preoccupied with being criticised or rejected socially;
- inhibited in novel social situations due to feelings of inadequacy;
- construes self as inept, unappealing and inferior to others;
- reluctant to engage in new activities that might prove embarrassing.

As a consequence of these traits, those suffering from Avoidant Personality Disorder may have difficulty in interpersonal interactions because they are over-vigilant in their appraisal of the behaviour of those with whom they interact. They will appear shy, lonely and isolated. Within occupational settings they may avoid activities that involve interactions with others, avoidance that can affect their progress in the work place.

Avoidant Personality Disorder — basic facts Avoidant Personality Disorder is equally common among males and females.

The prevalence of the disorder is estimated to be between 0.5% and 5.0% in the general population and can be as high as 10% in outpatient settings (see Table 23.2). Onset may be evident from childhood difficulties, including a fear of strangers and new situations. Shyness is a common precursor; however, the majority of shy children do not develop the disorder. The disorder is particularly problematic during late adolescence and early adulthood when the capacity to develop new relationships is particularly key. It is frequently comorbid with other personality disorders, including Borderline, Schizotypal, Schizoid and Paranoid.

Dependent Personality Disorder

The key defining features of Dependent Personality Disorder are an excessive need to be taken care of, and a fear of abandonment which frequently leads to submissive or clinging behaviour. To meet the diagnostic criteria individuals must meet four or more of the following:

- indecisive without excessive advice and reassurance;
- requires others to take on responsibility for major aspects of his/her life;
- fearful about expressing disagreement with others, through fear of disapproval;
- difficulty in initiating projects, because of lack of confidence;
- excessive need for nurturance; may volunteer to do unpleasant activities;
- distressed when alone; fears being unable to care for self;
- urgently seeks new relationship when a relationship is terminated;
- preoccupied with fears of abandonment.

As a consequence of these traits, those suffering from Dependent Personality Disorder may have difficulty in close relationships, in which they will tend to seek protection from a dominant partner. Their view of self is frequently characterised by pessimism and doubt; criticism merely serves to reinforce their negative self-evaluation. They may avoid positions of responsibility because they are frightened of making mistakes.

Dependent Personality Disorder — basic facts Dependent Personality Disorder is equally common in males and females. The prevalence of the disorder is estimated to be between 1.0% and 2.2% in the general population; no adequate estimates are available for other settings (see Table 23.2). It is frequently comorbid with other personality disorders, including Borderline, Avoidant and Histrionic.

Obsessive–Compulsive Personality Disorder

The key defining features of Obsessive–Compulsive Personality Disorder are preoccupations with mental and personal control, perfectionism and orderliness at the cost of efficiency, openness and flexibility. To meet the diagnostic criteria individuals must meet four or more of the following:

- preoccupied with details, rules, etc. so that the primary purpose of activity is lost;
- perfectionism interferes with the completion of tasks;
- over-focused on work to the exclusion of friendships and leisure;
- overly conscientious, scrupulous and inflexible about ethics and morality;

- hoards objects even though they lack sentimental value;
- reluctant to delegate tasks unless they are completed exactly to their standard;
- miserly approach to both self and others;
- rigid and stubborn.

As a consequence of these traits, those suffering from Obsessive–Compulsive Personality Disorder may have occupational difficulties because they cannot start key tasks, they may become frustrated and angry in situations that they cannot control, and they may be particularly concerned with dominance and submission in relationships.

Obsessive–Compulsive Personality Disorder — basic facts Obsessive–Compulsive Personality Disorder is twice as common in males as females. The prevalence of the disorder is estimated to be between 1.7% and 2.2% in the general population, and can be as high as 10% in outpatient settings (see Table 23.2). Comorbidity with other personality disorders is rare.

Personality disorder not otherwise specified

DSM-IV provides a final category of personality disorder that may be diagnosed if the individual does not meet the criteria for any of the above personality disorders but meets a mixture of criteria from a number of disorders and, in addition, experiences significant distress or impairment in different areas of functioning.

Other DSM definitions for personality disorder

Understanding of personality disorders is still developing, and thus research criteria have been provided in the DSM manuals to promote research and understanding of other forms of personality pathology. Within the current edition two disorders have been described: Depressive Personality Disorder and Passive–Aggressive Personality Disorder.

Depressive Personality Disorder

The key defining features of Depressive Personality Disorder are depressive thoughts and behaviour as indicated by five or more of the following criteria:

- mood is dominated by dejection, gloom and an absence of joy, happiness, or cheerfulness;
- believes self to be worthless, inadequate; low self-esteem;
- overly critical and derogatory of self;
- broods and worries;
- negativistic judgements of others;
- pessimistic;
- feels guilt and remorse.

Passive–Aggressive (Negativistic) Personality Disorder

The key defining feature of Passive–Aggressive (Negativistic) Personality Disorder is a passive resistance to reasonable demands made of the individual in social or occupational settings. The disorder is indicated by the presence of four or more of the following criteria:

- passively resists fulfilling routine social and occupational tasks;
- believes that they are unappreciated or misunderstood;
- sullen and argumentative;

- criticises and scorns authority with no foundation;
- expresses resentment and envy towards more fortunate;
- persistent complaints of personal misfortune;
- alternates between contrition and hostile defiance.

UNDERSTANDING THE AETIOLOGY — RISK FACTORS FOR PERSONALITY DISORDER

Given the comparative recency of systematic nosologies of personality disorders it is perhaps not surprising that there are no comprehensive, empirically supported theories of aetiology. Paris (1993) indicated that the aetiology of personality disorders is unlikely to be underpinned by simple, linear, mono-causal processes; complex interactive processes among variables derived from various conceptual domains are likely to be at the core of the aetiology. Understanding this is particularly difficult because personality disorders emerge as the result of a number of processes which occasionally may be synergistic, amounting to more than the sum of the parts, some within the individual and some in society; it is not a static process; and key risk factors are likely to be drawn from many domains. Indeed, in his review, Paris (1993) extracted evidence from the biological, psychological and social domains and proposed a comprehensive biopsychosocial model for the development of personality disorders. We will consider the evidence for risk factors at different levels of abstraction.

Genetic influences

Studies of normal personality have long established the importance of genetic influences (Plomin et al 1994); their importance in regard to disorders of personality is less clear. A primary difficulty is the absence of clear definitions of phenotype, which are prerequisites for the establishment of inheritance; misdiagnosis and overlapping diagnostic categories will inevitably lead to spurious estimates of inheritance (Jang & Vernon 2001). Given the limitations of current diagnostic systems for personality disorders, there is limited knowledge of genetic influences. Summarising current knowledge derived from twin studies of personality functioning, Jang & Vernon (2001) contended that there are two broad findings.

- First, 40–50% of phenotypical variation can be attributed to additive genetic factors, little variation can be attributed to shared environmental factors, and the remaining variation relates to non-shared environmental factors.
- Second, the most replicable results are achieved when the Five-Factor Model of personality is used (FFM; Costa & McCrae 1992). This model measures five domains of personality functioning described as neuroticism, extraversion, openness to experience, agreeableness and conscientiousness.

Fewer twin studies have been carried out with regard to personality pathology, and these have focused on traits rather than diagnostic categories. Two studies are of note. DiLalla et al (1996) examined the heritability of Minnesota Multiphasic Personality Inventory (MMPI) dimensions in pairs of twins reared apart and recruited in the general population. Heritability estimates ranged from 28% (Paranoia), through 34% (Social Introversion) to 61% (Psychopathic Deviate). Jang et al (1996) reported the heritability of aspects of the Dimensional Assessment of Personality Problems (DAPP). Heritability estimates ranged from 35% (Rejection), through 49% (Cognitive distortions) to 53% (Narcissism) and 56% (Callousness).

Molecular genetic approaches have been applied in attempts to identify the actual alleles causing behaviour. Cloninger (1986) developed a model whereby candidate genes were identified and predictions made about the neurochemical basis of normal and abnormal personality; it was postulated that four traits of temperament would be underpinned by distinct monoamine neurotransmitter systems: dopamine for novelty seeking, serotonin for harm avoidance, noradrenaline (norephinephrine) for reward dependency and persistence. Empirical evidence has not supported the simple model; however, it has served as an important stimulus to work in this area. An overview of the molecular genetics and personality disorder can be found in Herbst et al (2000).

In conclusion, while there is some evidence of genetic contribution to personality disorder the inadequacy of diagnostic systems means that personality disorders remain phenotypically and genotypically obscure.

Biological influences

Explorations at the biological level, with the consideration of both neurotransmitters and neuropsychological structure and functioning, have implicated various risk factors for personality pathology. Of the neurotransmitters, serotonin (5HT) has been the most heavily researched. There is compelling and consistent evidence of an inverse association between 5HT and both impulsivity and aggression (Coccaro 2001). Virkkunen et al (1987) demonstrated that impulsivity may be most central. By comparing concentrations of 5HIAA (a serotonin metabolite) in CSF among impulsive arsonists suffering from Borderline Personality Disorder with concentrations among normal volunteers and impulsive violent offenders, they found that the arsonists and the violent offenders had similar levels of CSF 5HIAA: levels that were considerably lower than the normal volunteers. Pharmacological challenge studies have generally supported the role of 5HT in aggressive behaviour (Siever & Trestman 1993), as have studies of platelet receptor markers (Coccaro et al 1997).

Neither the role of noradrenaline (NA) nor that of dopamine (DA) has received substantial study in relation to personality disorders. There is limited evidence currently for the role of these neurotransmitters in relation to personality disorder (Coccaro 2001).

The growth of structural imaging procedures has yet to impact markedly on the study of personality disorders; the majority of studies has focused on Schizotypal Personality Disorder. The available studies suggest a reduced volume in temporal lobes and hippocampus, with increased ventricular size in the frontal lobes (Coccaro 2001).

Raine et al (2000) examined structural differences in the prefrontal cortex of a group of men in the community diagnosed with Antisocial Personality Disorder. Using magnetic resonance imaging they found that the Antisocial Personality Disorder group had a reduction in prefrontal grey matter compared with controls.

It is important to emphasise that these biological differences should not be assumed to be a consequence of genetics; they may be a consequence of experience, including experience in the womb. A clear illustration of this point comes from the famine studies. In the winter of 1944–1945 sections of the Dutch population were systematically starved by the occupiers because of their assistance to the Allies. It has been demonstrated that severe nutritional deficiency in the first or second trimester of intrauterine life increased the risk of developing Antisocial Personality Disorder (Neugebauer et al 1999). Other intrauterine insults have been considered. Wakschlag et al (2002) indicated that available evidence was consistent with the hypothesis that maternal smoking during pregnancy results in an elevated risk for the onset of antisocial behaviour. However, Silberg et al (2003) have recently contended that these results are more likely to be the consequence of the transmission of a latent tendency to develop conduct disorder rather than a direct effect of maternal smoking.

Early experiences

Within the field of personality disorder it has long been held, by authors from distinct theoretical positions, that early experiences are key in the ontogenesis of these disorders (e.g. Adler 1985, Millon & Davis 1996), yet, as Paris (2001) has argued, the evidence is not compelling. Risks are often construed as causal without adequate evidence (Kraemer et al 1997). Early adversities that are commonly reported by those in clinical samples only lead to significant pathology among a minority of those experiencing similar adversity within community populations (e.g. Brown & Harris 1978, Cooke 1981). Most individuals are resilient; consistent with a stress–diathesis model, only those with underlying vulnerabilities develop pathological states (Zuckerman 1999). Thus, early experience may trigger disorder, the nature of the disorder being shaped by the diatheses; this model accounts for the non-specificity of risk factors, the same risk factors being implicated in many disorders.

A variety of early adversities has been linked to the ontogenesis of personality disorder; we will consider three broad domains: social stressors, childhood abuse and dysfunctional families.

Social stressors

Increases in the prevalence of both Antisocial and Borderline Personality Disorder in contemporary society have been attributed to social stressors (Robins et al 1991, Millon 1993). Robins et al (1991), reporting on the Epidemiological Catchment Area study, argued that the lifetime prevalence of Antisocial Personality Disorder would increase from 3.7% to 6.4% by the time that members of the youngest cohort were over 30 years of age. A variety of explanations have been posited. Breakdown in stable relationships and the traditional social structures that suppress traits such as impulsivity may have a role. Also, a relative diminution in the availability of secure attachments may result in affective instability (Linehan 1993).

Childhood abuse

Sexual abuse in childhood has been frequently viewed as a causal risk factor for some forms of personality disorder (Hermann & van der Kolk 1987), with Borderline Personality Disorder being viewed as a complex form of PTSD. Reviewing this research, Paris (2000) argued that three conclusions can be drawn: first, sexual abuse during childhood is only one of several important risk factors for personality disorder; second, sexual abuse may be most clearly linked to Borderline Personality Disorder; third, this link appears to be important only in a subgroup of those suffering from Borderline Personality Disorder.

The evidence with regard to physical abuse is less clear and less consistent. Associations between physical abuse and the development of Antisocial Personality Disorder have been reported (Pollock et al 1990); however, it is difficult to disentangle the effects of abuse from parental psychopathology (Robins 1966). The role of parental psychopathology is considered below.

Dysfunctional families

Parental psychopathology Personality disordered individuals generally have parents and other relatives with psychopathology (Siever & Davis 1991); the influence of parental psychopathology is most evident for impulsive disorders. Robins (1966) found that having a psychopathic father was a key risk factor that remained important even when other co-occurring risks were controlled for. With regard to Borderline Personality Disorder, first-degree relatives have an elevated risk of 'impulsive spectrum' disorders, including Antisocial and Borderline Personality Disorder, substance abuse as well as mood disorders (e.g. Silverman et al 1991). The effects may be evident early; in a recent study paternal Antisocial Personality Disorder was reported to be associated with an increased odds of conduct disorder (OR = 5.27, p = 0.001), particularly among male offspring (OR = 8.55, p = 0.03) (Foley et al 2001).

Family disruption. Samples of males and females suggest that the prevalence of family breakdown during childhood is higher in those who suffer from personality disorders than in those who do not (Paris et al 1994a, 1994b). Disruption is more frequently posited as significant for Borderline Personality Disorder than other disorders.

Parenting practices. The notion that personality disorders may result from negative parenting practices is long rooted in psychodynamic theories, including attachment theory (Bowlby 1969) and theory of self pathology (Kohut 1997). One difficulty in researching this area is the retrospective nature of most of the research. Critically, it has been demonstrated that there is a heritable component to self-report of childhood experiences (Plomin & Bergeman 1991). Nonetheless, Brewin et al (1993) contended that if sufficient safeguards are put in place, including careful interviewing techniques, it is possible to retrospectively identify childhood adversity accurately.

McCord & McCord (1964) linked the development of psychopathy to parental neglect and erratic punishment. Marshall & Cooke (1998) demonstrated specificity of effect, with family stressors being linked to the interpersonal and affective aspects of the disorder, while social stressors during childhood were linked to the behavioural aspects. Longitudinal work has indicated that symptoms of personality disorder develop more frequently among children who have been grossly neglected or abused (Johnson et al 1999).

Cultural influences

The culture of a particular population is the sum of work and thought expressed or produced by members of that population, including their social practices, beliefs, institutions, and arts (Rogler 1999, Lopez & Gaurnaccia 2000). Although it is a reflection of people and the ecological and socio-economic contexts in which they live, at the same time culture exerts a profound influence on individual behaviour, cognition and emotion (Fiske 1995). In addition to influencing normal or non-pathological behaviour, culture can play an important role in the development and expression of mental disorder through pathogenic or pathoplastic mechanisms (Rogler 1993, 1996, Mezzich et al 1996, Alarcon et al 1998, Cooke & Michie 1999, Lopez & Gaurnaccia 2000, Cooke et al 2003). While some mental disorders have a strong pan-cultural core (i.e. a high degree of syndromal stability across cultures), others are specific or unique to a particular culture (i.e. culture-bound syndromes) (Draguns 1973, 1986).

Personality disorders are mental abnormalities characterised by chronic disturbances in relating to self, others and the environment (World Health Organization 1992b, APA 1994, 2000). Because personality is inherently relational in nature, manifested largely (some would argue even primarily) in the interpersonal sphere, culture may have a greater impact on personality disorders than on most other forms of mental disorder (Alarcon et al 1998, Cross & Markus 1999). Because complex and manifold social processes encourage interpersonal behaviours consistent with important norms and values (Weisz et al 1987, Weisz & McCarty 1999), personality disorders may tend to be an exaggeration of prevalent patterns of adaptation within a society (Draguns 1973, 1986, Alarcon et al 1998).

There has been considerable debate concerning the impact of culture on the expression of psychopathic personality disorder (also known as antisocial or dissocial personality disorder). Anthropological evidence suggests that psychopathic personality disorder is found across cultures (Cooke 1996), but it has been speculated that the disorder may be more prevalent in highly individualistic cultures (Hare 1993, Lykken 1995, Paris 1998). Collectivistic cultures promote the development of an interdependent self-identity, one in which the concept of self includes relationships with others; in contrast, individualistic cultures promote the development of self-identity that is independent of relationships with others (Cross & Markus 1999). Consequently, characteristics such as distinctiveness, status, self-confidence, honour, competition, and freedom from obligations to others are highly valued in individualistic cultures. Extreme manifestations of these characteristics may include conceit, manipulativeness, irresponsibility, pathological dominance, and aggressiveness (Wilson & Herrnstein 1985, Harpending & Draper 1988, Mealey 1995, Nisbett & Cohen 1996) — characteristics that resemble symptoms of psychopathic personality disorder contained in diagnostic criteria such as the Psychopathy Checklist–Revised (PCL-R; Hare 1991), DSM-IV (APA 1994, 2000) and ICD-10 (WHO 1992a).

Cooke & Michie (1999) demonstrated considerable variation in both the expression and prevalence of psychopathy, as measured by the PCL-R when Scottish and North American samples were compared. Cooke et al (2003) demonstrated that, while the affective deficits associated with psychopathy were stable across cultures, the expression of the interpersonal and behavioural features varied substantially across settings. Although most information on cross-cultural effects comes from the research on psychopathy, cultural effects are likely to affect all the personality disorders.

CATEGORICAL VERSUS DIMENSIONAL MODELS OF PERSONALITY DISORDER

Whether personality disorders should be classified using categorical or dimensional systems remains a key issue for researchers in this field, reflecting concern in other areas of psychiatric nosology (Brugha 2002, Endler & Kovovski 2002). The publication of DSM-III and DSM-IV led to increased interest in research in personality disorders; however, several major problems with clinical approaches to personality disorder were identified (Costa & Widiger 1994, Zimmerman 1994, Widiger & Sanderson 1995). A primary difficulty is that existing nosologies were based on the opinions of practitioners from a multitude of theoretical backgrounds, and these categorical nosologies lacked empirical support. As Schroeder et al (1994) expressed it:

> [C]onceptions of personality disorders are largely the consensus of experts who base their decisions on traditional clinical concepts and clinical experience. Consequently, classifications of personality disorders consist of relatively unstructured lists of diagnoses that reflect multiple theoretical perspectives within the clinical tradition. They do not incorporate, to any significant degree, accumulated empirical knowledge. ... The consequence of these developments is that current classifications tend to lack explicit structure and clear conceptual underpinnings. (p. 117)

A second problem is that the standard categorical systems fail to capture important information about the nature and severity of symptoms present in a given case. For example, there are 93 different ways in which a person can receive a diagnosis for Borderline Personality Disorder and 149 495 616 by which they can receive a diagnosis for Antisocial Personality Disorder in DSM-IV, even if one ignores the issue of symptom severity (Widiger & Sanderson 1995).

Third is the problem of comorbidity. DSM-IV encourages the diagnosis of more than one personality disorder in a given case. Research indicates that most individuals who suffer from a personality disorder meet the diagnostic criteria for two or three separate disorders; indeed, only about 15% of patients meet criteria for a singleton personality disorder (Costa & Widiger 1994, Stuart et al 1998). This may be due to flaws in the DSM conceptualisation of personality disorders (e.g. the inclusion of disorders that do not exist in nature, or the incorrect assumption of a categorical structural model) or flaws in the DSM criteria for these disorders (e.g. inordinate length or complexity, reliance on symptoms of poor sensitivity or specificity). Whatever the reason, the high degree of observed comorbidity seriously complicates research and clinical practice. If a patient meets criteria for more than one personality disorder, should treatment target all of them separately, those symptoms common to all the disorders, or only the primary disorder? And, if the latter, which criteria should be used to specify which personality disorder is primary and which secondary?

One potential solution to these problems, proposed by those familiar with the traditions of personality psychology, is the adoption of an empirically based dimensional structural model (Widiger & Frances 1994, Widiger & Sanderson 1995). Using dimensional models, it is possible to summarise rich symptom-level information efficiently and reliably. Comorbidity is not a concern within dimensional models, as there is no assumption that distinct and separate personality disorders ('types') exist.

Although there is general consensus that dimensional models of personality disorder are superior to categorical models in almost every respect, there is no agreement concerning which of the numerous possible dimensional models is preferable. Dimensional models differ in three important respects:

- first, whether they focus on phenotypic or 'surface' traits as compared with genotypic or 'source' traits;
- second, whether they focus on a relatively small number of general or 'higher-order' dimensions as compared with a relatively large number of more specific or 'lower-order' dimensions;
- third, whether they assume the traits are independent or 'orthogonal' dimensions compared with correlated or 'oblique' dimensions.

Two models illustrate these differences. The Five-Factor Model (FFM) was originally developed to describe normal personality, but more recently has been applied to personality disorder. Excellent overviews are provided by Costa & Widiger (1994) and Wiggins (1997). Within the FFM, five broad, bipolar, orthogonal dimensions are necessary and reasonably sufficient to account for the associations among phenotypic aspects of personality (Table 23.3). The dimensions can be defined as follows:

- Neuroticism is a tendency to be emotionally unstable and experience negative affect.
- Extraversion is a tendency to be energetic and sociable.
- Agreeableness is a tendency to be warm and non-confrontational.
- Conscientiousness is a tendency to be responsible and organised.
- Openness to experience is a tendency to value the exploration of new feelings and ideas over traditionalism (Costa & McCrae 1992).

Each broad dimension comprises a number of specific lower-level facet traits. The dimensions and their facets have been explicated over the course of decades by numerous investigators via factor analysis of data from tests of normal personality. One noteworthy strength of the FFM is that it subsumes another empirically based dimensional model, the Interpersonal Circle; another is its cross-cultural generalisability (Wiggins 1997).

The second model is the Dimensional Assessment of Personality Pathology (DAPP) developed by Livesley and colleagues (e.g. Livesley et al 1989, 1992, Schroeder et al 1994). These researchers chose a 'bottom-up' approach, which focuses primarily on lower-level traits and only secondarily on broad, general dimensions. In the DAPP model, 18 oblique dimensions are considered necessary and reasonably sufficient to describe the domain of personality pathology. The dimensions were identified by factor analysis of data obtained from comprehensive measures of personality disorder symptomatology. Subsequent analyses have examined the phenotypic and genotypic structure of the 18 dimensions (Livesley et al 1998), identifying four broad, orthogonal factors that parallel the FFM in many respects (Table 23.4). Other investigators have independently developed models similar to the DAPP in many respects (e.g. Clark et al 1994). However, at present there is little evidence examining the generalisability of the DAPP across cultures.

Numerous assessment procedures based on dimensional models of personality disorder are available for use in research and clinical practice. Both self-report inventories (Costa & McCrae 1992) and structured interviews (Trull et al 1998) have been developed to measure FFM dimensions. The same is true for the DAPP (Schroeder et al 1994) and similar models (Clark 1993). These procedures have good reliability and validity and provide highly detailed information, which makes them useful both in research and clinical practice. These procedures ask respondents to report specific behaviours, experiences and attitudes, rather than symptoms, and thus they appear to be less susceptible to bias than are measures based on categorical models of personality disorder.

ASSESSMENT AND DIAGNOSIS OF PERSONALITY DISORDER

Conceptual issues

In our view, at least six important principles should guide psychiatrists' decisions regarding the assessment and diagnosis of personality disorder. Below, we discuss these in some detail.

Personality disorder is a culture-bound concept Personality and personality disorder are defined and determined in relation to other cultural concepts such as self, abnormality and gender (Alarcon et al 1998, Cross & Markus 1999). Also, cultural customs differ markedly with respect to such things as interpersonal behaviour,

---

Table 23.3 A dimensional model of normal personality: the Five-Factor Model (FFM) as measured by the Revised NEO Personality Inventory

Factor	Facet scales
Neuroticism	Anxiety, hostility, depression, self-consciousness, impulsiveness, vulnerability
Extraversion	Warmth, gregariousness, assertiveness, activity, excitement-seeking, positive emotions
Openness	Fantasy, aesthetics, feelings, actions, ideas, values
Agreeableness	Trust, straightforwardness, altruism, compliance, modesty, tendermindedness
Conscientiousness	Competence, order, dutifulness, achievement striving, self-discipline, deliberation

After Costa & McCrae (1992).

Table 23.4 A dimensional model of personality disorder: factors and scales of the Dimensional Assessment of Personality Pathology – Basic Questionnaire (DAPP–BQ)

Factor	Scales
Neuroticism	Insecure attachment, anxiousness, diffidence, affective lability, narcissism, social avoidance, passive-oppositionality
Disagreeableness	Rejection, interpersonal disesteem, conduct problems, stimulus seeking, suspiciousness
Introversion	Intimacy problems, restricted expression, identity problems
Compulsivity	Compulsivity

After Schroeder et al (1994). Scales that were factorially complex appear under the factor on which they loaded highest. Two additional scales — Self-Harming Behaviors and Perceptual Cognitive Distortions — were not included in the factor analysis.

emotional expressiveness, religiosity and childrearing practices. This means that evaluators, as much as possible, should be familiar with critical features of their patients' culture and how these might influence the expression of personality disorder. It is impossible to assess and diagnose personality disorder independent of culture.

Personality disorder is a higher-order, inferential construct Personality disorder does not exist physically; rather, the concept is a (more or less) convenient fiction used to describe regularities in behaviour, affect and cognition (Bromley 1977, Livesley 2001). In this respect, it is similar to more familiar concepts such as climate, an inferential construct used to describe regularities in temperature, precipitation and so forth. The important point here is that evaluators' inferences regarding personality disorder will be reliable only to the extent that they are based on accurate information regarding their patients' patterns of behaviour, affect and cognition. It is impossible to assess and diagnose personality disorder without gathering data concerning multiple domains of functioning.

Personality disorder is inherently relational Symptoms of personality disorder are disturbances in one's relationships with self, others and the environment (Rutter 1987). As was noted by Schneider and many others since, this is one of the key features that distinguishes personality disorder from other forms of mental disorder: the former primarily causes distress in other people and may also cause personal distress; whereas the latter primarily causes personal distress and may also cause distress in others. Also, personality disorder may impair patients' insight into the nature and severity of their symptomatology, or may be associated with conscious attempts to distort their reports of symptomatology. One implication here is that evaluators' inferences regarding personality disorder will be reliable to the extent that they reflect the observations and perceptions of important members of their patients' social networks. Another implication is that there is no single 'truth' concerning patients' symptomatology; observers are likely to have perceptions of patients that differ from each other and from those of patients themselves. It is impossible to assess and diagnose personality disorder based solely on self-report.

Personality disorder reflects enduring patterns of dysfunction Personality disorder is a form of chronic mental disorder (Livesley 2001). Symptoms of personality disorder are rigid and maladaptive personality traits, not problems that are time-limited or context-specific. The implication here is that evaluators' inferences regarding personality disorder will be reliable to the extent that they reflect their patients' adjustment problems across times, across situations, and across interactions with various people. It is impossible to assess and diagnose personality disorder cross-sectionally.

Personality disorder symptomatology is diverse As discussed previously, researchers have described at least four or five high-order dimensions of personality disorder, comprising at least 16 or 18 basic symptoms dimensions and dozens or even scores of individual symptoms (Livesley 2001). Individual symptoms may differ from each other in severity, and also may fluctuate in severity over time. Indeed, there may be no clear line demarcating normal and abnormal personality. This means that evaluators' assessments and diagnoses will be useful to the extent that they are comprehensive, reflecting the diverse nature and severity of personality disorder symptomatology. It is impossible to capture the diversity of personality disorder using simple categorical or dimensional systems for assessment and diagnosis.

Personality disorder is independent of acute mental disorder Personality disorder may exist on its own or comorbid with acute mental disorder (Foulds 1965, Dolan-Sewell et al 2001). Distinguishing symptoms of the two can be a difficult task. Symptoms of other mental disorder may be comorbid with personality disorder symptomatology, but they can also mimic or mask personality disorder symptomatology. For example, acute dysthymia is observed frequently in people suffering from personality disorder. From a clinical perspective, the possibility of 'true' comorbidity makes good sense: It may reflect a common diathesis underlying the affective and personality disturbances; or it may reflect the existence of personality disturbance that caused psychosocial disturbance and led, directly or indirectly, to affective disturbance. But it is also possible that acute dysthymia mimics personality disorder, leading patients to over-report their adjustment problems in some domains of life functioning; or that it masks personality disorder, leading patients to under-report adjustment problems in other domains. The primary implication here is that evaluators should assess and diagnose personality disorder only as part of a comprehensive clinical investigation. It is impossible to assess and diagnose personality disorder without considering the potential impact of any comorbid mental disorder.

Summary

This brief discussion highlights the difficulties and complexities of assessing and diagnosing personality disorder. Even screening for the presence of personality disorder requires evaluators to consider a wide range of symptoms, primarily relational disturbances, inferred from reports reflecting multiple perspectives about regularities in affect, behaviour and cognition across time and situations; and these inferences should take into account contextual factors such as culture or comorbid acute mental disorder. Clearly, it is impossible to assess and diagnose personality disorder without exercising considerable professional judgement or discretion. In fact, it would seem that evaluators must be expert in the assessment and diagnosis of acute mental disorder before they can even begin to develop expertise in the assessment and diagnosis of personality disorder.

Measurement issues

Methods

Many different methods can be used to assess psychopathology.

Self-report methods include such things as interviews, self-ratings and questionnaires. The hallmark of self-reports is that they rely on patients to communicate information about their attitudes, experiences, thoughts, feelings, behaviour or self-appraisals. It should not be assumed naïvely that patients' self-reports are truthful; rather, they are a form of self-presentation that is, in turn, a function of self-perception, insight and compliance with the assessment process (e.g. Zimmerman 1994, Clark & Harrison 2001). As most self-report methods are administered orally or in writing, an assessment of literacy or fluency in the target language may be a prerequisite for their use. One strength of self-reports is that they are an economical and efficient way of collecting information. Another strength is that they are useful for gathering information about symptoms that are not publicly observable. A weakness is their failure to tap the perspectives of multiple people.

Observational methods rely on other people to communicate information about the attitudes, experiences, thoughts, feelings or behaviour of patients. These methods include clinician or peer reports and ratings. Again, it should not be assumed that observations are truthful; they are reports concerning the impact of patients on others and are a function of observers' knowledge of or familiarity with patients, as well as observers' perceptions, insight and compliance with the assessment process. An important strength of these methods is that evaluators can select people with the knowledge, skills or ability necessary to make observations. Another strength is that observational methods are an excellent way of assessing relational disturbances, especially when the observations of several people are aggregated. A weakness is that they cannot be used to gather information about the private or personal experiences of patients without their co-operation.

Performance methods involve evaluating the nature or success of patients' behaviour during the completion of specific tasks. They include such things as ability or achievement tests, in-vivo or simulated environment behaviour tests, and projective tests. These methods require co-operation with the assessment process, and also may require intact motor, language or literacy skills. An important strength is that they attempt to evaluate directly the products or consequences of personality organisation. A weakness is that, by definition, they reflect functioning at a specific time and in a specific context.

Psychophysiological methods evaluate physiological reactions to patients' perceptions of external stimuli. The physiological reactions include such things as changes in heart rate, blood pressure, cerebral blood flow, electrocortical or electrodermal functioning, and hormone levels. These methods may be invasive and require considerable co-operation from patients. Their primary strength is that they may permit relatively precise quantification of responses in highly controlled situations. Weaknesses include the fact that physiological measurements are often expensive and time-consuming to collect; also, they can be influenced by a host of nuisance factors, including physical health problems and the use of psychoactive medications, and also reflect the functioning of patients at a specific time and in a specific context.

Archival methods involve the evaluation of documents, records and other physical traces. They include such things as the review of hospital, school, employment, police or corrections files. These methods do not require the co-operation of patients, or any special skills and abilities on their part; however, they do require that patients have had the opportunity to be the subject of records or leave physical traces. A strength of archival methods is that they may permit the evaluation of behaviour over long periods of time. A weakness is that archives themselves — the ways in which information is obtained, stored, and retrieved — often change over time, thus introducing potential sources of error into the assessment process.

Structure and quantification

Regardless of the general type of method, assessment procedures vary with respect to structure. Structured procedures have fixed and explicit rules regarding how information is gathered, weighted or combined. In some cases, the structure is designed to permit information to be summarised in the form of categorical decisions or quantitative scores using flow charts or algorithms. Decisions or scores for individual patients may be interpreted with respect to those of a specific reference group, or with respect to an absolute standard or cutoff. These are sometimes referred to as *norm-referenced assessment* and *criterion-referenced assessment*, respectively. In contrast, the use of unstructured procedures gives evaluators considerable freedom with regard to gathering, weighting and/or combining information.

Structure and quantification can be helpful in many respects. First, they help to organise and set limits on the activities of the evaluator during the assessment process. Second, they attempt to reduce potential error and bias, or at least to reduce the number of sources of error and bias. Third, they facilitate the comparison of assessment findings across patients, evaluators and time. But these benefits come at the cost of flexibility. The limited room for the exercise of judgement and discretion may result in findings that are precise and reliable, but that lack validity and meaningfulness. Also, it may be impossible to use some structured assessment procedures with some patients, at some times, or in some circumstances. Finally, existing assessment procedures may not be relevant to the specific clinical issues under investigation.

Objectivity versus subjectivity

It is common, although somewhat misleading, to characterise assessment procedures as *objective* or *subjective*. Some commentators view information provided by patients as subjective and information provided by anyone else as objective; others view the findings of structured procedures as objective and the findings of unstructured procedures as subjective. But the use of any assessment procedure, and especially the interpretation of findings, requires evaluators either to exercise their own judgement or discretion or to accept that of other evaluators. In a sense, then, all assessment procedures are subjective; the only real question is who exercises how much judgement or discretion with respect to which aspects of the assessment process.

How should personality disorder be assessed?

There is no single 'best' way to assess psychopathology in general or, more specifically, personality disorder. Each assessment procedure has its strengths and weaknesses, including its own sources of error and bias. This is why *comprehensive clinical evaluations of personality disorder should integrate the findings of multiple assessment procedures*. When assessment findings are integrated, the strengths of a given procedure compensate for the weaknesses of others. The advantages of using multiple procedures will be most apparent when they are based on different assessment methods. For example, an assessment of personality disorder based primarily on several self-report procedures (say, three questionnaires and a structured diagnostic interview) will provide information that is systematically biased, relative to another that is based on a mixture of self-report, observational and archival methods (say, a questionnaire, a clinical rating scale and a review of medical records).

Of course, it is not a simple task to integrate the diverse and sometimes conflicting findings of different assessment procedures. But the fact that findings of various assessment procedures may diverge is not a problem; rather, disagreement is expected and, indeed, instructive. The evaluator's task is to analyse the nature and sources of such disagreement to see what substantive lessons, if any, can be learned about the personality of patients. This process of integration is sometimes referred to as *triangulation*. Triangulation is an inherently unscientific task, requiring evaluators to exercise judgement and discretion concerning how to weigh and combine information to reach final decisions regarding what should be done for the care of their patients.

Notwithstanding that there is no best single way to assess personality disorder and that each has strengths and weaknesses, it is certainly the case that some procedures are naturally better suited to the task than are others. The measurement concepts *method–mode match* and *method–function match* suggest that the selection of assessment procedures should be determined in part by the nature of the construct being evaluated and the nature of the decision(s) to be made. Taking into account the nature of personality disorder (i.e. the six principles discussed previously), and assuming that the evaluator's task is assessment and diagnosis to guide decisions regarding treatment, then self-report, observational and archival methods have obvious advantages relative to psychophysiological and performance methods. Specifically, self-report and observational methods may be superior for evaluating relational disturbances from multiple perspectives, whereas archival methods may be superior for evaluating regularities in relational disturbance over time and situations. The cross-sectional and dynamic nature of psychophysiological and performance methods means that, potentially, they could be used for evaluating short-term changes or fluctuations in personality disorder — although it is not clear, either theoretically or empirically, whether or how much personality disorder is expected to change over time.

Overview of procedures for assessing personality disorder

We have noted already that procedures for assessing personality disorder vary according to method, structure and quantification. But these procedures can also be distinguished in terms of two important features: the type of measurement model on which they are based and their scope. With respect to underlying measurement models, procedures may be divided into those based on *categorical models* of personality disorder, such as those from the DSM-IV or ICD-10, versus *dimensional models* of personality disorder, such as the Five-Factor Model or the models of Livesley (e.g. Livesley et al 1989) and Clark (e.g. Clark 1993). Of course, some procedures provide dimensional ratings within categorical diagnoses or categorical classifications based on dimensional ratings, but the underlying model is still either categorical or dimensional. With respect to scope, procedures may be further divided into those that are *comprehensive*, assessing the entire domain of personality disorder symptomatology, versus *focused*, assessing a small domain of symptoms corresponding to one or only a few categories or dimensions of personality disorder. In practice, procedures based on categorical models all are comprehensive in nature; it makes little sense to develop focused categorical measures, as they provide very limited information about patients.

In this section, we briefly describe the format of the most commonly used procedures for assessing personality disorder. Our goal here is to provide readers with an overview of the major procedures currently in use. Readers interested in more detail concerning the psychometric properties or validity of the procedures should consult detailed and excellent reviews by people such as Clark & Harrison (2001) and Kaye & Shea (2000). We do not summarise here the findings of empirical studies supporting the usefulness of each procedure; rather, the section concludes with general observations regarding the relevant research.

Comprehensive categorical procedures

Interview-based observer ratings A number of diagnostic interviews have been developed to assist the assessment of personality disorder. Focusing on procedures constructed according to the DSM-IV or ICD-10 criteria, these include the Diagnostic Interview for DSM-IV Personality Disorders (DIPD-IV; Zanarini et al 1996), the International Personality Disorder Examination (IPDE; Loranger 1999), the Structured Clinical Interview for DSM-IV Axis II Personality Disorders (SCID-II; First et al 1995), the Structured Interview for DSM-IV Personality Disorders (SIDP; Pfohl et al 1997), and the Personality Disorder Interview–IV (PDI-IV; Widiger et al 1995). Most are based on the DSM–IV categorical model of personality disorder, although the IPDE is based on the ICD-10 categorical model. The interviews range from highly structured to semi-structured. They are organised thematically or topically (according to domain of psychosocial functioning) in the IPDE and symptomatically (according to the symptom or disorder they are designed to tap) in the DIPD-IV and SCID-II; in the other interviews, both thematic and symptomatic versions are available. On average, the interviews contain about 100 questions, with thematically organised interviews being somewhat shorter. Evaluators rate the presence and severity of individual symptoms based on the patient's responses, although most of the interviews also allow evaluators to consider and integrate collateral information. Administration of the interviews typically requires about 60 to 120 minutes, and averages about 90 minutes; the IPDE, SCID-II and SIDP-IV can be used with screening tests to reduce administration time. Note that the interviews generally assume that evaluators have conducted an assessment of acute psychopathology prior to assessing personality disorder.

Self-report measures Again focusing on procedures constructed according to the DSM-IV criteria, several self-report measures were developed solely for the assessment of personality disorder, including the Coolidge Axis II Inventory (CATI; Coolidge & Merwin 1992), the Personality Diagnostic Questionnaire–IV (PDQ-IV; Hyler 1994), and the Wisconsin Personality Disorder Inventory for DSM-IV (WISPI-IV; Klein et al 1993). In contrast, the third edition of the Millon Clinical Multiaxial Inventory (MCMI-III; Millon et al 1997) was designed as a broad-band measure of psychopathology, including the DSM-IV personality disorders. There are no inventories in wide use developed according to the ICD-10 criteria. The items are declarative statements concerning experiences or attitudes related to symptoms of personality disorder, and patients are asked to indicate, using a fixed response format, the extent to which they agree with the statements. The inventories range in length from 85 items for the PDQ-IV to 214 for the WISPI-IV; administration typically requires 30 to 60 minutes.

Comprehensive dimensional procedures

Interview-based observer ratings No interviews of personality pathology based on dimensional models are in widespread use. Livesley has developed an interview version of the Dimensional Assessment of Personality Pathology–Brief Questionnaire (DAPP-BQ; Livesley & Jackson 2000), but it is unpublished and used infrequently.

Self-report measures Although comprehensive self-report measures of normal personality traits are common, there are relatively few measures designed specifically to provide a comprehensive assessment of personality pathology according to trait models. Existing procedures include the DAPP-BQ (Livesley & Jackson, *in press*), the Inventory of Interpersonal Problems–Big 5 Version (IIP-B5; Trapnell & Wiggins 1990), the Personality Psychopathology–Five (PSY-5; Harkness & McNulty 1994), and the Schedule of Nonadaptive and Adaptive Personality (SNAP; Clark 1993). The DAPP-BQ, PSY-5 and SNAP were constructed empirically, using a 'bottom-up' approach: scales were constructed by analysing the statistical associations among a large pool of items reflecting aspects of personality pathology. In contrast, the IIP-B5 was constructed theoretically, using a 'top-down' approach: items and scales were constructed to assess systematically major domains of personality pathology, and then the scales were refined in light of statistical analysis. The inventories range in length from 100 items for the IIP-B5 to 290 for the DAPP-BQ; typically, administration requires about 30 minutes for the IIP-B5 and an hour for the other inventories. The exception here is the PSY-5, which comprises a subset of items from the second edition of the Minnesota Multiphasic Personality Inventory (MMPI-2; Butcher et al 1989) and therefore requires about 90 to 120 minutes to administer. The IIP-B5 and PSY-5 yield scores on five major dimensions of personality disorder, whereas the DAPP-BQ and SNAP yield scores on multiple lower-order scales (18 and 15, respectively) comprising four higher-order dimensions.

Focused dimensional procedures

Interview-based observer ratings For evaluators who require in-depth assessment of a single personality disorder, a number of interview-based observer rating procedures have been developed, including the Revised Diagnostic Interview for Borderlines (DIB-R; Zanarini et al 1989), the Diagnostic Interview for Narcissism (DIN; Gunderson et al 1990), and the Hare Psychopathy Checklist–Revised (PCL-R; Hare 1991, 2003) and its Screening Version (PCL:SV; Hart et al 1995). Each of these procedures is designed to assess the full range of symptomatology associated with the disorder it assesses, including but not limited to DSM-IV or ICD-10 criteria. The procedures require the evaluator to rate the presence and severity of various symptoms — ranging in number from 12 on the PCL:SV to 33 on the DIN — based on responses to the interview. The interviews for the DIB and DIN are quite structured, whereas those for the PCL-R and PCL:SV are only loosely structured. Also, collateral information is required for making PCL-R and PCL:SV ratings; indeed, they can be made solely on the basis of collateral information, if necessary. Administration of these procedures typically requires between 60 and 120 minutes or more.

Self-report measures Numerous self-report measures are designed to assess specific personality disorders or specific domains of personality pathology. These include the Borderline Features scale of the Personality Assessment Inventory (PAI; Morey 1991), the Interpersonal Dependence Inventory (Hirschfeld et al 1977), the Narcissistic Personality Inventory (Raskin & Hall 1979), and the Schizotypal Personality Questionnaire (Raine 1991). For reasons that are not entirely clear, there is a bewildering number of self-report measures designed to assess antisocial (psychopathic or dissocial) personality disorder, including the Aberrant Self-Promotion scale (Gustaffson & Ritzer 1995), the Antisocial Features scale of the PAI (Morey 1991), the Antisocial Personality Questionnaire (Blackburn & Fawcett 1999), the Hare and

Levenson Self-Report Psychopathy Scales (Hare 1985; Levenson et al 1995), the Psychopathic Personality Inventory (Lilienfeld & Andrews 1996). Most of these are questionnaires of moderate length, typically including about 50 to 150 items from multiple subscales and requiring about 15 to 30 minutes to complete.

Reliability and validity of procedures — general observations

There is some research evaluating the reliability and validity of all these procedures, although the number of studies ranges from a handful for some instruments to scores — even hundreds — for others, particularly the SCID-II, MCMI-III and PCL-R. One general finding is that psychometric evaluations based on classical test theory indicate most of the procedures have achieved only moderate levels of internal consistency, interrater and test–retest reliability (e.g. Zimmerman 1994, Kaye & Shea 2000, Clark & Harrison 2001). Few have been subjected to intensive evaluations based on generalisability theory or modern test theory that could provide strong tests of reliability, as well as bias due to age, culture and gender; noteworthy exceptions here are the PCL-R and PCL:SV (e.g. Cooke & Michie 1997, 1999, Cooke et al 1999, Hare 1991, 2003). A second general finding is that most of the measures have limited concurrent validity. The agreement among various interview-based ratings and among various self-report measures typically also is moderate or moderate-to-high; but agreement across methods — that is, between interview-based ratings and self-report measures — is low to moderate (e.g. Zimmerman 1994, Kaye & Shea 2000, Clark & Harrison 2001). In summary, psychiatrists can rest assured that most of the procedures they might use can yield some useful information, although that information must be considered general or crude in nature.

TREATMENT OF PERSONALITY DISORDER

Nature of treatment

Treatments for personality disorders can be divided into two main classes: pharmacological and psychosocial. Most treatments are focused in nature, targeting specific symptom clusters; however, some psychosocial treatments are not specific to any particular personality disorders or personality disorder symptoms.

In turn, psychosocial treatments vary according to theoretical orientation, treatment modality and setting. Theoretical orientation refers to the underlying model of pathology and mechanism of change; some of the major orientations include supportive, psychoeducational, psychodynamic, cognitive-behavioral and interpersonal approaches. Treatment modality refers to the format in which the treatment is delivered, such as individual, couple or family, and group therapy. Finally, setting refers to the context in which the treatment is delivered, and may include outpatient, inpatient, or partial hospitalisation.

These treatments are not necessarily delivered independently. Indeed, the use of multiple treatments for a given patient is the rule rather than exception, based on 'the belief, which is based on both clinical experience and research evidence, that powerful treatment combinations are required to change integrated patterns of behavior and internal personality structure' (Piper & Joyce 2001 p. 324).

Effectiveness of treatment

Far more has been written about the effectiveness of treatment for personality disorders than actually is known about the topic. Although scores of potentially relevant articles have been published in the past fifty years, there is no substantial body of scientifically sound research on the treatment of people with personality disorders. Indeed, very few studies meet minimal criteria for methodological adequacy accepted in the field of psychotherapy outcome evaluation (e.g. Chambless & Ollendick 2001).

The existing research literature suffers from a number of problems (e.g. Coccaro 2001, Markovitz 2001, Piper & Joyce 2001). First, *most researchers are unclear about the goal or target of the treatments they evaluated.* Specifically, there is confusion in the literature concerning whether the goal of treatment is to reduce symptoms of personality disorder or to reduce symptoms despite personality disorder. The former goal is to achieve remission in patients with personality disorders by the end of treatment. In contrast, the latter goal is the significant reduction of specific symptoms (e.g. anxiety) or problem behaviours (e.g. substance abuse) associated with personality disorder, regardless of the diagnostic status of patients before or after treatment.

Second, studies have used *inconsistent concepts and measures of personality disorder.* These include a variety of diagnostic interviews, self-report inventories, and clinical assessments based on institutional records, based on different dimensional or categorical models. As a consequence, it is very difficult to compare the findings from various studies.

Third, the studies were hampered by a *failure to control for heterogeneity within treatment groups.* The studies ignored between-subject differences in the nature and severity of personality disorder symptomatology. The studies also ignored comorbid psychopathology, both acute mental disorder and personality disorders, as well as other risk factors, such as employment status, marital status and so forth. The failure to assess and control for heterogeneity may have obscured important findings.

Fourth, the studies typically had *inadequate definition and implementation of treatment.* The vast majority focused on treatments that have never been described or manualised, so it is impossible to know precisely which therapeutic interventions were used. Most studies did not take proper steps to ensure and evaluate treatment integrity. Few studies have paid attention to therapeutic process variables that might have shed light on mechanisms of change.

Fifth, the studies suffered from a *lack of adequate control groups.* Many studies did not include any kind of control group at all, and sample sizes tended to be reasonably small. Some studies included no-treatment or comparative treatment ('treatment as usual') control groups, but did not randomly assign offenders to these groups. A few studies attempted to offset the absence of random assignment by matching treated and control offenders *post hoc* on selected variables, but these groups were not equivalent with respect to other potentially important variables. The bottom line is that only a handful of studies used a true experimental design, i.e. one in which treatment and control groups were formed prior to treatment using random assignment and in which group equivalence with respect to theoretically important variables was evaluated.

Sixth, the studies were characterised by *severely restricted outcome criteria.* Most focused exclusively on symptom or diagnostic status at the end of treatment or a single follow-up time, rather than evaluating a broad range of measures related to psychosocial adjustment at multiple points in time. Broad outcome criteria might include sense of well-being, isolated dysfunctional behaviours, integrated patterns of behaviour, and internal personality structure (e.g. Piper & Joyce 2001).

Finally, in most studies there was a *lack of attention to developmental factors.* Some research has examined the treatment of characteristics related to personality disorder in children or adolescents, but there is no good evidence that personality disorder per se exists prior to adulthood, let alone that it can be measured reliably or in a manner comparable to that for personality disorder in adulthood. Even most studies of adults typically have ignored developmental changes throughout early, middle and late adulthood.

In light of these limitations, it is not possible to reach any firm conclusions regarding the effectiveness of treatment for personality disorders. Nevertheless, important trends are apparent in the literature and provide some guidance for treatment planning. We turn now to a discussion of the various forms of treatment for personality disorder, commenting on effectiveness where evidence exists. Readers interested in more detail should consult Livesley (2001).

Psychosocial treatments

Supportive

Supportive therapy is a specific form of treatment in which the therapist 'uses direct measures to ameliorate symptoms and maintain, restore, or improve self-esteem, adaptive skills, and psychological function' (Pinsker et al 1991 pp 221–222). It is typically delivered individually, although it can be delivered in group format. It tends to be non-specific in nature.

The mechanism of change for supportive therapy is believed to be the acquisition of new knowledge that leads to improvements in adaptive behaviour, accomplished through 'identification with or introjection of an accepting, well-related therapist' (Winston et al 2001 p. 345). A variety of specific techniques may be employed by the therapist, most of which involve active listening, providing advice and information, bolstering healthy defences and encouraging problem-focused coping.

Unfortunately, 'very little has been published on supportive psychotherapy specifically for personality disorders' (Winston et al 2001 p. 355).

Psychoeducational

In many respects, psychoeducational treatment can be conceptualised as supportive treatment that is provided to the families of patients, rather than to the patients themselves. It typically is delivered in family format, although it also can be delivered individually, in couple format, or in group format. It is most likely to be useful when focused in nature.

Psychoeducational treatment is founded on the belief that family interactions exert an important influence on the course of personality disorder, playing 'a key role in creating or perpetuating a maladaptive pattern [of] interaction', and that 'through a better understanding of the disorder, families will be able to learn and modify their responses to the maladaptive behaviors of their relatives with personality disorder' (Ruiz-Sancho et al 2001 p. 465).

Empirical support for this approach for personality disorders is very limited.

Psychodynamic

Psychodynamic treatment is based on the assumption that the unconscious urges, conflicts, introjects and structures believed to underlie personality disorder can be ameliorated through experiencing interactions and relationships with, or under the supervision of, a skilled therapist in controlled circumstances. Numerous forms of psychodynamic treatment have been developed, including a 'host of short-term dynamic therapies . . . though none are explicitly oriented to the treatment of personality disorder' (Piper & Joyce 2001 p. 326). Psychodynamic treatment is most often delivered individually, although it can be delivered in couple, family or group format. It is non-specific in nature.

Empirical support for this approach for personality disorders is very limited.

Cognitive-behavioural

Behavioural treatment of personality disorder attempts to change maladaptive behaviour by exploiting learning processes such as operant conditioning and modelling. Cognitive therapy for personality disorder, in contrast, is a 'schema-centred psychotherapy based on an information-processing model of psychopathology' (Cottraux & Blackburn 1995 p. 377). Cognitive-behavioural treatment (CBT) is a general term that refers to therapies that blend diverse elements of these two approaches. CBT may be delivered individually, in couple or family format, or in group format. It is specific in nature, comprising a wide range of techniques and procedures for various problems.

Research indicates that CBT is a potentially useful primary or secondary treatment for a variety of problems related to personality disorder (e.g. Rice & Harris 1997b, Piper & Joyce 2001). For example, social skills training programmes may help to remediate the interpersonal communication and assertiveness deficits observed in a wide range of serious personality disorders, especially DSM-IV Cluster A disorders. For people with impulsivity-related problems such as educational and vocational deficits or chronic hostility and aggression — a trait commonly found among people who meet criteria for DSM-IV Cluster B personality disorders — life skills programmes may be of assistance. For people with problems related to anxiety, depression, and affective lability, who are likely to meet criteria for DSM-IV Cluster C personality disorders, individual or group treatment programmes that teach emotion management skills may be useful. A major problem with behavioural treatment is that, despite behaviour change, 'often, there is minimal change in associated attitudes and beliefs and minimal generalization across associated behaviors and situations' (Piper & Joyce 2001 p. 337)

One form of treatment, known as Dialectical Behaviour Therapy (DBT; Robins et al 2001) is particularly noteworthy here. DBT was developed initially as a way of reducing impulsive, self-harmful behaviour in patients with borderline personality disorder by helping them to manage their emotional dysregulation. It includes behavioural techniques such as skills training, contingency management, cognitive modification, and exposure to emotional cues (Piper & Joyce 2001). It is the only form of treatment for personality disorder which has been deemed 'empirically validated' by independent reviewers (Chambless &

Ollendick 2001). One limitation is that relief of subjective distress has been limited (Piper & Joyce 2001).

Interpersonal

Interpersonal treatment seems, on the surface, ideally suited to personality disorders in light of their relational nature. Interpersonal theory posits that people may develop characteristic maladaptive styles of relating that are self-reinforcing, but that can be altered by interactions with others that force patients to engage in new patterns of behaviour in controlled settings. Interpersonal treatment can be delivered individually, but may be most effective when delivered in couple, family or group format. As MacKenzie (2001) observed, 'The group situation provides a unique context in which interpersonal phenomena can be enacted within a boundaried space' (p. 498). Interpersonal treatment may also be most effective when delivered in partial hospitalisation or inpatient settings, where the physical context facilitates the establishment of new rules for interaction and where a variety of adjunctive treatments may be available. Treatment of the latter sort is often referred to as milieu therapy, the essence of which is 'the patient's experience of interacting with others in a structured communal setting' (Piper & Joyce 2001 p. 329).

Although research on couple, family and group treatment for personality disorders is limited, there is substantial evidence supporting the effectiveness of milieu therapy (Piper & Joyce 2001). According to Piper & Joyce (2001), 'milieu treatments offer a comprehensive intervention "package" and capitalize on the patients' shared group experience. These elements likely work singly and in combination to promote benefit across a range of outcome indices' (p. 331).

Pharmacological treatment

Treatment of borderline personality disorder

Nefazodone, selective serotonin reuptake inhibitors (SSRIs), and serotonin and noradrenaline reuptake inhibitors (SNRIs) — which act at least in part via $5HT_2$ (serotonin-2) antagonism — appear to be the treatments of choice at present for borderline personality disorder (Coccaro 2001, Markovitz 2001). Reversible monoamine oxidase inhibitors (MAOIs) and opiate antagonists have potential due to apparent symptom reduction or low lethality, but require more systematic evaluation. Mood stabilisers such as lithium and anticonvulsants, antidpressants such as tricyclics and MAOIs, and typical and atypical antipsychotics are less effective, poorly tolerated, or highly lethal in overdose. Markovitz (2001) recommends nefazodone for most patients with borderline personality disorder, but SSRIs or SNRIs (in particular venlafaxine) for those with prominent obsessive–compulsive symptoms. Although a limited improvement in global symptomatology is common, most of the agents appear to be effective primarily in reducing impulsive behaviour, especially impulsive aggression and impulsive self-harm (Coccaro 2001, Markovitz 2001), as well as affective instability and somatic complaints. Research suggests that the same medications may also be effective in treating the impulsivity associated with antisocial personality disorder, but no good data are available to support this speculation. One problem is that pharmacotherapy is likely to be a long-term treatment, as 'reductions in effective dosages result in relapses' (Markovitz 2001 p. 487).

Treatment of schizotypal personality disorder

Several researchers have examined the effectiveness of low doses of antipsychotic agents in the treatment of schizotypal personality disorder, symptoms of which also may be found in schizoid, paranoid, and borderline personality disorder. In general, the research suggests that 'there may be an acute response . . . but long-term efficacy is doubtful' (Markovitz 2001 p. 485). More recent research suggests that SSRIs may be useful with schizotypal personality disorder patients who present with obsessive–compulsive symptoms.

Summary

Based on the limited evidence available, psychosocial treatments for personality disorder appear to be most effective when, like milieu therapies, they 'involve combinations of treatments' (Piper & Joyce 2001 p. 337). An inference from the literature reviewed here is that combined treatment may be most effective when it includes supportive and interpersonal treatments, and when delivered (at least in part) in group format. An untested but sensible assumption is that psychosocial treatments are not 'one size fits all' but rather should be matched to patients based on their personality characteristics, such as quality of object relations and psychological mindedness (Piper & Joyce 2001).

Pharmacological treatments have shown some promise in the management of certain personality disorder symptoms (Siever & Davis 1991), although 'there are few studies that address pharmacotherapy of personality disorder, let alone which symptom cluster groups respond best to which medications' (Markovitz 2001 p. 487). Medications may be used as the primary form of treatment in some cases, but should be considered as a secondary or adjunctive therapy for people receiving psychosocial treatments, as clinical experience suggests that concurrent pharmacotherapy may facilitate motivation for and compliance with psychosocial treatments.

PERSONALITY DISORDER AND THE LAW

Mental disorder and the Law

Mental illness has been recognised in medicine, and law, for millennia. If a mental illness causes substantial cognitive or volitional impairment, the law may deem the person incapable of making rational choices and therefore non-culpable (i.e. not responsible and undeserving of punishment) for past, current or future acts (Verdun-Jones 1989). In other words, mental illness may be considered a mitigating factor in forensic arenas. The fact that people are no longer considered agents, exercising free will, may be used to justify decisions to detain or incapacitate them for their own safety or for the safety of the general public. There are, however, reasonable grounds to believe that mental illnesses may remit (they are, after all, acute in nature), and if this happens it is generally the case that people's full rights and freedoms are returned to them.

Personality disorder came to be recognised in psychiatry only recently, in the late 19th and early 20th centuries (Berrios 1996). It was defined as a chronic disturbance of emotion or volition, or a disturbance of their integration with intellectual functions, that was distinct from both psychotic and neurotic illness and that resulted in socially disruptive behaviour. Although there was little agreement among alienists in the specific variants of personality disorder they identified, or in the names given to these disorders, there was general consensus that one important cluster was characterised by impulsive, aggressive and antisocial behaviour (Berrios 1996). For example, Schneider described 'labile', 'explosive', and 'wicked' psychopaths; Kahn described a cluster of 'impulsive', 'weak', and 'sexual' psychopaths; and Henderson described a cluster of psychopaths with 'predominantly aggressive' features.

The law quickly accepted the idea that personality disorder also can influence cognition and volition. For example, people suffering from personality disorder appear to be at increased risk for engaging in violent and other criminal behaviour. Personality disorder is, however, unlikely to impair cognition and volition substantially, and therefore people with personality disorders rarely are considered non-culpable for their acts. This is particularly true when the personality disorder is psychopathy (also commonly referred to as antisocial or dissocial personality disorder), reflecting characteristics such as impulsivity, irresponsibility, lack of empathy and remorse, and so forth (e.g. Hare 1996, Cooke et al 2004). A related concern is that personality disorder is, by definition, not likely to remit. If the personality disorder is not severe enough to be a mitigating factor in forensic decision making it may be considered, somewhat ironically, an aggravating factor, something that can be used to argue for harsher punishment or imposition of long-term social controls.

Legal relevance of personality disorder

Personality disorder and 'character'

Character is an important, if somewhat vague, concept in the law. For example, Anglo-American law holds that criminal proceedings should be reserved for situations in which there is no other way to express public condemnation or ensure public safety (Verdun-Jones 1989). A person who is charged with a relatively minor criminal offence but who is otherwise of 'good character' may be diverted out of the criminal justice system. This is especially true in the case of young people (juveniles; Melton et al 1997). Contrariwise, people with 'bad character' are not seen as appropriate candidates for diversion. Evidence of 'bad character' also may be entered in criminal of civil proceedings to call into question the credibility of a person's statements or testimony, or in family law disputes to argue that a person may be an unfit parent (Lyon & Ogloff 2000). Bad character generally is defined as a tendency toward deceitfulness, minimisation or denial of responsibility and lack of remorse for past misdeeds, lack of empathy, irresponsibility and a history of committing antisocial and aggressive acts. At least at the extremes, then, bad character clearly resembles personality disorder, especially psychopathic (antisocial, dissocial) personality disorder.

Personality disorder and decision-making capacity

Adjudicative competency Consideration of accuracy and fairness in criminal proceedings requires that defendants are able to communicate about and appreciate, at least to a limited extent, the nature and the possible consequences of the charges against them when dealing with police and courts (Roesch et al 1996, 1999, Melton et al 1997). In some jurisdictions, the law further requires that people are capable of using this understanding to make a rational decision (Roesch et al 1996). People who are judged to have a mental illness that renders them incom-petent to make decisions about their legal defence may be hospi-talised and treated involuntarily until they become competent, or if the charges are relatively minor and they present no undue risk to public safety they may be diverted out of the criminal justice system altogether.

In most Anglo-American jurisdictions, courts have considered personality disorder and determined that, as a general rule, it does not sufficiently impair adjudicative competence so as to render people incompetent (Verdun-Jones 1989, Melton et al 1997). This is because symptoms of personality disorder are unlikely to result in gross impairments of thought and speech or in grossly irrational perceptions of and beliefs about the external world. Only substantial impairment is likely to result in adjudicative incompetence, in part because the law expects that people can be represented by attorneys who are, of course, expert in criminal proceedings and who will spend considerable time and effort working on behalf of their clients (Roesch et al 1996).

Criminal responsibility   In Anglo-American law, a criminal offence comprises two elements: commission of a forbidden act (the *actus reus*) with negligent, reckless or maleficent intent (the *mens rea*). Both elements must be proven in court to convict a defendant (Verdun-Jones 1989, Blackburn 1993, Carson 1995, Golding et al 1999). When deciding whether the *actus reus* element exists, the law presumes that a person who acts has done so freely and voluntarily, with the opportunity to have considered the consequences of the act. This presumption is rebuttable, however. The law acknowledges that mental disorder (e.g. delirium and severe dissociative states) may lead people to act when not in a state of full consciousness or in an involuntary manner, a condition sometimes referred to as automatism. When deciding whether *mens rea* exists, the law presumes that a person had the ability to understand the nature and consequences of the act and that the act was wrong (Verdun-Jones 1989, Golding et al 1999). This pre-sumption is also rebuttable. The law acknowledges that mental dis-order (e.g. psychosis and dementia) may lead people to have beliefs or perceptions so irrational that they did not understand what they were doing or that what they were doing was wrong. When defen-dants are found not guilty on account of mental disorder, they usually are hospitalised until they are no longer mentally ill or no longer present a risk to public safety (Golding et al 1999).

Defining the nature and degree of the impairment that must exist before a person is found not criminally responsible on account of mental disorder has proved difficult. The legal defini-tion varies across jurisdictions and even within jurisdictions over time, partly in reaction to governmental and public concerns that mentally ill people should not escape sanctions for criminal behav-iour. What seems clear from research (Steadman et al 1993) is that the insanity defence is raised in only a tiny fraction of criminal cases — somewhere between about 1 in 100 and 1 in 1000 cases in which people are charged with serious crimes. As many as half of these cases never go to trial, because the prosecution and defence agree that defendants were not responsible when they committed the acts. Furthermore, people found not guilty on account of mental disorder often spend more time in the hospital than they would have spent in prison had they been found guilty. There seems little reason for concern that large numbers of men-tally ill people are 'getting away with murder'.

Although the law (somewhat grudgingly) accepts that a small number of people with mental illness — primarily those with psy-choses — will be found not criminally responsible on account of mental disorder, it is loath to accept this for people with personal-ity disorders. Yet people with personality disorders have, on occa-sion, successfully raised the insanity defence (Steadman et al 1993, Melton et al 1997, Golding et al 1999). In an effort to prevent this, the law has tried to narrow the scope of the legal test for criminal responsibility by increasing the severity of the requisite cognitive or volitional impairment. This strategy involves specifying that the mental disorder must result in cognitive (as opposed to emotional or volitional) impairment, and that the impairment must be severe (Verdun-Jones 1989). It is relatively easy for people with personality disorders to argue that their mental disorder results in emotional impairment (e.g. the intense and labile affect characteristic of borderline personal disorder, or the generalised affective deficits characteristic of psychopathy) or in volitional impairment (e.g. the impulsivity characteristic of borderline and psychopathic personality disorder), but difficult to argue that their mental disorder results in severe cognitive impair-ment (except, perhaps, the persecutory ideation or perceptual disturbances found in some cases of schizotypal personality disorder).

Competency to consent to treatment   Competency to consent to medical or psychological treatment is, in many respects, parallel to adjudicative competency (Applebaum & Grisso 1995, Roesch et al 1996). The law requires that people are able to com-municate about the decision and have at least a basic understand-ing of the possible risks and benefits of treatment options. Once again, in some jurisdictions, there may be a further requirement that people be able to use this understanding to make a rational decision (Roesch et al 1996). People who are judged to have a mental illness that renders them incompetent to make decisions about treatment may be treated or hospitalised involuntarily, with their decision-making powers transferred to family members, guardians or healthcare professionals. Only a substantial impair-ment of cognition will result in a finding of incompetence, in part because the law expects that people's welfare typically is protected by physicians or other professionals who are expert in healthcare and who are bound by professional ethics to act in the best inter-ests of their patients (Applebaum & Grisso 1995). Symptoms of personality disorder, however, are unlikely to result in such severe impairment.

Personality disorder and risk for criminality and violence

General sentencing issues   As discussed earlier, mental disorder that influences cognition or volition but does not sub-stantially impair them may be considered an aggravating factor in sentencing for criminal offences. There are two possible ratio-nales for this. One is based on the notion of specific deterrence, which refers to the idea that criminal sentences are punishments meted out against specific individuals that can be used to change their future behaviour. People with personality disorders, it could be argued, have demonstrated that they were not deterred by the usual social mechanisms and therefore may be in need of a special warning or reminder that criminal behaviour will not be tolerated by the courts. The second rationale is to ensure the pro-tection of public safety. People with personality disorders may require special controls — ranging from intensive supervision in the community, through electronic monitoring, to incarceration — to manage effectively their increased risk for future crime and violence.

Indeterminate sentencing   Some jurisdictions allow for the indeterminate (i.e. indefinite) commitment of people found guilty of repeated and serious criminal offences, especially sexual offences, who also are believed to be at high risk for future violence (Griffiths & Verdun-Jones 1994, Melton et al 1997). Such laws are based primarily on the principle of protection of public safety. Personality disorders (such as psychopathy) or symptoms of personality disorder (such as impulsivity, callousness or lack of remorse) often are considered to be *prima facie* grounds for determining that an individual presents a high risk for violence (MacLean 2000).

Civil commitment   Civil commitment allows for the involuntary hospitalisation and/or treatment of people who suffer from a mental disorder that impairs their ability to care for themselves (e.g. to meet their nutritional, hygiene or health needs) or that causes them to be a high risk for suicide or violence. The most common statutes provide for the short-term (several weeks to several months) commitment of individuals who present an imminent risk (Melton et al 1997). The expectation is that people will receive treatment and be released either to the least restrictive alternative or altogether as soon as their mental disorder is in remission or as soon as they no longer present an imminent risk. It is usually the case in law or, if not, in practice that the only people subject to civil commitment of this sort are those suffering from a severe mental illness (Melton et al 1997). Personality disorder may be explicitly excluded from the legal definition of mental disorder; even if not, it is unlikely to be considered a factor that results in imminent risk.

Another type of civil commitment that is becoming increasingly common is one designed for the indeterminate (several years to lifetime) commitment of people with mental disorder that makes them a long-term risk for violence — specifically, in some jurisdictions, sexual violence (Schlank & Cohen 1999, Janus 2000, MacLean 2000). Given the focus on long-term risk, it is not surprising that personality disorder is a major focus of indeterminate commitment laws. People committed in this manner are subject to or may request periodic reviews (typically at least once per year) to determine whether they may be released to a less restrictive alternative or freed altogether due to remission of the mental disorder or reduction in violence risk. Indeterminate civil commitment laws are controversial because they often are targeted at prison inmates who are completing a lengthy sentence and nearing their time for release into the community; thus, it is argued, they constitute a second punishment for offences committed many years previously (Janus 2000).

Within the United Kingdom personality disorder and risk to others has become a central, if controversial, concern in recent years. Within England and Wales, individuals who have been described as 'dangerous people with severe personality disorder' (DSPD) will be subject to new legislation (Department of Health 2000). Legal restraints will be placed on those who show significant disorder of personality *and* who present a significant risk of causing serious physical or psychological harm to others. In addition — critically — the risk that these individuals pose must be *functionally* linked to their personality disorder. The establishing of a functional link is fundamental if decisions regarding preventative detention are to be compatible with Article 5 (Right to liberty and security) of the European Convention of Human Rights. Within Scotland, personality disorder — in particular, psychopathic personality disorder — will be a factor in determining whether an individual should be subject to an Order of Life-long Restriction (MacLean 2000).

Issues in the forensic assessment of personality disorder

High prevalence of personality disorder

Regardless of whether psychiatrists adopt a categorical or a dimensional model, their assessments are complicated by the high prevalence of personality disorder in forensic settings (Trestman 2000, Hart 2002). For example, between 50% and 80% of all incarcerated adult offenders meet the diagnostic criteria for antisocial personality disorder (Hare 1983, Robins et al 1991); if one considers all the personality disorders contained in the DSM-IV or ICD-10, then the prevalence rate may be as high as 90% (Neighbors 1987). Of course, from the dimensional perspective things are even worse: every offender has traits of personality disorder; the only question is, how severe are the traits? Triers of fact may be unaware that personality disorder is pandemic in forensic settings and place undue weight on or draw unwarranted conclusions from the diagnosis. Psychiatrists should attempt to provide a context for diagnoses of personality disorder in three ways. First, they should explicitly acknowledge its high prevalence (e.g. 'Mr X meets the DSM-IV diagnostic criteria for antisocial personality disorder, which is found in about 50% to 80% of all incarcerated adult offenders'). Second, they should characterise it in terms of relative severity (e.g. 'My assessment of Mr X using the PCL-R indicates that he has traits of psychopathic personality disorder much higher than those found in healthy adults, but only average in severity relative to incarcerated adult male offenders'). Third, they should explain what they believe to be its legal relevance in the case at hand (e.g. 'In my opinion Mr. X poses a high risk for future sexual violence relative to other sexual offenders that is due at least in part to a mental disorder, specifically a severe antisocial personality disorder characterised by extreme impulsivity and lack of empathy').

Inchoate diagnoses

A special issue here concerns diagnosis in cases where the individual being evaluated manifests symptoms of personality disorder but does not meet the criteria for any specific disorder. It is common for clinicians to diagnose such patients as suffering from traits of one or more personality disorders (e.g. 'Axis II: Histrionic and Narcissistic traits, moderate severity') or from a rare or unspecified personality disorder (e.g. 'Axis II: Personality disorder, Not Otherwise Specified'). In civil settings, this practice makes sense. Alerting others to the possibility that a patient suffers from personality disorder may help them to plan or deliver treatments more effectively. The costs of false positive and false negative diagnoses are relatively small and roughly equal. In forensic settings, though, the routine diagnosis of personality disorder traits or unspecified personality disorders can have serious repercussions. Triers of fact may not realise that such diagnoses may reflect relatively minor adjustment problems on the part of the patient (especially in light of the high prevalence of personality disorder in forensic settings, as discussed previously) or significant uncertainty on the part of the evaluator. They may also not be aware that the reliability and validity of these diagnoses is highly questionable. Psychiatrists should keep in mind that what to them may be a rather minor part of their overall diagnostic formulation may be used in forensic decision making as grounds for something as serious as indeterminate commitment or capital sentencing. Accordingly, forensic psychiatrists should be very cautious — or even avoid altogether — making diagnoses of personality disorder traits or unspecified personality disorders. Those who do so should be prepared to justify their diagnoses in light of the general definition of personality disorders (e.g. WHO 1992, APA 1994, 2000) and in light of the specific symptoms present in the case at hand. Forensic psychiatrists also should acknowledge the uncertain reliability and validity of their diagnoses.

Causal role of personality disorder

An evaluator's opinion that a person suffers from personality disorder is, in itself, not of much interest in forensic decision making. As noted previously, the personality disorder is relevant only if the evaluator's opinion is that it *causes*, at least in part, some impairment of competency or elevated risk for criminality and violence *in this individual*. The unwarranted assumption of causality may render an opinion inadmissible because it is deemed to be irrelevant, not probative, or more prejudicial than probative. Psychiatrists should make explicit their opinions regarding the causal role played by personality disorder with respect to the relevant legal issue, whether impairment or risk. They should also acknowledge that such opinions are ultimately professional rather than scientific in nature — that is, based on inference and speculation, not on the direct application of scientific principle or procedures.

Diagnostic significance of antisocial behaviour

A history of antisocial behaviour may be of considerable diagnostic significance in civil psychiatric settings, where only a minority of patients has been charged with or convicted of criminal offences. In the DSM-IV, the diagnostic criteria for antisocial personality disorder are based largely on such a history. Obviously, antisocial behaviour is of little diagnostic significance in many forensic settings, where virtually everyone has record of arrests (APA 1994). Psychiatrists should be careful not to over-focus on antisocial behaviour — especially on isolated criminal acts — when diagnosing personality disorders. By definition, personality disorders should be manifested across various domains of psychosocial functioning, across time, and across important personal relationships (WHO 1992, APA 1994). A person who engages in antisocial behaviour only of a specific type, only against a specific person, or only at specific times may not suffer from a personality disorder at all. For example, consider a 50-year-old man who suffers from a sexual deviation and exposes his genitals to teenage girls in public places several times per year, but who is otherwise well adjusted — has a relatively stable marriage, holds a steady job, has good peer relationships, and so forth. In this case, the sexual deviation accounts for all of the patient's antisocial behaviour; there is no need to infer the presence of a personality disorder or even traits of personality disorder. Other mental disorders commonly associated with specific patterns of antisocial behaviour include impulse control disorder such as kleptomania (stealing) and pyromania (fire-setting).

In conclusion, it is hoped that this chapter has raised awareness of personality disorders, clinical phenomena that while frequently ignored have significant consequences for our patients, their families and society as a whole.

REFERENCES

Adler G 1985 Borderline psychopathology and its treatment. Jason Aronson, New York

Alaracon R D, Foulks E F, Vakkur M 1998 Personality disorders and culture: clinical and conceptual interactions. Wiley, New York

American Academy of Psychiatry and the Law 1995. American Academy of Psychiatry and the Law ethical guidelines for the practice of forensic psychiatry [On-line]. Internet: http://aapl.org/ethics.htm

APA 1980 Diagnostic and statistical manual of mental disorders, 3rd edn. American Psychiatric Association, Washington, DC

APA 1987 Diagnostic and statistical manual of mental disorders, 3rd edn. American Psychiatric Association, Washington DC

APA 1994 Diagnostic and statistical manual of mental disorders, 4th edn. American Psychiatric Association, Washington, DC

APA 2000 Diagnostic and statistical manual of mental disorders: text revision. American Psychiatric Association, Washington, DC

Applebaum P, Grisso T 1995 The MacArthur Treatment Competence Study (1): Mental illness and competence to consent to treatment. Law and Human Behavior 19:105–126

Bernstein D P, Useda D, Siever L J 2001 Paranoid personality disorder. In: Livesley W J (ed) The DSM-IV personality disorders. Guilford, New York, p 45–57

Berrios G E 1996 The history of mental symptoms: descriptive psychopathology since the nineteenth century. Cambridge University Press, Cambridge

Blackburn R 1993 The psychology of criminal conduct: theory, research and practice. Wiley, Chichester

Blackburn R, Fawcett D 1999 The Antisocial Personality Questionnaire: An inventory for assessing personality deviation in offender populations. European Journal of Psychological Assessment 15:14–24

Blanchard J J, Gangestad S, Brown S A, Horan W P 2000 Hedonic capacity and schizotypy revisited: a taxometric analysis of social anhedonia. Journal of Abnormal Psychology 109:87–95

Blashfield R K, McElroy R A 1987 The 1985 journal literature on the personality disorders. Comprehensive Psychiatry 28:536–546

Bowlby J 1969 Attachment. Hogarth, London

Brewin C R, Andrews B, Gotlib I H 1993 Psychopathology and early experiences: a reappraisal of retrospective reports. Psychological Bulletin 114:82–98

Bromley D B 1977 Personality description in ordinary language. Wiley, London

Brown G W, Harris T O 1978 Social origins of depression: a study of psychiatric disorder in women. Tavistock, London

Brugha T 2002 The end of the beginning: a requiem for the categorization of mental disorder? Psychologcal Medicine 32:1149–1154

Bull R, Carson D C (eds) 1995 Handbook of psychology in legal contexts. Wiley, Chichester

Butcher J N, Dahlstrom L, Graham J R et al 1989 Minnesota Multiphasic Personality Inventory–2. University of Minnesota Press, Minneapolis

Carson D C 1995 Criminal responsibility. In: Bull R, Carson D C (eds) Handbook of psychology in legal contexts. Wiley, Chichester, pp 277–289

Chambless D L, Ollendick T H 2001 Empirically supported psychological interventions: controversies and evidence Annual Review of Psychology 52:685–716

Clark L A 1993 Manual for the Schedule of Non-adapative and Adaptive Personality. University of Minnesota Press, Minneapolis

Clark L A, Harrison J A 2001 Assessment instruments. In: Livesley W J (ed) Handbook of personality disorders: theory, research, and treatment. Guilford, New York, p 277–306

Clark L A, Vorhies L, McEwen J L 1994 Personality disorder symptomatology from the Five-Factor Model perspective. In: Costa P T, Widiger T A (eds) Personality disorders and the Five-Factor Model of personality. American Psychological Association, Washington, DC, p 95–116

Cleckley H 1976 The mask of sanity, 5th edn. Mosby, St Louis

Cloninger C 1986 A unified biosocial theory of personality and its role in the development of anxiety states. Psychiatric Developments 3:167–226

Coccaro E F 2001 Biological and treatment correlates. In: Livesley W J (ed) Handbook of personality disorders: theory, research and treatment. Guilford, New York, p 124–135

Coccaro E F, Kavoussi R, Sheline Y I et al 1997 Impulsive aggression in personality disorder correlates with 5-HT2A receptor binding. Neuropsychopharmacology 16:211–216

Coid J W 2003 Epidemiology, public health and the problem of personality disorder. British Journal of Psychiatry 182:3–10

Committee on Ethical Guidelines for Forensic Psychologists 1991 Specialty guidelines for forensic psychologists. Law and Human Behavior 15:655–665

Compton W M, Helzer J E, Hwu H G et al 1991 New methods in cross-cultural psychiatry: psychiatric illness in Taiwan and the United States. American Journal of Psychiatry 148:1697–1704

Cooke D J 1981 Life events and syndromes of depression in the general population. Social Psychiatry 16:181–186

Cooke D J 1996 Psychopathic personality in different cultures: what do we know? What do we need to find out? Journal of Personality Disorders 10:23–40

Cooke D J 1998 Cross-cultural aspects of psychopathy. In: Millon T, Simonsen E, Birket-Smith M, Davis R D (eds) Psychopathy: antisocial, criminal and violent behavior. Guilford, New York, p 260–276

Cooke D J, Michie C 1997 An Item Response Theory evaluation of Hare's Psychopathy Checklist. Psychological Assessment 9:2–13

Cooke D J, Michie C 1999 Psychopathy across cultures: North America and Scotland compared. Journal of Abnormal Psychology 108:55–68

Cooke D J, Michie C 2001 Refining the construct of psychopathy: towards a hierarchical model. Psychological Assessment 13:171–188

Cooke D J, Michie C, Hart S D, Clark D 2003 Searching for the pancultural core of psychopathy. (Under review)

Cooke D J, Michie C, Hart S.D, Clark D 2004 Reconstructing psychopathy: clarifying the significance of antisocial and socially deviant behavior in the diagnosis of psychopathic personality disorder. Journal of Personality Disorders (in press)

Cooke D J, Michie C, Hart S D, Hare R D 1999 The functioning of the Screening Version of the Psychopathy Checklist–Revised: an item response theory analysis. Psychological Assessment 11:3–13

Coolidge F L, Merwin M M 1992 Reliability and validity of the Coolidge Axis II Inventory: a new inventory for the assessment of personality disorders. Psychological Assessment 59:223–238

Costa P T Jr, McCrae R R 1992 Revised NEO Personality Inventory (NEO PI-RTM) and NEO Five-Factor Inventory (NEO-FFI). Psychological Assessment Resources, Inc Odessa, Fl

Costa P T, Widiger T A 1994 Introduction: personality disorders and the five-factor model of personality. In Costa P T, Widiger T A (eds) Personality disorders and the Five-Factor Model of personality. American Psychological Association, Washington, DC, p 1–12

Cottraux J, Blackburn I 1995 Thérapies cognitives des troubles de la personalité. Paris

Cross S E, Markus H R, 1999 The cultural constitution of personality. In: Pervin L A, John P O (eds) Handbook of personality. Guilford, New York, p. 378–396

Department of Health 2000 Reforming the Mental Health Act. Department of Health, London

Desjarlais R, Eisenberg L, Good B, Kleinman A 1995 World mental health: problems and priorities in low income countries. Oxford University Press, Oxford

DiLalla D L, Carey G, Gottesman I I, Bourgeois J A 1996 Heritability of MMPI personality indicators of psychopathology in twins reared apart. Journal of Abnormal Psychology 105:491–499

Dolan-Sewell R T, Krueger R F, Shea M T 2001 Co-occurrence with syndrome disorders. In: Livesley W J (ed) Handbook of personality disorders: theory, research, and treatment. Guilford, New York, p 84–104

Draguns J G 1973 Comparison of psychopathology across cultures: issues, findings, directions. Journal of Cross-cultural Psychology 4:9–47

Draguns J G 1986 Culture and psychopathology: What is known about their relationship. Australian Journal of Psychology 38:329–338

Dutton D G, Bodnarchuk M A, Kropp P R et al 1997 Client personality disorders affecting wife assault post-treatment recidivism. Violence and Victims 12:37–50

Edens J F, Hart S D, Johnson D W et al 2000 Use of the personality assessment inventory to assess psychopathy in offender populations. Psychological Assessment 12:132–139

Endler S E, Kovovski N L 2002 Personality disorders at the crossroads. Journal of Personality Disorders 16:487–502

First M B, Spitzer R L, Gibbon M et al 1995 The Structured Clinical Interview for DSM-III-R personality disorders (SCID-II), II: Multi-site test–retest reliability study. Journal of Personality Disorders 9:92–104

Fiske A P 1995 The cultural dimensions of psychological research: method effects imply cultural mediation. In: Shrout P E, Fiske S T (eds) Personality research method and theory: a festschrift honoring Donald W Fiske. Erlbaum, Hillsdale. NJ, p 271–294

Foley D L, Pickles A, Simonoff E et al 2001 Parental concordance and comorbidity for psychiatric disorder and associated risks for current psychiatric symptoms and disorders in a community sample of juvenile twins. Journal of Child Psychology and Psychiatry 42:381–394

Forth A E, Brown S L, Hart S D, Hare R D 1996 The assessment of psychopathy in male and female noncriminals: reliability and validity. Personality and Individual Differences 20:531–543

Foulds G 1965 Personality and personal illness. Tavistock, London

Golding S, Skeem J, Roesch R, Zapf P 1999 The assessment of criminal responsibility: current controversies. In: Hess A K & Wiener I B (eds) Handbook of forensic psychology, 2nd edn. Wiley, New York, p 379–408

Griffiths C T, Verdun-Jones S N 1994 Canadian criminal justice, 2nd edn. Harcourt Brace, Toronto

Gunderson J G, Ronningstam E F, Bodkin A 1990 The diagnostic interview for narcissistic patients. Archives of General Psychiatry 47:676–680

Gustaffson S B, Ritzer D R 1995 The dark side of normal: a psychopathy-linked pattern called aberrant self-promotion. European Journal of Personality, 9:1–37

Hare R D 1983 Diagnosis of antisocial personality disorder in two prison populations. American Journal of Psychiatry 140:887–890

Hare R D 1985 A comparison of procedures for the assessment of psychopathy. Journal of Consulting and Clinical Psychology 53:7–16

Hare R D 1991 The Hare Psychopathy Checklist – Revised. Multi-Health Systems, Toronto

Hare R D 1993 Without conscience: the disturbing world of the psychopaths among us. Pocket Books, New York

Hare R D 1996 Psychopathy: a clinical construct whose time has come. Criminal Justice and Behavior 23:25–54

Hare R D 1998 The Hare PCL-R: Some issues concerning its use and misuse. Legal and Criminological Psychology 3:101–122

Hare R D 2003 The Hare Psychopathy Checklist – Revised, 2nd edn. Multi-Health Systems, Toronto

Harkness A R, McNulty J L 1994 The Personality Psychopathology Five (PSY-5): issues from the pages of a diagnostic manual instead of a dictionary. In: Strack S, Lorr M (eds) Differentiating normal and abnormal personality. Springer, New York, p 291–315

Harpending H, Draper P 1988 Antisocial behavior and the other side of cultural evolution. In: Moffitt T E, Mednick S A (eds) Biological contributions to crime causation. Marinus Nijhoff, Boston

Hart S D, Hare R D 1997 Psychopathy: assessment and association with criminal conduct. In: Stoff D M, Brieling J, Maser J (eds) Handbook of antisocial behavior. Wiley, New York, p 22–35

Hart S D, Forth A E, Hare R D 1991 The MCMI-II as a measure of psychopathy. Journal of Personality Disorders 5:318–327

Hart S D, Cox D N, Hare R D 1995 Manual for the Hare Psychopathy Checklist – Revised: Screening Version (PCL:SV). Multi-Health Systems, Toronto

Herbst J H, Zonderman A B, McCrae R R, Costa P T 2000 Do the dimensions of the Temperament and Character Inventory map a simple genetic architecture? Evidence from molecular genetics and factor analysis. American Journal of Psychiatry 157:1285–1290

Hermann J van der Kolk B A 1987 Traumatic antecedents of borderline personality disorder. In: van der Kolk B A (ed) Psychological Trauma. American Psychiatric Association, Washington, DC, p 111–126

Hirschfeld R M A, Klerman G L, Gough H G et al 1977 A measure of interpersonal dependency. Journal of Personality Assessment 41:610–618

Hogan R E, Johnson J A E, Briggs S R E 1997 Handbook of personality psychology. Academic Press, San Diego

Hyler S E 1994 Personality Diagnostic Questionnaire-IV (PDQ-IV). New York State Psychiatric Institute, New York

Jang K L, Vernon P A 2001 Genetics. In: Livesley W J (ed) Handbook of Personality Disorders: theory, research and treatment. Guilford, New York, p 177–195

Jang K L, Livesley W J, Vernon P A, Jackson D N 1996 Heritability of personality disorder traits: a twin study. Acta Psychiatrica Scandinavica 94:438–444

Janus E S 2000 Sexual predator commitment laws: lessons for law and the behavioral sciences. Behavioral Sciences and the Law 18:5–21

Johnson J G, Cohen P, Brown J et al 1999 Childhood maltreatment increases risk for personality disorders during early adulthood. Archives of General Psychiatry 56:600–606

Kalus O, Bernstein D P, Siever L J 1995 Schizoid personality disorder. In: Livesley W J (ed) The DSM-IV Personality Disorders. Guilford, New York, p 58–70

Kaye A L, Shea T M 2000 Personality disorders, personality traits, and defense mechanisms. In: Rush A J, Pincus H A, First M B (eds) Handbook of psychiatric measures. American Psychiatric Press, Washington, DC, p 713–749

Kendler K S, Hewitt J 1992 The structure of self-report schizotypy in twins. Journal of Personality Disorders 6:1–17

Klein M H, Benjamin L S, Rosenfeld R et al 1993 The Wisconsin Personality Disorders Inventory: development, reliability, and validity. Journal of Personality Disorders 7:285–303

Kohut H 1997 The restoration of the self. International Universities Press, New York

Kraemer H C, Kazdin A E, Offord D R et al 1997 Coming to terms with the terms of risk. Archives of General Psychiatry 54:337–343

Lenzenweger M F 1999 Deeper into the schizotypy taxon: on the robust nature of maximum covariance analysis. Journal of Abnormal Psychology 108:182–187

Levenson M R, Kiehl K A, Fitzpatrick C M 1995 Assessing psychopathic attributes in a non-institutionalized population. Journal of Personality and Social Psychology 68:151–158

Lilienfeld S O & Andrews B P 1996 Development and preliminary validation of a self-report measure of psychopathic personality traits in non-criminal populations. Journal of Personality Assessment 66:488–524

Linehan M M 1993 Cognitive-behavioural treatment of Borderline Personality Disorder. Guiford, New York

Livesley W J 1998 The phenotypic and genotypic structure of psychopathic traits. In: Cooke D J, Forth A E, Hare R D (eds) Psychopathy: theory, research and implications for society. Kluwer, Dordrecht, p 69–81

Livesley W J 2001 Conceptual and taxonomic issues. In: Livesley W J (ed) Handbook of personality disorders: theory, research, and treatment. Guilford, New York, p 3–38

Livesley W J, Jackson D 2000 Dimensional assessment of personality pathology. Sigma Press, Port Huron, Mich

Livesley W J, Jackson D, Schroeder M L 1989 A study of the factorial structure of personality pathology. Journal of Personality Disorders 3:292–306

Livesley W J, Jackson D, Schroeder M L 1992 Factorial structure of traits delineating personality disorders in clinical and general population samples. Journal of Abnormal Psychology 101:432–440

Livesley W J, Jang K L, Vernon P A 1998 Phenotypic and genotypic structure of traits delineating personality disorder. Archives of General Psychiatry 55:941–948

Lopez S T, Gaurnaccia P J J 2000 Cultural psychopathology: uncovering the social world of mental illness. Annual Review of Psychology 5:571–598

Loranger A M 1999 International Personality Disorder Examination. Psychological Assessment Resources, Odessa, Fl

Loranger A W, Sartorius N, Andreoli A et al 1994 The International Personality Disorder Examination: the World Health Organization/Alcohol, Drug Abuse, and Mental Health Administration international pilot study of personality disorders. Archives of General Psychiatry 51:215–224

Lykken D T 1995 The antisocial personalities. Erlbaum, Hillsdale, NJ

Lyon D, Ogloff J R P 2000 Legal and ethical issues in psychopathy assessment. In: Gacono C (ed) The clinical and forensic assessment of psychopathy: a practitioner's guide. Erlbaum, Mahwah NJ, p 139–173

McCord W, McCord J 1964 The psychopath: an essay on the criminal mind. Van Nostrand, Princeton, NJ

MacKenzie K R 2001 Group psychotherapy. In: Livesley W J (ed) Handbook of personality disorders. Guilford, New York, p 497–526

MacLean R (Chairman) 2000 Report of the Committee on Serious Violence and Sexual Offenders. Scottish Executive, Edinburgh

Markovitz P 2001 Pharmacotherapy. In: Livesley W J (ed) Handbook of personality disorders. Guilford, New York, p 475–495

Marshall L, Cooke D J 1998 The childhood experiences of psychopaths: a retrospective study of familial and societal factors. Journal of Personality Disorders 13:211–225

Mattia J I, Zimmerman M 2001 Epidemiology. In: Livesley W J (ed) Handbook of Personality Disorders: theory, research, and treatment. Guilford, New York, p 107–123

Mealey L 1995 The sociobiology of sociopathy: an integrated evolutionary model. Behavioral and Brain Sciences 18:523–599

Melton G B (ed) 1985 Nebraska symposium on motivation, vol. 33: The law as a behavioral instrument. University of Nebraska Press, Lincoln

Melton G B, Petrila J, Pothress N G, Slobogin C 1997 Psychological evaluations for the courts: a handbook for mental health professionals and lawyers, 2nd edn. Guilford, New York

Mezzich J E, Kleinman A, Fabrega H, Parron D L 1996 Culture & psychiatric diagnosis: a DSM-IV perspective. American Psychiatric Association, Washington, DC

Millon T 1993 Borderline personality disorder: a psychosocial epidemic. In: Paris J (ed) Borderline personality disorder: etiology and treatment. American Psychiatric Press, Washington, DC

Millon T, Davis R D 1996 Disorders of personality DSM-IV and beyond, 2nd edn. Wiley, New York

Millon T, Davis R, Millon C 1997 Millon Clinical Multiaxial Inventory–III (MCMI-III) manual, 2nd edn. National Computer Systems, Minneapolis

Morey L 1997 Personality diagnosis and personality disorders. In: Hogan R E, Johnson J, Briggs S (eds) Handbook of Personality Disorder. Academic Press, San Diego, p 919–946

Morey L C 1991 The Personality Assessment Inventory professional manual. Psychological Assessment Resources, Odessa, Fl

Neighbors H 1987 The prevalence of mental disorder in Michigan prisons. DIS Newsletter 4:8–11

Neugebauer R, Hoek H W, Susser E 1999 Prenatal exposure to wartime famine and development of antisocial personality disorder in early adulthood. Journal of the American Medical Association 282:455–462

Nisbett R E, Cohen D 1996 Culture of honor: the psychology of violence in the South. Westview Press, Oxford

Ottoson H, Ekselius L, Grann M, Kullgren G 2002 Cross-system concordance of personality disorder diagnosis of DSM-IV and diagnositic criteria for research of ICD-10. Journal of Personality Disorders 16:283–292

Paris J 1993 Personality disorders: a biopsychosocial model. Journal of Personality Disorders 7:255–264

Paris J 1998 Personality disorders in sociocultural perspective. Journal of Personality Disorders 12:289–301

Paris J 2001 Psychosocial adversity. In: Livesley W J (ed) Handbook of Personality Disorders: theory, research, and treatment. Guilford, New York, p 231–241

Paris J, Zweig-Frank H, Guzder J 1994a Psychological risk factors for borderline Personality Disorder in female patients. Comprehensive Psychiatry 35:305

Paris J, Zweig-Frank H, Guzder J 1994b Risk factors for borderline personality disorder in male outpatients. Journal of Nervous and Mental Disease 182:375–380

Pfohl B, Black D W, Zimmerman M 1997 Structured interview for DSM-IV personality (SIDP-IV). American Psychiatric Press, Washington, DC

Pilkonis P A, Blehar M C, Prieh R F 1997 Research directions for the personality disorders, Part 1. Journal of Personality Disorders 11:201–204

Pinel P 1962 A treatise on insanity. Hafner, New York (Original published 1801)

Pinkster H, Rosenthal R N, McCullogh L 1991 Dynamic supportive psychotherapy. In: Crit-Christoph P, Barber J P (eds) Handbook of short term dynamic psychotherapy. Basic Books, New York, p 220–247

Piper W E, Joyce A S 2001 Psychosocial treatment outcomes. In: Livesley W J (ed) Handbook of personality disorders. Guilford, New York, p 323–343

Plomin R, Bergeman C S 1991 The nature of nurture: genetic influences on "environmental" measures. Behavioral and Brain Sciences 14:373–427

Plomin R, Owen M J, McGuffin P 1994 The genetic basis of complex human behaviors. Science 264:1733–1739

Pollock V E, Briere J, Schneider L et al 1990 Childhood antecedents of antisocial behavior: parental alcoholism and physical abusiveness. American Journal of Psychiatry 147:1290–1293

Raine A 1991 The SPQ: a scale for the assessment of schizotypal personality based on DSM-III criteria. Schizophrenia Bulletin 17:555–564

Raine A, Benishay D 1995 The SPQ-B: a brief screening instrument for schizotypal personality disorder. Journal of Personality Disorders 9:346–355

Raine A, Lencz T, Bihrlc S et al 2000 Reduced prefrontal gray matter volume and reduced autonomic activity in antisocial personality disorder. Archives of General Psychiatry 57:119–127

Raskin R N, Hall C S 1979 A narcissistic personality inventory. Psychological Reports 45:590

Rice M E, Harris G T 1997a Cross-validation and extension of the Violence Risk Appraisal Guide for child molesters and rapists. Law and Human Behavior 21:231–241

Rice M E, Harris G T 1997b Mentally disordered offenders: what research says about effective service. In: Webster C D, Jackson M A (eds) Impulsivity: theory, assessment and treatment Guilford, New York

Robins C, Ivanoff A M, Linehan M M 2001 Dialectical behavior therapy. In: Livesley W J (ed) Handbook of personality disorders. Guilford, New York, p 437–459

Robins L N 1966 Deviant children grown up: a sociological and psychiatric study of sociopathic personality. Williams & Wilkins, Baltimore

Robins L N, Tipp J, Przybeck T 1991 Antisocial personality. In: Robins L N, Regier D (eds) Psychiatric disorders in America: the Epidemiologic Catchment Area study. Free Press, New York, p 258–290

Robins L N, Tipp J, Przybeck T 1991 Psychiatric disorders in America. In: Robins L N, Regier D A (eds) Antisocial personality disorder. Free Press, New York, p 258–290

Roesch R, Hart S D, Zapf P 1996 Conceptualizing and assessing competency to stand trial: implications and applications of the MacArthur treatment competence model. Psychology, Law, and Public Policy 2:96–113

Roesch R, Zapf P, Golding S, Skeem J 1999 Defining and assessing competency to stand trial. In: Hess A K, Wiener I B (eds) Handbook of forensic psychology, 2nd edn. Wiley, New York, p 327–349

Rogler L H 1993 Culturally sensitizing psychiatric diagnosis: a framework for research. Journal of Nervous and Mental Disease 191:401–408

Rogler L H 1996 Framing research on culture in psychiatric diagnosis: the case of the DSM-IV. Psychiatry 49:145–155

Rogler L H 1999 Methodological sources of cultural insensitivity in mental health. American Psychologist 54:424–433

Ronningsham E F 1999 Nacisstic personality disorder. In: Millon T, Blaney P H, Davis R D (eds) Oxford textbook of psychopathology. Oxford University Press, Oxford, p 674–693

Ruiz-Sancho A M, Smith G W, Gunderson J G 2001 Psychoeducational approaches. In: Livesley W J (ed) Handbook of personality disorders. Guilford, New York, p 460–474

Rutter M 1987 Temperament, personality and personality disorder. British Journal of Psychiatry 150:443–458

Schlank A, Cohen F (eds) 1999 The sexual predator: law, policy, evaluation, and treatment. Civic Research Press, Kingston, NJ

Schneider K 1958 Psychopathic personalities, 9th edn. Cassell, London (Original published 1923)

Schroeder M L, Wormworth J A, Livesley W J 1994 Dimensions of personality disorder and the five-factor model of personality. In: Costa P T, Widiger T A (eds) Personality disorders and the Five-Factor Model of personality. American Psychological Association, Washington, DC, p 1–12

Siever L J, Davis K L 1991 A psychobiological perspective on the personality disorders. American Journal of Psychiatry 148:1647–1658

Siever L J, Trestman R L 1993 The serotonin system and aggressive personality disorder. International Journal of Clinical Psychopharmacology, 8(suppl 2):33–39

Silberg J L, Parr T, Neale M et al 2003 Maternal smoking during pregnancy and risk to boys' conduct disturbance: an examination of the causal hypothesis. Biological Psychiatry 53:130–135

Silverman J D, Pinkham L, Horvath T B et al 1991 Affective and impulsive personality disorder traits in the relatives of patients with borderline personality disorder. American Journal of Psychiatry 148:1378–1385

Slovenko R 1997 Civil competency. In: Hess A K, Wiener I B (eds) Handbook of forensic psychology, 2nd edn. Wiley, New York, p 151–167

Steadman H J, McGreevy M A, Morrissey J et al 1993 Before and after Hinckley: evaluating insanity defense reform. Guilford, New York

Stuart S, Pfhol B, Battaglia M et al 1998 The co-occurrence of DSM-III-R personality disorders. Journal of Personality Disorders 12:302–315

The cultural constitution of personality. In: Pervin L A, John P O (eds) Handbook of personality. Guilford, New York, p 378–396

Trapnell P D, Wiggins J S 1990 Extension of the Interpersonal Adjective Scales to include the Big Five dimensions of personality. Journal of Personality and Social Psychology 59:781–790

Trestman, R. L 2000 Behind bars: personality disorders. Journal of the American Academy of Psychiatry and the Law 28:232–235

Trull T J, Widiger T A E, Useda D et al 1998 A structured interview for the assessment of the five factor model of personality. Psychological Assessment 10:229–240

Tyrer P, Simmonds S 2003 Treatment models for those with severe mental illness and comorbid personality disorder. British Journal of Psychiatry 182:15–18

Verdun-Jones S N 1989 Criminal law in Canada: cases, questions and the code. Harcourt Brace Jovanovich, Toronto

Virkkunen M, Nuutila A, Goodwin F W, Linoila M 1987 Cerebrospinal fluid monoamine metabolite levels in male arsonists. Archives of General Psychiatry 44:247

Wakschlag L S, Pickett K E, Cook E et al 2002 Maternal smoking during pregnancy and severe antisocial behavior in offspring: a review. American Journal of Public Health 92:966–974

Weissman M M 1993 The epidemiology of personality disorders: a 1990 update. Journal of Personality Disorders 7:44–62

Weisz J R, McCarty C. A 1999 Can we trust parents' reports in research on cultural and ethnic differences in child psychopathology? Using the bicultural family design to test parental culture effects. Journal of Abnormal Psychology 108:598–605

Weisz J R, Suwanlert S, Chaiyasit W, Walter B R 1987 Over and undercontrolled referral problems among children and adolescents from Thailand and the United States: the Wat and Wai of cultural differences. Journal of Consulting and Clinical Psychology 55:719–726

WHO 1992a International classification of diseases and causes of death, 10th edn. World Health Organization, Geneva

WHO 1992b The ICD-10 classification of mental and behavioural disorders: clinical descriptions and diagnostic guidelines. World Health Organization, Geneva

Widiger T A, Frances A J 1994 Toward a dimensional model for the personality disorders. In Costa P T, Widiger T A (eds) Personality disorders and the Five-Factor Model of personality. American Psychological Association, Washington, DC, p 19–39

Widiger T A E, Rogers J J 1989 Prevalence and comorbidity of personality disorders. Psychiatric Annals 19:132–136

Widiger T A, Sanderson C J 1995 Toward a dimensional model of personality disorders. In: Livesley W J (ed) The DSM-IV personality disorders. Guilford, New York, p 433–458

Widiger T A E, Mangine S, Corbitt E et al 1995 Personality Disorder Interview–IV: A semistructured interview for the assessment of personality disorders, Psychological Assessment Resources, Odessa, FL

Wiggins J S 1997 In defense of traits. In: Hogan R E, Johnson J, Briggs S (eds) Handbook of personality psychology. Academic Press, New York, p 97–117

Wilson J Q, Herrnstein R J 1985 Crime and human nature. Simon & Schuster, New York

Winston A, Rosenthal R N, Muran J C 2001 Supportive psychotherapy. In: Livesley W J (ed) Handbook of personality disorders. Guilford, New York, p 344–358

Wolff S, Chick J 1980 Schizoid personality disorder. Psychological Medicine 10:85–100

Zanarini M, Gunderson J G, Frankenburg F R, Chauncey D L 1989 The Revised Diagnostic Interview for Borderline: discriminating borderline personality disorder from other Axis II disorders. Journal of Personality Disorders 3:10–18

Zanarini M, Frankenburg F R, Sickel A E, Yong L 1996 Diagnostic interview for DSM-IV personality disorders. Harvard University Press, Cambridge, Mass

Zimmerman M 1994 Diagnosing personality disorders: a review of issues and research methods. Archives of General Psychiatry 51:225–245

Zuckerman, M 1999 Vulnerability to psychopathology: a biosocial model. American Psychological Association, Washington, DC

24 | Learning disability

Walter J Muir

INTRODUCTION

Learning disability (LD), considered as a field within which psychiatrists seek to practice, continues to change at a bewildering pace. The term itself is unsatisfactory, and no more informative than the epithet 'mental illness' is as a term for the multitude of distressing psychiatric conditions that can affect the individual. It is also a source of confusion — most other countries adopt the term mental retardation, and, in countries dominated by the classifications of DSM-IV, learning disability commonly refers to specific disorders of learning in those who do not necessarily have an intellectual impairment. And yet, as with 'mental handicap' before it, LD has passed into our language as the term we currently use to describe the complex intellectual and social condition that affects a substantial group of people. Most of the previous nomenclatures have become viewed as opprobrious, sometimes with good reason, others largely through the way society has treated and alienated people with LD. The history behind this nosology has been dealt with before (Muir 1998). What is usually important to people with LD is not the terminology used but whether they are recognised and respected as individuals in their own right, whether the doctor can remember their first and second names. Cognitive disability does not diminish the moral status of any individual, no matter how severe that disability, and this status is enshrined by our common humanity. The philosophical and other arguments for (and against) the proposition that our common humanity insists that we have respect for every individual with LD have been well addressed by Byrne (2000).

That LD is a descriptive term, not a disorder in itself, is the central theme of this chapter. It is only by understanding the proximate causes that have cognitive outcomes that we can progress to separate out and study the different life trajectories of individuals with LD so as to make predictions about outcomes, about susceptibilities and strengths, about interventions that are useful to the person. Each syndrome has features that not only distinguish it from others but also determine how these will change and develop over time. Nearly forty years ago Leo Kanner (1964 in his *History of the Care and Study of the Mentally Retarded*) entitled a chapter 'From homogeneity to heterogeneity', noting the changes from the unitary idea of the early 19th century which recognised only one specific type of disorder associated with LD (congenital hypothyroidism, then termed cretinism), through to a wide range of conditions including Down syndrome (DS) by the turn of the century. This trend has now become a huge flood, and behind this flood lies the march of molecular genetics. There are approaching a thousand genetic syndromes alone that are associated with LD, with no sign of the pace of discovery slackening. This phenomenon is certainly not restricted to LD (Childs 2001). The gene pool is highly mutable — it has to be so in order to maintain the genetic flexibility that underpins much of the homeostatic capacity of a species. Mutations are essential and frequent — they provide the necessary substrates for adaptive responses to environmental change and stress. It is not surprising then that many will not be adapted to the environment at any given time — these we often regard as deleterious. Mankind has also increased its homeostatic capacity through cultural and social mechanisms; we can alter the environment so that many previously severely incapacitating conditions have had their effects reduced, sometimes eliminated. This is of course a major function of medicine. Phenylketonuria (PKU) is an autosomal recessive disorder (prevalence around 1:15 000) caused by a gene mutation disrupting a key enzyme that converts phenylalanine to tyrosine. Unchecked phenylalanine accumulates to toxic levels, and formerly it was often associated with severe LD, epilepsy, microcephaly, and in some cases repeated self-injury. Knowledge of its genetic basis led to the elimination of phenylalanine from the diet of individuals so affected with a marked effect — intellectual impairment has been drastically reduced. So important was this discovery that the inhibition test devised by Guthrie was one of the earliest perinatal screening programmes for a genetic disease and still continues. The rate of mutation for PKU has not decreased however, but the mutation is now much more congruent with survival (Lindee 2000).

For the majority of conditions, however, the cognitive disability is not open to such interventions, the aim is to maximise the person's potential within the restrictions that the disability imposes, and to detect and treat other coexisting conditions. Among these, psychiatric illness and behavioural disorder are those that most concern the psychiatrist. When these arise in the setting of specific disorders, then they are affected by the shared characteristics of the group of individuals, as well as by their individual variations, including those due to previous history and experience. It is not only the genetic foundations of these syndromes that are being clarified, however; how they affect developmental neurobiology is now much better understood for many, with disorders of neuronal division and patterning, neuronal migration and neuronal maturation, and examples of these are discussed below. In addition, infections, toxins and trauma still continue to take a huge worldwide toll, and their associations with LD are outlined.

LD requires a broad knowledge base drawn from a diverse set of disciplines: child health and paediatrics, psychology, neurology, genetics and ageing. The repertoire of the psychiatrist in learning disabilities has narrowed with the closure of most of the large LD hospitals, and they are no longer responsible for the bulk of primary care. However, as the interdisciplinary nature of LD practice expands, there is a great need to understand the person beyond the limiting concept of LD. This chapter focuses where possible on recent research; this is not to minimise the importance of the corpus of older work on which it is based, but space constraints mean that a focus has to be set. The older literature is covered in previous editions of the *Companion*.

CURRENT DEFINITIONS OF LEARNING DISABILITY

The most widely used clinical approaches to defining LD are similar in requiring a triad of features: intellectual impairment, problems with social or personal adaptive functioning and an onset before the age of 18 years. DSM-IV-TR (APA 2000) uses a multiaxial system very similar to that promoted by the American Association on Mental Retardation criteria (AAMR 1992). The AAMR criteria use the same three basic constructs as DSM-IV-TR but are more complex, with extensive definitions of patterns and degrees of support-needs covering ten different domains. Both these systems are an advance in that LD (mental retardation) is no longer classified as a primary disorder but placed correctly as a descriptive category. Thus, using DSM-IV-TR, a hypothetical person may have a disorder on axis I, and also mental retardation on axis II. If they also had epilepsy, this would be coded as for other general medical conditions on axis III. Axis IV would be used to describe problems in someone with autism and LD, for example, who also has difficulties in the psychosocial/environmental domains such as a disrupted social support network due to bereavement, or life transition problems that often occur around school leaving age. Axis V is based on a global assessment of function scale, and since it refers to a supposed continuum between mental health and illness, it is rather more difficult to relate to the person who has LD without a given mental illness. In spite of the usefulness of the multiaxial approach, DSM-IV-TR still permits a non-axial approach, placing (unfortunately) mental retardation back as a specific disorder.

The tenth revision of the International Statistical Classification of Diseases and Related Health Problems (ICD-10) lists mental retardation among the mental and behavioural disorders (WHO 1992, 1993). It is not multiaxial, nor has a strict age criterion other than that impairment must occur during the developmental period, but does use the same IQ banding structure as DSM-IV-TR. However, the need for support is used as one of the indicators when differentiating mild from severe LD, and it also allows that overall functioning may change with time — so subdefining LD depends on current state. Any other disorders that are present generate an independent additional code. Recently the International Classification of Functioning, Disability and Health (ICF or ICIDH-2) has described aspects of interactions between person and environment and individual functioning that can be used to enrich ICD-10 descriptions (WHO 2001). Overall, however, the DSM-IV-TR approach is probably the most useful and emphasises the need to search for and define the proximate cause(s) of which LD is the outcome (King et al 2000a).

Intellectual impairment

The use of IQ measures in the definition of LD is controversial. However, there needs to be a degree of intellectual functioning that is statistically below the population average as a necessary, but not in itself sufficient, criterion. The use of a cut-off value of 70 (two standard deviations below the mean) is not a problem; the problem is largely how the psychological instruments available estimate this. DSM-IV-TR and ICD-10 qualify the value of 70 with word 'approximately', and the AAMR 'approximately 70–75'. IQ scores are not precise, with an error range of near ± 5 points. Thus the concept of 'borderline' LD has emerged, but its practical utility is limited. There are strong sociocultural influences in IQ testing, which affect the choice of instrument, and thus comparability. In spite of these difficulties, IQ measures are still useful. The divisions into mild, moderate and severe, whilst based on IQ measures alone, reflect definite gradations in adaptive ability, which, in turn, have major influences on independence, communication, self-care and dependency on others (reflected for instance in the differing levels and types of services needed to provide for patients' social and health needs). DSM-IV-TR maintains the category of profound LD, although pragmatically it is difficult to distinguish it from many with severe LD, and the validity of formal IQ tests at this level is open to doubt. Clinically, it is probably best to consider three levels — mild, moderate and severe — and their clinical and social outcomes (Table 24.1), without overt emphasis on IQ boundaries. The AAMR definition, in fact, does away with IQ boundaries in subclassification altogether, using instead categories based on levels of support needed: intermittent, limited, extensive and pervasive. These support levels often equate to people who meet the IQ-based definitions mild, moderate or severe LD but emphasise that the IQ spectrum is a continuum and that the needs-based approach may be much more relevant to the person's care and well-being.

The overall IQ of a given population changes over time, leading to temporal differences in those who would be classified as having LD if it were the sole criterion. Again, this especially applies to those in the grey zone between mild LD and those without LD. It is thus essential that other criteria be involved in the definition.

Problems with adaptive functioning

Limitations in social or personal adaptation are also required for a diagnosis of LD to be made. In fact these are usually the presenting features that lead to investigation of intellectual functioning. These are usually expressed as problems in communication or the use of speech, the ability to self-care, interpersonal and other social relationships. Many children who obtain formal IQ estimates around 70 fulfil full roles as adults in society. There is no need to describe them as having a disability or handicap within the cultural norms of a given society although they are statistically different on IQ testing. This fact explains why the administrative prevalence of LD is usually far less than the number of people with IQ test scores less than 70.

Age at onset

This third criterion reflects the aetiological nature of conditions that generate LD; they are neurodevelopmental and are apparent during infancy, childhood or adolescence. Eighteen years is used as the cut-off — again arbitrarily, since the development of the nervous system is not complete at this time. Myelination completes at around 30 years of age, and the brain continues to change throughout life. The age criterion is thus partly administrative but does help differentiate the cognitive impairments inher-

Table 24.1 Features associated with various severities of learning disability

Severity of learning disability	IQ score ranges commonly used to subdivide a population into the gradations of severity	Approximate functional equivalent mental age in the general population	Percentage of total population affected*	Associated features	Notes
Mild	69–50	12–9	1.5–2	Adaptive functioning usually mildly impaired, but in specific situations dysfunction may be in excess of that expected on the basis of IQ measures. Communication skills may be mildly affected, with specific educational difficulties	IQ changes in large part due to similar polygenic factors determining IQ in general population. Association with lower social class of parents. Sometimes called 'subcultural' or 'cultural-familial'. But increasing number of specific aetiologies being discovered
Moderate	49–35	<9–6	Up to 0.5 combining moderate and severe (excess over expected values due to organic pathologies)	Significant problems with day-to-day functioning. Communication often affected, with difficulties in the use of language	Overlaps with above but, as the disability becomes more severe, the number of specific organic pathologies increases
Severe	34 and less	<6		Major adaptive problems. Structured verbal communication may be absent. High care needs, little awareness of personal dangers. In the most severe, all body functions may be compromised, with double incontinence, severe feeding difficulties, inability to walk etc.	Vast majority associated with detectable organic pathology in uterine, peri- or postnatal period.
(Profound)	(<20)	(<3)	(0.05)		(Profound disability is in brackets here as the distinction from severe has doubtful value)

* Figures are approximate averages summarised from a number of prevalence studies.

ent to conditions associated with LD from those due to brain injury in adults, which have a different profile and require different types of management and treatment. Although many conditions are detected early, some, even apart from trauma or severe encephalopathies that can strike at any age, may not develop until teenage years. Neuronal ceroid lipofuscinoses (NCL or Batten disease) are a group of relatively rare but tragic hereditary neuronal storage disorders (0.1 to 7 per 100 000) that involve progressive visual loss, epilepsy and a dementia in a previously normally developing child or adolescent (Wisniewski 2001). Juvenile NCL becomes clinically apparent at 4–10 years of age whereas 'adult' NCL can be manifest anywhere in the range 15–50 years and is thus a condition where association with LD depends on the exact age at onset.

PREVALENCE OF LEARNING DISABILITY

It is difficult to give accurate estimates of how many people have LD. The current AAMR upper cutoff of an IQ of 75 had the potential to include up to 2.8% of the population (IQ 71–75) (MacMillan et al 1995). The AAMR upper limits have varied from 84 in the fifth (1961) revision, which retained the concept of borderline retardation (IQ 68–84), through 67 in the sixth revision and 70 in the eighth, emphasising the difficulties in comparing data across time (Leonard & Wen 2002). Epidemiological studies also have tended to dichotomise LD into two groups around the IQ 50 point, which does not marry exactly with the various formal clinical definitions.

Epidemiological studies usually give most weight to the intellectual deficit, which has the simple merit of being quantifiable, but almost completely ignore important adaptive factors, and so tend to be over-inclusive. Estimates should state whether the prevalence relates to a specific age-band, as the incidence will be cumulative during the childhood years. Gissler et al (1998) found the cumulative incidence of LD overall to be 6.1 per 1000 children between the ages of 0 and 7 years). For children between the ages of 6 and 16 a large-scale study in Western Australia that used multiple ascertainment methods gave a prevalence rate of 14.2 per 1000 (Leonard et al 2003). Age-banded prevalences seem to indicate a peak at about 14 years, falling thereafter, but it is difficult to say whether this represents a true differential mortality or increased ascertainment while the child is still in the school system. The easiest measure of intellectual impairment is still IQ testing, and although the pattern of strengths and weaknesses within the overall test result are perhaps more important, the global score with its limitations is largely used to define the subgroups of LD.

Mild LD

The statistical definition of LD where an IQ of 70 is the cutoff, predicts that 2–3% of the population have LD. The figure is inflated by the numbers with severe LD due to specific organic factors. It has long been known that the distribution of IQ in the population is not Gaussian, most easily explained by the lower tail of the curve comprising two overlapping distributions — the 'two-group' interpretation. The numerically larger group is that defined by the Gaussian tail (i.e. the expected 2.27% of the population with IQ < 70), and this has been called 'sociocultural' LD, or 'physiological' LD on the assumption that it is determined by similar multifactorial influences to those contributing to IQ levels > 70. In practice, differential mortality and diagnostic differences mean that this estimate is too high, and a widely accepted figure is around 1–2%. Short forms of the standard Wechsler Adult Intelligence Scale are highly correlated with results using the entire test, and their ease of use may facilitate more accurate population estimates (Nagle & Bell 1995). Prevalence estimates for mild LD are sometimes surprisingly low, indicating the difficulty in defining caseness. In Gothenburg children a level of only 4 per 1000 was reported, in Northern Finland 5.5 per 1000. Other estimates have been as high as up to 85 per 1000. While acknowledging these problems, a figure of 10 to 11 per 1000 would seem reasonable.

Previously it was assumed that the cognitive impairment in mild LD was largely due to a combination of polygenic inheritance patterns with other environmental factors. Thus, for most, a specific cause was not thought to be identifiable. Although this is still the case for the majority of people with mild LD, it is clear that a specific cause can be identified for a substantial, and increasing, minority. Scandinavian studies have shown that in 50% of mild LD no cause could be attributed (assumed polygenic). Around 15–20% had perinatal hypoxia, and congenital causes were present in 10%. Around 5% have a defined genetic syndrome (including DS), and around the same number had fetal alcohol syndrome. The data from developing or low-income countries is sparse, and many who would be identified as having a mild LD in the West would be culturally accepted elsewhere and thus not come to notice. However it has been shown to have the same association with low socio-economic status in Bangladesh (Islam et al 1993).

'Sociocultural' aspects of mild LD

A very consistent finding in LD epidemiological research has been the relationship between mild LD (largely that of unknown-cause or 'isolated' LD) and low socio-economic status. Although this certainly holds for mild LD, any relationship to severe LD is unclear, with some studies showing no effect (Stromme & Magnus 2000) and others finding a relationship (Croen et al 2001). Mild LD is known to be over-represented in families from social class IV and also associates with large sibship size, room overcrowding, low income, and maternal educational level.

IQ scores are not stable over time, and the intellectual development of the individual is highly complex and plastic. The older surmise that brain neurons are unable to divide in adult life has been shown incorrect, at least for the hippocampus (van Praag et al 2002). IQ is, however, heritable. Twin studies (Bouchard et al 1990) showed high concordance in IQ between twins reared together and apart, but relate largely to twins with normal IQ. Twin studies have also shown that IQ heritability and the heritability of brain grey and white matter volume are highly correlated and possibly influenced by the same mechanisms, linking IQ with brain architecture (Posthuma et al 2002). Adoption studies, albeit with methodological shortcomings (Horn et al 1979), compared the IQ of children who were adopted within a few days of birth, and the IQ of their biological and adoptive mothers. The heritability was high for young children but became less for older children. The children were largely adopted into affluent homes, and the adoptive parents had IQ scores well above average.

The implication is that LD to a partial extent at least might be modifiable by social interventions, or more specifically the amelioration of social and educational disadvantage. There have been a number of trials aiming to alter cognitive outcome by removing the sociocultural and educational disadvantages for children with mild LD. A comprehensive intervention programme for low-birth-weight infants (another strong risk factor for LD) during the first 3 years of life seemed to increase the intellectual development measured at 3 years (Blair et al 1995), but longer-term outcomes are awaited. A programme for early educational and social intervention for children from disadvantaged families has been followed up to the age of 15 and compared with a control group without such interventions, with encouraging results (Campbell & Ramey 1995). Such findings, if confirmed, have profound implications for the support and care of children at risk of mild LD

Although sociocultural influences are important, biological factors may have been underplayed in the past, and up to 45% of people with mild LD may have definite organic factors including subtle chromosome rearrangements and perinatal insults from toxins such as alcohol. Thus estimates of the importance of polygenic factors and social disadvantage may have to be revised downwards, although it is clear that they are crucial factors in most mild LD.

Severe LD

Roeleveld et al (1997) gave an overall prevalence figure of 3–4 per 1000 for children with moderate or more severe LD, consistent with other work including figures for adult populations. This represents around 10–20% of the total number of people with LD. The excess at more severe levels of disability is due to organic or pathological factors, with a cluster of disorders of definable aetiology, including genetic causes and environmental agents such as hypoxia, toxins, trauma and infections. Some who have disorders such as autism, cerebral malformation syndromes and cerebral palsy without, as yet, a defined cause, are assumed to have definite biological factors in their genesis. Overall, 50–80% have a definite known cause. A large study of nearly 12 000 individuals with LD in Taiwan showed a genetic basis in nearly 55% with severe LD (Hou et al 1998). Of the known chromosomal abnormalities, 83% had DS, 12% fragile X syndrome, and a smaller but significant proportion had contiguous gene syndromes. The predominance of DS among the known causes is clear from nearly all populations studied. The rates of non-genetic causes such as the fetal alcohol syndrome are much more variable, and it is important to remember that there is still a large group of people for whom no cause can be assigned.

In developing countries the prevalence of severe LD is much higher, over 5 per 1000, and in some specific areas such as the very poor urban areas of Lahore in Pakistan it can be dramatically so: 22 per 1000 (Durkin 2002). The causation again is mixed, with infections, environmental toxins such as lead, and nutritional deficiencies all playing a role. Interestingly, some genetic causes seem to be actually more common in developing countries (e.g. hereditary thalassaemia and sickle cell disease), and, because of the high birth rate, DS prevalence can be up to three times that seen in developed countries.

ASSESSMENT AND A LIFESPAN APPROACH TO LEARNING DISABILITY

Psychiatrists often have difficulties in assessing and understanding the patient with LD, problems that increase with the severity of the patient's intellectual impairment. For people with very mild LD with good communication skills the interview in itself does not differ significantly from a referral of someone without LD. The issue of whether a person in the borderline area has LD can generate friction between services. A demarcation that incorporates the global IQ of 70 marries with the current definitions even if this may seem unnecessarily restrictive at a deeper level. With most referrals, however, the assessment is far more complex, and there is probably no area in psychiatry that so necessitates a multidisciplinary approach. The person generally needs more time than others to respond to questions, a limited attention span may also significantly prolong the interview. Three things stand out, all interrelated: the person's

- basic level of understanding,
- ability to communicate,
- particular developmental history in the widest sense.

An extended series of interviews/meetings with the patient may be needed, and information gathered from multiple sources — such as family, carers, social work and other health professionals — to facilitate diagnosis of coexisting problems. These problems may be situation dependent, requiring visits to home, work or educational establishment. Observational recordings are often important; they may use objects or behaviours as communication devices, or in some cases they may find that learned sign language (modified British sign languages such as Makaton or Signalong) is easier than the spoken word. Families and long-term carers are often the best interpreters. A wide-ranging developmental history is crucial to understanding why a particular behaviour set or apparent psychiatric disorder has occurred at any particular time — after all, LD affects a person's whole life from childhood and requires a lifespan approach.

The family and LD

A child with LD is usually cared for by his family, whose own needs can go unrecognised in the face of those of the child. Most children with LD are not intolerable management problems, and most parents wish to keep the child at home, but increasingly it is not inevitable that the parents will always wish to care for their children at home. There are several route markers on the road to adulthood that can cause concern for the family.

Diagnosis The most obvious marker is when the child is diagnosed as having LD. The family may have suspected this,

observing the delay in milestones before the physician. The phases of adaptation to the diagnosis parallel grief reactions, going through shock, denial, anger and eventual adaptation. The stress on the family can be very high, and maternal coping strategies and her own levels of social support are important determinants of the child's eventual self-sufficiency. There can be other effects on family life, notably on the stability of marriage and perceived life satisfaction. For siblings there may be role reversal, with a younger sibling adopting a care role for an older one with LD.

Schooling is the next family milestone. Mainstream schooling is the usual wish, but parents can have great difficulty in accepting that a child may be failing in such circumstances and needs special educational provision. Although assisted learning at normal schools is an educational goal, the reality is that it is not universally available, and chronic class failure may be detrimental and delaying to the child who needs a specifically adapted educational curriculum.

Adolescence In adolescence, behavioural and emotional difficulties are as apparent in the person with LD as in any other teenager. Often these are interpreted as challenging behaviours to be treated, rather than as an intrinsic part of the development of emotional maturity. The difficulties may be more intense because of problems in communication, or may have a temporal lag, lasting into the subsequent decade.

Adulthood The last phase is the transition to adulthood and ageing. The transition is not only personal but also one of service provision. The health services for the child are usually unified under paediatrics, but those for adults are diverse, and co-ordinated by general practitioners. The transition is also a time of 'letting go' for parents, with its implied increased risk taking, and it is often harder for them to do so with their adult 'child' with LD than with their other children. The parents (or siblings after bereavement) remain the main carers for many adults with LD, and with dual ageing, older parents usually become most concerned about the future for their child when they are not around, but are faced with conflicting feelings, as the relationship is as important a source of support to them as it is to the child. Much tact and understanding is needed in discussions of future placements and social skills training, building up to the time when the parent is no longer able to care through incapacity or death. Younger parents, however, mostly consider that a future independent life for their child is feasible. School programmes are now designed with independence in mind, with self-care and work skill development as well as self-travel and the use of community facilities. To ensure success the parents must play a full role, and it is essential for them to be involved in participating in the assessment and choice of the future home for their child.

Bereavement can precipitate apparent behavioural problems. Not only do people with LD recognise death, they go through a grieving process that may appear aberrant because of the different communication styles used to express their emotions and feelings. The degree of understanding which shapes the concept of death and dying may be related to the level of cognitive development, as proposed by Piaget, rather than the actual age of the person. Group work with others who have been bereaved may be helpful, but individual support is often needed.

Ageing Finally there are issues associated with ageing and LD. Previously a 'healthy survivor' effect occurred, with most learning-disabled people who survived to an advanced age having mild LD. Severe LD still carries an increased risk of early mortality but, as in the general population, there has been an increasing shift to the right in the age distribution. The changing cohort makes the data confusing. A large US study showed increased cardiovascular disability load with age and high mortality from cardiovascular disease even though overall the group had low cardiovascular risk indices (Janicki et al 2002). There were also age-related increases in musculoskeletal disorders and respiratory disease. Cooper (1999a) has shown that where dementia occurs, even without DS, there is a marked increase in the number of associated physical conditions.

CONDITIONS ASSOCIATED WITH LEARNING DISABILITY

Non-genetic conditions

This is a misnomer; no disorder is totally without genetic influences of some sort. However, for many conditions, non-genetic factors play a predominant role. Some disorders that used to have very damaging outcomes are now much less common, at least in developed countries. One example is the congenital rubella syndrome caused by maternal rubella infection during pregnancy that, at its most severe, could lead to multiple congenital abnormalities, multi-system sensory impairment, and seizure disorder coupled to severe LD. However, we may still encounter people with such profound disabilities as adults, and there is still a yearly incidence of new cases in the UK. Similarly the brain damage associated with once common infections (e.g. tuberculous encephalitis/meningitis) is now rare. Major improvements in the management of neural tube defects, especially open spina bifida, make the LD that was often the consequence of ascending infection almost a thing of the past. However, there are still all too many cases that are due to infections, to toxins, or to metabolic disturbances. It is noteworthy that, worldwide, iodine deficiency is still the most common preventable cause of LD (Hetzel 1988).[31]

Severe prematurity

The consequences of severe prematurity are being increasingly realised, especially in relation to cerebral palsy, which in itself in many cases is associated with LD. Cerebral palsy can be defined as a cluster of conditions that show non-progressive motor impairment secondary to disorders of brain development. It is the most common developmental motor disorder of children, with a prevalence rate around 2–3 per 1000. Seventy percent of children with cerebral palsy will have one or more major developmental impairment, mainly LD and visual impairment, thus the overlap is large. Over the last twenty to thirty years the prevalence may have been increasing (Schendel et al 2002).

Intrauterine infections are now thought to play an important role in early labour and thus severe prematurity. Chronic chorioamnionitis or systemic maternal infections may act through neonatal encephalopathy. With advances in neonatology the survivability of the severely premature infant has increased dramatically in developed countries, but some of the less desired outcomes are also becoming apparent. Intrauterine infections may also play a role in cerebral palsy and LD in term or near-term infants, but the situation is less clear. The most commonly isolated organisms in preterm labour are ureaplasma, mycoplasma and fusobacteria species. The roles of chlamydia and viral infections, including cytomegalovirus and herpes simplex, are less certain in chronic chorioamnionitis, although they are thought to play roles in neurological damage at term. For the preterm the major damage seems to be in the white matter, as revealed by ultrasound and MRI studies. In an ultrasound study of children born preterm, 60% of those with large white-matter lucencies (parenchymal white-matter lesions or enlargement of the ventricles, and in particular periventricular leucomalacia) had LD (Holling & Leviton 1999). MRI studies are limited in sample size but tend to confirm these findings. Regional brain volumes in the sensorimotor cortex, the putamen and the corpus callosum correlated with full scale IQ, and specific grey-matter deficits (e.g. hippocampal volume) are found which correlate with measures of memory (Isaacs et al 2000). One current aetiological theory invokes cytokine damage (interleukins, tumour necrosis factor alpha, macrophage inflammatory protein) as a final common pathway to brain injury for a variety of mechanisms, including infections, hypoxic insults, and damage due to toxins. Animal models have revealed that alterations to the cytokine cascade as part of the inflammatory response can have a marked effect on the extent of neuronal damage that occurs; an imbalance between the degree of fetal inflammatory cytokine response and the protection offered by growth factors may be important, especially in the late second trimester.

Infections

These remain an important cause of LD in addition to any role in the very premature. They are still an enormous cause of disability in low-income countries, and many are now preventable. Rubella is epidemic in many developing countries in spite of the fact that it is preventable by vaccination. In some populations syphilis is still present at a high rate. Although in Western countries congenital syphilis is rare, this is not the case elsewhere, and deafness and LD are often the important sequelae for the child. The meningites still cause damage. *Haemophilus influenzae* (type B) is preventable, and vaccination has proved effective in developed countries. With vaccination against meningococcal strains now also possible, it is to be hoped that the tragic outcomes of such infections can also be reduced in frequency. The encephalites, uncommon in developed countries, still take an enormous toll in the third world. Measles encephalitis is not only a major cause of LD and sensory impairment but also of mortality in the under-fives in low-income countries. In Asia, Japanese encephalitis is a major problem with similar outcomes (Committee on Nervous System Disorders in Developing Countries 2001). Vertical infection of the fetus with the human immunodeficiency virus is possible in up to 40% of carrier mothers. The outcome can be severe, and the infant may have microcephaly, seizure and movement disorders and severe LD in the worst case.

Non-infective environmental agents and toxins

The classical fetal neurotoxin is lead, and that severe LD can follow acute lead encephalopathy has been known for over a hundred years. Only in the last thirty years however have the long-term effects of lower lead levels been realised, with a continuum of dose-related consequences from frank encephalopathy through to subtle impairments of cognition, growth and hearing. The diagnostic trigger level for blood lead in children has fallen six-fold since the 1960s. Mercury poisoning was highlighted as a cause of severe LD by the well-known Japanese Minamata Bay incident (methylmercury poisoning through contaminated fish) in the

1950s. Like lead, there is continued concern about the effects of lower levels of mercury in various areas of the world. The issue for both is one of prevention through removal of such metals from the environment. This is also applicable to other man-made or distributed toxins, especially PCBs (polychlorinated biphenyls), which can lead to wide-ranging cognitive deficits in children exposed in utero.

Certain maternal behaviours are now well known to be risk factors. The fetal alcohol syndrome is a major cause of mild LD in some populations, and it is likely that it will be increasingly recognised as an important factor (American Academy of Pediatrics 2000). Some studies indicate that subtle deficits in language and comprehension may result from even socially acceptable levels of alcohol intake during pregnancy. Alcohol is also passed into the breast milk. Maternal smoking is now recognised as a factor in low infant birth weight (another risk factor for LD) and may independently have direct effects on fetal neurological development. Among prescribed drugs, both cocaine and cannabis use in pregnancy have been associated with LD in the child. It should also be remembered that many, and sometimes essential, prescribed medications can have marked effects on the developing nervous system. Some associations with LD have become so clear that epithets have been attached — one example is the fetal valproate syndrome in association with this common antiepileptic therapy. Nutritional deficiencies are still very common in low-income countries. Iodine deficiency and thyroid dysfunction leading to congenital hypothyroidism has already been mentioned (Haddow et al 1999). Parasitical infection leading to chronic iron deficiency anaemia affecting the child in utero and beyond is extremely common and has also been linked to poor cognitive performance. It is likely that many more correlations could be made, but there is an unfortunate dearth of research in this area.

Specific disorders of the developing nervous system

Building a central nervous system is a highly complex process. It has long been known the morphological shaping of the brain occurs in a definite sequence of anatomical events, and recently there have been major advances in our understanding of the biological events determining the timing and the position of developing neurons and how these relate to the micro- and macro-architecture, especially of the cerebral cortex. The abnormal brain, and in particular specific syndromes that produce LD, have thrown light on the genetic basis of normal brain development, and we are starting to make sense of disorders of neuronal positioning. In some of these conditions the gross anatomy of the brain may be normal, and it is only at the microscopic level that definite abnormalities occur. It is likely that many further such syndromes will be uncovered in the next few years and they will play an increasing role in our understanding of the basis of LD. Thus, although some of these disorders are rare it is important to review our current state of knowledge.

Shaping the developing nervous system

The brain develops through a well-choreographed dance of migrating cells from distant origins; eventually neurons with similar properties are grouped into discrete anatomical systems, brain nuclei and, most clearly, the laminar patterns that evolve in the developing cerebral, cerebellar and limbic cortices. Cortical neurons do not develop in situ, but in special regions deep in the brain where mitosis and patterning (broadly cell fate specification) activity is active. They have been estimated to travel up to one thousand cell body lengths to reach their final site where they undergo differentiation. So developing neurons must proliferate, they must move, and they must differentiate. As well as proliferation, selective neuronal death (apoptosis) also plays a major role in shaping the nervous system. All these processes require a complex series of time-dependent gene activations and deactivations, the secretion of signalling molecules that set off protein signalling interactions (extra- and intracellular cascades) as well as signalling by cell–cell interactions. Neurons do not move unguided. Glial cells grow and form a scaffold along which neurons can ascend, and glial disorders can affect brain development in profound ways. Extracellular matrix components act as signals to both glia and neurons; movement of neurons is a process of differential adhesion, weaker at the rear and stronger at the leading edge — cell adhesion molecules and intracellular contractile filaments play an important role. Although the phases overlap and in some areas are reversed in the temporal sequence, it is a useful simplification to envisage three types of events:

- mass divisions of partly undifferentiated neuronal precursors;
- the movement of these to their final destinations;
- the differentiation of precursors into neurons with the selective formation and pruning of their axonal systems and dendritic contacts by intrinsic and extrinsic inputs.

It is the last process that is most influenced by the external environment and is the basis for the modulation by sensory and feedback motor excitations. It has most clearly been demonstrated by elegant studies on visual cortical development in recent decades — examining how sensory input modulates the visual cortical columnar arrangements, and the effects of sensory deprivation during important temporal developmental windows. The final stage is probably the most important determinant of cognitive individuality and ability to respond to neurological challenge, but presupposes an intact cortical system on which to act. Current thinking about the fragile X syndrome suggests that, at least in part, the problems may lie in this final stage (see p. 549). The correct achievement of the first two stages, however, is also vitally important in preventing cognitive disability.

Disorders of cell proliferation and patterning — holoprosencephaly

Holoprosencephaly is another of those conditions originally thought homogeneous but now known to be an end result of a large number of processes (Muenky & Beachy 2001). In its milder forms it may go unnoticed, and so prevalence estimates are probably conservative (1 per 16 000). In its most severe form it manifests as a failure of the cerebral hemispheres to separate and of the surrounding midface to undergo midline division, resulting in single cerebrum, single midline eye, single nostril, etc. Very severe forms are not compatible with life (but are a relatively common form of fetal loss); mild forms exist where a single midline incisor tooth or hypertelorism are the only visible features. LD can likewise vary from very severe to absent.

Most cases are due to chromosomal abnormalities, but the study of sporadic cases has revealed mutations in several important signalling genes. One of these is termed (unfortunately) sonic hedgehog (*SHH* gene found on human chromosome 7q36) since mutations in the fruit fly homologue lead to spiky outgrowths on the larval belly. In vertebrates the protein produced by the sonic hedgehog gene (Shh) is involved at several stages of nervous system development, including the control of right–left asymmetry and the dorsoventral patterning of the central nervous system. The first discovered function was revealed by its distribution in the early embryo: it was present in the two main signalling centres — the notochord and the floor plate — which are involved in the formation of the neural tube. Shh, by repressing or stimulating various transcription factors, regulates the specific proliferation and patterning of neural cell progenitor types down the neural tube. It also acts more anteriorly to induce dopamine neurons in the midbrain and serotonergic neurons in the developing forebrain as well as being involved in the proliferation and differentiation of cells in the cerebellum and retina (Marti & Bovolenta 2002). Shh is a secreted protein that needs to be cleaved to an active form then modified by addition of a cholesterol unit. Some features of the Smith–Lemli–Opitz syndrome (multiple dysmorphic features and CNS hypoplasia), where abnormalities of cholesterol biosynthesis occur, may relate to Shh dysfunction. Shh binds transmembrane receptors on the neural precursors. Again the non-human derived nomenclature may sound strange — two proteins 'patched 1 and 2' normally interact with a third, 'smoothened' to tonically inhibit the latter's function. Shh de-represses the system by preventing patched's action. Disruption of the genes involved can lead to tumours, indicating in yet another way that SHH is important in controlling cell proliferation. The eventual signal in the cell is via a system of proteins produced by *GLI* genes (name derived from glioma). CREB-binding protein (CBP) is a transcriptional coactivator now thought to interact with GLI3. CBP is abnormal in Rubenstein–Taybi syndrome, where LD is linked to dysmorphic features: syndactyly and short stature, broad thumbs and big toes, and increased risk of neurodevelopmental tumours (Petrij et al 2001). The genotype–phenotype link between these features and disorders of the SHH system remains to be confirmed, but it is likely that there are biological links between Rubenstein–Taybi and holoprosencephaly. It is clear that further links to other LD syndromes are likely to be revealed as the complex cascades of signalling are unravelled.

Disorders of neuronal migration — the lissencephalies

Strictly, lissencephaly simply means 'smooth brain'. Like so many conditions associated with LD it is heterogeneous in origin. Basically all lissencephalies involve varying degrees of altered brain gyral formation (and its corollary, sulcal formation), accompanied by a thickening of the cerebral cortex. At its most severe the whole cortex may be affected, with a resulting severe LD, seizure disorder, cortical blindness and motor paralysis. In the mildest forms only small areas of the cortex may be included: pockets of misplaced neurons, focal neuronal heterotopia, which may be rather common (one quarter of childhood epilepsy may be associated with them). The cells involved in the lissencephalies all migrate from the ventricular neuroepithelium, and this to some extent validates the grouping. Three-quarters of the lissencephalies have been found to be due to mutations in one of two genes: *LIS1* and *DCX* (otherwise known as *doublecortin*) (Ross & Walsh 2001).

The involvement of *LIS1* was first detected in the study of Miller–Dieker syndrome, characterised by severe LD, a character-istic facial appearance (thickened upper lip, upturned nose, tall forehead, narrowing of the intertemporal distance), and classical lissencephaly. Over 60% of children with Miller–Dieker syndrome have visible, and most of the rest submicroscopic, deletions on chromosome 17 (at 17p13.3). Thus this may be a contiguous gene syndrome where more than one gene suffers hemizygous deletion due to the chromosome abnormality. Smaller deletions or point mutations at the same locus produce the isolated lissencephaly sequence which is neurologically very similar to Miller–Dieker but without the facial features. Both conditions disrupt *LIS1*, which maps to this region, and recently *LIS1* has been shown to be identical to the beta subunit of platelet-activating factor acetylhydrolase (PAFAHB1). The soluble protein product of *LIS1* binds tubulin and may modulate microtubule organisation, promoting movement of microtubule segments via the intracellular dynein motors important to neuronal cell movement.

Another related lissencephaly was found to have X-linked inheritance. Manifest in males it is clinically similar to the isolated lissencephaly sequence, but usually to a somewhat less severe degree. In females the symptoms are milder — a seizure disorder may be associated with cognitive disability of varying degree, and up to one-quarter of subjects may have normal intellectual levels. Most cases are sporadic, although a few families with severely affected males and mildly affected females have been described. The condition has been shown to be due to disruptions (protein truncation/nonsense mutations or missense mutations) in a gene called *Doublecortin* (*DCX*) at Xq22.3-q23, which is only expressed in the central and peripheral nervous systems. Its protein binds tubulin, and since it interacts with lis1 protein in vitro, they probably interact in vivo in microtubule control. Disruption of *DCX* leads to an inverted pattern of cortical neuronal lamination (normally the youngest cells are most external, migrating past older cells leading to a six-layered structure; *DCX* mutations lead to an 'inside-out' arrangement with an apparent 'double' layer). Both lis1 protein and doublecortin may act with other intra- and extracellular effector molecules including those in the reelin system and the Abl kinase family. Thus the pattern is set of series of parallel but interacting signalling mechanisms that co-operate to control neuronal migration.

The reelin system was named after the movement disorder it produces in a mutant mouse strain (*reeler*). In mice the gene controls the expression of a large secreted protein, reelin, that is only produced by certain cell groupings in the developing brain, more especially the cerebral cortex marginal zone. It binds migrating neurons via receptors (VLDL-receptor and APOE-receptor 2) inducing an intracellular phosphorylation cascade involved in defining the correct position of the neuron within the forming brain (Rice & Curran 2001). The human homologue of reelin is termed *RELN*, and mutation is associated with the lissencephaly/cerebellar hypoplasia syndrome type-b (LCHb), where a thickened cortex, pachygyria and a very abnormal hippocampus is associated with gross cerebellar hypoplasia with absence of the usual folia. Reelin itself links into a large number of other control systems, and the study of other genes involved will generate new candidates for LD-associated syndromes.

Behavioural phenotypes

A phenotype is the observable (either clinical or biological) features that consistently arise with a given genotype. That behaviour could be a phenotype has been controversial, especially to those holding a view that behaviours do not have genetic determinants, or that these are open to such temporal environmental and learning changes as to be insignificant in comparison. However, recently, it has become more accepted that certain behavioural patterns have strong innate underpinnings. The classical association was with self-mutilating behaviours seen in the rare Lesch–Nyhan syndrome (Hall et al 2001), an inborn error of purine metabolism (Nyhan 1997), but can be extended readily, e.g. to the hyperphagia associated with Prader–Willi syndrome. By definition, psychotic disorders are diagnosed by behavioural and communication features, and if these are felt to be largely genetically determined then these also could be considered to be behavioural phenotypes. The cognitive features involved in the dementia associated with DS have also been described as a behavioural phenotype. It is obvious that varying degrees of genetic determination can occur, as with other phenotypic features of a genotype, leading to a variable presentation. That certain genotypes can also contribute towards a, sometimes variable, behavioural pattern (or, perhaps more correctly, cognitive responses that are manifest as behaviour) is also reasonable. The concept prompts us to look for behavioural and cognitive outcomes as well as readily observable physical changes as part of the clinical constellation of a disorder.

Genetic syndromes associated with LD

Many conditions associated with LD have been shown to have genetic origins. We now know the human complement of genes from the draft sequencing of the human genome, and the next stage, where their detailed sequence will be found, is certain to lead to even more findings relevant to LD. A survey of the most important conditions is therefore important; they provide insights into all aspects of LD as well as illustrating increasingly-varied mechanisms of inheritance. The older classical patterns that were described by Mendel are probably exceptional; more complex genetics, with partial penetrance, with varied phenotypes arising from the same genotype, and with varied genotypes giving rise to similar clinical outcomes, is probably the rule. Genetic underpinnings also give us one way to start reclassifying LD, unifying cognitive outcomes on the basis of the interactions of underlying genetic profiles with environmental influences. Understanding the genetic basis of the conditions is necessary to understanding how environment can modulate them, and thus the design of interventions that can maximise the person's potential in spite of the prior genetic loading. A conceptual framework can be introduced based on the type of mutation that is involved in the disorder. Mutations are changes in the sequence of DNA in chromosomes and are necessary to maintain the adaptive richness of the genetic endowment. It is useful to order mutations by scale. It happens that the largest-scale mutations — those where a whole chromosome is duplicated or absent — include the most common genetic condition associated with LD:DS. Next down in scale are the partial duplications and deletions of chromosomes, which include the partial monosomies that produce conditions such as Cri-du-chat and the Wolf–Hirschhorn syndrome. Continuing through small interstitial deletions (that give rise to contiguous gene syndromes) and rearrangements, including those in the telomeric region of chromosomes, eventually the smallest mutations, those involving DNA sequence changes within a single gene, are reached. Figure 24.1 gives examples of some of these different orders of mutation.

Chromosomal abnormalities and LD

Human chromosomes have been studied for over one hundred years, but it was only in the 1950s that the correct human somatic and meiotic counts were established. Improvements in cell culture techniques and histology, especially stains that bound DNA, heralded an era of discovery in which chromosome abnormalities were found in association with a wide variety of clinical conditions associated with LD. At first these were largely numerical abnormalities, or large-scale rearrangements. Stains were subsequently developed that bound differentially within normal chromosomes revealing a striped banding that could be used as a grid-map to describe and position a host of other abnormalities; classical chromosome banding still lies at the heart of clinical cytogenetic services today. More recently, molecular methods combining DNA-manipulation techniques with fluorescent labelling have identified changes not seen under light microscopy, and direct DNA amplification by the polymerase chain reaction has changed the way conditions such as fragile X syndrome are diagnosed.

Figures 24.2 and 24.3 illustrate LD-associated chromosomal abnormalities.

- First, numerical abnormalities of autosomes and sex chromosomes may occur, e.g. DS due to trisomy 21. Absence of an entire chromosome is termed a monosomy, the commonest being Turner syndrome where only one X chromosome is present.
- A second group are partial chromosomal duplications or deletions. The whole of a chromosome arm may be lost, e.g. the short arm of chromosome 5 in Cri-du-chat syndrome. There are also smaller, usually interstitial, deletions that underlie the contiguous gene syndromes. Duplications are rare and usually of small chromosomal segments.
- A third group comprises translocations, where two chromosome regions break, with subsequent transfer and fusion of the pieces to the other breakpoint. This may be between two separate chromosomes (reciprocal translocation) or between the fragments from separate arms of a single chromosome (pericentric inversion). Occasionally a fragment will invert within a single chromosomal arm (paracentric inversion). Reciprocal translocations are often without effect when they are inherited in a balanced form, but the unbalanced form results in partial monosomy and trisomy of the respective chromosomes involved and may be lethal in utero, resulting in miscarriage. If the breakpoints disrupt genes, then the reciprocal balanced form may have clinical effects.
- A fourth group involves isochromosome formation. The centromere splits abnormally, leading to loss of one arm. This is made up by the duplication of the remaining arm, forming a chromosome with two identical arms symmetrical about the centromere.
- A final group can be considered as a catch-all for other abnormalities such as rare ring chromosomes and the more common small supernumerary marker chromosomes (chromosome fragments which retain their viability through the presence of an active centromere; the most common is a much attenuated chromosome 15).
- Mosaicism refers not directly to a chromosomal abnormality but to the presence of more than one clonal cell line in a given tissue. Mosaicism is especially common with sex chromosome numerical abnormalities.

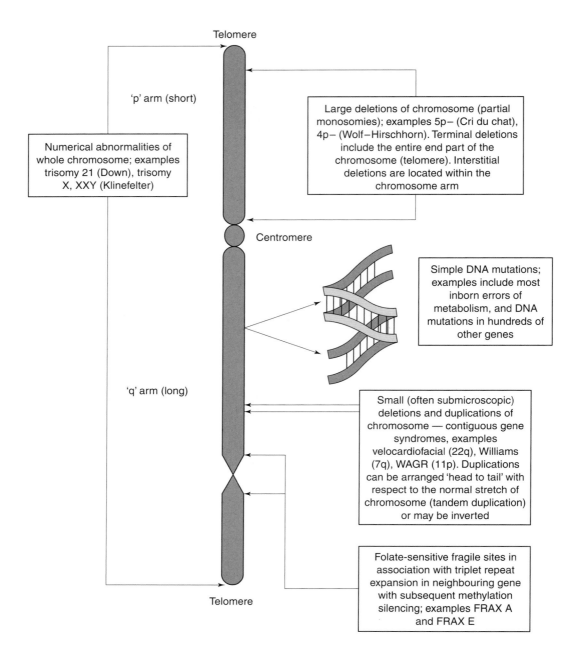

Telomere

'p' arm (short)

Numerical abnormalities of
whole chromosome; examples
trisomy 21 (Down), trisomy
X, XXY (Klinefelter)

Large deletions of chromosome (partial
monosomies); examples 5p– (Cri du chat),
4p– (Wolf–Hirschhorn). Terminal deletions
include the entire end part of the
chromosome (telomere). Interstitial
deletions are located within the
chromosome arm

Centromere

Simple DNA mutations;
examples include most
inborn errors of
metabolism, and DNA
mutations in hundreds of
other genes

'q' arm (long)

Small (often submicroscopic)
deletions and duplications of
chromosome — contiguous gene
syndromes, examples
velocardiofacial (22q), Williams
(7q), WAGR (11p). Duplications
can be arranged 'head to tail' with
respect to the normal stretch of
chromosome (tandem duplication)
or may be inverted

Folate-sensitive fragile sites in
association with triplet repeat
expansion in neighbouring gene
with subsequent methylation
silencing; examples FRAX A
and FRAX E

Telomere

Fig. 24.1
Examples of genetic conditions that have learning disability as part of their phenotype, in relation to chromosomal events that accompany
them. (The representation of the chromosome is schematic.) Then various conditions are discussed further in the text.

Trisomies   Classical chromosomal abnormalities are common and found in around 0.6% of newborn infants (1 per 200). Most are trisomies, which occur in at least 0.36% of all live births (autosomal trisomies 0.12%; sex chromosome aneuploidies 0.24%) and in over 25% of spontaneous abortions. Thus they are the leading cause of pregnancy loss. In first-trimester spontaneous abortions recognised as such they may account for 50–60%. Trisomies of the large chromosomes are rare, usually lethal in utero, occurring more frequently in early spontaneous abortions. The survivability of a trisomy to term depends on the gene count of the chromosome rather than on its overall size. The human genome map shows that chromosome 21 is especially gene poor in relation to

its overall size, whereas the slightly smaller chromosome 22 is much more gene dense and is rarely seen in trisomy in the liveborn. Trisomy of low-gene-density chromosomes, and especially 13, 18, 21 and the sex chromosomes (which are a special case) are compatible with a full-term pregnancy. Patau syndrome (trisomy 13: colobomata and other eye malformations, facial clefting, polydactyly, severe LD) and Edward syndrome (trisomy 18: micrognathia, multiple dysmorphisms including rocker bottom feet, severe LD) are associated with severe congenital abnormalities. Children with trisomy 13 usually die around 4–6 months of age, with few surviving into the first years of life. Trisomy 18 is also lethal, and most die in the first year. Trisomy 16 is of interest in

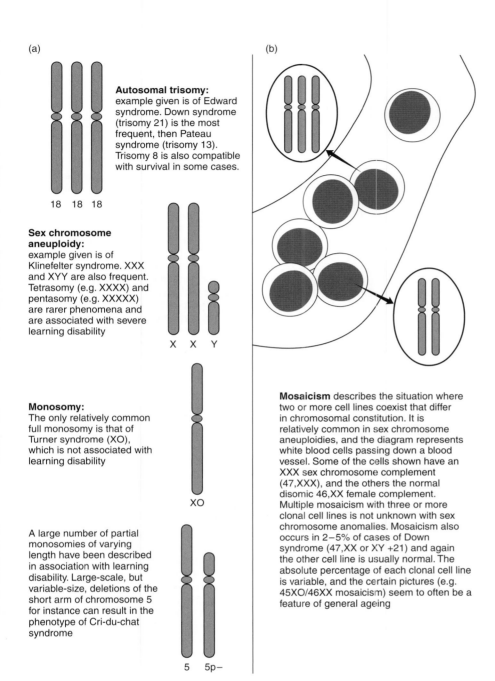

(a)

Autosomal trisomy: example given is of Edward syndrome. Down syndrome (trisomy 21) is the most frequent, then Pateau syndrome (trisomy 13). Trisomy 8 is also compatible with survival in some cases.

18 18 18

Sex chromosome aneuploidy: example given is of Klinefelter syndrome. XXX and XYY are also frequent. Tetrasomy (e.g. XXXX) and pentasomy (e.g. XXXXX) are rarer phenomena and are associated with severe learning disability

X X Y

Monosomy: The only relatively common full monosomy is that of Turner syndrome (XO), which is not associated with learning disability

XO

A large number of partial monosomies of varying length have been described in association with learning disability. Large-scale, but variable-size, deletions of the short arm of chromosome 5 for instance can result in the phenotype of Cri-du-chat syndrome

5 5p–

(b)

Mosaicism describes the situation where two or more cell lines coexist that differ in chromosomal constitution. It is relatively common in sex chromosome aneuploidies, and the diagram represents white blood cells passing down a blood vessel. Some of the cells shown have an XXX sex chromosome complement (47,XXX), and the others the normal disomic 46,XX female complement. Multiple mosaicism with three or more clonal cell lines is not unknown with sex chromosome anomalies. Mosaicism also occurs in 2–5% of cases of Down syndrome (47,XX or XY +21) and again the other cell line is usually normal. The absolute percentage of each clonal cell line is variable, and the certain pictures (e.g. 45XO/46XX mosaicism) seem to often be a feature of general ageing

Fig. 24.2
(a) Trisomies and monosomies of chromosomes. (b) Mosaicism.

that its occurrence seems almost entirely related to maternal age. Trisomy 8 is being increasingly described, especially with newer methods of fetal investigation and diagnosis, but the fetus rarely survives until birth. There is an excess of male fetuses, and mosaicism is usual. In surviving trisomy 8 there is a moderate degree of LD. However, in terms of both numbers affected, and the importance to the specialist in the psychiatry of LD, trisomy 21 or DS holds first place; this is discussed at length in the following section. Numerically the individual trisomies of the sex chromosomes are next in rank.

Partial trisomies, involving duplication of a segment of the chromosome or an entire chromosome arm, are known for many chromosomes; those of 4p, 5p, 6p, 7q, 9p, 10p 10q, 11q, 12p, 13q, 14q, 15q and 20p, although rare, are the most important. Deletion of a whole autosome is usually lethal. A partial deletion leads to monosomy of that segment of the chromosome, and partial monosomy of 4p, 4q, 5p, 9p, 11q, 12p, 13q, 18p, 18q, 21p and 21q have been described. The unifying features of all these relatively rare syndromes are LD of varying degrees, and growth retardation. With the advent of more sensitive fluorescent hybridisation studies of karyotype, new syndromes in association with more restricted chromosomal rearrangements are being regularly described.

DOWN SYNDROME

Recognisable descriptions of Down syndrome (DS) have been present for hundreds of years. However, the first detailed description of the condition was by James Langdon Down in 1866, who

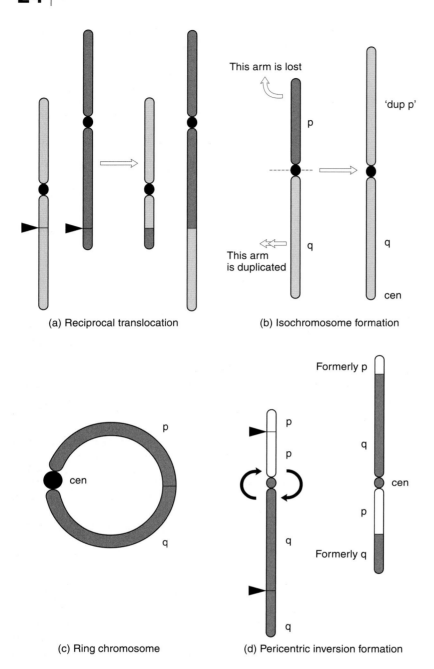

(a) Reciprocal translocation

This arm is lost

p

'dup p'

This arm
is duplicated

q

q

cen

(b) Isochromosome formation

p

cen

q

(c) Ring chromosome

Formerly p

p
p

q

cen

p

q

Formerly q

q

(d) Pericentric inversion formation

Fig. 24.3
(a) Reciprocal translocation between chromosomes. These can occur between autosomes or between autosomes and sex chromosomes. When segregated to germ cells they may produce partial trisomies and monosomies (unbalanced) forms in the offspring, or the balanced rearrangement may persist which may be without clinical effect unless a breakpoint directly disrupts a gene. (b) Formation of an isochromosome. An error during cell division leads to abnormal centromere splitting with loss of one arm of a chromosome (here it is the short arm) and duplication of the remaining arm. The X chromosome is often that involved in isochromosome formation. (c) Ring chromosome formation — there has been fusion at the ends (telomeres) of the individual arms of a single chromosome. This usually results in some loss of chromosomal material with resultant gene loss, and, although a rare condition, learning disability is a common co-occurrence. (d) Pericentric inversion — which can be conceptualised as a reciprocal translocation but within a single chromosome, although the mechanics are far from clear for either. A pericentric inversion of chromosome 2 near the centromere is fairly common (1:13 000) but without a clear phenotype associated. Paracentric inversions are inversions of stretches of material within a given chromosomal arm.

used the term 'Mongolian idiocy' to characterise certain clinical features that occurred in combination with, on average, a moderate degree of LD. Down was also a pioneer of early medical photography and took the first photographs of subjects with the syndrome. The original epithet with its incorrect and racial assumptions of origin has been abandoned (Ward 1998).

Not only were the clinical features of DS clearly demonstrated early on, so also were associated risk factors. Shuttleworth in 1909 showed those with DS tended to be the youngest in their sibships, and this was clearly associated with advanced maternal age. A variety of causes were later put forward to account for the development of DS — from maternal alcoholism, tuberculosis to hypothyroidism — but since the 1950s it has been clear that nearly all cases result from an extra full or partial chromosome.

The origins of trisomy 21

Waardenburg in 1932 suggested that non-disjunction of 'genetic factors' could be a cause of DS. Lejeune and his colleagues in 1959 demonstrated an extra acrocentric chromosome in fibroblasts of people with DS, and simultaneously Jacobs and her group in Edinburgh demonstrated the same finding in bone marrow cells. Studies since then encompassing a wide variety of populations have shown that DS is almost exclusively associated with an extra copy of chromosome 21. The trisomy usually occurs de novo, and DS is the most common example of a genetic condition that is not inherited.

Non-disjunction is the failure of segregation of chromosomes during cell division so that one daughter cell will have an extra chromosome and the other one less. Monosomy 21 is not often seen, and most cases are presumed to be lethal to the cell. However trisomy 21 is often compatible with survival to term. Meiotic cell division forms gametes in two stages. Recombination or crossing over of DNA occurs during meiosis I, and is marked by the formation of specific structures called chiasma that bridge between the chromosomes. Changes in the rate and/or position of exchanges as marked by chiasmata are a feature of human trisomies. Molecular studies of trisomy 21 have shown that the extra chromosome is maternal in over 90% of cases, and around 75% of errors occur at the first meiotic division. Chiasma numbers are decreased, with around 40% showing no chiasmata at all. Where they do occur, it is between the distal long arms and they are thought to be less efficient than those more proximal on the chromosome (Hassold et al 2000). With second meiotic division errors the first-division chiasmata numbers are actually increased, especially proximally. Thus too few or too many chiasmata at maternal division-I increase the risk of trisomy 21. Paternal meiotic errors leading to trisomy 21 may act through similar mechanisms, although most such are at meiosis-II (60%). In around 5% of cases of trisomy 21 the error is thought to be mitotic rather than meiotic. For most then the error is maternal and a key question is how altered chiasma formation relate to maternal age effects. Women in their 40s have at least a fifteen-fold increase in risk compared with women in their 20s. One possibility is that the ageing ovum becomes less efficient at processing abnormal configurations, with perhaps a double-hit phenomenon where ageing oocyte factors interact with a predisposition to abnormal chiasma formation.

Nearly 95% of people with DS have full trisomy 21 (karyotype is 47,XX,+21 or 47,XY,+21). Robertsonian translocations between acrocentric chromosomes account for another 5%. Some of these (around 45%) are due to a Robertsonian fusion chromosome, (usually between chromosomes 14 and 21) being inherited from a balanced carrier parent (if the carrier was the mother, she would have a karyotype of the form 45,–14,–21,XX, +rob(14;21)), leading to trisomy for the long arm of chromosome 21, which contain the majority of chromosome 21 (depending on the whether the fusion is mono- or di-centric, a small short-arm component may be present). Clinically there is full DS. The small short arms of acrocentric chromosomes contain many repetitive sequences and extensive sequence homology that may relate to their tendency to form fusion chromosomes. The fusion and its normal homologue are able to pair during meiosis. Other Robertsonians arise de novo, and most are maternal in origin. Robertsonian formation does not seem related to maternal or paternal age, and their relative contribution to DS decreases with maternal age. The situation is even more complex in that proximal 21q loci usually show a great deal of homozygosity, even if the parent's chromosomes were heterozygous for alleles in this region. A familial balanced carrier of a Rob(21;21) fusion is especially unfortunate as all offspring will have DS (monosomy 21 being unviable).

A further 5% of people with DS will have two cell lines in their body, one with full trisomy 21 and one with a normal karyotype (47,XY,+21/46,XY for example). Such mosaicism may arise from loss of a chromosome 21 in a trisomic cell early in embryogenesis, or result from an early mitotic non-disjunction. Mosaicism is a complex phenomenon with varying percentages in different cell lines (e.g. lower in lymphocytes than fibroblasts) and varies with time within the same cell line.

Table 24.2 summarises the various genetic abnormalities underlying DS.

Prevalence and mortality of DS

Although variation occurs from country to country, DS is still common at around 1:600 to 1:1000 newborns. The age-related risk is well known, but, since most babies are born to younger mothers, so most DS children will be born to younger mothers. In developing countries where the birth rate is higher, the absolute numbers are greater. For service development and clinical planning purposes it is also important to look at numbers of people with DS in different age cohorts, as the ageing of the general population is mirrored in LD. In fact today there are twice as many DS adults as DS children. A case-finding survey found 343 persons in community settings in the Lothian Region of Scotland (population 850 000), of whom 139 were over 36 years old (Fig. 24.4). These are minimum numbers, and 30–40% of these will be showing some clinical signs of dementia. These figures are broadly comparable with other surveys done in Lanarkshire and Ayrshire.

The number of DS adults is projected to increase and peak at least 50% above 1990 levels in the first two decades of this millennium. Survival is still lower for people with DS than the general population. In a large US study of mortality data on nearly 18 000 people with DS, median age at death increased from 25 years old in 1983 to 49 years old in 1997. This rate of 1.7 years increase per year of the study was highly significant (Yang et al 2002). During the same period the median age at death in the general population increased by only 3 years (73 to 76). The largest increase came in the early 1990s with a striking reduction in the proportion of deaths in DS children under 5 years. Congenital heart disease took its toll at all ages, with a peak

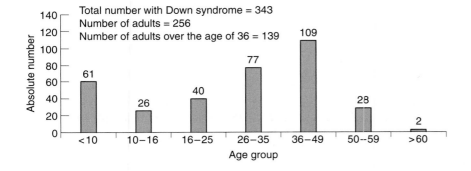

Fig. 24.4
Down syndrome — numbers by age in Lothian, Scotland (population about 800 000).

Table 24.2 Genetic abnormalities underlying Down syndrome

Genetic variant of Down syndrome	Chromosomal complement in parents	Chromosomal complement in person with Down syndrome	Percentage of people with Down syndrome
Full trisomy 21	Usually 46,XX and 46,XY	47,XX +21 or 47,XY +21	95%
Robertsonian translocation: Chromosomes 13, 14, 15, 21 and 22 have very small short arms (acrocentric) with satellite and alphoid sequence DNA but little coding DNA. Fusion between two such chromosomes at the centromere (centric fusion) yields a composite chromosome with long arms from each of the contributing acrocentrics.	Can be as above (around 50% for those involving chromosome 13–15 and 96% of the others) or one parent may be a carrier of a balanced rearrangement e.g. 45,XY, −14, −21, t(14;21) 45,XX, −21, −22, t(21;22) 45,XX, −13, −21, t(13;21) 45,XX, −15, −21, t(15;21) 45,XY, −21, −21, t(21;21) (sometimes written as e.g. 45,XY, rob(14;21)) The first two are the most common, the homologous recombination is rare	Down syndrome will result from inheritance of the unbalanced chromosome complement, for instance: 46,XY −14, t(14;21) In such cases there are two normal chromosome 21s in addition to the long arms of 21 inherited from segregation of the Robertsonian derivative chromosome. The alternative unbalanced form where chromosome 14 is (in essence) in trisomy is not usually compatible with survival to term	<5%
Unbalanced derivative arising where one parent has a balanced reciprocal autosomal translocation	e.g. 46,XX, t(2;21)(p11;p11) as a hypothetical example The parent may also have a normal karyotype and the rearrangement occur de novo in the child	Inherits the unbalanced form 46,XY, der(21) – the der 21 replaces the normal chromosome 2, and trisomy of the long arm results	Very rare
Mosaicism	Usually normal	e.g. 46,XX / 47,XX +21 Can coexist with both full trisomy 21 and with a Robertsonian translocation	Around 2%

standardised mortality odds ratio (SMOR) of 85.5 (95% CI) between the ages of 20 and 29 and a numerical peak (2980 deaths) under 10 years old. Respiratory associated conditions were also very prominent, with a peak SMOR of 14.3 between the ages 50 and 59 and a numerical peak of 1632 deaths in the same band. Presenile dementia had a peak SMOR of 116 between 40 and 49, indicating its great relative importance with a numerical peak of 430 in the 50–59 band. In contrast, malignancies apart from leukaemias and testicular cancer were underrepresented at all ages. In spite of the improvements it is clear that people with DS are still at substantially increased risk of early death.

Prenatal screening for DS

Up to 80% of DS children are born to women under 35 years of age. Maternal age considerations are thus only one factor in preventing DS. In the UK, routine maternal screening occurs for those over 35 years, but this is not the case for younger mothers. It is difficult to reliably identify specific changes in the maternal age-related incidence of DS, and there is a great variability in birthrates from year to year. For reasons that are not clear, there may also be an increased rate of DS babies in mothers under 20 years. The most commonly used marker for fetal DS is lowered maternal serum alpha fetoprotein level (AFP). DS fetal liver has a lowered AFP production. Recently a combination of AFP, human chorionic gonadotrophin (HCG) and urinary unconjugated oestratriol has been used to calculate the risk for a younger mother

of carrying a fetus with DS. More invasive is ultrasound-guided fetal cell sampling from amniotic fluid (amniocentesis: 15–22 weeks, 0.5% loss risk). The main indication for this is advanced maternal age. In addition to a karyotype, DNA tests for fragile X and other conditions can also be made. Chorionic villus sampling (CVS) obtains placental tissue trans-cervically or trans-abdominally, and also has an increased fetal loss risk. Its main advantage is that it is done earlier (10–12 weeks). Very early CVS has occasioned some reports of fetal limb abnormalities. Combining first and second trimester serum testing has been reported to increase the detection rate (to 85%) and decrease the false positive rate (to 1%) and may lead to a decrease in the need for invasive testing (Wald et al 1999). Much current effort centres on isolating fetal cells that leak into maternal peripheral blood and PCR amplifying fetal DNA or detecting anomalies by fluorescent methods. The technology could be developed as a primary screen with a secondary quadruple hormone screen (all above-mentioned hormones and inhibin A) (Roizen 2001). Advanced ultrasound methods, especially colour doppler imaging, have led to an increasing detection rate of systemic abnormalities associated with fetal DS, e.g. cardiac and gastrointestinal abnormalities (especially duodenal atresia). More subtle variations such as thickening of the nuchal skin fold and cystic hygromas may have higher sensitivity. Nicolaides's group were able to show that 55% of major cardiac/great vessel abnormalities were associated with fetal nuchal translucency at 10–14 weeks gestation (Hyett et al 1999).

Clinical features of DS

DS is a multisystem disorder, and almost every organ-system in the body can be involved. It is important to have some working knowledge of these, since the interplay between the various systems can be extensive.

The classical clinical features

Not everyone with DS will have all clinical features or to the same degree. For instance a protruding tongue is present in under 50%, the 'diagnostic' transverse palmar crease in 53%. Even the most consistent feature, upslanting palpebral fissures, is restricted to 80% (Epstein 2001). Differential growth in DS is especially clear in the head shape and facial features. Head circumference is reduced slightly at birth. At about 6 years it is 2 SD below normal. Markedly reduced anteroposterior head diameter (brachycephaly) develops after birth. The maxilla is also decreased in size relative to the mandible. The bridge of the nose may be underdeveloped and the eyes closer together, with the characteristic slope and presence of an epicanthic fold. Specific non-CNS changes in DS are given in Table 24.3.

Table 24.3 Specific physical conditions associated with Down syndrome	
Specific system or developmental area	Annotation
Growth	*Generalised growth disturbance.* At birth the infant is slightly smaller than normal. Mean height for adult men is around 1.5 m and women 1.4 m. Growth is reduced more in the limbs than trunk. Rate of growth may differ at different ages, and in spite of the reduced stature the intrinsic bone development seems normal. Height at 10 years (as in general population) predicts final adult height. Plasma growth hormone is not reduced, but serum insulin-like growth factor (IGF-1) is increased during the first 2 years, then remains at a constant level throughout life rather than showing the normal two-fold difference between adult and childhood levels. IGF-2 levels are normal. Treatment with growth hormone increases the mean growth velocity and both IGF-1 and IGF-2 levels, suggesting the growth impairment may be a specific rather than a general effect. However, growth hormone treatment does not alter head size or affect the level of learning disability, and it is *not* recommended unless a specific and pathological lack of growth hormone can be demonstrated. *Over 30% of both sexes* tend to be overweight, and in one sample nearly 50% were *obese*. This related to living at home rather than in supported accommodation, suggesting a social factor. However Down syndrome individuals have a lower resting (not active) metabolic rate, and they also tend to be less active than their peers overall, and the link between body mass index and diet is not strong.
Respiratory tract	*Hypopharynx is narrowed* with an increased risk of sleep apnoea, especially in the young. Psychological disturbance, e.g. excessive daytime restlessness / behavioural difficulties, in association with snoring can indicate this diagnosis, for which remedial treatments are available
Joints and muscle tone	*Neck joints* have been a focus of attention for young adults and adolescents. Atlanto-axial joint instability is associated with transverse ligament weakness, but only symptomatic in 1.5%. X-ray diagnosis can be difficult, requiring repeated films from different views. It may be seen in up to 13% on X-ray, but intervention is controversial. In general it should not overtly restrict physical activity, save in those sports where there is a high risk of neck strain. In a few cases death in association with medical procedures has occurred (including tracheal intubation and physical restraint). The Down syndrome newborn has a striking *muscular hypotonia* (perhaps a universal feature). Involuntary reflexes that participate in forming the background muscle tone are reduced in intensity, as well as voluntary muscle control such as handgrip. It is worsened by coexisting congenital cardiac disease. The decrease in tone is probably central in origin and continues in older children to a lesser but still significant degree. Hypotonus and feeding difficulties during the neonatal period are important correlates of early mortality.
Skin	*Characteristic developmental anomalies* formerly played a key part in diagnosis. Dermatoglyphs of the palm and sole show ulnar loops on the second finger, and an arched tibial pattern on the hallucis of the foot. A transverse palmar crease is often marked. These represent developmental problems that occur during the third month in utero. Skin itself is soft in children with Down syndrome, the hair is often soft and fine, but has a tendency to dryness in adults. The circulation to the extremities is often poor and acrocyanosis in cold weather is frequent.
Congenital anomalies: heart and gastrointestinal tract	*Congenital heart disease* in 40–50% of children — still a leading cause of infant mortality, which requires early detection and treatment if pulmonary hypertension is to be avoided. Anomalies of the venous inflow tract lead to a variety of outcomes (in approximate rank frequency: atrioventricular canal, ventricular septal defect, atrial septal defect, tetralogy of Fallot and patent ductus). Operations for these are no different from those in other children save for complete atrioventricular septal defect, which tends to be complex and has a higher early and late mortality. The echocardiogram can reveal most defects. *Gastrointestinal anomalies* are less prevalent and variable. Incidence of congenital duodenal stenosis or atresia is strikingly raised to near 300 times that in the general population, but the indications for treatment are the same.

continued

Table 24.3 Continued	
Specific system or developmental area	Annotation
Vision/hearing	*Eye* — squints in up to 20%, which may require surgical correction. Myopia and other refractive errors present in over one-third. Preserving visuospatial learning in children with Down syndrome is vital, so correction of such abnormalities is essential. Later cataracts become common. Keratoconus (acute and painful corneal inflammation with scarring and the formation of a cone-shaped protrusion) is rarer but sight threatening. Two peaks of incidence: one in late teenage years, and one after 40 years. *Hearing* — otitis media affects many children; may be exacerbated by structural anomalies of the ear. Most children have a unilateral or bilateral hearing loss to some degree, which is added to by later onset of sensori-neural deafness. The more profoundly disabled can find using corrective hearing aids and spectacles difficult, but, since they facilitate communication, efforts should be made. The provision of appropriate specialist audiometry services can help greatly.
Haematology/immunology	*Deficiencies in immunological competence/surveillance* may be a common denominator for several disorders, including infections, haematological tumours and endocrine disturbances. Infection, especially pneumonia, is still the leading cause of death in Down syndrome. Although B lymphocytes appear to have normal morphology there is a tendency to raised levels of IgG and IgM antibodies, save in newborns where they may be decreased. Cell-mediated immunity is altered, with a small decrease in T lymphocyte numbers (esp. T helper cells). Thymus is often severely dysmorphic, with associated T cell maturation delay releasing an excessive proportion of immature cells. A high frequency of transient leukaemoid reactions occur in newborn, and the white cells involved always seem to be fully trisomic for chromosome 21. The risk of true leukaemia is also raised in both children and adults. In the first year acute non-lymphocytic leukaemia predominates. In later years the spectrum of types is similar to that in the general population, but there are massively increased risks for myelodysplastic syndrome (relative risk 175) and acute megakaryocytic leukaemia (relative risk 600). The treatment response in people with Down syndrome may differ, and methotrexate may be toxic at even standard doses.
Endocrine system	*Probably related to immune disturbance* is an increased prevalence of *autoimmune thyroid dysfunction* (usually hypothyroidism) at all ages. Microsomal antibodies can be detected in the infant, and seroconversion from euthyroid to compensated hypothyroid to full illness can occur throughout life. Some cases are congenital, but most are of later onset, and the presence of thyroid antibodies is variable. However, up to 20% of adolescents and adults with Down syndrome may suffer from it, and it is a crucial differential diagnosis to be eliminated in the presentations of behavioural disturbance, depression and dementia in these age groups. Screening is advised for children on a regular basis, and for adults a 2-yearly screen is suggested, but is not yet universal. *Diabetes mellitus* is also more prevalent (esp. type I) and again is postulated to have an autoimmune basis.
Reproductive system	*Men with Down syndrome* due to full trisomy 21 are usually infertile (only one documented case of a man with Down syndrome fathering a child). This is not the case for mosaic trisomy 21, and offspring both normal and with Down syndrome have been reported. Spermatogenic arrest of varying degrees leads to an average lowered sperm count. Cause is unknown. In contrast over 20 women with Down syndrome are known to have had children, and slightly less than half of these had Down syndrome in turn. However, there may also be a slowing of follicular development in the ova, with some women completely failing to ovulate. Another reproductive change is that the menopause occurs on average 5 years early in women with Down syndrome

The central nervous system in DS

Neuroanatomy

On average, brain weight is decreased by 10–20%, with reduced fronto-occipital length. Other changes are subtler and variable: decreased gyral count, cortical thinning, underdeveloped cerebellar mid-lobe. Neuronal heterotopias occur in cerebellar white matter and vermis, indicating neuronal migration problems. Neuronal numbers are decreased in a patchy fashion, in cerebellum, locus coeruleus and basal forebrain. Individual neuron morphology is also altered, with abnormal dendrite formation. There are anomalies in neuron-associated cells, including glial cell enlargement. The development of the brain in DS involves abnormal degrees of neuronal differentiation, abnormal cortical lamination and a decrease in the number of neurons eventually formed.

Cultured fetal neurons show normal initial differentiation but subsequent degeneration and programmed cell death (apoptosis). There is also dendritic atrophy (at least in visual cortex) which continues into adult life. These mechanisms suggest problems at all levels of brain maturation — proliferation, neuronal migration, and differentiation. Apoptosis may involve defects in the mechanisms that scavenge cellular free radicals. Such defects may also predispose to dementia. Free-radical excess is a key candidate hypothesis for the development of Alzheimer's disease in the normal population, and one of the tri-allelic genes on chromosome 21 is superoxide dismutase, which performs a scavenging function. The presence of pathological features of Alzheimer's disease, including neurofibrillary tangles and amyloid-containing plaques, is well documented and found in practically all individuals with DS over the age of 35 who have had postmortems. The brain distribution of these lesions is similar to that of Alzheimer's disease of the normal population (the clinical dementia is further discussed below). The substrate on which the dementia develops is certainly not normal, however; e.g. the hippocampus in DS has rather specific changes with a doubling of cells (thought to be astroglia) that stain positive for a protein marker termed S100.

Neurochemistry

In the fetus with DS the activity of choline acetyltransferase is normal but the number of muscarinic receptors is reduced. Pharmacologically, a well-reported peripheral neurological effect is atropine hypersensitivity. In adults there may be an increased turnover of central monoamines unrelated to cognitive decline.

Cognitive changes associated with DS

Intellectual disability becomes apparent during the first few months of life, and increases as the child becomes older, as measured by progressive delay in attaining developmental milestones. The earliest milestones, such as smiling at faces, may be delayed only for a few months, but later milestones, especially language-related items such as the ability to form a sentence of three words, may be delayed for up to 2 years. These delays are group averages, and for individual children changes may be more difficult to elicit. Cognitive decline starts within the first year and is almost continuous from then until 10 years. After the first decade the intellectual disability tends to remain relatively static or only slowly progresses, with some late teenagers showing a phase of improvement followed by a period of stability until the decline with advancing years, in many cases accelerated by dementia. As most studies have focused on children, there are much fewer reports on the stability or otherwise of cognitive abilities of adults without dementia. At around 5 years most children have test scores in the high-moderate to mild range of LD, and early educational and psychological interventions may be a key to maintaining this. The variability in intellectual attainment is well demonstrated by children with full DS having test scores in the normal (low average) range. There is evidence that parental educational levels, partly reflecting their IQs, are related to the degree of intellectual disability in DS children. About 60–75% of DS children have impairments in language production more severe than their mental age would predict, 20–35% had language comprehension and production on par with their mental age, and only 5% had deficits in both areas (Miller et al 1999). Vocabulary skills develop more quickly than syntax, and there is a deficit in expressive language.

Early intervention and intellectual and social achievement in DS

DS children brought up in their own homes do better than those in institutions or foster care. One study showed an increase of over 17 IQ points at the age of around 10 if the child is brought up at home (Ludlow & Allen 1979). In the comparative longitudinal survey reported by Shepperdson (1995a) the attainment levels were linked to the social class of the parents, and also higher for children of younger mothers who gave greater stimulation. However, a single measure such as IQ very inadequately describes the profile of disability experienced in DS. Some consensus findings are emerging from studies of the neuropsychological strengths and weaknesses. There seems to be a preservation of

visuomotor skills and co-ordination (Thase et al 1984). Wishart, in an important series of experiments, found that infants with DS tended to use avoidance as a strategy for coping with cognitive psychological challenges, rather than try and use extant problem-solving skills. In fact infants became more skilled in avoidance with age. They also showed significant deficits of motivation — with very variable test–retest scores, failing on items they previously passed on. These motivational and behavioural profiles are important in designing for the education of the child (Wishart 1995). Haxby (1989) found that young DS adults, without confounding medical problems, did better on tests of short-term memory based on visual and spatial (Corsi's block-tapping tests) rather than verbal tasks. Other adults with non-specific learning disabilities showed the opposite effect. Wang & Bellugi (1994) compared groups of adolescents with DS and William's syndrome, confirming that those with DS were worse at the digit span test, and better on block tapping. Young DS adults also performed better on tests of manual dexterity and sequencing of movements. The relative deficit in auditory short-term memory may be important in overall attainment, and is compounded by the hearing problems to which children and DS adults are susceptible. A detailed speech, language and hearing assessment should take place in any educational intervention programme for DS, and strategies used that combine written and oral communication. Computer-based teaching could be helpful in this context. Early language interventions should centre on encouraging attempts at communication regardless the mode used (Miller et al 1999), and speech therapy may be needed especially to promote the development of expressive language.

Psychiatric disorders in DS

DS adults are affected by the same variety of psychiatric disorders and comorbidities as the general population. In a study of over two hundred adults, psychiatric disorders (WHO criteria) occurred at a rate approaching 30% (Prasher 1995).

Affective disorders and DS

Overall prevalence figures vary. Collacott et al (1992) found a high incidence of depression (11%) (all types of depression included), nearly three times greater than in a matched LD control group. Myers & Pueschel (1991) found psychiatric disorders of some form in nearly 18% of children and 27% of DS adults; 6% had major depressive disorder. They noted that depression tends to present with marked biological features, with prominent sleep disturbance, psychomotor slowing or agitation. Much less apparent are cognitive associates such as loss of interest in day-to-day activities, poor concentration, or thoughts of guilt and worthlessness. Suicidal thoughts are uncommon. Hallucinations (auditory and visual), however, may occur in a substantial percentage (Myers & Pueschel 1995). The relative paucity of cognitive and subjective symptoms of depression can make differential diagnosis difficult. The functioning of those with depressive illness seems poorer than matched groups, with continuing problems in adaptive behaviour even after recovery. In Prasher's study, symptoms were still present a year after the initial episode, suggesting a relatively poor prognosis for some (Prasher & Hall 1996). The main alternatives are dementia, physical disorders including hypothyroidism, and bereavement reactions. Dementia and depression may coexist, and some have suggested a definite relationship between the two in DS (Burt et al 1992). Although Prasher's findings sound a warning, the clinical impression is that the therapeutic response to conventional antidepressants is usually good, with some evidence that those acting on the serotonergic system are preferable. Although bipolar disorder is not common in DS, previous reports suggesting that DS adults did not exhibit mania are unsupported, and a series of reports has shown that the clinical features are similar to bipolar disorder in the non-DS learning-disabled population (Cooper & Collacott 1993).

Other disorders

- *Autism.* Myers & Pueschel (1991) suggested a comorbidity rate with autism of 1%. A more recent study in Birmingham put the rate at nearer 7% (Kent et al 1999). The apparent increase in the prevalence of autism in the general population is controversial, and the same factors may apply here.
- *Abnormal bereavement reactions.* These are relatively common in DS adults. There are two contributing factors. First, the maternal ageing effect means many parents are older when their child is born; second, and more importantly, the adult with DS is usually looked after by his or her parents no matter what age they are.
- *Schizophrenia.* Schizophrenia and DS was described as long ago as 1959, by Neville. Although it is not commonly diagnosed, and must be differentiated from hallucinations in depression or psychotic features in the early stages of dementia, small-scale studies suggest that a chronic negative outcome is not common (Cooper et al 1995).
- *Other conditions.* Many other disorders have been reported in DS, including obsessive–compulsive disorder (Prasher & Day 1995) and Tourette syndrome, but their incidence is uncertain. However, many ritualistic and compulsive behaviours in DS have similarities to those seen in learning-disabled people without DS, and differentiation from autism can be difficult if the person has a moderate or severe degree of LD (Evans & Gray 2000).

Dementia

DS and Alzheimer's disease   Langdon Down noted that a female patient developed dementia in her 50s (Ward 1998). In 1876, only 10 years after the first report of DS, Fraser and Mitchell in Edinburgh noted the co-occurrence. The pathological features of Alzheimer's disease were described at postmortem in an adult with DS by Struwe in 1929. Plaques and neurofibrillary tangles occur in the brains of almost 100% of older DS adults, and the anatomic distribution of these lesions is similar to that seen in Alzheimer's disease in elderly subjects without LD. The pathology is, however, acting on a differently prepared substrate. MRI studies indicate a smaller hippocampal but not amygdala volume in DS adults without dementia (Aylward et al 1999a). In those with dementia, however, both structures are smaller than in subjects without dementia.

The anatomic changes of Alzheimer's disease can begin as early as the second decade of life in DS, and have even been described in a 12 year old, but not apparently in younger children. The main component of the amyloid in DS is amyloid βA4 protein with 42 amino acid residues ($A\beta_{42}$), coded for by the amyloid precursor protein (*APP*) gene on chromosome 21, mutations in which are the cause of a class of relatively rare early-onset familial dementia

in the general population. APP exists in three isoforms. In DS fetal brain there is an almost five-fold increase in the expression of the APP-695 variant, and a four-fold increase in the APP-751 and APP-770 forms. The latter two isoforms have structures suggesting that they may act as protease inhibitors, and levels are increased in the hippocampus and striatum of DS adults. In plasma of DS adults the $A\beta_{42}$ form of amyloid is increased, as is the less common $A\beta_{40}$ form. Interestingly, if DS adults are divided into those with and without dementia the $A\beta_{42}$ isoform is specifically increased by a further 26% in the dementia group. The levels of $A\beta_{42}$ but not $A\beta_{40}$ varied with the *ApoE* genotype, suggesting a specific role for the former in the pathology (Schupf et al 2001). APP's part in the development of pathology is still unclear, and there must be some mechanism to explain why the plaques and tangles do not, on average, appear until the third decade, whereas the levels are persistently high throughout life. Teller et al (1996) showed that the abnormal accumulation of $A\beta_{42}$ occurs from the 21st week in utero, long before the formation of any plaques, right through to the 61st year of life — a situation not seen in matched controls. Normally the APP is processed into $A\beta_{40}$ with only small amounts of $A\beta_{42}$ produced. However, in DS the $A\beta_{42}$ peptide is present even in the absence of amyloid plaques. They suggested that in DS a mechanism exists to degrade this protein, preventing it aggregating, and it may be this mechanism that fails with age rather than the protein deposition into plaques being the proximate cause of the disease.

Another candidate on chromosome 21 is the Copper–Zinc-requiring superoxide dismutase (SOD) gene (*CuZnSOD*) that lies close to the *APP* gene. SOD is a free radical scavenger, forming hydrogen, which is then the substrate for other enzymes to form water. Defective metabolism of reactive oxygen species is a feature of fetal DS neurons. Duplication of SOD in itself is not essential to cognitive impairment but occurs in nearly all DS subjects. Apoptosis may link the biology to the pathology of dementia in both the general population and DS adults. Caspase, an apoptosis-associated enzyme and caspase-cleaved APP product, are found in neurons showing granulovacuolar degeneration in the hippocampal CA1 region in DS brains (Su et al 2002). Gliosis is also prominent in DS, and the gene coding for glial calcium-binding protein subunit (S100β) is also found on chromosome 21. Interleukin 1, a cytokine produced by macrophages, which promotes gliosis, is also involved in the cellular regulation of APP uptake. Interleukin-1-containing cells are markedly increased in DS, and it may link the defective immune response of DS to the regulation of already aberrantly expressed proteins. It is likely that many or all of these factors interact to create the histological changes and the temporal sequence of the disease.

Prevalence of dementia   The incidence is age-related, and follow-up studies show that over the age of 40 around 10% of DS adults per year will develop clinical signs of dementia. This predicts an overall prevalence of clinical dementia at around 40% for all DS adults over 40, correlating well with the numbers found in practice. For a presenile dementia, this represents a considerable number of affected people, and DS is probably the single most common cause.

Clinical dementia in DS adults   Clinical dementia does not occur as frequently as the histopathological changes, and prevalence reports range widely, from 6% to 75%. A large Irish survey of DS adults (285 subjects; 35–74 years) found a rate of 13.3%, and the dementia group had a mean age of 54.7 years (Temple et al 2001). In those over 40 who presented with functional decline in an American adult DS residential centre, 21% had clinical signs of Alzheimer's disease (Chicoine et al 1998). For those over 50 years of age, this figure increases; Van Buggenhout et al (1999) found 42%. The overall trend is clear, differences probably reflecting diagnostic criteria/tests used, and cohort effects in a period where the longevity for DS has markedly changed. At the turn of the century the average life expectancy with DS was around 9 years. Now nearly 15% of DS men and 20% of women are over 55, with most of this change occurring since 1960. The effects of normal ageing in DS must be separated from those of Alzheimer's pathology. It is unfortunate that the term 'premature ageing' is rather widely applied to any ageing phenomena in DS, when in fact most evidence to support the concept is (circularly) based on Alzheimer's neuropathology. The problem is compounded by the difficulty of applying standard dementia diagnostic criteria in DS adults, and a presentation that may highlight features that are atypical of dementia in the general population. Longitudinal studies show that DS adults over 50 show adaptive behaviour deterioration at a greater rate than comparison LD groups (Zigman et al 1996) and that this adaptive loss is global rather than specific. Older studies of DS adults found little evidence for deterioration in cognitive measures, including short-term memory, but any clinical Alzheimer's-type dementia was usually an exclusion criterion, and they focused on younger adults below 50 years. Studies with wider age spread show definite declines, especially in tasks involving planning and attention (Das et al 1985).

It is not possible at present to predict who will develop dementia, although some studies have tried. Changes in neuropsychological measures and in the timing of auditory event-related potentials over a 2-year time period have been described. Recently, a modified form of the selective reminding test suggested long-term recall is affected up to 1 year before the appearance of clinical signs (Krinsky-McHale et al 2002). An increase in P300 waveform latency may predict dementia before clinical signs are apparent (Muir et al 1988). However, the common hearing loss of older DS subjects makes such tests difficult. Biological and psychological markers may be more useful. The genetic polymorphisms associated with the *ApoE* gene (chromosome 19) may be predisposing factors for dementia. The gene product binds to amyloid-β peptide in the plaques and tangles. The commonest allele in Western populations is ApoEε3. Being homozygous or heterozygous for the less common ApoEε4 leads to an increased risk and decreased age-at-onset of late-onset forms of Alzheimer's dementia in the general population. Schupf & Sergievsky (2002) reviewed the data indicating that apolipoprotein E may modulate the age when clinical symptoms of dementia appear, concluding that, in DS, ApoEε4 was a risk factor for earlier onset and ApoEε2 protective, as in the general population. The original level of cognitive functioning may also help in predicting the dementia risk. Controlling for a variety of variables (but in a small sample set) suggested that higher initial cognitive levels reduce dementia risk (Temple et al 2001).

The place of imaging in diagnosis is not clear, partly because of lack of normative data. CT scans can be difficult to interpret until clinical signs are very obvious, although one small study indicates that temporal lobe oriented views might be useful (Lawlor et al 2001).

Clinical features and diagnosis of dementia At present it is often not easy to make an early diagnosis. For the DSM-IV-TR diagnosis of any form of dementia, there must be a demonstrable deterioration in short-term and later long-term memory, along with a worsening ability to focus attention and maintain personal orientation. The DS adult is very different in many aspects from non-LD populations with presenile or old-age dementia. The metabolic and genetic background differs, but so also does their upbringing, education, language acquisition, work placements and social support structure. Thus dementia acts on a different substrate, and can be expected to produce different effects in most areas of functioning. Memory change may not be the initial symptom; difficulties in multiple areas of function occur and deteriorating self-care skills seems the commonest, followed by loss of social and language skills and then memory loss. In younger DS adults a frontal lobe presentation with marked behavioural disturbance may be an early feature. This may also be present in older adults but usually here accompanied by detectable memory loss. Various behavioural difficulties are very common (including wandering) and may occur de novo or may represent an exacerbation of long-term behaviours. Psychotic features such as auditory and visual hallucinations are quite frequent and may be early, although the degree of LD may make their interpretation difficult. Depression is common, either as a result of, or comorbid with, dementia, and a treatment trial may be required to resolve the issue. Other behavioural changes include general motor slowing, a decrease in motivation levels and interest in previous pursuits. Altered language use may be an early sign. The vocabulary may become restricted, with increased repetitiveness or in some cases the onset of mutism. 'Organic' features again may occur early, and it is especially notable that late-onset features in the cognitively normal person may be presenting features in DS: incontinence, mobility impairment and epilepsy. The course of dementia varies, but is often rapid. In some cases death may occur within 6 months of initial diagnosis, in others the course runs several years. In late stages the person may be completely immobile and doubly incontinent.

In the assessment the establishment of baseline level of functioning is important, but may be a difficult and at present often retrospective process. Testing instruments include structured observer ratings (reviewed by Deb & Braganza 1999) in combination with more specific psychological scales such as Vineland or the Severe Impairment Battery. A longitudinal approach is needed, sometimes over an extended period, to pick up subtler early changes. There are still no tests, however, that alone permit a definitive diagnosis. In adults with milder LD the Mini Mental State Examination modified to suit the person's abilities has been found helpful when combined with longitudinal measures. Clinical work-up must be extensive, making full use of information from key informants at work and at home, as well as clinical, physical and psychological examination of the person themselves. Brain imaging, including CT and MRI scans, to be useful needs to be repeated but then can clearly show changes typical of Alzheimer's disease.

Epilepsy, dementia and DS Unlike for other causes of LD, epilepsy in DS is not common save in the very young and in association with dementia. Although it can occur without dementia the adult onset of epilepsy should be regarded as a serious occurrence demanding further investigation. Grand mal epilepsy may occur in both early and late dementia, but myoclonic epilepsy is more common. There may be a diurnal pattern, with a prominence of the fits on awakening. Although the usual antiepileptic medications are useful, the epilepsy is sometimes difficult to treat (Tangye 1979). The usual recourse is sodium valproate provided the liver function is adequate; lamotrigine and carbamazepine sometimes make things worse. The DS adult who develops myoclonic epilepsy usually has a much more rapid deterioration than others with dementia.

Differential diagnosis The differential diagnoses are mostly treatable — depression, hypothyroidism, bereavement reactions — and should always be considered. Less common are anaemias (both iron-deficient and folate-deficient), and chronic coeliac disease is over-represented in DS adults and children. Depression and anxiety are common in DS adults and are the mental health disorders that are most commonly unrecognised. Functional mental health problems, physical disorders and dementia may all coexist, and vigorous treatment of amenable conditions may be needed to resolve the issue. There is some evidence that DS adults with dementia are at greater risk of developing hypothyroidism than those without dementia (Percy et al 1990).

Treatment and management After the diagnosis of dementia is confirmed, the psychiatrist has a role to play in working with and supporting the family or carers, treating the behavioural or psychiatric components of the condition, and also advising on the suitability of the particular environments that the person encounters. Many of the current care settings are not an environment compatible with dementia. For example, adult training/resource centres serve large numbers of changing clients, noise levels are often high, and open-plan design can lead to increased confusion and behaviour disturbance. Much can be done to create smaller, quieter areas within such settings, maintaining placement continuity while creating a much less sensory-threatening environment. Similarly, hospitals usually have high ambient noise levels, multiple staff changes and, to the already confused, present an additional source of fear and disorientation. Sadly, eventual nursing home or hospital placement often occurs for the wrong reasons, at the wrong stage of the illness, because of the lack of appropriate alternatives. Care of the elderly wards are not age-generic and may distance the person from the appropriate social work and specialist healthcare services for LD adults. Although management is largely supportive, there is interest in anticholinesterases. Two small trials of donepezil have been undertaken. Prasher's group conducted a pilot placebo-controlled double-blind parallel-group trial, but, perhaps understandably for an early trial in LD, only on thirty subjects with DS and dementia. They showed that the drug was relatively safe and well tolerated, but the numbers were too small to show significant changes (Prasher et al 2002). Larger trials are at present underway. There is, in fact, no a-priori reason that someone with DS and early dementia should not receive anticholinesterase medication after full clinical investigation, as would any other person with a presenile dementia.

Dementia and the family Dementia is a tremendous stress for the family or carers, especially parents, who themselves may be experiencing problems of ageing. Janicki described this as 'two generation ageing', an inversion from the normal situation where the children usually look after the parent sufferer. Attempts should be made to maintain the home placement and support parents in the immediate practical aspects of healthcare, and in making plans for future care. Carers are especially troubled by restlessness, loss of speech, incontinence and wandering, and these behavioural problems need careful management. Parents are also very concerned as to who will look after their son/daughter when they themselves die, whether or not the person suffers from dementia. After parental loss, it is still the family that usually look after the person with DS (usually the siblings, most often a sister, take over the role of carer). In the final stages, health needs may be overwhelming, and there is a great need for specialist respite/terminal care. Hospice terminal care facilities have proved useful for some, and studies on good palliative care practice for people with LD are beginning, but clinically the general practitioner is generally adept at palliative care.

Sexual development in DS and its problems

Sexuality and sexual expression is as much part of normal development for the DS adolescent as it is for anyone else. The sexual development of men with DS seems to follow a normal course, with the development of primary and secondary sexual characteristics. DS girls start menstruating at around the same age as others, and cycles are usually regular with regular ovulation (Scola & Pueschel 1992). However, most DS men have reduced sperm counts — a problem of unknown cause, spermatogenesis arrest varies from very mild to complete. Men with mosaic DS however are fertile and have been known to have children. Women with full trisomy 21 can be fertile (over 24 children have been reported). Some have problems, however, with ovulation or slowed follicle growth.

The development of sexuality during adolescence is often a major issue for both the person with DS and their carers. Shepperdson (1995b) described longitudinal studies on two cohorts of young people with DS: a group born in the 1960s and followed up during teens and mid-twenties, and a group born in the 1970s who were then seen in their teens. Although the carers of adolescents born in the 1970s appeared more permissive, carers of both cohorts were rarely in favour of parenthood for people with LD. Over half thought that sterilisation might be appropriate in certain circumstances. Although two-thirds of both groups felt sex education was appropriate for teenagers, only one-third of carers in the first cohort felt it appropriate to adults. Although, superficially, attitudes seem changed, such views are still unfortunately common today. Sex education is appropriate for young people with DS, and they should learn about forming relationships, marriage, heterosexuality and homosexuality, as well as the mechanistic aspects of intercourse and body function. The LD in combination with increased independence makes them vulnerable to abuse and exploitation, and dealing with such risks should be a part of any educational programme. Community LD nurses who develop a specialist interest in sex education/sexual health can be useful in adult education.

THE X CHROMOSOME AND LEARNING DISABILITY

The X chromosome is especially important to our understanding of LD. In 1897 Johnson reported that, on the basis of the US census of 1890, 24% more men than women had LD. Both Luxenburger in 1932 and Penrose's classic 1938 study confirmed this in institutional populations. Initially it was thought that increased male aggressiveness led to notification and institutionalisation, but the same excess is seen outside hospitals. The overall male gender relative risk for all LD is near 1.7, for mild LD alone is around 1.9, and for severe LD somewhat less at 1.4 (Croen et al 2001). An increased male susceptibility to neonatal injury partly contributes; low birthweight male infants have a higher mortality than females, and recently an association between birth-weight and IQ has been shown for males (Matte et al 2001). However, most of the male bias is due to X chromosome abnormalities. The human genome sequence reveals that 3.75% of all genes are on the X chromosome, and the X chromosome seems to be predisposed to disorders affecting cognition. Even assuming some disorders presently regarded as independent are part of the phenotypic spectrum of single mutations, in the premier genetic database, Online Mendelian Inheritance in Man, over 200 of almost 1000 conditions associated with LD are X-linked (Zechner et al 2001).

The unusual genetics of the X chromosome

Only one X chromosome is fully active in any cell. This is the case no matter how many X chromosomes are present. Man is a sexually dimorphic animal, and some means of ensuring equivalent gene dosage is needed. In all cells of normal females, one X chromosome exists in a densely packaged inactive state, the heterochromatic Barr body, created in the late blastocyst embryonic stage. Specific mechanisms are involved in both X chromosome inactivation and also in 'counting' the number of X chromosomes present, so that all are inactivated save one in any given karyotype (Avner & Heard 2001). Both these functions are located in a region called XIC (X inactivation centre, Xq13.3). In this complex a gene, *XIST* (X inactive-specific-transcript), produces an RNA (Xist) which coats its own chromosome. *XIST* on the X chromosome that is to remain active is transcriptionally silenced. Before the coating occurs, all X chromosomes in the cell express Xist at low levels, but it has a short half-life. The events that trigger inactivation increase the stability of Xist, possibly dependent on a certain level of accumulation being reached. Wheras Xist coating by itself is insufficient to maintain inactivity, a secondary process involving hypermethylation and the recruitment of hypoacetyled chromatin-associated proteins (histones H3 and H4) fixes the chromosome in the inactive state. This inactivation, once begun, is a spreading process, responding to chromosome-specific DNA signals (probably long interspersed nuclear elements, LINEs) that act as inactivation boosters. Certain regions (low LINE density) are spared and continue to remain active on the 'inactive' X. With respect to inheritance they behave like autosomal regions and are termed 'pseudoautosomal'.

Counting and the identification of which X chromosome is to be inactivated require distinct, poorly understood mechanisms separate from inactivation itself. Counting may involve low levels of a blocking factor sufficient to bind only one XIC in a cell. The correct autosome count is also necessary to the inactivation process, and in the triploid state (cells with 69 chromosomes, normally lethal in utero) the extra X chromosome is not inactivated. The pattern of X-inactivation in human cells is random, producing a paternal and maternal X active mosaic. Human extra-embryonic tissues, however, only express maternal X, suggesting imprinting of the paternally inherited X that may be important in some disorders. Usually the mosaic pattern in females allows around 50% of cells to express paternal-sourced X and 50% maternal-sourced X. Only maternal-sourced X exist in men, so they are fully affected by X-linked conditions whereas women vary in clinical expression. At the extremes, an apparently non-random inactivation may occur by chance, resulting in the full disorder in some women, while at the other extreme there is no detectable effect. In some conditions there is a truly non-random inactivation, e.g.

some families with Lesch–Nyhan syndrome have multiply-affected females. Another, commoner, type of non-random inactivation can occur in identical female twins that explains some of the clinical twin discordance in X-linked disorders.

Sex chromosome aneuploidies

These are numerical anomalies of X or Y. All excess X chromosomes when present are inactivated. Thus phenotypic consequences must be due to the higher copy number of the pseudoautosomal genes that escape inactivation. Abnormalities of the number of sex chromosomes are not uncommon, at over 1:500 live births (1:400 men; 1:600 women). The Y chromosome harbours few genes, and only aneuploidies leading to an increased X chromosome number show a strong association with LD. Females with Turner's syndrome (XO) do not have LD; in fact, mosaicism (around 25%) may confer a slightly higher than normal IQ. The clinically important aneuploidies have the karyotypes 47,XXY, 47,XXX and 47,XYY. Various mosaic karyotypes (the other cell line usually being normal) are also found. Higher number aneuploidies are well described but rare (Willard 2001).

Klinefelter syndrome

Klinefelter syndrome (47,XXY; 1:500 to 1:1000 men) is a relatively common and important condition, but still with an extensive prenatal loss (50% of all 47,XXY conceptions, 1:300 spontaneous abortions). The non-disjunction is nearly 50% paternal and 50% maternal in origin. Seventy-five percent of the maternally derived cases show a maternal age effect, and most paternally derived cases are associated with advanced paternal age. Klinefelter's original clinical description in 1942 pre-dated cytogenetic analysis, and his cohort was later found to include men who did not have XXY. The key criteria are now held to be an XXY karyotype and male hypogonadism. Diagnosis often occurs at puberty, with varying development of secondary sexual characteristics along with small testes, or through referral to an infertility clinic. Around 90% have scant facial hair, and gynaecomastia occurs in about 50%. The adult with Klinefelter's syndrome is usually around 4 cm taller than average (with especially long lower limbs) and with an asthenic body build. The average IQ (adults) is around 90, and also a substantial percentage of those with 47,XXY fall into the LD range — usually mild, with most having IQs above 60. Specific learning disorders are common, although the usual delay in diagnosis predicates against early intervention. In adolescents, verbal comprehension is decreased whereas performance IQ may be in the normal range. The postulated relationship of Klinefelter's syndrome to psychiatric disorders, especially psychoses, was based on the studies in institutions, and the true relationship is uncertain. No association was found when information from large cytogenetic and psychiatric databases was cross-linked in Denmark (Mors et al 2001); however, it is unclear whether this incorporated data on LD.

Trisomy X

The karyotype 47,XXX is found in around 1:1000 women. Generally there is little clinical evidence to suggest physical abnormality (a slight increase in height may occur, but this is also partly correlates with parental height). However up to 70% have specific learning disorders and LD is over-represented due to the slight decrease in average IQ. Some women have reduced fertility, but most do not, and their children have normal karyotypes. There are reports of an increased incidence of schizophrenia, not necessarily associated with LD, and some evidence for behavioural changes during the transition from adolescence to adulthood (Harmon et al 1998).

47,XYY males

Again, this occurs in around 1:1000 men. There are even fewer physical correlates than trisomy X (overall height is increased), and yet XYY has gained a controversial status out of proportion to its clinical importance. Studies on populations of men in maximum-security psychiatric hospitals in the 1960s seemed to show an excess of XYY carriers as well as XXY (Witkin et al 1976). These studies lacked adequate comparison groups, and the high prevalence of XYY in the general population casts doubts on inferences relating XYY to criminal behaviour. Average IQ may be very slightly lower than in the normal population, which may play a small part in a general increase in behavioural problems.

Sex chromosome polysomies, and other abnormalities

Where the number of X chromosomes and/or Y chromosomes increases further the phenotype is often severe. X chromosome tetrasomy (48,XXXX) and pentasomy (49,XXXXX) are rare but well described. 48,XXXY and 49,XXXXY are more common. Generally there is a marked LD, and a variety of physical abnormalities. The greater the number of X chromosomes, the more profound the LD. These extra X chromosomes are entirely maternal in origin, and are all inactivated, and the phenotype is a consequence of increased copy number of genes escaping inactivation. Ring X and supernumerary marker chromosomes derived from the X chromosome are usually also associated with LD. In some cases they may fail to inactivate, due to lack of XIC, or sometimes a failure to express Xist even when the gene is present. In these cases all regions of the X chromosome are expressed from both copies (a functional disomy), not just the pseudoautosomal, and the phenotype is severe.

Dynamic mutations — the fragile X syndrome

It has been long known that the male excess of LD could be familial. In 1943 Martin & Bell described a family where 11 men had a common set of clinical features including LD, and other similar families were reported over the next two decades. In 1971 Turner and her group suggested grouping cases where X-linked LD was the only clinical feature. In 1969 Lubs showed that under specific culture conditions (thymidine/folate deprivation) a cytogenetic marker became visible on the X chromosome in four LD members of one X-linked family. However it was not until the late 1970s that Sutherland and others realised this finding to be an important diagnostic tool. The anomaly shows up in a percentage of lymphocytes as a faintly staining constricted region near the end of the long arm of X (Xq27.3). Its apparently tenuous nature led to the appellation 'fragile site' and it is one of three such on X chromosome (termed FRAXA; the others are FRAXE and FRAXF; all are folate sensitive). Rare fragile sites are also found on autosomes, largely without clear clinical consequences (Sutherland & Baker 2000). There are also several 'common' fragile sites on X

of no clinical significance, including FRAXD, which, lying near FRAXA, can cause confusion. Over 80 common fragile sites are found through the genome, but their clinical significance is unclear. The presence of other fragile sites close to FRAXA led to an initial prevalence overestimate. Turner's early Australian reports for instance suggested around 1:2500 men and 1:4000 women. The discovery of the gene that is disrupted in association with the cytogenetic marker led to diagnostics directly based on DNA analysis, and the rate was revised downwards to around 1:4000–4500 men and 1:8000–9000 women, but this is still a very common inherited cause of LD.

The genetics of fragile X syndrome

Early work revealed several unusual features of inheritance that did not follow classical Mendelian lines, including a very low penetrance compared with other X-linked disorders. In the 1980s Sherman and her colleagues studied over a hundred families with fragile X syndrome and found that the daughters of women who must be obligate carriers of the gene mutation were at much greater risk of LD than daughters of unaffected male carriers ('normal transmitting males'). Further, they could identify fragile X chromosomes (by karyotyping or inferred from intellectual impairment) in only around half of female obligate carriers. In pedigrees it was noted that LD seemed to be more severe in younger generations — they displayed genetic anticipation, and in fragile X this was termed the Sherman Paradox. The answer to this paradox came with the identification and sequencing of the underlying gene, designated FMR1 (fragile X mental retardation gene 1), and its associated mutation in 1991. It is now clear that disruption of this gene alone is sufficient to cause fragile X syndrome. The gene has 17 exons, spanning around 38 kbp of DNA. Over 95% of cases of fragile X are associated with a very long linear sequence of multiply repeated DNA nucleotide base pair triplets — Cytosine–Guanine–Guanine or Guanine–Cytosine–Cytosine, dependent on the strand that is chosen (Warren & Sherman 2001). This is more readily written as $(CGG)n$ where n is the number of repeated triplets. This non-coding DNA sequence is found in the 5′ untranslated end of the FMR1 gene near the promoter and is very variable in size in the population. On average around 29 triplets exist (range of 6 to 52) and these have no effect on gene function. However, in men with full fragile X syndrome the copy number of the triplet is huge, ranging from over 230 to well over 1000, representing 690 to over 3000 extra bases of DNA. Cells do not permit such a large repeat in the FMR1 gene region to persist without modification. The cytosine residues of GC pairs in the repeat, nearby CpG island and gene promoter are highly methylated enzymatically, accompanied by de-acetylation of chromosome-associated histone proteins. Proteins recruited to the area include the methyl cytosine binding protein type MECP2, which is disrupted in Rett syndrome and other MRX disorders (see below), linking these to Fragile X. These alterations lead to an architectural compaction of the chromosomal region, preventing access of DNA polymerase and resulting in transcription failure. The gene is silenced and no mRNA produced. Transcription failure of FMR1, preventing production of its associated protein FMRP (fragile X mental retardation protein), is the cause of the disorder, not the repeat presence itself. Rare individuals with full fragile X syndrome phenotype have been reported with other FMR1-silencing disruptions such as gene deletions, intragenic mutations, even a single base pair mutation.

Table 24.4 Fragile X syndrome — size of base pair triplet repeat in *FMR1* gene, classification and stability, and phenotypic outcome

Size of repeat in terms of number (*n*) of triplets — (CGG)*n*	Classification	Clinical phenotype
6–60	Stable; the normal situation; not prone to expansion	None
60–200	Unstable; prone to expansion through a female meiosis	Largely no effect; controversially, some specific cognitive changes at the upper end of the premutation range
Over 200	Full expansion repeat size, unstable if passed through a further female meiosis	Fragile X syndrome

That the repeat itself is not causal is further emphasised by studies of transformed cell lines carrying the fragile X mutation where blocking histone deacetylases and methylation enzymes can reactivate the gene (Chiurazzi & Neri 2001). However, as a possible therapy, this approach is limited since translation as well as transcription seems suppressed in full mutation carriers.

The origins of the repeat are beginning to be understood. Repeat size can increase by up to 10–20 times between generations as a natural event. Most likely this is due to slippage in the DNA replication mechanism, with the repeated motif more likely to form hairpin loops and other structures that predispose to replication errors. A polarity exists, with repeats added at the 3′ end (i.e. during the final stage of repeat replication). Repeats of around 60–200 triplets are highly unstable but only when transmitted through the female germline, where massive further expansion occurs. In the general population the size of the repeat can be used to indicate its stability, and three classes of repeat size are generally recognised (Table 24.4).

Repeats have an important fine structure. A normal-size repeat of 30 or so CGG triplets will have a few (1–3) interspersed AGG triplets. These break up the tract of CGG triplets and in doing so confer increased stability. Mutations that remove the AGG repeats increase the length of 'perfect' CGG sequence and also the risk of meiotic instability. Premutations need to have at least 50 uninterrupted CGG repeats before they will expand to a full mutation, but shorter lengths of 'perfect' CGG sequence may also increase the likelihood of smaller intergenerational expansion, especially if the tract is closer to the 3′ end of the sequence.

In women, when repeat length is within the premutation range, then in around 50% cases with 60–80 triplets, and in nearly 100% with over 90 triplets, an expansion to a full mutation occurs in germ cells. In contrast in male carriers there is usually no further expansion. In some X-containing sperm there may be a contraction in repeat size, which is actually more likely with larger premutations. These sex differences explain the unusual inheritance patterns seen in families. The change from premutation to full mutation probably occurs pre-zygotically, that is in the developing gametes themselves. Ova obtained from females who have full fragile X syndrome show a further expansion in repeat size. The observation that somatic tissues in those with full fragile X syndrome are often mosaic for the repeat expansion is now thought to be due to contraction of repeat size in such tissues rather than the outcome of a post-zygotic expansion event. The mechanisms of the enormous expansions are not yet fully clear, but may involve very large-scale replication slippage, with extra CGG triplets added at the 3′ end. DNA repair enzymes exist to excise such repeated sequences, but the effectiveness of one of these, FEN1, is reduced in proportion to the size of large hairpin loops (Henricksen et al 2000). Factors also act on repeat length in the male germline, but in the opposite direction. Sperm from males with full fragile X show only X-premutations. Oostra's group has shown that cells from the early fragile X fetus have the full mutation, but by the 17th week only the premutation exists, indicating a true contraction of repeat size (Malter et al 1997).

In the families of subjects with fragile X syndrome the size of the repeated triplet thus varies. Normal transmitting males and obligate carrier females have premutations between 60 and 200 repeats, only unstable when passed from mother to a child. Thus daughters of normal transmitting males will have a premutation of much the same size as their father. However, when they pass this X chromosome to their offspring, then full expansion occurs and around half their sons have full fragile X syndrome and half their daughters are heterozygous full-mutation carriers.

The functions of FMRP

The *FMR1* gene produces a 4.4 kbp mRNA that codes for the FMRP protein. The individual mRNAs of the 17 exons are spliced together in alternate ways to form a series of different RNA molecules (spliceforms) and so different protein isoforms. FMRP has mRNA-binding regions (these motifs are termed KH domains and an RGG box). Such binding sites may be highly relevant to cognitive outcome — in a patient with full fragile X syndrome and severe LD due to a single point mutation of FMR1, the mutation lay directly in a KH domain. The RGG box has been shown to bind a subgroup of mRNAs with specific structures (G-quartets) (Brown et al 2001). The sequestering and suppression of translation of this type of mRNA may be a clue to FMRP's normal function. FMRP is synthesised in ribosomes in neuronal cell bodies and also in the vicinity of synapses in dendrites. In mice where the murine equivalent of *FMR1* has been experimentally silenced (mouse 'knock-outs') the dendritic spines on neurons are immature in form, perhaps indicating a slowing of maturation rather than a fixed phenomenon, since the synaptic changes may resolve over time.

Neuronal and brain changes in fragile X syndrome

Relatively few postmortem studies of fragile X syndrome have looked directly at neuronal architecture. In full fragile X males the neuronal count is normal but the dendritic structure in the cerebral cortex is aberrant, with long, thin, immature spines that are more numerous than in controls. In-vitro experiments using pinched-off and resealed presynaptic neuronal processes (the 'synaptoneurosome') show that dendrites synthesise proteins, including FMRP directly in the synaptic regions, a process essential to correct developmental synaptogenesis. Synaptogenesis in excessive initial amounts with subsequent removal/pruning forms the mature connectivity arrangements needed to process later sensory input, as was well shown for visual cortex in the classical studies of Hubel & Wiesel during the 1960s and 1970s, and more recently for other cortical sensory areas. A second subsequent stage of cortical synaptogenesis and pruning is directly regulated by sensory input and has been described in both sensory and motor cortex. Direct protein synthesis in the presynaptic zone is probably highly important to such synaptic plasticity. In synaptoneurosomes, FMRP synthesis is increased by glutamate-induced neuronal excitation, and the mechanism is absent in synaptoneurosomes derived from murine *FMR1* knockout tissues (Greenough et al 2001). Such elegant studies suggest that fragile X syndrome might be an example of a disorder that acts at the final stages of brain development.

MRI imaging (both males and females) indicates hippocampal changes, but results are inconsistent. One explanation of this may be age-related — studies on younger individuals tend to show an age-related increase in the volume of the hippocampus, whereas older individuals have shown an age-related decrease. Other abnormalities repeatedly reported in full fragile X males include decreased size of posterior cerebellar vermis, and increases in fourth ventricle, lateral ventricle and caudate (Eliez et al 2001). Abnormal cerebellar vermis has also been reported in some studies of autism; however, there is no increased comorbidity with autism

in fragile X, and the clinical picture, although showing superficial similarities and certain autistic-type behaviours, has important differences, including a less severe overall delay in social skills in fragile X. Further the autistic behaviours do not relate to the expressed levels of FMRP, which is deficient in fragile X syndrome (Bailey et al 2001). More information may result from future functional MRI studies. For example, a small study of 14 full fragile X females showed increased activation of the anterior prefrontal cortex and absence of expected activation of the inferior/superior parietal lobe compared with controls during a psychological task (a counting Stroop inhibition task of executive function) (Tamm et al 2002).

Screening issues and the place of the dynamic mutation in the population as a whole

DNA-based methods are replacing karyotyping in fragile X diagnosis. The mutation can be sized on a gel after restriction enzyme digestion of DNA, or detected by direct amplification using PCR. Many individuals who may have fragile X remain to be screened, and this is most apparent in adults with LD. A recent institutional survey found fragile X in 3.5% of all residents (Van Buggenhout et al 2001). Thus testing of adults as well as children is an important area. If there are physical features and/or a family history of LD, it is important to test for fragile X and obtain genetic counselling for the family. The current American College of Medical Genetics recommendations for testing are given in Table 24.5.

Table 24.5 Fragile X syndrome — simplified indications for diagnostic testing adapted from American College of Medical Genetics guidelines*

Whom to test?	Important features	Features that lower the threshold for testing	Other points
Males and females	• With learning disability • and/or other developmental delay • and/or autism	• Any phenotypic characteristics of fragile X syndrome • Family history of fragile X • Family history of undiagnosed learning disability	• DNA testing is now method of choice • If there is a confirmed family history of fragile X syndrome then DNA analysis alone is sufficient • Fragile X testing should otherwise be done as part of a full genetic evaluation
Persons seeking genetic/reproductive counselling	• With a family history of fragile X syndrome • or with a family history of undiagnosed learning disability		
Fetuses of known carrier mothers			• Prenatal testing follows the positive carrier test in mother • NB: CVS is sometimes ambiguous
Person with a positive cytogenetic result	With atypical clinical features		
Person with negative or uncertain cytogenetic result	With strong clinical features		

CVS, chorionic villus sampling.
* Working Group of the Genetic Screening Subcommittee of the Clinical Practice Committee, American College of Medical Genetics 1994 Fragile X syndrome: diagnostic and carrier testing. American Journal of Medical Genetics 53:380–381.

Screening DNA for fragile X does not eliminate the need for an additional general karyotype. Chromosomal abnormalities have been detected as, or more, frequently than fragile X in individuals referred for fragile X screening (Warren & Sherman 2001). Prenatal screening is possible but controversial especially with female fetuses, when prediction of outcome is limited. There has been some concern that the methylation status of the repeat may not be adequately ascertained by CVS, and some recommend amniocentesis to confirm hypermethylation as well as repeat expansion. With new technologies the situation is rapidly changing. Antibodies that directly bind FMRP may be useful diagnostic tools, especially in those cases of fragile X not associated with repeat expansion.

Direct DNA examination of DNA has also helped define the population prevalence of the varying mutation subtypes. The dynamic mutation is found in every ethnic population so far studied, although the average repeat length differs between groups. In contrast the position of intercalated AGG sequences seems very conserved and an ancestral form $(CGG)_9AGG$ $(CGG)_9AGG(CGG)_9$ suggested. The premutation shows a sex bias (around 1:1000 men, 1:400 women) compatible with proposed mechanisms of repeat expansion. In certain genetically isolated populations such as Finland there is good evidence for a founder effect (common ancestor); in others, including the UK and USA, the premutation does not have the same diversity of variants found in the full mutation, suggesting different expansion/contraction rates between populations or that a true equilibrium between premutation and full mutation has not yet been reached in some populations. Proportions in French Canadians from Quebec are similar to those in British and American populations, but relate to a different haplotype, and there are still many unanswered questions about how the mutation evolves in populations.

For an X-linked condition the apparently low rate of new mutations and evidence for a founder effect (common ancestor) is unusual, but clear in Swedish and Finnish families. It appears that the premutation can be carried silently over many generations. At first this seems to conflict with the high frequency of the condition, but there also may be a slow 'creep' in size of the premutation over generations. Marker haplotypes close to the mutation can be used, as well as the sequence of the mutation itself, to follow the disorder within families. These markers show linkage disequilibrium in a variety of populations. Thus French ancestors may have been different from the Finnish and Swedish who may have shared at least one common ancestor. UK studies show a wider diversity of haplotypes, and evidence for a common ancestor is not so strong. A different process may account for UK evolution, with occasional stepwise 'jumps' upward in premutation size. These population differences make generalisations about the absolute numbers of premutation carriers difficult. However, a very large Quebec study examined mutation size in over 10 000 females (Rousseau et al 1995). Premutations of 66 triplets or over were found in around 1:500 females, with a similar frequency for 55 to 63 triplets. From these figures the predicted full mutation child carriage rate is around 1:2900.

Clinical features of the fragile X syndrome

Physical features of full mutation carriers   Features found in full fragile X males are very variable and overlap considerably with the normal population (Table 24.6). The most consistent are

Table 24.6   Common physical features in adults with fragile X syndrome

Phenotypic feature	Approximate percentage of adult cases showing feature
Macro-orchidism	90
Elongated face	80
Prominent ears / cupped ears	65
High arched palate	60
Flat feet	60
Hyperextensible digital joints	48

an elongated face, enlarged testicles and ears. All these are more apparent after puberty. Up to 20% of children may show no obvious physical features, save some cupping of the ears. A squared chin often accompanies the long face. Ear prominence is especially noticeable in Caucasians, less so in other ethnic groups. Testicular volume may be dramatically increased up to and over 120 ml; the average is around 45 ml. Gonadotrophin levels and spermatogenesis seem normal, however. The growth trajectory is interesting. An increased average childhood height is replaced, after an early onset of puberty (when testicle size increases) between the ages of 10 and 12 years, with a decreased adult height. Both the growth changes and the adult facial features suggest problems with pituitary or hypothalamic function. A disorder of connective tissue may account, in part, for the large, prominent (anteverted) ears, and also for other, less consistent findings including a smooth 'velvet-like' skin, hyperextensible finger joints, flat feet and mitral valve prolapse. Mild macrocephaly is a relatively consistent feature. Around a third experience recurrent gastro-oesophageal reflux (with vomiting) during infancy; during childhood recurrent mid ear infections and sinusitis are common. Twenty percent have seizure disorder and up to one-third have squints. Full fragile X females are protected against the full clinical expression by random X inactivation. The cognitive deficit correlates with the extent of physical features, and, in the most severely affected, physical features are similar to those of males (obviously excepting macro-orchidism), with the same relation between puberty and expression.

Physical features of premutation carriers   The most striking physical associates of the premutation are the high incidence of premature ovarian failure (POF) in women — in 16% before the age of 40 (Allingham-Hawkins et al 1999) — and Parkinsonism in older men (Hagerman et al 2001). Both features seem specific to the premutation and are not replicated in protomutation or full mutation carriers. Tentatively they may relate the *FMR1* mRNA to FMRP ratio, which is higher in premutation carriers than controls. Female premutation carriers also have an increased rate of fragile-X-linked general physical features, with greater jaw and ear prominence.

LD and the behavioural phenotype of fragile X syndrome

LD is usually the first feature detected in male children with fragile X, but varies from severe to very mild. On average it is moderate, but with important changes over the lifespan. Early reports that preschool boys did not show LD-range IQ have been challenged, but what is not in question, and consistently shown in multiple independent studies, is that a decline occurs, probably starting as early as middle childhood. Most male adults with fragile X will test within the moderate to severe range of LD. The specific cognitive contributions to the overall IQ score are not uniform. In a prospective study (Bailey et al 1998) consistently higher scores on motor and adaptive performances were seen than on cognition and communication. Underlying these outcomes are deficits in short-term memory (with specific features; for sentences it is worse than objects), visuomotor co-ordination and arithmetical ability. Related to the storage problem is a deficit in processing information that requires action in a sequential rather than simultaneous fashion. Full fragile X females on average show a decrease of 10–20 IQ points, placing many in the learning disabled range, and many others have specific learning disorders. Unlike in men, there is no suggestion as yet of IQ decline, but there is evidence for similar weaknesses on specific skills such as arithmetic, and on tests of executive function, spatial ability and visual memory (Bennetto et al 2001). In fact the deficits in executive function have been well replicated and are not simply explained by the lowered IQ.

In addition to LD a behavioural phenotype has been described. In full mutation males, hand flapping or waving, and other repetitive mannerisms are common, and similar features noted in fragile X women. Like the men, fragile X women also tend to be shy and anxious. Communication difficulties include conversational rigidity and perseveration, and a 'cluttered' and over-detailed form of speech has been noted. Small-scale studies have indicated a raised incidence of mood and personality disorders, including schizotypal personality. There are also areas of great relative strengths. Domestic and daily living skills are especially well preserved and often improve in adults.

Shyness, social anxiety, gaze avoidance and poor peer group relations, and the mannerisms have suggested an overlap with autism in both men and women. There are differences, and detailed analysis of speech patterns suggests that they differ between fragile X and autism. Autistic features indistinguishable on testing from non-fragile-X autism may exist in a subgroup of fragile X children (Rogers et al 2001), but the subsequent temporal course of cognitive changes is not the same (Fisch et al 2002). Whether the link is coincidental comorbidity or a true biological link is still uncertain. Neurological and imaging findings, however, suggest that there may be a true overlap between the conditions.

Cognitive and behavioural changes associated with the premutation

Although relatively well researched, earlier results linking the premutation with cognition are controversial. Reported work has almost entirely focused on premutation females. Overall, premutation carriers are not more frequent in children in special education placements or in LD patients, and the consensus is that LD per se is not associated with having a premutation. Case reports can suffer from selection bias, and studies on larger groups of premutation carriers have produced confusing findings. At present the best interpretation is that cognitive and social behaviours are also unaffected by the presence of a permutation (Mazzocco 2000). One interesting, replicated finding is a high lifetime prevalence rate of depression in premutation-carrying mothers of fragile X children. This is not fully explained by the stress of bringing up a child with a developmental disability, as the age at onset of depression predated the age at which LD in the child was diagnosed.

Treatments and interventions for the person with fragile X and their family.

No treatment exists for the primary disorder in fragile X at present, but treatment of associated conditions is essential. Vision and hearing need to be carefully monitored to maximise the person's potential, and all therapeutic interventions need to make the most of the adaptive strengths present with fragile X. Cardiac and other physical problems may be open to intervention and speech and language therapy may be needed to improve communication. The various behavioural components need careful assessment. In some the hyperactivity may respond to metamphetamine or similar stimulants. However, at present most strategies follow those used for people with LD in general. For parents, having a fragile X child is a major life event; supportive family therapy and counselling may be needed not only for the immediate, but also the extended family. Genetic counselling if accepted by the family is often useful, and early access should be encouraged. The risk estimates for daughters who may carry a premutation need to be considered. Until we know more about the underlying biological and developmental mechanisms involved in fragile X, however, we do not have any specific therapies. Therefore it is still the understanding of the profile of LD in fragile X that is of most help in maximising their educational potential. In fact identifying particular constellations of weaknesses, strengths and developmental trajectories is the way forward for all LD-associated syndromes.

Other important LD-associated conditions with definite physical or dysmorphic syndromes (MRXS — X-linked mental retardation, syndromic forms)

An increasing number of other syndromes are being defined by their association with abnormalities on the X chromosome (Chelly & Mandel 2001). Disorders once thought separate in spite of overlapping phenotypes are now being linked at the genetic level. For example at least four neurological disorders — X-linked callosal agenesis, MASA syndrome, X-linked hydrocephalus and the complicated spastic paraplegia syndrome type 1 — are now known to be due to mutations in the human *L1* gene that encodes a cell adhesion molecule (L1CAM). These are now grouped as the CRASH syndrome (an acronym of Corpus callosal hypoplasia, mental Retardation, Adducted thumbs, Spastic paraplegia and Hydrocephalus). One example, Rett syndrome, is worth considering in some detail.

Rett syndrome

Rett syndrome, although rare, is important as it has revealed novel mechanisms underlying LD conditions. Its aetiology also forms conceptual bridges between the biology of fragile X and that of various MRX disorders. Rett syndrome is an X-linked dominant genetic disorder, with a prevalence of around 1:10 000 to 1:15 000. A short-lived plateau, then a rapid deterioration in motor and speech abilities, follows a period of apparently normal development lasting 6–28 months. There are subsequent age-related changes, with a secondary plateau lasting for years being succeeded by a late motor system deterioration. Rett first described the syndrome in Austria in 1966. He mentioned some clinical features that resembled autism (stereotyped hand wringing and waving movements that replaced purposeful activity) as well as a progressive dementia, gait disturbance and loss of facial

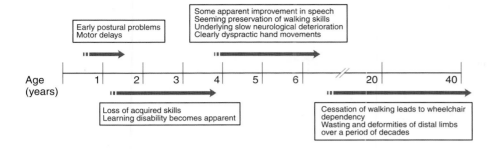

Fig. 24.5
Typical time course of symptoms in Rett syndrome. The four classical phases are illustrated, with a guide to the expected times of appearance of the features.

expressiveness. In the early stages it may be confused with Batten's disease, Angelman syndrome or autism (through communication loss), but there are diagnostic tests for the first two and for Rett syndrome itself. The sex linkage explains the female predominance; the few males described with Rett syndrome have severe neonatal encephalopathy. The time course and age-related features of the disorder are illustrated in Figure 24.5.

Physical and behavioural phenotypes are associated with Rett syndrome. A primary criterion is a deceleration in head growth rate after initially normal growth, which eventually results in significant microcephaly. Although reports of hormonal deficiencies are inconsistent, overall growth is also slowed. Gait and trunk movement apraxias are also primary features, starting at around 1–4 years. Many girls also have a relative slowing of foot growth, resulting in very small hypoplastic feet by adolescence that are very prone to trophic skin changes and acrocyanosis. Later progressive changes in lower-limb innervation patterns occur with fixation of the feet in a rigid, supine and often asymmetric flexure (Hagberg 2002). Scoliosis is also common and variable. A double curve develops progressively around primary school age, and its neurological consequences may require rapid surgical intervention. GI manifestations such as reflux and swallowing problems are frequent, can be serious, and may represent autonomic pathology. Over 90% have epilepsy with seizures usually beginning around 4 years. These may decrease in frequency and severity after teenage years.

Cognitive and behavioural features are prominent. An initially normally developing child looses purposeful hand movements, which are replaced by near continuous stereotyped wringing and twisting whilst awake. Any learned speech, even babbling used as communication, is lost. Most (85%) preschool children have disturbed sleep with night wakening coupled to paroxysmal or continuous laughter. Older girls may have episodes of violent screaming unexplained by detectable physical pain. Breath holding and hyperventilation occur, sometimes alternating, and other episodic phenomena include bruxism and air swallowing. By school age, intense staring to gain eye contact may represent an attempt at communication. Most important, however, are progressive phases of cognitive deterioration leading eventually to severe LD. Girls with Rett syndrome often live into adulthood, but there is a decreased average lifespan (30–40 years) although there have been reports of women up to 78 years. There is a raised risk of sudden death partly attributed to problems with cardiac conduction. Cognitive skills may be preserved much more than motor systems with age, suggesting premature physical ageing.

The brain in Rett syndrome In Rett syndrome the brain is around 15–30% smaller than in an age-matched control. Pathological signs of degenerative changes, demyelination or inflammatory changes are absent, and the overall picture resembles a developmental arrest in infancy. There are some specific features. The earliest reports by Rett and his colleagues showed a decrease in substantia nigra melatonin. This and associated striatal abnormalities may play a role in the movement disorder. Later studies showed a decrease in the number and arborisation of dendrites and a lack of dendritic spines of layer III and V pyramidal cells, especially in the frontal cortex, but also in inferior temporal cortex and hippocampus. This pattern seems unique to Rett syndrome, and is compatible with arrested cortical maturation. Biological markers (such as MAP2 and COX2) of the period of dendritic development and synaptic pruning are absent in the areas involved. In contrast to the apparent arrested development in the cerebrum, MRI studies indicate cerebellar degenerative changes with progressive loss of Purkinje cells (Armstrong 2002). Neurotransmitter findings have been conflicting. A finding of increased in CSF glutamate has been replicated, however, and in younger patients an increase in glutamate and NMDA receptors has been shown, which changes to a reduction in older subjects (Blue et al 1999).

The genetics of Rett syndrome, and men with Rett syndrome Most cases (80%) of Rett syndrome are due to sporadic mutations in the gene *MECP2* (coding for methyl-CpG-binding protein type 2) at Xq28, and over two hundred different mutations in this gene have been described. *MECP2*, like most X chromosome genes, is normally expressed from only one chromosome of the pair in females. Thus the expression of Rett syndrome depends on the number of X chromosomes without the mutation that are inactivated, and there is a spectrum of severity in the female phenotype. In some cases when inactivation is skewed towards the mutated chromosome the clinical features are mild, and this mechanism also explains the variable phenotype in those rare families where the condition is inherited.

MeCP2 binds to 5-methylcytosine residues that are found in CpG dinucleotides, including those of CpG islands and the promoter regions of genes. On binding to promoters a complex of other proteins are recruited, including histone de-acetylases and a co-repressor protein. This complex initiates a series of events leading to heterochromatin becoming compacted, which represses downstream gene transcription. This sequence has already been noted to have a role in the fragile X, and *MECP2* is a key regulator of many genes. *MECP2* mutations seem to arise mainly in the paternal germline (around 70%) (Girard et al 2001). This (rather unexpectedly) explains most of the predominance of women with the disorder, rather than intrauterine lethality in male fetuses. One possible explanation is that maternal germ cells are much less methylated (at CpG dinucleotides) than male, and methylation increases the risk of deamination and mutation. Methylated CpG sequences are mutation 'hotspots' in germ cells, and there are more of them in male germ cells. There is in fact a cluster in and around the *MECP2* gene. Rare cases of *de novo* maternal mutations and the even rarer situation where Rett syndrome runs in families have shown that when males do inherit the disrupted gene the consequences are severe, with profound developmental delay, microcephaly, hypotonia and seizure disorder leading to death in the first few years. Scanning here has indicated diffuse abnormality or apparently normal findings. Several reports exist of men with Klinefelter's syndrome who meet all the criteria for Rett syndrome. In these cases it can be predicted that random X inactivation will produce a mosaic picture (in addition to the clonal mosaicism common in sex chromosome abnormalities), leading to a less severe outcome. The features are similar to those in girls with Rett syndrome (Hammer et al 2002).

LD-associated conditions with no physical or dysmorphic manifestations (MRX disorders — X-linked mental retardation, non-syndromic forms)

In addition to disorders where LD is associated with physical features, reports of familial X-linked disorders where cognitive disability and behavioural features are the only outcome abound. Synonyms for these include MRX (mental retardation X-linked, non specific) and non-specific or non-syndromic XLMR (X-linked mental retardation). In spite of the narrowed phenotype when compared with MRXS disorders, linkage studies on such families have shown them to be a very heterogeneous group. However, large-scale collaborative research has mapped many within the X chromosome, and for at least ten the genes have been identified. Mutations in some genes are restricted at present to single or a few families. However, this will probably change as more cases of MRX are examined.

FRAXE and the FMR2 syndrome

FRAXE, a fragile site around 600 kbp from FRAXA, is also associated with a GCC repeat expansion. The associated disorder has much in common genetically with the fragile X but clinically the syndrome is different with only mild LD or simply speech delay and specific reading and writing disorders (IQs 50–85) (Gecz 2000). The IQ does not decline with age, and no other clear features have been described. The prevalence is uncertain; estimates of 1:50 000 to 1:100 000 are largely based on screening LD populations, and the true carriage frequency may be higher. The gene responsible, *FMR2*, was identified from analysis of a submicroscopic deletion that contained the FRAXE site in a FRAXE patient. The full expansion (over 250 repeats) leads to a methylation-dependent silencing of *FMR2*. *FMR2* is a large gene with 22 exons that show complex splicing patterns. Its protein, FMR2, is present at high levels in the hippocampus (granule cell layer), the neocortex, and cerebellar Purkinje cells (Miller et al 2000), and its concentration in the cell nucleus makes it a potential transcription factor (Hillman & Gecz 2001).

Other MRX disorders

Alpha-GDQ is a protein that suppresses the hyperexcitability of cortical pyramidal cells. It is one of a series of RabGTPases involved in neurotransmission. Mutations in its gene, *GDI1* at Xq28, occur in several MRX families. Another neuronal signalling

pathway is the RhoGTPase system. Genes for three different proteins in this pathway have been shown to be disrupted in a subset of MRX families. The (unfortunately named) oligophrenin gene (*OPHN1*) is expressed in neurons and glia, and its protein stimulates GTPase activity important in the dynamics of the neural growth cone. PAK3 (p21-activating kinase-3 gene) is also mutated in some families, and the protein regulates neuronal cytoskeleton functions. *ARHGEF3* gene codes for a protein (cool-2) that is again involved in the control of neuronal cytoskeletal movements. These and other recent discoveries on the X chromosome are listed in Table 24.7.

MRX and MECP2

As well as Rett syndrome it is now known that different mutations in *MECP2* are involved in a broad range of MRX syndromes. In men the resulting LD is usually moderate to severe, but in women it may be mild. Expressive language can be affected, and there are reports of psychiatric symptoms including auditory and visual hallucinations in some men. In one family bipolar disorder was associated with LD, pyramidal and parkinsonian features, and macro-orchidism (PPM-X syndrome) (Klauck et al 2002). The hallmark regression of Rett syndrome is not seen in MRX-associated *MECP2* disorders. In total the number of affected individuals with *MECP2* mutations who have LD may be (at least) as high as the total number with the fragile X, making them a very important new class of LD-associated conditions (Couvert et al 2001).

CONTIGUOUS GENE SYNDROMES

Contiguous gene syndromes (CGSs) constitute another important class of disorders associated with LD, and only recently have we begun to understand their aetiologies. The common feature is a chromosomal abnormality, most often a deletion but sometimes a duplication, whose visibility is at or just below the threshold of the light microscope. They usually require specialised imaging techniques for their detection — in particular the increased sensitivity of karyotype methods provided by fluorescent in-situ hybridisation (FISH) or direct DNA analysis. Since these methods are relatively new, many more CGSs remain to be discovered and current prevalence figures are not necessarily helpful. The chromosomal abnormality is small on the scale of the whole chromosome (usually less than 3–5 Mbp) but large enough to encompass at least several genes; thus these mutations are differentiated from the single-gene disorders such as the MRXS and MRX conditions described above, and large-scale abnormalities such as trisomies and partial monosomies. Only a few syndromes will be discussed in depth. They can broadly be grouped into four classes (Table 24.8).

Deletions of non-imprinted autosomal regions

Williams syndrome

Williams syndrome (or Williams–Beuren syndrome; 1:20 000 to 1:50 000 live births) was first described in 1961 for subjects with a characteristic facial presentation ('elfin' face; peri-orbital fullness, star or lacy iris pattern, anteverted nostrils, long philtrum and prominent lips). An infantile hypercalcaemia may be present, and

Table 24.7 Some proteins involved in X-linked learning disability

MRXS and MRX examples not mentioned in detail in main text	Gene product / gene locus	Notes
Coffin–Lowry syndrome (severe learning disability)	Serine/threonine protein kinase / Xp22 (*RSK2* gene)	Males and some expression in females. Characteristic dysmorphisms. Some mutations lead to a much milder learning disability. Chromatin structure may be defective
ATR-X syndrome (severe learning disability)	Helicase protein – wide range of cellular functions including DNA repair / Xq13 (*helicase-2* gene)	Mental retardation with thalassaemia syndrome. Males, very rarely females have any features. Chromatin structure may be defective
Lesch–Nyhan syndrome (severe learning disability)	Enzyme in purine metabolism pathway / Xq26-27.2 (*HPRT* gene)	Severe self-mutilation. Reduction in dopaminergic neuronal systems associated with significant decrease in size of caudate and putamen
MASA syndrome (severe learning disability)	Neural cell adhesion molecule / Xq28 (*L1CAM* gene)	**M**ental retardation, **A**phasia, **S**huffling gait, **A**dducted thumbs. X-linked hydrocephalus is major but not constant part of syndrome. CRASH syndrome is a synonym (**C**allosal hypoplasia, **R**etardation, **A**dducted thumbs, **S**pastic paraplegia, **H**ydrocephalus)
Hunter syndrome	Mucopolysaccharide metabolism enzyme / Xq28 (*IDS* gene)	Variable degree of learning disability in males. About 30% are due to deletions. Affected females are due to skewed X inactivation
Duchenne muscular dystrophy	Sarcolemma membrane associated protein / Xp21.2 (*Dystrophin* gene)	Mild learning disability in some cases (18% of boys have IQ < 70). Progressive muscle wasting
Norrie disease	Possible growth factor / Xp11.4 (*NDP* gene)	Mild learning disability, but a deterioration occurs over time. Deteriorating vision leads to blindness
MRX Type 60 (including MRX family 60 and cytogenetically abnormal patients)	Oligophrenin / Xq12 Possible signalling protein in RhoGAP series (*OPHN1* gene)	Up to 0.1% of learning disability
MRX type 46 (including family MRX46)	Cytoskeleton activity regulating protein / Xq26 (*ARHGEF6* gene)	Up to 1% of learning disability
MRX Type 3	Protein involved in synaptic vesicle function / Xq28 (*RABGDIA* gene)	Up to 1% of learning disability

heart valve abnormalities are frequent. IQ is very variable (mean 58, range 20–106) with 75% of children in the LD range. Most others have specific learning disorders, but IQ may not be static and there are indications of a decrease over time. Great interest has centred on the cognitive profile that is hidden by global IQ measures. There is a relative (sometimes severe) weakness in visuospatial constructive ability, with strengths in the auditory rote memory and language. Visuospatial construction involves the ability to envisage an object as a set of parts, and, when given these parts, an ability to reconstruct the object. Williams syndrome children find this very difficult but adolescents and adults less so. Compared with DS children matched on age and global IQ, those with Williams syndrome are much worse at copying even simple geometrical objects. They tend to focus on parts of objects rather than the whole. Visual perception seems normal, and they can correctly linguistically describe visually presented material. A behavioural phenotype has also been described. There is a characteristic type of social behaviour: highly sociable, over friendly, but at the same time susceptible to significant social anxiety, easily distractible, more excitable, more prone to negative moods. The most characteristic of these are the increased likelihood of approaching others spontaneously and the increased

distractibility, the other features being common to many LD-associated disorders (Mervis & Klein-Tasman 2000). These features have been interpreted on the basis of theories of social knowledge acquisition and usage, especially the 'theory of mind'. The social-perceptual component is preserved (ability to make judgements of others' mental state based on facial/body expressions which relate to affective processes) while the social-cognitive domain (false-belief tasks, etc.) is impaired. Only 20% of younger Williams syndrome children are successful at false-belief tasks.

The genetics of Williams syndrome   There is a microdeletion within the long arm of chromosome 7 (del(7)(q11.23q11.23)). Nearly all cases are sporadic, with a few rare autosomal-dominant families. The deletion consistently spans a region of 2 Mbp of DNA, and specific low-copy-number repeat DNA sequences that bracket the region may facilitate unequal crossing-over, leading to the deletion which removes a series of genes (at least 16). The parental source of the deletion seems unimportant. One gene, *elastin*, accounts for the great vessel problems, and perhaps also the hoarse voice and prematurely ageing skin. Other genes of interest in the region include *LIM kinase-1*, which may be involved in the visuospatial problems.

Table 24.8   Contiguous gene syndromes associated with learning disability

Contiguous gene syndrome grouping	Syndrome	Chromosomal locus	Notes
Autosomal microdeletion syndromes	Monosomy 1p36	1p36	Common (1: 10 000), variably LD
	Microdeletion cri-du-chat	5p15	Deletions usually macroscopic; see main text
	Microdeletion Wolf–Hirschhorn	4p16	Deletions usually macroscopic; see main text
	Williams	7q11.23	See main text
	Langer–Giedion	8q24.1	71% have LD, multiple exostoses of cartilage
	Potocki–Shaffer	11p11.2	Variable LD, multiple exostoses
	WAGR	11p12–14	**W**ilms tumour, **A**niridia, **G**enitourinary, mental **R**etardation; presentation depends on deletion size
	Rubenstein–Taybi	16p13.3	Facial/digital anomalies
	Smith–Magenis	17p11.2	Facial anomalies. Behavioural phenotype includes hyperactivity and self-injury. Rather common (1: 25 000)
	Miller–Dieker	17p13.3	Facial anomalies and type 1 lissencephaly
	DiGeorge/VCF	22q11.2	See main text
Autosomal microdeletion syndromes, with imprinting effects	Prader–Willi	15q11.2–13	See main text
	Angelman	15q11.2-13	See main text
Autosomal microduplication syndromes	Dup 17p11.2	17p11.2	Mild to no LD. Only described in a few patients so far
X chromosome microdeletion syndromes	Kallman / steroid sulfatase	Xp22.3	Where the deletion involves the steroid sulfatase gene all men have mild LD
	Duchenne Muscular Dystrophy region microdeletions	Xp21	Variable LD
	Choroderaemia region microdeletions	Xq21	Very rare. Variable LD, sometimes without the eye problems

The Velocardiofacial / Di George syndrome

This (1:4000 live births) is the most common CGS so far detected., and it has been suggested as one cause of the association between LD and schizophrenia. A characteristic facial appearance (receding jaw, wide spaced eyes, broad nose root, midface hypoplasia with hypernasal speech, occult cleft palate, external ear anomalies) accompanies conotruncal cardiac abnormalities in the velocardiofacial syndrome (VCFS), and also absent thymus and hypocalcaemia in the more severe form called Di George syndrome. LD is usually mild to moderate, some have no LD but specific learning disorders. There have been frequent reports of an association with schizophrenia and affective psychoses (both bipolar and major depressive disorders) (Murphy et al 1999). In a study of 26 patients with VCFS and psychiatric illness, Carlson's group found a high prevalence of attention deficit hyperactivity disorder and bipolar disorder in children and adolescents. All six adults had bipolar disorder, four with paranoid and grandiose delusions. Twenty-three of the patients had the classical microdeletions on chromosome 22 (Carlson et al 1997). The link with schizophrenia has been replicated (Murphy & Owen 2001), but its importance is hard to quantify. In one study of consecutive referrals no cases were found in over two hundred patients with developmental delay, but a microdeletion found in 2 of 16 patients with psychosis without LD, a very high rate (Waite et al 2002). MRI imaging of 11 adults with schizophrenia and VCFS showed white matter foci in 90%, midline anomalies in 45%

and cerebral atrophy or ventricular enlargement in around 54% (Chow et al 1999). The white matter hyperintensities were found in another small study of 10 patients where septum pellucidum and cerebellar abnormalities were also described (van Amelsvoort et al 2001).

The genetics of Velocardiofacial/Di George syndrome
Most subjects have a microdeletion in chromosome 22 (del(22) (q11.2q11.2)). The deletion is usually on the verge of light-microscope visibility, and careful high-resolution banding reveals presence in most cases. However, there are now standard techniques for FISH analysis, or the deletion can be detected using PCR. The common deletion is around 3 Mbp long and bracketed by low-copy-number repeat DNA sequences that predispose to unequal crossing-over and deletion formation. Chromosome 22 is a 'hot-spot' for such abnormalities. Cat-eye syndrome (a rare condition where colobomata, craniofacial and heart abnormalities coexist with very mild to moderate LD) is normally due to a tetrasomy of a region of the short arm down to 22q11. This is usually due to an extra small supernumerary marker chromosome (inv dup(22)) but can also result from a direct duplication leading to partial trisomy. Cat-eye syndrome clinically overlaps with the der(22) syndrome which is due to non-disjunction of a constitutional t(11;22) translocation leading to a partial trisomy of chromosomes 11 and 22 (McDermid & Morrow 2002). Although a large number of genes are deleted in VCFS, many of the affected tissues are derived from the embryonic pharyngeal arches. Neural crest cells are involved in the formation of these and their derivative structures,

and neural crest cell migration problems may underlie many VCFS features. A mouse model with a deletion of over 24 genes has been made (mimicking the minimal deletion size in humans). It only takes four human genes to be reinserted to produce an almost complete phenotype rescue. Of these *TBX1* (a human T-box gene and potent transcription factor) is the most interesting as its known functions have the most explanatory power for the heart, endocrine and dysmorphic features. However, any role in cognitive and psychiatric symptoms is uncertain.

Contiguous gene syndromes in imprinted autosomal regions

Prader–Willi and Angelman syndromes

The LD-associated syndrome with the clearest behavioural phenotype is probably Prader–Willi. It is not common (1:10 000 to 1:20 000 live births) but usually readily distinguished from other disorders. Langdon Down noted the physical appearance and the hyperphagia, made the earliest photographic record, and labelled the syndrome 'polysarcia' (Ward 1998). Prader, Labhart and Willi described the clinical features in detail in 1956, and the eponym was created for them. Prader–Willi syndrome has recordable features even in the fetus. Fetal movements and activity are delayed in onset and diminished in extent throughout pregnancy. Especially in mothers who have had previously normal pregnancy, a marked decrease in fetal activity should alert the clinician to the possibility of the condition. At birth and in the neonate there is severe hypotonia and hyporeflexia, which may impair feeding. Other features are less consistent at birth (visible hypogonadism in both sexes, facial appearance and a peculiar cry) but develop during infancy and childhood. Most children are slow to grow, and there is a relative decrease in hand and especially foot growth. The eyes are almond shaped, and there may be squints. The bi-frontal diameter of the face is narrowed. Other reported features include relative depigmentation (said to be confined to those where the syndrome is caused by deletions). Prader–Wiili adults are small relative to others in their family.

The eating disorder   Body leptin levels are elevated even before the onset of any eating disorder, indicating a relative increase in infantile body fat. The eating disorder begins between 18 months and 5 years. There is an intense preoccupation with food. Most children show abdominal stretch marks from about 6 years. Itching may lead to pruritus. If unchecked the food-craving behaviour results in morbid obesity. Individuals report a constant hunger and a lack of satiety (they also rarely vomit). In addition to the increased food intake a lowered metabolic rate and decreased physical activity level contribute to a rapid weight gain. They may hide food and gorge themselves on it; they may also eat foodstuff otherwise considered unappetising — rotten food, dog food, etc. The rate of eating is usually not higher than normal, however, but feeding continues for an extended period. If uncontrolled the weight gain is dramatic and damaging. Alimentary diabetes and cardiac failure due to insufficiency are common and the usual cause of early death. Although older adults (some over 60) have been reported, the survival is rarely beyond 30 years of age without major obesity reduction. With strict control, survival may be near normal.

Cognitive, other behavioural and psychiatric manifestations   LD is usually mild, but very variable in range from severe to absent. In those without LD, specific learning disorders usually occur. They perform better on tasks of visuomotor discrimination than on auditory verbal processing. In addition to the eating disorder, compulsive behaviours are very common (Dimitropoulos et al 2000). Ritualistic and repetitive traits are seen which are not food related. Over 50% may show hoarding behaviours or repeatedly rearrange objects. Self-injury may occur — most commonly skin picking, which is seen at some time in up to 70% of people with Prader–Willi. It can be severe to the point of bleeding. As adults the risk of psychotic illness, especially affective or cyclical forms, is markedly increased. Although affective disorder is very commonly associated with general LD, 100% of older adults in a recent study with the uniparental disomic origin of Prader–Willi syndrome (see below) were psychotic with hallucinations. Although the numbers were small, hallucinations were restricted to this subgroup (Boer et al 2002).

Angelman syndrome   (1:15 000 live births) is grouped here with Prader–Willi syndrome on the basis of their related genetics. The clinical conditions are very different, however. Slow head growth results in microcephaly, and LD is severe (speech does not usually develop) with seizure disorder (80%). The facial appearance is distinctive, with a prominent jaw and wide mouth, the gait is ataxic, and there is a behavioural phenotype of paroxysmal outbursts of laughter unrelated to prevailing affect or environment, and a tendency to tongue thrusting. The brain shows abnormal choroidal pigmentation, and distinctive electroencephalograph discharges occur. Not all body systems are equally affected (e.g. there has been a report of pregnancy).

The genetics of Prader–Willi and Angelman Syndromes
Both syndromes are due to microdeletions or gene mutations on the long arm of chromosome 15 at the same point (15q11–13). The very different outcomes arise from the complex genetics of this region. Certain genes are expressed from only one chromosome of the pair; which particular chromosome depends on the parental origin. The parental 'stamp' (imprint) is maintained by epigenetic effects, which almost certainly involve differential methylation. In Prader–Willi around 70% have a microdeletion (del(15)(q11.2q13); around 4 Mbp) on the chromosome 15 inherited from their father. Some genes in this deleted segment are only expressed by the paternal-sourced chromosome, and so their proteins will be entirely absent. Of these genes, *SNRPN* (encodes small nuclear ribonucleoprotein polypeptide N), and a second genetic unit within it termed *SNURF* (SNRPN upstream reading frame) play a key role. This complex unit has embedded within it smaller genes that code for small nucleolar RNAs (snoRNAs). The protein encoded by *SNRPN* can bind of another group of RNAs, small nuclear RNAs, which may regulate mRNA splicing activity. However, rare individuals where Prader–Willi is due to a chromosomal translocation breakpoint within the region have narrowed the critical interval and suggest that snoRNA genes may play a more important role in the core phenotype (Gallagher et al 2002). Their function is at present unknown, and other genes probably modify the syndromic features.

Angelman syndrome is also usually due to a microdeletion (70%) at exactly the same point on chromosome 15, but this time on the maternal-sourced chromosome, implying deletion of gene(s) normally active solely on the maternal chromosome. The key gene is *UBE3A*, which encodes an ubiquitin-protein ligase. This gene does not show imprinted expression in cultured human cells, but discrete areas of in-vivo human brain (Purkinje cells, hippocampal neurons, olfactory mitral cells) only express the maternal allele. The molecular basis for such tissue-specific paternally derived chromosome silencing is unclear, but may be signalled through alternative spliceforms of the gene's mRNA (Jiang et al 1999). The protein encoded by *UBE3A* has multiple functions, including down-regulating a cytoplasmic initiator of apoptosis (p53). Increased p53 may contribute to later aspects of the disorder. More than *UBE3A* may be involved, and an adjacent GABA-A receptor gene cluster has been implicated in the severity of the epilepsy seen with a full deletion. As well as microdeletions there are other rare mechanisms leading to Prader–Willi or Angelman. Uniparental disomy (UPD) arises when both chromosomes of the pair originate from the same parent. This may be due to one parental gamete containing both chromosomes of the pair and the other gamete neither (gamete complementation); another mechanism involves the creation of a trisomy and subsequent loss of one of the chromosomes (trisomy rescue); finally a monosomy may be 'corrected' by duplication to a disomy. There is evidence for the second type in some Prader–Willi cases. UPD resulting in two copies of maternal-sourced chromosome 15s will result in the Prader–Willi syndrome, and two paternal-sourced chromosomes in Angelman, as the active imprinted genes are absent in these situations. A third mechanism involves the apparatus creating the imprint itself. Errors in an imprinting centre in the region can lead to a failure to establish an imprint of the correct parental kind. Thus a chromosome 15 inherited from a father with an imprinting mechanism defect may carry a maternal imprint (technically the grand-maternal imprint is maintained), leading to both chromosome 15s in the child having a maternal imprint. Although these effects give insights into the formation of differential methylation patterns and UPD formation, they make diagnostics rather complex! Around 30% of Prader–Willi cases have no deletion; of these about 28% have maternal UPD. A small number have imprinting centre mutations or are carriers of a chromosomal translocation that breaks in the Prader–Willi critical region. For Angelman the situation is not quite the reverse; paternal UPD only accounts for around 5% and more often shows a complete chromosome duplication suggesting monosomy rescue; 3% will have an imprinting centre mutation; 5% have a direct mutation in the *UBE3A* gene; the others have no identifiable defect of chromosome 15 and may be phenocopies of the syndrome with a locus elsewhere in the genome.

SYNDROMES OF MIXED OR UNCERTAIN AETIOLOGY ASSOCIATED WITH LEARNING DISABILITY

Autism

Autism has recently had a high profile, especially on two fronts: the apparently massive increase in prevalence, and claims of associations with infant vaccination programmes. Both concepts are highly controversial. The first may be largely due to an increased awareness of the condition, and re-definition of many people whose problems were not understood or simply not acknowledged. The second (a link to triple-vaccination for mumps, measles and rubella or MMR) in spite of consistent lack of evidence in rigorous epidemiological surveys still continues to occupy much public and media attention. It is not proposed to discuss the latter issue in this chapter.

Pervasive developmental disorder, in the DSM-IV classification, embraces autistic disorder, childhood disintegrative disorder, Rett syndrome, Asperger syndrome, and unspecified forms of autism.

Rett syndrome has already been described; Asperger syndrome is not associated with LD. Unfortunately there is no clear evidence for causal links between the other pervasive developmental disorders that are associated with LD, and autism itself is probably heterogeneous in origin. At present a multitude of theories exist to explain the origin and development of autism from psychodynamic constructs, psychological dysfunctions, through biological and genetic diatheses. Autism is of major concern to the adult psychiatrist in LD. Early assumptions of a good cognitive outcome for autistic children after treatment of the supposed psychogenic disturbance have not been validated, and 50–60% of autistic children have LD that persists into adulthood.

Autism was first described in 1943 by Leo Kanner, who proposed five components:

- 'a profound lack of affective contact with other people';
- 'an anxiously obsessive desire for the preservation of sameness';
- 'a fascination for objects which are handled with skill in fine motor movements';
- 'mutism or a kind of language that does not seem intended to serve interpersonal communication';
- 'the retention of an intelligent physiognomy and good cognitive potential manifested, in those who can speak, by feats of memory, or in the mute children, by their skill on performance tests'.

Wing pointed out that Kanner, did not perceive LD as integral to the syndrome, instead explaining failure on IQ tests on a lack of cooperation (Wing 1991). Bertelheim in 1956 believed the prime cause of autism was an unloving and threatening relationship with the parents in the earliest years — the so-called 'refrigerator mother'. Kanner (who first suggested a genetic basis) felt he could detect autistic traits in the child's parents that could contribute to this supposed abnormal bonding. The idea that the mother and her upbringing of the child is the root cause of the autism has probably been as damaging as Bateson's theories of the double-bind as a cause of schizophrenia. There is no evidence that parents of autistic children are less affectionate or caring than others, and even at its conception the idea could not explain why other children in the family were completely normal.

The terms 'childhood schizophrenia' and 'childhood psychosis' used as synonyms for autism have also created confusion. The term 'autistic', meaning autistic aloneness or social withdrawal, was first proposed by Bleuler as one of the primary diagnostic symptoms of schizophrenia. However, psychodynamic origins of autism were questioned in the early 1960s, and it is now clear that autism is a disorder of developmental neurobiology and associated developmental psychology with a strong genetic background. Autism is not a variant of schizophrenia. However, autism's first entry into classification schemes for childhood disorders (ICD-8, in 1967) was as a schizophrenia subgrouping. True childhood schizophrenia is a distinct and very rare disorder, properly introduced into classification by DSM-III. There is no place now for 'infantile psychosis', and 'infantile autism' should also be abandoned, as the person grows into a teenager and adult with autism.

Definitions of autism in the major classification systems

Current definitions centre on dysfunction in three main areas: two-way social interactions, communication, and restricted,

Table 24.9 ICD-10 and DSM-IV-TR definitions used in autism

Classification	Social domain	Language domain	Behavioural domain
ICD-10	**Interaction deficits** Inadequate appreciation of social cues	**Language skills** Lack of appropriate use of whatever language skills that have developed	**Behaviour patterns** Stereotyped and repetitive patterns of behaviour, interests and activities. In children especially there may be a specific attachment to unusual objects. Motor stereotypies may occur such as handflapping and rocking movements
	Lack of adjustment of behavioural response in accordance with social context Marked problems in establishing and maintaining two-way relationships	Lack of appropriate response to other people's verbal and non verbal cues Restricted tonality of speech with unusual or little use of emphasis, cadence or accompanying gestures	Rigidity and routine to wide range of daily activities Resistance to change in above areas.
DSM-III-TR	**At least two items from social interaction impairment list**	**At least one item from qualitative impairments in communication list**	**At least one of the following restricted, repetitive and stereotyped patterns of behaviour, interests and activities**
	Marked impairment of multiple non-verbal behaviours, such as eye-to eye contact, facial expressiveness, body posture, and gestures used to regulate social interaction	They do not develop, or show a delay in developing, spoken language, which is not accompanied by attempts to compensate through other ways of communicating, e.g. by gestures, or signing, or imitation	An all encompassing preoccupation with one or more stereotypes and restricted pattern of interest, abnormal in intensity or focus
	Fail to develop relationships appropriate to their developmental level with their peer group Limitation in ability to spontaneously seek out and share enjoyments, interests or achievements with other people	Where speech has developed adequately they have a marked impairment in the ability to initiate or sustain a conversation. They show a stereotyped and repetitive use of language, or idiosyncratic and peculiar language	They have an apparently inflexible adherence to specific and (seemingly) non-functional routines or rituals There are stereotyped and repetitive motor mannerisms
	Fail to reciprocate appropriately in social or emotional interactions	They lack varied spontaneous make-believe play or social imitative play appropriate to their level of development	They have a persistent preoccupation with parts of objects

repetitive behaviour. ICD-10 (WHO 1992) created a group of pervasive developmental disorders that included childhood autism (F84.0) and atypical autism (F84.1) within a larger grouping of disorders of psychological development (others were Rett syndrome, Asperger syndrome and overactivity disorder with LD and stereotyped movements). ICD-10 also requires an onset before the age of 3 in addition to the triad. This definition mirrors that found in DSM-IV-TR (APA 2000) for autistic disorder, which created a well-defined set of diagnostic criteria, and it is useful to consider these here. A total of at least six items from three groups is needed for diagnosis. With DSM-IV, autistic disorder moved from being an Axis II to an Axis I disorder, in part due to the increasing acceptance of its developmental and neurobiological origins. LD is not required for its diagnosis, and when present, is classed as an Axis II associated condition. A synopsis of current definitions is given in Table 24.9.

The changing epidemiology of autism

Estimates of autism prevalence very much depend on the diagnostic criteria used. It has sometimes been over-diagnosed in LD children and adults, especially those in long-stay institutions who showed some features resembling autism, including stereotyped movements and rigid and repetitive behaviours. However, studies on hospitalised subjects have shown that up to one-third have autistic spectrum disorders with a tendency to also have severe behavioural difficulties.

In a review of 23 epidemiological surveys of autism (1966–1998; over 4 million people surveyed, identifying 1533 cases) the median prevalence was 5.2:10 000 (Fombonne 1999). However, it was found that prevalence rates significantly increased with publication year, and if only surveys from 1989–98 were considered the rate increased to 7.2:10 000. The numbers of males affected was greatly increased if LD was present, but overall the male:female ratio was 3.8:1, strongly implying sex-linked effects (assuming no diagnostic bias towards males). Some studies indicate that it is most pronounced in those with mild LD. Perhaps a specific group of X-linked conditions leads to a subset of autism with mild LD. Overall LD is found in 60% of subjects, much lower than the 80% previously reported, and some recent studies suggest even lower comorbidity. Most of this effect is due to the increased numbers of new diagnoses in people without LD, and autism's importance as an LD-associated condition remains as strong as ever. In 6% of people with autism a specific medical condition of possible aetiological relevance was present, tuberous sclerosis being especially common. There were no associations with social class for autism as a whole (Kanner had believed it to be associated with higher parental social class), but a more recent study has indicated increased maternal education (as well as male sex and being one of multiple births) as a risk factor (Croen et al 2002). Grouped together, all pervasive developmental disorders had a prevalence (minimum) of 18.7:10 000, or in other words nearly 1:500 — a very high rate. Wing & Potter (2002), in an important review, updated the evidence and showed a continued annual rise in autism incidence in preschool children as well as in age-banded prevalences. For autism alone prevalences of 60:10 000 have now been reported. No environmental cause (including MMR) has been confirmed by replicated scientific investigations, but there is strong evidence that genetic factors are a major influence. It is likely that most of the rise in both incidence and prevalence figures is due to an increased awareness of autism as a condition and changes in the definitions used to classify it and its spectrum disorders. The question of whether there has been a true rise is difficult to answer.

The clinical features of autism in association with LD

Most behavioural changes associated with autism require the development of complex abilities in children, and thus the diagnosis of autism is rarely made in the youngest years, often not until the child is around 4 years old. The implication that autism was present at an earlier age is usually based on a retrospective analysis of the developmental history (it is even more difficult if LD coexists). Early studies indicated little that discriminated infants who would later develop autism from others. However, a recent analysis of videotapes of 1-year-olds suggests subtle differences in the amount of looking at others and orientation to their own names between typically developing children, those later developing autism, and children with LD alone (Osterling et al 2002). At 18 months autistic children start to show specific problems in social interactions. The clinical picture is highly variable, and the atypical case can seem more common than the classical picture, especially when there is also severe LD. It is clear that autism is not restricted to childhood but continues throughout life. When associated with LD, this can cause immense social problems for the person and their family. The LD may show a specific profile with verbal IQ significantly less than performance. However, this relates to LD severity and is much less apparent as IQ approaches or enters the normal range (Ozonoff et al 2000). More clearly, there is a remarkably consistent skill on the Block Design subset of the WAIS, which may relate to theory of mind, and a weakened central coherence may lead to a tendency to organise cognitive processing in a localised and part-oriented fashion (Happé 2000).

The following descriptions relate to the person who has both autism and significant LD. Social difficulties can vary from aloneness and indifference to the social presence of others, through to a highly passive stance in social interaction. Gaze avoidance (stressed in early descriptions), is often inconsistent, instead there may be inappropriate eye contact, sometimes staring for long periods. The structure of the social interaction is disorganised; the person may use social cues and body language inappropriately; for instance, one person breaks into song or whistles at odd points in a conversation whilst staring directly; at first glance this is over-friendly and welcoming, but later seen as a stereotyped and an inappropriate approach to making initial contact. In children, any play that exists is not influenced by other children and does not display normal degrees of imaginative development. Speech may never develop, especially with severe LD but sometimes also in those whose overall IQ is much greater. Mutism can be disconcerting in the high-functioning person, although the facial expression of emotions may be relatively intact. The severity of speech disorder relates to the severity overall of autistic symptoms. Where speech develops it can be very repetitive, sometimes echolalic, with a narrow range of topics. However, within these topics ideas are often surprisingly developed, giving the impression of an obsession with intrinsic detail and facts. Stereotyped movements are also more prominent with severe LD, but mannerisms and tic-like activity can be seen even with mild LD. When one questions the person, he may report these as having a purpose or meaning themselves. Hand flapping, gazing and body rocking are very common. Some repetitively spin around, sometimes with their hands outstretched. Especially with severe LD, self-injurious behaviour, head-banging, face-slapping and other forms may be very distressing and difficult to manage. There is often a fascination for objects, which may form part of the mannerisms, e.g. the twirling of sticks or feathers in the hand. Other objects may be collected obsessively and hoarded, e.g. records, cards, envelopes, which must be arranged in special patterns. There can be a preoccupation with a temporal routine: they must rise at a specific time, must go to certain places at definite times of the day, and incorporate rituals and mannerisms around a specific timetable. In at least some there is also an increased need for personal space.

Attempts to change such behaviours by psychological interventions, or even physical limitation of activity, have not been highly successful, and often seem to cause a great deal of anguish and meet with exceptional resistance from the autistic person. One view holds that we should accept that the autistic person has specific environmental and temporal needs, that, within limits, should be permitted, rather than engaging in anxiety-provoking efforts to alter them.

The biology and genetics of autism

The autism phenotype is probably an outcome of many different underlying disorders. Numerically, only a few may predominate, but most aetiological studies are trying to interpret a heterogeneous condition. Further, most research has been on children, and longitudinal studies through adulthood are much less common.

The brain in autism; structural and imaging studies Early postmortem studies revealed Purkinje and granule cell loss in the cerebellar vermis and limbic and paralimbic cortices (Bauman & Kemper 1985). In the limbic system, in particular the hippocampus and amygdala, there are also cytoarchitectural abnormalities, with decreased neuronal size, denser neuronal packing and reduced dendritic tree complexity. These suggest an arrested early neuronal development, conceptually linking autism with other LD-associated conditions. Overall brain size in autism is increased, and MRI studies suggest this results from enlargement of the cerebellum (Hardan et al 2001) and basal ganglia (Sears et al 1999). Imaging also yields evidence for a limbic system abnormality that persists through life, with amygdala and hippocampus significantly smaller in adolescents with autism without LD (Aylward et al 1999b). The hippocampal area dentata is significantly smaller than normal, and this abnormality is present in varying age groups (Sears et al 1999). Amygdala and medial temporal lobe involvement is interesting given their proposed core role in the theory of mind (Siegal & Varley 2002). Functional MRI studies are now being conducted, and initial results show temporal lobe hypoperfusion (Boddaert & Zilbovicius 2002).

Neurochemistry of autism Such abnormalities might be expected to influence neurotransmitter systems. Platelet serotonin has repeatedly been shown to be increased in autism, but this is not specific and is found in other people with LD. Attempts to link this to candidate genes such as the serotonin transporter have been inconsistent, and double-blind cross-over trials of serotonin-lowering agents have not shown consistent effects on symptoms. CSF endorphins have also been reported as increased. Based on animal studies, stereotypies and mannerisms have suggested dopaminergic hyperactivity, but differences in dopamine metabolite level are inconsistent in autism. Nevertheless, antipsychotics are sometimes useful in reducing stereotypies in LD in general.

Genetics and autism Genetic factors operate in autism, and the male bias suggests a sex-linked component in at least a subset. Familial autism is also well known. The autism rate in siblings of a proband is near 3%, and this increases when other cognitive changes such as language impairments are considered. Diagnostic widening to include atypical autism and Asperger syndrome increases the rate to 6%, and for all forms of pervasive developmental disorder, 7%. The concordance rate for monozygotic twins (65%) is much higher than for dyzygotic (0%), implying a major genetic component with environmental modification (Pericak-Vance 2002).

Physical illnesses involving the brain occur in many autistic people, especially those with more severe LD. They include tuberous sclerosis, untreated phenylketonuria, neurofibromatosis, and neuronal (temporal lobe) damage caused directly by infections such as congenital rubella and herpes simplex, or indirectly via immune mechanisms as with cytomegalovirus. It is unclear whether these associations are real or coincidental, but it is reasonable to assume that some will be true phenocopies. In spite of such multiple aetiologies there has been some success in identifying genomic loci that may contain susceptibility genes for autism (Folstein & Rosen-Sheidley 2001). The male excess is relevant to suggestions of an association with fragile X, though an excess of triplet expansions is not found in autism per se (Margolis et al 1999). A large collaborative linkage study of families and sib-pairs multiply affected by autism yielded some evidence for a locus on the long arm of chromosome 7 (International Molecular Genetic Study of Autism Consortium 2001). A similar result has been reported for chromosome 2q (Buxbaum et al 2001). Chromosomal abnormalities (interstitial duplications of chromosome 15q in the Prader–Willi deletion region) have also been reported in autism (Cook et al 1997), and genetic association studies implicated chromosome 15. Recently, DNA

deletions from 5 to over 260 kbp have been found in several chromosomes in multiply affected families (Yu et al 2002).

Psychological approaches to understanding autism

Our limited knowledge about the neural processes involved in communication and social interactions, although expanding, still restricts the testability of psychological models, and the idea that a single common process underlies the three areas of difficulty in autism may be over-simplistic.

The central coherence model proposes a deficit in the ability of people with autism to synthesise (gestalt) parts into a whole design, so that they focus on parts (Happé 2000). There may also be deficits in executive functioning, cognitive control mechanisms (working memory, attention shifting, suppression of innate responses, etc.) that systematise lower-level behaviours. A dysfunction would result in rigidity and inability to readily switch mental set. This model would explain repetitive mannerisms and social engagement problems. Certainly, people with autism find it difficult to complete executive function tests such as the Tower of Hanoi.

The model with the greatest current explanatory power is the 'theory of mind', which relates to the domain of social cognition. People with autism have difficulties in attributing mental states as part of the self or independently as belonging to others — in other words difficulties in developing cognitive representations of abstract concepts (such as self and non-self) essential to socialisation, communication and imagination. Autistic children fail on items such as the Sally-Ann task designed to test the ability to make secondary abstractions about mind-sets, tests that DS children of comparable mental age can cope with. It seems they fail to recognise that the mind-set is a representation or model of the real world that people hold, not a faithful carbon copy that is common to all. However, performance on 'theory of mind' tasks is also related to language ability and executive function, and it is difficult to dissect out linguistic and executive control problems from cognitive misrepresentation (Tager-Flusberg 2001). The social cognitive skills that underlie the 'theory of mind' arise in later infant years, and develop over the next few years, paralleling the emergence of social deficits in autistic children. Many autistic adolescents still cannot view stimuli within a social framework. It is likely that central coherence, executive dysfunction and problems with the development of social cognition are not mutually exclusive and interact to produce the complex social, linguistic and behavioural problems that emerge in autism.

Associated behavioural and psychiatric problems

Repetitive behaviours are especially prominent in people with autism and more severe LD. A need for sameness encompasses many aspects of their lives. The mannerisms and routines need to be repeated in specific ways, in specific places and at specific times. They may only wear the same specific type of clothes, which have to be laid out for them in the correct order. The same questions may be asked again and again, and they may misinterpret the meanings of both questions and responses. There may be attach-ments to specific objects, and collection and hoarding activities. Some seem to enjoy endlessly manipulating objects — pieces of string, magazines that may be collected or alternatively constantly ripped up and so on. Most behaviours that are interpreted by others as difficult in autism occur when changes are made in the predictable routines of day-to-day life. Aggression or self-injury is usually a response to fear or associated anxiety, either fear of change or as a reaction to change underway. Many have a strong temporal sense; things must happen and people must behave in a predictable way.

Problems with communication, especially lack of speech, can lead to the use of other ways of imparting the person with autism's concerns, such as screaming. Understanding any true meaning to such outbursts (otherwise labelled as temper tantrums) is important. Some need specific environments. Hyperacusis has often been described in autism, and they also may have difficulty in filtering multiple, competing sensory stimuli (cocktail party effect). Some require greatly increased personal space compared with others, and this can require limiting the numbers of people around the person. The introduction of new environments and routines is best done over a long timescale, with gradual changes in day-to-day living building up to the eventual goal. The needs of someone with autism are very different from those of others, and the concept of normalisation does not usually mean that they should be forced to adopt the norms of general society. They have a right to have their own specific needs met, implying the design of appropriate environments and routines.

Psychiatric problems are common and increase in teens and adulthood. Bipolar disorder and major depressive disorder have been reported as starting in adolescence, as well as an increase in the severity of some behavioural symptoms such as obsessions, and an apparent lack of motivation. Anxiety disorders, as part of the spectrum or distinct, are very common. There are no reports of an increase of schizophrenia, but neither is the risk reduced, and co-occurrence is seen in clinical practice. The management of such severe psychiatric disorders in people with autism is problematic. Psychotic features destroy the internal predictability that the person with autism needs, and severe anxiety and aggression may result from their great difficulties in interpreting hallucinations and delusions.

Specific therapies

The main aim with children who have both LD and autism is to allow as full an education as possible. Facilitating language acquisition may need a highly individualised educational programme, whether within a normal school or in a special educational setting. The emphasis is on matching the environment to the child rather than force-fitting. Behavioural disorders may interfere with learning, and the full co-operation of the family is needed for successful resolution. Behavioural therapies may have to operate on a one-to-one basis, and although the person may readily exist within a group (including group living), there may be little constructive interaction. The general treatment focus is on developing and generalising social skills and expressive language and in using task analysis to aid day-to-day living (Matson et al 1996). The interventions should occur in the person's natural environment, and identifying and tackling the pivotal behaviours around which others evolve is helpful. For autistic people at all ages the management of change can be difficult. Change can be of three basic sorts: change in living environment, change in the temporal structure of the daily routine, and change in social contacts and carers. The effects of the last are often forgotten when the person is living in supported accommodation away from home. High staff turnover may lead to increased behavioural difficulties. Even though there may be difficulty in forming relationships, the person with autism has a need for relationship consistency.

Drug therapies have a limited role. Antipsychotics may reduce anger and irritability in some children, facilitating language development. Only studies of haloperidol have been replicated, but there are concerns about the long-term consequences of its use in children. Recently a large, multicentre, randomised, double-blind study of risperidone against placebo was conducted in over a hundred children and adolescents (5–17 years old) with autism who also had severe tantrums, aggression or self-injurious behaviour (McCracken et al 2002). Eight weeks of risperidone significantly reduced the irritability score of the Aberrant Behaviour Checklist, a commonly used assessment tool in LD. At least 69% of the active compared with 12% of the placebo group had a positive response (a 25% decrease in irritability scores) and an improved or very much improved rating on the Clinical Global Impressions Severity Scale. In two-thirds the improvement was maintained 6 months after the start of therapy. Although these results are important and encouraging, there were side-effects including a significant mean weight gain of on average 3 kg (compared with 0.8 kg on placebo) and less dramatic but significant increases in appetite, fatigue, drowsiness and salivation. Long-term movement disorders (including tardive dyskinesia) are a significant risk with antipsychotics in this group. In adults with autism and LD, antipsychotics are used widely, often as a last resort to reduce behaviour disturbances, especially aggression and self-injury, as well as their conventional use in treating coexisting psychiatric illness. Antipsychotics are probably helpful in a subgroup of people with autism, especially to reduce agitation when enforced change occurs, but should be regularly reviewed, and it is better to try and examine environmental factors to see if these can be met and a routine maintained. Risperidone in part acts on the serotonergic system. Trials of specific serotonin reuptake inhibitors (SSRIs), however, have produced inconsistent results, but SSRIs help in individual cases. One study suggests they may be specific to a subgroup of autistic children (DeLong et al 2002). Of over 120 children (2–8 years) treated with fluoxetine for 5–75 months, around 69% had a favourable response with significant improvements in socialisation and interpersonal contact including language use and non-verbal appropriateness. As in most drug studies in autism, those with the highest cognitive functioning did best. Among responders, two optimal dose ranges seemed to be present. One group needed up to 8 mg per day, and the other a much higher dose of 20–40 mg per day. Fluoxetine response also correlated highly with a family history of major affective disorder in first- or second-degree parental relatives, especially bipolar disorder. In fact 68% of all the children and 85% of the treatment-responders had a first degree relative with major depression. A more puzzling association was with high family achievement, but this also correlated with major depression in the families, and again especially bipolar disorder. A correlation was also found between treatment response and early preoccupation with letters and numbers ('hyperlexia'). A variety of other treatments have been tried in autism, from naltrexone to secretin, but replicable findings are few.

DISORDERS THAT COEXIST WITH LEARNING DISABILITY

Psychiatric disorders

The nomenclature where psychiatric disorders coexist with LD has become confused. Dual diagnosis, widely used in LD psychiatry to describe this, can also mean coexistence of substance abuse and psychiatric disorder. There are a wide variety of comorbidities, and it probably makes most sense to spell out clearly, whenever possible, the two (or more) conditions that are present.

Psychiatric illness in people with LD has been described since the mid-19th century. Hurd in 1888 had noted its presence in people with mild LD especially where a genetic liability existed. Tredgold in 1908 also noted mental illness at some time in up to 50% of people with LD. The mid- to late-20th century, however, saw a loss of interest in the association; the creation of large LD institutions with low levels of psychiatric input may have been a factor (Došen & Day 2001). Recently the situation has changed again, perhaps stimulated by the drive to community care. It is generally accepted that not only do psychiatric disorders occur in people with mild LD, they can also be diagnosed in those with severe LD, and many psychiatric disorders have a much higher prevalence than in the general population. A continuing problem lies with diagnostic overshadowing, occurring when one diagnosis leads to the exclusion or non-detection of a coexisting condition. In the extreme case all disorders are subsumed under the term LD or are thought to be aetiologically secondary to it (the old concepts of primary and secondary handicaps) (Jopp & Keys 2001). When behaviour disorders are also included, high levels of LD-associated psychiatric morbidity are seen at all ages. Rutters group's Isle of Wight studies in 1970 showed half of children with IQs under 70 had a psychiatric disorder compared with 7% of those with normal IQ. More recent reports confirm this. In New South Wales (Einfeld & Tonge 1996), over 40% of children aged 4–18 had severe emotional or behavioural disorder or psychiatric disorder. For adults the overall prevalence is around 30–40%, and since people with LD are part of an overall ageing population, psychiatric morbidity does not fall with age so dramatically as formerly (where there was a 'healthy survivor' effect). In the older group non-DS dementia is especially common (20%) (Cooper 1999b).

Psychiatric assessment schedules and diagnostic instruments

Early studies suffered from a lack of adequately validated rating scales for psychiatric disorder in those with intellectual disability, but several structured and semi-structured instruments are now available for research use. For people with mild LD and good communication skills the widely used schedule for affective disorders and schizophrenia (Endicott & Spitzer 1978) in its various forms has been used in several studies, and straddles the area between LD and the normal population. Schedules specifically devised for use in LD include the Psychopathology inventory for Mentally Retarded Adults (PIMRA; Senatore et al 1985) (self report and informant versions), the Diagnostic Assessment for the Severely Handicapped (DASH; Matson et al 1991) (severe and profound with emotional disorders), and the Psychiatric Assessment Schedule for Adults with Developmental Disabilities (PAS-ADD; Costello et al 1997). With regard to diagnostic criteria there are problems and inconsistencies in the way both DSM-IV and ICD-10, and also the specific guide for LD ICD-10-MR (WHO 1996), classify the various psychiatric and developmental conditions associated with LD. The Royal College of Psychiatrists (2001) has produced Diagnostic Criteria for LD (DC-LD) that better address the issues in moderate to severe LD, which should improve research consistency and, one hopes, also

clinical diagnosis. It includes conditions not easily described by the classical systems such as attention-deficit hyperactivity disorder in LD adults and various problem behaviours. A series of axes define a hierarchical approach to diagnosis, and this is given in synopsis form in Table 24.10.

Including personality disorders and problem behaviours may appear controversial but is in fact useful — a systematic classification of behaviours in particular has been greatly needed. Through its focus on adults, its approach to diagnosis in severe LD and its inclusion of a systematised approach to behavioural disorders, DC-LD is likely to be very useful to psychiatrists in LD whether based on clinical interview of the patient or on the use of structured questionnaires.

Schizophrenia

Kraepelin described a condition of 'propfschizophrenie' in people where dementia praecox arose in a setting of pre-existing intellectual impairment. He stated that dementia praecox could be diagnosed in 7% of people with LD, that the psychosis had a very early onset and that the pathological process involved in this actually led to the LD. Bleuler later denied that any true association existed, a concept that persisted. Limited genetic approaches also tended to reduce the relationship. Kallman's group in 1940 claimed no increase in the rate of schizophrenia in families of LD patients. The two conditions were still thought to be mutually exclusive even after psychodynamic aetiological theories of psychotic illness were on the wane — it was supposed that most people with LD did not have the necessary communication skills to permit such cognitively complex disorders. If 'schizophrenia' is an epithet applied only to the surface communication abnormality then this is true, but we usually mean that an underlying biological disorder is also present. There is no reason to suppose that people with severe LD are immune, rather the clinical presentation is modified by the presence of the intellectual impairment. It is possible that some medication-responsive 'behavioural' disorders in people with severe LD may fall into this class, especially if there is also a family history of psychosis. However, there are dangers in classifying on the basis of treatment response, and until a biological or molecular marker is found the area will remain grey. Schizophrenia prevalence is raised in mild LD on average to 3%, which is much higher than that in the general population (Doody et al 1998). When it is considered that this is likely to be an underestimate (most studies excluded severe LD), then its importance cannot be overstated.

Clinical features

In mild LD, schizophrenia presents in a similar way as in the general population. The main danger is in misattributing obvious psychotic symptoms to an underlying behavioural disorder, especially where behavioural outbursts arise from the psychopathology. The corollary, the incorrect diagnosis of schizophrenia on the basis of a primary behavioural disturbance, is also not uncommon. Partly to exclude such biases the time taken to make a diagnosis may be much longer than in the general population.

Auditory hallucinations are the most common symptom and present in around 90%. However, as in the general population, hallucinations occur in all sensory modalities, and careful questioning often elicits visual hallucinations (Meadows et al 1991). The content rather than the form of hallucinations is determined by the LD, and they relate more to the developmental than to the

Table 24.10	DC-LD classification system		
DC-LD axis	Typology	Specific comments	General notes
Axis I	**Severity of learning disability** Mild Moderate Severe Profound	 IQ 50–69 IQ 35–49 IQ 20–34 IQ less than 20	As in ICD-10 there is no concept of borderline learning disability
Axis II	**Cause of learning disability** Unknown origin Infections and parasitical diseases Endocrine, nutritional and metabolic diseases Mental and behavioural disorders Diseases of the nervous system Perinatal conditions Congenital malformations / deformities, chromosomal abnormalities Injury, poisoning, other external causes	 Includes specific meningitis, encephalitis Includes the inborn errors of metabolism Rett syndrome included here Includes non-specific meningitis, etc. Includes fetal / placental traumas, maternal conditions, extreme low birthweight or prematurity, congenital infections	Codings are used which match relevant ICD-10 categories
Axis III	**Psychiatric disorders** Level A Level B Level C Level D Level E	 *Developmental disorders* Autism; other pervasive developmental disorders; specific developmental disorders *Psychiatric illness* Dementia; non-affective psychotic disorders, including schizophrenia and schizoaffective disorder; affective disorders; anxiety disorders; phobias; obsessive–compulsive disorders; eating disorders; hyperkinetic disorders of adults *Personality disorders* *Problem behaviours* Verbally aggressive behaviour; physically aggressive behaviour; destructive behaviour; self-injurious behaviour; sexually inappropriate behaviour; oppositional behaviour; wandering *Other disorders*	This gives a DC-LD-specific coding to each but cross links this to the nearest ICD-10 and DSM-IV codes

DC-LD, Diagnostic Criteria for Learning Disability (Royal College of Psychiatrists 2001).

chronological age, and to social factors (e.g. peer group and carer interactions). The content may be simple commands or statements that the person is bad, has done some wrong, or is urged to do something that he knows to be incorrect. People with LD are often more cognitively pliable than others. They seek to please, and will agree that 'voices' could not really happen, only to have the 'voices' return immediately the interviewer leaves. A similar superficial denial of delusions can also be deceptive. Delusions may be simple in form, partly attributable to a reduction in life experience and opportunity ('psychosocial masking'). On the other hand they may be difficult to interpret and appear cognitively bizarre. Again the fixity of the delusion may appear open to question. The person may agree with the interviewer that the delusional ideas can not possibly be true, only to describe them again to the next person who asks.

The emphasis must be on a consistent approach to collating information from the individual and others, examining the problem over a period of time. This will also buffer the clinician against the misreading of the many cognitive misunderstandings and unusual responses that are naturally part of LD. Most people talk to themselves at some time; people with LD frequently do when there is apparently no one else there, but this can be a cognitive style rather than psychopathology. Formal thought disorder is less common in people with LD (although not unknown), as are thought echo, delusional perception, passivity phenomena and thought withdrawal. The apparent reduction may be due to a difficulty in explaining these experiences to the interviewer. Thought blocking is as difficult to interpret as in the general population. Again a consistent approach over a period of time will help distinguish attention changes due to true hallucinations rather than to intrinsic attentional deficits. It is important also to assess whether there is a consistent relationship between the phenomenology and the person's mood state, and this again often takes time.

With increasing LD severity there is a greater behavioural overlay to symptoms; the key features in distinguishing them from underlying behavioural problems lie in their time course, where they arise without known precipitants including a multitude of simple to complex physical complaints and recent environmental or carer changes. Some support for a psychotic base to some non-precipitant-induced behaviours comes from a study using the DASH schedule in people with severe LD who were said to have schizophrenia — significantly increased scores in domains indicating reality distortion and disorganisation occurred compared with a control group without the diagnosis (Cherry et al 2000). Sometimes, however, a trial of neuroleptics is necessary where an unspecified functional psychosis is suspected in a person with severe LD, even if it cannot resolve the issue as to the presence of schizophrenia.

Aetiology

As in the general population the cause of schizophrenia is unknown, but genetic factors play an important role, and imaging studies have advanced our understanding of the disease process. The schizophrenia–LD association is highly familial, probably due to strong genetic factors. In one study where the comorbid group was carefully ascertained and compared against controls with schizophrenia alone or LD alone, the incidence of schizophrenia in a first- or second-degree relative was higher when the proband had comorbid LD than when he had schizophrenia alone (Doody et al 1998). Comorbidity also tended to occur in excess in the families of comorbid probands. Overall the comorbid group had a similarly raised incidence of pure LD in their families to that of the LD control group. MRI scans in these subjects showed that the comorbid group more closely resembled controls with schizophrenia than LD controls (Sanderson et al 1999). In particular, although overall brain size of LD controls was smaller than the others, the relative amygdala–hippocampus size was greater bilaterally than in comorbid or schizophrenic groups, where size was reduced, especially in the former. One interpretation of these findings is that the comorbid group represents a very early onset and more severe form of schizophrenia whose sole childhood manifestation is LD. This concept is not new and has been around since at least the time of Kraepelin, but has never been adequately tested. Schizophrenic symptomatology per se had its onset at a similar age in both comorbid and schizophrenic groups. For those admitted to maximum security settings there seems to be an earlier age at onset in the comorbid patients compared with general schizophrenic patients, but the reasons for admission to such units are complex and do not always relate to an increased severity of a condition (Doody et al 2000). Relating historical variables to structural findings proved more difficult (Sanderson et al 2001). Obstetric complications were more common in the comorbid group than in the schizophrenic group, but whether this is a cause or outcome of the disorder is not certain. Other aetiologies associated with comorbid schizophrenia and LD have already been mentioned — velocardiofacial syndrome, and some disorders of the X chromosome. It is likely that the origins are heterogeneous, CGSs are typically sporadic in origin and would not explain the commonness of a family history of this disorder.

Affective disorders

Bipolar disorder

Bipolar disorder appears more frequent in LD adults, although prevalence reports vary from as little as 1% to as high as 12%. Some groups feel that there is no increase (Došen & Day 2001), but significant misdiagnosis as behavioural disorder has occurred in the past, especially for those with severe LD. Further confusion has arisen by the failure to separate recurrent major depressive disorder from bipolar disorder (continuing the older grouping of both disorders as manic depressive illness). A recent, small scale, community prevalence study using structured instruments for diagnosis found around 2% had mania or hypomania, and 3% depression (Deb et al 2001).

Clinical features   The age at onset tends to be earlier than in the general population. During the manic phase of the illness overactivity and lack of sleep can be prominent, but the patient does not always easily express a clear elevation of mood. Instead irritability and aggressive outbursts are more common. Pressure of speech may occur, but complex speech disturbances such as clang associations and punning are rare. Psychotic features, e.g. simple grandiose delusions, are not uncommon, especially in those with mild LD (Reid 1972). An excess of the rapid-cycling bipolar disorder has been suggested, but an ascertainment bias may exist, since the association with severe aggressive outbursts would make admission more likely (Ballinger 1997). In clinical practice, however, cyclical and rapid alterations in mood state are often encountered, with multiple episodes of affective disorder in a relatively short space of time. The tendency to rapid-cycling is associated with an earlier age at onset (Vanstraelen & Tyrer 1999). Catatonic symptoms (stupor, mutism, waxy flexibility) are sometimes seen, and catatonia, as in the general population, may be a severe variant of bipolar illness rather than schizophrenia, especially where the stupor alternates with an excited phase. Previously it was considered that mania did not occur in people with DS; this has now clearly been shown not to be the case and its prevalence is probably similar to that in other people with LD. In fact all forms of bipolar disorder, including rapid-cycling, have been described in DS.

Aetiological factors   There has been little research here, but a recent association with Prader–Willi syndrome is important (Boer et al 2002). Of 15 adults with Prader–Willi, 7 had a psychiatric disorder that was either bipolar or depressive in type. Five out of the 8 adult patients with uniparental disomy (UPD), but only one patient with a deletion, also had clear psychotic features. In a separate 15-year longitudinal follow-up study of 53 children and adults with Prader–Willi syndrome 8 individuals developed a psychiatric illness, 4 of the deletion subjects had a bipolar disorder, 2 had transient psychoses, both the UPD patients had cycloid psychoses (Descheemaeker et al 2002). If results from such studies are confirmed, they mark an important association between genes on chromosome 15 and affective disorders.

Major depressive disorder

The symptoms of depression are common in those with LD, and the biological features assist diagnosis in those with more severe LD. In 285 adult outpatients with LD, around 9% had a depressive disorder or dysthymia (Stavrakaki 1999), lower than some reported figures for the general population. LD often modifies depressive symptoms, and under-diagnosis may be present again. Certain behaviours (hyperactivity and wandering, mutism, unexplained temper tantrums, etc.) not seen in depression in the general population may be symptomatic of depression in this group ('depressive equivalents'). Aggression may also be a prominent feature of depression, especially with severe LD.

Clinical features   The biological features are helpful. Sleep disturbance (usually lack of sleep or a disturbed sleep pattern with night-time wakening) and appetite changes are frequent. Weight gain may be as common as weight loss. Although low mood is common even with severe LD, irritability may be a more prominent feature, and changes in the levels of prevailing behaviours are as important as new onset of these; self-injury, temper outbursts, altered self-care and other skill levels, even the development of incontinence anew. The need to differentiate such symptoms from dementia is clear, especially in a person with DS, or a person over 65 with LD, while remembering that the coexistence of dementia and depression is not uncommon. A treatment trial may be needed to resolve the issue. Somatisation of symptoms is common — the person may, for instance, complain of headaches, stomach pains, and excessive fatigue. Suicidal thoughts and acts occur mainly in those with mild LD, and overall they are not frequently reported. A time chart of sleep, activity pattern, eating and cyclical changes in mood associates (aggressive, self-injurious behaviour, sexual behaviour, irritability, anhedonia, apathy and withdrawal) as well as observed mood changes can help establish diurnal or other circadian rhythms and point to the diagnosis. The differential diagnosis is sometimes very difficult in the severely disabled. Dementia, metabolic and endocrine disturbances, and the side-effects of the many medications that are often prescribed are among some of the alternatives. In adult women with severe LD, disruption associated with the menstrual cycle must be considered, and a painful premenstrual period or menses themselves can be mistaken for mood disorder.

Other disorders

- Generalised *chronic anxiety disorder*, often difficult to distinguish from depression, with which it may coexist, is not rare in both LD adults and children, and low self-esteem is common in both conditions. In mild LD the prevalence of brooding, somatisation and sleep disturbance may be increased over the condition in the general population (Masi et al 2000). In more profound disability it may manifest as temper outbursts and other symptoms that have been also considered as depressive equivalents. Where autism coexists with LD, severe anxiety is a relatively common response to any change in routine or environment. In fact a search for aetiological factors is important in any anxiety disorder; physical disorders, post-traumatic stress induced by physical or sexual abuse, and bereavement reactions can play a role.
- *Abnormal grief reactions* are in fact common and often misinterpreted by carers (Hollins & Esterhuyzen 1997).
- *Obsessive–compulsive disorder* has been little studied but, like all other mental illnesses, also occurs in people with LD. The main differential diagnosis is from the rituals of autism. The cognitive self-interpretation of symptoms in obsessive–compulsive disorder is not usually seen in autism.
- *Phobic disorders* are common — 4% in one recent small study (Deb et al 2001) — and often specific, such as animal phobias. More generally, panic disorder and social phobia can

be found and have been seen in the early stages of dementia of DS.

- *Personality disorder* in people with LD is a controversial concept. Reid & Ballinger (1987) considered it present in over 20% of a hospitalised group with mild to moderate LD. It is difficult to separate features such as passiveness and dependence from the symptom cluster that characterises LD itself, and one needs to be on very certain grounds since personality disorder diagnoses often lead to exclusion from services. On the other hand, there has been considerable reluctance to use the diagnoses even where warranted in those with mild LD, and a balance needs to be struck, and unnecessary treatments or interventions avoided (Hurley & Sovner 1995).
- *Attention deficit/hyperactivity disorder* is common in children and adults with LD, with up to 20% meeting diagnostic criteria. Stimulant medications may help those with mild LD, but their effectiveness in the many children and adults who have only partial symptoms, and in people with severe or profound LD, has not yet been shown.

Treatment issues

Pharmacotherapy

Antipsychotics are extensively used in treating both psychiatric and behavioural disorders. The dearth of properly constituted and controlled trials of interventions used in LD has complex origins (Oliver et al 2002). Recently, issues around informed consent, diverse service configurations leading to access difficulties, and unclear boundaries between social services and healthcare have all played a role, as has the increased time needed to collect data from people with LD. A review of antipsychotic use in LD found only one randomised trial, reporting on only two cases and published over forty years ago (Duggan & Brylewski 1999). In most cases, therefore, prescribing practice has been to generalise results from the treatment of psychiatric disorders in the non-LD population. In clinical practice, with respect to medication dosage, this is usually quite acceptable. It is important to avoid misinterpreting side-effects as having other origins (e.g. behavioural), and careful monitoring for drug interactions is needed since many will also be on antiepileptic medication; many psychotropics lower seizure threshold. However co-therapy with both antiepileptic and psychotropic medication is often necessary and, with close supervision by an experienced psychiatrist, is usually successful.

Prior to the era of hospital closure the number of LD psychiatrists was proportionately very small, but prescription rates were high, and psychoactive medications prescribed to up to 50% of the population. This has continued. In one North American study 50% of patients in community resources received more than one psychotropic medication, and 4% over four (Burd et al 1991). While such prescribing may be unusual, on average around 30% of those known to community services receive psychotropics, and it does highlight the ubiquity of their use. The chief indications are schizophrenia or a schizophreniform psychosis (about 50% of prescriptions). However, a significant minority (23%) do not have a psychosis, the use here often being to control a behavioural disorder. Long-term central consequences of typical and atypical antipsychotics in people with significant pre-existing cognitive impairment have not been investigated. Short-term movement disorders may be confused with intrinsic stereotypies, but more chronic parkinsonism and tardive dyskinesia can usually be clearly demarked.

Treatment of schizophrenia Most advice follows that for treatment in the general population. Where treatment is elective, a full prior blood screen, physical examination and an ECG is required. At the very least these should be repeated at yearly intervals. A review of past therapies and responses is advisable both before starting any medication and at regular intervals thereafter. For emergency control of an acute psychosis, a typical antipsychotic such as haloperidol may be combined, if necessary, with a short-acting benzodiazepine. An atypical antipsychotic is first choice for the longer-term treatment. Risperidone and olanzapine are usually well tolerated, but weight gain can be a problem. Thioridazine was formerly widely used both in small doses for its presumed anti-anxiety effect and in larger doses in the treatment of psychotic illness. However, recent concerns about its possible cardiac toxicity have meant that many have had to be changed over to atypical antipsychotics. Clinical experience has shown that withdrawal of medication from people with LD needs to be done more slowly than in the general population; they may benefit from a cross-over period where two medications are prescribed, one reducing and one increasing in dose. In severe drug-refractory illness clozapine can help, although the regular blood monitoring requirements may pose problems, especially in those with more severe LD who may not understand or comply with regular venepuncture. Routine anticholinergic use is not often needed. Most people are quite happy to take medication orally, and the former widespread use of depot medication is now less common.

Even with current levels of community care a person in the acute phase of schizophrenia with LD often needs hospitalisation for stabilisation. Ideally this would be in specialist inpatient LD settings. Although a person with mild LD can be managed successfully in a general adult psychiatry ward, the staff may feel untrained in the support of the needs deriving from the patient's LD. Specialist LD psychiatric support to the clinical teams is essential in such cases. The person with moderate to severe LD and psychosis is inappropriately served by general psychiatric services, and there remains a continuing need for acute specialist treatment settings for this group — a fact not always clearly recognised in LD hospital closure programmes.

Therapies for depression The usual first choice is an SSRI, and there is little to choose between them (Ruedrich et al 2001). As in the general population the adequate dosage needs (up to the maximum tolerable with respect to side-effects) and the adequate treatment duration usually ensure response. Tricyclics are second-line, although the overdose risk is much less with LD. The side-effects are more prominent, and tricyclics may lower epilepsy threshold more than SSRIs. Trials of antidepressant therapy may be appropriate in those with severe LD and depressive equivalent symptoms/biological features that are not responsive to other interventions, even when the subject is not able to report a clear subjective depressive mood. In fact Reid's seminal study showed that this group was especially likely to respond to antidepressants (Reid 1972). In severe depression ECT should be considered, and it is underused in people with LD. One caveat is DS, where the anaesthetist should be aware of the rare possibility of atlanto-axial instability with any neck manipulation, especially in younger individuals. Another clear indication for ECT is where catatonic symptoms are prominent. In such cases it is usually rapidly effective.

Drugs that stabilise mood Lithium has long been used to stabilise mood swings in people with LD. Often in the past this was used in cases of otherwise intractable cyclical behavioural disturbance as well as clear bipolar disorder, or recurrent major depressive disorder. Lithium, in the UK, is also licensed for use in controlling aggressive outbursts, although any superiority over behavioural interventions has not been shown. It is likely that where it has been successful there has been an underlying major affective disorder. In DS the increased risk of hypothyroidism means that its use should be carefully monitored. Patients with LD are also susceptible to its renal effects, and polydipsia or polyuria always requires investigation. Antiepileptic medications are also widely used for mood control. With the prevalence of epilepsy in those with LD there is a great deal of experience in their use. Carbamazepine can be used on its own or combined with lithium to achieve the desired effect. Doses are as for the control of epilepsy. Valproic acid is said to be more effective in rapid cycling bipolar illness (King et al 2000b). Other newer antiepileptics such as lamotrigine may have a use in selected cases, but there is as yet no real evidence for or against their usefulness as mood stabilisers in LD.

Medications for anxiety disorders Medications are really second-line after a thorough search for environmental and social precipitating and maintaining factors. Small doses of SSRIs are often effective (in generalised anxiety, and especially in social phobia) and do not engender tolerance seen with benzo-diazepines. However, careful short-term prescribing of benzodiazepines can be useful, especially as an adjunctive therapy to psychological and cognitive interventions. Direct sedation for short periods may be needed to help the patient get through medical or dental interventions. Traditionally, benzodiazepines (especially temazepam) have been used, and if usage is kept to as small a dose as needed they are very helpful.

For sleep disorders a behavioural approach to regulating sleep patterns and the avoidance of daytime somnolence is often more effective than medication. The use of long-acting benzodiazepines has decreased in recent years, and newer very short-acting medications such as zopiclone may be helpful, but again for limited periods of time. There have been some reports that melatonin may help regulate sleep patterns in children with autism and LD.

Psychotherapy and cognitive behavioural therapy in adults with LD

One school of thought proposed that LD is often a consequence of emotional or psychological abuse, rather than that the two situations simply coexist (e.g. Sinason 1992). However, the outcomes of severe deprivation are not identical with LD. Dynamic psychotherapy has had rather little use in LD and most of the attempts have been with emotionally disturbed children with LD and/or their families; the theoretical constructs are more developed than the clinical practice. Many psychotherapists shy away from the field because of the difficulties in communication and the problem of maintaining a strictly confidential therapeutic relationship with the patient in a milieu where disclosure of therapy to carers is often expected. A form of object relations therapy has been developed by Gaedt (1995), and Došen (2001) has pioneered a maturational system combining ideas from Piaget, Mahler, Erikson and Bowlby based on psychosocial and cognitive staging and applied this to the treatment of depression and other mental illness in children with severe LD. However, it is fair to say that the practical use of such therapies is limited largely to an adjunctive nature at present.

Cognitive-behavioural approaches have been more widely successful, provided the problems of comprehension, self-reporting of cognitions and self-regulation can be overcome (Kroese 1997). This is often the case for people with mild or moderate LD, and the treatment can form a useful adjunct to pharmacotherapy, especially in the management of depression and dysthymic disorder. Cognitive distortions in general are common, in particular those of placing things into extreme categories — all good or all bad, completely acceptable or totally unwanted, and so on. The lack of subtlety in categorisation is also felt to underlie some of the behaviours shown by people with LD who commit sex offences, and cognitive-behaviour therapy has an important place in their management.

BEHAVIOURAL DISORDERS

Maladaptive behaviours ('challenging behaviours') are very prevalent in both LD children and adults. A survey of over two thousand adults showed 64% to have at least one behaviour disorder (Smith et al 1996). Behavioural disorder in fact is used to describe a vast range of problems from minor antisocial behaviours leading to some disruption of day-to-day living up to serious aggressive outbursts. By definition those that are outwardly directed are challenging if they transgress a social boundary or rule, and thus are context dependent. Self-injury is much more likely to be challenging in any social context. Severe challenging behaviour may occur in 10–16% of LD individuals. Behavioural disorders are a common reason for psychiatric referral, but their analysis and management usually requires a joint multidisciplinary approach. A set of criteria for defining when a given behaviour has become a problem is given in Box 24.1.

Box 24.1   Definitions of challenging behaviour

Challenging behaviour*
- At some time must have caused more than minor injuries to themselves or others or destroyed their immediate living or working environment
- At least weekly had a behaviour that required intervention by others or placed them in physical danger, or caused damage that could not be rectified immediately or caused at least an hour's disruption
- Cause over a few minutes disruption at least daily

Severe challenging behaviour†
- Occur at least once a day
- Usually prevent participation in programmes/activities appropriate to person's ability level
- Usually require physical intervention by one or more staff members
- Would usually lead to major injury to either individual or others

---
* After Quereshi H 1994 The size of the problem. In: Emerson E, McGill P, Mansell J (eds) Severe learning disabilities and challenging behaviours: designing high quality services. Chapman & Hall, London, p 17–36.
† After Emerson E, Kiernan C, Alborz A et al 2001 The prevalence of challenging behaviours: a total population study. Research in Developmental Disabilities 22:77–93.

It is difficult to separate challenging behaviour from psychiatric illness, and indeed the definition of mental illness in classification schemes such as DSM-IV could as easily encompass behavioural disorder in those with LD as it does conduct disorders of children. At present the level of true comorbidity between psychiatric and behavioural disorder is uncertain. Certainly the rate of antipsychotic and antidepressant use is high in those with behavioural disorders, and aggressive outbursts and self-injury have been considered as depressive equivalents in those with severe disability. A full psychiatric assessment is an important part of the work-up of behavioural disorder, and this should also include screening for autism or other pervasive developmental disorder. The person's ability to interpret the behaviour is also important. It is often found in people with mild LD that the nature of the behaviour in itself is fully understood, but that there is a complete lack of insight into the chain of events that the behaviour has set in progress and its persisting effect on others. Such insight difficulties are intrinsic to the nature of LD and have generally led to a different legislature around behavioural disturbance in LD. Capacity generally decreases with LD severity, and it would be difficult to maintain that a person with severe LD was fully responsible for his or her actions.

Being a social construct, behavioural disorder can take a huge number of forms and is highly context and culture sensitive. The usefulness of a catalogue of such behaviours is uncertain, but a pragmatic scheme based on the form of the behaviour can help conceptualise some of the difficulties. Table 24.11 gives such a scheme; this is by no means comprehensive and has no implied relationship to any aetiological factors; it is roughly structured into increased severity of danger to the person or others.

Multiple behaviours may co-occur in the same person or emerge at different times; the duration and intensity of each may vary considerably. Persistent antisocial behaviours are often very wearing for both the person and their carers. Sometimes they are environmentally determined, but the concept that most were due to institutionalisation is contradicted by their persistence after discharge from hospital and their prevalence in those never hospitalised. At the other extreme, severe physical violence, although fortunately rare, is probably the major limiting factor in community provision for people with LD, especially if there are no identifiable factors that predict outbursts. Self-injurious behaviour can range from simple skin picking through to severe eye gouging, head banging and face beating. Repetitive self-injury and self-mutilation is perhaps the most distressing of all the problems that present to psychiatrists in LD. It is much more common in people with severe LD, and here it is associated with the presence of other challenging behaviours such as noisiness, overactivity, irritability and stripping.

The causes of behavioural disorders

All factors tend to interact, so that one particular type of behaviour may relate to different causal mechanisms at different times; often a causal factor can never be clearly identified, especially in those with severe LD. Many of the most difficult behaviours follow a maturational pattern. They are first exhibited when the person is a child, sometimes preschool, and gradually become more pronounced and persistent with age. This is especially so with temper outbursts — eventually the parents are unable to physically manage them, and secondary referral occurs. During teenage years, problems can be further exacerbated by the devel-

Table 24.11 A suggested typology of behavioural problems

Form of behaviour	General area	Some specific examples
Persistent antisocial behaviours	Noise related	General repeated shouting, screaming
	Elimination related	Anal poking, faecal smearing (not related to constipation)
	Food related	Vomiting, deliberate choking, food smearing (not related to GI disorder)
	Property related	Persistent misuse of facilities — e.g. leaves taps running, gas or electricity left on, without memory disturbance
		Minor thefts
	Absconding	Persistent running away
Persistent aggressive behaviours	Directed against property	Destruction of furnishings and windows, belongings, clothes
	Directed against others	Verbal threats
		Isolated nipping, scratching, punching, kicking, biting, throttling, throwing objects at person
		Outbursts combining elements of these
		Outbursts using weapons of some form
	Directed against self	Skin picking, hand or arm biting with injury
		Head or body slapping and punching with injury
		Ingestion of inedible and dangerous objects
		Head banging with injury
		Self injury using external objects

opmental and emotional changes that are associated with puberty, and they persist into adulthood. Such an enduring pattern is very familiar to those working with people with LD, and it may be considered an innate feature, what Read has termed 'organic behaviour disorder' which is modulated rather than caused by social or environmental factors (Read 1997).

Biological factors

The behavioural phenotype concept tries to relate clusters of behaviours with particular clinical syndromes. Some of these have been discussed already in the sections on DS and autism. Lesch–Nyhan syndrome, a very rare X-linked recessive metabolic disorder (mutations in hypoxanthine phosphoribosyltransferase gene) is associated with striking degrees of self-mutilation. At birth such children appear healthy, but by 3–4 months dystonias become apparent, later developing into spasticity, choreiform movements and transient hemiparesis. At around 2 years a severe self-mutilation emerges with lip, buccal and finger biting. These begin suddenly and can be clinically distinguished from self-injury associated with autism (Hall et al 2001). The postmortem finding of reduced synaptic basal ganglia and substantia nigra dopamine (but not other monoamines) suggested that dopaminergic dysfunction underlies the self injury. However, both pharmacological and behavioural interventions have produced similarly disappointing results, and most people who self-injure do not have this syndrome. Other neurochemical theories include central serotonergic and opiate dysfunctions. However, since these have also been implicated in autism, there is a need to distinguish those who have this and also self injure from those who do not. The other classic behavioural syndrome is that of Prader–Willi syndrome (see p. 557), where self-injury is common in addition to hyperphagia.

Psychological factors

The idea, derived from operant conditioning, that both behaviour disorder symptoms and the ways of modifying them are learned and maintained by positive or negative reinforcers, lies behind many psychological management approaches. The initial reinforcer of a behaviour may be apparently unrelated to the eventual one. Reinforcers are divided into primary ones (e.g. food, drink, pain) associated with basic biological needs, and secondary ones that result from a pairing with primary reinforcers. Social reinforcers (praise, pleasant environments, aversive stimuli, etc.) are generally thought to be secondary in type. A careful behavioural analysis is needed to clarify these, but finding the antecedents of behaviour is often difficult, and any specific behaviour may generalise beyond the original inducing stimuli and reinforcers. However, it is important to try to understand both the origin of the behaviour, the original and current maintaining factors and any meaning it has for the person. Meaning has often been neglected, with the focus on changing the behaviour rather than viewing it as a form of communication. It is also important to consider whether the behaviour is a consequence of physical, emotional or sexual abuse, whether by family, carers or other people with LD. Other inducing stimuli include undetected/untreated pain, or physical illness. Social reinforcers, both positive and aversive in type, have often been shown to be maintaining factors. The linking of unwanted behaviours to positive reinforcements such as warm social responses, or concern, often leads to the person being labelled as attention-seeking, and ignored, rather than a focus being made on the cause of the anomalous responses.

Environmental factors

The living situation can be important in maintaining a behaviour or preventing the adoption of alternative, acceptable behaviours. Long-stay hospitals were often an under-stimulating and over-populated environment reducing the opportunity to develop the skills required to alter behaviours that may themselves be an ethological response to living in very large groups. Smaller group settings are usually much more successful, but there is a danger that staffed individual placements may also reduce the necessary opportunities to develop peer-appropriate social skills. Although there is often a good response to many low-level behaviour disorders in community settings, a substantial improvement in severe behavioural disorders is not so clear, and other reinforcers may be acting. Some environmental needs, such as stability and continuity of day-to-day living patterns and adequate personal space based on individual needs, may be lacking in community placements and may also contribute to behavioural problems. The concept that a very rich and stimulating environment is always best may not hold for people with severe LD — over- as well as under-stimulation may be detrimental.

Assessment and treatment

The clinical psychologist and psychiatrist need to work together on diagnosis and management. A screen should be carried out for psychiatric disorder either as a primary cause of the disturbance or coexistent. With severe LD a family history of psychiatric disorder, cyclical components to the behaviour pattern, and more specific indicators such as depressive equivalents may assist diagnosis. Physical problems, e.g. incontinence, constipation, infections, epilepsy, endocrine disturbances and sources of pain should be assessed and treated. Sensory impairments and how the living environment affects these should be considered. Communication restrictions may mean that the behaviour is a way of attracting attention. Where there are no, or limited, verbal skills, some can use Makaton or Sign-Along, sign languages devised for people with LD, and the psychiatrist may need an interpreter (e.g. an experienced carer or a speech and language therapist). Detailed behavioural diaries, the aberrant behaviour checklist (ABC) or other psychometric instruments can chart the periodicity and event-relatedness of the behaviours.

Treatments should address the possible causes, stimuli and reinforcers, and the environment in which the behaviour occurs. In general, outcomes are better for people with mild LD, where teaching anger management and self-management skills, and the self-monitoring of unwanted behaviours, can be combined with operant interventions to replace unwanted with desired responses. Interventions in severe LD are more difficult. A behavioural treatment programme that works within a specialist setting is often much more difficult to implement and maintain within the restrictions of the person's own home or place of work.

Physical restraint was formerly widely used as a treatment modality rather than an emergency protective measure, especially in those with severe self-injurious behaviour. Nowadays this is not generally viewed as acceptable. In the UK, aversive procedures have no place in treatment, but restraints of one form or another are still unfortunately sometimes urgently needed to prevent dangerous consequences of behaviours. Restraints can be mechanical (e.g. protective headgear to prevent the consequences of head banging), or physical restraint by others (e.g. brief period arm restraint to prevent self beating of the face). A third type of intervention is that of removing the person deliberately to a non-dangerous environment. Various forms of this have been used in the past under the label of 'time out'. When a person is placed in a situation that they are unable to exit by their own free will then this is really always a form of seclusion whatever the environment. Ethical questions arise around often conflicting requirements of the duty to care and protect the individual against harm and allowing them freedom to exercise their free will. Recently there have been questions as to any superior efficacy of imposed restraint when compared with other methods, as well as moral questions as to acceptability.

Positive programming methods such as those devised by La Vigna use non-aversive programmes based on the teaching of skills functionally equivalent or related to target behaviours to establish a more socially appropriate repertoire. They can be combined with other psychological approaches based on the analysis of operant conditioning effects. Drug treatments are still widely used. Neuroleptics are the most common, but the use of anti-depressants, especially SSRIs, and mood stabilisers is also widespread. As an adjunctive therapy to other approaches they have their place. Good practice would advocate periodic attempts at dose reduction, and this applies equally to atypical antipsychotics, about whose long-term consequences we are as yet unclear. Complete drug washout, in hospital if necessary to ensure safety, may help those on high doses of medication for long periods.

FORENSIC ISSUES IN LEARNING DISABILITY

Most issues relevant to LD are dealt with in the chapter on forensic psychiatry in this volume. In essence there are two important areas: specific associations between LD and offending, and issues around legal process and consent.

Offending and LD

While many studies have shown that people with intellectual impairment are overly common within the criminal justice system, it is not clear whether they all meet the full criteria for LD, and some suggest that it is intellectual disadvantage rather than LD that is over-represented (Fraser 2002). Estimates of those with learning problems range up to 8% of those attending police stations (of whom 40% had special schooling), with 14% of this group also having a mental health disorder (Barron et al 2002). Similar prevalence rates have been reported for prisoners and for those serving probation orders. As would be expected, most of this population has mild LD, and there is little to distinguish most offences from those occurring in the general population. They may place themselves at risk, however, due to a lack of understanding of society's norms and conventions and chronic low self-esteem. They are also more likely to give false confessions. The person with mild LD often comes from a socially disadvantaged living situation, and such circumstances are associated with increased risk of offending. There are other balances towards and against the detection of offences — they are more likely to be detected and apprehended on the one hand, but carers often have a much higher threshold of acceptance of behavioural disturbance on the other. Because of their intrinsic profound difficulties in understanding the rules of society, people with severe LD should not be classed as offenders, and diversion from the system is the norm via mental health legislation. Because of the disability, such acts that would otherwise be classified as exhibitionism or public masturbation in the general population have completely different origins. Unfortunately, it is still the case that non-LD specialists can misinterpret such problems, leading to a great deal of distress for all those involved.

Specific offence types and LD

Previously, two offences were held as more common in people with mild LD — sex offending and arson. However, both these associations may, at least partly, have suffered from selection bias. Previous studies often focused on inpatient and especially maximum-security or special-hospital populations, and certainly a hospital order is more likely for an offender with LD.

Within the total group of *sex offenders*, however, people with LD are more likely to have committed sexual offences across many categories with a wider range of victims and especially against younger children and male children (Blanchard et al 1999). They are also more likely to have been sexually abused themselves in childhood (Lindsay et al 2001). There may be a persistent denial or minimisation of the seriousness of the offence, which makes it difficult to engage in direct therapies. Cognitive-behavioural approaches are currently the best strategies, although the treatment duration may need to be very long. There is little evidence for the efficacy of anti-libidinal medications. Re-offending rates are difficult to interpret and selectively reported. Many studies have shown worryingly high rates of re-offending (40–72% for sex offences), but much less in smaller groups undergoing specific treatments. Re-offending may relate to the length of therapy; shorter durations lead to more re-offending. Re-offending and re-conviction is actually a problem across the spectrum for people with LD. In those discharged from medium-secure units the rates are 30–85%.

Deliberate fire setting has again been consistently linked to LD in those referred for hospital treatment, but any true association is still unclear. The group seems to be younger — late teens to early adults — and mainly male. Arson is a very serious offence in which the danger to others is exceptionally high. Treatments again may need to be very long term; placement options and treatment programmes are often very expensive and under-evaluated.

Comorbidity in offenders with LD

Where a significant psychiatric disorder is already present, then the person is often already known to the local LD services, and their risk of misplacement will be lessened. In medium-secure units for offenders with LD, O'Brien (2002) reported that 40% have a formal psychiatric disorder, usually an autistic spectrum disorder or schizophrenia. A study on behalf of the National Autistic Society found that a minimum of 2.5% of the population of the three English special hospitals had an autistic spectrum disorder (Hare et al 2000).

LD and the law

The status of LD within current legislation is changing. There has been recent debate on whether LD should be considered as a mental disorder at all. It still remains useful, however, to distinguish those with LD who are at risk due to LD alone (rather than a coexisting mental illness or behavioural disorder), although the framework for such protection has moved from hospital to community. The use of a hospital as a place of safety used to protect a person with severe LD without any other coexisting condition has decreased markedly. In Scotland the Incapable Adults (Scotland) Act is representative of such change, and allows the appointment of a welfare attorney, sometimes with wide-ranging powers, where representation of the person's interests is under question. It has also regulated the complex issue of consent, which is linked to *capability* (formerly termed competence). Capability is not all or nothing; a person can understand at different levels, and the concept is socioculturally bound (Jenkins 1998). However, there are now clearer guidelines as to how a practitioner may proceed whether the consent is to do with therapeutic interventions or allowing a person to take part in a research study.

The appropriate adult

people with LD are especially vulnerable when they stand accused, are witness to, or victims of a crime. They may be readily confused, especially with the stress of the situation, and may easily make self-incriminatory, erroneous or conflicting statements. The person must be helped to understand the concepts of arrest, caution, charging and questions, and to know their rights to contact a lawyer and relative if detained. In the UK the standard adversarial system in court compounds the situation. The 'appropriate adult' scheme was devised to assist in such situations. The appropriate adult is a trained person (training involves police, psychiatric, legal and social work professionals) and facilitates the process of interview for both the individual and the police. The appropriate adult should be present when a person is charged. Attendance is especially important if the person is to be searched or intimately examined, especially if there is any indication that the person has been sexually abused or assaulted. During interview they are not a substitute for a lawyer, nor expected to provide emotional support, but would indicate when a line of questioning was likely to lead to unreliable answers, read any documents or statements signed by the person, and note on this anything felt to be inaccurate. They would also advise on the need for medical assistance, or rest periods. The appropriate adult's role is not that of an advocate, who has a much wider remit to provide emotional support, to interpret and be a voice for the person with LD, and to be an active participant in safeguarding the person's rights, interests and feelings.

EPILEPSY AND LEARNING DISABILITY

Taken together, epilepsy and LD are the most common conditions (both affecting at least 2% of the population) that involve the nervous system, and they frequently coexist. Epilepsy may occur in 30–40% of hospitalised LD patients. It tends to mirror the degree of neurological damage, being more prevalent in severe LD. A seizure disorder may affect around 5:1000 children at some time, and severe intractable epilepsy, especially with repeated status attacks, may be a cause of LD itself. However, the overall prognosis for epilepsy has improved and most children without LD with epilepsy will be seizure free as adults. The prognosis is not so good for people with LD, where seizures are often severe and multiple in form, but even here the newer antiepileptic medications can be very effective.

Aetiology

In about 25% the cause is unknown. For the rest the wide variety of causes mirrors that of the LD — infections, trauma and genetic/metabolic conditions. Many mechanisms have been proposed to lead to hyperexcitability of neurons, and in the hippocampus and other cortical areas injury leads to aberrant axonal sprouting which may cause epileptogenesis (McNamara 1999). Epilepsy is often variably present in syndromic LD, paralleling the incomplete penetrance of many other phenotypic features. For instance 18% of those with fragile X have seizure disorder, nearly always beginning after 2 years of age. In other syndromes epilepsy is also age dependent. In DS, epilepsy incidence has two peaks: one in early childhood and the other in older subjects in association with dementia. In some autistic patients epilepsy can begin in later teenage or early adult years. The series of disorders associated with disruption of cerebral cortex formation (lissencephalies, double cortex, heterotopias) are characteristically associated with epilepsy. The seizure type and frequency may change over time. In the various autosomal dominant forms of tuberous sclerosis, early infantile spasms may later be replaced with generalised tonic–clonic seizures and simple or complex partial seizures. The cerebral hamartomas are very dysplastic and highly epileptogenic. Other neurocutaneous syndromes, including Sturge–Weber and neurofibromatosis, are also associated with epilepsy.

Diagnostic pitfalls

Epilepsy is the clinical event associated with an underlying excessive and abnormal neuronal discharge. Two or more seizures that are not initiated by an immediately identifiable cause are usually required for diagnosis. Some manifestations of epilepsy may be behavioural and difficult to distinguish from non-epileptic behaviours. Temporal lobe seizures can produce a variety from limited tics and stereotypies through to complete motor automatisms and psychosis-like behaviour. On the other hand many abrupt-onset voluntary and involuntary behaviours may be misinterpreted as epileptic in nature, for example aggressive outbursts and nystagmus. Conversely, during the peri-ictal period, continuing subclinical epileptiform activity can cause confusion and aggression. The most useful aid to correct diagnosis is high-quality clinical observation and description of the seizures. Imaging (especially MRI) may be useful in some cases to detect specific brain lesions. In LD practice the acquisition of an electroencephalograph is common, but it needs careful and specialist interpretation to be useful,

and it is often affected by frequently prescribed psychotropic medications.

Treatments

Treatment of the multiple forms of epilepsy may be difficult. Carbamazepine and valproate remain the usual mainstays in clinical LD practice. They are also useful where a mood disorder coexists with epilepsy. Phenytoin is now less widely prescribed, but still useful in difficult cases; its therapeutic window is narrow, and an apparently increased seizure rate may be due to too high as well as too low a level. A host of newer antiepileptic drugs are now available and often very helpful in adjunctive control of refractory partial epilepsy (and some as monotherapies). Vigabatrin is known to be associated with visual field defects and only used if all other lines of therapy have failed. The psychiatrist should be aware that typical neuroleptics will reduce the seizure threshold, and atypicals have a variable effect. They are in no way contraindicated but cautious prescribing must be observed. A brief resumé of current treatments is given in Table 24.12.

Antiepileptics should all be used only with full knowledge of their possible interactions with each other and with other therapies. Status attacks or serial repeated seizures are a medical emergency. Rectal diazepam will usually control the situation, but intravenous benzodiazepines (diazepam or lorazepam) may be needed (used in a hospital with full resuscitation facilities) and oxygen required for cyanosis. Midazolam as a nasal or intra-oral spray has been shown to be effective in controlling status in children, but is not yet licensed in the UK for adults. It offers the promise of an easier and much less invasive route for control. Paraldehyde still has a place in some paediatric settings. Overall the management of complex epilepsy associated with LD is best done by specialist epilepsy services for people with LD, which have been successfully established with clinics based in health centres or

Table 24.12 General guide to seizure disorders and their therapies			
Seizure group	Subtypes	Typical first-line medications	Typical adjunctive medications
Generalised seizure group	Tonic–clonic	Carbamazepine Valproate Lamotrigine Phenytoin	
	Absence (petit mal)	Valproate Ethosuximide	
	Myoclonic	Valproate Lamotrigine Clonazepam Ethosuximide	
	Atypical absence, tonic, atonic (usually children)	Valproate Phenytoin Lamotrigine Clonazepam Ethosuximide	
Partial (or focal or localised) seizure group	Simple and complex	Carbamazepine Valproate Lamotrigine Phenytoin	Topiramate Tiagabine Gabapentin Levtiracetam (Vigabatrin)

general practices. The psychiatrist in LD with extensive experience of epilepsy management often has a lead role in developing these.

THE FUTURE FOR THE PSYCHIATRIST IN LEARNING DISABILITY

The changing nature of psychiatry of LD

The era of large hospital facilities for people with LD is now rapidly drawing to a close. This is to the benefit of our patients — one bald fact may sum things up: in 1971, single wards in a Scottish large hospital held up to 86 men. Today the maximum ward size in the same service is eight (and this is probably at the upper limit of what is reasonable). The current recommendation is four treatment and assessment beds for every 100 000 population — a huge difference from the thousands of beds that previously existed. Of all the psychiatric disciplines, we have turned from being the most hospital based to the most community based. This has seen a major shift in the psychiatrist's role — no longer can we be the 'generalist' for all our patients, controlling every part of their lives from near birth to death. The place is now in the specialist management of psychiatric and behavioural disorders associated with LD. There may even be a need for subspecialisms — in forensic aspects of LD, in the problems of ageing, the difficulties of autism and especially the psychiatry of children with LD. There is probably little need for involvement in the management of physical problems of people with LD. Profound multiple disability (previously 'profound special needs') with severe cortical sensory impairment, quadriplegia, feeding difficulties (through to parenteral gastric feeding) and complex epilepsy may all be better managed by professionals with training in physical and rehabilitation medicine. In saying this, however, there are still too few interested or skilled in working with such adults, whose numbers are rising with the much reduced child mortality. LD psychiatrists may have an educational function here and also to general hospital medicine, which increasingly cares for adults with LD. Liaison psychiatric services for LD already exist in some areas, have been welcomed and made an impact where they exist, and should develop further.

The changing locus of care

Smaller domestic-type environments are beneficial to all people with LD, no matter the severity; and, for people with mild disabilities, proper social skills training and support systems can allow many to live in unstaffed or minimally staffed accommodation — in other words their own homes. In fact the hospital population was always a small percentage of those with LD, and most people have always lived in the community. What is now apparent is a community movement of young adults away from families to stay in their own homes or homes with staffed support. Day care is also changing from the large adult training or resource centre to individualised work and support projects. Social work's function is altering; no longer are they the main direct care support service given that the voluntary and private sector is increasing substantially. Community care is much more costly than hospital care, and the current trend to smaller or single-person units even more so. There is also a danger that the cost of care for individuals with very severe behavioural difficulties may swamp finite local resources. Placement breakdown in such cases is a

major factor in readmission to hospital and one source of bed blocking as community services struggle to find an alternative. With restricted LD capacity, general psychiatric services or resources may by default become increasingly involved in the care of people with mild LD. The psychiatrist is usually now part (not necessarily the lead) in a community LD team. Other professions — social work, clinical psychology, speech and language therapy, physiotherapy, occupational therapy, and dietetics — are all as important as psychiatry and nursing, and more and more are forming subspecialties within their own disciplines. The team is more often based at a locality general practice than a hospital, and interaction between primary care and LD psychiatry has markedly increased.

The changing nature of LD

Perhaps the most important change with relevance to psychiatry is our increasing understanding of the basic processes and conditions that lead to LD. The very rapid pace of change should lead to new prognostic and therapeutic understandings. In some ways the psychiatrist in LD is still the true generalist; thousands of conditions lead to the cognitive outcomes in his or her patients. The delineation and study of the natural histories and individual trajectories of these conditions is the next step for us.

REFERENCES

AAMR 1992 Mental retardation: definition, classification and systems of supports. American Association on Mental Retardation, Washington, DC

Allingham-Hawkins D J, Babul-Hirji R, Chitayat D et al 1999 Fragile X premutation is a significant risk factor for premature ovarian failure: the International Collaborative POF in Fragile X study—preliminary data. American Journal of Medical Genetics 83:322–325

American Academy of Pediatrics 2000 Committee on Substance Abuse and Committee on Children With Disabilities. Fetal alcohol syndrome and alcohol-related neurodevelopmental disorders. Pediatrics 106:358–361

APA 2000 Diagnostic and statistical manual of mental disorders: DSM-IV, Text revision. American Psychiatric Association, Washington, DC

Armstrong D D 2002 Neuropathology of Rett syndrome. Mental Retardation & Developmental Disability Research Review 8:72–76

Avner P, Heard E 2001 X-chromosome inactivation: counting, choice and initiation. Nature Reviews Genetics 2:59 67

Aylward E H, Minshew N J, Goldstein G et al 1999a MRI volumes of amygdala and hippocampus in non-mentally retarded autistic adolescents and adults. Neurology 53:2145–2150

Aylward, E H, Li Q, Honeycutt N A et al 1999b MRI volumes of the hippocampus and amygdala in adults with Down's syndrome with and without dementia. American Journal of Psychiatry 156:564–568

Bailey D B Jr, Hatton D D, Skinner M 1998 Early developmental trajectories of males with fragile X syndrome. American Journal on Mental Retardation 103:29–39

Bailey D B Jr, Hatton D D, Skinner M, Mesibov G 2001 Autistic behavior, FMR1 protein, and developmental trajectories in young males with fragile X syndrome. Journal of Autism & Developmental Disorders 31:165–174

Ballinger C B 1997 Affective disorders. In: Read S T (ed) Psychiatry in learning disability. W B Saunders, London, p 216–236

Barron P, Hassiotis A, Banes J 2002 Offenders with intellectual disability: the size of the problem and therapeutic outcomes. Journal of Intellectual Disability Research 46:454–463

Bauman M, Kemper T L 1985 Histoanatomic observations of the brain in early infantile autism. Neurology 35:866–874

Bennetto L, Pennington B F, Porter D et al 2001 Profile of cognitive functioning in women with the fragile X mutation. Neuropsychology 15:290–299

Blair C, Ramey C T, Hardin J M 1995 Early intervention for low birthweight, premature infants: participation and intellectual development. American Journal on Mental Retardation 99:542–554

Blanchard R, Watson M S, Choy A et al 1999 Pedophiles: mental retardation, maternal age, and sexual orientation. Archives of Sexual Behavior 28:111–127

Blue M E, Naidu S, Johnston M V 1999 Development of amino acid receptors in frontal cortex from girls with Rett syndrome. Annals of Neurology 45:541–545

Boddaert N, Zilbovicius M 2002 Functional neuroimaging and childhood autism. Pediatric Radiology 32:1–7

Boer H, Holland A, Whittington J et al 2002 Psychotic illness in people with Prader Willi syndrome due to chromosome 15 maternal uniparental disomy. Lancet 359:135–136

Bouchard T J Jr, Lykken D T, McGue M et al 1990 Sources of human psychological differences: the Minnesota Study of Twins Reared Apart. Science 250:223–228

Brown V, Jin P, Ceman S et al 2001 Microarray identification of FMRP-associated brain mRNAs and altered mRNA translational profiles in fragile X syndrome. Cell 107:477–487

Burd L, Fisher W, Vesely B N et al 1991 Prevalence of psychoactive drug use among North Dakota group home residents. American Journal on Mental Retardation 96:119–126

Burt D B, Loveland K A, Lewis K R 1992 Depression and the onset of dementia in adults with mental retardation. American Journal on Mental Retardation 96:502–511

Buxbaum J D, Silverman J M, Smith C J et al 2001 Evidence for a susceptibility gene for autism on chromosome 2 and for genetic heterogeneity. American Journal of Human Genetics 68:1514–1520

Byrne P J 2000 Philosophical and ethical problems in mental handicap. Macmillan, Basingstoke

Campbell F A, Ramey C T 1995 Cognitive and school outcomes for high-risk African-American students at middle adolescence. American Educational Research Journal 32:743–772

Carlson C, Papolos D, Pandita R K et al 1997 Molecular analysis of velo-cardio-facial syndrome patients with psychiatric disorders. American Journal of Human Genetics 60:851–859

Chelly J, Mandel J L 2001 Monogenic causes of X-linked mental retardation. Nature Reviews Genetics 2:669–680

Cherry K E, Penn D, Matson J L, Bamburg J W 2000 Characteristics of schizophrenia among persons with severe or profound mental retardation. Psychiatric Services 51:922–924

Chicoine B, McGuire D, Rubin S S 1998 Specialty clinic perspectives. In: Janicki M P, Dalton A J (eds) Dementia, aging, and intellectual disabilities: a handbook. Brunner-Mazel, Philadelphia, p 278–293

Childs B 2001 The inborn error and biochemical individuality. In: Scriver C R et al (eds) The metabolic & molecular bases of inherited disease. McGraw-Hill, New York, p 129–153

Chiurazzi P, Neri G 2001 Pharmacological reactivation of inactive genes: the fragile X experience. Brain Research Bulletin 56:383–387

Chow E W, Mikulis D J, Zipursky R B et al 1999 Qualitative MRI findings in adults with 22q11 deletion syndrome and schizophrenia. Biological Psychiatry 46:1436–1442

Collacott R A, Cooper S A, McGrother C 1992 Differential rates of psychiatric disorders in adults with Down's syndrome compared with other mentally handicapped adults. British Journal of Psychiatry 161:671–674

Committee on Nervous System Disorders in Developing Countries 2001 Neurological, psychiatric and developmental disorders: meeting the challenge in the developing world. Institute of Medicine, Washington, DC

Cook E H Jr, Lindgren B, Leventhal B L et al 1997 Autism or atypical autism in maternally but not paternally derived proximal 15q duplication. American Journal of Human Genetics 60:928–934

Cooper S A 1999a The relationship between psychiatric and physical health in elderly people with intellectual disability. Journal of Intellectual Disability Research 43:54–60

Cooper S A 1999b Psychiatric disorders in elderly people with developmental disabilities. In: Bouras N (ed) Psychiatric and behavioural disorders in developmental disabilities and mental retardation. Cambridge University Press, Cambridge, p 212–225

Cooper S A, Collacott R A 1993 Mania and Down's syndrome. British Journal of Psychiatry 162:739–743

Cooper S A, Duggirala C, Collacott R A 1995 Adaptive behaviour after schizophrenia in people with Down's syndrome. Journal of Intellectual Disability Research 39:201–204

Costello H, Moss S, Prosser H, Hatton C 1997 Reliability of the ICD 10 version of the Psychiatric Assessment Schedule for Adults with Developmental Disability (PAS-ADD). Social Psychiatry & Psychiatric Epidemiology 32:339–343

Couvert P, Bienvenu T, Aquaviva C et al 2001 MECP2 is highly mutated in X-linked mental retardation. Human Molecular Genetics 10:941–946

Croen L A, Grether J K, Selvin S 2001 The epidemiology of mental retardation of unknown cause. Pediatrics 107:E86

Croen L A, Grether J K, Selvin S 2002 Descriptive epidemiology of autism in a California population: who is at risk? Journal of Autism & Developmental Disorders 32:217–224

Das J P, Divis B, Alexander J et al 1995 Cognitive decline due to aging among persons with Down syndrome. Research in Developmental Disabilities 16:461–478

Deb S, Braganza J 1999 Comparison of rating scales for the diagnosis of dementia in adults with Down's syndrome. Journal of Intellectual Disability Research 43:400–407

Deb S, Thomas M, Bright C 2001 Mental disorder in adults with intellectual disability 1: Prevalence of functional psychiatric illness among a community-based population aged between 16 and 64 years. Journal of Intellectual Disability Research 45:495–505

DeLong G R, Ritch C R, Burch S 2002 Fluoxetine response in children with autistic spectrum disorders: correlation with familial major affective disorder and intellectual achievement. Developmental Medicine & Child Neurology 44:652–659

Descheemaeker M J, Vogels A, Govers V et al 2002 Prader-Willi syndrome: new insights in the behavioural and psychiatric spectrum. Journal of Intellectual Disability Research 46:41–50

Dimitropoulos A, Feurer I D, Roof E 2000 Appetitive behavior, compulsivity, and neurochemistry in Prader–Willi syndrome. Mental Retardation & Developmental Disabilities Research Reviews 6:125–130

Doody G A, Johnstone E C, Sanderson T L et al 1998 'Pfropfschizophrenie' revisited Schizophrenia in people with mild learning disability. British Journal of Psychiatry 173:145–153

Doody G A, Thomson L D, Miller P, Johnstone E C 2000 Predictors of admission to a high-security hospital of people with intellectual disability with and without schizophrenia. Journal of Intellectual Disability Research 44:130–137

Došen A 2001 Developmental–dynamic relationship therapy. In: Došen A, Day K (eds) Treating mental illness and behavior disorders in children and adults with mental retardation. American Psychiatric Press, Washington, DC, p 415–427

Došen A, Day K 2001 Epidemiology, etiology and presentation of mental illness and behavior disorders in persons with mental retardation. In: Došen A, Day K (eds) Treating mental illness and behavior disorders in children and adults with mental retardation. American Psychiatric Press, Washington, DC, p 3–24

Duggan L, Brylewski J 1999 Effectiveness of antipsychotic medication in people with intellectual disability and schizophrenia: a systematic review. Journal of Intellectual Disability Research 43:94–104

Durkin M 2002 The epidemiology of developmental disabilities in low-income countries. Mental Retardation & Developmental Disabilities Research Reviews 8:206–211

Einfeld S L, Tonge B J 1996 Population prevalence of psychopathology in children and adolescents with intellectual disability, II: Epidemiological findings. Journal of Intellectual Disability Research 40:99–109

Eliez S, Blasey C M, Freund L S et al 2001 Brain anatomy, gender and IQ in children and adolescents with fragile X syndrome. Brain 124:1610–1618

Endicott J, Spitzer R L 1978 A diagnostic interview: the schedule for affective disorders and schizophrenia. Archives of General Psychiatry 35:837–844

Epstein C J 2001 Down syndrome (trisomy 21). In: Scriver C R et al (eds) The metabolic & molecular bases of inherited disease. McGraw-Hill, New York, p 1223–1256

Evans D W, Gray F L 2000 Compulsive-like behavior in individuals with Down syndrome: its relation to mental age level, adaptive and maladaptive behavior. Child Development 71:288–300

Fisch G S, Simensen R J, Schroer R J 2002 Longitudinal changes in cognitive and adaptive behavior scores in children and adolescents with the fragile X mutation or autism. Journal of Autism & Developmental Disorders 32:107–114

Folstein S E, Rosen-Sheidley B 2001 Genetics of autism: complex aetiology for a heterogeneous disorder. Nature Reviews Genetics 2:943–955

Fombonne E 1999 The epidemiology of autism: a review. Psychological Medicine 29:769–786

Fraser W I 2002 Forensic learning disabilities: the evidence base. Executive summary. Journal of Intellectual Disability Research 46(suppl 1):1–5

Gaedt C 1995 Psychotherapeutic approaches in the treatment of mental illness and behavioural disorders in mentally retarded people: the significance of a psychoanalytic perspective. Journal of Intellectual Disability Research 39:233–239

Gallagher R C, Pils B, Albalwi M, Francke U 2002 Evidence for the role of PWCR1/HBH-85 C/D box small nucleolar RNAs in Prader–Willi syndrome. American Journal of Human Genetics 71:669–678

Gecz J 2000 The FMR2 gene, FRAXE and non-specific X-linked mental retardation: clinical and molecular aspects. Annals of Human Genetics 64:95–106

Girard M, Couvert P, Carrie A et al 2001 Parental origin of de novo MECP2 mutations in Rett syndrome. European Journal of Human Genetics 9:231–236

Gissler M, Hemminki E, Louhiala P, Jarvelin M R 1998 Health registers as a feasible means of measuring health status in childhood—a 7-year follow-up of the 1987 Finnish birth cohort. Paediatric & Perinatal Epidemiology 12:437–455

Greenough W T, Klintsova A Y, Irwin S A et al 2001 Synaptic regulation of protein synthesis and the fragile X protein. Proceedings of the National Academy of Sciences of the USA 98:7101–7106

Haddow J E, Palomaki G E, Allan W C et al 1999 Maternal thyroid deficiency during pregnancy and subsequent neuropsychological development of the child. New England Journal of Medicine 341:549–555

Hagberg B 2002 Clinical manifestations and stages of Rett syndrome. Mental Retardation & Developmental Disabilities Research Reviews 8:61–65

Hagerman R J, Leehey M, Heinrichs W et al 2001 Intention tremor, parkinsonism, and generalized brain atrophy in male carriers of fragile X. Neurology 57:127–130

Hall S, Oliver C, Murphy G 2001 Self-injurious behaviour in young children with Lesch–Nyhan syndrome. Developmental Medicine & Child Neurology 43:745–749

Hammer S, Dorrani N, Dragich J et al 2002 The phenotypic consequences of MECP2 mutations extend beyond Rett syndrome. Mental Retardation & Developmental Disabilities Research Reviews 8:94–98

Happé F 2000 In: Baron-Cohen S, Tager-Flusberg H, Cohen D (eds) Understanding other minds: perspectives from autism and developmental cognitive neuroscience. Oxford University Press, Oxford, 203–221

Hardan A Y, Minshew N J, Harenski K, Keshavan M S 2001 Posterior fossa magnetic resonance imaging in autism. Journal of the American Academy of Child & Adolescent Psychiatry 40:666–672

Hare D J, Gould J, Mills R, Wing L 2000 A preliminary study of individuals with autistic spectrum disorders in three special hospitals in England. National Autistic Society, London

Harmon R J, Bender B G, Linden M G, Robinson A 1998 Transition from adolescence to early adulthood: adaptation and psychiatric status of women with 47,XXX. Journal of the American Academy of Child & Adolescent Psychiatry 37:286–291

Hassold T, Sherman S, Hunt P 2000 Counting cross-overs: characterizing meiotic recombination in mammals. Human Molecular Genetics 9:2409–2419

Haxby J V 1989 Neuropsychological evaluation of adults with Down's syndrome: patterns of selective impairment in non-demented old adults. Journal of Mental Deficiency Research 33:193–210

Henricksen L A, Tom S, Liu Y, Bambara R A 2000 Inhibition of flap endonuclease 1 by flap secondary structure and relevance to repeat sequence expansion. Journal of Biological Chemistry 275:16420–16427

Hetzel B S 1988 Iodine-deficiency disorders. Lancet i:1386–1387

Hillman M A, Gecz J 2001 Fragile XE-associated familial mental retardation protein 2 (FMR2) acts as a potent transcription activator. Journal of Human Genetics 46:251–259

Holling E E, Leviton A 1999 Characteristics of cranial ultrasound white-matter echolucencies that predict disability: a review. Developmental Medicine & Child Neurology 41:136–139

Hollins S, Esterhuyzen A 1997 Bereavement and grief in adults with learning disabilities. British Journal of Psychiatry 170:497–501

Horn J M, Loehlin J C, Willerman L 1979 Intellectual resemblance among adoptive and biological relatives: the Texas adoption project. Behavior Genetics 9:177–201

Hou J W, Wang T R, Chuang S M 1998 An epidemiological and aetiological study of children with intellectual disability in Taiwan. Journal of Intellectual Disability Research 42:137–143

Hurley A D, Sovner R 1995 Six cases of patients with mental retardation who have antisocial personality disorder. Psychiatric Services 46:828–831

Hyett J, Perdu M, Sharland G et al 1999 Using fetal nuchal translucency to screen for major congenital cardiac defects at 10–14 weeks of gestation: population based cohort study. British Medical Journal 318:81–85

International Molecular Genetic Study of Autism Consortium 2001 A genomewide screen for autism: strong evidence for linkage to chromosomes 2q, 7q, and 16p. American Journal of Human Genetics 69:570–581

Isaacs E B, Lucas A, Chong W K et al 2000 Hippocampal volume and everyday memory in children of very low birth weight. Pediatric Research 47:713–720

Islam S, Durkin M S, Zaman S S 1993 Socioeconomic status and the prevalence of mental retardation in Bangladesh. Mental Retardation 31:412–417

Janicki M P, Davidson P W, Henderson CM et al 2002 Health characteristics and health services utilization in older adults with intellectual disability living in community residences. Journal of Intellectual Disability Research 46:287–298

Jenkins R 1998 Culture, classification and (in)competence. In: Jenkins R (ed) Questions of competence: culture, classification and intellectual disability. Cambridge University Press, Cambridge, p 1–24

Jiang Y, Lev-Lehman E, Bressler J 1999 Genetics of Angelman syndrome. American Journal of Human Genetics 65:1–6

Jopp D A, Keys C B 2001 Diagnostic overshadowing reviewed and reconsidered. American Journal on Mental Retardation 106:416–433

Kent L, Evans J, Paul M, Sharp M 1999 Comorbidity of autistic spectrum disorders in children with Down syndrome. Developmental Medicine & Child Neurology 41:153–158

King B H, Hodapp R M, Dykens E M 2000a Mental retardation. In: Sadock B J, Sadock V A (eds) Kaplan & Sadock's comprehensive textbook of psychiatry. Lippincott Williams & Wilkins, Philadelphia, p 2587–2613

King R, Fay G, Croghan P 2000b Rapid cycling bipolar disorder in individuals with developmental disabilities. Mental Retardation 38:253–261

Klauck S M, Lindsay S, Beyer K S et al 2002 A mutation hot spot for nonspecific X-linked mental retardation in the MECP2 gene causes the PPM-X syndrome. American Journal of Human Genetics 70:1034–1037

Krinsky-McHale S J, Devenny D A, Silverman W P 2002 Changes in explicit memory associated with early dementia in adults with Down's syndrome. Journal of Intellectual Disability Research 46:198–208

Kroese, B S 1997 Cognitive-behaviour therapy for people with learning disabilities: conceptual and contextual issues. In: Kroese B S, Dagnan D, Loumidis K (eds) Cognitive-behaviour therapy for people with learning disabilities. Routledge, London, p 1–15

Lawlor, B A, McCarron, M, Wilson, G, McLoughlin M 2001 Temporal lobe-oriented CT scanning and dementia in Down's syndrome. International Journal of Geriatric Psychiatry 16:427–429

Leonard H, Wen X 2002 The epidemiology of mental retardation: challenges and opportunities in the new millennium. Mental Retardation & Developmental Disability Research Review 8:117–134

Leonard H, Petterson B, Bower C, Sanders R 2003 Prevalence of intellectual disability in Western Australia. Paediatric & Perinatal Epidemiology 17:58–67

Lindee M S 2000 Genetic disease since 1945. Nature Reviews Genetics 1:236–241

Lindsay W R, Law J, Quinn K 2001 A comparison of physical and sexual abuse: histories of sexual and non-sexual offenders with intellectual disability. Child Abuse & Neglect 25:989–995

Ludlow J R, Allen L M 1979 The effect of early intervention and pre-school stimulus on the development of the Down's syndrome child. Journal of Mental Deficiency Research 23:29–44

McCracken J T, McGough J, Shah B et al 2002 Risperidone in children with autism and serious behavioral problems. New England Journal of Medicine 347:314–321

McDermid H E, Morrow B E 2002 Genomic disorders on 22q11. American Journal of Human Genetics 70:1077–1088

MacMillan D L, Gresham F M, Siperstein G N 1995 Heightened concerns over the 1992 AAMR definition: advocacy versus precision. American Journal on Mental Retardation 10:87–95

McNamara J O 1999 Emerging insights into the genesis of epilepsy. Nature 399:A15–22

Malter H E, IBer J C, Willemson R et al 1997 Characterization of the full fragile X syndrome mutation in fetal gametes. Nature Genetics 15:165–169

Margolis R L, McInnis M G, Rosenblatt A, Ross C A 1999 Trinucleotide repeat expansion and neuropsychiatric disease. Archives of General Psychiatry 56:1019–1031

Marti E, Bovolenta P 2002 Sonic hedgehog in CNS development: one signal, multiple outputs. Trends in Neurosciences 25:89–96

Masi G, Favilla L, Mucci M 2000 Generalized anxiety disorder in adolescents and young adults with mild mental retardation. Psychiatry 63:54–64

Matson J L, Gardner W I, Coe D A, Sovner R 1991 A scale for evaluating emotional disorders in severely and profoundly mentally retarded persons. Development of the Diagnostic Assessment for the Severely Handicapped (DASH) scale. British Journal of Psychiatry 159:404–409

Matson J L, Benavidez D A, Compton L S et al 1996 Behavioral treatment of autistic persons: a review of research from 1980 to the present. Research in Developmental Disabilities 17:433–465

Matte T D, Bresnahan M, Begg M D, Susser E 2001 Influence of variation in birth weight within normal range and within sibships on IQ at age 7 years: cohort study. British Medical Journal 323:310–314

Mazzocco M M 2000 Advances in research on the fragile X syndrome. Mental Retardation & Developmental Disabilities Research Reviews 6:96–106

Meadows G, Turner T, Campbell L et al 1991 Assessing schizophrenia in adults with mental retardation: a comparative study. British Journal of Psychiatry 158:103–105

Mervis C B, Klein-Tasman B P 2000 Williams syndrome: cognition, personality, and adaptive behaviour. Mental Retardation & Developmental Disabilities Research Reviews 6:148–158

Miller J F, Leddy M, Leavitt L A 1999 Improving the communication of people with Down syndrome. Paul H Brookes, Baltimore

Miller W J, Skinner J A, Foss G S, Davies K E 2000 Localization of the fragile X mental retardation 2 (FMR2) protein in mammalian brain. European Journal of Neuroscience 12:381–384

Mors O, Mortensen P B, Ewald H 2001 No evidence of increased risk for schizophrenia or bipolar affective disorder in persons with aneuploidies of the sex chromosomes. Psychological Medicine 31:425–430

Muenke M, Beachy P A 2001 Holoprosencephaly In: Scriver C R et al (eds) The metabolic & molecular bases of inherited disease. McGraw-Hill, New York, p 6203–6230

Muir W J 1998 Learning disability. In: Johnstone E C, Freeman C P, Zealley A K (eds) Companion to psychiatric studies, 6th edn. Churchill Livingstone, Edinburgh, p 597–647

Muir W J, Squire I, Blackwood D H et al 1988 Auditory P300 response in the assessment of Alzheimer's disease in Down's syndrome: a 2-year follow-up study. Journal of Mental Deficiency Research 32:455–463

Murphy K C, Owen M J 2001 Velo-cardio-facial syndrome: a model for understanding the genetics and pathogenesis of schizophrenia. British Journal of Psychiatry 179:397–402

Murphy K C, Jones L A, Owen M J 1999 High rates of schizophrenia in adults with velo-cardio-facial syndrome. Archives of General Psychiatry 56:940–945

Myers B A, Pueschel S M 1991 Psychiatric disorders in persons with Down syndrome. Journal of Nervous & Mental Disease 179:609–613

Myers B A, Pueschel S M 1995 Major depression in a small group of adults with Down syndrome. Research in Developmental Disabilities 16:285–299

Nagle R J, Bell N L 1995 Clinical utility of Kaufman's "amazingly" short forms of the WAIS-R with educable mentally retarded adolescents. Journal of Clinical Psychology 51:396–400

Nyhan W L 1997 The recognition of Lesch–Nyhan syndrome as an inborn error of purine metabolism. Journal of Inherited Metabolic Diseases 20:171–178

O'Brien G 2002 Dual diagnosis in offenders with intellectual disability: setting research priorities: a review of research findings concerning psychiatric disorder (excluding personality disorder) among offenders with intellectual disability. Journal of Intellectual Disability Research 46(suppl 1):21–30

Oliver P C, Piachaud J, Done J et al 2002 Difficulties in conducting a randomized controlled trial of health service interventions in intellectual disability: implications for evidence-based practice. Journal of Intellectual Disability Research 46:340–345

Online Mendelian Inheritance in Man. http://wwwncbinimnihgov/omim/

Osterling J A, Dawson G, Munson J A 2002 Early recognition of 1-year-old infants with autism spectrum disorder versus mental retardation. Development & Psychopathology 14:239–251

Ozonoff S, South M, Miller J N 2000 Asperger disorder: cognitive, behavioral, and early history differentiation from high-functioning autism. Autism: the International Journal of Research & Practice 4:29–46

Percy M E, Dalton A J, Marcovich V D et al 1990 Autoimmune thyroiditis associated with mild "subclinical" hypothyroidism in adults with Down syndrome: a comparison of patients with and without manifestations of Alzheimer disease. American Journal of Medical Genetics 36:148–154

Pericak-Vance M A 2002 The genetics of autism. In: Plomin R, DeFries J C, Craig I W, McGuffin P (eds) Behavioral genetics in the postgenomic era APA Books, Washington, DC, p 267–288

Petrij F, Giles R H, Breuning M H, Hennekam R C M 2001 Rubenstein–Taybi syndrome. In: Scriver C R et al (eds) The metabolic & molecular bases of inherited disease. McGraw-Hill, New York, p 6167–6182

Posthuma D, De Geus E J, Baare W F et al 2002 The association between brain volume and intelligence is of genetic origin. Nature Neuroscience 5:83–84

Prasher V P 1995 Prevalence of psychiatric disorders in adults with Down's syndrome. European Journal of Psychiatry 9:77–82

Prasher V P, Day S 1995 Brief report: obsessive–compulsive disorder in adults with Down's Syndrome. Journal of Autism & Developmental Disorders 25:453–458

Prasher V P, Hall W 1996 Short-term prognosis of depression in adults with Down's syndrome: association with thyroid status and effects on adaptive behaviour. Journal of Intellectual Disability Research 40:32–38

Prasher V P, Huxley A, Haque M S 2002 A 24-week, double-blind, placebo-controlled trial of donepezil in patients with Down syndrome and Alzheimer's disease—pilot study. International Journal of Geriatric Psychiatry 17:270–278

Read S G 1997 Organic behaviour disorder. In: Read S G (ed) Psychiatry in learning disability. W B Saunders, London, p 129–149

Reid A H 1972 Psychoses in adult mental defectives. I: Manic depressive psychosis. British Journal of Psychiatry 120:205–212

Reid A H, Ballinger B R 1987 Personality disorder in mental handicap. Psychological Medicine 17:983–987

Rice D S, Curran T 2001 Role of the reelin signaling pathway in central nervous system development. Annual Review of Neuroscience 24:1005–1039

Roeleveld N, Zielhuis G A, Gabreels F 1997 The prevalence of mental retardation: a critical review of recent literature. Developmental Medicine & Child Neurology 39:125–132

Rogers S J, Wehner D E, Hagerman R 2001 The behavioral phenotype in fragile X: symptoms of autism in very young children with fragile X syndrome, idiopathic autism, and other developmental disorders. Journal of Developmental & Behavioral Pediatrics 22:409–417

Roizen N J 2001 Down syndrome: progress in research. Mental Retardation & Developmental Disabilities Research Reviews 7:38–44

Ross M E, Walsh C A 2001 Human brain malformations and their lessons for neuronal migration. Annual Review of Neuroscience 24:1041–1070

Rousseau F, Rouillard P, Morel M L 1995 Prevalence of carriers of premutation-size alleles of the FMRI gene—and implications for the population genetics of the fragile X syndrome. American Journal of Human Genetics 57:1006–1018

Royal College of Psychiatrists 2001 DC-LD Diagnostic criteria for psychiatric disorders for use with adults with learning disabilties/mental retardation. Royal College of Psychiatrists/Gaskell, London

Ruedrich S, Noyers-Hurley A D, Sovner R 2001 Treating mental illness and behavior disorders in children and adults with mental retardation. In: Došen A, Day K (eds) Treating mental illness and behavior disorders in children and adults with mental retardation. American Psychiatric Press, Washington, DC, p 201–226

Sanderson T L, Best J J, Doody G A et al 1999 Neuroanatomy of comorbid schizophrenia and learning disability: a controlled study. Lancet 354:1867–1871

Sanderson T L, Doody G A, Best J et al 2001 Correlations between clinical and historical variables, and cerebral structural variables in people with mild intellectual disability and schizophrenia. Journal of Intellectual Disability Research 45:89–98

Schendel D E, Schuchat A, Thorsen P 2002 Public health issues related to infection in pregnancy and cerebral palsy. Mental Retardation & Developmental Disabilities Research Reviews 8:39–45

Schupf N, Sergievsky G H 2002 Genetic and host factors for dementia in Down's syndrome. British Journal of Psychiatry 180:405–410

Schupf N, Patel B, Silverman W et al 2001 Elevated plasma amyloid beta-peptide 1–42 and onset of dementia in adults with Down syndrome. Neuroscience Letters 301:199–203

Scola P S, Pueschel S M 1992 Menstrual cycles and basal body temperature curves in women with Down syndrome. Obstetrics & Gynecology 79:91–94

Sears L L, Vest C, Mohamed S et al 1999 An MRI study of the basal ganglia in autism. Progress in Neuropsychopharmacology & Biological Psychiatry 23:613–624

Senatore V, Matson J L, Kazdin A E 1985 An inventory to assess psychopathology of mentally retarded adults. American Journal of Mental Deficiency 89:459–466

Shepperson B 1995a Two longitudinal studies of the abilities of people with Down's syndrome. Journal of Intellectual Disability Research 39:419–431

Shepperson B 1995b The control of sexuality in young people with Down's syndrome. Child: Care, Health & Development 21:333–349

Siegal M, Varley R 2002 Neural systems involved in "theory of mind". Nature Reviews Neuroscience 3:463–471

Sinason V 1992 Mental handicap and the human condition. Free Association Books, London

Smith S, Branford D, Collacott R A et al 1996 Prevalence and cluster typology of maladaptive behaviors in a geographically defined population of adults with learning disabilities. British Journal of Psychiatry 169:219–227

Stavrakaki C 1999 Depression, anxiety and adjustment disorders in people with developmental disabilities. In: Bouras N (ed) Psychiatric and behavioural disorders in developmental disabilities and mental retardation. Cambridge University Press, Cambridge, p 175–187

Stromme P, Magnus P 2000 Correlations between socioeconomic status, IQ and aetiology in mental retardation: a population-based study of Norwegian children. Social Psychiatry & Psychiatric Epidemiology 35:12–18

Su J H, Kesslak J P, Head E, Cotman C W 2002 Caspase-cleaved amyloid precursor protein and activated caspase-3 are co-localized in the granules of granulovacuolar degeneration in Alzheimer's disease and Down's syndrome brain. Acta Neuropathologica (Berlin) 104:1–6

Sutherland G R, Baker E 2000 The clinical significance of fragile sites on human chromosomes. Clinical Genetics 58:157–161

Tager-Flusberg H 2001 A re-examination of the theory of mind hypothesis of autism. In: Burack J, Charman T, Yirmiya N et al (eds) The development of autism: perspectives from research and theory. Erlbaum, Mahwah, NJ p 173–193

Tamm L, Menon V, Johnston C K et al 2002 fMRI study of cognitive interference processing in females with fragile X syndrome. Journal of Cognitive Neuroscience 14:160–171

Tangye S R 1979 The EEG and incidence of epilepsy in Down's syndrome. Journal of Mental Deficiency Research 23:17–24

Teller J K, Russo C, DeBusk L M et al 1996 Presence of soluble amyloid beta-peptide precedes amyloid plaque formation in Down's syndrome. Nature Medicine 2:93–95

Temple V, Jozsvai E, Konstantareas M M, Hewitt T A 2001 Alzheimer dementia in Down's syndrome: the relevance of cognitive ability. Journal of Intellectual Disability Research 45:47–55

Thase M E, Tigner R, Smeltzer D J, Liss L 1984 Age-related neuropsychological deficits in Down's syndrome. Biological Psychiatry 19:571–585

van Amelsvoort T, Daly E, Rbertson D et al 2001 Structural brain abnormalities associated with deletion at chromosome 22q11: quantitative neuroimaging study of adults with velo-cardio-facial syndrome. British Journal of Psychiatry 178:412–419

Van Buggenhout G J, Trommelen JC, Schoenmaker A et al 1999 Down syndrome in a population of elderly mentally retarded patients: genetic-diagnostic survey and implications for medical care. American Journal of Medical Genetics 85:376–384

Van Buggenhout G J, Trommelen J C, Brunner H G et al 2001 The clinical phenotype in institutionalised adult males with X-linked mental retardation (XLMR). Annals of Genetics 44:47–55

van Praag H, Schinder AF, Christie BR et al 2002 Functional neurogenesis in the adult hippocampus. Nature 415:1030–1034

Vanstraelen M, Tyrer S P 1999 Rapid cycling bipolar affective disorder in people with intellectual disability: a systematic review. Journal of Intellectual Disability Research 43:349–359

Waite S J, Thomas N S, Barber J C 2002 Absence of 22q11 deletions in 211 patients with developmental delay analysed using PCR. Journal of Medical Genetics 39:e18

Wald N J, Watt H C, Hackshaw A K 1999 Integrated screening for Down's syndrome on the basis of tests performed during the first and second trimesters. New England Journal of Medicine 341:461–467

Wang P P, Bellugi U 1994 Evidence from two genetic syndromes for a dissociation between verbal and visual-spatial short-term memory. Journal of Clinical & Experimental Neuropsychology 16:317–322

Ward O C 1998 John Langdon Down: a caring pioneer. Royal Society of Medicine Press, London

Warren S T, Sherman S L 2001 The fragile X syndrome. In: Scriver C R et al (eds) The metabolic & molecular bases of inherited disease. McGraw-Hill, New York, p 1257–1289

WHO 1992 The ICD-10 classification of mental and behavioural disorders: Clinical descriptions and diagnostic guidelines. World Health Organization, Geneva

WHO 1993 The ICD-10 classification of mental and behavioural disorders: Diagnostic criteria for research. World Health Organization, Geneva

WHO 1996 ICD-10 guide for mental retardation. World Health Organization, Geneva

WHO 2001 International classification of functioning, disability and health. World Health Organization, Geneva

Willard H F 2001 The sex chromosomes and X chromosome inactivation. In: Scriver C R et al (eds) The metabolic & molecular bases of inherited disease. McGraw-Hill, New York, p 1191–1211

Wing L 1991 The relationship between Asperger's syndrome and Kanner's autism. In: Frith U (ed) Autism and Asperger's syndrome. Cambridge University Press, Cambridge, p 93–121

Wing L, Potter D 2002 The epidemiology of autistic spectrum disorders: is the prevalence rising? Mental Retardation & Developmental Disabilities Research Reviews 8:151–161

Wishart J G 1995 Cognitive abilities in children with Down syndrome: developmental instability and motivational deficits. In: Epstein C J, Hassold T, Lott I T et al (eds) Etiology and pathogenesis of Down syndrome. Wiley-Liss, New York, p 57–91

Wisniewski K E 2001 Pheno/genotypic correlations of neuronal ceroid lipofuscinoses. Neurology 57:576–581

Witkin H A, Mednick S A, Schulsinger F et al 1976 Criminality in XYY and XXY men. Science 193:547–555

Yang Q, Rasmussen S A, Friedman J M 2002 Mortality associated with Down's syndrome in the USA from 1983 to 1997: a population-based study. Lancet 359:1019–1025

Yu C E, Dawson G, Munson J et al 2002 Presence of large deletions in kindreds with autism. American Journal of Human Genetics 71:100–115

Zechner U, Wilda M, Kehrer-Sawatzki H et al 2001 A high density of X-linked genes for general cognitive ability: a run-away process shaping human evolution? Trends in Genetics 17:697–701

Zigman W B, Schupf N, Sersen E, Silverman W 1996 Prevalence of dementia in adults with and without Down syndrome. American Journal on Mental Retardation 100:403–412

25 | Psychiatric disorders in childhood and adolescence

Peter Hoare

This chapter has three sections: psychiatric disorders in childhood; psychiatric disorders in adolescence; and psychiatric aspects of learning disability in childhood and adolescence. Not surprisingly, there is considerable overlap and continuity between childhood and adolescence, so that disorders with an adolescent predominance will be discussed in the second section of the chapter.

PSYCHIATRIC DISORDERS IN CHILDHOOD

INTRODUCTION

Child psychiatry is concerned with the assessment and treatment of children's emotional and behavioural problems. These problems are very common, with prevalence rates of 10–20% in several community studies. The majority of disturbed children are not seen by specialist psychiatric services but by general practitioners, community doctors and paediatricians along with other professionals such as teachers and residential care staff. Consequently, knowledge about the range and variety of emotional and behavioural problems shown by children is important for all doctors involved in the care of children. The everyday work of the paediatrician provides clear evidence of the stressful effects of illness on the psychological well-being and adjustment of children and their families.

For the psychiatrist in training, knowledge of child development and experience in child psychiatry are important for several reasons. First, it demonstrates that childhood experiences are influential in the development of the adult personality. Second, it provides an explanation for the continuity or discontinuity of psychopathology between childhood and adult life. Third, it shows the ways in which parental psychiatric illness can adversely affect the child's development. The last can happen either directly through the effects on the parent–child relationship or indirectly through the child's exposure to deviant parental role models. For both these reasons, the child is at greater risk of becoming disturbed. Fourth, it provides the basis on which to evaluate the significance or otherwise of childhood experience in the development of adult psychopathology. Finally, it gives the trainee the competence to assess families and their functioning.

Psychiatric disturbance in childhood is most usefully defined as an abnormality in at least one of three areas: emotions, behaviour or relationships. It is *not* helpful to regard these abnormalities as strictly defined disease entities with a precise aetiology, treatment and prognosis. Rather, it is preferable to regard them as deviations or departures from the norm, which are distressing to the child or to those involved with his welfare. Although child psychiatric disorders do not conform to a strict medical model of illness, it does not follow that these disorders are trivial or unimportant. Some disorders such as autism or conduct disorder have major implications for the child's development and adaptation in adult life.

In childhood, the distinction between disturbance and normality is imprecise. Isolated symptoms are common and not pathological. For example, many children will occasionally feel sad, unhappy or have temper tantrums. This does not mean that they are disturbed. Disturbance is characterised by the number, frequency, severity and duration of symptoms rather than by the type of symptomatology. In addition, disturbed children rarely present with unequivocal pathological symptoms such as hallucinations or delusions, whereas symptoms such as unhappiness and lying are common and not diagnostic. In clinical practice, it is often more important to establish why the child is the focus for concern rather than to adopt the more narrow perspective of whether the child is disturbed or not.

Another important feature of psychiatric disturbance in childhood is that several, as opposed to single, factors contribute to the development of disturbance. This makes assessment and treatment more difficult, so that an essential prerequisite for successful treatment is the correct evaluation of the relative contribution of the different aetiological factors. Aetiological factors are usually categorised into two groups: constitutional and environmental. The former includes heredity factors, intelligence and temperament. The three major enviornmental influences are the family, schooling and the community. Another factor, physical illness or handicap, if present, can have a profound effect on the child's development and on his vulnerability to disturbance.

Three other considerations are of general importance in understanding children's behaviour: the situation-specific nature of behaviour; the impact of current stressful events; and the role of family. Children's behaviour varies markedly in different situations; that is, it is situation specific. For instance, a child may be a major problem at school but not at home, or vice versa. Consequently, there may well be an apparent discrepancy between accounts of the child's behaviour from parents and from teachers. The most likely explanation for this discrepancy is that the demands and expectations upon the child in the two situations are different. It is therefore essential to obtain several independent accounts about the child's behaviour wherever possible in order to derive a more accurate and realistic assessment of the problem. This situation-specific nature of the behaviour has implications for treatment, as it is important to explain to parents and to teachers the reasons for the discrepancy, thereby lessening the likelihood of misunderstanding.

Children are immature and developing individuals whose capacities and coping skills change markedly during childhood. Childhood is also a period of life characterised by change, challenge and the necessity for adaptation. Consequently it is not surprising that symptoms of disturbance may arise at times of stress when the demands on the child are excessive. Recent research (Goodyer 1990) has shown that life events are associated with an increased psychiatric morbidity among children, a finding similar to that reported for adults. Some stresses such as the birth of a sibling or starting school are of course normal and inevitable, whereas others, such as marital break-up or life-threatening illness, are serious, with long-term implications for the child's well-being.

The child may, however, cope successfully with the stress, thereby enhancing the child's self-esteem and confidence. Alternatively, the child may be overwhelmed, responding with the development of symptomatic behaviour. The latter may involve regressive behaviour (i.e. behaving in a more immature, dependent fashion) or more specifically maladaptive behaviour (e.g. aggression, excessive anxiety or withdrawal). A crucial feature of assessment is the identification of stressful factors that may be contributing to the problem, as this will influence treatment strategies and also the prognosis.

The family is the most potent force for the promotion of health as well as for the development of disturbance in the child's life. Assessment of parenting qualities, the marital relationship and the quality of family interaction are essential components of child psychiatric practice. It is a frequent observation that it is the parents who are disturbed and not the child. One consequence of this observation is that in many cases the focus of treatment is likely to be the parents, or the whole family, rather than the child. Indeed, in many instances the main emphasis of treatment is the promotion of normal healthy family interaction as much as in the amelioration of disturbed behaviour.

Finally, many disturbed children do not complain about their distress nor admit to problems, but rather it is their parents or other adults involved with their care who bring the child to the attention of professionals. Disturbed children more commonly manifest their distress or unhappiness indirectly through symptoms such as abdominal pain, aggression or withdrawal. Direct questioning of the child during the initial interview is unlikely to reveal the true extent of the child's feelings or the degree of his distress. Sensitive observations during the interview and the use of indirect techniques such as play are necessary to elicit a more accurate view of the child's feelings. This is only likely to be successful once a relationship of trust has been established between the child and the doctor.

NORMAL AND ABNORMAL PSYCHOLOGICAL DEVELOPMENT

Children are developing individuals. They are not small adults. A 2-year-old is very different to a 12-year-old, whereas an adult aged 25 may not differ that much from a 35-year-old. During childhood, the child undergoes a remarkable transformation from a helpless, dependent infant to an independent self-sufficient individual with his own views and outlook, capable of embarking on a career and living separately from his family. Knowledge about the *mechanisms*, *processes* and *sequences* underlying these events is

necessary in order to understand the nature of psychological disturbance in childhood. This knowledge also helps to define more clearly what is age-appropriate behaviour and to distinguish the pathological from the normal. This section has three parts: developmental theories, developmental psychopathology and personality development.

Developmental theories

It is useful to define some terms at the outset, as they are often used interchangeably. *Growth* refers to the incremental increase of a characteristic; *maturation* to those phases of development that are mainly due to innate or endogenous factors; and *development* to those changes in the organism's structure and behaviour that are systematically related to age. Many behaviours (for example walking and talking) have a substantial maturational component, whereas others (for instance emotional and social development) are strongly influenced by environmental factors. The continuous interaction between maturational and environmental factors throughout childhood helps to mould the personality development of the child.

Developmental theories (Table 25.1) tend to focus on at least one of the following areas: cognitive, emotional or social. They differ widely in theoretical orientation, in the supporting empirical evidence and in the relative importance attributed to experience in influencing development. No single theory is satisfactory, so that most clinicians utilise some parts of the various theories to explain different aspects of development. The theories are usually described as stage theories, implying that they regard development as a series of recognisable phases of increasing complexity through which the child progresses

Cognitive development

In 1929, the Swiss psychologist Piaget proposed a comprehensive theory of cognitive development. Many of his conclusions were based on experiments conducted on his own children over a number of years. Piaget has had a tremendous impact on educational concepts and teaching, particularly in primary schools over the last 30 years. More recently, the theoretical basis and validity of Piaget's conclusions have been questioned by further empirical studies (Bee 1999). Despite these criticisms, his views remain the most comprehensive account of cognitive development.

Piaget's theory is set within a biological framework. In order to survive, the individual must have the capacity to adapt to the demands of the environment. Cognitive development is the result of interaction between the individual and the environment. Four factors influence cognitive development: increased neurological maturation, enabling the child to appreciate new aspects of experience and to apply more complex reasoning as he gets older; the opportunity to practise newly acquired skills; the opportunity for social interaction and to benefit from schooling; and the emergence of internal psychological mechanisms or *structures* that allow the child to construct a successively more complex cognitive model based on maturation and experience.

Piaget describes two types of intellectual structure: *schemas* and *operations*. The former are present at birth, the latter arise during childhood. *Schemas* are internal representations of some specific action, for instance sucking or grasping, whereas *operations* are internal rules of a higher order which have the distinctive feature that they are *reversible*, as, for example, multiplication is reversible

Table 25.1   Summary of cognitive, emotional and social development

	Age in years				
	0	2	6	9	12+
Cognitive (Piaget)	*Sensorimotor* Differentiates self from objects Begins to act intentionally Achieves object permanence	*Pre-operational* Learns to use language and to represent objects by image and words Thinking is egocentric (unable to see other viewpoint) and animistic (everything has feelings including inanimate objects)	*Concrete operational* Thinking is more logical and less egocentric Achieves conservation of number (age 6), volume (age 7) mass (age 8) Able to arrange objects in rank order		*Formal operational* Able to think in abstract manner about propositions and hypotheses
Emotional (Freud)	*Oral* Main concern is initially with satisfaction of basic needs such as hunger Later on, attachment to caregiver	*Anal* Co-operative activity with caregiver Satisfaction with increased self-control and achievement	*Phallic* Learns to interact with peers, often leads to rivalry Aware of own sexuality causing Oedipal conflict, resolved by identification with the same sex parent Conscience begins to form	*Latency* Reduced sexual interest with main concerns about peer relationships and position within peer group	*Genital* Revival of earlier conflict, especially sexual conflict Four main tasks: separation from parents, sexual role, career choice, identity
Social & personality development	Social smiling (8 wks)	Attachment (6 mths) Stranger anxiety (10 mths)	Co-operative play (3 yrs)	Strong preference for same sex friends with stereotyped expectations (6–7 yrs)	Enduring relationships (8 yrs onwards)
	Erikson's stage of trust vs mistrust	*Erikson's stage of autonomy vs shame and doubt*	*Erikson's stage of initiative vs guilt*	*Erikson's stage of industry vs inferiority*	*Erikson's stage of identity vs role diffusion*

by division. There are two ways whereby the child adapts his cognitive structure to the demands of the environment: *assimilation* and *accommodation*. The former refers to the incorporation of new objects, thoughts and behaviour into existing structures, whereas the latter describes the change of existing structures in response to novel experiences. The child attends and learns most when his environment has a degree of novelty that challenges his curiosity but is not so strange that it becomes too confusing.

Piaget describes four main phases: *sensorimotor*, *pre-operational*, *concrete operational* and *formal operational*. The age range given for each stage is the average, though this can vary considerably depending upon intelligence, cultural background or socioeconomic factors. However, the order is assumed to be the same for all children. Schemas predominate in the sensorimotor and pre-operational stages, whereas operations predominate in the concrete operational and formal operational stages.

- *Sensorimotor stage (birth–2 years)*. Initially, behaviour is dominated by innate reflexes such as feeding, sucking or following, hence the name for this period. Gradually, the infant realises the distinction between *self* and *non-self*, namely where his body ends and the world outside begins. The infant also realises that his behaviour can influence the environment, so that intentional and purposeful behaviour begins. Finally, the infant achieves *object permanence* whereby he recognises

that an object still exists even although it is no longer visible.

- *Pre-operational stage (2–7 years)*. Language development greatly facilitates cognition, so that the individual begins to represent objects by symbols and words. Thinking is, however, *egocentric* and *animistic*. The former refers to the child's tendency to regard the world solely from his own position, along with the inability to see a situation from another point of view. Animistic thinking describes the child's tendency to regard everything in the world as endowed with feelings, thoughts or wishes. For instance, the moon is watching over you when you sleep, the child says 'naughty door' when he bangs into the door.

The child has problems with the principles of conservation for number, volume and mass. The essential principle underlying conservation is that the number, volume or mass of an object are not changed by any visual alteration in their display or appearance. For instance, the child readily believes that the more widely spaced of two rows of counters has more counters than a denser packed row, or that there is more water in a tall beaker when it has been poured there from a shorter, more squat beaker.

The child also believes that every event has a preceding cause, rejecting the concept of chance or coincidence. Again, the child's moral sense is rigid and inflexible, so that punishment is invariable, irrespective of the circumstances. The child's concept of illness is radically different to that of the adult, with illness seen as a consequence for misdeeds, a punishment for a misdemeanour.

- *Concrete operational stage (7–12 years).* Thinking becomes more logical and less dominated by immediate perceptual experience or by changes in appearance. Conservation of number, volume and mass is successively achieved during this period. The child becomes less egocentric, capable of seeing events from another person's standpoint. The child is able to appreciate and utilise reversibility, for example if 2 and 2 equals 4, then 4 minus 2 must equal 2.
- *Formal operational stage (12 years and upwards).* This stage represents the most complex mode of thinking. Its main characteristics are the ability to think in an abstract fashion, to formulate general rules and principles and to devise and test hypotheses, an approach similar to that used in mathematics or in a scientific investigation. An example of such reasoning is the following: Joan is fairer than Susan; Joan is darker than Anne. Who is the darkest? (Answer: Susan). Prior to the formal operational stage, the child would require the aid of dolls to solve this problem. It should be pointed out that not everyone achieves this stage of thinking, even as an adult! The content of thinking also alters markedly with an emphasis on the hypothetical, the future and ideological issues.

Critical comment on Piaget   Recently, the Piagetian model has been criticised extensively for the lack of evidence to support the existence of the internal structures necessary for the concrete and formal operational stages. Alternative non-Piagetian explanations for a child's inability to carry out conservation tasks successfully before a certain age have also been put forward (Matthews 1994). These criticisms are substantial, but they do not detract from the major conceptual contribution that Piaget has made to knowledge about cognitive development in children.

Recent developments in cognitive theory   Psychologists and psychiatrists have become increasingly interested in the development and application of cognitive theory to the understanding and treatment of psychiatric disorders (Hawton et al 1995, Johnstone 1998). The main principles underlying this theory are that an individual's beliefs about (a) himself, (b) the future and (c) the world influence his mood and behaviour, an idea similar in some ways to the Piagetian concept of schemas. When a person is depressed, his thoughts are self-defeating and he commits certain cognitive errors. Two common types of cognitive error are *personalisation* and *dichotomous thinking*. The following two statements are examples of these two errors respectively: 'The reason my parents separated is all because of me' and 'I'm no good at tennis, so I'm bound to be useless at any other sport'.

A major extension of these ideas in childhood is the notion of the *self-concept*. By the age of 6 or 7 years, most children have very definite and clear ideas about themselves and their qualities. For example, they are able to compare themselves to other children with respect to popularity, attractiveness, scholastic ability and so on. Self-concept is a construct similar to that of a schema in Piaget's theory. Another important facet of self-concept is the favourable or unfavourable evaluation that the child makes of himself, an aspect called *self-esteem*. Children with high self-esteem appear to do better in school, regard themselves as in control of their own destiny, have more friends and get along better with their families (Bee 1999).

Emotional and social development

Sigmund Freud developed the most comprehensive theory about emotional development, while Erikson (1965), also a psychoanalyst, applied psychoanalytic concepts within a social and cultural framework. Freudian theory emphasises the biological and maturational components of development with an invariable sequence to development for everyone. Like Piaget, it is a stage or phase theory with the individual progressing successively through each phase. A major criticism of Freudian theory is that its concepts do not lend themselves readily to scientific investigation, so that it is difficult to prove or disprove the validity of the theory.

Freud proposed that an individual goes through five stages prior to adulthood, namely *oral, anal, phallic, latency* and *genital*. These terms refer to the major developmental task or potential conflict that the individual has to achieve or resolve during this period. Table 25.1 describes the important features of the different stages; e.g. during the phallic stage, the Oedipal crisis arises. At this time (around 3–4 years), the child becomes aware of his own sexual feelings and also that he is attracted in a sexual manner to the parent of the opposite sex. Moreover, the child is simultaneously aware that the parent of the same sex is a rival for the attention of the other parent. The conflict arises because the child is caught between the desire for one parent and the wrath of the other. The conflict is successfully resolved by the child identifying with the parent of the same sex, thereby eliminating the rivalrous feelings.

Erikson's major contribution has been to place psychoanalytic concepts in a social and cultural dimension (see Table 25.1). For Erikson, the most important task for the individual is to achieve a coherent sense of identity, a balanced and mature appraisal of one's abilities and limitations, with a recognition of the importance of previous experience and with realistic expectations for the future. Such a task occupies the individual throughout his lifetime. The individual passes through a series of developmental stages, all of which are polarised into two extremes: one successful and adaptive and the other unsuccessful and maladaptive. The two poles of the first stage are *trust* and *mistrust*. The former refers to the child's belief that the world is safe, predictable, and that he can influence events towards a favourable outcome, whereas a sense of mistrust implies a world that is cruel, erratic and unable to meet his needs. The role of the caregiver, usually the mother, is crucial to the achievement of a successful outcome. Erikson also believed that the individual carries forward the residues of earlier stages into the present, thereby giving the past an influence on contemporary behaviour. Erikson's writings are a compelling and coherent account of development. A major weakness is, however, the lack of empirical evidence to support the conclusions.

Development of social relationships

A characteristic of human beings is their predisposition to establish and maintain social relationships (Bee 1999). Although Freud and Erikson refer to social relationships, it is only with the recent elaboration of *attachment theory* by Bowlby (1969) and by Ainsworth (1982) that a plausible theory for this phenomenon has been described. Attachment theory proposes that social relationships develop in response to the mutual biological and psychological needs of the mother and the infant. Mother–infant interaction promotes social relationships. Each member of the dyad has a repertoire of behaviour that facilitates interaction: the infant by crying, smiling or vocalisation; the mother by facial expression, vocalisation or gaze. A mother can regulate the infant's state of alertness: for instance rocking or stroking to soothe the child, or talking or varying facial expression to stimulate the child.

The term *attachment* describes the infant's predisposition to seek proximity to certain people and to be more secure in their presence. Bowlby maintained that there is a biological basis to this behaviour, as it has been found extensively in other primates as well as in most human societies. It has considerable survival and adaptive value for the species, as it enables the dependent infant to explore from a secure base and also to use the base as a place of safety at times of distress. From 6 months onwards, infants develop selective attachment to people, usually the mother initially, but not exclusively to her. This first relationship is regarded as the prototype for subsequent relationships, so that its success or failure may have long-term consequences. Clinicians distinguish between *secure attachment* and *anxious attachment*, with the former referring to healthy and the latter to potentially unsatisfactory relationships.

Bonding refers to the persistence of relationships over time, namely the child's capacity to retain the relationship despite the absence of the other individual. Much of the infant's behaviour promotes the development of attachments by ensuring close proximity and interaction with the mother. These ideas have many implications for obstetric and paediatric practice, for the reduction of stress associated with hospitalisation and for possibly explaining the origins of non-accidental injury to children.

Other aspects of development

Gender and sex role concepts   Gender identity is a part of self-concept, but the development of the child's understanding about 'boyness' or 'girlness', the sex role concept, is a more elaborate process. Children usually acquire *gender identity* (correctly labelling themselves and others) by about the age of 2 or 3 followed by *gender stability* (permanence of gender identity) by about 4 years old. *Gender constancy* (gender identity unalterable by change in appearance) appears around 6 years, similar to other conservation-like concepts. Children show clear evidence of sex role stereotyping from an early age, with an excessively rigid concept for a brief period around 6 or 7 years. Freudian theory explains these findings on the basis of identification whereby the child imitates the same-sex parent, thus acquiring appropriate sex-typed behaviour. Alternative explanations emphasise the importance of social reinforcement and of cognition whereby the child acquires a schema about the respective roles and behaviour of boys and girls.

Moral development   The acquisition of moral or ethical values is an important aspect of the socialisation of children. Freud and Piaget have both described how this process happens. Freudian theory maintains that the superego or conscience develops during the phallic stage around 4 to 5 years. At this time, the child is identifying strongly with the same-sex parent in order to resolve the Oedipal conflict and in consequence acquires parental values and prohibitions. In contrast, Piaget hypothesises a much more gradual or stage-like sequence to the acquisition of moral values. The child around the age of 3 years bases his judgement on the outcome rather than the intention of an act, with an emphasis on punishment following from a misdemeanour. Subsequently, the child adopts a more conventional morality based upon con-

formity with family values. Finally, the adolescent derives a personal value system that combines his own idiosyncratic values with those of his family and of society with the intention of achieving the 'greatest good for the greatest number'.

Developmental psychopathology

This long-winded phrase refers to two important dimensions necessary to evaluate children's behaviour: first, whether the behaviour is age appropriate (the developmental aspect), and second, whether the behaviour is abnormal (the psychopathological). For example, separation anxiety is a normal phenomenon among children between 9 months and 4 years approximately, whereas it would be abnormal in a child aged 6 years.

The threefold division of disturbance into abnormalities of behaviour, emotions or relationships provides a useful way to analyse disturbance. Many behavioural problems can be conceptualised in terms of deficits or excesses. For instance, children with encopresis or enuresis can be regarded as having failed to acquire the skills necessary for toileting. Similarly, the aggressive child is showing excessive belligerent or assertive behaviour at an inappropriate time. This approach also has implications for treatment, as the latter is often based on behavioural techniques designed to increase certain behaviours or alternatively to eliminate others.

Anxiety is central to the understanding of emotional disturbance. It has physical manifestations such as palpitations or dry mouth as well as psychological such as fear or apprehension. Anxiety is a normal, indeed essential, part of growing up. It may occur in many situations: in response to external threat; new or strange situations; or in response to the operation of conscience. Anna Freud (1936) developed the concept of *defence mechanisms* to explain how the individual dealt with excessive anxiety. This response is entirely healthy and appropriate in many situations, only becoming maladaptive when it is used exclusively or excessively, thereby preventing the individual from learning how to cope with a normal amount of anxiety. Common defence mechanisms include *denial, rationalisation, regression* and *displacement*. Denial is the process where the child refuses to accept the psychological implications of a particular event or situation. For instance, a child refuses to admit to stealing, even when the theft is obvious, as the resultant loss of self-esteem and the sense of guilt make this impossible. Rationalisation is when the child attempts to justify or minimise the psychological consequences of an event. 'I don't really like football, so that I am not bothered about playing for the team' is an example of the way in which the child may deal with a failure to gain selection for the school team. Regression occurs when a child behaves in a more developmentally immature manner, often at times of stress, for example becoming enuretic at the start of primary school. Displacement is the transfer of hostile or aggressive feelings from their original source onto another person, for instance getting angry with a sibling rather than with an adult.

Social relationships are often impaired among disturbed children. This may be a primary failure in some instances, such as autism, or more commonly a secondary phenomenon. Children with neurotic or conduct disorders are usually isolated and unpopular with their peer group as they have either excluded themselves or have alternatively been excluded as a result of their deviant behaviour. In addition, the behaviour usually brings them into conflict with parents or other adults such as teachers.

Personality development

Childhood is the time during which personality is formed. Wordsworth's aphorism 'the child is father to the man' is substantially true. Personality is a broad concept referring to the enduring and uniquely individual constellation of attributes that distinguish one person from another. It comprises cognitive, emotional, motivational and temperamental attributes that determine the individual's view about himself, his world and the future. Throughout childhood, the various elements interact with each other to mould the child's personality. Moreover, this process occurs in the context of the child's life experiences, particularly within the family, and also subsequently in the world outside the family. Healthy personality formation is an important prerequisite for satisfactory adjustment during childhood and also during adult life.

Personality is influenced by two main factors: constitutional and environmental. A third factor — illness or handicap — if present, can have a profound effect on the child. Constitutional factors include intelligence and temperament. The former describes the individual's ability to think rationally about himself and his environment, while the latter refers to the individual's characteristic style or approach to new people or situations, his level of activity and prevailing mood. These temperamental traits influence the child's response to his environment and also shape the range and variety of his experiences.

The main environmental influences are the family, schooling and the community. The family is the most powerful force for promoting healthy development as well as for causing severe disturbance in a child's life. Families fulfil many functions for children including: the satisfaction of basic physical needs such as food and shelter; the provision of love and security; the development of social relationships with adults and peers; the promotion of cognitive and language skills; the experience of appropriate role models and socialisation; and the acquisition of ethical and moral values.

Schooling has three main roles for children: the attainment of scholastic skills; the promotion of peer relationships; and the acceptance of adult authority outside the family. The community, through the quality of housing and the availability of resources, also has a considerable influence on the child's development. Finally, physical handicap or illness, when present, exert a major effect on personality development. This arises not only from the direct restrictions or limitations that they may impose on the child's abilities or activities, but more commonly and importantly, through indirect effects on the child's self-esteem, from over-protectiveness by the parents and from poor social relationships with siblings and peers.

GENERAL FEATURES OF PSYCHIATRIC DISTURBANCE

Diagnostic classification

A single cause is rarely responsible for the development of disturbance. The usual pattern is for several factors to be involved, with a broad distinction into constitutional and environmental factors. The important constitutional factors are intelligence and temperament, whilst current life circumstances, the family, schooling and the community are the major environmental influences. One consequence of this multiple causation is that it is not possible to devise a diagnostic classification on the basis of aetiology, as the relative contribution of each factor is often unclear.

Diagnostic practice is therefore descriptive or phenomenological, with three main categories of abnormality: *emotions*, *behaviour* and *relationships*. In addition, these abnormalities should be of sufficient severity that they impair the individual in his daily activities and/or cause distress to the individual or to those responsible for his well-being. A commonly used definition of disturbance is as follows: an abnormality of emotions, behaviour or relationships which is sufficiently severe and persistent to handicap the child in his social or personal functioning and/or to cause distress to the child, his parents or to people in the community.

The two commonest systems are the ICD-10 (WHO 1992) and DSM-IV (APA 1994). DSM-IV is used extensively in North America, whereas ICD-10 is popular in the United Kingdom. The two systems have similar underlying principles with an emphasis on a clinical-descriptive approach to diagnosis. An important difference between ICD-10 and DSM-IV is that the latter allows for more than one diagnosis, whereas ICD-10 prefers a single diagnosis. Box 25.1 shows a convenient classification of the important psychiatric syndromes in childhood. Conduct disorder is characterised by severe, persistent, socially disapproved of behaviour such as aggression or stealing that often involves damage to or destruction of property and is unresponsive to normal sanctions. The main feature of emotional disorder is a subjective sense of distress, often arising in response to stress. This group is further divided into phobic, anxiety, obsessional, conversion states and severe reactions to stress. Many disturbed children show a mixture of emotional and behavioural symptoms, so that a mixed category is clinically useful. An important source of confusion between the two classificatory systems is the terminology relating to hyperkinetic disorders in ICD-10 and attention deficit hyperactivity disorder in DSM-IV. Although both systems have the same core features (overactivity, impulsivity and inattention), the different names imply that the two systems regard the main abnormality differently, namely hyperactivity for ICD-10 and inattention for DSM-IV. The situation is further complicated by the popular usage of another term to describe this group of disorders, namely attention deficit disorder (ADD). Disorders of social functioning comprise conditions such as selective mutism and attachment disorders. Pervasive developmental disorders include autistic spectrum disorder, Rett's syndrome and childhood disintegrative disorder. The miscellaneous group contains a diverse group of problems such as encopresis, enuresis and developmental disorders. Other important but uncommon conditions such as schizophrenia and mood disorders are categorised in a similar fashion to that for adults, providing that the diagnostic criteria are fulfilled.

Box 25.1 Classification of important psychiatric syndromes in childhood

- Conduct disorders
- Emotional disorders
- Mixed disorders of conduct and emotions
- Hyperkinetic disorders (ICD-10) or attention deficit hyperactivity disorder (DSM-IV)
- Disorders of social functioning
- Tic disorders
- Pervasive developmental disorders
- Miscellaneous disorders: encopresis, enuresis, sleep disorders and eating disorders

---

Epidemiology of disturbance

Epidemiological research in the UK over the past 30 years has provided important information about the frequency and distribution of disturbance throughout childhood and adolescence (Rutter et al 1970a), the differences between urban and rural areas (Rutter et al 1975), the effects of illness and handicap on vulnerability to disturbance (Rutter et al 1970b) as well as providing clues about the relative importance of various aetiological factors (Rutter et al 1975).

Most studies have shown prevalence rates of between 10% and 20% depending on the criteria for deviance. The first and most influential study was the Isle of Wight study (IOW) carried out by Rutter and his colleagues (1970a). Using a strict definition of disorder, they found rates of approximately 7% among 10–11-year-old children. Follow-up of these children into adolescence indicated a prevalence rate of around 7%, with more than 40% of the children with conduct disorder still having major problems. Disorders arising for the first time during adolescence were more adult-like in presentation, with a preponderance of females. Over 80% of the disorders were in the emotional, conduct or mixed categories. Emotional disorders were more common among girls, with anxiety as the commonest type. By contrast, conduct disorders, and to an important extent mixed disorder, were more common among boys, with an association with specific reading retardation. A comparative study of 10-year-olds living in London (Rutter et al 1975) showed a rate of disturbance over twice that on the IOW. This study also showed that the difference in prevalence rate was entirely accounted for by the increased frequency of predisposing factors among children and their families in London compared with those on the IOW. These factors were family discord, parental psychiatric disorder, social disadvantage and inferior quality of schooling.

The IOW study (Rutter et al 1970b) also showed that children with chronic illness or handicap had much higher rates of disturbance than healthy children. For instance, children with a central nervous disease such as epilepsy or cerebral palsy had a rate over five times that of the general population, while children with other illnesses such as asthma or diabetes were twice as likely to be disturbed as healthy children. A more recent epidemiological study carried out by the Department of Health in the UK (Meltzer & Gatward 2000) on 10 000 children aged 5–15 years found a very similar prevalence rate and range of disturbance as the IOW study, namely an overall prevalence rate of 10%, with conduct disorder (5%), emotional disorder (4%) and attention deficit disorder (1%) the main diagnostic categories. The survey also confirmed that adverse social circumstance, chronic illness and learning difficulties were still important risk factors for disturbance.

Studies of preschool children, most notably by Richman et al (1982), have found that about 20% of children have significant behaviour problems, with 7% classified as severe. Follow-up studies of these children indicated that about 60% persisted, most commonly among overactive boys of low ability. An important association was found between language delay and disturbed behaviour. Finally, problems were more likely to persist when there was marital discord, maternal psychiatric ill health and psychosocial disadvantage such as poor housing or large family size.

ASSESSMENT PROCEDURES

Assessment is more time consuming in child psychiatry than in other branches of paediatrics. It has three components: history taking and examination; psychological assessment; information about the child and family from other professionals.

History taking and examination

This has many similarities to traditional methods, though with important modifications. Interview skills are essential to the elucidation, understanding and treatment of emotional and behavioural problems in children. Points of general importance include:

- clarification about the nature of the problem and the reason for referral;
- obtaining adequate factual information;
- observing and eliciting emotional responses and attitudes about past events and about behaviour during the interview;
- establishing trust and confidence of the child and family;
- providing the parents with a summary of problems and a provisional treatment plan at the end of the initial interview.

There are no absolute rules about interviewing, indeed flexibility is essential. However, the following guidelines are useful:

- The interview room should be large enough to seat the family comfortably and also to allow the children to use the play material in a relaxed manner.
- Avoid having a desk between the interviewer and the family, i.e. put the desk against the wall of the interview room.
- Do not spend the interview writing down notes but rather encourage eye-to-eye contact, taking the minimal notes necessary.
- The play material must be suitable for a wide age range and include crayons and paper, jigsaws, simple games, books (provides a rough estimate of reading ability), doll's house, play telephones and miniature domestic and zoo animals.
- The play material should be gradually introduced as appropriate and not left around in a haphazard manner.
- Interview parents and young children together.
- Older children and adolescents like to be seen separately from parents at some point during interview.
- Older children and adolescents are able to talk about problems openly once trust in the interviewer has been established.
- Too-direct questions usually elicit denial from the child, so that open-ended questions are much more preferable.

The interview should provide the information listed in Box 25.2 (bold type indicates essential facts).

Formulation

At completion of the assessment, the clinician should be able to make a formulation. This is a succinct summary of the important features of the individual case. The formulation consists of the following:

- statement of main problems;
- diagnosis and differential diagnosis;
- relative contribution of constitutional and environmental factors to the aetiology;
- probable short-term and long-term outcome;
- further information required (including special investigations);
- initial treatment plan.

Box 25.2   Information to be elicited in interview in child psychiatry

1. **Presenting problem(s); frequency; severity; onset; course; exacerbating/ameliorating factors; effect on family; help given so far**
2. Other problems or complaints
   a. General health: eating, sleeping, elimination, physical complaints, fits or faints
   b. Interests, activities and hobbies
   c. **Relationship with parents and sibs**
   d. Relationship with other children, special friends
   e. Mood: happy, sad, anxious
   f. Level of activity, attention span, concentration
   g. Antisocial behaviour
   h. **Schooling: attainments; attendance; friendships; relationship with teachers**
   i. Sexual knowledge, interests and behaviour (when relevant)
3. **Any other problems not previously mentioned**
4. Family structure
   a. **Parents: ages; occupations; current physical and psychiatric state; previous physical and psychiatric history**
   b. Sibs: ages; problems
   c. Home circumstances
5. Family function
   a. Quality of parenting: mutual support and help; level of communication and ability to resolve problems
   b. Parent–child relationship: warmth, affection and acceptance; level of criticism, hostility and rejection
   c. Sibs' relationship
   d. Pattern of family relationships
6. Personal history
   a. Pregnancy and delivery
   b. Early mother–child relationship: post-partum depression; early feeding patterns
   c. Temperamental characteristics: easy or difficult, irregular, restless baby and toddler
   d. Developmental milestones
   e. **Past illnesses and injuries; hospitalisation**
   f. Separations greater than one week
   g. Previous schooling
7. **Observation of child's behaviour and emotional state**
   a. **Appearance: nutritional state; signs of neglect or injury**
   b. Activity level; involuntary movements; concentration
   c. Mood: expressions or signs of sadness, misery, anxiety
   d. Reaction to and relationship with the doctor: eye contact; spontaneous talk; inhibition and disinhibition
   e. Relationship with parents: affection/resentment; ease of separation
   f. Habits and mannerisms
   g. Presence of delusions, hallucinations, thought disorder
8. Observation of family relationships
   a. Patterns of interaction
   b. Clarity of boundaries between parents and child
   c. Communication
   d. Emotional atmosphere of family: mutual warmth/tension, criticisms
9. Physical examination
   a. Screening neurological examination
      (i)   Note any facial asymmetry
      (ii)   Eye movements: ask child to follow a moving finger and observe eye movement for jerkiness, unco-ordination
      (iii) Finger–thumb apposition: ask child to press the tip of each finger against the thumb in rapid succession; observe clumsiness, weakness
      (iv)   Copying pattern; drawing a man
      (v)   Observe grip and dexterity in drawing
      (vi)   Observe visual competence when drawing
      (vii) Jumping up and down on the spot
      (viii) Hopping
      (ix)   Hearing: capacity of child to repeat numbers whispered 2 metres behind him
   b. Further medical examination (if relevant).

Bold type indicates essential facts.

The formulation should be included in the case notes, thereby providing the clinician with a record of his views at referral.

Psychological assessment

Psychological assessment carried out by a child psychologist is a valuable part of the overall assessment of a child's problems in some situations. It can provide information about three aspects of development: general intelligence, educational attainments and special skills. Assessment is usually based upon the administration of standardised assessment tests. These are either norm referenced or criterion referenced. The former compares the child's ability with other children of the same age, whereas the latter is on a pass/fail basis, for instance whether he can tie his shoelaces. Ideally, the test items should have good discriminatory value (distinguish between children of different ability), be reliable (give similar results when repeated) and valid (in agreement with other independent evidence). An important aspect of the assessment is that the tasks are carried out in a standardised fashion, thereby increasing reliability and validity.

Intellectual ability

Developmental assessment in infancy and early childhood   The commonly used tests are the Bailey's Scales (Bailey 1993), Griffiths Mental Development Scales (Huntley 1996) and the Kaufman Assessment Battery for Children (K-ABC) (Kaufman & Kaufman 1983).

Assessment of general intelligence among school-age children   The most popular test is the Wechsler Intelligence Scale for Children, Revised Form (WISC-R) (Wechsler 1992). This covers an age range from 6 to 16 years. Ten subtests are usually used, measuring different aspects of the child's ability. Commonly, the tests are divided into 'verbal' and 'performance' categories yielding a 'verbal IQ' and a 'performance IQ'. The 'verbal' subtests commonly used are *information, comprehension, arithmetic, similarities* and *vocabulary*, whilst the 'performance' tests are *picture completion, picture arrangement, block design, object assembly* and *coding*. Each subtest has a mean score of 10, so that combining the 10 tests gives a 'full scale' IQ of 100 with a standard deviation of 15. The 'normal' distribution of the test scores means that it is possible to state that 66% of children will be within the IQ range 85–115, 95% within IQ range 70–130, 99% within IQ range 55–145. Other tests used include the Stanford–Binet (Thorndike et al 1986) and the British Ability Scales (BAS) (Elliott 1996).

Educational attainment

There are two commonly used reading tests: the WORD (Wechsler Objective Reading Test) (Rust 1995) and the Neale Analysis of Reading Ability (Neale 1989). The former measures basic reading, comprehension and spelling skills, whilst the latter provides information about speed, accuracy and comprehension of reading. The scores on the Neale test can be transformed into reading ages of so many years and months, for instance 6 years 11 months. The subtest scores of the WISC-R or the BAS can be used as a guide to mathematical ability.

Specific skills

The Reynell Developmental Language Scales (Reynell 1985), Bender Motor Gestalt Test and the Vineland Social Maturity Scale are examples of tests to assess the child's acquisition of certain abilities and skills. These are often helpful with some specific problems.

Limitations of assessment

Caution should always be exercised in the interpretation of test results. It is wrong to attribute undue significance to a single result, most often done with the IQ score. Many factors influence test results, including fatigue, poor testing conditions and the use of inappropriate tests. The results should be evaluated in the context of the overall assessment and the report from the child psychologist. A great deal of harm, upset and distress can arise for a child when he is incorrectly classified or labelled as too able or too dull on the basis of an unreliable psychological assessment.

Additional information

A distinctive feature of child psychiatry practice is the importance attached to obtaining independent evidence about the child's behaviour. This is for two reasons: first, a child's behaviour varies from one situation to another, so that it is helpful to have information about the child's behaviour in several contexts; second, parental accounts of the child's behaviour are likely to be distorted in many cases, as it is the parents who are disturbed rather than the child. Consequently, an important part of assessment is to obtain reports from other professionals involved with the family such as schools, health visitors or general practitioners. Another common practice is the use of questionnaires to supplement information provided by referrers and other more formal reports. Several questionnaires (Achenbach 1991, Richman et al 1982, Rutter et al 1970a) have been devised to assess different age ranges and have satisfactory psychometric properties. Until recently, the most extensively used questionnaires for schoolage children in the UK have been the Rutter parents' and teachers' scales, also known as Rutter A and Rutter B, respectively. These scales have established reliability and validity as well as classifying children into neurotic or emotional, conduct or antisocial and mixed categories. Over the past 5 years, the Strengths and Difficulties Questionnaire (SDQ) (Goodman 1997) has become more popular, as it assesses pro-social behaviour as well as disturbed behaviour.

DISORDERS IN PRESCHOOL CHILDREN

Except for rare but severe disorders such as childhood autism, psychiatric disorders in this age group are mostly deviations or delays from normality rather than a psychiatric illness as such. Moreover, the child's behaviour and development are so influenced by the immediate surroundings that it is often the environment rather than the child that is responsible for the problems.

Aetiology

Four types of factors contribute to problems in varying degrees in the individual case: temperamental factors; physical illness or handicap; family psychopathology; and social disadvantage. The New York Longitudinal Study (Thomas et al 1968) showed clearly that children with certain types of temperamental characteristics — the so-called 'difficult child' and the 'slow to warm up child' profiles — were more likely to develop problems. Again, physical illness or handicap can reduce activity, directly or indirectly affect developmental progress and increase parental anxiety, all of which potentiate the likelihood of behavioural disturbance. Parental psychiatric illness, marital disharmony and poor parenting skills are examples where disturbance in the parents adversely affects the child's behaviour. Several authors (Brown & Harris 1978, Richman et al 1982) have shown high rates of depression among mothers with pre-school children. Social disadvantage such as poor housing or inadequate recreational facilities increases the risk of disturbance among pre-school children (Richman et al 1982).

Frequency of problems

Table 25.2 shows the prevalence of common problems among 3- and 4-year-olds in the general population (Richman & Lansdown 1988).

Problems are mainly about eating, sleeping and elimination, with a marked decrease in wetting and soiling over a 1-year period. Affective symptoms such as unhappiness and relationship problems are much less common, but probably more significant. Community studies (Richman et al 1982) indicate that 20% of children are regarded by their mothers as having problems, with 7% rated as severe.

Common problems

This section discusses those problems that are particularly frequent among pre-school children, whilst others such as soiling which occur in older children as well are discussed later in the chapter.

Temper tantrums

Tantrums usually arise when the child is thwarted, angry or has hurt himself. They can occur in isolation or as part of a wider problem. They comprise a variety of behaviours, including screaming, crying, often with collapse onto the floor and banging of feet. A child can be aggressive towards other people around him, but the child rarely injures himself. Most tantrums 'burn themselves out', so that specific intervention is not necessary. If it

Table 25.2 Problem behaviours in 3- and 4-year-olds		
Behaviour	3-year-olds (%)	4-year-olds (%)
Poor appetite	19	20
Faddy eater	15	24
Difficulty settling at night	16	15
Waking at night	14	12
Overactive and restless	17	13
Poor concentration	9	6
Difficult to control	11	10
Temper	5	6
Unhappy mood	4	7
Worries	4	1
Fears	10	12
Poor relationships with siblings	10	15
Poor relationships with peers	4	6
Regular day wetting	26	8
Regular night wetting	33	19
Regular soiling	16	3
From Richman & Lansdown (1988).		

Box 25.3   Common characteristics of abused children and their families

Risk characteristics of the abused child:
- Product of unwanted pregnancy
- Unwanted child in the family
- Low birth weight
- Separation from mother in neonatal period
- Mental or physical handicap
- Habitually restless, sleepless or incessantly crying
- Physically unattractive.

Risk characteristics of the parent(s):
- Single parent
- Young
- Abused as a child
- Low self-esteem
- Unrealistic expectations of the child and his development
- Inconsistent or punishment-orientated discipline.

Risk characteristics of social circumstances:
- Low income or unemployment
- Social isolation
- Current stress such as housing crisis, domestic friction, exhaustion or ill-health
- Large family

is, then the following points are useful: if necessary, restrain from behind by folding arms around child's body; minimise any additional attention to the child; and only respond and praise when behaviour is back to normal.

Feeding problems

They range in severity from a minor problem such as the finicky child to the severe disabling problem of non-organic failure to thrive. Minor problems will usually respond to patient and attentive listening to the parents' concerns, counselling and specific advice. Severe non-organic failure to thrive (prevalence 2%) is a complex problem requiring comprehensive assessment and a large amount of time and resources to remedy (Skuse et al 1992). Several factors are responsible in most cases, including poor mother–child relationship, often in the context of more widespread emotional and social deprivation, and factors in the child, including temperamental factors and an aversion to feeding. *Pica*, the ingestion of inedible material such as dirt or rubbish, is a normal transitory phenomenon during the toddler period. Persistent ingestion is found amongst learning disabled, psychotic or socially deprived children. Lead poisoning, though always mentioned, is a possible but uncommon danger from pica.

Sleep problems

These are common, with up to 20% of 2 year olds waking at least five times per week (Richman et al 1982, Morrell 1999). The two most frequent problems are reluctance to settle at night and persistent waking up during the night. Several factors contribute to the problem, including adverse temperamental characteristics in the child, perinatal problems and maternal anxiety. It is also important to distinguish between those factors responsible for the onset of the problem and those for maintaining the problem. Medications such as trimeprazie or promethazine are frequently prescribed, but side-effects often outweigh any advantages. The only real indication is to provide a brief respite for the parents as

well as ensuring that the child has an uninterrupted night's sleep. The most successful management is a behavioural strategy. Richman & Lansdown (1988) provide a useful summary of these techniques. More recently, there have been case reports of the successful use of melatonin to treat sleep disorders among visually and neurologically impaired children (Jan et al 1994). This has now been extended to other groups of children with sleep problems, with some success.

Sleep problems in older children are discussed in the Miscellaneous section.

PSYCHIATRIC ASPECTS OF CHILD ABUSE

Originally this was restricted to the 'battered baby syndrome', but it has now been extended to include physical abuse, sexual abuse, emotional abuse and neglect. This section will concentrate on the psychiatric aspects in childhood, whilst adolescent aspects are discussed in the second section of this chapter. It is also important to remember that the different components of child abuse are frequently present in the same child and family and that many comments about detection, management and treatment apply equally to all aspects of child abuse.

Physical abuse

Diagnostic awareness and suspicion are the key elements in the detection and recognition of physical abuse. Box 25.3 summarises the common characteristics of abused children and their families, although the most important factor to recognise is that child abuse can occur in any family irrespective of social class, ethnic group or religious affiliation.

Management

Most cases of child abuse do not require the involvement of a child psychiatrist, as the principal concerns are the protection of the child, practical support for the family and help with parenting skills. The child psychiatrist can make a useful contribution in two ways: first, to act as an outside consultant on various aspects of management and treatment to the other professionals and agencies working with the family; and second, to provide individual and/or family therapy for the child, the parents or the family depending upon the assessment.

In addition to the immediate effects, child abuse may have medium-term and long-term sequelae. Many abused children continue to be exposed to emotional abuse and neglect throughout their childhood, so that they often show symptoms of disturbance such as unhappiness, wariness, lack of trust, low self-esteem and poor peer relationships. This childhood experience in turn predisposes abused children to become abusing parents as adults.

Sexual abuse

This has continued to be a major source of public and paediatric concern over the past decade. Several factors have contributed to this concern: it is a common event affecting 12–17% of females and 5–8% males according to several epidemiological surveys (Stevenson 1999); it is traumatic for the child, giving rise to major distress at the time of its occurrence; but equally importantly acts as a predisposing factor for psychiatric disorder later in life. Indeed, a history of sexual abuse in childhood is a very common finding among women referred to adult psychiatric services.

Complex psychological processes contribute to the development of psychopathology, as attitudes to sexuality are shaped in a dysfunctional manner by the abuse. Also, the individual has a sense of betrayal, powerlessness and stigmatisation leading to shame, guilt and low self-esteem. One consequence of this process is that sexual abuse can present in a wide variety of ways from the physical, e.g. vaginal discharge, to the psychological, such as anxiety, aggression or encopresis. It is therefore crucial to be aware that unexplained or atypical symptoms may be the presenting complaint for a child with a current or past history of sexual abuse.

The child psychiatry team has a more clearly defined role in the management of sexual abuse, as interviewing skills, psychotherapeutic expertise and the use of specialist equipment (anatomically accurate dolls) are often necessary at the detection and also during the treatment stage of management. Detailed accounts of this work including the use of the anatomical dolls, are well described in several books, e.g. that by the Great Ormond Street child sex abuse team (Bentovim et al 1988) and the APSAC Handbook (Briere et al 1996).

Emotional abuse

This term has been introduced to describe the severe impairment of social and emotional development resulting from repeated and persistent criticism, lack of affection, rejection, verbal abuse and other similar behaviour by the parent(s) to the child. Affected children display a variety of symptoms: low self-esteem; limited capacity for enjoyment; severe aggression; impulsive behaviour.

Neglect

This varies markedly, ranging from a relative inadequacy and incompetence in providing basic shelter, love and security for the child to a severe failure in the provision of basic essentials, often combined with emotional and social deprivation.

Munchausen's syndrome by proxy

This remarkable variant of physical abuse (Eminson & Postlethwaite 1999) often occurs against the same background of parental psychopathology and social disadvantage as other forms of abuse. The role of the child psychiatrist is usually confined in most cases to offering counselling for the parents and/or family therapy when indicated.

PERVASIVE DEVELOPMENTAL DISORDERS

Historically, these disorders were classified under childhood psychoses, as they are severe and disabling with clear-cut abnormalities (Cohen & Volkmar 1997, Gillberg 1995). However, autistic children do not experience hallucinations or delusions, key features of a psychotic disorder, and moreover have had the abnormalities from early infancy. For these reasons, ICD-10 and DSM-IV have separated out childhood autism and related conditions from other psychotic conditions in childhood into a new diagnostic category called pervasive developmental disorders. In clinical practice, most people recognise that autistic disorders comprise a spectrum of disabilities (autistic spectrum disorders) with childhood autism at the severe end and Asperger's syndrome at the mild end. Rett's syndrome and disintegrative disorder are also included in the pervasive developmental disorders category.

Childhood autism

Kanner's (1943) original description of 11 children with 'an extreme autistic aloneness' has not been improved upon with its astute observation of 'inability to relate in an ordinary way to people and to situations' and 'an anxiously obsessive desire for the maintenance of sameness'. Subsequently, opinions have fluctuated about the diagnosis, aetiology and treatment. Most authorities now agree that three features are essential to the diagnosis: general and profound failure to develop social relationships; language retardation; and ritualistic and compulsive behaviour. Additionally, these abnormalities should be manifest before 30 months.

Prevalence

Previous epidemiological studies in childhood have found prevalence rates of 4 per 10 000, increasing to 20 per 10 000 when individuals with severe mental retardation and some autistic features are included. Boys are three times more frequently affected than girls. However, a much more recent study (Chakrabarti & Fombonne 2001) found a rate of 16 per 10 000 for autistic disorder and 46 per 10 000 for other pervasive developmental disorders. It remains to be seen whether these new findings are replicated elsewhere.

Clinical features

Impaired social relationships Parental recollections of infancy often reveal that as an infant the child was slow to smile, unresponsive and passive with a dislike of physical contact or affection. Contemporary social deficits include the failure to use eye-to-eye gaze and facial expression for social interaction, rarely seeking others for comfort or affection, rarely initiating interaction with others, a lack of empathy and of co-operative play. The children are aloof and indifferent to people.

Language abnormalities Language acquisition is delayed and deviant with many autistic children never developing language (approximately 50%). When present, language abnormalities are many and varied, including immediate and delayed echolalia (repetition of spoken word(s) or phrase(s)), poor comprehension and use of gesture, pronominal reversal (the use of the third person when 'I' is meant) and abnormalities in intonation, rhythm and pitch.

Ritualistic and compulsive behaviour Common abnormalities are rigid and restricted patterns of play, intense attachments to unusual objects such as stones, unusual preoccupations and interests (timetables, bus routes) to the exclusion of other pursuits and a marked resistance to any change in the environment or daily routine. Tantrums and explosive outbursts often occur when any change is attempted.

Other features Autistic children often exhibit a variety of stereotypies including rocking, finger twirling, spinning and tiptoe walking. They are often overactive with a short attention span. Seventy percent of autistic children are in the retarded range of intelligence, with only 5% having an IQ above 100. Occasionally, some have remarkable abilities in isolated areas, for instance computation, music or rote memory. About 20% will develop epilepsy during adolescence, though not usually severe.

Association with other conditions Autistic behaviour occurs in some patients with a diverse group of conditions including the fragile X syndrome, rubella, phenylketonuria, tuberous sclerosis, neurolipoidoses and infantile spasms (Lord & Rutter 1994). More recently, Rett's syndrome, with its marked autistic features, has been described (Hagberg 1993).

Aetiology

Most people favour an organic basis because neurological abnormalities are common, there is an association with epilepsy and various neurological syndromes, an increased rate of perinatal complications, and there is a greater concordance rate among monozygotic compared with dizygotic twins (Rutter & Schopler 1988, Lord & Rutter 1994). Application of investigative techniques such as CT, MRI and positron emission tomography are beginning to reveal abnormalities in the frontal lobe region, with distinctive deficits on tests of executive function (Pennington & Ozonoff 1996). The relationship between autism and the fragile X syndrome is also unclear, as the different rates in the various studies may be a reflection of the degree of mental handicap rather than of any aetiological significance. A most interesting psychological perspective on the autistic deficit is provided by the work of Baron-Cohen (1995) and Hobson (1993). On the basis of sophisticated cognitive experiments with autistic children, they propose that the primary deficit in autism is a lack of empathy, namely an inability to perceive and interpret emotional cues in social situations.

Treatment

The explanation of the diagnosis is a vital first step in helping parents to accept the presence of handicap with the consequent lessening of parental guilt about aetiology. Counselling and advice are likely to be necessary throughout childhood. Lord & Rutter (1994) suggested that treatment aims should have four components:

- the promotion of normal development;
- the reduction of rigidity and stereotypies;
- the removal of maladaptive behaviour;
- the alleviation of family stress.

Behavioural methods, including operant conditioning and shaping, are the most likely ways to achieve some success with the first three aims, whilst counselling is important for the fourth. Special schooling, where the child's special social and educational needs are recognised, is very beneficial, sometimes on a residential basis. Drugs do not have an important part in management.

Outcome

Many autistic individuals are unable to live independently, with only 15% looking after and supporting themselves as adults. Many were placed previously in institutions for the learning disabled, though government policy now favours community care. Autistic children with an IQ of at least 70, receiving proper education and coming from middle-class families do better than other groups. In most individuals there is some improvement in social relationships, though many are still handicapped. Parents often find it helpful to join a voluntary society such as the National Society for Autistic Children.

Other pervasive developmental disorders

Asperger's syndrome / schizoid personality

This condition, originally described by Asperger (1944), shows some similarities to childhood autism in that there is an impairment of social relationships with a lack of reciprocal social interaction and a restricted repertoire of interests and activities. However, the children differ diagnostically from those with childhood autism in two important respects: there is no general intellectual retardation; and the language development is normal. Other characteristics include male preponderance and poor motor co-ordination with marked clumsiness. The condition is now regarded as one of the autistic spectrum disorders (Gillberg 1995) with the impairment in social relationships persisting into adult life.

The term 'schizoid' personality of childhood was coined by Wolff & Chick (1980) to describe a small number of children with unusual but distinctive personality characteristics, similar in some ways to children with Asperger's syndrome. These 'schizoid' children were described as aloof, distant and lacking in empathy. Other features include: obstinate and aggressive outbursts when under pressure to conform, often at school; undue rigidity; sensitivity to criticism; and unusual interests to the exclusion of everything else. More recently, Wolff (1991) has argued from follow-up studies of these children that they form a separate diagnostic category, the schizoid personality of childhood, similar to but distinct from childhood autism and Asperger's syndrome. As adults, Wolff (1991) found that they showed features of the schizotypal disorder.

Rett's syndrome

In 1966 Rett described 22 learning-disabled children, all girls who had a history of regression in development and displayed strikingly repetitive movements of the hands. He thought that the children were autistic with progressive spasticity, and proposed that diffuse cerebral atrophy was the underlying cause. A more recent review (Hagberg 1993) has indicated this syndrome is more common than previously thought, with a prevalence rate of 1 per 15 000 among girls.

Clinical features   The condition which has only been described in girls shows a characteristic clinical picture: a period of normal development upto around 18 months followed by a rapid decline in developmental progress and the rapid deterioration of higher brain functions.

Over the following 18 months, there is evidence of severe dementia, a loss of purposeful hand movements, jerky ataxia and acquired microcephaly. After this rapid decline, the condition may stabilise with no further progression for some time. Subsequently, more neurological abnormalities appear, including spastic paraplegia and epilepsy.

Aetiology   Rett originally believed that high levels of ammonia were responsible for the condition, though subsequent studies have not confirmed this observation. The most commonly proposed explanation is that it is due to a dominant mutation on one X chromosome, and that the condition is non-viable in the male.

Prognosis   The majority of children are left profoundly retarded with severe neurological impairments. Many succumb to intermittent infections or to the underlying neuropathological disorder.

Disintegrative disorder

Clinical features   This term refers to a group of conditions characterised by normal development until around four years of age followed by profound regression and behavioural disintegration, loss of language and other skills, impairment of social relationships and the development of stereotypies (Corbett et al 1977, Lord & Rutter 1994). It can follow from a minor illness or from a more definite neurological disease such as measles encephalitis. The prognosis is poor because of the underlying degenerative pathology in many cases. Most individuals are left with severe learning disability.

Other related conditions

Many children with learning disability show some autistic features. In clinical practice, it is often difficult to know whether they fulfil the criteria for pervasive developmental disorder in addition to that for intellectual retardation. It is clear that there is a wide diversity in the severity of these 'autistic features', so that it is often arbitrary whether the label childhood autism is applied to these children. Many of them also show features of hyperactivity and aggression. For these reasons, ICD-10 has made two additional categories: overactive disorder associated with mental retardation and stereotyped movements; and pervasive development disorder unspecified.

EMOTIONAL DISORDERS

The primary abnormality is a subjective sense of distress due to anxiety that can be expressed overtly, as in anxiety disorders, or covertly as in somatisation or conversion disorders. This group of disorders is similar in many respects to neurotic disorders in adults. They are further divided into the following categories: anxiety and phobic states; obsessional disorders; conversion disorders, dissociative states and somatisation disorders; and reaction to severe stress and adjustment disorders. Many children often show a mixed pattern of symptoms, so that a clear-cut distinction into a single category is not possible. The Department of Health 2000 study (Meltzer & Gatward 2000) found a prevalence rate of 4% with an equal gender prevalence. Prognosis is generally favourable as many problems arise from an acute stress, so that the problems should resolve once the stressful effects lessen.

Anxiety states

Clinical features

This is the commonest type of emotional disorder. Anxiety has physical and psychological components, with the former referring to palpitations and dry mouth and the latter to the subjective sense of fear and apprehension. Somatic symptoms, particularly abdominal pain, are common. Again, many symptoms represent the persistence or exaggeration of normal developmental fears, ranging in severity from an acute panic attack to a chronic anxiety state over several months. Predisposing factors include temperamental characteristics, over-involved and over-concerned parents and the 'special child syndrome'. The latter refers to children who are treated differently by their parents. This may arise in several circumstances — for instance the child is much wanted, previous ill health during pregnancy or infancy — resulting in 'anxious' attachment between the child and parents. In turn, 'anxious' attachment may lead the parents to inadvertently reinforce normal fears and anxieties.

Treatment

Several approaches, including individual, behavioural and family therapy, are used, often in combination depending upon the assessment and formulation. The newer SSRIs (selective serotonin reuptake inhibitors) such as buspirone have been shown to be effective in clinical trials, and are preferable to benzodiazepines.

Phobic states

Clinical features

Phobias are common and normal among children. For instance, toddlers are fearful of strangers, whereas adolescents are anxious about their appearance or weight. Pathological fears often arise from ordinary fears that are exacerbated by parental and/or social reinforcement. A phobia is defined as a fear of a specific object or situation, for instance dogs or heights. Its characteristics are that it is out of proportion to the situation, is irrational, is beyond voluntary control and leads to avoidance of the feared situation. This avoidance behaviour is the main reason why the fear is maladaptive, as it leads to increasing restriction and limitation of the child's activities.

Treatment

A behavioural approach using graded exposure to the feared situation is the most commonly used treatment. The rationale of this approach is that continued exposure to the feared stimulus reduces the anxiety associated with the stimulus, thereby decreasing avoidance behaviour. The success of this method often depends on the ability of the therapist to devise a treatment programme that provides gradual exposure without inducing too much anxiety. Occasionally, anxiolytic drugs are used in conjunction with this behavioural approach.

School refusal

This term, also known as school phobia, refers to the child's irrational fear about school attendance (Berg 1992). It is also known as the masquerade syndrome as it can present in a variety of disguises, including abdominal pain, headaches or a viral infection. The child is reluctant to leave home in the morning to attend school, in contrast to the truant who leaves home but does not arrive at school. It occurs most commonly at the commencement of schooling, change of school, or the beginning of secondary school.

Most cases can be understood in terms of the following three mechanisms, often in combination:

- separation anxiety, whereby the child and/or the parent are fearful of separation, of which school is an example;
- a specific phobia about some aspect of school such as travelling to school, mixing with other children, or some part of the school routine, for instance some subjects, gym, or assembly;
- an indication of a more general psychiatric disturbance such as depression or low self-esteem, which is more frequent among adolescents.

Typically, most school refusers have good academic attainments, are conformist at school, but oppositional at home. School refusal can present acutely or insidiously, often becoming a chronic problem in adolescence.

Treatment

The initial essential step is to recognise the condition itself, and hence to avoid unnecessary and extensive investigations for minor somatic symptoms or to advise prolonged convalescence following a minor illness. For the acute case, early return to school with firm support for the parents and liaison with the school is the most successful approach. For the more intractable cases, extensive work with the child and parents, along with a graded return to school is advisable. A specific behavioural programme for the phobic aspects may be necessary as well as the use of anxiolytic drugs in some instances. The chronic problem often requires a concerted approach, sometimes involving a period of assessment and treatment at a child psychiatric day or inpatient unit. Many clinicians use family therapy to tackle the major relationship problems that exist in some cases.

Outcome

Two-thirds usually return to school regularly, whilst the remainder, usually adolescents from disturbed families, only achieve erratic attendance at school at best. Follow-up studies have found that approximately one-third continue with neurotic symptoms and social impairment into adult life.

Obsessive–compulsive disorders

Definition

An obsession is a recurrent, intrusive thought that the individual recognises is irrational but cannot ignore. A compulsion or ritual is the behaviour(s) accompanying these ideas, the aim of which is to reduce the associated anxiety.

Clinical features

Most children display obsessional symptoms to a minor degree at some time, for instance avoiding cracks on paving stones or walking under ladders. They have no significance. It is when the behaviour interferes with ordinary activities that it amounts to a disorder. Common obsessional rituals are hand washing and dressing. Obsessional thoughts often have a foreboding quality, for instance that 'something could happen' to a parent or sibling, that he might die, or get run over. The rituals are maintained, though maladaptive, because they produce temporary reduction in anxiety (Fig. 25.1). Commonly, the child involves other members of the family in the performance of rituals, so that the child assumes a controlling role within the family. The disorder is rare (community prevalence 0.3%) but commoner among older children and adolescents, with an acute or gradual onset. In addition to anxiety symptoms, many children have depressive features.

Treatment

Behavioural methods, particularly response prevention, are successful in eliminating the obsessive–compulsive behaviour. Response prevention consists of training the child to become aware of the cues that trigger the symptom and then using distraction techniques to make the performance of the ritual impossible. Recent clinical trials (Shafran 2001) have shown that SSRIs such as paroxetine or sertraline are effective in their own right, but more importantly are very valuable as part of a combined

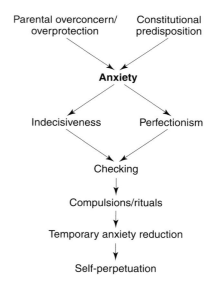

Fig. 25.1
Development of obsessive–compulsive behaviour.

medication–behavioural treatment package. Involvement of other members of the family, whether specifically in family therapy or to assist the child in the elimination of rituals, is necessary. Some cases require inpatient admission.

Outcome

Two-thirds do well, with the remainder continuing to have problems, usually in a fluctuating fashion.

Conversion disorders and dissociative states

Clinical features

These are rare in childhood. Conversion disorder is the development of physical symptoms, usually of the special senses or limbs, without a pathological basis in the presence of identifiable stress and/or affective disturbance. The emotional conflict is said to be 'converted' into physical symptoms which are less threatening to the individual than the underlying psychological conflict. A dissociative state is the restriction or narrowing of consciousness by psychological causes, for example amnesic or fugue states. It is, however, extremely dangerous to diagnose the condition solely by the exclusion of organic disease, as follow-up studies have found that a minority subsequently develop definite organic illness. There should always be positive psychological reasons to explain the development of the symptoms. Common reasons include major life events or stresses for the child, a similar illness among other family members/peers or an underlying depressive disorder.

Minor degrees of these disorders are extremely common and frequently occur as a transitory phenomenon during the course of many illnesses. The more general term 'abnormal illness behaviour', similar to the physician's phrase 'functional overlay', has been coined to describe the situation when the individual persists with or exaggerates symptoms following an illness.

Treatment

Successful treatment depends upon the recognition that the symptoms are 'real' for the child. Psychic pain is just as distressing as physical pain. Anger and confrontation are unhelpful. A firm sympathetic approach with little attention to the symptom per se as well as avoiding rewarding the symptom is the best strategy. Allow the child to give up the symptoms with good grace, often providing the child with some face-saving reason for improvement. Identify and treat any affective disturbance. The outcome is good for an individual episode, though other psychological problems may persist.

Somatoform disorders

Clinical features and management

Many children complain of somatic symptoms that do not have a pathological basis (Garralda 1996). Common symptoms are abdominal pain, headaches and limb pains with community prevalence rates of approximately 10%. This condition is usually managed by general practitioners, though it sometimes results in a referral for a specialist opinion. Management involves the minimum necessary investigation to exclude any pathology, the identification of any stressful circumstances and a sensitive explanation of the basis for the symptoms. The prevention of restrictions and the active encouragement of normal activities are essential.

When the somatic symptoms are persistent, chronic and involve several systems of the body, ICD and DSM use the term somatisation disorder. Whilst it is doubtful whether this disorder occurs in childhood, there is no doubt that persistent unexplained physical complaints are a common reason for children being taken to see the doctor. In many cases, there is clear evidence of underlying anxiety or recent stressful events. (See p. 607 for chronic fatigue syndrome.)

Reaction to severe stress and adjustment disorders

This group of disorders arises in response to an exceptionally stressful event or to a significantly adverse life change. The clinical features of the different syndromes vary considerably, with a preponderance of affective symptoms in most cases.

Adjustment disorder

Definition This is a maladaptive response occurring within 3 months of an identifiable psychosocial stressor. The maladaptive response must be of sufficient severity to impair daily activities such as schooling, hamper social relationships and be greater than expected given the nature of the stressor. Finally, the reaction must not last longer than 6 months.

Clinical features By definition, the symptoms vary, with ICD and DSM recognising more than six categories. Clinical practice shows that anxiety and depressive symptoms, often combined, are the most frequent categories. Common stressors include parental divorce, unemployment, family illness or family move.

Predisposing factors Age has different effects depending on the type of stressor. For instance, separation is more upsetting for a younger child than for an adolescent, whereas a loss of or change in a heterosexual relationship is far more important for an adolescent than for a younger child. Boys are also more vulnerable to the adverse effects of stress than girls. Temperamental characteristics such as 'difficult' or 'slow to warm up' style probably influence susceptibility as well. Again, the child's previous experience and repertoire of coping skills affect the response to the current stressor. For instance, if the child has successfully coped with adversity in the past, resilience and the ability to withstand the present situation are enhanced. Finally, the family, particularly the parents, can magnify or minimise the impact of a stressor, depending on their resourcefulness and coping style.

Outcome By definition, the disorder can only last for 6 months, after which time the diagnostic category must change. The more important clinical consideration is not the change in diagnostic category, but the adverse effect that chronic or repeated stresses can have on the child's long-term adjustment.

Post-traumatic stress disorder (PTSD)

The 'epidemic' of disasters that some British children have been involved with over the past 20 years (the capsize of the ferry *Herald of Free Enterprise*, the sinking of the cruise ship *Jupiter*, the PanAm Lockerbie air crash and the crushing disaster at the Hillsborough football stadium) have made clinicians acutely aware of this syndrome. Clinicians are now familiar with the wide symptomatology often found, and have also become involved in treatment programmes to reduce the distress both in the immediate aftermath and also in the long term.

Definition This disorder arises following exposure to a stressful event of an exceptionally threatening or catastrophic nature that would cause pervasive distress in almost anyone. The events include accidents or disasters as well as more personal traumas such as witnessing a murder, a rape or torture. In clinical practice, children who have been sexually abused commonly present with symptoms falling within the diagnostic category of PTSD.

Clinical features These include 'flashbacks' (the repeated re-enactment of the event with intrusive memories, dreams or nightmares); a sense of detachment, 'numbness' and emotional blunting; irritability, poor concentration and memory problems. Following disasters, many survivors often experience an increased awareness of danger, a foreshortened view of the future ('only plan for today'), a feeling of 'survivor' guilt (self reproach about own survival, whilst companions died) and acute panic reactions.

Yule (1994) indicates that 30–50% of children show significant psychological morbidity following disasters, with symptoms persisting for several months.

Individual vulnerability factors Important modifying factors are probably age, previous experiences, current life situation and the availability of help. Though cognitive immaturity may protect the child from appreciating the implications of a disaster, it may also be a disadvantage, as the child may not be given the opportunity to talk about the event. The child's previous experience of stressful events and their outcome, successful or otherwise, are likely to influence the response to the disaster.

Similarly, coexisting adverse circumstances such as family disharmony or school problems reduce the child's capacity to cope with the new situation.

Management Though most research is anecdotal rather than systematic, the available evidence (Yule 1994) suggests that post-disaster 'debriefing' sessions on an individual or group basis are helpful. Specific counselling sessions to help a child deal with phobic, anxiety or depressive symptoms are frequently necessary as well. Cognitive/behavioural approaches are particularly suitable for this pattern of symptoms.

MOOD DISORDERS

Mood disorders are discussed in the section on psychiatric disorders in adolescence (p. 601).

CONDUCT DISORDER

Clinical features

This is usually defined as persistent antisocial or socially disapproved of behaviour that often involves damage to property and is unresponsive to normal sanctions. The IOW study (Rutter et al 1970a) found a prevalence rate of 4% when the mixed disorder category was included as well, with a marked male predominance (at least 3:1). There is no independent criterion for deviancy, as social and cultural values determine the seriousness or otherwise attached to antisocial behaviour. Consequently, most clinicians would add the criterion of impairment, namely an adverse effect on the child's daily life or development, before applying the diagnostic lable of conduct disorder.

Common symptoms include temper tantrums, oppositional behaviour, overactivity, irritability, aggression, stealing, lying, truancy, bullying and wandering away from home/school. Delinquency (a legal term for a person committing an offence against the law) is a frequent feature among older children and adolescents. Stealing, vandalism, arson and firesetting are common forms of delinquency (male:female ratio is 10:1).

Traditionally, a distinction has been made between socialized and unsocialized behaviour. The former describes behaviour that is in accord with peer group values, but contrary to those of society, for instance antisocial gang behaviour such as stealing and vandalism. Unsocialised antisocial behaviour implies more disturbed behaviour, as it is often done alone against a background of parental rejection or neglect and poor peer relationships. Learning difficulties, especially specific reading retardation, occur more commonly among children with conduct disorders. This is a further reason why schooling is unpopular and a source of discouragement for these children. Additionally, many children with conduct disorder have affective symptoms such as anxiety or unhappiness, as well as low self-esteem and poor peer relationships. When these symptoms are prominent, it is often appropriate to classify the disorder as mixed, implying both emotional and behavioural symptomatology.

Aetiology

Four factors — the family, the peer group, the neighbourhood and constitutional — make some contribution in most cases, but the family is usually the most important. Families of children with conduct disorder are characterised by a lack of affection and by rejection, marital disharmony, inconsistent and ineffective discipline, parental violence and aggression. The families are often of large size, which aggravates the problems of supervision and care. Constitutional factors present in some cases include low intelligence and learning difficulties, along with adverse temperamental features such as overactivity and impulsiveness. Oppositional peer group values are an important feature in older children and adolescents. Many children with conduct disorder live in areas of urban deprivation with poor schooling. The intractable and chronic nature of these problems is a major reason for the continuation of conduct disorder into adolescence and adult life.

Treatment

Help for the family, either by counselling for the parents or by family therapy, is often used. More recently, specific intervention programmes aimed at promoting positive parenting have been developed with good outcomes in the short term at least (Webster-Stratton & Herbert 1993). Educational support through remedial teaching or the provision of special education can be important in some cases. For many families, however, the role of psychiatric services is limited, with practical support with rehousing in order to alleviate social disadvantage the most important contribution.

Prognosis

Continuity into adult life is common with over 50% having problems as adults. Bad prognostic features are many and varied symptoms, problems at home and in the community and anti-authority and aggressive attitudes.

HYPERACTIVITY AND ATTENTION DEFICIT SYNDROMES

Clinical features

Considerable controversy surrounds the diagnostic terms hyperkinetic disorder (HKD), attention deficit hyperactivity disorder (ADHD) and attention deficit disorder (ADD) (Gillberg 1995, Taylor et al 1998). HKD is the category used by ICD-10, which is the diagnostic system mainly used in the UK. This emphasises the importance of pervasive overactivity (i.e. present in all situations) as a diagnostic feature. By contrast, North American psychiatrists use DSM-IV, which has the diagnostic category of ADHD. The latter stresses inattentiveness as a key symptom rather than overactivity. The different diagnostic practices probably explain the wide variation in prevalence rates (from 1% to 10%) found in epidemiological studies. Despite the difference in terminology, the two systems agree upon the same three core features: *overactivity, impulsivity* and *inattentiveness.*

Current UK practice has changed radically over the past 10 years, so that most UK psychiatrists use the term ADD rather than HKD. One consequence of this change has been the dramatic increase in the prescription of methylphenidate, with the annual rate rising from 180 000 in 1991 to 1.5 million by 1995.

Another controversy concerns the existence of comorbidity among children with ADD symptoms, which in turn is linked to the conceptual argument about whether disorders are categorical or dimensional. Traditional UK clinical practice prefers a single as opposed to several concurrent diagnoses. For instance, if a child is overactive, they may be classified as HKD or conduct disorder, but not both. By contrast, North American practice allows, or even encourages, more than one diagnosis, namely the overactive child could have ADD and conduct disorder. Unfortunately, current evidence is unable to provide a definite answer about the best approach. This difference in diagnostic approach is another reason for the divergent prevalence rates in epidemiological studies.

In conclusion, it is probably best to regard overactivity as a symptom, rather than a diagnostic term, that can occur in many clinical situations:

- a symptom of ADHD, HKD or ADD;
- a feature of many children with conduct disorder;
- a reflection of developmental delay on its own or in association with general intellectual retardation;
- one extreme of normal temperamental variation;
- an uncommon response to high anxiety or tension;
- a symptom of childhood autism;
- rarely, as a reaction to some drugs, for example barbiturates or benzodiazepines.

Treatment of attention deficit disorder

The recent MTA Study (MTA Co-operative Group 1999) and the report from the National Institute for Clinical Excellence (NICE 2000) have provided the clearest evidence and guidance, respectively, about the most effective treatment package. Most people would advocate a multimodal approach involving drug treatment, a psycho-educational and parenting skills programme, and individual or group work with the child. The MTA Study showed that 80% of children improved significantly on methylphenidate, with improvement persisting over the 14-month trial period. There appeared little convincing evidence that a combined approach involving drug and behavioural treatments significantly improved the outcome, but it must be remembered that the MTA study was carried out in the USA where diagnostic practices are different.

Methylphenidate (up to 60 mg daily in divided doses) is the commonest prescribed drug in the UK, whereas dexamphetamine (up to 30 mg daily) is more popular in the USA and Australasia. Both drugs are equally effective and have a similar side-effect profile, but dexamphetamine has a longer time course of effect. Stimulant drugs seem to work through an increase in dopamine levels in the frontal lobes. The common side-effects of both drugs are loss of appetite and night-time insomnia with abdominal pain, headache, tearfulness and tics less common. It is debatable whether stimulants have any long-term effect on growth or the exacerbation of tics, but careful monitoring is advisable. A long-acting form of methylphenidate, Concerta XL, was given a UK licence in 2002. It seems to be as effective as three times daily dosage methylphenidate and to have a similar side-effect profile (Pelham et al 2001). The once daily dosage of Concerta XL offers several potential advantages; in particular, it avoids the necessity of a lunchtime dose of methylphenidate, which is a major source of embarrassment for older children and adolescents at school.

Tricyclic antidepressants such as imipramine or nortriptyline are also an effective alternative treatment, and are used when the child is unresponsive to stimulants, side-effects are disabling or there is a depressive component to the child's symptoms. There are also open-label studies with clonidine, particularly for aggressive symptoms, but there have been case reports of sudden death due to cardiac arrhythmias, so that an ECG prior to commencement of treatment is essential. Pemoline, which has the considerable advantage of a once daily dosage, has now been withdrawn in the UK on account of fears about hepatic toxicity.

Behavioural techniques, parental counselling and the alteration and manipulation of the child's environment, particularly at school, to reduce and minimise distraction are important components of most treatment programmes. An alternative approach adopted by some clinicians has been the use of exclusion diets on the basis that the child is allergic to certain substances, commonly tartrazine. Evidence for the efficacy of these exclusion diets other than as a placebo response is unconvincing, though Egger et al (1992), using a sophisticated methodological design, showed that children with severe hyperactivity and learning disability did respond. It is, however, unclear whether these results would apply to children of normal intelligence with less severe problems who make up the majority of children with ADD.

Outcome

Hyperactivity and attention deficits lessen considerably by adolescence, though other major problems such as learning difficulties and behaviour problems persist. A substantial minority continue to have problems in adult life, mainly of an antisocial nature. There is also increasing evidence for the efficacy of methylphenidate in adults in whom the diagnosis of attention deficit disorder had been missed in childhood or who have continued on treatment from childhood (Biederman et al 1993, Spencer et al 1995).

DISORDERS OF ELIMINATION

Enuresis

This term refers to the involuntary passage of urine in the absence of physical abnormality after the age of 5 years. It may be nocturnal and/or diurnal. Bed wetting continuously, though not usually every night, since birth is termed primary enuresis, whereas when there has been a 6-month period of dry beds at some stage, recurrence of bed wetting is termed secondary or onset enuresis. Diurnal enuresis is much less common than nocturnal, but more common among girls and among children who are psychiatrically disturbed. Depending upon definition, approximately 10% of 5-year-olds, 5% of 10-year-olds and 1% of 18-year-olds have nocturnal enuresis. The majority of children with nocturnal enuresis are not psychiatrically ill, though a substantial minority, approximately 25%, have signs of psychiatric disturbance.

Aetiology

A combination of individual factors such as positive family history (approximately 70%), lower intelligence, psychiatric disturbance and small bladder capacity along with environmental factors such as recent stressful life events, large family size and social disadvantage are present in most cases.

Treatment

It is important to exclude any physical basis for the enuresis by history, examination and, if necessary, investigation of the renal tract. Assuming no physical pathology, the most important initial step is to minimise the handicap, namely to point out to the parents the very favourable natural outcome of the condition, and to relabel the child's enuresis as immaturity rather than laziness or wilfulness. A star chart, the accurate recording of enuresis plus positive reinforcement for dry nights, provides an accurate baseline as well as a successful treatment in its own right. An enuresis alarm is successful with older co-operative children. The success of this approach is probably because the child becomes more aware of the sensation of a full bladder along with the encouragement from parents for dry nights. The modern alarms are extremely compact, and do not require a pad placed between the sheets, thereby increasing patient compliance considerably. It is useful to combine an alarm with a star chart. Drugs such as desmopressin and imipramine are very effective at stopping enuresis, though the major limitation is that the enuresis recurs when they are stopped. Most paediatricians believe that it is wrong to prescribe potentially lethal drugs such as imipramine for a benign condition such as enuresis, so that desmopressin is the preferred drug treatment.

Soiling and encopresis

Most children are clean and continent of faeces by their fourth birthday. Encopresis is usually defined as the inappropriate passage of formed faeces, usually onto the underwear, in the absence of any physical pathology after 4 years of age. Soiling, the passage of semi-solid faeces, is often used synonymously with encopresis. Symptoms vary widely in severity, ranging from slight staining of underwear to encopresis with the smearing of faeces onto the walls. It is uncommon, with a community prevalence among 8-year-olds of 1.8% for boys and 0.7% for girls. Psychiatric disturbance is common among children with encopresis. Enuresis may also be present.

Clinical features

Figure 25.2 shows a convenient way to classify encopresis, with a broad distinction into children who retain faeces with eventual overflow incontinence and those who deposit faeces inappropriately on a regular basis. Some children have never achieved continence, a situation called continuous or primary encopresis, whilst others have had periods of cleanliness followed by relapse, the so-called discontinuous or secondary encopresis. Figure 25.2 also lists the common different patterns of interaction found among children with encopresis and their parents. For instance, children with retentive encopresis have often been subjected to coercive and obsessional toilet training practices, so that the encopresis is seen as a reaction, often of anger or aggression, towards this practice. Similarly, many children with continuous non-retentive encopresis come from disorganised chaotic families where regular training and toileting are not the norm. Again, encopresis can arise in some children as a response to a stressful situation. Finally, encopresis can reflect poor parent–child relationship, often longstanding, and usually associated with other aspects of psychiatric disturbance. The clinical picture is often, however, not as clear-cut, with the different elements each making some contribution. There may be a previous history of constipation and occasionally of anal fissure.

Treatment

A physical aetiology such as Hirschsprung's disease must be excluded before commencement of psychiatric treatment. The assessment must include an account of previous treatments and, most importantly, the current attitude of the parents and the child to the problem. Treatment has two aims: the promotion of a normal bowel habit and the improvement of the parent–child relationship. Initially, a bowel washout and/or microenemata may be necessary to clear out the bowel. Judicious use of bowel smooth muscle stimulants (Senokot), stool softeners (Dioctyl) and bulk agents (lactulose) is helpful for the child with retention. Again, suppositories are often useful from time to time. This should also be combined with parental and child education about the dietary importance of fibre. The psychological component

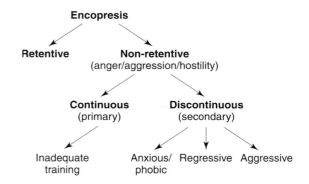

Fig. 25.2
Types of encopresis and their psychopathology. Three patterns are common: primary, retentive and secondary.

includes behavioural (star chart) and individual psychotherapy to gain the co-operation and trust of the child along with parental counselling or family therapy to modify attitudes and hostile interactions between the child and his parents.

Prognosis

It usually resolves by adolescence, though other problems may persist. Occasional case reports of persistence into adult life have been published.

MISCELLANEOUS DISORDERS

Developmental disorders

Language disorders

Children with language disorders are more vulnerable to disturbance, mainly because of the associated anxiety and embarrassment caused by the disorder. Specific language delay (5–6/1000) is twice as common in boys than girls, with a strong association with large family size and lower social class. Richman et al (1982) found that approximately 25% of 3-year-olds with specific language delay had behavioural problems.

Stuttering, an abnormality of speech rhythm consisting of hesitations and repetitions at the beginning of syllables or words, is a normal, though transitory phenomenon, occurring at around 3–4 years of age. When it persists (approximately 3% of the general population), often due to inadvertent parental attention, it leads to anxiety and low self-esteem.

Selective mutism This is not strictly a language disorder, as the main problem is the child's refusal to talk in certain situations, most commonly at school, rather than an inability to speak. Mild forms of the disorder are common but transitory, usually at the commencement of schooling, while the severe form has a prevalence rate of about 1 per 1000. Other features include a previous history of speech delay, excessively shy but stubborn temperament and parental overprotectiveness.

A combination of behavioural and family therapy techniques to promote communication and the use of speech is most commonly used, though some cases require inpatient assessment. Fluoxetine had been shown to be effective in an open trial of children with selective mutism and comorbid anxiety disorder (Dummit et al 1996). Prognosis is good for approximately 50%, with failure to improve by the age of 10 years a poor prognostic sign.

Reading difficulties

Though mainly of educational concern, the paediatrician or child psychiatrist may get involved because of the associated behavioural or emotional problems. The two main types are first, general reading backwardness, when the retardation is a reflection of generalised intellectual delay, and second, specific reading retardation when the attainment in reading is significantly behind the expected level after controlling for age and intelligence. The problem is 'significant' when the delay is at least 2 years. Dyslexia is a concept similar to specific reading retardation, implying a neuropsychological substrate for the specific reading difficulties. The use of this term is contentious, so that the more bland expression 'specific reading retardation' is preferred by many clinical psychologists.

The aetiology is multifactorial, involving genetic, social, perceptual and language deficits. A noteworthy feature is the strong association between specific reading retardation and conduct disorder, with the behaviour problem most likely arising secondary to the frustration and disillusionment associated with the reading difficulty. Treatment involves a detailed psychometric assessment of the problem by a psychologist followed by an individualised remedial programme carried out by a specialised teacher in collaboration with the psychologist. Help with the behavioural problem is also necessary in order to prevent more serious problems arising during adolescence.

Habit disorders

Tics and Tourette's syndrome

Tics are rapid, involuntary, repetitive muscular movements, usually involving the face and neck: for instance blinks, grimaces and throat clearing. Simple tics occur as a transitory phenomenon in about 10% of the population with boys outnumbering girls three to one and with a mean age of onset around 7 years. They range in severity from simple tics involving head and neck through to complex tics extending to the limbs and trunk and finally to Tourette's syndrome. The latter comprises complex tics accompanied by coprolalia (uttering obscene words and phrases) and echolalia (the repetition of sounds or words). Like stammering, tics are made worse at times of stress and may be exacerbated by undue parental concern. The differential diagnosis of tics in childhood is principally from chorea, where the movements are less co-ordinated and predictable, not stereotypic in form and cannot be suppressed.

Other features of tic disorder are a positive family history and a previous history of neurodevelopmental delay. Many tics resolve spontaneously, but those that persist can be extremely disabling and difficult to treat.

Treatment Several approaches are used singly or in combination, depending on the assessment. Medication is effective, but should be reserved for severe cases. Haloperidol is the most common drug used for Tourette's syndrome, but pimozide and clonidine are alternative drugs. Many children with simple tics respond to explanation and reassurance along with advice for the parents. Individual and/or family therapy may be indicated when anxiety and tension are clearly exacerbating the problem. Behaviour therapy in the form of relaxation and or massed practice can also be helpful.

Prognosis Simple tics have a good outcome with complete remission, whereas in Tourette's syndrome the condition fluctuates in a chronic manner with 50% continuing with symptoms into adult life.

Sleep disorders

Sleep disorders in preschool children are discussed on page 588.

Night terrors

The usual pattern is for the child to wake up in a frightened, even terrified state, not to respond when spoken to, nor appear to see objects or people. Instead, he appears to be hallucinating, talking to and looking at people/things not actually present. The child may be difficult to comfort, with a period of disturbed behaviour and altered consciousness lasting up to 15 minutes, occasionally longer. Eventually the behaviour settles, with or without comfort, and the child goes back to sleep, awakening in the morning with no recollection of the episode. The latter point is invaluable in helping to allay parental anxiety about the episodes. Night terrors arise from stage 4 or deep sleep. The peak incidence is between 4 and 7 years, with a continuation of 1–3% into older children. It is also helpful to identify and ameliorate any identifiable stresses that may occasionally contribute to the problem. Lask (1988) has described an apparently successful novel behavioural approach relying on waking the child 15 minutes prior to the expected time of the night terror. Drugs such as benzodiazepines or tricyclics have also been used successfully.

Nightmares

These are frightening or unpleasant dreams, occurring during REM (rapid eye movement) sleep. The child may or may not wake up, but there will be a clear recollection of the dream if he does wake up and also in the morning. There is no period of altered consciousness or inaccessibility as with night terrors. Again, daytime anxieties and/or frightening television programmes in the evening may be contributory factors.

Sleepwalking (somnambulism)

The child, usually aged between 8 and 14 years, calmly arises from his bed with a blank facial expression, does not respond to attempts at communication and can only be awakened with difficulty. The child is in a state of altered consciousness at the deep level of sleep (stages 3 or 4). Any contributory anxiety should be treated as well as giving the parents some advice about the safety and protection of the child during these episodes.

PSYCHOLOGICAL EFFECTS OF ILLNESS AND DISABILITY

Approximately 15% of children have some form of chronic illness or disability. The IOW study (Rutter et al 1970b) showed clearly that this group of children was much more at risk for disturbance: a rate of 33% for children with chronic illness affecting the central nervous system, 12% for children with chronic illness not affecting the central nervous system and only 7% among the general population. The IOW study also showed that children with chronic illness or disability had the same range of disorders as other disturbed children, thereby implying that the mechanisms involved with this increased morbidity are probably indirect and non-specific rather than direct and specific to each illness or disability. They can cause psychological stress on the child and family not only at the time of diagnosis but also in the long term. These effects are now discussed with regard to the child himself and to other family members, though the two effects interact with each other.

Effects on the child

Three aspects are important: the acquisition of skills and outside interests; the development of self-concept; and the development of adaptive coping behaviour. Many illnesses or disabilities inevitably restrict the child's ability or opportunity to acquire everyday skills and to develop interests and hobbies. For example, cerebral palsy causes movement and motor problems, diabetes imposes dietary restrictions, asthma imposes limitations on exercise, and epilepsy necessitates the avoidance of some activities such as cycling or swimming. Additionally, educational problems are common among this group of children for a variety of reasons including increased absence from school, specific learning difficulties, especially among children with epilepsy, and low expectations from parents and teachers.

Illness and disability can adversely affect the child's self-concept in several ways through the effects on the child's body image and self-esteem. Many children have a distorted view of their body, seeing the disability as very prominent or disfiguring. These ideas can often be reinforced by comments from parents or peers. Self-esteem can also be reduced by the child's distorted cognitive appraisal of the situation, which in turn leads to a pessimistic view about himself and the future. This is particularly likely and also potentially very disabling among older children and adolescents.

Successful adaptation to a disability depends upon the acquisition of a range of coping behaviours and defence mechanisms to lessen anxiety to a manageable level. Effective coping strategies include regulating the amount of stress into containable amounts, obtaining information, rehearsing the possible outcomes of treatment and assessing the situation from several viewpoints. Parents, nursing staff and paediatricians have an important role in promoting this repertoire of skills for children with a disability. Additionally, defence mechanisms such as denial, rationalisation and displacement can be helpful for the child during the initial stages of adjustment to the illness or disability.

Effects on the parents

Parents respond in different ways both in the short term and also in the long term. Most parents eventually achieve some degree of adaptation, though for a minority maladaptive behaviour patterns emerge and are persistent. The common parental response is that of overprotection whereby the parent(s) is unable to allow the child to experience the normal disappointments and upsets inevitable during childhood, so that the child leads a 'cotton wool' existence. Less frequently, the parent(s) may be rejecting and indifferent to the child because the child's disability is so damaging to the parents' self-esteem or because the disability has exacerbated an already precarious parent–child relationship. Overprotection and rejection are sometimes combined together in the parental reaction to a child's disability.

The parents may also find it difficult to provide appropriate discipline and control, as they irrationally fear that such control may aggravate the child's condition. For example, parents of children with epilepsy may think that thwarting the child's demands may induce an epileptic fit.

Finally, the stress of coping with the child's condition may exacerbate parental marital disharmony, though in a minority it may paradoxically unite them as they face the adversity together.

Effect on siblings

This can manifest itself in several ways: the oldest sibling may be given excessive responsibility, such as for looking after the disabled sib; the sibs may lose friendships because they are reluctant to bring their friends home in case their disabled sib is an embarrassment; and finally, the sibling's own developmental needs may be neglected, with consequent resentment and frustration.

Breaking bad news to parents

This distressing but inevitable aspect of paediatrics is required in various circumstances, such as the birth of a child with Down syndrome or with the diagnosis of cystic fibrosis. Unfortunately, most undergraduate and postgraduate training includes very little teaching about this important subject. Though the details vary for each case, the general principles given in Box 25.4 are important.

Reactions to hospitalisation

Admission to hospital is a common experience during childhood, with approximately 25% admitted by the age of 4 years. For most children, this is a short admission for a brief treatable illness, whilst a minority (approximately 4%) remain in hospital for at least a month. While most parents and their children cope successfully with the admission, some, particularly those with repeated admissions for minor illnesses, show evidence of disturbance which may in turn have been the reason why the child was admitted in the first place.

Admission to hospital can have adverse effects in the short term as well as in the long term. The contributory factors can be grouped under three headings:

- the child and family;
- the nature of the illness;
- the attitudes and practices of the hospital and its staff.

Important factors within the child and family include age, temperament of the child, previous experience of hospital, previous parent–child relationship and current family circumstances. Children aged between 1 and 4 years are particularly stressed by separation from familiar figures. Similarly, children with adverse temperamental characteristics, such as poor adaptability or irregularity of habits, are more vulnerable. If the child had a favourable experience when in hospital previously, this will ease the burden for any subsequent admission. If the parent–child relationship was poor prior to admission, hospitalisation is likely to exacerbate this problem because of the additional stress. Adverse family circumstances, for instance financial, may also be aggravated by admission.

The nature of the illness, particularly the associated pain or the necessity for painful procedures, influences the child's response. Again, an acute admission is likely to be more stressful than an elective procedure.

The attitudes of the staff and hospital practices can minimise considerably the distress for the child. Helpful and favourable aspects include good rooming-in facilities, adequate preparation for painful or unpleasant procedures, and nursing and medical staff trained to minimise distress and to offer comfort when required. The ward should be organised so that parents and sibs are encouraged to visit as well as ensuring the ready availability of playleaders and teachers. Medical and nursing staff should also have access to social work resources as well as to psychological and psychiatric services. Finally, joint liaison between the medical and psychiatric team and the establishment of a staff support group to enable staff to discuss their own anxieties about working in a stressful environment are likely to be beneficial.

TREATMENT METHODS

Several factors are usually responsible for the development of disturbance, so that it is unlikely that one treatment method will resolve the problem. All treatment approaches also rely upon common elements that are not only necessary but also essential for a successful outcome. These elements include active co-operation between the therapist and the child and family, agreement between them about the aims of treatment, and a mutual trust to enable these aims to be achieved. Again, the relative efficacy of different treatments is not clearly established, so that the choice of treatment is often a reflection of the therapist(s)' training and experience rather than an absolute indication in any particular instance. Careful analysis of the factors listed in Box 25.5 is therefore necessary in order to devise an effective treatment programme. The formulation of the problem along the four dimensions shown in Box 25.5 provides the basis on which to decide the programme.

The three main types of treatment approach available are *drug treatment*, *the psychotherapies* and *liaison* or *consultation work*. The latter refers to the common practice whereby the child psychiatrist or a member of the psychiatric team does not have direct contact with the referred child, but rather helps those involved with the child to understand and modify the child's behaviour. Psychotherapies are those treatments that use a variety of psychological techniques to ameliorate disturbance. They include individual therapy, behaviour therapy, family therapy and group therapy as well as counselling and advice for parents.

Drug treatment

This has increasing importance in child psychiatry (Kutcher 1997) Table 26.3 summarises the important indications and side-effects of various drugs used in child psychiatry.

Box 25.4	Breaking bad news to parents

- Information should be given by the most senior and experienced doctor involved with the child's care.
- Both parents must be seen together if at all possible, as this reduces misinformation and allows the parents to be mutually supportive from the outset.
- Allow adequate time for the interview (not 10 minutes at the end of a ward round).
- Privacy is essential not only as a matter of courtesy and dignity but also because it allows parents to express their emotions more freely.
- Begin the interview by asking the parents to tell you what they know about the problems.
- Tell parents frankly and honestly in simple and non-technical language the nature of the problem, explaining the reasons for the investigations and the basis for the diagnosis.
- Encourage the parents to ask questions (by asking them some open-ended questions).
- Emphasise the positive as well as the negative aspects of the diagnosis, for instance the child will be able to have physiotherapy and special equipment, will be able to go to school and to receive effective control for pain.
- Facilitate the expression of emotions by the parents, namely respond sympathetically and sensitively to the parent(s)' distress and crying.
- Make a definite offer of a further appointment to talk things over again.
- Many parents find it helpful to continue the discussion with a nurse or social worker after the interview.

Psychotherapies

These are a very common treatment approach in child psychiatric practice.

Individual psychotherapy

Though there are several theoretical orientations, including psychoanalytic (Freud 1946) and Rogerian (Reisman 1973), the

---

Box 25.5 Factors influencing a treatment programme

1. Individual
   a. Physical illness or disability
   b. Intellectual ability
   c. Type of symptomatology
2. Family
   a. Developmental stage (for instance a family with preschool children or one with adolescents)
   b. Psychiatric health of parents
   c. Marital relationship
   d. Parenting qualities
   e. Communication patterns within the family
   f. Ability to resolve conflict
   g. Support network, for instance availability of the extended family
3. School
   a. Scholastic attainments
   b. Child's and parents' attitudes to the authority of the school
   c. Peer relationships
4. Community
   a. Quality of peer relationships and of role models
   b. Neighbourhood and community resources.

---

therapist has nevertheless the same therapeutic tasks (Lanyardo & Horne 1999). These are:

- to develop a trusting, non-judgemental relationship with the child;
- to enable the child to express his feelings and thoughts;
- to understand the meaning of the child's symptoms, including his behaviour during the therapeutic session;
- to provide the child with some understanding and explanation for his behaviour.

The indications for individual psychotherapy are not clearly established, though most usually it is for children with a neurotic or reactive disorder rather than for those with a constitutionally based disorder. For younger children the medium for communication is play such as sand play or through drawing, whilst for older children verbal exchange and discussion are possible.

Behavioural psychotherapy

This approach is based upon the application of the findings from experimental psychology, particularly learning theory, to a wide range of problems such as enuresis, encopresis, tantrums and aggression (Herbert 1996). Its characteristics are as follows:

1. Define problem(s) objectively with reference to the Antecedents, the Behaviour itself and the Consequences (the ABC approach).
2. Emphasise current behaviour rather than past events.
3. Set up hypotheses to account for the behaviour.
4. Establish a pre-treatment baseline to determine the frequency and severity of the problem.
5. Devise behavioural programmes on an individual basis to test the hypothesis.

Table 25.3 Drug treatment in child psychiatry

Drug	Usage	Comment
Anxiolytics	Anxiety / phobic conditions	Short-term adjunct to behaviour treatment
Antipsychotics		
Phenothiazines (e.g. chlorpromazine)	Schizophrenia / ADD	Extrapyramidal side-effects common
Butyrophenones (e.g. haloperidol)	Complex tics / Tourette's syndrome	Extrapyramidal side-effects common
Newer antipsychotics (e.g. risperidone, olanzapine)	Schizophrenia	Fewer side-effects
Tricyclics		
Imipramine, nortriptyline	Second line of treatment for ADD	Useful when an affective component present
Clomipramine	Obsessive–compulsive disorder	Long-term usage often necessary
SSRIs (fluoxetine, paroxetine, sertraline)	Probably first choice for depressive disorder	Better compliance, with fewer side-effects
Stimulants Methylphenidate, dexamphetamine	ADD	80% effective. Side-effects closely monitored
Hypnotics (melatonin)	Persistent sleep disorder	Sometimes used for sleep problems associated with ADD
Lithium	Recurrent bipolar affective disorder	Close supervision of blood level and for signs of toxicity
Laxatives e.g. bulk-forming (methylcellulose), stimulants (senna), softener (Dioctyl)	Encopresis with constipation	Facilitates formation and passage of faeces
Central α-agonist (e.g. clonidine)	Unresponsive Tourette's syndrome	Sedation and rebound hypertension

ADD, attention deficit disorder; SSRI, selective serotonin reuptake inhibitor

6. Evaluate the outcome of treatment programmes.
7. Tackle one problem at a time.

As with other psychotherapies, success depends upon the establishment of a trusting relationship with the patient and the close supervision of the treatment programme together with the involvement of teachers and parents in many cases.

Cognitive behavioural therapy (CBT)

This is used increasingly with older children and adolescents for a variety of conditions including anxiety, depression and anorexia nervosa (Kendall 1999). The central premise is that the individual's cognitive distortions are responsible for the symptoms and the disorder, so that therapy is designed to change cognitions through a collaborative approach between the therapist and the patient. Usually the treatment lasts about 12 sessions. The early part of the treatment is devoted to teaching the patient to recognise their cognitive distortions, and then training them to devise alternative and more healthy interpretations of the situation. This is combined with 'homework tasks' between sessions in order to put into practice the new ideas or responses to situations that they find difficult.

Family therapy

This is a popular treatment approach now. The rationale underlying family therapy is that the child's disturbed behaviour is symptomatic of the disturbance within the family as a group. There are many different theoretical approaches and techniques (Gorrell Barnes 1994), but all usually involve interviewing the whole family on each occasion for about one hour. Most family work is short term, lasting about 6 months, with approximately monthly sessions. The emphasis is on current behaviour, verbal and non-verbal, observed during the session rather than on past events. The main aim is to improve communication within the family, so that dysfunctional patterns of behaviour are replaced by more healthy and adaptive behaviour.

Group therapy

Older children and adolescents often benefit from group therapy when the aim is to improve interpersonal relationships, particularly with the peer group, using a variety of theoretical models (for instance psychodynamic and social skills).

Supportive psychotherapy and counselling

The former is frequently used for the child with chronic illness or disability when the focus may be the child or the parents. It is especially beneficial at the time of diagnosis and also in the long term when the implications of the disability become more evident. Parental counselling is also used to help the parents understand their child's behaviour problems, the factors that may have led to them and that are responsible for their continuation, along with an emphasis on the parent–child relationship and the improvement of parenting skills. Counselling may therefore help the parents to devise and implement a behavioural programme to modify the child's behaviour as well as to promote normal development.

Liaison and consultation psychiatry

This is a collaborative approach between the child psychiatry team and the professionals directly involved with the child, for instance hospital staff, teachers or residential care staff, in order to help these professionals understand the child's disturbed behaviour, their own possible contribution to the problem and to suggest ways to improve the situation (Lask 1994). Although the child psychiatrist may see the referred child in the first instance, subsequent contact is usually with the staff rather than with the child. This approach can also include the establishment and supervision of a staff support group whose aim is to look at the attitudes and emotional responses of the staff towards the behaviour shown by the children under their care.

PYSCHIATRIC DISORDERS IN ADOLESCENCE

This section has two parts: adolescent psychological development and adolescent psychiatric syndromes.

ADOLESCENT DEVELOPMENT

Adolescence is the transition between childhood and adult life. Four maturational tasks must be accomplished successfully to ensure a favourable outcome:

- the attainment of independence;
- the establishment of a sexual role and orientation;
- the self-control of aggressive and oppositional impulses;
- the achievement of self-identity.

Though these tasks are not necessarily complete nor entirely resolved by the end of adolescence, the adolescent should have made substantial progress with these tasks. Three tasks — independence, sex role and orientation, sex role and orientation, self-control of aggressive and oppositional impulses — refer to specific aspects of psychological development, whereas the fourth, self-identity, is a global term referring to that sense of uniqueness or individuality that distinguishes one person from another. Erikson (1965) believed that the attainment of a stable self-identity during adolescence is the prerequisite for successful adult adjustment. Important components of self-identity for Erikson are 'sexual identity' and 'career identity'. The Eriksonian unsuccessful outcome of adolescent conflict is 'identity diffusion', where the person lacks clear goals and direction in the fulfilment of individual ambition.

Adolescent development is commonly divided into four phases:

- the pre-adolescent phase (11–13 years);
- early adolescence (13–15 years);
- mid-adolescence (15–17 years);
- late adolescence (18 years onwards).

The main features of the pre-adolescent phase are the onset of biological puberty and an increased interest in peer relationships and teenage pursuits. Early adolescence is characterised by the critical questioning of parental values combined with an uncritical acceptance of peer group views. The establishment of a separate sexual and social identity occurs during mid-adolescence. The individual explores and develops their own gender and sexual role. The development of social relationships outside the family enables the individual to have their own social network as well as altering the basis of their relationship with their parents. Later adolescence is focused on the career or work choice along with the expression of the sexual role through more-satisfying and enduring relationships.

Determinants of adolescent adjustment

Though the same general factors influence development and adjustment in adolescence as in earlier periods, brief mention will be made of those that are of particular relevance.

Previous childhood experience(s) Unsatisfactory earlier experience(s) and relationships, particularly the child–parent(s) relationship, are major factors affecting predisposition to adjustment during adolescence. The individual's capacity to withstand the inevitable stresses of adolescence and also their resilience are greatly impaired when the outcome of earlier experiences was unsatisfactory. Adverse childhood experience is an important vulnerability factor in adolescent breakdown.

Family psychopathology Parental psychopathology such as marital disharmony or parental psychiatric illness has a powerful influence on children's behaviour throughout childhood, but even more so during adolescence, when conflicts over discipline, control and autonomy are normal and unavoidable. Parental disagreements and disunity on these matters greatly exacerbate the difficulties.

Schooling Common problems are: academic failure with scholastic subjects; poor motivation and disillusionment with schooling; conflicts over authority with teaching staff.

Peer group Peer group values and pressure exert enormous influence on the adolescent, so that contact with and membership of a deviant peer group can lead to major problems in school, for instance truancy, or in the community, for instance delinquency or vandalism.

Chronic illness or handicap The normal adolescent drive for self-appraisal and self-identity leaves the disabled or handicapped adolescent feeling isolated and different from his peers, a most distressing experience. Early childhood feelings of acceptance and tolerance by peers are replaced by those of exclusion and separateness, with a reluctance or inability to gain peer group acceptance. The adolescent often deals with these feelings of anger and frustration by denial or minimalisation of the seriousness of his condition. This can result in poor compliance with medication or reckless exposure to dangerous situations.

Interviewing and assessment of adolescents

Though the earlier part of the chapter discussed the general principles of interviewing and assessment, it is helpful to mention some specific points relating to adolescence. Flexibility in approach is essential for successful interviewing. In general, the older the adolescent and the more serious or intimate the problem, the greater the necessity for a separate interview with the adolescent. Usually, this is combined with a family interview in order to complete the assessment.

Many adolescents are reluctant, confused or anxious attenders, so that the clinician must clarify and explain the purpose, sequence and duration of the assessment procedures at the outset. Respect for the adolescent's maturity, the right to privacy and confidentiality must be acknowledged clearly. The distinction between 'family business' and 'individual business' must be emphasised to the adolescent and to the parents. Adolescent anxieties about 'see-ing the shrink' or being 'treated like a child' must be addressed and talked through. The individual interview may allow the clinician to conduct a thorough assessment of the mental state, though careful phrasing of questions about sexual or psychotic phenomena is essential in order to avoid a dismissive denial and a further increase in anxiety and confusion.

Silence and refusal to talk during the interview are common and often difficult to overcome. The clinician can use three tactics to deal with this problem: it can be pointed out that the silence is just as difficult for the interviewer as it is for the adolescent; there will be the opportunity and time to talk through difficult topics now or alternatively on another occasion; and finally, to terminate the interview when necessary to prevent prolonged or undue tension.

Family interviews are often not only part of the assessment procedure but also of the treatment plan. Sometimes, however, it is more appropriate to interview the parents and the adolescent together rather than the whole family.

ADOLESCENT PSYCHIATRIC SYNDROMES

These are divided into three categories:

- those disorders persisting from earlier childhood;
- new disorders arising during adolescence;
- those disorders with features special to adolescence.

Prior to the discussion of these topics, brief comment will be made about the prevalence of psychiatric disorders in adolescence.

Prevalence

This varies widely from 10% to 20% depending upon the population studied, the diagnostic criteria and the age group. Most studies do, however, show a consistent pattern with respect to gender ratio, urban versus rural differences and the range of clinical syndromes. In contrast to earlier childhood, when psychiatric disorder is more common among boys, the adolescent period shows a shift towards an equal gender ratio in early adolescence followed by a subsequent female preponderance in late adolescence and adult life. Prevalence rates in urban populations are at least twice those for rural populations. Schizophrenia, major affective disorder, suicide and attempted suicide, anorexia and substance misuse all begin to appear with some frequency during adolescence, whereas encopresis or enuresis decrease markedly.

Persistent childhood disorders

Childhood disorders are more likely to continue into adolescence when one or more of the following are present:

- a major constitutional factor to the syndrome;
- the adverse circumstances responsible for the onset of the disorder are still present;
- perpetuating or maintaining factors are prominent.

The follow-up study of 10-year-old children in the Isle of Wight study (Rutter et al 1975) showed that 40% of the disorders had persisted into adolescence, with a strong continuity for boys with conduct disorder and associated educational problems. This section now discusses the factors responsible for the persistence of some disorders into adolescence from earlier childhood.

Conduct disorder

The oppositional and defiant character of conduct disorder means that it is very likely to be exacerbated by the rebellious and anti-authoritarian nature of ordinary adolescent behaviour. Childhood predictors of persistent conduct disorder are: early onset of symptoms; extensive and varied symptomatology; and severe aggressive behaviour. Adverse temperamental characteristics combined with continued exposure to deviant family psychopathology such as deficient and ineffective parenting, marital disharmony or parental psychiatric illness are thought to be important factors maintaining the conduct disorder. The persistence of the frequently associated learning disorders is another source of frustration and disillusionment for the adolescent, producing conflict with the teachers and reluctance to attend school.

Emotional disorders

Generally, emotional disorders have a good prognosis, often because they arise in response to some identifiable but remedial stress. Consequently, emotional disorder persisting into adolescence implies a more serious underlying cause. The school refusal syndrome is the most likely condition to show continuity from early childhood. It may reappear at the transfer from primary to secondary school, or early on during secondary schooling. Previous history of separation difficulties, for instance at the start of nursery or primary school and/or an overdependent relationship between the child and parent(s), are commonly found. The increased necessity for independence, autonomy and assertiveness at secondary school may prove too much for the vulnerable adolescent.

Childhood autism

The overt autistic-like behaviour and overactivity prominent in younger children with the disorder often decrease during adolescence, but the majority are still profoundly impaired in social and communication skills, with a marked apathy and lack of empathy. Educational and learning disabilities are very evident. Epilepsy also develops in about 15% of individuals, with a greater risk when severe mental retardation is also present.

Attention deficit disorder

The overactivity usually decreases during adolescence, but persistent problems with antisocial behaviour, impulsivity, recklessness, distractibility and learning disorders mean that the adolescent with attention deficit disorder is likely to remain disturbed.

New disorders arising during adolescence

These can be divided into two categories: those related to the stress of adolescence, and major adult-like disorders arising in adolescence.

Stress-related adolescent disorders

During adolescence, the distinction between normal and abnormal behaviour is often imprecise, so that it is more important to understand why the adolescent's behaviour is such a cause of concern rather than whether the behaviour fulfils the criteria for a disorder in a diagnostic classification system. In many cases, conflict often arises between the adolescent and the parents over independence and control issues. Allied with the pressure from peers, this often leads the adolescent to engage in antisocial or conduct disordered behaviour. Delinquency, vandalism and out of control behaviour are common, sometimes mixed with a pattern of alcohol or drug misuse. Persistent antisocial disorder often culminates in criminal behaviour and arrest by the police. Coexistent family problems with a limited capacity to resolve issues also contribute to the severity of the disorder. Eventually, it may be necessary for the adolescent to leave the family home and to provide him with alternative care arrangements, for instance with foster parents or community carers. Another solution sometimes adopted by the adolescent is to run away from home. Although the majority of runaways eventually return home, a minority stay away and become involved with the homeless subculture found in large cities.

The common neurotic or emotional responses to adolescent stress are affective symptoms such as irritability, lability of mood and anxiety symptoms, particularly related to social situations or mixing with peers. The latter may sometimes lead to marked social withdrawal. School refusal may sometimes present for the first time during early adolescence, when it represents a combination of adolescent stress and the revival of an earlier overdependent parent–child relationship. The increased need for independence and autonomy posed by the demands of secondary school precipitates an avoidance response to school attendance from the adolescent. The anxiety symptoms often masquerade themselves as physical complaints such as headaches or abdominal pain. The prompt exclusion of organic pathology with a minimum amount of investigation is essential in order to prevent the secondary elaboration of physical symptomatology. Delay in the recognition of the underlying psychological basis for the problem greatly exacerbates the difficulties. The prognosis is not good for a significant minority of adolescents, with up to a third failing to maintain regular school attendance. Poor prognosis is usually a sign of more serious underlying family psychopathology. Follow-up studies into adult life have shown that anxiety or agoraphobic symptoms are present in about 20% (Berg 1992).

Obsessive–compulsive disorder (OCD) sometimes begins during adolescence, when its occurrence can be seen as a maladaptive response to the stress of adolescence. There is often a history of earlier childhood obsessional and anxiety traits. The key element in the maintenance and exacerbation of the disorder is usually the willingness of the family to participate in the ritualistic behaviour. SSRIs such as sertraline or fluvoxamine have been shown to be effective in reducing OCD symptoms, but more importantly they are particularly effective when combined with cognitive-behaviour therapy (King et al 1998).

Major adult-like disorders arising in adolescence

Three categories of disorder — schizophrenia, mood disorders and anorexia nervosa — begin to occur with increasing frequency during adolescence.

Schizophrenia   This is a rare disease during childhood. Even during adolescence, it has a frequency of less than three per 10 000. Symptoms are usually classified into two groups: positive and negative. Positive symptoms comprise delusions (fixed, false beliefs), hallucinations (a perceptual experience in the absence of the relevant sensory stimulus) and distortions of thinking (thought insertion and withdrawal). Negative symptoms include social withdrawal, emotional blunting, apathy, lack of motivation, poverty of speech and slowness of thought. The usual presentation is insidious rather than florid, with a gradual social withdrawal and increased internal preoccupation. Dysphoric symptoms are common, so that a diagnosis of affective disorder is sometimes made. The adolescent is often able to conceal his bizarre ideas from parents and peers. However, it is the presence of increasingly unpredictable and erratic behaviour that indicates something more serious is occurring. The possibility of drug misuse is an important alternative diagnostic possibility.

Aetiology There is good evidence of a genetic component, with approximately 20% of relatives having the disease (Hollis 2000). The Maudsley long-term follow-up study of early-onset psychosis (Hollis 2000) showed that one-third had significant pre-morbid social difficulties affecting the ability to make and retain friends. There was also a downward shift in intelligence, with a mean IQ of 85. The disorder tends to run a chronic course with only a minority making a full symptomatic recovery — only 12% of patients in the Maudsley study were in remission at 6 months. The best prognostic indicator was the clinical state at that time.

Treatment This must be comprehensive, including drug treatment with antipsychotics, individual and family therapy as well as help with education. Traditional antipsychotics such as chlorpromazine and haloperidol are effective, particularly for positive symptoms, but side-effects such as extrapyramidal side-effects and drowsiness adversely affect compliance. Consequently, the newer antipsychotics such as risperidone and olanzapine, with their low side-effect profile, are now the drugs of first choice. When treatment with first-line drugs is ineffective, serious consideration should be given to clozapine. This drug has been shown to be effective for treatment-resistant schizophrenia in adults, and promising case reports have been published for adolescents. There must be careful screening and monitoring for side-effects, particularly for blood dyscrasias, when clozapine is used.

Finally, bad prognostic features include poor premorbid functioning, negative symptoms and a long period of untreated illness.

Depression as a symptom / syndrome Depression has been recognised as a syndrome in adults for a long time because of its characteristic constellation of symptoms, response to treatment and outcome. The depressed mood or dysphoria has qualities other than just simple sadness or unhappiness. Rather, it is the inability to derive pleasure or satisfaction from daily life (anhedonia) or to be able to respond emotionally to ordinary events. Other features of the syndrome are cognitive disturbances, behavioural changes and alterations in physiological functions. The cognitive disturbances are primarily cognitive distortions around oneself (self-blame, self-reproach, guilt and worthlessness), the world (helplessness and despair about one's life situation) and the future (hopelessness and despondency about the future). The behavioural changes range from marked agitation to withdrawal and stupor, while the physiological changes are poor appetite, weight loss and disturbed sleep pattern.

In adolescence, depression can present in the following ways:

- as a transient mood state;
- as a symptom in other psychiatric disorders, for instance anxiety states;
- as a symptom in physical illnesses, for instance infectious mononucleosis;
- as part of a symptom complex in major depressive disorder.

Epidemiological studies have shown an increasing prevalence of depressive symptomatology from childhood to adolescence. Rutter et al (1976) found that adolescents had experienced feelings of misery and depression (40%), self-deprecation (20%) and suicidal thoughts (7%) at one time or another. Comprehensive accounts can be found in Park & Goodyer (2000) and Goodyer (2001).

Depressive disorders Both the ICD and DSM classifications now state that depression in children and adolescents should have the same features as that in adults. They recognise the following core features: abnormal depressed mood for at least 2 weeks; marked loss of interest or pleasure in almost all activities; decreased energy or increased fatigue. Additional features include: loss of confidence and self-esteem; unreasonable feelings of guilt or self-reproach; suicidal thoughts; poor concentration and indecisiveness; psychomotor agitation or retardation; sleep disturbance; and loss of appetite.

Aetiology There is no adequate theory for child or adolescent depression, but there is some support for each of the two main theories: genetic and environmental. Evidence for a genetic component comes from twin, adoption and family studies, though the size of the effect is not known. Environmental theories range from the traditional psychoanalytic perspective, to the adverse impact of life events, to the cognitive theory of Beck et al (1979). The latter regards the individual's negative view of himself, the world and the future as the cause of the depression, though clearly these cognitions could be seen as a consequence of the depressed mood rather than the cause.

Assessment This involves detailed and sensitive interviewing of the adolescent, usually alone, as well assessment of the adolescent and the family. Family assessment is useful for two reasons: the adolescent's behaviour can be seen in the context of current family functioning; and other sources of stress for the adolescent or family may be identified. Physical symptoms are frequently found among depressed adolescents, though the findings are not specific as anxious adolescents often have physical symptoms as well. The differential diagnosis must involve the distinction between normal sadness or unhappiness, other psychiatric conditions with depressive symptomatology, for instance anorexia nervosa, or physical illnesses such as infectious mononucleosis or influenza.

Treatment A comprehensive treatment package is most likely to be most effective. Components include drug treatment, individual and family therapy and the reduction or lessening of stressful circumstances. The relative emphasis and sequence of treatments are dependent upon assessment.

Drug treatment is most likely to be effective for adolescents who are most severely affected and have a disturbance of physiological functions such as appetite, sleep or weight. SSRIs are the drugs of choice because of the low side-effect profile. Emslie et al (1997) have shown the superiority of fluoxetine to placebo in a well-conducted randomised controlled trial.

The purpose of individual therapy varies widely depending on the assessment and therapeutic style of the clinician. The common aims of an individual approach are: to establish a trusting relationship with the adolescent; to enable the adolescent to feel understood and accepted; and to allow the adolescent to disclose their concerns and anxieties including suicidal thoughts. Beyond these core aims, the therapeutic approach is varied, ranging from psychodynamically insight-orientated psychotherapy to cognitive-behavioural therapy.

Work with the family is often undertaken more to improve communication between members of the family rather than to specifically treat family dysfunction. Family sessions are extremely useful at the start of treatment as a way to discuss events of emotional significance that may have happened recently but have not been talked through, for instance a family illness or a bereavement. These sessions also provide the opportunity to discuss ways to reduce any overt source of stress or anxiety for the adolescent. Common sources of stress include lack of friends, bullying or teasing at school and the adolescent's sense, usually distorted, of academic failure at school.

Bipolar disorder or manic–depressive psychosis   ICD and DSM use similar criteria for the diagnosis of bipolar disorder whether in adolescents or adults; the following points summarise the main criteria.

- A disorder characterised by repeated episodes, that is two or more, in which the subject's mood and activity are significantly disturbed. This disturbance consists on some occasions of an elevation of mood with increased energy and activity (mania or hypomania), and on others of a lowering of mood with decreased energy and activity (depression).
- Recovery is characteristically complete between episodes.
- Manic episodes usually begin abruptly, lasting from 2 weeks to 4 or 5 months, whilst depressive episodes often last longer.

Clinical features   A hypomanic or depressive episode is equally common as the first manifestation of a bipolar illness, with subsequent episodes more likely to be hypomanic than depressive. A depressive episode shows similar features to other depressive illnesses except that it tends to be more severe with a pronounced disturbance in physiological functioning and frequent suicidal thoughts.

The main feature of the hypomanic episode is an elevated, expansive or irritable mood, with the other aspects understandable in terms of the elevated mood. The common features are: increased physical activity or physical restlessness; increased talkativeness; difficulty in concentration and distractibility; less need for sleep; increased sexual energy; mild spending sprees or other types of reckless behaviour; and increased sociability or over-familiarity. A manic episode causes severe disruption to the individual's life. The increased talkativeness becomes a 'pressure of speech' with flight of ideas (rapid switching of ideas based on a literal rather than a logical association, for instance rhyming or punning). The social disinhibition and recklessness can have a devastating effect on the individual's life. Cases with early onset have a worse prognosis with more frequent episodes, rapid cycling and a greater risk of suicide.

Though uncommon, several organic conditions can mimic a hypomanic episode. These include infections (encephalitis), endocrine (hyperthyroidism), neurological (repeated seizures, head trauma), brain tumour (meningioma, glioma), medication (steroids) and substance misuse (alcohol and amphetamine/LSD misuse).

Management   A depressive episode should be managed in a similar manner to other depressive episodes: that is, SSRIs, individual and family support. ECT may need to be considered for a severaly depressed and/or suicidal patient.

The hypomanic episode is often harder to manage, as it usually requires inpatient admission, measures to ensure the safety and protection of the patient and also drug treatment. The most useful drug for an acute episode is haloperidol (dosage 0.05 mg/kg/day in three divided doses). It is usually necessary to supplement this medication with anti-Parkinsonian drugs such as benzhexol or orphenadrine. An acute dystonic reaction such as an oculogyric crisis or acute torticollis can occur when treatment is commenced. Consequently, it is essential to observe closely the initiation of the medication.

Lithium carbonate is also effective in the acute episode, though its effect has a slower onset. Lithium is more useful as a prophylactic medication for individuals who have had several episodes. Its introduction should be carefully supervised and monitored. There have been no controlled trials of the effectiveness of lithium in the prevention of further episodes in children or adolescents. Lithium has, however, been shown to be less effective among individuals with a rapid cycling disorder, features common among adolescents with bipolar disorder. Other drugs such as carbamazepine and sodium valproate have been used in the treatment of previously drug resistant manic episodes in adults, but there is insufficient evidence to evaluate their efficacy for adolescents with bipolar disorder.

Prognosis   Most individuals usually recover from an acute episode. For individuals with repeated episodes, poor prognostic features include the absence of a precipitating factor, a family history of recurrent illness and the continuation of some symptoms between acute episodes.

Suicide   This is extremely rare below the age of 12 years, with an increase during adolescence to approximately 30 cases per million per year (Shaffer & Piancentini 1994). It is more common in males with no trend in social class. Males tend to use violent methods such as hanging or jumping from high buildings or bridges, whilst females have a preference for self-poisoning. Shaffer & Piancentini (1994) identified four types of personality characteristics among adolescents who commit suicide: irritable and over-sensitive to criticism; impulsive and volatile; withdrawn and uncommunicative; and perfectionist and self-critical. They also found that some evidence for an increased psychiatric disturbance in the family and that a 'disciplinary crisis' was the most common reason precipitating the suicide.

Attempted suicide   This is common, with a rate of four per thousand per year among 15–19-year-olds. Females are three times more likely than males to make an attempt, and there is an excess among lower socio-economic groups. Not surprisingly, the families show evidence of marital disharmony, maternal psychiatric ill health, particularly depression, and paternal personality disorder. About 50% of adolescents show some evidence of psychiatric disorder, usually depression. In older adolescents, there is often a history of alcohol or drug misuse and running away from home. Social isolation and poor peer relationships are also common.

The most common method is an overdose of non-opiate analgesics such as aspirin or paracetamol, probably related to their easy availability. The severity of the overdose varies markedly from a few tablets taken impulsively to swallowing the contents of a bottle of analgesics. The attempt often follows a row with a boyfriend or a serious dispute with the parents over discipline. The adolescent may have threatened to take an overdose on previous occasions, and about 50% have consulted their general practitioner in the month prior to the overdose.

A crucial part of management is the assessment of future suicide risk. This depends on three factors: the circumstances of the attempt, the patient's current mental state and their attitude to the future. Detailed questioning about events prior to the attempt are necessary as well as a 'blow by blow' account of the attempt. The latter includes infromation about the degree of planning, whether anybody else was present and any action taken after the attempt.

The identification of any difficulties at home or at school is also important.

The presence of significant depressive symptoms and pessimism about the future are predictors of continued suicide risk. It is important to enquire whether the overdose has altered the adolescent's or family's attitude to their current difficulties and their resolve to improve the situation. An assessment of the coping strategies and the capacity for change within the family is important in order to make a more realistic judgement about the future. Finally, there should be some agreement about future plans and any further contact between the adolescent, the family and the relevant professional agencies.

Treatment depends on the assessment and clinical judgement. The majority of adolescents do not require specialist psychiatric follow-up, though clearly they must know how to access psychiatric services in order to arrange further help when necessary. The indications for more specialised help include: the seriousness of the attempt; the presence of definite depressive disorder or persistent suicidal ideas; poor family circumstances and social support; and the limited capacity of the family for change. A small number may require inpatient psychiatric care, particularly the older adolescent. Follow-up psychiatric contact often involves individual counselling for the adolescent as well as family sessions to improve communication and the capacity to resolve disagreements.

There have been few systematic follow-up studies, though clinical impression suggests that those with definite psychiatric disorder or adverse social or family circumstances are more likely to be 'repeaters'.

Anorexia nervosa and related disorders   Anorexia nervosa is a disorder of older female adolescents, with a prevalence rate of 1% among 15–19 year olds (Lask & Bryant-Waugh 1999). It does, however, occur among prepubertal children. The core features are:

- self-induced starvation and weight loss;
- a strong desire to be thinner, and a marked fear of weight gain;
- a distorted body image (for instance feeling fat when emaciated)
- a body mass index < 17.5.

Clinical features   The presentation is varied, sometimes mimicking physical illness or the consequences of weight loss and starvation. The history is of prolonged self-imposed starvation. Dieting often begins following a chance remark about size or shape, or alternatively as a group behaviour with other adolescent girls. Food portions at mealtimes are reduced, and some meals such as breakfast or lunch are skipped entirely with the total elimination of high calorific foods such as sweets, puddings or cakes. The individual derives satisfaction from the weight loss, which in turn is a further incentive for weight loss. Parents and other adults are often complimentary and pleased at this initial weight loss. More extreme and rigid dieting is then self-imposed to meet the target for further weight reduction. Appetite and hunger pains are prominent, but the prospect of further weight loss is a powerful motivator. Only when the illness is well established does the anorexia and nausea over food become apparent. Interest and participation in exercise and athletic activities often parallel the dieting in the belief that these activities will enhance weight loss. Later on, excessive laxative use begins in order to reduce weight further.

Despite an increasingly thin physique, the adolescent refuses to accept her emaciated status, still believing and perceiving herself as fat or overweight. The distorted body image is often the first indication to the parents that the adolescent has a serious illness. Increasing arguments over food and its consumption, combined with an implacable refusal to eat, convince the parents that urgent medical help is required. Often, the adolescent is initially referred to a paediatrician or an endocrinologist in order to exclude a physical basis to the problem rather than accepting a psychological basis for the weight loss.

Physical examination usually shows an individual who is bright and alert despite the evident emaciation. Prominent cheekbones, sunken eyes, bones protruding through the skin, dry skin and hair, with blue cold hands and feet are common features. Severe emaciation is accompanied by the appearance of fine downy hair or lanugo hair on the face, limbs and trunk, with a slow pulse rate, low blood pressure and hypothermia. Most biochemical investigations are normal, but low gonadotrophin levels with high growth hormone and cortisol levels are sometimes found. Although anorexia is the most likely diagnosis, other psychiatric disorders such as depression, obsessive–compulsive disorder or schizophrenia may need to be excluded.

Aetiology   Almost as many theories have been proposed as the number of people who have researched the condition, with individual, family or societal factors prominent in most explanations. Review of the premorbid personality characteristics of anorexics shows them to be conformist, conscientious, compliant and high achieving. Issues over autonomy and independence are core issues for anorexics, with control over food intake the only available means to preserve self-identity and independence. Similar conflicts over autonomy and independence have been observed among families with an anorectic member, but whether this is cause or effect is unclear. Again, over the past 40 years, society's view about female attractiveness has veered towards the thin end of the spectrum, so that the 'pursuit of thinness' is a major issue for many women.

Management   The severity of the condition varies widely, so that treatment includes outpatient and inpatient management with an emphasis on a 'multimodal' approach. The latter implies that a variety of treatment strategies such as individual, family or cognitive therapies are used, often concurrently or sequentially, dependent on assessment. Recognition and acknowledgement of the problem are the first crucial steps in management. The nature and seriousness of the condition highlighted by the avoidance of food and the irrational ideas about eating must be explored thoroughly in order to establish a therapeutic alliance with the adolescent and the family. Only when the latter has occurred is it possible to commence a specific treatment programme.

The next stage is the alteration of eating habits in order to restore weight loss and to correct nutritional deficiencies. Advice and collaboration with a dietician are important from the outset, particularly for any nutritional deficiencies. A target weight, usually around the average for the age and height, should be agreed upon along with the appropriate daily calorific intake to ensure its attainment. Only minimal concessions to food fads or preferences should be allowed, and there should be a standard protocol for regular weight checks.

If the patient is in hospital, the nursing care and support are the most important aspects of management. The nursing staff have to win the co-operation of the adolescent for the treatment plan. They must also be vigilant about food hoarding and surreptitious vomiting. Treatment programmes usually involve a graded series of privileges dependent upon satisfactory weight gain. Once the target weight is attained, the diet should be modified, so that age-appropriate weight gain continues. Inpatient programmes often involve nursing staff supervising family meals at home during weekend leave.

Working with the family has two aims: to provide educational advice about the disorder; and to improve communication patterns within the family. Individual and group work is also useful, but drug treatment is not indicated unless there is a specific treatable disorder such as comorbid depression. Russell et al (1987) in a randomised intervention study into the effectiveness of family versus individual therapy found that family therapy was better than individual therapy in the prevention of relapse among anorexics under 18 years of age who had had the illness for less than 3 years. An important limitation of this study was that only 65% of the 80 patients completed the intervention programme.

In many ways, the easiest part of the treatment programme, particularly with inpatients, is the restoration of weight loss. A more challenging aspect is the restructuring of the adolescent's and family's attitude to food and their pattern of interaction. Regular supervision, support and contact are essential to maintain progress and keep up morale. Very often a compromise has to be made between an ideal resolution of the problem and a realistic appraisal of the adolescent's and family's capacity to change.

Outcome Results from follow-up studies vary widely according to inclusion criteria, outcome measures and length of follow-up. Despite these problems, outcome appears to fall into three categories: one-third good, one-third intermediate and one-third poor. There is a 10% mortality in the long term, with malnutrition and suicide accounting for most deaths. Poor prognostic factors are an early age of onset, coexistent psychiatric disorder and poor family functioning.

Bulimia nervosa This has three key features: recurrent binges and purges, a lack of control and a morbid preoccupation with weight and shape. It is rare in the prepubertal period, but becomes increasingly common in older adolescents and young adults, when it is often associated with depression. Most patients are of normal weight. The most serious medical concern is potassium depletion from frequent vomiting. The patient's lifestyle is often chaotic, so that the first aim of treatment is to establish some structure and boundaries for the patient. Dependent on assessment, a combination of individual, cognitive-behavioural and family work is appropriate in most cases.

Two new types of eating disorder have recently been described: *food avoidance emotional disorder* and *pervasive refusal syndrome*. The former is a disorder of emotions in which food avoidance is a prominent symptom along with other affective symptoms such as depression, anxiety or phobias. There is often a previous history of food fads or food restrictions, but the symptoms do not meet the criteria for anorexia nervosa. The validity and independence of this syndrome has, however, not yet been established.

Pervasive refusal syndrome is a severe life-threatening syndrome characterised by pervasive refusal to eat, drink, talk, walk or engage in any self-care skills. The patients are markedly under-weight with an adamant refusal to eat or drink, which ultimately becomes life threatening. Although they fulfil some criteria for anorexia nervosa, the pervasiveness of the symptomatology makes this diagnosis inappropriate. They require prolonged and exten-sive inpatient nursing care in order to maintain vital body func-tions. Most patients are girls with some suggestion that previous traumatic sexual abuse, often involving violence, may have been responsible for the precipitation of the disorder. Most make a sat-

isfactory physical recovery, but the long-term psychiatric adjustment is not yet known.

Special topics

Chronic fatigue syndrome

This has attracted widespread media coverage because of the controversy surrounding aetiology and treatment (Wright et al 2000). It is usually defined as a severe disabling fatigue affecting physical and mental functioning accompanied by myalgia, mood and/or sleep disturbance. Accurate prevalence figures are difficult to obtain, but are probably about 1 in 2000. Clinic samples tend to be adolescents aged 11–15 years, with more girls and from a higher socio-economic grouping.

Two-thirds of patients have had a previous viral infection, but not usually of the Epstein–Barr type. This leads to fatigue which results in a reduction in physical activity, leading to more fatigue on undertaking any physical activity. The situation is reinforced by parental and personal beliefs about causation, so that a state of inactivity and fatigue become established.

Management involves a through assessment to exclude comorbid psychiatric disorder such as depression, but keeping investigations to an agreed minimum. The establishment of mutual trust and a collaborative approach with the adolescent and the parents are essential to a good outcome. Individual cognitive and family work combined with a structured incremental rehabilitation strategy (a graded exercise programme) are the best way to make progress and limit further incapacity. A co-ordinated plan for school and social reintegration is also necessary.

Outcome is varied depending on the initial severity, but three-quarters have made a reasonable recovery after 2 years.

Substance misuse

This ranges from the readily available and legal substances such as tobacco or alcohol to the more uncommon and illegal substances such as heroin or cocaine. Though the latter give rise to more public concern, there is little doubt that cigarette smoking and excessive alcohol consumption have a far more deleterious effect on the health of the population as a whole. A recent survey of over 7000 15- and 16-year-olds in the UK (Miller & Platt 1996) found that almost everyone had drunk alcohol, 30% had smoked cigarettes in the previous 30 days and 43% had at some time used illicit drugs. High levels of smoking were associated with a poorer school performance, and smoking was more common among girls. Adolescents are, however, only rarely referred to psychiatric services because of their smoking or alcohol habits.

Solvent abuse (glue sniffing) Ashton (1990), reviewing the available literature, estimated that 5–10% of adolescents have at some time inhaled solvents, with 0.5–1% regular users. Since 1971, the death rate from solvent overdose has risen from two per annum to over 100 per annum recently. Solvent abusers have the follow-ing characteristics: male gender; peak adolescent usage between 13 and 15 years; and more common among lower socio-economic groupings, minority ethnic groups and disrupted families.

Inhaled substances include many everyday items such as adhesives, aerosols, dry-cleaning fluids and cigarette lighter fuel. The substances are inhaled through paper bags, saturated rags or by direct inhalation. It is often done as a group activity in the socio-economically disadvantaged areas of large cities, with regular solitary sniffing a cause for more serious concern. The immediate effect is euphoria followed by confusion, perceptual distortion, hallucinations and delusions. The regular user is often able to titrate the 'sniffs', so that a pleasantly euphoric state is maintained for several hours. The characteristic appearance of red spots around the mouth is highly suggestive of solvent abuse.

Sudden death during inhalation can occur from anoxia, respiratory depression, trauma or cardiac arrhythmia. The latter accounts for over half the deaths, whilst anoxia, usually from inhalation of vomit, is responsible for over 10% of deaths. Accidents or suicide attempts during the intoxication are another cause of death, particularly with toluene adhesives. Long-term effects include neurological damage (peripheral neuropathy, encephalopathy, dementia and fits) as well as renal and liver damage.

Most solvent abusers do not come into contact with psychiatric services, unless they are referred following hospital admission with acute intoxication. School-based educational programmes and community-resource initiatives are more likely to be beneficial in the long-term. The encouragement of retailers and shop owners to enforce the restrictions on the sale of solvents is also useful. A number of solvent abusers are referred for psychiatric assessment, usually when the abuse is seen as part of more widespread individual or family psychopathology. In the long-term, most adolescents do not persist with the habit, but a minority progresses onto more addictive drugs such as heroin or cocaine.

Other substances   These include 'soft' drugs such as cannabis (marijuana) or 'hard' drugs such as amphetamines, cocaine, heroin, lysergic acid diethylamide (LSD) and designer drugs such as 'Ecstasy'. The effects are euphoric and relaxing in the short term, but apathy and inertia occur with chronic use. Most individuals do not progress from cannabis to other more seriously addictive drugs, and its consumption is not indicative of underlying psychological disturbance.

Hard drug consumption is a far more serious problem with deleterious effects on physical and psychological well-being and also from the risk of physical or psychological dependence. In addition to euphoric and pleasurable effects, most of these drugs can produce acutely distressing symptoms such as panic, fright or hallucinations. This can result in suicidal behaviour or an increased risk of accidents. Long-term use, for example with amphetamine or cocaine, can precipitate a florid psychotic episode with hallucinations, usually visual, and paranoid delusions. Psychological withdrawal symptoms such as an unbearable craving for a 'fix' and physical withdrawal symptoms such as nausea, vomiting and diarrhoea make stopping the drug extremely difficult. Physical neglect and malnutrition are also common and exacerbate the problems. The necessity for a regular supply of the drug means that the individual resorts frequently to stealing or crime to support the addiction. The practice of needle-sharing is a major health hazard with HIV infection a strong possibility. Referral of the adolescent to a specialist treatment centre and support for the parents are essential to prevent the serious social and psychological problems inevitable with long-term drug misuse.

Sexual problems

Two topics are discussed: sexual abuse and sexual offenders in adolescence; and gender identity disorders.

Sexual abuse and sexual offenders in adolescence   Sexual abuse can present in two ways, direct disclosure of abuse or indirect manifestations of abuse. The same principles of practice and management apply to adolescents as to children (see child section of the chapter), but some special features are important (Briere et al 1996). Open disclosure by the adolescent is often accompanied by the plea for complete confidentiality and no further action. Clearly this guarantee cannot be given, and the adolescent must be counselled about the necessity for an open investigation and the need for a child protection conference.

Indirect manifestations of abuse are twofold: sexually related behaviour and psychiatric symptomatology. Sexually related manifestations include pregnancy, venereal disease and promiscuity. The last often arises because the adolescent relates too readily to adults in a sexual manner as a result of the earlier experience of sexual abuse by an adult. Paradoxically, the promiscuous behaviour may also lead some adults to disbelieve the adolescent's claims of abuse or to believe that the adolescent was responsible for the initiation of the sexual contact. Psychiatric presentations of abuse are numerous, with distress a prominent feature. Common presentations include depression, deteriorating school performance or attendance, suicidal behaviour and running away from home.

Help for the sexually abused adolescent has two aims: the protection of the adolescent from further abuse and the provision of therapy to lessen the psychological trauma of the abuse. The first aim is usually achieved by ensuring that the perpetrator is no longer living at home and/or does not have contact with the adolescent. A wide range of therapies is used, including individual counselling and support, family therapy or group therapy. Group therapy has become extremely popular recently. This approach has several advantages: the adolescent realises that other adolescents have had a similar experience; the adolescent has the opportunity to discuss and share their feelings with other adolescents who are in a similar predicament; and the adolescent may feel less stigmatised. The group approach is probably less successful when the predominant feeling of the adolescent is betrayal. In this instance, it is more useful to offer individual psychotherapy to enable the adolescent establish trust with the therapist, so that disclosure and discussion can occur in a confidential setting.

A more recent development has been the provision of treatment strategies for adolescents who have committed sexual offences. The latter include exhibitionism or indecent exposure as well as sexual abuse of other, usually younger, children. The treatment programme(s) involves an assessment of the offender's sexual knowledge and attitudes as well as their social skills and relationships. Treatment programmes use a variety of approaches, often in combination, including social skills training, sex education and cognitive-behavioural approaches.

General identity disorders

Society's attitudes towards sexuality have been changing in recent years, so that a more open discussion about sexual values and behaviour is possible with greater tolerance and less stigma associated with homosexuality whether in males or females (Di Ceglie 2000). Homosexual behaviour in some form or another is quite common during the pre-adolescent and adolescent years, occurring in approximately 20% of boys and 10% of girls. It appears to be a transitory pattern of behaviour, as estimates of adult male and female homosexuality are 3% and 1.5%, respectively. Whilst homosexuality per se is most unlikely to be a reason for psychiatric referral, anxiety and depression associated with doubts about the homosexual role are occasionally sufficiently severe to warrant referral.

Clinicians are more likely to be involved with children or adolescents who have a gender identity disorder. A core distinction is made between individuals who display anomalous gender role behaviour and those with gender identity disorder. Anomalous gender role behaviour is the individual's preference for interests, activities and clothes normally associated with the opposite gender. For example, effeminate boys prefer girls' style of clothing and to play with dolls, whilst 'tomboy' girls like aggressive contact games and boys' style of clothing.

By contrast, the essential feature of the gender identity disorder is the persistent wish to be of the opposite gender. This is confirmed by the frequent expression of this wish and by extensive anomalous gender role behaviour including cross-dressing. During adolescence, referral is often sought for problems associated with cross-dressing, homosexual behaviour and social ostracism from peers. Trans-sexualism or the wish for permanent change of gender assignment can also become an issue.

The search for aetiological factors in gender identity disorder has not been fruitful, with no convincing evidence for chromosomal, physiological or endocrine abnormalities. Most clinicians believe that several psychosocial factors acting in combination are responsible. The initial parental tolerance of the anomalous sexual behaviour followed by subsequent acceptance and reinforcement is a common finding among referred patients, together with an over-dependent maternal–child relationship.

Treatment strategies for gender identity disorder include individual and family therapy, parental counselling and behaviour therapy. The most important aspect of treatment is to define and agree goals with the parents and the child. Clinic studies (Zuker & Bradley 1995) indicate that the earlier treatment is commenced the better the prognosis. Behavioural programmes with attainable short-term goals are much more likely to be successful than more ambitious plans. Minimising anomalous gender behaviour such as cross-dressing, and the promotion of gender-appropriate behaviour, are the basis of the intervention strategies. Treatment of coexisting individual and family psychopathology is also beneficial. Finally, the long-term follow-up of 66 effeminate boys (Zuker & Bradley 1995) found that three-quarters were bisexual or homosexual as adults.

PSYCHIATRIC ASPECTS OF LEARNING DISABILITY IN CHILDHOOD AND ADOLESCENCE

Introduction

Child psychiatrists are likely to become involved with children with learning disability in several different ways. Sometimes, they are responsible for the provision of the specialist medical care for these children, but more commonly they are asked for advice from other professionals about the emotional and behavioural problems that are quite frequent in this group of children.

Terminology

Many terms such as 'mental subnormality' or/and 'mental handicap' have been used in the past. ICD and DSM use IQ (intelligence quotient) or mental age as the basis for classification.

IQ is defined as (mental age/chronological age) × 100. The mean or average IQ is therefore 100 with a standard deviation of 15. The normal or Gaussian distribution of intelligence means that approximately 2.5% of individuals are two standard deviations below the mean, corresponding to an IQ of 70. This is usually taken as the dividing point between the normal range of intelligence and mental retardation. ICD and DSM have four categories of mental retardation: mild (IQ 50–69 approximately); moderate (IQ 35–49 approximately); severe (IQ 20–34 approximately); profound (IQ less than 20). The other important defining criterion is that there should be evidence of social impairment and limitation in the individual's daily activities and self-care skills. Despite the use of the term 'mental retardation' by the ICD and DSM classification systems, most professionals in the UK prefer the term 'learning disability', hence its usage in this chapter.

Psychiatric aspects of learning disorder in children and adolescents with learning disability

Prevalence

The Isle of Wight study (Rutter et al 1970b) found that approximately one-third of children with learning disability showed signs of disturbance, with the rate rising to 50% among moderate to severely retarded children. The children exhibited the same range of disturbance as children of normal ability but in addition three disorders were much more frequent: childhood autism, pervasive hyperkinetic disorder and severe stereotyped movement disorder. Self-injurious behaviour and pica were also more frequent.

Aetiology

It is important to distinguish between the factors responsible for disorders occurring in mildly learning disabled children and those with moderate to severe disability. Children with mild learning disability probably have the same risk factors as children of average ability — that is adverse temperamental characteristics, specific learning disorders and family psychopathology — but to a greater extent. The last factor is particularly important, as parents of children with mild learning disability are also likely to be within the lower range of intellectual ability. Consequently, their parenting capacity may be limited, with inconsistent discipline and control prominent features. In addition, this may be combined with marital disharmony and socio-economic disadvantage, so that the vulnerability to psychiatric disturbance is considerably increased among this group of children.

By contrast, brain damage is an important causative factor among children with severe learning disability. Several studies (Rutter et al 1970a, b) have found that half the children with moderate to severe mental retardation have demonstrable brain damage. This increases the risk of psychiatric disturbance in several ways: loss of specific functions or skills; active disruption or dysfunction of normal brain activity; and the increased risk of epilepsy. Children with moderate to severe learning disability are also more likely to have specific learning difficulties that further increase vulnerability. In addition, adverse temperamental characteristics such as impulsivity, distractibility or overactivity are more common among this group of children. The psychosocial consequences of handicap for the child and the family also constitute a factor in some cases, though its importance is difficult to quantify.

Psychiatric syndromes specifically associated with moderate to severe retardation

Childhood autism

80% of children with childhood autism have an IQ less than 70. Many clinicians distinguish individuals who have classical childhood autism from those with severe learning disability and some autistic features. The latter include stereotypies, mannerisms and deficits in comprehension and expressive language. These symptoms, which are quite common among learning disabled children, tend to occur in isolation, so that the individual does not fulfil the diagnostic criteria for childhood autism. Clinical practice and research findings do not however provide clear cut criteria to decide the dividing line between childhood autism and severe learning disability with autistic features. Consequently, clinicians tend to have their own personal preferences in terminology and classification.

Autistic behaviours are also features of some syndromes associated with mental retardation such as tuberous sclerosis, rubella, fragile X syndrome and infantile spasms. In some cases, for instance rubella, the autistic behaviour seems to be a response to the coexisting sensory deficit rather than the separate occurrence of childhood autism. Finally, individuals with extremely uncommon neurodegenerative diseases such as subacute sclerosing panencephalitis or with disintegrative disorder often show autistic-like stereotypic behaviour.

Hyperkinetic syndrome / attention deficit disorder

Like autistic behaviour, overactive or hyperkinetic behaviour is common among children with severe learning disability. In most cases, the overactivity occurs in some situations but not others, with the overactivity reflecting an immaturity in behaviour and language skills. A much smaller but nevertheless significant number of children with severe learning disability do show pervasive hyperactivity with other features of that syndrome including distractibility, impulsivity and aggressive behaviour.

Stereotypic and self-injurious behaviour

Stereotypic movements such as body rocking or hand-flapping have been reported as frequently as 40% in mild to severely mentally retarded children. Self-injurious behaviour such as headbanging, biting of limbs or eye gouging is much less common but more potentially harmful and also difficult to eradicate. It often arises in an individual of very limited ability whose surroundings and immediate environment provide little or minimal stimulation. The Lesch–Nyhan syndrome is particularly associated with the development of self-mutilating behaviour.

Murphy (1985) reviewed the treatment methods for these intractable and destructive behaviours. Protective devices such as helmets, treatment with major tranquillisers such as haloperidol and behavioural approaches have all been used with some success. A real disadvantage with drug treatment is that once started it is difficult to stop, so that the individual can remain on a drug for several years, often with an increasing dose over time. A behavioural approach is more likely to produce long-lasting benefits, but it is more time consuming to carry out and more demanding of staff co-operation.

Pica

The ingestion of inedible substances is a transitory phenomenon among normal toddlers and is even more common among children with severe learning disability. The main adverse consequence of this behaviour is lead intoxication from the licking of objects. Faecal smearing and ingestion can occur among some severely retarded children, particularly those with an additional sensory handicap such as blindness.

Learning disability syndromes associated with specific behavioural characteristics

Traditionally, children with certain learning disability syndromes have been said to show a characteristic behavioural or personality profile, though contemporary opinion is more sceptical about such association.

Down syndrome Children with this syndrome are often described as sociable, musical, contented and easy going, features they share with their siblings. Overall, these children have a slightly increased rate of disturbance, with a minority showing aggressive and oppositional behaviour, usually associated with Down syndrome due to a translocation trisomy.

Phenylketonuria Untreated, these children develop severe learning disability with autistic and hyperkinetic behaviour prominent. Successful dietary treatment usually results in normal growth and development, but treated children have a greater risk of psychiatric disturbance, with overactivity, distractibility and restlessness common.

Lesch–Nyhan syndrome This sex-linked disorder of purine metabolism, occurring only in boys, is associated with an extrapyramidal movement disorder including chorea and athetosis, severe learning disability and self-injurious behaviour. The latter is extremely difficult to treat and eliminate.

Prader–Willi syndrome The main behavioural feature is the explosive outbursts associated with dietary restriction frequently imposed to control the voracious appetite and accompanying obesity.

Hydrocephalus Children with hydrocephalus were previously described as showing the 'cocktail party' syndrome. This is characterised by a verbosity in their speech and a superficiality or shallowness to the content of their conversation. The early detection and treatment of hydrocephalus have now produced a reduction in morbidity, so that these features are less commonly seen.

Management

Many professionals including paediatricians, teachers and psychologists are likely to be involved in the provision of care for children with learning disability and their families. A multidisciplinary approach to assessment and treatment is vital. Different aspects of management are important at various stages during the child's life.

Breaking the news

This topic is discussed more fully in the child section of the chapter, so that only brief comments are made here. The ability to communicate bad news in a sensitive manner is a skill rarely taught to medical students or junior doctors. Many parents complain justifiably that the initial interview with the doctor was unsatisfactory and distressing. Tact, sympathy and time are essential to enable the parent(s) to begin to grasp and understand the implications of the situation. Honest discussion combined with an emphasis on the hopeful aspects are the important prerequisites for a satisfactory interview.

Promotion of normal development

Parents should be encouraged from the outset to develop the social, self-care and educational skills of their child to the maximum. A 'normalisation' and 'optimalisation' strategy is the basis to the approach. Specific treatment packages, for example the Portage scheme, are helpful in enabling the parents to set realistic targets for their child.

Treatment of medical and behavioural problems

Advice from neurologists, physiotherapists and occupational therapists is important in the management of the neurological deficits frequently present among this group of children. Behavioural problems are managed in a variety of ways including medication (for hyperactivity and aggressive outbursts), protective devices (for excessive headbanging) and operant or time-out procedures (for maladaptive behaviour).

Educational needs

Parents need advice from an early stage about the most appropriate educational provision. A specialised pre-school nursery is vital, and should be combined with a plan for later special educational placement. Some children may benefit from attendance at schools for children with communication or autistic-like disorders.

Genetic counselling

This is clearly essential for all parents, especially when a specific syndrome is identified

Long-term casework and support

Clinical experience and practice suggest that many families find this type of help invaluable in the long-term. The identification of a key professional worker who coordinates the care plan for the child is very useful. A social worker or a professional from a voluntary organisation with counselling skills is often the person best placed to fulfil this role.

Outcome

Treatment programmes with their emphasis on maximising potential, minimising adverse effects and integrating the child into the community are the best approach. Despite cognitive impairment, behaviour problems can be reduced by treatment programmes, and families learn to adapt satisfactorily. The policy of the UK government is to close institutions for individuals with learning disability and to integrate them into the community in order to promote better long-term adjustment.

REFERENCES

Achenbach T 1991 Integrative Guide for the 1991 CBCL/41-18, YSR and TRF Profiles. University of Vermont, Burlington, Vt

Ainsworth M 1982 Attachment: retrospect and prospect. In: Parkes C M, Stevenson-Hinde J (eds) The place of attachment in human behaviour. Basic Books, New York

APA 1994 Diagnostic and Statistical Manual of mental disorders, 4th edn. American Psychiatric Association, Washington, DC

Ashton C 1990 Solvent abuse: little progress after twenty years. British Medical Journal 300:135–136

Asperger H 1944 'Die Autistischen psychopathen' im kindesalter. Archive für Psychiatrie und Nervenkrankheiten 117:76–136

Bailey N 1993 Bailey's Scales II. Psychological Corporation, San Antonio, Tx

Baron-Cohen S 1995 Mindblindness. MIT Press, London

Beck A, Rush A, Shaw B, Emery G 1979 Cognitive therapy of depression. Wiley, New York

Bee H 1999 The developing child, 9th edn. Harper, New York

Bentovim A, Elton A, Hildebrand J et al 1988 Sexual abuse within the family. Wright, London

Berg I 1992 Absence from school and mental health. British Journal of Psychiatry 161:154–166

Biederman J, Faraone S, Spencer T et al 1993 Patterns of comorbidity, cognition, and psychosocial functioning in adults with attention deficit hyperactivity disorder. American Journal of Psychiatry 150:1792–1798

Bowlby J 1969 Attachment and loss, vol 1: Attachment. Hogarth Press, London

Briere J, Berliner L, Buckley J 1996 The ASPAC Handbook on child maltreatment. Sage Publications, Thousand Oaks, Ca

Brown G, Harris T 1978 Social origins of depression. Tavistock, London

Chakrabarti S, Fombonne E 2001 Pervasive developmental disorders in pre-school children. Journal of the American Medical Association 285:3094–3098

Cohen D, Volkmar F 1997 A Handbook of Autism and Pervasive Developmental Disorders. Wiley, Chichester

Corbett J, Harris R, Taylor E, Trimble M 1977 Progressive disintegrative psychosis of childhood. Journal of Child Psychology and Psychiatry 18:211–219

Di Ceglie D 2000 Gender identity disorder in young people. Advances in Psychiatric Treatment 6:458–467

Dummit E, Klein R, Tancer N et al 1996 Fluoxetine treatment of children with selective mutism. Journal of the American Academy of Child and Adolescent Psychiatry 35:615–621

Egger J, Stolla A, McEwan L 1992 Controlled trial of hyposensitisation in children with food-induced hyperkinetic syndrome. Lancet 339:1150–1153

Elliott C 1996 British Ability Scales Second Edition (BASI II). National Foundation for Educational Research/Nelson, Windsor

Eminson M, Postlethwaite R 1999 Munchausen by proxy: a practical approach. Butterworth-Heinemann, Oxford

Emslie G, Rush J, Weinberg W et al 1997 A double blind, randomised, placebo-controlled trial of fluoxetine in child and adolescents with depression. Archives of General Psychiatry 54:1031–1037

Erikson E 1965 Childhood and society. Penguin, London

Freud A 1936 The ego and the mechanisms of defence. Hogarth Press, London

Freud A 1946 The psychological treatment of children. Imago, London

Garralda E 1996 Somatisation in children. Journal of Child Psychology and Psychiatry 37:13–33

Gillberg C 1995 Clinical child neuropsychiatry. Cambridge University Press, Cambridge

Goodman R 1997 The Strengths and Difficulties Questionnaire: a research note. Journal of Child Psychology and Psychiatry 38:581–586

Goodyer I 1990 Life experiences, development and childhood psychopathology. Wiley, Chichester

Goodyer I 2001 The depressed child and adolescent: developmental and clinical perspectives, 2nd edn. Cambridge University Press, Cambridge

Gorrell Barnes G 1994 Family therapy. In: Rutter M, Taylor E, Hersov L (eds) Child and adolescent psychiatry: modern approaches, 3rd edn. Blackwell, Oxford

Hagberg B 1993 Rett's syndrome—clinical and biological aspects. MacKeith Press, London

Hawton K, Salkovskis P, Kirk J, Clark D 1995 Cognitive behaviour therapy for psychiatric problems: a practical guide, 2nd edn. Oxford University Press, Oxford

Herbert M 1996 ABC of behavioural methods. British Psychological Society, Leicester

Hobson P 1993 Autism and the development of mind. Lawrence Erlbaum, Hove

Hollis C 2000 Adolescent schizophrenia. Advances in Psychiatric Treatment 6:83–92

Huntley M 1996 Griffiths Mental Development Scales from birth to two years. Association for Research on Infant and Child Development, London

Jan J, Espezel H, Appleton P 1994 The treatment of sleep disorders. Developmental Medicine and Child Neurology 36:97–107

Johnstone E C 1998 Schizophrenia. In: Johnstone EC, Freeman CPL, Zealley AK (eds) Companion to psychiatric studies 6th edn, Churchill Livingstone, Edinburgh, p 369–397

Kanner L 1943 Autistic disturbances of affective contact. The Nervous Child 2:217–250

Kaufman A, Kaufman N 1983 Kaufman Assessment Battery for Children (K-ABC). American Guidance Service, Circle Pines, Mn

Kendall P 1999 Child and adolescent therapy: cognitive-behavioral procedures. Guilford Press, New York

King R, Leonard H, March J et al 1998 Practice parameters for the assessment and treatment of children and adolescents with obsessive–compulsive disorder. Journal of the American Academy of Child and Adolescent Psychiatry 3:27S–47S

Kutcher S 1997 Child & adolescent psychopharmacology. Saunders, Philadelphia

Lanyardo M, Horne A 1999 A handbook of child and adolescent psychotherapy. Routledge, London

Lask B 1988 Novel and non-toxic treatment for night terrors. British Medical Journal 297:592

Lask B 1994 Paediatric liaison work. In: Rutter M, Taylor E, Hersov L (eds) Child and adolescent psychiatry: modern approaches, 3rd edn. Blackwell, Oxford

Lask B, Bryant-Waugh R 1999 Anorexia nervosa and related eating disorders in childhood and adolescence, 2nd edn. Psychology Press, Hove

Lord C, Rutter M 1994 Autism and other pervasive developmental disorders. In: Rutter M, Taylor E, Hersov L (eds) Child and adolescent psychiatry: modern approaches, 3rd edn. Blackwell, Oxford

Matthews S 1994 Cognitive development. In: Bryant P, Colman A (eds) Developmental psychology. Longman, London

Meltzer H, Gatward R 2000 Mental health of children and adolescents in Great Britain. The Stationery Office: London

Miller P, Platt M 1996 Drinking, smoking and illicit drug use among 15 and 16 year olds in the United Kingdom. British Medical Journal 313:394–397

Morrell J 1999 The infant sleep questionnaire: a new tool to assess infant sleep problems for clinical and research purposes. Child Psychology & Psychiatry Review 4:20–26

MTA Co-operative Group 1999 Fourteen-month randomised clinical trial of treatment strategies for Attention Deficit Hyperactivity Disorder. Archives of General Psychiatry 56:1073–1086

Murphy G 1985 Update—Self-injuring behaviour in the mentally handicapped. Association for Child Psychology and Psychiatry Newsletter 7:2–11

Neale M D 1989 Neale Analysis of Reading Ability Test, 2nd edn. National Foundation for Educational Research/Nelson, Windsor

NICE 2000 The clinical effectiveness and cost effectiveness of methylphenidate for hyperactivity. National Institute for Clinical Excellence, London

Park R, Goodyer I 2000 Clinical guidelines for depressive disorders in childhood and adolescence. European Child and Adolescent Psychiatry 9:147–161

Pelham W E, Gnagy E M, Burrowes-Maclean L et al 2001 Once-a-day Concerta methylphenidate versus 3-times-daily methylphenidate in laboratory in natural settings. Pediatrics 107:1–15

Pennington B, Ozonoff 1996 Executive functions and developmental psychopathology. Journal of Child Psychology and Psychiatry 37:51–88

Reisman J M 1973 Principles of psychotherapy with children, 2nd edn. Wiley, New York

Reynell J 1985 Reynell Developmental Language Scales. Second Revision NFER, Windsor

Richman N, Lansdown R 1988 Problems of pre-school children. Wiley, Chichester

Richman N, Stevenson J, Graham P 1982 Pre-school to school: a behavioural study. Academic Press, London

Russell G, Szmukler G, Dare C, Eisler I 1987 An evaluation of family therapy in anorexia nervosa and bulimia nervosa. Archives of General Psychiatry 44:1047–1056

Rust J 1995 Wechsler Individual Achievement Tests. Psychological Corporation, San Antonio, Tx

Rutter M, Schopler E (eds) 1988 Autism: a reappraisal of concepts and treatment. Plenum Press, New York

Rutter M, Tizard J, Whitmore K 1970a Education, health and behaviour. Longmans, London

Rutter M, Graham P, Yule W 1970b A neuropsychiatric study of childhood. Clinics in Developmental Medicine, nos 35/36, SIMP/Heinemann, London

Rutter M, Yule B, Quinton D et al 1975 Attainment and adjustment in two geographical areas. III: Some factors accounting for area differences. British Journal of Psychiatry 126:520–533

Rutter M, Graham P, Chadwick O, Yule W 1976 Adolescent turmoil: fact or fiction? Journal of Child Psychology and Psychiatry 17:35–56

Shaffer D, Piancentini J 1994 Suicide and attempted suicide. In: Rutter M, Taylor E, Hersov L (eds) Child and adolescent psychiatry: modern approaches, 3rd edn. Blackwell, Oxford

Shafran R 2001 Obsessive–compulsive disorders in children and adolescents. Child Psychology and Psychiatry Review 6:50–58

Skuse D, Wolke D, Reilly S 1992 Failure to thrive. Clinical and developmental aspects. In: Remschmidt H, Schmidt M (eds) Child and youth psychiatry, European perspectives, vol II: Developmental psychopathology. Hans Huber, Stuttgart

Spencer T, Wilens T, Biederman J 1995 A double-blind crossover comparison of methylphenidate in adults with childhood-onset attention deficit hyperactivity disorder. Archives of General Psychiatry 52:434–443

Stevenson J 1999 Treatment of sequelae of child abuse. Journal of Child Psychology and Psychiatry 40:89–112

Taylor E, Sergeant J, Doepfner M 1998 Clinical guidelines for hyperkinetic disorder. European Child and Adolescent Psychiatry 7:184–200

Thomas A, Chess S, Birch H 1968 Temperament and behaviour disorders in childhood. New York University Press, New York

Thorndike R, Hagen E, Sattler J 1986 Stanford Binet Intelligence Scale, 4th edn. Psychological Corporation, San Antonio, Tx

Webster-Stratton C, Herbert M 1993 Troubled families—problem children. Wiley, Chichester

Wechsler D 1992 Manual for the Wechsler Intelligence Scale for Children, 3rd UK edn (WISC-III UK). Psychological Corporation, Kent

WHO 1992 The ICD-10 classification of mental and behaviour disorders: clinical descriptions and diagnostic guidelines. World Health Organization, Geneva

Wolff S 1991 Schizoid personality in childhood and adult life. III: The childhood picture. British Journal of Psychiatry 159:629–635

Wolff S, Chick J 1980 Schizoid personality in childhood: a controlled follow-up study. Psychological Medicine 10:85–100

Wright B, Partridge I, Williams C 2000 Management of chronic fatigue syndrome in children. Advances in Psychiatric Treatment 6:145–152

Yule W 1994 Posttraumatic stress disorder In: Rutter M, Taylor E, Hersov L (eds) Child and adolescent psychiatry: modern approaches, 3rd edn. Blackwell, Oxford

Zucker K, Bradley S 1995 Gender identity disorder and psychosexual problems in children and adolescents. Plenum press, New York

26 | Old-age psychiatry

Neil Anderson, Alan Jacques

INTRODUCTION

In Britain 15.9% of the population was aged over 65 years in 2001. The male-to-female ratio falls steadily from 1:1.1 in the 65–69 year age band to 1:2.6 at over 85 years (patients will therefore generally be referred to as female). Table 26.1 shows how the elderly population has expanded during the 20th century. For the first time ever, people aged 60 years and over now constitute a larger proportion of the population than children under 16. Today, women of 80 represent not a group of elite survivors but half their original birth cohort (Grundy 2002). The very elderly group, the 'old-old', will continue to expand for several further decades, whereas the 'young-old' population has already peaked, though there will be a further rise when people born in the postwar 'baby boom' enter old age. In other developed countries the pattern is similar, and in developing countries the average life expectancy has already dramatically risen from around 41 years in the early 1950s to a projected estimate of 70 years by 2020 (WHO 1998). The projected age distribution of the UK population in the period 2001–2071 is shown in Figure 26.1.

Only 5% of the total elderly population of Britain lives in any type of institutional care. More than a quarter of older people suffer from mental disorder — an estimated 10% with dementia and 16.3% with other mental illness (Bartels 2002) — so psychiatric illness is a community problem. Nearly half the older female population and a quarter of the older male population who live at home live alone, and the availability of potential carers is lessening with smaller family size, increased social mobility and changes in working practices, especially among women, so patients are often relatively isolated compared with their younger counterparts. On the other hand, about 65% of psychiatric hospital residents in Britain are aged over 65 years, and this figure may increase in the future.

Despite its growing importance, old age psychiatry is still in some areas an underdeveloped specialty. Some services are still plagued by bed blocking, inadequate staffing levels and poor morale. The pessimism and carelessness of 'ageism' or 'gerontophobia' can occasionally infect even the most enthusiastic services. Nevertheless, considerable success has been achieved in transforming a 'back-ward' non-specialty to a subject of major clinical, teaching and research interest.

HISTORY

The idea that elderly psychiatric patients might need separate attention first arose in the late 1940s. The gradual increase in older age groups (due to better housing, nutrition and social conditions during their childhood in the late 19th century) led to an increase in the elderly population of the long-stay wards of mental hospitals. Most of these patients were presumed to be suffering from 'senile dementia', but inevitably some had other, reversible conditions. Roth's (1955) simple demonstration that five diagnostic groups of elderly patients (senile dementia, arteriosclerotic dementia, delirium, depression and late paraphrenia) had different prognoses for discharge and survival showed the importance of accurate diagnosis. Psychogeriatric assessment wards for the elderly (Robinson 1975) began to be set up in the 1950s in a few hospitals, and the idea gradually spread.

In the 1960s, problems of waiting lists for long-term care and assessment wards, and of 'misplacement' of dementing patients in medical wards (Kidd 1962), preoccupied psychiatrists. One solution was the development of day hospitals as an alternative to admission. Unfortunately it has not been proven that day hospitals either avoid or delay admission (Greene & Timbury 1979, Eagles & Gilleard 1984, Murphy 1994) although they may relieve carer stress (Rolleston & Ball 1994, Rosenvinge et al 1994).

The 1970s was a decade of plans for coping with the population explosion of elderly people (Department of Health and Social Security 1972, Scottish Home and Health Department 1979). The concepts of relief admission (to relieve carers in a crisis) and respite admission (regular, preplanned breaks from caring) were introduced and, together with specialist EMI (elderly mentally infirm) homes for dementia sufferers in some areas (de Zoysa & Blessed 1984, Norman 1987), began to show that continued increases in long-stay hospital provision might not be necessary.

In the 1980s the burgeoning of private sector nursing and residential homes, some specialising in dementia, meant that in many areas unsatisfactory accommodation in old asylums was closed down. Increased interest in community care led to patchy development of sitter services, non-hospital day care and attempts at multiagency care planning.

Paralleling this slow evolution of services was an equally slow growth of old-age psychiatry as a specialty. The first consultants with a special interest in the field were appointed in the 1950s, a special section of the Royal College of Psychiatrists was founded in the 1970s, academic posts were created in the 1980s, specialist journals such as the *International Journal of Geriatric Psychiatry* were founded, and in 1989 the Department of Health accorded the profession specialty status.

The 1990s saw further extension of these developments and currently the specialty of old-age psychiatry is perhaps undergoing more change than at any time since its inception. The shift away from provision of long-stay care by hospitals has focused the

Table 26.1 Population trends and projections for the United Kingdom 1901–2021

Year	Population (millions)		
	65–74 years	75–84 years	85 years
1901	1.28	0.47	0.06
1931	2.46	0.84	0.11
1951	3.69	1.56	0.22
1971	4.76	2.16	0.49
1991	5.07	3.13	0.90
2001	4.94	3.29	1.13
2011	5.50	3.48	1.35
2021	6.55	4.04	1.59
% increase 1901–2001	285	600	1800
% increase 2001–2021	32	23	41

Adapted from Office for National Statistics (2003).

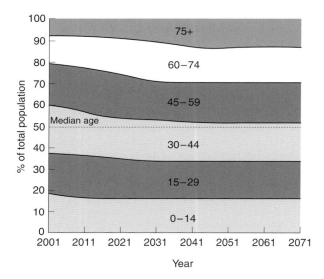

Fig. 26.1
Projected age distribution of the UK population, 2001–2071.
Source: National Statistics website (www.statistics.gov.uk). Crown copyright material is reproduced with the permission of the controller of HMSO.

old-age psychiatry team even more than in the past on diagnosis, assessment, acute treatment and rehabilitation, with outreach to the community and to those living in care homes. It is still unclear to what extent good community care as envisaged in legislation (Department of Health/Department of Social Security 1989) can replace institutional care for dementia (Challis & Davies 1986), as much of the effect of the changes in the past 25 years has been to replace one type of long-stay institutional care (in hospital) with another (in residential and more especially nursing homes). There is still a long way to go to achieve equitable, responsive and truly needs-led care for older people with dementia (Alzheimer Scotland Action on Dementia 2000) and other mental illnesses, and it is hoped that progress can now be made following an awakening of government interest in reforming care for the nation's elderly (Audit Commission 2000, Scottish Executive 2002). A seminal move was the recommendation by the Royal

Commission on Long Term Care (1999) that free personal care should be available to all elderly people that need it. Unfortunately, only the Scottish Parliament has complied with this report, the remaining legislature in the United Kingdom adopting a more limited view that only nursing care be free. Recent government policies commending joint working with colleagues in social services, housing and other care sectors only prescribe what most old-age psychiatrists have been doing for years, although they have been helpful in making joint commissioning and funding of services a reality in some areas of the country. Details can be found at http://www.doh.gov.uk/scg/sap/ and http://www.scotland.gov.uk/health/jointfutureunit/. In the meantime old-age psychiatry's maturity has been marked by a huge growth in research publications and in textbooks (Copeland et al 2002, Jacoby & Oppenheimer 2002).

THE OLD-AGE PSYCHIATRY SERVICE

Catchment area

Most old-age psychiatrists believe that a defined catchment area for a service is not only desirable but also essential. Care is provided locally for patients and relatives who may find travel difficult, 'boundary disputes' between services are unlikely, and some attempt at planning the use of scarce resources is possible. There are inevitable inequalities between areas that are rich and poor in resources, or between active, optimistic teams and passive, pessimistic teams; though such differences may lessen with better education and audit. However, the catchment area principle has stood the test of time.

Age limit policy

Clear, carefully negotiated age policies on dementia and on 'functional' disorders are vital for good relationships between old-age psychiatry and other specialties. Although old-age services increasingly take referrals for diagnosis of early-onset dementia the younger patients do not fit easily with their elderly counterparts. Younger patients and their carers tend to fall unsatisfactorily between specialties, and it is not surprising that their experience of care tends to be a negative one (Luscombe et al 1998). Their numbers are sufficient for a dedicated regional service with sessional consultant input, but this tends to be the exception rather than the rule (Royal College of Psychiatrists 2000).

A comprehensive approach

In the few areas which offer pure dementia services, staff recruitment and morale may pose problems. Debates about segregation or integration of dementia sufferers have been prolonged. Old long-stay hospital wards were often examples of segregation at its worst, suffering from 'back-ward' mentality, distant from relatives and familiar territory, and rarely visited by outsiders. Meacher's broadside (1972) against some specialist EMI homes was an early plea for integration of dementia sufferers with the non-demented elderly. Rabins (1986) and Norman (1987) have emphasised the merits of 'segregated' dementia services, which can provide a separate environment where staff build up special skills and patients feel safe from the frequently stigmatising attitudes of their fit contemporaries. Wilkin et al (1985) concluded that there might be a 'right mix' for any integrated institution. Residential homes which had over about 30% of dementing residents appeared less successful than those with lower percentages.

In old-age psychiatry services, similar conflicts of interest between 'organic' and 'functional' patients are found. Referrals, workload and service provision tend to be skewed toward those with dementia, and there is the risk that the considerable needs of older people with other psychiatric illnesses are neglected.

Multidisciplinary teamwork

The multiple problems of older patients require multiple assessment and treatment skills. Psychiatric expertise should be backed up by readily available advice from colleagues in old-age medicine, and access to other specialist medical services. The multidisciplinary team of doctors, clinical psychologist, community psychiatric nurses (CPNs — in some areas based in primary care, but nevertheless most important members of the team), hospital nurses, occupational therapist, physiotherapist, social worker and pharmacist should regularly attend patient reviews in respite and long-stay care as well as in the day hospital and assessment wards. Good access to speech and language therapy and to dietetic, podiatry and dental services are essential.

The practice of inviting relevant outsiders to multidisciplinary discussions on particular patients is becoming more widespread, encouraged by the development of the Care Programme Approach. Such 'network meetings' may involve the patient herself if she is able to participate, and any of: relatives, other friends or neighbours, home help, voluntary sector staff, area team social workers, housing agency representatives, general practitioner, primary care nurses, solicitor, police and clergy. The clinician needs to balance the good practice of gaining and disseminating appropriate information with the paramount importance of patient confidentiality.

A range of services

Domiciliary assessment

Most referrals come from general practitioners, and consultants customarily see patients in their own homes. General practitioners (Audit Commission 2000), old age psychiatrists (Orrell & Katona 1998) and patients (Jones et al 1987) favour domiciliary assessment, and there is evidence as to its cost effectiveness (Aquilina & Anderson 2002). Visiting a patient in her own home not only provides better information on the social circumstances of the patient, her practical abilities and family relationships, but it avoids the disturbing or artificial effect of outpatient clinics, and usually starts the psychiatrist on a better footing with the patient. It often allows useful contact with relatives, though lack of privacy to interview the patient on sensitive topics, or the interference of a 'helpful' relative, can lessen the value of the visit. Domiciliary assessment should help avoid hasty decisions and unnecessary admission. In some areas other members of the multidisciplinary team contribute to domiciliary assessment, and in a few areas the multiagency approach of the 'dementia team' is used.

Outpatient clinics

Only some services run traditional outpatient clinics. These help to overcome the few limitations of domiciliary visiting. More

privacy can be accorded to patient or informants. Physical examination and investigations can be carried out and a medical opinion obtained.

Memory clinics first developed in North America in the 1970s and subsequently in the United Kingdom in the early 1980s. They originally took the form of open-access clinics, often designed to facilitate recruitment of those with early cognitive impairment into research trials. Their structure and function have evolved and they are now a feature of many old-age psychiatry services. Most operate a multidisciplinary model involving assessment, investigation, diagnosis, information giving and support (Lindesay et al 2002a). Such a system may overcome the reluctance of general practitioners to refer patients with possible early dementia, allows differential diagnosis which would otherwise be neglected, and gives some reassurance to the 'worried well'. Luce et al (2001) found that patients seen at a memory clinic were significantly younger than those referred to a traditional old-age psychiatry service, less cognitively impaired and had a wider range of diagnoses.

Day hospital

Despite the lack of evidence regarding their effectiveness, day hospitals are now an integral part of most old-age psychiatry services. In some, mainly rural, districts facilities are shared with old-age medicine and other services, or 'mobile' day hospitals have been developed. The trend in day hospitals in recent years has been away from providing social care for patients with milder dementia. This role is being increasingly taken over by local day centres, run by social services, voluntary or private organisations, thus allowing day hospitals to concentrate on their diagnostic, assessment, treatment and rehabilitative functions, and to offer long-term intensive support to those who need nursing care with multidisciplinary back-up. These tasks can only be carried out if there is active clinical review of the patients who attend, otherwise lengthy waiting lists develop and the end result is 'institutional' day care delivered by professionals whose skills could be put to better use. Close working relationships with those in the community who provide day care assist the transition of the patient from one service to the other.

Flexibility in day care is essential if the actual needs of patients and carers are to be met. For carers in employment, for example, a 5-day day hospital may mean that they know where their relative is while they are working, but gives them no respite from caring when they are at home. In many areas, evening or weekend day care is now being offered, while 'night hospital' has been developed in one or two places.

Day hospital care can help effectively in the management of affective disorders and psychosis in the community. For dementia, it has been shown to be highly acceptable to carers (Gilleard et al 1984b), and it may be that, if sufficiently intensive and flexible, it can prevent admission to hospital.

Assessment beds

Dementing patients should be assessed in a separate ward from the 'functional' group, though there are of course some patients with both types of disorder and some who need considerable assessment before it is clear which category of bed is most suitable, so flexibility is required. Since domiciliary and day hospital assessment have become the norm, and as respite care has reduced the load of crisis admissions to short-stay wards, the need for assessment beds for dementia is lessening. Only a few patients need inpatient diagnosis. Some can benefit from inpatient treatment of specific behaviour problems. Draper (2000) found mixed results when he reviewed the evidence concerning the effectiveness of inpatient care. Although 50% of patients with behavioural problems in dementia improved sufficiently to be able to return home and over 75% of those with depression were significantly improved on discharge, staff tended to be more satisfied with the outcome than patients or their carers. If resources are used efficiently and the discharge of patients waiting for longer-term care is not unnecessarily delayed, then the need for dementia assessment beds proper is perhaps as low as 0.3 per 1000 of the population over 65 years of age.

Respite beds

Respite for carers is of course an essential function of much domiciliary and day care. Residential respite care is most suited for dementing patients who live with their carers. A few patients are confused or develop minor infections as a result of the move, so respite care away from home is often unsuitable for patients who live alone.

A choice of respite services is now available in most areas, including: holidays for groups of couples arranged by the Alzheimer organisations (the Alzheimer's Society for England, Wales and Northern Ireland, and Alzheimer Scotland – Action on Dementia); 'fostering' breaks with specially trained families; residential or nursing home care; and geriatric and psychiatric hospital care for those who need nursing. The system is most helpful if admissions come at regular intervals, planned with the relatives so that each break comes *before* the stress of caring becomes too great, rather than giving relief *after* a crisis. In severe cases this may mean that the patient spends half (or even more) of her time in hospital and half at home with day hospital support. If respite care is well planned very few patients fail to return home. A clear contract between the hospital and relatives avoids unplanned 'ditching' of patients.

Because hospital respite care developed rapidly without central planning it was, by necessity, fitted into available spaces. The beds may be in either assessment or long-stay wards, and neither is entirely satisfactory. Some respite admissions can be seen as short-term or intermittent assessment admissions, and there is a trend to redesignate respite beds accordingly. An alternative is to have specially designated and designed small wards for respite care. Whatever the title, there is a need for a significant number of these beds for people with major nursing needs, perhaps up to 0.8 beds per 1000 of the population over 65 years of age. A useful concept is of a dementia resource centre, a small local unit providing support, day care and respite care in one place. Another innovation is 'respite at home', where care is provided in the patient's own home, thus minimising disruption to her routine, though this may not be a satisfactory solution for a cohabiting carer who needs a more complete break.

Continuing care

The need for long-term hospital care for those with functional disorders is very small. Residential homes or other supported accommodation are able to cater for most who cannot return home after admission, with the exception of the few psychotic or chronically depressed patients who make no response to drug treatments or have intractable side-effects. If there were equitable access to the types of supported accommodation available for younger people with severe and enduring mental illness then the numbers of elderly patients requiring continuing hospital care would be even smaller.

There is still a place for continuing multidisciplinary hospital care for dementia associated with major behaviour disturbance. Nursing and residential homes are unlikely, unless highly specialised, to be able to tolerate such residents (Capewell et al 1986). Better training and greater numbers of staff, regular support by consultants, CPNs and other psychiatric team members, judicious drug treatments, and the promise of admission if a difficult situation does not improve, should enable such patients to survive longer in non-hospital care. Some services even offer 'respite care' for homes. A small number of hospital beds, and certainly less than the old norms of 3/1000 elderly for England and Wales (Department of Health and Social Security 1972, already reduced to around 2.5/1000 by the RCP/RCPsych report of 1989) or 5/1000 for Scotland (Scottish Home and Health Department 1979) should suffice, depending on local conditions. Here and elsewhere in service planning the 'balance of service' model is most important. If beds are provided in another service sector, even if their core function is slightly different, then the need for hospital beds will be less. Similarly, community provision, if sufficiently intensive, along with regular respite services, can lessen the need for long-stay hospital care. But if these alternatives are not available the burden of care will inevitably fall on hospital provision. The concept of NHS nursing homes or 'Domus' units (Lindesay et al 1991) is one way forward in ensuring specialist dementia care for those who need it. Whatever the solution, and in whatever setting it is provided, the very poor standard of continuing care that continues to exist for many older people with mental illnesses needs urgent attention and investment (Ballard et al 2001).

Liaison psychiatry

Older people occupy almost two-thirds of general hospital beds, and prevalence rates of up to 53% for depression, 35% for dementia and 61% for delirium are reported (Holmes et al 2002). Psychiatric illness is poorly detected and under-treated by general hospital staff. Only 2–4% of those who are psychiatrically unwell in general hospitals are referred to an old-age psychiatrist, though this constitutes between a quarter and a third of all referrals. Organic disorder accounts for around 60% of referrals, and it is likely that patients with depression are particularly neglected — perhaps because they do not present the same behavioural disturbances or placement problems. The value of a separate old-age psychiatry liaison service has been shown by Scott et al (1988) and Swanwick et al (1994). The special diagnostic and treatment skills of the old-age psychiatrist and his knowledge of local services allow patients to be more effectively treated in the medical wards, enable better discharge planning and help avoid unwise disposal or unnecessary long-term care. In a good liaison service, which makes itself readily available, most referrals will be for diagnosis and advice, rather than for transfer.

Liaison old-age medicine

Significant physical illness may be present in around half of the patients admitted to an acute old-age psychiatry ward, and this, rather than the psychiatric diagnosis, tends to predict a greater length of stay (Draper 2000). In many cases such illness will contribute to the psychiatric disorder, or interfere with treatment or rehabilitation. Readily available advice from an old-age physician in the outpatient clinic, day hospital and wards can be very helpful, and can minimise the transfer of patients between the services.

Joint activities

To overcome the problems of overlap between psychiatric and medical services (Murdoch & Montgomery 1992), and to help each other with difficult patients, some centres have developed the concept of joint working (Pitt & Silver 1980, Aire 2002). Part of the service is managed together by the two specialties, as in a joint assessment ward, joint day hospital or joint long-stay care. The patients involved will be both physically and mentally disabled, or require further assessment to determine which service should become responsible. The logical consequence is a 'department of care of the elderly' in which all facilities are shared.

Links with community services

Old age psychiatrists are very aware that their patients do not depend on the efforts of the psychiatric service alone if they are to be maintained in the community. A wide network of caring agencies and professions is also involved (Table 26.2). General practitioners are central to case finding, assessment and treatment of elderly people with mental disorders. CPNs provide continuing assessment and treatment services, and in some areas are introducing intensive home nursing care. Home care services and home helps are rightly said to be the backbone of community care. In their different ways primary care nurses also contribute greatly, though they have traditionally concentrated their efforts on the physically disabled. Care needs assessment and management in the community have been the particular responsibility of social workers since 1993. Social services departments may provide or purchase from others day care, respite care and other services. Recent legislation promoting partnership between health and social work services, and establishing Primary Care Trusts in England and Wales that have powers to commission services, is likely to have a significant influence on service provision and delivery for older people. Workers in a growing number of voluntary organisations offer advice, support, counselling, and sitter, day care or other respite services. Some housing associations have recently been developing extra-care housing for dementia sufferers. The recent decline in the private sector's involvement in nursing home care is matched by their increasing involvement in providing home support services.

In the last 20 years great initiative has been shown in developing alternative forms of care for older people with psychiatric disorders. An effective old-age service spends much of its efforts on liaising with agencies who share the care of patients living in the community, and on supporting them, whether in care planning, training and support of staff, project development, or just by paying them a regular visit. Two particular models of co-operation have been developed: the mental health liaison meeting and the community dementia team.

The mental health liaison meeting

Representatives of the various agencies covering a particular community meet regularly, usually monthly, and discuss those

Table 26.2 Community services for elderly people with psychiatric disorders	
Service	Potential providers
Informal support and supervision	Family, friends, neighbours, shopkeepers, police, clubs, church groups, 'sitting' circles
Home help	Social services Private agencies
Sitting services, day or night	Voluntary agencies Private, including nursing agencies A few hospitals and social services departments
Meals on wheels	Social services Voluntary agencies
Aids, adaptations and safety	District nurses Occupational therapists (community or hospital based) Housing agencies Gas and electricity companies
Incontinence care	District nurses and health visitors, some specialist incontinence nurses Laundry services (social services or community health)
Day care	Social services Voluntary agencies Private agencies
Respite care	Informal carers Social services Voluntary agencies Private agencies
Long-term care at home	Informal carers All agencies
Planning and coordination of care — the 'key worker'	Informal carers Social workers Community psychiatric nurses Health visitors General practitioners

patients with mental disorders who are of mutual interest to at least two of them. Such meetings help in care planning, avoid overlaps or gaps in care, and are mutually supportive and educative. Patients may be referred between the services. The meetings also develop a political role. Gaps in service provision become obvious, and ideas about how to fill these gaps can be pursued. The liaison group is an efficient, effective and remarkably cheap method of organising care in the community, though it may challenge the rigid application of the social work lead role in care management. Such groups can provide the structure for developing the Care Programme Approach for those with especially complex care needs.

The community dementia team

A dementia team (Lodge & McReynolds 1985) is also a multiagency group, and is formed by representatives of the relevant bodies, usually by secondment or special appointment. After local consultation and advertisement, it provides an open-access point for people in the community who are worried about dementia in themselves, their relatives or those they care for professionally (cf. the 'memory clinic' concept, but here the emphasis is on care planning rather than diagnosis). Inevitably most referrals come from professionals, but informal referral of patients who would otherwise fail to come to the attention of mainstream services is encouraged. A particular member of the team, who may come from any of the agencies involved, is selected to make an initial assessment and may become the 'key worker' for that patient and family over the succeeding months or years, introducing the patient to the services she needs, and providing continuing support. Such teams have not always succeeded. Referral rates may be low and, to be effective, they need to be able to have direct access to the necessary services.

Links with care homes

Between 30% and 80% of residents in care homes are likely to suffer from dementia, and perhaps 40% suffer from significant depressive symptoms (Ames 1990, Godlove et al 2000). The quality of care in such home varies enormously; often it is not good, though no worse than that in continuing care wards of hospitals (Ballard et al 2001). Due to improvements in community care over the last decade that have quite properly supported older people in their own homes for longer, care home residents now represent a frailer, more dependent and more cognitively impaired group. Links between the old-age psychiatry service and care homes may be informal or formal. Jackson & Lyons (1996) found regular visits to cares homes were well received by staff, reduced the need for urgent domiciliary consultations and hospital admission and appeared to be highly cost-effective. CPNs or clinical psychologists may provide a regular advice and support service, particularly where hospital patients are discharged to the homes. Formal training sessions by doctor, CPN or clinical psychologist and formal liaison groups are found in a few areas.

Partnership with carers

Carers' groups have always been part of normal day hospital practice. Now carers' groups run by the Alzheimer organisations, social services and other community-based organisations are commonplace. Carers form an essential part of the treatment team in dementia, having much information to provide about the patient, and wishing to be involved in decisions which are made throughout the illness. In day and respite care the psychiatric team is truly 'sharing care' with relatives and needs to recognise this. Carers are also a valuable source of feedback in evaluating and planning services, though their views may not necessarily be the same as those of patients (Dening & Lawton 1998)

Community bias

Attention in old age psychiatry has now moved away from the problems of seemingly endless waiting lists for long-stay care to the opportunities of community care coupled with, if anything, brief contact with hospital (Challis et al 2002). This trend is welcomed by almost all patients and most families. Indeed, long-term care of patients with dementia is more and more being seen as the responsibility of extra-care housing and care homes. More formal integration between health services and the various statutory and non-statutory agencies providing community care is likely to occur over the coming years. The implications of this shift in care arrangements for all involved, including the taxpayer, are the subject of continuing political debate in all developed countries.

INTERVIEW METHODS

Interviewing the patient

Interviewing older psychiatric patients requires special skills.

Normal changes of ageing

In response to the almost universal slowing of all mental processes, the interviewer must slow his pace and learn patience. Older people tend to be more cautious in their responses to questions, so the interviewer may need to be more encouraging than for a younger patient, and use more multiple-choice or forced-choice questions. A tendency to greater introspection makes some older people more reticent about personal problems than is the norm for younger generations. A 'transference' effect may add to this. Inevitably, the interviewer is considerably younger than the patient, and may be treated as an inexperienced person, who needs to be protected from unpleasant reality.

In addition, 'countertransference' attitudes may interfere with the interviewer's willingness to ask personal questions of someone who could be their grandparent. Some doctors seem to believe that elderly people have inevitably led sheltered lives. They therefore avoid important questions about alcohol or sexual behaviour. Even worse is the still prevalent tendency to infantilise elderly people. This can have strange effects on interviewers, who fail to explain the interview process, 'speak down' to the patient, assume that she lacks understanding, general knowledge or wisdom, ignore her right to make or be involved in decisions, or speak to her relatives as if they were her parents. Some older people prefer a formal approach to interviewing. On the other hand, many become less inhibited than younger adults are about touch, probably because it has less obvious sexual connotations. Not only a shake of the hand, but holding the hand and other reassuring bodily contact is often both acceptable and helpful.

Older people of the present generation sometimes have surprisingly fatalistic, ageist attitudes towards illness. This affects not only patients themselves but also their families and even professional carers, who may treat quite serious symptoms as evidence of 'just old age', fail to report them or underplay their significance. Persistence may be required to elicit the full clinical picture.

Difficulty with or dislike of change is also common. This may be a real biological aspect of ageing or may be culturally determined. Introducing new concepts or new activities can lead to considerable resistance, most obvious when the doctor is recommending a course of action or therapy. Considerable time and gradual persuasion may be necessary to get the patient to consider even quite simple changes. Major changes such as accepting a home help for the first time or leaving home may be met in the first instance by total resistance.

Disabilities

Disabilities, often unconnected with the patient's psychiatric disorder, may interfere with the interviewing process. Impairment of hearing is the most common, and, if not recognised, can easily lead to misdiagnosis of mental impairment. Access to a voice amplifier or communicator is essential. In severe cases it is necessary to write questions or use behavioural evidence of the mental state. Visual impairment brings difficulties with certain tests. Like deafness it may not be mentioned by a proud or self-conscious patient, and so is misconstrued. Patients who are physically ill, fatigued or in discomfort may not concentrate, so questioning will have to be simple, repetitive and carefully explained. Parkinson's disease leads to mumbled speech, slow responses and impaired affective reactivity, which hinders interviewing and can tempt the interviewer to diagnose depression or dementia wrongly.

Mental impairment

Impaired comprehension entails the interviewer having to explain carefully the rationale, content and duration of the interview. These explanations will have to be repeated several times for patients who show poor concentration, forgetfulness or suspiciousness. Difficulty with attention span, receptive dysphasia, poor vocabulary and grammar, impaired comprehension and abstract thinking all mean that questions or instructions should use simple words and simple one-clause sentences, dealing with only one item at a time, avoiding abstractions. It is not unusual for a patient to recall only the beginning (primacy effect) or the end (recency) of a long sentence. Retention of an instruction to be carried out in the future ('future memory') is likely to be impossible. Since attention and concentration are often impaired it is usually necessary to intersperse short periods of questioning with more informal talk. A patient whose impairment of simple mental tasks is being revealed will need the reassurance of a spell of interesting reminiscence before new embarrassment is caused. Patients with expressive dysphasia may need assistance from the interviewer, who guesses what words she is trying to say, or uses prompt cards. Considerable skill and inventiveness is required to interview a patient who has no idea that the interviewer is a doctor, has severe receptive dysphasia or has no insight into her condition. Skill is also required in dealing with the defensive patient who has developed the ability to sidetrack interviewers into repetitive reminiscence to cover amnesia.

Interviewing informants

In general psychiatry it is usual for the patient to be able to give enough information about the history to allow accurate diagnosis. This is much less true in old-age psychiatry. In organic disorders, interviewing the patient can rarely give a reliable or comprehensive history. Even at very early stages of dementia, sufferers fail to time-code information properly, so that vital questions about the natural history of the illness cannot be answered. However, the patient's history should not be ignored. Her attitude to her illness is important in assessing insight, working out treatment strategy and predicting compliance. And she may have more knowledge of some details than even her close relatives have. Furthermore, some patients do not have any available informant, or their informants themselves may have dementia or other disabilities.

It is important, even in severe dementia, to ask the patient's permission before seeing the relative. Relatives (and professionals) often need to be reminded that they are not legally in charge of the patient, even though they may feel or act 'in loco parentis'. The doctor must also remind himself that he is the patient's advocate as well as trying to help the relatives. He may have to balance the distress of an exhausted relative who is demanding help against strong resistance from the patient who does not believe that any help is needed.

The relatives' history itself may be inaccurate, either because they wish to emphasise their need for help, or because they wish to carry on caring without outside intrusion. Clarifying questions are very important, to pin down the exact time when a symptom started, or how often it has been obvious. These details are most important in diagnosis and in assessing what action is needed.

A useful procedure with informants for a patient who may have dementia is:

- Explain the purpose, structure and timing of this interview, and of the interview with the patient.
- Details of relevant past history, personality, abilities and medical history will provide a baseline which is essential to diagnosis, and gives some currently relevant information.
- Obtain the general history of the mental decline and enough information to indicate that the impairment is *global*. Pin down timing as accurately as possible and clarify whether the process has been acute, gradual or irregular. Information from relatives may be as important as mental testing of the patient and other investigations in suggesting a diagnosis of dementia. A standardised questionnaire such as the Information Questionnaire on Cognitive Decline in the Elderly (IQCODE, Jorm & Jacomb 1989) may be helpful.
- Using a problem checklist, such as Table 26.3 or that of Gilleard (1984), list the problems experienced by the relatives, patient and others. There may be as many as 15–20 dementia-related problems for one patient. Clarify the seriousness, circumstances, timing, frequency, consequences and variations of each problem separately and record any treatment or management strategies which have been tried. Review the problem list with the relative and ask them if any other significant problems have been omitted. This essential part of the interview enables the relative to feel that all their concerns have been covered; yet the whole process has been quick and effective. The extensive Present Behavioural Examination (PBE) of Hope & Fairburn (1992) concentrates on the various 'non-cognitive' symptoms of dementia and is useful for research purposes.
- Ask about current supports, make a timetable of regular visitors or outings during the week and establish how long the patient can be left alone. This locates gaps and overlaps in care and support.
- Check that the patient is in receipt of appropriate benefits and enquire into arrangements for managing her finances. It is important to know if formal arrangements are in place such as a welfare or financial attorney appointed under the Adults With Incapacity (Scotland) Act 2000.

MENTAL STATE EXAMINATION

Much of the mental state examination is, as in younger patients, composed of information gathered during history taking, by observation of the patient's behaviour and from responses to questions. Organic mental testing (Hodges 1994) is central to much of the work of the old-age psychiatrist. A few points are worth stressing:

Table 26.3 A short check-list of potential problems in dementia

Problem	Examples
Memory impairment	Forgets appointments
	Forgets to change clothes, wash, go to the toilet
	Forgets to eat, take tablets
	Loses possessions
Disorientation	Time, day or night
	Around house
	Recognising family or other visitors
Needs physical help	Dressing
	Washing, bathing
	Toileting
	Eating
	Housework
	Mobility
Risks in the home	Falls
	Fire from cigarettes, cooker, heating
	Flooding
	Letting strangers in
	Wandering out
Risks outside	Driving, road sense
	Gets lost
Apathy	Little conversation
	Lack of interest
	Poor self-care
Poor communication	Dysphasia
Repetitiveness	Questions or stories
	Actions
Uncontrolled emotion	Distress
	Anger or aggression
	Demands for attention
Uncontrolled behaviour	Restlessness, day or night
	Vulgar table or toilet habits
	Undressing
	Sexual disinhibition
	Shop lifting
Incontinence	Urine
	Faeces
	Inappropriate excretion
Emotional reactions	Depression
	Anxiety
	Frustration
	Embarrassment or withdrawal
Other reactions	Suspiciousness
	Hoarding
Mistaken beliefs	Still at work
	Parents or spouse still alive
Decision making	Indecisiveness
	Easily influenced
	Poor judgement
	Refuses help
Burden on family	Disruption of social and family life
	Distress, guilt, rejection
	Family discord

From Jacques & Jackson 2000.

- The principles of history taking from older people, particularly about explanation, pace, breaks from questions and simplicity of communication apply equally to mental testing.
- Cognitive testing must be handled sensitively. A simple explanation of the rationale for such tests, acknowledging their potential to appear infantilising or stressful to the patient, usually helps them proceed smoothly. Firing a series of questions at a patient with dementia without heeding her increasing distress is liable to provoke a catastrophic reaction, in which she becomes emotionally overwhelmed and terminates the interview in a distressed, tearful or angry manner. Dispersing the process of cognitive testing throughout the interview may be less challenging to the patient.
- Standardised tests help to a degree but, as with any information, they require careful clinical interpretation. The most frequently used test is probably the Mini-Mental State Examination (MMSE) (Folstein et al 1975). Although it has attracted much criticism it does achieve a balance of acceptable brevity while covering a reasonable range of cognitive functions (Burns et al 1998). It does not examine fronto-subcortical executive functioning, so additional tests are required to detect these deficits in patients who may have vascular cognitive impairment, Parkinson's disease or frontotemporal dementia. It also has significant floor and ceiling effects so it is insufficiently discriminatory for those with either very mild or very severe impairment. Perhaps the most common mistake is to rely on the raw score without interpreting it in light of clinical information. Many patients in the earliest stages of dementia will score well above the standard cut-off of 23 or 24 out of 30. The Addenbrooke's Cognitive Examination (ACE) (Mathuranath et al 2000) is a newer tool designed for use in routine clinical practice, that more comprehensively assesses memory, fluency and language. The Alzheimer's Disease Assessment Scale — Cognitive and Non-Cognitive Sections (ADAS-Cog and ADAS-Non-Cog) (Rosen et al 1984) is a lengthier instrument that is frequently used by researchers, especially to measure change in cognitive function in drug trials.
- No individual item tests only one function. For example, to ask 'What day is it today?' can lead to information about receptive dysphasia, general comprehension, immediate memory, recent memory, motivation and affect, expressive ability, hearing and sight as well as telling how orientated the person is. The serial sevens test may reveal dyscalculia or dysphasia as well as poor concentration. Very non-specific tests such as clock drawing (Shulman et al 1986) can be invaluable.
- Impairments can interact. A patient who has significant receptive dysphasia will be unable to participate in other mental tests which involve spoken questions or commands; this must not be taken to mean that she is impaired in these respects. Poor attention or low mood may interfere with all testing.
- Although some standard questions are useful, imagination and flexibility are also essential. For example, questions about general knowledge, remote memory and new learning must all be varied according to the individual's premorbid intelligence, education, interests and experience. And, as information emerges, the doctor may need to employ additional tests to explore, say, parietal lobe function or dysphasia.
- A patient's performance may vary from time to time. Mood, motivation, fatigue, time of day, and her attitude to the

particular examiner may all make the difference between good and bad performance in tests. The doctor should never assume that what she has presented to him is how she always is. Mental state examination gives a tiny snapshot of her whole mental condition. Indeed, variations in presentation at different times provide useful information for both diagnosis and functional assessment.

- The mental state examination is carried out for diagnostic purposes or to monitor progress. It is not an assessment of the practical needs of the patient. That is a separate exercise.

FURTHER INVESTIGATIONS

Rating scales

Intellectual rating scales, such as the MMSE, the ACE, the information–orientation section of the Clifton Assessment Procedure for the Elderly (CAPE, Pattie & Gilleard 1979) or Hodkinson's Abbreviated Mental Test (1973), provide a general rating of mental impairment which can be used to assess severity or chart progress or decline. They are widely used as screening tests but are not diagnostic. They are reasonably sensitive for mental impairment, but not very specific. The ADAS-Cog (see above) is used in research, and the Severe Impairment Battery (SIB, Saxton et al 1990) has been devised for assessment of cognitive function in severe dementia.

Ratings of behaviour using scales such as the Crichton Behaviour Rating Scale (Robinson 1975), the behaviour section of the CAPE, and the REPDS (Fleming & Bowles 1994) are in regular use. Again these are not in any way diagnostic, and many of the items they test could relate to a variety of illnesses or disabilities. They do, however, give some estimate of severity of general impairment, after diagnosis has been carried out, and can be used to chart changes or to predict the level of care needed by the patient (Pattic & Gilleard 1976). Derived from the more extensive PBE, the Manchester and Oxford Universities Psychopathological Assessment of Dementia (MOUSEPAD, Allen et al 1996) measures psychiatric symptoms and behavioural changes in patients with dementia. These symptoms are also evaluated by the Neuropsychiatric Inventory (NPI, Cummings et al 1994), which has been used in several drug trials in dementia.

Standard depression rating scales are not very appropriate to old-age psychiatry, as questions about biological symptoms will not clearly distinguish depressive from physical illness. The Geriatric Depression Scale (GDS, Yesavage et al 1983) and the Cornell Scale for depression in dementia (Alexopoulos et al 1988) have been specifically developed for use in elderly and dementing populations respectively.

The Problem Checklist and Strain Scale was devised by Gilleard (1984) to measure carers' views and experiences. Although many others have followed, none is better than Gilleard's original scale.

Outcome measures are now frequently used to determine the effect of clinical interventions. The Health of the Nation Outcome Scales (HoNOS) have been adapted for use in an elderly population (HoNOS 65+, Burns et al 1999a, 1999b)

Research interview schedules

Two major instruments were introduced in Britain in the 1980s: the Geriatric Mental State Schedule (GMSS) of Copeland et al (1986), which links with the AGECAT computerised diagnostic programme, and the Cambridge Diagnostic Examination (CAMDEX) of Roth et al (1986), both covering the major diagnoses of old-age psychiatry. These have made epidemiological surveys more reliable and valid, and have provided a common language for researchers. They are not for routine use, but can be useful in examining difficult cases.

Neuropsychological assessment

Neuropsychological assessment can be an extremely useful adjunct to examination, clarifying thinking, providing more detail about particular impairments, and adding weight for or against a particular diagnosis. It is particularly useful in assessing those with milder cognitive impairment where the diagnosis of dementia may be in doubt and those who have an unusual or contradictory range of impairments. The subject has been reviewed by Woods (1999) and Morris et al (2000).

Activities of daily living (ADL)

The psychological abilities examined in mental state or psychological testing represent only a sample of brain activity that may be affected by brain damage. Behaviour rating scales give some evidence of other impairments, but the most practically useful evidence comes from assessment of the 'activities of daily living'. This is the special province of the occupational therapist, and is best carried out on a visit to the patient's own home, rather than in an artificial 'ADL suite'. Improved performance under scrutiny, performance anxiety, variations with mood, motivation, time of day and the relationship with the therapist must be taken into consideration when interpreting the results. The Barthel Index is widely used to summarise ADL information (Wade & Collin 1988).

Physical examination, blood tests and other investigations

Screening of older people in the community has generally brought little success in case finding, but screening of groups of elderly people at special risk of physical illness has been much more productive. Elderly patients with any major psychiatric diagnosis are such a group. It is far more likely that exacerbating factors rather than reversible causes of mental impairment or mood disturbance are found on screening. Thyroid dysfunction, vitamin B_{12} deficiency, impaired glycaemic control and the presence of vascular risk factors including hypertension and hypercholesterolaemia are all commonly discovered. The results of routine screening tests affected patient management in 13% of consecutive patients being evaluated for dementia in one study (Chui & Zhang 1997). Table 26.4 lists some possible tests and the rationale behind their use.

The electroencephalogram (EEG) still has some place in old-age psychiatry, but mainly in the diagnosis of possible fits and Creutzfeldt–Jakob disease (CJD).

Computed tomography (CT) scanning is now widely available, and modern scanners perform a head CT in less than 30 seconds, making them much more user friendly. Routine access to magnetic resonance imaging (MRI) and single photon emission CT (SPECT) is more variable for old-age psychiatrists, and these are lengthier and potentially distressing procedures for confused or anxious people. The use of positron emission tomography (PET)

Table 26.4 Investigations and some differential diagnoses in old age psychiatry

Test	Which patients	Possible diagnoses
Physical examination	All	Exclude any contributing physical problem, detect vascular risk factors, e.g. hypertension, carotid bruits
Full blood count	All	Infection, alcohol problems, anaemia
ESR	All	Infections, inflammatory disease, tumours
Urea and electrolytes	All	Uraemia, metabolic disorders, electrolyte disturbance secondary to drugs, e.g. diuretics, SSRIs
Liver function tests	All	Alcohol problems, drugs effects, secondary tumours
Thyroid function tests	All	Hypothyroidism, hyperthyroidism
Calcium and phosphate	All	Parathyroid disorders, metastatic bone disease
Midstream urine	All	Infection
Glucose	All	Diabetes
Chest X-ray	If indicated, especially in smokers and heart disease	Tumours, cardiac failure
ECG	Indicated if risk of conduction disorder, especially prior to treatment with AChEI, antipsychotics or antidepressants	Cardiac arrhythmias or ischaemia
Vitamin B_{12} and folate	If indicated by raised MCV	B_{12} and folate deficiency
Syphilis serology	No longer routine; may be indicated if risk of past exposure	Tertiary syphilis
HIV testing	Only if indicated due to risk of past exposure	AIDS dementia complex
Autoantibody screen	Few selected patients	Cerebral vasculitis
Copper studies	Very few selected patients	Wilson's disease
Heavy metal screen	Very few selected patients	Heavy metal poisoning
Lumbar puncture	Few selected patients	Encephalitis
EEG	Selected patients only	Creutzfeldt–Jakob disease, temporal lobe epilepsy
CT scan	Younger patients (< 65-years) and those with focal neurological signs or unusual history, e.g. rapid decline, early gait disturbance and urinary incontinence, impaired or fluctuating conscious level	Primary or secondary tumour, subdural haematoma, normal pressure hydrocephalus
MRI scan	Few selected patients	Vascular dementia, posterior fossa tumour
SPECT scan	Selected patients	Frontotemporal dementia (most dementias have characteristic but non-diagnostic pattern which may aid diagnosis in difficult cases)

AChEI, acetylcholinesterase inhibitor; MCV, mean corpuscular volume.

and functional MRI (fMRI) is largely confined to research. Scans are not perfect diagnostic tools, are relatively expensive and, in the case of SPECT and PET, invasive. Practice varies according to the specialty of the clinician, the patient population seen and the ease of access to scanning facilities, but for most old-age psychiatrists they are not routine investigative tools. The sense of this practice is emphasised by the fact that probably 95% of dementias in old age are of the more common types. A scan should be performed when there are unusual clinical features or courses, specific reasons to suspect a space-occupying lesion, subdural haemorrhage or hydrocephalus, or a particularly difficult differential diagnosis. The incidence of structural lesions is greater in younger patients who have cognitive impairment, and so it is sensible that all such patients under the age of 65 receive a scan. The typical neuroimaging findings in dementia are shown in Table 26.5. Neuroimaging has also revealed cerebrovascular lesions in patients with late-onset depression. Scans rarely alter their management, but the discovery of extensive vascular changes may provide an explanation for treatment resistance in some cases and alert the clinician to the heighten risk of dementia in the future.

THERAPIES

Psychodynamic psychotherapy

Many older patients do not suit or show interest in explorative psychotherapy, and many psychotherapists are reluctant to take on older clients (Murphy 2000). Until recently, therapists tended to agree that brief, problem-solving therapy related to current life difficulties was more likely to be relevant and effective, although such a view may be changing. Garner (2002) and others consider that many of the losses, adjustments and unresolved issues that accompany late life are well suited to a psychodynamic approach. Although some older people are resistant to change, others view time as being of the essence at their advanced stage of life, and are committed to therapy that will bring resolution to long-standing psychic conflict and enhance their remaining years.

The psychodynamic issues that are relevant to older people differ from those which preoccupy young adults (Brink 1979, Knight 1996). Coming to terms with the losses of old age and with

Table 26.5 Typical neuroimaging findings in dementia

	Structural imaging (CT and MRI)	Functional Imaging (SPECT)
Alzheimer's disease	Generalised cerebral atrophy and ventricular enlargement Reduced medial temporal lobe width on angled CT view Serial MRI scans show progressive medial temporal lobe atrophy May be minor periventricular white-matter changes	Temporoparietal hypoperfusion
Vascular dementia	Infarct(s) Extensive periventricular and deep white-matter lesions	Patchy multifocal pattern of hypoperfusion
Dementia with Lewy bodies	Generalised ventricular enlargement Relative preservation of medial temporal lobe structures May be white-matter changes similar to those in AD but less extensive than in VaD	Occipital hypoperfusion Reduced D_2 receptor and dopamine transporter density
Frontotemporal dementia	Frontal lobe atrophy	Frontal hypoperfusion

AD, Alzheimer's disease; VaD, vascular dementia.

decreasing independence and increasing dependence is often central. This is particularly difficult for active, independent personalities who have never anticipated such changes. Coming to terms with the past is also likely to be relevant, typical issues being regrets, renunciation of hopes, forgiveness or lack of forgiveness of perceived wrongs, and putting past preoccupations into perspective (Butler 1963). Although for many people reminiscence is an entirely enjoyable experience, some achieve that enjoyment by idealisation and denial, and others fail to find happiness in their recollections or are entrenched in bitterness. Erikson's (1963) counterpoint of 'ego integrity' versus 'despair' is relevant here.

Changed relationships and power structures in the family and among friends may cause both external and internal conflicts, and family therapy is a growing interest. Previously held expectations of old age may cause a variety of problems. Many had expected that they would be surrounded by a family who have instead moved away physically or emotionally. Many looked forward to activities which they are kept from by disability or illness. Most are unprepared for the fact that old age can last for a very long time (average expectation of life at the age of 65 years is now 16 years for a man and 19 years for a woman). Personal and social attitudes to ageing may conflict. Older persons who wish to 'disengage' may find themselves at odds with those around them who think continuing activity and engagement are important. Conversely, those who wish to be working, physically energetic or sexually active may meet with disapproval from family and friends who expect them to 'retire'.

Psychological therapies

Clinical psychologists have recently begun to show a greater interest in treating older people (Stokes & Goudie 1990, Woods 1999) and have successfully applied cognitive and behaviour therapy techniques in treating anxiety, phobias, depression and sexual problems. Some fear that learning-based theories may have less value because older people tend to be more rigid psychologically and less inclined to change, but there is ample evidence that older

people can continue to learn. In a study of the effectiveness of cognitive-behavioural psychotherapy, Walker & Clarke (2001) found older adults with a wide range of illnesses missed far fewer sessions and improved more quickly than a comparable younger group.

Psychology has also contributed much to the treatment of people with dementia, from the use of memory management (Wilson & Moffat 1992) and specific examples of behaviour modification to evaluation of more general therapies (Woods 1999). Whatever approach is taken, it is vital not to lose sight of the previous and current personal experiences of the person with dementia. Kitwood (1997) advocates a person-centred approach to care, based on the idea that until recently most people with dementia have been surrounded by a malignant social psychology which damaged them as much or more than their illness. When caring for those with dementia we must treat the person, not the disease.

Reality orientation (RO)

This originated as a resocialisation technique in the back wards of American mental hospitals, but became metamorphosed into a treatment for dementia. It was enthusiastically embraced by staff in day care, residential homes and wards, partly because it was optimistic. But the optimism became excessive, RO was used as a universal 'therapy' whether it suited individual patients or not, and eventually it got a bad name. Research (Brook et al 1975, Holden & Woods 1988) shows that the principle of encouraging orientation can help some patients in some aspects of their mental state, but perhaps only verbal orientation. Active involvement of the patient, and learning which makes use of procedural memory, are particularly effective. 'Classroom RO' has probably now had its day, but as a '24 hour' technique RO may be useful in dealing with disorientation, mistaken ideas and distorted memories.

Reminiscence

This is less a specific therapy than a general principle (Butler 1963, Norris 1986, Thornton & Brotchie 1987) that older people often gain satisfaction, confidence and a sense of identity from reminiscing. Those with dementia may find reminiscence particularly satisfying. Lack of recent memory and helplessness in the present make them fall back on remote memories in a search for identity and security. Of course their stories may be fragmentary or repetitive, but good reminiscence therapy allows for this and helps the person expand from the merely stereotyped. Photographs, slides and films, old objects, old songs and dances, 'theatre' where the person 'performs' old work or domestic activities, handling old objects, and visits to the person's school, childhood home or other familiar scenes have all been effectively used. However, like reality orientation, reminiscence is not for all. For some, old memories evoke only sadness, regret or bitterness which they would rather avoid and may not be able to work through.

Validation therapy

This technique was introduced to escape from some of the impersonal excesses of 'classroom' style reality orientation (Feil 1993). It looks to the emotional state which underlies a patient's disoriented speech and behaviour. If she talks of wanting her mother, is it because she is feeling insecure, and would be helped by reassuring emotional or physical contact? If she wants to go off to work, is it because she is bored, and would benefit from exercise or activity? Although popular, there is no research evidence of its effectiveness.

Multisensory therapy

This therapy originated in the Netherlands in the field of learning disability (as 'snoezelen') but in recent years has been much in vogue for patients with dementia. It is postulated that disturbed behaviour in dementia occurs because the patient is deprived of meaningful sensation due to her physical, sensory and cognitive impairments compounded by an unstimulating environment. Multisensory therapy usually takes place in a dedicated room where the patient experiences an assortment of visual, auditory, olfactory and tactile stimuli produced by a variety of means including fibreoptic lighting, bubble-tubes, a projector and the use of aromatherapy oils, calming music and textured surfaces. The evidence that it is effective is largely anecdotal and it may be that money invested in expensive equipment is better spent on staff training and maintaining a suitably stimulating environment throughout the day.

Psychopharmacology

The changes in drug absorption, pharmacodynamics and activity with age are complicated. From the practical point of view certain principles are of day-to-day use:

- Most research in pharmacology and therapeutics has until recently been carried out on younger subjects. Check that any statements about a drug are relevant to older people.
- The body's ability to handle drugs changes in various ways with the process of ageing, but not in any absolute sense. Age is not in itself a contraindication to any drug.
- The normal interpersonal variation in drug metabolism and effects is greater in old age. One person may both need and tolerate large doses of a particular drug, while another, apparently similar, person may obtain the same therapeutic

effect with a lower dose, and even that low dose may cause harmful side-effects.
- Because of this great variability, it is important to start most drugs at a very small dose and build up gradually, particularly when using drugs with long half-lives or persistent metabolites.
- Gradual reduction in renal function and in some hepatic enzymes is the norm in old age, so drugs which are cleared by these pathways need particular care.
- Due to the relative increase in body fat in older people, lipophilic drugs, which include most psychotropics, have an increased volume of distribution and increased half-life as fat acts as a reservoir for these drugs. A reduction in body water leads to an increased concentration of water-soluble compounds such as alcohol. Nutritional deficiencies can cause hypoalbuminaemia resulting in an increased serum concentration of the active drug.
- Side-effects of drugs may appear at much lower doses than in younger patients, and in some cases at well below the therapeutic dose for that patient. Patients with dementia with Lewy bodies (DLB) are at particular risk. There are also a few elderly schizophrenic patients who seem unable to tolerate therapeutic doses of any antipsychotic drug without major parkinsonian side-effects, though the introduction of atypical agents has lessened their number.
- Even simple or mild side-effects may have disastrous consequences. Mild postural hypotension from an antidepressant can lead to a fractured femur, and mild anticholinergic effects can cause severe urinary retention or constipation.
- Drug interactions are common, partly because of some doctors' penchant for polypharmacy. The assessment of any elderly patient should include a careful listing of all her medications. In many cases cutting or stopping drugs, simplifying schedules or changing to safer equivalents will lead to improvement in some or all of her symptoms (Findlay et al 1989).
- It may not be clear what drugs the patient is actually taking, and compliance can be a major problem. Again polypharmacy may be responsible. The patient may have a cupboard full of drugs whose purpose she does not understand, or which she has forgotten about. The drug list which the general practitioner has may not be the list of drugs that the patient is taking. Patients who are being treated both at home and in a day hospital or respite ward are in particular danger of mix-up and poor communication about changes. It is good practice, where possible, to provide clear instruction and counselling, and to monitor compliance carefully.

DELIRIUM

Incidence

Delirium as a consequence of physical illness or toxic effects is more common in elderly people than in younger age groups (Lindesay et al 2002b). It affects between 10% and 15% of patients aged over 65 years on admission to medical wards, with a further 10–40% developing delirium during the course of their stay in hospital (Bucht et al 1999, Fann 2000). Unknown numbers suffer delirious states at home. The incidence may be high partly because elderly people are more prone to have one or more physical illness, and to be taking one or more drug. In addition the ageing brain is more susceptible to insult, perhaps involving the cholinergic and noradrenergic systems, which are important in cognition and the wake–sleep cycle. Those with dementia are especially susceptible to superadded delirium (Hodkinson 1973, Inouye & Charpentier 1996).

Causes

Delirium is often multifactorial in aetiology. A number of risk factors have been found to predispose to delirium, including visual impairment, severe physical illness, pre-existing cognitive impairment, biochemical evidence of dehydration, age more than 80 years, being male, having a fracture, and having an abnormal serum sodium (Schor et al 1992, Inouye et al 1993, O'Keefe & Lavan 1996). A more recent meta-analysis (Elie et al 1998) revealed pre-existing dementia, severe medical illness, alcohol misuse and prior physical dependency as significant risk factors for delirium in medical and surgical patients.

Although there are many possible precipitants of delirium (see Box 26.1) it is important to bear in mind commonplace causes such as infection, pain and constipation before subjecting the individual to more extensive and invasive investigation. Delirium is also a side-effect of a wide variety of drugs, particularly opiates, benzodiazepines and those with anticholinergic properties (Tune et al 1992). Not only psychotropic medication, but also the cumulative anticholinergic burden of many drugs commonly prescribed for medical conditions in the elderly, such as H_2 antagonists, warfarin, digoxin and antiparkinsonian agents, may precipitate delirium. Alcohol and benzodiazepine withdrawal should always be considered, and head injury, with the possibility of subsequent subdural haemorrhage, may not be reported. Even a move ('translocation') can cause temporary delirium, though this is probably only true of those with an early or latent dementia.

Some patients suffer from more than one potential cause of the delirium. In some cases, particularly of possible stroke or transient ischaemic attack, the cause of the delirium may remain obscure even after scanning. Disentangling possible delirium in a dementia sufferer may be even more difficult. An acute change in mental state, or the emergence of one or more of the characteristic features (see below) should suggest possible delirium, but may be simply due to further progress in the illness, particularly in multi-infarct dementia or dementia with Lewy bodies (DLB).

Clinical features

The core features of delirium include:

- acute onset;
- fluctuating course;
- impaired attention;
- altered level of consciousness;
- sleep disturbance;
- disorganised thinking;
- evidence of an underlying cause.

The characteristic variability of delirium means that a doctor's assessment does not necessarily reflect the patient's mental state over the whole day. Family or nursing reports of delirious symptoms at other times of day or night must be taken seriously. The classic picture of the agitated, frightened and over-aroused patient

---

Box 26.1 Possible causes of delirium

Intracranial
- Vascular
  — Transient ischaemic attack
  — Cerebral infarction or haemorrhage
  — Subarachnoid haemorrhage
- Head injury
  — Concussion
  — Subdural haemorrhage
- Infection
  — Meningitis
  — Encephalitis
  — Cerebral abscess
  — Cerebral malaria
- Epilepsy
  — Post-ictal states
  — Status epilepticus due to generalised or complex partial seizures
- Neoplasm
  — Primary
  — Secondary, e.g. breast, lung
- Autoimmune disorders
  — Cerebral vasculitis

Extracranial
- Infection
  — Most commonly urinary tract and respiratory
  — Cellulitis
  — Septicaemia
  — Viral infections: influenza, herpes zoster, HIV
  — Subacute bacterial endocarditis
- Hypoxia
  — Primary: pneumonia, pulmonary oedema, COPD, pulmonary embolism
  — Secondary: anaemia, cardiac failure, carbon monoxide poisoning, silent myocardial infarction
- Metabolic disturbance
  — Renal failure
  — Hepatic failure
  — Hyper- and hyponatraemia
  — Hyper- and hypoglycaemia
  — Hypercalcaemia
  — Acidosis
  — Hypercapnia
- Endocrine disorder
  — Hyper- and hypothyroidism
  — Hyper- and hypoparathyroidism
  — Addisonian crisis
- Vitamin nutritional deficiencies
  — Thiamine — Wernicke's encephalopathy
  — Vitamin B_{12} and folic acid — pernicious anaemia
  — Nicotinic acid — pellagra
- Other physical problems (all common causes of delirium in the elderly, especially in the oldest age groups)
  — Constipation
  — Pain
  — Urinary retention
  — Hypothermia

Toxins
- Drugs
  — Anticholinergics
  — Antidepressants — especially tricyclics, but delirium seen with all antidepressants
  — Antipsychotics
  — Benzodiazepines
  — Anticonvulsants

Box 26.1   Continued

- — Antiparkinsonian drugs
- — Steroids
- — Antihypertensive drugs, especially methyl dopa and beta blockers
- — Digoxin
- — Non-steroidal anti-inflammatory drugs
- — Opiates
- — H₂ antagonists, especially cimetidine
- — Some antibiotics
- Other toxins
  - — Heavy metals: lead, arsenic, mercury
  - — Carbon monoxide

Withdrawal states
- Alcohol
- Drugs
  - — Benzodiazepines
  - — SSRIs

Table 26.6   Clinical features which tend to distinguish delirium from dementia. Global mental impairment is common to both conditions

Delirium	Dementia
Rapid onset	Slowly progressive
Acute medical cause	Slowly progressive cause
Clouding of consciousness	Clear consciousness
Sleep disturbance	Normal sleep pattern, but 'clock' may be wrong
Irregular variability	Tends to be worse towards evening but otherwise stable
Restlessness and unease	Usually settled apart from aimless wandering or searching
Affect laden visual perceptual disturbances	Hallucinations less common and not usually disturbing
Lability of affect and distress	Lability less common

---

may be seen more often in younger age groups and drug/alcohol withdrawal states. The delirious elderly individual may more commonly be dull, apathetic and withdrawn (O'Keefe & Lavan 1999).

Delirium should not be regarded as a brief condition from which there is invariably full recovery. Significant delirium may be fatal in up to one-third of cases (Rabins & Folstein 1982). Many elderly patients take several weeks to recover even after treatment of the underlying cause. Patients who do not instantly recover after their physical state or investigations have apparently returned to normal should not be prematurely diagnosed as suffering from dementia. Even when a delirious state has fully abated, persisting cognitive dysfunction may be commoner than previously thought. Treloar & Macdonald (1997) found that although many patients showed a degree of reversibility to their cognitive impairment, only a few regained their premorbid cognitive functioning. Other studies have confirmed that patients with delirium have an enhanced risk of subsequently developing dementia (Kobeinsson & Jonsson 1993, Cole & Primeau 1993).

Differential diagnosis

Dementia   The classical distinction between delirium and dementia (Table 26.6) is an important but not absolute guide; features of delirium can appear during dementia, particularly if progress is rapid, and especially in DLB. Many cases of delirium have few or none of the distinguishing features except for the acute course.

Affective disorders and psychosis   Delirium can be mistaken for a functional psychiatric disorder. The psychomotor retardation or agitation that often accompany delirium in the elderly may be wrongly attributed to a depressive illness. Those with delirium tend to have labile mood compared with the more pervasive affective changes seen in a mood disorder. In general, the cognitive changes seen in depression tend to be overshadowed by the disturbance in mood and behaviour, whereas in delirium the reverse is more often the case. Abnormalities in perception and thought processes tend to fluctuate and be rather fragmentary in delirium. It is rare to experience the systematised delusions which are more suggestive of schizophrenia. In delirium, visual illusions and hallucinations are liable to predominate over the auditory phenomena more commonly seen in psychotic illness.

Management

As at all ages the treatment of delirium is the treatment of the cause. Secondary medical problems arising during the delirium, such as anaemia, hypoxia or electrolyte imbalance, should be corrected. A review of the patient's drug prescription sheet will identify drugs that may be exacerbating matters and which should be discontinued. Care needs to be paid to ensure adequate hydration and nutrition. All authorities rightly emphasise the importance of psychological support and appropriate environmental management (Flacker & Marcantonio 1998, APA 1999, Lindesay et al 2002b). Key interventions in this respect include:

- reducing understimulation and maximising the clarity of perceptions, while avoiding overstimulation;
- minimising the unfamiliarity of the environment;
- minimising disorientation;
- reassurance that the illness is physical and temporary, and that any hallucinations are really being experienced by the patient, but will soon disappear;
- maintaining an emotionally calm environment.

Drug treatment should be the last thing on the treating doctor's mind, but judicious use of medication may be necessary for those who are severely disturbed, or whose sleep pattern is severely disrupted. There is little evidence base to guide the clinician and no placebo-controlled trials. Haloperidol remains the most widely used drug but should always be started in low dose. There is increasing interest in the use of atypical antipsychotics (Schwartz & Masand 2002). Benzodiazepines may result in paradoxical disinhibition and are best reserved for delirium caused by alcohol and drug withdrawal, where they are the treatment of choice. Acetylcholinesterase inhibitors have theoretical promise for the treatment of delirium (Wengel et al 1998) but they have not yet been fully evaluated for this purpose. However, they are probably the treatment of choice for delirium associated with DLB (Samuel et al 2000).

Hospital is not the best environment for an elderly delirious patient, and home treatment should always be considered, though the need for investigation and supervision may make admission necessary. As with dementia, no branch of medicine has sole responsibility for the treatment of delirium. Most patients quite rightly go to medical wards. Liaison psychiatric help is often needed for differential diagnosis and for advice on associated behaviour problems. Some advocate a specialised delirium service (Wahlund & Bjorlin 1999) but this would not help the many patients in general medical or surgical wards whose delirium goes undiagnosed. Above all, a high index of suspicion is necessary: any elderly patient with an acute change in his or her mental state should be assumed to have a delirium until proven otherwise.

DEMENTIA

Epidemiology

Henderson (1986) pointed to considerable difficulties in conducting community surveys of dementia:

- defining the population: are residents in care included or not?
- allowing for differing age structures of different populations;
- differential survival in different populations;
- using a valid diagnostic test — most simple tests measure impairment at the time of interview, only one of the steps in diagnosis; comprehensive tests are laborious to administer;
- estimating mild dementia — many surveys give estimates for moderate and severe cases only;
- differentiating between Alzheimer's Disease (AD) and other dementias.

Jorm et al (1987; Fig. 26.2) suggested from a meta-analysis of the many epidemiological studies of dementia that the prevalence rises exponentially with age, doubling with each successive period of

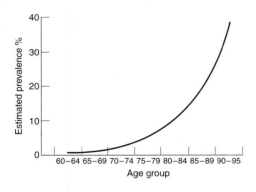

Age group	Estimated prevalence %
60–64	0.7
65–69	1.4
70–74	2.8
75–79	5.6
80–84	10.5
85–89	20.8
90–95	38.6

Fig. 26.2
Prevalence rates of dementia by 5-year age intervals for baseline population, pooled from selected studies (adapted from Jorm et al 1987). The graph can probably be extrapolated to younger age groups, but rates in the over-90s may level out, and almost certainly do not continue to rise exponentially.

5.1 years, as shown by the classic Newcastle study (Kay et al 1964) and more recent studies (Hofman et al 1991, Ritchie & Kildea 1995, Lobo et al 2000). Overall prevalence for populations over 65 ranges from 2% to 7% for moderate and severe dementia, with great variability in the figures for mild cases. In a chronic illness like dementia, incidence is low compared with prevalence, with figures around 1.0–1.5% being typically reported from elderly community samples. Epidemiological studies now concentrate on finding risk factors for the individual illnesses which cause dementia, only old age being a general risk factor. The median age for suffering from dementia in developed countries is about 82 years.

Because of the anticipated growth in older age bands the number of sufferers will rise (though there is growing evidence that prevalence does not continue its exponential rise beyond 90–95 years; Ritchie & Kildea 1995). Absolute numbers are uncertain, but the percentage rise in a particular community can be estimated, using Jorm's formula. In some areas of Britain there will be an increase of nearly 20% in the number of dementia sufferers in the next 10 years. The service needs of these extra sufferers and their carers are more important than absolute numbers or percentage increases, and local service planners need reliable estimates. The pool of available caring younger people is diminishing because of changes in population structure and social mobility, and because patients' children are increasingly likely to be either working or elderly and frail themselves.

About 70% of elderly dementia sufferers in Britain live in private houses, so the emphasis has always been on community care. About half of those living at home are living with close relatives, who may be coping with a severely disabled or disturbed individual. Slightly less than half are on their own, and the focus of attention is on the risks of independent living.

Assessment

Identification

O'Connor et al (1988) found that general practitioners knew of roughly 80% of severe dementia sufferers, but they were aware of only 30% of mild sufferers. A more recent study revealed two-thirds of patients with dementia go unrecognised within the primary-care system (Valcour et al 2000). This is perhaps not surprising given the fatalistic attitudes towards dementia that continue to prevail in general practice. The Audit Commission Report *Forget Me Not* (2000) found that almost half of all GPs surveyed did not consider it important to diagnose dementia as early as possible, many feeling there was no point in looking for an incurable disease. Regular primary care visits to those aged over 75 years and the use of simple screening instruments such as the Mini Mental State Examination (Iliffe et al 1991b) may improve these figures. There now exist evidence based guidelines to help clinicians (Eccles et al 1998, Knopman et al 2001). Memory clinics and the advent of drug therapies have encouraged more to come forward early. Increasingly now, patients wish to know and discuss their diagnosis, but there remains a reluctance from both relatives and professionals to disclose a diagnosis of dementia. Sullivan & O'Conor (2001) reviewed the evidence concerning differing points of view towards disclosure of diagnosis, and suggested that attitudes among the general public may now be changing, with the overwhelming majority of younger people preferring to be told a diagnosis of AD. However, there is still a great deal of pessimism about help for dementia, which, together with stigma, lack of insight, ignorance of services and isolation from services that could identify the problem, conspires against early presentation. Further work is also required on how best to enlighten patients and their carers, who will vary greatly in how they respond to information about dementia (Proctor et al 2002). It should now be the norm that patients are sensitively offered the opportunity to hear of and discuss their diagnosis and the follow-up available to support them in the post-diagnosis period.

Diagnosis of the syndrome

The essential steps in diagnosis are:

1. demonstrating a global mental impairment compared with that individual's previous normal performance;
2. showing that this impairment has been gradually progressive over a period of some months;
3. ruling out other causes of a similar clinical picture.

These steps require a clear history from the patient and informants, a full mental state examination and, at the very least, some simple screening investigations. The most common mistakes are to rely only on the mental state examination, to use only tests of orientation instead of demonstrating global impairment, and to fail to talk to another informant. The assessment of dementia should be seen as a process as described in Box 26.2.

Both ICD-10 and DSM-IV stipulate that in addition to memory impairment, which is almost always found in dementia, there is decline in other cognitive domains evidenced by changes such as disturbance in language, praxis, executive functioning and personality, and a decline in social and practical functioning. These changes must represent a change and occur in clear consciousness. These criteria are summarised in Box 26.3.

Box 26.2   Assessment process in patient with suspected dementia

- History from patient (largely for baseline, insight and attitudes)
- History from informants (for background, baseline, evidence of impairment and course)
- Seek evidence of:
  — General forgetfulness
  — Misplacing items or forgetting names of close family members
  — Repetitiveness
  — Disorientation to time and place — getting lost
  — Failure to cope with previous routine tasks
  — Poor self care
  — Emotional changes: anxiety, depression, irritability, shallowness of mood, apathy
  — Personality change
  — Change in behaviour — unusual behaviour, risky behaviour, social withdrawal
  — Psychotic symptoms
- Baseline information re premorbid personality, intelligence, abilities
- Mental state examination including cognitive assessment
- Physical examination and routine screening investigations
- Assessment of activities of daily living
- Problem list
- Cause of problem

Box 26.3   The dementia syndrome (ICD-10 and DSM-IV)

- Multiple cognitive deficits (which must include memory impairment)
- Functional impairment
- No evidence of delirium
- Change from previous level
- Duration of > 6 months*

* ICD-10 only.

Neuroimaging can be helpful in aiding diagnosis, but undue weight should not be placed on such investigation; a carefully taken history with the benefit of an informant and a clinical examination of the patient remain the most valuable tools in diagnosis and differential diagnosis of dementia. The typical imaging findings in different subtypes of dementia are summarised in Table 26.5. Townsend et al (2002) and O'Brien & Barber (2000) provide useful reviews of this area.

Some, but by no means all, patients are now presenting in the early stages of dementia when diagnosis can be more difficult. A 'wait and see' approach is reasonable with such individuals, asking the patient to return for repeat assessment in 3–6 months, when there may be more evidence of progressive deterioration. Alternatively, detailed neuropsychological assessment can be useful in delineating more precisely the nature and extent of cognitive impairment.

Differential diagnosis

The differential diagnosis of dementia in an elderly patient includes the following.

Normal old age   There remains debate regarding the cognitive profile of normal elderly people in the community. Although crystallised intelligence (the end product of accumulated information gained over a lifetime) may only decline in late old age, episodic memory and cognitive speed begin to decline in early adulthood. This deterioration is probably universal, but poor health, hypertension, poorer education and presence of the *ApoE* ε4 allele predict increased risk and amount of cognitive decline (Christensen 2001). Longitudinal studies of ageing do not identify a single point of transition between 'normal' ageing and dementia (Whalley 2002). It may not be possible to differentiate conclusively the very earliest stages of dementia from normal old age; and difficulties are further compounded in people with life-long mental impairment, those who are deaf and those with communication problems because of stroke. It is now increasingly postulated that there may be a continuum along a spectrum of cognitive impairments between normal old age and dementia.

Mild cognitive impairment   More recently, the concept of mild cognitive impairment has developed. Previous descriptions of variants of ageing, such as 'benign senescent forgetfulness' (Kral 1962), 'age associated memory impairment' (Crook et al 1986) and 'age associated cognitive decline' (Levy 1994) suggested that there is a form of benign impairment which does not progress to dementia. Mild cognitive impairment defines an intermediate state between normal ageing and dementia, characterised by subjective complaints of poor memory accompanied by objective evidence of such impairment but in the absence of frank dementia (Peterse et al 2001a). The criteria for amnesic mild cognitive impairment

---

Box 26.4   Criteria for amnesic mild cognitive impairment

- Memory complaints, preferably corroborated by informant
- Impaired memory function for age and education
- Preserved general cognitive function
- Intact activities of daily living
- No evidence of dementia

---

are listed in Box 26.4. Other types of mild cognitive impairment exist where single domains other than memory (e.g. language) are affected. It is important to recognise and take seriously those with mild cognitive impairment, as such individuals are at higher risk of subsequently developing dementia, one estimate giving a rate of between 10% and 15% per year (Petersen et al 2001b).

Chronic brain damage which is not progressive   This is often quite reasonably called dementia, but the non-progressive nature of the damage following head injury or other insults and the possibility of some gradual improvement makes care planning a very different matter in the two conditions. It is important to differentiate them.

Delirium   See above.

Korsakov's syndrome   An alcohol history is essential in all cases. The restriction of impairment to recent memory and some frontal lobe damage, with relative sparing of immediate memory and other intellectual functions, should be suggestive, and MRI scanning may be helpful.

Pseudodementia of depression   See section on affective disorders.

Pseudodementia of physical illness   There is some overlap and realistic lack of clarity between this term and the term 'reversible dementia'. Is, for example, secondary mental impairment in a hypothyroid patient a true dementia which is reversible or an 'artefact' of the illness? In practice it does not matter, since treatment of the thyroid problems in either case will cure the 'dementia'. Unfortunately, it is more common for thyroid disorder and dementia to coexist as completely unconnected problems.

Diagnosis of the cause

It is unclear what proportion of the elderly dementing population suffers from each of the many causes of dementia. Clinical and postmortem studies alike are liable to bias, depending on whether they use community or hospital samples and their age structure. Clinical differentiation of AD from vascular dementia (VaD) and dementia with Lewy bodies (DLB) is not reliable, with many apparently mixed cases. Even at postmortem there are debates about definitions. It is probable, however, that over 95% of elderly patients suffer from the common forms of dementia — AD, VaD and DLB — and that AD is the most common cause, perhaps accounting for over two-thirds of all sufferers.

Alzheimer's disease

In AD, cognitive decline is insidious in onset and gradual in progression. The most usual presenting scenario is that the patient has become increasingly and pervasively forgetful of new information as testified by their own account or that of an informant. Language disturbance may be an early feature, progressing from initial subtle word-finding difficulties to a fluent aphasia with word substitutions or paraphrasias. Lexical and grammatical abili-

ties may become increasingly impoverished and general comprehension progressively more impaired. Complex tasks that previously presented no difficulty are undertaken less well, leading to a decline in social, domestic and personal functioning. Non-cognitive symptoms such as mood disturbance, personality change and psychotic symptoms are common and are discussed later. Roth (1986) and others have noted differences between 'old-old' type 1 and 'young-old' type 2 AD. Pathological and neurochemical evidence suggests that in older patients damage is more topographically restricted, and more limited to the acetylcholine system. There are less obvious differences between older AD sufferers and normal people of the same age in their cholinergic systems, in psychological tests and in their expectation of life (Christie & Train 1984). Although it has been traditionally held that younger cases pursue a more malignant course, the time from onset of dementia to death decreases with advancing age. Brookmeyer et al (2002) found mean survival times of almost 9 years in those diagnosed at age 65 compared to $5\frac{1}{2}$ years in 75 year olds and only 3 years in those aged 90. Of course, the relative reduction in lifespan is greater for younger people. It is also possible to explain some apparent differences between older and younger sufferers using the concept of 'cerebral reserve'. If older people have less reserve then smaller amounts of cerebral damage will emerge earlier and have greater clinical effects.

Diagnosis is largely on clinical grounds. The NINCDS–ADRDA criteria (Box 26.5) provide good descriptions of definite, probable and possible AD and have been widely used in research (McKhann et al 1984).

Genetic testing   The identification of the apolipoprotein E (*ApoE*) ε4 allele as a 'dose-dependent' risk factor for late-onset AD and of the ε2 allele as a protective factor have been well established (Corder et al 1993, Strittmatter et al 1993). However *ApoE* allele testing is not in routine use in current clinical practice. The absence of the ε4ε4 genotype does not preclude a diagnosis of AD, and its presence does not inevitably lead to AD, so testing cannot be used predictively and its use is not recommended in asymptomatic individuals (Post et al 1997). Box 26.6 summarises the current knowledge of genetic influences in familial AD (covering all age groups). There is a place for genetic testing in the few people with a family history of early-onset dementia where there is thought to be an autosomal-dominant mode of inheritance. An up-to-date list of all known mutations in the three genes associated with familial AD can be found at http://molgen-www.uia.ac.be/ADMutations. Other risk factors which have been implicated are summarised in Box 26.7.

Neuroimaging   Jobst et al (1998) have suggested that measurement of the width of the medial temporal lobe on CT is a sensitive and specific marker for differentiating AD from normal controls, although its usefulness in differentiating between different types of dementia has been questioned (O'Brien et al 2000). MRI studies in those with early AD consistently demonstrate atrophy of the medial temporal lobe structures, especially the hippocampus and entorhinal cortex. Fox and his colleagues (2001) have shown that serial scans can be useful to measure disease progression and detect atrophy in presymptomatic individuals. Numerous studies have suggested that temporoparietal hypoperfusion seen with SPECT scanning may be useful in diagnosing AD during life (Quality Standards Subcommittee of the American Academy of Neurology 1994). The combination of CT and SPECT brings about greater sensitivity and specificity in diagnosis (Jobst et al 1998).

Box 26.5   NINCDS–ADRDA criteria for the clinical diagnosis of Alzheimer's disease

I. Criteria for diagnosis of PROBABLE Alzheimer's disease:
  - Dementia established by clinical examination, and documented by a standard test of cognitive function (e.g. Mini-Mental State Examination, Blessed Dementia Scale, etc.) and confirmed by neuropsychological tests
  - Significant deficiencies in two or more areas of cognition: for example, word comprehension and task-completion ability
  - Progressive deterioration of memory and other cognitive functions
  - No loss of consciousness
  - Onset from age 40 to 90, typically after 65
  - No other diseases or disorders that could account for the loss of memory and cognition

II. A diagnosis of PROBABLE Alzheimer's disease is supported by:
  - Progressive deterioration of specific cognitive functions: language (aphasia), motor skills (apraxia) and perception (agnosia)
  - Impaired activities of daily living and altered patterns of behaviour
  - A family history of similar problems, particularly if confirmed by neurological testing
  - The following laboratory results:
    ■ Normal lumbar puncture
    ■ Normal or non-specific findings on EEG. Evidence of cerebral atrophy in a series of CT scans

III. Other features consistent with PROBABLE Alzheimer's disease:
  - Plateaux in the course of illness progression
  - CT findings normal for the person's age
  - Associated symptoms, including: depression, insomnia, incontinence, delusions, hallucinations, weight loss, sex problems, and significant verbal, emotional, and physical outbursts
  - Other neurological abnormalities, especially in advanced disease: including: increased muscle tone and a shuffling gait

IV. Features that decrease the likelihood of PROBABLE Alzheimer's disease:
  - Sudden onset
  - Such early symptoms as: seizures, gait problems and loss of vision and coordination

V. Clinical diagnosis of POSSIBLE Alzheimer's disease
  - Dementia with variations in onset or course
  - Single progressive cognitive deficit
  - Presence of systemic or other brain disorder

VI. Clinical diagnosis of DEFINITE Alzheimer's disease
  - Clinical diagnosis of AD
  - AD neuropathology at biopsy or autopsy

NINCDS–ADRDA, National Institute of Neurological and Communicable Disease and Stroke–Alzheimer's Disease and Related Disorders Association

---

Box 26.6   Genetic risk factors for Alzheimer's disease

Early-onset familial Alzheimer's disease (EOFAD)
  - Age of onset of symptoms is before the age of 60–65
  - Autosomal-dominant familial AD represents only approximately 5% of all AD cases
  - Three genes, inherited in an autosomal-dominant fashion, have been identified and are thought to be responsible for 30–50% of familial AD

The *APP* gene
  - β-amyloid precursor (*APP*) gene on chromosome 21 has an important role in the formation of amyloid found in senile plaques in AD
  - *APP* has an autosomal dominant pattern of inheritance, and all known mutations to the *APP* gene are fully penetrant. This means that each child of affected individuals has a 50% chance of inheriting the gene mutation, and, if they do inherit it, they will get AD if they live through the age of risk
  - The age of risk is 40–65 years
  - The *APP* gene and its mutations have been found in only 43 families worldwide

The Presenilin genes
  - Presenilin gene one (*PS-1*) is located on chromosome 14, and presenilin gene two (*PS-2*) is located on chromosome 1
  - Mutations of these two genes are inherited in an autosomal dominant pattern and are fully penetrant
  - All those individuals who have the mutation will get AD
  - The normal function of the presenilin genes is unclear, but they may interact with the *APP* gene to organise traffic along neurons
  - There are 127 different mutations in *PS-1* and 9 mutations in *PS-2*
  - Onset of AD in *PS-1* gene mutations occurs between ages 30 and 55
  - Onset of AD in *PS-2* gene mutations occurs in the age range 40–75
  - 70% of all the *PS* gene mutations are found in only single patients or families and in no other unrelated patients. This means that a new patient with AD who undergoes a screen for the known mutations in *PS-1* or *PS-2* will likely have a negative result even when they have a mutation of the presenilin genes

Late-onset Alzheimer's disease (LOAD)
  - One gene, apolipoprotein E (ApoE) influences susceptibility to LOAD
  - Different alleles of ApoE are called 'susceptibility polymorphisms'. This means that no single allele is necessary or sufficient to cause the disease, and everyone has some age-dependent risk for AD, depending on which alleles of the gene they carry
  - The ApoE gene has three alleles or forms, designated as ε2, ε3 and ε4. Every individual inherits two alleles, one from each of their parents. It is the ε4 allele that is associated with a higher relative risk of AD and an earlier age of onset of AD
  - The presence of the ε2 allele is associated with a lower relative risk and older age of onset of AD
  - 20–30% of the general population has at least one copy of the ε4 allele
  - 45–60% of AD cases are associated with ε4
  - The presence of one ε4 allele confers an estimated 29% risk of getting AD. Those people with two ε4 alleles, i.e. who are homozygous for the allele, are at even greater risk of developing AD

Other tests   The search for a peripheral marker for AD continues. None has been found to be universally satisfactory, although cerebrospinal fluid assays showing low levels of Aβ$_{42}$ and high levels of tau have shown most promise (Ronald and Nancy Reagan Research Institute of the Alzheimer's Association and the National Institute on Aging Working Group 1998).

Box 26.6 Continued

- Approximately 2–3% of the general population is homozygous for the ε4 allele, whereas homozygotes represent 12–15% of AD patients
- Not all people homozygous for the ε4 allele get AD, and likewise, you can have AD without having the ε4 allele at all
- The *ApoE* gene acts primarily to modify the age at which susceptible people will develop AD. This has been determined by observing sibling pairs who have the same mutations in the *APP* gene but different alleles for *ApoE*. The sibling with an ε4 allele will develop AD earlier than their sibling without an ε4 allele. This appears to hold true for mutations of *PS-1* and *PS-2* as well

---

Box 26.7 Risk and protective factors for non-familial Alzheimer's disease

Risk factors
Proven
- *Age* — Advanced age is by far the most important risk factor
- *Family history* — Risk is around 3.5-fold greater in those who have a first-degree relative with AD, which equates to a risk between 1 in 5 and 1 in 6 that the relatives of patients with AD will develop the disease
- *Down syndrome* — People with Down syndrome always develop Alzheimer's disease pathology before the age of 40 years, although a decline in functioning is often not seen until a much later age
- *ApoE ε4* — The ε4ε4 genotype is associated with a much higher risk of AD compared with the ε3ε3 genotype (around 15 times in Caucasians), while the ε2ε4 and ε3ε4 genotypes are associated with a somewhat higher risk (around three times in Caucasians). The ε4 allele is less common in Orientals than in Caucasians, which might account for the lower incidence of AD reported in some Oriental studies
Likely
- *Female sex* — Even controlling for longevity, women are at increased risk of AD, possibly due to hormonal factors
- *Vascular risk factors* — There is now increasing evidence of a positive association between AD and vascular risk factors such as insulin-dependent diabetes, hypertension and smoking
- *Educational status / premorbid intelligence* — Education is related to intelligence. Poor education, especially in males, has been shown to increase the risk of developing AD. The notion that this is simply due to better-educated individuals' greater ability to compensate for cognitive changes of AD has been challenged by the seminal Nun study which revealed that low linguistic ability in early life was a strong predictor of AD. In this study there was a direct association between poor linguistic ability in early life and later neuropathological changes of AD, leading to the hypothesis that the poorer linguistic ability of those who went on to develop AD was in fact a very early manifestation of the disease (Snowdon et al 1996)
Possible
- *Head injury* — Studies showing a positive association between head trauma and later AD may have been adversely affected by recall bias of informants. One recent study using independently documented evidence in US war veterans did show a twofold increased risk of AD (Plassman et al 2000). There may be a synergistic effect between head injury and *ApoE* ε4

Box 26.7 Continued

- *Depression* — Depressive symptoms have been shown to predict later cognitive decline (Yaffe et al 1999). Associated high levels of cortisol may result in neuronal death. It may be, however, that depression is merely an early manifestation of AD
- *Herpes simplex virus* — Itzhaki et al (1997) reported that the presence of herpes simplex virus type 1 (HSV-1) DNA in the brain, together with possession of the *ApoE* ε4 allele, is a strong risk factor for AD
- *Family history of Down syndrome or Parkinson's disease* — Studies have revealed a familial aggregation of Down syndrome and Parkinson's disease with AD, suggesting that there may be shared susceptibility gene(s) underlying these diseases (van Duijn et al 1991)
Not proven
- *Aluminium* — A recent review has concluded that, as yet, there is not enough evidence to support a link between AD and exposure to aluminium in drinking water, antiperspirants and antacids (Rondeau 2002)
- *Electromagnetic fields* — Earlier work by Sobel et al (1996) suggesting an association with occupations involving exposure to electromagnetic fields from electric motors have not been confirmed by more recent studies (Li et al 2002)
- *Maternal age* — The evidence is conflicting — both old and young maternal ages have been found by different studies to increase the risk of AD in offspring

Protective factors
Possible
- *ApoE ε2* — The *ApoE* ε2 allele is possibly protective against AD, although the evidence is not conclusive
- *Anti-inflammatory drugs* — A meta-analysis suggested that the risk of AD was halved in those who took NSAIDs and reduced by one-third by the use of steroids (McGeer et al 1996)
- *Oestrogen* — Yaffe et al (1998) estimated that the risk of AD was reduced by around 30% in women who took oestrogen replacement therapy. However, women who take oestrogen may differ in other respects, such as having a higher level of education. As with anti-inflammatory drugs, randomised controlled trials will provide the ultimate test of whether oestrogen replacement therapy is protective
- *Premorbid education and intelligence* — Superior premorbid intellect and education may protect against AD
- *Exercise* — Lindsay et al (2002) and others found regular physical activity protected against AD

Vascular dementia

The terminology and concept of vascular dementia (VaD) are currently becoming more controversial and uncertain. Although usually still cited as the second commonest cause of dementia after AD by many, there is now a growing body of opinion challenging the very entity as commonly understood (Bowler & Hachinski 2000, Stewart 2002). Much of the difficulty lies in current diagnostic criteria for both AD and VaD. Existing systems used to diagnose AD may identify an overly pure subset of patients since they specifically exclude potentially important causal factors such as vascular disease, including cortical strokes, which are common in AD. It is also not clear if this exclusion also extends to the more subtle vascular changes that can now be detected by neuroimaging.

Box 26.8   Features of subcortical dementia

- Executive dysfunction
- Poor verbal fluency
- Psychomotor slowness
- Perseveration
- Inattention
- Memory loss characterised by poor retrieval and intact recognition
- Apathy and depression
- Mild focal neurological signs
- Short stepping gait (marche à petit pas)
- Dysarthria
- Pseudobulbar palsy
- Extrapyramidal features

Equally, the diagnostic criteria for vascular dementia, such as the NINDS–AIREN criteria (Román et al 1993), have been criticised for borrowing too heavily on those for AD by giving undue weight to the neuropsychological profile of memory loss found in AD. While memory impairment is seen in vascular dementia, the most characteristic deficits are those of frontal and subcortical dysfunction. Blinkered focus on the normal profile of memory loss seen in AD and overlooking executive dysfunction could result in many of those with cognitive changes due to cerebrovascular disease being missed at a stage where addressing vascular risk factors could potentially help modify disease progression.

VaD often results in a subcortical dementia. Although specific descriptions such as Binswanger's disease and lacunar state (état lacunaire) have been used to describe various pathological and clinical presentations, these conditions probably represent a single entity (Román 2002) which may also subsume more subtle white-matter ischaemia. Common clinical manifestations of subcortical dementia are listed in Box 26.8.

Other criticisms of the traditional strict dichotomy between AD and VaD include the poor reliability of the classical stepwise course in differentiating AD and VaD (Fischer et al 1990), the association of vascular risk factors with AD (Stewart 1998, de la Torre 2002), evidence that post-stroke dementia tends to follow an AD like course (Kokmen et al 1996), the low inter-rater reliability and poor correlation between different diagnostic schedules used in VaD (Chui et al 2000, Gold et al 2002), postmortem evidence of high rates of mixed dementia (Holmes et al 1999) and the finding that cerebrovascular pathology at autopsy is usually associated with neuropathological evidence of AD (Hulette et al 1997).

It has therefore been argued (Bowler 2002, Rockwood 2002) that the concept of vascular dementia should be replaced with one of vascular cognitive impairment (VCI), a much broader description encompassing all forms of cognitive dysfunction due to cerebrovascular disease. VCI is intended to include those that do not yet have functional impairment (and so could not be said to have a dementia syndrome according to current classification) and also emphasises the different neuropsychological profile seen in cerebrovascular disease.

Although there is dispute concerning the usefulness of vascular dementia as a discrete entity, there are a number of dementia syndromes in which cerebrovascular damage is the primary pathology. These are listed in Box 26.9.

Vascular dementia and Alzheimer's disease may therefore have more that links them than separates them. It is likely that pure AD

Box 26.9   Specific vascular dementia syndromes

Genetic disorders

- *Cerebral autosomal dominant arteriopathy with subcortical infarcts and leukoencephalopathy (CADASIL)* — CADASIL first appears after the third decade of life, often with multiple episodes of migraine with aura, and progresses in one decade with recurrent cerebral infarcts in the absence of important risk factors for cerebrovascular disease, resulting in dementia, usually with a pseudobulbar palsy. Infarcts result from thickening and fibrosis of the walls of small and medium penetrating arteries. CADASIL is caused by mutations in the *Notch3* gene on chromosome 19
- *Hereditary cerebral haemorrhage with amyloidosis–Dutch type (HCHWA-D)* — HCHWA-D is an autosomal-dominant disorder in which there is amyloid deposition in the meningocortical microvasculature resulting in recurrent lobar haemorrhages
- *Familial British dementia with amyloid angiopathy* — This autosomal dominant disorder, characterised by amyloid angiopathy, parenchymal amyloid plaque deposition and neurofibrillary degeneration, has been described in a large British family of more than 300 members spanning 9 generations. It is associated with a point mutation in the *BRI2* gene on chromosome 13
- *Hereditary endotheliopathy with retinopathy, nephropathy and stroke (HERNS)* — An autosomal-dominant syndrome of generalised vasculopathy described in a Chinese American family. Renal, skin and gastric biopsies demonstrate systemic basement membrane abnormalities
- *Fabry's disease* — An X-linked recessive lysosomal storage disorder caused by a deficiency of α-galactosidase A, resulting in intracellular accumulation of globotriasylceremide, leading to painful neuropathy with progressive renal, cardiovascular and cerebrovascular damage. Men are predominantly affected in mid-life, but many female carriers may also have symptoms, including increased risk of stroke
- *Mitochondrial myopathy, encephalopathy, lactic acidosis, and stroke-like episodes (MELAS)* — Usually presents in childhood with myopathy, migraine, focal vascular events and seizures. Eye, cardiac and gastrointestinal systems may also be involved. Maternal relatives may have a partially expressed disorder. A mutation in mitochondrial transfer RNA is responsible in many cases

Other disorders

- *Strategic single infarct* — Dementia related to stroke is associated with higher mean tissue loss, infarct number and location. (Gorelick 1997). Dominant thalamic and angular gyrus infarcts, bilateral infarcts, deep frontal infarcts and left hemisphere infarcts can result in dementia
- *Other conditions associated with cerebrovascular pathology and secondary dementia*
  - Buerger's disease
  - Neurosyphilis
  - Polyarteritis nodosa
  - Polycythaemia rubra vera
  - Subdural haematoma
  - Systemic lupus erythematosus

---

and pure VaD are rare entities and that mixed pathology is far more common than previously thought (Korczyn 2002). Furthermore, the interaction between the vascular component and other pathologies more than doubles the rate of progression of dementia (Snowden et al 1997, Heyman et al 1998). Alzheimer would perhaps not have been surprised at this confluence of ideas, since his original patient had autopsy findings suggesting arteriosclerosis.

Dementia with Lewy bodies

Lewy bodies are eosinophilic inclusion bodies composed of abnormally phosphorylated neurofilament proteins aggregated with ubiquitin and α-synuclein. In Parkinson's disease, Lewy body formation and neuronal loss occur in the brainstem nuclei, particularly the substantia nigra, leading to the characteristic movement disorder. In dementia with Lewy bodies (DLB), Lewy bodies (which are morphologically different from those in the brainstem) are also found in the cerebral cortex, where they have a predilection for the limbic and neocortical structures. Acetylcholine is markedly depleted as a result of degeneration in the brainstem and basal forebrain cholinergic projection neurons. Some Alzheimer type changes are also present, senile plaques more so than neurofibillary tangles. Minor vascular disease occurs in approximately one-third of cases.

DLB may be the second commonest form of dementia, accounting for 15–20% of both community and hospital cases (Weiner et al 1996, Holmes et al 1999). DLB can be seen to lie on a spectrum between Parkinson's disease and AD (Campbell et al 2001), although within that there is a second continuum between Parkinson's disease, Parkinson's disease with dementia and DLB (McKeith & Burn 2000). There are internationally recognised criteria for diagnosing DLB (McKeith et al 1996) which have been shown to be as diagnostically accurate as those for AD and VaD (McKeith et al 2000b). Many cases may in the past have been diagnosed as of Alzheimer or vascular type, and many research findings may therefore have been based on impure samples. The typical characteristics of DLB are summarised in Box 26.10. It should be noted that these may not all be present and that DLB can exist in the absence of parkinsonism if other diagnostic features are present.

The recent discovery of a point mutation in the α-synuclein gene as a rare cause of familial Parkinson's disease has led to the finding that α-synuclein is the major component of Lewy bodies. DLB can be seen as a member of a family of α-synucleinopathies that also includes Parkinson's disease and multiple system atrophy (Spillantini & Goedert 2000).

Other causes of dementia

Metabolic and other 'medical' causes, often reversible, may be detected by simple screening tests (Table 26.4); but thyroid dysfunction and vitamin B_{12} and folate deficiencies are usually coincidental findings rather than causes of the dementia. Secondary or primary brain tumours and non-metastatic effects present more often to neurologists than to psychiatrists. The main rarer causes of dementia of which an old-age psychiatrist needs to be aware are described in Box 26.11.

Management of dementia

Estimation of severity

Although there have been many attempts to grade dementia into three or more categories (Hughes et al 1982, Reisberg et al

---

Box 26.10   Clinical characteristics of dementia with Lewy bodies

- Age at onset: 50 to 83 years
- Age at death: 68 to 92 years
- Sex distribution: Slight excess of males
- Mean survival time: Similar to that of AD but a subgroup show more rapid progression with death in 1 to 2 years
- Rate of progression: Cognitive functioning worsens at the same rate as in AD. Parkinsonism also progresses in a similar fashion to that seen in Parkinson's disease: approximately 10% decline per year
- Clinical features
  - *Fluctuating cognitive performance and degree of alertness.* Variations may be marked within a day and on a day-to-day basis and help distinguish DLB from other dementia where more minor fluctuation is seen. Transient and severe disturbances can be mistaken for a transient ischaemic attack
  - *Spontaneous motor features of parkinsonism.* Up to 70% patients have parkinsonism. Bradykinesia, limb rigidity and gait disturbance are the most common features. Tremor is seen less often than in Parkinson's disease
  - *Visual hallucinations and other psychiatric symptoms.* Visual hallucinations are present in approximately two-thirds of patients. In addition, depression is found in up to 40% of cases, and auditory hallucinations occur more frequently than in AD
  - *Falls and syncopal episodes* occur in up to a third, most likely due autonomic nervous system involvement
  - *Neuroleptic sensitivity.* Approximately half of all patients with DLB show extreme sensitivity to antipsychotic drugs which is associated with a two- to threefold increase in mortality. Severe reactions can precipitate irreversible parkinsonism, further impair conscious level and induce autonomic disturbances reminiscent of neuroleptic malignant syndrome. Atypical antipsychotics do not have a greatly more favourable side-effect profile in DLB

Adapted from McKeith & Burn (2000), Leverenz & McKeith (2002) and McKeith (2002).

1982), they have been unsuccessful because of the complexity of the illness. Staging has anyway little practical significance for the sufferer or carers, who are more interested in practical problems. For example, wandering may be severe at mild stages, when the patient is physically fit and partially aware of her situation, and mild at severe stages, when she is frail and unmotivated. Severity is best rated using one of the simpler rating scales. In earlier stages neurocognitive rating scales are appropriate; later, behaviour and non-cognitive (affective, psychotic or neurological) assessments are more useful. Burns et al (1999c) have produced a helpful compendium of the myriad of rating scales now used in old-age psychiatry.

Listing problems

The causes of symptoms in dementia are extremely complicated.

First, there are gradual losses of function. Some are simple and progressive losses of clearly localised brain functions such as recent memory impairment, agnosias and dyspraxias, the various

---

Box 26.11 Other causes of dementia in late life

Alcoholic dementia (Oslin et al 1998)
- Arguably, one of the commonest causes of dementia in many societies
- Advancing age, rather than duration of alcoholism, probably represents main risk of developing cognitive impairment
- Predominance of frontal lobe dysfunction but more widespread cortical deficits also seen
- Alcohol may be risk factor that increases susceptibility to dementia — either directly or via other known risk factors such as head injury and hypertension
- With abstinence, gradual resolution of cognitive impairment may occur over months and years

Frontotemporal dementia (FTD) (Kertesz and Munoz 2002, Snowden et al 2002)
- Second commonest form of primary degenerative dementia after AD
- Only a minority have neuropathological changes of Pick's disease, hence the broader term FTD is preferred
- Onset usually between ages 45 and 65 years although can present in both younger and older age groups
- Equal sex distribution
- Core features consist of insidious onset and gradual progression, early decline in social and interpersonal conduct, emotional blunting and early loss of insight
- Supportive features include mental rigidity, distractibility, hyperorality, perseveration and stereotypy of talk or behaviour, progressive reduction of speech output, echolalia with preserved praxis, spatial orientation and receptive speech
- Physical signs include early incontinence, primitive reflexes, late akinesia, rigidity and tremor, and low and labile blood pressure
- Mean survival of 8 years

Huntington's disease (HD) (Naarding et al 2001)
- Onset typically in mid life, although can present in seventh or eighth decade
- Autosomal dominant inheritance with 100% penetrance
- HD caused by expansion of a trinucleotide repeat beyond 35 repeats in *huntingtin* gene located on short arm of chromosome 4
- Clinical features characterised by triad of:

Motor symptoms
- — Involving voluntary movement: bradykinesia, rigidity, gait disturbance, dysarthria and dysphagia
- — Involving involuntary movement: chorea, athetosis, dystonia, myoclonus and motor restlessness

Cognitive impairment
- — Predominantly subcortical dementia
- — Impairment of memory, calculation, verbal fluency, visuospatial functioning and executive functioning
- — Aphasia, agnosia and apraxia uncommon

Psychiatric phenomena
- — May precede onset of movement disorder or cognitive impairment
- — Major depressive illness most common; schizophrenia-like picture seen in a minority
- — Behaviour and personality change common. Typical features include apathy, aggression, irritability and poor impulse control
- Structural imaging shows dilated ventricles, often particularly affecting frontal area. May be atrophy of the head of the caudate
- Dynamic imaging reveals hypometabolism in caudate and putamen
- Slow progression to death over 10 to 20 years, aspiration pneumonia or suffocation often being terminal events

Normal-pressure hydrocephalus (Hakim et al 2001, Bret et al 2002)
- Triad of cognitive impairment, gait disturbance and urinary incontinence
- Causes include subarachnoid haemorrhage, trauma and meningitis, although many cases are idiopathic
- CT or MRI scan reveals ventricular enlargement out of keeping with more minor cerebral atrophy
- CSF pressure is raised but only intermittently, typically at night
- Treatment by insertion of ventriculoperitoneal shunt is of variable benefit — gait disturbance more likely to improve than dementia

Creutzfeldt–Jakob disease (CJD) (See UK Creutzfeldt–Jakob Disease Surveillance Unit website for more details — http://www.cjd.ed.ac.uk)

Sporadic CJD
- Commonest of the human prion diseases but is very rare, affecting approximately one person per million
- Occurs due to spontaneous conversion of the normal prion protein to a pathogenic form
- Affects middle-aged and elderly individuals
- Presents as a rapidly progressive dementia with myoclonus and often with visual or cerebellar problems
- Typical EEG findings of triphasic periodic complexes at approximately one per second
- Death usually occurs within 6 months

Variant CJD
- Occurs most probably due to transmission of infection from BSE in cattle to humans via food
- Infected individuals much younger than in sporadic CJD, with average age of onset of around 27
- Most cases present with psychiatric symptoms and persistent painful sensory symptoms, and subsequently develop a cerebellar syndrome with gait and limb ataxia
- Cognitive impairment often appears late in the clinical course but progresses with the development of severe cognitive impairment and a state of akinetic mutism in the majority of cases
- Myoclonus develops in the majority of patients and in some is preceded by choreiform movements, but typical EEG appearances of CJD are absent
- The course of the illness is longer, typically around 1 year

CJD can also occur very rarely due to autosomal dominant transmission of an abnormal *PrP* gene and iatrogenically from use of infected surgical instruments or receiving contaminated human growth hormone

Box 26.11 Continued

Progressive supranuclear palsy (Rajput & Rajput 2001, Pastor & Tolosa 2002)
- Variable age of onset, mean 63 years. Slight male preponderance
- Clinical features include gait instability, frequent falls, rigidity, erect posture with retrocollis, infrequent blinking and later dysarthria and dysphagia
- Typical vertical gaze palsy may not develop until later in the illness
- Early psychiatric features include bradyphrenia (mental slowing), irritability, social withdrawal and fatiguability
- Emotional incontinence or depression also seen
- Frontal lobe dysfunction may be striking but severe dementia is rare
- Median survival is less than 10 years

AIDS dementia complex (ADC) (Clifford 2002)
- Subcortical dementia with cognitive decline and motor slowing
- Associated with significant immunodeficiency and therefore tends to present late in the disease
- Incidence has fallen to less than 10% of AIDS patients since the introduction of highly active antiretroviral therapy (HAART). However, in HAART-treated patients, ADC has declined less than other complications and so ADC now represents a greater proportion of AIDS-defining clinical events

dysphasias and, later, harder neurological signs. Others seem to be due to more generalised damage, such as the impairment of abstract thinking, remote memories and intelligence.

Second, there is the loss of standards, judgement, conscience, self-control and planning ability commonly found in frontal lobe disorder and relating to the 'executive' and monitoring functions of the brain. Loss of inhibition on cognition, action and feeling can lead to disturbed behaviour, particularly at mild and moderate stages. Similar mechanisms explain loss of control of the bladder and, later, the bowel, emergence of primitive reflexes, some psychotic symptoms and fits.

Third are the reactions of the patient to her illness. There is a growing interest in exploring and understanding the experiences of people who suffer dementia (Goldsmith 1996, Wilkinson 2001). Insight and emotions decline only gradually and sufferers retain into quite late stages some ability to react, though these reactions become distorted by other impairments and by disinhibition. Estimates of the prevalence of depression vary greatly but rates of 10–20% in those with AD and 20–30% in vascular dementia are not unlikely (Newman 1999). Anxiety is common, and paranoid reactions and hoarding of possessions may occur. Covering up the embarrassment of the condition, and social withdrawal, are probably the most common reactions. Some sufferers may sense the frightening disintegration of personality. When insight is lost, the patient may react to what she sees as unnecessary intrusions into her life, since she feels entirely competent. Later she is likely to become more passive and may end her days in a mildly disinhibited euphoria quite out of keeping with the seriousness of her condition.

Fourth, family interactions contribute to the problems of dementia. The family is aware of and remembers all the impairments and disturbances of the patient. They are likely to experience grief for the loss of her mental powers and personality and be more distressed than she is about her embarrassing behaviour, while simultaneously coping with the burden of her physical and psychological care and arranging services which can feel like an intrusion into family life. Worse still, they are likely to get no thanks from the increasingly withdrawn or egocentric patient. When other relatives and friends desert the patient out of embarrassment, it is no wonder if the now isolated remaining carer is very distressed on occasions, and that the relationship between carer and patient may become disturbed, with effects on the patient's behaviour.

Carers

Caring for a dementia sufferer is not usually a role taken on by choice. The research on stress among caring relatives has been well reviewed by Morris et al (1988) and more recently by Dunkin & Anderson-Hanley (1998) and Burns & Rabins (2000). The majority of carers are female, either spouses, daughters or daughters-in-law. Of the 40% of carers who are male, most are husbands, with sons constituting only a small number. The burden of caring at home can be enormous. As many as 65% of close carers of day hospital attenders (Gilleard et al 1984a) experience distress at levels equivalent to a psychiatric case. Donaldson et al (1997) have emphasised the effect of 'non-cognitive' symptoms in the patient on the stress felt by carers. Early-onset dementia is associated with even higher levels of carer burden (Freyne et al 1999). Those from minority ethnic backgrounds (Patel et al 1998) and other groups such as lesbian and gay carers looking after their partner (Ward 1999) may feel marginalised and excluded by statutory and voluntary services.

Whether this strain is tolerable to the carer or not depends somewhat on the patient's symptoms, but more on the nature of the carer's previous relationship with the patient (Gilhooley 1984). Other important factors include the support that the carer feels she receives from her family and others, the services and financial assistance she receives and her methods of coping, some lifelong, some learnt during the experience of caring. Levin et al (1994) and others have shown that carers generally feel better when their relative finally moves into longer term care.

Support for carers is of cardinal importance in the management of dementia. First, along with the patient, they need to be clearly informed of the diagnosis. This may bring enormous relief if they have been blaming the sufferer for laziness or obstinacy, or themselves for impatience or lack of concern. Then they need to be educated fully about the problems which dementia may bring and the services and benefits which are available, using talks and literature (HEBS 1996, Mace & Rabins 1999, Brotchie 2003). They need moral support, practical advice from others and the feeling that they are not alone in caring. Carers' groups are invaluable, though not for everybody. Stress management techniques may be useful, and counselling may help in coping with grief or with disturbances to family and social life. There is considerable scope to use family and individual therapies to help carers develop their coping skills (Richardson et al 1994, Marriott et al 2000). The particular needs of families from differing ethnic groups and of younger carers need to be catered for in any catchment area service. Most of all, all families will need regular, planned respite. Finally, when the patient dies the support should not end.

It is important to assess also the ability of the patient to understand and make decisions on matters such as finances, care and medical treatment.

If all these aspects are covered in discussions with the patient, the caring relatives and others who know her, it is likely that a comprehensive list of problem titles can be prepared (see Table 26.3). In practice, much of the management of dementia consists of trying to find explanations and solutions to the problems on the individual's problem list. Estimates of the frequency of individual problems in dementia (e.g. Sunderland et al (1988), Burns et al (1990b) and Ballard et al (1996) on *mood disorders*; Berrios & Brook (1985), Burns et al (1990a) and Ballard & Oyebode (1995) on *psychotic symptoms*) have not been entirely successful, as so much depends on which population of sufferers is studied. Other research usefully analyses the nature and causes of behaviour disturbances in detail (e.g. Morris et al (1989) and Keene & Hope (1996) on *eating disorders*; Hope et al (1994) on *wandering*; Stokes (1987), Ware et al (1990) and Patel & Hope (1993) on *aggression*; and Stokes (1986) on *screaming and shouting*).

Treatment of the cause of dementia

Ideally, treatment should address the cause of the neuronal damage in dementia. At present this is not possible except in the relatively few cases of reversible dementia. However, the last few years have witnessed significant advances in both the pharmacological and non-pharmacological management of dementia.

Pharmacological treatment of AD

Acetylcholinesterase inhibitors (Bullock 2001, Bonner & Peskind 2002) Acetylcholinesterase inhibitors (AChEIs) were the first drugs licensed specifically for AD. The three AChEIs currently available — donepezil, rivastigmine and galantamine — have been endorsed by the National Institute for Clinical Excellence (2001) for use in mild to moderate AD. Approximately 40–50% of patients respond to treatment, although only a few do so dramatically, the majority showing a more modest benefit of relative stability or slower decline. Improvement occurs across the spectrum of impairments seen in AD; the various trials undertaken have shown efficacy in enhancing not only cognition but also non-cognitive symptoms, quality of life and ability to perform activities of daily living. Efforts to predict which patients will do well with AChEI treatment have not been successful; all patients with mild to moderate AD deserve a trial of treatment, providing there are no significant contraindications and compliance can be ensured. The benefits of AChEIs have been shown in trials to continue for at least 1 year; clinical experience suggests a more prolonged response may be seen. The main adverse effects seen are due to the cholinergic effect on the gastrointestinal tract and include nausea, vomiting and diarrhoea. These effects are dose dependent and may recede with time. Other side-effects include weight loss, agitation and insomnia. Because of their cholinergic enhancing effects, caution is warranted when prescribing AChEIs for those with significant bradycardia or cardiac conduction defects, prostatism, airways obstruction and peptic ulcer disease. Slow dose titration also helps lessen the incidence of adverse effects.

Although the three AChEIs have many similarities they differ to some extent in their pharmacology. Donepezil is highly selective for acetylcholinesterase (AChE) whereas rivastigmine also inhibits butyrylcholinesterase (BuChE). As AD advances, the level of AChE falls and that of BuChE increases, but the clinical significance of the relative selectivity of the drugs is not known. Donepezil and rivastigmine are both non-competitive reversible inhibitors of AChE, although the mechanism of action of rivastigmine is sometimes referred to as pseudoirreversible because the duration of AChE inhibition it produces is longer than its half-life. Galantamine is a competitive and reversible AChEI which also potentiates cholinergic nicotinic neurotransmission by allosterically modulating nicotinic acetylcholine receptors. This additional mechanism of action produces increased amounts of acetylcholine in the synapse by a direct effect on presynaptic release. Again, the clinical relevance of galantamine's dual action is not known. Both donepezil and galantamine are metabolised by the liver whereas rivastigmine is metabolised by brain, hepatic and intestinal cholinesterases and is renally excreted. Perhaps the main clinically pertinent difference between the three AChEIs is in their half-lives. Donepezil, which has a half-life of 72 hours, can be given in a once daily dose, which aids compliance especially in those who live alone; rivastigmine and galantamine have half-lives of 8 hours and 7 hours, respectively, and so must be given twice daily.

The decision to discontinue an AChEI depends on a variety of factors. If a patient cannot tolerate the drug, then the decision is straightforward. An alternative AChEI may be tried, as individual patient reaction to different AChEIs varies and is not entirely predictable (although rivastigmine does tend to have higher rates of gastrointestinal disturbance). Lack of response to treatment after a trial period is also clearly a reason for stopping the drug. A minimum of 3 months should be allowed to elapse before determining efficacy, but many advocate a trial of 6 months treatment, as there appear to be some patients who are 'late responders'. The most difficult decision concerns when to stop treatment in those who have had an initially favourable response. Protocols that suggest discontinuation beyond a certain point (such as a decline in cognition coupled with a global impression of deterioration) or event (such as entry to permanent care) bring some objectivity, although the decision is essentially a clinical one that the patient is no longer benefiting from treatment. A phased withdrawal of treatment may determine whether the drug is still helping the patient; if there is a noticeable deterioration the drug can be restarted, though this does not always result in improvement. When response to an AChEI is eventually lost, patients usually decline quickly and lose any early benefit gained from the drug. It is generally agreed that AChEIs are not disease-modifying agents and do not alter the overall prognosis of AD.

Although AChEIs are currently only licensed for mild to moderate AD, they may also have positive effects on cognition, function and behaviour in those with more advanced illness (Feldman et al 2001).

Memantine Glutamate is a major excitatory neurotransmitter whose effects are mediated by a variety of receptor types, one of which is the *N*-methyl-D-aspartate (NMDA) receptor, which is found in high density in the hippocampus and cortex. In dementia, it is believed that excitotoxic reactions due to chronic release of glutamate ultimately lead to neuronal death. Memantine (Jarvis & Figgitt 2003) is an NMDA receptor antagonist which blocks excitotoxic glutamate activity. It has been used for over a decade in Germany to treat dementia and has recently received approval in the UK for use in moderate to severe AD, in which it has been shown to reduce decline in functional abilities and in overall clinical state (Reisberg et al 2003). Memantine is a remarkably well-tolerated drug. Dizziness, headache, agitation, insomnia and diarrhoea are the main adverse effects, although in clinical practice these are rarely of major importance. The introduction of a drug to treat more severe dementia, and its impact on already stretched services, raises significant ethical and economic questions regarding risks and benefits.

Vitamin E Following an influential trial in the United States (Sano et al 1997), vitamin E, an inexpensive and relatively safe antioxidant, has gained increasing popularity as a treatment for AD and potentially other dementias. High doses (1000–2000 IU) may slow progression of AD, although further confirmatory studies are awaited.

Gingko biloba Gingko biloba is a traditional Chinese herbal medicine made from the leaves of the maidenhair tree that has gained great popularity in recent years as a cognitive enhancer. Le Bars and colleagues' trial (1997) gained significant publicity when it showed a modest benefit in favour of gingko over placebo in AD and VaD, although drop-out rates were high. More recent work has cast doubt on the beneficial effects of gingko (Van Dongen et al 2000) and it should be remembered that the manufacture and supply of gingko and other herbal products is not subject to the same controls as for pharmaceutical medicines. Also, gingko is not without its possible side-effects, concerns having been expressed with regard to its potential for causing significant bleeding.

Oestrogen Oestrogen has a host of effects on the brain, including neurotrophic, anti-inflammatory and antioxidant activity. Postmenopausal women taking hormone replacement therapy may have reduced risk or delayed onset of AD (Tang et al 1996), though women who take hormone replacement differ in other ways from their counterparts who do not. The promise shown by earlier studies that oestrogen replacement may be of benefit in AD has not been borne out by more recent work (Mulnard et al 2000), and at present hormone replacement therapy cannot be recommended for use as a treatment for AD. Cholerton et al (2002) have reviewed this area in detail.

Anti-inflammatory drugs The finding of inflammatory markers at postmortem in the brains of patients with AD has led to interest in the use of anti-inflammatory drugs as potential treatments for AD. The story is unfortunately the familiar one of the promise of early studies not being replicated by later more rigorous work. Trials with traditional non-steroidal anti-inflammatory agents (Rogers et al 1993, Stewart et al 1997, Scharf et al 1999) have produced mixed results, and a recent study which also included one of the newer selective cyclo-oxygenase-2 inhibitors showed no benefit for either naproxen or rofecoxib in mild to moderate AD (Aisen et al 2002). Similarly, prednisolone has been shown to be ineffective in preventing decline in AD (Aisen et al 2000). Interest remains in these drugs, although the focus of attention has shifted to their use to delay the onset of AD in cognitively intact individuals.

HMG-CoA reductase inhibitors ('statins') Vaughan (2003) reviewed the evidence that patients treated with statins have a reduced incidence of dementia. The observational studies to date may have been subject to bias, and prospective trials which are currently underway should help to clarify the usefulness of these agents in slowing cognitive decline in dementia.

Anti-amyloid strategies The finding by Schenk et al (1999) that immunisation of transgenic mice with synthetic human $A\beta_{42}$

prevented amyloid plaque formation in younger mice and resulted in a reduction in the extent and progression of AD-like pathology in older animals raised the exciting prospect that immunisation against β-amyloid may be an effective means of treating AD. Unfortunately trials in humans had to be halted because some subjects developed inflammatory changes in the central nervous system, so the potential for this area of research is uncertain.

Other strategies to treat Alzheimer's disease A variety of other approaches are being studied to determine their effect in AD and other dementias. Chelation therapy using clioquinol, α- and γ-secretase inhibitors, neurotrophic agents, gene therapy and stem cell therapy are all in various stages of development.

Specific strategies for vascular dementia At present, there are no drugs licensed in the UK for the treatment of VaD, although there is emerging evidence that AChEIs may have a therapeutic effect in dementing illnesses where there is a significant contribution from cerebrovascular disease (Bowler 2002). Memantine has also been shown to be of benefit in VaD (Orgogozo et al 2002, Wilcock et al 2002). A surprising gap in evidence-based practice is that, despite the widespread prescription of aspirin for VaD, there is no firm evidence, either positive or negative, of aspirin's effects in patients with established VaD. (Williams et al 2003). Nimodipine (a calcium channel blocker), nootropic agents such as piracetam and other drugs including hydergine and pentoxifylline have all shown some efficacy in VaD but not to a sufficient extent to warrant their routine use.

Despite the relative paucity of concrete evidence for many of the above pharmacological interventions, there is much that can be done to lessen morbidity and mortality in VaD. Recurrent stokes and coronary artery disease are prevalent in these patients. Treating hypertension, prescribing statins for hyperlipidemia and giving anti-platelet drugs to those who have a history of stroke disease reduce the risk of further stroke and may thus slow the progression of dementia. In those with atrial fibrillation, warfarin should be considered. Patients with significant carotid artery stenosis (> 75%) may benefit from surgery. Other vascular risk factors such as smoking and diabetes should similarly be addressed.

Pharmacological management of dementia with Lewy bodies The treatment of patients with DLB presents particular challenges. Consideration should first be given to addressing factors that may be exacerbating psychotic symptoms. It is often necessary to balance delicately the benefits and adverse effects of drugs used to treat parkinsonism. Barber et al (2001) suggest that, if clinically indicated, a reduction/withdrawal of antiparkinsonian drugs could be tried in the following order: anticholinergics, amantadine, selegeline, dopamine agonists and levodopa preparations. Antipsychotics should be avoided if at all possible because of their propensity to cause severe adverse effects. Approximately 50% of patients with DLB who receive antipsychotics experience significant adverse effects including sedation, immobility, rigidity, postural instability, falls and increased mental impairment. Withdrawal of the offending antipsychotic does not always lead to improvement, and such patients have a two- to threefold increase in mortality (McKeith et al 1992). Although atypical antipsychotics may be thought to offer theoretical advantages, they too carry risks of significant extrapyramidal and cognitive side-effects. If antipsychotic treatment is initiated, this should only be done by a specialist, at very low dose and preferably as an inpatient.

Fortunately, alternative treatment strategies now exist for DLB without the hazards of neuroleptic sensitivity. AChEIs may now be considered the drug of choice for the management of both cognitive and psychotic symptoms in DLB (McKeith et al 2000a, Wesnes et al 2002). Adverse effects are similar to those seen in AD, and exacerbation of parkinsonian symptoms is rare.

DLB can be associated with a REM sleep behaviour disorder which is characterised by the loss of normal muscle atonia and by vivid dreams. Clonazepam, which potently abolishes REM sleep, may be useful in such instances. Patients with DLB and neurological symptoms seem to respond less well to levodopa than those with Parkinson's disease, but if there are significant motor symptoms a cautious trial of levodopa should be considered.

Behavioural and psychological symptoms of dementia

Alzheimer, in his classic description of the disease that later came to bear his name, made only passing reference to cognitive impairment in his patient; his portrayal was one of marked neuropsychiatric disturbance (Alzheimer 1906). For most patients, carers and clinicians a significant amount of the burden and challenge of dementia lies in managing the troublesome behavioural and psychological aspects of dementia. A consensus statement issued by the International Psychogeriatric Association recommended replacing the overly restrictive term 'behavioural disturbance' with 'behavioural and psychological symptoms of dementia (BPSD)' to encompass all symptoms of disturbed perception, thought, mood or behaviour that frequently occur in patients with dementia (Finkel & Burns 2000). Such symptoms are rarely pure in nature and seldom occur in isolation; very frequently cognitive, psychological and behavioural processes appear enmeshed. The elderly woman with AD who has significant memory impairment may forget where she has put her handbag. It is not difficult to understand how she becomes suspicious that others have stolen her bag, subsequently reports that she has seen intruders in her home, culminating in her 'wandering' out of her house in the middle of the night in a fearful and distressed state.

BPSD are common, occurring at any given point in time in up to two-thirds of people with dementia in the community, with half of those affected experiencing serious disturbance (Lyketsos et al 2000). Higher rates are seen in those in institutional care. Various BPSD can occur at different stages of the illness; depression often occurs early on whereas apathy and aggression tend to be features of the later stages of dementia. The preponderance of particular symptoms may vary in different types of dementia, frontotemporal dementia being characterised by disinhibition whereas psychotic symptoms are more common in DLB.

The emergence of BPSD is often one of the main triggers to institutionalisation (O'Donnell et al 1992), and such symptoms result in greater carer burden than the functional or cognitive deficits of dementia (Coen et al 1997). A recent estimate suggested that BPSD contribute approximately 30% of the cost of caring for an individual with AD (Beeri et al 2002). The development of BPSD is also associated with a worse prognosis and a more rapid rate of illness progression (Paulsen et al 2000).

Although disinhibited or poorly judged behaviour may have an organic basis, it is nevertheless influenced by environment, circumstances and the individual's own predisposition and earlier life experiences. For this reason encouraging normal behaviour can have dramatic effects on patients who otherwise seem to be uncontrollable. Patients' emotional reactions to early dementia should not be dismissed as part of the illness, but listened to with empathy. In some early cases, talking directly about the diagnosis will be both possible and reassuring. As public awareness of dementia grows and stigma disappears, more will wish to know their diagnosis and its consequences. Later, of course, there is a limit to the usefulness of repeated reassurance of any sort. Sometimes the best response to recurrent distress is to change the subject gently, or engage the patient in other activities. The outraged, insightless patient requires skilful and imaginative handling.

Simple behaviour modification techniques, altering the reactions of others rather than trying to alter the patient's behaviour directly, can be effective. A labile aggressive man may be more placid with his wife if she realises that his anger is not intended, and so learns to react in an unemotional way. It is also valuable to attempt to understand the behaviour from the patient's perspective. An aphasic cognitively impaired man who poorly comprehends his environment may feel threatened by the hurried attempts of a busy nurse to help him bathe; a slower, more careful explanation with the use of non-verbal cues, such as showing him the bath full of water, may prevent him hitting out in frightened distress. Knowledge of a patient's background and habits will also bring understanding to behaviours initially mistaken as simply inherent to the dementia. The Polish woman who becomes agitated and cries inconsolably when the transport arrives to take her to day care may find the experience reminiscent of being taken away from her home many years ago as a prisoner of war. The reassuring presence of her husband for the first few trips may help her settle more easily into her new environment.

Such commonsense approaches without recourse to drug treatment should always be implemented, and pharmacological intervention reserved only for those who have more severe BPSD. It is also necessary to ask if the symptom warrants intervention. It may well be necessary to attempt to improve the disturbed sleep pattern of a patient who is being looked after by an exhausted spouse, but if the individual is in nursing home care one must question the need to intervene at all. A first step should be to seek and exclude simple remediable physical causes for BPSD such as pain, constipation and infection. The non-pharmacological management of BPSD is summarised in Box 26.12. Although the evidence base in this field is sparse, empirical data are now emerging and have been reviewed by Teri et al (2002).

Traditionally, antipsychotic drugs have been used to control disturbed behaviour in dementia, but meta-analyses have shown that conventional antipsychotics help only 18% to 26% more patients than placebo (Schneider et al 1990, Lanctot et al 1998). There has probably been overuse of these drugs, for example in nursing homes (McGrath & Jackson 1996), they may even worsen mental impairment (McShane et al 1997) and stopping the drugs may bring improvement (Findlay et al 1989). Sometimes small doses of antipsychotic drugs are both safe and effective, but often, for example in repetitive shouters, such large doses are necessary to quieten that major side-effects occur. When specific antipsychotic effects are required, say for hallucinations or marked aggression, atypical antipsychotic drugs, with potentially fewer side-effects, are favoured. There is now evidence to support the use of low doses of risperidone (De Deyn et al 1999, Katz et al 1999, Brodaty et al 2003) and olanzapine (Street et al 2000) in treating BPSD. Efficacy should be evaluated after 4–6 weeks. As many BPSD pursue a phasic course a trial of withdrawing the antipsychotic in those who do improve should be attempted after around 3 months; a significant number of patients will not need to recommence the drug.

Depression is common in dementia, occurring in 20% of patients in the community (Ballard et al 1996) with higher rates

Box 26.12   Non-pharmacological management of behavioural and psychological symptoms of dementia — points to consider

General principles
- Always exclude physical cause first
- Non-drug treatment should always be considered first line
- Needs to be practical, inexpensive and possible for carers to implement
- Be consistent
- Preserve dignity
- Encourage normal behaviour
- Avoid punishment

Physical environment
- Keep it as familiar, constant and stress free as possible
- Environment should be age appropriate
- Careful design and good staffing is better than physical security
- Buildings for people with dementia should
  — make sense
  — help them find their way
  — provide a therapeutic environment
  — provide a safe environment
  — provide good facilities for staff

Temporal environment
- Use routine and anchor points
- Keep it stable
- Timing of activities — may be better in late afternoon when agitation is more of a problem
- Attend to sleep hygiene

Sensory functions
- Normal changes that occur with ageing affect both vision and hearing
- Further compounded by dementia
- Routinely evaluate vision and hearing and correct as necessary
- Avoid abstract/noisy designs
- Mirrors may be confusing
- Highly contrasting colours aid differentiation
- Use of soft lighting and calm colours
- Carpets can absorb sound
- Reduce extraneous noise
- Music can be calming

Behavioural interventions
- Identify target symptom(s)
- Assess the significance of the symptom
- Gather information about symptom
- Identify what happens before after and after symptom
- Set realistic goals and make plans
- Be consistent
- Encourage normal behaviour
- Avoid punishment
- Encourage caregivers to reward themselves and patient for achieving goals
- Continually evaluate and modify plans

Example of how to deal with aggression
- Intervene early
- Keep patient away from provoking situations
- Reassuring and gentle voice
- Calm, slow approach from the front
- Non-threatening posture
- Use touch judiciously
- Distract the person
- Don't argue
- Maintain calm environment
- Avoid physical restraint
- Summon help if necessary

Example of how to deal with depression
- Increase and encourage enjoyable activity
- Promote sense of purpose, meaning, autonomy
- Address isolation and loneliness
- Maintain a bright and cheerful environment
- Individualise approach to patient — what does she enjoy?
- Attention to carer's mental and physical health

in nursing home residents. A high index of suspicion is necessary, as patients with dementia may be less able to articulate their inner mood state, and many of the other signs of affective disorder, such as withdrawal, agitation, loss of appetite and sleep disturbance, may be wrongly attributed to progression of dementia. Despite the widespread prescription of antidepressants in dementia, there have been few rigorous studies evaluating their effectiveness (Bains et al 2003). The risks of tricyclic antidepressants generally outweigh their benefits in this patient group, and selective serotonin reuptake inhibitors (SSRIs) or one of the other newer antidepressants are generally preferred because of their more favourable side-effect profile. Possible serotonergic mechanisms in repetitive behaviour have led to the use of antidepressants such as fluoxetine and trazodone. Emotional lability can also respond very well to an SSRI.

The anticonvulsants carbamazepine and sodium valproate have been shown to significantly reduce agitation and aggression in dementia (Tariot et al 1998, Porsteinsson et al 2001) although these drugs are not without side-effects and are generally reserved for second line management.

Benzodiazepines are best avoided other than for brief management of marked agitation or distressing insomnia. Their chronic prescription often results in further mental and functional impairment, inappropriate sedation and ataxia with the inherent risk of falls. If sedation is required, especially at night, trazodone may be helpful. Melatonin has attracted interest as a possible treatment for insomnia and evening restlessness ('sundowning') although the results of recent trials have not been encouraging (Haffmans et al 2001, Serfaty et al 2002).

The International Psychogeriatric Association has published a comprehensive guide to BPSD which can be found online at http://www.ipaonline.org/ipaonlinev3/ipaprograms/bpsdrev/toc.asp.

Losses

The normal losses of old age are further compounded by dementia. A decline in memory is accompanied by impairment in the skills required for day-to-day living. More abstract but nonetheless important losses include the loss of role, status, esteem and autonomy that may accompany dementia. The sufferer should be encouraged to use her remaining abilities to the full. Where there are gaps in her ability, the task is to fill those gaps so that she is not struggling helplessly. Gap fillers relate to all aspects of daily living, ranging from a phone call to remind her to get up in the morning to full nursing care. The carer's imagination and the experience of other carers are the most helpful guides. Sometimes a modest amount of retraining is possible. A patient who has recently forgotten how to use her cooker may be retrained after the device has been simplified, and so gain a few more months of independence. Patients who are repeatedly distressed by constantly rediscovering the death of their spouse may be helped by repeated but sensitive exposure to the facts of the death.

Environment

For patients who live at home it is often necessary to 'treat' the environment. This may mean providing reminders and aids around the house, or reducing risks from gas and electrical appliances. Similar principles apply to the design of homes and wards for dementing residents. Ideally, dementia sufferers should be in an environment which combines homeliness, privacy and individuality with compensation for lost abilities and a reasonable level of stimulation, while allowing freedom to move about under good observation (Lawton 2001, Hoskins & Marshall 2002).

Physical care

Because of their age, most people with dementia suffer from concurrent medical conditions (Volicer & Hurley 1997) but they may forget physical symptoms, be unable to communicate them or suffer anosagnosia or autotopagnosia. Patients must be treated in this respect (though not in others) rather like infants. The only outward evidence of illness may be restlessness, a deterioration in mental state or frank delirium. Poor medical care leads to both physical and psychiatric problems.

Dementia, decision making and the law

Impairment of comprehension, insight, memory, reasoning, judgement, conscience, motivation and communication make it inevitable that dementing patients are less able to make either day-to-day or major decisions from early in the illness. At first the person with dementia will be entirely competent, but gradually her competence to make some decisions or judgements will be more and more doubtful, until she becomes legally incapable (BMA / The Law Society 1995).

In addition she may be more or less suggestible as a result of her illness, and the motives of families and financial advisers may not always be entirely altruistic. Her ability to communicate her views will be impaired to some extent. It is nearly impossible to define exactly when the patient becomes unable to understand enough to decide for herself. And it is perfectly possible to be competent in one area, such as whether to accept help at home, and not another, such as whether to sell one's house.

Much will depend on the patient's level of understanding of her current situation. It is very likely that at the beginning of the illness she will be able to understand the diagnosis. At later stages the clinician will need to judge how best to give the necessary information to help decision making.

In all areas of decision making the choice for a dementia sufferer is:

- She takes her own decisions.
- She gives an advance directive about what should happen if she should become incapable of making the necessary decisions.
- She arranges to hand them over to others because she feels unable to handle them herself.
- Decisions are taken over from her through a legal process, because she is not only unable to manage them herself, but is also unable to direct other people to manage for her.

Capacity is the ability to make decisions based on a number of factors, which need to be taken into account in assessment:

- *information* — given at a level appropriate to the person's ability to understand;
- *understanding* — comprehending and believing the information given;
- *reasoning* — weighing up the evidence to reach a decision;
- *voluntariness* — freedom from undue influence from others;
- *consistency* — reliability in achieving the same decision on different occasions;
- *communication* — ability to express views sufficiently, using an interpreter or communication aids if necessary.

A patient's expressed views are an amalgam of previously held views ('substitute judgement'), present views expressed in words or actions and passive 'behavioural' consent. Many cannot express their views even if they hold them. Many become excessively apathetic or suggestible. The consequence of all this is that there are decisions which theoretically only the patient herself can ever take but which she may become effectively incapable of taking. In such a circumstance the views of relatives may be assumed to be more important. Relatives have no legal right (unless through a legal process) to take decisions for incapable patients, although doctors and others sometimes informally give them such rights. Professionals, and to a lesser extent relatives, may be protected by the common law if their actions can be shown to benefit the patient and to do no harm ('best interests'), though this is gradually less so as the arguments for personal autonomy become increasingly powerful, except in emergency situations.

In Britain, the law on incapacity separates financial issues from issues of care and treatment. Most of the common and statute law regarding control of finances, testamentary capacity, guardianship or admission under the Mental Health Act, and consent to treatment was not developed with dementia sufferers in mind. This resulted in unwieldy and sometimes quite inappropriate legislation being adapted by ingenious lawyers and doctors to manage problem areas in those with dementia. However, in recent years there has been considerable legislative progress in Scotland, but not, as yet, in England and Wales. The Adults With Incapacity (Scotland) Act 2000 was the first major piece of legislation passed by the new Scottish Parliament and it represents a major step forward in enabling decisions to be made concerning those who lack capacity. Similar law reform, with an emphasis on decision-specific capacity, has been proposed in other parts of the United Kingdom (Lord Chancellor's Department 1999).

The powers of a mental health guardian, the responsible medical officer, the Court of Protection (England and Wales) and the Office of Care and Protection (Northern Ireland) are defined in law. In Scotland the Office of the Public Guardian has a statutory duty to monitor all financial interventions under the Adult's With Incapacity (Scotland) Act 2000, with the local authority having similar duties which also extend to welfare interventions.

Finances

One of the great advantages of early diagnosis of dementia is that it gives the sufferer the chance to appoint an agent to collect benefits, grant power of attorney to someone she trusts, or to make or update her will. The old age psychiatrist may be called in to declare whether someone is competent to make such decisions, but all too often this occurs after the event. In England, Wales and Northern Ireland where she has not given advance directions, the patient has to depend on arrangements such as Department of Social Security appointeeship or the Court of Protection. There are considerable gaps in the current legal framework to protect people with dementia from potential financial abuse from unscrupulous relatives or others. In Scotland, a relative or others with a genuine interest (but not the local authority) can apply to the Public Guardian to access the funds of the person with dementia in order to manage her day-to-day finances. For more complex financial matters, it would be necessary to apply to the Sheriff court for financial guardianship.

Restraint

Conflict may arise between a patient's wish to move about autonomously and the fears of relatives or professionals about her safety. Restricting the right to drive a car is often seen as relatively uncontroversial (Bahro et al 1995) but others disagree. O'Neill (2002) emphasises the need to balance more accurately the risk to the driver and others from continuing to drive against the potential adverse effects on heath, welfare and functioning as a result of ceasing driving. In the care of older people in general, and those with dementia in particular, a variety of restraining practices have been developed. However, physical and mechanical restraints, the use of drug treatment as a form of restraint, locking the doors of care facilities, surveillance cameras in care and living areas, electronic tagging and 'passive' alarms have all been subject to considerable criticism. The 'best interests' argument has often been used to justify such measures, but in the unequal power relationship between dementia sufferers and their carers, this can be tantamount to justifying impersonal treatment or even frank neglect or abuse. Protection from risk is also frequently cited as a reason for limiting an individual's freedom but it is necessary to acknowledge that life is never risk free and some degree of risk-taking is an essential part of good care. A thorough analysis of the risks to which an individual is exposed is part of good practice, considering not only methods of minimising risk but weighing up the potential harm of both intervening and not intervening. Where a patient with dementia is actively and consistently objecting to advice from carers which would restrict her freedom the powers of the Mental Health Act or the Adults With Incapacity (Scotland) Act 2000, including admission and guardianship, should always be considered. If these powers are seen as too draconian in a particular case, those caring for the patient need to be very aware of the potential for abuse of their power over a vulnerable adult and the distress likely to be caused by restraint in her 'best interests'. A thoughtful analysis of the issues involved in restraint, and guidance on good practice has been produced by the Mental Welfare Commission for Scotland (2002).

Medical treatment

The Mental Health Act covers medical treatment only where it can be seen as treatment for mental disorder. In England and Wales, doctors and other professionals who prescribe or administer medical, surgical or other investigation or treatment do so 'in good faith', in accordance with professional expectations, and with the protection of the common law where its principles would suggest that it would be neglectful if the treatment were necessary but was not given. This is all very well in life-saving treatment in early dementia and where everybody is agreed. If there are disagreements or uncertainties about the necessity of the treatment the patient's voice may be missing from the discussion, and a domineering relative or a strong doctor might override other views. Full consultation, a second opinion if necessary, clear recording of decisions and in difficult cases referral to a court procedure are the essentials of good practice in this area. In Scotland, the Adults With Incapacity (Scotland) Act 2000 allows treatment to be given to safeguard or promote the physical or mental health of an adult who is unable to consent. The doctor responsible for treatment must follow the general principles of the Act:

- The intervention or treatment must be necessary to achieve anticipated benefits.
- It must be the minimum effective intervention.
- The person's past and present wishes and feelings must be taken into account.
- Relevant others such as relatives and carers should be consulted.
- The exercise of residual capacity should be encouraged.

Special provisions apply where others such as welfare attorneys and welfare guardians with powers relating to medical treatment have been appointed under the Act. There is legal mechanism in place to resolve disputes, which includes a right to a second opinion and ultimately recourse to the Court of Session if necessary. The use of non-emergency force or detention is not permitted under the Act. A patient actively refusing or resisting necessary psychiatric treatment would require detention under the Mental Health (Scotland) Act 1984.

Terminal care

Terminal care in dementia is a particularly sensitive subject. At this stage the patient cannot contribute to discussions about how far investigation or treatment should proceed. It is normal practice to consider any previously expressed wishes of the patient, to consult with relatives and staff caring for her, but for the doctor to make the decision to treat or not on the basis of her present quality of life, expectation of recovery and level of distress. Following a number of legal cases, advance directives (often misleadingly called 'living wills'), by which a person declares that they do not wish to be actively treated under certain conditions, are now seen as legally binding in England, Wales and Northern Ireland. Any doctor failing to comply with an advance directive could be held legally liable. Any decision to withdraw or withhold life-prolonging treatment, including artificial hydration and nutrition, should be made only after wide consultation with the multidisciplinary team, relatives and carers. It is incumbent upon the doctor to ascertain if at all possible the patient's previously held views. Excellent guidance is now available to assist clinicians with these difficult decisions (BMA 2001, GMC 2002b). Active euthanasia for dementing people is difficult even to conceive of, since the patient's request would, to be valid, necessarily have been made before the dementia began, probably several years before the event, and it is almost impossible for an individual to predict what their own experience of dementia would be. Consent by relatives could hardly be valid, and the suspicion might be that relatives and staff were motivated by impatience at caring, when a more appropriate response would be to try to improve the lot of the vulnerable sufferer.

Research

This is another controversial and difficult area (Brooke 1988, Berghmans & ter Meulen 1995). Here there is rarely the protection of necessity. Even in therapeutic research, it is hard to argue that the patient will necessarily be better off as a result, and the argument that fellow patients may benefit later is difficult to sustain. The discussions, explanations and consent which ethics committees rightly demand in all research on patients will be impracticable beyond the early stages. Some have got round this problem by concentrating their efforts on the earliest stages of the illness. Others have suggested an important role for ethics committees or emphasise the possible use of advance directives or proxy decision making. In Scotland, the Adults With Incapacity Act permits research on those incapable of giving consent only if *all* the following criteria apply:

- Similar research cannot be carried out on capable adults.
- The research is to obtain knowledge of causes, diagnosis, treatment or care of the adult's incapacity.

- There will be real and direct benefit to the adult (unless research will contribute to significant understanding or will benefit others with similar incapacity).
- The adult does not express unwillingness to participate.
- Ethics committee approval is obtained.
- There is no or minimal foreseeable risk or discomfort to the adult.
- Consent has been obtained from any guardian, welfare attorney or nearest relative.

Similar principles are emphasised by the General Medical Council (GMC 2002a) but many contentious questions remain and the subject deserves wide debate both by psychiatrists, lawyers and the public.

Advocacy

In response to some of the deficiencies of the law and to the risk that vulnerable dementing patients may be exploited or neglected, or not have their views represented, the concept of advocacy has been introduced. Family and professionals of course act as advocates in many cases but, where the patient is isolated or at particular risk, there is virtue in having someone whose sole function is to represent her in seeking help or benefits, in discussions about decisions, or in commenting on standards of care. The appointment of a lay advocate, perhaps through an Alzheimer association, may be appropriate. Law reformers need to address the peculiar needs of insightless patients who desperately need advocacy but would reject it if offered.

Case conference In the absence of an adequate legal framework or developed advocacy, the best practice, when there is debate about a dementing patient's competence and if she may be at risk in any way, is to hold a case conference involving all concerned. This helps avoid compulsory measures in most cases, while encouraging creative thinking about ways of reducing risks or helping her come to rational decisions. Case conferences must never, however, be used to bully vulnerable patients or reluctant carers.

PSYCHOSIS

'Old' psychosis — the 'graduate' population

The advent of antipsychotic drugs in the 1950s and the subsequent move towards deinstitutionalisation led to a progressive decrease in the long-stay schizophrenic population of psychiatric hospitals, the so-called 'graduates'. It is only in the last decade that these previously neglected individuals have received appropriate acknowledgment (Abdul-Hamid et al 1998, Rodriguez-Ferrera & Vassilas 1998, Palmer et al 1999). Elderly chronic schizophrenic patients are now more likely to be found in the community, often living alone or in hostel accommodation which cannot always offer the physical or psychiatric nursing care which they need. Others are inappropriately placed in nursing homes where many of the other residents suffer from dementia and the staff may not have the necessary psychiatric skills to care for those with enduring psychotic illness.

A decline in basic daily living skills such as feeding, dressing and bathing is commonly witnessed over time in patients with schizophrenia (Friedman et al 2002, Velligan et al 1997). Negative symptoms predominate and cognitive functioning also deteriorates in those with schizophrenia as they age. This is even more marked in elderly institutionalised patients whose illness runs a chronic course (Harvey et al 1999). Unsurprisingly, those with the greatest neuropsychological impairment tend to have more negative symptoms and do worse overall. However, others who have criticised such studies for concentrating on a non-representative sample of chronically institutionalised patients, emphasise that only a small group of ageing schizophrenics experience significant cognitive decline (Heaton et al 2001). Other studies have shown that patients living outwith a hospital setting do better (Rossler et al 1999, Trieman et al 1996), although this is not a universal finding (Harvey et al 1998). Such a contradiction is simply explained by the fact that it is the quality of the environment that is of paramount importance. The Royal College of Psychiatrists (2002) have produced guidance regarding good practice with this group of patients.

'New' psychosis — late-onset schizophrenia and very late-onset schizophrenia-like psychosis

Controversy concerning the classification of schizophrenia-like and paranoid disorders in older people has persisted for centuries (Naguib 1992). Aubrey Lewis (1970) reminded us that the words paranoia and paranoid have entered common parlance. He and others (Munro 1988) make the point that both psychiatrists and laymen use the term very loosely.

In 1909, in the eighth edition of his *Lehrbuch*, Kraepelin identified a group of patients with chronic fantastic delusions and hallucinations developing at a relatively old age (over 40 years) who did not show over time the steady progressive mental decline to dementia praecox. Although he coined the term paraphrenia to describe such patients, the actual concept of such an illness is in fact much older and figures in French psychiatry where the term délire hallucinatoire chroniques persists in current classification (Pichot 1982). Mayer (1921) followed up Kraepelin's series of paraphrenic patients and found that 50 out of 78 had become schizophrenic. Munro (1991) cited this as one of the main reasons for what he described as the half-hearted attitude toward paraphrenia that then ensued. He pointed out that many of the remaining patients were still acceptably paraphrenic and not schizophrenic.

Roth & Morrisey (1952) revived interest in paraphrenia when they used the term 'late paraphrenia' to describe a group of older patients with a well-organised system of delusions, with or without hallucinations, existing in the setting of a preserved personality and affective response. Roth later made it very clear that the term that he was using, which broadly conformed to Kraepelin's earlier description, was a descriptive one which did not make any implications concerning aetiology or prognosis (Kay & Roth 1961). Unfortunately, the similarity to Kraepelin's terminology served to confuse future discussion. Late paraphrenia was never proposed to be equivalent to paraphrenia, and Kraepelin did not regard late age of onset as a feature of paraphrenia.

Manfred Bleuler (1943) first described 'late-onset schizophrenia' as occurring in individuals over the age of 40 without organic brain disease and having symptoms indistinguishable from schizophrenia arising at an earlier age. This concept influenced German literature whilst Roth and Morrisey's views held sway in the United Kingdom.

More recently, as increasing evidence has been gathered, a greater consensus has been achieved regarding the classification, phenomenology, aetiology and treatment of psychotic illnesses arising in late life. In 1998 the International Late-onset Schizophrenia Group developed a consensus statement based on published evidence. Two diagnostic categories were recognised: late-onset schizophrenia (with onset between 40 and 59 years) and very late-onset schizophrenia-like psychosis, which was considered to be distinct from schizophrenia (Howard et al 2000)

Epidemiology

Old age psychotic disorder is not common. The point prevalence of paranoid ideation in older people has been estimated to be 4–6% (Chistenson & Blazer 1984, Henderson et al 1998, Forsell & Henderson 1998), but most of these patients will have dementia. The peak incidence of schizophrenia in males is between the ages of 15 and 30 years, and male hospital admission rates fall through old age, but for women a later peak has been found and admission rates rise in the eighth and ninth decades. Just under one-quarter of patients with schizophrenia present after the age of 40 (Harris & Jeste 1988), and the 1-year prevalence rate for those between the ages of 45 and 64 is 0.6% (Keith et al 1991). Population studies of those over the age of 65 have revealed low community prevalence rates of schizophrenia in older people of between 0.1% and 0.5% (Kua 1992, Castle & Murray 1993, Copeland et al 1998). If the figures for late-life psychosis are added to those from younger people the lifetime risk is roughly equal between the sexes, but with more of the risk for females occurring in late life.

Aetiology

Some aetiological factors support the link with schizophrenia but others suggest specific environmental factors.

Sex All studies of late-life schizophrenia reveal a marked preponderance of women. In Kay & Roth's series (1961) the sex ratio for old-age schizophrenia was 9:1 for females to males, though others have found it as low as 4:1. Even allowing for the excess of elderly women in the community this is a very striking sex difference. The later the age of onset, the greater the proportion of women affected. It has been postulated that this is due to an agerelated fall in the number of dopamine D_2 receptors, with men starting life with a relatively greater number but loosing them at a greater rate with increasing age, leaving older women with a relative excess of D_2 receptors (Wong et al 1984). It has also been suggested that the antidopaminergic effect of oestrogen may protect women before the menopause (Seeman 1982). However, since late-onset psychoses commonly arise for the first time approximately 20 years after the menopause, falling ovarian oestrogen levels are unlikely to play a direct aetiological role in determining the onset of paraphrenia. Rather, withdrawal of oestrogen represents the end of an exclusively female protection against the risk of cerebrovascular disease, which men have experienced earlier in life (Howard et al 1994a). It may be that various psychosocial and environmental stressors contribute to the emergence of psychosis in later life but these factors have not been systematically studied in older people.

Genetics The genetic contribution to schizophrenia decreases with increasing age of onset in probands (Castle & Howard 1992). A positive family history of schizophrenia is commoner in those whose illness commences in early life or middle age (Jeste et al 1997). Indeed, two studies reported no increased prevalence of schizophrenia in the relatives of patients developing schizophrenia in later life (Howard et al 1997, Brodaty et al 1999). Attempts to link late-onset psychosis to HLA antigen subtype (Naguib et al 1987) or apolipoprotein E genotype (Howard et al 1995a) have not been successful.

Personality Kay & Roth (1961) found that 45% of patients had life-long paranoid or schizoid personality traits, and that this factor was independent of genetic and sensory causes. Premorbid educational, occupational and social functioning is generally less impaired compared with those with early-onset schizophrenia (Castle et al 1995, Jeste et al 1997).

Sensory deprivation Deafness has been shown to be associated with old-age schizophrenia in 25–40% of cases (Kay & Roth 1961, Post 1966, Cooper 1976). Visual impairment is less commonly relevant. Prager & Jeste (1993) have proposed that some of the association is due to suboptimal correction of the sensory deficits.

Social isolation All studies have found that the great majority of these patients are socially isolated. They are often unmarried, divorced or separated, or they married late and had few children. Their personality may have also led to isolation, and deafness increases this tendency. It is possible that some of this isolation is a consequence rather than a cause of the illness.

Life events Some studies have shown a preponderance of life events preceding late-onset schizophrenia. However, in many cases the isolation and suspiciousness of the sufferer delay referral, so that events before onset are unclear or modified by paranoid misinterpretation.

Organic factors Non-specific diffuse structural brain changes analogous to those seen in early-onset schizophrenia, such as ventricular enlargement, are found on CT scanning (Naguib & Levy 1987, Burns et al 1989) and MRI scans (Corey-Bloom et al 1995, Jeste et al 1998). Focal structural abnormalities are also similar to those in younger patients, including reduced volume of the left temporal lobe (Howard et al 1995) and superior temporal gyrus (Pearlson et al 1993). Although focal cerebrovascular changes have been reported in the brains of those with late life psychosis (Almeida et al 1995b), studies that carefully exclude those with organic cerebral disorder do not reveal an excess of such abnormalities (Howard et al 1995b, Symonds et al 1997). Temporal and frontal hypoperfusion have been reported in functional imaging studies (Miller et al 1992, Sachdev et al 1997). Neuroreceptor studies using PET have not clearly shown abnormalities in the number or function of dopamine D_2 receptors in late-onset schizophrenia. Patients with late-onset schizophrenia demonstrate a number of neuropsychological deficits, including impairment of executive functioning, learning, motor skills and verbal ability, that are qualitatively and quantitatively different from the cognitive dysfunction of dementia (Almeida et al 1995a). The relationship of the organic changes to the cognitive impairment seen, or to outcome, is unclear (Hymas et al 1989). Some evidence would suggest a spectrum of disorders, with at one end a pure delusional disorder associated with organic changes and at the other hallucinosis associated with sensory deprivation (Flint et al 1991 using CT, Howard et al 1994b using MRI). It is has been postulated that different fundamental mechanisms underlie psychosis occurring at different ages. Schizophrenia developing in early adult life may be seen as a neurodevelopmental disorder, whereas neurodegenerative changes may be of greater aetiological significance in psychotic illnesses occurring in older people (Arnold 2001).

Clinical features

The onset is usually insidious, and in the past some cases of late-onset delusional disorder have been thought of as personality developments in schizoid or suspicious individuals rather than true psychosis. Resistance to help because of lack of insight may prevent diagnosis for years after the first psychotic experiences.

Persecutory delusions tend to dominate the clinical picture, although delusions of reference and control and those of a hypochondriacal, grandiose, erotic and jealous nature are also often present. Howard et al (1992) describe partition delusions occurring in up to two-thirds of patients with very late-onset schizophrenia-like psychosis; such patients believe that people, animals, material or radiation can pass through a structure that would normally constitute a barrier to such passage. Hallucinations are most commonly auditory, but olfactory hallucinations, somatic hallucinations of electricity or rape and visual hallucinations, usually of flashes, also occur. In some patients, perhaps 10–20%, only delusions are present, as in Kraepelin's *paranoia* (1919), or 'persistent delusional disorder', though some of these may have organic brain lesions (Flint et al 1991). Typical first-rank symptoms are found in about 30% of cases. These may include experiences of intrusion into the thoughts or body of the sufferer. Complaints of intrusions into her personal space in the sense of house or property are much more typical. An important consequence of this is that when the patient is admitted to hospital or moves house to escape from her persecutors, the symptoms may temporarily disappear (Post 1966). This can give the impression that the symptoms were exaggerated at home, or that the patient is now cured. However, a return visit home, or time to settle into a new personal space in hospital or a new house brings a resurgence of symptoms. Typical negative symptoms are uncommon, and indeed patients often preserve strong paranoid personality traits, making management difficult.

Despite the evidence of neuropsychological deficits on formal testing, most patients continue to function apparently well within the limits of their psychosis. They are proud of their continuing mental alertness and see this as protection against their persecutors. Possibly no more than expected develop dementia in the long run. If dementia does develop, the psychotic symptoms may 'dissolve' and antipsychotic treatment is no longer needed.

Depression secondary to the persecutions is not uncommon, and causes difficulties in differentiating old age schizophrenia from affective or schizoaffective disorders. The more usual reaction is of outrage and anger. The patient retaliates against her persecutors, who are likely to be unsuspecting neighbours. Calling in the police or a solicitor is as likely as calling in the doctor, and lack of insight usually leads the patient to suggest that the neighbours rather than she need treatment.

Treatment

Antipsychotic drugs are effective in old-age schizophrenia and delusional disorder (Jeste et al 1996, Maixner et al 1999, Bouman & Pinner 2002), and long-term treatment is necessary. Christie (1982) has shown the quite dramatic effect on the need for hospital long-stay care by comparing 1970s figures with Roth's figures from the 1940s (Roth 1955). Compliance is a problem, and the psychiatrist may have to resort to indirect means to persuade the patient to take drugs. Some patients have a trusted 'ally' who can persuade them. A community psychiatric nurse (CPN) who gradually gets to know her can become such an ally. Suggestions that the drug will help her 'cope with the persecution better' or 'will put the problem into the background' may help. Few patients have enough insight to feel that treatment is fully justified. Compliance is not helped by the tendency of antipsychotic drugs to produce more side-effects the older the patient. Due to their better tolerability, atypical antipsychotics are now generally preferred over their older counterparts, but there is dearth of robust trial data in this group of patients (Arunpongpaisal et al 2003). The few studies that have been carried out in older adults tend to make no distinction between the varying causes of psychosis in older people; until there are good randomised controlled trials, we must extrapolate from studies in younger adults and older people with dementia or non-specific psychosis. The different atypical antipsychotics each have their own drawbacks: olanzapine has the potential for anticholinergic side-effects, while risperidone may have a greater propensity to cause extrapyramidal side-effects. Quetiapine is theoretically the least likely to cause parkinsonism. Age is not a contraindication to clozapine treatment but it is poorly tolerated by older people and there is an age-related increase in risk of agranulocytosis (Wahlbeck et al 1999). Depot treatment is tolerated by some patients and is easier to monitor over a long period but carries the risk of greater parkinsonian side-effects. The recent availability of long-acting preparations of atypical antipsychotics has generated interest that they may be more suitable than traditional depots for older patients, although further experience and evaluation is required before their place in clinical practice can be determined. Relieving isolation and deafness have also been proposed as possible treatments.

Other conditions with paranoid or hallucinatory symptoms

The differential diagnosis of paranoid symptoms and of hallucinations in old age is complicated, and there is considerable overlap between some of the conditions.

Secondary paranoid states A variety of organic cerebral conditions and treatment with steroids, antiparkinsonian or other drugs can sometimes produce psychotic phenomena without obvious mental impairment. History and investigation of the patient's physical state are important in all cases of paranoid psychosis.

Delirium The psychotic symptoms of delirium may be mistaken for symptoms of a primary paranoid psychosis. The acute time-course, relation to physical illness, evidence of cognitive impairment, and characteristic symptoms of delirium (see Table 26.6) should help to differentiate the disorders. In delirium, visual hallucinations are more common than auditory hallucinations, whereas the reverse is the case in schizophrenia.

Dementia Paranoid and other psychotic symptoms are common in dementia (Ballard & Oyebode 1995). Paranoid ideas may be a reaction to memory impairment in a sensitive individual, or may relate to the basic disease process. Agnosias, receptive dysphasia, impairment of comprehension and other related disorders may explain misinterpretations, which lead on to more fixed paranoid ideas. Visual hallucinations have traditionally been ascribed to delirium occurring in the course of VaD, but are now more clearly linked to a diagnosis of DLB (see Box 26.10).

Paranoid ideas and hallucinatory experiences in dementia are usually relatively transient and ill formed. They respond, though often incompletely, to antipsychotic medication.

Affective disorders Psychotic symptoms are common in both severe depressive illness and in hypomania in old age. The admixture of symptoms helps to differentiate, as does the affective colouring of the experiences. A curious phenomenon is the persistence of psychotic symptoms between episodes in some patients with a long history of recurrent affective disorder.

Schizoaffective disorder Post (1971) described a number of cases who did not fit into either the description of paranoid psychotic illness or affective illness, but who were intermediate in clinical features, aetiology and outcome.

Hallucinations of sensory deprivation Berrios & Brook (1984) suggested that visual hallucinations without marked paranoid ideas might be a non-specific phenomenon in elderly patients, linked to visual impairment rather than to any particular diagnosis. The 'visions' are of people, animals or scenes and the patient has a degree of or even complete insight. If there is no other associated psychiatric or cognitive disorder then the term *Charles – Bonnet syndrome* is appropriate (Menon et al 2003). Teunisse et al (1995) studied a large group of these patients and confirmed the association with visual sensory deprivation and old age. Some may prove to have DLB. Small doses of antipsychotic drugs may help but they are often only partially effective. Anticonvulsants have also been suggested as an appropriate treatment. Optimising visual functioning as much as possible, reassurance, appropriate stimulation and company often help when drugs do not, and such approaches should be used in all patients.

An auditory equivalent of this phenomenon, musical hallucinations (Berrios 1990), occurs in those with hearing impairment.

AFFECTIVE DISORDERS

Affective disorders in older people tend to be more heterogeneous in aetiology and presentation than those presenting in earlier life. Difficulties in diagnosis and management may arise from ageist attitudes of clinicians and the public who erroneously assume that to be old is to be miserable. Older people may deny depression or perceive it as shameful, adding to under-recognition and lack of treatment. Comorbid medical conditions, cognitive impairment, multiple life events and losses, most especially bereavement, and the tendency of some older people to somatise further complicate matters. Continued efforts are required to heighten both public and professional awareness that depression in later life represents frank illness with significant morbidity and is not just an understandable and normal reaction to growing older.

Depression

Epidemiology

The prevalence of depression in a given population may say more about the methods of study than the frequency of treatable morbidity (Blazer 1999). Problem areas in epidemiological studies of late-life depression include differing age cohorts studied, exclusion of those in care, or of those with dementia and physical illness, the uncertain status of bereavement reactions, the use of hierarchical diagnostic systems and instruments only validated on younger subjects, definition of illnesses and caseness and biological symptoms in physical illnesses. Studies consistently demonstrate that the prevalence of depressive symptoms far exceeds that of depressive illness or syndromal depression. Major depression affects only 1–3% of older people but, when all clinically relevant depressive syndromes are considered, studies reveal rates of up to 35% (Beekman et al 1999). Longitudinal studies of the natural history of affective disorder show a general trend for episodes to occur more frequently and to last longer (Zis & Goodwin 1970, Cutter & Post 1982). Depression in all age ranges is more common in women, and this finding is also borne out by studies in older people. Those that are widowed or separated appear to be more at risk than those that are married or who have never married, although marriage appears to be a more protective for men than women (Prince et al 1999).

Aetiology

Genetic factors are much less important causally in affective disorder beginning in late life (Young & Klerman 1992) with the prevalence of a positive personal history decreasing linearly with increasing age of onset (Van Ojen et al 1995). Physical illness and disability are significantly associated with depression in older people, the personal meaning and associated handicap of ill health being of more importance than any particular pathology (Prince et al 1997a). In community studies of major depression, Murphy (1982) and Prince et al (1997b) showed the importance of life events, illness and lack of a confiding relationship. An absence of supports and perceived loneliness were strongly associated with depression. The many losses to which elderly people are susceptible explain the relatively high prevalence of milder depressions, though sufferers may hesitate to complain because such losses are expected (Parkes 1964).

Broadly defined depression does not decrease in prevalence with advancing age. However, the genetic contribution to depression is less in older subjects, necessitating a search for other aetiological factors. Over recent years, there has been increasing evidence that vascular disease may be of importance in the genesis of depression in older people, particularly those whose illness arises for the first time in later life. (Alexopoulous et al 1997, Baldwin & O'Brien 2002). It is well recognised that depression is a common consequence of cortical stroke disease (Kotila et al 1998, Pohjasvaara et al 1998) and vascular dementia (Newman 1999). More subtle cerebrovascular disease can be detected by cerebral imaging, MRI studies revealing an excess of white-matter hyperintensities (O'Brien et al 1996). It is hypothesised that vascular damage to fronto-subcortical circuitry results in a so-called vascular depression that tends to be of later onset and characterised by more executive dysfunction and psychomotor retardation and by less depressive ideation (Alexopoulous et al 1997). Such patients have a poorer response to treatment (O'Brien et al 1998, Simpson et al 1998) and may have a higher risk of developing dementia (Hickie et al 1997).

Shulman & Post (1980), Stone (1989) and Broadhead & Jacoby (1990) have emphasised that new cases of mania are often related, perhaps causally, to brain disease, at least in men. A link between onset of depressive illness in elderly men and a later diagnosis of abdominal cancer has been postulated, though not all are agreed.

Clinical features

Younger and older people who are depressed differ less often in symptomatology than is commonly believed. The stereotypes of somatic preoccupation, hypochondriacal complaints and marked agitation that have been previously reported arose from studies of inpatients, and such features probably were markers of more severe illness. The data concerning delusional depression is conflicting, with some authors reporting increased rates in older people (Brodaty et al 1993, Meyers & Alexopoulos 1988) whereas others have found no difference compared with younger subjects (Nelson et al 1989). Those with late-onset 'vascular' depression tend to present with apathy and loss of motivation and may be less likely to complain of depressed mood.

Atypical presentations of depressive disorder are relatively common. The most debated is *pseudodementia*, or *depressive dementia*. Measurable intellectual impairment is often found during late-life depressions, and although this may return to normal after treatment, such patients are subsequently at greater risk of developing dementia (Alexopoulos et al 1993). Moreover, depressive symptoms without apparent cognitive impairment predict the later development of cognitive decline and dementia (Geerlings et al 2000, Paterniti et al 2002), especially in those with persistent and more severe depressive symptomatology. The following list of clinical features (adapted from Wells 1979) distinguishing pseudodementia from dementia is helpful:

- past history of depressive illness;
- depressed mood;
- diurnal variation in mood;
- other biological symptoms;
- islands of normality;
- exaggerated presentation of symptoms.

Chronic, more minor depressive symptomatology is often poorly recognised and under-treated in older people. Studies reveal that late-onset dysthymia has much in common with major depression, suggesting the existence in late life of a single condition along a continuum (Devanand et al 2000).

Differential diagnosis

Dementia As well as the problem of pseudodementia, there are often difficulties in distinguishing the social withdrawal, lack of self-care and apathy of early dementia from depression. Depression during dementia causes particular difficulties (Ballard et al 1996). If there is doubt a trial of antidepressants is advisable.

Depression associated with physical illness Depression in older people is commonly associated with a range of physical conditions such as stroke disease, Parkinson's disease, cancer, cardiac disease, arthritis, infection and endocrine dysfunction. Painful illness is a particular risk factor for depression. Mood disorder is also a side-effect of many drugs used in elderly patients (Box 26.13). Every new case of depression requires a full medical

---

Box 26.13   Drugs that can cause organic mood disorder

Antihypertensive drugs	Antiparkinsonian drugs
• Beta-blockers	• L-dopa
• Methyldopa	• Amantadine
• Reserpine	Psychotropic drugs
• Clonidine	• Antipsychotics
• Nifedipine	• Benzodiazepines
Steroids	Miscellaneous
Analgesics	• Sulphonamides
• Opioids	• Digoxin
• Indomethacin	• Tetrabenazine

history, including alcohol and drugs, physical examination and screening investigations.

The diagnosis of affective disturbance after a stroke is difficult, most of all in patients with communication problems. Previous studies that linked lesions in the left frontal cortex to depressive symptoms have been criticised for not including a representative sample of patients, and more recent investigators have concluded that the risk of depression is not associated with either the hemisphere or the location of the stroke (Carson et al 2000, Rao 2000). Apparent depression following a stroke may be due to emotional lability, reactive distress, organic apathy or lack of motivation and side-effects of drugs (House et al 1991). Lability is particularly common and may respond to small doses of antipsychotic drugs or, more specifically and sometimes dramatically, to antidepressants such as fluoxetine.

Differentiating depression and mild parkinsonism is sometimes difficult, as retardation and a downcast expression occur in both conditions. Poor communication may impede examination. The picture is confused further because the side-effects of antiparkinsonian drugs include delirium, hallucinations, depression, elation and sexual disinhibition, paranoid states and even obsessional symptoms.

Distress due to environmental factors The contribution of the vicissitudes of life and its inherent stresses often need to be addressed. Poor housing, poverty, social isolation and unsatisfactory relationships may all result in understandable upset. Indeed, such factors make depression more likely and their presence should not lead to the pernicious diagnosis of 'no mental illness', although they may need to be tackled in their own right. Finally the possibility of previous sexual abuse or other past traumas should not be overlooked.

Treatment

Antidepressant drug treatment Salzman et al (2002) and Wilson et al (2003) have comprehensively reviewed the recent literature. Their findings emphasise the efficacy of all the major classes of antidepressant in treating older people. In clinical practice, SSRIs and other newer antidepressants now tend to be favoured over tricyclic antidepressants. The evidence that they have fewer side-effects is slight, although it may be that such side-effects are less hazardous. If older antidepressant agents are to be used (and it has been suggested that they may be more effective in the most severe illnesses) then careful supervision is essential when starting these drugs and adjusting doses, with daily lying and standing blood pressure measurement if possible. For a significant number however, the cardiovascular, anticholinergic and antiadrenergic side-effects of tricyclic antidepressants preclude their use. Some clinicians still use traditional monoamine oxidase inhibitors as second-line drugs with good effect, even in major depression, though delayed postural hypotension may be a problem. Depression with psychotic features responds poorly to antidepressant drugs alone, combined treatment with an antipsychotic or electroconvulsive therapy being required. With all antidepressants, small starting doses, gradual increases and prolonged trial periods of up to 2 months are required. Jacoby & Lunn (1993) propose that medication should continue for 2 years or more after recovery. The high risk of recurrence of illness with all its detrimental effects on health and well-being means that many old-age psychiatrists pragmatically recommend indefinite prophylaxis. Lithium augmentation and other combination treatments are worth trying in intractable cases and have been reviewed by Baldwin (1996).

Electroconvulsive therapy (ECT) Problems with antidepressant drugs have persuaded many clinicians that ECT has an important part to play in the treatment of late-life depression, as a first-line treatment in severe illness, and where drugs are contraindicated, fail or have undesirable side-effects. Flint & Gagnon (2002) reviewed the literature and concluded that it is a safe and effective treatment for major depression in old age, with a good response in 70–90% of cases, although a recent Cochrane review reminds us that there is little in the way of good randomised studies (Van der Wurff et al 2003). Unilateral placement of electrodes carries a lower risk of post-ictal confusion at the expense of probably being less effective. Unfortunately, as many as 50% of patients relapse within 6 to 12 months following a course of ECT despite continued antidepressant medication. There is little to guide the clinician in choosing appropriate antidepressant treatment in such situations; lithium, psychological approaches and continuation ECT are all possibilities. Dementia is not a contraindication to ECT if coexisting depression warrants its use. Coexisting medical problems, including ischaemic heart disease, chronic airways disease, epilepsy, having a pacemaker and being on warfarin, are usually not a barrier to ECT although, as with all patients, careful anaesthetic assessment is required.

Psychological treatment of depression The increasing evidence that cognitive-behavioural therapy and interpersonal psychotherapy are effective in treating depression in older adults is reviewed by Areán & Cook (2002). The additive effects of antidepressant medication and psychotherapy may be superior to either treatment alone, especially in preventing relapse. In reactive depressions, counselling, for example from the Cruse bereavement counselling service or other agencies, can be helpful. In intractable depression, ongoing support is vital, and discussing practical difficulties may bring some relief.

Psychosocial intervention is valuable in all those with depression, but especially those with less severe or chronic illness who may have persistent practical difficulties, relationship problems or are socially isolated.

Prognosis

Although there has been some dispute regarding the long-term prognosis of depression in older people, recent studies which have followed up patients for several years (Sharma et al 1998, Denihan et al 2000, Beekman et al 2002) suggest a tendency to chronicity and relapse, which becomes increasingly evident over time. Mortality is high, around 30% of community patients dying over 3 years, confirming the association between depression and physical ill-health. As few as one-quarter of patients remain consistently well for at least 5 years after initial diagnosis, with almost one-third having persistent depressive symptomatology. The remainder tend to follow a relapsing remitting course. Many of these individuals are poorly diagnosed or poorly treated, and Baldwin (2000) persuasively argues that with appropriate treatment the prognosis of late-life depression improves and should be no worse than that of younger patients.

Bipolar disorder and mania

Although it is generally believed that the incidence of mania declines with age, there appears to be two peak periods for the onset of mania: one in early adult life and another in old age. The manic illnesses of these two groups may differ in aetiology, many of those who become unwell for the first time in old age having associated cerebral pathology, most often vascular disease with right hemispheric lesions predominating (Braun et al 1999). Such organic factors probably explain why patients with late-onset mania have a lower incidence of family history of affective disorder. Studies of elderly bipolar patients suggest that they experience a relatively late age of onset of approximately 50 years, with around half first having a depressive episode. Such patients can have a very long latent period before their first manic episode. Shulman et al (1992) found a mean gap of 15 years between the first episodes of depression and mania, with one-quarter of patients experiencing a latency of at least 25 years.

Treatment of bipolar disorder and mania

Antipsychotic drugs should be used in the same way as for younger patients, though in age-appropriate doses. Atypical antipsychotics are now increasingly used to treat mania in old age. Lithium can be used as first-line treatment or as a prophylactic mood stabiliser. Clearance of lithium declines steadily in later life. Equivalent doses lead to higher blood levels, and relatively low blood levels can lead to toxic effects. For these reasons it must be administered with considerable care, and in lower doses than for younger patients. Blood levels of 0.4–0.6 mmol/l may be effective, and over-enthusiastic attempts to aim for higher serum concentrations carry a significant risk of toxicity. Regular thyroid and renal function checks are most important in this age group, and the lithium level should be retested if there is any intercurrent infection, or change in drug treatment, especially the concomitant prescription of thiazide diuretics, ACE inhibitors or non-steroidal anti-inflammatory agents.

Because of the low therapeutic index of lithium the use of anticonvulsants as mood stabilisers in older people has increased in recent years. Valproic acid and, to a lesser extent, carbamazepine are being used increasingly as first-line treatments. Reports of experience with newer anticonvulsants in older people, such as gabapentin and lamotrigine, are limited mainly to positive anecdote.

SUICIDE AND DELIBERATE SELF-HARM

Suicide

In Britain, around 20% of all suicides are by older people, despite the fact that only 15% of the population is over 65 years in age. The rate declined in the 1960s due to detoxification of the gas supply, and there has been a further significant reduction in the last two decades. The exception is elderly men, where rates have remained fairly static (Cattell 2000). Rates for men are roughly three times those for women, and continue to increase with advancing age, while the female rate may gradually fall. Until recently elderly men were the most likely age group to end their life by suicide but now, in the United Kingdom, young males have higher rates. Older women, however, continue to have the highest rates across the lifespan.

The main factors which predict late-life suicide include not only age and male sex, but also physical illness (estimates range from 35% to 85% of cases), social isolation, widowed or separated status, alcohol abuse and, most especially, depressive illness and a past history of depression. In Barraclough's (1971) classic series 87% of

those over 65 years had an affective disorder, and others more recently have confirmed the overwhelming contribution of depression to suicide in older people (Conwell et al 1996). Elderly people are less likely to spontaneously voice suicidal ideation, but hypochondriacal complaints, insomnia, weight loss and feelings of hopelessness and guilt are associated with future completed suicide and should alert the clinician to the likely presence of a depressive illness. Physical illness, particularly painful illness, is an important antecedent to suicide, the risk probably being due again to associated depression. Barraclough emphasised that around 80% of suicides had contacted their general practitioner in the 3 months before death, but Cattell & Jolley (1995) found somewhat lower rates of contact and low rates of onward referral to psychiatric services. Attempts to reduce the rate of suicide by restricting the availability of lethal methods such as firearms or potentially fatal drugs seem to be especially successful in older people, but the most effective strategy is to effectively recognise and treat depression (Conwell 2001).

Deliberate self-harm

In contrast, deliberate self-harm (DSH) is relatively uncommon in older age groups, contributing only about 5% to the total (Hawton & Fagg 1990). The male to female ratio is much more even than in younger people. Instances of DSH in older people are more likely to represent failed suicide rather than being gestures of distress, interpersonal difficulties or personality problems. Draper (1996) emphasised that the factors associated with DSH in old age were similar to those associated with completed suicide, and relationship problems may be important in some cases. Depression, somatisation, hypochondriasis and physical illness have all been associated with DSH in the elderly. Compared with younger individuals, repetition of DSH occurs less frequently in older people but subsequent completed suicide is more common (Hepple & Quinton 1997).

All suicidal behaviour in the elderly should be taken seriously, and depressive illness should be suspected. Of course, there are also some personality-disordered individuals who have habitually harmed themselves over many years and continue to do so.

NEUROSIS

Prevalence

It is not always recognised that depression and anxiety problems are overall more prevalent in old age than dementia. Epidemiological studies of neurosis are beset with methodological difficulties. Differing case-finding methods, arguments about definition of syndromes, the issue of 'caseness', the boundary between personality and neurotic disorders, and the correct classification of 'depressive neurosis' are but some of the pitfalls. Kessell & Shepherd (1962) showed that while there was no great decline in community prevalence in neurosis in older people, and general practitioner attendances for neurotic disorders fell little, there was a marked fall in referrals to psychiatrists. Elderly people with neurotic disorders probably accept their complaints more readily, and general practitioners may be reluctant to refer on, perhaps considering such disorder to be 'just old age'. Estimates of prevalence range between 1% and 10% (Eastwood & Corbin 1985). Saunders et al (1993) found rates of clinical neurosis of 2.5% but there may also be a penumbra of 'subcases', perhaps a further 15%. Male prevalence rates are always lower, and there have been suggestions that rates may decline in the very old age groups. Most studies find 'old' and 'new' cases to be roughly equal in frequency.

Clinical features

Bergmann (1978) examined a group of subjects with late-onset neurosis and found that most had symptoms of anxiety or depression. Anxiety symptoms may be generalised or may present as panic attacks or phobias (Lindesay 1991). A particular phobia, uncommon in younger people but relatively common in the elderly, has been named *space phobia* by Marks (1981). Agoraphobics experience anxiety in crowded places, while space phobics become anxious in open spaces where they have no supports to hold on to. They usually have few background neurotic traits, and have had some physical illness or accident which has led them to fear falling or lack confidence in their mobility. They often become housebound. They respond relatively poorly to both physiotherapy and behaviour therapy.

Aetiology

By factor analysis of background variables Bergmann showed that physical illness, a feeling of loneliness (as distinct from actual isolation), impaired self-care and 'anxiety-prone' or 'rigid, insecure' personality traits contributed to the development of new cases of neurosis in old age. More recent studies come to similar conclusions, adding an emphasis on the role of life events.

Differential diagnosis

Obsessional disorders, eating disorders, hypochondriasis or abnormal illness behaviour rarely emerge for the first time in late life. New symptoms suggestive of any of these disorders should make the clinician think first of other diagnoses, using a hierarchical approach.

Physical illness   Patients who feel ill but cannot identify clear symptoms may present pseudoneurotic symptoms, or present their symptoms in an exaggerated fashion. An apparent eating disorder is much more likely to be caused by serious physical illness than by a late-onset neurosis, though rare cases of primary eating disorder do occur (Cosford & Arnold 1992). Kay & Bergmann (1966) found that one of the best predictors of mortality in older psychiatrically ill patients was a physical complaint. Because of the predominance of physical symptoms many patients may present to cardiologists, neurologists or gastroenterologists rather than psychiatrists.

Acute or chronic brain disease   Disinhibitory mechanisms can lead to the emergence or magnification of neurotic personality traits or symptoms.

Affective disorder   Depressive illness, hypomania or a mixed affective disorder can present in old age with pseudoneurotic symptoms, and there is considerable comorbidity between depressive illness and anxiety (Flint 1994). In particular, the complaint of hypochondriasis, which only rarely begins as a neurotic disorder in later life, is much more likely to be caused by a depressive illness.

Personality disorder   By definition, personality disorder does not arise de nove in fate life. Behavioural disturbance, 'histrionic' conduct and 'acting out' behaviour all suggest organic illness or depression until proven otherwise.

Treatment

Those with long-standing neurotic illness will be likely to require continuing treatment which has been effective. Given the likely causal factors in 'new' late-life neurosis, treatment of these cases should aim at resolving, or helping the patient come to terms with, problem issues such as physical ill health, losses or loneliness. Cognitive-behavioural therapy has been shown to be effective in elderly patients with depression, generalised anxiety, phobic disorders, panic disorder, prolonged grief and obsessive–compulsive disorder (Lindesay 2002). Benzodiazepines should in general be avoided. SSRIs have anxiolytic and anti-panic properties, and a trial of antidepressant medication is often indicated, certainly if there is any hint of depression. The traditional use of low-dose tricyclic antidepressants for anxiety symptoms has nothing to commend it. Drug and psychological approaches should not be seen as mutually exclusive.

SUBSTANCE MISUSE IN OLDER PEOPLE

Alcohol problems

Prevalence

Johnson (2000) has reviewed the epidemiology of alcohol problems in old age. Around 40% of older people are abstainers, with women more likely to be teetotal than men. Those who do drink take on average less than younger people. Cohort effects play a large part in this, and current cohorts may be gradually raising the levels of intake (Bennett et al 1995). Premature mortality in heavy drinkers may contribute to the lower rates of alcohol consumption in the elderly. However, many individual elderly people do cut down their alcohol intake. As an individual ages, tolerance to alcohol is likely to decrease, because of reduction in important liver enzymes and changes in the response of the brain to alcohol. The same dose of alcohol produces higher blood levels, more intoxication and more adverse effects. Financial considerations also play a part; elderly people are often relatively poorer than they were when of working age. Furthermore, at present there are social pressures against drink among many, but not all, elderly groups, and many social activities for older people are not associated with drinking as they would be for younger people.

As might be expected the prevalence of heavy drinking is lower than in younger people (Saunders et al 1989). Defining the numbers who have alcohol problems is difficult, for there is probably considerable under-reporting. Often the relevant questions are simply not asked, in the mistaken belief that older people, and especially older women, rarely drink. Luttrell et al (1997) found that screening questionnaires and a high mean corpuscular volume were insensitive tools for detecting alcohol misuse in the elderly. Although the female rate of problem drinking remains significantly below the male rate, older women are slightly more likely than their male counterparts to develop alcohol problems for the first time in later life (Blow 2000). Recent changes in the drinking habits of younger women will change this pattern in the future.

New and old cases of alcohol abuse tend to show some differences (Rosin & Glatt 1971, Atkinson 1994). In late-onset cases family history is not as great a factor as in younger cases. Risk factors in late-onset cases include female gender, higher socio-economic class, precipitating life events (including not only losses but also sudden access to excess time and money at retirement) and physical ill health. These 'new' cases are more 'neurotic' in type, with less evidence of a background personality disorder, and they often involve a history of social or heavy (but not dependent) drinking in their younger years. The misuse of alcohol tends to be milder, and may fluctuate more, with greater chance of spontaneous remission.

Alcohol problems may also be a symptom of or a reaction to psychiatric illness, though this is not the explanation for most 'new' cases. The older person with depression or mild dementia may begin drinking heavily for the first time in her life, and here cause and effect can be difficult to disentangle. Alcohol-related dementia remains a controversial subject, but in all cases of dementia enquiry about past alcohol consumption is essential. Korsakov's syndrome is, of course, a common finding in 'old' cases, including the important subgroup of 'graduates' who were admitted with the Korsakov syndrome in middle age.

Treatment

The link between practical problems and recent onset allows greater optimism about treatment, which can focus on the person's circumstances and social milieu. Brief intervention in the form of simple advice to cut down on drinking may be all that is required in mild 'at risk' cases (Blow 1999). For heavier drinkers and those who are alcohol dependent, an ideal approach is to combine individual support and education with age-specific group work (Atkinson et al 1998). Treatment is assisted by the availability of non-drinking social activities, by the absence of social stigma about abstinence and by a greater willingness among families to control an elderly person's finances in order to control her drinking. Effects of alcohol on the older person's physical state and mobility further encourage abstinence.

People who have abused alcohol over many years may also cut down their intake. But it is also quite common for their drinking to continue along the pattern of earlier years, and the associated physical or psychiatric problems continue or intensify. Those in lodgings and hostels may be particularly at risk.

Drug abuse

Drug abuse is not a major problem among older people except in relation to prescribed drugs such as benzodiazepines, opiates and other analgesics, occasionally barbiturates and other 'older' drugs, and less obvious drugs of abuse, particularly laxatives. Petrovic et al (2002) found that chronic elderly benzodiazepine users were typically widowed females with dysthymia and anxiety who were predisposed to alcohol dependence and had borderline personality traits. Abuse of 'street' drugs by older people is likely to gradually increase as a problem over the next decades as a cohort effect.

It is sometimes felt that withdrawal of drugs of dependence from an older person is cruel, as they have 'not long to go'. However, falls, dysphoria and cognitive dysfunction are often associated with these drugs in the older patient, and abstinence may greatly improve a person's quality of life. The greatest arguments arise over hypnotics in patients who show no obvious adverse effects but are clearly psychologically dependent.

SEXUAL PROBLEMS IN OLDER PEOPLE

In his helpful review of sexual dysfunction in old age, Phanjoo (2000) reminds us that the sexual behaviour of older people is more often the target of jocularity or ridicule than the subject of serious scientific research. Good physical health, the availability of a partner and a regular and stable pattern of sexual activity earlier in life predict the maintenance of a healthy sex life in old age. Sexual activity and interest declines with age, although approximately one-third of those over 65 years continue to be sexually active (Dello Buono et al 1998). Older men report more interest in sex than women, although around half are moderately or completely impotent (Feldman et al 1994). Physiological changes, drugs and illness, particularly cardiovascular disease, diabetes, arthritis and prostatic surgery can make intercourse more difficult, and even though these may be temporary problems for one or other partner, reinstituting sexual relations after a break can be a major problem. Sildenafil is effective in both non-organic and organic erectile failure, but it is contraindicated in those taking nitrates.

Some dementia sufferers begin to make sexual demands on their partners after years of lack of interest, or show disinhibited sexual interest in other adults or children (Haddad & Benbow 1993a, 1993b). Indiscriminate sexual behaviour by a resident in a care home or ward can cause considerable distress among staff and relatives.

Despite the prevalence of sexual problems in older people they rarely come to attention. Out of a total of 3340 people seen by Phanjoo in his sexual problems clinic in Edinburgh, only 54 were over the age of 65 and all of them were male. Doctors and others may have to overcome a 'countertransference' difficulty in addressing sexual problems in people who could be their parents or grandparents. This may interfere with questioning and therapy, especially where subjects such as extramarital relationships, cross-generation relationships or homosexuality are concerned.

PERSONALITY

Normal changes of old age

In the past, social gerontology has been divided between those who believed that it was normal for older people to *disengage* from social life and activities and become more introspective, a process sometimes seen as a preparation for death, and those who stressed the benefits of continued *engagement* in physical and mental activity. Both theories have been replaced by an emphasis on *continuity*, that is, that ageing individuals usually retain the attitudes, interests and styles of relating which have made up their personality throughout life. However, whether for biological, psychological or social reasons, it is commonly found that cautiousness, introversion and obsessionality do tend to increase with age, but there is great interpersonal variation. Those who had these characteristics as lifelong traits may adjust to old age relatively easily.

People who had disordered personalities in younger years rarely come to psychiatric attention, except as residents in homes and hostels, where their egocentricity, impulsiveness or lack of concern for the consequences of their actions make them less than ideal residents. 'Mellowing' is said to occur in some with antisocial personality disorder in later life, although there may also be attrition due to excess mortality. Long-term follow-up studies of antisocial personality disorder to late life and borderline personality disorder to middle age suggest improvement occurs, although data concerning the late-life course of borderline personality disorder is lacking (Agronin & Maletta 2000). Certainly, some explanation, as yet unforthcoming, is required to account for the lack of such traits in older patients when they are relatively prevalent in younger age groups. There is the concern that these problems may become more evident in tomorrow's elderly population. Those with lesser degrees of personality disorder are only likely to see psychiatrists if they suffer another psychiatric disorder or in response to adverse life events.

During the decades of old age, many planned or unplanned changes occur in family and other relationships, social circumstances and housing. It is unlikely that all will be entirely consonant with the individual's personality characteristics. At a time when change is becoming more difficult to cope with, major problems can arise. The independent-minded individual who develops parkinsonism or a stroke where outside help becomes essential may be a very 'bad' patient, resenting the dependent position, reacting violently against any hints of infantilisation and so responding poorly to attempts at rehabilitation. She may present to the liaison psychiatrist as depressed, but the depression hides an underlying resentment of her predicament.

Personality disorder and illness

Personality disorders are generally found in around 5–10% of older people in epidemiological studies (Abrams 1996). Some elderly people present with an exaggeration of previous personality traits, even to the point of caricature. It is frequently assumed that this is a part of the normal ageing process, but it may be a manifestation of psychiatric illness, including depressive illness, hypomania or paranoid psychosis; or of organic (especially frontal lobe) disorder, other brain damage, or early dementia without obvious global impairment. Personality disorder is lifelong by definition, and therefore personality *change* or *exaggeration* in old age demands an explanation. A careful history is essential, concentrating particularly on lifelong traits of personality, the time sequence of changes, their relationship to important life events and other possible symptoms of illness. Neuroimaging is appropriate in cases of apparent personality change where organic disorder is a possibility.

'Senile squalor'

Clark et al (1975) and Macmillan & Shaw (1966) described elderly people who seemed to become by choice reclusive and eccentric in old age, and could end up living in squalor. Many seemed oblivious of the conditions they were living in and were very resistant to help. Many of Clark's group were physically ill and half of them died after admission to hospital. In Macmillan & Shaw's group there was a preponderance of psychiatrically ill people. A variety of names have been used to describe these patients, such as senile squalor syndrome and Diogenes syndrome. A related, probably obsessive problem of compulsive collecting, which can also lead to squalor, is called *syllogomania*. It is likely that elderly people may live in squalor for very varied reasons, including unrecognised physical illness, frontal lobe dysfunction due to early dementia or other organic disorder (Orrell et al 1989), other psychiatric illness, alcohol or drug misuse and lifelong eccentricity of personality. Halliday et al (2000) criticise earlier studies for relying on a skewed group of hospital patients. In their community sample of people living in squalor, over half were younger than 65, with males of lower socio-economic class predominating. They found high rates of mental illness in younger

people, whereas those that were older were more likely to have significant physical problems rather than mental illness. They emphasised that squalor should be seen as a proxy of a range of physical and mental disorders rather than a rare syndrome due to reclusiveness or an eccentric personality.

OLDER PEOPLE WITH LEARNING DISABILITY

A growing number of people with learning disability are entering old age. Cooper (1997) found 69% of those over the age of 65 with learning disability had a coexistent mental illness, predominantly mood disorders and dementia. Although neuropathological changes of AD in those with Down syndrome are almost universal by the age of 40, not all have neuropsychological evidence of dementia. Other factors, such as *ApoE* status may be important in this regard. Holland et al (1998) found prevalence rates of AD increased from 3.4% to 10.3% to 40% in the 30–39, 40–49 and 50–59 year age groups. The expansion of community care for people with learning disability means that most will be living at home, perhaps with very elderly relatives, or in supported accommodation. The difficult decisions about who should take responsibility for this small but growing and important group need further debate.

LEGAL CONSIDERATIONS

The elderly mentally disordered offender

Accurate statistics concerning the number of elderly offenders are hard to come by, as often their crimes may go unreported or undetected, and if they do attract attention, the police and the courts can be unreasonably lenient, due either to an ageist belief that older people are inevitably less responsible for their actions or to a protective paternalism. Courts may feel that harrowing trials are not appropriate for relatively frail elderly people, and cautioning by the police is relatively common. An elderly person fits uncomfortably into a criminal justice system geared to managing young offenders. This set of attitudes can act against elderly people. It removes their right to answer accusations made against them, and may brand them as sick or incapable when they are in fact perfectly well and responsible for their actions. It also leaves the victims of crime with no redress.

Although rates of offending among older people remain very low, both the absolute numbers of convictions in older people and the rates relative to younger people are increasing: 0.7% of convictions in England and Wales in 1993 were in the over-59s; by 1998 the number had risen to 1.2% (Fazel & Jacoby 2000). The numbers of male prisoners aged 60 years and over more than doubled to 1.7% in the period from 1983 to 1998. Older offenders have higher rates of dementia and affective psychosis, and lower rates of schizophrenia and personality disorder than their younger counterparts, although personality disorder is still common in older inmates (Fazel & Grann 2002).

Elderly people who have traffic accidents, shoplift, are violent or make disinhibited sexual advances to others require careful assessment for early dementia and other disorders, though unfortunately they may not be referred for reports. The same is true of older people who are putting themselves at risk without necessarily committing any crime. Incautious drivers, wanderers, people who make repeated complaints about their neighbours can all come to the attention of police, but no further action is taken.

The same ageist and paternalistic attitudes that are shown to the elderly criminal can infect the legal system when the older person is the victim of crime. This can relate to violence in the home, bogus workmen or accusations of stealing by home helps. The older person's evidence is taken as less valid than that of a younger person, and investigations are not pursued as vigorously as they should be.

Abuse of and by elderly people

Elderly victims of abuse by family or other carers are the subject of increasing concern (Eastman 1984). Carers' groups often discuss angry and violent feelings once the group has become cohesive (Homer & Gilleard 1990). Figures are difficult to interpret, because definitions of abuse vary greatly, and underreporting is likely. At its broadest, abuse can include irritability and verbal abuse, physical neglect, financial exploitation, sexual abuse as well as direct physical assault. Objective evidence of physical abuse is difficult to assess in elderly people prone to falls or those who bruise easily. The problem of whom to believe is particularly thorny when the possible victim is dementing. Vulnerable elderly people can also be victims of abuse by those whose job it is to care for them. Financial exploitation by solicitors, neglectful treatment by doctors, undue restraint in institutions, physical aggression and sexual abuse by nursing or other care staff all need considerably more attention than they get at present.

Psychiatrically ill elderly people may also become verbally abusive, or physically or sexually aggressive towards their informal and formal carers. In close relationships carers may find it difficult to discuss such problems openly. Once again, carers' groups are helpful.

Prevention is the best approach to problems of abuse. It is essential that all agencies involved in the care of vulnerable people work together in partnership to ensure those at risk are identified and protected by appropriate policy, procedure and practice. Such an approach is detailed in the recent commendable guidance *No Secrets* issued by the Department of Health (2000). Better training and support of staff and informal carers is vitally important (Pritchard 1995). The value of regular visits by relatives, senior nursing staff, medical staff and students to long-stay wards and care homes should not be underestimated. Openness in discussing the mixed feelings that caring for elderly people induces should be encouraged. Respite from caring is most important of all.

REFERENCES

Abdul-Hamid W, Holloway F, Silverman M 1998 The needs of elderly chronic mentally ill — unanswered questions. Aging & Mental Health 2:167–170

Abrams R 1996 Personality disorders in the elderly. International Journal of Geriatric Psychiatry 11:759–763

Agronin M E, Maletta G 2000 Personality disorders in late life. Understanding and overcoming the gap in research. American Journal of Geriatric Psychiatry 8:4–18

Aisen P S, Davis K L, Berg J D et al 2000 A randomized controlled trial of prednisone in Alzheimer's disease. Neurology 54:588–593

Aisen P, Schafer K, Grundman M et al 2002 Results of a multicenter trial of rofecoxib and naproxen in Alzheimer's disease. Neurobiology of Aging 23(suppl 1):1569 (abstract)

Alexopoulos G S, Abrams R C, Young R C, Shamonian C A 1988 Cornell scale for depression in dementia. Biological Psychiatry 23:271–284

Alexopoulos G S, Meyers B S, Young R C et al 1993 The course of geriatric depression with 'reversible dementia': a controlled study. American Journal of Psychiatry 150:1693–1699

Alexopoulos G S, Meyers B S, Young R C et al 1997 'Vascular depression' hypothesis. Archives of General Psychiatry 54:915–922

Allen N H P, Gordon S, Hope T, Burns A 1996 Manchester and Oxford universities scale for the psychopathological assessment of dementia (MOUSEPAD). British Journal of Psychiatry 169:293–307

Almeida O P, Howard R J, Levy R et al 1995a Cognitive features of psychotic states arising in late life (late paraphrenia). Psychological Medicine 25:685–698

Almeida O, Mullen R, Graves P et al 1995b White matter abnormalities in the brains of patients with late paraphrenia and the normal community living elderly. Biological Psychiatry 38:86–91

Alzheimer A 1906 Über einen eigenartigen schweren Er Krankungsprozeß der Hirnrinde. Neurologisches Centralblatt 23:1129–1136

Alzheimer Scotland Action on Dementia 2000 Planning signposts for dementia care services. Alzheimer Scotland Action on Dementia, Edinburgh

Ames D 1990 Depression among elderly residents of local-authority residential homes: its nature and the efficacy of intervention. British Journal of Psychiatry 156:667–675

APA 1994 Diagnostic and statistical manual of mental disorders, 4th edn. American Psychiatric Association, Washington, DC

APA 1999 Practice guidelines for the treatment of patients with delirium. American Psychiatric Association, Washington, DC

Aquilina C, Anderson D 2002 Domiciliary clinics, II: A cost minimisation analysis. International Journal of Geriatric Psychiatry 17:945–949

Areán P A, Cook B L 2002 Psychotherapy and combined psychotherapy/pharmacotherapy for late life depression. Biological Psychiatry 52:293–303

Arie T 2002 Health care of the elderly: the Nottingham model. In: Copeland J R, Abou-Saleh M, Blazer D (eds) Principles and practice of geriatric psychiatry. Wiley, Chichester

Arnold S E 2001 Contributions of neuropathology to understanding schizophrenia in late life. Harvard Review of Psychiatry 9:69–76

Arunpongpaisal S, Ahmed I, Aqeel N, Suchat P 2003 Antipsychotic drug treatment for elderly people with late-onset schizophrenia (Cochrane Review). In: The Cochrane Library, Issue 2. Oxford: Update Software

Atkinson R 1994 Late onset problem drinking in older adults. International Journal of Geriatric Psychiatry 9:321–326

Atkinson R M, Turner J A, Tolson R L 1998 Treatment of older adult problem drinkers: lessons learned from the 'Class of '45'. Journal of Mental Health & Aging 4:197–214

Audit Commission 2000 Forget me not – mental health services for older people. Audit Commission, London. Online: http://www.audit-commission.gov.uk

Bahro M, Silber E, Box P, Sunderland T 1995 Giving up driving in Alzheimer's disease: an integrative therapeutic approach. International Journal of Geriatric Psychiatry 10:871–874

Bains J, Birks J S, Dening T R 2003 Antidepressants for treating depression in dementia. In: The Cochrane Library, Issue 2. Oxford: Update Software

Baldwin R C 1996 Treatment resistant depression in the elderly: a review of treatment options. Reviews in Clinical Gerontology 6:343–348

Baldwin R C 2000 Poor prognosis of depression in elderly people: causes and actions. Annals of Medicine 32:252–256

Baldwin R C, O'Brien J 2002 Vascular basis of late-onset depressive disorder. British Journal of Psychiatry 180:157–160

Ballard C, Oyebode F 1995 Psychotic symptoms in patients with dementia. International Journal of Geriatric Psychiatry 10:743–752

Ballard C G, Bannister C, Oyebode F 1996 Depression in dementia sufferers. International Journal of Geriatric Psychiatry 11:507–515

Ballard C, Fossey J, Chithramohan R 2001 Quality of care in private sector and NHS facilities for people with dementia: cross sectional survey. British Medical Journal 323:426–427

Barber R, Panikkar A, McKeith I G 2001 Dementia with Lewy bodies: diagnosis and management. International Journal of Geriatric Psychiatry 16:12–18

Barraclough B 1971 Suicide in the elderly. In: Kay D W K, Walk A (eds) Recent developments in psychogeriatrics. Headly, Ashford, p 87–97

Bartels S J 2002 Quality, costs, and effectiveness of services for older adults with mental disorders: a selective overview of recent advances in geriatric mental health services research. Current Opinion in Psychiatry 15:411–416

Beekman A T F, Copeland J R M, Prince M J 1999 Review of community prevalence of depression in later life. British Journal of Psychiatry 174:307–311

Beekman A T F, Geerlings S W, Deeg D J H 2002 The natural history of late-life depression: a 6-year prospective study in the community. Archives of General Psychiatry 59:605–611

Beeri M S, Werner P, Davidson M, Noy S 2002 The cost of behavioral and psychological symptoms of dementia (BPSD) in community dwelling Alzheimer's disease patients. International Journal of Geriatric Psychiatry. 17:403–408

Bennett N, Jarvis L, Rowlands D et al 1995 Living in Britain. HMSO, London.

Berghmans R I P, ter Meulen R H J 1995 Ethical issues in research with dementia patients. International Journal of Geriatric Psychiatry 10:647–651

Bergmann K 1978 Neurosis and personality disorder in old age. In: Isaacs A D, Post F (eds) Studies in geriatric psychiatry. Wiley, Chichester

Berrios G E 1990 Musical hallucinations: a historical and clinical study. British Journal of Psychiatry 156:188–194

Berrios G E, Brook P 1984 Visual hallucinations and sensory delusions in the elderly. British Journal of Psychiatry 144:652–664

Berrios G E, Brook P 1985 Delusions and the psychopathology of the elderly with dementia. Acta Psychiatrica Scandinavica 72:296–301

Blazer D 1999 EURODEP Consortium and late-life depression. British Journal of Psychiatry 174:284–285

Bleuler M 1943 Die spatschizophrenen krankheitsbilder. Fortschritte der Neurologie Psychiatrie 15:259–290

Blow F C 1999 The effectiveness of an elder-specific brief alcohol intervention for older hazardous drinkers. The Gerontologist 39:569

Blow F C 2000 Treatment of older women with alcohol problems: meeting the challenge for a special population. Alcoholism: Clinical and Experimental Research. 24:1257–1266

BMA 2001 Withholding and withdrawing life-prolonging treatment: guidance for decision making, 2nd edn. British Medical Association, London. Online: www.bmjpg.com/withwith/ww.htm

BMA/The Law Society 1995 Assessment of mental capacity: guidance for doctors and lawyers. British Medical Association, London

Bonner L T, Peskind E R 2002 Pharmacologic treatments of dementia. Medical Clinics of North America 86:657–674

Bouman W P, Pinner G 2002 Use of atypical antipsychotic drugs in old age psychiatry. Advances in Psychiatric Treatment 8:49–58

Bowler J V 2002 The concept of vascular cognitive impairment. Journal of the Neurological Sciences 203–204:11–15

Bowler J V, Hachinski V 2000 Criteria for vascular dementia: replacing dogma with data. Archives of Neurology 57:170–171

Braun C M, Larocque C, Daigneault S, Montour-Proulx I 1999 Mania, pseudomania, depression, and pseudodepression resulting from focal unilateral cortical lesions. Neuropsychiatry, Neuropsychology, & Behavioral Neurology 12:35–51

Bret P, Guyotat J, Chazal J 2002 Is normal pressure hydrocephalus a valid concept in 2002? A reappraisal in five questions and proposal for a new designation of the syndrome as 'chronic hydrocephalus'. Journal of Neurology, Neurosurgery & Psychiatry 73:9–12

Brink T L 1979 Geriatric psychotherapy. Human Sciences Press, New York

Broadhead J, Jacoby R 1990 Mania in old age: a first prospective study. International Journal of Geriatric Psychiatry 5:215–222

Brodaty H, Harris L, Peters K et al 1993 Prognosis of depression in the elderly: a comparison with younger patients. British Journal of Psychiatry 163:589–596

Brodaty H, Sachdev P, Rose N et al 1999 Schizophrenia with onset after age 50 years, I: Phenomenology and risk factors. British Journal of Psychiatry 175:410–415

Brodaty H, Ames D, Snowdon J et al 2003 A randomized placebo-controlled trial of risperidone for the treatment of aggression, agitation, and psychosis of dementia. Journal of Clinical Psychiatry 64:134–143

Brook P, Degun G, Mather M 1975 Reality orientation, a therapy for psychogeriatric patients: a controlled study. British Journal of Psychiatry 127:42–45

Brooke H 1988 Consent to treatment and research. In: Hirsch S R, Harris J (eds) Consent and the incompetent patient. Gaskell/Royal College of Psychiatrists, London

Brookmeyer R, Corroda M M, Curriero F C, Kawas C 2002 Survival following a diagnosis of Alzheimer disease. Archives of Neurology 59:1764–1767

Brotchie J 2003 Caring for someone who has dementia. Age Concern England, London.

Bucht G, Gustafson Y, Sandberg O 1999 Epidemiology of delirium. Dementia and Geriatric Cognitive Disorders 10:315–318

Bullock R 2001 Drug treatment in dementia. Current Opinion in Psychiatry 14:349–353

Burns A, Rabins P 2000 Carer burden in dementia. International Journal of Geriatric Psychiatry 15:9–13

Burns A, Carrick J, Ames D, Levy R 1989 The cerebral cortical appearance in late paraphrenia. International Journal of Geriatric Psychiatry 4:31–34

Burns A, Jacoby R, Levy R 1990a Psychiatric phenomena in Alzheimer's disease, I: Disorders of thought content. British Journal of Psychiatry 157:72–75

Burns A, Jacoby R, Levy R 1990b Psychiatric phenomena in Alzheimer's disease, III: Disorders of mood. British Journal of Psychiatry 157:81–85

Burns A, Brayne C, Folstein M 1998 Mini-Mental State: a practical method for grading the cognitive state of patients for the clinician. M. Folstein, S. Folstein and P. McHugh, Journal of Psychiatric Research (1975) 12:189–198. International Journal of Geriatric Psychiatry 13:285–294

Burns A, Beevor A, Lelliott P et al 1999a Health of the nation outcome scales for elderly people (HoNOS 65+). British Journal of Psychiatry 174:424–427

Burns A, Beevor A, Lelliott P et al 1999b Health of the nation outcome scales for elderly people (HoNOS 65+). Glossary for HoNOS 65+ score sheet. British Journal of Psychiatry 174:435–438

Burns A, Lawlor B, Craig S 1999c Assessment scales in old age psychiatry. Martin Dunitz, London

Butler R N 1963 The life review: an interpretation of reminiscence in the aged. Psychiatry 26:65–76

Campbell S, Stephens S, Ballard C 2001 Dementia with Lewy bodies: clinical features and treatment. Drugs & Aging 18:397–407

Capewell A E, Primrose W R, MacIntyre C 1986 Nursing dependency in registered nursing homes and long term care geriatric wards in Edinburgh. British Medical Journal 291:1719–1721

Carson A J, MacHale S, Allen K et al 2000 Depression after stroke and lesion location: a systematic review. Lancet 356:122–126

Castle D, Howard R 1992 What do we know about the aetiology of late-onset schizophrenia? European Psychiatry 7:99–108

Castle D J, Murray R M 1993 The epidemiology of late-onset schizophrenia. Schizophrenia Bulletin 19:691–700

Castle D J, Abel K, Takei N, Murray R M 1995 Gender differences in schizophrenia: hormonal effect or subtypes? Schizophrenia Bulletin 21:1–12

Cattell H 2000 Suicide in the elderly. Advances in Psychiatric Treatment 6:102–108

Cattell H, Jolley D 1995 One hundred cases of suicide in elderly people. British Journal of Psychiatry 166:451–457

Challis D, Davies B 1986 Case management in community care. Gower, Aldershot

Challis D, Reilly S, Hughes J et al 2002 Policy, organisation and practice of specialist old age psychiatry in England. International Journal of Geriatric Psychiatry 17:1018–1026

Cholerton B, Gleason C E, Baker L D, Asthana S 2002 Estrogen and Alzheimer's disease: the story so far. Drugs & Aging 19:405–427

Christensen H 2001 What cognitive changes can be expected with normal ageing? Australian & New Zealand Journal of Psychiatry 35:768–775

Christenson R, Blazer D 1984 Epidemiology of persecutory ideation in an elderly population in the community. American Journal of Psychiatry 141:1088–1089

Christie A B 1982 Changing patterns in mental illness in the elderly. British Journal of Psychiatry 140:154–159

Christie A B, Train J D 1984 Changes in the pattern of care for the demented. British Journal of Psychiatry 144:9–15

Chui H, Zhang Q 1997 Evaluation of dementia: a systematic study of the usefulness of the American Academy of Neurology's Practice Parameters. Neurology 49:925–935

Chui H C, Mack W, Jackson J E 2000 Clinical criteria for the diagnosis of vascular dementia: a multicenter study of comparability and interrater reliability. Archives of Neurology 57:191–196

Clark A N G, Mankiker G D, Gray I 1975 Diogenes syndrome: a clinical study of gross neglect in old age. Lancet i:366–373

Clifford D B, 2002 AIDS dementia. Medical Clinics of North America 86:537–550

Coen R F, Swanwick G R, O'Boyle C A, Coakley D 1997 Behaviour disturbance and other predictors of carer burden in Alzheimer's disease. International Journal of Geriatric Psychiatry 12:331–336

Cole M G, Primeau F J 1993 Prognosis of delirium in elderly hospital patients. Canadian Medical Association Journal 149:41–46

Conwell Y 2001 Suicide in later life: a review and recommendations for prevention. Suicide and Life-Threatening Behavior 31:32–47

Conwell Y, Duberstein P R, Cox C 1996 Relationships of age and axis I diagnoses in victims of completed suicide: a psychological autopsy study. American Journal of Psychiatry 153:1001–1008

Cooper A F 1976 Deafness and psychiatric illness. British Journal of Psychiatry 129:216–226

Cooper S A 1997 Epidemiology of psychiatric disorders in elderly compared with younger adults with learning disabilities. British Journal of Psychiatry 170:375–380

Copeland J R M, Dewey M E, Griffiths-Jones H M 1986 Computerized psychiatric diagnostic system and case nomenclature for elderly subjects: GMS and AGECAT. Psychological Medicine 16:89–99

Copeland J R M, Abou-Saleh M T, Blazer D G 1994 Principles and practice of geriatric psychiatry. Wiley, Chichester

Copeland J R M, Dewey M E, Scott A et al 1998 Schizophrenia and delusional disorder in older age: community prevalence, incidence, comorbidity and outcome. Schizophrenia Bulletin 24:153–161

Copeland J R, Abou-Saleh M, Blazer D (eds) 2002 Principles and practice of geriatric psychiatry, 2nd edn. Wiley, Chichester

Corder E H, Saunders A M, Strittmatter W J 1993 Gene dose of apolipoprotein E type 4 allele and the risk of Alzheimer's disease in late onset families. Science 261:921–923

Corey-Bloom J, Jernigan T, Archibald S et al 1995 Quantitative magnetic resonance imaging of the brain in late-life schizophrenia. American Journal of Psychiatry 152:447–449

Cosford P, Arnold E 1992 Eating disorders in later life: a review. International Journal of Geriatric Psychiatry 7:491–498

Crook T H, Bartus R T, Ferris S H et al 1986 Age-associated memory impairment: proposed diagnostic criteria and measures of clinical change — Report of a National Institute of Mental Health workgroup. Developmental Neuropsychology 2:261–276

Cummings J L, Mega M, Gray K 1994 The neuropsychiatric inventory: comprehensive assessment of psychopathology in dementia. Neurology 44:2308–2314

Cutter N R, Post R M 1982 Life course of illness in untreated manic-depressive illness. Comprehensive Psychiatry 23:101–115

De Deyn P P, Rabheru K, Rasmussen A et al 1999 A randomized trial of risperidone, placebo, and haloperidol for behavioral symptoms of dementia. Neurology 53:946–955

De la Torre J C 2002 Vascular basis of Alzheimer's pathogenesis. Annals of the New York Academy of Sciences 977:196–215

De Zoysa A S R, Blessed G 1984 The place of the specialist home for the elderly mentally infirm in the care of mentally disturbed old people. Age & Ageing 13:218–223

Dello Buono D, Zaghi P C, Padoani W et al 1998 Archives of Gerontology and Geriatrics 6:155–162.

Denihan A, Kirby M, Bruce I, Cunningham C, Coakley D, Lawlor BA 2000 Three-year prognosis of depression in the community-dwelling elderly. British Journal of Psychiatry 176:453–457

Dening T, Lawton C 1998 The role of carers in evaluating mental health services for the elderly. International Journal of Geriatric Psychiatry 13:863–870

Department of Health/Department of Social Security 1989 Working for patients. HMSO, London

Department of Health 2000 No secrets: guidance on developing and implementing multi-agency policies and procedures to protect vulnerable adults from abuse. Department of Health, London. Online: http://www.doh.gov.uk/scg/nosecrets.htm

Department of Health and Social Security 1972 Services for mental illness related to old age. HMSO, London

Devanand D P, Turret N, Moody B J et al 2000 Personality disorders in elderly patients with dysthymic disorder. American Journal of Geriatric Psychiatry 8:188–195

Donaldson C, Tarrier N, Burns A 1997 The impact of the symptoms of dementia on caregivers. British Journal of Psychiatry 170:62–68

Draper B 1996 Attempted suicide in old age. International Journal of Geriatric Psychiatry 11:577–587

Draper B 2000 The effectiveness of old age psychiatry services. International Journal of Geriatric Psychiatry 15:687–703

Dunkin J J, Anderson-Hanley C 1998 Dementia caregiver burden: a review of the literature and guidelines for assessment and intervention. Neurology 51:53–60

Eagles J M, Gilleard C J 1984 The functions and effectiveness of a day hospital for the demented elderly. Health Bulletin (Edinburgh) 42:87–91

Eastman M 1984 Old age abuse. Age Concern England, London

Eastwood R, Corbin S 1985 Epidemiology of mental disorders in old age. Recent Advances in Psychogeriatrics 1:17–33

Eccles M, Clarke J, Livingstone M et al 1998 North of England evidence based guidelines development project: guideline for the primary care management of dementia. British Medical Journal 317:802–808

Elie M, Cole M G, Primeau F G, Bellavance F 1998 Delirium risk factors in elderly hospitalised patients. Journal of General Internal Medicine 13:204–212

Erikson E 1963 Childhood and society. Triad Granada, London, p 241–242

Fann J R 2000 The epidemiology of delirium: a review of studies and methodological issues. Seminars in Clinical Neuropsychiatry 5:64–76

Fazel S, Grann M 2002 Older criminals: a descriptive study of psychiatrically examined offenders in Sweden. International Journal of Geriatric Psychiatry 17:907–913

Fazel S, Jacoby R 2000 The elderly criminal. International Journal of Geriatric Psychiatry 15:201–202

Feil N 1993 The validation breakthrough: simple techniques for communicating with people with 'Alzheimer's type dementia'. Health Professions Press, Baltimore

Feldman H, Gauthier S, Hecker J et al 2001 A 24-week, randomized, double-blind study of donepezil in moderate to severe Alzheimer's disease. Neurology 57:613–620

Feldman H A, Goldstein I, Hatzichristou D G et al 1994 Impotence and its medical and psychosocial correlates: results of the Massachusetts Male Aging Study. Journal of Urology 151:54–61

Findlay D J, Shamara J, McEwen J et al 1989 Double-blind controlled withdrawal of thioridazine treatment in elderly female inpatients with senile dementia. International Journal of Geriatric Psychiatry 4:115–120

Finkel S I, Burns A (eds) 2000 Behavioural and psychological symptoms in dementia: a clinical and research update. International Psychogeriatrics 12 (suppl 1)

Fischer P, Gatterer G, Marterer A et al 1990 Course characteristics in the differentiation of dementia of the Alzheimer type and multi-infarct dementia. Acta Psychiatrica Scandinavica 81:551–553

Flacker J M, Marcantonio E R 1998 Delirium in the elderly: optimal management. Drugs & Aging 13:119–130

Fleming R W, Bowles J 1994 How, when and why to use the REPDS. University of Western Sydney: MacSearch

Flint A 1994 Epidemiology and comorbidity of anxiety disorders in the elderly. American Journal of Psychiatry 151:640–649

Flint A J, Gagnon N 2002 Effective use of electroconvulsive therapy in late-life depression. Canadian Journal of Psychiatry/Revue Canadienne de Psychiatrie 47:734–741

Flint A J, Rifat S I, Eastwood M R 1991 Late-onset paranoia: distinct from paraphrenia? International Journal of Geriatric Psychiatry 6:103–109

Folstein M F, Folstein S E, McHugh P R 1975 Mini-mental state. Journal of Psychiatric Research 12:189–198

Forsell Y, Henderson A S 1998 Epidemiology of paranoid symptoms in an elderly population. British Journal of Psychiatry 172:429–432

Fox N C, Crum W R, Scahill R I et al 2001 Imaging of onset and progression of Alzheimer's disease with voxel-compression mapping of serial magnetic resonance images. Lancet 358(9277):201–205

Freyne A, Kidd N, Coen R, Lawlor B A 1999 Burden in carers of dementia patients: higher levels in carers of younger sufferers. International Journal of Geriatric Psychiatry 14:784–788

Friedman J I, Harvey P D, McGurk S R et al 2002 Correlates of change in functional status of institutionalized geriatric schizophrenic patients: focus on medical comorbidity. American Journal of Psychiatry 159:1388–1394

Garner J 2002 Psychodynamic work and older adults. Advances in Psychiatric Treatment 8:128–135

Geerlings M I, Schoevers R A, Beekman A T 2000 Depression and risk of cognitive decline and Alzheimer's disease: results of two prospective community-based studies in The Netherlands. British Journal of Psychiatry 176:568–575

Gilhooley M L M 1984 The impact of caregiving on caregivers: factors associated with the psychological wellbeing of people supporting a dementing relative in the community. British Journal of Psychological Medicine 57:35–44

Gilleard C J 1984 Living with dementia: community care of the elderly mentally infirm. Croom Helm, London

Gilleard C J, Belford H, Gilleard E et al 1984a Emotional distress amongst the supporters of the elderly mentally infirm. British Journal of Psychiatry 145:172–177

Gilleard C J, Gilleard E, Whittick J E 1984b Impact of psychogeriatric day hospital care on the patient's family. British Journal of Psychiatry 145:487–492

GMC, 2002a Research: the role and responsibilities of doctors. General Medical Council, London. Online http://www.gmc-uk.org/standards/default.htm

GMC, 2002b Withholding and withdrawing life-prolonging treatments: good practice in decision-making. General Medical Council, London. Online: http://www.gmc-uk.org/standards/default.htm

Godlove Mozley C, Challis D, Sutcliffe C et al 2000 Psychiatric symptomatology in elderly people admitted to nursing and residential homes. Aging & Mental Health 4:136–141

Gold G, Bouras C, Canuto A et al 2002 Clinicopathological validation study of four sets of clinical criteria for vascular dementia. American Journal of Psychiatry 159:82–87

Goldsmith M 1996 Hearing the voice of people with dementia. Kingsley, London

Gorelick P B 1997 Status of risk factors for dementia associated with stroke. Stroke 28:459–463

Greene J G, Timbury G C 1979 A geriatric psychiatry day service: a five year review. Age & Ageing 8:49–53

Grundy E 2002 Demography of the old: implications for recent trends. In: Copeland J R, Abou-Saleh M, Blazer D (eds) Principles and practice of geriatric psychiatry. Wiley, Chichester

Haddad P, Benbow S 1993a Sexual problems associated with dementia, part 1: Problems and their consequences. International Journal of Geriatric Psychiatry 8:547–551

Haddad P, Benbow S 1993b Sexual problems associated with dementia, part 2: Aetiology, assessment and treatment. International Journal of Geriatric Psychiatry 8:631–637

Haffmans P M J, Sival R C, Lucius S A P et al 2001 Bright light therapy and melatonin in motor restless behaviour in dementia: a placebo-controlled study. International Journal of Geriatric Psychiatry 16:106–110

Hakim C A, Hakim R, Hakim S 2001 Normal-pressure hydrocephalus. Neurosurgery Clinics of North America 12:761–773

Halliday G, Banerjee S, Philpot M, Macdonald A 2000 Community study of people who live in squalor. Lancet 355:882–886

Harris M, Jeste D 1988 Late-onset schizophrenia: an overview. Schizophrenia Bulletin 14:39–55

Harvey P D, Howanitz E, Parrella M et al 1998 Symptoms, cognitive functioning, and adaptive skills in geriatric patients with lifelong schizophrenia: a comparison across treatment sites. American Journal of Psychiatry 155:1080–1086

Harvey P D, Parrella M, White L et al 1999 Convergence of cognitive and adaptive decline in late-life schizophrenia. Schizophrenia Research 35:77–84

Hawton K, Fagg J 1990 Deliberate self-poisoning and self-injury in older people. International Journal of Geriatric Psychiatry 5:367–373

Heaton R K, Gladsjo J A, Palmer B W et al 2001 Stability and course of neuropsychological deficits in schizophrenia. Archives of General Psychiatry 58:24–32

HEBS 1996 Coping with dementia: a handbook for carers. Health Education Board for Scotland, Edinburgh

Henderson A S 1986 The epidemiology of Alzheimer's disease. British Medical Bulletin 42:3–10

Henderson A S, Korten A E, Levings C et al 1998 Psychotic symptoms in the elderly: a prospective study in a population sample. International Journal of Geriatric Psychiatry 13:484–492

Hepple J, Quinton C 1997 One hundred cases of attempted suicide in the elderly. British Journal of Psychiatry 171:42–46

Heyman A, Fillenbaum G G, Welsh-Bohmer K A et al 1998 Cerebral infarcts in patients with autopsy-proven Alzheimer's disease: CERAD, part XVIII. Consortium to Establish a Registry for Alzheimer's Disease. Neurology 51:159–162

Hickie I, Scott E, Wilhelm K, Brodaty H 1997 Subcortical hyperintensities on magnetic resonance imaging in patients with severe depression — a longitudinal evaluation. Biological Psychiatry 42:367–374

Hodges J R 1994 Cognitive assessment for clinicians. Oxford University Press, Oxford

Hodkinson H M 1973 Mental impairment in the elderly. Journal of the Royal College of Physicians 7:305–317

Hofman A, Rocca W A, Brayne C et al 1991 The prevalence of dementia in Europe: a collaborative study of 1980–1990 findings. Eurodem Prevalence Research Group. International Journal of Epidemiology 20:736–748

Holden U P, Woods R T 1988 Reality orientation: psychological approaches to the 'confused' elderly. Churchill Livingstone, Edinburgh

Holland A J, Hon J, Huppert F A et al 1998 Population-based study of the prevalence and presentation of dementia in adults with Down's syndrome. British Journal of Psychiatry 172:493–498

Holmes C, Cairns N, Lantos P, Mann A 1999 Validity of current clinical criteria for Alzheimer's disease, vascular dementia and dementia with Lewy bodies. British Journal of Psychiatry 174:45–50

Holmes J, Bentley K, Cameron I 2002 Between two stools: psychiatric services for older people in general hospitals. Report of a UK survey. University of Leeds, Leeds. Online: http://www.leeds.ac.uk/medicine/divisions/psychiatry/lpopreport.pdf

Homer A C, Gilleard C 1990 Abuse of elderly people by their carers. British Medical Journal 30:1359–1362

Hope T, Patel V 1993 The assessment of behavioural phenomena in dementia. In: Burns A (ed) Ageing and dementia: a methodological approach. Edward Arnold, London, p 221–236

Hope T, Tilling K M, Gedling K et al 1994 The structure of wandering in dementia. International Journal of Geriatric Psychiatry 9:149–155

Hoskins G, Marshall M 2002 Expect more: making a place for people with dementia. In: Jacoby R, Oppenheimer C (eds) Psychiatry in the elderly. Oxford University Press, Oxford

House A, Dennis M, Mogridge L et al 1991 Mood disorders in the year after first stroke. British Journal of Psychiatry 158:83–92

Howard R, Castle D, O'Brien J et al 1992 Permeable walls, floors, ceilings and doors. Partition delusions in late paraphrenia. International Journal of Geriatric Psychiatry 7:719–724

Howard R, Almeida O, Levy R 1994a Phenomenology, demography and diagnosis in late paraphrenia. Psychological Medicine 24:397–410

Howard R, Almeida O, Levy R et al 1994b Quantitative magnetic resonance imaging volumetry distinguishes delusional disorder from late onset schizophrenia. British Journal of Psychiatry 165:474–480

Howard R, Dennehey J, Lovestone S et al 1995a Apolipoprotein E genotype and late paraphrenia. International Journal of Geriatric Psychiatry 10:147–150

Howard R, Mellers J, Petty R et al 1995b Magnetic resonance imaging volumetric measurements of the superior temporal gyrus, hippocampus, parahippocampal gyrus, frontal and temporal lobes in late paraphrenia. Psychological Medicine 25:495–503

Howard R J, Graham C, Sham P et al 1997 A controlled family study of late-onset non-affective psychosis (late paraphrenia). British Journal of Psychiatry 170:511–514

Howard R, Rabins P V, Seeman M V et al 2000 Late-onset schizophrenia and very-late-onset schizophrenia-like psychosis: an international consensus. American Journal of Psychiatry 157:172–178

Hughes C P, Berg L, Danziger W L 1982 A new clinical scale for the staging of dementia. British Journal of Psychiatry 140:566–572

Hulette C, Nochlin D, McKeel D et al 1997 Clinical-neuropathologic findings in multi-infarct dementia: a report of six autopsied cases. Neurology 48:668–672

Hymas N, Naguib M, Levy R 1989 Late paraphrenia – a follow-up study. International Journal of Geriatric Psychiatry 4:23–29

Iliffe S, Haines A, Gallivan S et al 1991b Assessment of elderly people in general practice: social circumstances and mental state. British Journal of General Practice 41:9–12

Inouye S K, Charpentier P A 1996 Precipitating factors for delirium in hospitalised elderly persons. Journal of the American Medical Association 275:852–857

Inouye S K, Viscoli C M, Horowitz R I et al 1993 A predictive model for delirium in hospitalised elderly medical patients based on admission characteristics. Annals of Internal Medicine 119:474–481

Itzhaki R F, Lin W R, Shang D et al 1997 Herpes simplex virus type 1 in brain and risk of Alzheimer's disease. Lancet 349:241–244

Jackson G A, Lyons D 1996 Psychiatric clinics in residential homes for the elderly. Psychiatric Bulletin 20(9):516–518

Jacoby R, Lunn D 1993 How long should the elderly take antidepressants? A double-blind placebo-controlled study of continuation/prophylaxis therapy with dothiepin. Old Age Depression Interest Group. British Journal of Psychiatry 162:175–182

Jacoby R, Oppenheimer C (eds) 2002 Psychiatry in the elderly, 3rd edn. Oxford University Press, Oxford

Jacques A, Jackson G A 2000 Understanding dementia, 3rd edn. Churchill Livingstone, Edinburgh

Jarvis B, Figgitt D P 2003 Memantine. Drugs and Aging 20:465–476

Jeste D V, Eastham J H, Lacro J P et al 1996 Management of late-life psychosis. Journal of Clinical Psychiatry 57:39–45

Jeste D V, Symonds L L, Harris M J et al 1997 Nondementia nonpraecox dementia praecox? Late-onset schizophrenia. American Journal of Geriatric Psychiatry 5:302–317

Jeste D V, McAdams L A, Palmer B W et al 1998 Relationship of neuropsychological and MRI measures to age of onset of schizophrenia. Acta Psychiatrica Scandinavica 98:156

Jobst K A, Barnetson L P D, Shepstone B J 1998 Accurate prediction of confirmed Alzheimer's disease and the differential diagnosis of dementia: the use of NINCDS-ADRDA and DSM IIIR criteria, SPECT, X-ray CT and ApoE4 in medial temporal lobe dementias. International Psychogeriatrics 10:271–302

Johnson I 2000 Alcohol problems in old age: a review of recent epidemiological research. International Journal of Geriatric Psychiatry 15:575–581

Jones S J, Turner R J, Grant J E 1987 Assessing patients in their own homes. Bulletin of the Royal College of Psychiatrists 11:117–119

Jorm A F, Jacomb P A 1989 The information questionnaire on cognitive decline in the elderly (IQCODE): socio-demographic correlates, reliability, validity and some norms. Psychological Medicine 19:1015–1022

Jorm A F, Korten A E, Henderson A S 1987 The prevalence of dementia: a quantitative survey of the literature. Acta Psychiatrica Scandinavica 76:465–479

Katz I R, Jeste D V, Mintzer J E et al 1999 Comparison of risperidone and placebo for psychosis and behavioral disturbances associated with dementia: a randomized, double-blind trial. Risperidone Study Group. Journal of Clinical Psychiatry 60:107–115

Kay D W K, Roth M 1961 Environmental and hereditary factors in the schizophrenias of old age (late paraphrenia) and their bearing on the general problem of causation in schizophrenia. Journal of Mental Science 107:649–686

Kay D W K, Beamish P, Roth M 1964 Old age mental disorders in Newcastle upon Tyne. British Journal of Psychiatry 110:146–158

Kay D W K, Bergmann K 1966 Physical disability and mental health. Psychosomatic Research 10:3–12

Keene J M, Hope T 1996 The microstructure of eating in people with dementia who are hyperphagic. International Journal of Geriatric Psychiatry 11:1041–1049

Keith S J, Regier D A, Rae D S 1991 Schizophrenic disorders. In: Robins L N, Reiger D A (eds) Psychiatric disorders in America: the Epidemiologic Catchment Area Study. Free Press, New York, p 33–52

Kertesz A, Munoz D G 2002 Frontotemporal dementia. Medical Clinics of North America 86:501–518

Kessell N, Shepherd M 1962 Neurosis in hospital and general practice. Journal of Mental Science 108:159–166

Kidd C B 1962 Misplacement of the elderly in hospital. British Medical Journal 2:1491–1495

Kitwood T 1997 Dementia reconsidered: the person comes first. Open University Press, Milton Keynes

Knight B R 1996 Psychotherapy of older adults. Sage, Thousand Oaks

Knopman D S, DeKosky S T, Cummings J L et al 2001 Practice parameter: diagnosis of dementia (an evidence-based review). Report of the Quality Standards Subcommittee of the American Academy of Neurology. Neurology 56:1143–1153

Kobeinsson H, Jonsson A 1993 Delirium and dementia in acute medical admissions of elderly patients in Iceland. Acta Psychiatrica Scandinavica 87:123–127

Kokmen E, Whisnant J P, O'Fallon W M et al 1996 Dementia after ischemic stroke: a population-based study in Rochester, Minnesota (1960–1984) Neurology 46:154–159

Korczyn A D 2002 Mixed dementia — the most common cause of dementia. Annals of the New York Academy of Sciences 977:129–134

Kotila M, Numminen H, Waltimo O, Kaste M 1998 Depression after stroke: results of the FINNSTROKE Study. Stroke 29:368–372

Kraepelin E 1919 Dementia praecox and paraphrenia. Barclay R M (transl). Churchill Livingstone, Edinburgh

Kral V 1962 Senescent forgetfulness: benign and malignant. Journal de l'Association Medical Canadien 86:257–260

Kua E H A 1992 Community study of mental disorders in elderly Singaporean Chinese using the GMS-AGECAT package. Australian and New Zealand Journal of Psychiatry 26:502–506

Lanctot K L, Best T S, Mittmann N et al 1998 Efficacy and safety of neuroleptics in behavioral disorders associated with dementia. Journal of Clinical Psychiatry 59:550–561

Lawton M P 2001 The physical environment of the person with Alzheimer's disease. Aging & Mental Health 5 (suppl 1):S56–64

Le Bars P L, Katz M M, Berman N et al 1997 A placebo-controlled, double-blind, randomized trial of an extract of Ginkgo biloba for dementia. Journal of the American Medical Association 278:1327–1332

Levin E, Moriarty J, Gorbach P 1994 Better for the break. HMSO, London

Levy R 1994 Aging-associated cognitive decline. Working Party of the International Psychogeriatric Association in collaboration with the World Health Organization. International Psychogeriatrics 6:63–68

Leverenz J B, McKeith I G 2002 Dementia with Lewy bodies. Medical Clinics of North America 86:519–535

Lewis A J 1970 Paranoia and paranoid: a historical perspective. Psychological Medicine 1:2–12

Li C Y, Sung F C, Wu SC 2002 Risk of cognitive impairment in relation to elevated exposure to electromagnetic fields. Journal of Occupational & Environmental Medicine 44:66–72

Lindesay J 1991 Phobic disorders in the elderly. British Journal of Psychiatry 159:531–541

Lindesay J 2002 Neurotic disorders. In: Jacoby R, Oppenheimer C (eds) Psychiatry in the elderly. Oxford University Press, Oxford

Lindesay J, Briggs K, MacDonald A, Herzberg J 1991 The Domus philosophy: a comparative evaluation of a new approach to residential care for the demented elderly. International Journal of Geriatric Psychiatry 6:727–736

Lindesay J, Marudkar M, van Diepen E, Wilcock G 2002a The second Leicester survey of memory clinics in the British Isles. International Journal of Geriatric Psychiatry 17:41–47

Lindesay J, Rockwood K, Macdonald A 2002b Delirium in old age. Oxford University Press, Oxford

Lindsay J, Laurin D, Verreault R et al 2002 Risk factors for Alzheimer's disease: a prospective analysis from the Canadian Study of Health and Aging. American Journal of Epidemiology 156:445–453

Lobo A, Launer LJ, Fratiglioni L et al 2000 Prevalence of dementia and major subtypes in Europe: a collaborative study of population-based cohorts. Neurologic Diseases in the Elderly Research Group. Neurology 54:S4–S9

Lodge B, McReynolds S 1985 The use of multidisciplinary assessment by the community dementia team. Age Concern, Leicester

Lord Chancellor's Department 1999 Making decisions. The government's proposals for making decisions on behalf of mentally incapacitated adults. (Cm 4465). The Stationery Office, London. Online: http://www.lcd.gov.uk/family/mdecisions/indexfr.htm

Luce A, McKeith I, Swann A et al 2001 How do memory clinics compare with traditional old age psychiatry services? International Journal of Geriatric Psychiatry 16:837–845

Luscombe G, Brodaty H, Freeth S 1998 Younger people with dementia: diagnostic issues, effects on carers and use of services. International Journal of Geriatric Psychiatry 13:323–330

Luttrell S, Watkin V, Livingston G et al 1997 Screening for alcohol misuse in older people. International Journal of Geriatric Psychiatry 12:1151–1154

Lyketsos C G, Steinberg M, Tschanz J T, 2000 Mental and behavioral disturbances in dementia: findings from the Cache County Study on Memory in Aging. American Journal of Psychiatry 157:708–714

Mace N L, Rabins P V 1999 The 36-hour day: a family guide to caring for persons with Alzheimer disease, related dementing illnesses, and memory loss in later life. Johns Hopkins University Press, Baltimore

McGeer P L, Schulzer M, McGeer E G 1996 Arthritis and anti-inflammatory agents as possible protective factors for Alzheimer's disease: a review of 17 epidemiologic studies. Neurology 47:425–432

McGrath A M, Jackson G A 1996 Survey of neuroleptic prescribing in residents of nursing homes in Glasgow. British Medical Journal 312:611–612

McKeith I G 2002 Dementia with Lewy bodies. British Journal of Psychiatry 180:144–147

McKeith I G, Burn D 2000 Spectrum of Parkinson's disease, Parkinson's dementia, and Lewy body dementia. Neurologic Clinics 18:865–883

McKeith I G, Perry R H, Fairbairn A F et al 1992 Operational criteria for senile dementia of Lewy body type (SDLT). Psychological Medicine 22:911–922

McKeith I, Del Ser T, Spano P et al 2000a Efficacy of rivastigmine in dementia with Lewy bodies: a randomised, double-blind, placebo-controlled international study. Lancet 356:2031–2036

McKeith I G, Ballard C G, Perry R H et al 2000b Prospective validation of consensus criteria for the diagnosis of dementia with Lewy bodies. Neurology 54:1050–1058

McKeith I G, Galasko D, Kosaka K et al 1996 Consensus guidelines for the clinical and pathologic diagnosis of dementia with Lewy bodies (DLB): report of the Consortium on DLB international workshop. Neurology 47:1113–1124

McKhann G, Drachman D, Folstein M 1984 Clinical diagnosis of Alzheimer's disease: report of the NINCDS–ADRDA work group under the auspices of Department of Health and Human Services Task Force on Alzheimer's disease. Neurology 34:939–944

McShane R, Keene J, Gedling K et al 1997 Do neuroleptic drugs hasten cognitive decline in dementia? Prospective study with necropsy follow up. British Medical Journal 314:266–270

Macmillan D, Shaw P 1966 Senile breakdown in standards of personal and environmental cleanliness. British Medical Journal 2:1032–1037

Maixner S M, Mellow A M, Tandon R 1999 The efficacy, safety, and tolerability of antipsychotics in the elderly. Journal of Clinical Psychiatry 60 (suppl 8):29–41

Marks I 1981 Space phobia: syndrome or agoraphobic variant? Journal of Neurology, Neurosurgery & Psychiatry 44:387–390

Marriott A, Donaldson C, Tarrier N, Burns A 2000 Effectiveness of cognitive-behavioural family intervention in reducing the burden of care in carers of patients with Alzheimer's disease. British Journal of Psychiatry 176:557–562

Mathuranath P S, Nestor P J, Berrios G E et al 2000 A brief cognitive test battery to differentiate Alzheimer's disease and frontotemporal dementia. Neurology 55:1613–1620

Mayer W 1921 Über paraphrene Psychosen. Zeitschrift für die Gesamte Neurologie und Psychiatrie 71:187–206

Meacher M 1972 Taken for a ride. Longman, London

Menon G J, Rahman I, Menon S J, Dutton G N 2003 Complex visual hallucinations in the visually impaired: the Charles Bonnet Syndrome. Survey of Ophthalmology 48:58–72

Mental Welfare Commission for Scotland 2002 Rights, risks and limits to freedom. Mental Welfare Commission for Scotland, Edinburgh. Online: http://www.mwcscot.org.uk/publications/goodpractice/rights.pdf

Meyers B S, Alexopoulos G 1988 Age of onset and studies of late-life depression. International Journal of Geriatric Psychiatry 3:219–228

Miller B L, Lesser I M, Mena I et al 1992 Regional cerebral bloodflow in late-life-onset psychosis. Neuropsychiatry, Neuropsychology & Behavioural Neurology 5:132–137

Morris C H, Hope R A, Fairburn C G 1989 Eating habits in dementia: a descriptive study. British Journal of Psychiatry 154:801–806

Morris R G, Morris L W, Britton P G 1988 Factors affecting the emotional wellbeing of the caregivers of dementia sufferers: a review. British Journal of Psychiatry 153:147–156

Morris R G, Worsley C, Matthews D 2000 Neuropsychological assessment in older people: old principles and new directions. Advances in Psychiatric Treatment 6:362–372

Mulnard R A, Cotman C W, Kawas C et al 2000 Estrogen replacement therapy for treatment of mild to moderate Alzheimer disease: a randomized controlled trial. Journal of the American Medical Association 283:1007–1015

Munro A 1988 Delusional (paranoid) disorders. Canadian Journal of Psychiatry 33:399–404

Munro A 1991 A plea for paraphrenia. Canadian Journal of Psychiatry 36:667–672

Murdoch P S, Montgomery E A 1992 Revised guidelines for collaboration between physicians in geriatric medicine and psychiatrists of old age. Psychiatric Bulletin 16:583–584

Murphy E 1982 Social origins of depression in old age. British Journal of Psychiatry 141:135–142

Murphy E 1994 The day hospital debate. International Journal of Geriatric Psychiatry 9:517–518

Murphy S 2000 Provision of psychotherapy services for older people. Psychiatric Bulletin 24:181–184

Naarding P, Kremer H P H, Zitman F G 2001 Huntington's disease: a review of the literature on prevalence and treatment of neuropsychiatric phenomena. European Psychiatry 16:439–445

Naguib M 1992 Paranoid disorders. In: Arie T (ed) Recent advances in psychogeriatrics. Churchill Livingstone, Edinburgh

Naguib M, Levy R 1987 Late paraphrenia: neuropsychological impairment and structural brain abnormalities on computed tomography. International Journal of Geriatric Psychiatry 2:83–90

Naguib M, McGuffin P, Levy R et al 1987 Genetic markers in late paraphrenia: a study of HLA antigens. British Journal of Psychiatry 150:124–127

National Institute for Clinical Excellence 2001 Guidance on the use of donepezil, rivastigmine and galantamine for the treatment of Alzheimer's disease. National Institute for Clinical Excellence, London

Nelson J C, Conwell Y, Kim K, Mazure C 1989 Age at onset in late-life delusional depression. American Journal of Psychiatry 146:785–786

Newman S C 1999 The prevalence of depression in Alzheimer's disease and vascular dementia in a population sample. Journal of Affective Disorders 52:169–176

Norman A 1987 Severe dementia: the provision of longstay care. Centre for Policy on Ageing, London

Norris A 1986 Reminiscence. Winslow Press, London

O'Brien J, Barber B 2000 Neuroimaging in dementia and depression. Advances in Psychiatric Treatment 6:109–111

O'Brien J T, Ames D, Schweitzer I 1996 White matter changes in depression and Alzheimer's disease: a review of magnetic resonance imaging studies. International Journal of Geriatric Psychiatry 11:681–694

O'Brien J, Ames D, Chiu E et al 1998 Severe deep white matter lesions and outcome in elderly patients with major depressive disorder: follow up study. British Medical Journal 317:982–984

O'Brien J T, Metcalfe S, Swann A et al 2000 Medial temporal lobe width on CT scanning in Alzheimer's disease: comparison with vascular dementia, depression and dementia with Lewy bodies. Dementia & Geriatric Cognitive Disorders 11:114–118

O'Connor D W, Pollitt P A, Hyde J B et al 1988 Do general practitioners miss dementia in elderly patients? British Medical Journal 297:1107–1110

O'Donnell B F, Drachman D A, Barnes H J et al 1992 Incontinence and troublesome behaviors predict institutionalization in dementia. Journal of Geriatric Psychiatry and Neurology 5:45–52

O'Keefe S T, Lavan J N 1996 Predicting delirium in elderly patients: development and validation of a risk stratification model. Age & Ageing 25:317–321

O'Keefe S T, Lavan J N 1999 Clinical significance of delirium subtypes in older people. Age & Ageing 28:115–119

O'Neill D 2002 Driving and psychiatric illness in later life. In: Jacoby R, Oppenheimer C (eds) Psychiatry in the elderly. Oxford University Press, Oxford

Office for National Statistics 2003 Annual abstract of statistics. The Stationery Office, London

Orgogozo J M, Rigaud A S, Stoffler A et al 2002 Efficacy and safety of memantine in patients with mild to moderate vascular dementia: a randomized, placebo-controlled trial. Stroke 33:1834–1839

Orrell M, Katona C 1998 Do consultant home visits have a future in old age psychiatry? International Journal of Geriatric Psychiatry 13:355–357

Orrell M, Sahakian B J, Bergmann K 1989 Self-neglect and frontal lobe dysfunction. British Journal of Psychiatry 155:101–105

Oslin D, Atkinson R M, Smith D M, Hendrie H 1998 Alcohol related dementia: proposed clinical criteria. International Journal of Geriatric Psychiatry 13:203–212

Palmer B W, Heaton S C, Jeste D V 1999 Older patients with schizophrenia: challenges in the coming decades. Psychiatric Services 50:1178–1183

Parkes C M 1964 The effects of bereavement on physical and mental health: a study of the case records of widows. British Medical Journal 2:274–279

Pastor P, Tolosa E 2002 Progressive supranuclear palsy: clinical and genetic aspects. Current Opinion in Neurology 4:429–437

Patel N, Mirza N R, Lindblad P, Samaoli O 1998 Dementia and minority ethnic older persons. Managing care in the UK, Denmark and France. Russell House, Lyme Regis

Patel V, Hope T 1993 Aggressive behaviour in elderly people with dementia: a review. International Journal of Geriatric Psychiatry 8:457–472

Paterniti S, Verdier-Taillefer M-H, Dufouil C, Alperovitch A 2002 Depressive symptoms and cognitive decline in elderly people: longitudinal study. British Journal of Psychiatry 181:406–410

Pattie A H, Gilleard C J 1976 The Clifton assessment schedule: further validation of a psychiatric assessment schedule. British Journal of Psychiatry 129:68–72

Pattie A H, Gilleard C J 1979 Manual of the Clifton assessment procedures for the elderly (CAPE). Hodder & Stoughton, Sevenoaks

Paulsen J S, Ready R E, Stout J C et al 2000 Neurobehaviors and psychotic symptoms in Alzheimer's disease. Journal of the International Neuropsychological Society 6:815–820

Pearlson G D, Tune L E, Wong D F et al 1993 Quantitative D2 dopamine receptor PET and structural MRI changes in late-onset schizophrenia. Schizophrenia Bulletin 19:783–795

Petersen R C, Stevens J C, Ganguli M et al 2001a Practice parameter: early detection of dementia: mild cognitive impairment (an evidence-based review). Report of the Quality Standards Subcommittee of the American Academy of Neurology. Neurology 56:1133–1142

Petersen R C, Doody R, Kurz A et al 2001b Current concepts in mild cognitive impairment. Archives of Neurology 58:1985–1992

Petrovic M, Vandierendonck A, Mariman A et al 2002 Personality traits and socio-epidemiological status of hospitalised elderly benzodiazepine users. International Journal of Geriatric Psychiatry 17:733–738

Phanjoo A L 2000 Sexual dysfunction in old age. Advances in Psychiatric Treatment 6:270–277

Pichot P 1982 The diagnosis and classification of mental disorders in French speaking countries: background, current views and comparison with other nomenclatures. Psychological Medicine 12:475–492

Pitt B, Silver C P 1980 The combined approach to geriatrics and psychiatry: evaluation of a joint unit in a teaching hospital district. Age & Ageing 9:33–37

Plassman B L, Havlik R J, Steffens D C et al 2000 Documented head injury in early adulthood and risk of Alzheimer's disease and other dementias. Neurology 55:1158–1166

Pohjasvaara T, Leppavuori A, Siira I et al 1998 Frequency and clinical determinants of poststroke depression. Stroke 29:2311–2317

Porsteinsson A P, Tariot P N, Erb R et al 2001 Placebo-controlled study of divalproex sodium for agitation in dementia. American Journal of Geriatric Psychiatry 9:58–66

Post F 1966 Persistent persecutory states of the elderly. Pergamon, Oxford

Post F 1971 Schizo-affective symptomatology in late life. British Journal of Psychiatry 118:437–445

Post S G, Whitehouse P J, Binstock R H et al 1997 The clinical introduction of genetic testing for Alzheimer disease: an ethical perspective. Journal of the American Medical Association 277:832–836

Prager S, Jeste D V 1993 Sensory impairment in late-life schizophrenia. Schizophrenia Bulletin 19:755–772

Prince M J, Harwood R H, Blizard R A et al 1997a Impairment, disability and handicap as risk factors for depression in old age. The Gospel Oak Project V. Psychological Medicine 27:311–321

Prince M J, Harwood R H, Blizard R A et al 1997b Social support deficits, loneliness and life events as risk factors for depression in old age. The Gospel Oak Project VI. Psychological Medicine 27:323–332

Prince M J, Beekman A T, Deeg D J et al 1999 Depression symptoms in late life assessed using the EURO-D scale. Effect of age, gender and marital status in 14 European centres. British Journal of Psychiatry 174:339–345

Pritchard J 1995 The abuse of older people. Kingsley, London

Proctor R, Martin C, Hewison J 2002 When a little knowledge is a dangerous thing . . .: a study of carers' knowledge about dementia, preferred coping style and psychological distress. International Journal of Geriatric Psychiatry 17:1133–1139

Quality Standards Subcommittee of the American Academy of Neurology 1994 Practice parameters for diagnosis and evaluation of dementia (summary statement). Neurology 44:2203–2206

Rabins P V 1986 Establishing Alzheimer's disease units in nursing homes: pros and cons. Hospital & Community Psychiatry 37:120–121

Rabins P, Folstein M 1982 Dementia and delirium: diagnostic criteria and fatality rates. British Journal of Psychiatry 140:149–153

Rajput A, Rajput A H 2001 Progressive supranuclear palsy: clinical features, pathophysiology and management. Drugs & Aging 18:913–925

Rao R 2000 Cerebrovascular disease and late life depression: an age old association revisited. International Journal of Geriatric Psychiatry 15:419–433

Reisberg B, Ferris S H, de Leon M J, Crook T 1982 The global deterioration scale for assessment of primary degenerative dementia. American Journal of Psychiatry 139:1136–1139

Reisberg B, Doody R, Stoffler A et al 2003 Memantine in moderate-to-severe Alzheimer's disease. New England Journal of Medicine 348:1333–1341

Richardson C A, Gilleard C, Lieberman S, Peeler R 1994 Working with older adults and their families: a review. Journal of Family Therapy 16:225–240

Ritchie K, Kildea D 1995 Is senile dementia "age-related" or "ageing-related"? — evidence from meta-analysis of dementia prevalence in the oldest old. Lancet 346:931–934

Robinson R A 1975 The assessment centre. In: Howells G (ed) Modern perspectives in the psychiatry of old age. Churchill Livingstone, Edinburgh

Rockwood K 2002 Vascular cognitive impairment and vascular dementia. Journal of the Neurological Sciences 203–204:23–27

Rodriguez-Ferrera S, Vassilas C A 1998 Older people with schizophrenia: providing services to a neglected group. British Medical Journal 317:293–294

Rogers J, Kirby L C, Hempelman S R et al 1993 Clinical trial of indomethacin in Alzheimer's disease. Neurology 43:1609–1611

Rolleston M, Ball C 1994 Evaluating the effects of brief day hospital closure. International Journal of Geriatric Psychiatry 9:51–53

Román G C 2002 Vascular dementia revisited: diagnosis, pathogenesis, treatment, and prevention. Medical Clinics of North America 86:477–499

Román G C, Tatemichi T K, Erkinjuntti T et al 1993 Vascular dementia: diagnostic criteria for research studies. Neurology 43:250–260

Ronald and Nancy Reagan Research Institute of the Alzheimer's Association and the National Institute on Aging Working Group 1998 Consensus report of the Working Group on: 'Molecular and Biochemical Markers of Alzheimer's Disease'. Neurobiology of Aging 19:109–116

Rondeau V 2002 A review of epidemiologic studies on aluminum and silica in relation to Alzheimer's disease and associated disorders. Reviews on Environmental Health 17:107–121

Rosen W G, Mohs R C, Davis K L 1984 A new rating scale for Alzheimer's disease. American Journal of Psychiatry 141:1356–1364

Rosenvinge H P, Woolford J E, Martin A 1994 Evaluation of extension of a psychogeriatric day hospital to open on Saturdays. International Journal of Geriatric Psychiatry 9:764–765

Rosin A J, Glatt M M 1971 Alcohol excess in the elderly. Quarterly Journal of Studies on Alcohol 32:53–59

Rossler W, Salize H J, Cucchiaro G et al 1999 Does the place of treatment influence the quality of life of schizophrenics? Acta Psychiatrica Scandinavica 100:142–148

Roth M 1955 The natural history of mental disorder in old age. Journal of Mental Science 101:281–301

Roth M 1986 The association of clinical and neurobiological findings and its bearing on the classification and aetiology of Alzheimer's disease. British Medical Bulletin 42:42–50

Roth M, Morrisey J 1952 Problems in the diagnosis and classification of mental disorders in old age. Journal of Mental Science 98:66–80

Roth M, Tym E, Mountjoy C Q 1986 CAMDEX: a standardised instrument for the diagnosis of mental disorders in the elderly with special reference to early detection of dementia. British Journal of Psychiatry 149:698–709

Royal College of Physicians of London and Royal College of Psychiatrists 1989 Care of elderly people with mental illness. Royal College of Physicians, London

Royal College of Psychiatrists 2000 Services for younger people with Alzheimer's disease and other dementias. Council Report CR 77. Royal College of Psychiatrists, London

Royal College of Psychiatrists 2002 Caring for people who enter old age with enduring or relapsing mental illness ('graduates'). Council Report 110. Royal College of Psychiatrists, London

Royal Commission on Long Term Care 1999 With respect to old age: long term care — rights and responsibilities. The Stationery Office, London. Online: http://www.royal-commission-elderly.gov.uk

Sachdev P, Brodaty H, Rose N, Haindl W 1997 Regional cerebral blood flow in late-onset schizophrenia: a SPECT study using 99mTc-HMPAO. Schizophrenia Research 27:105–117

Salzman C, Wong E, Wright B C 2002 Drug and ECT treatment of depression in the elderly, 1996–2001: a literature review. Biological Psychiatry 52(3):265–284

Samuel W, Caligiuri M, Galasko D et al 2000 Better cognitive and psychopathologic response to donepezil in patients prospectively diagnosed as dementia with Lewy bodies: a preliminary study. International Journal of Geriatric Psychiatry 15:794–802

Sano M, Ernesto C, Thomas R G et al 1997 A controlled trial of selegiline, alpha-tocopherol, or both as treatment for Alzheimer's disease. The Alzheimer's Disease Cooperative Study. New England Journal of Medicine 336:1216–1222

Saunders P, Copeland J, Dewey M et al 1993 The prevalence of dementia, depression and neurosis in later life: the Liverpool MRC-ALPHA study. International Journal of Epidemiology 22:838–847

Saunders P A, Copeland J R M, Dewey M E 1989 Alcohol use and abuse in the elderly: findings from the Liverpool longitudinal study of continuing health in the community. International Journal of Geriatric Psychiatry 4:103–108

Saxton J, McGonigle-Gibson K, Swihart A et al 1990 Assessment of severely impaired patients: description and validation of a new neuropsychological test battery. Psychological Assessment 2:298–303

Scharf S, Mander A, Ugoni A et al 1999 A double-blind, placebo-controlled trial of diclofenac/misoprostol in Alzheimer's disease. Neurology 53:197–201

Schenk D, Barbour R, Dunn W et al 1999 Immunization with amyloid-beta attenuates Alzheimer disease-like pathology in the PDAPP mouse. Nature 400:173–177

Schneider L S, Pollock V E, Lyness S A 1990 A meta-analysis of controlled trials of neuroleptic treatment in dementia. Journal of the American Geriatrics Society 38:553–563

Schor J D, Levkoff S E, Lipsitz L A et al 1992 Risk factors for delirium in hospitalised elderly. Journal of the American Medical Association 1992:827–831

Schwartz T L, Masand P S 2002 The role of atypical antipsychotics in the treatment of delirium. Psychosomatics 43:171–174

Scott J, Fairbairn A, Woodhouse K 1988 Referrals to a psychogeriatric consultation–liaison service. International Journal of Geriatric Psychiatry 3:131–135

Scottish Executive 2002 Adding life to years. Report of the expert group for the healthcare of older people. Scottish Executive, Edinburgh. Online: http://www.scotland.gov.uk/publications/recent.aspx

Scottish Home and Health Department 1979 Scottish health authorities' priorities for the eighties. HMSO, Edinburgh

Scottish Home and Health Department 1989 Scottish health authorities' review of priorities for the eighties and nineties. HMSO, Edinburgh

Seeman M 1982 Gender differences in schizophrenia. Canadian Journal of Psychiatry 27:107–111

Serfaty M, Kennell-Webb S, Warner J et al 2002 Double blind randomised placebo controlled trial of low dose melatonin for sleep disorders in dementia. International Journal of Geriatric Psychiatry 17:1120–1127

Sharma V K, Copeland J R M, Dewey M E et al 1998 Outcome of the depressed elderly living in the community in Liverpool: a 5-year follow-up. Psychological Medicine 28:1329–1337

Shulman K, Post F 1980 Bipolar affective disorder in old age. British Journal of Psychiatry 136:26–32

Shulman K I, Shedletsky R, Silver I L 1986 The challenge of time: clock drawing and cognitive function in the elderly. International Journal of Geriatric Psychiatry 1:135–140

Shulman K I, Tohen M, Satlin A et al 1992 Mania compared with unipolar depression in old age. American Journal of Psychiatry 149:341–345

Simpson S, Baldwin R C, Jackson A, Burns A S 1998 Is subcortical disease associated with a poor response to antidepressants? Neurological, neuropsychological and neuroradiological findings in late-life depression. Psychological Medicine 28:1015–1026

Snowden J S, Neary D, Mann D M A 2002 Frontotemporal dementia. British Journal of Psychiatry 180:140–143

Snowdon D A, Kemper S J, Mortimer J A et al 1996 Linguistic ability in early life and cognitive function and Alzheimer's disease in late life. Findings from the Nun Study. Journal of the American Medical Association 275:528–532

Snowdon D A, Greiner L H, Mortimer J A et al 1997 Brain infarction and the clinical expression of Alzheimer disease. The Nun Study. Journal of the American Medical Association 277:813–817

Sobel E, Dunn M, Davanipour Z et al 1996 Elevated risk of Alzheimer's disease among workers with likely electromagnetic field exposure. Neurology 47:1477–1481

Spillantini M G, Goedert M 2000 The alpha-synucleinopathies: Parkinson's disease, dementia with Lewy bodies, and multiple system atrophy. Annals of the New York Academy of Sciences 920:16–27

Stewart R 1998 Cardiovascular factors in Alzheimer's disease. Journal of Neurology, Neurosurgery & Psychiatry 65:143–147

Stewart R 2002 Vascular dementia: a diagnosis running out of time. British Journal of Psychiatry 180:152–156

Stewart W F, Kawas C, Corrada M, Metter E J 1997 Risk of Alzheimer's disease and duration of NSAID use. Neurology 48:626–632

Stokes G 1986 Screaming and shouting. Winslow Press, London

Stokes G 1987 Aggression. Winslow Press, London

Stokes G, Goudie F 1990 Working with dementia. Winslow Press, London

Stone K 1989 Mania in the elderly. British Journal of Psychiatry 155:220–224

Street J S, Clark W S, Gannon K S et al 2000 Olanzapine treatment of psychotic and behavioral symptoms in patients with Alzheimer disease in nursing care facilities: a double-blind, randomized, placebo-controlled trial. The HGEU Study Group. Archives of General Psychiatry 57:968–976

Strittmatter W J, Saunders A M, Schmechel D et al 1993 Apolipoprotein E: high-avidity binding to β-amyloid and increased frequency of type 4 allele in late-onset familial Alzheimer's disease. Proceedings of the National Academy of Sciences of the USA 90:1977–1981

Sullivan K, O'Conor F 2001 Should a diagnosis of Alzheimer's disease be disclosed? Aging & Mental Health 5:340–348

Sunderland T, Alterman I, Yount D 1988 A new scale for the assessment of depressed mood in demented patients. American Journal of Psychiatry 145:955–959

Swanwick G R J, Lee H, Clare A W, Lawlor B A 1994 Consultation–liaison psychiatry: comparison of two service models for geriatric patients. International Journal of Geriatric Psychiatry 9:495–499

Symonds L L, Olichney J M, Jernigan T L et al 1997 Lack of clinically significant gross structural abnormalities in MRIs of older patients with schizophrenia and related psychoses. Journal of Neuropsychiatry & Clinical Neuroscience 9:251–258

Tang M-X, Jacobs D, Stern Y et al 1996 Effect of oestrogen during menopause on risk and age at onset of Alzheimer's disease. Lancet 348:429–432

Tariot P N, Erb R, Podgorski C A et al 1998 Efficacy and tolerability of carbamazepine for agitation and aggression in dementia. American Journal of Psychiatry 155:54–61

Teri L, Logsdon R G, McCurry S M 2002 Nonpharmacologic treatment of behavioral disturbance in dementia. Medical Clinics of North America 86:641–656

Teunisse R J, Cruysberg J R, Verbeek A, Zitman F G 1995 The Charles–Bonnet syndrome: a large prospecive study in the Netherlands. A study of the prevalence of the Charles–Bonnet syndrome and associated factors in 500 patients attending the University Department of Ophthalmology at Nijmegen. British Journal of Psychiatry 166:254–257

Thornton S, Brotchie J 1987 Reminiscence: a critical review of the empirical literature. British Journal of Clinical Psychology 26:93–112

Townsend B A, Petrella J R, Doraiswamy P M 2002 The role of neuroimaging in geriatric psychiatry. Current Opinion in Psychiatry 15:427–432

Treloar A, Macdonald A J 1997 Outcome of delirium diagnosed by DSM-III-R, ICD-10 and CAMDEX and derivation of the reversible cognitive dysfunction scale among acute geriatric inpatients. International Journal of Geriatric Psychiatry 12:609–613

Trieman N, Wills W, Leff J 1996 TAPS Project 28: does reprovision benefit elderly long-stay mental patients? Schizophrenia Research 21:199–208

Tune L, Carr S, Hoag E, Cooper T 1992 Anticholinergic effects of drugs commonly prescribed for the elderly: potential means for addressing risk of delirium. American Journal of Psychiatry 149:1393–1394

Valcour V G, Masaki K H, Curb J D, Blanchette P L 2000 The detection of dementia in the primary care setting. Archives of Internal Medicine 160:2964–2968

Van der Wurff F B, Stek M L, Hoogendijk W L, Beekman A T F 2003 Electroconvulsive therapy for the depressed elderly (Cochrane Review). In: The Cochrane Library, Issue 2. Oxford: Update Software

Van Dongen M C J M, Van Rossum E, Kessels A G H et al 2000 The efficacy of ginkgo for elderly people with dementia and age-associated memory impairment: new results of a randomized clinical trial. Journal of the American Geriatrics Society 48:1183–1194

Van Duijn C M, Clayton D, Chandra V et al 1991 Familial aggregation of Alzheimer's disease and related disorders: a collaborative re-analysis of case-control studies. EURODEM Risk Factors Research Group. International Journal of Epidemiology 20 (suppl 2):S13–20

Van Ojen R, Hooijer C, Jonker C et al 1995 Late-life depressive disorder in the community, early onset and the decrease of vulnerability with increasing age. Journal of Affective Disorders 33:159–166

Vaughan C J 2003 Prevention of stroke and dementia with statins: effects beyond lipid lowering. American Journal of Cardiology 91:23B–29B

Velligan D I, Mahurin R K, Diamond P L et al 1997 The functional significance of symptomatology and cognitive function in schizophrenia. Schizophrenia Research 25:21–31

Volicer L, Hurley A C 1997 Physical status and complications in patients with Alzheimer disease: implications for outcome studies. Alzheimer Disease and Associated Disorders 11(suppl 6):60–65

Wade D T, Collin C 1988 The Barthel ADL index: a standard measure of physical disability. International Disability Studies 10:64–67

Wahlbeck K, Cheine M, Essali A, Adams C 1999 Evidence of clozapine's effectiveness in schizophrenia: a systematic review and meta-analysis of randomized trials. American Journal of Psychiatry 15:990–999

Wahlund L A, Bjorlin G A 1999 Delirium in clinical practice: experience from a specialized delirium ward. Dementia & Geriatric Cognitive Disorders 10:389–392

Walker D A, Clarke M 2001 Cognitive behavioural psychotherapy: a comparison between younger and older adults in two inner city mental health teams. Aging and Mental Health 5:197–199

Ward R 1999 Waiting to be heard — dementia and the gay community. Journal of Dementia Care 8:24–25

Ware G J G, Fairburn C G, Hope R A 1990 A community-based study of aggressive behaviour in dementia. International Journal of Geriatric Psychiatry 5:337–342

Weiner M F, Koss E, Wild K V et al 1996 Measures of psychiatric symptoms in Alzheimer patients: a review. Alzheimer Disease and Associated Disorders 10:20–30

Wells C E 1979 Pseudodementia. American Journal of Psychiatry 136:895–900

Wengel S P, Roccaforte W H, Burke W J 1998 Donepezil improves symptoms of delirium in dementia: implications for future research. Journal of Geriatric Psychiatry & Neurology 11:159–161

Wesnes K A, McKeith I G, Ferrara R 2002 Effects of rivastigmine on cognitive function in dementia with lewy bodies: a randomised placebo-controlled international study using the cognitive drug research computerised assessment system. Dementia & Geriatric Cognitive Disorders 13:183–192

Whalley L J 2002 Brain ageing and dementia: what makes the difference? British Journal of Psychiatry 181:369–371

WHO 1992 The ICD-10 classification of mental and behavioural disorders. World Health Organization, Geneva

WHO 1998 Population ageing — a public health challenge. World Health Organization factsheet. Online. http://www.who.int/health_topics/ageing/en/

Wilcock G, Mobius H J, Stoffler A 2002 A double-blind, placebo-controlled multicentre study of memantine in mild to moderate vascular dementia. International Clinical Psychopharmacology 17:297–305

Wilkin D, Hughes B, Jolley D 1985 Quality of care in institutions. In: Arie T (ed) Recent advances in psychogeriatrics. Churchill Livingstone, Edinburgh

Wilkinson H 2001 The perspectives of people with dementia. Jessica Kingsley, London

Williams P S, Rands G, Orrel M, Spector A 2003 Aspirin for vascular dementia. The Cochrane Library, Issue 2. Oxford: Update Software.

Wilson B A, Moffat N 1992 Clinical management of memory problems. Chapman & Hall, London

Wilson K, Mottram P, Sivanranthan A, Nightingale A 2003 Antidepressants versus placebo for the depressed elderly (Cochrane Review). In: The Cochrane Library, Issue 2. Oxford: Update Software

Wong D F, Wagner H N, Dannals R F et al 1984 Effects of age on dopamine and serotonin receptors measured by positron tomography in the living human brain. Science 226:1393–1396

Woods R T 1999 Psychological assessment of older people. In: Woods R T (ed) Psychological problems of ageing: assessment, treatment and care. Wiley, Chichester.

Yaffe K, Sawaya G, Lieberburg I, Grady D 1998 Estrogen therapy in postmenopausal women. Journal of the American Medical Association 279:688–695

Yaffe K, Blackwell T, Gore R et al 1999 Depressive symptoms and cognitive decline in nondemented elderly women: a prospective study. Archives of General Psychiatry 56:425–430

Yesavage J A, Brink T L, Rose T L 1983 Development and validation of a geriatric depression screening scale: a preliminary report. Journal of Psychiatric Research 17:37–49

Young R, Klerman G 1992 Mania in late life: focus on age at onset. American Journal of Psychiatry 149:867–876

Zis A P, Goodwin F K 1970 Major affective disorder as a recurrent illness. Archives of General Psychiatry 36:835–839

27 | Suicide and deliberate self-harm

George Masterton, Jonathan Cavanagh

SUICIDE

Definition

Suicide is not a diagnosis, rather it is a verdict or category of death which is broadly defined by the following requirements:

- The death was unnatural.
- It was the result of the victim's own actions.
- The victim intended to kill himself.

There can be doubts at all three stages of this process (Farmer 1988), particularly in regard to the motive of a person who cannot be interviewed.

Determination

Countries vary in how suicide is determined, which makes national comparisons of suicide statistics unreliable. In Britain, for instance, the English system relies on the coroner, who investigates every case where violent or unnatural death is suspected. A verdict is reached at a public inquest, where self-inflicted deaths are recorded as a suicide, an accident, or, if undecided, an open verdict is reached. Variation occurs not only among courts, but between a coroner and his deputy (Barraclough 1978) and within the same court and jury with different coroners (O'Donnell & Farmer 1995). In Scotland, there is rarely a formal or public inquiry; the police investigate sudden, suspicious or unnatural deaths, and the procurator fiscal, on behalf of the Crown Office, determines whether a self-inflicted death is categorised as an accident, a suicide, or it is undetermined whether the death was an accident or suicide. The Scottish verdict is based on the evidence indicating that suicide was the most probable and reasonable explanation, whereas the coroner must apply a stricter test, that suicide has been proved by the evidence. It is argued that the higher suicide rates in Scotland compared with England and Wales probably more accurately reflect the true rate (Pounder 1991).

With a few exceptions such as hara-kiri, death by suicide has been disowned and despised by society. It was well into the 20th century before attempting suicide was decriminalised in Britain, and up to two hundred years ago English law stated that individuals who committed suicide and their spouses should 'forfeit all chattels real and personal which he has in his own right', which resulted in penury for the victim's family.

From the 17th century, sympathetic coroners sought to avoid returning verdicts of suicide, and this humanitarian trend has continued to the present day with efforts being made to spare the feelings of relatives from the guilt and anguish that a suicide frequently generates. Since 1975, when Lord Chief Justice Widgery ruled on an appeal against a coroner's verdict of suicide, this has been reinforced by the legal requirement for conclusive proof before suicide is established (Dolman 1994). The consequence is that most research into suicide includes the victims of undetermined deaths, although the characteristics of these individuals lie midway between those of suicides and accidents in many respects (Holding & Barraclough 1978). When psychiatrists have investigated the Crown's decisions, there is a consensus that between a third and a half of probable suicides are categorised as accidental or undetermined deaths (O'Donnell & Farmer 1995).

Epidemiology

Basic statistics

There is a worldwide lack of consistent, common nomenclature and classification procedures for suicide. There is also a lack of operationalised definitions and reliable valid measures of key terms. Neither ICD-10 nor DSM-IV have specific entries for suicidal acts. Suicide is the endpoint of a complex series of biological, psychological/psychiatric and sociological factors and processes. The pathways to suicide can be described under these headings, but ultimately the pathway is unique to the individual. There are known risk factors and increasingly recognised protective factors. These tend to be consistently observed globally albeit with some cultural variations.

Global picture

Across the European region there is a geographical pattern to suicide. The lowest rates are seen in southern European countries, followed by those in the north-west, including the UK and the Netherlands. Higher rates are prevalent in the Scandinavian countries and those countries which form the 'belt' of Europe, i.e. France and Belgium in the west, through Switzerland, Austria and Hungary to Russia in the east. This order has remained virtually unchanged for the last century although the overall per-period averaged rate has increased.

Table 27.1 gives some data on the prevalence of suicide in various countries. While evidence suggests that prevalence continues to vary in accordance with international differences in traditions, customs, religious practice and other influences, it appears that the strength of these differences is decreasing and that there is increasing homogenisation among nations. The situation is, however, more complex than this. In the USA, suicide rates fell by 14% in the decade 1990–1999 (Moscicki 2001); its position in the international league table of suicide fell from 8th to 11th. By contrast, in China, there was a substantial increase in the rate of suicide, especially in young females living in a rural environment. The individual nature of suicide lends itself to ethnic and cultural influence. For example, the observed rise among young rural females in China contrasts with the rise in young males (mostly urban) in Scotland (see below) over the same period.

UK changes

The rising suicide rates observed during the 1970s and 1980s in England and Wales reversed in both genders from 1990 to 1997 (McClure 2000). Further, rates of undetermined deaths also fell in both genders over the same time period. However, the rate among young males remains disproportionately high despite the overall pattern of decreases. The declining suicide rate in England and Wales contrasts with Scotland, where there has been a rise in suicides of more than 70% in the last 30 years, and no recent reversal in trends among young adult men, such that suicide is now the cause of more deaths of young males than road traffic accidents. More than 50% of the 600 suicides per annum in Scotland are now in males under 45 years of age. Importantly, the Scottish rates are twice as high as those in England and Wales. Interestingly, female suicide rates in Scotland have fallen since the 1970s and are currently one-third of the male rate. However, the proportion of females under 45 who kill themselves in Scotland is still twice that of the per-annum rate in England and Wales.

Age and gender

Suicide increases as a function of age (Vaillant & Blumenthal 1990). It is rare in children under 12; it increases after puberty, and the incidence continues to increase with each adolescent year (Moens 1990). A change in the picture occurs from late adolescence onwards with a divergence in the age–mortality relationship. This can be seen in two parameters: between countries and between genders within a country.

There are two ways of analysing age–mortality relationships. The first method is age–suicide-mortality correlation. Using this technique, the highest suicide rates are among older men in almost all European countries. The rate among females is more variable, peaking at a younger age (45–64) in some countries, notably Scandinavia. The majority of European countries, nevertheless, demonstrate a strong direct correlation between age and suicide. The other technique uses proportional mortality rates. The rank order of suicide in the range of causes of death decreases with increasing age. If all age groups are taken together, then suicide ranks as the 9th or 10th cause of death in most European countries. This translates to roughly 1% of all female deaths and 2% of all male deaths.

There are important changes in the epidemiology of suicide. There has been a real increase in youth suicide in the last 20 years. In industrialised nations there has been an increase in male rates within all age groups but most worryingly in the younger cohorts, which show mean changes of 70+% in the period 1970–1986. In women this phenomenon is evident to a lesser extent, with an increase of 40+% in the 15–29-year-old group. However, in several countries, e.g. Canada and the USA, there has been a decrease in the female rate.

Table 27.1	Prevalence of suicide in various countries
Country	Pattern
Australia	Highest youth rate in industrialised world: 16. per 100 000 in 15–24-year group
Germany	Decline 1989–1991 from 18.4 to 17.5 per 100 000. Sex rate stable at 2.2: 1 male:female. Higher rate in former East Germany
Denmark	Good records. One of Europe's highest rates. Majority are males aged 30–59 years. Greatest increase is in females aged 40–54 years. In last 70 years, male rate has risen by 3% to 33.5 per 100 000 and females by 58% to 17.2 per 100 000
Brazil	Poor records. Highest incidence is in 25–44-year group; increasing trend is in 15–24-year group
Japan	Rate falling; no longer regarded as 'honourable'. Peak in 1986 of 21.2 per 100 000 now falling. Most cases in 55 and over group, Worrying trends — doubling of rate in 10–14 year group within a year
USA	Controversy over rates doubling in last 20 years; these figures relate especially to males. Recent figures are more encouraging: in the decade 1990–1999 suicide rates fell by 14% and the position of the USA in the international league table of suicide fell from 8th to 11th
China	Substantial increase in rate of suicide, especially in young females living in a rural environment (Phillips et al 2002)
Netherlands	Fall of 10% overall since 1985. Most cases in elderly men, but rates in 30–39-year-old males have increased
France	Among the highest in Europe. Upward trend over last 10 years from 16 per 100 000 to 20.1 per 100 000. May reflect underestimation. Male:female = 3:1. Rates in males 30–34 years doubled and increased by 50% in 20–29-year-olds in 20 years. Higher in rural than in urban centres

Gender is one of the most frequently replicated predictors for suicide. Qin et al (2000) conducted a time-matched nested case–control study using Danish longitudinal register databases to obtain 811 suicide cases and 79 871 controls. They found that a history of hospitalised mental illness was the most powerful predictor of suicide for both genders. Unemployment, retirement, being single and sickness absence were significant risk factors for men, whereas having a child less than 2 years old was significantly protective for women. The relative risks for suicide differed between genders according to psychiatric admission status and being the parent of a child under 2 years. However, adjustment for these factors did not eliminate the gender difference in suicide risk. They concluded that risk factors for suicide differed by gender, and gender differences could not be explained by differential exposure to known risk factors.

Methods

Methods of committing suicide have been categorised as nonviolent (drugs and poisons) and violent (all other methods). The most common methods vary among nations, cultures and age groups, between sexes and over time. In general, violent methods are more commonly employed by males and by the mentally ill. In Britain, suicides by hanging and by poisoning with vehicle exhaust fumes account for two in three male suicides but only one in three women; over half of female suicides are attributed to drug overdoses. Suicides involving firearms are associated with men, while suffocation using a plastic bag is more common among women. Two modes show an age rather than a sex bias: jumping from a high place among young adults, and drowning among older victims.

Studies of cohorts of victims based on the violent method by which they ended their lives have revealed interesting features about suicidal behaviour and factors that determine the method employed. One example is self-immolation, where there are associations with a particular mental illness (schizophrenia), an independent cultural element (Asian-born women) and combined homicide–suicide (Prosser 1996). A study of survivors of attempted suicide by deliberately throwing themselves in front of London Underground trains found most of these individuals suffered from severe mental illness and were currently in treatment; the method was determined not only by its perceived dangerousness but by its ready availability, and often there was little or no planning involved (O'Donnell et al 1996). A comparison of men who committed suicide by hanging, using a firearm or non-domestic gas, found differences among the groups that indicate that impulsive traits, the type of mental illness, the presence of physical illness, and the social and forensic background, influenced the selection of method — and hence might act as potential indicators of suicidal tendency in an individual (De Leo et al 2002).

Methods are subject to fashion. There are well-known suicide 'hot spots' such as Beachy Head and the Golden Gate Bridge, with victims sometimes travelling hundreds of miles to end their life at a special place. Suicides may follow the death of an idol, particularly if this has been by suicide, when the method may be copied. Mass suicides occasionally occur, often in the setting of an isolated and extreme religious sect, although forensic examination usually reveals a mixture of suicides and homicides among these victims. In suicide pacts, which account for 1 in 40 suicides, the couple invariably choose the same method, which is more likely to be poisoning by car exhaust fumes (Brown & Barraclough 1997). Murder–suicides are not uncommon, with 20% of partner homicides being followed by the suicide of the perpetrator.

An important consideration is whether suicides can be prevented by reducing the availability of potentially more lethal methods. Between 1945 and 1965 carbon monoxide poisoning by domestic gas accounted for around 40% of suicides in men and 60% in women. The detoxification of town gas during the 1960s prevented the 'head in the gas oven' suicide, and a corresponding fall in the total number of suicides by about one-third occurred (Kreitman 1976). The same phenomenon has been reported recently in England and Wales, with the 10–15% fall in the suicide rates in men and women from 1990–1997 being mainly attributed to a 60% fall in deaths caused by vehicle exhaust gases, as a result of the widespread use of catalytic converters (McClure 2000). In the USA, states with the strictest handgun control laws have the lowest rates of suicide involving firearms, and as there is almost no compensatory increase among other methods, these states also have the lowest suicide rates overall (Lester & Murrell 1982).

There has been debate in Britain about whether employing newer, less toxic antidepressants in place of the tricyclic antidepressants would contribute to suicide prevention, notwithstanding such poisoning deaths accounted for less than 5% of suicides. A recent prospective study paradoxically found rates of presentation to hospital with deliberate self-harm were significantly higher among patients who were prescribed SSRIs compared with tricyclics, with the antidepressant being taken in overdose in less than one-third of cases (Donovan et al 2000). This is in line with a population-based study that found only one in seven suicide victims who were taking antidepressants employed the drug to end their life (Jick et al 1995), with no difference in the suicide rates by antidepressant compound after other variables were taken into account.

It is likely that some patients' lives will be saved by restricting access to lethal methods. However a Finnish study has confirmed that suicide victims who had survived an earlier attempt usually switched to a more lethal method to achieve their aim, so that restricting one lethal method will not prevent suicide in a person with strong intent (Isometsa & Lonnqvist 1998).

Risk factors

These are often quoted without due care for the individual nature of suicide risk and without due attention to the methodological shortfalls which surround much of suicide research, such as the lack of controlled or longitudinal studies. The other element of the risk calculation is protective factors. There are a variety of models of suicide and much debate both about these models and how suicide rates might be reduced.

- The *stress diathesis model* of suicidal behaviour is concerned with stressors and predisposing factors. Typical stressors include: mental disorder, alcohol and drug misuse; medical illness; adversity. The diathesis or predisposition to suicidal behaviour may be a key element in understanding why one person with depressive illness kills himself whereas another with the same illness does not. Diatheses could be genetic, early adverse experience(s) or chronic illness (Mann 1998).
- The *hierarchical model* of suicide is primarily concerned with the relative contribution of factors to overall risk of suicide and is divided into primary, secondary and tertiary risk factors. Primary factors involve mental disorder and healthcare; secondary factors are separate from illness and are concerned with adverse aspects of everyday life, e.g. isolation and loss; tertiary factors are mainly demographic and are often immutable, e.g. male gender. Primary factors are seen as powerful predictors of suicide and do not require the presence of secondary or tertiary factors to remain active. Secondary factors are powerful in the presence of primary factors but are weak alone. Tertiary factors are of very low predictive power in the absence of primary or secondary factors (Rhimer 1996).
- A more complex general pathway to suicide has been constructed to include primary prevention (predisposing factors, e.g. psychiatric diagnosis, suicide history, age, gender and social difficulties); secondary prevention (predictors and risk factors, e.g. affective disorder, alcohol and drug abuse, impulsivity and cognitive rigidity, isolation and relationship/work disruption); feedback loops (protective factors, e.g. treatment, physical well-being, hopefulness and coping skills, social support); tertiary prevention (trigger factors, e.g. suicide attempt, low levels of the serotonin metabolite 5HIAA, physical illness, hopelessness, stress and object loss) (Maris 2002).

A relatively simple model of the relationship of various risk factors is sketched in Figure 27.1

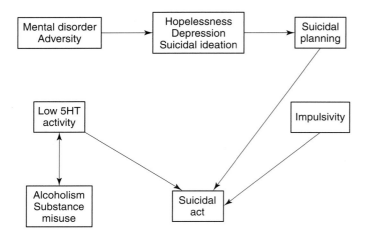

Fig. 27.1
A model of the relationship of various risk factors.

Social variables

The first classification of sociological variables operating in suicide was proposed by Emil Durkheim. Three suicide types were identified: anomic, egoistic and altruistic. Anomie occurs when the normal cohesive bonds in a social group are weakened, so that the usual standards which guide in times of stress are lost. The egoistic variety refers to individuals being separated from their social group and losing their sense of belonging to a community, so that the mores of that society no longer influence them. The altruistic form, as the term implies, refers to ending one's own life for a greater good. It is important to note that explicit distinction between the three varieties, especially between anomic and egoistic, is not always possible. Social isolation, subjective sense of loss of contact and loss of values are prominent characteristics of those who die by their own hand. Durkheim proposed that factors which increase social integration decrease suicide. Lester (1996) reviewed the birth and marriage rates of ten countries from 1900 to 1988 and found that the birth rates were more strongly and consistently associated with suicide rates, supporting Durkheim's hypothesis.

Modern social variables which have been extensively evaluated in suicide research include unemployment, social marginalisation and isolation, and economic variables such as recession and poverty. Heikkinen et al (1995) studied social factors associated with suicide and found that several varied across age groups among completed suicides. In comparison with the general population, victims were more commonly never married (especially men aged 30–39) or were divorced or widowed (especially women aged 60–69). Victims were more often living on their own, although living with parents was more common among young males, who also had a greater incidence of psychiatric admission. Social isolation, accompanied by alcohol misuse, was particularly common among middle-aged males. While many of these features replicate sociological findings in suicide, the authors highlighted the fact that some social variables might be consequences of the victim's psychopathology and excessive alcohol use. Gender-related psychopathology and alcohol misuse could be seen as confounders, and future studies may reveal more if these are taken into account.

Whitely et al (1999) investigated the association between suicide and measures of deprivation and social fragmentation in the UK. They found that mortality from suicide and all other causes increased with increasing deprivation score, social fragmentation score and abstention from voting in all age and gender groups. Suicide was most strongly related to social fragmentation, whereas deaths from other causes were more closely related to deprivation scores. The relation between social fragmentation and suicide was largely independent of deprivation score, whereas the association with the deprivation score was generally reduced after adjustment for fragmentation. It was concluded that suicide was more strongly associated with social fragmentation than with poverty.

With respect to adverse life events, uncontrolled studies have identified potential precipitants to suicide: interpersonal loss and conflict; financial difficulties; the effects of physical illness (Rich et al 1988). Comparative studies of life events and suicide with general population controls have found an excess risk of suicide in the 4–5 years following bereavement of spouse or parent, especially in males. In a psychological autopsy study comparing suicide cases with living controls matched for age, gender and mental illness, Cavanagh et al (1999) found that cases had significantly more adverse life events than controls in terms of interpersonal family adversity and physical ill-health.

Cheng et al (2000) examined the interaction between psychosocial and psychiatric risk factors for suicide. They identified five major risk factors: loss events, suicidal behaviour in first-degree relatives, major depression, emotionally unstable personality disorder and substance abuse. However, only loss events and a family history of suicidal behaviour retained their independent effects after adjusting for the effects of the other three factors. This study highlights the independent effects of mental disorder and loss events. It also raises the question of cause and effect; that is, are loss events causes or consequences of mental disorder? The investigation of pathways to suicide is required to explore these questions.

Unemployment is often reported to be a significant variable (Platt 1984, Pritchard 1988). Although the causal mechanism is not fully understood, it may be that the trigger is the demoralisation, depression and despair associated with being jobless (Warr 1987). In young men such pressure may be experienced more acutely as they seek to establish an independent adult identity. The association between increased male suicide rates and unemployment is not unexpected in view of the known 'depressive' reaction and poorer health associated with being out of work, especially over a prolonged period (Platt 1984, Warr 1987, Platt & Kreitman 1990). The demands placed on men and women by a changing society, altered roles and changing social norms can be interpreted as a form of anomie. The loss of hope associated with prolonged unemployment creates a culture of hopelessness that may exacerbate the stresses upon those who are economically and psychologically vulnerable. Such individuals are often the first among the victims of socio-economic recession.

An association between age, socio-economic grouping and suicide was found in a study of suicide and undetermined death in the UK. There was a concentration of suicide and undetermined deaths in the middle age groups of the lower socio-economic category. Taking into account methodological considerations, these results could be explained in terms of the downward social drift associated, among other things, with long-term unemployment (Kreitman et al 1991).

The evidence to date shows that suicide results from a complex interaction of biological, psychological, social and situational/personal factors. Several sociodemographic factors characterise those who commit suicide, including the finding that suicide is more common in males and in those who are unmarried, separated, widowed or divorced (Buda & Tsuang 1990). Decreased social integration, increased social isolation and unemployment have also been shown to be significant interacting variables.

Biological variables in suicide

The biology of suicide is a growth area in research, encompassing investigation of neurotransmitter function, neuroimaging and genetics.

Neurotransmitters The most replicated finding in suicide biology is the lower CSF concentrations (< 92.5 nmol/l) of the serotonin metabolite 5HIAA. There are also indications that suicidal behaviour is associated with a deficit in transmission of serotonin (5HT). Other findings among those who die by suicide include a decrease in 5HT transporter sites, an increase in $5HT_{1A}$ and $5HT_{2A}$ receptors, smaller serotonergic neurons and more numerous, but less functional, neurons (Table 27.2). In summary, dysfunction of monoaminergic neurotransmission has been impli-

cated in suicidal behaviour (Roy 1994), based on postmortem studies of the serotonergic and, to a lesser extent, noradrenergic systems. It is difficult to control for the confounding variables associated with postmortem findings. They can only be a snapshot of brain function at the moment of death and are subject to genetic effects, developmental and early life processes, associated psychiatric disease and treatment for this, environmental stressors and artefacts of postmortem delay. Research in this area is still dominated by studies with small sample sizes, multiple paradigm testing and retrospective designs. Overall, results from biological studies in this area represent continuing research and experimentation and are not yet at the stage of providing clinical tools.

Aggression, violence and suicide Aggression is an inner state and violence is an overt act. Suicide can be seen as both aggressive and violent. In challenge tests to measure serotonin indirectly — e.g. prolactin response to fenfluramine — patients with the highest aggression scores have been reported as having the lowest prolactin responses, implying that aggression and serotonergic activity are negatively associated.

Table 27.2 Biological variables of suicide

Authors	Biological variables	Findings
Asberg et al 1976	5HIAA	Depressed patients with low CSF 5HIAA made more suicide attempts than other depressed patients
Mann et al 1989	5HT/5HIAA	No evidence for greater reduction in violent rather than non-violent suicides
Mann et al 1994	5HT/5HIAA	Postmortem brain tissue from suicide victims; modest reduction in brainstem 5HT and 5HIAA — independent of diagnosis
Arango et al 1996	Noradrenaline (norepinephrine)	Neuronal reduction in locus coeruleus in completed suicides versus controls? Specific to suicide or also associated with depression
Arango et al 1990 Biegon & Israeli 1988 Mann et al 1986	β-adrenoceptors	Increased binding to β-adrenoceptors in cortex of suicides versus controls
De Paermentier et al 1990 Little et al 1993 Stockmeier & Meltzer 1991	β-adrenoceptors	Did not concur with β-receptor findings above
Arango et al 1993 Meana & Garcia-Sevilla 1987	α-adrenoceptors	Increased binding in cortex of suicides
Gross-Isseroff et al 1990		Decreased α-receptor binding
Garcia-Sevilla et al 1996	Imidazoline receptors	Adrenergic receptors in brain and platelets. Platelet subtypes show upregulation in depression. Brain subtypes show downregulation in suicide victims
Arato et al 1989	CRF	Increased CRF concentration in CSF of suicide victims
Nemeroff et al 1988	CRF	Decreased receptor density in frontal cortex of suicide victims attributed to downregulation of CRF binding sites due to CRF hypersecretion by the hypothalamus
Banki et al 1987	CRF	No differences in CSF CRF concentrations between suicidal and non-suicidal depressed patients
Sundman et al 1997	GABA	No differences in the ligand binding of GABA receptors in frontal cortex of suicides and normal controls postmortem.
Linkowsky et al 1983 Linkowsky et al 1984	TSH	Lower TSH response to TRH in depressed patients who subsequently die by their own hand. Many inconsistencies and contradictions in the literature
Muldoon et al 1990	Cholesterol	Long-term follow-up of effect of cholesterol-lowering drugs — significant increase in suicide accidents and violence. Questions as to causal link. Hypotheses on biological plausibility, i.e. lower neuronal lipid viscosity and knock-on effect on 5HT receptor availability

CRF, corticotrophin-releasing factor; CSF, cerebrospinal fluid; GABA, γ-aminobutyric acid; 5HIAA, 5-hydroxyindole-acetic acid; 5HT, 5-hydroxytryptamine; TRH, thyrotrophin-releasing hormone; TSH, thyroid-stimulating hormone.

Genetic studies Classical genetic techniques such as twin and adoption studies have been pursued. Roy et al (1991) reported that monozygotic twin suicides showed a greater concordance than those of dizygotic twins, a finding which held for twins who attempted as well as for those who completed. Ingraham & Kety (2000) showed that 4–5% of adoptive parents of people who killed themselves also took their own lives compared with only 0.7% of controls.

Clinical variables

One of the early cohort studies examining mental illness among those who commit suicide found over 90% of the 100 cases could be diagnosed as having a mental disorder (Barraclough et al 1974). Of these, 70% were depressed, 15% were alcohol dependent and 3% were schizophrenic. The findings of this study implied that suicide is rare among those with good mental and physical health and is most strongly associated with depression and alcoholism. These results were mirrored by the results of Cheng et al (2000) from a different cultural setting. In a case-controlled study in East Taiwan, 97–100% of the sample suffered from mental illness prior to suicide. Again the two most prevalent disorders were depression and alcoholism and the most common comorbid pattern was depression accompanied by substance abuse.

Psychological autopsy The major obstacle to an understanding of suicide is that the victim cannot be interviewed and the reason directly ascertained. One solution has been the development of psychological autopsy. This technique is based upon a combination of interviews of those closest to the deceased and an examination of corroborating evidence from sources such as hospital and general-practice case-notes, social work reports and criminal records. From this information an assessment is made of the victim's mental and physical health, personality, experience of social adversity, and social integration. The aim is to produce as

full and accurate a picture of the deceased as possible with a view to understanding why they killed themselves. Psychological autopsy is the most direct technique currently available for determining the relationship between particular risk factors and suicide. This type of intensive approach not only provides direct information but also aids the interpretation of studies employing other techniques (Hawton et al 1998).

A systematic review of 154 psychological autopsy studies (Cavanagh et al 2003) found that mental disorder was the most strongly associated variable of those that have been studied. Cavanagh et al also calculated population attributable fractions (PAFs) which estimate the proportion of cases (e.g. suicides) in a population that can be attributed to the exposure (e.g. mental disorder) and can be interpreted as the fraction of cases in a population that could be avoided by reducing or eliminating the exposure. The PAFs suggest that between a half and three-quarters of suicides could be avoided were it possible to have completely effective treatment, or prevention, of mental disorders. Similarly, a meta-analysis of studies examining the mortality associated with mental disorders (Harris & Barraclough 1997) found that of 44 disorders considered, 36 had a significantly raised standardised mortality rate (SMR) for suicide. They concluded that all mental disorders, with the exception of dementia and learning disability, are risk factors for suicide. A summary of Harris & Barraclough's findings (Table 27.3) provides an overview of the SMRs associated with the main psychiatric diagnoses (an increased SMR is statistically significant when the lower 95% confidence interval is greater than 100). Another psychological autopsy study carried out in Northern Ireland (Foster et al 1997) confirmed the finding that around 90% of suicide victims suffered from an Axis I and/or Axis II mental disorder. Most studies have described affective disorder as having the strongest association with suicide, followed by substance/alcohol misuse and schizophrenia.

Table 27.3 An abbreviated summary of standardised mortality rates (SMRs) associated with psychiatric diagnoses

	Observed	Expected	SMR	95% CI
Organic disorders (incl. epilepsy, dementia and LD)				
Total	264	79.45	332	293–375
Substance use (Incl. alcohol)				
Total	1095	190.63	574	541–609
Functional disorders				
Anorexia nervosa	25	1.11	2252	1458–3325
Bulimia nervosa	1	0.08	1250	32–4465
Major depression	351	17.25	2035	1827–2259
Mood disorders (NOS)	377	23.41	1610	1452–1781
Bipolar disorder	93	6.18	1505	1225–1844
Dysthymia	1436	118.45	1212	1150–1277
Schizophrenia	1176	139.13	845	798–895
Brief reactive psychosis	1081	70.33	1537	1447–1631
OCD	3	0.26	1154	238–3372
Panic disorder	9	0.90	1000	457–1898
Anxiety neurosis	151	24.00	629	533–738
Neurosis	85	22.87	372	297–460
PD	30	4.24	708	477–1010
Somatisation	2	0.38	526	64–1901
All mental disorders	5787	478.53	1209	1178–124

From Harris & Barraclough (1997).
LD, learning disability; OCD, obsessive–compulsive disorder; NOS, not otherwise specified; PD, personality disorder.

Box 27.1	Main correlates of suicide in major depression

- Greater severity of illness
- Self-neglect
- Impaired concentration/memory
- Hopelessness
- Alcohol abuse
- Mood cycling
- History of suicidal behaviour

Box 27.2	Main correlates of suicide in non-major depression

- Male sex
- Comorbid substance abuse
- Younger age
- Limited contract with health services

Box 27.3	Main correlates of suicide in bipolar affective disorder

- Relatively early in course of illness
- Current major depressive episode or mixed affective state
- Recent adverse life events

Affective disorders   The main correlates of suicide and affective disorders are given in Boxes 27.1 to 27.3. Barraclough et al (1974), Barraclough & Pallis (1975) and Modestin & Kopp (1988) found insomnia, impaired memory and self-neglect as well as greater overall severity of illness to be more common among depressed suicide victims. Fawcett and colleagues' (1990) prospective cohort study identified two main groups of predictors: short-term and long-term. The former comprised anhedonia, anxiety, impaired concentration and alcohol abuse; the latter featured hopelessness, mood cycling and a history of deliberate self-harm.

In bipolar disorder, the majority (79%) experience a major depressive episode immediately before death. A minority have mixed states, which has been linked to especially high suicide risk (Goodwin & Jamison 1990, Strakowski et al 1996). Adverse life events constitute risk factors for both deliberate self-harm and suicide itself (Paykel & Dowlatshani 1988).

Hopelessness   The relationship between extreme pessimism or hopelessness and suicidal intent has traditionally been regarded as a close one (Beck et al 1975), and clinical strategies for alleviating hopelessness have been found to be useful for countering the suicidal crisis (Beck et al 1979). What is unclear is whether hopelessness is the crucial cognitive aspect in suicidal thinking. One study which examined this issue concluded that self-reported 'unusual thinking' was found to be the most important predictor of various aspects of suicidal intent in their sample (Mendonca & Holden 1996). Unusual thinking was defined as a cognitive distortion which involves feelings of loss of control over one's thoughts. This finding implies that this aspect of cognitive distortion may be an important predictor and thus its evaluation may be integral to the assessment of suicidal ideation and risk. However, unusual thinking is regarded as a state linked to current risk rather than a trait variable such as pessimistic attitude, problem-solving rigidity or perfectionism, all of which

have been implicated in the long-term risk of suicide (Linehan et al 1987).

Substance abuse   The San Diego Suicide Study investigated young suicides. It was set up partly because the predictive power of known variables in relation to suicide is poor and because, more than any other disorders, substance abuse and depression are associated with suicide. One element of this study was the examination of relationships between interpersonal and other stressors on the one hand and diagnoses of substance abuse and depression on the other. It was demonstrated that interpersonal loss or conflict occurred more frequently near the time of death for substance abusers with or without depression than for those with affective disorder alone. These results, which are consistent with other studies, suggest there may be differences in the manner in which suicidal individuals with substance abuse and those with affective illness respond to external stressors (Rich et al 1988). More specifically, suicide associated with alcoholism and substance abuse may be preceded more often by interpersonal loss and conflict during the 6 weeks before death. There is evidence that those dependent on alcohol or other substances are confronted with a broader range of stressors than those with mood or anxiety disorder who experience conflicts/arguments and attachment disruptions (Duberstein et al 1993).

Alcohol   Alcoholism correlates with an increased risk of suicide (Box 27.4). Murphy & Wetzel (1990) reviewed the world literature and concluded that the lifetime risk varied according to the type of treatment received:

- 2.2% for alcoholics with a history of outpatient treatment;
- 3.4% for those with a history of inpatient treatment.

This represents a lifetime risk twice that of the general population and 60–120 times that of those without psychiatric illness in the general population. Examining cohort studies of suicides indicates that about 20% of the samples have an alcohol problem.

Schizophrenia   Schizophrenia correlates with an increased risk of suicide, with this risk estimated at 10–15% of patients (Black et al 1985). Several risk factors appear with regularity in the literature. These include (Box 27.5) young age and male sex; previous deliberate self-harm; comorbid depression — there is consistent evidence of association between depression and suicide in schizo-

---

Box 27.4	Main correlates of suicide in those with alcohol problems

- Male sex
- Longer duration of problems
- Single/divorced/widowed
- Currently drinking
- Presence of depressive symptoms

Box 27.5	Main correlates of suicide in schizophrenia

- Young and male
- Relapsing pattern of illness
- Past history of depression
- Current depressive illness / comorbid with depression
- Recent discharge from inpatient care to outpatient care
- Social isolation in the community
- Relatively good insight into illness

---

phrenia. Schizophrenic victims have been shown to present with depressed mood, as well as other features of depression, during their index admission to hospital. However, they are not more likely to fulfil criteria for major depression. They tend to exhibit the psychological features of depressive illness, e.g. hopelessness, but fewer of the somatic features (Drake & Cotton 1986).

There is evidence that patients with insight into their illness are at greater risk of suicidal behaviour (Cotton et al 1985). These individuals develop a sense of hopelessness and demoralisation, leading to suicidal behaviour. Accordingly, improving awareness of illness should be tempered with caution with regard to the effects of such increased awareness on the patient's risk of suicide.

Suicide in special groups

Psychiatric patients Psychiatric hospital inpatients are known to be at high risk of suicide (Appleby 1992; see Box 27.6). The National Confidential Inquiry into Suicide and Homicide by People with Mental Illness has identified inpatients as a priority group for whom service recommendations are most required, and has recommended that the risk assessment skills of clinical staff should be strengthened (Appleby et al 1999). Suicide by psychiatric hospital inpatients was strongly associated with suicidal ideas or acts of self-harm preceding or during admission. Five predictors had adjusted likelihood ratios greater than two: recent bereavement, presence of delusions, suicidal ideation, chronic mental illness and family history of suicide.

Barraclough & Pallis (1975) asked which type of depressive commits suicide. They found signicantly more of the suicides were unmarried, lived alone and had a history of deliberate self-harm. These characteristics were also found in a subsequent case–control study of risk factors for suicide in psychiatric patients (Roy 1982). Roy's study indicates that depression needs to be recognised and treated, especially in those with other high-risk factors. The immediate period when changing from inpatient to outpatient care is one of increased risk for suicide.

Risk factors for the psychiatric inpatient population have been the focus of renewed attention. In a case–control study, those psychiatric inpatients at particular risk had previously exhibited suicidal behaviour, suffered from schizophrenia, were admitted involuntarily and lived alone (Roy & Draper 1995). There is further evidence which contends that, once age, sex and diagnosis are controlled for in discharged psychiatric patients, the

conventional risk factors of being unmarried, being unemployed, living alone, substance misuse and previous deliberate self-harm, are common to cases and controls and may be characteristic of people with mental illness generally. The suicide rate in patients discharged from hospital has been reported to be at its highest in the first month after discharge, which emphasises the need for targeted care after discharge, especially against a background trend of reduced number of inpatient beds and shorter inpatient stay in hospital (Geddes & Juszczak 1995).

A problem with most risk factors is that they are relatively common in all psychiatric patient groups. They correlate well with suicide but predict it badly. Taken together, however, they offer some help in identifying high-risk subjects within an already high-risk population. More usefully, there appear to be two major vulnerability points in an episode of illness: the initial acute phase when the patient is at home and admission may be contemplated; and the period of recovery when they may be discharged earlier than was once conventional clinical practice, perhaps at a time of incomplete recovery.

Pregnancy and the puerperium During pregnancy and in the first postnatal year women have a low risk of suicide despite having increased rates of psychiatric morbidity. Motherhood appears to act as a protective factor against suicide — and concern for dependants in a general sense may provide an important focus for preventative measures in the clinical setting (Appleby 1991). This finding provides an important balance to the assumption that suicide risk is determined solely by the mental state and psychiatric history. Social factors must be taken account of, particularly from the viewpoint of preventative measures (Kendell 1991).

Suicide in young people The suicide rate among young people has been a cause of particular concern over the last thirty years. Appleby et al (1999) explored the characteristics of people aged under 35 who commit suicide. A number of highly significant clinical, social and interpersonal differences between suicides and controls were found. Factor analysis identified two groups of variables within each of these three domains which were independently linked to suicide: acute, severe mental disorder and chronic disorder of behaviour; rootlessness and social withdrawal; chronic and recent interpersonal problems. Similarly, Hawton et al (1999) investigated the characteristics of a series of consecutive suicides in under-25-year-olds. Their findings revealed that more individuals were of lower social class and unemployed than in the local population. Hanging and carbon monoxide poisoning were the most frequent methods of suicide, and Co-proxamol was the drug most often used in overdose. Previous self-harm had occurred in 44.8%; half of these were multiple repeaters, and 80% had self-harmed within the previous year. Little support was found for an earlier finding of increasing frequency of general practitioner visits shortly before death. Only 22.4% of individuals were in the care of psychiatric services. Both these studies emphasised the need for a broad-based approach to suicide prevention in the young.

Farmers Farmers are recognised as having the occupation with the highest suicide rate among UK occupational groups, and have been a topic of specific study (Hawton et al 1998b). Apart from the long-term decline in the industry, it has been suggested that the explanation for the high suicide rate may lie in farmers' ease of access to dangerous methods. Hawton et al (1998b) examined data on 719 deaths in farmers of both genders in England and Wales between 1981 and 1993 in which a verdict of suicide or an open verdict was recorded. Of 702 deaths in male

---

Box 27.6 Features which might increase the risk of suicide in psychiatric patients

- *Mental state:* psychosis, depressed mood, hopelessness, suicidal ideas, suicidal content to psychotic phenomena, communication of intent
- *Past history:* previous parasuicide, history for years, several admissions, ? long history with recent change
- *Social / demographic:* living alone, single / divorced features widowed, unemployed male, young
- *Current episode:* acute relapse, recent discharge, inpatient or recent outpatient, recent transition in care
- *Ward and staff:* staff hostility to patient, high staff or patient turnover, low morale, insufficient observation facilities, inadequate staff expertise

From Appleby (1992).

farmers, firearms were involved in 40%, which was considerably greater than firearm use among male victims in the general population. During the study period there was a reduction in firearm death rates, particularly after 1989 when legislation on firearm ownership, registration and storage was strengthened — and there were also fewer farming suicides after this date. By the end of the study period, hanging had overtaken firearms as the commonest method.

Physical health variables

An increased risk of suicide has been associated with many physical illnesses, particularly chronic neurological, gastrointestinal, cardiovascular and malignant disorders. The relative risk of committing suicide among patients with cancer of all types is 2.5 (Allebeck & Bolund 1991). Some well-known associations are indirect, for instance the link between suicide and peptic ulceration is almost entirely explained by coexisting alcohol dependence.

Thinking that particular diseases and drugs are associated with increased suicide risk produces a false dichotomy; it is more useful to think in general terms about features that are linked to increased risk (Box 27.7). Physical ill health is a significant factor in 25–75% of suicides, the higher figures being reported in studies of suicide among cohorts of older victims. In a review of 100 cases of suicide among elderly people, 65% had significant physical illness and 23% had been medical inpatients within the preceding year (Cattell & Jolley 1995). There is a strong relationship between physical ill health and depression or subclinical distress (Mayou & Hawton 1986), and although these emotional disorders are usually mild, it is likely that this factor largely mediates the association between physical ill health and suicide.

Protective factors

Less attention has been paid to clinical features that might protect against the emergence of suicidal behaviour. An important question to bear in mind is not so much why people want to commit suicide, but why they want to live. An attempt to tap into these factors has been made using the Reasons for Living Inventory, a self-report instrument measuring beliefs that might contribute to the inhibition of suicidal behaviour. The six factors included in this are easy to remember in assessing any suicidal patient: survival and coping beliefs, responsibility to family, child-related concerns, fear of suicide, fear of social disapproval, and moral objections to suicide. Malone et al (2000) explored reason for living during a major depressive episode and found that the

---

Box 27.7 Factors associated with a disease or drug side-effect that increase the likelihood of suicide

- Mood disorder, especially depression, emotional lability
- Motor overactivity, e.g. agitation, akathisia
- Disinhibition, reduced impulse control
- Severe chronic or recurrent pain that is inadequately controlled
- Disfigurement, especially in women
- Severe disability, especially loss of mobility
- Extensive sick role limitations, e.g. loss of job, family role
- Prospect of a degenerating disease without hope of recovery

---

subjective perception of stressful life events may be more pertinent to suicidal expression than the objective quantity of such events. In addition, a more optimistic perceptual set may modify against hopelessness. It was suggested that an assessment of reason for living should be included in the evaluation of suicidal patients. Cavanagh et al (1999) in a case–control study which controlled for age, gender and mental disorder, found that the living controls had significantly more care of whatever kind than the cases who had committed suicide. The protective role of engagement in care must be considered in any assessment of suicidality.

Management

Most psychiatrists will encounter suicides among their patients and will have to manage the aftermath of the event, particularly if the death occurred in an inpatient (Hodelet & Hughson 2001). All unnatural deaths, whether definite suicides or not, must be reported to the statutory authorities — the procurator fiscal in Scotland and the coroner in England and Wales. The police will have to investigate the death on behalf of the Crown, so a death certificate cannot be issued and a postmortem examination will be required. In Scotland the Mental Welfare Commission should be informed of all suicides among psychiatric patients, irrespective of whether or not they are detained under mental health legislation. Psychiatrists should also provide details when requested to the National Confidential Inquiry into Suicides and Homicides by People with Mental Illness.

Consideration must be given to the relatives who have to cope with the untimely death and the inevitable statutory procedures (and delays). Of course their emotional process is one of grief, but the nature and circumstances of the death predispose to extreme or atypical reactions, profound guilt or anger, and an increased risk of deliberate self-harm or suicide among the bereaved. Helping the family has to be carefully handled, sensitive and responsive to their wishes.

The emotional impact on the individual who found the body or inadvertently caused the death must also be borne in mind. Post-traumatic stress disorder (PTSD) may develop in these circumstances. Among train drivers involved in railway suicides PTSD occurred in 17% and other mental illnesses in a further 23% (Farmer et al 1992).

Giving staff who were involved in the care, discovery or attempted resuscitation of the victim an opportunity to share their experiences is usually helpful, and may reduce the risk of PTSD. Staff need this debrief within 2–3 days, in a safe, non-judgemental environment — a task that is separate from the audit of such deaths that should become a routine part of clinical practice. The audit, or suicide review, should take place one or two months later in a planned way, and preferably with an external chairperson, primarily to establish whether there are learning points. A report should be prepared for healthcare trust management, statutory authorities and members of the team. Finally, consultants must be aware of the potentially very stressful effect of a patient suicide on their trainees (Yousaf et al 2002) and themselves, and they should seek to address this, principally through the support of colleagues, if necessary.

Prevention

Despite all the uncertainties, confusion and controversy surrounding suicidal behaviour, suicide prevention has been high on the mental health agenda for the past decade, not only in Britain but internationally. The main problem with preventing suicide is that it remains a rare and unpredictable event, even among patients who are known to be at high risk. Suicidal intent is not constant; it waxes and wanes, often suddenly and unexpectedly. Further, the risk can be greater when the patient is becoming ill, or is recovering, or has recovered from illness rather than when the disorder is severe. The difficulty in predicting suicide even among likely victims is illustrated in an American study of patients with mood illness who were admitted to a psychiatric hospital. A statistical model determined risk based on established factors such as previous suicide attempts, suicidal ideation and outcome at discharge, but this failed to pinpoint with 50% probability any of the 46 patients who committed suicide, and only one victim at 15% probability — i.e. at the same likelihood of suicide as for depressive illness (Goldstein et al 1991). Further, the changing epidemiology of suicide has reduced the potential opportunity for doctors to intervene, as young men who commit suicide are less likely to have consulted their general practitioner in the weeks leading up to their death, or to be in contact with psychiatric services (Hawton et al 1999).

Another doubt is whether medical intervention can prevent suicide even when high risk is identified. The debate was fuelled by 'the Gotland study' (Rutz et al 1989). The purpose of this study had been to test the effect of increasing general practitioners' knowledge about the diagnosis and treatment of patients with affective disorders, and the suicide rate on the island was monitored primarily to ensure the treatment strategies did not increase the risk for individual patients. To the contrary, the investigators found suicides fell from an average 11 per year in 1982–1984 to 4 in the year of the study, a finding that was not mirrored by a reduction in Sweden as a whole. The suicide rate returned to normal in subsequent years (Rutz et al 1992). The Gotland study had major drawbacks, not least that the base population was only 56 000 and its effect was fleeting, but its significance has been considerable, and perhaps mainly symbolic — that if doctors learned to identify high-risk patients and treat their mental illnesses energetically, an appreciable impact on the suicide rate would follow.

No intervention has been demonstrated to be effective in well-conducted clinical trials, so espousing that medical interventions could prevent suicide not only has no evidence base, but runs the risks of raising false expectations among the public and encouraging grieving relatives to blame healthcare professionals inappropriately. On the other hand, sometimes a leap of faith is necessary, and complacent or slipshod practice may make the difference between life and death, even if it cannot be proved. Irrespective of their position, all medical authorities agree that it is impossible to prevent all suicides and that medical considerations are but one element of the strategy.

Measures that could form part of a comprehensive suicide prevention strategy (Gunnell & Frankel 1994) broadly fall into two categories:

- population-based measures, which can be subdivided into method-targeted, group-targeted and general;
- high-risk individual-focused measures.

Population-based measures are principally aimed at reducing the availability of lethal methods: for instance by detoxifying town gas and curbing prescriptions of barbiturates in the past; and, in recent years, by the widespread introduction of catalytic converters and by packaging over-the-counter paracetamol in smaller quantities.

Tighter gun control laws, the design of underground trains and the monitoring or restriction of access to hot spots are similar strategies. Group-targeted approaches involve focusing on high-risk populations such as farmers (Malmberg et al 1999) and prisoners (Gore 1999), while general measures include policies to tackle homelessness and unemployment, and media reporting and portrayal of suicide.

Focusing on high-risk individuals, identifying them and neutralising the factors that make them at high risk of suicide is the key, practical, medical strategy — and of course the very high frequency of mental disorder among suicide victims justifies this effort (Mortensen et al 2000). The National Confidential Inquiry into Suicide and Homicide by People with Mental Illness represents a sustained, co-ordinated response to this challenge. Its findings and clinical recommendations have been widely disseminated in two reports — Safer Services (Appleby et al 1999) and Safety First (Appleby et al 2001) — and this has quickly become the 'gold standard' against which service provision, and perhaps more tellingly, service failures, will be measured.

DELIBERATE SELF-HARM

Terminology

There has been difficulty agreeing a suitable term to define presentations of self-injury and self-poisoning that have not resulted in death. 'Attempted suicide' is widely used by the media and general public, although Kessel argued over thirty years ago that this term was not merely misleading but was wrong and ought to be discarded, as an intent to die applied in less than half these presentations (Kessel 1965). 'Parasuicide' is defined as an act of deliberate self-injury or self-poisoning which mimics the act of suicide but does not result in a fatal outcome; the term indicates a behavioural analogue of suicide but without conveying a psychological orientation towards death (Kreitman 1977). While dissociating the behaviour from a specific motive, the fact that 'suicide' remained in the term caused confusion, although it has been retained for the international study being undertaken in Europe since 1989 (Platt et al 1992, Michel et al 2000). The term (non-fatal) deliberate self-harm avoids all reference to suicide, and merely describes the common end-point of aberrant behaviour that is the basis for study. Deliberate self-harm (DSH) is widely used by the Royal College of Psychiatrists (Royal College of Psychiatrists 1994) and government bodies (Department of Health and Social Security 1984) — and it is the preferred term for this chapter.

Features

The core features of DSH, which were agreed for a proposed ICD-10 definition, are:

- The behaviour is self-initiated and non-habitual.
- Self-harm is intended.
- The act results, or may result, in injury and possibly death to the individual.

Excluded by this definition are acts of self-harm where the intent is pleasure or experiment, where injury occurs accidentally, and where the person lacks capacity to understand the meaning or consequences of their behaviour. Factitious disorders, in which deliberate self-injury often occurs, are distinguished from DSH by the elements of intentional deception and the simulation or induction of disease. Other forms of self-injurious behaviour which are not considered under the rubric of DSH are habit disorders such as trichotillomania, bingeing and self-induced vomiting, and repeated 'delicate' self cutting. Medical presentations where injury results from intentional non-compliance (such as a patient with diabetes deliberately withholding their insulin or a patient with chronic renal failure refusing to continue on haemodialysis), would fall within this definition but are generally regarded as distinct.

Basic statistics

The epidemiological study of DSH is dogged by the fact that no country collects national data on DSH. Thus, it is not possible to correlate national trends with those for suicide. What can be done is to examine data from studies which looked at specific groups of cases of DSH in well-defined sample areas over several years (Kreitman 1977, Kreitman & Schreiber 1979, Diekstra 1982, Hawton & Goldacre 1982). What these studies demonstrate is that hospital discharge rates for DSH by young people showed a marked increase in tandem with their suicide rates in the period 1965–1980 (Diekstra 1996). On the basis of results from these studies and others, it is apparent that the trends of suicide and DSH rates were similar.

Kessler et al (1999), as part of the National Comorbidity Study in the USA, examined non-fatal suicidal behaviour among a nationally representative sample of 5877 adults aged 15–54 over the period 1990–1992 and found that 13.5% reported lifetime suicidal ideation and 4.6% overall had made a suicide attempt. Weissman et al (1999) reported the results of nine independent studies covering over 4000 people in USA, Canada, Puerto Rico, Europe (France and Germany), Lebanon, Taiwan, Korea and New Zealand. The lifetime prevalence rates for suicidal ideation varied considerably from 2.1% in Lebanon to 18.5% in New Zealand, while lifetime DSH rates ranged from 0.7% in Lebanon to 5.9% in Puerto Rico.

In the most recent UK survey of non-fatal suicidal behaviour among adults aged between 16 and 74, Meltzer et al (2002) reported the following:

- Suicidal ideation — overall, 14.9% had considered suicide at some point in their life, 3.9% during the last year and 0.4% during the past week. Women considered suicide more often than men across all age groups, while suicidal ideation was commoner among the young: 17% in the 16–44 years group in contrast to 6% in the 65–74 group.
- Suicide attempts — overall, 4.4% had attempted suicide in their lifetime and 0.5% in the past year, again with an age gradient as for ideation. However, only 2% of respondents stated that they had deliberately harmed themselves without suicidal intent.

Methods

In the UK, poisoning by drugs accounts for 90% of all hospital presentations of DSH. Of the remainder, two-thirds present with cutting of the wrist(s) or arm(s), while all other methods account for the remaining 3–4%. These proportions have remained constant in Britain over many years and are similar in Scotland (Edinburgh) and England (Oxford) (Platt et al 1988). In the WHO/EURO study, presentations as a result of a drugs overdose occurred most frequently in the British centre (Oxford) — 85% of males and 91% of females — compared with a median and range in the other 11 countries of 66% (51–80%) for males and 82% (72–91%) for females (Michel et al 2000). There was considerable national variation in other methods employed, with some interesting local findings that might inform suicide prevention strategies, such as pesticide poisoning presentations accounting for about 20% of cases in the Hungarian centre.

There are important temporal trends apparent in the drugs used for overdoses by patients seen at British hospitals, which are due largely to changes in prescribing practices. Barbiturate hypnotics and methaqualone accounted for 40% of admissions to Edinburgh's Regional Poisoning Treatment Centre during the late 1960s, but were superseded by the benzodiazepines during the 1970s (Proudfoot & Park 1978) and had virtually ceased as a method of poisoning by the mid-1980s (Platt et al 1988). Likewise, benzodiazepine self-poisoning peaked at over 40% of referrals in the late 1970s, fell gradually during the early 1980s and then steeply, following curbs in prescribing, so that during the 1990s less than 20% of presentations involved these compounds (Hawton & Fagg 1992, McLoone & Crombie 1996). However, from 1981 to 1993, hospital presentations of paracetamol self-poisoning increased fourfold in Scotland (McLoone & Crombie 1996). The same trend was apparent in Oxford: in 1978–1979 paracetamol accounted for 17% of cases of self-poisoning; by 1983–1984 this had risen to 28% (Platt et al 1988) and in 1995 to 53% of all overdoses (Hawton et al 1997). Curiously, self-poisoning as a result of the other well-known over-the-counter analgesic, aspirin, remained constant throughout this period.

The popularity of paracetamol, particularly among younger patients, was of particular concern because of its serious medical complications. Indeed most patients admitted to liver transplant units because of fulminant hepatic failure have taken paracetamol overdoses, and this poses major ethical dilemmas because transplantable organs are a scarce resource and adequate psychiatric assessment is often prevented by encephalopathy (O'Grady et al 1991). In an attempt to stem the morbidity and mortality of paracetamol poisoning in particular, legislation was passed in September 1998 which limited the pack sizes of paracetamol, salicylates and their compounds when sold over the counter. The success of this strategy is still too early to judge, but the findings of the first major review are promising, with a 21% fall in paracetamol-related deaths, a 48% fall in aspirin-related deaths and a spectacular reduction by 66% in liver transplant rates for paracetamol poisoning in England (Hawton et al 2001).

Motives

The reasons why a patient self-harms are varied, usually multiple, and sometimes complex or even mutually contradictory; nevertheless it is important to establish the key motives (Box 27.8) to form an appropriate management plan. The motives patients report on assessment after DSH may not be what they would have said when they decided to harm themselves or during the act. Often the patient may genuinely not know what their prime motive was, particularly when the act was impulsive and in a setting of intoxication with alcohol or drugs (and alcohol is a factor in half the presentations). Some acutely suicidal patients will set out to trivialise their act to gain another opportunity to kill themselves if they manage to avoid detection. On the other hand,

Box 27.8 Motives associated with deliberate self-harm
• Wish to die • Trial by ordeal • Time out • Cry for help • Communication with others • Unbearable symptoms

Box 27.9 Environmental variables associated with deliberate self harm
• Adverse life events, especially interpersonal relationship difficulties • Unemployment • Socio-economic adversity

some patients may justify their act by infusing it with a degree of seriousness and life threat that is out of keeping with the circumstances surrounding their presentation.

Bearing these factors in mind, the main reasons patients offer for an act of DSH are as follows:

• *To die.* Wanting to die is cited as a motive by about 50% of patients who are hospitalised (Bancroft et al 1976) — but much less often by psychiatrists (Bancroft et al 1979). The same findings apply to adolescents (Hawton et al 1982a). Ambivalence about death is reported more often than an unequivocal intent to die, and this may be expressed as indifference about survival.

• *Trial by ordeal.* Again reflecting ambivalence, patients may test the benevolence of fate by gambling with their life, usually by harming themselves in circumstances in which someone may or may not discover them. Survival is then interpreted as a sign of destiny or of divine intervention, and the patient may proceed to address the problems that precipitated the act.

• *Time out.* Patients may harm themselves in a blind reaction to obtain respite from acute or chronic social difficulties, and the unpleasant thoughts and feelings these have engendered.

• *Cry for help / 'cri du coeur'.* The intent here is to enlist the assistance and sympathy of other people such as a disenchanted partner or family, or authorities such as the police or housing, usually after more acceptable methods have failed. In practice this motive is uncommon, its exaggerated importance arising from the fact it fits readily into the stereotype of DSH patients as inadequate and manipulative.

• *Communication with other people.* This is a motive reported by about 30% of DSH patients admitted to hospital (Bancroft et al 1976). These interpersonal acts take two basic forms: either the expression of a powerful emotion, particularly anger but also guilt or love, to another person or people; or ascertaining how someone regards them through their reaction to the act.

• *Unbearable symptoms.* Escape from intolerable symptoms, by death if necessary, is not uncommon and needs to be distinguished from accidental overmedication for symptom relief. The most common reasons are inadequately controlled pain and/or insomnia. Panic, akathisia, constipation and fatigue are other symptoms that may lead to DSH.

Social variables

The social variables which appear to operate most frequently in DSH include adverse life events and socio-economic factors, notably unemployment (Box 27.9).

Life events

Situational crises have long been accepted as important precursors to DSH (Kessel 1965, Lukianowicz 1972). For example, there

have been reports which have found that those who deliberately harmed themselves had experienced the recent death of a parent more commonly than other psychiatric patients (Birtchnell 1970) or suffered a variety of separations (Levi et al 1966). However, there has been a dearth of studies which have used controlled comparison of both healthy and psychiatrically ill individuals. A notable exception to this (Paykel et al 1975) found that the events encountered by those who self-harm are different from those of controls in amount, type and temporal distribution. Generally, those who self-harm experience substantially more events than the general population, with the type of event reported most often being interpersonal relationship disputes. There is evidence that those who harm themselves deliberately report more life events than depressed controls, but of a specific sort. Those who self-harm reported more events of a threatening nature, for example: more undesirable but not more desirable events; more uncontrolled events but not more controlled ones; and more events major and intermediate in upset but not more minor in upset. Paykel and colleagues concluded that these events of a threatening nature are more closely linked to DSH than to the onset of a depressive episode. Serious physical illness of self or of a close family member was also reported more often than by controls. The entrance or exit of someone from the social environment was more frequent before an episode of DSH than in the general population. As far as the timing of life events was concerned, Paykel et al found that there was a peak in the month before the episode of DSH. Overall, their findings indicate a strong and immediate relationship between episodes of DSH and adverse life events.

Unemployment

The relationship between economic instability or recession and suicidal behaviour has been a source of dispute for many years. On the relationship between DSH and unemployment, there has been a preponderance of studies using a cross-sectional design. They have shown that significantly more people who self-harm are unemployed than would be expected among the general population (Hawton et al 1982b), and DSH rates among the unemployed are always considered higher than among those in work (Bancroft et al 1975, Kessel et al 1975). Caution must be exercised in ascribing causal links, as it is likely that DSH results from the complex interaction of many factors. Clinical experience, for example, suggests that many males who self-harm lead chronically marginalised existences with lives characterised by irregular employment, petty crime, excessive alcohol consumption and loneliness. However, the role of unemployment as a major contributing factor to this situation must not be underestimated. Unemployment leads to increased interpersonal strife, hopelessness and depression, social isolation, financial hardship, loss of self-esteem. Consequently, the likelihood of an adverse event, for example loss or argument with a partner, leading to an act of DSH is greater in the context of unemployment (Platt 1984). Hawton & Rose (1986) indicate that unemployment may worsen risk factors for DSH. In order to tease out the variables, more research is needed in the context of evidence that the long-term unemployed are at a significantly higher risk of DSH.

Clinical variables

In a UK-wide survey of non-fatal suicidal behaviour (suicidal thoughts, suicide attempts, and DSH without suicidal intent) among adults aged 16–24, Meltzer et al (2002) found that at least 40% of respondents with panic, phobic symptoms, depressive ideas, obsessions and compulsions had lifetime suicidal thoughts. The corresponding proportion in the symptom-free group was 5%. In the UK survey, of those having significant levels of psychiatric symptoms (panic, phobia and depressive ideation) 20% had made a suicide attempt in their lifetime in contrast with 1% of the symptom-free population. Specifically, 25% of those with depressive symptoms had at one time attempted suicide compared with 2% of those with no such symptoms. In those diagnosed with a possible psychotic disorder approximately two-thirds had thought about suicide and just over 50% had attempted it. Four percent of the non-alcohol-dependent group had, at one time, thought about suicide. This proportion increased to 9% among those moderately dependent and rose to 27% of the severely dependent. Those who were dependent on drugs other than cannabis were around five times more likely than the non-dependent group ever to have attempted suicide (20% vs 4%). Twenty-three percent of those with phobic disorder had harmed themselves at some time. A lifetime rate of 30% for DSH was found among those with three or more neurotic disorders (including depression). Similarly, approximately 25% of those with a psychotic diagnosis had deliberately harmed themselves (without suicidal intent). Again, a significant increase in the rates of DSH was noted with increasing levels of alcohol or drug dependence.

Few studies of DSH have been based on well-defined operationalised criteria for mental disorders. One study (Suominen et al 1996) interviewed consecutive cases of DSH over 6 months and found that 98% had at least one Axis I diagnosis, with depressive syndromes more common in women and alcohol dependence more common in men. They concluded that a high proportion of DSH patients suffered from comorbid mental disorders and that comorbidity appears to play an important role in DSH, as is the case in completed suicide. Another case–control study found that, of those who made a serious attempt, 90% had a mental disorder at the time of the attempt and that there were high rates of mood disorders, substance abuse, conduct disorder or antisocial personality disorder, and non-affective psychosis. The relationship between psychiatric morbidity and suicide risk varied with age and gender. The incidence of comorbidity was high, with 57% of those who made serious suicide attempts having two or more disorders. Also, the risk of a suicide attempt increased with increasing psychiatric morbidity, i.e. those with two or more disorders had odds of serious attempts that were 90 times the odds of those with no psychiatric disorder (Beautrais et al 1996). So, it can be concluded that those who make serious attempts have high rates of mental disorder and of comorbid disorders and that subjects with high levels of psychiatric comorbidity have higher risk of serious suicide attempts.

Major depression

An examination of the risk of DSH in those inpatients with major depression found that the first 3 months after the onset of an episode of major depression and the first 5 years after the onset of major depression represented the highest risk period for attempted suicide, independent of the severity or duration of the depression. There is also some evidence which suggests that familial and genetic factors, early loss experiences and comorbid alcoholism may be associated (Malone et al 1995). Controversy surrounds whether there are clinically meaningful differences between depressed patients who deliberately harm themselves and those who do not. Large, representative case-controlled studies are required to discover whether such differences exist.

Most depressed patients who made a suicide attempt did so within the first 12 months of the depressive episode (Vieta et al 1992). The timing of suicidal behaviour in the course of major depression may indicate whether depression is a precipitant for 'latent' suicide attempters to cross the threshold to overt suicidal behaviour. If there is a biopsychological vulnerability for suicidal behaviour, then suicide attempters should manifest overt suicidal behaviour after exposure to the same or less duration and severity of depression as compared with non-attempters. Evidence indicates that, despite at least comparable levels of depression, non-attempters appear to tolerate severe depression without crossing the threshold into suicidal behaviour, whereas suicide attempters exceed the threshold during a similar depressive syndrome (Malone et al 1995). The extent to which age and duration of affective illness interact with the risk of DSH is another area under investigation. The view that the risk of DSH is highest in the early stages of the illness and decreases as the illness progresses has been challenged by results which indicate that the risk of DSH is unchanged in all age groups and throughout all stages of untreated illness (Ahrens et al 1995).

In a meta-analysis, Lester (1993) highlighted two possible trends of suicidal behaviour in unipolar and bipolar illness: an excess of subsequent completed suicides in unipolar depression and an excess of subsequent DSH in bipolar illness. Investigating suicidality in bipolar illness is beset by the major problem of which descriptive constructs are used, i.e. dimensional constructs based on symptom severity or categorical constructs which divide syndromes into discrete entities. While it is accepted that suicidality is more common in the depressive rather than the manic phase of bipolar illness, the risk in mixed states is less clear. In a study which analysed the relationship between suicidality and the affective state of bipolar patients, the severity of concurrent depressive symptoms in mania, i.e. a mixed affective state, rather than the presence of a depressive syndrome, was associated with suicidality in bipolar patients (Strakowski et al 1996).

Ultimately, depression is the most common psychiatric disorder in DSH patients and in those who commit suicide. Haw et al (2002) examined the treatment received by DSH patients with depression and their progress following DSH. Their results were as follows. Before the index episode of DSH, 37% of patients were receiving treatment from the psychiatric services and a further 33% were receiving treatment for mental health problems from their general practitioner; 49% were prescribed antidepressants (in therapeutic dosages in 94%). After the episode of DSH 89% were offered treatment with the psychiatric services, either as a new referral or continuation of treatment they were receiving prior to DSH. Of the patients who were followed-up, 36% remained in contact with the psychiatric services, 52% showed poor compliance with recommended treatment and 60% no longer fulfilled the diagnostic criteria for depression. Almost one-third reported a further episode of DSH during the follow-up period. The conclusion from this study was that all patients presenting following DSH need to be carefully screened for depressive illness. It also indicates a need for randomised controlled studies to be conducted on DSH patients with depression to determine which treatments are effective.

Personality disorder

One study which examined suicidal behaviour in those with major depression and comorbid personality disorder concluded that those with borderline personality disorder symptoms are at risk for serious suicide attempts. The presence and severity of Axis II personality disorder has been positively related to indicators of suicidality (Corbitt et al 1996). This supports previous research findings that the presence of personality disorder may increase the risk of suicidal behaviour, especially in borderline personality disorder. Group differences also supported previous findings that major depression with comorbid borderline personality disorder carries a higher risk for attempted suicide than major depression alone. Therefore, it is important to consider the severity of comorbid Cluster B personality disorder characteristics (see Ch. 23) when assessing suicide risk in those with major depression, even those who have not been categorised as having a personality disorder. This provides a salutary warning contradicting the clinical folklore that those with borderline personality disorder tend to make frequent, trivial suicidal gestures which are not highly life-threatening. Recent research findings suggest that if borderline personality disorder is comorbid with depressive disorder it can lead to serious suicide attempts. Research supports the hypothesis that the higher levels of suicidality findings in borderline personality disorder are due to a vulnerability for suicidal behaviour in these patients. The threshold for such behaviour is lowered in the presence of comorbid stressors such as major depression (Malone et al 1993).

In a recent study Haw et al (2001) explored the nature and prevalence of psychiatric and personality disorders in self-harm patients. They found that ICD-10 psychiatric disorders were diagnosed in 92% of patients, with comorbidity of psychiatric disorders in 47%. The most common diagnosis was affective disorder (72%). Personality disorder was identified in 46% of patients interviewed at follow-up, with comorbidity of psychiatric and personality disorder in 44%. This study confirms that psychiatric and personality disorders, and their comorbidity, are common in DSH patients.

Substance abuse

Aggression, impulsivity and comorbid Cluster B Axis II personality disorder are reproducible trait-related predictors of suicidal behaviour in adolescence (Brent et al 1994), and those who have these trait-related features have greater risk of comorbid alcohol and substance abuse which may also contribute to lowering the threshold for suicidal behaviour. Research comparing depressed alcoholics with non-depressed alcoholics and depressed non-alcoholics found that depression with alcoholism was associated with greater suicidality, implying that alcoholism can also lower the threshold for suicidality or is associated with other factors which underlie a lower threshold (Cornelius et al 1996).

Alcohol use has been found to increase the risk of suicidal behaviour in both alcoholic and non-alcoholic populations and is associated with about 50% of all suicides (Frances et al 1987). There is extensive use of alcohol in connection with DSH. The use of alcohol also adds to the potential danger of an overdose of psychotropic drugs because alcohol increases their toxicity; clinically, it is not unusual for unconsciousness to be attributed to alcohol alone, thus delaying medical treatment for the overdose. Indeed in the WHO/EURO study, alcohol alone accounted for 17% of male DSH presentations and 12% of female DSH presentations (Michel et al 2000).

The association of alcohol intoxication and suicidal risk has been extensively reported (Barraclough et al 1974, Goldney 1981). Among those receiving hospital treatment for the sequelae of DSH, 40–75% of males and 12–50% of females had taken alcohol at the time of the act or up to 6 hours before it (Goldney 1981, Hawton et al 1989). In a study of DSH in which alcohol was involved in an accident and emergency setting, the consumption of alcohol just before or at the time of an episode of DSH was found to be more common among young or socially isolated men with a past history of DSH. This group was less often referred to a psychiatrist, and their risk of suicide was judged to be less serious. At the end of a 5-year follow-up period, 3.3% had killed themselves, and the suicide mortality in the year following the initial attempt represented a 51-fold higher risk compared with that of the local general population; they were therefore a group at greater risk (Suokas & Lonnqvist 1995).

Psychosis

Generally, the clinical risk factors consistently associated with suicidal behaviour in patients with psychosis are: depression, hopelessness and severity of illness (Drake & Cotton 1986, Roy 1986, Addington & Addington 1992). Other clinical and demographic variables have less consistent associations, perhaps because samples have been composed of consecutive admissions and therefore vary in the distributions of illness stage and treatment experience. With regard to bipolar patients with psychotic symptoms, who have a high risk of completed suicide, a study of index admissions found they had a significantly reduced risk of DSH (Goldstein et al 1991).

On comparing schizophrenic and depressed patients, one study found that positive symptoms predicted later suicidal activity for the schizophrenic group. Deficit or negative symptoms such as psychomotor retardation, concreteness, etc. predicted later suicidal activity only for the depressed group. The general adequacy of overall functioning predicted later suicidal activity for both diagnostic categories (Kaplan & Harrow 1996).

Factors specific to women

A variety of social risk factors including divorce, illegitimacy, unemployment, family factors, education, income and other factors which affect the status of women, probably influence the prevalence of DSH among females. There is also evidence of a special relationship between premenstrual syndrome (PMS) and mood disorder (Rubinow & Schmidt 1987) in that women with PMS have a greater lifetime prevalence of affective disorder (Mackenzie et al 1986). A recent study examining the relationship between PMS and DSH found that those reporting suicidal ideas during the premenstrual phase were more commonly college students and working women rather than housewives. Depressive premenstrual syndrome symptoms were significantly more often reported by women who had suicidal ideas than those without (Chaturverdi et al 1995).

The relationship between childhood sex abuse and DSH in women was examined in a group of women who met criteria for borderline personality disorder. The vast majority of those with a history of at least two DSH episodes reported a history of some form of childhood sexual abuse. Moreover, this group engaged in acts of DSH which were more medically serious and with greater suicidal intent than those who reported no such abuse (Wagner & Linehan 1994). Asking about childhood trauma is important when examining any case of DSH, but it may have important predictive value in the case of women with borderline personality disorder. Similarly, sexual assault is associated with an increased lifetime rate of DSH (Davidson et al 1996).

Assessment

Current guidance remains that 'the consultant who has charge of the patient whether in the Accident and Emergency Department or in a ward will be responsible for ensuring that a full physical assessment is made and that before patients are discharged from hospital, a psychosocial assessment is carried out by staff specifically trained for this task' (Department of Health and Social Security 1984). This requirement took into account research which demonstrated that DSH patients who were assessed by non-psychiatrists did not appear to be at greater risk of subsequent repetition or suicide. However, the reality has been that patients were often not assessed by staff with adequate training and supervision in psychosocial assessment (including junior psychiatrists) (Owens & House 1995). A national survey of practice found little movement towards the recommendations (Butterworth & O'Grady 1989), and it was widely accepted that DSH services were in a state of disarray.

This led to an important consensus statement on minimum standards for service provision in regard to the general hospital management of adult DSH (Royal College of Psychiatrists 1994), which took into account that DSH patients might be assessed in the accident and emergency department or on an inpatient ward, and the assessment might be undertaken by psychiatric or general medical staff. The key recommendation was that each service should establish a self-harm services' planning group with a multidisciplinary membership. This group would determine specifications, policies and minimum quality; it would supervise a designated self-harm specialist clinical team, organise training and monitor the service, by audit of the case notes and aftercare arrangements. While ambitious and perhaps unrealistic in their scope, these recommendations were undoubtedly valuable. In particular they established a framework on which the assessment and management of individual patients could be based.

Surveys since this publication have found little change. A prospective review of the DHS service in four major English teaching hospitals found that 46% of the patients had had no psychosocial assessment at any time during their hospital contact: the authors concluded justifiably that these services 'remain in disarray' (Kapur et al 1998). More recently, a postal survey of all healthcare trusts in England, with a 65% response rate, found that service provision 'falls substantially below' the recommendations, with 40% of trusts having no documented policy and 58% not

having the self-harm services planning group that was the cornerstone of the College guidelines (Slinn et al 2001).

Purpose of the assessment

The purpose of the psychosocial assessment is to identify among DSH patients those who have a psychiatric illness, a high suicide risk, or potentially remediable coexisting problems such as substance misuse, interpersonal or social difficulties. The principles are those of any emergency psychiatric assessment, hence an exhaustive account of interview procedures is unnecessary. The element that is different, in terms of emphasis, is the evaluation of suicide risk, of which there are four components.

Assessing suicide risk

Recognised risk factors The sociodemographic and clinical factors associated with repetition of DSH and suicide are widely known (Box 27.10). They are of limited clinical value: they represent a statistical stereotype and, with the exception of past episodes of DSH being a useful predictor of further episodes, they have proved uniformly poor predictors of outcome in the short term. Further, these factors rarely enable the clinician to plan interventions that will reduce the risk. However, entirely disregarding established risk factors would be a mistake, mainly because their presence should act as a warning sign to the clinician that a more intensive assessment is warranted, particularly if the apparent risk seems low.

Suicidal intent An essential element in assessing suicide risk is to establish a factual account of the act itself, as well as the patient's expectations and motives. Scales of suicidal intent have been developed for use by clinical staff undertaking assessments, the most widely used being the Beck Suicide Intent Scale (Beck et al 1974). While suicidal intent is associated with medical lethality (Power et al 1985), its usefulness in predicting outcome is poor (Pallis et al 1984); it is most helpful among patients who make repeated high-intent attempts (Pierce 1981). It is also unclear how useful the dangerousness of the attempt is in predicting outcome (Hawton 1987). Plainly patients who opt for violent methods are more like-

---

Box 27.10 Features that predict suicide or repeat deliberate self-harm

Suicide
- Male sex
- Older age
- Living alone; socially isolated
- Previous DSH
- Physical illness
- Mental illness
- Substance misuse

Repeat DSH
- Unemployed
- Lower social class
- Criminal record
- Previous DSH
- High suicidal intent
- Hopelessness
- Past psychiatric history
- Substance misuse
- Non-compliance

ly to die, but this outcome may reflect greater impulsivity, copycat activity, cultural factors and ready availability rather than greater intent.

Present mental state Assessing the current psychiatric state adequately requires first and foremost a responsive and co-operative patient who is fit for interview, i.e. not drowsy, intoxicated or distressed by symptoms like pain or vomiting. Other requirements include sufficient time, a suitable milieu, the opportunity to reassess if necessary, and finally a good collateral informant, who becomes essential when the patient is unco-operative or unfit.

The approach should be methodical, serious and sensitive. In general the topic of suicidal ideation should not be broached until rapport has been established. The precise wording and directness of the initial enquiry is a matter of opinion and style; however, this should be flexible, depending on the patient's age, culture and emotional state as well as the perceived threat of suicide. Although silences should be sanctioned, unanswered questions must be returned to later on, perhaps expressed in another way. Ambiguous comments must be clarified: remarks like 'I don't want to live' or 'there is no future for me' may or may not indicate suicidal ideation; it all depends on their context. Where doubt exists or increased risk is established or suspected, asking more than once during the interview and repeating the enquiries at subsequent interviews become essential. Indicating willingness to listen to such thoughts, then or later facilitates this process. It is neither valid nor acceptable to regard suicidal risk as present or absent on the basis of a one-off enquiry such as 'Do you feel suicidal?'.

Plainly the presence of mental disorder is important to establish. Particular attention needs to be paid to indicators of depressive illness, and hopelessness has been established as an important predictor of eventual suicide in depressed patients (Beck et al 1985). Other depressive features which distinguished depressed patients who committed suicide from those who did not included insomnia, impaired memory, self-neglect and delusions; contrary to popular belief psychomotor retardation was not protective (Barraclough & Pallis 1975).

Among patients with schizophrenia, those who committed suicide were more likely to be depressed, and/or to report hopelessness or fear of mental disintegration. They also tended to have high non-delusional expectations of themselves and had struggled to adjust to their illness. Finally, the presence of akathisia and the abrupt discontinuation of medication may also increase the risk of suicide (Hawton 1987). These features probably explain why suicide among patients with schizophrenia occurs particularly in the early years of their illness and during what appears to be a quiescent phase.

With alcoholism, the majority of patients who killed themselves were concurrently depressed (Barraclough et al 1974); the same applied for patients with neurotic conditions (Sims & Prior 1978). Particularly among younger patients, personality disorder characterised by impulsivity, aggressiveness and lability of mood is prominent. Of course such individuals often abuse alcohol or drugs.

Social support Adverse social circumstances contribute to an increased risk of repetition or suicide, so it is essential to establish the circumstances from whence the patient came and, more often than not, to which they will return. Patients who live alone — particularly if this is not through choice, such as following rejection by the family or the death of a partner — are at greater risk, partly because they have nobody to seek help on their behalf or to supervise any treatment they require. This group is particularly a problem with first presentations when the circumstances are not already known to the general practitioner or the mental health or social services.

Homicide risk

Finally, when assessing suicide risk it should become automatic practice to consider the potential risk to others as well — as indeed the risk of suicide or DSH should be considered in patients who are primarily regarded as a threat to other people (Royal College of Psychiatrists 1996). Classically, the risk to others is associated with the baby of a woman who has postnatal depression, but suicide following murder is not rare and is certainly not confined to puerperal women. It is most important where children or other dependants are involved, and particularly when the break-up of a relationship is a prominent factor in the presentation.

Management

Management is determined by the outcome of the psychosocial assessment, the wishes of the patient and their family, and the availability of appropriate resources. For patients who are already known to services, communicating with the key worker and teeing up an appointment may be all that is required if the patient has not deteriorated to the extent that more intensive intervention is warranted.

DSH can be problem-solving rather than problem-indicating behaviour, so there is not always a need for further intervention. Self-harm may have a cathartic effect: for instance, the prevalence of mental disorder fell from 60% to 40% during the following week in one study in which there had usually been no other treatment (Newson-Smith & Hirsch 1979). However, others have found problem resolvers did improve on many psychological measures, yet their repetition rate was the same as those whose problems were not resolved (Sakinofsky et al 1990).

It has long been known that DSH patients have a very poor compliance rate with psychiatric follow-up, with non-attendance remaining likely even when the appointment was offered for 1–3 days later (Owens et al 1991), but a study of their consultation behaviour in primary care found DSH patients were, if anything, less likely to miss appointments than matched controls (Gorman & Masterton 1990). Hence the need for follow-up, and the acceptability and appropriateness of the arrangements are crucial considerations. Sixty percent (Newson-Smith & Hirsch 1979) to 92% (Haw et al 2001) of DSH patients have been found to have a mental disorder. Haw's study in particular found substantial psychiatric morbidity, with, notably, 70% of cases having an affective disorder, half of which were severe or psychotic. The management of patients with severe mental illness and high suicide risk is usually straightforward, in that inpatient care, under a compulsory detention order if necessary, is often the only viable option. Paradoxically, less severe presentations can prove more difficult propositions, particularly given the tendency of suicidal ideation to fluctuate.

Patients in this category may still warrant a period of inpatient psychiatric assessment, given the limitations of a single interview at a point of crisis, but the widespread pressure on psychiatric admission beds and the understandable reluctance of patients to be admitted means that other options may have to be used. For many of these patients a day hospital assessment or early outpatient appointment with the psychiatric service is appropriate, although in some services specialist psychiatric nurses have been employed to follow-up selected patients (Evans et al 1992). The nurse's role has been extended to undertake cognitive behavioural problem solving, with a reduction in depression, suicidal ideation and target problems — and possibly a reduction in repeat DSH (Salkovskis et al 1990).

If psychiatric follow-up is undertaken, the first appointment must take place within a few days of discharge; preferably it should be community based, with domiciliary visiting if necessary. Given that many patients have brief and mild mood disorders, in which case antidepressant medication confers little or no benefit, the prescription of antidepressant treatment should be restricted to those patients who have persisting moderate or severe mood illness. In these circumstances it is obviously sensible to take precautions that reduce the risk of the patient overdosing with prescribed medication. The patient's compliance with past treatment, the toxicity of the drug and the prescribing arrangements should all be taken into account. Weekly prescriptions have been advocated, particularly when antidepressants with greater fatal toxicity are being used, but this arrangement is only worthwhile if there is somebody at home to supervise the taking of the drug, as the isolated individual can quickly stockpile a lethal quantity.

Interventions to prevent repeat DSH

Specific psychological interventions to reduce the risk of repeat DSH and suicide have been the subject of a recent systematic review (Hawton et al 1998a). The samples in all studies were too small to show a statistically significant reduction in the repetition rate; the conclusions were that treatment consisting of brief, focused problem-solving therapy, brief cognitivebehaviour therapy (CBT) or interpersonal therapy (IPT) improved the patient's sense of well-being, reduced the level of psychiatric symptoms and probably reduced the rate of repetition, whereas intensive follow-up conferred no additional benefit. Most studies also reported a reduction in social problems, together with an improvement in social adjustment. In a subsequent study Guthrie and colleagues reported a dramatic reduction in repetition, from 28% to 9% ($p < 0.01$), which they attributed to their intervention (brief psychodynamic IPT) (Guthrie et al 2001).

There are two other elements a DSH service should offer: a contact arrangement in the event of crisis, and established links or referral routes to the social services and non-statutory agencies. Regarding a contact arrangement, the Bristol Green Card Scheme first demonstrated that when 'first-timers' were given a contact card which enabled them to have immediate access to on-call junior psychiatric staff, the repeat DSH admission rate was halved compared with controls although only 15% of the group used the scheme (Morgan et al 1993); but a further study in which repeaters were included found no overall benefit, and indeed found an 85% increase in repetition among repeaters against a modest reduction among first-timers (Evans et al 1999). This type of support will help some patients, perhaps more likely to be first-timers (Evans et al 1999), and if such systems are not available then the patient should be informed about the Samaritans: this is an organisation which has a vital role to play in helping the suicidal but is often disregarded by hospital services. Discussion and agreement with the patient on an arrangement for dealing with a recurrence of suicidal ideation or impulses should be a routine part of management.

Given that many DSH presentations are linked to interpersonal and social problems which lie outwith the scope of the hospital service, the satisfactory management of these patients often depends on establishing contact with community resources. An exhaustive list of the possibilities would be tiresome — the service ought to be able to put patients in touch with reputable counsellors and organisations, and should have recognised ways of dealing with common, serious problems such as homelessness, domestic violence, sexual abuse, substance misuse and bereavement.

While hospital staff may tend to trivialise DSH, it should be remembered that for many patients this act is of great personal significance, a bridge between life and death, and the doctor or nurse who undertakes their psychosocial assessment has a chance, which may be fleeting, to influence the outcome.

Prognosis

The outcome following an act of DSH is traditionally considered in terms of repeat DSH and suicide, but other causes of death are also of interest.

Repeat deliberate self-harm

British reports over the past thirty years have consistently found the proportion of first-timers among all DSH hospital admissions in the range 40–60%, which implies that about half the admissions involve repeaters (Kreitman & Casey 1988). Studies report 1–2-year follow-up rates of repeat admission in the range 12–26%, with a median of 16% (Table 27.4). In a recent systematic review of outcome the 1-year repetition rate was found to be 15% (Owens et al 2002).

Repetition is much more likely to occur early; for example Bancroft & Marsack (1977) found 10% of their sample had their first repeat within the first 3 months, 6% in the following 9 months and only a further 2% during the second year. The authors postulated three patterns of repetition were occurring: chronic repetition arising because of recurrent crises; bursts of repetition during periods of stress; and one-off repetition in severe crisis. Kreitman & Casey (1988) subdivided repeaters into 'minor repeaters', who had a lifetime history of 2–4 episodes, and 'major/grand repeaters' who had a lifetime history of 5 or more episodes. They found that

Table 27.4 UK outcome studies for hospital admission following repeat deliberate self-harm (n = 200)			
Study	Follow-up period (years)	Sample size	Repeated admission (%)
Hall et al 1998	1	8304	12
Hall et al 1998	13	8304	32
Owens et al 1994	1	992	12
Wilkinson & Smeeton 1987	1–2	1376	19
Bancroft & Marsack 1977	1	690	16
Kreitman 1977	1	847	16
	1	910	17
	1	1052	17
Buglass & Horton 1974	1	2809	16
Greer & Bagley 1971	1–2	204	26

Table 27.5   Suicide following deliberate self-harm (n = 200)

	Sample size	Follow-up (years)	Rate (%)
UK studies			
Hall et al 1998	8304	13	2.6
Hawton & Fagg 1988	1959	8	2.8
Pierce 1981	500	5	2.6
Buglass & Horton 1974	2809	1	0.8
Greer & Bagley 1971	204	1.5	2.0
Buglass & McCulloch 1970	511	3	3.3
Studies elsewhere			
De Moore & Robertson 1996	1223	18	6.7
Nordentoft et al 1993	974	10	10.6
Suokas & Lonnqvist 1991	1018	5	3.2
Ekeberg et al 1991	934	5	4.0
Nielsen et al 1990	207	5	11.6
Beck & Steer 1989	413	5–10	4.8
Rygnestad 1988	253	5	8.3

repeaters outnumbered first-episode patients among men and were marginally less frequent among women, while grand repeaters accounted for 1 in 6 men and 1 in 8 women. Repeaters with over 20 admissions accounted for 4.3% of all DSH patients in a Scottish linked data study (Hall et al 1998). Hence the multiple repeater is no rarity. Much less common are patients who are admitted frequently within a short space of time: patients with bursts of three or more admissions within a week accounted for less than 1% of the individuals admitted as a result of DSH over a 6-year period (Stocks & Scott 1991).

Suicide

The rate of death by suicide following an act of DSH is considerably increased. Studies vary in the proportion of patients who go on to commit suicide, with UK studies consistently reporting lower rates than other countries (Table 27.5). The UK results are certainly underestimates, given the constraints already described in reaching a verdict of suicide; in Hawton & Fagg's (1988) study the observed against expected rate of deaths was 23.7 for suicides, 40.2 for undetermined causes and 18.6 for accidents due to poisoning, which accords with these restrictions. A consistent finding is that the highest risk of suicide is in the first few years after DSH, and especially during the first year. However, these patients continue to be at greater risk of suicide compared with the general population for at least 20 years, and probably for the rest of their lives (De Moore & Robertson 1996). In their systematic review, Owens et al (2002) estimated the risk of suicide following DSH as between 0.5% and 2% after 1 year and above 5% after 9 years.

Other causes of death

Hawton & Fagg (1988) found that deaths from natural causes were more than double the expected number, the excess being greater among females and associated with accidents (other than due to poisoning), endocrine disorders (especially diabetes), nervous disorders and respiratory disorders. Nordentoft et al (1993) also found deaths from natural causes were 2–3 times the expected rate in a cohort of 974 patients followed up for 10 years,

with the excess being most marked among younger men. Alcohol-related conditions, digestive disorders, sudden unexplained deaths and a ragbag of single cases of rare diseases were associated. Hall et al (1998) confirmed excess deaths among DSH patients from natural causes (especially neurological, endocrine and gastrointestinal disorders) as well as three- or fourfold increases from accidents and homicides.

REFERENCES

Addington D E, Addington J M 1992 Attempted suicide and depression in schizophrenia Acta Psychiatrica Scandinavica 85:288–291

Ahrens B, Berghofer A, Wolf T, Muller-Oerlinghausen B 1995 Suicide attempts, age and duration of illness in recurrent affective disorders. Journal of Affective Disorders 36:43–49

Allebeck P, Bolund C 1991 Suicides and suicide attempts in cancer patients. Psychological Medicine 21:979–984

Appleby L 1991 Suicide during pregnancy and in the first postnatal year. British Medical Journal 302:137–140

Appleby L 1992 Suicide risk in psychiatric patients: risk and prevention. British Journal of Psychiatry 161:749–758

Appleby L, Shaw J, Amos T, McDonnell R 1999 Safer services: Report of the National Confidential Inquiry into Suicide and Homicide by People with Mental Illness. The Stationery Office, London

Appleby L, Shaw J, Sherrat J et al 2001. Safety first: Five-year report of the National Confidential Inquiry into Suicide and Homicide by People with Mental Illness. Department of Health, London

Arango V, Ernsberger P, Marzuk P M et al 1990 Autoradiographic demonstration of increased serotonin 5-HT 2 and beta adrenergic receptor binding sites in the brain of suicide victims. Archives of General Psychiatry 47:1038–1047

Arango V, Ernsberger P, Sved A F, Mann J J 1993 Quantitative autoradiography of alpha 1 and alpha 2 adrenergic receptors in the cerebral cortex of controls and suicide victims. Brain Research 630:271–282

Arango V, Underwood M D, Mann J J 1996 Fewer pigmented locus coeruleus neurons in suicide victims: preliminary results. Biological Psychiatry 39:112–120

Arato M, Banki C, Bissette G, Nemeroff C 1989 Elevated CSF CRF in suicide victims. Biological Psychiatry 35:355–359

Asberg M, Traskman L, Sjostrand L 1976 Monoamine metabolites in CSF and suicidal behaviour. Archives of General Psychiatry 33:1193–1197

Bancroft J, Marsack P 1977 The repetitiveness of self-poisoning and self-injury. British Journal of Psychiatry 131:394–399

Bancroft J, Skrimshire A, Reynolds F 1975 Self-poisoning and self-injury in the Oxford area: epidemiological aspects 1969–1973. British Journal of Preventive and Social Medicine 29:170–177

Bancroft J, Skrimshire A M, Simkins 1976 The reasons people give for taking overdoses. British Journal of Psychiatry 128:538–548

Bancroft J, Hawton K, Simkin S et al 1979 The reasons people give for taking overdoses: a further inquiry. British Journal of Medical Psychology 52:353–365

Banki C, Bissette J, Arato M et al 1987 CSF CRF-like immunoreactivity in depression and schizophrenia. American Journal of Psychiatry 144:873–877

Barraclough B M 1978 Reliability of violent death certification in one coroner's district. British Journal of Psychiatry 132:39–41

Barraclough B, Pallis D J 1975 Depression followed by suicide: a comparison of depressed suicides with living depressives. Psychological Medicine 5:55–61

Barraclough B, Bunch J, Nelson B, Sainsbury P 1974 A hundred cases of suicide: clinical aspects. British Journal of Psychiatry 125:355–373

Beautrais A L, Joyce P R, Mulder R T et al 1996 Prevalence and comorbidity of mental disorders in persons making serious suicide attempts: a case–control study. American Journal of Psychiatry 153:1009–1014

Beck A T, Steer R A 1989 Clinical predictors of eventual suicide: a 5- to 10-year prospective study of suicide attempters. Journal of Affective Disorders 17:203–209

Beck A T, Herman I, Schuyler D 1974 Development of suicidal intent scales. In: Beck A T, Resnik H L P, Lettieri D (eds) The prediction of suicide. Charles Press, Maryland, p 45–56

Beck A T, Kovacs M, Weissman A 1975 Hopelessness and suicidal behaviour: an overview. Journal of the American Medical Association 234:1146–1149

Beck A T, Rush A J, Shaw B F, Emery G 1979 Cognitive therapy for depression; a treatment manual. Guilford Press, New York

Beck A T, Steer R, Kovacs M, Garrison B 1985 Hopelessness and eventual suicide: a 10 year prospective study of patients hospitalised with suicidal ideation. American Journal of Psychiatry 145:559–563

Biegon A, Israeli M 1988 Regionally selective increases in beta adrenergic receptor density in the brains of suicide victims. Brain Research 442:199–203

Birtchnell J 1970 The relationship between attempted suicide, depression and parent death. British Journal of Psychiatry 116:307–313

Black D W, Warrak G, Winokur G 1985 The Iowa record linkage study I–III. Archives of General Psychiatry 42:71–88

Brent D A, Johnson B A, Perper J et al 1994 Personality disorder, personality traits, impulsive violence and completed suicide in adolescents. Journal of the American Academy of Child and Adolescent Psychiatry 33:1080–1086

Brown M, Barraclough B 1997 Epidemiology of suicide pacts in England and Wales, 1988–92. British Medical Journal Psychiatry 315:286–287

Buda M, Tsuang M T 1990 The epidemiology of suicide: implications for clinical practice. In: Blumenthal S J, Kupfer D J (eds) Suicide over the life cycle: risk factors, assessment and treatment of suicidal patients. American Psychiatric Association Press, Washington, DC, p 17–38

Buglass D, Horton J 1974 The repetition of parasuicide: a comparison of three cohorts. British Journal of Psychiatry 125:168–174

Buglass D, McCulloch J W 1970 Further suicidal behaviour: the development and validation of predictive scales. British Journal of Psychiatry 116:483–491

Butterworth E, O'Grady T J 1989 Trends in the assessment of cases of deliberate self-harm. Health Trends 21:61

Cattell H, Jolley D J 1995 One hundred cases of suicide in elderly people. British Journal of Psychiatry 166:451–457

Cavanagh J T O, Owens, D G C, Johnstone, E C 1999 Suicide and undetermined death in South East Scotland: a case control study using the psychological autopsy method. Psychological Medicine 29:1141–1149

Cavanagh J T, Carson A, Sharpe M, Lawrie S, 2003 Psychological autopsy studies of suicide: a systematic review. Psychological Medicine 33:395–405

Chaturverdi S K, Chandra P S, Gururaj G et al 1995 Suicidal ideas during the premenstrual phase. Journal of Affective Disorders 34:193–199

Cheng A T A 1995 Mental illness and suicide. Archives of General Psychiatry 52:594–603

Cheng A T, Chen TH, Chen C C, Jenkins R 2000 Psychosocial and psychiatric risk factors for suicide: case-control psychological autopsy study. British Journal of Psychiatry 177:360–365

Corbitt E M, Malone K M, Haas G L, Mann J J 1996 Suicidal behaviour in patients with major depression and comorbid personality disorders. Journal of Affective Disorders 39:61–72

Cornelius J R, Salloum I M, Day N L et al 1996 Patterns of suicidality and alcohol use in alcoholics with major depression. Journal of Alcoholism, Clinical and Experimental Research 20:1451–1455

Cotton P, Drake R, Gates C 1985 Critical treatment issues in suicide among schizophrenics. Hospital and Community Psychiatry 36:534–536

Davidson J R T, Hughes D C, George L K, Blazer D G 1996 The association of sexual assault and attempted suicide within the community. Archives of General Psychiatry 53:550–555

De Leo D, Evans R, Neulinger K 2002 Hanging, firearm and non-domestic gas suicides among males: a comparative study. Australian and New Zealand Journal of Psychiatry 36:183–189

De Moore G M, Robertson A R 1996 Suicide in the 18 years after deliberate self harm: a prospective study. British Journal of Psychiatry 169:489–494

De Paermentier F, Cheetham S C, Crompton M R et al 1990 Brain beta adrenoceptor binding sites in antidepressant-free depressed suicide victims. Brain Research 525:71–77

Department of Health and Social Security 1984 The management of deliberate self-harm. HN(84) 25 DHSS, London

Diekstra R F W 1982 Epidemiology of attempted suicide in the EEC. In: Wilmotte J, Mendlewicz J (eds) New trends in suicide prevention. Bibliotheca Psychiatrica, Karger, Basel, p 1–16

Diekstra R F W 1996 The epidemiology of suicide and parasuicide. Archives of Suicide Research 2:1–29

Dolman W F G 1994 The ceroner's response. In: Jenkins R, Griffiths S, Wiley I et al (eds) The prevention of suicide. HMSO, London, p 135–139

Donovan S, Clayton A, Beeharry M et al 2000 Deliberate self harm and antidepressant drugs. British Journal of Psychiatry 177:551–556

Drake R, Cotton P 1986 Depression, hopelessness and suicide in chronic schizophrenia. British Journal of Psychiatry 148:554–559

Duberstein P R, Conwell Y, Caine E D 1993 Interpersonal stressors, substance abuse and suicide. Journal of Nervous and Mental Disorders 181:80–85

Ekeberg O, Ellingsen O, Jacobsen D 1991 Suicide and other causes of death in a five-year follow-up of patients treated for self-poisoning in Oslo. Acta Psychiatrica Scandinavica 83:432–437

Evans M, Cox C, Turnbull G 1992 Parasuicide response. Nursing Times 88:34–36

Evans M, Morgan H, Hayward A, Gunnell D 1999 Crisis telephone consultation for deliberate self-harm patients: effects on repetition. British Journal of Psychiatry 175:23–27

Farmer R 1988 Assessing the epidemiology of suicide and parasuicide. British Journal of Psychiatry 153:16–20

Farmer R, Tranah T, O'Donnell I, Catalan J 1992 Railway suicide: the psychological effects on drivers. Psychological Medicine 22:407–414

Fawcett J, Scheftner W A, Fogg L et al 1990 Time-related precipitators of suicide in major affective disorders. American Journal of Psychiatry 147:1189–1194

Foster T, Gillespie K, McClelland R 1997 Mental disorders and suicide in Northern Ireland. British Journal of Psychiatry 170:447–452

Frances R, Franklin J, Flavin D 1987 Suicide and alcoholism. American Journal of Drug and Alcohol Abuse 13:327–341

Garcia-Sevilla J A, Escriba P V, Sastre M et al 1996 Immunodetection and quantitation of Imidazoline receptor proteins in platelets of patients with major depression and in brains of suicide victims. Archives of General Psychiatry 53:803–810

Geddes J R, Juszczak E 1995 Period trends in rate of suicide in first 28 days after discharge from psychiatric hospital in Scotland, 1968–1992. British Medical Journal 311:357–360

Goldney R 1981 Alcohol in association with suicide and attempted suicide in young women. Medical Journal of Australia 2:195–197

Goldstein R B, Black D W, Nasrallah A, Winokur G 1991 The prediction of suicide: sensitivity, specificity, and predictive value of a multivariate model applied to suicide among 1906 patients with affective disorders. Archives of General Psychiatry 48:418–422

Goodwin F K, Jamison K R 1990 Manic depressive illness. Oxford University Press, Oxford

Gore S 1999 Suicide in prisons. British Journal of Psychiatry 175:50–55

Gorman D, Masterton G 1990 General practice consultation patterns before and after intentional overdose: a matched control study. British Journal of General Practice 40:102–105

Greer S, Bagley C 1971 Effect of psychiatric intervention in attempted suicide. British Medical Journal 1:310–312

Gross-Isseroff R, Dillon K A, Fieldust S J, Biegon A 1990 Autoradiographic analysis of alpha-1 noradrenergic receptors in the human brain postmortem. Archives of General Psychiatry 47:1049–1053

Gunnell D, Frankel S 1994 Prevention of suicide: aspirations and evidence. British Medical Journal 308:1227–1233

Guthrie E, Kapur N, Mackway-Jones K et al 2001 Randomised controlled trial of brief psychological intervention after deliberate self poisoning. British Medical Journal 323:135–138

Hall D, O'Brien F, Stark C et al 1998 Thirteen year follow-up of deliberate self-harm, using linked data. British Journal of Psychiatry 172:239–242

Harris E C, Barraclough G 1997 Suicide as an outcome for mental disorders. British Journal of Psychiatry 170:205–228

Haw C, Hawton K, Houston K, Townsend E 2001 Psychiatric and personality disorders in deliberate self-harm patients. British journal of Psychiatry 178:48–54

Haw C, Houston K, Townsend E, Hawton K 2002 Deliberate self-harm patients with depressive disorders: treatment and outcome Journal of Affective Disorders 70(1):57–65

Hawton K 1987 Assessment of suicide risk. British Journal of Psychiatry 150:145–153

Hawton K, Fagg J 1988 Suicide, and other causes of death, following attempted suicide. British Journal of Psychiatry 152:359–366

Hawton K, Fagg J 1992 Trends in deliberate self poisoning and self injury in Oxford, 1976–1990. British Medical Journal 3–4:1409–1411

Hawton K, Goldacre M 1982 Hospital admission for adverse effects on medical agents (mainly self-poisoning) among adolescents in the Oxford region. British Journal of Psychiatry 141:166–170

Hawton K, Rose N 1986 Unemployment and attempted suicide among men in Oxford. Health Trends 18:29–32

Hawton K, Cole D, O'Grady J, Osborn M 1982a Motivational aspects of deliberate self poisoning in adolescents. British Journal of Psychiatry 141:286–291

Hawton K et al 1982b Adolescents who take overdoses; their characteristics, problems and contact with helping agencies. British Journal of Psychiatry 140:118–123

Hawton K, Fagg J, McKeown S 1989 Alcoholism, alcohol and attempted suicide. Alcohol 24:3–9

Hawton K, Houston K, Shepperd R 1999 Suicide in young people. British Journal of Psychiatry 175:271–276

Hawton K, Fagg J, Simpkin S et al 1998b Methods used for suicide by Farmers in England and Wales. British Journal of Psychiatry 173:320–324

Hawton K, Fagg J, Simkin S 1997 Trends in deliberate self-harm in Oxford, 1985–1995 British Journal of Psychiatry 171:556–560

Hawton K, Arensman E, Townsend E et al 1998a Deliberate self-harm: systematic review of efficacy of psychosocial and pharmacological treatments in preventing repetition. British Medical Journal 317:441–447

Hawton K, Townsend E, Deeks J et al 2001 Effects of legislation restricting pack sizes of paracetamol and salicylate on self poisoning in the United Kingdom: before and after study. British Medical Journal 322:1203–1207

Heikkinen M E, Isometsa E T, Marttunen M H et al 1995 Social factors in suicide. British Journal of Psychiatry 167:747–753

Hodelet N, Hughson M 2001 What to do when a patient commits suicide. Psychiatric Bulletin 25:43–45

Holding T A, Barraclough B M 1978 Undetermined deaths — suicide or accident? British Journal of Psychiatry 133:542–549

Ingraham, L J, Kety S S 2000 Adoption studies of schizophrenia. American Journal of Medical Genetics 97(1):18–22

Isometsa E, Lonnqvist JK 1998 Suicide attempts preceding suicide. British Journal of Psychiatry 173:531–535

Jick S S, Dean A D, Jick H 1995 Antidepressants and suicide. British Medical Journal 310:215–218

Kaplan K J, Harrow M 1996 Positive and negative symptoms as risk factors for later suicidal activity in schizophrenics versus depressives. Suicide and Life-Threatening Behaviour 26:105–121

Kapur N, House A, Creed F et al 1998 Management of deliberate self-poisoning in adults in four teaching hospitals: descriptive study. British Medical Journal 316:831–832

Kendell R E 1991 Suicide in pregnancy and the puerperium. British Medical Journal 302:126–127

Kessel A, Nicholson A, Graves G, Krupinski J 1975 Suicidal attempts in an outer region of metropolitan Melbourne and in a provincial region of Victoria. Australian and New Zealand Journal of Psychiatry 9:255–261

Kessel N 1965 Self-poisoning I. British Medical Journal 2:1265–1270, 1336–1340

Kessler R C, Borges G, Walters E E 1999 Prevalence of and risk factors for lifetime suicide attempts in the National Comorbidity Survey. Archives of General Psychiatry 56(7):617–626

Kreitman N 1973 Social and clinical aspects of suicide and attempted suicide. In: Forrest A (ed) A companion to psychiatric studies. Churchill Livingstone, Edinburgh, vol 1, p 38–63

Kreitman N 1976 The coal gas story. British Journal of Preventive and Social Medicine 30:86–93

Kreitman N 1977 Parasuicide. Wiley, London

Kreitman N, Casey P 1988 Repetition of parasuicide: an epidemiological and clinical study. British Journal of Psychiatry 153:792–800

Kreitman N, Schreiber M 1979 Parasuicide in young Edinburgh women, 1968–75. Psychological Medicine 9:469–479

Kreitman N, Carstairs V, Duffy J 1991 Association of age and social class with suicide among men in Great Britain. Journal of Epidemiology and Community Health 45:195–202

Lester D 1993 Suicidal behaviour in bipolar and unipolar affective disorders: a meta-analysis. Journal of Affective Disorders 27:117–121

Lester D 1996 Testing Durkheim's theory of suicide: a comment (letter.) European Archives of Psychiatry and Clinical Neuroscience 246:112–113

Lester D, Murrell M E 1982 The preventive effect of strict gun control laws on suicide and homicide. Suicide and Life-Threatening Behaviour 12:131–140

Levi L D, Fales C H, Stein M et al 1966 Separation and attempted suicide. Archives of General Psychiatry 15:158–164

Linehan M M, Camper P, Chile J A, 1987 Interpersonal problem solving and parasuicide. Cognitive Therapy Research 11:1–13

Linkowski P, Wettere J, van Kerkhofs M 1983 Thyrostrophin response to thyrostimulin in affectively ill women: relationship to suicidal behaviour. British Journal of Psychiatry 143:401–405

Linkowski P, Wettere J, van Kerkhofs M 1984 Violent suicidal behaviour and the TRH-TSH test: a clinical outcome test. Neuropsychobiology 12:19–22

Little K Y, Clark T B, Ranc J, Duncan G E 1993 Beta adrenergic receptor binding in frontal cortex from suicide victims. Biological Psychiatry 34:596–605

Lukianowicz N 1972 Suicidal behaviour: an attempt to modify the environment. British Journal of Psychiatry 121:387–390

McClure GMG 2000 Changes in suicide in England and Wales, 1960–1997. British Journal of Psychiatry 176:64–67

McGlashan T H 1987 Borderline personality disorder and unipolar affective disorder; long-term effects of comorbidity. Journal of Nervous and Mental Disorders 175:467–473

Mackenzie T B, Wilcox K, Baron H 1986 Lifetime prevalence of psychiatric disorders in women with premenstrual difficulties. Journal of Affective Disorders 10:15–19

McLoone P, Crombie I K 1996 Hospitalisation for deliberate self-poisoning in Scotland from 1981 to 1993: trends in rates and types of drugs used. British Journal of Psychiatry 169:81–85

Malmberg A, Simkin S, Hawton K 1999 Suicide in farmers. British Journal of Psychiatry 175:103–105

Malone K M, Haas G L, Sareney J A, Mann J J 1993 Familial effects on attempted suicide and depression. American Psychiatric Association annual meeting, San Francisco, Ca, NR 119

Malone K M, Haas G L, Sweeney J A, Mann J J 1995 Major depression and the risk of attempted suicide. Journal of Affective Disorders 34:173–185

Malone K M, Oquendo M A, Haas GL et al 2000 Protective factors against suicidal acts in major depression: reasons for living. American Journal of Psychiatry 155(7):1084–1088

Mann JJ 1998 The neurobiology of suicide. Nature Medicine 4:25–30

Mann J J, Stanley M, McBride P A, McEwen B S 1986 Increased serotonin-2 and beta adrenergic receptor binding in the frontal cortices of suicide victims. Archives of General Psychiatry 43:954–959

Mann J J, Arango V, Marzuk P M et al 1989 Evidence for the 5-HT hypothesis of suicide: a review of post-mortem studies. British Journal of Psychiatry 155(suppl.8):7–14

Mann J J, Underwood M D, Arango V 1994 Postmortem studies of suicide victims. In: Watson S J (ed) Biology of schizophrenia and affective disease. Raven, New York

Maris R W 2002 Suicide. Lancet 360:319–326

Mayou R, Hawton K 1986 Psychiatric disorder in the general hospital. British Journal of Psychiatry 149:172–190

Meana J J, Garcia-Sevilla J A 1987 Increased alpha adrenoceptor density in the frontal cortex of depressed suicide victims. Journal of Neural Transmission 70:377–381

Meltzer H, Lader D, Corbin T et al 2002, Non-fatal suicidal behaviour among adults aged 16–74 in Great Britain. Office of National Statistics, The Stationery Office, London

Mendonca J D, Holden R R 1996 Are all suicidal ideas closely linked to hopelessness? Acta Psychiatrica Scandinavica 93:246–251

Michel K, Ballinari P, Bille-Brahe U et al 2000 Methods used for parasuicide: results of the WHO/EURO Multicentre Study on Parasuicide. Social Psychiatry and Psychiatric Epidemiology 35:156–163

Modestin J, Kopp W 1988 Study on suicide in depressed in-patients. Journal of Affective Disorders 15:157–162

Moens G F G 1990 Aspects of the epidemiology and prevention of suicide. Leuven University Press, Leuven

Morgan H G, Jones E M, Owen J H 1993 Secondary prevention of non-fatal deliberate self harm: the green card study. British Journal of Psychiatry 163:111–112

Mortensen P B, Agerbo E, Ericson T et al 2000 Psychiatric illness and risk factors for suicide in Denmark. Lancet 355:9–12

Moscicki E 2001 Epidemiology of suicide. In: Goldsmith S (ed) Risk factors for suicide. National Academy Press, Washington, DC, p 1–4

Muldoon M, Manuck S, Mathews K 1990 Lowering cholesterol concentrations and mortality: a quantitative review of primary prevention trials. British Medical Journal 301:309–314

Murphy G E, Robins E 1967 Social factors in suicide. Journal of the American Medical Association 199:303–308

Murphy G E, Wetzel R D 1990 The lifetime risk of suicide in alcoholism. Archives of General Psyhiatry 47:383–392

Nemeroff C, Owens M, Bissette G 1988 Reduced CRF binding sites in the frontal cortex of suicide victims. Archives of General Psychiatry 45:577–579

Newson-Smith J G B, Hirsch S R 1979 Psychiatric symptoms in self-poisoning patients. Psychological Medicine 9:493–500

Nielsen B, Wang A G, Bille-Brahe U 1990 Attempted suicide in Denmark, IV: a five-year follow-up. Acta Psychiatrica Scandinavica 81:250–254

Nordentoft M, Breum L, Munck L K et al 1993 High mortality by natural and unnatural causes: a 10 year follow up study of patients admitted to a poisoning treatment centre after suicide attempts. British Medical Journal 306:1637–1641

O'Donnell I, Farmer R 1995 The limitations of official suicide statistics. British Journal of Psychiatry 166:458–461

O'Donnell I, Farmer R, Catalan J 1996 Explaining suicide: the views of survivors of serious suicide attempts. British Journal of Psychiatry 168:780–786

O'Grady J G, Wendon J, Tan K C et al 1991 Liver transplantation after paracetamol overdose. British Medical Journal 303:221–223

Owens D, House A 1995 Assessment of deliberate self-harm in adults. Advances in Psychiatric Treatment 1:124–130

Owens D, Dennis M, Jones S et al 1991 Self-poisoning patients discharged from accident and emergency departments: risk factors and outcome. Journal of the Royal College of Physicians of London 25:218–222

Owens D, Dennis M, Read S, Davis N 1994 Outcome of deliberate self-poisoning: an examination of risk factors for repetition. British Journal of Psychiatry 165:797–801

Owens D, Horrocks J, House A 2002 Fatal and non-fatal repetition of self-harm: systematic review. British Journal of Psychiatry 181:193–199

Pallis D J, Gibbons S, Pierce D W 1984 Estimating suicide risk among attempted suicides, II: Efficiency of predictive scales after the event. British Journal of Psychiatry 144:139–148

Paykel E S, Dowlatshani D 1988 Life events and mental disorder. In: Fisher S, Reason J (eds) Handbook of life stress, cognition and health. Wiley, Chichester, p 241–263

Paykel E S, Prusoff B A, Myers J K 1975 Suicide attempts and recent life events. Archives of General Psychiatry 32:327–333

Phillips M R, Yang G, Zhang Y et al 2002 Risk factors for suicide in China: a national case-control psychological autopsy study. Lancet 360(9347):1728–1736

Pierce D W 1981 The predictive validation of a suicide intent scale: a five year follow-up. British Journal of Psychiatry 139:391–396

Platt S 1984 Unemployment and suicidal behaviour: a review of the literature. Social Science & Medicine 19:93–115

Platt S, Kreitman N 1990 Long-term trends in parasuicide and unemployment in Edinburgh 1968–1987. Social Psychiatry and Psychiatric Epidemiology 25:56–61

Platt S, Hawton K, Kreitman N et al 1988 Recent clinical and epidemiological trends in parasuicide in Edinburgh and Oxford: a tale of two cities. Psychological Medicine 18:405–418

Platt S, Bille-Brahe U, Kerhof A et al 1992 Parasuicide in Europe: the WHO/EURO multicentre study on parasuicide, I: Introduction and preliminary analysis for 1989. Acta Psychiatrica Scandinavica 85 97–104

Pounder D J 1991 Changing patterns of male suicide in Scotland. Forensic Science International 51:79–87

Power K G, Cooke D J, Brooks D N 1985 Life stress, medical lethality, and suicidal intent. British Journal of Psychiatry 147:655–659

Pritchard C 1988 Suicide, gender and unemployment in the British Isles and the EEC 1974–85. Social Psychiatry and Psychiatric Epidemiology 23:85–89

Prosser D 1996 Suicides by burning in England and Wales. British Journal of Psychiatry 168:175–182

Proudfoot A T, Park J 1978 Changing pattern of drugs used for self-poisoning. British Medical Journal 1:90–93

Qin P, Agerbo E, Westergard-Neilsen N et al 2000 Gender differences in risk factors for suicide in Denmark. British Journal of Psychiatry 177:546–550

Rhimer Z 1996 Strategies of suicide prevention focus on health care. Journal of Affective Disorders 39:83–91

Rich C L, Motooka M S, Fowler R C, Young D 1988 Suicide by psychotics. Biological Psychiatry 23:595–601

Roy A 1982 Risk factors for suicide in psychiatric patients. Archives of General Psychiatry 39:1089–1095

Roy A 1986 Depression, attempted suicide and suicide in patients with chronic schizophrenia. Psychiatric Clinics of North America 9:193–207

Roy A 1994 Recent biological studies on suicide. Suicide and Life-Threatening Behaviour 24:10–14

Roy A, Draper R 1995 Suicide among psychiatric hospital in-patients. Psychological Medicine 25:199–202

Roy A, Dejong J, Lamparski D et al 1991 Depression among alcoholics. Archives of General Psychiatry 48:428–432

Royal College of Psychiatrists 1994 The general hospital management of adult deliberate self-harm: a consensus statement on standards for service provision. CR 32. Royal College of Psychiatrists, London

Royal College of Psychiatrists 1996 Assessment and clinical management of risk of harm to other people. CR53. Royal College of Psychiatrists, London

Rubinow D R, Schmidt P J 1987 Mood disorders and the menstrual cycle. Journal of Reproductive Medicine 32:389–394

Rutz W, von Knorring L, Walinder J 1989 Frequency of suicide on Gotland after systematic postgraduate education of general practitioners. Acta Psychiatrica Scandinavica 80:151–154

Rutz W, von Knorring L, Walinder J 1992 Long term effects of an educational programme for general practitioners given by the Swedish Committee for the Prevention and Treatment of Depression. Acta Psychiatrica Scandinavica 85:83–88

Rygnestad T 1988 A prospective 5-year follow-up study of self-poisoned patients. Acta Psychiatrica Scandinavica 77:328–331

Sakinofsky I, Roberts R S, Brown Y et al 1990 Problem resolution and repetition of parasuicide: a prospective study. British Journal of Psychiatry 156:395–399

Salkovskis P M, Atha C, Storer D 1990 Cognitive behavioural problem solving in the treatment of patients who repeatedly attempt suicide: a controlled trial. British Journal of Psychiatry 157:871–876

Sims A, Prior P 1978 The pattern of mortality in severe neuroses. British Journal of Psychiatry 133:299–302

Slinn R, King A, Evans J 2001 A national survey of the hospital services for the management of adult deliberate self-harm. Psychiatric Bulletin 25:53–55

Stockmeier C A, Meltzer H Y 1991 Beta adrenergic receptor binding in frontal cortex of suicide victims. Biological Psychiatry 29:183–191

Stocks R, Scott A I F 1991 What happens to patients who frequently harm themselves? A retrospective one-year outcome study. British Journal of Psychiatry 158:375–378

Strakowski S M, McElroy S L, Keck P E, West S A 1996 Suicidality among patients with mixed and manic bipolar disorder. American Journal of Psychiatry 153:674–676

Sundman I, Allard P, Eriksson A, Marcusson J 1997 GABA uptake sites in frontal cortex from suicide victims and in aging. Neuropsychobiology 35:11–15

Suokas J, Lonnqvist J 1991 Outcome of attempted suicide and psychiatric consultation: risk factors and suicide mortality during a five-year follow-up. Acta Psychiatrica Scandinavica 84:545–549

Suokas J, Lonnqvist J 1995 Suicide attempts in which alcohol is involved; a special group in general hospital emergency rooms. Acta Psychiatrica Scandinavica 91:36–40

Suominen K, Henriksson M, Suokas J et al 1996 Mental disorders and comorbidity in suicide. Acta Psychiatric Scandinavica 94:234–240

Vaillant G E, Blumenthal S J 1990 Introduction: suicide over the life cycle–riser factors and lifespan development. In: Blumenthal S J, Kupfer D J (eds) Suicide over the life cycle. American Psychiatric Press, Washington, DC p 1–16

Vieta E, Nieto E, Gasto C, Cirera E 1992 Serious suicide attempts in affective patients. Journal of Affective Disorders 24:147–152

Wagner A W, Linehan M M 1994 Relationship between childhood sexual abuse and topography of parasuicide among women with borderline personality disorder. Journal of Personality Disorders 8:1–9

Warr P 1987 Unemployment and mental health. Oxford University Press, Oxford

Weissman M M 1993 The epidemiology of personality disorders: a 1990 update. Journal of Personality Disorders 7(suppl 1):44–62

Weissman M M, Bland R C, Canino G J et al 1999 Prevalence of suicide ideation and suicide attempts in nine countries. Psychological Medicine 29:9–17

Whitely, E, Gunnell D, Dorling D, Davey Smith G 1999 Ecological study of social fragmentation, poverty and suicide. British Medical Journal 319:1034–1037

Wilkinson G, Smeeton N 1987 The repetition of parasuicide in Edinburgh 1980–1981. Social Psychiatry 22:14–19

Yousaf F, Hawthorne M, Sedgwick P 2002 Impact of patient suicide on psychiatric trainees. Psychiatric Bulletin 26:53–55

28 Psychiatry in relation to other areas of medicine

Michael Sharpe

This chapter is devoted to a consideration of how our understanding of the nature and treatment of the psychiatric disorders considered elsewhere in this book has to be adapted if it is to be successfully applied to the detection, diagnosis, assessment and management of patients attending non-psychiatric medical services. The chapter is organised as follows:

1. Introduction and overview;
2. The presentation of psychiatric disorder in medical settings;
3. The coexistence of psychiatric and medical conditions;
4. General principles of management;
5. Specific psychiatric disorders, including somatoform disorders and their management;
6. Psychiatric services for patients attending general medical services.

The chapter should be read in conjunction with others in this book, especially the chapters on deliberate self-harm and organic disorders.

INTRODUCTION AND OVERVIEW

Conceptual issues

It is useful to begin by considering what we mean by 'psychiatric disorder', how it differs from 'medical conditions', and the implications of this distinction.

Body and mind

Psychiatric disorders are, in a literal sense, simply those syndromes defined in the psychiatric diagnostic classifications of ICD-10 and DSM-IV. The designation of an illness as psychiatric (as opposed to medical or surgical) simply means that it has been traditionally regarded as lying within the scope of that subspecialty of medicine. However, further assumptions have been made. Psychiatric disorders have generally been assumed to be 'mental' in nature. The allocation of certain illnesses to a 'mental' as opposed to a 'physical' category has reflected the absence of known bodily pathology, and a tendency for the illness to present with disturbed mental states and behaviour, or both. The underlying assumption of this dichotomous classification, that disorders of the mind can be meaningfully separated from disease of the body, and that mental illnesses are consequently fundamentally different entities from physical ones, has been called mind–body dualism. The idea of mind–body dualism is commonly attributed to the writings of the philosopher Descartes. So-called Cartesian dualism has and continues to exert a profound influence on Western medical thinking, several aspects of which are illustrated below. It is especially important that the psychiatrist working in general medical settings be aware of the various manifestations of dualism if he or she is to avoid falling into the traps they give rise to.

Conceptual dualism By and large a dualistic approach works adequately well in day-to-day practice; patients who present with psychological problems are assumed to have 'psychopathology' and receive psychiatric treatments whereas those presenting with somatic symptoms are considered to have somatic pathology and are treated medically or surgically. Practical difficulties arise however when clinical problems do not fit readily into this dichotomous scheme. The two principal problems are shown in Table 28.1.

Somatisation refers to the problem that is posed by patients who present with somatic symptoms with no evidence of somatic pathology. These patients may fall into *neither* major category of illness. It is unclear whether their illness should be categorised as a somatic one (with presumed but unidentified somatic pathology) or as a psychological one (with assumed psychopathology). One common solution is to allocate these patients to psychiatry by proposing that their somatic symptoms are in fact a reflection of psychopathology, the somatic manifestation occurring because of a process called 'somatisation'. Somatisation is a theoretical device to explain how psychological states can manifest as somatic symptoms. It was originally proposed by a psychoanalyst (Steckel 1943). In recent times the value of this concept has been questioned, both because it remains unproven and because it is potentially unhelpful clinically — for example if it encourages neglect of the patient's somatic symptoms in favour of a search for psychopathology. Such an approach is frequently rejected by patients as both a denial of their somatic illness experience and an unwelcome accusation of mental illness. The main alternative solution is to regard such patients as genuinely medical on the assumption that they have actual, albeit undetected, somatic pathology. This alternative approach also has disadvantages. Although it is more congruent with the patient's illness experience, it may lead to relentless medical investigation and an inaccurate and unhelpful assumption that they have disease pathology that can only be treated medically or surgically. In practice neither approach is sustainable, leading to uncertainty about whether the patient should be best regarded as medical or psychiatric. This often results in their being rejected by both medicine and psychiatry and being relegated to a medical 'no man's land'. The confusion, controversy and conflict that results has been particularly well illustrated by both medical and lay literature about the condition called chronic fatigue syndrome (CFS) or myalgic encephalomyelitis (ME) (Sharpe 2002).

Table 28.1 The traditional 'dualistic' categories of mental and physical illness

	Mental symptoms	Somatic symptoms
Bodily pathology	*Comorbidity*	Medical condition
No bodily pathology	Psychiatric condition	*Somatisation*

Comorbidity is the second major problem and is posed by patients who have *both* prominent psychological symptoms and definite somatic pathology. These patients consequently fall into both medical and psychiatric categories of illness. This coexistence of medical and psychiatric conditions is referred to as 'comorbidity'. The concept of comorbidity is controversial as it leads to the conclusion that the patient's experience of a unitary illness is divided into two separate illnesses. In practice, it may be unhelpful in that the patient who is considered to have separate medical and psychiatric diagnoses may not be adequately treated by either specialty, a focus on either the medical or the psychiatric aspect of their illness leading to neglect of the other. Perhaps the most prominent example of this problem is the widespread neglect of depression in patients with medical disease (Sharpe et al 2003).

Classificatory dualism A consequence of this conceptual dualism is a classificatory dualism — that is, the existence of entirely separate although overlapping classifications for psychiatric and medical conditions that each focus on different aspects of the patient's illness. An example is the case of a patient with medically unexplained gastroenterological symptoms: a focus on the somatic complaints may lead to a 'medical' diagnosis of irritable bowel syndrome, and a focus on their mental symptoms to a 'psychiatric' diagnosis of generalised anxiety disorder. Which do they really have? The overlapping classification of symptoms leads to uncertainty about which diagnosis the symptoms should count toward. Another example is a patient who has had a stroke and who complains of the somatic symptom of fatigue, should fatigue be regarded as a manifestation of the stroke or of a depressive disorder? The choice of medical or psychiatric diagnosis will in practice depend on the preference and theoretical orientation of the doctor.

Moral dualism It is important to be aware that conceptual and classificatory dualisms are not value free: there is also a moral aspect to dualism — that is, psychiatric and medical diagnoses have different moral implications in the eyes of both the public and of many medical practitioners. Medical disorders are, by and large, regarded as unfortunate failures of the bodily machinery that are beyond the person's responsibility and control. Consequently, they attract the sympathy of others to the unfortunate victim. Psychiatric disorders on the other hand are often regarded as illnesses of mind, which represent a failure of the faculties of reason and self-control. They carry the implication not of being a victim but of a failure of will, and consequently of culpability, associations that encourage a response not of sympathy but of fear and contempt (Kirmayer 1988). This stigma associated with psychiatric diagnosis and treatment may have a strong influence on how a patient presents, to whom they are referred, and how they are subsequently managed. Psychiatrists working in non-psychiatric settings should not underestimate the effect of such stigma on their patients, their treatments and their colleagues and, of course by association, on how they themselves are regarded by both patients and by their non-psychiatric colleagues.

Organisational dualism Conceptual, classificatory and moral dualism give rise to an organisational dualism. Organisational dualism is the division of medical services and specialities into separate medical/surgical and psychiatric organisations. Medical and psychiatric services are not only professionally and organisationally distinct but often are actually geographically separated. These organisational divisions make 'joined up', 'integrated' or 'holistic' care of patients almost impossible. Indeed, many of the practical difficulties encountered in the management of patients who may be regarded as having psychiatric disorders but who are attending general medical services arise from this separation of services. Although the degree to which this is acknowledged is limited, one response to this problem has been the establishment of so-called liaison (linking) psychiatry services to general hospitals (see below).

Beyond dualism

New scientific knowledge, such as the demonstration of a neural basis to many psychiatric disorders, is rendering crude dualistic thinking increasingly untenable. Recent evidence for the effect of psychiatric disorder on the outcome of medical conditions (Frasure-Smith et al 1993) has highlighted its negative implications for the practical management of patients. Consequently, dualism is increasingly being replaced by the alternative hypothesis that mind and brain are best regarded as simply two sides of the same coin — the mind/brain (Granville-Grossman 1993) — rather than as separate entities. The implications of such a paradigm shift (Sharpe & Carson 2001) are potentially enormous and have not yet been fully realised. It implies that 'psychiatric disorders' are no more distinct from 'medical conditions' than the nervous system is from the rest of the body. Hence, not only is psychiatry rapidly becoming less 'brain-less' but medicine will also have to become less 'mind-less' (Eisenberg 1986).

For the present, however, the legacy of dualism continues to shape everyday medical thinking and practice. Patients' illnesses are separated into medical and psychiatric with separate knowledge bases and distinct systems of care. It is important that the psychiatrist working in medical settings is aware of the problems that result and of ways to address them. A major pitfall for the psychiatrist more used to specialist psychiatric practice is to feel that there is nothing that he can do for patients whose symptoms do not fit neatly into standard psychiatric diagnostic categories. The often-quoted statement 'no formal psychiatric diagnosis, patient discharged' is both ill-informed and unhelpful. Such behaviour ignores the fact that psychiatric diagnoses are merely constructions to guide treatment (Scadding 1996). In practice the psychiatrist can often contribute usefully to the patient's care by applying psychiatric management skills, even if no clear diagnosis can be made. That is because management is often guided as much by a case formulation as by diagnosis. One important contribution that the psychiatrist can make is to ensure that not only biological, but also psychological and social aspects of the patient's illness are considered in every case. This is the so-called biopsychosocial approach proposed by George Engel (1977). It offers the psychiatrist working in a medical setting a useful basis for safe and effective practice that frequently adds both to the understanding of the case and to the patient's management. The factors to consider in a biopsychosocial formulation are shown in Box 28.1.

| Box 28.1 | Factors to consider in a biopsychosocial formulation |

Box 28.1   Factors to consider in a biopsychosocial formulation

- **Biological**
  — Disease
  — Physiology
- **Psychological**
  — Cognition
  — Mood
  — Behaviour
- **Social**
  — Interpersonal
  — Social & occupational
  — Healthcare system

Table 28.2   Relative prevalence of psychiatric disorders in various medical settings

	General practice	Casualty	Medical /surgical Outpatients	Inpatients
Adjustment	++	+++	++	+++
Depression/anxiety	++	++	+++	+++
Somatoform	+	++	+++	++
Delirium	−	+	−	+++
Alcohol abuse	++	+++	++	+++
Psychosis	+	+	−	−

−, rare; +, uncommon; ++, common; +++, very common.

A further elaboration is to divide factors into those that predisposed the patient to the illness, those that precipitated or triggered it and those that perpetuate it. The last group of factors comprises the most important targets for intervention in established cases. An example of the use of such a formulation is shown in Table 28.5. The other factors are potentially important in primary prevention.

Psychiatric disorder in medical settings

Characteristics of psychiatric disorder in medical settings

Patients seen in non-psychiatric medical services who nonetheless merit psychiatric attention are likely to differ from those seen in a specialist psychiatric service in their presentation, in the occurrence of coexisting medical conditions and in the type of psychiatric diagnosis they are likely to receive.

Presentation   Patients seen in medical services who require psychiatric attention are, perhaps not surprisingly, more likely to have presented with somatic than with psychological symptoms; for example, the patient who meets criteria for a depressive disorder may have presented with bodily pain. Alternatively, they may have presented with a problem in medical management or with poor compliance with medical treatment, such as poorly controlled insulin-dependent diabetes mellitus. Finally, they may present with a behaviourally induced medical condition: for example because of overdose, the effect of excess alcohol intake or because of other forms of self-harm. In all these cases, the presence of features of a psychiatric diagnosis may not be obvious, unless they are specifically sought.

Coexistence of medical conditions   Patients with psychiatric disorder seen in medical services, especially in general hospitals, often have coexisting medical conditions. Such medical/psychiatric comorbidity has important implications for how we understand the aetiology of a patient's psychiatric disorder and how we manage it. For example, a patient who has had a stroke that has given rise to a depressive disorder (see below) may present particular difficulties in psychiatric management because the medical condition may impair their ability to tolerate antidepressant medication.

Psychiatric diagnoses prevalent in medical settings   The relative prevalence of the various types of psychiatric diagnosis encountered in medical settings is different from that seen in those attending specialist psychiatric services. Adjustment disorders, depression, anxiety, somatoform disorders and alcohol problems are the psychiatric diagnoses most commonly made in primary

care and in medical outpatient services; while acute organic psychiatric disorders, especially delirium, are particularly common among medical and surgical inpatients. Conversely, the functional psychoses of schizophrenia and bipolar affective disorder, which form such a large part of specialist psychiatric work, are relatively uncommon in medical settings. This relative prevalence of diagnosis by setting is illustrated in Table 28.2.

The importance of psychiatric disorder in medical settings

Psychiatric disorder is not only a cause of suffering to medical patients but also has major implications for the management and prognosis of their medical condition. Non-disease aspects of the patient's illness, which includes 'psychiatric disorder', can magnify the disability resulting from medical conditions, complicate the medical management, lead to poorer outcome and also greatly increases the consumption of general medical as well as psychiatric resources (Katon & Ciechanowski 2002). These aspects of the patient's illness are also a common reason why non-psychiatric doctors find as many as a quarter of their patients 'difficult to help' by the application of standard disease-based medical management alone (Sharpe et al 1994).

The principles of psychiatric treatment in medical settings

The effective treatment of psychiatric disorder in medical settings is based on that described elsewhere in this book. However, it also requires that the factors described above be taken into account. It requires an awareness of the differing presentations, a consideration of the possibility of interactions between psychiatric drugs and the medical conditions and their treatments, an appreciation of the importance of the medical context when providing treatment, and a capacity to collaborate effectively with non-psychiatric physicians.

THE PRESENTATION OF PSYCHIATRIC DISORDER IN MEDICAL SETTINGS

In medical settings, patients who would benefit from psychiatric management commonly do not present with typical psychological symptoms. More commonly they present with medically unexplained somatic symptoms, with illness disproportionate to demonstrable disease, with problems in medical management and with behaviourally induced medical conditions.

Presentation as medically unexplained or 'functional' somatic symptoms

Terminology

A large number of terms have been coined to describe an illness that presents somatically but is inadequately explained by somatic pathology. These include:

- medically unexplained somatic symptoms;
- medical symptoms not explained by organic disease;
- functional somatic symptoms;
- somatisation symptoms;
- hysterical (conversion) symptoms;
- hypochondriasis;
- somatoform symptoms.

The profusion of terms and an examination of each indicate that none is ideal. As described above, 'somatisation' implies a 'psychological' origin for the somatic symptoms and is of dubious validity. Other terms such as hysteria and hypochondriasis also carry clear historical theoretical baggage. The more neutral descriptive terms such as 'medically unexplained somatic symptoms' and 'medical symptoms not unexplained by organic disease' are preferable but are effectively non-diagnoses. The modern ICD and DSM psychiatric classifications use the term 'somatoform'. Although claimed to be theoretically neutral this term (meaning mental disorder in somatic form) clearly has echoes of somatisation. Recently a case has been made for the rehabilitation of the term 'functional' for such symptoms. Although in medical circles this word is now often used to imply 'mental' or 'hysterical', its original meaning in the late 19th century was of a disturbance of brain function, as opposed to structure. This less dualistic term also seems to be more acceptable to patients and consequently provides a non-stigmatising and potentially scientifically accurate rationale for both behavioural and antidepressant drug treatments (Stone et al 2002).

Relative frequency of somatic presentation

An American population survey found that a quarter to a third of the population had been severely troubled with symptoms such as pain and fatigue at some time in their lives and that in one-third of these cases the symptoms remained unexplained by somatic pathology. They could therefore be regarded as functional symptoms (Kroenke & Price 1993). In primary care, one in five new consultations are functional somatic symptoms (Goldberg et al 1988). In hospital practice, functional somatic symptoms are among the commonest reasons for referral from primary care. The somatic symptoms of fully one-third of all patients seen in gastroenterology, neurology and cardiology clinics remain best described as functional at the time of discharge (Hamilton et al 1996).

Patients with specific patterns of functional symptoms tend to cluster in medical specialties according to the organ system to which their symptoms appear to relate; hence, abdominal and bowel symptoms predominate in gastroenterology clinics, headache in neurology clinics and chest pain and palpitations in cardiac clinics. However, there is now an increasing acceptance that a separation of

Box 28.2   Medical functional syndromes
• Irritable bowel syndrome
• Non-cardiac chest pain
• Hyperventilation syndrome
• Chronic fatigue syndrome
• Fibromyalgia syndrome
• Chronic pain
• Tension headache

these specialty-associated 'functional somatic syndromes', such as irritable bowel syndrome, tension headache and noncardiac chest pain, may be artificial, and that these conditions overlap both with each other and with depression and anxiety syndromes (Wessely et al 1999).

Making a diagnosis

When making a diagnosis in a patient who has presented somatically there are three important pitfalls to beware. First, a presentation with somatic symptoms does not necessarily imply a diagnosis of somatoform disorder (see below). In fact, a diagnosis of depressive and anxiety disorders (especially panic disorder) is more likely. Second, a diagnosis of a psychiatric disorder does not exclude the possibility that the patient also has a medical condition: the patient's symptoms may be subsequently explained by somatic pathology that was missed at initial assessment, or somatic pathology may explain some of the patient's symptoms but not others. Third, the medical classificatory scheme of functional somatic syndromes should not be regarded as excluding a psychiatric diagnosis, but only as alternative descriptive labels for the same conditions. The common functional medical disorders are listed in Box 28.2.

In the absence of a satisfactory non-dualistic classification for functional somatic symptoms, that is shared by both medicine and psychiatry, the best working solution is for the clinician to note both the relevant medical and psychiatric diagnoses. For example a combined diagnosis of irritable bowel syndrome/generalised anxiety disorder may be more useful than either alone.

The importance of functional somatic symptoms

Although in many cases functional somatic symptoms are mild and transient, in a significant minority of patients they represent an important clinical problem. The associated disability may be severe and the outcome poor. Furthermore, the presentation to disease-oriented medical services may lead to repeated investigation without benefit, and at considerable cost. For example a Danish study found that the small number of patients who, during an 8-year period, were admitted at least 10 times to general hospitals for functional somatic symptoms, consumed 3% of the entire budget for admissions to non-psychiatric hospital departments (Fink 1992). Such inappropriate medical investigation and treatment is not only expensive to the healthcare system but may also result in iatrogenic harm to the patient.

Neglect of depressive and anxiety disorders as a cause of somatic symptoms

Medical practitioners may not be aware that pain and fatigue are common symptoms of depression (Mathew et al 1981) and that breathlessness, muscle pain dizziness and palpitation are common in anxiety and panic (Katon 1996). Consequently, in a large proportion of cases where the patient has presented somatically, the psychiatric diagnosis is missed entirely. Effective recognition and management of somatically presenting psychiatric disorder therefore has the potential not only to reduce the patient's distress and disability but also to achieve significant savings in the overall cost of their medical care and to improve the overall quality of healthcare.

Presentation as disproportionate symptoms or disability

Another type of presentation where psychiatric management may be appropriate is where a patient's illness or disability seems disproportionate to the disease they have. This sort of presentation is sometimes referred to as exaggerated or abnormal illness behaviour.

Illness behaviour

A patient may be regarded as manifesting 'abnormal' illness behaviour if he behaves as if medically ill when he is not, or as more ill than the severity of the somatic pathology suggests (Pilowsky 1969). Examples are severe disability, frequent attendance for medical care, the unnecessary use of equipment such as wheelchairs, and exaggerated claims for financial benefits. The term 'abnormal illness behaviour' is a qualification of the sociological concept of 'illness behaviour' used to describe the behaviour and social role of the ill person (Mechanic 1986). It is controversial because it begs the question of what is 'normal' illness behaviour. Consequently it tends to be applied subjectively and is often perceived as pejorative. While it may sometimes be appropriately used to describe a clinical presentation, care should be taken to remember that it is not a diagnosis. The diagnoses most commonly associated with abnormal illness behaviour are depressive, anxiety and somatoform disorders. In such cases it is presumed that the illness behaviour is not consciously motivated. There are other cases where there is good evidence that the patient has deliberately feigned or manufactured somatic symptoms and signs. If aimed at obtaining medical care this may merit a diagnosis of factitious disorder. If aimed at obtaining a personal advantage such as money, the person is not deemed psychiatric ill but may be described as a malingerer. In practice this distinction can be difficult to make, and accusations of malingering should be made with care, if at all (Sharpe 2003).

Presentation as problems in medical management

Problems in medical management, either disturbed behaviour or poor adherence to treatment, may require psychiatric intervention.

Disturbed behaviour

Disturbed behaviour is a common presentation in medical as it is in psychiatric settings. However, in the former situation it is more likely to indicate a diagnosis of personality disorder, substance misuse, delirium or adjustment disorder than a psychosis. Delirium is especially common in the inpatient setting and must always be suspected. It is discussed more fully in Chapter 17.

Poor adherence to and refusal of treatment

Failure to adhere to the physician's recommended treatment is common. It is, however, less common for patients to actively refuse the treatment recommended by their physician. The most common reason for such refusal is of course simply patient choice. However, in an important minority of such cases the patient's judgement may have been influenced by a psychiatric disorder. For example, elderly patients with ischaemic heart disease who also have depression adhere less well to their recommended drug regimens (Carney et al 1995). The question of whether psychiatric disorder is influencing a patient's judgement is of even greater importance when life-saving treatment is refused or positive help to die (physician-assisted suicide) is requested. A determination of the patient's competence or capacity to make the decision and a psychiatric assessment is essential in all such cases (Sullivan & Youngner 1994) (see also Ch. 30).

Presentation as behaviourally induced medical conditions

Perhaps the most conspicuous example of a behaviourally induced illness is deliberate self-harm (DSH), most commonly by overdose of drugs. DSH is one of the most common reasons for a patient to be admitted to a general hospital medical unit and for a general hospital inpatient to be referred to a psychiatrist. In some cases the DSH is related to depressive disorder, personality disorder or substance misuse, in many others it is not. The problem of DSH is examined in more detail in Chapter 27. Further consideration of the role of behavioural factors in the aetiology of medical conditions reveals that they play a key role in the aetiology of many more, including lung cancer, cirrhosis of the liver, HIV infection and heart disease. This observation offers substantial opportunities for the prevention of disease by interventions that modify risk behaviour. Such interventions clearly raise major political and practical issues, and the potential they offer remains largely untapped.

COEXISTENCE OF A PSYCHIATRIC AND A MEDICAL CONDITION

The other major problem highlighted in the introduction was that of cases in which the patient's illness is described in such a way that it is deemed to represent both a medical and a psychiatric disorder, i.e. medical/psychiatric comorbidity.

Terminology and classification

The psychiatric disorders most commonly comorbid with medical conditions are adjustment, depressive, anxiety, substance misuse and organic mental disorders. In order to examine the issues and implications associated with such comorbidity, depression is used as an example.

The current classifications of psychiatric disorder offer two different ways of recording medical/psychiatric comorbidity. The first is to code the medical condition separately from the psychiatric disorder. In DSM-IV, which is multiaxial, psychiatric disorder is recorded on Axis 1 and the comorbid medical condition on Axis 3. (The ICD-10 classification is not fully currently multiaxial but also suggests that comorbid medical conditions be recorded.) The second way of coding comorbidity refers to circumstances where the psychiatric disorder is judged to be a *direct consequence* of the medical condition. The psychiatric diagnosis of 'mental disorder due to a general medical condition'. In DSM-IV and 'organic mental disorders' in ICD-10 is then applicable. The use of these special diagnoses for comorbid depression and anxiety is, however, controversial. This is because, while it is likely that a medical condition such as a stroke *can* give rise to depression by means of a direct action on the nervous system, it is doubtful in practice whether a reliable decision about the aetiology of the patient's depression can be made simply on the basis of a clinical assessment. Furthermore, a firm diagnosis of 'organic' mood disorder, as opposed to one of simple mood disorder, has disadvantage for the patient if it leads to a neglect of important psychological and social aspects of aetiology and management. Therefore, whereas the above categories may be appropriate for delirium, in the case of other psychiatric diagnoses such as depression it is probably wise to use the multiaxial method to record comorbidity and to only use the special diagnostic categories described above sparingly, if at all (see below).

Conceptual and research issues

The psychiatrist must be aware of the conceptual difficulties comorbidity presents both for research and in clinical practice. These result from problems in the definition of psychiatric disorder in the medically ill, from the importance of factors other than the disease itself in causing psychiatric disorder and from difficulties measuring the association between psychiatric disorders and medical conditions.

Defining psychiatric disorder in the medically ill

The first problem arises from the criteria used to define psychiatric disorder. These symptom descriptions have been derived from psychiatric populations and are not necessarily valid for the medically ill. For example, how are we to interpret somatic symptoms such as weight loss, which may be a manifestation of disease pathology such as cancer but may also be regarded as part of the criteria for a depressive disorder. Four main methodological approaches have been employed in order to address this problem (Kathol et al 1990):

- The psychiatric diagnostic criteria are simply applied *unmodified*; symptoms are counted toward the psychiatric diagnosis whatever their cause is believed to be (the inclusive approach).
- The diagnostic criteria are applied unmodified, but a judgement is made in each case about the *aetiology of individual symptoms*; they are only counted if they are judged not to be caused by the medical condition (the aetiological approach).
- The standard criteria are modified to *exclude* those symptoms such as weight loss that might be caused by a medical condition (the exclusive approach).
- The criteria that have been developed in psychiatric populations are *redefined*; new criteria are developed specifically for use in the medically ill (the substitution approach).

Each of these approaches has its merits but none is more obviously correct than another. The simplest approach is to apply the psychiatric diagnostic criteria unmodified (the inclusive approach)

while being aware of the consequent risk of overdiagnosis. A useful discussion of these problems is provided by House (1988).

Patients attending medical care may not be typical of those with the disease in the general population Patients with a given medical condition seen in medical settings may have a higher prevalence of psychiatric disorder than those in the community because patients with psychiatric disorder are more likely to be hospitalised and receiving medical treatment and also because medical treatment including hospitalisation itself may cause psychiatric disorder.

Illness factors other than the disease pathology cause psychiatric disorder While medical conditions are generally defined in terms of objectively demonstrable abnormalities in bodily organs, other non-disease factors are relevant and may be more important determinants of whether they develop a psychiatric disorder. These include:

- the duration and course of the medical condition;
- the meaning of the medical condition for the patient;
- the effect on the patient's social and occupational context.

Drawing conclusions about the association between medical and psychiatric diagnoses simply by assessing the prevalence in patients who share disease pathology is simplistic and may be misleading.

The prevalence of comorbidity

Despite the problems described above, it is reasonable to conclude from the available literature that persons who have a medical condition are more likely than persons without a medical condition to have a psychiatric disorder (Weyerer 1990). Furthermore, some medical conditions appear to have a stronger association with psychiatric disorder than others. For example, the prevalence of depressive disorder is particularly high among patients with heart disease and neurological disorders (approximately 25%), but only just higher than that in the general population in patients with hypertension and diabetes (nearer 15%) (Wells et al 1988).

Aetiology

Why should persons with medical conditions be more likely to have psychiatric disorder? There are four main possible reasons:

- coincidence;
- common causation;
- the psychiatric disorder caused the medical condition;
- the medical condition caused the psychiatric disorder.

Coincidence Both physical disease and psychiatric disorder are common in the general population. In clinical practice, it is common to see patients whose psychiatric disorder appears to be unrelated to their medical condition. For example in as many as a quarter of patients with depression and a medical condition, the depression was present before the onset of the medical condition (Moffic & Paykel 1975).

Common causation Both the psychiatric disorder and the medical condition may share a common cause. For example, stressful life events in a vulnerable person may precipitate both a stroke (House et al 1990) and a depressive illness (Emmerson et al 1989).

Psychiatric disorder causes the medical condition Psychiatric disorders can certainly cause medical conditions. The most clearly established examples are those in which the patient's behaviour has produced direct physical damage as described above.

The question of whether psychiatric disorder and personality traits can cause medical conditions by mechanisms other than by influencing behaviour is much more controversial. A failure to establish the hypothesis proposed by psychosomatists working in the 1930s and 1940s that certain personality types were prone to specific medical conditions such as asthma (Alexander 1950) has led to caution in more recent aetiological speculation. Modern research has instead attempted to elucidate the possible mechanisms whereby psychological factors could directly influence physical health. An example is the link between the nervous system and the immune system, an area of research called psychoneuro-immunology (Kiecolt-Glaser & Glaser 1989). At present, however, there is little convincing evidence that depression and anxiety are major factors in the initial aetiology of most medical conditions. There is, however, very good evidence that comorbid depression and anxiety can influence the outcome of existing medical conditions such as ischaemic heart disease (Frasure-Smith et al 1993), stroke (Morris et al 1993) and most other chronic medical illnesses.

The medical condition and its treatment cause the psychiatric disorder The development of a medical condition may cause the predisposed individual to develop a psychiatric disorder. This may be a consequence of: (a) a direct biological effect on the central nervous system; (b) a psychological reaction; (c) the social consequences.

A direct biological mechanism The following criteria are listed in DSM-IV as being useful in deciding whether the psychiatric disorder in question can be regarded as being directly biologically caused by the medical condition:

- an organic cause (disease, drug) is present;
- the organic cause was present before the psychiatric disorder;
- treatment of the organic cause results in relief of the psychiatric symptoms;
- the psychiatric disorder is atypical in some way (e.g. lack of family history);
- there is evidence from the literature that the medical condition in question can cause psychiatric disorder by an established biological mechanism.

These requirements are easily met for clearly organic disorders such as delirium. Their value when applied to other disorders such as anxiety and depression is less clear (see above). A medical condition may be considered more likely to cause psychiatric disorder by a biological mechanism if it affects the nervous system either structurally or chemically. Medical conditions that do affect the central nervous system and that can probably cause depression via a biological mechanism include:

- *endocrine conditions*
  — Cushing's syndrome
  — hypothyroidism
- *neurological conditions*
  — Parkinson's disease
  — stroke
  — multiple sclerosis
  — advanced cancer
  — brain damage or injury.

A variety of drug treatments also have the capacity to cause psychiatric disorders by their action on the nervous system. Many drug treatments commonly used in medicine are known to cause depression. Important examples include:

- steroids;
- H₂ receptor antagonists, e.g. cimetidine;
- antihypertensive drugs, e.g. beta-blockers.

A psychological reaction It is easy to understand how a medical condition could give rise to a psychiatric disorder by acting as a psychological stressor. In such cases, the critical factor is the *meaning* of the condition to the patient. For example, it is not surprising that the person who learns that he or she has developed cancer may become depressed, and that depression is more likely to develop in persons who believe their disease to be incurable (Alexander et al 1993). Similarly, patients with skin disease are more likely to be depressed if they regard the skin disease as disfiguring, regardless of the objective severity of their condition (Wessely & Lewis 1989). In general, medical conditions are more likely to cause depression if they are *perceived* by the patient as disfiguring, disabling or potentially fatal. Medical and surgical treatments can also have major psychological effects on a patient's mental state. Examples include major investigations and procedures such as genetic counselling, surgery, radiotherapy and drug therapy.

A reaction to social consequences The meanings a person attaches to his medical condition will be influenced by social factors. These in turn reflect the reaction of persons other than the patient to the observed diagnosis, symptoms and disability. One major social factor that may lead to depression after diagnosis of a medical condition is loss of status, often associated with loss of employment. In addition some medical conditions (such as AIDS) are associated with social stigma (Goldin 1994) that may have a major impact on the individual. Medical treatment also has a social impact, and medical consultation and hospital admission are significant and stressful events for many patients.

The patient and his social situation For any given medical condition, it is only a minority of patients who will develop associated psychiatric disorder. Individual vulnerability is therefore an important risk factor. For affective and anxiety disorders the constitutional factors predisposing to emotional disorders in the general population also apply to the medically ill. Of risk factors for depression, perhaps the most easily identifiable is demonstrated vulnerability as evidenced by a family or personal history of psychiatric disorder (Cassano & Fava 2002). As with depression in general, the social context and especially the degree of support the person enjoys are important. Lack of social support has been repeatedly found to be an important risk factor for adverse emotional reactions to medical conditions such as cancer (Godding et al 1995).

Summary

In practice, rather than trying to decide whether an individual patient's psychiatric disorder is biologically, psychologically or socially caused, it is more useful to seek evidence for each of these categories of aetiological factors in every case. This has been called the biopsychosocial approach (see above). The areas to assess in this way should include not only the medical condition and its treatment, but also the premorbid characteristics of the individual and his social situation. The factors that may be regarded as risk factors for the development of psychiatric disorder in the medically ill are:

- *The medical condition*
  — involves the central nervous system;
  — is negatively perceived (threat or loss).
- *The treatment*

— affects the central nervous system;
— is disfiguring or disabling.
- *The person*
  — has a previous history of psychiatric disorder.
- *The social context*
  — offers a lack of social support;
  — implies loss of status and stigma.

GENERAL PRINCIPLES OF MANAGEMENT

In this section the general principles of the management of psychiatric disorder in general medical settings are outlined. The special features of the medical context relevant to psychiatric management are examined and the issues of detection, assessment and treatment reviewed. It is important to note that relatively few patients with psychiatric disorder attending medical services currently receive any specific treatment for it and to consider what the obstacles are to implementing more effective management.

Obstacles to effective management

Potential obstacles to effective psychiatric treatment include those given below.

Failure of detection

The first obstacle to the effective management of patients with psychiatric disorder is a low rate of detection. There are a number of reasons for this: the patient may present with somatic complaints; the doctor may focus attention on medical aspects of the patient's complaints, which may distract him from concern with the psychiatric disorder; and the setting may deter the patient from disclosing psychological symptoms. And whereas the psychiatrist must be mindful that it is often appropriate for the treatment of the medical condition to take priority over psychiatric treatment, in some cases it is not. For example a complaint of pain may lead to a focus on medical causes while a coexisting and aetiologically important major depressive disorder, the treatment of which may reduce or even eliminate the pain, is ignored (Von Korff & Simon 1996). Improved management of psychiatric disorder in medical settings therefore depends on better detection.

Failure to perform adequate assessment and treatment

Even if detected, psychiatric disorder may not be adequately assessed and treated. Two commonly held attitudes may prevent the physician actively assessing and treating the psychiatric disorder. First, it may be regarded merely as a result of the medical condition and consequently, but wrongly, viewed as requiring no specific treatment. This surprisingly widely used argument can be countered by asking whether it is necessary to treat 'understandable' bleeding in a patient who has suffered trauma. Second, the physician may erroneously believe that psychiatric treatment would be ineffective in any case, and is therefore pointless. This may be countered with evidence. These attitudes are compounded by a lack of psychiatric training, expertise, time and facilities in the non-psychiatric parts of the healthcare system, as well as by unwillingness to make a potentially stigmatising diagnosis.

Medical undergraduate teaching devotes relatively little attention to these aspects of medicine and only a minority of doctors receive relevant postgraduate training. Furthermore, doctors working in general medical services often feel under pressure and regard psychiatric assessment as too time consuming. Often there is a lack of basic facilities for psychiatric assessment, such as a private interview rooms. There is also likely to be a shortage of treatment resources such as adequately trained cognitive behaviour therapists. Finally, both patient and doctor may wish to avoid the stigma that a psychiatric diagnosis and the acceptance of psychiatric treatment imply. Strategies intended to improve psychiatric assessment and treatment in medical settings will have to address all these obstacles.

Effective psychiatric management in the medical context

The first consideration for the effective detection, assessment, and treatment of psychiatric disorder outside specialist psychiatric settings is an appreciation of the special characteristics of the medical context. As can be seen from the foregoing, the psychiatrist working in this setting cannot simply transplant a standard psychiatric approach. Essential modifications include the following.

Addressing the medical patient's concerns It is likely that the patient will be more concerned about his medical state (whether an established medical condition or an unexplained somatic symptom) and its management than about his psychiatric state — a factor to which the psychiatrist must be sensitive if she is to obtain his co-operation. Not infrequently, the patient will express reluctance to see a psychiatrist at all. Therefore, whatever the reason for the assessment, it is wise to begin the interview by taking time to explain the reasons for the consultation and to elicit the patient's concerns about his somatic complaints and medical treatment before going on to ask about psychological symptoms.

Other doctors and nurses The medical patient is under the care of non-psychiatric physicians, nursing and other staff, and their co-operation is essential. Providing a positive explanation for a psychiatric assessment is a necessary preliminary, and the collection of information about the patient from these informants is essential. Once assessment is completed, those concerned with the patient's ongoing management require a detailed explanation of the diagnosis in plain English and practical guidance about their own role in the psychiatric management. A brief written note is rarely sufficient and frequently results in the psychiatrist's suggested treatment plan, however appropriate, being ignored (Huyse et al. 1990).

Facilities Although the facilities for psychiatric assessment and treatment are often poor, the psychiatrist should persevere in finding an appropriately private and undisturbed place to interview the patient. Any suggestions that the patient be given psychological therapy must take account the actual availability of skilled therapists, and may require that the psychiatrist takes responsibility for this aspect of the patient's treatment. If psychotropic drug treatment is recommended, it is necessary to check that the drugs are readily available; frequently they are not, and an unanticipated delay may result while they are ordered from the pharmacy.

Follow-up It is usually desirable to carry out a follow-up consultation to check on the patient's progress. The psychiatrist should not simply rely on others who may lack the necessary skill to monitor the patient's mental state.

Detecting psychiatric disorder

As with all medical diagnoses the most important requirement is for the assessing doctor to have a high 'index of suspicion' based on an awareness of the prevalence of and risk factors for psychiatric disorder as described above. The practical task of detection may be aided by systematic screening procedures.

Questionnaires One approach to screening is the use of questionnaires. These may be administered in pencil and paper form or by other mean such as touch screen computer. Examples of aspects of illness screened for and associated questionnaires are:

- depression and anxiety — Hospital Anxiety and Depression Scale (HAD) (Zigmond & Snaith 1983);
- alcohol misuse — Alcohol Use Disorder Identification Test (AUDIT) (Barbor et al 1992);
- cognitive impairment — Mini Mental State Examination (MMSE) (Folstein et al 1975);
- 'quality of life' — Medical Outcomes Study Short Form (SF-36 and SF-12) (Ware & Sherbourne 1992).

Interviews An alternative to the questionnaire is simply to add a few questions to the routine medical and nursing assessment of every patient. Interviews for use in the medical setting need to be relatively brief. For example, simply asking the patient if he has suffered depressed mood may be as useful as giving him a questionnaire to measure depression (Van Hemert et al 1993).

Assessment, diagnosis and formulation of psychiatric disorder

Once screening has indicated a probable psychiatric disorder, it is necessary to make a diagnosis. Full diagnostic interviews are of course time consuming, but 'cut-down' versions have been developed specifically for use in medical settings. An example is the PRIME-MD interview, which can be conducted in minutes (Spitzer et al 1994). Assessment requires more than diagnosis; an assessment of the person, his concerns and his social context and of any comorbid medical condition is also necessary. The assessment may be usefully summarised as a diagnosis supplemented by a formulation, which covers biological, psychological and social aspects of the problem (see Box 28.1 and Table 28.5).

Treatment of psychiatric disorder

The usual principles of psychiatric management can be applied in the medical setting as long as attention is paid to contextual issues outlined above. Treatment may be considered in relation to the factors identified in the biopsychosocial formulation (Table 28.3)

Pharmacotherapy There are several complications in the use of pharmacotherapy for psychiatric disorder in medical patients.

Table 28.3 A biopsychosocial treatment plan: example of interventions		
Main factors	Subfactors	Interventions
Biological	Disease	Medical care
	Physiology	Antidepressant drugs
Psychological	Cognition	Explanation
	Mood	Treat depression/anxiety
	Behaviour	Encourage normal behaviour
Social	Interpersonal	Explain to family
	Social & occupational	Encourage activity
	Healthcare system	Ensure appropriate care

Patients may not wish to take 'psychiatric drugs', they may be intolerant of them or the drugs may be contraindicated by the patient's medical condition or ongoing medical treatment. Therefore, care must always be taken to explain to the patient the need and rationale for prescribing such agents. One way is to emphasise the understandability of distress in the context of a medical condition. Another is to explain how such drugs act to normalise brain function in those under stress. It is also important to check for potential contraindications and treatment interactions by using appropriate reference sources such as the *British National Formulary* (www.bnf.org). It is desirable to begin treatment with a lower dose of the drug than is usual in general psychiatric practice, and to choose short-acting agents in case of adverse reaction.

Psychological therapy Psychological treatments lack the potential of drug therapy to cause adverse effects and interactions. However, some patients (and their physicians) may be reluctant to accept an explicitly 'psychological' treatment. Time devoted to explaining the nature and relevance of this form of treatment as a means to help the patient to cope with the medical problem is well spent. Simple psychological interventions such as information giving are of value for patients with alcohol problems (Chick 1991) and could be profitably extended to other conditions. More elaborate therapies, especially cognitive behaviour therapy (CBT), have a proven role in the management both of comorbid emotional disorder and a wide range of somatoform disorders (see below).

Compulsory treatment Patients may occasionally have to be given treatment for disturbed behaviour associated with a psychiatric disorder (such as an attempt to harm themselves) without their consent. In such cases, the application of legal powers of compulsory treatment may be considered. It must be remembered that in most countries such legislation cannot usually be used to force a person to have medical treatment unless (a) they have a mental disorder and (b) the treatment is directed at the relief of that disorder (see also Ch. 30).

Summary

Seven key points for the general psychiatric management of medical patient are the following.

- Liaise with those providing general medical care.
- Ensure relevant medical conditions have been adequately treated.
- When assessing the patient, start by addressing the somatic complaints, only then widening discussion to include psychological symptoms and social stressors.
- Make a psychiatric diagnosis if appropriate and always supplement this with a biopsychosocial formulation.
- Explain the need for psychiatric treatment in a way that is acceptable and understandable to the patient and his physician.
- Take account of the patient's medical condition and management when choosing psychiatric treatment and discuss this with his medical attendants when necessary.
- Ensure that appropriate psychiatric treatment is actually implemented.

SPECIFIC PSYCHIATRIC DISORDERS AND THEIR TREATMENT

The psychiatric disorders most commonly encountered in medical settings are reviewed below. The specific management outlined for the disorders is a supplement to general aspects of management outlined above.

Reactions to stressors

Reactions to stress can be broadly divided into acute, persistent and chronic forms. In medically ill patients the onset or exacerbation of disease, as well as hospitalisation and treatment, are also potent stressors that can produce marked psychological reactions.

Acute stress reactions are transient but severe reactions and are common in patients who have suffered acutely stressful events, such as accidents. The patient with an acute stress reaction is likely to be aroused and anxious and may become disturbed in behaviour. The patient may also deny the reality or implications of what has happened, so that the adverse psychological reaction is delayed. Denial of the medical diagnosis is a coping mechanism that may complicate the management of conditions such as cancer (Greer 1992).

Adjustment disorders are longer-lasting disorders usually manifest as depressed or anxious mood and may also lead to disturbed behaviour and to poor compliance with medical treatment. The symptoms of distress often wax and wane in accordance with improvements and deteriorations in the medical condition, and successes and failures in its treatment. For example, distress in patients having haemodialysis for renal failure has been noted to fluctuate in association with problems occurring in treatment (Reichsman & Levy 1973). Adjustment reactions are, by definition, usually transient, but a proportion of patients who manifest them will go on to develop more persistent psychiatric disorders, usually depression. In practice, the precise boundary between adjustment disorder and established mood disorder can be hard to draw.

Post-traumatic stress disorders are persistent emotional responses to a past event that was perceived as life threatening (for example a serious road accident or invasive medical procedure). The onset may be weeks to months or more after the trauma. The key symptoms are the repeated reliving of the event in images or other sensory modalities ('flashbacks') and nightmares, as well as chronic anxiety, insomnia and tendency to avoid reminders of the trauma. This disorder has been described in a significant proportion of persons who have experienced severe accidents such as car crashes (Mayou 2002). It is also increasingly recognised to be a potential complication of acute medical illness and its treatment (Shalev et al 1993).

Management of reactions to stressors

Most emotional reactions to accidents, acute illness and their medical treatment are transient and require no specific treatment other than ensuring that the patient has adequate and accurate information. More persistent or severe reactions are more likely in persons who have a previous history of psychiatric disorder. Such persons should therefore be regarded as being 'at risk'. Attempts to prevent the development of later problems by giving all patients counselling or 'psychological debriefing' early after a trauma do not seem to be effective (Wessely & Bisson 2001). Established disorders should however be treated with either antidepressant drugs and/or psychological therapy (see Ch. 16).

Mood disorders

Mood disorders are classified as either bipolar or unipolar; and, if unipolar, are further subclassified on the basis of severity and persistence. ICD-10 subdivides unipolar depression into mild, moderate and severe forms and DSM-IV into major depression and a chronic milder form termed dysthymia (see also Ch. 20). The prevalence of depressive disorder identified in surveys of medical populations depends on the threshold of severity used and the particular group of patients assessed. Differing practices for the differentiation of adjustment disorder from established mood disorder contribute to variations in quoted rates. Nonetheless, general conclusions can be drawn:

- The prevalence of more severe depressive disorder (usually defined as DSM major depression) is approximately 5% in primary care, 5–10% in medical outpatients, and 10–20% in medical inpatients (Katon & Schulberg 1992).
- When milder forms of depression are included the overall rate is two to three times higher than for major depression (Katon & Schulberg 1992).
- Chronic depressive states such as dysthymia are particularly common in patients with chronic medical conditions (Howland 1993).

The depressive disorder of many hospitalised medical patients resolves after discharge without any specific psychiatric treatment. However, continuing depression occurs in 10–20% and is associated with persistence of the medical condition and with ongoing social problems (Mayou et al 1991). Depressive disorder is particularly important in medical patients as it not only represents considerable distress but also amplifies disability and increases the cost of medical care (see above).

Management of mood disorders

The first stage of effective management of depression in the medically ill is detection and diagnosis. Once a depressive disorder has been diagnosed, management is based either on pharmacological treatment with an antidepressant agent or on psychological treatment, usually CBT. Relatively few randomised trials have examined the effectiveness of such treatments specifically in medical populations. However a review of the available trials shows that antidepressants are effective in treating depression in patients with significant coexisting medical conditions (Gill & Hatcher 1999) as well as in those who present with medically unexplained somatic complaints (O'Malley et al 1999). There is less evidence for the effectiveness of psychological treatments for patients with comorbid depression, although they have been shown to be effective for somatic presentations of depression (Guthrie 1996). A combination of antidepressant drugs and psychological therapy may be particularly effective in relieving major depressive disorder, including that occurring in patients with comorbid medical conditions (Katon et al 1996).

Anxiety disorders

Anxiety disorders are common in medical settings but, like depression, the precise prevalence reported from surveys depends on both the threshold of severity required and the sample of patients studied. Furthermore, if a hierarchical approach to diagnosis, which subsumes anxiety under depression, is employed, anxiety is under-diagnosed (see Ch. 21). The main subtypes of anxiety disorders are paroxysmal anxiety or panic, generalised anxiety and phobic anxiety.

Panic disorder is a frequent cause of presentation to medical services. This is perhaps not surprising for a condition in which fear of dying and multiple somatic symptoms are core features. Panic is a particularly common cause of the somatic complaints of dizziness, paraesthesiae, breathlessness, palpitations and chest pain and is a common accompaniment of hypochondriasis (Sherbourne et al 1996). Panic is particularly common in patients with non-cardiac chest pain, in whom anxiety may not be as prominent as the somatic symptoms (Fleet et al 1998).

Generalised anxiety disorder is also common in medical patients. It may present with fatigue, widespread aches or worry about disease. It has been relatively neglected in research, and its contribution to functional somatic symptoms, disability and excessive use of medical services may have been underestimated (Sherbourne et al 1996).

Specific phobias may interfere with medical treatment and investigation. Blood injury or needle phobias pose particular problems in medical and surgical care. This is particularly the case for conditions requiring frequent injections, such as insulin-dependent diabetes mellitus. Claustrophobia may prevent patients accepting CT and MRI scans.

Management of anxiety disorders

The information physicians and surgeons give to patients about their symptoms may be an important determinant of subsequent anxiety. For example physicians who correctly address the illness concerns of patients with irritable bowel syndrome achieve a greater reduction in the patient's anxiety than those who do not (van Dulmen et al 1995). Established anxiety states are managed using psychological treatments or with antidepressant drugs (see Ch. 21) although, as with depression, there are few evaluations of therapy specifically in medical populations. Benzodiazepines can be particularly useful, especially for brief effective relief of anxiety, such as during anxiety-provoking medical procedures. However, caution must be exercised in their prolonged use as it may lead to dependence (see Ch. 15).

Somatoform disorders

Somatoform is a term given to a group of psychiatric disorders in DSM-IV and ICD-10 that present in a way that suggests a medical condition (mental disorders in a somatic form — see above). Patients with somatoform disorders present more commonly to primary-care and secondary-care physicians rather than to psychiatrists, although some are subsequently referred for a psychiatric opinion when no disease explanation is found.

History of somatoform disorders as a category

The category of Somatoform Disorder was introduced into DSM-III as one of the new categories to replace the broad concept of neurosis, which had been removed in that edition (Editorial 1982). It was a response to the challenge of classifying those patients, previously diagnosed as neurotic, who had functional somatic symptoms but who lacked the psychological symptoms of depression and anxiety. Central to the somatoform concept was the newly formulated syndrome of Somatisation Disorder. This somatoform category also covered a disparate group of clinical problems: Conversion Disorder (arbitrarily separated from dissociative disorder), Hypochondriasis, and Psychogenic Pain

Disorder. In addition, there was a small residual category, Atypical Somatoform Disorders. There were minor changes to these subcategories in DSM-IIIR and DSM-IV. There was, however, one major change — the introduction of a new category of Undifferentiated Somatoform Disorder to provide a home for the very large numbers of patients with functional somatic symptoms who did not fall within the existing more specific categories. ICD-10, which was developed in parallel with DSM-IV, shares many of the underlying assumptions and principles. There are however some differences in the organisation of the somatoform category, in the precise diagnostic criteria and in its inclusion in a broader category of 'neurotic, stress-related and somatoform disorders'.

The somatoform diagnoses

The ICD-10 and DSM classifications of somatoform disorders are shown in Table 28.4. Both classifications include Somatisation Disorder, Hypochondriasis, and Pain Disorder. ICD-10 also includes the category of Somatoform Autonomic Dysfunction (with the relevant organ system specified), which DSM does not. DSM-IV includes Conversion Disorder and Body Dysmorphic Disorder as Somatoform Disorders; whereas in ICD-10 Conversion Disorders are listed under Dissociative Disorders, and Body Dysmorphic Disorder is included under Hypochondriacal Disorder. DSM has the large catchall category of Undifferentiated Somatoform Disorder. It is also notable that ICD-10 retains the old term Neurasthenia as a diagnosis, for a chronic fatigue state, whereas there is no such condition in DSM-IV; similar patients would be allocated to one differentiated somatoform disorder (with the symptom of fatigue) in DSM.

These discrepancies between the classifications reflect a general lack of consensus on both the overall grouping of somatoform disorders and specific criteria for these diagnoses. The individual diagnoses are considered in more detail below.

Somatisation disorder (Briquet's syndrome) was intended to describe those patients, usually women, who present with long histories of multiple medically unexplained somatic complaints. Definitions of the disorder require that the patient have a history of more than a certain number of lifetime functional somatic

Table 28.4 The classifications of somatoform disorders in DSM-IV and ICD-10	
DSM-IV	ICD-10
Somatoform disorders	*Somatoform disorders*
Somatisation disorder	Somatisation disorder
Undifferentiated somatoform disorder	Undifferentiated somatoform disorder
Pain disorder	Persistent somatoform pain disorder
Hypochondriasis	Hypochondriacal disorder (includes body dysmorphic disorder)
Body dysmorphic disorder	
Somatoform disorder NOS	Somatoform autonomic dysfunction
Conversion disorder	Somatoform disorder unspecified
	Dissociative (conversion) disorders
	Disorders of movement and sensation
	Other neurotic disorders
	Neurasthenia

symptoms for which they have seen a physician. The frequency of functional symptoms is continuously distributed in the general population; the setting of a specific number (4 to 13 have been used) serves merely to define a threshold for the purpose of case definition. The prevalence of somatisation disorder found in the general population is 1–4% and in medical settings 10–20%, depending on which case definition is used to define the disorder. There are strong associations between Briquet's syndrome and both personality disorder and affective disorder. Indeed many of the symptoms are appropriately regarded as the somatic symptoms of depression and anxiety. Although the cause of somatisation disorder is unknown, a tendency for the disorder to run in families (Guze 1993) has been observed, suggesting a genetic factor. There is, however, also an association with childhood deprivation and abuse (Morrison 1989). For established cases, it seems likely that iatrogenic factors such as excessive investigation and inappropriate medical treatment may also play a part in maintaining the disorder. There is no treatment of proven efficacy, although these are being developed. The prognosis is very poor.

Dissociative/conversion disorder is the modern equivalent of hysteria. The essential difference from other somatoform disorders is a clear 'alteration or loss of physical functioning', with deficits in motor or sensory function that are unexplained by a medical condition and are not intentionally produced (as they are in factitious disorder). Classical conversion symptoms, such as inability to move an arm or blindness, continue to be seen in modern specialist medical practice, especially neurology. The aetiology is unknown, although there is evidence that hysteria is triggered by stress and trauma (both psychological and physical) in vulnerable persons.

The reason why the conversion symptoms take a particular form (such as blindness) is also unclear. While from a psychodynamic perspective the symptom was assumed to symbolise the patient's predicament — for example inability to speak in someone with a conflict about speaking out (House & Andrews 1988) — it seems more likely that the presentation is shaped by the patient's personal experience of medical illness and by social and cultural factors. Hence it has been argued that hysteria has changed its form over time and now manifests in more 'subtle' and socially acceptable ways such as by the general weakness of chronic fatigue syndrome rather than by paralysis (Shorter 1992). Such a conjecture is intriguing but of course difficult to test.

The prognosis for acute conversion symptoms is good. However, once established, they can be enduring, and patients may become chronically disabled and even wheelchair bound (Davison et al 1999). A much quoted study suggested that most patients initially diagnosed as having conversion disorder, eventually turned out to have neurological disease (Slater 1965). This conclusion was widely accepted, perhaps because it resonated with medical prejudice. Subsequent studies have however shown it to be untrue (Mace & Trimble 1996).

Specific somatic symptoms (pain and fatigue) may occur as a sole or predominant complaint, as well as occurring together with many others, as is the case in patients with somatisation disorder. The current psychiatric classifications have singled out the symptom of pain and have dignified it with the diagnosis of 'somatoform pain disorder'. Unexplained pain is extremely common in medical patients, common sites being the back, abdomen, pelvis and muscles. Widespread pain complaints may also be diagnosed as the functional medical syndrome of fibromyalgia (Wolfe 1990).

Fatigue as a symptom is singled out only by ICD-10. If it occurs in the absence of a depressive or anxiety diagnosis, it may merit a diagnosis of Neurasthenia. In DSM-IV, however, chronic fatigue enjoys no special status and simply falls into the residual category of undifferentiated somatoform disorder (with fatigue as the symptoms). Chronic fatigue states may also be diagnosed as the functional medical syndrome of Chronic Fatigue Syndrome (CFS) (Fukuda et al 1994). The aetiology of these specific somatoform disorders is uncertain, but both chronic pain and chronic fatigue have a strong association with both previous and current depressive disorder. Both chronic fatigue and chronic pain are frequently both persistent and profoundly disabling.

Hypochondriasis (health anxiety) is an anxious preoccupation with the possibility that one has, or may have, a serious (usually fatal) disease, based on a misinterpretation of somatic symptoms, that persists despite adequate medical evaluation and reassurance. Anxiety and depressive symptoms are common in such patients, and it has been suggested that hypochondriasis should not be considered as a diagnosis but only as a manifestation of depression (Kenyon 1964) or of anxiety (Salkovskis & Warwick 1986). The association with these syndromes is strong, but there are a sizable number of patients who meet criteria for hypochondriasis but not for depression or anxiety disorder (Appleby 1987). Clinically a dimensional approach in which the degree of anxiety, depression and hypochondriacal concern are assessed and described separately is often more useful than an attempt to determine which of these aspects of the patient's illness is primary and which secondary. Occasionally, hypochondriacal concerns may be delusional and a diagnosis of psychotic disorder appropriate.

The prevalence of established hypochondriasis in medical outpatients has been estimated as approximately 5%, although transient hypochondriacal states are more common (Barsky et al 1990). As well as depression and anxiety, the aetiology includes persistent fears about vulnerability to severe illness (Barsky & Wyshak 1989). Once hypochondriasis has developed, repeated reassurance seeking about the absence of disease from doctors and others may actually perpetuate the problem (Warwick & Salkovskis 1985). The outcome is variable. However, severe and untreated hypochondriacal states have a poor prognosis.

Body dysmorphic disorder, previously known as dysmorphophobia, is regarded as a subtype of hypochondriasis by ICD-10 but classified separately in DSM-IV. The essential characteristic is that the person is concerned about a defect in their appearance for which there is inadequate objective evidence (Veale et al 1996). The disorder is relevant to medicine insofar as persons afflicted by it often attend doctors, especially plastic surgeons, in order to seek the desired alteration of their appearance. Whilst minor dissatisfaction with appearance is extremely common, severe morbid preoccupation (for example with shape of nose or size of breasts) is relatively rare. As with hypochondriasis, these concerns may occasionally become delusional in intensity. Body dysmorphic disorder may be associated with repeated presentation to plastic surgery and dissatisfaction with the outcome.

Somatoform autonomic dysfunction is an ICD-10 category describing patients who present with concerns about symptoms that are the result of autonomic arousal rather than disease and includes 'cardiac neurosis', irritable bowel syndrome and hyperventilation. Its utility remains unclear and it appears to be little used.

Undifferentiated somatoform disorder is designed as a residual category but is very common in community surveys (Escobar et al 1987). It is really only a description of a symptom and adds little.

Criticisms of the concept of somatoform disorders

The category of somatoform disorder has come in for considerable criticism.

It is an artificial grouping of conditions purely on the basis that, although considered psychiatric, they tend to present to medical specialists. Is that a useful basis for a classification? Some say it is, because it usefully focuses attention on a group of similar presentations. Others argue that the grouping of somatoform disorders is spurious and that many of the subcategories would have a more comfortable home elsewhere in the classifications. For example, it has been suggested that somatisation disorder is better regarded as a personality disorder (Bass & Murphy 1995) and hypochondriasis as an anxiety disorder (Warwick & Salkovskis 1990).

The terminology is unacceptable to patients and many reject the diagnostic terms. Somatoform is seen as conveying medical doubt about the genuineness of the suffering without offering the prospect of care. While valid, this criticism is not unique to this category.

The concept is essentially dualistic and implies that symptoms are of psychogenic origin. This does not do justice to our current understanding of aetiology, which identifies multiple cases and does not simply dichotomise cause into psychogenic and somatogenic categories (see above). This issue is exemplified by the increasing acceptance that pain cannot be meaningfully classified as having either somatogenic or psychogenic causes (Sharpe & Williams 2001).

In practice the category leads to the under-diagnosis of depression and anxiety, as a diagnosis of somatoform disorder obscures the important association of functional somatic symptoms with anxiety and depressive disorders. There is practical merit in this argument although the fault lies not with the classification (which explicitly excludes patients with depressive and anxiety disorders from the somatoform category) but with sloppy practice in interpreting it.

The concept is culture bound and does not readily translate to cultures which have more holistic views of the mind and the body (for example, the current Chinese classification is based on DSM but specifically excludes the somatoform disorder category). It could be regarded as unfortunate that the international use of DSM (and ICD) promotes a dualist approach within cultures which currently have considerably more integrated concepts about all forms of illness and disease.

The somatoform disorders do not map onto the widely used general medical classification of functional syndromes, preferred by physicians, which has greater face validity. We might ask whether medically unexplained somatic symptoms should feature in a psychiatric classification at all. Arguably, they should insofar as psychiatrists, particularly those working in general hospitals, are asked to help diagnose and manage them.

The categories are of limited utility in directing treatment. However, it is arguable that a diagnosis of hypochondriasis implies specific management.

The future of somatoform disorders

It is clear that there need to be changes in our conceptualisation of, terminology for and classification of these problems. Decisions about the relative importance of aetiological or descriptive principles, comorbidity, and whether we use dimensions or categories, are all fundamental to the classification as a whole. What is clear is that any new classification of somatoform disorders will have to be both genuinely aetiologically neutral and use terms that are more acceptable to patients that those we have now.

Suggestions for using the current classification

As the somatoform disorder classification is not likely to be revised for some time we need to use what we have most effectively. The following are suggestions:

- It is most useful for the clinician to use *both* medical functional syndrome diagnosis *and* psychiatric diagnosis, rather than choosing one or the other. For example, such a combined diagnosis might be 'irritable bowel syndrome/hypochondriasis'.
- It is also helpful to add a formulation to highlight the main aetiological factors. The perpetuating factors are especially important targets for treatment. An example is shown in Table 28.5.
- When it comes to explaining the symptoms to the patients the word 'functional' has the advantages over somatoform of being both generally acceptable to patients and also allowing for the application of treatments that 'alter nervous function', such as psychological and behavioural interventions and psychotropic drugs.

Management of somatoform disorders

Management should be based on an appropriate assessment. This requires diagnosis and the construction of an aetiological formulation. An example for a patient with hypochondriasis is shown in Table 28.5. Treatment can then be targeted at multiple perpetuating factors.

Table 28.5 Example biopsychosocial formulation: a patient with hypochondriasis

Main factors	Subfactors	Predisposing	Precipitating	Perpetuating
Biological	Disease Physiology		Acute minor illness	Somatic symptoms of anxiety
Psychological	Cognition Mood Behaviour	Memory of brother's death Tendency to anxiety	Fear of death Acute anxiety	Chronic anxiety Reassurance seeking
Social	Interpersonal Social & occupational Healthcare system		Reassurance Loss of occupation Investigation	Reassurance Loss of occupation Investigation

A *positive explanation* of the symptoms to patient and family that takes the reality of the patient's somatic experience of symptoms as its starting point is essential, as described above. This should include practical advice about how to cope, such as ending the search for 'miracle cures' and the importance of returning to as normal and active a life as possible. It should then lead on to a positive rationale for treatment aimed at correcting the real but potentially reversible functional disturbances underlying the patient's somatic symptoms.

Antidepressant drugs have been shown to have a role in reducing many unexplained complaints, especially pain (O'Malley et al 1999). Furthermore these agents are effective whether or not the patient is depressed and are usefully considered as having a wide range of action on somatic symptoms as well as relieving depressed mood

Psychological treatments, especially cognitive behaviour therapy are superior to conservative medical care for a range of unexplained somatic complaints (Kroenke & Swindle 2000). In practice these treatments are best given by therapists used to working with medical patients; an approach based on that given to psychiatric patients often neglects the patient's somatic symptoms and medical concerns.

Physical rehabilitation services can be useful for patients with chronic severe disability, especially for patients with chronic pain and fatigue and for conversion disorders.

No treatment may be appropriate for some chronically disabled patients who, after consideration of the options, to not want to make changes. Acceptance of chronic disability rather than repeated and unproductive argument about the need for treatment can improve the doctor's relationship with the patient in such cases. Infrequent but long-term follow-up can often help to avoid iatrogenic damage and can sometimes be associated with gradual but positive changes in the patient's functioning.

Factitious disorders and malingering

Factitious disorders and malingering are conditions in which the patient deliberately feigns or otherwise manufactures symptoms (such as abdominal pain) and signs (such as haematemesis by swallowing and then regurgitating animal blood) with the aim of being regarded as sick and being given medical treatment (see below) (Sutherland & Rodin 1990). Factitious disorder is a psychiatric diagnosis and differentiated from malingering, which is not, on the basis that in the latter there is an obvious goal for the behaviour other than medical care (such as avoiding an exam). Both are differentiated from somatoform disorders, which are conditions in which the patient is considered not to have deliberately produced his symptoms. In practice, these distinctions are often not clear-cut.

Patients presenting with factitious disorder may be dramatic, dishonest and have extensive medical knowledge. They may also use an actual bodily abnormality such as a scar as evidence to support their story, for example of an abdominal condition that has required previous emergency surgery. Severe cases who move from hospital to hospital have been described as having Münchausen's syndrome, after Baron von Münchhausen who told fantastic tales of his exploits (Asher 1951). Factitious disorder is relatively rare but memorable because of the degree of difficulty it creates for doctors.

Management of factitious disorders

Usual management is first to prevent iatrogenic harm by stopping investigation and treatment, and then to combine confrontation of the patient with the evidence that they are deliberately creating signs of illness (e.g. evidence of self injection), with the offer of psychological help. This is only rarely accepted, however.

'Organic' mental disorder

These are disorders grouped on the basis that they result from demonstrable cerebral dysfunction. They are discussed in detail in Chapter 17. ICD-10 retains this term but it has been eschewed in DSM-IV (in order to avoid the implication that other disorders are not organic). All organic disorders are more commonly encountered in medical than in psychiatric settings. The most important is delirium associated with medical conditions and their treatment and with substance misuse.

Delirium is the term for a general syndrome of transient impairment of consciousness and cognitive function. It is more common in elderly inpatients where it may afflict as many as a quarter (Francis et al 1990). In most cases the delirium will result from the effect on the central nervous system of a coexisting medical condition or its treatment. It is especially common in the elderly and in those with pre-existing cognitive impairment. It is important because it is associated with a poorer medical outcome and with a greater length of stay in hospital.

Dementia is a major problem in the population and consequently for general medical services. As elderly persons are increasingly represented among hospital patients, the prevalence of dementia in the general hospital has increased. The most difficult task is often to differentiate dementia from delirium.

Other organic disorders are common in those with cerebral disease. These include the effect of damage to specific parts of the brain such as the frontal lobes. The symptoms may result from damage or from seizure activity. Misdiagnosis of such medical conditions as functional psychosis may occur and results in a lost opportunity for effective medical treatment (e.g. such as in the case of an operable cerebral tumour). Mood syndromes or *organic mood disorders* may occur because of a direct effect of a medical condition on the brain (but see comorbidity above).

Management of organic disorders

A prerequisite of management is detection. The diagnosis may be missed even if the patient is assessed. There are three common reasons for this: first, the cognitive impairment typically fluctuates (it is usually worse at night), and a 'snapshot' assessment may miss it; second, the patients may present with mood changes rather than confusion, leading to a misdiagnosis as mood disorder; third, cognitive impairment in an elderly patient may be incorrectly diagnosed as dementia when in fact it is of recent onset. A careful history from an informant and, if necessary, repeated assessments will often overcome these difficulties.

Once the diagnosis has been made it is essential to ensure that remediable medical causes have been sought and addressed. It is particularly important to suspect alcohol withdrawal, as this may explain the delirium and also indicates a risk of seizures and of Wernicke–Korsakoff syndrome. Treatment for the latter (with thiamine) can prevent the development of permanent memory impairment (Zubaran et al 1997). The other important management task is to limit potential damage to the patient (and to others). Close nursing observation and sedation may be required to prevent wandering and accidents. Nursing in a side room will minimise disruption to others (Brown & Boyle 2002).

Substance misuse disorders

Substance misuse is described in more detail in Chapter 18. A history of substance misuse is very common among patients seen in medical settings. Intoxication is a common cause of casualty attendance, and the behavioural effects, such as accidents, and complications such as liver damage are a cause of medical illness.

Alcohol misuse is the most common substance misuse disorder. Alcohol problems are encountered particularly frequently in accident and emergency departments. The problem is greater in males, and as many as 20% of male medical admissions are problem drinkers (Orford et al 1992).

Other substances commonly misused include opiates and psychostimulants. Presentation may be because of intoxication, withdrawal, or associated disease. Drug misusers are most likely to be encountered in inner-city casualty departments where they may present with disturbed behaviour, medical complications of misuse, or demands for drugs. The demands for drugs may be explicit, or implicit with a complaint of pain.

Management of substance misuse

The rate of detection of substance misuse without specific screening is low, but is improved by a systematic approach including specific questions, physical examination and appropriate investigations (Persson & Magnusson 1988). The physician is in a particularly good position to provide education about the adverse effects of substance misuse and to use the patient's concern for his health as a motivating factor for behavioural change. Simple advice and education can have a worthwhile effect on alcohol intake (Chick 1991). Similarly for patients who misuse other drugs, it is useful to give information, practical help to those who wish to abstain, and advice on harm limitation for those who do not. The management of severe pain in opiate users is a particular challenge. If the pain is genuine, it is helpful to find out their opiate intake from their prescriber. They may require much higher doses of opiates than usually required

Psychotic disorders

These are discussed in Chapter 19. Non-delirious psychosis is encountered in general medical settings relatively rarely, and most of such cases are known to psychiatric services. However, psychotic individuals may occasionally present with somatic complaints that may be bizarre in nature (such as 'my bowels are rotting'). New psychotic states occasionally arise during inpatient treatment and are often transient.

Management of psychotic disorders

Management may require the use of antipsychotic drugs and the application of compulsory powers to either enforce treatment in a medical ward but more often to enable removal to a psychiatric ward.

Other disorders

Eating disorders (see Ch. 22) are occasionally encountered in medical settings. They may be a cause of unexplained symptoms such as vomiting or weight loss or may severely complicate the management of a medical condition such as diabetes mellitus. If severe they require well-co-ordinated medical and psychiatric care.

Sexual problems are also common in medical patients, where they may result either from the medical conditions or its treatment (Hawton 1984). They are frequently neglected but are important to patients and may be a reason for non-adherence to treatments.

PSYCHIATRIC SERVICES FOR GENERAL MEDICAL SETTINGS

In an effort to improve the management of patients with psychiatric disorder who are attending non-psychiatric settings, attempts have been made to improve the level of psychiatric expertise available. One approach has been to educate the physicians working in these settings; another is to have psychiatrists or other mental health workers become directly involved in the care of medical patients.

Primary care

In primary care, efforts have focused on improving the management of patients with depressive disorder and with medically unexplained somatic complaints.

Recognition has been tackled by training physicians in interview methods, especially in the eliciting of depressive symptoms in patients who present somatically and by the systematic use of screening questionnaires (Pignone et al 2002). However, studies have found that this approach alone does not necessarily produce better patient outcomes (Gilbody et al 2001). Improvement in the outcome of patients successfully treated for depression appears to also require the involvement in the patients' care of a professional trained in psychiatric treatment (Von Korff et al 2001).

For functional somatic symptoms the problem is so large that most of the work on this topic has focused on attempts to improve the ability of primary-care doctors to engage and manage such patients themselves. Early studies show promise (Morriss & Gask 2002), and the findings of randomised trials that will examine the effectiveness of various training packages are awaited.

Secondary and tertiary care

Similar approaches have been attempted in general hospitals. Progress has been made in training medical specialists to elicit and recognise depressive disorder in specific areas such as oncology (Parle et al 1997). However, both the biomedical focus of hospital physicians' work and the time pressure under which they work are obstacles to the widespread adoption of this approach. There is therefore a case for systematic screening of patients here also, for example by using computer touch-screen-administered questionnaires (McLachlan et al 2001).

Specialist services

In order to improve the treatment of psychiatric illness in general hospitals, a number of small, dedicated general hospital psychiatric departments have been established specifically for this purpose. These units have been devoted principally to the management of conspicuous psychiatric morbidity, especially deliberate self-harm (see Ch. 27) and to the management of obvious psychiatric emergencies in inpatients, rather than to the systematic detection and management of the full range of psychiatric disorder encountered in general hospitals. Two principal ways of working have been described: 'liaison', which involves meeting with medical staff and discussing both general management issues and the management of individual patients; and 'consultation', which is the giving of opinions on individual referred patients. Most services now use a combination of both approaches and are referred to as consultation–liaison or C-L services in the USA and simply as liaison psychiatry or psychological medicine services in the UK. The staff usually includes a consultant psychiatrist together with a clinical psychologist and specialist nursing staff.

Are these services effective? The studies that have set out to demonstrate the overall effectiveness of generic C-L services in improving the outcomes of medical inpatients have so far failed to do so (Goldberg 1992, Levenson et al 1992). However, small trials of more targeted services for conditions such as pelvic pain (Blake et al 1998) and chronic fatigue syndrome (Sharpe et al 1996) have been able to demonstrate substantial benefits. More and larger trials of targeted interventions are clearly required.

Medical–psychiatric units

A further development has been the establishment of medical–psychiatric (or 'Med-Psych') inpatient units for those patients with both severe medical and psychiatric illnesses (Kathol 1994). These units are staffed by physicians trained in both general medicine and general psychiatry. Anyone who has been involved in the management of a patient with both a severe medical condition and a significant psychiatric disorder (such as severe debility in a woman with anorexia nervosa) will immediately see the potential value of such a facility. However, they require specially trained staff and are likely to have only a small number of beds, so great care needs to be taken in selection of patients admitted to them. There are no such units outside the USA.

Future developments

Future trends in the development of psychiatric liaison services are likely to include:

- a greater focus on outpatients and on primary care;
- the development of closer collaborative working with physicians — e.g. joint clinics;
- the greater use of specialist nurses to deliver treatments;
- an increased focus on reducing excess medical costs and inappropriate use of medical services.

Summary points

- Psychiatric disorder in medical settings often presents as somatic symptoms or as problems with medical care.
- The most common diagnoses encountered are depression, anxiety, somatoform disorders, alcohol misuse, and delirium.
- The coexistence of a medical condition and a psychiatric disorder (comorbidity) is common and may complicate the management of both.
- Psychiatric treatments are effective in medical patients with psychiatric disorder, but management needs to take into account both the patient's medical conditions and treatment and the medical setting.

The role of primary care, the relationship between specialist hospital liaison psychiatry and general psychiatry services, and the question of who pays for the care of patients with unexplained somatic symptoms and with medical psychiatric comorbidity will no doubt continue to generate argument and controversy. However, the interface between psychiatry and other areas of medicine is likely to remain a clinically important one and to become increasingly central to the future of psychiatry as a medical specialty.

SUGGESTED READING

Creed F, Guthrie E (eds) 1996 Seminars in liaison psychiatry. Royal College of Psychiatrists, London

Mayou R A, Bass C, Sharpe M (eds) 1995 Treatment of functional somatic symptoms. Oxford University Press, Oxford

Mayou R A, Sharpe M, Carson A C (eds) 2003 The ABC of psychological medicine. BMJ Books, London

Royal College of Physicians and Royal College of Psychiatrists 2003 The psychological care of medical patients: a practical guide. Report of a joint working party. Royal College of Physicians of London

REFERENCES

Alexander F 1950 Psychosomatic medicine: its principles and applications. Norton, New York

Alexander P J, Dinesh N, Vidyasagar M S 1993 Psychiatric morbidity among cancer patients and its relationship with awareness of illness and expectations about treatment outcome. Acta Oncologica 32:623–626

Appleby L 1987 Hypochondriasis: an acceptable diagnosis? British Medical Journal 294:857

Asher R A J 1951 Munchausen's syndrome. The Lancet i:339–341

Barbor T F, de la Fuente J R, Saunders J, Grant M 1992 AUDIT: The alcohol use disorders identification test. World Health Organization, Geneva

Barsky A J, Wyshak G 1989 Hypochondriasis and related health attitudes. Psychosomatics 30:412–420

Barsky A J, Wyshak G, Klerman G L, Latham K S 1990 The prevalence of hypochondriasis in medical outpatients. Social Psychiatry and Psychiatric Epidemiology 25:89–94

Bass C, Murphy M 1995 Somatoform and personality disorders: syndromal comorbidity and overlapping developmental pathways. Journal of Psychosomatic Research 39:403–427

Blake F, Salkovskis P M, Gath D et al 1998 Cognitive therapy for premenstrual syndrome: a controlled trial. Journal of Psychosomatic Research 45:307–318

Brown T M, Boyle M F 2002 Delirium. British Medical Journal 325:644–647

Carney R M, Freedland K E, Eisen S A et al 1995 Major depression and medication adherence in elderly patients with coronary artery disease. Health Psychology 14:88–90

Cassano P, Fava M 2002 Depression and public health: an overview. Journal of Psychosomatic Research 53:849–857

Chick J 1991 Early intervention for hazardous drinking in the general hospital. Alcohol & Alcoholism Supplement 1:477–479

Davison P, Sharpe M, Wade D, Bass C 1999 "Wheelchair" patients with nonorganic disease: a psychological inquiry. Journal of Psychosomatic Research 47:93–103

Editorial 1982 Goodbye neurosis? The Lancet i:29

Eisenberg L 1986 Mindless and brainless in psychiatry. British Journal of Psychiatry 148:497–508

Emmerson J P, Burvill P W, Finlay Jones R, Hall W 1989 Life events, life difficulties and confiding relationships in the depressed elderly. British Journal of Psychiatry 155:787–792

Engel G L 1977 The need for a new medical model: a challenge for biomedicine. Science 196:129–196

Escobar J I, Burnam M A, Karno M et al 1987 Somatization in the community. Archives of General Psychiatry 44:713–718

Fink P 1992 The use of hospitalizations by persistent somatizing patients. Psychological Medicine 22:173–180

Fleet R P, Dupuis G, Marchand A et al 1998 Panic disorder in coronary artery disease patients with noncardiac chest pain. Journal of Psychosomatic Research 44:81–90

Folstein M F, Folstein S E, McHugh P R 1975 Mini-Mental State. Journal of Psychiatric Research 12:189–198

Francis J, Martin D, Kapoor W N 1990 A prospective study of delirium in hospitalized elderly. Journal of the American Medical Association 263:1097–1101

Frasure-Smith N, Lesperance F, Talajic M 1993 Depression following myocardial infarction. Impact on 6-month survival. Journal of the American Medical Association 270:1819–1825

Fukuda K, Straus S E, Hickie I B et al 1994 Chronic Fatigue Syndrome: a comprehensive approach to its definition and management. Annals of Internal Medicine 121:953–959

Gilbody S M, House A O, Sheldon T A 2001 Routinely administered questionnaires for depression and anxiety: systematic review. British Medical Journal 322s:406–409

Gill D, Hatcher S 1999 A systematic review of the treatment of depression with antidepressant drugs in patients who also have a physical illness. Journal of Psychosomatic Research 47:131–143

Godding P R, McAnulty R D, Wittrock D A et al 1995 Predictors of depression among male cancer patients. Journal of Nervous & Mental Disease 183:95–98

Goldberg D, Bridges K, Duncan-Jones P, Grayson D 1988 Detecting anxiety and depression in general medical settings. British Medical Journal 297:897–899

Goldberg D P 1992 The treatment of mental disorders in general medical settings. General Hospital Psychiatry 14:83–85

Goldin C S 1994 Stigmatization and AIDS: critical issues in public health. Social Science in Medicine 39:1359–1366

Granville-Grossman K 1993 Mind and body. In: Lader M H (ed) Handbook of psychiatry, vol 2. Cambridge University Press, Cambridge

Greer S 1992 The management of denial in cancer patients. Oncology 6:33–36

Guthrie E 1996 Emotional disorder in chronic illness: psychotherapeutic interventions. British Journal of Psychiatry 168:265–273

Guze S B 1993 Genetics of Briquet's syndrome and somatization disorder: a review of family, adoption, and twin studies. Annals of Clinical Psychiatry 5:225–230

Hamilton J, Campos R, Creed F 1996 Anxiety, depression and the management of medically unexplained symptoms in medical clinics. Journal of the Royal College of Physicians of London 30:18–20

Hawton K E 1984 Sexual adjustment of men who have had strokes. Journal of Psychosomatic Research 28:243–249

House A 1988 Mood disorders in the physically ill — problems of definition and measurement. Journal of Psychosomatic Research 32:345–353

House A O, Andrews H B 1988 Life events and difficulties preceding the onset of functional dysphonia. Journal of Psychosomatic Research 32:311–319

House A O, Dennis M, Mogridge L et al 1990 Life events and difficulties preceding stroke. Journal of Neurology, Neurosurgery & Psychiatry 53:1024–1028

Howland R H 1993 General health, health care utilization, and medical comorbidity in dysthymia. International Journal of Psychiatry in Medicine 23:211–238

Huyse F J, Strain J J, Hammer J S 1990 Interventions in consultation/liaison psychiatry, Part II: Concordance. General Hospital Psychiatry 12:221–231

Kathol R G 1994 Medical psychiatry units: the wave of the future. General Hospital Psychiatry 16:1–3

Kathol R G, Mutgi A, Williams J et al 1990 Diagnosis of major depression in cancer patients according to four sets of criteria. American Journal of Psychiatry 147:1021–1024

Katon W 1996 Panic disorder: relationship to high medical utilization, unexplained physical symptoms, and medical costs. Journal of Clinical Psychiatry 57 (suppl 10):11–18

Katon W, Ciechanowski P 2002 Impact of major depression on chronic medical illness. Journal of Psychosomatic Research 53:859

Katon W, Schulberg H 1992 Epidemiology of depression in primary care. General Hospital Psychiatry 14:237–247

Katon W, Robinson P, Von Korff M et al 1996 A multifaceted intervention to improve treatment of depression in primary care. Archives of General Psychiatry 53:924–932

Kenyon F 1964 Hypochondriasis: a clinical study. British Journal of Psychiatry 100:478–488

Kiecolt-Glaser J K, Glaser R 1989 Psychoneuroimmunology: past, present, and future. Health Psychology 8:677–682

Kirmayer L J 1988 Mind and body as metaphors: hidden values in biomedicine. In: Lock M, Gordon D (eds) Biomedicine examined. Kluwer, Dordrecht, p 57–92

Kroenke K, Price R K 1993 Symptoms in the community: prevalence, classification, and psychiatric comorbidity. Archives of Internal Medicine 153:2474–2480

Kroenke K, Swindle R 2000 Cognitive-behavioral therapy for somatization and symptom syndromes: a critical review of controlled clinical trials. Psychotherapy & Psychosomatics 69:205–215

Levenson J L, Hamer R M, Rossiter L F 1992 A randomized controlled study of psychiatric consultation guided by screening in general medical inpatients. American Journal of Psychiatry 149:631–637

Mace C J, Trimble M R 1996 Ten-year prognosis of conversion disorder. British Journal of Psychiatry 169:282–288

McLachlan S A, Allenby A, Matthews J et al 2001 Randomized trial of coordinated psychosocial interventions based on patient self-assessments versus standard care to improve the psychosocial functioning of patients with cancer. Journal of Clinical Oncology 19:4117–4125

Mathew R J, Weinman M L, Mirabi M 1981 Physical symptoms of depression. British Journal of Psychiatry 139:293–296

Mayou R A 2002 Psychiatric consequences of motor vehicle accidents. Psychiatric Clinics of North America 25:27–41, vi

Mayou R A, Hawton K E, Feldman E, Ardern M 1991 Psychiatric problems among medical admissions. International Journal of Psychiatry in Medicine 21:71–84

Mechanic D 1986 The concept of illness behaviour: culture, situation and personal predisposition. Psychological Medicine 16:1–7

Moffic H S, Paykel E S 1975 Depression in medical in-patients. British Journal of Psychiatry 126:346–353

Morris P L, Robinson R G, Andrzejewski P et al 1993 Association of depression with 10-year poststroke mortality. American Journal of Psychiatry 150:124–129

Morrison J D 1989 Childhood sexual histories of women with somatization disorder. American Journal of Psychiatry 146:239–241

Morriss R K, Gask L 2002 Treatment of patients with somatized mental disorder: effects of reattribution training on outcomes under the direct control of the family doctor. Psychosomatics 43:394–399

O'Malley P G, Jackson J L, Santoro J et al 1999 Antidepressant therapy for unexplained symptoms and symptom syndromes. Journal of Family Practice 48:980–990

Orford J, Somers M, Daniels V, Kirby B 1992 Drinking amongst medical patients: levels of risk and models of change. British Journal of Addiction 87:1691–1702

Parle M, Maguire P, Heaven C 1997 The development of a training model to improve health professionals' skills, self-efficacy and outcome expectancies when communicating with cancer patients. Social Science & Medicine 44:231–240

Persson J, Magnusson P H 1988 Comparison between different methods of detecting patients with excessive consumption of alcohol. Acta Medica Scandinavica 223:101–109

Pignone M P, Gaynes B N, Rushton J L et al 2002 Screening for depression in adults: a summary of the evidence for the U.S. Preventive Services Task Force. Annals of Internal Medicine 136:765–776

Pilowsky I 1969 Abnormal illness behaviour. Psychological Medicine 42:347–351

Reichsman F, Levy N 1973 Problems in adaptation to maintenance haemodialysis: a four year study of 25 patients. Archives of Internal Medicine 130:859–865

Salkovskis P M, Warwick H M 1986 Morbid preoccupations, health anxiety and reassurance: a cognitive-behavioural approach to hypochondriasis. Behaviour Research and Therapy 24:597–602

Scadding G 1996 Essentialism and nominalism in medicine: logic of diagnosis in disease terminology. The Lancet 348:594–596

Shalev A Y, Schreiber S, Galai T, Melmed R N 1993 Post-traumatic stress disorder following medical events. British Journal of Clinical Psychology 32:247–253

Sharpe M 2002 The English Chief Medical Officer's Working Parties' report on the management of CFS/ME: Significant breakthrough or unsatisfactory compromise? Journal of Psychosomatic Research 52:437–438

Sharpe M 2003 Distinguishing malingering from psychiatric disorders. In: Halligan P W, Bass C, Oakley D A (eds) Malingering and illness deception. Oxford University Press, Oxford

Sharpe M, Carson A J 2001 "Unexplained" somatic symptoms, functional syndromes, and somatization: Do we need a paradigm shift? Annals of Internal Medicine 134:926–930

Sharpe M, Williams 2001 Treating patients with hypochondriasis and somatoform pain disorder. In: Turk D C, Gatchel R J (eds) Psychological approaches to pain management. Guilford, New York

Sharpe M, Mayou R A, Seagroatt V 1994 Why do doctors find some patients difficult to help ? Quarterly Journal of Medicine 87:187–193

Sharpe M, Hawton K E, Simkin S et al 1996 Cognitive behaviour therapy for the chronic fatigue syndrome: a randomized controlled trial. British Medical Journal 312:22–26

Sharpe M, Allen K, Strong V et al 2004 Major depression in outpatients attending a regional cancer centre: screening, prevalence and unmet treatment needs. British Journal of Cancer 90:314–320

Sherbourne C D, Jackson C A, Meredith L S et al 1996 Prevalence of comorbid anxiety disorders in primary care outpatients. Archives of Family Medicine 5:27–34

Shorter E 1992 From paralysis to fatigue: a history of psychosomatic illness in the modern era. Free Press, New York

Slater E O 1965 Diagnosis of hysteria. British Medical Journal 1:1395–1399

Spitzer R L, Williams J B, Kroenke K et al 1994 Utility of a new procedure for diagnosing mental disorders in primary care: the PRIME-MD 1000 study. Journal of the American Medical Association 272:1749–1756

Steckel W 1943 The interpretation of dreams. Liveright, New York

Stone J, Wojcik W, Durrance D 2002 What should we say to patients with symptoms unexplained by disease? The "number needed to offend". British Medical Journal 325:1449–1450

Sullivan M D, Youngner S J 1994 Depression, competence, and the right to refuse lifesaving medical treatment. American Journal of Psychiatry 151:971–978

Sutherland A J, Rodin G M 1990 Factitious disorders in a general hospital setting: clinical features and a review of the literature. Psychosomatics 31:392–399

van Dulmen A M, Fennis J F, Mokkink H G et al 1995 Doctor-dependant changes in complaint related cognitions and anxiety during medical consultations in functional abdominal complaints. Psychological Medicine 25:1011–1018

Van Hemert A M, Hawton K E, Bolk J H, Fagg J R 1993 Key symptoms in the detection of affective disorders in medical patients. Journal of Psychosomatic Research 37:397–404

Veale D, Boocock A, Gournay K et al 1996 Body dysmorphic disorder: a survey of fifty cases. British Journal of Psychiatry 169:196–201

Von Korff M, Simon G 1996 The relationship between pain and depression. British Journal of Psychiatry Supplement 168:101–108

Von Korff M, Katon W, Unutzer J et al 2001 Improving depression care: barriers, solutions, and research needs. Journal of Family Practice 50(6):E1

Ware J E, Sherbourne C D 1992 The MOS 36-item short-form health survey. Medical Care 30:473–481

Warwick H M, Salkovskis P M 1985 Reassurance. British Medical Journal 290:1028

Warwick H M, Salkovskis P M 1990 Hypochondriasis. Behaviour Research & Therapy 28:105–117

Wells K B, Golding J M, Burnam M A 1988 Psychiatric disorder in a sample of the general population with and without chronic medical conditions. American Journal of Psychiatry 145:976–981

Wessely S, Bisson J 2001 Brief psychological interventions ("debriefing") for trauma-related symptoms and prevention of post traumatic stress disorder. Cochrane Database of Systematic Reviews, Issue 1

Wessely S, Lewis G H 1989 The classification of psychiatric morbidity in attenders at a dermatology clinic. British Journal of Psychiatry 155:686–691

Wessely S, Nimnuan C, Sharpe M 1999 Functional somatic syndromes: one or many? The Lancet 354:936–939

Weyerer S 1990, Relationships between physical and psychological disorders. In: Sartoris N et al (eds) Psychological disorders in general medical settings. Hogrefe and Huber, Toronto, p 34–46

Wolfe F 1990 Fibromyalgia. Rheumatic Disease Clinics of North America 16:681–698

Zigmond A S, Snaith R P 1983 The hospital anxiety and depression scale. Acta Psychiatrica Scandinavica 67:361–370

Zubaran C, Fernandes J G, Rodnight R 1997 Wernicke–Korsakoff syndrome. Postgraduate Medical Journal 73:27–31

The relationship between crime and psychiatry

Derek Chiswick, Lindsay D G Thomson

INTRODUCTION

This chapter is about the relationship between crime and mental disorder, the forensic aspects of certain psychiatric disorders, risk assessment, the clinical aspects of certain crimes, and the mentally disordered offender in the criminal justice system.

Biological basis for crime

In 2000, police in England and Wales recorded 5.2 million crimes. Figures from the British Crime Survey (2002) suggest that only half of all offences are reported to the police and a quarter are recorded. Crime is therefore common. A third of men, and 9% of women, born in 1953 were convicted of an offence by the age of 46, though two-thirds of their offences were committed by 8% of the male population (Home Office 2001). Crime is an activity of teenagers and young adults; the rates peak at 18–20 years for males. Females account for about 1 in 5 offenders, and their peak age for offending is 2–3 years earlier than for males. Theft in its various forms, car crimes and criminal damage account for over 80% of recorded crimes.

Before considering the association between individual psychiatric disorders and crime, we will briefly consider the biological basis for criminal behaviour generally. For an activity as common, and yet diverse, as crime, most observers agree that explanations must be multifactorial in type, and that postulating a single mental condition as the 'cause' of criminal behaviour would be absurd. No biological explanation for criminal behaviour has withstood scientific analysis. Nonetheless, researchers continue to seek evidence of a criminal trait and to explore whether biological factors make a contribution to criminal behaviour.

Farrington (1993) has drawn attention to the range of factors that contribute to criminal behaviour (Box 29.1). To these we can add the inconsistencies of the criminal justice system in which detection, arrest, prosecution and conviction are variables that will have a major influence on who is and is not ultimately classified as 'criminal'.

Can psychiatry have anything of value to say about the concept of criminality? The clinical approach to criminology has become unfashionable. It has its roots in psychoanalytical theory, and its tenets have been based on detained and therefore the largely 'unsuccessful' offenders. More significantly it is scarred by Lombrosian beliefs, that criminals can somehow be identified, whether it be by the shape of their head or by other stigmata of degeneration associated with the eugenics movement of the early 20th century. However, two developments have re-ignited interest in the biological component of criminality. First is the opportunity afforded by research developments in molecular genetics, and second is the policy espoused by the UK government that it intends to introduce preventive detention for those identified as having a dangerous severe personality disorder (see p. 723).

Genetics, personality, psychopathy and intelligence

Attempts to identify the genetics of antisocial behaviour have been bedevilled by the different concepts of antisocial behaviour. In other words, 'what is the relevant condition the genetics of which we need to study?'. Psychiatrists tend to seek diagnostic categories such as conduct disorder or antisocial personality disorder. Criminologists regard antisocial behaviour as any behaviour that is against the law, perhaps with distinctions for frequency and types of offending. Personality psychologists conceptualise personality traits based on attitudes, beliefs or preferences that are said to indicate an inclination to take advantage of or to harm others. Finally there are strong proponents of the concept of psychopathy as a disorder distinct from antisocial personality disorder, in which diminished capacity for remorse and poor behavioural control are present (Hare 1991). Moffitt (2002) emphasises the importance of regarding antisocial behaviour as a normally distributed continuum; the most reliable genetic research is based on gathering data about a wide range of antisocial behaviours over a period of observation that is long enough for the research cohort to exhibit that behaviour.

In an important recent review Moffitt (2002) concludes that the most reliable research produces estimates of around 0.5 for the heritability of antisocial behaviour. Indeed a meta analysis of 51 twin and adoption studies yielded an estimated heritability of 0.41. This finding that 50% of persistent antisocial behaviour is attributable to genetic factors would fit with a behaviour that is normally distributed in the population. The role of assortative mating in concentrating these genes that drive excessive antisocial behaviour is of course crucial. Heritability of antisocial behaviour appears to be slightly higher in males than in females.

Is the heritability of violent behaviour the same as that for antisocial behaviour? The research evidence cannot provide an answer; there are major methodological problems in measuring violence. According to criminal record data, violent behaviour has a low base rate, and conviction records are, in any case, a poor indicator of 'true violence'. There is probable heritability for violent behaviour but it cannot be determined at present.

There is a long-established link between low intelligence and delinquency (Rutter & Giller 1983). The inference that this

---

Box 29.1   Factors that influence offending

- Genetic factors
- Personality and impulsivity
- Intelligence
- The natural history of offending behaviour
- Family influences
- Peer influence
- Schools
- Socio-economic deprivation
- Community influences
- Ethnicity

From Farrington (1993).

---

results from an increased likelihood of duller offenders being caught is not borne out by research. The finding holds for self-reported, as well as recorded, offending even though offending by less intelligent youngsters is more likely to be 'missed' in self-report research. Low intelligence is probably related to general neuropsychological deficits, particularly the ability to manipulate abstract concepts. Conversely, high intelligence may be protective for high-risk children, giving them the opportunity to escape from a ghetto background. The interaction of biological and social disadvantage is encapsulated in a disturbing study of 14 juveniles on death row in America (Lewis et al 1988). The youths showed serious central nervous system deficits, low intelligence and multiple psychotic symptoms. Five had been sodomised by a relative, and nearly all came from violent families.

Molecular genetics and brain dysfunction

A natural consequence of finding significant heritability is to search for the expression of the genes at molecular level. The wide distribution of antisocial behaviour disorder in the community suggests that many genes of small effect are likely to play a part, rather than the popular misconception that there is a 'gene for crime'. An association reported in the 1960s of an extra Y chromosome in some offenders was later shown to be an invalid finding (Borgaonkar & Shah 1974).

The finding of a single point gene mutation in a Dutch family in which the male members were seriously violent and aggressive caused much interest (Brunner et al 1993). Attention focused on the gene responsible for producing monoamine oxidase A (MAOA), an enzyme involved in the metabolism of serotonin. Caspi et al (2002) studied the link between the genotypes producing high and low levels of MAOA activity in the brain and antisocial behaviour in 500 boys. Boys with low levels of MAOA activity were significantly more likely to be antisocial but only if they had also been maltreated and abused as children. The interaction between the genetic variant and the environment was crucial in the association with antisocial behaviour. Gene–environment interaction was similarly important in a Danish study of 397 males followed from birth to early adult life. A subgroup with early neuromotor deficits who also had unstable families showed more than twice the adolescent disturbance and adult criminality than subgroups with either neuromotor deficits or family instability alone (Raine et al 1996).

Emotional impairment giving rise to poor socialisation is a cardinal feature of the diagnostic criteria for psychopathy.

Neuroimaging studies have shown that amygdala and possibly orbitofrontal cortical dysfunction is associated with psychopathy (Blair 2003). It is postulated that the processes of aversive conditioning and instrumental learning, both necessary in acquiring socialisation, are impaired. Numerous studies have shown that persistent and pervasive aggressive and disruptive behaviours in children under 11 years are strongly associated with antisocial behaviours in adolescent and adult life.

Finally, evidence of a genetic basis for criminal behaviour has obvious social and legal implications. So far, the admissibility of such evidence in cases coming before the courts in America and elsewhere has met with varying success. The XYY syndrome has been introduced but failed as a defence in five major American cases; in Australia, France and Germany it may have been a factor affecting sentence in some cases (Denno 1996). Of more interest is the case of Stephen Mobley, who in 1991 shot and killed a pizza store manager in Georgia during an armed robbery. On the basis of his personal, criminal and family history, his lawyer requested the court that he undergo testing for a possible genetic absence of MAOA. The court refused the testing and Mobley awaits execution on death row; repeated appeals have been based on other legal issues.

CRIME AND MENTAL DISORDER

Some people with a psychiatric disorder may behave in a criminal manner, and some offenders have psychiatric disorders. Crime and psychiatric disorder is therefore a legitimate area for psychiatric study, but attempts to understand what, if any, is the relationship between crime and psychiatric disorder are fraught with problems. These arise for five principal reasons:

- Crime is a man-made concept; it is whatever a society chooses at any particular time to decree as unlawful. The classifications of crime change within the same country over time (e.g. in the UK in relation to abortion, homosexual acts and prostitution), and they vary from country to country.
- The use of a person's criminal record as a measure of his offending is unreliable: most crime is unreported and undetected. It is also impossible to glean the nature and gravity of an offence simply from its statutory description. Indecent assault, for example, may be the merest contact between perpetrator and victim or a sexual attack of homicidal intensity. Classification of the degree of violence in an assault is an inexact science.
- Most research is based on captive populations of offenders (and patients) because this is more easily conducted. There are no systems for the routine psychiatric examination of court-based samples. Thus criminals in prison are more likely to be studied than either criminals in the community or criminals who are never caught. Extrapolating findings from such samples may be misleading. Self-report studies and criminal surveys of community samples are of greater value and are beginning to be reported. Similarly, psychiatric research cohorts in this field have tended to be on inpatient rather than community-based samples. It may not be possible to generalise findings from these restricted samples. Cohorts which include, where appropriate, undetected sufferers of psychiatric disorder in the community are preferable.

Table 29.1 Studies of psychiatric morbidity in prisoners

Authors	Measures	Prisoners	Results
Gunn et al (1991)	CIS	1769 male convicted	2% psychosis* 6% neurotic disorder* 23% drug/alcohol abuse[†]
Cooke (1994)	SADS-L	247 male remand/convicted	7.3% major psychological disorders* 32% neurotic disorder* 38% alcohol dependence[†] 20.6% drug abuse/dependence[†]
Davidson et al (1995)	CIS	389 male remand	2.3% psychosis* 24.8% neurotic disorder* 22% alcohol abuse/dependence[†] 73% drug abuse/dependence[†]
Brooke et al (1996)	SADS-L	750 male remand	5% psychosis* 26% neurotic disorder* 38% drug/alcohol misuse[†]
Birmingham et al (1996)	SADS-L	548 male remand	4% psychosis* 22% minor psychological disorder* 32% alcohol abuse/dependence[†] 33% drug misuse/dependence[†]
Singleton et al (1998)	CIS-R SCAN	1250 male remand	10% psychosis 59% neurotic disorder* 58% alcohol abuse[‡] 51% drug dependence[‡]
Singleton et al (1998)	CIS-R SCAN	1121 male convicted	7% psychosis* 40% neurotic disorder* 63% alcohol abuse[‡] 43% drug dependence[‡]

* Point prevalence.
[†] Lifetime diagnosis.
[‡] Present in past year.
CIS, Clinical Interview Schedule; CIS-R, Clinical Interview Schedule – Revised; SADS-L, Schedule for Affective Disorders and Schizophrenia – Lifetime Version; SCAN, Schedules for Clinical Assessment in Neuropsychiatry

- Great care must be taken before extrapolating findings from one population to another. The relation between crime and mental disorder is affected by overall rates of crime, the operation of the criminal justice system, social policy in respect of offenders, and the nature and the provision of healthcare and social care for mentally disordered people. These factors differ between countries and in different areas of the same country; they also vary over time within individual countries. Conclusions must therefore be considered in the context of prevailing circumstances.
- Use of standardised diagnostic criteria in research on offender populations is a relatively recent development. Older studies tended to group together all diagnostic categories, often including personality disorders and substance misuse disorders within a single category of 'mentally disordered'.

While bearing in mind the limitations imposed by these factors, it is convenient to consider the relationship between crime and mental disorder by examining:

- the extent of mental disorder among offenders;
- the criminality of psychiatric populations;
- the manner in which specific psychiatric disorders might sometimes be associated with criminal acts.

Mental disorder in offenders

Mental disorder in prison populations

The total prison population in the United Kingdom is heading towards 100 000. Psychiatric morbidity in both the remanded (i.e. those awaiting trial) and sentenced prison populations has been found to be significantly higher than in the community, although findings vary depending on the population sampled and instruments used. See Table 29.1 (Bartlett et al 2001).

A recent systematic review (Fazel & Danesh 2002) of 23 000 prisoners in 12 countries showed 4% had a psychotic illness and 10% had a major depressive disorder; 47% of male and 21% of female prisoners had an antisocial personality disorder. Findings from prisons in America indicate that the number of inmates with a psychotic illness or depression is equal to twice the number of all patients currently in American psychiatric hospitals.

The presence of a mental illness is one of the factors likely to lead an accused person to be remanded in prison rather than be granted bail. Prisoners may also develop mental illness during their period of remand or sentence. Although it is possible to treat mental illness in prison, the standard of psychiatric care is likely to fall far short of that available in the National Health Service (Reed

2003). The mentally disordered offender has been depicted as the 'revolving door psychiatric patient' of the 1990s (Birmingham 1999). Treatment in the absence of the prisoner's consent is not permitted. Where a prisoner requires treatment in hospital this is possible under mental health legislation (see Table 29.2). Problems may arise in obtaining a suitable psychiatric bed, and there are significant delays in effecting transfers to hospitals (Reed 2003).

Suicide in prison Suicide in prison is an issue of major concern (see Box 29.2). The rate of prison suicide is eight times that of the young male community population, although direct comparisons are difficult because of lack of studies using appropriate controls (Royal College of Psychiatrists 2002). More than 14% of prison suicides take place in the prison healthcare centre (Reed 2003). A newly introduced prison suicide risk reduction strategy in UK prisons has emphasised the importance of multidisciplinary assessment and management. There has been a cultural shift away from segregation and strip cells to supportive, non-isolating care for prisoners with an identified risk of self-harm.

Female prisoners Women in prison show higher rates of neurotic conditions, personality disorder and substance abuse than men (Maden et al 1990). They are less likely than male prisoners to be serving a sentence for violence or burglary but are more likely to have committed a drug offence, theft, fraud or deception. Prison has become a receptacle for some very disturbed women with severe personality disorders, many of whom have previously been rejected for admission to secure hospital facilities (Gorsuch 1999).

In an endeavour to tackle mental health problems some prisons have established mental health teams. Some run day programmes for vulnerable or mentally disordered offenders; their success is dependent on clarity of purpose, a multidisciplinary approach and sufficient resources (Bartlett et al 2001). Comorbid substance abuse and personality disorder is common in this population.

Table 29.2   Mental Health Act 1983 — authority to transfer prisoners to psychiatric hospital

Provision Number in 2000–01*	Act & Section Authority	Recommendation	Psychiatric grounds for transfer from prison to hospital	Duration Appeal
Transfer direction. Removal to hospital of prisoners: chiefly those on remand or detained under immigration legislation *n* = 21	MHA 1983 S.48 Home Secretary must be of the opinion, having considered the public interest and the circumstances of the case, that the transfer is expedient	Two fully registered medical practitioners (one approved under S.12 as having special experience in the diagnosis or treatment of mental disorder)	Suffering from a mental illness or severe mental impairment of a nature or degree which makes detention in hospital for medical treatment appropriate and that the need for such treatment is urgent	Period of remand or until return to prison/ detention centre. Immediate right of appeal to Mental Health Review Tribunal on transfer
Transfer direction. Removal to hospital of convicted prisoners *n* = 14	MHA 1983 S.47 Home Secretary	Two fully registered medical practitioners (one approved under S.12 as having special experience in the diagnosis or treatment of mental disorder)	Suffering from a mental illness, psychopathic disorder, mental impairment or severe mental impairment of a nature or degree to make detention in hospital for medical treatment appropriate. If the case is of psychopathic disorder or mental impairment then such treatment must be likely to alleviate or prevent a deterioration of the condition	6 months, renewable for a further 6 months and thereafter annually. RMO can discharge from detention. Right of appeal to Mental Health Review Tribunal within first 6 months of transfer and on each renewal of detention
Restriction direction. Restriction on discharge of remand or sentenced prisoners transferred to hospital S.47 + S.49 *n* = 214[†] S.48 + S.49 *n* = 210[†]	MHA 1983 S.49 Mandatory for remand prisoners (not civil or immigration detainees) Otherwise at discretion of Home Secretary. Decision based on public safety and length of sentence to serve			S.48 until court deals fully with case. S.47 until return to prison or expiry of sentence (can then be converted to equivalent of a hospital order) Appeal as S.47 or S.48

* Department of Health (2001a).
[†] Johnson & Taylor (2002).
RMO, responsible medical officer.

Box 29.2	Prison suicide
High risk	• Remand prisoners
	• First 3 months of imprisonment
	• History of self harm — 25% male and 40% female prisoners
Method	• Asphyxiation commonest
Number	• 100/year in UK
Suicide risk reduction strategy	• Anti-bullying measures
	• Staff-training programmes
	• Screening of all admissions to prison
	• Confidential prisoner listener schemes
	• Multidisciplinary assessment and decision making
	• Active response for families, prisoners and staff following a suicide

Drug and alcohol programmes and some specific interventions such as anger management have been developed to assist prisoners with these problems, but access is limited and the provision is not uniform.

Criminality in psychiatric populations

The traditional view

Criminal behaviour, particularly violence, by the mentally ill has become a major public issue in the Western world. In the context of an increasing crime rate the public has identified the mentally ill as a significant contributory factor (Appleby & Wessely 1988, Levey & Howells 1995). The UK government has responded by emphasising public protection as the paramount issue in its mental health policies. The question 'how criminal are people with psychiatric disorder?' can never be answered with certainty, and any answer requires qualification. As a proportion of all psychiatric admissions, the number of patients admitted compulsorily as a consequence of an offence is tiny. In 2000–01 there were 1300 hospital admissions in England and Wales under Part III (the criminal provisions) of the Mental Health Act 1983; this represents approximately 5% of all compulsory admissions to hospitals (Department of Health 2001a). During a 3-year period between 1996 and 1999 a confidential inquiry into suicides and homicides identified 164 homicides committed by people with symptoms of mental illness at the time of the killing (Department of Health 2001b). The mentally ill perpetrators accounted for 15% of the total number of killings in the period under study.

Early research in this area concentrated on arrest rates in former psychiatric patients. These were shown to be equal to or only marginally higher than those of the general population, or only higher for certain offences. However, when arrest rates of former mental hospital patients were compared with samples matched for demographic variables, the differences disappeared (Monahan & Steadman 1983). Thus a somewhat sanguine view of the relation between mental illness and violent offending prevailed for many years. It was held that the well-established factors associated with offending, such as poverty, criminality in the family, poor parenting, school failure, and hyperactivity and antisocial behaviour in childhood, were powerful factors that overshadowed any effect due to mental illness (West 1988).

A reappraisal

In the last decade there has been a reappraisal driven by the fact that new research has shown clear associations between violence and certain diagnostic groups (Monahan & Steadman 1994, Wessely 1997). For example there are high rates of serious mental illness, particularly schizophrenia, in prisoners remanded in custody (see above), high rates of violence by mentally ill people before admission to hospital (MacMillan & Johnson 1987, Humphreys et al 1992) and during their admission (Tuninger et al 2001). Better research has demonstrated clearer relationships between various psychiatric disorders and offending behaviour. This research has been based on:

• large and comprehensive samples;
• reliable psychiatric case registers to identify admissions;
• research diagnostic criteria for defining psychiatric disorders;
• measurement of non-recorded as well as recorded crime;
• lengthy periods of follow-up or data collection.

There have been three principal research methods population surveys, birth cohort studies and longitudinal studies. The most significant of these are summarised in Table 29.3

Epidemiological surveys of community populations and birth cohort studies have the advantages of unbiased population cohorts, inclusion of never-treated cases, robust diagnostic interviewing schedules, and self-report in addition to formal hospital and criminal records for information. Two American population studies showed that violence was six times more common in people with a diagnosis of schizophrenia (Swanson et al 1990), and that violence was more likely in those with current psychotic symptoms irrespective of whether or not they had ever been hospital patients (Link et al 1992).

Three Scandinavian studies of birth cohorts have found an association between schizophrenia and violence. Hodgins (1992) conducted a 30-year follow-up of 15 117 people born in Stockholm in 1953. Men with a major mental disorder were 2.5 times more likely to have a criminal record than men without, and four times more likely to have been convicted of violence. For women the increased likelihood was five and 27 times, respectively. Broadly similar findings were reported by Tiihonen et al (1997), who followed up 12 058 births in Northern Finland over 26 years. The strongest association between mental disorder and offending was with alcohol-related conditions, but men with schizophrenia or a psychotic mood disorder were up to nine times more likely than controls to have committed a crime of violence.

By far the most comprehensive birth cohort study is by Hodgins et al (1996) of all 0.36 million people born in Denmark between 1944 and 1947 and followed up until aged 43. The researchers were able to utilise the high-quality information available in the Danish psychiatric and criminal registers. Those who had been hospitalised had higher rates of offending. Although this was an 'ever-hospitalised' cohort, and therefore did not include less disordered cases, these patients will have spent most of their lives in the community rather than in hospital. In this respect the patients are typical of those currently seen by psychiatric services. The relative risk estimates for commission of a violent crime in various diagnostic categories are shown in Table 29.4. The likelihood of a person with a major mental disorder committing a violent crime was increased nearly 4.5 times in men and 8.5 times in women compared with controls. These relative risk rates were substantially lower than in those with admissions for mental

Table 29.3   Studies of psychiatric disorder and offending

Author	Country	Type of study	Offending measured by	Principal findings
Swanson et al (1990)	USA	Population: 10 000 people in community	Self-report	Higher rates of violence in substance misuse, affective and schizophrenic disorders
Stueve & Link (1997)	Israel	Population: 2678 young adults in community	Self-report	High association with psychotic and bipolar disorders while controlling for substance abuse disorders
Link et al (1992)	USA	Population: sample of New York residents	Self-report	Association between violent crime and mental disorder
Hodgins (1992)	Sweden	Birth cohort: all births in 1953	Criminal records	Association between violent crime and mental disorder
Tiihonen et al (1997)	Finland	Birth cohort: all births in 1966	Criminal records	Association between violent crime and mental disorder
Hodgins et al (1996)	Denmark	Birth cohort: all citizens born 1944–47	Criminal records	Association between violent crime and all forms mental disorder
Lindqvist & Allebeck (1990)	Sweden	Longitudinal: 644 discharged patients for 17 years	Criminal records	No association between mental disorder and serious violence
Steadman et al (1998)	USA	Longitudinal 1136 discharged patients for 12 months	Self-report and informant	Increased violence only in those abusing alcohol or drugs

Table 29.4   Danish 1944–47 birth cohort study (Hodgins et al 1996) — relative risk estimates of at least one violent crime between 1978 and 1990

Psychiatric disorder	Female ($n = 158\ 799$)	Male ($n = 165\ 602$)
Major mental disorder	8.66	4.48
Mental retardation		
Antisocial personality	11.81	7.65
disorder	12.15	7.20
Drug use disorder	15.08	8.67
Alcohol use disorder	14.87	6.68
Other mental disorders	3.97	3.15

retardation, antisocial personality disorder or substance misuse disorders.

Longitudinal studies follow up the offending careers of former psychiatric patients. Lindqvist & Allebeck (1990) found crimes of violence (mostly minor) were four times higher among 644 patients in Stockholm, treated for schizophrenia and followed up for 17 years, than among controls. Belfrage (1998) has suggested there may have been loss of data concerning more serious violent crimes. Collecting accurate information about subsequent violence is crucial and was addressed in the large MacArthur Violence Risk Assessment Study by Steadman et al (1998). The researchers interviewed 1136 patients discharged from acute inpatient units in three North American cities. They supplemented self-report by speaking to an informant, usually the carer of the discharged patient. Interviews were conducted every 10 weeks for 1 year. Matched community controls were interviewed once. Results showed:

- subjects who did not abuse alcohol or drugs were no more violent than controls;
- subjects were, however, more likely than controls to abuse alcohol or drugs;
- this accounted for increased violence in the first 20 weeks post-discharge only;
- after 20 weeks there was no difference between subjects and controls;
- 86% of violence by subjects was directed at family members or friends.

Observers have commented (Link & Stueve 1998) that symptom remission in the first 12 months after discharge may account for the low level of violent behaviour.

Dual diagnosis   Comorbid alcohol and drug misuse is widespread in patients with major mental illness. Comorbidity of this type has been widely reported in samples of psychiatric patients in secure settings (Corbett et al 1998). Other studies and reviews point to the extremely high risk rates in those with dual diagnoses of mental illness and substance misuse (Soyka 2000). In a Finnish study, schizophrenia with secondary alcohol misuse increased the risk of homicide by 17 times in men and 80 times in women (Eronen et al 1996a). It is not known whether there is any specific reason for the increased violence in dual diagnosis patients or whether it arises from a combination of male gender, associated antisocial personality traits, severe psychopathology or treatment resistance.

Public perception

Serious violence, particularly homicide by a psychiatric patient, causes widespread concern and media scrutiny. Since 1994 the government in England and Wales has required that an independent inquiry follows any homicide by a person who has been in contact with psychiatric services. The attendant publicity, with its focus on an individual case, has done little to improve services (Peay 1996) and has probably increased the stigma associated with mental illness. The inquiries have also fostered a public perception that de-institutionalism and community care have in some way been responsible for a massive rise in such homicides. Using Home Office data Taylor & Gunn (1999) have demonstrated that the number of people with a mental illness committing homicide between 1957 and 1995 has remained remarkably constant each year. Over that period, psychiatric homicides, as a proportion of all homicides, have fallen by 3% each year. A Canadian study (Stuart & Arboleda-Florez 2001) also found a very small contribution by the mentally ill to societal violence in general. Unfortunately, public perception is in the opposite direction.

Summary

The key points in the relationship between psychiatric disorder and criminal behaviour are summarised in Box 29.3.

Specific psychiatric disorders and criminal acts

Schizophrenia The phenomena of schizophrenia and their association with offending have attracted relatively little research. Most investigations are of acting on delusions. Of 20 people who had pushed strangers on to New York's subway tracks, 10 were influenced by delusions or hallucinations (Martell & Dietz 1992). Taylor found that 47% of a cohort of psychotic prisoners described psychotic motivation, usually delusions, for their offences; passivity, religious and paranormal delusions were particularly noted (Taylor 1993).

In a study that supplemented the patient's account with that of an informant, Buchanan et al (1993) found that 50% of their sample reported acting on delusions in the previous week, though rarely with violence. Patients who reported acting on delusions were more likely to have sought further evidence for their beliefs, reduced the conviction of their belief when challenged and registered accompanying affective symptoms.

Almost all types of delusions have in various studies been said to indicate a potential for violence; there are major methodological problems relating chiefly to accurate identification of phenomena. The presence of acute symptoms may be more important than their nature (Humphreys et al 1992); the early years of the illness seem to produce more violence than the later years (Hafner & Boker 1982). Evidence on the role of command hallucinations in violent acts is conflicting. A study of patients detained in a secure hospital found that command hallucinations were associated with acts of self-harm rather than with violence to others (Rogers et al 2002). Other variables, such as the concept of 'threat-control-override' (Link & Stueve 1994), have been postulated. Psychotic symptoms are more likely to result in violence, it is claimed, when symptoms cause a feeling of personal threat or the intrusion of thoughts that can override self-controls; this can be measured on a simple scale.

Violence by people with schizophrenia has a contextual element. A fully independent life is rarely compatible with having schizophrenia. Reliance on family, carers, health and social care staff, and housing and welfare agencies is likely to impinge significantly on daily life. Shelter, warmth and nourishment may not be easily obtained. Crime and violence even when attributable to psychotic symptoms need to be considered in this wider context.

Affective disorders In clinical practice major affective disorder in association with crime is less commonly encountered than is schizophrenia. Grandiosity of mood and disinhibition in mania and hypomania commonly leads to public disorder and driving offences or fraud from failure to pay for restaurant and hotel bills. Less commonly there may be a serious sexual or violent crime. The confidential inquiry into suicides and homicides (Department of Health 2001b) reported a diagnosis of affective disorder in 8% of the 1600 people convicted of homicide.

> **Box 29.3 Summary of relationship between psychiatric disorder and offending**
>
> - Major mental illness increases the likelihood of acquiring a criminal conviction for a violent crime by about eight times, and for any crime by about 30 times
> - The increased likelihood is modified by local influences such as the crime rate and sociodemographic variables
> - Antisocial personality disorder and substance misuse disorders have greater association with offending than does any major mental illness
> - Dual diagnosis, particularly including a substance misuse disorder, may be more relevant than any single category of mental illness
> - Most offending by those with mental illness is minor in degree
> - Where serious violence occurs it is likely to be directed at a family member or carer
> - Psychiatric homicides, as a proportion of all homicides, fell by 3% each year between 1957 and 1995

The role of depressive disorders in offending behaviour is controversial and probably rare (Guze 1976). The literature on shoplifting and depression is largely historical; a study of 1649 shoplifters in Montreal found 1% who were suffering from depression or bipolar disorder (Lamontagne et al 1994). Of greater significance is the rare but well-recognised phenomenon of extended or altruistic homicide in which a depressed person (usually a parent) kills one or more family members (usually including a child) and then commits or attempts suicide (Stroud 1997). Given the frequency of depression and the rarity of altruistic homicide it seems an impossible task to identify these cases in advance.

Personality disorder Surveys of offender populations always find high rates of personality disorder; this is expected, as offending will often be a component in reaching the diagnosis. The confidential inquiry into suicides and homicides (Department of Health 2001b) reported a diagnosis of personality disorder in 29% of the 231 perpetrators who received any type of psychiatric diagnosis.

The situation is further complicated by the confusing clinical and legal terminology in relation to psychopathic disorder. The term that appears in the Mental Health Act 1983 has a legal definition and refers to a disorder that results in abnormal aggression or serious irresponsibility. It became a legal entity in the 1950s, replacing its predecessor, the moral imbecile (Home Office & Department of Health and Social Security 1975). It is therefore incorrect to assume that the disorder defined in law 50 years ago is the equivalent of any particular category of psychiatric disorder in current use. In practice, 'pure forms' of antisocial personality disorder are uncommon in patients admitted in the legal category of psychopathic disorder; there is often overlap with other categories of personality disorder, together with other Axis I diagnoses and multiple psychiatric symptoms (Coid et al 1999).

In the last 10 years offenders in the category psychopathic disorder constitute a vanishing proportion of those ordered to hospitals by courts. The reasons are self-evident. There are serious clinical difficulties in measuring change in personality-disordered patients while they are detained in secure settings, and in making decisions about discharge (Norton & Dolan 1995). Follow-up studies show that psychopathic disorder patients discharged from secure hospitals re-offend at twice the rate of those with mental illness (Bailey & MacCulloch 1992, Steels et al 1998). There are difficulties in moving such patients on to other settings after periods of treatment in secure conditions, and lack of supervision conditions on discharge is associated with re-offending. Given this fragile therapeutic background, the government's intention to introduce new laws for the detention of dangerous people with severe personality disorders arises from the perceived need for public protection rather than any therapeutic expectations.

Multiple personality disorder (MPD) is a clinical diagnosis confined to American forensic practice. A report concerning a 'case' in an English court cautioned psychiatrists not to 'collude with the MPD phenomena' by looking for further alters or investigating those that 'appear' (James & Schramm 1998).

Neuroses Neurotic symptoms are common in offenders, but it is unusual to find a causal relationship between an offence and a disorder that satisfies ICD-10 diagnostic criteria for a neurotic, stress-related or somatoform disorder. Whether an offence is attributed to the effects of post-traumatic stress disorder or to an underlying personality disorder may depend on whether a transverse or longitudinal view of the offender's psychopathology is taken. Neurotic conflicts, as distinct from disorder, may play a speculative role in any offending behaviour, e.g. shoplifting, fire-setting or sexual offending. West (1988) has given a perceptive account of the role of individual psychopathology in crime.

Learning disability Over the last 30 years there has been a major reduction in the admission of offenders with learning disability from the courts, though an unknown number may have dual diagnoses and be detained in the category of mental illness. Early literature contained grossly exaggerated prevalence figures for 'feeble-mindedness' among offenders (Walker & McCabe 1973). Offending by the learning disabled does not occur in a vacuum; it is subject to all the influences which typically affect offending, i.e. unstable families, poor parenting, socio-economic disadvantage, educational underachievement and substance misuse. The Stockholm 1953 birth cohort study (Hodgins 1992) found a significant association between special schooling and subsequent offending.

Property offending predominates, but the range of offences committed is wide. There is some evidence to support increased arrest rates among the learning disabled (Robertson 1988). Crimes of serious violence may be less common, but arson and sexual offences were over-represented in studies of hospital-based cohorts (Day 1994). Sexual offending by people with a learning disability is usually opportunistic with low specificity in the age and sex of the victim (Green et al 2002).

Alcohol and substance abuse The relationship between abuse of alcohol or drugs and crime is complex and not necessarily causal, even though problems of abuse are almost endemic among offender populations, and offending is common in those with alcohol and drug problems. The majority of male and half of the female prisoners in the UK misuse alcohol (Singleton et al 1998). One in 10 men and 1 in 4 women in prison have been regular users of opiates or stimulants before imprisonment (Maden et al 1990, 1991). More than a third of prisoners in Scotland have injected drugs, and the majority of these have injected in prison (Dye & Isaacs 1991).

Alcohol consumption has been implicated in family violence, child abuse, rape and other sex offences (Lindqvist 1991) and homicide (Rada 1975, Department of Health 2001b). Similar findings were reported from Finland, where 39% of men and 32% of women convicted of homicide had diagnoses of alcoholism

(Eronen et al 1996b). Occasionally, offending may be associated with the neuropsychiatric sequelae of alcoholism, such as delirium tremens or alcoholic hallucinosis. Chronic drinkers with multiple social handicaps form a large proportion of the short-sentence populations in most prisons. Many receive their only medical care when in prison.

Organic conditions In theory disinhibition and impaired judgment, characteristic of organic brain disease, may lead to minor crimes of dishonesty or sexual offences. In practice elderly sexual offenders rarely have psychiatric or organic disorders (Clark & Mezey 1997). Elderly offenders convicted of other crimes have high rates of alcohol misuse. In younger men, offending may be associated with any cause of organic brain disease such as head injury or Huntington's chorea.

Epilepsy Epilepsy is a rare contributory factor to offending. Twenty-five years ago Gunn (1977) reported an increased prevalence of epilepsy in prisoners compared with the general population but not with a population showing the same socioeconomic disadvantage from which the prison population is typically drawn. Gunn's sample of epileptic prisoners showed no excess rates for crimes of violence. The most likely explanation for any excess, if present, is that the socio-economic and psychosocial correlates of epilepsy are similar to those for crime in general. Serious violence as an ictal phenomenon is exceedingly rare.

Pathological jealousy and other disorders of passion Delusional syndromes characterised by pathological feelings of jealousy, love or entitlement are commonly associated with criminal behaviour. Pathological (or morbid) jealousy is the most common. Normal jealousy can generate criminal behaviour, and the distinction between normal and pathological jealousy cannot be defined in scientific terms. Indeed assessment of jealousy is difficult because it may be:

- a normal but transient response to infidelity in a partner;
- a preoccupation in an insecure individual;
- a feature of a personality disorder, e.g. paranoid, narcissistic or antisocial;
- a complication of alcohol dependence;
- an overvalued idea without psychotic features;
- a delusion in the setting of a psychotic illness.

The syndrome classically described by Shepherd (1961) involves repeated, often violent, questioning, checking and following of the partner. There are attempts to force a 'confession'. Elaborate delusional beliefs lead to searches for 'evidence' of infidelity by the partner. The treatment is that of the underlying condition.

More difficult to assess are the remaining jealousies which Mullen (1993) refers to as normally or pathologically reactive. A pathological reaction is manifested by exaggerated responses that come to dominate personal functioning and relationships. It is commonly related to problems in personality development. Offending behaviour occurs in all types of jealousy, including normal reactive jealousy. Careful assessment is crucial and requires appraisals of premorbid personality, the relationship with the partner, and the nature of the provoking incident or behaviour. The couple are often disparate in terms of social skills, educational attainment or occupational status. The syndrome has a high association with violence and homicide. Both partners need to be made aware of the risks, and often separation is required; this clearly does not eliminate the risk of further violence.

The delusional conviction of being loved by someone who is identified but unattainable, usually by reason of their social class or importance, is the basis of erotomania or de Clérambault's syndrome. Pursuing the object of the delusion and repeatedly pestering them by telephone, by letter and with gifts is typical. Some erotomanics 'arrange' holidays or weddings with their victims. The condition is rare but surfaces in forensic populations as a result of criminal acts secondary to the delusion (Taylor et al 1983). Menzies et al (1995) found that multiple delusional objects and a history of other antisocial behaviour were predictive of future violence. The syndrome has various aetiologies (schizophrenic and affective), though it can present as a single delusional disorder (Segal 1989). It is only one of a number of behaviours that may be associated with stalking (Kamphius & Emmelkamp 2000), a behaviour that is recognised as an offence in the Protection from Harassment Act 1997. Laws of this type are more effective with non-mentally-ill stalkers (McGuire & Wraith 2000).

The conviction of having been wronged by others (e.g. a doctor or lawyer or employer) and of consequent entitlement to redress is the basis of morbid querulousness. The convictions dominate, usually in fluctuating outbursts, the lives of sufferers, who may hound their victims with letters, distribute leaflets, daub walls and write to newspapers and members of parliament. Often they are declared 'vexatious litigants' and become banned from using the courts. There is a high likelihood of assaults on the perceived 'wrongdoer' or damage to his or her property. As with other disorders of passion, there are various aetiologies (Rowlands 1988).

Factitious illness by proxy This term (also known as Münchausen syndrome by proxy) correctly describes a situation rather than a psychiatric disorder (Bools 1996). The behaviour is the fabrication of symptoms in, or the injury of, a child by its carer (usually mother) who then presents the child to a doctor or other agency for treatment. Bools describes a wide range of injurious behaviours from verbal fabrications and tampering with specimens and charts to poisoning, smothering and withholding of nutrients. The condition may be a factor in child abuse and has been implicated in acts of serial killings by healthcare workers. Underlying psychiatric conditions include personality disorders (particularly antisocial and borderline types), somatisation, affective and eating disorders and substance misuse.

Special groups

Young offenders Nearly half the offenders under 16 years old serving custodial detention in excess of 12 months have committed murder, manslaughter, arson, rape or wounding. The remainder have committed robbery or burglary, nearly always having previous similar convictions. Bailey (1995) has emphasised that young offenders convicted of serious crimes have high rates of previous psychiatric contact, substance misuse, previous criminality, mental illness within the family and parental marital conflict. However, those convicted of homicides appear to have low rates of psychopathology (Dolan & Smith 2001).

Elderly offenders Elderly offenders constitute less than 1% of the offending population, but they have high rates of psychiatric disorder and their number is increasing (Yorston 1999). Older men may commit any type of crime, but those imprisoned are more likely than younger men to have committed a crime of dishonesty or a sexual crime (Jacoby 1997). Needham-Bennett et al (1996) studied 50 consecutive police referrals of offenders aged over 60 to a community service. Shoplifting accounted for 63% of offences, and 28% of the sample scored as 'cases' on a computerised diagnostic screening device for the elderly.

Ethnic minorities Black people are over-represented among those in local authority care, young offender institutions and prisons. In a survey of secure forensic services Coid et al (2000) found rates of admission for black men to be 5.6 times that of white men, and 2.9 for black women compared with white women. The authors concluded that this results from a combination of socio-economic disadvantage and a lack of effectiveness in community services to prevent escalating dangerous behaviour in mentally ill African-Carribeans.

RISK ASSESSMENT AND MANAGEMENT

In psychiatry the term risk is applied to the likelihood of an adverse event such as suicide, self-harm, self-neglect, non-compliance, substance misuse, side-effect development, relapse or violence. Risk of harm to others is the primary concern in assessing and treating mentally disordered offenders.

Research into the evaluation of risk has been considerable, and several risk assessment tools have now been developed. The object of risk assessment is not simply to label an individual as a high, medium or low risk of future violence but to identify those risk factors, such as alcohol abuse, amenable to change and to assist the clinician in developing a plan of treatment in which risk management is central. Risk is a dynamic concept that changes with time, place, people and mental state. The risk of harm to others can therefore be reduced but not eliminated. Systems and services to assess and manage risk are essential. These are illustrated in Box 29.4.

A number of factors are known to increase the risk of harm to others. A study examining differences between patients with schizophrenia within and without a high security psychiatric hospital found that high security patients tended to be male and single (Miller et al 2000). They had poorer school achievement, lower premorbid intelligence and worse occupational levels. They were more likely to have a family history of alcohol abuse, to have had police contact and to have attempted suicide. They had less frequent but longer psychiatric admissions, and more current and lifetime schizophrenic symptoms.

Study results vary, particularly on psychiatric rather than criminogenic findings, but factors generally associated with increased risk of violence in people with mental disorders are described in Box 29.5

Development of risk assessment instruments

The standard psychiatric history and examination with information from third-party sources contains all the elements of a modern risk assessment. In spite of this, a review of research on the accuracy of clinical risk assessment found that clinicians were correct in their

---

Box 29.4 Systems and services to manage risk

- Staff training
- Referral and/or screening process to identify those requiring assessment
- Risk assessment
- Communication of assessment results
- Risk management and ongoing reassessment
- Immediate response to adverse events
- Documentation

Box 29.5   Factors associated with increased risk of violence in people with mental disorder

- History of previous violence
- Adverse childhood experiences
- Behavioural problems in childhood
- Social instability — poor employment record, disturbed relationships
- Substance abuse
- History of self harm
- History of impulsive behaviour
- History of poor compliance or response to treatment
- Presence of
  - persecutory delusions
  - command hallucinations
  - passivity
  - irritability
  - anger
  - hostility
  - suspiciousness
  - lack of insight
  - specific threat(s)
  - identified precipitant(s) / stressor(s)

---

prediction of violent behaviour on only one out of three occasions (Monahan 1981). More recent work, however, suggests that the accuracy of these clinical predictions has improved (Gardner et al 1996, McNiel et al 1998). This may be due to increased awareness of factors associated with violence and clearer guidance on the clinical assessment and management of risk of harm to other people (e.g. Royal College of Psychiatrists 1996).

Concerns about the validity, reliability and transparency of clinical risk assessment led to research into the use of actuarial methods in the prediction of violence. These are statistical methods that examine potential violence-predicting variables and, by use of logistic regression, select those variables with the greatest predictive power. These variables are weighted according to their predictive power and combined to give a total risk assessment score. The actuarial approach has been criticised because it is based on historical factors that cannot change with clinical intervention. Furthermore, there is an inevitable false-positive rate, that is an incorrect prediction of future violence (e.g. 45% for the Violence Risk Appraisal Guide). Caution must be exercised as to the applicability of a risk assessment instrument in the individual to be assessed. Monahan et al (2001) refer to questionable validity generalisation: that is whether an instrument developed in one setting is relevant to another, for example whether an instrument developed in a North American high-security psychiatric hospital is of use in a European prison. Furthermore, the clinician must consider whether any rare or protective risk factors overrule an actuarial risk assessment. For example, a patient assessed as a low risk of future violence who makes a direct threat against a specific individual, or a patient with a high risk prediction who becomes physically disabled. These criticisms have lead to the development of a structured clinical approach to risk assessment that combines actuarial risk assessment with clinical and risk factors.

Receiver Operating Characteristic Analysis (ROC) is often used to assess the predictive accuracy of risk assessment instruments. It plots sensitivity (true positive rate) against 1 minus specificity (false-positive rate) for a series of cut off points on a scale predicting future violence. The statistical result is shown as the

area under the curve (AUC), and this indicates the accuracy of the test: zero area equals a perfect negative prediction, 0.50 (straight line) a chance prediction, and 1.0 a perfect positive prediction. The greater the AUC, the greater the probability that a randomly selected violent patient will have been assessed as a higher risk for future violence than a randomly selected non-violent patient.

Risk assessment instruments

Table 29.5 lists some of the risk assessment instruments developed for use in different populations. Two instruments for use with mentally disordered offenders are discussed in detail below.

Violence risk appraisal guide (VRAG)

The violence risk appraisal guide (Quinsey et al 1998) was designed to assess risk of violence in mentally disordered offenders. It was developed from a study of high-security psychiatric patients ($n = 618$) in Canada. Box 29.6 (p. 712) contains the twelve factors identified as being collectively most predictive of violence, and these were given positive and negative weightings (shown in parentheses).

The scoring of some of these items appears clinically counterintuitive; for example schizophrenia is scored negatively. This has arisen because the population on which the instrument was developed contained two large diagnostic groups: schizophrenia and psychopathy. Their comparison lead to schizophrenia appearing to be a protective factor. The VRAG gives detailed instructions for the rating of each item. Items are totalled (range – 26 to 38) and each score placed within one of nine 'bins'. Each bin has a recorded estimated probability for violent recidivism at 7- and 10-year follow-up. For example, bin 2 (score –21 to –15) 8% probability of violence at 7 years and 10% at 10 years; bin 6 (score +7 to +13) 44% and 58%, respectively; and bin 9 100% for both time periods.

The VRAG has been validated largely in North American samples. A recent study in a Scottish prison sample (Cooke et al 2001) found a reasonable predictive validity similar to other studies (AUC 0.67 for violent recidivism and 0.66 for violent incidents in prison).

Historical, clinical, risk management–20 (HCR-20)

The HCR-20 (Webster et al 1997) is designed for use in settings containing people with possible mental illness or personality disorder and a likely history of violence. It was developed from a literature review of factors associated with violence and from

---

Box 29.6   Violence Risk Appraisal Guide

1. Lived with both biological parents until age 16 (–)
2. Elementary school maladjustment (+)
3. History of alcohol problems (+)
4. Marital status (single +)
5. Criminal history score for non-violent offences (+)
6. Failure on prior conditional release (+)
7. Age at index offence (young +)
8. Victim injury at index offence (–)
9. Female victim (–)
10. Diagnosis of personality disorder (+)
11. Diagnosis of schizophrenia (–)
12. Psychopathy Checklist — Revised score (+)

Table 29.5 Risk assessment instruments

Title	Authors	Target population	Purpose
Violence Risk Appraisal Guide (VRAG)	Quinsey et al 1998	Mentally disordered offenders	Actuarial measure of violent recidivism
Historical Clinical Risk–20 (HCR-20)	Webster et al 1997	Mentally disordered offenders	Structured clinical approach to examine risk of violent recidivism
Violence Risk Scale (VRS)	Wong & Gordon in press	Violent offenders	Dynamic measure of change in risk
Sexual Offender Risk Appraisal Guide (SORAG)	Quinsey et al 1998	Sex offenders	Actuarial measure of violent (*not* sexual) recidivism
Sexual Violence Risk–20 (SVR-20)	Boer et al 1997	Sex offenders	Structured clinical approach to examine risk of sexual offending
Sex Offender Needs Assessment Rating (SONAR)	Hanson & Harris 2001	Sex offenders	Actuarial measure of change in risk of sexual violence
Rapid Risk Assessment for Sexual Offence Recidivism (RRASOR)	Hanson 1997	Sex offenders	Actuarial screening instrument to predict sexual offending recidivism
Structured Anchored Clinical Judgement (SACJ)	Hanson & Thornton 2000	Sex offenders in prison or with police contact	Actuarial screening instrument to predict sexual offending recidivism
Static – 99	Hanson & Thornton 1999	Male sexual offenders over 18 years of age	Actuarial scale for assessing long-term risk of sexual recidivism
Spousal Assault Risk Assessment Guide (SARA)	Kropp et al 1995	Male or female perpetrators of actual, attempted or threatened physical harm against a current or former partner in an intimate sexual relationship	Structured clinical risk assessment tool for evaluating risk of spousal assault
Level of Service Inventory — Revised (LSI-R)	Andrews & Bonta 1995	Offenders in prison or under probation	Structured clinical risk/needs assessment tool to assess risk of recidivism
Offender Group Reconviction Scale (OGRS)	Copas & Marshall 1998	Offenders in prison or under probation	Actuarial scale to predict likelihood of reconviction 2 years after release or community sentence
Risk Assessment Guidance Framework (RAGF)	SWSIs 2000	Offenders — for use mainly by social workers	Structured clinical guidelines for assessing risk of reconviction, criminogenic needs and risk of harm to others
Reconviction Prediction Score (RPS)	Ward 1987	Offenders — Parole Board assessment	Actuarial tool to assess risk of reconviction 2 years after release from prison
Risk of Reconviction (ROR)	Copas et al 1996	Offenders — Parole Board assessment	Actuarial tool to predict risk of re-offending (any or serious) after release for a maximum of 2 years
Offender Assessment System (OASys)	Home Office 2002a	Offenders in prison or under probation	An aid to professional judgement
Iterative Classification Trees (ICTs)	Monahan et al 2001	Civil psychiatric patients in community settings	To assign patients to risk prediction groups based on actuarially determined algorithms. Uses a model of 5 repeat ICTs with different initial variables to improve accuracy

experienced clinical opinion. It combines an actuarial and clinical approach and is a dynamic instrument with 20 items; see Box 29.7 Each item is scored from 0 to 2 indicating the absence, possible or partial presence, or definite presence of each factor. The authors advocate that clinically this scale should be used as an aide memoire, but for research purposes the scores can be summed. The HCR-20 has been validated in criminal justice, civil and forensic psychiatric populations both in North America and to a lesser degree in Europe. Cooke et al (2001) in a Scottish prison sample found an AUC of 0.64 for violence in prison and 0.69 for violent recidivism.

Risk management

Following risk assessment the clinician should organise a management plan that increases safety and reduces any identified risk. Decisions to be taken are illustrated in Box 29.8.

Sharing of information is essential for good risk management. Usually this is done within a multiprofessional team and confidentiality is not an issue. Many countries, however, allow for confidentiality to be breached when disclosure is necessary to protect an individual, and when the risk is real and involves potential violence.

Box 29.7   HCR-20 assessment items

Historical items
1. Previous violence
2. Young age at first violent incident
3. Relationship instability
4. Employment problems
5. Substance use problems
6. Major mental illness
7. Psychopathy
8. Early maladjustment
9. Personality disorder
10. Prior supervision failure

Clinical items
1. Lack of insight
2. Negative attitudes
3. Active symptoms of major mental illness
4. Impulsivity
5. Unresponsive to treatment

Risk management items
1. Plans lack feasibility
2. Exposure to destabilisers
3. Lack of personal support
4. Non-compliance with remediation attempts
5. Stress

HCR-20, Historical, Clinical Risk Management–20 (Webster et al 1997).

Box 29.8   Risk management decisions

- Appropriate location of patient
- Use of mental health legislation
- Use of a restriction order
- Need for secure setting
- Level of observation
- Use of medication
- Management of aggressive behaviour
- Requirement for specific therapies, e.g. alcohol and drug relapse prevention
- Need for community supports — housing, employment, education, social
- Needs of carers for education and support
- Information sharing
- Content of care plan with specified staff for each action point, agreed review mechanism and dates, and response plan in event of deterioration or crisis
- Use of a monitoring system, such as the Care Programme Approach
- Feasibility of care plan
- Review of any critical incidents

Systems to support risk management include the Care Programme Approach (CPA). This is a formalised method of good clinical practice requiring a multidisciplinary assessment of health and social care needs, an agreed, recorded care plan with an identified co-ordinator, and systematic review.

Risk assessment instruments are there to assist the clinician in decision-making and risk management. Clinicians must be aware of the criticisms and limitations of these instruments. They are not an alternative to a thorough psychiatric assessment or a substitute for a psychiatric court report. Clinicians should resist the pressure to complete scales for every aspect of assessment. Risk assessment instruments, particularly those following a structured clinical approach, can, however, usefully focus clinical assessment of risk.

Offences and offenders

Every crime is a unique event in which offender, victim and circumstances interact in a manner that is 'special' for that particular episode. The offender brings his life experiences, attitudes, beliefs, personality, the effects of any psychiatric disorder and of any alcohol or substance he or she might have used to a particular set of circumstances. In this section we examine the range of offences that may be committed.

Homicide

The homicide rate has increased annually in England and Wales over the last 40 years, and in 2000–01 there were 850 killings, which included the crimes of murder, manslaughter and infanticide (Home Office 2001). All defendants charged with murder are examined for the purpose of a psychiatric report. The legal definition of murder is 'the unlawful killing of any reasonable creature under the Queen's peace, with malice aforethought, death occurring within a year and a day of the act'.

Approximately half the male, and nearly 75% of female, victims are usually known to their killers. Nearly half of the women killed in 2000–01 were killed by a current or former partner or lover. Death other than by means of a sharp or blunt instrument, brute force or strangulation is unusual.

For statistical purposes homicide is normal where the outcome is conviction for murder, or for manslaughter other than by reason of diminished responsibility (see below). 'Abnormal' murder comprises convictions for manslaughter due to diminished responsibility (the majority of abnormal homicides), infanticide, homicide in a failed suicide pact, and legal findings of insanity. On this basis, in England, abnormal homicides accounted for less than 1 in 6 killings (Home Office 2001). Findings of diminished responsibility are falling as the homicide rate rises; in recent years diminished responsibility has applied in less than 5% of homicides.

Legal verdicts (e.g. of diminished responsibility) do not depend on research-based diagnostic criteria. Studies using such criteria in countries with low rates of homicide confirm an association between some psychiatric disorders (antisocial personality disorder, alcohol misuse and schizophrenia, but not affective disorders or learning disability) and homicide (Eronen et al 1996b). The association with mental disorder is even stronger in women who commit homicide (Eronen 1995). Suicide of the suspect before coming to trial occurs in less than 10% of cases. A study of homicide–suicide in the north of England found these were mostly men who had killed wives, children or both. The most common factors were ending of relationships, depression and jealousy; in nearly a third of cases alcohol abuse contributed (Milroy 1995).

In practice, psychiatric findings in abnormal homicide usually relate to a domestic or family killing with a background of any one or more of the following: interpersonal strife, jealousy, substance misuse, chronic ill health in victim or suspect and, where mental illness is present, either psychotic or depressive disorder (see Box 29.9). Even in homicides by the mentally ill there is usually a large contextual component; the nature of the relationship between victim and killer, the victim's behaviour and situational factors may all have contributory roles in the homicide. Sometimes the homicide is the mercy-killing of a chronically disabled parent,

---

Box 29.9 Psychiatric aspects of homicide

- As number of homicides in UK rises, proportion classified as 'abnormal' is falling
- Diminished responsibility applies in less than 5% of homicides
- Usually a domestic or family killing
- Killing of stranger by mentally ill perpetrator is unusual
- Often chronic interpersonal problems, alcohol or substance misuse, or chronic ill health in victim or perpetrator
- Mental illness, if present, is usually psychotic or depressive disorder
- Alcohol or substance abuse at time of homicide is common
- May be followed by act of self-harm
- Perpetrator commonly reports the crime

---

child or spouse. Infants under the age of 1 year are at the greatest risk of death by homicide, and 60% of victims are killed by their mothers. Some of these are the victim of a mentally ill parent (d'Orban 1979, McGrath 1992) but others have their origins in situational, relationship and personality problems (Resnick 1969, Scott 1973). Many of these, together with younger child victims, are killed in circumstances associated with chronic ill treatment, battering or neglect (Cordess 1995).

The killing of parents or siblings is the rarest form of family homicide. An association between matricide and schizophrenia has been frequently described (Green 1981, Clark 1993) but may owe as much to opportunity as it does to the psychopathology of the disorder. Many adult schizophrenic sons live with, or are dependent on, their mothers; in the setting of these, often strained, relationships mothers can easily become the target of any aggression (Chiswick 1981).

Where the victim is a stranger, it is unusual to find any evidence of mental illness in the accused. An exception is the rare instance when a person with schizophrenia identifies a stranger as a victim on the basis of psychotic phenomena. Sexual or sadistic murder of a random victim is rare, though such cases attract wide publicity, particularly when the killings are of a serial type. Grubin (1994a) compared a group of sexual murderers with non-homicidal rapists. The murderers were isolated men with few, if any, intimate relationships in their lives. They did not otherwise greatly differ from the rapists and did not meet the stereotypical picture of the sadistic killer described by Brittain (1970).

Sexual offences

Sexual offences account for less than 1% of all notifiable offences; since 1985 the rate of increase in sexual offences has been equal to that of recorded crime in general — about 4% per year. Sex offenders are almost exclusively men among whom mental illness is not prevalent. There is no absolute relationship between any particular type of sexual offence and any particular type of sexual disorder; none should ever be assumed or implied. A man who sexually assaults a child may or may not be a paedophile, and a person convicted of the offence of indecent exposure may or may not be an exhibitionist.

Sexual offences and sexual offenders are widely heterogeneous. Sexual offences have precise legal definitions, but the same offence (e.g. indecent assault) may conceal a wide range of behaviours. This heterogeneity makes it impossible to arrive at a useful classification of sexual offenders. Indeed Grubin & Kennedy (1991) have argued that, until we have such a classification, it is

pointless to talk of the 'psychiatry' of sex offending. Such classifications as we have are usually based on one particular facet of the offence or the offender. Most reflect the personal bias of their creator. Few have been tested for validity, reliability or practicability. They are usually based on a confusing mishmash of offence behaviour, imputed motivation, type of victim, personality traits and psychological or psychodynamic theory. The following is a brief account of some of the more common sexual offences, with particular reference to any psychiatric aspects.

Rape Approximately 600 men are convicted of rape each year, while some 8500 offences were recorded by the police in 2000–01; in the last decade the number or reported rapes has increased nearly threefold (Home Office 2001). The Criminal and Public Order Act 1994 introduced the specific crime of male rape; 650 such offences were recorded in 2000–01 by police.

Rape is a sexual crime not a psychiatric disorder; therefore there can be no satisfactory clinical classification of rapists. Traditional classifications based on categories such as violent, sadistic or sexual rape depend largely on the perspective of the researcher and have not been shown to have inter-rater reliability (Knight & Prentky 1989). Robust definition and focused application is required if these types of behavioural classifications are to have any value. Studies of convicted (and usually imprisoned) rapists find they are predominantly young men with poor social backgrounds and education. There is usually an overrepresentation of people from black ethnic minorities (Dietz 1978). Most rapists have criminal records, often for violence and up to a third for sex offences. However, in all these respects they are not greatly different from other prisoners (West 1993).

While some rapists describe sadistic fantasies and 'try-outs' prior to offending, the significance of these phenomena is uncertain (Grubin 1994b). Sadistic fantasy is common in men but it is probably the combination with social isolation and an impaired capacity for empathy that distinguish those who put sadistic fantasy into practice.

Incest and other sexual behaviour with children For legal purposes incest is sexual intercourse (vaginal) within a forbidden relationship. In the last decade the number of recorded crimes of incest has fallen from 400 to 100. Legally, incest requires proof of penetration: much intrafamilial sexual abuse falls short of penetration. In England (though not in Scotland) step relationships do not come within the legal definition of incest. Therefore prosecution for stepfather–daughter sexual intercourse will be for a different crime. Sexual abuse by mothers of their sons is increasingly recognised. Family factors in incest have been emphasised, particularly findings of a dysfunctional family with generational blurring. Wives are often absent, incapacitated or unavailable or they commonly have a passive or dependent role in the family. Family pathology often coexists with pathology in the father.

Up to 30% of incest perpetrators have a sexual preference for children, nearly half having offended outside the family (Abel et al 1988). Other psychiatric features may be alcohol abuse and antisocial personality disorder. There are no consistent findings suggestive of low intelligence. A proportion of incest perpetrators have been victims of child sexual abuse. This appears to be more common in those with paedophilia, backgrounds of other crimes and in adolescent perpetrators (Hilton & Mezey 1996). Other sexual offences against children vary from minor indecency to violent sexual activity. Among adolescent boys the criminal behaviour is associated with poor social skills, physical unattractiveness and peer group isolation. Adult offenders are more likely to show features of paedophilia. Such men become skilled in targeting vulnerable children, grooming them with behaviour designed to increase their trust and then gradually increasing the degree of intimacy in the relationship. Emotional bribery is employed to maintain secrecy; they commonly refer to their behaviour as a 'secret game'.

Indecent exposure   In the last 2 years there have been fewer than 700 convictions each year for indecent exposure (Home Office 2001), and the annual rate of offending seems to be falling. Only a minority of episodes are reported, and an even smaller proportion result in conviction. Traditionally, offenders have been divided into those who are exhibitionists, with the features classically described in the 19th century by Lasègue (1877), and those whose exposing occurs in the context of drunkenness or a disinhibiting psychiatric disorder such as schizophrenia, hypomania, organic brain disorder or a learning disability.

Typically, exhibitionists (almost invariably men) expose their genitals to a female victim in a public but quiet location, or on public transport, or from their own home or car. They are sexually excited, often later masturbating to the image of the exposure. Few make any attempt to speak to or touch their victims. They are usually unable to explain their behaviour. It is known that a small proportion of exposers progress to more serious sexual crimes. Sugarman et al (1994) reviewed 210 cases and found subsequent more serious offending was associated with childhood conduct disorder, other criminal offences, and pursuing or touching the victim.

Psychiatric assessment of sexual offenders   Assessment of a person charged with, or convicted of, a sexual offence should be approached without preconceptions and with information from sources other than solely the accused. Establishing the presence or absence of a psychiatric disorder is a prerequisite, together with a detailed psychosexual history. In addition, assessment requires a consideration of the victim's behaviour and relationship (when present) to the accused, and situational factors such as the relevance of substance misuse by assailant and victim.

Psychotic illness in sexual offenders is unusual, though disinhibition due to a manic illness or to residual schizophrenia may occasionally be a factor. Rarely is the offence a direct response to delusional or hallucinatory symptoms (Smith & Taylor 1999). The men usually have records of other types of crime.

In practice few sex offenders are seen at times other than when they face criminal charges or are being considered for release from prison. The appropriateness of offering treatment, and the conditions under which it may be provided, must be balanced with the requirements of the criminal justice system. Those few patients with an underlying mental illness usually require treatment for that illness. For sex offenders who do not consider that they have any problem, who minimise their offending and who present to psychiatrists for statutory purposes, there is little prospect of treatment being either feasible or beneficial.

Re-offending and community treatment   There is a public perception that sex offenders always re-offend, and the political sensitivity of the issue is reflected in recent legislation. The Criminal Justice Act 1991 introduced mandatory supervision for certain sex offenders after release from prison. The Sex Offenders Act 1997 requires sex offenders discharged from prison or hospital to notify themselves to the police within 14 days of discharge. They must give the police their name, date of birth and home address and keep them notified of any changes in name or address. Under the Crime (Sentences) Act 1997 there is an automatic life sentence for a second serious violent or sexual offence, other than in exceptional circumstances.

Studies of re-offending have been reviewed by Grubin & Wingate (1996) and do not generally support the public's impression. Sexual reoffending occurred in 7–19% of released offenders (Marshall 1994). Grubin & Wingate point out the limitations of re-offending studies based on criminal records and the fact that longer periods of follow-up reveal higher rates of re-offending. Francis & Soothill (2000) followed up 7000 men convicted of a sex offence in 1973 for 21 years. Compared with the general male population, the sex offenders were seven times more likely to go on to commit a homicide. Nevertheless, re-offending rates of under 20% for sex offenders compare with rates of up to 80% for other offenders

Attempts to identify high-risk offenders have depended on gathering data of a demographic and historical type and seeking correlations with re-offending. The common variables with high correlations are childhood conduct disorder, parental instability, previous sex offending, early first conviction and a diagnosis of personality disorder (Grubin & Wingate 1996). These have predictive value for groups but not for the individual. As for their relevance for treatment, they are facts of history unamenable to change. In contrast, the factors that interest those who treat sex offenders are anger, self-esteem, social skills and victim empathy at the time when re-offending may take place. Thus the practical value of 'predictors' is limited.

Allam et al (1997) have described a programme for offenders undergoing community service; it is therefore targeted at less serious offenders. The programme attempts to address cognitive distortions, self-esteem and assertiveness, sexuality, the role of fantasy, victim empathy and relapse prevention techniques. The work is unevaluated but the treatment themes are familiar in other approaches to sex offender therapy. In Denmark until 1970 surgical castration was carried out on selected sex offenders. Since 1989 aggressive medical castration using antigonadotrophin in combination with antiandrogen preparations has been used (Hansen & Lykke-Olsen 1997).

Offences against property

Arson   Arson is among the leading causes of fires throughout the world (Geller 1992). It is a grave crime for which a sentence of life imprisonment can be imposed. The lawful form of the activity is a mark of public celebration. There were 50 000 episodes of arson reported to the police in 2000–01, a doubling in rate over 10 years. The clear-up rate is among the lowest for any crime. Studies based on captive populations of arsonists therefore probably exclude approximately 90% of people who commit the crime. As with other crimes, arson is multifactorial in origin, and arsonists are a widely heterogeneous group (Geller 1992, Barker 1994, Prins 1994a).

Most attempts to classify fire-setters have been based on assessment, or speculation, of their motivation; such classifications are bound to contain overlap between categories. Clare et al (1992) identified problems in classifications based on:

- arsonists' personal and social characteristics;
- typologies of motives (Barnett & Spitzer 1994, Prins 1994a);
- functional analysis of the behaviour.

All methods have deficiencies. Few studies have used adequate control groups, motivation is often complex and multifactorial, while behavioural analysis does not help identify the weight of particular contributory factors in any given case. An historical association between fire-setting and sexual psychopathology is not borne out in current practice or literature. The following are examples of fire-raising and should not be seen as mutually exclusive categories within an all-embracing classification.

- *Motivated fire-setting.* This is a deliberate act with the aim of a fraudulent insurance claim, engineering a change of housing, taking revenge in a broken relationship or failed business venture, or concealing another crime, e.g. murder or burglary.
- *Political fire-setting.* This is a group activity common at times of social unrest. Not all the perpetrators may be politically motivated.
- *Suicide by fire.* An epidemic of self-immolation, as an apparent political gesture, occurred in the late 1960s. It is possible that some of the subjects were mentally disturbed. This method of suicide is sometimes employed by prisoners.
- *Psychiatric disorder or organic brain disease.* Fire may be set by schizophrenics in response to psychotic phenomena, by people with a learning disability for reasons of excitement, and by substance abusers in states of intoxication, delirium tremens, alcoholic hallucinosis or drug-related psychosis.
- *No psychiatric disorder.* Fires may be set out of boredom or as a vague form of 'protest'.
- *Those with no motive.* Some fire-setters gain satisfaction from watching the fire and the subsequent emergency. They may act heroically, often being early on the scene and appearing to help the fire brigade. Such men sometimes gain employment as firemen or security guards. For some of these offenders the condition defined as pyromania in ICD-10 may be relevant.
- *Female fire-setters.* A comparison of imprisoned female fire-setters with other women in prison failed to show significant psychiatric or social differences between the two groups (Stewart 1993). Both had highly disturbed backgrounds, histories of abuse and unstable lives as adults.

Current classifications of fire-setters have not reached such sophistication that they provide a practical guide to treatment and prognosis. Individual assessment based on standard psychiatric examination together with full details of the fire-setting behaviour is necessary. Only a tiny proportion of fire-setters receive a psychiatric disposal in court; in the highly selected samples examined by psychiatrists, a mental illness may be present in 10–30% of cases (Puri et al 1995). Alcohol or other substance abuse is common, while mental illness, if present, is likely to be schizophrenia or an associated paranoid psychosis. Among the population of people with a learning disability in secure hospital settings, arson is a common index offence. Studies of prognosis give widely different re-offending rates for arson: from 4% to 30% (Soothill & Pope 1973, O'Sullivan & Kelleher 1987). In a Finnish follow-up study of 304 fire-setters who had pretrial psychiatric assessments, 40 had died within 2–15 years of the offence, 17 by suicide (Repo & Virkkunen 1997).

Shoplifting Shoplifting is a form of theft which is perpetrated on a massive scale with huge losses to the retail trade. Most shoplifting has nothing to do with any mental disorder. Gibbens et al (1971), in an early follow-up study of 532 women who had shoplifted 10 years earlier, found rates of subsequent psychiatric hospitalisation three times greater than expected. Depressive disorders were the most common, but a unitary causal model for the offence is often inadequate (Gudjonsson 1990).

The disorder of kleptomania has a place in ICD-10 and DSM-IV. It refers to the repeated failure to control an impulse to steal objects that are not required and are then often discarded, given away or hoarded. The condition is exceedingly rarely encountered in clinical practice. A study of 20 patients who met diagnostic criteria for kleptomania were all found to have lifetime diagnoses of major mood disorders; 16 had additional diagnoses of anxiety disorders and 12 of eating disorders (McElroy et al 1991). Depressed shoplifters typically make little effort to conceal their actions or to escape arrest. Shoplifting is often seen in association with substance abuse and residual schizophrenia. It may also occur in organic states or in states of absent-mindedness.

Child abduction

Abduction or stealing of a child is notified to police with increasing frequency; there were 500 reported incidents in 2000–01, but annual convictions are less than 70. The great majority are carried out by men in custody disputes with their partners. The abduction of a child by a stranger for sexual purposes is rare (d'Orban & Haydn-Smith 1985), but cases understandably receive wide publicity.

Baby stealing is almost invariably carried out by women. Most stolen babies are found fairly quickly and have usually been well cared for by their abductors. An early classification by d'Orban (1976) based on 24 cases remains useful. He described three types of offence:

- comforting offences by deprived women with backgrounds of immaturity, and often having had their own child taken into care;
- a manipulative offence by an older woman with personality difficulties but with a better social adjustment. Such women seek to manipulate a relationship by presenting the baby as their own;
- mentally ill women who steal a baby impulsively, with little or no planning, during a psychotic illness.

The risk of repetition is a real issue, particularly in the third group, in whom delusions concerning babies are often systematised.

Victims of crime

Current growth in crime rates brings a parallel growth in the numbers of victims. There is good evidence that being a victim is associated with psychiatric morbidity. This applies not only to victims of sexual abuse and sexual crimes but also to victims of violent and other offences. In 2001–02 the British Crime Survey (2002) reported that the risk of being a victim of a violent crime was 4%. Community surveys in America have reported even higher figures. Acute and longer-term psychiatric sequelae occur, including symptoms of fear, anger, guilt and irritability as well as recognised disorders such as adjustment reactions and post-traumatic stress disorder. Impaired capacity for intimate emotional relationships, increased impulsivity and risk-taking behaviour commonly develop (Mezey & Robbins 2000). The more profound effects are likely where there has been a perceived threat to life and a physical injury.

The effects of child sexual abuse are well recognised, though up to one-third of adult survivors report no long-term effects (Hilton

& Mezey 1996). Psychiatric morbidity is associated with abuse by a father or stepfather, violent sexual behaviour, penetrative sex and bizarre or repugnant sexual acts. Adult survivors of abuse show high rates of depression, guilt, low self-esteem, alcoholism, sexual problems, eating disorders, self-harm and further victimisation. Male survivors show similar psychiatric sequelae.

MENTALLY DISORDERED OFFENDERS AND THE CRIMINAL JUSTICE SYSTEM

De-institutionalisation of the mentally ill and community care have increased the contact between people with mental disorders and the criminal justice system. Mentally disordered offenders (MDOs) can be moved from the criminal justice system to mental health services at any stage of the criminal justice process. This does not prevent the legal process from progressing; it may do so either in tandem with an individual's psychiatric assessment and treatment, or at a later stage. Indeed prosecution of serious offenders can ensure the identification of an individual's true risk and access to appropriate services. Conversely, a patient can be returned to the criminal justice system from psychiatric services unless a final disposal is made solely to the latter. Clearly, involvement of mental health professionals with people in the criminal justice system is dependent on the existence of appropriate services and the recognition of mental health problems. Training of police, probation and prison officers, prosecutors and the judiciary is therefore essential.

In this chapter English and Welsh legislation is used to illustrate specific psychiatric legal defences, and powers to detain and treat MDOs. At the time of writing a new Mental Health Act is proposed (Department of Health 2002), although its future is uncertain.

Mental disorder and the police

Contact with the police can be the first step in accessing help for people with mental disorder, and as such the police have both a specific power and a statutory responsibility in managing and interviewing people with suspected mental disorder.

Place of safety

A police officer has the power under Section 136 of the Mental Health Act 1983 to remove a person found in a public place who appears to be suffering from a mental disorder and to be in immediate need of care or control to a place of safety for up to 72 hours. Over 2600 of these orders are used annually (Department of Health 2001a). A place of safety is locally agreed and is usually a hospital, social services building or a police station. In that location the detained individual is examined by a medical practitioner and any necessary arrangements made. Alternatively, if an individual has been arrested and taken to police cells, he can be assessed in that setting by a forensic medical examiner (usually a general practitioner) or duty psychiatrist.

Police interviews and false confessions

It is recognised that police interviews of adults with a mental disorder require careful attention because of potential problems with communication, lack of comprehension, delusional thinking, limited insight, emotional distress and suggestibility. In the last decade both the legal and public attitude to the possibility of a false confession has changed largely as a result of high-profile cases such as the Birmingham Six. Caution is particularly required in dealing with confessions made by individuals with a mental disorder. Such false confessions may arise directly from delusional beliefs, suggestibility, a desire to escape an immediate situation, or from a desire to comply. The presence of a mental disorder, however, does not always invalidate a confession. In cases of disputed confession, Gudjonsson & MacKeith (1996) advise an examination of:

- the circumstances surrounding a crime;
- the interaction between interviewer and suspect;
- the suspect's physical and mental health;
- the suspect's personality, including assessment of suggestibility and compliance.

A police officer may request an assessment of an individual's fitness to be interviewed. Medical or legal criteria do not currently exist for this, but factors to be considered include the individual's:

- understanding of the police caution after it has been fully explained;
- orientation in time, place and person, and recognition of key people present during the police interview;
- ability to understand the consequences of answers and likelihood of giving answers that can be seriously misconstrued by the court (Gudjonsson 2003).

If a detainee is found fit for interview but has a mental disorder, an appropriate adult must be present.

Appropriate adults

The Police and Criminal Evidence Act (PACE) 1984 and its accompanying Codes of Practice established a statutory requirement for mentally disordered suspects to be interviewed by the police in the presence of an appropriate adult. Appropriate adults are volunteers who ideally are experienced and/or trained in dealing with people with mental disorders. They are most frequently social workers or psychiatric nurses. They do not act in their professional role and must not be police employees. The role of the appropriate adult is to provide support and reassurance to a person with a mental disorder being interviewed by the police and to ease communication. The appropriate adult should ensure that a person with a mental disorder understands the legal process and the effect of his answers. He should neither advise the interviewee on how to answer any of the questions, object to any of the questions asked or prompt any identification of a suspect by a witness.

Research in England suggests that appropriate adults are used in between 0.2% and 2% of all police interviews. Estimates of the numbers of mentally disordered suspects being interviewed vary from 2% to 20%. In spite of the absence at police interview of an appropriate adult in some cases, the courts have been reluctant to dismiss or overturn a conviction for this reason (Nemitz & Bean 2001).

Mental disorder and court proceedings

Liaison services between the legal and psychiatric systems, and specific laws have been developed to ensure that MDOs are fairly and justly treated during legal proceedings.

Court diversion schemes

Modern health policy promotes early intervention and diversion from prosecution of MDOs (Home Office 1990, Scottish Office 1999). Court diversion schemes have been developed to ensure that MDOs appearing in court are identified and diverted to alternative services where appropriate. Chiefly, these schemes aim to detect people with psychosis or active suicidal ideation. The schemes vary: some offer a daily presence at court, screening referred cases or briefly checking custody notes; others an on-call service; and some a regular meeting between prosecution and forensic psychiatry services to determine pre-trial the suitability of a case for diversion. A diversion scheme requires a psychiatrist to complete the relevant detention process or to make recommendations to the court, and to gain access to hospital beds. In many schemes a psychiatric nurse carries out the initial screening.

In the UK these schemes have been shown to identify mental illness in prisoners, accelerate admission and avoid lengthy remands in custody but have not increased the overall numbers admitted to hospital from the criminal justice system (James 1999). As schemes become established, so the number of referrals tends to rise, although the proportion of people admitted remains fairly constant. In Glasgow Sheriff Court there was a 250% increase in referrals by the prosecution service to the local scheme between 1994 and 1998, although the proportion admitted fell from 46% (54 patients) to 15% (44). Consequently, doubts have been expressed about the efficient use of psychiatric time (White et al 2002). Each scheme requires clear referral criteria and education of referrers to prevent overload with inappropriate referrals.

Drug courts

The recognition of an association between substance abuse or mental disorder and crime has lead to the establishment in some areas of specialised drug or mental health courts. Eley et al (2002) reviewed the practice of one drug court established with the aim of reducing drug abuse and associated offending by offering treatment-based disposals to the court. This court deals with less serious offences and targets adults over the age of 20 with well-established, associated problems of drug misuse and offending. Potential candidates are identified by the prosecution service from the police report and screened for suitability. Following a positive recommendation the custody court can refer the case to the drug court if the individual pleads guilty. The case is then adjourned for 4 weeks to obtain a social enquiry report, drug action plan and drug testing. The drug court has the full range of disposals available to any court dealing with summary proceedings but can impose drug treatment and testing orders (DTTOs), probation orders with a condition of drug treatment, concurrent DTTOs and conditional probation orders, or deferred sentences. Cases are reviewed monthly and can be breached if non-compliant. Drug courts were introduced throughout England and Wales in 2000, and 4400 drug treatment and testing orders were commenced in 2001.

Fitness to plead

At times a defendant because of a mental disorder may lack the capacity to defend himself and is said to be unfit to plead. These cases typically involve people with a major mental illness or learning disability. There are five tests to determine fitness to plead, arising mainly from R v Pritchard (1836). See Box 29.10. A sixth criterion of ability to give evidence in a trial has been suggested following the abolition of a defendant's right to silence in police interviews and at court (Gray et al 2001). James et al (2001) in a study of 479 patients referred by courts for a psychiatric opinion found that the most important legal criteria in determining fitness to plead were ability to instruct a solicitor and to follow the proceedings in court. Positive symptoms of psychosis, in particular thought disorder and delusions, were significantly associated with unfitness to plead.

Unfitness to plead is a matter of relevance at the time of the trial. Some accused individuals are initially unfit to plead, but pre-trial treatment can reverse this. The law on fitness to plead is governed by the Criminal Procedure (Insanity) Act 1964 Section 4 as amended by the Criminal Procedure (Insanity and Unfitness to Plead) Act 1991 Section 2. The 1991 Act sets out a three stage process described in Box 29.11.

There are a number of options available to the court for disposal of a case if an individual is found to be unfit to plead. These options are the same as those available if a person is acquitted on the grounds of insanity at the time of an offence. See Box 29.12

The Home Secretary has the power to refer the case of an individual found unfit to be tried to the Court of Appeal. He can also remit for trial an accused person, found 'guilty' at the trial of facts and given a hospital order, who subsequently becomes well enough to be tried.

Box 29.10   Fitness to plead — criteria

A defendant must be able to:
- understand the charge(s)
- distinguish between a plea of guilty and not guilty
- instruct counsel
- follow proceedings in court
- challenge a juror (does not apply in Scotland)

Box 29.11   Fitness to plead — legal process

1. Finding of unfitness to plead recorded
2. Trial of the facts
   This is not a psychiatric issue; it is as near as possible to an ordinary trial. The evidence must prove beyond reasonable doubt that the accused carried out the alleged act
3. Facts are found
4. Disposal — one of four specified options

Box 29.12   Fitness to plead and insanity — disposal options

- *Admission order.* This is the equivalent of a hospital order with the possible addition of a restriction order. Both are *mandatory* in cases of *murder*.
- *Guardianship order.* This is appropriate in cases where care and protection are the main issues rather than treatment.
- *Supervision and treatment order.* Using this order an individual is supervised in the community by a social worker or probation officer for a maximum of 2 years, and given treatment provided by a doctor.
- *Absolute discharge with no order.*

In England the number of cases found unfit to plead and given a restriction order rose from under 10 to over 40 per year (Johnson & Taylor 2002). Pleas in bar of trial doubled in Scotland following the introduction of similar new insanity legislation with flexible disposals (Burman & Connelly 1999).

Psychiatric defences

Criminal conviction is dependent on evidence proving beyond reasonable doubt that the accused carried out the physical act of an offence (actus reus) and deliberately intended or risked a harmful outcome (mens rea). Children under the age of 10 in England and Wales (8 in Scotland) are assumed to be incapable of forming criminal intent. It is accepted that mental disorder can remove or reduce criminal responsibility, and this forms the basis for specific psychiatric defences. Drug and alcohol misuse are generally not considered grounds for a defence unless associated with involuntary intoxication or secondary problems such as an alcohol dementia or a drug-induced psychosis.

Insanity at the time of the offence Offences can be committed directly because of psychotic symptoms and altered thought processes. The legal system recognises this with the special defence of insanity set out in the Criminal Procedure (Insanity) Act 1964 Section 5 as amended by the Criminal Procedure (Insanity and Unfitness to Plead) Act 1991 Section 3. It is an individual's mental state at the time of the offence that is relevant. It is a separate legal process from fitness to plead, although it is possible for someone to be both unfit to plead and insane at the time of the offence.

In England and Wales the legal test is set by the 1843 McNaghten rules. There are two components to these: first, that the individual had at the time of the offence a mental disorder, and second, that this lead to the absence of mens rea (a guilty mind). In the words of the judgement that the '*accused was labouring under such a defect of reason, from disease of the mind, as not to know the nature and quality of the act he was doing, or if he did know it, that he did not know that what he was doing was wrong*'.

The burden of proof lies with the defence and is decided on the balance of probabilities. The defendant must prove:

- that he was suffering from a disease of the mind at the time of the crime,
- that this caused a defect of reason, and
- that the defect of reason robbed him of the capacity to either know what he was doing or know that it was wrong.

It is for the jury to decide with guidance from the trial judge on matters of law. It is recognised that the jurors' concept of insanity does not fit well with the legal or psychiatric constructs (Skeem & Golding 2001). Generally, people found not guilty on account of insanity have committed a serious violent offence, usually against a family member, when acutely psychotic (Nestor & Haycock 1997, Gibbons et al 1997).

Under the Criminal Procedure (Insanity and Unfitness to Plead) Act 1991 a wide range of options for disposal of a case is open to the Court following an acquittal on the grounds of insanity; see Box 29.12. Since this range of disposals became available in 1992 the number of insanity cases receiving a restriction order has remained constant at approximately eight per year (Johnson & Taylor 2002). In the Crown Court in 2000 there were 15 cases found not guilty by reason of insanity (Home Office 2002a).

Diminished responsibility Diminished responsibility is a legal defence available in murder cases to suggest a reduced degree of responsibility for the homicidal act. It originated in Scotland with the Dingwall case of 1867 and was introduced to English law by the Homicide Act 1957. It exists because a conviction for murder results in a mandatory life sentence. The psychiatric defence of diminished responsibility reduces a murder charge to manslaughter, and a full range of sentencing disposals is then available to the judge. Historically the concept has been used for other charges, and as recently as 1986 it was used in Scotland to reduce a charge of attempted murder to assault to severe injury (HMA v Blake) although the defendant died before an appeal against this verdict was considered.

The criteria for diminished responsibility are set out in Section 2 of the Homicide Act 1957:

Where a person kills or is party to the killing of another, he shall not be convicted of murder if he was suffering from such an abnormality of mind (whether arising from a condition of arrested or retarded development of mind or any inherent cause or induced by disease or injury) as substantially impaired his mental responsibility for his acts and omissions in doing or being a party to the killing.

Abnormality of mind was defined in R v Byrne (1960) as

a state of mind so different from that of ordinary human beings that the reasonable man would term it abnormal. It appears to us to be wide enough to cover the mind's activities in all its aspects, not only the perception of physical acts and matters and the ability to form a rational judgement as to whether the act is right or wrong, but also the ability to exercise will-power to control physical acts in accordance with that rational judgement.

Only the defence can raise the issue of diminished responsibility. The defendant must prove on a balance of probabilities three matters:

- that he was suffering from an abnormality of mind at the time of the crime;
- that the abnormality of mind resulted from one of the causes specified in Section 2 of the 1957 Act;
- that the abnormality of mind substantially impaired mental responsibility.

The case law on diminished responsibility is constantly changing. It is used most frequently in cases of psychosis and depression but has been used for personality disorder, premenstrual syndrome, mercy killings and battered wives syndrome (Mitchell 1997a). Voluntary intoxication with drugs or alcohol is usually not considered grounds for a diminished responsibility defence, although the original Dingwall case concerned a man suffering delirium tremens. A study of 101 cases referred to a regional secure unit between 1987 and 1994 found that female gender and absence of a criminal history made a successful diminished responsibility plea more likely (Mitchell 1997b).

In uncontested cases the judge can accept a plea of guilty to manslaughter on the grounds of diminished responsibility and can sentence as he sees fit. Where there is conflicting psychiatric evidence, a conviction for murder usually results. Of those convicted of Section 2 manslaughter, a small number receive a discretionary life sentence; others receive determinate prison sentences, hospital orders with or without restrictions, and some are placed on probation.

Infanticide By the 18th century the judicial execution of mothers who killed their babies had ceased. This leniency was formalised in the first infanticide act of 1922. The subsequent 1938 Infanticide Act states that *where a woman by any wilful act or omission causes the death of her child under the age of 12 months, but at the time of the act or omission the balance of her mind was disturbed by reason of her not having fully recovered from the effect of giving birth to the child or by reason of the effect of lactation consequent upon the birth of the child, then notwithstanding that the circumstances were such that but for this Act the offence would have amounted to murder she shall be guilty of an offence, to wit of infanticide, and may for such offence be dealt with and punished as if she had been guilty of the offence of manslaughter of the child.*

Reasons for infanticide include concealed, denied or unwanted pregnancy (usually neonaticide, i.e. killing the infant in the first 24 hours of life); loss of control and battering often associated with a deprived maternal childhood and poor current socio-economic circumstances; as well as mental disorder (Dobson & Sales 2000). In the 1990s there were on average four cases of infanticide per year in England and Wales, accounting for 0.7% of all homicides (Home Office 2002b). One-tenth of perpetrators went to prison for a period of less than 4 years, one-tenth was sent to a psychiatric hospital, and four-fifths were given a probation or supervision order. It is argued that the defences of diminished responsibility or insanity negate the need for the specific defence of infanticide.

Automatism An automatism is an act committed during a state of unconsciousness or grossly impaired consciousness. Such an act lacks mens rea or a guilty mind. Automatism was defined by the Court of Appeal as '*the state of a person who, though capable of action, is not conscious of what he is doing. . . . It means unconscious involuntary action, and it is a defence because the mind does not go with what is being done*' (Bratty v Attorney General for Northern Ireland 1963).

There are two types of automatism: a sane automatism leads to a full acquittal, whereas an insane automatism leads to a verdict of not guilty by reason of insanity. With the latter the judge can utilise the full range of disposals set out in the Criminal Procedure (Insanity and Unfitness to Plead) Act 1991 (Box 29.12). The difference between the two is based on whether the automatism or behaviour leading to the offence is likely to recur. The court's concern is primarily about public safety. Indeed, in the case of Regina v Burgess (1991) it was stated that 'if there is a danger of recurrence that may be an added reason for categorising the condition as a disease of the mind'.

Sane automatisms are considered to be singular events due to exogenous causes such as confusional states, hypoglycaemia, concussion or night terrors. Insane automatisms are viewed as events due to a disease of the mind which are likely to recur and which therefore require control of that individual to ensure public safety. They are said to be due to endogenous causes, and examples include sleepwalking and epilepsy. The distinction between internal and external causes is purely legal and makes no sense from a medical perspective. Indeed some, such as dissociative states, have been declared both sane and insane automatisms. All causes are associated with altered brain functioning, and some of the so-called sane automatisms, such as hypoglycaemia, may well recur.

Psychiatric court reports

A psychiatric report communicates a psychiatrist's opinion to the court and provides the background material from which that opinion arose. It assists the court in determining whether an individual has a mental disorder, the nature of any such disorder, its relationship to the (alleged) offence, and the presence of any mitigating circumstances. In addition it acts as a screening test for admission to psychiatric services. Gethins et al (2002) found that 20% of all patients referred for preparation of a medico-legal report to a regional forensic mental health service were subsequently admitted. A court may remand an individual to a prison hospital wing for the purpose of obtaining a psychiatric court report. It can also remand a defendant to hospital on bail for this purpose, although this provides staff with no powers to detain the accused if he insists on leaving. Alternatively, reports can be prepared on individuals on bail, in the community, or remanded to prison.

A psychiatrist asked to prepare such a report must know who is requesting it (defence, prosecution service, court officers) and why. There may be questions that the report's commissioner particularly wishes to be addressed such as fitness to plead. The psychiatrist must have access to all relevant available information such as the charge sheet, witness statements, police summary and criminal record. If these are not automatically made available, they must be requested. Preparation of a psychiatric court report involves detailed background reading of available legal and medical papers, interview of the patient, interview of informants (professional and personal), and consideration of the medico-legal issues involved. A psychiatric court report breaches a basic rule of medical practice — confidentiality. It is essential that this is made clear at the beginning of the patient interview.

The report's content is based largely on a standard psychiatric assessment with a particular emphasis on criminological history, and the index or alleged offence. If the report is being prepared pre-trial, statements on the patient's account of the alleged offence should comment on the patient's behaviour and use of alcohol and drugs prior to the alleged offence, and his ability to understand and remember. It should not be a recorded confession. If the psychiatrist is suggesting that the patient was insane at the time of the offence, then a more detailed account will be appropriate. The report must be an unbiased professional opinion and be easily understandable by a lay person. Any medical terms must be explained. Box 29.13 lists the information routinely contained in a psychiatric court report.

Box 29.13 Psychiatric court report

- Demographic details of accused person
- Charge(s)
- Court location and date
- Sources of data: patient interview, documents and case notes, other informants
- Circumstances of interview: where, when, length, subject's ability to comprehend and participate (brief statement only)
- Background history: birth, childhood, education, employment, relationships, current social circumstances
- Family history: psychiatric, substance abuse and criminality
- Medical history: physical and psychiatric
- Alcohol and drug misuse
- Previous convictions
- Alleged index offence
- Mental state examination
- Additional information, e.g. from a relative or carer
- Opinion
- Recommendations
- Name, designation and qualifications of writer

Most psychiatric reports are presented to court without it being necessary for the psychiatrist to attend. If details of the report require clarification, or there are conflicting psychiatric opinions, then attendance at court to give oral evidence will be required. An accurate, balanced and unbiased report is the essential basis for a successful witness appearance. This should be read several times in preparation for court and consideration given to likely questions. Medical terminology will need to be explained. Witnesses should ensure that they are aware of normal court proceedings and dress appropriately for a formal setting. Close attention is required to the questions asked, and these should be answered slowly and clearly. Expert witness courses are now commonly available and assist the psychiatrist in ensuring that his opinion is accurately presented.

Court disposals of mentally disordered offenders

Powers exist for courts to send MDOs to the care of psychiatric services. They become patients rather than prisoners. Table 29.6 describes the relevant legislation for England and Wales. Such legislation can be used pre-trial, or post-trial but pre-sentencing, for assessment and treatment; or as a final disposal. Formerly, final disposals were either to hospital or to the criminal justice system, with the exception of a probation order with a condition of psychiatric treatment which combined both. It is used mainly for offenders with substance abuse problems. There may be problems in the management of MDOs who fail to attend for appointments.

The introduction of a hospital and limitation direction order created a combined disposal of initial hospitalisation with a term of imprisonment. When psychiatric treatment in hospital has finished, the individual is transferred to prison unless the sentence period has expired. Initially, doubts were expressed regarding the ethics of such a disposal (Thomson 1999), but a study of psychiatrists' and judges' views in Scotland on the use of such orders suggests that this is changing (Darjee et al 2000, 2001). Many see this order as potentially useful in the treatment of comorbid mental illness and personality disorder. In England and Wales it is currently only available in cases within the legal category of psychopathic disorder.

Services for mentally disordered offenders

The guiding principles for the care of MDOs (Department of Health & Home Office 1992, Scottish Office 1999) have been established and widely accepted. MDOs should be cared for:

- with regard to quality of care and proper attention to the needs of individuals;
- as far as possible in the community rather than in an institutional setting;
- under conditions of no greater security than is justified by the degree of danger they present to themselves or others;
- in such a way as to maximise rehabilitation and their chances of sustaining an independent life;
- as near as possible to their own homes or families if they have them.

The successful management of MDOs is dependent on access to a range of services in different settings. In the UK the legislation exists to allow ease of movement between the criminal justice and health systems (see Tables 29.2 and 29.6), but sadly failure to identify need or, more commonly, lack of facilities may prevent appropriate placement and treatment.

A properly functioning forensic psychiatric service requires the following components.

- Staff and resources:
  — a multidisciplinary forensic mental health team with members drawn from psychiatry, nursing, social work, psychology and occupational therapy;
  — access to facilities for patients with special needs such as hearing impairment;
  — access to specific psychotherapeutic programmes for anger management, substance abuse, mental health education and offending behaviour;
  — a systematic approach to care planning, such as the Care Programme Approach, with clearly delineated problems and solutions, identified responsible staff, regular review arrangements and a crisis response strategy. Such a care plan incorporates risk assessment and management.
- Links and liaisons:
  — a liaison service to the police, prosecution services and courts to allow diversion of prisoners to psychiatric services, where required, for further assessment and/or treatment;
  — an established relationship with the local Probation Service to share information in the preparation of reports, to provide probation officers with advice and to jointly manage people on a probation order with attendance for psychiatric treatment as a condition;
  — a psychiatric service to local prisons;
  — a good relationship with general psychiatry and learning disability services to allow movement of patients between services as appropriate, and sharing of community resources such as day hospitals.
- Inpatient facilities — access to inpatient beds for assessment and treatment at the appropriate level of security: high, medium or low. There should be sufficient provision to allow ease of movement between these facilities dependent on security needs and to meet the needs of those requiring long-term medium- and low-security care. No definitive criteria exist to define a patient's need for varying levels of security. These clinical judgements are based on factors such as the seriousness of the index offence or behaviour, assessment of future risk of violence, likely response of identified risk factors to treatment, and probable length of stay.
- Community facilities:
  — access to a full range of community facilities such as supported accommodation, day hospital, work placements and support groups for users and carers;
  — a forensic community mental health team (FCMHT) for those patients being cared for in a non-institutional setting. Closure of psychiatric hospitals and the policy of care in the community have lead to the development of general CMHTs. A review of the literature has shown that CMHTs improve treatment satisfaction and may be associated with a reduction in death by suicide but have no overall effect on admission rates, length of inpatient stay, or overall outcome (Tyrer et al 2002). Intensive outreach has not been shown to reduce levels of violence in a randomised control trial of patients with schizophrenia in a general adult setting (Walsh 2001). While the intensive group had double the input of the control group, it may be that patients in the control group

Table 29.6 Court disposals of mentally disordered offenders

Provision Number/year	Act & Section Authority	Recommendation	Psychiatric grounds for order	Duration Appeal
Remand to hospital for report on accused person's mental condition

n = 150* | MHA 1983 S.35

Magistrates' or Crown Court | One fully registered medical practitioner (approved under S.12 as having special experience in the diagnosis or treatment of mental disorder) | Reason to suspect accused person has mental illness, psychopathic disorder, mental impairment, or severe mental impairment. Bed must be available within 7 days | 28 days, renewable every 28 days to a maximum of 12 weeks. Court can terminate earlier if appropriate

Can appeal against remand |
| Remand of accused person to hospital for treatment

n = 18* | MHA 1983 S.36

Crown Court (excludes murder charge) | Two fully registered medical practitioners (one approved under S.12 as having special experience in the diagnosis or treatment of mental disorder) | Mental illness or severe mental impairment of a nature or degree to make detention in hospital for medical treatment appropriate. Bed must be available within 7 days | 28 days, renewable every 28 days to a maximum of 12 weeks. Court can terminate earlier if appropriate

Can appeal against remand |
| Interim hospital order. Post-conviction but pre-final disposal, this order allows time to consider issues of diagnosis and treatability. About 70% receive a final hospital disposal (White et al 2001).

n < 160* | MHA 1983 S.38

Magistrates' or Crown Court | Two fully registered medical practitioners (one approved under S.12 as having special experience in the diagnosis or treatment of mental disorder and one employed by the specified hospital). | Mental illness, psychopathic disorder, mental impairment or severe mental impairment. Reason to suppose a hospital order may be appropriate. Bed must be available within 28 days | 12 weeks, renewable thereafter each 28 days to a maximum of 12 months

No right of appeal |
| Hospital order & guardianship order. Hospital order can only be used for offences punishable by imprisonment. Magistrates' court can make a hospital order without recording a conviction. Person must be 16 or over

n = 614† | MHA 1983 S.37

Magistrates' or Crown Court | Two fully registered medical practitioners (one approved under S.12 as having special experience in the diagnosis or treatment of mental disorder). Confirmation of admission arrangements from proposed responsible medical officer or hospital managers | Mental illness, psychopathic disorder, mental impairment or severe mental impairment of a nature or degree to make detention in hospital for medical treatment appropriate. If psychopathic disorder or mental impairment then such treatment must be likely to alleviate or prevent a deterioration of the condition. Or a mental disorder or a nature or degree that warrants reception into guardianship. Bed must be available within 28 days | 6 months, renewable for a further 6 months and thereafter annually. RMO can use leave of absence or discharge when appropriate

A patient can appeal to Crown Court against the initial imposition of this order. Right of appeal to mental health review tribunal in second 6 months and thereafter annually |
| Restriction order S.37 + S.41

n = 239† | MHA 1983 S.41 | One of the two doctors giving evidence for a S.37 must give oral evidence. | Must consider: nature of the offence, antecedents of offender, and risk to public | Without limit of time. Secretary of State must consent to any leave of absence, transfer or discharge

Can appeal against imposition of order to the Court of Appeal (Criminal Division). Right of appeal to mental health review tribunal in second 6 months and thereafter annually. Must be seen a minimum of every 3 years |

Table 29.6   Contiued

Provision Number/year	Act & Section Authority	Recommendation	Psychiatric grounds for order	Duration / Appeal
Hospital and limitation direction. A final disposal post-conviction. It combines a period in hospital and a term of imprisonment. If no response to treatment, transferred to prison to complete sentence	MHA 1983 S. 45A and 45B or Crime (Sentences) Act 1997 S.46	Two fully registered medical practitioners (one approved under S.12 as having special experience in the diagnosis or treatment of mental disorder). One must give oral evidence Confirmation of admission arrangements from proposed responsible medical officer or hospital managers. Admission within 28 days of direction	Psychopathic disorder. Appropriate to be detained in hospital for treatment. Such treatment is likely to alleviate or prevent a deterioration of the condition	Length of prison sentence. Annual report by RMO to Secretary of State.
n = 3 †	Crown Court			Can appeal against imposition of order to the Court of Appeal (Criminal Division)
Probation order with condition of treatment for mental condition	Criminal Justice Act 1991 S.9(1)3 and Schedule 1A	By doctor to whom offender will report under probation order (approved under S.12 as having special experience in the diagnosis or treatment of mental disorder)	Offender needs treatment for mental disorder but does not require detention	Length of probation order or if the order is breached. Offender must agree to a probation order
n = 699‡	Magistrates' or Crown Court			

* Department of Health (2001a).
† Johnson & Taylor (2002).
‡ Home Office (2002d).
RMO, responsible medical officer.

with a history of violence or other recognised risk factors were selectively given more intensive input.
- Support services and systems:
  - information technology to allow the forensic mental health team ease of access to records, data and activity levels;
  - national and local co-ordination to further the development of forensic mental health services in a cohesive manner;
  - public education strategy on mental disorders to combat stigma and fear, particularly regarding MDOs. Such stigma can result in the failure to develop a range of services, and this ironically can increase the risk to public safety.

Contentious issues

Homicide inquiries

All homicides by people with mental disorder have been followed by mandatory inquiries in England and Wales. Findings have been collated (Petch & Bradley 1997), and persistent themes include misdiagnosis, lack of follow-up, lack of communication between services, poor record keeping and delays. The problem has usually been a failure to act rather than a failure to assess. It has become a tenet of medical practice that new developments and interventions should be subject to audit. It is therefore surprising that few inquiries established any process to review implementation of their recommendations. It is currently proposed that the National Patient Safety Agency will undertake homicide inquiries, although the exact process has still to be determined. It is hoped that this Agency will foster a culture of learning from adverse events rather than a culture of blame.

Inquiries into high-security psychiatric hospitals

Sadly, in the last few years scandal has continued to be an issue in the care and treatment of MDOs. In particular, the Inquiry into the Personality Disorder Unit at Ashworth Special Hospital (Department of Health 1999) highlighted problems with lack of control, widespread distribution of pornographic material, and paedophilic activities. It recommended the closure of Ashworth Hospital (although this has not occurred). It also proposed a reviewable sentence with a specified tariff for convicted individuals who are found on pre-sentence assessment to be suffering principally from personality disorder and who present a substantial risk of causing harm to others. It was proposed that a reviewable sentence board would be able to renew a sentence for up to 2 years, or to grant an absolute discharge or a conditional discharge for a maximum period of 2 years. This recommendation has not been developed.

The Ashworth Inquiry also recommended a comprehensive review of the security arrangements at the three high-security hospitals in England (Ashworth, Broadmoor and Rampton). This review made 86 recommendations including the need to increase funding for resources for patients inappropriately placed in high-security psychiatric care, and to upgrade perimeter security at all three hospitals (Department of Health 2000). The latter has taken place although there had been no escapes from the hospital sites within the 5 years prior to the report.

Dangerous and severe personality disorder

In 1999 the Government published proposals on managing people it considered had a dangerous severe personality disorder

(DSPD) (Home Office & Department of Health 1999). The primary concern is public safety. The term DSPD is used to describe people with a recognised personality disorder who pose a high risk to other people because of serious antisocial behaviour resulting from their disorder. The Government estimated that approximately 1800 such people will have committed serious offences and be in prison or hospital and a further 500 may not have committed any recent offence and be in the community. There are four main components to the Government's policy:

- creation of powers for detention and continued supervision of DSPD individuals;
- improved identification and assessment;
- development of specialist approaches to detention and management;
- establishment of a research programme to support development of policy and practice.

Subsequently, the Government committed £125 million to the development of pilot DSPD units in prisons and special hospitals. Criticism has been made of the term DSPD as it fails to equate with any modern diagnostic classification system and fails to identify issues of comorbidity between personality disorder and other mental disorders. Haddock et al (2001) found that 75% of forensic psychiatrists were opposed to the use of DSPD to allow indeterminate detention in unconvicted cases.

New mental health legislation

Since 1999 the Government in England and Wales has consulted on new mental health legislation and published a Draft Mental Health Bill (Department of Health 2002). The term DSPD does not appear in the bill but the opportunity for preventive detention is contained in it. At the time of writing, the Bill has failed to appear in the 2003/2004 parliament's legislative programme, but ministerial statements appear to suggest that it will proceed in spite of considerable opposition.

Elsewhere in the UK different legislatures are proposing different solutions to the problems of dangerous offenders. In Scotland, the MacLean Committee (Scottish Executive 2000) reviewed the sentencing of serious violent and sexual offenders, including those with personality disorder. It recommended the creation of an order for lifelong restriction (OLR) for offenders who were likely to present an ongoing risk to public safety. This would be an indeterminate sentence to be followed by release on licence subject to agreed conditions with recall available if these were not met.

The MacLean report recommended the establishment of a risk management authority to monitor progress of individuals in custody, and to promote service, training, and research and development in the field of risk assessment and management. Specialist services would be developed in the community for high-risk offenders, including intensive supervision and surveillance using, for example, electronic monitoring. MDOs perceived as a high risk for violent or sexual recidivism would be given an OLR in conjunction with a hospital direction, the latter combining a period of hospitalisation and a term of imprisonment (Thomson 1999).

Legislation to establish a risk management authority and for the introduction of the OLR is now contained in the Criminal Justice (Scotland) Act 2002. Similarly, the Millan Committee reviewed the Mental Health (Scotland) Act 1984, including legislation for

MDOs. The Mental Health (Care and Treatment) (Scotland) Bill was subsequently passed by the Scottish Parliament in 2003.

REFERENCES

Abel G G, Becker J V, Cunningham-Rathner J et al 1988 Multiple paraphilic diagnoses among sex offenders. Bulletin of the American Academy of Psychiatry & Law 16:153–168

Allam J, Middleton D, Browne K 1997 Different clients, different needs? Practical issues in community-based treatment for sex offenders. Criminal Behaviour & Mental Health 7:69–84

Andrews D A, Bonta J 1995 The level of service inventory — revised manual. Multi-Health Systems Inc, Toronto

Appleby L, Wessely S 1988 The influence of the Hungerford massacre on the public opinion of mental illness. Medicine, Science & the Law 28:291–295

Bailey J, MacCulloch M 1992 Characteristics of 112 cases discharged directly to the community from a new special hospital and some comparisons of performance. Journal of Forensic Psychiatry 3:91–112

Bailey S 1995 Young offenders, serious crimes. British Journal of Psychiatry 167:5–7

Barker A 1994 Arson. A review of the psychiatric literature. Oxford University Press, Oxford

Barnett W, Spitzer M 1994 Pathological fire-setting 1951–1991: a review. Medicine, Science and the Law 34:4–20

Bartlett K, Thomson L D G, Johnstone E C 2001 Mentally disordered offenders: an evaluation of the "Open Doors" Programme at HM Prison, Barlinnie. Scottish Prison Service Occasional Paper Series 2/2001

Belfrage H 1998 A ten year follow up of criminality in Stockholm mental patients. British Journal of Criminology 38:145–155

Birmingham L 1999 Between prison and the community. The "revolving door psychiatric patient" of the nineties. British Journal of Psychiatry 174:378–379

Birmingham L, Mason D, Grubin D 1996 Prevalence of mental disorder in remand prisoners: consecutive case study. British Medical Journal 313:1521–1524

Bisson J I, Shepherd J P 1995 Psychological reactions of victims of violent crime. British Journal of Psychiatry 167:718–720

Blair R J 2003 Neurobiological basis of psychopathy. British Journal of Psychiatry 182:5–7

Boer D P, Hart S D, Kropp P R, Webster C D 1997 Manual for the Sexual Violence Risk – 20. Professional Guidelines for Assessing Risk of Sexual Violence. The Mental Health, Law and Policy Institute, Simon Fraser University, Vancouver

Bools C 1996 Factitious illness by proxy (Munchausen syndrome by proxy). British Journal of Psychiatry 169:268–275

Borgaonkar D S, Shah S A 1974 The XYY chromosome — male or syndrome? Progress in Medical Genetics 10:135–222

British Crime Survey 2002 Crime in England and Wales 2001/2002. Research, Development and Statistics Directorate, London

Brittain R P 1970 The sadistic murderer. Medicine, Science and the Law 10:198–207

Brooke D, Taylor C, Gunn J, Maden A 1996 Point prevalence of mental disorder in unconvicted male prisoners in England and Wales. British Medical Journal 313:1524–1527

Brunner H G, Nelen M, Breakfield X O et al 1993 Abnormal behaviour associated with a point mutation in the structural gene for monoamine oxidase A. Science 262:578–580

Buchanan A, Reed A, Wessely S et al 1993 Acting on delusions II: the phenomenological correlates of acting on delusions. British Journal of Psychiatry 163:77–81

Burman M, Connelly C 1999 Mentally disordered offenders and criminal proceedings: the operation of Part VI of the Criminal Procedure (Scotland) Act 1995. Central Research Unit, the Scottish Office, Edinburgh

Caspi A, McClay J, Moffitt T E et al 2002 Role of genotype in the cycle of violence in maltreated children. Science 297:851–854

Cherrett M 1996 Mentally disordered offenders and the police. Mental health review. Pavilion, London

Chiswick D 1981 Matricide. British Medical Journal 238:1279–1280

Clare I C, Murphy G H, Cox D, Chaplin E H 1992 Assessment and treatment of fire-setting: a single-case investigation using a cognitive-behavioural model. Criminal Behaviour and Mental Health 2:253–268

Clark C, Mezey G 1997 Elderly sex offenders against children: a descriptive study of child sex abusers over the age of 65. Journal of Forensic Psychiatry 8:357–369

Clark S A 1993 Matricide: the schizophrenic crime? Medicine, Science and the Law 33:325–328

Coid J W 1984 How many psychiatric patients in prison? British Journal of Psychiatry 145:78–86

Coid J W 1992 DSM-III diagnosis in criminal psychopaths: a way forward. Criminal Behaviour and Mental Health 2:78–94

Coid J, Kahtan N, Gault S, Jarman B 1999 Patients with personality disorder admitted to secure forensic psychiatry services. British Journal of Psychiatry 175:528–536

Coid J, Kahtan N, Gault S, Jarman B 2000 Ethnic differences in admissions to secure forensic psychiatry services. British Journal of Psychiatry 177:241–247

Cooke D 1994 Psychological disturbance amongst prisoners. Scottish Prison Service Occasional Papers. Report No. 3/1994. Scottish Prison Service, Edinburgh

Cooke D J, Michie C, Ryan J 2001 Evaluating risk for violence: a preliminary study of the HCR-20, PCL-R and VRAG in a Scottish prison sample. Scottish Prison Service, Glasgow

Copas J B, Marshall P 1998 The offender group reconviction scale: a statistical reconviction score for use by probation officers. Applied Statistics 47(1):159–171

Copas J B, Marshall P, Tarling R 1996 Predicting reoffending for discretionary conditional release. Home Office, London

Corbett M, Duggan C, Larkin E 1998 Substance misuse and violence: a comparison of special hospital inpatients diagnosed with either schizophrenia or personality disorder. Criminal Behaviour and Mental Health 8:311–321

Cordess C 1995 Crime and mental disorder 1. Criminal behaviour. In: Chiswick D, Cope R (eds) Seminars in practical forensic psychiatry. Gaskell, London, p 14–51

Darjee R, Crichton J, Thomson L D G 2000 Crime and Punishment (Scotland) Act 1997: a survey of psychiatrists' views towards the Scottish Courts "Hybrid Order". Journal of Forensic Psychiatry 11:608–620

Darjee R, Crichton J, Thomson L D G. 2001 Crime and Punishment (Scotland) Act 1997: a survey of judges' and sheriffs' views towards the Scottish Courts "Hybrid Order". Medicine, Science and the Law 42:76–86

Davidson M, Humphreys M S, Johnstone E C, Owens D G C 1995 Prevalence of psychiatric morbidity among remand prisoners in Scotland. British Journal of Psychiatry 167:545–548

Day K 1994 Male mentally handicapped sex offenders. British Journal of Psychiatry 165:630–639

Denno D W 1996 Legal implications of genetics and crime research. Ciba Foundation Symposium 194:248–264

Department of Health 1999 Executive summary of the Report of the Committee of Inquiry into the Personality Disorder Unit, Ashworth Special Hospital (Fallon Inquiry) CM 4194–1. HMSO, London

Department of Health 2000 Report of the review of security at the high security hospitals (Tilt report) 21651 1P 600 May 00 (ESP)

Department of Health 2001a In-patients formally detained in hospital under the Mental Health Act 1983 and other legislation, England:1990–1991 to 2000–2001. Statistical Bulletin 2001/28. Department of Health, London

Department of Health 2001b Safety first. Five-year report of the National Confidential Inquiry into Suicide and Homicide by People with Mental Illness. Department of Health, London

Department of Health 2002 Draft Mental Health Bill CM 5538–1. HMSO, London

Department of Health, Home Office 1992 Review of health and social services for mentally disordered offenders and others requiring similar services. Final summary report. CM 2088. HMSO, London

Dietz P E 1978 Social factors in rapist behaviour. In: Rada R T (ed) Clinical aspects of the rapist. Grune & Stratton, New York

Dobson V, Sales B 2000 The science of infanticide and mental illness. Psychology, Public Policy, and Law 6(4):1098–1112

Dolan M, Smith C 2001 Juvenile homicide offenders: 10 years' experience of an adolescent forensic psychiatry service. Journal of Forensic Psychiatry 12(2):313–329 d'Orban P T 1976 Child stealing: a typology of female offenders. British Journal of Criminology 16:275–281

d'Orban P T 1979 Women who kill their children. British Journal of Psychiatry 134:560–571

d'Orban P T, Haydn-Smith P 1985 Men who steal children. British Medical Journal 290:1784

Dye S, Isaacs C 1991 Intravenous drug misuse among prison inmates: implications for spread of HIV. British Medical Journal 302:1506

Eley S, Malloch M., McIvor G et al 2002 The Glasgow drug court in action: the first six months. Scottish Executive Social Research. The Stationery Office, Edinburgh

Eronen M 1995 Mental disorders and homicidal behaviour in female subjects. American Journal of Psychiatry 152:1216–1218

Eronen M, Tiihonen J, Hakola P 1996a Schizophrenia and homicidal behaviour. Schizophrenia Bulletin 22:83–89

Eronen M, Hakola P, Tiihonen J 1996b Mental disorders and homicidal behaviour in Finland. Archives of General Psychiatry 53:497–501

Farrington D P 1993 The psychosocial milieu of the offender. In: Gunn J, Taylor P J (eds) Forensic psychiatry, clinical legal and ethical issues. Butterworth-Heinemann, Oxford, p 252–285

Fazel S, Danesh J 2002 Serious mental disorder in 23 000 prisoners: a systematic review of 62 surveys. Lancet 359:545–550

Francis B, Soothill K 2000 Does sex offending lead to homicide? Journal of Forensic Psychiatry 11(1):49–61

Gardner W, Lidz C W, Mulvey E P, Shaw E C 1996 Clinical versus actuarial predictions of violence of patients with mental illnesses. Journal of Consultant Clinical Psychology 64(3):602–609

Geller J L 1992 Arson in review: from profit to pathology. Psychiatric Clinics of North America 15:623–645

Gethins E, Larkin E, Davies S, Milton J 2002 Medico-legal reports and gatekeeping: one year of referrals to a forensic service. Medicine, Science and the Law 42(1):71–75

Gibbens T C N, Palmer C, Prince J 1971 Mental health aspects of shoplifting. British Medical Journal 3:612–615

Gibbons P, Mulyan N, O'Connor A 1997 Guilty but insane: the insanity defence in Ireland 1850–1995. British Journal of Psychiatry 170:467–472

Gorsuch N 1999 Disturbed female offenders: helping the "untreatable". Journal of Forensic Psychiatry 10(1):98–118

Gray N, O'Connor C, Williams T et al 2001 Fitness to plead: implications from case-law arising from the Criminal Justice and Public Order Act 1994. Journal of Forensic Psychiatry 12(1):52–62

Green C M 1981 Matricide by sons. Medicine, Science and the Law 21:207–214

Green G, Gray N, Willner P 2002 Factors associated with criminal convictions for sexually inappropriate behavior in men with learning disabilities. Journal of Forensic Psychiatry 13(3):578–607

Grubin D 1994a Sexual sadism. Criminal Behaviour and Mental Health 4:3–9

Grubin D 1994b Sexual murder. British Journal of Psychiatry 165:624–629

Grubin D H, Kennedy H G 1991 The classification of sexual offenders. Criminal Behaviour and Mental Health 1:123–129

Grubin D, Wingate S 1996 Sexual offence recidivism: prediction versus understanding. Criminal Behaviour and Mental Health 6:349–359

Gudjonsson G H 1990 Psychological and psychiatric aspects of shoplifting. Medicine, Science and the Law 30:45–51

Gudjonsson G H 2003 The psychology of interrogations and confessions: a handbook. Wiley, Chichester

Gudjonsson G H, MacKeith J 1996 Disputed confessions and the criminal justice system. Maudsley Discussion Paper No. 2 Institute of Psychiatry, London

Gudjonsson G H, Hayes G D, Rowlands P 2000 Fitness to be interviewed and psychological vulnerability: the views of doctors, lawyers and police officers. Journal of Forensic Psychiatry 11(1):74–92

Gunn J 1977 Epileptics in prison. Academic Press, London

Gunn J, Maden A, Swinton M 1991 Treatment needs of prisoners with psychiatric disorders. British Medical Journal 303:338–341

Guze S B 1976 Criminality and psychiatric disorders. Oxford University Press, New York

Haddock A, Snowden P, Dolan M 2001 Managing dangerous people with severe personality disorder: a survey of forensic psychiatrists' opinions. Psychiatric Bulletin 25:293–296

Hafner H, Boker W 1982 Crimes of violence by mentally abnormal offenders. Oxford University Press, London

Hansen H, Lykke-Olsen L 1997 Treatment of dangerous sexual offenders in Denmark. Journal of Forensic Psychiatry 8:195–199

Hanson R K 1997 The development of a brief actuarial risk scale for sexual offence recidivism (User Report 97–04). Department of the Solicitor General of Canada, Ottawa

Hanson R K, Harris A J R 2001 A structured approach to evaluating change among sexual offenders. Sexual Abuse: a journal of research and treatment 13(2):105–122

Hanson R K, Thornton D 1999 Static 99: Improving actuarial risk assessments for sex offenders (User Report 1999–02). Department of the Solicitor General of Canada, Ottawa

Hanson R K, Thornton D 2000 Improving risk assessments for sex offenders: a comparison of three actuarial scales. Law and Human Behaviour 24(1):119–136

Hare R D 1991 The Hare Psychopathy Checklist – Revised. Multi-Health Systems, Toronto

Hilton M R, Mezey G C 1996 Victims and perpetrators of child sexual abuse. British Journal of Psychiatry 169:408–415

Hodgins S 1992 Mental disorder, intellectual deficiency, and crime: evidence from a birth cohort. Archives of General Psychiatry 49:476–483

Hodgins S, Mednick S A, Brennan P A et al 1996 Mental disorder and crime: evidence from a Danish birth cohort. Archives of General Psychiatry 53:489–496

Home Office Circular No. 66/90 Provision for mentally disordered offenders. Home Office, London

Home Office 2001 Criminal statistics England and Wales 2000. Cmnd 5312. Home Office, London

Home Office 2002a Offender Assessment System (OASys). www.crimereduction.gov.uk

Home Office 2002b Persons sentenced, or other outcome under the Mental Health Act 1983 or the Criminal Procedure (Insanity) Act 1983, all courts England and Wales 2000. Personal Communication. Administration of Justice Statistics (RDS). Home Office, London

Home Office 2002c Homicide statistics. Personal Communication. Administration of Justice Statistics (RDS). Home Office, London.

Home Office 2002d Probation statistics England and Wales 2001. National Statistics. Research, Development and Statistics Directorate, London

Home Office, Department of Health and Social Security 1975 Report of the committee on mentally abnormal offenders. Cmnd 6244. HMSO, London

Home Office, Department of Health 1999 Managing dangerous people with severe personality disorder. Proposal for policy development. Department of Health, London

Humphreys M S, Johnstone E C, MacMillan J F, Taylor P J 1992 Dangerous behaviour preceding first admission for schizophrenia. British Journal of Psychiatry 161:501–505

Jacoby R 1997 Psychiatric aspects of crime in the elderly. In: Jacoby R, Oppenheimer C (eds) Psychiatry in the elderly. Oxford University Press, Oxford, p 749–760

James D 1999 Court diversion at 10 years: can it work, does it work and has it a future? Journal of Forensic Psychiatry 10(3):507–524

James D, Schramm M 1998 "Multiple personality disorder" presenting to the English court: a case study. Journal of Forensic Psychiatry 9:615–618

James D V, Duffield G, Blizard R, Hamilton L W 2001 Fitness to plead. A prospective study of the inter-relationships between expert opinion, legal criteria and specific symptomatology. Psychological Medicine 31(1):139–150

Johnson S, Taylor R 2002 Statistics of mentally disordered offenders 2001: England and Wales. Bulletin. Offending and Criminal Justice Group, Home Office Research Development and Statistics Directorate, London.

Kamphius J H, Emmelkamp P M G 2000 Stalking — a contemporary challenge for forensic and clinical psychiatry. British Journal of Psychiatry 176:206–209

Knight R A, Prentky R A 1989 Classifying sexual offenders: the development and corroboration of taxonomic models. In: Marsh W, Laws R, Barbaree H (eds) Handbook of sexual assaults. Plenum, New York

Kropp P R, Hart S D 2000 The spousal assault risk assessment (SARA) guide: reliability and validity in adult male offenders. Law and Human Behaviour 24(1):101–118

Kropp P R, Hart SD, Webster C D, Eaves, D 1995 Manual for the spousal assault risk assessment guide, 2nd edn. British Columbia Institute on Family Violence, Vancouver

Lamontagne Y, Carpentier N, Hetu C, Lacerte-Lamontagne C 1994 Shoplifting and mental illness. Canadian Journal of Psychiatry 39:300–302

Lasègue C 1877 Les exhibitionnistes. L'Union Médicale Troisième Série 23:709

Levey S, Howells K 1995 Dangerousness, unpredictability and the fear of people with schizophrenia. Journal of Forensic Psychiatry 6:19–39

Lewis D O, Pincus J H, Bard B et al 1988 Neuropsychiatric, pseudoeducational and family characteristics of 14 juveniles condemned to death in the United States. American Journal of Psychiatry 145:584–589

Lindqvist P 1991 Homicides committed by abusers of alcohol and illicit drugs. British Journal of Addiction 86:321–326

Lindqvist P, Allebeck P 1990 Schizophrenia and crime: a longitudinal follow up of 644 schizophrenics in Stockholm. British Journal of Psychiatry 157:345–350

Link B G, Stueve A 1994 Psychotic symptoms and the violent/illegal behaviour of mental patients compared to community controls. In: J Monahan, H J Steadman (eds) Violence and mental disorder. University of Chicago Press, Chicago, p 137–159

Link B G, Stueve A 1998 New evidence on the violence risk posed by people with mental illness. Archives of General Psychiatry 55:403–404

Link B G, Andrews H, Cullen F T 1992 The violent and illegal behaviour of mental patients reconsidered. American Sociological Review 57:275–292

McElroy S L, Pope H G, Hudson J I et al 1991 Kleptomania: a report of 20 cases. American Journal of Psychiatry 148:652–657

McGrath P 1992 Maternal filicide in Broadmoor Hospital 1919–69. Journal of Forensic Psychiatry 3:271–297

McGuire B E, Wraith A E 2000 Legal and psychological aspects of stalking: a review. Journal of Forensic Psychiatry 11(2):316–327

MacMillan J F, Johnson A L 1987 Contact with the police in early schizophrenia: its nature, frequency and relevance to outcome of treatment. Medicine, Science and the Law 27:191–200

McNiel D E, Binder R L, Greenfield T K 1988 Predictors of violence in civilly committed acute psychiatric patients. American Journal of Psychiatry 145:965–970

McNiel D, Sandberg D, Binder R 1998 The relationship between confidence and accuracy in clinical assessment of psychiatric patients' potential for violence. Law and Human Behaviour 22:655–669

Maden A, Swinton M, Gunn J 1990 Women in prisons and the use of illicit drugs before arrest. British Medical Journal 301:1133

Maden A, Swinton M, Gunn J 1991 Drug dependence in prisoners. British Medical Journal 302:880

Marshall P 1994 Reconviction of imprisoned sexual offenders. Home Office Research and Statistics Department. Research Bulletin 36:23–29

Martell D A, Dietz P E 1992 Mentally disordered offenders who push or attempt to push victims onto subway tracks in New York City. Archives of General Psychiatry 49:472–475

Menzies R P, Federoff J P, Green C M, Isaacson K 1995 Prediction of dangerous behaviour in male erotomania. British Journal of Psychiatry 166:529–536

Mezey G C, Robbins I 2000 The impact of criminal victimization. In: Gelder M G, López-Ibor J J, Andreasen N (eds) New Oxford Textbook of Psychiatry, vol 2. Oxford University Press, Oxford, p 2084–2088

Miller P McC, Johnstone E C, Lang F H, Thomson L D G 2000 Differences between patients with schizophrenia within and without a high security psychiatric hospital. Acta Psychiatrica Scandinavica 102(1):12–18

Milroy C M 1995 Reasons for homicide and suicide in episodes of dyadic death in Yorkshire and Humberside. Medicine, Science and the Law 35:213–217

Mitchell B 1997a Putting diminished responsibility into practice: a forensic psychiatric perspective. Journal of Forensic Psychiatry 8(3):620–634

Mitchell B 1997b Diminished responsibility manslaughter. Journal of Forensic Psychiatry 8:101–117

Moffitt T E 2002 Review of the evidence: antisocial behaviour. In: Genetics and human behaviour: the ethical context. Nuffield Council on Bioethics, London, p 89–96

Monahan J 1981 The clinical prediction of violent behaviour. Government Printing Office, Washington, DC

Monahan J 1984 The prediction of violent behaviour: toward a second generation of theory and policy. American Journal of Psychiatry 141:10–15

Monahan J 1993 Mental disorder and violence: another look. In: Hodgins S (ed) Mental disorder and crime. Sage, London

Monahan J, Steadman H J 1983 Crime and mental disorder: an epidemiological approach. In: Tonry M, Morris N (eds) Crime and justice: an annual review of research. University of Chicago Press, Chicago

Monahan J, Steadman H J 1994 Violence and mental disorder. Developments in risk assessment. University of Chicago Press, Chicago

Monahan J, Steadman H J, Silver E et al 2001 Rethinking risk assessment. The MacArthur study of mental disorder and violence. Oxford University Press, New York

Mullen P E 1993 The crime of passion and the changing cultural construction of jealousy. Criminal Behaviour and Mental Health 3:1–11

Murray D J 1989 Review of research on re-offending of mentally disordered offenders. Research and Planning Unit Paper 55. Home Office, London

Needham-Bennett H, Parrott J, Macdonald A J D 1996 Psychiatric disorder and policing the elderly offender. Criminal Behaviour and Mental Health 6:241–252

Nemitz T, Bean P 2001 Protecting the rights of the mentally disordered in police stations: the use of appropriate adults in England and Wales. International Journal of Law and Psychiatry 24:595–605

Nestor P G, Haycock J 1997 Not guilty by reason of insanity: clinical and neuropsychological characteristics. Journal of American Academy of Psychiatry and the Law 25(2):161–171

Norton K, Dolan B 1995 Assessing change in personality disorder. Current Opinion in Psychiatry 8:371–375

O'Sullivan G H, Kelleher M J 1987 A study of fire-setters in the south west of Ireland. British Journal of Psychiatry 151:818–823

Peay J 1996 Inquiries after homicide. Duckworth, London

Petch E, Bradley C 1997 Learning the lessons from homicide inquiries: adding insult to injury? Journal of Forensic Psychiatry 8(1):161–184

Player E, Jenkins M 1994 Prisons after Woolf: reform through riot. Routledge, London

Prins H 1994a Fire-raising: its motivation and management. Routledge, London

Prins H 1994b Is diversion just a diversion? Medicine, Science and the Law 34:137–147

Puri B K, Baxter R, Cordess C C 1995 Characteristics of fire-setters. British Journal of Psychiatry 166:393–396

Quinsey V L, Harris G T, Rice M E, Cormier C A 1998 Violent offenders, appraising and managing risk. American Psychological Association, Washington, DC

Rada R 1975 Alcoholism and forcible rape. American Journal of Psychiatry 132:444–446

Raine A, Brennan P, Mednick B, Mednick S A 1996 High rates of violence, crime, academic problems, and behavioural problems in males with both early neuromotor deficits and unstable family environments. Archives of General Psychiatry 53:544–549

Reed J 2003 Mental health care in prisons. British Journal of Psychiatry 182:287–288

Repo E, Virkkunen M 1997 Outcome in a sample of Finnish fire-setters. Journal of Forensic Psychiatry 8:127–137

Resnick P J 1969 Child murder by parents. American Journal of Psychiatry 126:325–334

Robertson G 1988 Arrest patterns among mentally disordered offenders. British Journal of Psychiatry 153:313–316

Rogers P, Watt A, Gray N S et al 2002 Content of command hallucinations predicts self-harm but not violence in a medium secure unit. Journal of Forensic Psychiatry 13(2):251–262

Rowlands M W D 1988 Psychiatric and legal aspects of persistent litigation. British Journal of Psychiatry 153:317–323

Royal College of Psychiatrists 1996 Assessment and clinical management of risk of harm to other people CR 53. Royal College of Psychiatrists, London

Royal College of Psychiatrists 2002 Suicide in prisons CR 99. Royal College of Psychiatrists, London

Rutter M, Giller H 1983 Juvenile delinquency: trends and perspectives. Penguin, Harmondsworth

Scott P 1973 Parents who kill their children. Medicine, Science and the Law 13:120–126

Scottish Executive 2000 Report of the Committee on Serious Violent and Sexual Offenders (Ch: Lord MacLean). Scottish Executive, Edinburgh

Scottish Office 1999 Health, social work and related services for mentally disordered offenders in Scotland NHS MEL(1999)5. Scottish Office, Edinburgh

Segal J H 1989 Erotomania revisited: from Kraepelin to DSM-III-R. American Journal of Psychiatry 146:1261–1266

Shepherd M 1961 Morbid jealousy: some clinical and social aspects of a psychiatric symptom. Journal of Mental Science 107:687–753

Singleton N, Meltzer H, Gatward R 1998 Psychiatric morbidity among prisoners in England and Wales. Office for National Statistics, Government Statistical Service, London

Skeem J L, Golding S L 2001 Describing jurors' personal conception of insanity and their relationship to case judgements. Psychology, Public Policy and Law 7(3):561–621

Smith A D, Taylor P J 1999 Serious sex offending against women by men with schizophrenia. Relationship of illness and psychotic symptoms to offending. British Journal of Psychiatry 174:233–237

Social Work Services Inspectorate 2000 Management and Assessment of Risk in Social Work Services

Soothill K L, Pope P J 1973 Arson: a twenty year cohort study Medicine, Science and the Law 13:127–138

Soyka M 2000 Substance misuse, psychiatric disorder and violent and disturbed behaviour. British Journal of Psychiatry 176:345–350

Soyka M, Naber G, Volcker A 1991 Prevalence of delusional jealousy in different psychiatric disorders. An analysis of 93 cases. British Journal of Psychiatry 158:549–553

Steadman H J, Mulvey E P, Monahan J et al 1998 Violence by people discharged from acute psychiatric inpatient facilities and by others in the same neighborhoods. Archives of General Psychiatry 55:393–401

Steels M, Rony G, Larkin E et al 1998 Discharged from special hospital under restrictions: a comparison of the fates of psychopaths and the mentally ill. Criminal Behaviour and Mental Health 8(1):39–55

Stewart L A 1993 Profile of female firesetters. Implications for treatment. British Journal of Psychiatry 163:248–256

Stroud J 1997 Mental disorder and the homicide of children; a review. Social Work and Social Science Review 6:149–162

Stuart H L, Arboleda-Florez J E 2001 A public health perspective on violent offenses among persons with mental illness. Psychiatric Services 52(5):654–659

Stueve A, Link B G 1997 Violence and psychiatric disorders: results from an epidemiological study of young adults in Israel. Psychiatric Quarterly 68:327–342

Sugarman P, Dumughn C, Saad K et al 1994 Dangerousness in exhibitionists. Journal of Forensic Psychiatry 5:287–296

Swanson J W, Holzer C E, Ganju V K, Jono R T 1990 Violence and psychiatric disorder in the community: evidence from the epidemiological catchment area surveys. Hospital and Community Psychiatry 41:761–770

SWSIS 2000 Managing the risk: an inspection of the management of sex offender cases in the community. Social Work Services Inspectorate for Scotland, Edinburgh

Taylor P J 1993 Psychosis, violence and crime. In: Gunn J, Taylor P J (eds) Forensic psychiatry, clinical legal and ethical issues. Butterworth-Heinemann, Oxford, p 329–372

Taylor P J, Gunn J 1984 Violence and psychosis I — risk of violence among psychotic men. British Medical Journal 288:1945–1949

Taylor P J, Gunn J 1999 Homicides by people with mental illness: myth and reality. British Journal of Psychiatry 174:9–14

Taylor P J, Parrott J 1988 Elderly offenders: a study of age-related factors among custodially remanded prisoners. British Journal of Psychiatry 152:340–346

Taylor P, Mahendra B, Gunn J 1983 Erotomania in males. Psychological Medicine 13:645–650

Taylor R 1999 Predicting reconvictions for sexual and violent offences using the Revised Offender Group Reconviction Scale. Home Office, London

Thomson L D G 1999 Crime and Punishment (Scotland) Act 1997: relevant provisions for people with mental disorders. Psychiatric Bulletin 23:68–71

Tiihonen J, Isohanni M, Rasanen P et al 1997 Specific major mental disorders and criminality: twenty-six year prospective study of the 1966 northern Finnish birth cohort. American Journal of Psychiatry 154:840–845

Tuninger E E, Levander S, Bernce R, Johansson G 2001 Criminalit and aggression among psychotic in-patients: frequency and clinical correlates. Acta Psychiatrica Scandinavica 103(4):294–300

Tyrer P, Coid J, Simmonds S 2002 Community mental health teams (CMHTs) for people with severe mental illnesses and disordered personality. Cochrane Database of Systematic Reviews, Issue 3.

Walker N, McCabe S 1973 Crime and Insanity in England. Vol 2: New solutions and new problems. University of Edinburgh Press, Edinburgh.

Walsh E 2001 Reducing violence in severe mental illness: randomised controlled trial of intensive case management compared with standard care. British Medical Journal 323:1093–1098

Ward, D 1987 The validity of the reconviction prediction score. Home Office Research Study No 94. HMSO, London

Webster CD, Douglas K S, Eaves D, Hart S D 1997 HCR-20, Assessing risk for violence: version 2. Mental Health, Law and Policy Institute, Simon Fraser University, Vancouver

Wessely S 1997 The epidemiology of crime, violence and schizophrenia. British Journal of Psychiatry 170(suppl 32):8–11

West D J 1988 Psychological contributions to criminology. British Journal of Criminology 28:77–92

West D J 1993 Disordered and offensive behaviour. In: Gunn J, Taylor P J (eds) Forensic psychiatry, clinical, legal and ethical issues. Butterworth-Heinemann, Oxford, p 543

White T, Douds F, Henderson T, Anderson J 2001 Survey of the use of the interim hospital order in Scotland. Medicine, Science and the Law 41(1):63–71

White T, Ramsay L, Morrison R 2002 Audit of the forensic psychiatry liaison service to Glasgow Sheriff Court 1994 to 1998. Medicine, Science and the Law 42(1):64–70

Wong S, Gordon A (in press) Violence Risk Scale. Multi-Health Systems, Toronto

Yorston G 1999 Aged and dangerous. British Journal of Psychiatry 174:193–195

Law reports

Bratty v Attorney General for Northern Ireland (1963) Appeal Cases 386

HMA v Blake (1986) Scots Law Times 661

R v Burgess (1991) 2 WLR 120

R v Byrne (1960) 44 Criminal Appeal Rep 246

R v McNaghten (1843) 4 State Trials and Proceedings 847

R v Pritchard (1836) 7 C & P 303

30 | Legal and ethical aspects of psychiatry

Stephen G Potts, John H M Crichton

Psychiatric practice is as much a moral as a medical endeavour.
(Mechanic 1989)

INTRODUCTION

After at most 20 hours devoted to ethics in a decade or more of training, would-be psychiatrists might take issue with Mechanic. This is because ethical issues, while ever-present, remain implicit in most psychiatric encounters, only becoming explicit when brought to the surface by conflict.

Contrast two cases. Ms Smith is referred by her general practitioner to a local psychiatrist who runs a private practice in behavioural psychotherapy. She has an uncomplicated spider phobia which causes her distress and interferes with her everyday life. She understands the principles of graded exposure, complies with the programme she is set, and after the six sessions she initially contracted for, is happy to report a substantial improvement. Mr Jones, on the other hand, is arrested after behaving bizarrely in busy traffic, endangering himself and others. Social services have already been alerted by neighbours about the apparent neglect of his two young children. Examination shows him to be floridly psychotic, and he is transferred under the Mental Health Act to a local psychiatric hospital against his will. There he becomes increasingly agitated and requires forcible medication, to which he develops an acute dystonic reaction. It becomes clear that he has schizophrenia, which responds to drug treatment, but is aggravated by continuing use of cannabis. His psychiatrist regrets that resources are insufficient to allow him to be offered, in addition to drugs, the psychological treatment which is known to improve compliance with medication and reduce the risk of relapse.

Both types of case are common in psychiatric practice. While the ethical issues in the second case are multiple and manifest, at first glance there appear to be none raised by the first. This is because the ethical principles which govern all medical transactions, including both of these, are implicit, or embedded, but no less present, in the dealings between Ms Smith and her doctor. It is only when clinicians and commentators struggle to resolve conflicts, such as those raised in Mr Jones's case, that the principles involved are exposed, delineated and made explicit. Where there is no conflict between principles, they remain so hidden that it is easy to suppose them absent.

While these ethical principles underlie the whole of medicine, they lie closer to the surface in psychiatry than in many other disciplines. This means that some ethical issues, such as resource

allocation, are no different in psychiatry than in other medical specialities, while others, though shared with medicine generally, are highlighted in psychiatry because of its nature — an example being the potential for sexual abuse of the doctor–patient relationship. Finally, there is an important set of issues, such as involuntary commitment to hospital, which arise exclusively in psychiatry, although the principles which apply remain those in operation elsewhere. While all psychiatry takes place in a legal framework, the law, very properly, has more to say about this third group of issues, via mental health legislation and the common law.

In what follows we hope to set out the nature of these principles, their origins, in terms of history and philosophy, and their application within psychiatry. We will also discuss, in outline, the relevant legal issues, although the specifics will vary between jurisdictions.

HISTORICAL AND PHILOSOPHICAL BACKGROUND

Recent years have seen a dramatic expansion in the number and range of ethical controversies in medicine and psychiatry, with loudly voiced argument assailing the bewildered practitioner from all sides. Yet until the 1970s medical ethics meant little more in Britain than, first, the medical etiquette governing transactions between practitioners — for example, 'Any undisclosed division of professional fees is *unethical*' (BMA 1981, italics added) — and, second, exhortations to avoid alcohol (at least when on duty), adultery (at least with one's patients) and, above all, advertising. The lay public, and many practitioners, took the view that any more specifically *ethical* questions could be resolved by reference to the Hippocratic Oath. This short and ancient text contains absolute but unargued prohibitions against euthanasia, abortion, sexual relationships with patients and breach of confidentiality. The model of medicine it advances is that of an art whose secrets are passed from one generation of adepts to the next, via a kind of masonic apprenticeship, and in which the overriding principle is one of benevolent devotion to the sick. The oath cannot possibly guide psychiatrists struggling with today's issues, partly because they were unanticipatable by Hippocrates and his peers, but mainly because the oath is a blunt list of dos and don'ts without an argued basis which could be extended to modern practice. The hippocratic tradition lives on in the modern equivalent of the oath, the Declaration of Geneva (World Medical Association 1948), which jettisons the archaic language, but which is still so generally phrased as to be of little value in guiding particular

Table 30.1 Features and problems of contrasting moral theories	Deontology (absolutism)	Teleology (consequentialism, utilitarianism)
Main features	Rule based (Rights and duties determine action) Consequences irrelevant	Outcome based (Greatest good of greatest number determines action) Consequences all-important
Major problems	No procedure to resolve conflicts of rights What kinds of things have rights, and why?	No common scale of measurement Individual interests easily overridden for greater good

decisions. British medical schools have recognised this, if belatedly, in that none now requires its medical graduates to declare the oath, and the Declaration of Geneva has not generally been adopted as a replacement.

The best-known specifically psychiatric codes are the Declaration of Hawaii (World Psychiatric Association 1977), a two-page list of 10 guidelines, and the rather more detailed *Principles of Medical Ethics with Annotations Especially Applicable to Psychiatry* (APA 1973). Even this last document is not specific enough to answer many questions, and its principles are again set forth as an unargued list, like the 10 commandments but without their vigour of expression. ('A physician shall recognise a responsibility to participate in activities contributing to an improved community.') The problem, of course, with such unargued lists, is that they give no guidance on how to act when principles are in conflict: and it is in just such cases that guidance is most needed. Oaths and declarations are clearly not sufficient, but the psychiatrist who goes beyond them to the philosophy from which they emerge soon risks confusion. Moral philosophy is a huge and venerable discipline, as old as medicine itself. It is also an important living academic subject, represented on the campus of any self-respecting university, with all that implies for continuing disagreement. It is possible, however, to identify, at the risk of brutal oversimplification, two broadly competing camps within the subject as a whole: the deontological and the teleological traditions, whose main features and major problems are summarised in Table 30.1.

Deontology versus teleology

Deontology

Of the two, deontology is by far the older, taking its roots in a combination of Judeo-Christian theology and Ancient Greek philosophy, which were first fully synthesised 700 years ago in St Thomas Aquinas's *Summa Theologica* (Shapcote 1912–1936). Aquinas claimed that secular reason could arrive at the same moral laws as were handed down in religious precepts, and, particularly since Immanuel Kant in the late 18th century, the philosophy has been divorced from the theology to stand or fall independently. The term deontology derives from the Greek *deon* for duty, indicating the centrality of rules. Initially these were expressed primarily as *obligations*, akin to commandments, but, since the great revolutions of the 18th century, the more legalistic language of *rights* has taken precedence. By virtue of their status as human beings, people have rights, such as the rights to life, liberty and the pursuit of happiness enshrined in the American Declaration of Independence. It is generally (but not universally) acknowledged that rights and duties are correlate, so that granting someone a right confers a duty elsewhere, whether it falls on specific individuals, people in general, or institutions, including hospitals and the state. If I have a right to confidentiality, my doctor has a duty to observe it; if I have a right to life, everyone has a duty not to kill me; and if I have a right to medical treatment, the government has a duty to ensure its provision. There is no such thing as half a right or a partial duty: rights and duties act like trump cards (Dworkin 1977) and hold absolutely (hence *absolutism* as an alternative term for this philosophy). This is so whatever the consequences: 'though the heavens fall' in Anscombe's phrase (1981).

There are many difficulties in this outlook. Where do rights come from? What sort of entities possess them, and why? By virtue of what are they granted? When are they acquired: at conception, viability, birth, or later? Can they be lost, temporarily, as perhaps in delirium, or permanently, in dementia? On what grounds are they granted to the severely mentally handicapped but withheld from higher primates? More pressingly, what happens in situations where they appear to conflict, as in therapeutic abortion to save a woman's life? And how can it be right to ignore consequences so blithely?

Teleology

Teleology derives its name from the Greek *teleon*, purpose, and was elaborated by the 19th century English philosophers Jeremy Bentham and John Stuart Mill, each of whom owed much to their Scottish forebear, David Hume. Teleological morality is also called consequentialism or utilitarianism. The central concept is that, rather than rights, people have *interests*, whether these be concerns, desires or needs. Fulfilment or frustration of these interests is the ultimate source of value, good or bad. Teleology relies heavily on the assumption that it is possible to measure the various possible outcomes of moral choices in terms of pleasure or pain, happiness lost or gained, for all those affected; and that, via some unspecified kind of moral calculus, a decision can be arrived at by applying the much-abused slogan 'the greatest good of the greatest number' as the determining principle.

Although teleological views have become very powerful in recent moral philosophy, and by extension, in medical ethics, there are again major problems. The system depends vitally on the claim that it is possible to measure, on the same scale of value, such widely varying outcomes as an examination passed, a cup final won, or a healthy baby born to a healthy mother. No such measuring system has been developed, and it strains credulity to accept without demur that it ever could be. Furthermore, such a system carries with it the inescapable risk that the interests of individuals or minorities could too readily be sacrificed to the common good, if the stakes were high enough. As the philosopher Bernard Williams (Smart & Williams 1973) has put it, in such a system the individual matters no more than do individual petrol tanks in the statistics on national petrol consumption.

Derivative principles

The psychiatrist who seeks guidance by taking a course in moral philosophy will thus probably emerge asking more questions than he started with; but it is neither necessary nor possible to resolve age-old questions of moral theory in order to arrive at a measure of consensus on general, but not fundamental, ethical principles at a lower level. John Stuart Mill, for example, famously argued that the greatest good of the greatest number can best be served by giving people as much liberty (or autonomy, as we would now put it) as possible to decide for themselves how to order their lives, limited only by the effects of their choices on others (Mill 1859).

It is possible, therefore, to arrive at a general principle of respect for autonomy both within a rights-based, deontological, moral outlook (people have a right to privacy and self-determination, and others have correlative duties), and from a teleological perspective, via Mill's argument (people's interests are most likely to be fulfilled if their freedom to choose is maximised).

The philosopher R M Hare (1981) has argued that the basic dispute between deontology and teleology can be resolved by making the latter primary, and deriving from it, by arguments like Mill's, a basic set of rules. These then acquire a secondary, derivative, deontological force, which can be used to guide practical decision-making. Where conflicts between these rules arise, they are resolved by resort to primary teleological reasoning.

While they do not explicitly adopt this approach, Beauchamp & Childress, in their widely influential work (1994), argue for a brief set of four prima facie principles: respect for autonomy, beneficence, non-maleficence and justice. While important, they are not necessarily fundamental, and can be supported by a variety of different moral theories, which are likely to take different approaches to the resolution of any conflict between them. Nor is the list immutable: Gillon (1994), for example, has added the further requirement of concern for the principles' scope of application. Figure 30.1 shows how these principles might act as intermediary levels of ethical reasoning between individual doctor–patient encounters and abstract moral theory. The principles and their

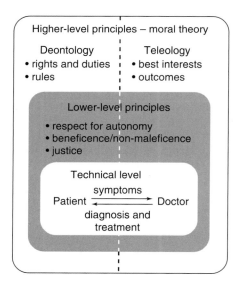

Fig. 30.1
Relationship between moral theory, lower-level principles and the clinical encounter.

applications will be examined further below. First, however, it is necessary to explore further the reasons for the dramatically increased interest in ethical issues in the last four decades.

A historical perspective

Abuses of psychiatry and the limits of paternalism

The increased interest in ethical issues cannot be explained by moral theory or derived principles; rather it reflects powerful social forces that impinge upon doctors, patients and the settings in which they meet. These forces need clarification.

Authors commonly cite new developments in medical technology as the primary driving force in generating interest in ethics. Although psychiatry lags behind other specialities in this respect, developments such as psychosurgery, electroconvulsive therapy (ECT), an ever-widening range of psychotropic drugs, brain-imaging techniques, and the identification of genetic tests for such conditions as Huntington's chorea have made it possible for psychiatrists to *do* a great deal more than hitherto, raising the inevitable question of whether they *should*. While undoubtedly relevant, technological development is not the only, or even the foremost, factor behind ethics' expansion. Much more important has been the attack, from several directions, on the benevolent paternalism implicit in the hippocratic model.

Paternalism was the key ethical principle underpinning the establishment of the county asylums in mid-19th-century Britain and their forerunner, the 'mad-houses'. People with mental illness from the mid-18th-century were cared for in a variety of 'mad-houses', which became subject to scrutiny in various parliamentary enquiries in the early 19th century. There was little legislation to govern the workings of 'mad-houses', and there were many publicised examples of abusive practices, especially involving the use of mechanical restraint. As an alternative to mechanical restraint, moral treatment was adopted in some of the more affluent 'mad-houses' (Porter 1987). Both methods of control were criticised at the time for being cruel. The county asylums, which were established together with strict legislative rules and guidelines to prevent malpractice, used the practices of the institution as a means of control. The newly established Lunacy Commission, among others, popularised the use of seclusion as an alternative to mechanical restraint. In turn, both use of seclusion and institutionalisation became subject to ethical concern (Barham 1992).

The activities of some German psychiatrists during the Second World War show, all too shockingly, how easily a benevolent paternalistic model may turn malevolent. Lifton (1986) and Barham (1992) describe how psychiatrists were at the forefront of the Nazi euthanasia campaign, from its beginnings well before the Second World War. Those patients they deemed *Lebensunwertes leben* — lives unworthy of life — were taken aside and murdered in their thousands. Even worse, this selective culling of schizophrenics, epileptics and the mentally handicapped served as the testing ground for methods, such as poison gas, which were later applied on a much wider scale in the wholesale slaughter of the Holocaust (Muller-Hill 1991). The motivation for this grotesque abuse of psychiatry appears to have been predominantly eugenic: the wish to preserve the purity of the race. No clearer illustration of the ease with which consequentialist reasoning can sacrifice the interests of individuals or minorities to a supposed higher good can be provided.

Although the abuses of the Nazi era are by far the worst, unchecked paternalism has an inbuilt tendency to overreach itself and turn malevolent. In the decades since, it has given rise to other abuses, all very different in their time, place and underlying motivation. From the 1950s to the 1980s, for example, the Soviet Union systematically abused psychiatry for political ends (Bloch & Reddaway 1977). A diagnosis not recognised elsewhere, sluggish schizophrenia, was defined so as to medicalise politically unacceptable dissident or reformist behaviour. Dissidents so labelled were detained in psychiatric hospitals and medicated against their will.

Although there were brave exceptions, many Soviet psychiatrists colluded with this practice. Some, no doubt, were well intentioned, and acted out of a belief in the validity of 'sluggish schizophrenia'. Others, more aware of the true nature of the diagnosis, turned a blind eye to its use, out of a mixture of political conformism, personal ambition, and fear of being labelled dissident themselves. It was only after a long campaign of criticism by Western psychiatrists, and the coming of *glasnost* and *perestroika*, that the practice ended.

Although the Nazi and Soviet abuses show that psychiatry is readily distorted in a totalitarian state, we should not complacently assume that it cannot also happen in a liberal democracy. Continuing concern about psychiatry in Japan (Harding 1991), the outrage that greeted the dumping of psychiatric patients in barbaric conditions on the Greek island of Leros (Ramsay 1990) and sporadic enquiries into conditions inside some British hospitals all attest to the need for continued vigilance. Nor should we forget the results of excessive therapeutic zeal. Between the end of the war and the development of effective psychotropic drugs in the 1950s, unmodified ECT, psychosurgery and insulin coma were the only effective physical treatments for serious mental illness. In the USA and Europe, well-intentioned but overenthusiastic use of these treatments became institutionalised, with the consequence that thousands of patients underwent inappropriate, unnecessary and dangerous physical procedures. The backlash against these excesses is still felt today in the profoundly negative public attitude to ECT, and the legislative barriers against its use in some American states. The initial overuse of a new intervention, followed by a rejecting overreaction, and then by due recognition of its proper place in treatment, is a pattern well recognised throughout medicine, but it seems to have been greatly exaggerated in the case of ECT and psychosurgery. No doubt this partly arose from the intense frustration engendered in psychiatrists responsible for large asylums with many disturbed patients and no effective treatment, but it was made more possible by the paternalistic attitude that the psychiatrists knew best, in which the patient's views were irrelevant.

The dawning recognition of the defects of paternalism grew from the civil liberties campaigns and the counterculture movement of the 1960s and subsequently. These movements, their aims embodied in the slogan 'Question authority', challenged the assumption that authority figures, including doctors and psychiatrists, could be trusted to act benevolently, replacing it with the contrary view that patients, like citizens in general, needed protection from the inherently (if unconsciously) malevolent tendencies of unrestrained authority, echoing Shaw's dictum that all professions are conspiracies against the laity. In other words they rejected the very notion of paternalism as a valid basis for civil society, and therefore for medicine and psychiatry.

Paternalism is thus now largely (but not completely) replaced by a contractarian model of the relationship between doctor and patient in which the participants are contracting equals, much as car owners and garage mechanics might be. There is an asymmetry of knowledge between mechanic and carowner, just as there is between doctor and patient, but there is no asymmetry of power. The mechanic is contractually obliged to undertake an accurate assessment of the presenting problem, to explain it to the owner to the owner's satisfaction, to propose the appropriate repair work, and then to abide by the owner's decision. In return the owner is obliged to provide payment, but he is free to accept or reject the mechanic's advice. The expertise might lie on one side of the transaction, but the choice, and more importantly the money, lies on the other, thus balancing the power relationship. Of course a great deal of medicine, and especially psychiatry, cannot be fitted to this model, and it distorts practice to assume that it can be. Nonetheless the model is now predominant, although paternalism retains a place where the patient's ability to choose for himself is impaired, as is often the case in psychiatry; it is paternalism that justifies the detention and treatment against his will of Mr Jones and others like him.

Antipsychiatry

A disconnected group of psychiatrists and others, influential beyond its size, and collectively known as the antipsychiatrists, went beyond the rejection of paternalism to deny altogether the validity of psychiatric diagnoses and therefore of treatment. Thomas Szasz is the first, foremost and longest-enduring. His central argument, stated in the title of his early work, *The Myth of Mental Illness* (1961), and reframed repeatedly since, is that mental illness, as a concept, has no validity. It is simply wrong, in his view, to medicalise mental distress and abnormal behaviour with a diagnostic label, and then to treat it: those who profess to do so are little more than frauds, acting as unwitting agents of social control. R D Laing's rather different argument — that schizophrenia is not so much a diagnosis as a sane response to an insane society, which psychiatrists protect via the labelling and segregation of dissenting victims — is expressed no less vigorously (Laing 1965). While these views still have their advocates, they are now less influential than when first promulgated, and have little influence on the day-to-day running of most psychiatric services.

Antipsychiatry views were also heavily influenced by a study of institutional psychiatric practice by the American sociologist Goffman (1961), who described the characteristics of a 'total institution' and the moral transformation of patients during their stay. Goffman's insights into the workings of institutions are often assumed to have a moral value of their own: not simply that moral change occurs in patients but that that change is morally wrong in itself. Another influence on the antipsychiatry movement was the writings of the French historican/philosopher Michel Foucault. He presented his views in a style which was novel and controversial. Much of what he wrote can be understood in metaphorical terms, and his theories have attracted wide and diverse interpretation. In Foucault's PhD thesis, the basis of his first book, there is an examination of mental disorder. The English reader is two steps away from the original work, *Histoire de la Folie*, since the thesis was shortened for publication and was then translated to *Madness and Civilisation* (Foucault 1967). Foucault clearly identifies psychiatric treatment as being a moral enterprise and reflects on the contemporary psychiatric approach, such as the use of medication, as being less transparent as a means of moral control compared with historical treatments. The ideologies of Foucault and Goffman, together with the antipsychiatrists, have been described as the 'ideologies of destruction', but their influence has been thought to have had a greater effect on the demise of the psychiatric asylum than on contemporary psychiatric practice (Jones 1993).

Fulford (1989) has mounted a spirited defence against the antipsychiatrists' charge that psychiatric diagnosis is inherently value-laden and therefore oppressive, intolerant of deviance and scientifically invalid. His argument has a much stronger philosophical (as opposed to polemical) grounding, and therefore a greater strength, than those of Szasz or Laing, whose positions he essentially turns on their heads. Szasz and Laing argue from analogy, claiming that since medical diagnoses are rooted in purely factual descriptions of organic pathology and its consequences, and since such descriptions are generally lacking in psychiatry, then psychiatric diagnoses cannot lay claim to the validity accorded their medical counterparts. Fulford shows, in our view convincingly, that medical diagnoses are no less value-laden than the psychiatric equivalents, and that it is simply false to claim that they rely universally on accounts of organic dysfunction; he thus rescues psychiatric diagnosis from the charge of scientific invalidity.

Nonetheless it is vitally important that psychiatry remains aware of the very real abuses committed in its name in the past, when psychiatrists clearly *did* act as agents of social control, in order to guard against this ever-present risk in the present and the future. It could be argued that one function of mental health legislation, beyond protecting the rights of patients, is to protect psychiatry against well-intentioned, but damaging, excursions beyond its legitimate boundaries. In this respect psychiatry clearly differs from other medical specialties.

THE FOUR-PRINCIPLES APPROACH

Respect for autonomy

Respect for a patient's autonomy always heads the various shortlists of prima facie ethical principles, reflecting the primacy of the contractarian model. According to this principle, patients should be treated as rational autonomous agents, making their own decisions about their lives. From it flow further lower-level requirements, including confidentiality and informed consent (see below). Respecting a patient's autonomy assumes that the patient's capacity to make rational choices is not impaired, temporarily or permanently, by mental or physical disorder (or, in the case of children, by immaturity). Many ethical problems in medicine generally, and especially in psychiatry, turn on this issue of capacity. Two sets of questions arise: those with a relatively narrow technical focus (What kinds of condition can limit a patient's capacity? How is capacity assessed? Is it a global matter, or can it be broken down to specific capacities for specific issues?); and those with a broader, more ethical dimension (Where capacity is limited, what principles then take over to guide action? The contractarian advance directive, the paternalism implied in a bestinterests standard, or the intermediate position afforded by a proxy judgement?).

Non-maleficence and beneficence

The Latin epithet *primum non-nocere*, meaning first (or above all) do no harm, has an obscure but ancient origin. It lives on in the clumsily labelled principle of non-maleficence, the requirement that doctors strive to avoid harming those in their care and their kin. Philosophers argue about the extent to which this principle can be separated from its correlate, the principle of beneficence (the requirement to do good or promote well-being), but it is clear that the primacy implied by the phrase 'above all' does not apply. If it did, no surgeon could ever operate because of the pain he might cause, and no psychiatrist could ever prescribe for fear of side-effects. In almost all therapeutic decisions, a judgement about the *balance* of burdens and benefits is made, non-maleficence and beneficence being as inseparable as the opposing sides of a coin. However, differing philosophical models of the interaction between doctor and patient lead to different views about how this balancing is to be done, and who does it.

In the contractarian/deontological model, there is an agreement, explicit or implicit, between doctor and patient. Acting benevolently and avoiding harm is what the doctor offers and the patient wants. They make a contract, which derives its binding power from the general duty to tell the truth and to keep promises, both of which originate in the the principle of respect for autonomy. Furthermore, the judgement about what constitutes benefit and harm, and how they are to be balanced, is the patient's. The doctor's role is to provide the patient with sufficient information to enable the patient to make a considered judgement according to his own view of the possible outcomes, and then to abide by the patient's choice. In the teleological model, acting benevolently and avoiding harm is fundamental, for it is the very root of *all* morality, medical decisions forming a particular subset. In principle at least, benefits and burdens can be assigned values on some common scale, and moral mathematics then determines the right action. However, given the lack of consensus on any such scale, heavy emphasis is placed on the patient's own valuations as those offering most accuracy. Again, therefore, the doctor is required to provide sufficient information to enable the patient to choose between the options before him according to his own ranking of burdens and benefits. Maximum benefit and minimum harm is most assured when patient autonomy, or, in Mill's term, liberty, is greatest.

The two models therefore yield similar lower-level views of the doctor–patient interaction, but in the contractarian model autonomy is paramount and beneficence/non-maleficence derivative, while in the teleological model the reverse is the case.

Justice

The justice referred to in this principle is not retributive, concerned with the punishment of wrongdoing, but distributive, concerned with the sharing out of losses and gains between individuals.

In the hippocratic tradition, represented in the Smith case above, the relationship between doctor and patient is dyadic and exclusive, and questions of justice do not arise. But medical encounters do not take place in a vacuum. The patient will often have a family, and he will always be a citizen; no man is an island. The doctor, a citizen too, will have other patients, and usually limited access to expensive tests and treatments. Doctor and patient are thus both located in a moral web of rights and responsibilities owed to other parties, and the strands of duty which link them to each other can be distorted and sometimes broken by the weight of moral burdens falling elsewhere in the web.

Sometimes these tensions are specfic and therefore stark, as when a nephrologist has two patients needing dialysis, but only the resources to treat one. Whom should he choose: the patient who is more likely to benefit, who is the more 'deserving', who has more dependants, who has more to offer society, who is younger, or whose condition is not self-inflicted? Psychiatry does not readily offer such dramatic dilemmas, and in truth they are rare in medicine generally. Usually the choices are less clear-cut, and lie not between specific individuals with competing claims on the same scarce resource, but between unidentified future patients with potential claims on different resources. For example, a psychiatric hospital may choose to delay resettling long-stay patients in community housing in order to liberate funds for an urgently needed alcohol detoxification project; or a health authority may limit the number of patients started on clozapine in order to pay for new anti-HIV drugs.

Questions of justice are not confined to matters of resource allocation. They also arise whenever a clinical decision confers potential burdens and benefits on people other than the patient, even when access to treatment is not limited. In Jones's case above, part of the justification for detaining him in hospital comes from the risks he poses to other (unidentified) members of the public who might be endangered by his bizarre behaviour in traffic; and part of the justification for medicating him against his will is the risk his disturbed behaviour poses to other (identified) patients and staff. The principle of justice requires attention to the means by which the benefits and burdens for the patient of detention and enforced medication are balanced against the benefits and burdens accruing to other people, whether they be his children, fellow patients or the public in general.

Consideration of the principles underpinning such choices and issues leads directly into unresolved debates about the best structure for a healthcare system, and, beyond this, to questions of *political* as well as moral philosophy. Deontological and teleological views are probably more at variance in this area than elsewhere in medical ethics. Deontology would imply, for example, that when patients compete for a scarce treatment, the only way to respect their rights is to choose between them at random. If one patient is elderly, unskilled, free of dependents and unlikely to benefit much from treatment, while another is young, with a dependent family, a valuable talent and a good prospect of cure, teleologists would decry the inefficiency and waste that follows from tossing a coin to choose between them.

In practice such decisions are usually made via a muddled mixture of teleological and deontological thinking, superimposed on long-standing but never justified custom and practice. The British NHS was founded on the principle of equal access to treatment, free at the point of need; but decisions about the relative budgets for cardiology and orthopaedics turn more on matters of local history and practical politics than they do on philosophy, however much cost-effectiveness data and teleological argument might be cited to choose between hearts and hips.

Scope

As Gillon has argued, even full consensus about the above four principles might not guarantee agreement about their application, because of differing views about their scope. Whose rights, whose interests are to figure in ethical deliberation: where and how are the limits to be set? The widely debated Oregon experiment is a case in point. After a long consultation period, the state of Oregon proposed a rank ordering of a long list of medical treatments and surgical procedures, in an attempt to determine which would, and which would not, be funded by public money. Unfortunately the orderings produced by various groups differed, sometimes considerably, raising the question: whose views count? Current patients, who know what it is like to suffer the condition in question? The general population, as potential patients, trying to imagine what it might be like? Medical staff, who know what it is like to treat such conditions, and who are more illness averse than the general population? Or the taxpayer, who pays for it all? Questions abound, but answers are few: a position familiar elsewhere in philosophy, but one on which, in this context, practical, real-world, decisions are based, sometimes with life and death consequences.

It is a common criticism of the four-principles approach that it gives no guidance about how to proceed when principles conflict. This reflects the principles' status as pragmatic, prima facie, lowerorder rules of thumb, derived ultimately from more abstract moral theory about which there is much less agreement. The four principles provide a common ground for moral debate between people of very different philosophical or religious outlooks, just as the same pitch can be used to play rugby or football. Those hoping for a set of universal binding rules governing all situations requiring moral choices will face inevitable disappointment, but they should not be surprised, given that we live in a pluralist democracy.

Applying the principles in legislation

There is a growing trend in British legislation to specify ethical principles at the outset of any new Act to help guide and interpret it. The clearest example of this is the Adults with Incapacity (Scotland) Act 2000 (see below), whose guiding principles specifically include respect for autonomy and beneficence. These principles are further elaborated in new mental health legislation in Scotland, which includes, for the first time in UK legislation, capacity criteria to justify detention for mental illness, in addition to dangerousness-based and needs-based criteria. The recommended principles for mental health legislation proposed by Millan (2001) again have their origin in the four-principles approach (Box 30.1).

Although, ideally, legislation which is based on capacity to justify compulsory detention, and which follows the principles above, appears ethically sound, there are practical difficulties in realising such an ideal. Governments will hesitate to approve legislation which is not first carefully costed. Although justice and reciprocity are sound principles, their cost is difficult to quantify. There are also particular problems with autonomy in a forensic psychiatric population: for example, a person charged with a serious offence might lack capacity to stand trial because of mental disorder, but retain sufficient capacity to refuse non-consensual treatment which might enable his participation in a fair trial.

In what follows, we hope to show how this principle-based approach might apply to various areas of ethical concern in psychiatry — namely, confidentiality, consent, capacity and compulsion — whether via the law or otherwise.

CONFIDENTIALITY

What I may see or hear in the course of the treatment, or even outside of the treatment, in regard to the life of men, which on no account must spread abroad, I will keep to myself, holding such things shameful to be spoken about.

Hippocratic Oath

The hippocratic adherence to confidentiality is absolute but unargued, with a complete lack of guidance to its scope of application. What are these things which must not be spread abroad? And is it really the case that on no account may confidentiality be breached? (Indeed it is possible to demonstrate the weakness of the oath by paraphrasing it: 'whatever should be kept secret, I will keep secret, because it should be kept secret.') While priests and lawyers still enjoy relationships with their clients which preserve this hermetically sealed notion of confidentiality, doctors do not. Questions of what clinical information doctors may (or may be obliged to) divulge, and under what circumstances, grow ever more complex, and require doctors to make judgements balancing patient autonomy against the interests of the patient himself, other individuals, or society in general.

The complexity of medical practice already means that large numbers of staff have access to potentially sensitive information held in a patient's casenotes. Add up the number of nurses, doctors, social workers, psychologists, occupational therapists, medical secretaries and administrative staff employed on a typical psychiatric ward: the total is unlikely to be less than 20. Add in the primary care staff to whom the discharge letter is sent, not to mention the general medical team who referred the patient, and the total rises further. It is not surprising that patients sometimes feel they lose control over sensitive information about their own lives when they enter psychiatric services; yet all these professionals have a legitimate need for access, if treatment is to be effective. Problems arise when patients seek to restrict the range of dissemination within this circle (refusing permission, for example, for the psychiatrist to communicate with the general practitioner, or divulging something on the condition that the nurses not be told), or when others outside this circle seek access to such information. Of course many disclosures of information occur with the patient's full knowledge and permission. Codes of practice have developed to guide this process, whereby any information passed on is the minimum necessary for the purpose at hand (such as ensuring payment by a health insurance company), and then only after the patient has given explicit written permission. Giving permission is not the same as conferring an obligation, however: there are circumstances in which the clinician may decline to pass on information at the patient's behest, if he feels it is detrimental enough to the patient's best interests.

More ethically interesting, however, are those cases in which confidentiality is breached in the face of opposition (or incapacity) on the part of the patient. It would be hard to construct a case where a capable patient's wish for confidentiality is overridden in the patient's own interest. If the patient is capable, then his autonomy is paramount, and he, not his psychiatrist, is the best judge of his own best interests. Where the patient lacks capacity (see below), then breaches of confidentiality may be justifiable in his best interest. A surgeon may need to be told, for example, that the semiconscious and unco-operative patient he is operating on for injuries sustained in a road traffic accident is heavily alcohol dependent, and likely to develop delirium tremens without appropriate postoperative treatment. The principle of beneficence/non-maleficence thus overrides the principle of respect for autonomy in circumstances such as these, at least until such time as the patient's capacity is restored. The same reasoning applies when divulging to others a depressed patient's suicidal ideation, in order to ensure his care in conditions of safety. In these cases the harm (breach of confidentiality) and the benefit (prevention of delirium tremens or suicide) accrue to the same person, the patient, and the temporary overriding of autonomy is generally readily justifiable. More troubling are those cases where the benefits involved accrue to someone else, raising the general issue of justice. Perhaps the most famous such case is that of Tarasoff (1976, see Box 30.2). Although the case was heard by California's Supreme Court, and is therefore not a precedent in other jurisdictions, it has influenced professional and legal attitudes in other US states and in Britain.

An unwelcome consequence of the ruling is to extend the psychiatrist's role as an agent of social control, and to impute to clinicians powers of predicting dangerousness they simply do not possess. It is significant that, after they were informed of Poddar's threats, the police arrested him, only to release him uncharged because he had committed no offence; no-one sued them.

Harm to third parties can come about in a variety of ways which fall short of direct threats to kill, raising the question of how severe the harm and what the level of risk must be before confidentiality is breached. In some areas the law imposes a statutory duty, and in others codes of practice apply. Examples include:

- the provisions of child protection legislation obliging professionals to report continuing abuse or neglect;
- the former (and widely ignored) duty to report drug-dependent patients to the Home Office;
- the requirement to report to the Driver and Vehicle Licensing Agency (DVLA) patients who are unfit to drive but ignore advice to stop.

In general, in such cases, the clinician's duty is not so much to warn and protect potential victims (who are sometimes identifiable, sometimes not) but to inform the relevant regulatory agencies, and the limits of the clinician's duty are well marked. Where there is no statutory provision, matters are much less clear-cut. The developing law relating to HIV and the acquired immune deficiency syndrome (AIDS) is a case in point. In some jurisdictions HIV infection is a notifiable disease, and a body of case law is slowly building up around HIV transmission. The question of whether knowingly infecting another with HIV is an offence, and if so what, is one that courts in Britain, Cyprus and elsewhere have recently grappled with: not far behind it will come the question of whether a therapist who becomes aware that her HIV-positive patient is continuing to have unprotected sex has a duty to warn his unsuspecting spouse.

In other cases it is not so much the patient's private behaviour that might pose risks, but his ability to function in a job which confers responsibility for the welfare and safety of others. A clinician's threshold for breaching confidentiality about a depressed airline pilot or a paranoid air traffic controller will clearly be lower than for a librarian or a shopkeeper, for example. Teleological reasoning readily accommodates such variations, even in the absence of an agreed scale of risk, but a deontologist will struggle to justify such a willingness to vary the threshold at which a duty is breached.

The duty to warn and protect third parties placed at risk by a patient's action confers on the clinician a kind of vicarious responsibility, which is at times burdensome. The burden has been increased further by the General Medical Council's recent clarification that doctors may also owe a duty of care to the patients of colleagues whose competence is threatened by illness. A surgeon who becomes aware that a colleague has developed a drink problem, and is operating while intoxicated, for example, is held to owe a duty to the colleague's patients, as well as his own, which requires him to report the situation in such a way as to bring it to an end.

Examples such as these show that we have come a long way from the view of confidentiality enshrined in the Hippocratic Oath as absolute and total. It is now seen as important but relative, contingent and overridable. Respecting confidentiality is only one among an ever-growing list of duties which the clinician must balance against one another. For further reading about confidentiality within the British context, Crichton (2001) discusses recent guidance from the General Medical Council and Royal College of Psychiatrists.

CONSENT

The law regarding consent to medical treatment makes it clear that any unconsented touching of a patient by a doctor may be both a civil wrong (a tort) and a criminal act (a battery). Doctors avoid action on these grounds in three ways: by reference to any relevant legislation, such as the Mental Health Act; by invoking common law rights and duties; or by showing the patient has consented to the treatment in question.

For some medical and psychiatric treatments (surgery, invasive procedures, ECT, entry into research projects), practice dictates that the patient must make explicit his consent by signing the requisite form. Elsewhere — that is, for nearly all psychiatric treatment — consent is implicit in the patient's attendance. Ms Smith, for example, is unlikely ever to be asked 'Do you consent to this programme of graded exposure for your spider phobia?'. The boundary separating treatments in need of explicit consent is erratically drawn, however. In British practice, a signed consent form would always be required before a biopsy of a brain tumour, sometimes before a lumbar puncture, but only rarely before magnetic resonance imaging. As a result of social pressures in the mid-1980s, blood tests for HIV status now require explicit consent, but other blood tests (including those for hepatitis B, which raise many of the same issues) do not.

Whether implicit or explicit, a patient's consent will not be valid unless he is informed, capable and free of duress. Given the asymmetry of knowledge and expertise described above, there is a requirement on the doctor to impart sufficient understandable and relevant information to the patient to enable a choice based on the patient's own judgement of the alternatives. Only then is the patient fully capable of acting autonomously. But what counts as relevant? And how much is sufficient? Various tests apply, including, in order of increasing rigour: that which would generally be divulged by a reasonable body of medical opinion; that which any reasonable patient would need and wish to know; and that which the particular patient in question would need and wish to know. British practice favours the former, after the Sidaway case (1983) of a woman who suffered paralysis after cervical spine surgery. She claimed damages on the grounds that if she had been informed beforehand of the small but definite risk of this complication (approximately 1%), she would not have consented; but her claim was dismissed, it being argued that there was no requirement upon doctors to divulge risks of this magnitude, and most generally did not.

Freedom from duress is an obvious element of valid consent but duress can range widely in degree, from the blatant, which is easily identified as such and therefore excluded, to the very subtle, which may never be thought of by patient or doctor as duress at all: for where lies the boundary between duress and persuasion?

Particularly frequent and problematic in psychiatry is the kind of duress applied by the doctor who tells his patient: 'We want you to stay on the ward and take this medication, Mr Roberts; and I'm afraid that if you don't we'll have to consider sectioning you'.

Of the three elements of consent, that raising most ethical issues, especially in psychiatry, is, however, capacity or competence, a complicated medical and legal concept which finds itself at the heart of many other ethical questions.

CAPACITY

The primacy of autonomy discussed above relies heavily, but usually invisibly, on the assumption that the patient has capacity to make choices about his treatment. Ethical debate tends to focus more on the issues raised if the patient is incapable, and his autonomy therefore impaired, than on what constitutes capacity. This implies that capacity is a dichotomous either/or phenomenon, and that there is consensus on how to assess it. Unfortunately this is not the case. Various definitions of capacity (and its constituent elements) can be offered, the common thread being capacity to make a personal, reasoned choice between alternatives. As such, it requires several subcapacities, including the ability to acquire, retain and understand information, and then to use it, together with personal preferences or valuations, to deliberate, make a reasoned choice, and then to communicate that choice, together with, where necessary, the reasoning behind it.

All these abilities are dimensional, not categorical, so capacity itself, being composed of them, cannot be otherwise: yet it is often discussed as if it were, and psychiatrists are regularly called in as the arbiters, especially in general hospitals. ('Does Mr Johnson have capacity to refuse transfusion/discontinue dialysis/decline chemotherapy?') This is partly because, in medicine as in law, patients are *deemed* capable until proven otherwise, and the burden of proof falls upon the clinician (or the courts) to demonstrate sufficient impairment of capacity for the matter at hand. Capacity may be eroded in a general way, as in a dementing illness, without ever being called into question, until a situation requiring a significant choice arises. If the patient is then declared incapable, it does not mean that he has just become so. Capacity is often erroneously thought of as being global, as well as dichotomous, so that a patient considered incapable in one area of his life is thereby so deemed in all other areas too. The psychiatrist who argues that, by virtue of his depression, Mr Johnson does indeed lack capacity to discontinue his dialysis, should not assume he also lacks capacity to make a will, manage his finances, or choose between steak and fish for dinner. The degree of evidence required to discharge the burden of proof varies between applications, as does the consequence of a judgement of incapacity. Capacity is thus *task-specific*: of course Mr Johnson can choose between steak and fish,

and even if he cannot manage his finances, he may retain the capacity to appoint a proxy to do it for him.

Questions of capacity therefore arise in a variety of arenas, including the criminal law, the civil law, the management of financial and other affairs, and medical treatment. Chapter 29 deals with the first, under such heads as fitness to plead, diminished responsibility, and the McNaughton Rules. The large literature on mentally disordered offenders which that chapter reviews tends to consider the concept of *responsibility* more central than capacity, although the two are closely related: the same factors which might lead to a defence of diminished responsibility may also call into question the defendant's capacity to stand trial at all (i.e. his fitness to plead) or to be punished. In this last context British psychiatrists are thankfully spared a particularly painful ethical dilemma imposed on some of our American colleagues: namely, the requirement that an offender who becomes mentally ill after being sentenced to death should receive psychiatric treatment to render him competent for execution.

As far as the civil law is concerned, capacity is most commonly questioned in regard to money: specifically the ability to make a will (testamentary capacity) and the management of one's assets while still alive. In order to be 'of sound disposing mind' the testator must understand what a will is, and must know the nature and extent of his property and the identities of those who might have a claim on it. He must be free of undue influence, and of mental disorder which might distort those of his judgements which are relevant to the making of the will. He need not be free of mental disorder entirely, however. An encapsulated delusional system, such as the belief that he is spied upon by police-appointed pigeons, need not intrude at all upon large areas of a patient's life, and indeed may be apparent only on direct questioning by a trained interviewer. Such a patient would be psychotic, and yet, at the same time, 'of sound disposing mind'.

Where a patient develops a mental illness, especially one which is chronic or irreversible, but may be expected to live for some time yet, the question of his capacity to manage his affairs naturally arises, particularly if those affairs are complex or he is wealthy. The test of capacity which applies is similar to that determining testamentary capacity, and is, once again, task-specific. For patients found incapable, a proxy, such as a family member or lawyer, may be appointed to act on his behalf to make financial decisions. Power of attorney is a legal instrument used to formalise the long-standing principle that whatever a person can legitimately do, he can appoint another to do on his behalf. Originally, however, power of attorney lapsed when capacity was lost. The recently developed durable power of attorney works differently: a proxy is appointed at a time when the patient retains capacity, but anticipates that his illness will erode it. The proxy's powers are not enacted at this stage, but spring into effect when the patient loses capacity, and remain in effect until the patient dies (or, less commonly, since the illness in question is usually dementia, recovers).

Where there is no suitable proxy, or where conflicts of interests might arise, more formal procedures are available, the details of which vary between jurisdictions. In England, for example, application may be made to the Court of Protection, who can provide a disinterested third party to manage the patient's affairs on a best-interests standard.

Medical treatment

For many years in the various jurisdictions that make up the British Isles, there has been concern about the legal basis by which the non-emergency medical treatment of incapable patients is undertaken. Valid consent from a capable patient clearly authorises treatment, whether emergency or otherwise, and protects the treating doctor against subsequent claims; and the common law concepts of necessity and duty of care both authorise and indeed *require* doctors to undertake emergency treatment of in incapable patient, on a best-interests standard. But what of a demented patient distressed by severe arthritis in her hip? She may well benefit from a hip replacement, but she cannot give valid consent. Who can? Relatives and carers are often asked to sign consent forms on behalf of the patient, but in most cases this process has no legal validity; it would, however, be a foolhardy surgeon who proceeded in the absence of, or in opposition to, family views.

Various efforts have been made to address this by extending durable powers of attorney to apply to medical treatment as well as financial matters, and by introducing advance directives. Such developments have arisen mainly out of the continuing debates on the subject of euthanasia. However, public anxiety about facing incurable pain in a terminal illness has been matched, and perhaps surpassed, by the widespread (and demographically justified) fear of a long twilight of decline, via dementia, to a life stripped to bare existence and maintained by medical interventions the patient is now incapable of refusing. In an attempt to reassert control over this much-feared indignity, the concept of a living will was first proposed in the late 1960s. Perhaps better known as an advance directive, this is a document drawn up by someone who is now capable and wishes to retain control over treatment decisions which might become necessary at some time in the future, when he might no longer be so. Different formats are available, the common feature being a list of interventions that prospective patients would accept or decline in variously specified circumstances (e.g. 'If I should develop a dementia or other incurable brain disease, then I would/would not — *delete as appropriate* — wish to have dialysis if it becomes necessary').

These documents are still much more widely used in the USA than in Britain, where argument rages about whether they should be legally binding, or whether they merely provide guidance to the doctor. The Voluntary Euthanasia Society recently proposed that a doctor who flouts the terms of a patient's living will should be made criminally liable and punishable with up to 2 years' imprisonment. The legislation that finally emerged did not go this far, and the extent to which British doctors *must* abide by a living will probably requires a test case for clarification — as does the appropriate action where a patient now demented and incompetent expresses a wish to continue living, in direct contradiction to the terms of a previously enacted living will.

Given their inflexibility, and the impossibility of ever drafting living wills sufficiently specific to cover all possible future medical scenarios, the alternative (or additional) use of healthcare proxies has much to recommend it. The medical counterpart of the durable power of attorney for financial matters, a proxy decision maker for healthcare, is usually a friend or family member nominated by a potential patient at a time when competent, who is empowered to take treatment decisions on the patient's behalf if, at some future time, he becomes incompetent to do so himself.

Ideally the proxy should apply a *substituted judgement* test to the decision at hand, and use her prior knowledge of the patient to determine what he would have wanted in the circumstances now prevailing.

The use of proxies is not without its difficulties, however. There is no reason to believe that the alternative *best-interests* test is necessarily any better applied by a proxy than by the doctors involved, and it may be difficult for the proxy to distinguish between substituted judgement, best interests, and the further question of what *she* would want for the patient. Furthermore, in cases where the proxy stands to benefit from any legacy, there is a potential conflict of interest which may complicate matters; and, where the proxy is of an age with the patient, and therefore vulnerable to the same risks of dementia, the question of the proxy's *own* competence may arise.

Perhaps the best way to minimise these complications is to adopt an instrument which combines the function of an advance directive and the nomination of a proxy, whose function it is to apply the terms of the advance directive in the light of her knowledge of the patient's preference and values.

New Scottish legislation: Adults with Incapacity (Scotland) Act 2000

The first major piece of legislation passed by the restored Scottish Parliament was the Adults with Incapacity (Scotland) Act 2000, though much of the preparation for the Act took place under previous arrangements for government north of the border. The essential feature of the legislation is that it establishes, for the first time in any part of Britain, a *statutory* authority to treat patients incapable of consenting for themselves. As in the forthcoming new Scottish Mental Health Act (see below) the Act lists a set of guiding principles underpinning its provisions, to aid patients, relatives and medical staff in applying them (see Box 30.3). The Act offers a significant role for healthcare proxies, although a less central place for advance directions.

From the point of view of the psychiatrist the Act carries the advantage that, while psychiatrists can assist in difficult cases, the assessment of capacity is seen as an integral part of the work of *all* medical practitioners. There are some uncertainties in operating the new Act (in particular the question of where lies the boundary with emergency treatment, which common law still justifies); and it may not yet be applied in Scotland to its full extent, but it seems likely to serve as a model for other jurisdictions both within the United Kingdom and more widely. (It is to be hoped, however, that other legislators find an alternative to the grating expression 'the adult'.)

Box 30.3   General principles of the Adults with Incapacity Act (Scotland) 2000

- **Benefit.** Any proposed treatment must be intended for the benefit of the patient
- **Minimum intervention.** The intervention considered must be the least restrictive alternative available
- **Adult's wishes.** There must be efforts to establish the adult's past and present wishes, and to take account of them
- **Consultation.** There must be consultation with 'relevant others', most importantly the family, carers and any appointed proxy
- **Exercise of residual capacity.** There must be efforts to encourage the adult to exercise such residual capacity as they still possess

---

COMPULSION

Questions of capacity to consent to treatment can arise for any kind of medical or surgical intervention; but specifically within psychiatry, ethical debates have long reverberated around the different issue of treatments or other measures (including simple incarceration) which patients might be *compelled* to undergo.

Development of mental health legislation

In the British context, prior to the 18th century there were few laws to regulate management of people with mental disorder. Historically, those with mental disorder were treated differently by the law, with their status in civil and criminal proceedings likened to that of a child. Plato suggested that those who were mentally unwell were the responsibility of their families, who should use whatever means they had to control them. There is evidence that this approach was followed in Roman law and in ancient English law. This early control of the mentally disordered was therefore capacity based — if someone because of illness was not able to make the decisions of an adult they should be treated as a child. Those with mental disorder only became widely incarcerated, in the British context, at the introduction of the Poor Law (1601), but even then allowances were made for those with mental disorder — lunatics were not subject to corporal punishment. The Vagrancy Act (1714) identified insane paupers as a distinct category and empowered local justices to apprehend lunatics who were 'furiously mad and dangerous' in a safe place. This gave rise to the 'mad-houses' of the 18th century. 'Dangerousness' was the first criteria which justified the statutory detention of the mentally disordered. There were concerns about the conditions in 'mad-houses' as early as 1754, when the Royal College of Physicians declined an invitation from a member of parliament to undertake inspections since this would be too difficult and inconvenient. Parliamentary enquiries were held in 1807 and 1815–16 into their conditions and heard a variety of witnesses, including a former apothecary at Warberton's 'mad-house' in London. He gave evidence describing prolonged restraint, theft, misuse of patient's property, beating, whipping, rape and 'mopping down' of incontinent patients (Porter 1987). Eventually in 1842 a regulatory authority was set up under Lord Shaftsbury. The Lunacy Commissioners would inspect without warning any 'mad-house' or asylum and could supervise any aspect of care. The Lunacy Act of 1845 began the building of county asylums across England and Wales. The legislative framework went on to develop throughout the 19th century and became ever more detailed and restrictive regarding the activities within asylums. The justification for detention was, in addition to dangerousness, simply the perceived medical need for such care. The activities of the Lunacy Commission and the tight legislative framework attempted to ensure that such paternalism remained beneficent, according to the standards of the day.

It was not until after the First World War that there were established psychiatric outpatient clinics to look after shell shocked former soldiers and eventually voluntary patients could be admitted to asylums. The Medical Treatment Act 1930 allowed voluntary and temporary hospital admission, and by 1938, 35% of patients in asylums were voluntary. Another major change in the care of the mentally disordered in Britain was in the 1950s, described by Jones (1993) as the three revolutions; psychological, pharmacological and legislative. The introduction of new psychological approaches,

such as the therapeutic community, and the introduction of effective pharmacological treatments, such as chlorpromazine, brought about a wave of optimism which was reflected in the Mental Health Act 1959. The Lunacy Act of 1890 had survived largely unchanged but it was decimated in length by the 1959 act. Admission procedures were streamlined, The Board of Control (the successor to the Lunacy Commission) was abolished and doctors were given wide powers of treatment over detained patients. Mental Health Review Tribunals were introduced in England and Wales to whom appeals against detention could be heard, but the justification for detention was still dangerousness and need. The 1959 Act could be seen as the triumph of medical paternalism, and such was the trust given to those in authority that many of the safeguards of an earlier age were withdrawn.

Mental health legislation in the 1960s and 1970s in Britain was increasingly seen as giving psychiatrists too much power and having too few safeguards. Civil libertarian lawyers and the arguments generated by the antipsychiatry movement influenced new mental health legislation in the early 1980s in Britain. That legislation, however, was merely a revision of the earlier act; it introduced greater safeguards and re-established in England and Wales the Mental Health Act Commission. Needs-based and dangerousness-based justifications, however, remained.

A growing trend in mental health legislation internationally over the last two decades has been the importance of autonomy in the justification to detain people with mental disorder. This is well described in the American context by Applebaum (1994). The trend is away from needs and dangerousness-based criteria towards capacity-based criteria to justify detention.

Justifying compulsion

The Jones case set out in the Introduction above is typical of those for which compulsory admission and treatment might be mooted. Jones has an acute florid psychotic illness, manifested by behaviour which poses direct and indirect risks to himself and to others, and by impaired insight, which calls into question his competence to refuse offers of help. In these circumstances beneficence (acting in what others, particularly psychiatrists, judge to be his best interests) and justice (acting out of concern for the rights and interests of others) together lead to the overriding of his autonomy, which would otherwise be paramount, and an order for compulsory admission to hospital.

This compulsion can be justified in either teleological or deontological terms. A teleologist would say that ordinarily a person is the best judge of his own interests, and for these reasons his autonomy should be respected, but, where his judgement is impaired by illness, others have to judge his interests on his behalf, at least temporarily. A deontologist would argue that autonomy is paramount, but can only be properly exercised by a competent moral agent; in circumstances where illness limits competence, then respect for autonomy requires the minimal necessary intervention in order to restore it. It can be argued, indeed, that Mr Jones has a *right* to be detained and treated against his will.

Set against this paternalistic approach, however, must be the recognition that deprivation of liberty is a harm, that supposedly benevolent institutions such as hospitals can be damaging, and that physical treatments such as drugs and ECT carry risks, including the risk of death. The principle of non-maleficence therefore requires that the procedures for compulsory detention and treatment have built-in safeguards, such as second opinions, rights of appeal and review, and specific time limits. Legislation varies between jurisdictions, but in general, the greater the potential harms, the more protection the patient is offered.

Risk assessment and management

Over the last decade there has been a shift away from the emphasis on the dangerousness of patients, to the broader concept of risk assessment and management. A key difference between these two concepts is that the risk of violence to others should be considered on a continuum rather than a 'yes/no' dichotomy. It has been recognised that there can be no single prediction of risk. Assessing the risk of an adverse outcome is a continual process and should be incorporated in the day-to-day management of mentally disordered people. The language of risk assessment and management was supposed to reduce the stigmatisation of the mentally disordered, particularly the mentally disordered offenders, but may have had the reverse effect. Only a few patients were given the label 'dangerous'; however, every psychiatric patient represents at least some degree of risk (as do members of the public who have never been and will not become psychiatric patients). In the British context concerns about violence of psychiatric patients coincided with the closure of large psychiatric institutions and the management of patients in the community. There were widespread fears about such a change. A number of high-profile cases re-enforced public stereotypes regarding the dangerousness of the mentally ill.

There are, however, contemporary concerns that the language of risk assessment and management has in itself created ethical problems, particularly regarding the doctor–patient relationship and the principle of beneficence. Current ethical concerns about this area are well summarised by Mullen (2002):

> If risk management is to emerge out of risk assessments; if risk management is to amount to more than coercion and incapacitation; if risk management is to be a legitimate activity for health professionals, then, assessments must focus on establishing those vulnerabilities contributing to offending which are open to modification through appropriate health related treatment.

Current English proposals to detain indefinitely some people with so-called dangerous severe personality disorder on the basis of risk assessment, including those who have not committed an offence, have given rise to particular ethical concern. Risk prediction can never be completely accurate, but it is sometimes presented in a way which appears overly scientifically robust. Then what should be the psychiatrist's role in the assessment of an individual which is likely to result in indeterminate incarceration with little likelihood of treatment? Some have argued that this is an impossible task for a professional who is also engaged in a therapeutic relationship. Instead it has been suggested that there should be 'forensicists', experts not in a treatment relationship, who could advise the courts. Such forensicists might limit their enquiries simply to case notes records rather than clinical interviews, which may have the appearance of a therapeutic interview to the mentally disordered individual but whose purpose is to justify indeterminate detention.

CONCLUSIONS

Psychiatry, more than any other branch of medicine, throws up a host of ethical issues, some of which intersect with the law as well as with clinical practice. The practising psychiatrist has always needed a familiarity with the relevant civil law and mental health legislation, though not, of course, to the level of a lawyer. Now, given the ever-increasing complexity of modern practice, the psychiatrist also needs a working knowledge of basic ethical principles, and an ability to reason ethically in areas where there is disagreement, though not, of course, at the level of the moral philosopher.

REFERENCES

Anscombe G E M 1981 The collected philosophical papers of G E M Anscombe, vol 3: Ethics, religion and politics. Basil Blackwell, Oxford

APA 1973 (revised 1988) Principles of medical ethics with annotations especially applicable to psychiatry. American Psychiatric Association, Washington, DC

Appelbaum P S 1994 Almost a revolution, mental health law and the limits of change. Oxford University Press, Oxford

Barham P 1992 Closing the asylum: the mental patient in modern society. England Books, London

Beauchamp T L, Childress J F 1994 Principles of biomedical ethics, 4th edn. Oxford University Press, New York

Bloch S, Reddaway P 1977 Russia's political hospitals: the abuse of psychiatry in the Soviet Union. Gollancz, London

BMA 1981 The handbook of medical ethics. British Medical Association, London

Crichton J H M 2001 Confidentiality: guidance from the General Medical Council and the Royal College of Psychiatrists. Journal of Forensic Psychiatry 12:671–676

Dworkin R M 1977 Taking rights seriously. Harvard University Press, Cambridge, Mass

Earns K 1993 Asylums and after: a revised history of mental health services from the early 18th century to the 1990s, Athlone Press, London

Eastman N 1997 The Mental Health (Patients in the Community) Act 1995: a clinical analysis. British Journal of Psychiatry 170:492–496

Foucault M 1967 Madness and civilisation: a history of insanity in an age reason. Translated from the French by R Howard. Tavistock, London

Fulford K W M 1989 Moral theory and medical practice. Cambridge University Press, Cambridge

Gillon R 1994 Four principles plus attention to scope. British Medical Journal 309:184–188

Goffman E 1961 Asylums: essays on the social situation of mental patients and other inmates. Anchor Books, New York

Harding T 1991 Mental health service delivery abuses in Japan. In: Bloch S, Chodoff P (eds) Psychiatric ethics, 2nd edn. Oxford University Press, Oxford

Hare R M 1981 Moral thinking: its levels, method and point. Oxford University Press, Oxford

Jones K 1993 Asylums and after: a revised history of mental health services from the early eighteenth century to the 1990s. Athlone Press, London

Laing R D 1965 The divided self. Penguin, Harmondsworth

Lifton R J 1986 The Nazi doctors: medical killing and the psychology of genocide. Basic Books, New York

Mechanic D 1989 Mental health and social policy, 3rd edn. Prentice-Hall, Englewood Cliffs, NJ

Mill J S 1859 On liberty. London. (Rapaport E (ed) 1978 Hackett Publishing, Indianapolis)

Millan B (Chairman) 2001 New directions: report on the review of the Mental Health (Scotland) Act 1984. Scottish Executive, Edinburgh

Mullen P V 2002 Introduction. In: Buchanan A (ed) Care of the mentally disordered offender in the community. Oxford University Press, Oxford

Muller-Hill B 1991 Psychiatry in the Nazi era. In: Bloch S, Chodoff P (eds) Psychiatric ethics, 2nd edn. Oxford University Press, Oxford

Porter R 1987 Mind-forg'd manacles: a history of madness in England from the restoration to the regency. Athlone Press, London

Ramsay R 1990 The scandal of Leros. British Medical Journal 300:688

Royal College of Psychiatrists 1993 Community supervision orders. Royal College of Psychiatrists, London

Shapcote L 1912–1936 The summa theologica (English translation). Burns, Oates, London, 22 vols

Sidaway 1983 Reported as (1985) 1 All ER 643

Smart J J C, Williams B A O 1973 Utilitarianism: for and against. Cambridge University Press, New York

Szasz T S 1961 The myth of mental illness. Harper & Row, New York

Tarasoff v Regents of The University of California 1976. Supreme Court of California Suppl 131 Report 14

World Medical Association 1948 General Assembly, Geneva. (Amended 1968, Sydney and 1983, Venice)

World Psychiatric Association 1977 (revised 1983) General Assembly, Hawaii

31 | Perinatal psychiatry

Siobhan MacHale, Roch Cantwell

Women are twice as likely as men to suffer from depression at some point in their lives, and are at greatest risk during their reproductive years. Contributory factors are likely to include not only the psychological and social challenges associated with childbearing and child-rearing, but also the marked neurohormonal alterations associated with pregnancy and parturition. The consequences of maternal mental illness may be severe. Suicide is now the leading cause of maternal death in the UK (RCOG 2001), and other psychiatric factors are implicated in a significant number of deaths in the first postnatal year. Furthermore, increasing evidence points to the detrimental effect of untreated maternal depression on infant development. Although the risk factors associated with severe postnatal mental illness are well known and preventative treatments are available, psychiatric services for women and their families at this time remain patchy and poorly coordinated.

PREGNANCY

Normal emotional changes during pregnancy

Pregnancy is a time of psychological change and challenge. For most women childbirth is an eagerly awaited event. Ambivalence about the pregnancy, health-related anxieties, role transition, concerns and fears about inability to cope (especially in first-time mothers) are, however, typical and normal.

- In the first trimester a woman may have increased emotional lability, which may be exacerbated by nausea, breast tenderness and other physical changes typical of early pregnancy.
- As pregnancy progresses, further bodily changes, alterations in sexual interest and anxieties about the delivery may all contribute to mood change.
- Late pregnancy may be associated with social withdrawal, and increased absorption and preoccupation with preparations for delivery and caring for the baby. Anxious and obsessional thoughts are not unusual, often focusing on the health of the baby.

Such emotional changes are bound up with the psychological adjustments necessary in pregnancy, but hormonal alterations may contribute. It is important to be able to distinguish these changes from those more clearly associated with mental illness.

Oates (1989) describes certain groups as having particular needs for increased support in relation to childbearing:

- very young, single and unsupported mothers, and women who themselves have poor experiences of mothering may be especially vulnerable; their own needs may conflict with those

of their babies, and early planning to provide appropriate support is desirable to help develop the woman's ability to care for her baby;
- older mothers who may have over-idealised expectations of pregnancy and delivery, and have problems adjusting to life changes after the birth;
- women with previous pregnancy loss;
- women who have undergone assisted conception;
- women with high-risk pregnancies or who required an emergency caesarean section.

Relationship with the partner

It is also relevant to consider the partner's adjustment to impending fatherhood. A lack of emotional support for the woman may contribute to both antenatal (prolonged hyperemesis) and postnatal (depression) difficulties. Violence may be used to resolve a crisis in male identity. Approximately 30% of domestic violence begins during pregnancy and often escalates in the postpartum period. In light of this, it has been recommended that women should be seen alone on at least one occasion during their antenatal care, enquiries about violence should be routinely included in the antenatal history, and information provided on legal rights and available supports. However, there is limited evidence to date that such responses benefit women (Jewkes 2002). Pregnant women who misuse alcohol or drugs, or who are depressed, are most likely to be at risk of domestic violence. The social circumstances and needs of women with mentally disordered partners must also be considered.

Couvade syndrome derives from the term 'couvade', an ancient custom whereby a new father took to his bed to be cared for by his recently delivered wife for a defined period of time. The syndrome, anecdotally known as 'sympathetic pregnancy', refers to the common experience of medically unexplained somatic symptoms in the expectant father during the pregnancy. They generally resolve on delivery. Epidemiological studies report couvade symptoms in 11–36% of pregnancies, predominantly affecting the gastrointestinal tract or presenting as headache or toothache. It is considered likely to be a somatic expression of anxiety, although psychodynamic explanations include identification with the fetus, ambivalence about fatherhood or parturition envy (Klein 1991). Psychotic cases of Couvade syndrome are very rare

Loss events specific to pregnancy

The most consistent vulnerability factor for developing psychiatric sequelae to pregnancy-related loss events is that of a past psychiatric history.

Infertility affects 10% of couples and has significant psychological effects for both men and women. These include low self-esteem, anger, depression and impotence, and marital breakdown is not uncommon.

Miscarriage, including ectopic pregnancies, may be associated with grief reactions, anxiety and depression at rates of up to four times the norm. For most women, these symptoms are greatest in the first 6 months and resolve spontaneously thereafter. Greater intensity of grief is found in women who had been pregnant for longer or who were childless. Frost & Condon (1996) have usefully reviewed the literature on the psychological consequences of miscarriage.

Termination of a pregnancy is not, of itself, associated with increased psychiatric morbidity. Risks are greater, however, for women with a past psychiatric history or those who have experienced some pressure to have a termination, whether from family, social pressures, or for medical reasons. There is an increased risk of depression and impaired bonding with the baby if the patient is denied their request for a termination of pregnancy. It is also important to be aware that a termination of pregnancy is as likely as childbirth to trigger an episode of puerperal psychosis in those predisposed (Gilchrist et al 1995).

Stillbirth after 22 weeks' gestation affects 0.5% to 1% of pregnancies, often triggering grief reactions, sexual dysfunction and marital breakdown. Non-evidence-based good practice guidelines widely disseminated across the UK have encouraged parents to see and hold their stillborn baby. These have recently been called into question by a case-matched control study suggesting that such contact is, in fact, associated with greater levels of anxiety and depression in the mother up to 1 year after the birth of the next baby (Hughes et al 2002). The authors themselves pointed out that a lack of randomisation, small numbers and primiparous controls were limiting factors. Nonetheless, good practice protocols may be over-applied at times of high anxiety for staff as well as patients, at the expense of listening to the patient.

Other loss events include *adoption* (relinquishment), in which guilt and grief are common, and *end of childbearing*. This includes sterilisation, which is regretted by 3% of patients, hysterectomy and the menopause.

Pseudocyesis

This is an increasingly rare condition whereby a woman mistakenly believes she is pregnant. This differs from a delusion, because of the presence of clinical signs which may include amenorrhoea, abdominal swelling, breast changes, nausea, uterine enlargement (to 6 weeks gestational size) and often the experience of fetal movements. Pathophysiological mechanisms may include the impact of stress on the hypothalamic-pituitary-adrenal (HPA) axis, constipation or weight gain, and movement of intestinal gas. However, a pathognomonic sign is the lack of navel flattening. In a review of the literature, vulnerability factors included recent pregnancy loss or infertility, combined with social isolation, naiveté and a focus on childbearing as a central female role (Whelan & Stewart 1990). With advances in pregnancy testing, it is now much less common. The differential diagnosis includes delusions of pregnancy, which can affect men and women and where there are no physical signs of pregnancy. It also differs from malingering, where pregnancy is deliberately simulated, for example to avoid imprisonment. Treatment requires supportive counselling and, occasionally, antidepressant medication.

Hyperemesis gravidarum

The reasons for severe and persistent nausea and vomiting in pregnancy remain poorly understood. Elevated levels of human chorionic gonadotrophin (HCG), changes in thyroid function and alterations in gastric motility and pH may play a part. Hyperemesis is more common in women with a history of gastrointestinal problems. Vomiting in the first trimester is associated with better adjustment to pregnancy and motherhood than for those without. If prolonged beyond the first trimester, however, it is associated with a sense of poor emotional support. Patients may become extremely distressed, resulting in a request for termination of the pregnancy. Treatment is symptomatic, aimed at correcting dehydration and metabolic disturbance, and reducing nausea. While it is unlikely that psychological distress acts as a sole precipitating factor, it often plays a role in maintaining and exacerbating symptoms. Case reports advocate the use of anxiety management techniques, including addressing concerns, relaxation training and desensitisation as part of the multidisciplinary management. Medical hypnosis has also been used to good effect.

Pica

Psychiatrists may also be asked to see patients with pica, the age-inappropriate eating of non-nutritive substances. It is important to consider cultural factors and risk of nutritional deficiencies. Clay eating may be associated with iron or zinc deficiency, while the eating of starch-based products may be linked with anaemia. Usually an educational approach is sufficient, although some women benefit from additional anxiety management techniques.

Psychiatric disorders arising in pregnancy

Although rates of psychotic disorder and suicide are reduced during pregnancy, accumulating evidence suggests that pregnant women have a similar risk of other forms of mental illness to those who are not pregnant. Any psychiatric illness may have its onset during pregnancy, although certain disorders may come to attention more frequently. This may be because of increased healthcare contact or due to a direct link with the pregnant state.

Adjustment disorders

These states of emotional disturbance, interfering with social functioning, arise when adapting to significant life change. Hence, they may be triggered by unwanted pregnancy, pregnancy loss, or other major changes occurring during pregnancy, e.g. separation from a partner or change in employment status. Patients may present with depressed mood, anxiety and feelings of inability to cope, or overwhelming irritability and frustration. Counselling or brief psychotherapy is often effective.

Adjustment disorder associated with *denial of pregnancy* affects 1 in 400 births. The clinical picture is often of a young or immature single female living with her parents. There is either a late or non-presentation of pregnancy, which may be due to concealment, lack of awareness or dissociation. The associated lack of antenatal care and increased risk of neonaticide lead to concerns for the welfare of both mother and baby.

Depressive and anxiety disorders

The previous emphasis of research literature on postnatal depression has recently been complemented by an emerging interest in the frequency and impact of depressive and anxiety disorders in the antenatal period. Depressive disorders of a severity to warrant specific pharmacological or psychological treatment occur in women with an approximate lifetime risk of 3–5%. Milder disorders may occur as frequently as 1 in 7–10. Therefore they may arise coincidentally during pregnancy. However, the same factors that give rise to adjustment disorders may also lead to the development of more severe depression. They are common in all women in the reproductive age group, and are equally as common in pregnant as non-pregnant, and during pregnancy as in the postnatal period. However, rates of deliberate self-harm and suicide are reduced in pregnancy to 5% of the expected rate, suggesting a protective effect (Appleby & Turnbull 1995).

The Avon longitudinal study of parents and children (ALSPAC) is a community-based project gathering prospective data from 14 000 pregnant women. The follow-up is ongoing, with a cohort of 10-year-old children to date. From this, Evans and colleagues have concluded that symptoms of depression are just as common and severe in the antenatal as the postnatal period (Evans et al 2001). Their use of a self-reporting instrument, the Edinburgh Postnatal Depression Scale (EPDS), which has not been validated for use during pregnancy, means that diagnostic studies are needed to confirm their results. However, clinical experience is supportive of their findings.

There is some interesting research suggesting that the possible effects of maternal mood on the fetus may depend on the gestational period.

- The experience of severe life events in the first trimester (at the time of organogenesis) has been linked to a 50% rise in rates of congenital abnormalities involving organs of cranial neural origin, such as cleft palate and cardiac malformations (Hansen et al 2000). Other evidence of a link between early antenatal anxiety and neurological development again derives from the ALSPAC cohort, which showed that high maternal anxiety at 18 weeks gestation predicted mixed handedness in the child.
- This contrasts with the links between raised anxiety in the third trimester (when neuronal connections are being formed) and increased risk of behavioural and emotional problems in the offspring at 4 years (O'Connor et al 2002). This association was not found with antenatal depression, and continued despite controlling for postnatal maternal anxiety. These latter results could, however, be explained by genetic transmission or biases in parental reporting, and, as yet, only tentative conclusions can be drawn about the potential fetogenic effects of antenatal stress.

More reliable data are available on obstetric outcomes, which consistently indicate links between antenatal distress and premature labour or intrauterine growth retardation (e.g. Hedegaard et al 1993). A number of pathophysiological mechanisms have been proposed, including increased uterine artery resistance and increased materno-fetal cortisol transfer.

Tokophobia is the phobic dread of labour and delivery. It may arise during the first pregnancy or be secondary to poor experiences of a previous delivery. Although well recognised as a problem by obstetricians, Hofberg & Brockington (2000) were the first to describe this as a distinct entity in a series of 26 cases. It may be a symptom of underlying depression or anxiety or have more distant antecedents, such as childhood sexual abuse or other sexual assault. These women often seek alternatives to vaginal delivery and, without an empathic professional presence, may see termination as their only option. Women who achieve their desired mode of delivery experience lower rates of psychological morbidity than those who are refused. *Severe needle phobia* may also be a barrier to good antenatal care. Early recognition and referral for psychological therapy, as well as close liaison between the obstetrician and psychiatrist, will help prevent crises in late pregnancy and childbirth.

Pre-existing psychiatric disorders

This category includes patients with

- pre-existing mental illness;
- learning disability;
- personality disorder.

It is important to emphasise that most mental disorders during pregnancy are mild and that pregnancy in itself may not be a problem. However, in those with pre-existing disorders, it may be that adjustment is more difficult, stress is dealt with inappropriately, and the patient's circumstances are particularly adverse. Some may lack a supportive partner, be impoverished, poorly compliant, self-neglecting or abused. Psychiatric disorder is not a contraindication to motherhood nor to effective, loving parenting. However, it is likely to be more problematic and require increased support during pregnancy, analogous to physical disability.

While the core disorder is difficult to change, we know that people with personality disorders cope less well with stressful situations and are more likely to develop comorbid mental illnesses which may not respond to treatment. Pregnancy and motherhood may represent just such increased stress, and women with personality problems are likely to require increased support to strengthen coping skills and prevent onset of mental illness. Maladaptive behaviours such as substance misuse or deliberate self-harm often lessen in pregnancy, due to maternal interest in the baby's welfare. If not reduced, however, there are particular concerns about the baby's welfare, and specialist expertise may be required.

Predicting the course of illness during pregnancy in women who suffer from pre-existing psychiatric disorder is fraught with difficulty. There are often specific concerns in deciding about the appropriateness of maintenance medication; for most women with enduring mental illness, such discussions should take place with their psychiatrist or general practitioner well in advance of conception. It hardly needs saying that the presence of mental illness per se does not mean a woman cannot make informed reproductive decisions. All too often, however, she is not given this opportunity. Mental health services, and ideally, specialist perinatal services, should be involved early in the antenatal care of women with these disorders. Good communication between the obstetric team, general practitioner and psychiatric team, alongside close collaboration with social services as appropriate, will optimise the perinatal outcomes for both mother and baby.

Bipolar affective disorder

Women with bipolar affective disorder are likely to be on maintenance therapy. There are teratogenic risks associated with most mood stabilisers, but a high risk of relapse on discontinuation. Pregnancy itself does not confer protection against relapse. Decisions regarding continuation of treatment should be made on an individual basis and always with the woman's fully informed involvement. Factors such as the previous natural history of the disorder (number, severity and time interval between episodes of illness) and response to previous treatment discontinuations, will help in reaching a decision on discontinuing maintenance treatment during pregnancy, reinstating it after the first trimester, or continuing throughout.

Pre-existing bipolar disorder is one of the greatest risk factors for puerperal psychosis — recent studies estimate that over 60% of women with bipolar disorder will experience relapse in the first 6 postnatal months if not taking mood-stabilising agents (Viguera et al 2000). Irrespective of decisions about medication during pregnancy, all women should be offered prophylactic medication (usually lithium) immediately following delivery. It is important to remember that, unlike with schizophrenia, there is little evidence that bipolar women are any less able to care appropriately for their children, except during the acute phase of the illness.

Schizophrenia

There is some evidence to suggest that the fertility of women with enduring severe mental illnesses such as schizophrenia is not dissimilar to that of the general population (Lane et al 1995). Their fertility may be increasing as a result of the increasing use of novel antipsychotic medications, which have a lower propensity to suppress ovulation. Women who switch from older drugs may not be aware of this and may place themselves inadvertently at risk of unwanted pregnancy. The outcome for a mother with schizophrenia who remains the primary carer for her child is often unfavourable, leading to great distress for the mother and for those (including health professionals) who support her. Appropriate supports, including social services, should be engaged at an early stage in pregnancy to ensure sufficient help is available to the mother and her family. It is often difficult for women with schizophrenia to cope with the frequent contact with health professionals during pregnancy, and there is a risk that they receive suboptimal care. Advance planning will also help reduce this risk.

Most women with schizophrenia will be on maintenance antipsychotic medication. The implications of relapse during pregnancy are severe for both mother and child, and, unless there are strong reasons to the contrary, treatment should continue, with appropriate monitoring, throughout pregnancy. In general, if antipsychotic medication is prescribed, high-potency drugs such as trifluoperazine are preferable because of lowered risk of hypotension. Difficult decisions may have to be made regarding the relative advantages and problems associated with continuing a well-established depot regimen or switching to oral medication, which has the advantage of increased flexibility of dosage and faster elimination should difficulties arise.

Depressive and anxiety disorders

The major issues relating to antenatal depressive illness have been outlined above. A past history of depressive illness is one of the strongest risk factors for antenatal depression, which in turn is predictive of postnatal depression (Box 31.1). 10% of pregnant women meet diagnostic criteria for depressive illness, but it remains under-diagnosed and treated.

Box 31.1 Factors associated with increased risk of antenatal anxiety or depression
• Past history of depression or anxiety disorder • Younger age • Previous stillbirth or miscarriage • Other life events

The available research suggests a variable impact of pregnancy on premorbid anxiety states. The possible anxiolytic impact of progesterone may be counterbalanced by the physiological changes in respiratory function during pregnancy, leading to an increased propensity to panic.

- Case-control and epidemiological data suggest that the pre-pregnancy severity of panic disorder is the best predictor of its course during pregnancy. Panic, as with other anxiety disorders, often worsens in the puerperium, even in those patients who have managed to discontinue anxiolytic medication during pregnancy.
- Most of the evidence available on obsessive–compulsive disorder (OCD) in pregnancy is gathered from retrospective studies or case reports. The perinatal period seems to increase the risk of onset or exacerbation of OCD. Generally there is a good response to treatment with SSRIs.
- There are few data available on the impact of pregnancy on generalised anxiety disorders or previous post-traumatic stress disorder (PTSD). An uncontrolled cohort study reported that 20% of women whose previous child was stillborn had PTSD in the third trimester of the subsequent pregnancy (Turton et al 2001). Associated risk factors were conception within 1 year of the stillbirth and a perceived lack of emotional support around the time of the loss. The majority of cases had remitted without treatment within 1 year of the subsequent delivery. Cases of PTSD following particularly traumatic deliveries have also been described.

Non-pharmacological treatments include *cognitive therapy* and *behavioural techniques* such as anxiety management, teaching the patient about the nature and genesis of symptoms, and engaging in relaxation exercises to reverse them. Drug treatments include SSRI antidepressants. Beta-blockers should be avoided given the potential risks of intrauterine growth retardation (IUGR) and adverse neonatal cardiorespiratory effects. The risks and benefits of prescribing medications during pregnancy or lactation are discussed below.

Eating disorders

Most studies suggest that eating disorder symptoms tend to improve in pregnancy. Conversely, the postnatal period tends to be associated with a worsening of symptoms, as well as an increased risk of postnatal depression. With regard to the impact of a pre-existing eating disorder on the pregnancy, the limited literature available suggests that women with active eating disorders are at increased risk of miscarriage, fetal abnormalities and smaller birth weights.

The fertility of *anorexic* women is reduced to one-third of normal. They also have an increased risk of obstetric complications including hypertension, forceps delivery and caesarean section and are more vulnerable to depressive illness. Additional areas of concern are the potential impact of insufficient nutritional intake on the developing fetus and problematic interactions around feeding during infancy.

Patients with *bulimia nervosa* may have reduced fertility if associated with polycystic ovarian disease. The nausea of early pregnancy may exacerbate pre-existing bulimia, and this needs to be considered in the differential diagnosis of hyperemesis gravidarum. In a retrospective study of 96 women who were actively bulimic during pregnancy, there was a reduction in bulimic behaviours with each trimester (Morgan et al 1999). Although one-third of the patients were no longer bulimic in the postnatal period, more than half of the sample reported a deterioration in symptoms to worse than pre-pregnancy levels. Those most vulnerable to relapse had

- a history of anorexia nervosa;
- an unplanned pregnancy;
- more severe symptoms at conception which persisted into the second trimester.

The authors suggest a greatly increased risk of postnatal depression, particularly if there is associated alcohol misuse or a history of anorexia and recommend that all postnatal bulimic women be screened for this.

Substance use disorders

Substance misuse is escalating in our society, with some of the greatest increases reported in young women of childbearing age. Such women with alcohol or drug problems often engage poorly with antenatal care, and their impaired physical health, as well as increased exposure to HIV and hepatitis, places them and their pregnancy at risk.

Alcohol Excessive use of alcohol is relatively rare in pregnancy As with other maladaptive behaviours, it tends to decrease during the antenatal period. Alcohol misuse may give rise to a number of physical complications for the woman, which may threaten or complicate pregnancy. These include nutritional deficiencies, liver and pancreatic disease. Withdrawal complications such as delirium tremens and seizures may also have adverse consequences. Excessive alcohol use is associated with disturbed organogenesis in early pregnancy, and intrauterine growth retardation and neurodevelopmental delay in later pregnancy. Other teratogenic effects include abnormalities of the cardiac and urogenital systems, as well as eye, ear and limb anomalies. The combination, *fetal alcohol syndrome* (FAS), was first described by Jones & Smith in 1973 (Box 31.2)

The classic triad of FAS as originally described did not include neurobehavioural problems. This led to the introduction of the term *fetal alcohol effects* (FAE), referring to behavioural problems presenting in children exposed to alcohol in utero but who do not show typical features of FAS. These children have better cognitive but similar behavioural problems and poor adaptability compared with children with FAS. There is some evidence that FAE may overlap with attention deficit disorders. The direct impact of alcohol on the fetus is unclear, as it is confounded by so many variables, including poor nutrition, cigarette smoking, other drugs and adverse social circumstances. However, it is likely that the more frequent the high-dose use of alcohol in pregnancy, the greater the fetal harm (Plant et al 1999). Babies of mothers who are alcohol dependent may also develop alcohol withdrawal symptoms after birth.

Other drug use effects vary depending on the properties of the specific drug, although it is important to recognise that patients

---

> **Box 31.2 Fetal alcohol syndrome**
>
> *Facial anomalies*
> - Short palpebral fissures
> - Premaxillary — long upper lip, flattened philtrum, flat midface, maxillary hypoplasia
>
> *Growth retardation*
> - Low birth weight
> - Decelerating weight gain disproportionate to nutritional deficits
> - Low weight:height ratio
>
> *Abnormal CNS development*
> - Microcephaly
> - Structural brain abnormalities
> - Neurological hard/soft signs — neurosensory deafness, impaired fine motor skills, impaired hand–eye coordination
>
> From Jones & Smith (1973)

---

may frequently use a combination of substances, and research in the area is not extensive. The possible link between exposure to benzodiazepines in early pregnancy and oral cleft anomalies was examined in a meta-analysis (Dolovich et al 1998). Pooled data from case-control studies showed an increased risk for fetal major malformations or oral cleft if the mother had been exposed to benzodiazepines in at least the first trimester. However, there was no such association in pooled data from cohort studies. Based on our current level of knowledge, the authors advise ultrasonography to look for visible forms of oral cleft in an exposed fetus. A summary of the evidence for the impact of particular drugs of misuse is given in Table 31.1.

Pregnant women who misuse drugs should receive specialist support, with the aim of stabilising, minimising or stopping their use. Abrupt discontinuation of drug use is not recommended. There is no good evidence at present to support maintenance prescribing of benzodiazepines during pregnancy. A review of the role of methadone emphasises the overall advantages to the fetus of methadone substitution of opiates, despite the potential for more prolonged withdrawal states (Ward et al 1999). Continued use of heroin suggests a bad prognosis. For women addicted to opiates:

- first-trimester stabilisation on methadone, without illicit drug use, is the aim;
- reduction is safest to consider in the second trimester;
- further stability of prescription in the last trimester is desirable to avoid triggering premature delivery.

Motivation to change is usually greatly increased during pregnancy, which, combined with increased healthcare input and support, may allow significant change at a crucial time. Early, proactive involvement of social work services is essential.

Medically unexplained symptoms (MUS) in pregnancy

Patients with a past history of MUS may present frequently with physical complaints during pregnancy. Somatoform disorders presenting with gastrointestinal symptoms such as abdominal pain or nausea are often managed very differently in pregnancy, because of a failure to take a careful history or review medical case notes. This is likely to result in multiple hospital admissions and unnecessary investigations if the underlying disorder is unrecognised. Factitious disorders may also present during pregnancy, e.g. factitious hyperglycaemia, vaginal bleeding or premature rupture of membranes.

Table 31.1 Possible effects on the fetus of substance misuse in pregnancy

Drug	Teratogenic effects	Fetal/neonatal effects	Neurobehavioural sequelae	Comments
Alcohol	Fetal alcohol syndrome Urogenital and cardiac malformations	IUGR Alcohol withdrawal symptoms	Fetal alcohol effects not attenuated by age	
Nicotine	No evidence	Miscarriage, IUGR, premature delivery	Unknown	Reduces placental blood flow
Benzodiazepines	Oral clefts	Withdrawal — mild: 'floppy infant' — severe: apnoeic episodes, impaired thermoregulation	Unlikely, data sparse	Withdrawal generally presents 10 days post delivery and may last for months
Cannabis	No conclusive evidence	Dose related IURG + premature delivery Withdrawal: jittery, crying, altered responses to light	Possible (slower visual responsiveness at 4 yr)	Strongly associated with alcohol and tobacco use
Amphetamines	Animals: CVS anomalies Humans: inconclusive	Miscarriage, IUGR, premature delivery Withdrawal: irritable, hypotonic, respiratory distress	Impaired scholastic ability at 14 yr	
Heroin	Unlikely	IUGR, decreased head circumference, premature delivery, raised PMR Withdrawal (affects 40–80%): tremor, sneezing, diarrhoea, impaired feeding, high pitched cry, seizures, coma	Impaired organisation and perception skills in preschool children	Postnatal environment more important than antenatal for developmental progess
Methadone	No evidence	IUGR, decreased head circumference, raised PMR, SIDS Withdrawal more severe and prolonged than with heroin (days to months)	Behavioural problems but not cognitive or social difficulties	Overall reduced adverse outcomes relative to heroin use
Cocaine	Possible orogenital and cranial anomalies	Intracranial haemorrhage, abruptio placentae, SIDS, IUGR, premature delivery Withdrawal less severe than with opiates	Impaired comprehension and expression language in 1–6 year olds	Non-dependent use not associated with adverse effects for infant

CVS, cardiovascular system; IUGR, intrauterine growth retardation; PMR, perinatal mortality rate; SIDS, sudden infant death syndrome.
NB: Many patients will be abusing a number of drugs concurrently.

The same issues arise as in usual management, but there are particular concerns with respect to subsequent child-care and a need to consider early involvement of social services. A review of the literature described a series of 18 case reports of Münchausen syndrome involving obstetric patients (Edi-Osagie et al 1997) but no systematic studies are available.

PUERPERIUM

Normal emotional changes in the puerperium

Postnatal blues

Postnatal or maternity blues affects 50–80% of women. This is a mild and self-limiting condition with onset typically in the first postnatal week (though generally not in the first couple of days), resolving within 1–2 weeks. The most common symptoms include labile mood, tearfulness, insomnia, fatigue and irritability. Preparation in antenatal classes, and reassurance and increased support from professionals, family and friends are all that is required,

but severe blues may progress to postnatal depression. Increased anxiety and depression in the third trimester predicts postnatal blues, but no association has been found with obstetric variables. Similarly, no replicated evidence exists to link postnatal blues with psychosocial variables. While it has been assumed that the rapid falls in oestrogen and progesterone occurring around the same time are responsible, research evidence to support this remains poor. Miller & Rukstalis (1999) have postulated that the blues represent a period of heightened emotional reactivity analogous to the oxytocin-related inducement of maternal behaviour in other mammals, and that it is therefore an adaptive and normal response which facilitates mother–infant attachment. This hypothesis awaits testing.

Psychiatric disorders arising in the puerperium

Classification of disorders relating to childbirth

Traditionally, disorders specific to childbirth have been divided into three categories: postnatal blues, postnatal depression and puerperal psychosis. Postnatal blues can, however, be regarded as a normal variation of emotional change occurring after childbirth. Since the original descriptions of postnatal depression and puerperal psychosis, there has been much debate about whether or not these conditions are distinct from depression and psychosis occurring at other times. ICD-10 only allows categorisation if criteria for other psychiatric disorders are not met, and DSM-IV, despite providing codings to denote a relationship to pregnancy or childbirth, also tends to play down any distinctive differences. It can be argued that this has led to under-recognition of these disorders, provides a barrier to effective research and communication, and ignores recent evidence in favour of distinctive features in aetiology, presentation and treatment. Recommendations for remedying this problem have emerged from a workshop on the classification of postnatal mood disorders (Paykel 1999).

Puerperal psychosis

Epidemiology and clinical features Psychotic disorders arise after 1 in 500–1000 births. Although the absolute risk for any woman is low, relative to other times in a woman's life, this period carries the highest risk (Fig. 31.1). A study examining first-episode bipolar disorder reported a seven-fold risk occurring in the 2nd to 28th day after delivery (Terp & Mortensen 1998). The illness has its onset in the early postnatal period, usually within the first month, but not commonly in the first 1–2 days. Organic causes are now very rare in the developed world. While the majority of cases are affective in nature, several studies describe atypical presenting features such as mixed affective state and confusion (Wisner et al 1994). Non-affective or schizophrenic presentations are much less common. Typically, the presentation is one of rapid fluctuations of mood (often a mixture of manic and depressive symptoms), perplexity, confusion and markedly altered behaviour. Ideas of self-

harm may be driven by delusions of guilt, self-worthlessness or hopelessness. Delusional ideas may arise in relation to the baby, and, while thoughts of harm concerning the baby or other children are rare, enquiry should always be made as part of the assessment.

With appropriate treatment most women will make a complete recovery but remain at very high risk of future puerperal episodes. The risk of future non-puerperal episodes may be even greater — estimated at over 60% in some studies.

Aetiology Several factors have been identified that significantly increase the risk of puerperal psychosis. Of greatest importance are:

- a past history of puerperal psychosis;
- a previous or family history (first or second degree relatives) of bipolar affective disorder.

Studies have consistently shown that women with a previous history of puerperal psychosis or bipolar disorder have a 20–30% risk of puerperal recurrence, but the risk rises to over 50% when family history is also a contributing factor. The strong association with bipolar disorder implies a genetic predisposition, and recent evidence has emerged of a specific familial risk for puerperal episodes in bipolar disorder (Jones & Craddock 2001). Attempts have been made to identify gene loci that may account for this risk, and variations at the serotonin transporter gene have been implicated. The characteristically dramatic, early presentation is also suggestive of a link with major hormonal changes after childbirth. It has been hypothesised that the rapid reduction in oestrogen levels is linked to the development of dopamine receptor supersensitivity, which in turn may trigger the onset of psychosis in genetically predisposed individuals (Wieck et al 1991). Apart from primiparity, no other obstetric factors have been consistently shown to increase risk of puerperal psychosis.

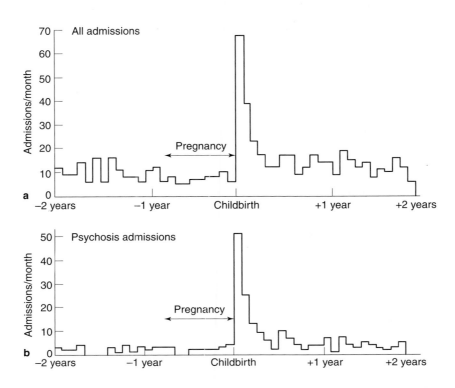

Fig. 31.1
Temporal relationship between psychiatric admission and childbirth: (a) all admissions; (b) psychosis admissions. (From Kendell et al 1987.)

Management Most patients will require admission to hospital, although some may be managed at home if specialised community services are available to provide intensive support for mother, baby and family. If facilities are available, her baby will usually accompany her, ensuring that mother and baby remain together during this critical attachment period. Where admission to a specialised mother and baby unit is not possible, decisions about admitting the baby are much more difficult and must take into account the impact of the mother's mental illness on her ability to act as main carer for her baby, the nature of other patients' illnesses and levels of disturbance, and ward structure and facilities in protecting and meeting the needs of the child.

While the evidence base for biological treatments specific to puerperal psychosis is poor, it is reasonable to extrapolate from knowledge of effective interventions for bipolar disorder occurring at other times. Pharmacological treatment consists of a combination of antipsychotic medication, antidepressants or mood stabilizers depending on the predominant symptoms. The issue of medication choice in relation to breast-feeding is dealt with below. Electroconvulsive therapy is an effective, safe and rapid treatment. Recovery usually takes place over a period of 1–2 months but there is great individual variation.

Postnatal depression

Epidemiology and clinical features In contrast to puerperal psychosis, non-psychotic depression often presents later in the postnatal period, with a peak occurrence at around 6 weeks. Early reports suggesting that the disorder might be specific to western cultures have not been borne out by recent research. While there is some evidence of an increase in the incidence of depression in the early postnatal weeks, a meta-analysis of the literature found that the overall prevalence of 10–15% in the first year is not very different from the prevalence of mild to moderate depression at any other time in a woman's life (O'Hara & Swain 1996). This apparent contradiction is explained by the finding that, on average, postnatal depressions have a shorter duration than those at other times. Untreated, however, more than 10% have a course running longer than 6 months. Similarly, the symptoms of depression in the postnatal period do not differ greatly from those at other times. Obsessional symptoms may be prominent and, while not occurring in a greater proportion of patients, are more frequent and distressing when they do occur. They may take the form of obsessional fears of causing harm to the baby. Much less commonly, there may be true infanticidal thoughts. Thoughts of self-harm are not uncommon and should be followed up with sensitive enquiry as to their depth and strength.

A recent review of the qualitative evidence distilled four essential themes from the mothers' experiences of postnatal depression (Beck 2002). These related to:

- an incongruity between expectations and reality of motherhood;
- a spiralling downward of negative feelings;
- a pervasive sense of loss of control, sense of self, and relationships;
- admitting a need for help, leading to reintegration and change.

Consequences for the child and family Untreated postnatal depression gives rise to disturbed mother–infant interaction and may result in adverse effects on child development. Depressed mothers give more negative responses in their interactions with their infants, and there may be a consequent detrimental influence on language skills, social and emotional development in the first year of life and insecure attachments at 18 months. In the longer term, evidence is mounting for ongoing cognitive impairment, especially in boys (Murray & Cooper 1997). These effects have been demonstrated up to the age of 11 years, and there appears to be a critical period in infant development, within the first year, where maternal depression, and the consequent disturbed mother–infant interaction, exerts this detrimental effect (Hay et al 2001).

There may also be associated adverse effects on other family members, with higher rates of depression reported in partners of postnatally depressed women. This in turn reduces the available compensatory supports for the child.

Aetiology Unlike puerperal psychosis, where risks are largely biological, *psychosocial factors* play a greater part in the development of postnatal depression (see Box 31.3). Those emerging from a meta-analysis (O'Hara & Swain 1996) of the evidence include:

- past history of depression;
- psychological problems during pregnancy;
- poor social support and marital relationship;
- recent adverse life events.

Less consistently, associations have been found with obstetric complications, a history of abuse, lower socio-economic status and perception of poor obstetric experience. Baby blues, if severe, may also increase risk, and there is an association between early lowered mood and the subsequent development of depressive symptoms. Unfortunately, these risk factors have low specificity and so cannot be used to accurately predict the development of depression in any one individual. It is also important to consider the effect of infant temperament on the mother, such that a particularly irritable or hypertonic baby may maintain or exacerbate a postnatal depressive episode.

Biological mechanisms are, however, important. A prior history of depression may of course exert its influence via biological or psychosocial mechanisms. One follow-up study compared postnatal depression, arising as the first episode of depression, with women who had postnatal depression following prior episodes of non-childbirth related depression. Those with 'pure' postnatal illness were at greater risk of subsequent postnatal episodes but

---

Box 31.3   Risk factors for postnatal depression and puerperal psychosis

Risk factors for postnatal depession
- Past history of depression
- Psychological problems during pregnancy
- Poor social support and marital relationship
- Recent adverse life events
- Severe baby blues

Weaker associations with:
- Obstetric complications
- History of abuse
- Lower socio-economic status
- Perception of poor obstetric experience

Risk factors for puerperal psychosis
- Past history of puerperal psychosis
- Pre-existing bipolar disorder
- Family history of puerperal psychosis or bipolar disorder

not of depression at other times, suggesting a specificity at least for a subtype of postnatal depression (Cooper & Murray 1995). Links have also been made to thyroid dysfunction either during pregnancy or in the postnatal period. Some studies have found an association with the presence of thyroperoxidase antibodies in pregnancy, but others have found no clear link. Oestrogen and progesterone changes occurring around parturition have also been suggested as possible triggers for postnatal depression, but no consistent abnormalities of sex hormones have been found.

Management The majority of depressions occurring at this time are mild and do not require specific psychiatric intervention. Most will be uncovered during routine postnatal screening by the general practitioner or health visitor. The provision of extra support and non-directive counselling by suitably trained primary healthcare workers (such as health visitors in the UK) has been shown in randomised trials to be effective in reducing depression when compared with routine care (Holden et al 1989, Wickberg & Hwang 1996). A variety of other psychological interventions have been described, but few demonstrate clear effectiveness. Cooper & Murray (1997) randomly assigned postnatally depressed women to one of three interventions (non-directive counselling, cognitive-behaviour therapy or dynamic psychotherapy) or routine primary care. They found an equally beneficial effect from each of the three interventions but, by 9 months, spontaneous recovery in the control group negated any differences. A further randomised trial showed benefits for an approach using interpersonal therapy (O'Hara et al 2000).

Other approaches demonstrated to be effective in randomised controlled trials include interventions providing help to the woman and her family. Support groups involving the woman and her partner have been shown to benefit both. Training the mother in infant massage produced improvements both in the woman's mood and in mother–infant interaction. These findings highlight the need to consider other members of the family when planning care.

In more severe disorders, or where psychological therapies are not available, drug treatments may be the preferred option. Studies have shown, however, that women with postnatal depression are often reluctant to consider antidepressant medication because of breastfeeding or concerns that side-effects will impair their ability to cope with childcare. Although it may be reasonable to assume that depression in the postnatal period will respond in the same way as depressions at other times, there are few investigations directed specifically at pharmacotherapies for postnatal depression. One randomised trial comparing cognitive-behavioural counselling with fluoxetine found an equal (though not additive) benefit from both (Appleby et al 1997). An open study judged sertraline to be a well-tolerated and effective treatment (Stowe et al 1995).

Suggestions of a link with hormonal changes have led some investigators to examine sex hormones as treatment. Despite early claims for a beneficial effect of synthetic progestogens, no conclusive evidence exists for their use, and they may, in fact, be associated with mood lowering. Oestrogen therapy was examined in a placebo-controlled trial in chronic, severe postnatal depression (Gregoire et al 1996). Oestrogen patches delivering 200 mg of 17 beta-oestradiol daily (with cyclical progesterone) were shown to bring about a faster and greater response. There is a need for caution, however, as there are significant risks associated with exogenous oestrogens in the early postnatal period. A Cochrane review of such treatments to date concludes that further research in this area is difficult because of these risks (Lawrie et al 2000).

Anxiety / obsessive–compulsive disorder

Pre-existing anxiety and panic disorder is likely to worsen in the postnatal period. If this history is known, preventative interventions (using SSRI antidepressants or cognitive-behaviour therapy) can be instigated prophylactically after delivery. There is also case report evidence of severe obsessional disorders arising postnatally (Sichel et al 1993). These are often associated with distressing thoughts of harm toward the infant and may lead to obsessional avoidance. Depressive symptoms usually follow. Again, SSRI antidepressants are effective in management.

Disorders of attachment

Brockington (1996) describes disturbances in mother–infant attachment manifesting as delayed development of the maternal response, hostility toward or rejection of the infant, as a significant area of neglect in perinatal psychiatry. Although usually associated with depressive symptoms, it may be independently related to unwanted pregnancy, infant temperament or illness, obstetric complications or other psychiatric disorder in the mother. Essential elements of care include maintaining mother–infant contact (unless there is clear risk to the child) and treating any underlying illness in the mother.

Infanticide

While child murder is more often committed by men than women, the younger the child, the more likely it is that the perpetrator will be the mother. Thus almost all cases of infanticide in the firs 24 hours (neonaticide) are caused by the mother, as are the majority of cases in the first 3 months of life (Oates 1997). Neonaticide is more commonly associated with young, inexperienced, single women and concealed pregnancies and deliveries. However, in mothers who kill their children after the first 24 hours, a significant minority suffer from severe mental illness, including puerperal psychosis, schizophrenia or depression, or from a personality disorder (D'Orban 1979). While infanticide is rare, it must always be considered as part of the risk assessment in women with postnatal mental illness. The safety of the child must be paramount in any management plan.

PSYCHOTROPICS DURING PREGNANCY AND BREASTFEEDING

Pregnancy

There is an understandable and justified caution about prescribing drugs to pregnant and breastfeeding women. Occasionally, however, there is need to relieve significant distress and disability in such women with mental illness. In addition, women of childbearing age are increasingly taking prescribed psychotropic medication at the time of conception, and sudden discontinuation may have its own attendant risks. General principles governing prescribing in pregnancy are outlined in Box 31.4.

Current evidence of adverse fetal effects is gleaned from case reports or retrospective analyses due to the ethical difficulties of conducting randomised controlled trials during pregnancy. While we can be more confident of evidence regarding major teratogenic effects and neonatal discontinuation symptoms, evidence remains scant in relation to prediction of long-term neurodevelopmental risk.

Drugs may also be less effective in pregnancy for a number of reasons.

- First, *physiological changes* increase the volume of distribution and renal clearance of drugs, resulting in altered pharmacokinetics. As a result, the dosages of certain drugs such as lithium and tricyclic antidepressants may require adjustment.
- Second, *reduced compliance* related to fears of harming the fetus means that up to 50% of pregnant women would not comply with a course of medication as prescribed by their doctor (Butters & Howie 1990). Therefore it is very important to engage in early, collaborative discussions with patients, ensuring thoughtful weighing of risks of fetal exposure against risks of discontinuation.

Drug treatments

Antidepressants Austin & Mitchell (1998) carried out a qualitative systematic review of the literature on adverse effects associated with the use of psychotropic medication in pregnancy. Of a total of 23 studies, 9 were prospective, with most of the reliable evidence relating to antidepressant medication. In the first trimester, they found no evidence of increased risk of major malformations or spontaneous abortion with most tricyclic and SSRI antidepressants. Both groups may be associated with a small increased risk of minor anomalies, prematurity and neonatal problems, although the studies were unable to discriminate between the impact of the depressive illness itself and potential drug effects. A tricyclic antidepressant (TCAD) or SSRI drug does not need to be withdrawn as a matter of routine in early pregnancy. It is important to consider the risks of sudden discontinuation of an antidepressant, including withdrawal phenomena (agitation, insomnia, anxiety and mood disturbance) and relapse of illness. Monoamine oxidase inhibitors are teratogenic in animals and, with little information from human studies available, should be avoided. There is also little information available on the impact of newer antidepressants such as venlafaxine or mirtezapine to date. In a well-controlled study of children exposed to fluoxetine or TCADs in pregnancy there was no evidence of impaired intelligence, growth, language or behavioural development over a 4-year follow-up period (Nulman et al 1997).

Antipsychotics The evidence is less comprehensive for antipsychotic drugs, with most data available for chlorpromazine and trifluoperazine. The majority of these studies relate to the low dose use of phenothiazines as an antiemetic in early pregnancy, with little information available on the impact of the higher doses necessary to treat psychotic illness. In a review of the literature on psychotropic drugs in pregnancy, the authors pooled the data from five studies of phenothiazine use (Altschuler et al 1996). They concluded that psychotic disorder itself may confer the greatest risk to the fetus, estimating a small increased risk of 0.4% of congenital anomalies directly due to the medication. There does not appear to be an effect on cognitive function in early childhood. In general, older preparations are preferable. Many consider that the reduced risks of side-effects, such as hypotension, with high-potency neuroleptics outweigh the potential risk of extrapyramidal symptoms requiring anticholinergic medication. Depot medication should be avoided if possible during pregnancy. However, the risks of discontinuation in women with schizophrenia are so significant that continuation throughout pregnancy may be warranted. Although preliminary data for olanzapine and clozapine are encouraging, there is currently insufficient information available to recommend their use in pregnancy.

Mood stabilisers Mood-stabilising drugs, such as lithium, carbamazepine and sodium valproate, which are used to prevent recurrence in women with bipolar affective disorder, have clear teratogenic risks. However, the risks for lithium have been overestimated in the past, based on retrospective data collection with a resultant bias toward reporting of abnormalities (Schou 1990). Lithium is associated with three times the risk of any congenital abnormality and an eight-fold risk of a cardiac malformation, particularly Ebstein's anomaly, a cardiac defect involving the tricuspid valve. However the absolute risk of this is estimated at 1 in 1000 pregnancies (0.1%). The UK National Teratology Information Service suggest that the average risk of congenital abnormalities (2–3%) rises to 10% in a woman taking lithium during pregnancy (Williams & Oke 2000). A woman taking lithium during her pregnancy therefore has a 90% chance of having a healthy baby. This needs to be counterbalanced against the consequences of discontinuation, which may be severe in women with unstable or frequently relapsing bipolar disorder. Individual judgement, with the woman making informed decisions on her care, should be made case by case under psychiatric supervision. A detailed ultrasound including fetal echocardiography should be carried out at 16–20 weeks if lithium is prescribed in the first trimester. If taken in later pregnancy there are potential risks of hypothyroidism, nephrogenic diabetes insipidus, polyhydramnios and 'floppy baby syndrome' in the neonate. Williams & Oke (2000) have developed a useful, clinically based algorithm on how to prescribe lithium during pregnancy.

Most of the evidence relating to the impact of alternative mood stabilisers in pregnancy comes from the literature on epilepsy. The risk of neural tube defects is greater with sodium valproate (risk 1–5%), especially at daily doses over 1 g, than with carbamazepine (risk 0.5–1%). Despite a lack of research in this area it has been suggested that high-dose folate (4 mg/day) prescription should be considered for all women of reproductive age who are taking these anticonvulsants (Taylor et al 2001). Other congenital malformations reported include cardiac and craniofacial anomalies. Synergistic teratogenicity seems to be a particular risk, affecting up to 1 in 6 pregnancies if multiple anticonvulsants are used, hence polypharmacy should be avoided. Maternal serum alpha-fetoprotein levels and a detailed ultrasound scan at 18 weeks should be carried out on pregnant women taking these medications. There are no reliable data regarding the use of lamotrigine in pregnancy to date, although animal studies have not shown evidence of teratogenic effects.

Beyond the first trimester, the main concerns relating to psychotropic prescribing are perinatal complications and potential long-term neurobehavioural sequelae. In most cases, symptoms of neonatal withdrawal or toxicity can be minimised by a slow reduction in dosage over the last month to 6 weeks, with reinstatement after delivery. Again this needs to be balanced against the risk of relapse around the time of delivery. All neonates exposed to such drugs should be monitored for withdrawal effects, which can be minimised by breastfeeding.

ECT is a very effective and relatively safe treatment for severe or psychotic depression during pregnancy, in both normal and high-risk pregnancies, when careful attention is paid to obstetric and anaesthetic factors. In a review of 300 case reports, Miller (1994) advises on appropriate preparations, including intravenous hydration, elevation of the patient's right hip and external fetal cardiac monitoring. They reported an overall low rate of ECT-related complications and no cases of premature labour.

Breastfeeding

The many benefits of breastfeeding for both mother and infant include enhanced maternal bonding, improved infant immunity, and reduced fetal withdrawal symptoms if a mother has taken psychotropic medication during the antenatal period. These need to be weighed against the advantages of bottle feeding, which leads to less disturbed sleep, increased practical support from others and the avoidance of transmitted drugs through breast milk. All psychotropic medication passes into breast milk, generally at 1% of the maternal serum level. In a recent review, Burt and colleagues found no controlled studies in this area and relied on case reports or small case series as a basis for their treatment guidelines (Burt et al 2001). There is also a dearth of information regarding the longer-term impact of such drugs on the developing infant.

There are a number of general clinical issues worth emphasising.

- Drugs or breastfeeding should be avoided if the baby is vulnerable by reason of prematurity or renal, hepatic, cardiac or neurological impairment.
- If possible, prescribe the medication as a single daily dose after the baby's longest feed and before its longest sleep.
- Close monitoring of the baby's behaviour as well as appropriate blood tests are necessary.
- Sedating medications should be avoided.

There is little evidence of short-term adverse effects on the breast-fed infant from TCAD (except doxepin) and SSRI antidepressants, and no contraindication to breastfeeding providing the baby is healthy and its progress monitored. However, sudden discontinuation of breastfeeding (or of the tablets by the mother) may lead to withdrawal symptoms in the infant. Paroxetine has the lowest milk/plasma ratio of the SSRIs but also the shortest half-life, increasing the risk of withdrawal effects in the infant if suddenly discontinued.

Given the same provisos, antipsychotic prescribing may also be compatible with breastfeeding. Again, lower doses of older drugs such as chlorpromazine, haloperidol or trifluoperazine are advised. Breastfeeding should be avoided with benzodiazepine use, unless the woman has taken this throughout pregnancy. In this case, breastfeeding will protect the infant against withdrawal symptoms. Women who require lithium should not breastfeed, because of the high concentration in breast milk leading to a risk of toxicity in the baby. Valproate or carbamazepine are the preferred mood stabilisers in a breastfeeding mother.

SCREENING AND PREVENTION

Antenatal screening

Puerperal psychosis

Antenatal screening for the specific risk factors associated with puerperal psychosis is straightforward. There are few other conditions in psychiatry where such high risk is concentrated in such a brief time period. All women should be asked about a past history of puerperal psychosis and past or family history of bipolar disorder at an early stage in their pregnancy. The best opportunity occurs when attending the initial booking clinic. Ideally, women with positive risk factors for puerperal psychosis should have antenatal psychiatric contact to assess risk and the value of prophylaxis.

Postnatal depression

Antenatal screening for postnatal depression is less effective, because of the poorer predictive value of the risk factors involved. However, where there is a previous history of depressive illness, whether or not associated with childbearing, the risk of subsequent postnatal depression is doubled — and even higher where the first depressive episode occurred postnatally (Cooper & Murray 1995). Women who are depressed during pregnancy, or who are at significant psychosocial disadvantage, should also be followed up more closely in the postnatal period.

Postnatal screening

Postnatal depression

In the postnatal period, it has become routine in the UK for health visitors to administer the Edinburgh Postnatal Depression Scale (EPDS) at two or three time points in the first 6–8 months. The EPDS is a simple 10-item self-report scale which reliably identifies women at high risk of developing depression (Cox et al 1987). There are several caveats to be observed when the EPDS is used in this way, most importantly that the scale is not a diagnostic instrument and that clinical judgement should always take precedence over any score obtained. Most health visitors are also trained in non-directive counselling techniques, employed in 'listening visits' to women at increased risk. Such extra visits have been shown to lower the rate of progression to depressive illness. To be effective, the EPDS should only be used as part of a programme of care by trained primary-care workers, where there are agreed criteria for its administration, interpretation of results, and referral on for intervention by secondary psychiatric services, where appropriate (National Screening Committee 2002, SIGN 2002).

Prevention

Puerperal psychosis

Two cohort studies have examined the use of lithium, given either in late pregnancy or immediately after delivery to prevent the onset of puerperal psychosis in high-risk women. Stewart et al (1991) in a small open study found that half the expected number developed a puerperal episode when given lithium in the immediate puerperium. A second study found that only 1 of 14 high-risk women who received mood stabilisers became ill compared with

8 of 13 untreated women (Cohen et al 1995). These impressive results have to be tempered by the open nature of the study designs. However, there is also evidence that bipolar women who discontinue lithium during pregnancy have very high rates of puerperal relapse (Viguera et al 2000).

Postnatal depression

There is no current evidence for effective interventions that could be given to all women to prevent the onset of postnatal depression. Measures that target high-risk women are mixed in their results. In one controlled study, first-time mothers identified antenatally as vulnerable to depression had significantly lowered EPDS scores following a parenthood educational programme (Elliot et al 2000). Beneficial effects have also been shown if high-risk women receive interpersonal therapy. However, no specific advantage has been shown for routinely providing home support workers, midwife managed care, postnatal check-ups or any of a range of antenatal interventions. Lastly, while an earlier, uncontrolled trial of antidepressants given prophylactically to prevent the onset of postnatal depression in high-risk women showed a beneficial effect, a recent placebo-controlled trial has not confirmed these findings (Wisner et al 2001).

CONFIDENTIAL ENQUIRY INTO MATERNAL DEATHS

The most recent *Confidential Enquiry into Maternal Deaths* (RCOG 2001) provides a timely reminder of the significance of perinatal illnesses. It identifies suicide as the leading cause of maternal death, once numbers from linkage studies are included. In contrast to female suicides at other times of life, suicides in the postnatal period are characterised by their violent nature (indicating a high degree of intent and likely presence of major mental illness) and wide social class distribution (not being biased toward those with lower socio-economic status). The significance of substance misuse as a contributing factor is also highlighted. Recommendations include:

- avoidance of the term 'postnatal depression' as a generic descriptor for all postnatal illness, as it may give false reassurance regarding the severity of previous episodes of illness;
- the importance of screening for past psychiatric disorder at booking clinics;
- the development of protocols for the management of women at risk of relapse or recurrence of severe mental illness in the postnatal period;
- the need for good communication between disciplines caring for women at this time;
- the availability of specialist perinatal psychiatric services to offer liaison, advice and treatment (including mother & baby admission facilities where appropriate) for all women with, or at risk of, severe postnatal mental illness.

This last recommendation has been influenced by the current ad hoc provision of dedicated services. Only approximately 12 units in the UK have the appropriate facilities and specialist expertise for admitting severely ill mothers and their babies. Research on mother–infant separation dating back more than 50 years demonstrates the clear detrimental effect on infant development (Bowlby 1977). While this cannot be automatically extrapolated to mentally ill mothers, neither do we have any evidence that separating mother and infant is beneficial for either, other than in exceptional cases where the mother may express infanticidal thoughts. Women and staff view the presence of their babies as helpful to their recovery. However, where there is a strong possibility of the mother not remaining the primary carer for her baby in the long run (for instance in some women with schizophrenia), joint admissions may be less helpful. More evaluative research is required in this area.

SUMMARY

Psychiatric disorders occurring coincidentially with or arising in relation to childbirth are common. They may be associated with serious morbidity for women and their families. In many cases effective preventative measures and treatments are available. There remain significant gaps, however, in our understanding of the aetiology of these conditions. A better understanding of hormonal and genetic influences would inform the development of novel treatments. In the immediate future, however, the greatest challenge is to improve rates of prevention, early detection and appropriate treatment for women and their families.

REFERENCES

Altschuler L, Cohen L, Szuba M et al 1996 Pharmacologic management of psychiatric illness during pregnancy: dilemmas and guidelines. American Journal of Psychiatry 153:592–606

Appleby L, Turnbull G 1995 Parasuicide in the first postnatal year. Psychological Medicine 25:1087–1090

Appleby L, Warner R, Whitton A, Faragher B 1997 A controlled study of fluoxetine and cognitive-behavioural counselling in the treatment of postnatal depression. British Medical Journal 314:932–936

Austin M, Mitchell P 1998 Psychotropic medications in pregnant women: treatment dilemmas. Medical Journal of Australia 169:428–431

Beck C 2002 Postpartum depression: a metasynthesis. Qualitative Health Research 12:453–472

Bowlby J 1977 The making and breaking of affectional bonds. I: Aetiology and psychopathology in the light of attachment theory. British Journal of Psychiatry 130:201–210

Brockington I 1996 Motherhood and mental health. Oxford University Press, Oxford

Burt V, Suri R, Altschuler L et al 2001 The use of psychotropic medications during breast-feeding. American Journal of Psychiatry 158:1001–1009

Butters L, Howie C 1990 Awareness among pregnant women of the effect on the fetus of commonly used drugs. Midwifery 6:146–154

Cohen L S, Sichel D A, Robertson L M et al 1995 Postpartum prophylaxis for women with bipolar disorder. American Journal of Psychiatry 152:1641–1645

Cooper P J, Murray L 1995 The course and recurrence of postnatal depression. British Journal of Psychiatry 166:191–195

Cooper P J, Murray L 1997 The impact of psychological treatments of postnatal depression on maternal mood and infant development. In: Murray L, Cooper PJ (eds) Postpartum depression and child development. Guilford Press, London

Cox J L, Holden J M, Sagovsky R 1987 Detection of postnatal depression: development of the 10-item Edinburgh Postnatal Depression Scale. British Journal of Psychiatry 150:782–786

Dolovich L, Addis A, Vaillancourt J et al 1998 Benzodiazepine use in pregnancy and major malformations or oral cleft: meta-analysis of cohort and case-control studies. British Medical Journal 317:839–843

D'Orban P T 1979 Women who kill their children. British Journal of Psychiatry 134:560–571

Edi-Osagie E, Hopkins R, Edi-Osagie N 1997 Munchausen's syndrome in obstetrics and gynaecology: a review. Obstetrical and Gynaecological Survey 53:45–49

Elliot S A, Leverton T J, Sanjack M et al 2000 Promoting mental health after childbirth: a controlled trial of primary prevention of postnatal depression. British Journal of Clinical Psychology 39:223–241

Evans J, Heron J, Francomb H et al 2001 Cohort study of depressed mood during pregnancy and after childbirth. British Medical Journal 323:257–260

Frost M, Condon J 1996 The psychological sequelae of miscarriage: a critical review of the literature. Australia & New Zealand Journal of Psychiatry 30:54–62

Gilchrist A, Hannaford P, Frank P, Kay C 1995 Termination of pregnancy and psychiatric morbidity. British Journal of Psychiatry 167:243–248

Gregoire A J, Kumar R, Everitt B et al 1996 Transdermal oestrogen for treatment of postnatal depression. Lancet 347:930–933

Hansen D, Lou H, Olsen J 2000 Serious life events and congenital malformations: a national study with complete follow-up. Lancet 356:875–880

Hay D F, Pawlby F, Sharp D et al 2001 Intellectual problems shown by 11-year-old children whose mothers had postnatal depression. Journal of Child Psychology and Psychiatry and Allied Disciplines 42:871–889

Hedegaard M, Henriksen T, Sabroe S, Secher N 1993 Psychological distress in pregnancy and preterm delivery. British Medical Journal 307:234–239

Hofberg K, Brockington I 2000 Tokophobia: an unreasoning dread of childbirth. British Journal of Psychiatry 176:83–85

Holden J M, Sagovsky R, Cox J L 1989 Counselling in a general practice setting: a controlled study of health visitor intervention in treatment of postnatal depression. British Medical Journal 298:223–226

Hughes P, Turton P, Hopper E, Evans C 2002 Assessment of guidelines for good practice in psychosocial care of mothers after stillbirth: a cohort study. Lancet 360:114–118

Jewkes R 2002 Preventing domestic violence. British Medical Journal 324:253–254

Jones I, Craddock N 2001 Familiality of the puerperal trigger in bipolar disorder: results of a family study. American Journal of Psychiatry 158:913–917

Jones K, Smith D 1973 Recognition of the fetal alcohol syndrome in early infancy. Lancet ii:999–1001

Kendell R, Chalmers J, Platz C 1987 Epidemiology of puerperal psychosis. British Journal of Psychiatry 150:662–673

Klein H 1991 Couvade syndrome: male counterpart to pregnancy. International Journal of Psychiatry in Medicine 21:57–69

Lane A, Byrne M, Mulvany F et al 1995 Reproductive behaviour in schizophrenia relative to other mental disorders: evidence for increased fertility in men despite decreased marital rate. Acta Psychiatrica Scandinavica 91:222–228

Lawrie T A, Herxheimer A, Dalton K 2000 Oestrogens and progesterones for preventing and treating postnatal depression (Cochrane review). In: The Cochrane Library, Issue 3. Update Software, Oxford

McElhatton P, Bateman D, Evans C et al 1999 Congenital anomalies after prenatal ecstasy exposure. Lancet 354:1441–1442

Miller L 1994 Use of electroconvulsive therapy during pregnancy. Hospital and Community Psychiatry 45:444–450

Miller L J, Rukstalis M 1999 Hypotheses about postpartum reactivity. In: Miller LJ (ed.) Postpartum mood disorders. American Psychiatric Press, Washington, DC

Morgan J, Lacey J, Sedgwick P 1999 Impact of pregnancy on bulimia nervosa. British Journal of Psychiatry 174:135–140

Murray L, Cooper P 1997 Effects of postnatal depression on infant development. Archives of Diseases in Childhood 77:99–101

National Screening Committee (accessed 15.12.02) http://www.nelh.nhs.uk/screening/adult_pps/postnatal_depression.html

Nulman I, Rovet J, Stewart D et al 1997 Neurodevelopment of children exposed in utero to antidepressant drugs. New England Journal of Medicine 336:258–262

Oates M 1989 Normal emotional changes in pregnancy and the puerperium. Baillières Clinical Obstetrics & Gynaecology 3:791–804

Oates M 1997 Patients as parents: the risk to children. British Journal of Psychiatry 170(suppl 32):22–27

O'Connor T, Heron J, Golding J et al 2002 Maternal antenatal anxiety and children's behavioural/emotional problems at 4 years. British Journal of Psychiatry 180:502–508

O'Hara M, Stuart S, Gorman L, Wenzel A 2000 Efficacy of interpersonal psychotherapy for postnatal depression. Archives of General Psychiatry 57:1039–1045

O'Hara M W, Swain A M 1996 Rates and risk of postnatal depression — a meta-analysis. International Review of Psychiatry 8:37–54

Paykel E S 1999 Classification of postpartum disorders in ICD 10 and DSM IV: recommendations prepared by Satra Bruck Workshop on Classification of Postnatal Mood Disorders. The Marce Society Newsletter 9

Plant M, Abel E L, Guerri C 1999 Alcohol and pregnancy. In: Macdonald (ed.) Health issues related to alcohol. Blackwell Science, Oxford

RCOG 2001 Why mothers die 1997–1999: the fifth report of the Confidential Enquiries into Maternal Deaths in the United Kingdom. Royal College of Obstetricians and Gynaecologists, London

Schou M 1990 Lithium treatment during pregnancy, delivery, and lactation: an update. Journal of Clinical Psychiatry 51:410–413

Sichel D A, Cohen L S, Dimmock J A, Rosenbaum J F 1993 Postpartum obsessive–compulsive disorder: a case series. Journal of Clinical Psychiatry 54:156–159

SIGN 2002 Guideline 60: Postnatal depression and puerperal psychosis. Scottish Intercollegiate Guidelines Network, Edinburgh (also available at www.sign.ac.uk/)

Stewart D E, Klompenhouwer J L, Kendell R F, van Hulst A M 1991 Prophylactic lithium in puerperal psychosis. British Journal of Psychiatry 158:393–397

Stowe Z N, Casarella J, Landry J, Nemeroff C B 1995 Sertraline in the treatment of women with postpartum depression. Depression 3:49–55

Taylor D, McConnell H, Duncan-McConnell D, Kerwin R (eds) 2001 The Maudsley 2001 prescribing guidelines, 6th edn. Martin Dunitz London

Terp I, Mortensen P 1998 Post-partum psychoses: clinical diagnoses and relative risk of admission after parturition. British Journal of Psychiatry 172:521–526

Turton P, Hughes P, Evans C, Fainman D 2001 Incidence, correlates and predictors of post-traumatic stress disorder in the pregnancy after stillbirth. British Journal of Psychiatry 178:556–560

Viguera A C, Nonacs R, Cohen L S et al 2000 Risk of recurrence of bipolar disorder in pregnant and nonpregnant women after discontinuing lithium maintenance. American Journal of Psychiatry 157:179–184

Ward J, Hall W, Mattick R 1999 Role of maintenance treatment in opioid dependence. Lancet 353:221–226

Whelan C, Stewart D 1990 Pseudocyesis — a review and report of six cases. International Journal of Psychiatry in Medicine 20:97–108

Wickberg B, Hwang C P 1996 Counselling of postnatal depression: controlled study on a population based Swedish sample. Journal of Affective Disorders 39:209–216

Wieck A, Kumar R, Hirst A D et al 1991 Increased sensitivity of dopamine receptors and recurrence of affective psychosis after childbirth. British Medical Journal 303:613–616

Williams K, Oke S 2000 Lithium and pregnancy. Psychological Bulletin 24:229–231

Wisner K L, Peindl K, Hanusa B H 1994 Symptomatology of affective and psychotic illnesses relating to childbirth. Journal of Affective Disorders 30:77–87

Wisner K L, Perel J M, Peindl K S et al 2001 Prevention of recurrent postpartum depression: a randomized clinical trial. Journal of Clinical Psychiatry 62:82–86

32 Sexual disorders

Gary Stevenson

INTRODUCTION

The human sexual response is a psychosomatic process, with the potential of both psychological and somatic processes contributing to sexual dysfunction, which in turn may provide a significant source of emotional and relationship dissatisfaction. Sexual disorders are among the more prevalent psychological disorders in the general population, but yet are generally under-reported by sufferers and under-recognised by clinicians. However, the introduction of newer and more effective pharmacological treatments for some sexual disorders, such as Viagra® for male erectile disorder, has rejuvenated interest in this arena by researchers, clinicians, and sufferers alike.

This chapter provides a brief overview of the topic by reviewing the current classification systems, the prevalence of, risk factors for, and the neurobiology relating to, sexual disorders. The diagnoses and management of the sexual dysfunctions, paraphilias, and gender identity disorders are then presented, followed by a discussion of issues relating to ageing, homosexuality, and sex therapy.

CLASSIFICATION OF SEXUAL AND GENDER IDENTITY DISORDERS

The classification of sexual disorders has evolved with each revision of the *Diagnostic and Statistical Manual of Mental Disorders* (DSM) of the American Psychiatric Association (APA) and the *International Classification of Diseases* (ICD) of the World Health Organization. The current classifications of sexual and gender identity disorders in DSM-IV and ICD-10 are given in Table 32.1. Current classification systems of sexual dysfunction are based on the 'sexual response cycle', as described by Masters & Johnson (1970) and Kaplan (1974), which consists of the theories of sexual desire, arousal, orgasm and resolution. Sexual dysfunction is viewed as 'a disturbance in the processes that characterise the sexual response cycle or by pain associated with sexual intercourse' in DSM-IV, and 'covers the various ways in which an individual is unable to participate in a sexual relationship as he or she would wish' in ICD-10. Primary sexual problems are classified as *dysfunctions* in DSM-IV when the disturbance causes marked distress or interpersonal difficulty, and the dysfunction is not better accounted for by another axis 1 disorder and is not due exclusively to the direct physiological effects of a substance or a general medical condition. The sexual dysfunctions may be subtyped as lifelong or acquired, generalised or situational, and due to psychological factors or a combination of factors. In contrast to the ICD-10,

DSM-IV groups all sexual function disorders together regardless of aetiology (including those caused by a general medical condition or substance-induced). ICD-10 separates Sexual Dysfunction, not caused by organic disorder or disease (F52), from Gender Identity Disorders (F64) and Disorders of Sexual Preference (F65). Unlike DSM-IV, ICD-10 has a category on excessive sexual drive, although no explicit research criteria are provided.

Criticisms of the current classification systems of sexual dysfunctions include the basic assumption that the sexual response cycle unfolds in a linear and discrete sequence, from desire to arousal to orgasm, whereas a more circular and interactive model is suggested to occur (Leiblum 2001). Furthermore, there are attempts to create parallels between male and female sexual complaints, with often a failure to recognise the emotional and interpersonal aspects of sexual exchange, aspects that may be more important to women than the actual genital response. The current classifications often fail to provide objective, operational definitions, but instead diagnosis is contingent on the disorder causing marked distress or interpersonal difficulty, and thus depends to a large degree on clinical judgement. In contrast to ICD-10, DSM-IV does not exclude the possibility that it is only the partner who is markedly distressed.

Suggestions for improved classification of sexual dysfunctions have been proposed (Vroege et al 1998). More recently, a multidisciplinary group of experts reported on consensus-based definitions for classification of female sexual dysfunctions (Basson et al 2000). This classification system follows the same general structure as the DSM-IV and ICD-10 with minor alterations and the inclusion of a new category of *non-coital sexual pain disorder*, but has been criticised by other researchers (Bancroft et al 2001).

PREVALENCE OF SEXUAL DYSFUNCTION

Published studies indicate that sexual difficulties are ubiquitous. Community samples indicate a current prevalence of 0–3% for male orgasmic disorder, 0–5% for erectile disorder and 0–3% for male hypoactive sexual desire disorder. Pooling current and 1-year figures provides community prevalence estimates of 7–10% for female orgasmic disorder and 4–5% for premature ejaculation (Simons & Carey 2001). Stable community estimates of the current prevalence of other sexual dysfunctions remain unavailable, while estimates obtained from primary care and sexuality clinic samples are generally higher.

In an anonymous UK postal questionnaire survey in a primary healthcare setting, 34% of male and 41% of female respondents

Table 32.1 classification of sexual and gender identity disorders

DSM-IV	ICD-10
Sexual dysfunctions	
• Sexual desire disorders	
Hypoactive sexual desire disorder	Lack or loss of sexual desire
Sexual aversion disorder	Sexual aversion and lack of sexual enjoyment
• Sexual arousal disorders	Excessive sexual drive
Female sexual arousal disorder	Failure of genital response
Male erectile disorder	
• Orgasmic disorders	
Female orgasmic disorder	Orgasmic dysfunction
Male orgasmic disorder	
Premature ejaculation	Premature ejaculation
• Sexual pain disorders	
Dyspareunia	Non-organic dyspareunia
Vaginismus	Non-organic vaginismus
• Sexual dysfunction due to a general medical condition	
• Substance-induced sexual dysfunction	
Paraphilias	*Disorders of sexual preference*
Gender identity disorders	*Gender identity disorders*

appeared more likely, with Hispanics less likely to have sexual problems compared with Whites.

With regard to *health and lifestyle risk factors*, those who experienced emotional or stress-related problems were more likely to experience sexual dysfunctions. Men with poor health had elevated risks for all categories of sexual dysfunction, but this was associated only with sexual pain for women. Falling household income was associated with an increased risk of sexual dysfunction for women, and erectile difficulties for men. Several sexual experience variables were important. Liberal sexual attitudes were associated with premature ejaculation in men. Men reporting any homosexual activity were more than twice as likely to experience premature ejaculation and low sexual desire. Arousal disorder in women was highly associated with an experience of sexual victimisation through adult–child contact or forced sexual contact, whilst male victims of adult–child contact were more likely to experience erectile dysfunction, premature ejaculation and low sexual desire. Men who reported sexually assaulting women were more likely to report erectile dysfunction.

In another study, erectile dysfunction was associated with increasing age, health status (cardiovascular disease, diabetes, disease-related medications, cigarette smoking) and emotional factors (depression and anger) (Feldman et al 1994). Depression is associated with reduced sexual desire, while both arousal and desire difficulties in men and women are associated with decreased physical and emotional satisfaction with the partner relationship (Rosen 2000).

HUMAN SEXUAL RESPONSE AND THE PSYCHOSOMATIC CIRCLE

As mentioned, current concepts of the human sexual response are based on those described by Masters & Johnson (1970) and Kaplan (1974), and consist of the stages of sexual desire, sexual excitement, orgasm, and resolution, although in clinical practice an integration of stages may be seen.

- *Sexual desire* is defined as the broad interest in sexual objects or experiences and is generally inferred from frequency of sexual thoughts, fantasies, wishes and interest in initiating and/or engaging in sexual experiences. Other factors such as attitudes, opportunity, partner availability, mood and health may impact.
- *Sexual excitement* refers to the subjective feeling of sexual pleasure and the accompanying physiological changes of penile erection and vaginal lubrication.
- *Orgasm* is characterised by a peak in sexual pleasure, accompanied by rhythmic contractions of the genital and reproductive organs, cardiovascular and respiratory changes, the release of sexual tension, and ejaculation in men.
- The final phase is *resolution*, with a sense of relaxation and well-being, including a refractory period for erection and ejaculation in men.

reported having a current sexual problem, with 52% of these stating that they would like to receive professional help for their problem, but only 5% had received such assistance (Dunn et al 1998). This compares with The National Health and Social Life Survey (NHSLS), a national probability sample of over 3000 adults living in US households, which indicated that in those individuals who reported any sexual activity with their partner in the previous 12-month period, the prevalence of sexual problems was 43% for women and 31% for men (Laumann et al 1999). For women these figures comprised a 22% prevalence for a low sexual desire category, 14% for arousal problems and 7% with sexual pain; for men, a 21% prevalence of premature ejaculation, 5% for erectile dysfunction and 5% for low sexual desire.

RISK FACTORS FOR SEXUAL DYSFUNCTION

Sexual dysfunctions are complexly determined and highly related to physical and psychosocial dimensions of a person's life. In the NHSLS a variety of risk factors were identified under demographic, health and lifestyle headings (Laumann et al 1999). *Demographic factors* that influence reported problems include gender, age, marital status, level of educational attainment, and ethnic race. For women, sexual problems tended to decrease with age, except for lubrication difficulties, which increase significantly at the menopause; for men, increasing age was associated with erectile difficulties and loss of sexual desire. Married individuals appeared at lower risk of experiencing sexual symptoms than their non-married counterparts. Higher educational attainment was correlated with less dysfunction for both sexes. Effects of race and ethnicity were more modest among both sexes although Blacks

Bancroft (1998) describes sexual function as a prime example of a psychosomatic process, and has schematically illustrated the interaction between the limbic system, spinal centres and the response to input from tactile and cognitive sources. These inputs result in bodily changes, while awareness of these, which can be exciting, anxiety-provoking or inhibitory, completes the cycle, as shown in Figure 32.1. Although factors may interrupt the cycle at many points, they may disrupt the system in a wider ranging manner to precipitate sexual dysfunction.

Other sex-response cycles have been proposed, as shown in Figure 32.2 (Basson 2001). Basson suggests that the willingness to experience arousal and subsequent desire stem from a wish to increase emotional intimacy. The increased sexual desire can facilitate mental processing of additional stimuli towards further arousal. The apparently spontaneous sexual desire (more often reported in younger men) drives the individual to seek out sexual stimuli, which influences the mind's processing of those stimuli. Central monitoring and processing of the sexual arousal response and of the emotional experience will further influence, either positively or negatively, the overall sex response. Enhanced emotional intimacy is achieved when the outcome is both physically and emotionally rewarding for the participants.

NEUROBIOLOGY OF SEXUAL FUNCTION

Physiological sexual arousal in males involves regulation of penile haemodynamics. The smooth muscles that line the sinusoidal spaces and the central artery of the penis are tonically contracted during the flaccid state, maintained by the sympathetic nervous system. Erection begins with smooth muscle relaxation mediated by non-adrenergic–non-cholinergic autonomic nerves that, together with the vascular endothelium, release nitrous oxide (NO) into the corpus cavernosum of the penis. The second messenger, cyclic guanosine monophosphate (cGMP), mediates the effect of NO that causes smooth muscle relaxation allowing the erectile bodies to fill with blood. The sympathetic nervous system is involved in emission and ejaculation. Detumescence occurs with the release of catecholamines during orgasm and ejaculation, with the sympathetic innervation mediating corporeal vasoconstriction. Centrally, penile erection is controlled by centres located in the thoracolumbar and lumbosacral regions of the spinal cord, with the higher centres located in the cortex, interhemispheric area, and the limbic region (Kandeel et al 2001).

Physiological sexual arousal in women begins with increased clitoral length and diameter, and vasocongestion of the vagina, vulva, clitoris, uterus and possibly the urethra. Pelvic nerve stimulation results in clitoral smooth muscle relaxation and arterial smooth muscle dilation, resulting in tumescence and extrusion of the clitoris and lubrication of the vaginal wall. NO may play an important role in relaxing clitoral corpus cavernosal smooth

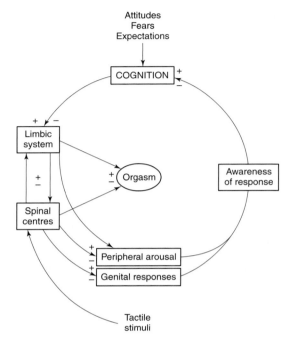

Fig. 32.1
The psychosomatic cycle of sex.

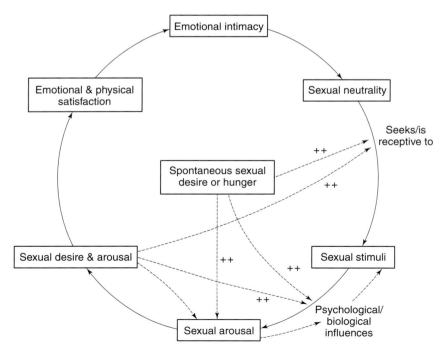

Fig. 32.2
An alternative depiction of the sex-response cycle. (Adapted from Basson 2001.)

muscle, and vasoactive intestinal peptide may play a role in the relaxation of vaginal tissue.

Endocrine, neurotransmitter and central nervous system influences on sexual function have been recently reviewed (Meston et al 2000) and are summarised below.

Endocrine influences

A certain level of testosterone is necessary for sexual desire in males, above which testosterone levels are unrelated to levels of sexual drive. Withdrawal of exogenous testosterone in hypogonadal men causes marked decrease in sexual interest and activity. Testosterone plays a role in nocturnal penile tumescence but whether it influences erectile responses to external stimuli is unclear. While sexual desire is influenced by androgen levels in women, androgens alone are not sufficient for the experience of sexual desire. The relation between testosterone level and sexual desire in premenopausal healthy women has produced inconsistent results although, with natural menopause, androgen levels are positively correlated with sexual interest.

Oestrogens and progesterone have little direct influence on sexual desire in either males or females. For men, oestrogen therapy has shown some effect in inhibiting sexual desire amongst sex offenders and in those who experience uncontrollable sexual urges. Oestrogen deficiency, as occurs with menopause, decreases genital vasoconstriction and lubrication and results in atrophy of the vaginal epithelium, which in turn may adversely effect sexual arousal and desire. In such cases, oestrogen replacement therapy has been shown to be effective.

Prolactin may have an inhibitory influence on sexual interest, while other studies suggest that levels of prolactin and oxytocin increase during sexual arousal. Excess cortisol can depress libido possibly via increased corticotrophin-releasing hormone. Most research on pheromones and sexuality in humans has centred on female reproductive cycle influences, although there is a suggestion that male pheromones increase the sexual attractiveness of men to women.

Neurotransmitter and neuropeptide influences

Nitric oxide is an essential component in the production of penile, and possibly clitoral, vasocongestion and tumescence. Sexual stimulation leads to NO production that stimulates the release of guanylate cyclase, which converts guanosine triphosphate to cGMP, which produces relaxation of smooth muscles of the penile arteries and corpus cavernosum, resulting in an increased blood flow into the penis. Sildenafil (Viagra®), a drug designed to treat erectile difficulties, prolongs the action of cGMP by inhibiting its metabolism by phosphodiesterase type 5.

Serotonin activation of the $5HT_2$ receptor impairs all stages of the sexual response in males and females, whereas stimulation of the $5HT_{1A}$ receptor facilitates sexual functioning. There is extensive literature on sexual dysfunction with the use of selective serotonin reuptake inhibitor (SSRI) antidepressants; this may, however, be useful in the treatment of premature ejaculation.

Dopaminergic agents (e.g. antiparkinsonian medication) have been reported to increase sexual desire and facilitate erection, whereas antipsychotic medications, which tend to decrease dopaminergic activity, have been reported to both impair erection or produce prolonged erections. Limited research conducted in females suggests a facilitatory role of dopamine on sexual desire and orgasm. It is noted that cocaine, which enhances dopamine activity by blocking the presynaptic autoreceptor, enhances sexual pleasure, but studies of cocaine addicts suggest that chronic cocaine use may impair sexual functioning.

In men, adrenergic activity plays a role in maintaining the penis in a flaccid state and in producing detumescence, with blockage of the α_1-adrenergic receptors producing an erection. By contrast, in women adrenergic activation facilities vasocongestion, and suppression of adrenergic activity impairs sexual arousal and orgasm. Noradrenaline (norepinephrine) levels increase during sexual activity in men; yohimbine, a drug that increases noradrenaline activity, has been shown useful in treating erectile dysfunction and anorgasmia.

The role of endogenous opiates in normal sexual functioning is unclear, but they may modulate the orgasmic response (Sathe et al 2001). Opioid abuse leads to sexual dysfunction, with withdrawal from opiates characterised by increased frequency of morning erections, spontaneous ejaculations, and a slow return of sexual drive. The mechanism by which opiates affect sexual functioning is unclear, but it may be via a decrease in the levels of circulating hormones, such as luteinising hormone and testosterone, and that it is the reduction in hormones that leads to sexual dysfunction. Opioid antagonists such as naloxone have been used to treat erectile dysfunction.

Acetylcholine facilitates penile erection via the relaxation of smooth muscles of the corpus cavernosum. One study of male diabetics with erectile failure suggests that acetylcholine-induced relaxation may be impaired in this group. Certain cholinergic agents have been reported to be useful in reversing antidepressant-induced erectile and ejaculation difficulties. There are a number of case studies in men reporting loss of libido and erectile failure associated with the H_2-antagonists cimetidine and ranitidine hydrochloride. These difficulties may result from a reduction in the uptake of testosterone. Finally, animal studies indicate an inhibitory influence of GABA on male sexual responding.

Central nervous system influences

The nucleus paragigantocellularis that projects directly to pelvic efferent neurons and interneurons in the lumbosacral spinal cord has been identified as important in male, and possibly female, orgasm. The periaquaductal grey area of the midbrain acts as a relay centre for sexually relevant stimuli. A SPECT study in right-handed men found an increase in right prefrontal cortex blood flow during orgasm. Hypersexuality has been associated with the bilateral removal of temporal lobes and following frontal lobotomy. Recently, PET scanning was used to identify the brain areas activated in healthy males during visually evoked sexual arousal. Results indicated a threefold pattern of activation: the bilateral activation of the inferior temporal cortex (a visual association area); the activation of the right insula and right inferior frontal cortex (paralimbic areas relating highly processed sensory information with motivation states); and the activation of the left anterior cingulate cortex (a paralimbic area known to control autonomic and neuroendocrine function).

SEXUAL DESIRE DISORDERS

Hypoactive sexual desire disorder (HSD)

HSD has been reported in approximately 30% of women and 15% of men in population-based studies, and thus represents one of the most common sexual disorders encountered, but remains one of the more difficult sexual dysfunctions to treat. DSM-IV defines HSD as 'persistently or recurrently deficient (or absence of) sexual fantasies and desire for sexual activity, which causes marked distress or interpersonal difficulty'. The diagnosis may be lifelong or acquired, generalised or situational, in type. The definition lacks objective behavioural criteria, however, and is thus based on clinical judgement, according to patient characteristics and life situation.

HSD appears to be age-related in both sexes, and is increasingly prevalent above the age of 60. Reduction in sexual desire may be related to:

- menstrual cycle changes;
- use of the oral contraceptive pill (which may lower androgen levels);
- alterations in oestrogen and prolactin levels postpartum;
- the presence of medical (e.g Parkinson's disease, post-stroke) and psychiatric disorders (especially depression);
- medications (antihypertensives, psychotropics, alcohol);
- the availability of a functional willing partner;
- marital harmony.

The treatment focus for *acquired* HSD may differ from that of *primary* HSD. It would be appropriate to treat any medical problem affecting desire, to alter prescribed medications to those with a lesser impact on sexual function, to discuss stress-management techniques, or to suggest social and partnership skills training. Androgen replacement therapy may be appropriate in hypogonadal men or postmenopausal women. The antidepressant bupropion has been shown to increase libido independent of its antidepressant properties, which may relate to a noradrenergic mechanism of action (Segraves et al 2001). There are reports of increased sexual desire in men following use of components derived from fertilised chicken's eggs! (Eskeland et al 1997).

There have been many psychotherapeutic approaches but few well-conducted trials. One prospective, non-controlled study of a community sample of 154 couples who underwent a modified Masters & Johnson (1970) treatment reported that, of those initially experiencing impaired sexual desire, 56% were rated as having their problem largely or completely resolved following treatment (Hawton & Catalan 1986). Active participation and motivation by the partner has a positive effect on treatment outcome. A controlled study, using a short-term cognitive-behavioural therapy (CBT) group treatment programme for HSD, resulted in reduced symptoms of HSD with improved overall cognitive, behavioural and marital functioning (Trudel et al 2001). Reports of orgasm consistency training in women, combined with a CBT approach aimed at increasing sexual satisfaction, intimacy and knowledge through expanding a couple's repertoire of sexual techniques and skills, indicated positive outcomes (Hurlbert 1993). A recent study (Hartmann et al 2002) suggested that a substantial level of at least subclinical psychiatric symptoms like mood disorders, low self-esteem and feelings of guilt, were present in women with HSD, thus re-emphasising the need for broadband treatment approaches where individual and interpersonal aspects can be taken into account simultaneously.

Sexual aversion disorder

This is defined in DSM-IV as 'the persistent or recurrent extreme aversion to, and avoidance of, all (or almost all) genital sexual contact with a sexual partner, which results in marked distress or interpersonal difficulty'. There are no prevalence figures available, but it is thought to be a rather rare disorder (Heiman 2002). When confronted with the sexual situation some individuals may experience panic attacks, and there may be impaired interpersonal relations often secondary to avoidance behaviours. Sixty-seven percent of patients with sexual aversion disorder referred to a specialist sexual disorders clinic reported a history of sexual abuse with high levels of emotional and physical abuse. In addition, more than two-thirds indicated having other compulsive or addictive problems (Carnes 1998).

SEXUAL AROUSAL DISORDERS

Female sexual arousal disorder (FSAD)

FSAD is defined in DSM-IV as 'the persistent or recurrent inability to attain, or to maintain until completion of the sexual activity, an adequate lubrication-swelling response of sexual excitement, which causes marked distress or interpersonal difficulties'. There are no consistent prevalence data for FSAD, and clinically it is rarely identified as separate from either sexual desire or orgasmic disorders. While the definition of FSAD emphasises physiological arousal, many women are unaware whether they are lubricating adequately or not, and hence it is a lack of subjective arousal which is generally complained of. An international consensus panel has proposed that this category should include a lack of subjective excitement (Basson et al 2000).

Findings from the NHSLS study (Laumann et al 1999) reported that approximately 20% of women aged 18–59 years reported difficulty in becoming lubricated during sexual stimulation. Increasing age, menopausal status, marital difficulties, anxiety and depression, have been found to be risk factors for this disorder. Investigators have suggested that in some women, sexual arousal problems may be associated with vascular and clitoral erectile insufficiency secondary to atherosclerotic vascular disease.

Currently, there are no psychological outcome data specifically related to FSAD as a separate diagnosis (Heiman 2002). There has been a report of some success in improving symptoms of FSAD with the use of a small, portable vacuum clitoral therapy device (Wilson et al 2001). Several different pharmacological agents have been investigated. Sildenafil citrate (Viagra®) has been shown to produce greater vaginal vasocongestion than placebo to sexually explicit stimuli in premenopausal women. However any genital physiological effect of sildenafil was not perceived as improving the sexual response in oestrogenised or oestrogen-deficient women with FSAD (Basson et al 2002), although it did appear to in a different study involving young premenopausal women. Currently, it remains unclear whether sildenafil might be effective for specific subgroups of women with sexual dysfunction. Other small studies have suggested a role for topical alprostadil (prostaglandin E_1) and oral phentolamine (peripheral non-selective alpha-blocker). A controlled study examining the effects of the NO precursor, L-arginine glutamate, and the α_2-blocker yohimbine, indicated increased physiological (but not subjective) sexual arousal compared with controls, in postmenopausal women with FSAD. In postmenopausal women hormone replacement therapy is generally the treatment of choice.

Male erectile disorder (MED)

DSM-IV defines MED as 'persistent or recurrent inability to attain, or to maintain until completion of the sexual activity, an adequate erection, and which is associated with marked distress or interpersonal difficulty'. The disorder can be classified as lifelong or acquired, generalised or situational. Community samples indicate a current prevalence of 0–5% for MED, the prevalence increasing with age, systemic disease and smoking. The prevalence of erectile disorder in older men ranges from 20% to 52% (Feldman et al 1994).

The aetiology of MED is often a combination of organic and psychological factors. MED is associated with depressive symptoms, panic disorder and perfectionism. Medications can induce erectile dysfunction by central or peripheral neurological blockade, or via stimulation of prolactin secretion, which may reduce testosterone concentration and action. Other causes of MED include systemic diseases (e.g. liver and renal failure, COPD, cancer, diabetes), vascular insufficiency (atherosclerosis or vasospasm), neurological and spinal cord disorders, and local penile diseases (e.g. congenital malformations, phimosis).

A wide range of treatment options for MED exists, including psychosexual counselling, pharmacological treatments and surgical intervention. Treatment should be individualised and directed at the identified aetiology (Kandeel et al 2001).

Treatments for male erectile dysfunction

The following treatments are available:

1. psychological and behavioural counselling;
2. drug therapy
   a. systemic medications
      (i) reproductive hormones
      (ii) sildenafil, tadalafil
      (iii) vasodilator agents (e.g. yohimbine, phentolamine)
      (iv) centrally acting drugs (e.g. trazodone, apomorphine, naltrexone)
   b. local vasoactive agents
      (i) intracavernous injections (e.g. papaverine, PGE_1 (alprostadil), phentolamine)
      (ii) topical applications
      (iii) urethral applications
3. non-surgical devices: (i) vacuum pump (ii) constrictor ring;
4. surgical treatment: (i) arterial revascularisation, (ii) venous ligation, (iii) repair of penile structural abnormalities and augmentation phalloplasty, (iv) phallic reinnervation, (v) penile prosthesis.

Psychological and behavioural counselling A wide range of psychological treatments have been reported, although the primary treatments are systematic desensitisation and general sex therapy, the latter including a combination of education, sensate-focus exercises and sexual communication skills. Treatment frequently reveals intense performance anxiety, and treatments which address interpersonal difficulties result in better outcomes than approaches that focus on problems in sexual functioning alone. Men with acquired MED tend to fare better than those with lifelong problems. Averaging across studies, approximately two-thirds of men appear satisfied with their improvement at follow-up. Psychosexual techniques that include setting of realistic couple goals, periodic psychosexual therapy follow-up, and continual utilisation of non-intercourse pleasuring sessions, have been advocated as relapse prevention strategies.

Drug therapies Drug therapies are based on the knowledge that the erectile state represents an equilibrium between pro-erectile and anti-erectile mechanisms that influence corporal smooth muscle tone. Promoting pro-erectile action can be achieved by either

- inducing smooth muscle relaxation through cell-receptor agonists or direct activators of tissue relaxant pathways (e.g stimulating cGMP or cAMP synthesis) or
- inhibiting the deactivation of smooth muscle relaxation pathways (e.g inhibition of phosphodiesterases, enzymes that inactivate cGMP or cAMP).

Suppressing anti-erectile action can be achieved by decreasing smooth muscle contraction through receptor antagonists of tissue contractile pathways (e.g α_1-adrenergic inhibitors). Treatment approaches may also be directed towards the central nervous system to either promote pro-erectile pathways or suppress anti-erectile pathways (Rowland & Burnett 2000).

Systemic medications. Treatment of hypogonadism will depend on its aetiology but may include the use of dopamine agonists, for example bromocriptine, for treatment of patients with hyperprolactinaemia. In some cases, treatment with androgen replacement may be appropriate.

Sildenafil (Viagra®) is a potent inhibitor of phosphodiesterase type 5 and prevents the breakdown of cGMP, which is the intracellular messenger that brings about smooth muscle relaxation. Such an effect potentiates erection during sexual stimulation. The production of cGMP is stimulated by the neurotransmitter NO, released from parasympathetic nerve endings in the corpora. Data from clinical trials indicate that about 70% of men with erectile dysfunction of all aetiologies will respond to the drug with improvement in the quality and frequency of erections. The commonest side-effects are headache, facial flushing, dyspepsia, digestive problems, priapism and alterations in colour vision, which is related to the limited inhibition of phosphodiesterase type 6, found in the retina. Sildenafil has a potential for interaction with nitrates and NO donors to cause hypotension, and hence is contraindicated in relevant patients.

Tadalafil (Cialis®) is a more specific inhibitor of phosphodiesterase type 5, with a shorter onset and longer duration of action than sildenafil. Treatment with tadalafil leads to successful intercourse even when attempted up to 36 hours after dosing. Headache and dyspepsia are the commonest side-effects, but with no significant effects on vision.

Yohimbine, an alkaloid derived from tree bark, facilitates erections by blocking central α_2-adrenoceptors and possibly by exerting peripheral adrenergic actions. Placebo-controlled studies have suggested the efficacy of yohimbine in treating MED due to psychogenic or mild organic aetiology. Adverse effects include hypertension, anxiety, tachycardia and headache.

Phentolamine induces relaxation of corpus cavernosum erectile tissue by direct antagonism of both α_1- and α_2-adrenergic receptors and by indirect functional antagonism via a non-adrenergic, endothelium-mediated effect, possibly through NO synthesis activation. It appears to have moderate efficacy, the main side-effects being headaches, facial flushing and nasal congestion.

Apomorphine, a dopaminergic agonist, when taken in the sublingual form was shown to induce erection in cases of psychogenic MED, although its usage appears limited by side-effects of nausea. Naltrexone, a long-acting opiate antagonist is reported to have improved erectile function in placebo-controlled studies.

Local vasoactive agents. Intracavernous injections act locally by promoting smooth muscle relaxation of the penile blood vessels. Papaverine, an opium alkaloid, prevents the inactivation of cAMP by acting as a non-specific phosphodiesterase inhibitor, and also blocks voltage-dependent calcium channels, resulting in smooth muscle relaxation. Papaverine injections produce a full erection in approximately half of patients, depending on the dose used and the underlying pathology. Patients with underlying arterial disease tend to require higher doses and have a lower rate of erectile response compared with patients with neurological disease. Prostaglandin E_1 (alprostadil) binds with specific receptors on smooth muscle cells, inducing tissue relaxation through a second messenger system. It also has an α_2-adrenergic blocking effect and hence has the potential of reducing sympathetic overtone in patients with psychogenic erectile dysfunction. The overall erectile response is about 70%. Phentolamine has a weak erectile-promoting effect when used alone but in combination with papaverine or prostaglandin E_1 potentiates their erectile effects. Dropout rates with intracavernous therapies range from 50% to 80%, the reasons including loss of efficacy, loss of sexual interest, preference for less invasive forms of treatment, or resumption of spontaneous erections probably via resolution of performance anxiety. These vasoactive therapies are contraindicated for men with psychological instability, a history of or risk for priapism, histories of severe coagulopathy or unstable cardiovascular disease. Risk of complications include priapism (less than 1% of men), with 10% of men experiencing penile fibrosis at the injection site, local haematoma and penile pain.

Prostaglandin E_1 has also been delivered intraurethrally as MUSE (medicated urethral system for erection). The overall response rate is approximately 40%, and erections are seldom completely rigid. The most common side-effects of MUSE include local urogenital pain (30% of patients) and minor urethral bleeding (5%), in addition to lower rates of hypotension, dizziness and priapism.

There is ongoing research into the topical application of vasoactive agents directly to the surface of the penis. The glans penis is the preferred site of application since the medication can enter the corpus spongiosum directly and then be absorbed much like drugs delivered into the urethra. There have been reports on the usage of minoxidil sulphate (a potassium channel opener), nitric oxide donors, prostaglandin E_1 and papaverine. Achieving a functional erection with topical application of these agents has been limited, and with more success in patients with psychogenic and neurogenic disorders than in those with vascular problems.

Other approaches. Non-surgical devices include vacuum pump erection devices and constrictive penile rings. Duration of erections induced by these methods should not be extended beyond 30 minutes because of the development of ischaemia. The vacuum constrictive device was found to be particularly effective in patients with partial impotence.

Penile prosthetic implants, of which there are several types, appear to produce patient satisfaction rates of 80%, with reported enhancement of sexual and non-sexual relationships between the partners after implant. Complications include device failure, infections and destruction of cavernosal tissue.

ORGASMIC DISORDERS

Female orgasmic disorder

This is defined in DSM-IV as 'persistent or recurrent delay in, or absence of, orgasm following a normal sexual excitement phase, which engenders marked distress or interpersonal difficulty'. It is noted that women exhibit a wide variability in the type or intensity of stimulation that triggers orgasm, and the diagnosis is based on a clinician's judgement that the woman's orgasmic capacity is less than would be reasonable for her age, sexual experience and the adequacy of sexual stimulation she receives. Some individuals are orgasmic with masturbation or sexual foreplay with a partner but are unable to achieve orgasm during intercourse. These problems are sometimes referred to as situational or secondary orgasmic dysfunction. Other individuals are unable to achieve orgasm through any means of stimulation and hence are referred to as anorgasmic, which is more prevalent in women than men. Orgasmic capacity in females increases with age, and is associated with sexual assertiveness and experience with masturbation. Female orgasmic disorder is a highly prevalent sexual dysfunction, with 15% of premenopausal and 35% of postmenopausal women reporting difficulties in population-based surveys. Relationship and psychological distress factors have been associated with secondary orgasmic dysfunction in women (Rosen 2000).

There are effective psychological treatments for this disorder though treatments are more effective for primary than secondary orgasmic problems. Across all comparison-controlled studies, directed masturbation was more effective than systematic desensitisation; and directed masturbation plus sensate focus was more effective than sensate focus alone (Heiman 2002). Whatever the success in achieving orgasm via masturbatory training, it begins to diminish as the woman moves from self-induced orgasm to partner-induced orgasm. However, over time, women demonstrate an increased capacity to achieve orgasm in partner-related as well as coital encounters. In addition, the prognosis appears more positive for women with lifelong orgasmic dysfunction than for women who acquire the dysfunction after a period of normal function. The worst outcome for an acquired dysfunction occurs when the problem results from psychological causes (e.g. relationship deterioration) which were not addressed in masturbatory training programmes (Segraves & Althof 2002).

Male orgasmic disorder (MOD)

This is defined in DSM-IV as 'persistent or recurrent delay in, or absence of, orgasm following a normal sexual excitement phase during sexual activity that the clinician, taking into account the person's age, judges to be adequate in focus, intensity and duration, and which causes marked distress or interpersonal difficulty.' Males can reach orgasm even when vascular or neurological conditions interfere with erectile rigidity, and in the absence of seminal emission. MOD is uncommon, occurring in only 3–10% of patients presenting with sexual dysfunction, with a higher prevalence noted in homosexual men (Simons & Carey 2001). In the most common form, a male cannot reach orgasm during intercourse although he can ejaculate from a partner's manual or oral stimulation. The condition may be associated with a variety of medical conditions (e.g. multiple sclerosis, prostatectomy), performance anxiety, fear of impregnation, and lack of desire or arousal.

There are no large-scale long-term controlled outcome studies of this condition. The objective of psychosexual treatment is to reduce the performance-induced anxiety, which can be achieved through implementation of a multiple-step treatment plan. Once the patient becomes orgasmic with self-stimulation, the presence and then participation of a partner are gradually introduced. Psychotherapy may also help the patient resolve his underlying conflicts (Kandeel et al 2001).

There is increasing recognition of *pharmacologically induced orgasmic disorders* in both men and women. This primarily refers to the SSRI class of drugs for which 9–40% of patients taking them report orgasmic disorder side-effects, with females reporting symptoms more often than males. Since the most common aetiology of anorgasmia is the intake of pharmacological agents, regaining the orgasmic sensation may be achieved with discontinuation of the inciting drug or substituting with an alternative psychotropic agent.

Premature ejaculation (PE)

This is defined in DSM-IV as 'persistent or recurrent ejaculation with minimal sexual stimulation before, on, or shortly after penetration and before the person wishes it, and which causes marked distress or interpersonal difficulty'. The clinician is required to take into account factors that affect duration of the excitement phase, such as age, novelty of the sexual partner or situation, and recent frequency of sexual activity but, in the absence of adequate norms, these considerations are subjective. Normally by age 18 years, 75% of men are able to control their ejaculation. PE is the most common male sexual dysfunction, with a prevalence of 25–40% of adult males in non-clinical samples, and a pooled community prevalence of 4–5% (Simons & Carey 2001). Men with PE are less likely to seek professional help for the problem than men with MED.

The motor component of the ejaculatory reflex involves both autonomic and somatic responses. Seminal emission results from activation of α_1-adrenergic neurons arising from the thoracolumbar region of the spinal cord. Cholinergic motor neurons of the pudendal nerve mediate ejaculation, associated with the subjective experience of orgasm. Ejaculation has been induced in men with spinal cord transections, indicating that the reflex can bypass central mediation. However, centrally mediated processes presumably play a modulating role, possibly via serotonergic systems. The timing of ejaculation is influenced by psychological processes such as attentional focus, cognitions and fantasy, and overall subjective sexual arousal. Sexual response in men without PE is characterised by parasympathetic dominance during erection but sympathetic dominance during ejaculation. However, men with PE may show heightened sympathetic activation very early in the sexual response cycle, slowing the erectile process and triggering the ejaculatory reflex prematurely (Rowland & Burnett 2000). Emotional stress factors, sexual anxiety and a history of urinary tract symptoms have been associated with PE (Laumann et al 1999).

Treatment of premature ejaculation

A variety of psychological approaches using various behavioural strategies have been used in the psychosexual treatment of PE. The basic procedure for the 'stop/start technique' was first described in 1956, in which the man is repeatedly brought to a high level of arousal and then stimulation is stopped just before ejaculation begins. This technique has been subsequently adapted to a 'stop/start/squeeze' sequence. Both techniques are employed in a graduated fashion. Other treatments have included pelvic-floor muscle rehabilitation with exercise training, electrostimulation, and biofeedback to help patients gain control of ejaculatory latency. Initial success rates of psychosexual-behavioural therapy range between 60% and 90%, which may fall to 25% 3 years after therapy.

Clinicians are increasingly turning to pharmacotherapy for treatment of PE. Approaches have included the application of anaesthetising ointments or creams directly to the glans penis to attenuate genital sensory input, thereby reducing ejaculation by up to several minutes (Choi et al 2000). A second approach employs intracavernosal injections of either prostaglandin or papaverine with phentolamine. This has improved the ejaculatory latency of men presenting with erectile dysfunction (Slob et al 2002). However, the most common pharmacological approach to treating PE involves the use of oral retardants of ejaculation, including clomipramine, SSRIs and alpha-adrenergic blockers. Although at antidepressant doses clomipramine induces erectile problems in about 20% of sexually functional men, at lower doses (25–50 mg) clomipramine is effective in delaying ejaculation by 2–6 minutes, for both daily dosing and when used 4–8 hours prior to intercourse. Ten to thirty percent of men do not respond, especially those who, prior to treatment, had ejaculation latencies of less than 1 minute. Most SSRIs tested have been moderately effective at fairly low dosages and have fewer side-effects than clomipramine, although the latter may be more effective. It is hypothesised that these medications act centrally at the $5HT_2$ receptor to inhibit serotonin reuptake, or via inhibiting peripherally-mediated ejaculation through the alpha-adrenergic system. Currently, there is no evidence that these medications can be discontinued without the PE returning. Alpha-adrenergic receptor blockers delay PE by a peripheral action, interrupting sympathetic activation in the pelvic region responsible for the peristaltic movement of the seminal fluid necessary for ejaculation. They appear effective in delaying ejaculation in about 50% of men with psychogenic PE, compared with 25% of men receiving placebo. Effects on ejaculation occur after 1–2 weeks of treatment. Autonomic-related side-effects are common (Cavallini 1995). Beta-blockers are not effective for PE. A recent study indicated the usefulness of sildenafil when compared with the as-needed use of clomipramine, sertraline, paroxetine and the pause–squeeze technique in the treatment of primary PE (Abdel-Hamid et al 2001).

SEXUAL PAIN DISORDERS

Dyspareunia

DSM-IV defines dyspareunia as 'recurrent or persistent genital pain associated with sexual intercourse in either a male or a female, which causes marked distress or interpersonal difficulty', and is not caused exclusively by vaginismus or lack of lubrication. Although the pain is most commonly experienced during coitus, it may also occur before or after intercourse and may result in the avoidance of sexual relationships. Several researchers are critical of the DSM-IV definitions and propose that dyspareunia (and vaginismus) should be conceptualised of as *pain disorders* that interfere with sexuality, rather than a sexual disorder characterised by pain (Binik et al 2002). According to the NHSLS data, 14% of women and 3% of men have experienced pain during sexual activity in the past year (Laumann et al 1999). The prevalence may be higher in post-menopausal women, while a lifetime prevalence of 0.2% has been noted in a random male population sample (Simons & Carey 2001).

A number of conditions, including hymenal scarring, pelvic inflammatory disease, vulvar vestibulitis and penile malformations, have been associated with dyspareunia, though there have been few controlled aetiological studies. Psychosocial factors, such as relationship discord and prior sexual abuse, have also been cited. There is some evidence that psychological factors, such as attribution and mood, influence reports of pain intensity. In addition, dyspareunia (and vaginismus) can be conditioned to the sexual situation involving a specific partner and not be apparent during a physical examination. Although many uncontrolled reports exist, there are no published randomised treatment outcome studies of general dyspareunia. Researchers have recently reported a randomised treatment outcome study comparing group CBT, surface electromyographic biofeedback, and vestibulectomy in the treatment of vulvar vestibulitis (a subcategory of dyspareunia). Although vestibulectomy was the most effective treatment with respect to pain outcome, it was not more effective with regard to frequency of intercourse and other psychosocial variables (Bergeron et al 2001).

Vaginismus

This is diagnosed as 'recurrent or persistent involuntary spasm of the musculature of the outer third of the vagina that interferes with sexual intercourse causing marked distress or interpersonal difficulty'. In some females even the anticipation of vaginal insertion may result in muscle spasm (DSM-IV). Alternative definitions which exclude the assumed vaginal muscle spasm, and suggest that pain may be an important aspect of the problem, have been proposed (Binik et al 2002). Vaginismus without concurrent dyspareunia appears to be a relatively rare condition, with community estimates ranging from 0.5% to 1% although with higher rates of 15–17% presenting at clinics (Simons & Carey 2001). Commonly cited factors for vaginismus are sexual abuse, negative sexual attitudes, sexual inexperience, and relationship difficulties, but none has been evaluated empirically. Distinction is made between *generalised* vaginismus, which refers to involuntary spasms in all situations, and *situational* vaginismus, in which some penetration is possible (e.g. insertion of a tampon). Secondary vaginismus is extremely common, particularly in women who have experienced vaginal pain caused by infections, surgery or chemical agents.

Most treatment models for vaginismus include gradual vaginal dilatation procedures combined with various forms of relaxation and anxiety reduction techniques, although, more recently, perineal biofeedback procedures have been used. Although there appears to be consensus concerning the success and overall positive treatment outcome for these techniques, neither has been investigated systematically. This need for randomised controlled trials to evaluate treatments which have produced positive results in uncontrolled evaluations has been noted (McGuire & Hawton 2002).

SEXUAL DYSFUNCTION RESULTING FROM A GENERAL MEDICAL CONDITION

According to DSM-IV, this is the presence of 'clinically significant sexual dysfunction that is judged to be due exclusively to the direct physiological effects of a general medical condition and which results in marked distress or interpersonal difficulty'. If psychological factors are felt to play a role in the onset, severity, exacerbation or maintenance of a sexual dysfunction, the diagnosis would be of the primary sexual dysfunction with the subtype 'due to combined factors'.

SUBSTANCE-INDUCED SEXUAL DYSFUNCTION

This is a clinically significant 'sexual dysfunction judged to be fully explained by the direct physiological effects of a substance (for example, a drug of abuse, a medication or toxin exposure) that results in marked distress or interpersonal difficulty'. The dysfunction may occur with impaired desire, arousal, orgasm or with sexual pain, and although the clinical presentation of the sexual dysfunction may resemble one of the specific primary sexual dysfunctions, the full criteria for one of those disorders need not be met.

A variety of chemical agents have been associated with sexual dysfunction. There are several mechanisms by which chronic alcohol abuse can cause sexual dysfunction, although the controlled evidence is in fact limited and concerns only male alcoholics. Some data suggest that in the absence of significant hepatic or gonadal failure in this group, sobriety may be compatible with normal sexual function. Narcotics diminish libido, which returns during drug-free periods. Cocaine and amphetamine use has been reported to cause increased libido and spontaneous erection, although chronic abuse of these agents results in decreased libido and other sexual dysfunctions. There is a high frequency of reported sexual dysfunctions, including decreased libido, erectile dysfunction and anorgasmia, while individuals are on antihypertensive agents, including spironolactone, reserpine, propranolol and verapamil. Among antihypertensive drugs, alpha-blockers, such as prazosin and labetalol, appear to have the lowest incidence of drug-induced sexual dysfunction, although they may be associated with ejaculatory inhibition.

Psychotropic medications may induce sexual dysfunction in any of the sexual phases. They may do so by non-specific sedation resulting in impaired arousal, hormonal effects (for example, prolactin elevation resulting in erectile dysfunction), or central or peripheral neurotransmitter effects. Most antidepressants have been reported to cause sexual dysfunction, with the possible exceptions of bupropion, mirtazapine and nefazodone (Ellison 1998). The SSRIs appear the worst offenders, producing reduced sexual desire in up to 55% of cases. Decreased genital sensitivity was reported by 28% of SSRI-treated women in one prospective study. In a further study, impotence emerged in 34% of men, the highest incidence being in those taking the more anticholinergic paroxetine. Delayed or absent orgasm can occur with antidepressant usage but are particularly prevalent with SSRIs, affecting 30–35% of men who took them in one prospective study. There are case reports of SSRIs occasionally producing increased sexual desire, and spontaneous orgasms with the more serotonergic antidepressants.

Antipsychotic-induced sexual dysfunction has been reported to correlate with prolactin elevation. Sexual desire decreased in about 37% of antipsychotic-treated patients, with higher rates for older age groups and with high-dose, low-potency neuroleptics. Phenothiazines are reported to inhibit erection in 20–44% of males. Antipsychotics can also inhibit orgasm, and thioridazine is reported to cause retrograde ejaculation into the bladder in up to half of patients. Most reports indicate that risperidone causes more sexual dysfunction than olanzapine, and that the sexual problems with risperidone appeared dose-related. There are reports of increased sexual desire with the use of testosterone and L-dopa, and the production of priapism with trazodone, prazosin (an α_1-receptor antagonist), phenothiazines, risperidone and SSRIs.

The management of psychotropic drug-induced sexual inhibition has been described (Clayton & Shen 1998). This includes:

- informing the patient about the possibility of sexual inhibition occurring before prescribing;
- waiting for remission or tolerance of sexual inhibition, with or without behaviour modification therapy;
- reducing the dosage while maintaining therapeutic efficacy; this has also included 'drug holidays', but will be less successful with drugs which have long elimination half-lives;
- switching the medication to one less likely to cause sexual inhibition; for example nefazodone and mirtazapine are less likely to induce sexual inhibition than SSRIs or tricyclic antidepressants;
- adjusting the concomitant non-psychotropic drugs — for example, among antihypertensives, ACE inhibitors are least likely to cause sexual inhibition, whereas among H_2-receptor antagonists, cimetidine has been most frequently implicated as causing sexual inhibition;
- adding agents to existing psychotropic medication. The only antidotes proven effective in double-blind trials are sildenafil and buspirone, although the latter result has not been replicated (Michelson et al 2000).

PARAPHILIAS

The paraphilias are defined in DSM-IV as 'a group of sexual disorders of at least 6-months duration, which cause significant distress or impair social, occupational or other important areas of functioning and which are characterised by recurrent, intense sexually arousing fantasies, sexual urges or behaviours generally involving (a) non-human objects (b) the suffering or humiliation of oneself or one's partner, or (c) children or other non-consenting individuals'. The paraphilias identified in DSM-IV are given in Box 32.1. The group 'paraphilia not otherwise specified' includes telephone scatologia (making obscene telephone calls), necrophilia, partialism (exclusive focus on part of the body), zoophilia, coprophilia (faecal involvement), klismaphilia (enemas), and urophilia (urine).

Many researchers have questioned the validity of the DSM-IV requirement that stress or functional impairment occur, as many patients and offenders experience the stress only upon disclosure of their crimes and not as a result of their condition. Although paraphilic behaviour has been reported secondary to a wide variety of neuropsychiatric disorders including temporal lobe epilepsy, post-encephalitic neuropsychiatric syndromes, septal lesions, frontal lobe tumours, bilateral temporal lobe lesions, and multiple sclerosis, sexually abnormal behaviour due to another disease process should not be included in this classification.

Although individuals may have combinations of these paraphilias, most individuals with paraphilic behaviour patterns have a

---

> **Box 32.1   Paraphilias (DSM-IV)**
>
> - *Exhibitionism*: Intense sexually arousing fantasies, sexual urges, or behaviours involving the exposure of one's genitals to a stranger
> - *Fetishism*: Intense sexually arousing fantasies, sexual urges, or behaviours involving the use of nonliving objects, not limited to articles of female clothing used in cross-dressing (as in transvestic fetishism) or devices designed for tactile genital stimulation
> - *Frotteurism*: Intense sexually arousing fantasies, sexual urges, or behaviours involving touching or rubbing against a nonconsenting person
> - *Paedophilia*: Intense sexually arousing fantasies, sexual urges, or behaviours involving sexual activity with a prepubescent child by a person at least 16 years old and at least 5 years older than the victim
> - *Sexual masochism*: Intense sexually arousing fantasies, sexual urges, or behaviours involving the act of being humiliated, beaten, bound, or otherwise made to suffer
> - *Sexual sadism*: Intense sexually arousing fantasies, sexual urges, or behaviours involving acts in which the psychological or physical suffering of the victim is sexually exciting
> - *Transvestic fetishism*: Intense sexually arousing fantasies, sexual urges, or behaviours in a heterosexual male involving cross-dressing
> - *Voyeurism*: Intense sexually arousing fantasies, sexual urges, or behaviours involving observing unsuspecting persons who are nude, disrobing, or in sexual activity
> - *Paraphilias not otherwise specified*

---

narrow range of behaviour which becomes a specialised and ritualised form of sexual arousal and gratification. There are numerous clinical descriptions of paraphilias, but perhaps the best known is *Psychopathia Sexualis*, first published in 1886 by Krafft-Ebing (1997). Depending on the specific practice, paraphilic behaviours may be performed alone as autoeroticism (which may lead to self-injury as in sexual masochism), or may be practised with a partner who may, or may not, be consenting. Many individuals with paraphilia become involved with work that allows them to be in contact with their preferred stimuli, or may preferentially focus on material that incorporates their preferred type of paraphilic stimulus.

As most of the research on paraphilias is derived from studies of convicted sex offenders the actual incidence and prevalence of the paraphilias is unknown. Most sexual offenders do not readily admit all their deviant behaviours, and many researchers believe that over 90% of paraphilic acts go undetected. Reported sexual crimes are increasing, however, with 30–70% of college-age females having been victimised in some fashion. The prevalence of people participating in some form of paraphilic or fetishistic behaviour is estimated at 5–30%, while approximately one-half of paraphilic individuals seen clinically are married. The APA have commented that, although paraphilia is rarely diagnosed, the ready availability of paraphilic books, photographs and paraphernalia on the commercial market would indicate a higher prevalence among the general public than might be suspected. Apart for sexual masochism where the sex ratio is estimated to be 20 males for each female, the other paraphilias are almost never diagnosed in females (Fedoroff et al 1999). However, discussions on internet chat groups indicate that some women participate in more of the activities than has been previously suspected (Agnew 2001).

The paraphilias most frequently presenting at specialised clinics are paedophilia, voyeurism and exhibitionism. Certain of the fantasies and behaviours associated with paraphilias may begin in childhood or early adolescence but become better defined and elaborated during adolescence and early adulthood. Elaboration and revisiting of paraphilic fantasies may continue over the lifetime of the individual but both the fantasies and the behaviours often diminish with advancing age in adults.

There is a lack of data on the epidemiology of the paraphilias, but numerous aetiological theories have been published (Maletzky 2002). These include the following.

- *Behavioural learning models* — these stress the primacy of early conditioning in the development of sexual deviations.
- *Critical stages model* — behaviour models have been augmented through the addition of research on proposed sensitivities in central nervous system development, with the suggestion that children may go through critical stages of growth when various aspects of sexuality develop. However, no objective verification of critical stages has yet been made.
- *Social learning models* — there is a suggestion that the culture in which offenders live is an important factor in increasing the likelihood of offending. Lack of parental (particularly paternal care), physical punishment, and frequent or aggressive sexual activity within the family may predispose children, through a deficiency in forming attachment bonds and lowered self-esteem, to begin sexual offending.
- *Addiction model* — deviant sexual activity acts as a drug substitute in filling some (unspecified) need. Some investigators suggest that the range of fantasies, urges and behaviours which can be considered 'addictive sexual disorders' can be readily identified in the DSM-IV as specific paraphilias, and suggest that subjects respond to treatment similar to that of chemical dependency involving individual and group work and attendance at 12-step programmes (Schneider & Irons 2001). Other authors disagree, and suggest that addiction models have not received empirical support and note that paraphilic deviations are more responsive to cognitive and behavioural therapy approaches than more standard addictions (Maletzky 2002).
- *The offender as victim* — this model suggests that offenders are revisiting and reliving their earlier traumas and perhaps identify with the aggressor. However, fewer than 30% of offenders were victims of sexual abuse before the age of 18, and these findings do not vary as a consequence of the type of offence.
- *Physiological models* — no replicated differences of sex hormone levels have yet been found between sexual offenders and non-sexual offenders, although it remains possible that in-utero hormonal levels may contribute to the nature and intensity of sexual drive later in life. CNS damage may destroy control mechanisms, resulting in disinhibition which has been associated with changes in sexual behaviour. However, CT scanning has not revealed structural changes in the majority of offenders. Studies from functional scanning are awaited.
- *Genetic factors* — chromosomal abnormalities have been implicated in the aetiology of atypical sexual behaviours and in those with gender dysphoric disorders, but there has been insufficient research in this field.

Thus, paraphilias are complex psychiatric disorders whose cause is unknown, and whether they represent an addiction, an obsessive–compulsive disorder, or a pattern of hypersexualism is still a matter of controversy (Bradford 2001).

Treatments for paraphilia

These have included surgery, psychotherapy and pharmacological approaches. There appears to be no evidence for the efficacy of neurosurgery for paraphilias, and the efficacy of castration is controversial (Gijs & Gooren 1996). In addition, neither castration nor neurosurgery are in accordance with current ethical norms.

Psychological treatment

Cognitive and behavioural therapies are now the standard psychotherapeutic interventions. The behavioural approaches include aversive conditioning, positive conditioning, and reconditioning (White et al 2002, Maletzky 2002). The aversive conditioning techniques include the following.

- *Electroshock*, with attempts to pair an unconditioned aversive stimulus with a deviant response in order to reduce the likelihood of that response occurring in the future. It has been largely replaced by other, more effective, aversive stimuli, particularly foul odours and tastes.
- *Covert sensitisation* in which the patient is first trained in relaxation techniques and then, in a relaxed state, is asked to visualise scenes of deviant sexual activity followed by an aversive event. Unfortunately, some patients demonstrate reductions in deviant arousal but no actual behaviour change.
- *Assisted covert sensitisation*, where the previous technique is augmented by introducing a foul odour at the point where aversive imagery begins. Variations on this technique have been employed in the majority of cognitive behavioural treatment programmes in recent years.
- *Minimal arousal conditioning*, which allows the placement of the aversive stimulus earlier in the response chain, when minimal arousal is present and before intense sexual pleasure is attained.
- *Aversive behavioural reversal*, where the offenders are faced with the reality of their own behaviours.
- *Covert sensitisation*, which contains elements of cognitive restructuring, empathy training, and aversive conditioning.

The positive conditioning techniques include:

- *social skills training*;
- *alternative behavioural completion*, which is based on the techniques of imagery desensitisation.

There are a number of reconditioning techniques:

- *Plethysmographic biofeedback*, where the plethysmograph (a type of penile strain gauge) is connected to an external light or sound device to provide feedback to the patient about his arousal level, thus teaching self-control.
- *Masturbation techniques* — pleasure in masturbation and climax are reinforcers of sexual behaviour, hence pairing fantasies of deviant sexual imagery with this reinforces deviant arousal. In 'fantasy change' the patient learns to change from deviant to non-deviant fantasies earlier in the masturbatory chain. In 'satiation' the patient is asked to masturbate to ejaculation only using non-deviant fantasies, and then following climax is asked to continue masturbating to deviant

fantasies, thus pairing deviant imagery with the period of minimal sexual arousal.

- *Sexual impulse control training* involves constructing obstacles early in the arousal chain, which may be more effective than designing interventions closer to the sexual pleasure of release.

Cognitive techniques include:

- *recognition and correction of cognitive distortions*;
- *relapse prevention strategies*;
- *empathy training*, which includes identification of the victim, the victimising act, the identification of harm, and role reversal.

Pharmacological treatment

Pharmacological treatments of paraphilias include psychotropic medications and hormonal treatments.

Psychotropic medications These have included trials of several conventional antipsychotic agents. In one study, benperidol was found to be significantly more effective than chlorpromazine and placebo in reducing sexual desire, but had no effect on sexual behaviour. There are reports on trials of lithium carbonate and buspirone. More common, however, is the use of the SSRIs and clomipramine, with studies providing evidence that these medications reduce deviant sexual fantasies, urges and behaviour. However the number of studies completed is still small, and no double-blind studies have been reported (Bradford 2001).

Hormonal treatment No psychotropic medication has been proven as powerful in clinical practice as the hormonal drugs medroxyprogesterone acetate (MPA) and cyproterone acetate (CPA) in reducing sexual drive. Although sexual arousability is heavily dependent on androgens, there is no evidence that persons with paraphilia have higher than normal androgen levels. The potentially beneficial effect of decreasing androgen action is thought to be derived from lowering sexual desire and sexual arousability (Gijs & Gooren 1996). Anti-androgens are known to decrease plasma testosterone, the intensity of sexual drive, erectile ability, ejaculate volume, spermatogenesis and sexual fantasies and dreams (Lothstein 1996).

MPA induces testosterone reductase in the liver, thereby decreasing circulating levels of testosterone, and blocks the secretion of FSH and LH. It does not compete with androgens at the androgen-receptor level and therefore, by definition, is not a true anti-androgen. CPA is a true anti-androgen, as well as having progestinic and anti-gonadotrophic effects, and is the most extensively studied anti-androgen in terms of a treatment for sexual deviation. CPA is a competitive inhibitor of testosterone and dihydrotestosterone at androgen receptors throughout the body, and it reduces the levels of FSH and LH. CPA decreases all types of sexual behaviour, including sexual fantasies, deviant sexual behaviour, masturbation, sexual intercourse, and it impacts on erections. Both MPA and CPA can be given orally or in long-acting depot form. Therapeutic changes usually start to occur after 1–3 weeks of administration, and by 4 months at the latest. There are relative medical contraindications for the use of CPA or MPA, most notably thromboembolic antecedents and diseases that affect the production of testosterone, such as renal failure, liver diseases, protein malnutrition, hypothalamic and pituitary dysfunction, and cancer chemotherapy. MPA and CPA have rarely been used in treating women suffering from paraphilias. The side-effects of MPA include weight gain, lethargy, nightmares, headache, nausea or vomiting, deep venous thrombosis, hyperglycaemia and leg cramps. The side-effects of CPA include gynaecomastia, thromboembolic phenomena, fatigue and depression. Both drugs probably cause bone mineral loss. Even if compliance is good, only 60–80% of men benefit from either drug.

Luteinising hormone-releasing hormone (LHRH) agonists have also been used to treat paraphilias. They overstimulate the hypothalamus, with initially an increase in GRH secretion and then a reduction to almost zero. Consequently, there is no gonadotrophin secretion and the levels of testosterone and dihydrotestosterone drop to castration levels. There have been limited clinical studies on the use of LHRH agonists. One uncontrolled observational study was on 30 men with severe long-standing paraphilia (25 with paedophilia) who received monthly injections of triptorelin and supportive psychotherapy. All men exhibited a reduction in paraphilic activities during therapy. Reported side-effects included hypogonadism, decreased bone mineral density associated with osteoporosis, and reductions in normal sexuality (Rosler & Witztum 1998). Depot leuprolide acetate resulted in a significant suppression of deviant sexual interests and behaviour in a further uncontrolled observational study of 12 patients with paraphilic disorders. The patients who were on long-term therapy, however, developed bone demineralisation suggesting that this is a significant side-effect of prolonged therapy (Krueger & Kaplan 2001).

On the basis of controlled studies there are strong indications that anti-androgens significantly reduce the intensity and frequency of sexual desire and sexual arousal. However, anti-androgens do not change the content of paraphilias, and most offenders treated with hormones show a rapid return to deviant arousal following the discontinuation of medication. It appears the damping effect of anti-androgens reduces the extent to which paraphilic desire disposes a person to paraphilic behaviour, creating room to treat the paraphilia with regard to its psychological content. Thus, it is important to combine hormonal treatment with cognitive and behavioural methods in a multimodal approach.

Outcome

Data on treatment efficacy of paraphilias have recently been published (Maletzky & Steinhauser 2002). This study was based on retrospective chart reviews of over 8000 clients entering treatment in a community-based sexual offender clinic, which employed a range of cognitive and behavioural techniques over the 25-year period from which the data were collected. More than 90% of participants were under judicial supervision for their offences, and the average duration of treatment was 21 months. Almost all participants were treated in individual therapy, although the majority also took part in group therapy. The treatment outcome data are presented in Table 32.2. The study is limited, however, by its retrospective nature, lack of inclusion of patients not available for follow-up in the data analyses, changing focus of applied therapies during the 25 years, and lack of comparison groups.

There have been no large outcome evaluations of single treatment techniques for paraphilic offenders. Hall (1995) conducted a meta-analysis of the treatment outcome literature for paraphilias and concluded that cognitive/behavioural treatments were significantly effective, with community-based treatments showing better effects than institutionally based treatment (confounded by seriousness of offence history). In addition, longer follow-ups led to more significant treatment effects when

Table 32.2 Treatment outcomes for paraphilias (n = 8156)

Category	n	Percentage meeting criteria for success*
Situational paedophilia, heterosexual	3312	95.6
Predatory paedophilia, heterosexual	1064	88.3
Situational paedophilia, homosexual	917	91.8
Predatory paedophilia, homosexual	796	80.1
Exhibitionism	1230	95.4
Rape	643	75.5
Voyeurism	83	93.9
Public masturbation	77	94.8
Frotteurism	65	89.3
Fetishism	33	94.0
Transvestic fetishism	14	78.6
Telephone scatologia	29	93.1
Zoophilia	23	95.6

* A treatment success was defined as an offender who: completed all treatment sessions; reported no covert or overt deviant sexual behaviour at the end of treatment or follow-up; demonstrated no deviant sexual arousal, defined as greater than 20% on the penile plethysmograph, at the end of treatment or at follow-up; had no repeat legal charges for any sexual crime at the end of treatment or at follow-up.

comparisons with control groups were available. A recent review has suggested that this previous meta-analysis had several shortcomings (White et al 2002). This review attempted to evaluate the effectiveness of anti-libidinal drugs and psychological treatments in reducing the target sexual acts, urges and thoughts by those who had been convicted of sexual offences or who exhibited disorders of sexual preference. They identified 431 citations but eventually included only three studies for analysis, therefore limiting its conclusions. The report authors concluded that anti-libidinal drug treatments should be used with caution as there appeared to be no trial-derived data to support or refute their use. They further suggested that the 'treatment of sex offenders requires fresh investigation and this should be done before subjecting numerous sex offenders to unproven and possibly harmful interventions and before coaxing the public into unrealistic expectations of what can currently be achieved with people who repeatedly sexually offend' (White et al 2002).

PARAPHILIA-RELATED DISORDERS

A number of investigators have reported on non-paraphilic hypersexual disorders. These sexual disorders are associated with personal distress or significant impairment in social role functioning. The major operational distinction between paraphilias and paraphilia-related disorders is that paraphilic sexual arousal is socially deviant, while paraphilia-related disorders represent excessive expressions of culturally tolerated heterosexual or homosexual behaviours (Kafka 2001). The common paraphilia-related disorders include compulsive masturbation, protracted promiscuity, pornography dependence, telephone sex dependence, cyber sex (Internet) dependence, and severe sexual desire incompatibility (in which excessive sexual desire in one partner produces sexual demands on the other partner that markedly interferes with the capacity to sustain that relationship). It is acknowledged that more empirically derived research categorising these disorders is required.

GENDER IDENTITY DISORDERS

The final diagnostic grouping subsumed under the chapter of sexual and gender identity disorders in DSM-IV is *gender identity disorder*, with the diagnostic criteria presented here in Box 32.2. Within ICD-10, gender identity disorders are placed in the chapter containing disorders of adult personality and behaviour. There, the gender identity disorders are subclassified as *transsexualism*, *dual-role transvestism* and *gender identity disorder of childhood*.

Gender identity disorder (GID) of childhood commences prior to puberty and is characterised by a persistent and intense distress about assigned sex together with the desire to be, or insistence that one is, of the opposite sex. There is a persistent preoccupation with the dress and/or activities of the opposite sex and/or repudiation of one's own sex, and sufferers may state that they find their genitalia disgusting. Boys may face ostracism from their peers, girls less so. The incidence of childhood GID is not firmly established, but in child clinic samples there are approximately five boys for each girl referred with this disorder, although this may partly reflect referral bias (Di Ceglie 2000). Children with GID may also present with separation anxiety, depression and emotional difficulties. Follow-up studies indicate that between one-third and two-thirds of boys with this disorder show a homosexual orientation during and after adolescence, but few exhibit transsexualism in adult life. The aetiology of childhood GID is likely to be multifactorial, and may include hereditary factors, in-utero hormonal influences, parental relationships, and attachment losses. The efficacy of psychotherapeutic approaches used with these children and families remains unproven (Di Ceglie 2000). There are Royal College of Psychiatrists (1998) guidelines on the staged use of hormonal and surgical interventions in these cases.

For adult males with GID some will be a continuation of childhood GID whilst others may present with the clinical presentation in early to mid-adulthood, often concurrent with transvestic fetishism. This late onset group may be more fluctuating in their degree of cross-gender identification, more ambivalent about

Box 32.2   Diagnostic criteria for gender identity disorders (DSM-IV)

1. A strong and persistent cross-gender identification (not merely a desire for any perceived cultural advantages of being the other sex)

   In children, the disturbance is manifested by four (or more) of the following:
   - repeatedly stated desire to be, or insistence that he or she is, the other sex
   - in boys, preference for cross-dressing or simulating female attire; in girls, insistence on only wearing stereotypical masculine clothing
   - strong and persistent preferences for cross-sex roles in make-believe play or persistent fantasies of being the other sex
   - intense desire to participate in the stereotypical games and pastimes of the other sex
   - strong preference for playmates of the other sex

   In adolescents and adults, the disturbance is manifested by symptoms such as:
   - stated desire to be the other sex
   - frequent passing as the other sex
   - desire to live or be treated as the other sex
   - conviction that he or she has the typical feelings and reactions of the other sex

2. Persistent discomfort with his or her sex or sense of inappropriateness in the gender role of that sex

   In children, the disturbance is manifested by any of the following: in boys, the assertion that his penis or testes are disgusting or will disappear, or assertion that it would be better not to have a penis, or aversion towards rough-and-tumble play and rejection of male stereotypical toys, games and activities; in girls, the rejection of urinating in a sitting position, assertion that she has or will grow a penis, or assertion that she does not want to grow breasts or menstruate, or marked aversion toward normative female clothing

   In adolescents and adults, the disturbance is manifested by symptoms such as preoccupation with getting rid of primary and secondary sex characteristics (e.g. request for hormones, surgery or other procedures to physically alter sexual characteristics to simulate the other sex) or belief that they were born the wrong sex

3. The disturbance is not concurrent with a physical intersex condition

4. The disturbance causes clinically significant distress or impairment in social, occupational or other important areas of functioning

established in their female role, are sexually attracted to males and regard themselves therefore as heterosexual, some do retain the attraction to women and thus regard themselves as lesbian women. The situation is broadly similar for female-to-male (FTM) individuals. A recent survey of FTM transsexuals indicated that they were not a homogeneous group; compared with non-homosexual FTMs, homosexual (relative to genetic sex) FTMs reported greater childhood gender non-conformity, preferred more feminine partners, experienced greater sexual rather than emotional jealousy, were more sexually assertive, had more sexual partners, had a greater desire for phalloplasty and had more interest in visual sexual stimuli. Both the homosexual and non-homosexual FTMs appeared not to differ in their overall desire for masculising body modifications, adult gender identity, or importance of partner social status, attractiveness or youth (Chivers & Bailey 2000).

Approximately 1 per 30 000 adult males and 1 per 100 000 adult females seek sex reassignment surgery. Hormone therapy and facial electrolysis may be introduced at an earlier stage than surgery. Hormone therapy involves oestrogens (possibly combined with progestogens) for the male-to-female, and androgens for the female-to-male. Oestrogens will probably induce breast growth, redistribution of body fat along more feminine lines, some change in skin texture and some slowing of facial and body hair growth. They may also suppress sexual interest and response. Androgens will increase muscle bulk, deepen the voice and increase body and facial hair growth. Clitoral enlargement occurs, often accompanied by an increase in sexual interest and response, and acne may be a problem. Surgery attempts to reconcile an individual's core identity and their physical characteristics. Surgical reassignment for the male transsexual includes penectomy, orchidectomy and vaginoplasty. A proportion of patients also require additional surgical services such as breast enlargement and laryngoplasty. Surgical reassignment for the female transsexual usually involves hysterectomy, oophorectomy, mastectomy and phalloplasty. Selection for surgery is regulated by international standards of care and includes psychiatric assessment and treatment for a minimum of 6 months to confirm diagnosis, exclude psychosis and assist in change of gender role. Criteria include a persistent wish (at least 2 years) to change gender and demonstrable ability to live adequately in the chosen gender role for at least a year by working and becoming self-supporting in that role. Although a number of transsexual people experience a successful outcome in terms of subjective well-being, cosmesis and sexual function, the actual evidence to support gender reassignment surgery is limited in that most studies are non-controlled or non-prospective in nature. They are also hampered by losses to follow-up and a lack of validated assessment measures.

In a controlled study investigating psychological and social change following surgical gender reassignment in male transsexuals, two groups of 20 selected male transsexuals were accepted for gender reassignment surgery. One group was offered early operation and therefore had surgery by follow-up 2 years later, while the second group was still awaiting operation at 2-year follow-up. Although the groups were similar initially, significant differences between them emerged at follow-up in terms of neuroticism and social and sexual activity, with benefits being enjoyed by the operated group (Mate-Kole et al 1990). For non-controlled studies, positive outcomes were reported in areas such as cosmetic appearance, sexual functioning, self-esteem, body image, socio-economic adjustment, family life, social relationships, psychological status and satisfaction.

sex reassignment surgery or likely to be sexually attracted to women and less likely to be satisfied after sex reassignment surgery (DSM-IV). Most of these adult presentations have a chronic course, but spontaneous remission has been reported.

In adult females transsexualism is less common, and in adult clinic samples, men outnumber women by about 3 to 1. Transsexualism in genetic females occurs predominantly in homosexual women, whereas presentations from gender-dysphoric genetic females who are sexually attracted to males is extremely rare (Chivers & Bailey 2000). The gender of the preferred sexual partner is not clearly predicted from the subject's gender identity, and in many cases the strength of the transsexual urge varies with the success or failure of the individual's ordinary sexual relationships. Whereas the majority of male-to-female transsexuals, when

Postoperative complications include haemorrhage, urethral stenosis, urinary incontinence, rectal fistulas, vaginal stenosis, and erectile tissue around the urethral meatus. There is also the thrombotic risk of oestrogen therapy. Serious postoperative incidents include requests for reversal, hospitalisation and suicide, with attempted suicide rates of 0–18% in uncontrolled studies published since 1980 (Wessex Institute for Health Research and Development 1998). Preoperative factors indicating a favourable outcome include (a) a reasonable degree of psychological stability with no history of psychosis, (b) successful adaptation in their desired role for at least 1 year, with convincing physical appearance and behaviour, (c) sufficient understanding of the limitations and consequences of surgery, and (d) preoperative psychotherapy in the context of a gender identity programme.

In 2002, transsexuals in the UK were granted the right to marry as a man or a woman and to apply for a new birth certificate in the gender of their choice, irrespective of whether they had undergone surgical reassignment.

PSYCHOLOGICAL AND BEHAVIOURAL DISORDERS ASSOCIATED WITH SEXUAL DEVELOPMENT AND ORIENTATION

ICD-10 includes this subheading under the chapter relating to disorders of adult personality and behaviour. It includes: *sexual maturation disorder* (where the individual suffers from uncertainty about his or her gender identity or sexual orientation, which causes anxiety or depression), *egodystonic sexual orientation* (in which the gender identity or sexual preference is not in doubt but the individual wishes it were different because of associated psychological and behavioural disorders), and *sexual relationship disorder* (the gender identity or sexual preference abnormality is responsible for difficulties in forming or maintaining a relationship with a sexual partner). ICD notes that sexual orientation alone is not to be regarded as a disorder.

SEXUAL FUNCTION AND AGEING

Ageing impacts on sexual function through both biological and psychological mechanisms.

Men

For males there is the gradual decrease in sexual responsiveness characterised by a prolongation of the time required to achieve full erection, and decrease in the effectiveness of psychic and tactile stimuli. The plateau phase is also prolonged, and the maintenance of erection requires continuing direct genital stimulation. Orgasm and the feeling of ejaculatory inevitability frequently becomes less intense, penile detumescence occurs more rapidly, and the refractory period is more prolonged. The ageing process is associated with decreased total serum and bioavailable testosterone concentration, decreased testosterone to oestradiol ratio, increased sex hormone-binding globulin leading to increased plasma protein binding of circulating testosterone, and decreased testosterone clearance. Several studies have confirmed the role of obesity in decline of androgen levels in ageing men. There is also a decline in the functional capacity of the hypothalamic–pituitary axis, and a decrease in the number of testicular Leydig cells (Kandeel et al 2001).

Women

For women the physical changes that may occur as a result of the menopause transition also have the potential to interfere with sexual functioning. Declining oestrogen levels result in vaginal dryness and atrophy, with loss of the elasticity of vagina and breasts. The clitoris undergoes shrinkage, with diminished engorgement during the desire and arousal phases, and a decline in the neurophysiological response. Decreased muscle tension may increase the time it takes for arousal to lead to orgasm, diminish the peak of orgasm and cause a more rapid resolution. Additionally, with advancing age the uterine contractions associated with orgasm may become painful (Kingsberg 2002). By the time most women reach their 60s their testosterone levels are half of what they were before age 40. Some perimenopausal women will notice an increase in sexual desire and activity, perhaps because their declining level of sex hormone-binding globulin frees up more testosterone. A clinical syndrome of *female androgen insufficiency* defined as a pattern of clinical symptoms in the presence of decreased bioavailable testosterone and normal oestrogen status, has been proposed. The clinical symptoms include impaired sexual function, mood alterations and diminished energy and wellbeing (Bachman et al 2002). In females, oestrogen replacement therapy will often prevent genital atrophy and preserve the epithelial integrity of urogenital tissues. Although the effects of oestrogen or androgen replacement therapy on sexual function remain speculative, sexual activity itself may be protective against the development of urogenital atrophy and associated female sexual dysfunction.

The 1998 National Council on Ageing Survey of older (60 years plus) Americans indicated that sexual activity plays an important role in relationships, with 48% of the over 60s reporting that they were sexually active (sex at least once per month) and over two-thirds of the respondents indicating that sex was an important component of their relationship with their partner. Good physical health, the availability of a partner and a regular and stable pattern of sexual activity earlier in life predict the maintenance of sexual activity in old age (Phanjoo 2000).

The NHSLS noted that the prevalence of sexual dysfunction in women, unlike that in men, tends to decline with age (Laumann et al 1999). Hypoactive sexual desire disorder is the most prevalent female sexual dysfunction for all women, and it is age more than menopausal status that is related to decreased sexual drive, which is impacted by declining testosterone levels. For many women, particularly postmenopausal, drive fades and is no longer the initial step in the sexual response cycle. Instead desire follows arousal, and many women begin to respond from a point of sexual neutrality (Basson 2001). Many postmenopausal women are abstinent because of their male partner's erectile difficulties or his decline in drive. Erectile failure is the commonest sexual problem encountered in older men, with 40% of men reporting mild to severe erectile dysfunction by age 40, increasing to 67% by age 70 in one study (Feldman et al 1994). The problem was associated with a significant number of physical problems and medication. However, despite high rates of sexual dysfunction, older people do not seek help for their sexual problems, for reasons that include ageism and an adoption of negative attitudes towards sexuality. It was reported that out of a total of 3340 patients seen over 25 years at the sexual problems clinic in Edinburgh, only 54 patients were over the age of 65; all were male, and two-thirds presented with erectile failure (Phanjoo 2000).

In addition to the physiological changes associated with the ageing process, other factors, including the increase in the prevalence of chronic illnesses, operative procedures and polypharmacy, can contribute towards the development of sexual dysfunction. Treatments for sexual dysfunction in older age follow similar principles to those in younger adults, with the addition of education about the physiological changes associated with ageing which may allow for reinterpretation of misattributions of sexual dysfunction in this age group.

HOMOSEXUALITY

Recently published community surveys from the Netherlands, USA, Australia and UK report the prevalence of homosexual practices in 1–2.8% of males and in 1.4–2.6% of females, but with each study employing differing definitions of homosexuality (Jorm et al 2002, Johnson et al 2001).

Homosexuality was removed as a diagnostic category from the DSM by the APA in 1973. Prior to this, homosexuality appeared a target for therapeutic intervention, including sexual reorientation therapy. There appears to be an ongoing debate whether homosexuality is a disorder, whether it should be treated and whether homosexuals can change during psychological treatment. The authors of a recent meta-analytic review of treatment of homosexuality noted that their study was not designed to defend the treatment of homosexuality or the identification of it as a disorder, but to assess whether treatment approaches had yielded therapeutic change empirically (Byrd & Nicolosi 2002). They identified 146 studies published prior to 1982, which used primarily behavioural interventions. Only 14 outcome studies were included in the meta-analysis, which indicated that treatment for homosexuality was significantly more effective than alternative treatment of control groups for *symptomatic* change in homosexuals. Few of these studies however had placebo-control groups (Byrd & Nicolosi 2002).

Studies examining sexual orientation and mental health have found a higher prevalence of anxiety, mood and substance-use disorders, suicidal ideation and attempts, in homosexual compared with heterosexual populations (Sandfort et al 2001, Gilman et al 2001). It is postulated that stresses due to stigmatisation and exposure to discriminatory behaviour lead to higher rates of mental disorders, as may the occurrence of victimisation and abuse especially during adolescence, with one recent survey concluding that adult minority sexual orientation is a risk indicator for positive histories of experiencing parental maltreatment during childhood (Corliss et al 2002). Various psychosocial factors may contribute to the higher rates of mental disorders, although a recent study indicated that there appeared to be little direct association with a wide range of quality of life, health and lifestyle variables (Horowitz et al 2001). Despite this, the risk of suicidal ideation and completed suicide among homosexuals is up to 13-fold greater than that of heterosexuals: somewhere between 20% and 42% of homosexual adolescents attempt suicide, with the attempts being generally more serious and more often fatal than those of their heterosexual counterparts (Lebson 2002).

Homosexuals experience sexual dysfunctions similar to those of their heterosexual counterparts, although it is unclear how common sexual problems are in this group (Bell 1999). In a study of 56 male homosexual couples with sexual dysfunctions, three major fears blocked homosexual men from seeking help for their sexual dysfunction: fear of health professionals' negative prejudice; fear of treatment failure; and fear of social exposure during or after the treatment process. One survey reported higher prevalence rates of sexual dysfunction, except premature ejaculation, in homosexual men compared with rates reported in heterosexual men (Rosser et al 1997). Painful receptive anal intercourse is a commonly reported sexual concern in homosexual men. One small study, comparing psychological factors associated with erectile dysfunction in a group of 15 heterosexual and homosexual men, indicated that the heterosexual men were significantly more likely to be affected by performance anxiety and showed higher levels of general anxiety, depression and lower levels of self-esteem than the homosexual group, who in turn appeared more affected by HIV anxiety, internalised homophobia and intimacy issues (Shires & Miller 1998).

PSYCHOLOGICAL THERAPIES FOR SEXUAL PROBLEMS

Over the past four decades, the treatment of sexual dysfunctions has moved from mainly a psychoanalytic approach, through a psycho-educational behavioural approach delineated by Masters & Johnson (1970), to the current mode of psychobiological therapies. Many couples or individuals with sexual dysfunctions may only require brief counselling, which includes both education and advice.

In 1970, Masters & Johnson published their results of a treatment module which consisted of physical examination, history taking, education, prescription of behavioural tasks, and counselling for intrapsychic or interpersonal issues that interfered with normal sexual functioning. The treatment was based on the sequential four-stage progression of arousal. The importance of psychogenic factors, particularly performance anxiety (the fear of future sexual failure based on a previous failure), in the aetiology and maintenance of sexual dysfunctions, and the amenability of most sexual disorders to a brief problem-focused treatment, was emphasised. They described the principle of 'sensate focus' exercises, in which couples were asked to accept limits to their lovemaking, the limits gradually being expanded when they managed a particular behavioural assignment without difficulty. Overall, the principles of sex therapy are those of behavioural psychotherapy in general, with a combination of behavioural, educational and psychotherapeutic components.

If sex therapy is required, factors indicating suitability include:

- the persistence of the sexual problems for at least a few months;
- the problem being caused or maintained by psychological factors;
- the couple's general relationship being reasonably harmonious;
- the couple showing reasonable motivation for treatment;
- there being no current active major psychiatric disorder nor serious alcohol or drug abuse;
- the female partner not being pregnant (Hawton 1995).

Treatment includes presentation of a formulation of the potential aetiological and maintaining factors, followed by a graded programme of homework assignments, with therapeutic work using cognitive, educational measures and other strategies.

General problems in a couple's relationship may have to be addressed in the context of sex therapy.

Studies that evaluated modifications of the original Masters & Johnson approach, which included daily treatment sessions with both partners and treatment by co-therapists (one of each gender), indicated that couples did as well when treated on a weekly basis and by a single therapist, the gender of whom was not related to outcome. The majority of patients continue to be seen in individual or couples therapy, despite the efficacy of a group format approach. A number of factors are associated with positive sex therapy outcome and include:

- the quality of the couple's general relationship, specifically the female partner's pre-treatment assessment of the relationship;
- the motivation of the partners, especially of the male partner;
- absence of serious psychiatric disorder in either partner;
- physical attraction between the partners;
- early compliance with the treatment programme homework assignments (Hawton & Catalan 1986, Hawton 1995).

Individuals without partners may also seek help for sexual dysfunction, and a number of studies have shown positive outcomes. One controlled study indicated that sexually dysfunctional men without partners responded well to behavioural group treatments; treatments that focused on their interpersonal problems resulted in better overall outcomes than treatments concentrating on problems in sexual functioning alone (Stravynski et al 1997).

Couples with sexual difficulties may also be helped by means of instruction manuals ('bibliotherapy'). This approach is possibly useful for couples who have no major relationship difficulties, although limited contact with the therapist (either by telephone or face-to-face) appears to be necessary for success in either couple, or individual, treatment (Hawton 1995). Results from a randomised waiting-list controlled clinical trial of cognitive-behavioural bibliotherapy were reported for 199 heterosexual couples with sexual dysfunction. The couples reported general improvement of their sexual problem, with fewer complaints of low frequency of sexual interaction, and benefits appeared related to treatment compliance. There did, however, appear to be a differential response, with female participants with vaginismus reporting fewer complaints post-treatment, but with more complaints of vaginal discomfort in those presenting with dyspareunia (Lankveld et al 2001).

REFERENCES

Abdel-Hamid I A, El Naggar E A, El Gilany A H 2001 Assessment of as needed use of pharmacotherapy and the pause-squeeze technique in premature ejaculation. International Journal of Impotence Research 13(1):41–5

Agnew J 2001 An overview of paraphilia. Venereology 14:148–156

Bachman G, Bancroft J, Braunstein G et al 2002 Female androgen insufficiency: The Princeton consensus statement on definition, classification, and assessment. Fertility and Sterility 77:660–665

Bancroft J 1998 Sexual Disorders. In: Johnstone E C, Freeman C P L, Zealley A K (eds), Companion to Psychiatric Studies, 6th edn. Churchill Livingstone, Edinburgh, p 529–550

Bancroft J, Graham C A, McCord C 2001 Conceptualizing women's sexual problems. Journal of Sex & Marital Therapy 27:95–103

Basson R 2001 Human sex-response cycles. Journal of Sex & Marital Therapy 27:33–43

Basson R, Berman J, Burnett A et al 2000 Report of the International Consensus Development Conference on Female Sexual Dysfunction: definitions and classifications. Journal of Urology 163:888–893

Basson R, McInnes R, Smith M D et al 2002 Efficacy and safety of sildenafil citrate in women with sexual dysfunction associated with female sexual arousal disorder. Journal of Womens Health & Gender-Based Medicine 11(4):367–377

Bell R 1999 ABC of sexual health: Homosexual men and women. British Medical Journal 318:452–455

Bergeron S, Binik Y M, Khalifé S et al 2001 A randomized comparison of group cognitive-behavioral therapy, surface electromyographic biofeedback, and vestibulectomy in the treatment of dyspareunia resulting from vulvar vestibulitis. Pain 91:297–306

Binik Y M, Reissing E, Pukall C et al 2002 The female sexual pain disorders: genital pain or sexual dysfunction. Archives of Sexual Behaviour 31(5):425–429

Bradford J M 2001 The neurobiology, neuropharmacology, and pharmacological treatment of the paraphilias and compulsive sexual behaviour. Canadian Journal of Psychiatry 46(1):26–34

Byrd A D, Nicolosi J 2002 A meta-analytic review of treatment of homosexuality. Psychological Reports 90:1139–1152

Carnes P J 1998 The case for sexual anorexia: an interim report on 144 patients with sexual disorders. Sexual Addiction & Compulsivity 5:293–309

Cavallini G 1995 Alpha-1 blockade pharmacotherapy in primitive psychogenic premature ejaculation resistant to psychotherapy. European Urology 28(2):126–130

Chivers M L, Bailey M 2000 Sexual orientation of female-to-male transsexuals: a comparison of homosexual and nonhomosexual types. Archives of Sexual Behaviour 29(3):259–278

Choi H K, Jung G W, Moon K H et al 2000 Clinical study of SS-cream in patients with lifelong premature ejaculation. Urology 55(2):257–261

Clayton D O, Shen W W 1998 Psychotropic drug-induced sexual function disorders: diagnosis, incidence and management. Drug Safety 19(4):299–312

Corliss H L, Cochran S D, Mays V M 2002 Reports of parental maltreatment during childhood in a United States population-based survey of homosexual, bisexual, and heterosexual adults. Child Abuse & Neglect 26(11):1165–1178

Di Ceglie D 2000 Gender identity disorder in young people. Advances in Psychiatric Treatment 6:458–466

Dunn K M, Croft P R, Hackett G I 1998 Sexual problems: a study of the prevalence and need for health care in the general population. Family Practice 15(6):519–524

Ellison J M 1998 Antidepressant-induced sexual dysfunction: review, classification, and suggestions for treatment. Harvard Review of Psychiatry 6:177–189

Eskeland B, Thom E, Svendsen K O B 1997 Sexual desire in men: effects of oral ingestion of a product derived from fertilized eggs. Journal of International Medical Research 25:62–70

Fedoroff J P, Fishell A, Fedoroff B 1999 A case series of women evaluated for paraphilic sexual disorders. Canadian Journal of Human Sexuality 8(2):127–140

Feldman H A, Goldstein I, Hatzichristou D G et al 1994 Impotence and its medical and psychosocial correlates: results of the Massachusetts Male Aging Study. Journal of Urology 151:54–61

Gijs L, Gooren L 1996 Hormonal and psychopharmacological interventions in the treatment of paraphilias: an update. Journal of Sex Research 33(4):273–290

Gilman S E, Cochran S D, Mays V M et al 2001 Risk of psychiatric disorders among individuals reporting same-sex sexual partners in the National Comorbidity Survey. American Journal of Public Health 91(6):933–939

Hall N G C 1995 Sexual offender recidivism revisited: a meta-analysis of recent treatment studies. Journal of Consulting and Clinical Psychology 63(5):802–809

Hartmann U, Heiser K, Ruffer-Hesse C, Kloth G 2002 Female sexual desire disorders: subtypes, classification, personality factors and new directions for treatment. World Journal of Urology 20(2):79–88

Hawton K 1995 Treatment of sexual dysfunctions by sex therapy and other approaches. British Journal of Psychiatry 167(3):307–314

Hawton K, Catalan J 1986 Prognostic factors in sex therapy. Behaviour Research and Therapy 24(4):377–385

Heiman J R 2002 Psychologic treatments for female sexual dysfunction: are they effective and do we need them? Archives of Sexual Behaviour 31(5):445–450

Heiman J R 2002 Sexual dysfunction: overview of prevalence, etiological factors, and treatments. Journal of Sex Research 39(1):73–78

Horowitz S M, Weis D L, Laflin M T 2001 Differences between sexual orientation behavior groups and social background, quality of life, and health behaviors. Journal of Sex Research 38(3):205–218

Hurlbert D F 1993 A comparative study using orgasm consistency training in the treatment of women reporting hypoactive sexual desire. Journal of Sex & Marital Therapy 19(1):41–55

Johnson A M, Mercer C H, Erens B et al 2001 Sexual behaviour in Britain: partnerships, practices, and HIV risk behaviours. Lancet 358:1835–1842

Jorm A F, Korten A E, Rodgers B 2002 Sexual orientation and mental health: results from a community survey of young and middle-aged adults. British Journal of Psychiatry 180:423–427

Kafka M P 2001 The paraphilia-related disorders: a proposal for a unified classification of nonparaphilic hypersexuality disorders. Sexual Addiction & Compulsivity 8:227–239

Kandeel F R, Koussa V K T, Swerdloff R S 2001 Male sexual function and disorders: physiology, pathology, clinical investigation, and treatment. Endocrine Reviews 22:342–388

Kaplan H S 1974 The new sex therapy. Brunner Mazel, New York

Kingsberg S A 2002 The impact of aging on sexual function in women and their partners. Archives of Sexual Behaviour 31(5):431–437

Krafft-Ebing 1997 Psychopathia sexualis: the case histories. Velvet Publications, London

Krueger R B, Kaplan M S 2001 Depot-leuprolide acetate for treatment of paraphilias: a report of twelve cases. Archives of Sexual Behavior 30:409–421

Lankveld, J J D M van, Everaerd W, Grotjohann Y 2001 Cognitive-behavioural bibliotherapy for sexual dysfunctions in heterosexual couples: a randomised waiting-list controlled clinical trial in the Netherlands. Journal of Sex Research 38(1):51–67

Laumann E O, Paik A M A, Rosen R C 1999 Sexual dysfunction in the United states: prevalence and predictors. Journal of the American Medical Association 281(6):537–544

Lebson M 2002 Suicide among homosexual youth. Journal of Homosexuality 42(4):107–117

Leiblum S R 1998 Definition and classification of female sexual disorders. International Journal of Impotence Research 10 (suppl 2): S104–S106

Leiblum S R 2001 Critical overview of the new consensus-based definitions and classification of female sexual dysfunction. Journal of Sex and Marital Therapy 27:159–168

Lothstein L M 1996 Antiandrogen treatment for sexual disorders: guidelines for establishing a standard of care. Sexual Addiction & Compulsivity 3(4):313–331

Maletzky B M 2002 The paraphilias: research and treatment. In: Nathan P E, Gorman J M (eds) A guide to treatments that work, 2nd edn p 525–557

Maletzky B M, Steinhauser C 2002 A 25-year follow-up of cognitive/behavioural therapy with 7,275 sexual offenders. Behavior Modification 26(2):123–147

Masters W H, Johnson V E 1970 Human sexual inadequacy. Churchill, London

Mate-Kole C, Freschi M, Robin A 1990 A controlled study of psychological and social change after surgical gender reassignment in selected male transsexuals. British Journal of Psychiatry 157:261–264

McGuire H, Hawton K 2002 Interventions for vaginismus (Cochrane review). In: The Cochrane Library, Issue 3, Update Software, Oxford

Meston C M, Frohlich P F 2000 The neurobiology of sexual function. Archives of General Psychiatry 57(11):1012–1030

Michelson D, Bancroft J, Targum S et al 2000 Female sexual dysfunction associated with antidepressant administration: a randomized, placebo-controlled study of pharmacologic intervention. American Journal of Psychiatry 157:239–243

Phanjoo A L 2000 Sexual dysfunction in old age. Advances in Psychiatric Treatment 6:270–277

Rosen R C 2000 Prevalence and risk factors of sexual dysfunction in men and women. Current Psychiatric Reports 2:189–195

Rosler A, Witztum E 1998 Treatment of men with paraphilia with a long-acting analogue of gonatropin-releasing hormone. The New England Journal of Medicine 338(7):416–422

Rosser B R S, Metz M E, Bockting W O, Buroker T 1997 Sexual difficulties, concerns and satisfaction in homosexual men: an empirical study with implications for HIV prevention. Journal of Sex & Marital therapy 23(1):61–73

Rowland D L, Burnett A L 2000 Pharmacotherapy in the treatment of male sexual dysfunction. Journal of Sex Research 37(3):226–243

Royal College of Psychiatrists 1998 Gender identity disorders in children and adolescents — guidelines for management. Council Report CR63. Royal College of Psychiatrists, London

Sandfort T G M, Graaf R de, Bijl R V, Schnabel P 2001 Same-sex sexual behavior and psychiatric disorders. Archives of General Psychiatry 58:85–91

Sathe R S, Komisaruk B R, Ladas A K, Godbole S V 2001 Naltrexone-induced augmentation of sexual response in men. Archives of Medical Research 32(3):221–226

Schneider J P, Irons R R 2001 Assessment and treatment of addictive sexual disorders: relevance for chemical dependency relapse. Substance Use & Misuse 36(13):1795–1820

Segraves T, Althof S 2002 Psychotherapy and pharmacotherapy for sexual dysfunctions. In: Nathan P E, Gorman J M (eds) A guide to treatments that work, 2nd edn, p 497–524

Segraves R T, Croft H, Kavoussi R et al 2001 Bupropion sustained release (SR) for the treatment of hypoactive sexual desire disorder (HSDD) in nondepressed women. Journal of Sex & Marital Therapy 27:303–316

Shires A, Miller D 1998 A preliminary study comparing psychological factors associated with erectile dysfunction in heterosexual and homosexual men. Sexual and Marital Therapy 13(1):37–49

Simons J S, Carey M P 2001 Prevalence of sexual dysfunctions: results from a decade of research. Archives of Sexual Behaviour 30(2):177–219

Slob A K, Verhulst A C M, Gijs L et al 2002 Intracavernous injection during diagnostic screening for erectile dysfunction; five-year experience with over 600 patients. Journal of Sex & Marital Therapy 28:61–70

Stravynski A, Gaudette G, Lesage A et al 1997 The treatment of sexually dysfunctional men without partners: a controlled study of three behavioural group approaches. British Journal of Psychiatry 170(4):338–344

Trudel G, Marchand A, Ravart M 2001 The effect of a cognitive-behavioural group treatment program on hypoactive sexual desire in women. Sexual and Relationship Therapy 16(2):145–164

Vroege J A, Gijs L, Hengeveld M W 1998 Classification of sexual dysfunctions: towards DSM-V and ICD-11. Comprehensive Psychiatry 39(6):333–337

Wessex Institute for Health Research and Development 1998 Surgical gender reassignment for male to female transsexual people, p 1–25

White P, Bradley C, Ferriter M, Hatzipetrou L 2002 Managements for people with disorders of sexual preference and for convicted sexual offenders (Cochrane review). In: The Cochrane Library, Issue 3, Update Software, Oxford

Wilson S K, Delk J R, Billups K L 2001 Treating symptoms of female sexual arousal disorder with the Eros-clitoral therapy device. Journal of Gender-Specific Medicine 4(2):54–58

33 | Disorders of sleep and wakefulness

David M Semple

INTRODUCTION

The nature of sleep has been one of the great mysteries of human existence. It has only been in relatively recent years that sleep and its disorders have become a true medical discipline. Interest began in the late 19th century, when Jean Baptiste E Gélineau published his work on 14 cases of hypersomnia in 1880, distinguishing primary from secondary hypersomnia, and coining the term 'narcolepsy' (Greek 'seized by somnolence'). In 1903 Santiago Ramón y Cajal and Francisco Tello's work on the morphological changes in reptilian brains during hibernation lead to a variety of neuronal theories of sleep. These culminated in the work of Constantine von Economo in patients dying from encephalitis lethargicans, following the 1917 epidemic. The idea that there were centres in the brain that controlled sleep caught the imagination of neuroscientists, focused attention on the hypothalamus, and laid the foundations for further neurophysiological and neuropathological research.

With the advent of the electroencephalogram (EEG), Hans Berger first showed in 1930 that cerebral electrical activity was different during sleep than in arousal, and in 1937 Alfred Loomis and colleagues described brainwave patterns of sleep that could be measured continuously. A major breakthrough came after the Second World War when Giuseppe Moruzzi and Horace Magoun discovered the relationship between the reticular formation of the brainstem and activation of the EEG during transitions from sleep to wakefulness.

The revolution in sleep research began with Nathaniel Kleitman's research on the relationship of rapid eye movements occurring regularly throughout sleep, and dreaming, which was published in *Science* in 1953. With his student, William Dement, he also described the typical 'architecture' of sleep in 1957. Dement also showed that the EEG during REM sleep had a characteristically desynchronised, 'active' pattern, a finding confirmed by Michel Jouvet in 1959. Jouvet described controlling centres in the brainstem, clarifying the role of pontine centres, and, in 1962, presented a clear neurophysiological framework for the generation of REM sleep, with its associated muscle atonia.

The first specific treatment for a sleep disorder came in 1959, following the work of Robert Yoss and David Daly, who introduced the use of Ritalin (methylphenidate hydrochloride) for narcolepsy. In 1965 sleep apnoea (or 'Pickwickian syndrome') was independently described by Henri Gastaut and colleagues in Marseilles, and Richard Jung and Elio Lugaresi in Bologna.

The publication of Allan Rechtschaffen and Anthony Kale's *Manual of Standardized Terminology, Techniques and Scoring System for Sleep Stages of Human Subjects* in 1968, the first classification of sleep disorders in 1979, and the introduction of surgery (e.g. tracheotomy and uvulopalatopharyngoplasty) or the continuous positive airway pressure apparatus (CPAP) for sleep apnoea, were all significant advances in the diagnosis and treatment of specific sleep disorders. Nowadays the presence of sleep centres and laboratories in general hospitals underlines the fact that the study of sleep is firmly established as a medical discipline.

THE BIOLOGICAL BASIS OF SLEEP

Wakefulness

Wakefulness implies awareness, of self and the environment, and the processing of incoming stimuli. A linked neuronal system, known as the reticular activating system (RAS) promotes wakefulness. This includes the reticular formation of the brainstem (ventral medullary, central pontine, and midbrain areas), posterior hypothalamus, subthalamus, basal forebrain (nucleus basilis of Meynert, septal nuclei, and diagonal band) and the reticular nuclei of the thalamus (ventromedial, intralaminar and midline thalamic nuclei). Sensory input (particularly acoustic and pain) reinforces the tonic activity in the RAS, maintaining wakefulness. The RAS is divided into two pathways: the dorsal pathway (brainstem via thalamus to cortex of the forebrain) and the extrathalamic pathway (subthalamus, posterior hypothalamus, and basal forebrain projecting directly to the whole cortical mantle).

EEG during wakefulness shows mainly low-amplitude, fast, intermixed, desynchronised waveforms. These are also seen during REM sleep, reflecting the fact that both are activated states where neuronal networks are ready to receive incoming information. In wakefulness this information comes mainly from the sensory system, whereas in REM sleep it is mainly internally generated.

Catecholamine- and acetylcholine-containing neurons modulate the activity of cortical and subcortical neurons during wakefulness. Glutaminergic neurons in the brainstem, thalamus and cortex are also excitatory. Other neuromodulators enhance wakefulness, including histamine, noradrenaline (norepinephrine)/drenaline (epinephrine), substance P, corticotrophin-releasing factor (CRF), glucocorticoids, thyrotrophin-releasing factor (TRF) and vasoactive intestinal peptide (VIP).

Synchronised (slow-wave) sleep

As the mechanism for the maintenance of wakefulness becomes less active, sleep-promoting neurons become active, resulting initially in slow-wave or synchronised sleep. The EEG shows high-voltage K complexes, sleep spindles, and high-voltage slow waves (in deep sleep). The generation of synchronised sleep involves a network composed of the solitary tract nucleus of the medulla, raphe nuclei of the brainstem, reticular thalamic nuclei, anterior hypothalamus, preoptic area, basal forebrain and orbitofrontal cortex.

As the activity of the RAS decreases, the thalamus begins to generate synchronous oscillations (sleep spindles — varying amplitude, 7–14 Hz, lasting 1–2 seconds). These are associated with blockade of afferent transmission through the thalamus and loss of consciousness. The reticular nucleus of the thalamus forms a neuronal sheet covering the rostral, lateral and ventral surfaces of the thalamus and acts as the synchronising pacemaker of the spindle oscillations. The principal neurotransmitter in this system is GABA (gamma-aminobutyric acid), and brainstem reticular cholinergic activation has a dampening effect on sleep spindle generation, erasing them during REM sleep and wakefulness.

Serotonergic neurons of the brainstem raphe dampen down sensory input and inhibit motor activity, allowing the emergence of slow-wave cortical activity and reinforcing resonant thalamocortical loops, associated with the generation of EEG delta waves. Only sufficiently strong stimuli, such as intense pain or loud noise, may bypass this gating of the thalamus, and lead to cortical arousal.

A number of other neurotransmitters have been shown to promote sleep (and conversely, their blockade promotes wakefulness). Adenosine receptors, found in the hypothalamus, are blocked by caffeine and other xanthines. GABA receptors are the site of benzodiazepine, barbiturate and alcohol action and are located on neurons in the reticular nucleus of the thalamus, the anterior hypothalamus, and the basal forebrain. The action of endogenous opiates, such as beta-endorphin, enkephalin and dynorphin, initiate and maintain sleep, perhaps because of their role in sensory modulation and analgesia. The recently discovered endocannabinoid receptors may help to explain the hypnotic effects of cannabinoids, the endocannabinoid anandamide, and other fatty acid amides (e.g. oleamide). Somatostatin causes analgesia, akinesia and depresses EEG activity. Other possible modulators of sleep include: alpha-melanocyte-stimulating hormone, prostaglandin D2, and uridine. Blood-borne factors have also been demonstrated to promote sleep. When insulin is injected intravenously, it produces slow-wave sleep, a fact utilised in early insulin coma therapy. The typical drowsiness that follows a heavy meal (postprandial sleep) occurs because of the release of cholecystokinin (which also produces satiety or appetite suppression) and bombesin from the gut. They act either directly on the periventricular regions of the brain, or indirectly through vagal afferents to the solitary tract nucleus of the brainstem. Muramyl peptides are produced by bacteria in the gut and are also sleep-inducing, either on their own or by secondary stimulation of interleukin 1. Promotion of sleep is clearly initiated by a wide variety of substances, with multiple influences and factors involved. Nevertheless, the brain regions where these substances ultimately have their effects are all part of the synchronised sleep-generating network.

Desynchronised (REM) sleep

Desynchronised or REM sleep has also been called 'paradoxic', 'active', or 'dream' sleep, and originates in the brainstem (pons and caudal midbrain). No single centre has been identified for the initiation of REM sleep, although the leading contender is the lateral portion of the nucleus reticularis pontis oralis, which lies ventral to the locus coeruleus. REM sleep has a number of characteristic features:

- *cortical desynchronisation* — due to activation of the central midbrain reticular formation;
- *hippocampal synchronisation* — generation of theta rhythms (4–10 Hz) by CA1 pyramidal cells in the dentate gyrus and medial entorhinal cortex;
- *muscle atonia* — sparing the oculomotor muscles and the diaphragm, due to activation of the magnocellular reticular nucleus (MRN) in the medial medulla (noradrenaline mediated), via the tegmentoreticular tract (TRT), by the perilocus coeruleus (PLC) area. The MRN inhibits the motor neurons via the reticulospinal tract (RST), with acetylcholine and glutamate as the principal neurotransmitters;
- *ponto-geniculo-occipital (PGO) spikes* — originate in the dorsolateral pontine tegmentum (or peribrachial X area), which borders the brachium conjunctivum. They reach the lateral geniculate nucleus and cortical areas, where they stimulate fragmentary imagery that we recognise as dreams. They can be triggered by cholinergic stimulation and inhibited by serotonin;
- *rapid eye movements* — rapid, saccadic, conjugate eye movements. Horizontal movements originate in the periabducens area of the dorsomedial pons, and vertical movements in the midbrain reticular formation. They are preceded by PGO waves and appear phasically throughout REM sleep, often associated with other motor events;
- *myoclonia (muscle twitches)* — brief clonic contractions of the facial muscles and the extremities appear in REM sleep, despite muscle atonia;
- *cardiorespiratory fluctuations* — increases in respiratory rate, heart rate, and variations in blood pressure due to phasic activation of centres in the medial and lateral parabrachial nuclei of the pons;
- *penile/clitoral erections* — unrelated to content of dreams;
- *thermoregulatory suspension* — weakening of the normal hypothalamic-mediated responses to changes in temperature;
- *other phenomena* — changes in cerebral blood flow and metabolism, variations in intracranial pressure, changes in the autonomic nervous system, reduced cardiac output, reduced urine volume, reduced sweating, and raised arousal threshold.

Dream generation appears central to REM sleep — it is reported by 85% of subjects woken from REM sleep. Sensory activation always includes the visual system, with auditory experiences reported in 65% of individuals, and spatial experiences (floating, flying, sinking) much less common. Other perceptions (touch, taste, smell) are rare, with pain almost never occurring. PGO waves originate from the pontine area and activate the lateral geniculate nuclei and forebrain systems. Increases in glucose metabolism have been observed in the visual cortex (presumably the substrate of visual dream experiences) and the motor cortex (consistent with reported dream experience on waking). Motor commands are not executed, because of muscle atonia during REM sleep; however, complex motor behaviours do rarely occur in the syndrome of REM sleep without atonia. The occurrence of motor-ineffectual non-random excitation of brainstem generators of complex motor behaviour (e.g. running, jumping) lead Hobson & McCarley (1977) to argue that the brain generates dreams as elaborations of these events, which are subjectively experienced (the 'activation-synthesis' hypothesis).

The effects on sleep of alterations in some neurotransmitters are summarised in Table 33.1.

Functional imaging studies of sleep in human subjects

Recently, functional imaging of regional brain activity has allowed the neural correlates of slow-wave sleep (SWS) and REM sleep to be examined in human subjects. During SWS, global cerebral glucose metabolism falls by about 20%, rising back to (or above)

Table 33.1	Effects of neurotransmitter alterations on sleep	
Neurotransmitter	Alteration	Effect
Acetylcholine	Increase	Induces REM sleep
	Decrease	Suppresses REM sleep
Dopamine	Increase	Promotes wakefulness
	Decrease	Variable effects
Noradrenaline (norepinephrine)	Increase	Promotes wakefulness Suppresses REM sleep
	Decrease	Reduces muscle atonia in REM sleep
Serotonin	Increase	Promotion of SWS, variable effects on REM sleep
	Decrease	Reduction in total sleep, particularly SWS
REM, rapid eye movement; SWS, slow-wave sleep		

waking levels during REM sleep (Heiss et al 1985, Buchsbaum et al 1989). Regional blood flow during SWS declines, proportional to slow-wave activity seen on EEG, in the rostral brainstem, thalamus, prefrontal and cingulate cortex (Hofle et al 1997, Macquet et al 1997). Regional blood flow increases during REM sleep are seen in the rostral brainstem, thalamus and limbic regions, with reduced blood flow in the prefrontal, posterior cingulate, and areas of the parietal cortex (Macquet et al 1996).

THE ARCHITECTURE OF SLEEP

Under normal circumstances, sleep follows a predetermined and well-organised pattern of stages and cycles (Rechtschaffen & Kales 1968).

Sleep stages

EEG patterns typical of the various stages are shown in Figure 33.1. The proportion of total sleep time occupied by each stage, and its variation with age, are given in Table 33.2.

Stage 1 (light sleep)

As wakefulness declines, posterior alpha activity disappears and slow theta (4–7 Hz) and delta (2–3 Hz) activity emerge in temporal and central areas, with occasional vertex waves. This lasts only a few minutes, and may recur briefly during the night during transitions in sleep stages or following body movements.

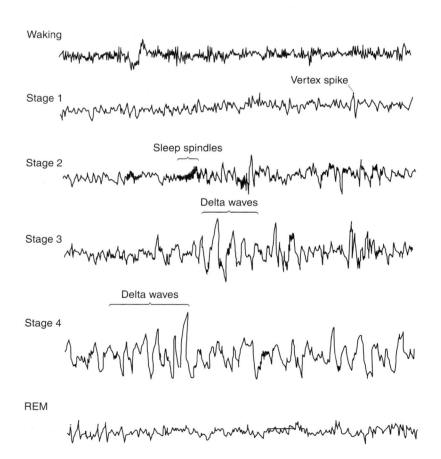

Fig. 33.1
EEG traces typical of the various stages of sleep. (Adapted from Rechtschaffen & Kales 1968.)

Stage 2

An increasing number of symmetrical high-voltage vertex waves with both a negative and a positive sharp component are seen (K complex). These arise both spontaneously or in response to sudden stimuli and are associated with 'sleep spindles' — waxing/waning fast activity (12–14 Hz), lasting 0.5 second, occurring maximally in a vertex location. After 15–30 minutes, high-voltage waves (> 75 mV) in the delta range (< 2 Hz) appear gradually in a semi-symmetrical distribution over both hemispheres. When this occurs greater than 20%, but less than 50%, of the time, this indicates the start of stage 3 sleep.

Stages 3 and 4 (delta sleep, slow-wave sleep)

Along with 20–50% delta waves, sleep spindles can occasionally be seen in stage 3. Stage 4 is defined by greater than 50% delta waves, and together stages 3 and 4 constitute slow-wave sleep, lasting for periods of 30–45 minutes, before reversion to stage 2.

REM sleep

A brief period of arousal marks the end of the first sleep cycle and the onset of REM sleep. Low-voltage, desynchronised activity is seen, associated with muscle atonia and episodic rapid eye movements (which may be preceded by notched, saw-tooth waves in the theta range over the vertex and frontal regions). Occasional bursts of EMG activity (myoclonia) may be seen in association with the phasic eye movements. Sleep spindles and K complexes are absent from REM sleep, and only rarely is alpha activity seen.

Sleep cycles

In a typical night 4 or 5 cycles of the sequential stages occur, each lasting 90–110 minutes (Fig. 33.2). As the night progresses, the amount of time spent in delta sleep decreases, with consequent increase in REM sleep. The first REM period may last only 5–10 minutes, whereas the last REM period, just before waking, may last up to 40 minutes (Pollack 1994). The total amount of sleep needed varies between individuals and throughout life. With the exception of rare individuals who need remarkably little sleep, total sleep time in adults is usually between 5 and 9 hours. REM sleep occupies 20–25% of total sleep time in all ages.

THE FUNCTIONS OF SLEEP

Although it may be tempting to advance a teleological theory of sleep as a necessary period of quiescence serving a restorative function, this view fails to accommodate the wealth of brain activity occurring whilst the individual sleeps. Nonetheless, physical and psychological restoration are undoubtedly key components of sleep's function. Equally, energy conservation, memory consolidation, emotional regulation, brain growth, and a variety of other biological functions, including maintenance of the immune system, must be accounted for in any theory (Rechstschaffen 1998). The conservation of REM sleep throughout life underlines an important role for this highly organised brainstem activity and is hypothesised by some commentators to relate to the consolidation of memories. Indeed, selective interruption of REM sleep has been shown to disrupt the acquisition of perceptual skills requiring repeated practice (Karni et al 1994).

SLEEP DEPRIVATION

Neuropsychological consequences

Sleep deprivation (SD) has been shown to have a variety of neuropsychological consequences. Attention, visual encoding and scanning, novel responses (May & Kline 1987), decision making

---

Table 33.2   Duration of sleep stages (as proportion of total sleep time) at various ages

Sleep stages	Childhood	Young adulthood	Old age
Arousals	Infrequent	5%	Frequent
REM	20–25%	20–25%	20–25%
Stage 1	Reduced	2–5%	Increased
Stage 2	45–55%	45–55%	Increased
Stage 3 (SWS)	Increased	3–8%	Reduced
Stage 4 (SWS)	Increased	10–15%	Reduced or absent
Total sleep time	10–12 hours	8–10 hours	6–8 hours

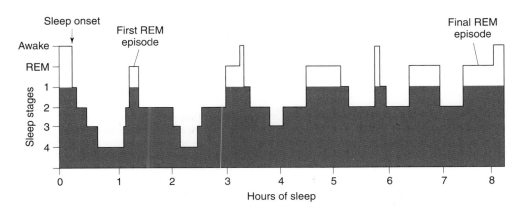

Fig. 33.2
Sleep cycles. (Adapted from Kales & Kales 1970.)

(Harrison & Horne 2000a), divergent thinking (Horne 1988), prolonged vigilance (Samkoff & Jacques 1991), reaction times (Jaskowski & Wlodarczyk 1997), temporal memory (recency) (Harrison & Horne 2000b) and speed in visual search tasks (De Gennaro et al 2001) are amongst the psychological measures affected. The negative effects of SD appear primarily to be in cognitive tasks requiring alertness, attention and contextually related novel responses — impairments which have a predominant prefrontal cortex (PFC) focus (Harrison & Horne 1998) and have been noted to be similar to those of normal aging (Harrison et al 2000).

Functional brain imaging in depressed patients

SD has been used successfully as an augmentative strategy in the treatment of depression, raising the question of how this novel treatment exerts its therapeutic effect. A recent review (Gillin et al 2001) of functional brain imaging studies in depressed patients treated with SD revealed relatively consistent findings. First, before SD, responders have significantly elevated metabolism compared with non-responders, and usually the normal controls, in the orbital medial prefrontal cortex, and especially in the ventral portions of the anterior cingulate cortex. Second, after SD these hyperactive areas normalise in the responders. The magnitude of the clinical improvement was significantly correlated with decreased local glucose metabolic rate or cerebral blood flow in three studies. These results are consistent with some (but not all) functional brain imaging studies of antidepressant medications in depressed patients. Results from a SPECT study using a radioactively labelled D2 receptor antagonist (IBZM) suggest that the antidepressant benefits of sleep deprivation are correlated with endogenous release of dopamine (Ebert et al 1994).

The pro-psychotic nature of sleep deprivation

The pro-psychotic effects of SD have been known for many years, and indeed SD was used to study 'experimental' or 'model' psychosis in the 1960s (Heinemann 1966, Spadetta & Caruso 1968, Vojtechovsky et al 1969). Interest has waxed and waned over the years, and more recently the pro-psychotic nature of SD has been highlighted again by reports implicating SD as a significant factor in the causation of: delirium and frank psychosis in postoperative patients (Sveinsson 1975, McGuire et al 2000), paranoid psychosis associated with sleep apnoea (Berrettini 1980, Lee et al 1989), transient psychosis in servicemen (Kudriavtsev & Korolev 1992), delusional disorders in solitary navigators (Devillieres et al 1996), and mania (Wright 1993).

A role for the prefrontal cortex in SD-mediated effects?

Similarities have been noted between the neuropsychological effects of SD and the symptoms cluster associated with hebephrenic schizophrenia, chronic depression and, to some extent, normal ageing (Horne 1993). The correlation between prefrontal cortex dysfunction and diminished human slow-wave sleep (hSWS) in these different conditions is interesting, but does not necessarily imply aetiology, as it could simply be the effect of more general sleep loss. There is clearly more to schizophrenia and depression than deficits in prefrontal cortex functioning; however, a change in prefrontal cortex functioning (and associated diminution of hSWS)

might account for some of the central clinical symptoms, either as a primary or secondary effect.

The putative role of monoaminergic mechanisms

It is hypothesised that SD may have similar neurobiological effects to psycho-stimulants such as amphetamine and cocaine, mediated through enhancement of monoaminergic release (particularly dopamine and serotonin) (Ebert & Berger 1998). Evidence to support this view comes from various clinical observations such as improvement in motor symptoms of Parkinson's disease following SD (Reist et al 1995), increased eye-blink rates (a possible correlate of central dopamine activity) after SD in depressed patients (Ebert et al 1996), the prevention of the antidepressant effects of SD by amineptine (a dopamine agonist) (Benedetti et al 1996), and worsening of delusional depression after SD (Benedetti et al 1999).

DISORDERS OF SLEEP

Classification of sleep disorders
DSM-IV and ICD-10

Because the specific pathophysiological mechanisms underlying many of the sleep disorders are, as yet, poorly understood, there are notable differences in the way that DSM-IV and ICD-10 classify sleep disorders. DSM-IV uses three broad categories: 'primary sleep disorders', 'sleep disorders related to mental disorders' and 'other sleep disorders'. In ICD-10, sleep disorders appear in three different locations: 'mental and behavioural disorders' (Box 33.1), 'diseases of the nervous system and sense organs', and 'symptoms, signs, and ill-defined conditions'.

The international classification of sleep disorders — revised (ICSD-R)

This has been developed with wide international consultation, in an attempt to standardise diagnoses in both clinical and research settings. The original classification of sleep disorders — the Diagnostic Classification of Sleep and Arousal Disorders — was published in the journal *Sleep* in 1979 and focused on cardinal symptoms (insomnia, hypersomnia, sleep phase disorders, and parasomnias). This was superseded by the 1990 International Classification of Sleep Disorders, which has now been further revised in 1997 (ASDA 1997). There are four major divisions of the sleep disorders: dyssomnias, parasomnias, medical/psychiatric

---

Box 33.1 ICD-10 — Nonorganic sleep disorders

- Nonorganic insomnia
- Nonorganic hypersomnia
- Nonorganic disorder of the sleep–wake schedule
- Sleepwalking (somnambulism)
- Sleep terrors (night terrors)
- Nightmares
- Other nonorganic sleep disorders
- Nonorganic sleep disorder, unspecified

From ICD-10, Chapter V: Mental & behavioural disorders

Box 33.2   ICSD-R (1997) classification outline

Dyssomnias
- Intrinsic sleep disorders
- Extrinsic sleep disorders
- Circadian rhythm sleep disorders

Parasomnias
- Arousal disorders
- Sleep–wake transition disorders
- Parasomnias usually associated with REM sleep
- Other parasomnias

Sleep disorders associated with mental, neurological, or other medical disorders
- Associated with mental disorders
- Associated with neurological disorders
- Associated with other medical disorders

Proposed sleep disorders

ICSD-R, International Classification of Sleep Disorders – Revised

---

sleep disorders, and proposed sleep disorders. These are further subdivided into categories related to common causative factors or characteristic symptoms and signs (Box 33.2)

Clinically, patients tend to present with three common types of complaint: insomnia (not getting enough sleep or feeling 'unrefreshed'), hypersomnia (feeling excessively sleepy during the day or sleeping too much), or a parasomnia (other sleep-related problem). The clinician also has to distinguish between primary sleep disorders and those which have arisen secondary to psychiatric, neurological or other medical disorders (including drug-related problems).

ASSESSMENT OF SLEEP DISORDERS

Sleep history

In taking a sleep history it is essential in most cases to obtain an account from the patient's bed partner, or from an informant such as a parent or carer. The main areas covered should include the following.

- The presenting complaint(s):
  — onset, duration, course, current frequency, severity, effects on everyday life;
  — pattern of symptoms, timing, fluctuations, exacerbating/relieving factors, environmental factors, relevant current stressors;
  — the usual daily routine: waking (time, method, e.g. alarm, natural), usual morning routine, usual daily activities (start and finish times), any daily naps (when, for how long), preparation for bed, time of going to bed, time of falling asleep, activities in bed (TV, reading, sex), description of sleep (including behaviour whilst asleep, dreams/nightmares, frequent wakening and how this is dealt with, satisfaction with quality of sleep);
  — whether tired/sleepy during the day: general alertness, when/if sleep occurs (particularly at times when patient is active — meal times, walking, driving, operating machinery), effects on work/social activities, any periods of confusion, any episodes of collapse.

- Family history.
- Past and current history of medical or psychiatric problems.
- Drug and alcohol history:
  — general review of any regular medications taken (for alerting/sedating effects), including 'timing' of administration;
  — specific questions regarding caffeine-containing drinks (tea, coffee, soft drinks), smoking, alcohol and other recreational drugs (sedatives, analgesics, cannabis, amphetamines, cocaine, etc.).
- Previous treatment:
  — types of treatment tried, benefits/usefulness, problems/side-effects.
- Third party information:
  — occurrence of snoring/gasping/choking/stopping breathing while asleep;
  — occurrence of muscle twitches, limb movement, unusual behaviours while asleep;
  — whether these occur every night or with any clear pattern;
  — any recent mood changes;
  — any recent change in use of drugs or alcohol.

Sleep diary

The use of a sleep diary to record information related to sleep–wake pattern over a 2-week period may clarify any pattern or particular factors that may be present. The information recorded will include an account of the daily activities, the pattern of sleeping, meal-times, consumption of alcohol/caffeine/other drugs, exercise, and daytime sleepiness/napping.

Video recording

The recording of sleep-related behaviours can be a useful component of assessment, particularly for the parasomnias. This is integrated into sleep studies performed in a sleep laboratory, but where such facilities are not available, or where hospital admission may be impractical, the use of home videos may be equally as informative.

Actigraphy

Actigraphy is a means of quantifying both circadian sleep–wake patterns and to identify movement disorders occurring during sleep. A piezoelectric motion sensor, usually incorporated into a wristwatch-like unit, collects data on movement over several days, for later computer analysis. Actigraphy may be useful in assessing circadian rhythm sleep disorders, jet lag, paediatric sleep disorders, and monitoring leg movements during the day and night (e.g. in 'restless leg syndrome' or periodic movements of sleep). It may also help in shift-work studies, or in monitoring the persistence of movement disorders (e.g. parkinsonian tremor) during sleep.

Polysomnography

This is a generic term for a variety of physiological recording methods and techniques employed in the diagnosis of sleep disorders in a sleep laboratory. A basic polysomnogram comprises the EEG, electro-oculogram (EOG), and electromyogram (EMG). Other parameters may be added as needed, including electrocardiogram (ECG), respiratory monitoring (nasal/oral airflow, diaphragm

EMG), oximetry (oxygen saturation), actigraphy, penile tumescence, and oesophageal pH (for oesophageal reflux). Recording may be complemented by the use of audio and video recording to assess nocturnal behaviours, vocalisations and snoring. Time coding of all these measures allows temporal correlations to be made of the various parameters. Less complex portable systems are now available and allow the recording of sleep stages, cardiorespiratory functions, and oximetry in the patient's own home or in other medical settings (e.g. intensive care unit).

Basic polysomnography allows the scoring of sleep stages and the compiling of a hypnogram. Daytime recordings may also be performed and are interpreted as a continuum of nocturnal recordings. As the characteristics of daytime sleep are modulated by nocturnal sleep, isolated daytime recordings are of little value. The 'first-night' effect is a well-described phenomenon seen in some individuals during sleep recording. Sleep tends to have long latencies, be fragmented, have reduced efficiency (often with reduced SWS), and demonstrate frequent position changes. The second night, and any subsequent, recordings tend to better reflect the patient's normal sleep pattern. In general, one night of testing, followed by a daytime multiple sleep latency test (MSLT) is sufficient to diagnose most conditions.

Polysomnography is indicated only in a small number of clinical situations (Box 33.3). Information obtained from polysomnography is scored using the criteria of Rechtschaffen & Kales (1968) for sleep staging. Sleep apnoea events are classified, measured and tabulated along with episodes of oxygen desaturation, arousals, ECG changes, EEG abnormalities (including seizure activity), leg movements and other parameters (snoring, body position, behaviours, vocalisations and other movements.) A number of different terms are used to describe the characteristics of sleep, including sleep continuity (total time in bed, total sleep time, total time awake, number of awakenings, sleep efficiency), non-REM sleep measures (total and percentage time in stages 1–4 sleep, total SWS) and REM sleep measures (REM latency, total and percentage time in REM sleep). Some of these terms are defined in Box 33.4.

Multiple sleep latency test (MSLT)

This test was devised to assess daytime somnolence, but also helps in identifying daytime REM sleep, for example in narcolepsy. The patient is put to bed at 2-hour intervals starting at 8 a.m. with 4–5 segments recorded (lasting 20 minutes if no sleep is recorded, or 15 minutes after the first epoch of sleep). The objective is to measure sleep latency. In adults (but not children) a mean sleep latency of 5 minutes or less, indicates a pathological level of daytime somnolence, 5–10 minutes is 'indeterminate' but may reflect a primary psychiatric disorder, and over 10 minutes is regarded as normal. The ICSD-R suggests specific MSLT criteria for a diagnosis of narcolepsy (see section on hypersomnia). Daytime REM sleep may also occur following the discontinuation of REM-suppressing drugs, in sleep apnoea, and as a normal finding in shift-workers. For this reason, the MSLT should always be preceded by a nocturnal polysomnogram, and the timing of recording should correspond to the individual's usual activity–rest cycle.

INSOMNIA

Insomnia is a common complaint, more frequent in women than men, greater in the elderly, and with an estimated prevalence of about 30% in the general population. ICD-10 specifies the following criteria for a diagnosis of clinically significant insomnia:

- difficulty falling asleep, maintaining sleep, or poor quality of sleep;
- sleep is disturbed at least 3 days/week, for at least 1 month;
- preoccupation with lack of sleep and excessive concern, day and night, over the consequences;
- sleep disturbance causes marked personal distress or interferes with social and occupational functioning.

Using these criteria, the prevalence of clinically significant insomnia is around 6%. A wide variety of conditions may result in insomnia (Box 33.5), and in this section we consider the causes defined by the ICSD-R as 'intrinsic' and 'extrinsic', excluding those caused by organic factors (e.g. a neurological or other medical condition), psychoactive substances, or medication, which are discussed in later sections.

Intrinsic causes

Psychophysiological insomnia

Most patients presenting to primary care with insomnia qualify for this diagnosis. There is difficulty initiating and maintaining sleep, and clear evidence of somatised tension-anxiety associated with

---

Box 33.3   **Indications for polysomnography**
Insomnia / hypersomnia • Sleep apnoea syndromes • Narcolepsy • Periodic limb movements of sleep   *Parasomnias* • REM sleep behaviour disorder • Mixed / multiple (REM / non-REM) parasomnias   *Other* • Assessment of treatment benefits (e.g. CPAP) • Suspected nocturnal epilepsy • Serious cases of sleep-related violence • Validation of reported sleep complaint
CPAP, continuous positive airway pressure apparatus

Box 33.4   **Definitions of terminology**
• *Sleep latency*: time from 'lights out' to onset of sleep • *REM sleep latency*: time from onset of sleep to first REM sleep episode • *Non-REM sleep latency*: Time from onset of sleep to first non-REM sleep episode • *Total sleep time (TST)*: time in sleep from onset to end • *Total time in bed (TIB)*: time spent in bed, including periods when awake • *Sleep efficiency (SE)*: percentage of time in sleep relative to total time spent in bed or total time recorded (TIB/TST × 100) • *Arousal*: partial awakening of < 30 seconds duration, with associated increased muscle tone and movement • *Awakening*: return to wake stage of > 30 seconds duration

Box 33.5   Differential diagnosis of insomnia

Intrinsic causes
- Psychophysiological insomnia
- Sleep state misperception
- Idiopathic insomnia
- Sleep apnoea syndromes
- Periodic limb movement disorder
- Restless legs syndrome

Extrinsic causes
- Inadequate sleep hygiene
- Environmental sleep disorder
- Altitude insomnia
- Adjustment sleep disorder
- Limit-setting sleep disorder
- Sleep-onset association disorder
- Food allergy insomnia
- Nocturnal eating (drinking) syndrome
- Hypnotic-dependent sleep disorder
- Stimulant-dependent sleep disorder
- Alcohol-dependent sleep disorder

Circadian rhythm disorder
- Delayed sleep-phase syndrome
- Advanced sleep-phase syndrome

Medical disorder
- Arousals related to pain (arthritis, peptic ulcer, headache)
- Respiratory disorders (COPD, cystic fibrosis, asthma)
- Diabetes (nocturnal hypoglycaemia / diarrhoea, painful neuropathy)
- Parkinson's disease
- Endocrine disorders (Addison's disease, Cushing's syndrome)

Psychiatric disorder
- Depression
- Bipolar affective disorder
- Anxiety / panic disorder
- Generalised anxiety disorder
- Post-traumatic stress disorder
- Anorexia nervosa
- Schizophrenia

Substance abuse
- Stimulants (amphetamine, cocaine, caffeine, nicotine)
- Withdrawal (alcohol, cannabis, opiates, benzodiazepines)
- Prescribed medication
- Antidepressants (MAOIs, SSRIs, venlafaxine, reboxetine)
- Antiparkinsonian drugs
- Beta-blockers
- Bronchodilators (aminophylline, theophylline, pseudoephedrine)
- Corticosteroids
- NSAIDs (high dose)
- Stimulants (dexamphetamine, methylphenidate)
- Thyroid hormones
- Withdrawal from hypnotics or opiates
- Other, e.g. chemotherapy agents, clonidine, verapamil, digoxin (toxicity), anabolic steroids

Idiopathic insomnia

A lifelong inability to obtain adequate sleep that is presumed to be due to an abnormality of the neurological control of the sleep–wake system. This is a rare disorder, and most sleep disturbances in childhood are associated with behavioural–psychological issues, not with idiopathic insomnia.

Sleep apnoea syndromes

- *Obstructive sleep apnoea syndrome (Pickwickian syndrome)* is characterized by repetitive episodes of upper airway obstruction that occur during sleep, usually associated with a reduction in blood oxygen saturation. It is most common in middle-aged, overweight males, with an estimated prevalence of 1–2% of the population. Symptoms include daytime somnolence, loud snoring and a dry mouth.
- *Central sleep apnoea syndrome* with cessation or decrease of ventilatory effort during sleep is more common in the elderly, but can also occur in isolation with degenerative neurological disorders. Snoring is intermittent and not as loud as in obstructive sleep apnoea. It is only considered pathological when the events are sufficiently frequent to disturb sleep or result in hypoxaemia or cardiac changes.
- True *'Ondine's curse'*, the total inability to breathe while asleep, is extremely rare and usually takes the form of *central alveolar hypoventilation syndrome* with marked hypoxaemia.

Polysomnography is required for the formal diagnosis of these disorders, assessment of severity, and measurement of the impact on sleep architecture and oxygen saturation levels. Symptoms may be improved by weight loss, the avoidance of sedative drugs, and reduction of alcohol consumption. The most widely used treatment is 'continuous positive airway pressure' (CPAP) or 'bi-level positive airways pressure' (Bi-PAP). Mild obstructive sleep apnoea may benefit from the use of an oral appliance (e.g. the 'sleep and nocturnal obstructive apnoea redactor', SNOAR). More aggressive treatments for severe cases involve surgical interventions such as nasal reconstruction, tonsillectomy, uvulopalatopharyngoplasty, bimalleolar advancement, and rarely tracheostomy.

Periodic limb movement (in sleep) disorder (PLMS)

Periodic episodes of repetitive and highly stereotyped limb movements occur during sleep. It appears to be rare in children and progresses with advancing age to become a common finding in up to 34% of patients over the age of 60 years. It may occur in up to 15% of patients with insomnia, may be exacerbated by tricyclic antidepressants and lithium, and should be differentiated from normal 'sleep starts' (see the section on parasomnias). The patient is usually unaware of the problem, although the bed partner may report kicking movements. There is associated daytime somnolence and diagnosis requires polysomnography.

Restless legs syndrome (Ekbom syndrome)

This is characterised by unpleasant, often painful sensations in the lower extremities, particularly on sleep onset, which significantly interfere with the ability to get to sleep. Movement (walking, stamping) or stimulation of the legs (rubbing, squeezing, hot showers, hot packs, ointments) may help relieve symptoms, and there is an association with PLMS. Most cases are idiopathic or

sleep. Apprehension about falling asleep constitutes a conditioned factor (learned sleep prevention) and patients actually sleep better when away from home.

Sleep state misperception

A disorder in which a complaint of insomnia or excessive sleepiness occurs without objective evidence of sleep disturbance.

familial, and symptoms are exacerbated by caffeine, fatigue or stress. Associated medical conditions include: rheumatoid arthritis, uraemia, pregnancy, iron deficiency anaemia, folate deficiency, hypothyroidism, poliomyelitis, peripheral neuropathy (e.g. diabetes), chronic myelopathy, and Parkinson's disease. It may also be caused by antidepressants, phenothiazines, lithium, calcium channel blockers, or withdrawal from sedatives and opiates. It should not be confused with antipsychotic-induced akathisia. In childhood, it is sometimes mistaken for ADHD.

Extrinsic causes

Common causes

- *Inadequate sleep hygiene* encompasses a wide range of daily living activities that are inconsistent with the maintenance of good quality sleep and full daytime alertness (e.g. coffee consumption, frequent late nights). Independently these practices may not produce a clinically significant insomnia; however, their contribution to the disruption of the normal sleep–wake schedule may be additive. Identifying each factor, and taking steps to eliminate or minimise their effects, may be sufficient to manage the problem.
- In *environmental sleep disorder*, sleep disturbance occurs due to factors such as heat, cold, noise, light, excessive movement of bed partner, danger, allergens, hospitalisation and unfamiliar surroundings.
- *Adjustment sleep disorder* occurs due to emotional arousal caused by acute stress, conflict or environmental change.

Childhood problems

- *Limit-setting sleep disorder* has an estimated prevalence of 5–10% and is due to inadequate enforcement of bedtimes, with resultant stalling or refusal to go to bed at an appropriate time.
- *Sleep-onset association disorder* occurs mainly in children aged 6 months to 3 years, declining thereafter. Sleep onset is impaired by the absence of a certain object (e.g. favourite toy) or set of circumstances.
- *Nocturnal eating (drinking) syndrome* is characterised by recurrent awakenings, with the inability to return to sleep without eating or drinking. It has an estimated prevalence of 5% in children aged 6 months to 3 years, showing a marked decrease after weaning.

Others

- *Altitude insomnia* is an acute insomnia, usually accompanied by headaches, loss of appetite, and fatigue, which occurs following ascent to high altitudes in the absence of administered oxygen. Symptoms are seen in 25% of individuals who ascend to 2000 metres above sea level and in the majority of individuals above 4000 metres.
- *Food allergy insomnia* is a disorder of initiating and maintaining sleep, caused by an allergic response to food allergens.

Management

Education

There are many myths surrounding sleep, and the clinician should be able to educate the patient about the stages of sleep, sleep cycles, changes in sleep patterns with age, and the nature of particular sleep problems.

Sleep hygiene

This encompasses two important general strategies for the successful management of sleep disorders: good sleep habits and stimulus control.

Good sleep habits In order to maximise the chances of a good night's sleep a number of practical measures can be employed:

- Ensure the bedroom is quiet (closing windows and doors, sound-proofing or ear-plugs may help), dark (particularly during the summer) and comfortably warm.
- Allow time (about 30 minutes) to 'wind down' before going to bed (e.g. reading, watching television, listening to music or having a warm bath).
- Avoid caffeine-containing drinks after about 4 p.m., and nicotine at least for an hour before bed.
- Exercise regularly (but not late at night).
- Take a 'tryptophan' snack (warm milk or other milky drink).
- Avoid taking naps during the day, or confine a daily nap (no more than 40 minutes) to the early afternoon.
- Set aside a time during the day to think over problems or make plans.

Stimulus control Often individuals with insomnia engage in activities, such as eating, watching television, studying or thinking over problems, whilst in bed. Stimulus control attempts to change these behaviours so that bed is only associated with sleep. General advice includes:

- Go to bed only when sleepy.
- With the exception of sexual activity, no other activity should occur whilst in bed.
- If sleep does not occur, the individual ought not to remain in bed for more than 10–20 minutes, but should get up and go to another room (without turning on all the lights), returning to bed only when feeling sleepy.
- Establish a regular time to get up, with no more than 1 hour's variation (even at weekends and during holidays).

Relaxation training

The regular practice of relaxation techniques during the day may help to provide patients with the means to reduce general arousal, which can be used if necessary whilst in bed.

Sleep restriction

For fragmented sleep, a sleep restriction strategy may help to reduce the total time spent in bed and improve the quality of sleep by 'consolidation'. There are a number of steps to sleep restriction, and completion of the programme requires motivation and encouragement:

- The patient should keep a sleep diary for 5–14 days to allow the calculation of total sleep time (TST) and sleep efficiency (SE):
  — TST = (total time spent in bed) – (hours spent awake during the night).
  — SE = (TST × 100) / (total time spent in bed).
- For the first few nights of a sleep restriction programme the patient spends only the same number of hours in bed as the

average TST for the past week. No naps are allowed, although the patient may feel more tired initially.

- The patient continues to keep a sleep diary, and when the calculated mean SE for 5 nights reaches 85% or better, they are allowed to go to bed 15 minutes earlier.
- The procedure is repeated with increases of 15 minutes if the mean SE remains 85% or better, or decreases of 15 minutes if the mean SE falls below 85%, until a satisfactory amount of sleep is achieved.

Medication

Despite the prevailing public perception that insomnia is best treated by the use of a 'sleeping tablet', prescribing should be the last option, rather than the first. The Committee on the Safety of Medicines (CSM) advise that hypnotics should only be used to treat insomnia when it is severe, disabling, or subjecting the individual to extreme distress. It is critical, before a hypnotic is prescribed, that the cause of insomnia is established, possible underlying factors are addressed, and any primary medical or psychiatric disorder is treated. Ideally hypnotics should be used as short-term adjuncts to other forms of therapy and prolonged administration should be avoided.

Intermediate-acting *benzodiazepines* (e.g. temazepam) are effective in initiating, maintaining and consolidating fragmented sleep, avoiding the 'hang-over' effects of longer-acting compounds and the 'rebound insomnia' of shorter-acting ones. An interrupted course is best (i.e. 5 nights with medication, 2 without), and they should not be continued for more than 4 weeks. Benzodiazepines may worsen sleep apnoea and should not be given to patients unless the respiratory syndrome is controlled by other means (e.g. CPAP). Clonazepam has been shown to be particularly effective in reducing cortical arousals associated with periodic limb movement (PLMS) disorder and may also be used in combination with other preparations (e.g. antiparkinsonian medication: sinemet, bromocriptine and opiates) in restless legs syndrome. Alternatives include *zopiclone, zolpidem* or *zaleplon*, which may be associated with fewer problems of tolerance, dependence or withdrawal than the benzodiazepines, *chloral hydrate*, or sedative antidepressants (particularly for depressed patients with associated insomnia).

HYPERSOMNIA (EXCESSIVE DAYTIME SOMNOLENCE)

There are a number of different forms of hypersomnia. Individuals may complain of:

- 'sleep attacks', i.e. recurrent daytime sleep episodes that may be refreshing or unrefreshing;
- 'sleep drunkenness', i.e. prolonged transition to a fully aroused state on waking;
- lengthening of night-time sleep;
- almost constant excessive daytime sleepiness;
- or even recurrent periods of more or less permanent sleep lasting several days over several months.

Epidemiological surveys suggest the prevalence of hypersomnia to be as high as 15% (Ohayon et al 2002). Diagnosis and management may be particularly relevant when the individual works in an industry or profession where vigilance and concentration are essential (e.g. hospital workers, pilots, train drivers, the military).

Box 33.6   Hypersomnia — differential diagnosis

Dyssomnia — intrinsic
- Narcolepsy
- Recurrent hypersomnia
- Idiopathic hypersomnia
- Post-traumatic hypersomnia
- Sleep apnoea syndromes
- Periodic limb movement disorder

Dyssomnia — extrinsic
- Insufficient sleep syndrome
- Hypnotic-dependent sleep disorder
- Alcohol-dependent sleep disorder
- Toxin-induced sleep disorder

Circadian rhythm disorder
- Time zone change (jet lag) syndrome
- Shift-work sleep disorder
- Delayed sleep-phase syndrome
- Advanced sleep-phase syndrome
- Non-24-hour sleep–wake syndrome

Medical disorder
- Neurological disorders
- Infectious disorders
- Metabolic disorders
- Endocrine disorders

Psychiatric disorder
- Mood disorders

Prescribed medication
- Anticonvulsants
- Antidepressants
- Antiemetics
- Antihistamines
- Antiparkinsonian drugs
- Antipsychotics
- Anxiolytics / hypnotics
- Other, e.g. clonidine, methyldopa, prazosine, reserpine, scopolamine, progestogens

---

ICSD-R provides a framework for the differential diagnosis of hypersomnia (Box 33.6), and in this section we consider the 'intrinsic' and 'extrinsic' causes.

Intrinsic causes

Narcolepsy

Originally described by Gélineau in 1880, narcolepsy is the most common neurological cause of hypersomnia, with an estimated prevalence of 0.047% (Ohayon et al 2002). It affects men and women equally, can begin before the age of 10 years or as late as 50 years, but usually occurs before the age of 25 years (70–80%). Yoss & Daly's (1957) classical 'tetrad' of symptoms — excessive sleepiness, cataplexy, sleep paralysis, and hypnagogic hallucinations — are suffered by only a minority of patients. Excessive daytime sleepiness and associated cataplexy (sudden bilateral loss of muscle tone triggered by a strong emotional reaction) are by far the most common complaints. Other REM sleep phenomena also occur, but are not necessary for the diagnosis to be made. These include sleep paralysis and hallucinations on falling asleep (hypnagogic) or waking up (hypnopompic, less common). Sleep may also be disturbed by frequent awakenings, sleep-talking and REM-related sleep behaviours.

Diagnosis is usually made clinically. Sleep attacks in narcolepsy are usually irresistible and refreshing, whereas in other forms of hypersomnia they tend to be more frequent, of longer duration, easier to resist, and unrefreshing. The attacks also tend to occur in unusual and often dangerous situations, and disturbances and shortening of nocturnal sleep are more common.

Where there is uncertainty it is worthwhile performing HLA (human leucocyte antigen) typing and polysomnography. Studies have shown a strong association between HLA-DR2 haplotypes coded on chromosome 6 and narcolepsy: HLA DQB1*0602 and DQA1*0102 are found in up to 85–95% of individuals, compared with 12–38% in the general population (Mignot et al 1997, Kadotani et al 1998).

Polysomnography involves a nocturnal evaluation followed by the multiple sleep latency test (MSLT). In many cases sleep-onset REM periods are seen with excessive cycles of REM sleep and frequent awakenings. The ICSD-R suggests criteria for a diagnosis of narcolepsy should include: sleep latency of 10 minutes or less, REM sleep latency of 20 minutes or less, MSLT demonstrating a mean sleep latency of 5 minutes or less, and two or more sleep-onset REM periods.

Management Narcolepsy is usually a chronic condition, although some of the symptoms may improve or remit. Poor quality of sleep tends to persist, and treatments are directed towards the most troublesome symptoms:

- *Daytime somnolence* — regular naps or use of stimulants (methylphenidate, methamphetamine, mazinol, pemoline, modafinil) (Thorpy 2001).
- *Cataplexy* — usually controlled by tricyclic or SSRI antidepressants (some evidence for newer antidepressants, e.g. venlafaxine, nefazodone, mirtazepine). Abrupt withdrawal of tricyclics and other antidepressants should be done cautiously, as sudden cessation may potentially cause cataplectic episodes, or even 'status cataplecticus'.
- *REM-related symptoms, hypnagogic/hypnopompic hallucinations*, and *sleep paralysis* — REM-suppressing antidepressants, benzodiazepines (e.g. clonazepam) and possibly gamma-hydroxybutyrate (GHB).

Recently, Lin & colleagues (1999) have shown that canine narcolepsy is caused by a mutation of the hypocretin 2 (*Hcrtr2*) gene. Reports are already beginning to emerge of hypocretin deficiency in human narcolepsy (Mieda & Yanagisawa 2002), and it is likely this will be a focus for future treatments.

Recurrent hypersomnia

The best known in this group of rare disorders is the '*Kleine–Levin syndrome*'. Originally described by Willi Kleine in 1925 and subsequently by Max Levin in 1936, the eponym was coined by Critchley and Hoffman in 1942 for this syndrome of 'periodic somnolence and morbid hunger'. It occurs almost exclusively in male adolescents, usually follows a course of decreasing frequency of attacks, and may persist for many years before complete cessation.

Diagnosis is made clinically on the basis of the cardinal features: periods lasting from days to weeks of attacks of hypersomnia accompanied by excessive food intake (megaphagia). Other behavioural symptoms include sexual disinhibition (which may appear compulsive in nature), and a variety of psychiatric symptoms such as confusion, irritability, restlessness, euphoria, hallucinations, delu-

sions and schizophreniform states. Attacks may occur every 1 to 6 months and last from 1 day to a few weeks. Between attacks the patient recovers completely, and the syndrome may be easily mistaken for other neurological, metabolic or psychiatric disease.

Symptoms of hypersomnia are usually treated using stimulants, which are only effective for short periods of time. When episodes are sufficiently frequent to cause major disruption of social or occupational functioning, preventative measures may be tried. Limited success is cited for the use of mood-stabilising/anticonvulsant medication (e.g. lithium, carbamazepine, valproate).

Menstrual-related hypersomnia

This is characterised by excessive daytime sleepiness preceding menstruation, with detectable alterations in polysomnography when symptomatic. The aetiology of the condition is unknown, and no clear hormonal differences have been found. Treatment is reserved only for symptomatic periods and generally involves the use of stimulants (Billiard et al 1975).

Idiopathic hypersomnia

Roth first described this disorder in 1976, distinguishing polysymptomatic and monosymptomatic forms. In polysymptomatic cases, nocturnal sleep is prolonged (10 hours or more), with sleep drunkenness on waking, and constant or recurrent excessive daytime sleepiness associated with frequent, unrefreshing naps. The monosymptomatic form simply comprises excessive daytime sleepiness. The condition has a chronic course and may have marked impact on social and occupational functioning. Diagnosis tends to be clinical, and polysomnography may help to exclude sleep apnoea, periodic limb movement disorder, or upper airways resistance syndrome. Treatment is similar to narcolepsy, although naps are best avoided as they are unrefreshing.

Post-traumatic hypersomnia

The prevalence of this condition is unknown, and it is more usual that, following head injury or concussion, patients complain of insomnia rather than hypersomnia. Pathologically, lesions implicated in this condition generally involve the brainstem (the tegmentum of the pons or thalamic projections) or the posterior hypothalamus.

Sleep apnoea syndromes and periodic limb movement disorder

These are discussed in the section on insomnia.

Extrinsic causes

Insufficient sleep syndrome

This refers to persistent failure to obtain sufficient nocturnal sleep required to support normally alert wakefulness. This condition is common in the general population, particularly among parents of young children, doctors, students, long-distance lorry drivers, and other occupations where 'unsociable' long hours of work are commonplace. Periods of excessive sleepiness are concentrated in the afternoon and early evening. Rest days are usually characterised by late rising from bed and frequent naps. Individuals report reduced productivity, difficulty in concentration/attention, low mood/

irritability, and somatic symptoms (usually gastrointestinal or musculoskeletal). Treatment is directed towards scheduling increased time asleep, either at night or with regular short naps during the day.

CIRCADIAN RHYTHM SLEEP DISORDERS

In this group of disorders patients may present with either complaints of insomnia or excessive daytime sleepiness. As well as a comprehensive history, the use of a 14-day sleep wake chart will aid in the diagnosis. Actigraphy may also allow objective measurement of the rest–activity cycle, and polysomnography is rarely needed.

ICD-10 specifies the following criteria for a diagnosis of 'disorder of the sleep–wake schedule'.

- Sleep–wake schedule is not in synchrony with the sleep–wake schedule of the cultural environment or society.
- Hypersomnia occurs during the waking period and insomnia during the sleep period nearly every day for at least 1 month or for recurrent shorter periods of time.
- Sleep difficulties cause marked distress or interfere with social or occupational function.

Differential diagnoses ought to include poor sleep hygiene, depression, drug (particularly stimulants or sedatives) and alcohol misuse, and physical conditions (e.g. dementia, head injury and recovery from coma).

According to ICSD-R, circadian rhythm sleep disorders comprise six distinct syndromes, which can be divided into extrinsic and intrinsic causes (Box 33.7).

Extrinsic causes

Time zone change (jet lag) syndrome

Symptoms include varying degrees of difficulties in initiating or maintaining sleep, daytime fatigue, reduced daytime alertness and performance, feelings of apathy, malaise or depression, and somatic symptoms (usually related to gastrointestinal function, muscle aches, or headaches).

Shift work sleep disorder

Adaptation to a change in shift-work schedule usually takes 1–2 weeks, however rotating day/night shifts may present particular

---

> **Box 33.7   ICSD-R (1997) dyssomnias — circadian rhythm sleep disorders**
>
> - Time zone change (jet lag) syndrome
> - Shift work sleep disorder
> - Irregular sleep–wake pattern
> - Delayed sleep phase syndrome
> - Advanced sleep phase syndrome
> - Non-24-hour sleep–wake disorder
> - Circadian rhythm disorder not otherwise specified
>
> ICSD-R, International Classification of Sleep Disorders – Revised

---

difficulties. Often sufferers consult with somatic complaints rather than the underlying disorder of sleep.

Intrinsic causes

Irregular sleep–wake pattern

In some individuals sleep occurrence and waking behaviour are very variable. This leads to considerable disturbance of the normal sleep–wake cycle, and patients present with complaints of inadequate nocturnal sleep and daytime somnolence/frequent napping. Although the idiopathic form is rare, it is associated with Alzheimer's disease, head injury, developmental disorders, and hypothalamic tumours.

Delayed sleep phase syndrome (DSPS)

The late appearance of sleep (typically around 2 a.m.), but with normal total sleep time and architecture, is found in some individuals. This may lead to complaints of sleep-onset insomnia and difficulty awakening at the desired time in the morning. The cause of such a delay in sleep onset is unknown, although in some cases there is a history of head injury. Usually the condition presents in adolescence and runs a continuing course until old age. Individuals may adapt to the condition by taking evening or night jobs. It should be distinguished from sleep phase delay caused by poor sleep hygiene, where daytime somnolence may be a problem in the afternoons, whereas in true delayed sleep phase syndrome patients complain of feeling sleepy or sub-alert first thing in the morning.

Advanced sleep phase syndrome (ASPS)

The opposite of DSPS, this syndrome leads to complaints of evening sleepiness, early sleep onset (e.g. 6–8 p.m.), and early morning wakening. This syndrome may be confused with depression (due to early morning wakening), particularly in elderly patients where prevalence is greater. In contrast to depression, sleep is continuous, without awakenings, the person feels refreshed, and total sleep time is normal for age.

Non-24-hour sleep–wake disorder

Very rarely, some individuals have a greater than 24-hour sleep–wake period. This leads to a chronic steady pattern of 1–2 hour daily delays in sleep onset and wake times when they attempt to conform to conventional schedules. Every few weeks they will have an 'in-phase' period when they will be free of symptoms, and this ought to alert the physician to the presence of this rare condition. There is a reported association with schizoid personality traits and, although the prevalence in the blind is unknown, one survey of blind individuals revealed a high incidence of sleep–wake complaints, with 40% of the respondents recognising a cyclical pattern to their symptoms.

Management

General measures

Education about the nature of sleep and establishing good sleep habits is particularly important for shift-work sleep disorder in which alcohol, nicotine and caffeine may be used to self-medicate symptoms. Other advice for shift-workers should emphasise: the maintenance of regular sleep and mealtimes whenever possible, the use of naps to limit sleep loss, and, when sleeping during the day, the minimisation of environmental factors (noise, light, other interruptions) that may interfere with sleep.

Chronotherapy

For DSPS, establishing a regular waking time, with only 1 hour's variability at weekends and holidays, may help initially. If this is unsuccessful, 'phase-delay' methods may be employed to achieve a phase shift of the sleep–wake cycle (Czeisler et al 1981). This involves establishing a 27-hour day to allow progressive delay of the usual onset of sleep by about 3 hours in each sleep cycle. Sleep should only be permitted for 7–8 hours, with no napping. The disruption to the person's normal routine caused by undergoing this regimen (which may take 5–7 days to complete) requires appropriate measures to be taken to ensure other family and work commitments are attended to. An alternative strategy is to advise the individual to remain awake at the weekend for one full night, and to go to bed the next evening 90 minutes earlier than usual. Sleep periods should again be limited to 7–8 hours, with no napping. The procedure can then be repeated each weekend until a normal bedtime is achieved.

Similarly, for ASPS, slowly delaying sleep onset with gradual increments of 15 minutes may be effective. 'Phase-advance' methods may also be used for the treatment of ASPS (Moldofsky et al 1986). In this therapy the patient goes to bed 3 hours earlier each night until the sleep cycle is advanced back to a normal bedtime. Although this strategy is often successful, it may be difficult to implement, particularly in elderly patients.

Luminotherapy

Light therapy includes both the use of bright light (2500–10 000 lux) with ultraviolet rays filtered out, and light restriction. The basis of therapy is the assumption that the bright light acts by suppressing melatonin (which is sleep-promoting) (Lewy et al 1980). In DSPS, exposure to bright light is scheduled on waking to prevent morning lethargy, usually 2 hours daily for 1 week. Adjunctive light restriction after 4 p.m. may also be helpful. In ASPS, exposure to bright light is recommended 2 hours before scheduled bedtime, to delay this to a more sociable time. Evidence for the effectiveness of light therapy in the rarer intrinsic circadian rhythm disorders of sleep is lacking, but it may have a role in the management of shift-work schedules and the treatment of jet-lag (Terman et al 1995).

Medication

The entrainment of circadian rhythms through the use of appropriately timed short-acting benzodiazepines (e.g. triazolam) has been advocated, particularly for the treatment of jet lag (Buxton et al 2000). Melatonin has been advocated for the treatment of jet lag syndrome. The most recent Cochrane Database systematic review supports the use of melatonin (0.5–5 mg) to prevent or reduce jet lag, in travellers flying across five or more time zones, particularly in an easterly direction, and especially if they have experienced jet lag on previous journeys (Herxheimer & Petrie 2002).

PARASOMNIAS

Parasomnias include unusual behaviours and motor acts with or without autonomic changes that accompany sleep. Sometimes the events occur when arousal is incomplete, or they are associated with REM sleep. Other episodes may arise during the transition form sleep to wakefulness, from wakefulness to sleep, or in transitions between sleep stages. The often 'bizarre' nature of the parasomnias frequently leads to their being misdiagnosed as psychiatric disorders, particularly if they appear temporally related to stressful situations. This may in turn lead to inappropriate treatment, with associated problems including exacerbation of the parasomnia. Often there will be associated psychological distress or psychiatric problems secondary to the parasomnia. Rarely there may also be forensic implications, where there is a history of sleep-related violence.

The ICSD-R subdivides parasomnias according to the sleep stages they occupy (see Box 33.8), and in this section arousal disorders, sleep–wake transition disorders and parasomnias of REM sleep are discussed.

Arousal disorders (or parasomnias of non-REM sleep)

Confusional arousals ('sleep drunkenness')

These are characterised by confusion during and following arousals from sleep, typically non-REM sleep, in the first part of the night. Repeated confusional arousals are almost universal in young children before the age of about 5 years, becoming less common in older childhood. They are fairly rare in adulthood, usually occurring in the context of sleep deprivation, exacerbated

---

Box 33.8 ICSD-R (1997) — parasomnias

Arousal disorders
- Confusional arousals
- Sleepwalking
- Sleep terrors

Sleep–wake transition disorders
- Rhythmic movement disorder
- Sleep starts
- Sleep talking
- Nocturnal leg cramps

Parasomnias usually associated with REM sleep
- Nightmares
- Sleep paralysis
- Impaired sleep-related penile erections
- Sleep-related painful erections
- REM sleep-related sinus arrest
- REM sleep behaviour disorder

Other parasomnias
- Sleep bruxism
- Sleep enuresis
- Sleep-related abnormal swallowing syndrome
- Nocturnal paroxysmal dystonia
- Sudden unexplained nocturnal death syndrome
- Primary snoring
- Infant sleep apnoea
- Congenital central hypoventilation syndrome
- Sudden infant death syndrome
- Benign neonatal sleep myoclonus
- Other parasomnia not otherwise specified

by alcohol or other depressant drugs. They are associated with sleep apnoea syndromes, narcolepsy, and idiopathic hypersomnia. They may also occur in the context of encephalopathy, and need to be carefully differentiated from acute confusional states. Individuals appear disorientated, incoherent, hesitant and slow. Nonetheless, they walk about, get dressed, and even perform complex motor behaviours. Although unusual, it is possible that violence, assault, and even homicide (Klawans 1991) may occur, due to a distorted perception of reality, but obvious planning or premeditation is not possible, and the acts appear more irrational than malicious (Bonkalo 1974). Differential diagnoses include sleep terrors, somnambulism, and REM sleep behaviour disorder.

Management Measures to prevent the patient from falling into deep, prolonged SWS will be helpful. These include the avoidance of sleep deprivation, restricted use of alcohol and other sedative drugs, and sleep hygiene measures to avoid wakening in the first third of the night.

Sleepwalking (somnambulism)

Characterised by complex, automatic behaviours (automatisms) such as aimless wandering, attempting to dress or undress, carrying objects, eating, urinating in unusual places, and rarely driving a car. The eyes are usually wide open, appear glassy, and the person may talk incoherently (somniloquy). Communication is usually impossible. Serious accidents may occur, such as falling down the stairs or exiting through a window. Activity never appears intentional or planned, and only rarely does aggressive behaviour occur (Broughton et al 1994). The person is usually easily returned to bed, falls back into normal sleep, and has no recollection of the episode the following morning. If awakened during the episode, the individual appears confused and disorientated. If any dream content is present, it tends to be fragmented and without a specific theme. Up to 17% of the general population report at least one episode of sleepwalking in childhood, with a peak age of 4–8 years. It occurs much less frequently in adults (with prevalence estimates ranging from 1% to 15%), but there is evidence of familial incidence (Kales et al 1980). Precipitating factors are similar to those for confusional arousals, and some authors regard somnambulism similarly as an arousal disorder, characterised by cortical blockade without motor inhibition (light non-REM sleep). The differential diagnoses include confusional arousal, episodic wandering, epileptic fugue states, and REM sleep behaviour disorder in the elderly. Episodes of variable duration usually occur 15–120 minutes after sleep onset, but may occur at other times. EEG typically shows light, non-REM sleep, with episodes sometimes preceded by hypersynchrony of generalised (non-epileptic) high-voltage delta waves.

Management The main aim of management is to protect the patient from coming to harm (e.g. closing windows, locking doors, sleeping downstairs). Relaxation techniques and attempting to minimise stressors may reduce the frequency of occurrence. Sleep hygiene measures and avoidance of sleep deprivation will also be beneficial. Medication is reserved for patients who have frequent episodes with high-risk behaviours and consists of small doses of a benzodiazepine (e.g. diazepam 2–10 mg) at night-time.

Sleep terrors (parvor nocturnes, incubus)

Sleep terrors are characterised by sudden awakening out of deep sleep accompanied by loud screaming. Occasionally the person will sit up rapidly, and there is associated autonomic arousal. Sometimes frenzied activity occurs, which may lead to injury. Episodes usually last for 10–15 minutes, with evident increase in muscle tone and resistance to physical contact. If wakened, the individual appears confused and incoherent, but soon falls asleep, wakening the next morning with no memory of the event. In children, sleep terrors usually occur in the first third of the night; however, in adults, they can occur at any time of night. Prevalence is approximately 3% in children, and around 1% in adults, with increased frequency in males and evidence for heritability (Kales et al 1980). Deep, prolonged SWS is a predisposing factor, precipitated by fever, sleep deprivation and depressant medication. Differential diagnoses include nightmares and nocturnal epilepsy. Abrupt wakening out of stage 3 or 4 sleep is seen on EEG, with generation of alpha activity, usually in the first third of the night. Partial arousals out of SWS, occurring up to 10–15 times in one night, are also seen even when a full episode is not recorded.

Management If the episodes are frequent (more than once a week), specific management should include: reassurance of the individual (and partner/parents) of the benign character of the disorder, attempts to reduce daytime stressors and any other precipitating factors, and pharmacological treatment with a low-dose benzodiazepine (e.g. diazepam 2–5 mg) at night.

Sleep–wake transition disorders

Rhythmic movement disorder

Characteristically stereotyped, repetitive movements involving large muscles, usually of the head and neck, typically occur immediately prior to sleep and are sustained into light sleep. They are common in young children, with some form of rhythmic activity found in about 60% of all infants at the age of 9 months. Occurrence declines, so that by 18 months the prevalence is around 25%, and by 4 years it is only 8%. They occur more frequently in boys, and common forms include headbanging ('jactatio capitis nocturna'), head rolling and body rocking. When seen in infancy, they are generally not associated with developmental problems or psychopathology. In older children or adults this is not the case, and sometimes the movements may become so violent that traumatic head injury results. Polysomnography reveals rhythmic movement artefacts during light non-REM sleep, without evidence of epileptiform activity.

Management This is unnecessary in most cases, and parents can be reassured that in the majority of infants the disorder will resolve by around the age of 18 months. If the disorder leads to injury or socially disruption, medication may be used (e.g. low-dose benzodiazepine or antidepressant), with variable reported success.

Sleep starts ('hypnic jerks')

These occur at sleep onset and present as sudden abrupt contractions of muscle groups, usually the legs, but sometimes also involving the arms, neck or even the entire body. Sleep starts are essentially a universal component of the sleep-onset process, with a reported prevalence of 60–70%, although often they are not recalled. When wakened by jerks, an individual may have the feeling of falling in space ('siderealism'). Sometimes this feeling is so intense and frightening that it can lead to fear of going to sleep, with subsequent sleep onset difficulties. Other conditions that may cause a similar presentation include nocturnal myoclonic jerks, fragmentary myoclonus, nocturnal leg myoclonus/periodic leg movements of sleep, and the rare 'startle disease' or hyperekplexia syndrome (myoclonus occurs following minor stimuli both during wakefulness and sleep). Polysomnography reveals occasional vertex waves with associated muscular contraction.

Management Treatment is usually unnecessary. If there is significant interference with sleep, measures such as avoidance of stimulants (e.g. caffeine, nicotine), and the use of a small dose of clonazepam at night, may be helpful.

Sleep talking (somniloquy)

Sleep talking is the common uttering of words or sounds during sleep. There is no subjective awareness of the event, and speech is generally devoid of meaning. Rarely, emotionally charged long 'tirades' occur with content related to the person's occupation or preoccupation. It may be associated with confusional arousals, sleep terrors, and REM sleep behaviour disorder. Brief partial arousal during non-REM sleep is usually seen on EEG in about 60% of cases. Less commonly, somniloquy may occur during REM sleep, if related to dream content, or in association with another disorder of REM sleep.

Management Unless the problem is leading to disruption of sleep in a bed partner, or is a secondary symptom of other sleep pathology, treatment is rarely necessary.

Nocturnal leg cramps

Nocturnal leg cramps are sensations of painful muscular tightness or tension, usually in the calf, but occasionally in the foot, occurring during sleep, and which awaken the sufferer. Symptoms of nocturnal leg cramps have been identified in up to 16% of healthy individuals, and may be associated with a variety of problems including excessive muscular activity, dehydration, diabetes, arthritis, pregnancy and Parkinson's disease. It is more commonly seen in the elderly, and ought to be differentiated from periodic leg movements of sleep, muscle spasm due to spasticity following stroke, or other neurological causes of muscle spasticity.

Management Treatment is reserved for severe, recurrent symptoms. Measures such as heat, massage, stretching, or quinine sulphate (325 mg nocte) may be effective.

Parasomnias usually associated with REM sleep

Nightmares

Nightmares are frightening dreams that usually awaken the sleeper from REM sleep, without associated confusion. Approximately half of adults admit to having at least an occasional nightmare, which may be preceded by a frightening or intense real-life traumatic event. Frequent nightmares (one or more a week) occur in about 1% of the adult population. Differential diagnoses include sleep terrors and REM sleep behaviour disorder. Characteristic findings on EEG are of increased REM density, lasting about 10 minutes, terminated by an awakening, usually in the second half of the night.

Management Treatment is usually unnecessary, unless episodes are frequent, distressing, or causing a major disturbance to the individual's carers or bed partner. General measures include the avoidance of stress, discontinuation of drugs that may potentially promote nightmares (Box 33.9), and principles of sleep

Box 33.9 Drugs leading to reports of vivid dreams and nightmares
• Baclofen
• Beta-blockers (atenolol, propanolol)
• Clonidine
• Digoxin toxicity
• Famotidine
• Indomethacin
• Methyldopa
• Nalbumetone
• Nicotine patches
• Pergolide
• Reserpine
• Stanozolol
• Verapamil
• Withdrawal (alcohol, barbiturates, benzodiazepines, opiates, and other hypnotics)
From Bazire (2001).

hygiene. REM-suppressing drugs, such as antidepressants, may be helpful, but should be used cautiously as sudden discontinuation may lead to exacerbation of the problem with REM-rebound.

Sleep paralysis

Sleep paralysis is the frightening experience of being unable to perform voluntary movements either at sleep onset (hypnagogic or predormital form) or upon awakening (hypnopompic or postdormital form), either during the night or in the morning. As an isolated phenomenon, it is reported to occur at least once in the lifetime of 40–50% of normal individuals, and to be associated with sleep-deprivation. As a chronic complaint, it is much less common. Differential diagnoses include narcolepsy and periodic hypokalaemia (described in adolescents, following a high carbohydrate meal, and with low serum potassium during the attack). Familial sleep paralysis does occur, but is exceptionally rare. Polysomnography shows atonia in peripheral muscles (as seen in REM sleep) despite desynchronised EEG with eye movements and blinking (i.e. awake). H-reflex activity is also abolished during an episode (as in REM sleep).

Management Improvement of sleep hygiene, particularly avoidance of sleep deprivation, may help to prevent episodes occurring. For persistent problems, the use of REM-suppressant medication (e.g. clomipramine 25 mg, or an SSRI) can be beneficial.

REM sleep behaviour disorder (RSBD)

This is a relatively rare sleep disorder that occurs predominantly in older males. There is usually a history of bizarre acts occurring during sleep. Loss of usual muscle atonia during REM sleep leads to the appearance of motor activity, ranging from twitches, jerks and restlessness, to complex organised motor behaviours. If awakened, individuals report vivid, often violent, dream content. The motor behaviours can be viewed as 'dream-enactment' and may often lead to injury of the person or their bed partner. The disorder is often associated with degenerative neurological disorders (e.g. Parkinson's disease) and narcolepsy. Some consider RSBD to be an early sign of neurological disease that manifests fully several years later, hence a full neurological examination should be performed. It is rarely associated with other psychiatric disorders, but may be induced or aggravated by psychiatric drugs (e.g. antidepressants), cessation/misuse of REM-suppressing agents (e.g. alcohol, amphetamine, cocaine), or severe stress related to traumatic experiences. Differential diagnoses include sleepwalking, sleep terrors, nocturnal dissociative disorders, nocturnal epilepsy, obstructive sleep apnoea, states of intoxication, and malingering. Polysomnography shows elevated submental EMG tone and/or excessive phasic submental/limb EMG twitching during REM sleep, in the absence of EEG epileptiform activity.

Management Initial management should be to ensure a safe sleeping environment for both the patient and the sleeping partner. Elimination of any factors that might be inducing or aggravating the condition, and treatment where possible of any primary neurological, medical or psychiatric disorder, should be considered. If symptoms persist and are problematic, then use of clonazepam (0.5–1.0 mg nocte) is the treatment of choice, effectively controlling both behaviours and dreams, with good evidence of long-term safety and sustained benefit (Schenk & Mahowald 2002).

Other REM-sleep-related disorders

A number of other disorders are recognised in ICSD-R as relating to REM sleep, but occur rarely. Erectile dysfunction, including *impaired sleep-related penile erections*, and *sleep-related painful erections*, should be differentiated from other causes of erectile dysfunction, such as phimosis, where daytime sexual arousal is also affected. *REM sleep related sinus arrest* is a cardiac rhythm disorder characterized by sinus arrest during REM sleep in otherwise healthy individuals. Little information is available on the prevalence of this disorder, because in most cases the condition is asymptomatic and presumably undiagnosed.

SLEEP DISORDERS ASSOCIATED WITH PSYCHIATRIC CONDITIONS

Almost all psychiatric disorders disrupt the normal sleep wake cycle. Although the biological basis for this is almost certainly related to the pathogenesis of the particular psychiatric illness, it is usually manifest in altered levels of arousal or associated anxiety. There are some characteristic changes on polysomnography, but these are not diagnostic (see Table 33.3). The problem of differentiating a primary sleep disorder from a psychiatric cause is complicated further by the concomitant use of psychiatric drugs (see the section on the effects of drugs and alcohol on sleep). Equally, sleep deprivation may have its own psychological consequences, or may precipitate the onset of a psychiatric illness, particularly a manic episode. In general, successful management of the primary psychiatric disorder is the treatment of choice, although selection and timing of medication may well be influenced by the accompanying sleep-related symptoms. General sleep hygiene measures and the judicious use of hypnotics may also be helpful

Major affective disorders

Alterations in sleep are central symptoms in the mood disorders. Initial insomnia, frequent waking (for often prolonged periods),

Table 33.3 Polysomnographic finding in psychiatric disorders

Disorders	Findings
Major affective disorders	• Loss of SWS (first half of night) • Increased REM sleep • Reduced REM sleep latency
Anxiety disorders	• Increased stage 1 sleep • Reduced SWS • Reduced REM sleep (normal latency)
Schizophrenia	• Equivocal findings for reduced REM latency and reduced SWS
Dementia	• Increased sleep latency • Reduced total sleep time • Increased fragmentation of nocturnal sleep

early morning waking, vivid or disturbing dreams, and daytime fatigue are frequently seen in major depressive disorder. Occasionally, hypersomnia may be a feature in 'atypical' cases, bipolar affective disorder, and 'seasonal affective disorder'. Episodes of mania may be characterised by marked insomnia and a decreased need for sleep.

Anxiety disorders

In general, anxiety disorders commonly disrupt the normal sleep pattern, leading to insomnia, which may be triggered by an acute stressful event, initial insomnia, frequent waking, reduced total sleep time, and early morning waking. In panic disorder, 'sleep-related' attacks may occur with associated intense fear, feelings of impending doom, autonomic arousal, and somatic symptoms. There may be fear associated with going to sleep and subsequent avoidance behaviour that may present as 'insomnia'. They may be differentiated from similar symptoms seen in 'night terrors' because patients are alert during the episodes of panic. Night terrors also have their onset in childhood, and are not accompanied by daytime anxiety. Nightmares are easily distinguished because of their intense dream content and early morning occurrence. Of note, however, recurrent distressing dreams related to a traumatic event are a feature of post-traumatic stress disorder (PTSD).

Schizophrenia

Given the 'similarities' between psychotic phenomena (hallucinations, reality distortion, bizarre delusional ideation) and the dream state, investigators originally expected to see sleep abnormalities in patients with schizophrenia. One hypothesis was that REM sleep 'intrusions' during wakefulness might explain the occurrence of psychotic symptoms. Some animal models support this hypothesis, with the demonstration of hallucinatory behaviour associated with PGO waves intruding into states of wakefulness (and SWS), which can be eliminated with antipsychotic medication. Because of the difficulty in directly identifying PGO waves in humans, it has so far proved impossible to either confirm or refute this hypothesis. As discussed previously, more recent hypotheses regarding the pro-psychotic nature of sleep deprivation, point to the correlation between prefrontal cortex dysfunction and diminished SWS. Patients with schizophrenia have been shown to have a decrease in SWS, with amplitude reduction, which may be corrected with antipsychotic medication (Kaplan et al 1974). Other studies have related these findings to negative symptoms or enlarged lateral ventricles (van Kammen et al 1988). A recent study of drug-naïve patients with schizophrenia, however, did not demonstrate any abnormalities of SWS or REM sleep, suggesting that at least some findings may be related to medication or to differences in patients with acute, rather than chronic symptoms (Lauer et al 1997). Indeed, one of the early findings in schizophrenic populations was a differential effect, on REM sleep rebound following REM suppression, between acute schizophrenia, where there was no REM sleep rebound, and chronic schizophrenia, where there was exaggerated rebound (Zarcone et al 1975). Clinically, patients with schizophrenia do demonstrate increased nocturnal wakefulness and daytime somnolence. It is often difficult to disentangle the effects of medication, active positive symptoms, persistent negative symptoms, and disorganised behaviour.

Dementia

Normal ageing brings about characteristic changes in sleep architecture, with increased sleep latency, reduced total sleep time, loss of SWS, frequent arousals leading to fragmentation of nocturnal sleep, and an increase in daytime napping. Other sleep disorders, for example sleep apnoea syndromes and periodic limb movements of sleep, occur more frequently in the elderly population. Dementia generally causes further increases in sleep latency, further reductions in total sleep time, and increased fragmentation of nocturnal sleep, in proportion to the severity of the illness (Bliwise 1993). Disorders of normal circadian rhythm are also commonly seen, with a characteristic 'sundown syndrome' of confusion and agitation at bedtime. Some studies suggest that the cholinergic deficits seen in Alzheimer's disease may cause reductions in both SWS and REM sleep (Vitiello et al 1992).

SLEEP DISORDERS ASSOCIATED WITH MEDICAL DISORDERS

The contribution of medical disorders to disturbance of sleep and wakefulness ought not to be overlooked when assessing patients who present with symptoms of a sleep disorder. Medical disorders, particularly neurological disorders, may directly affect brain areas essential to the maintenance of a normal sleep–wake pattern. Other ways in which sleep may be disturbed include indirect mechanisms, such as metabolic disturbance, causes of anoxia, pain or discomfort, and the effects of drugs used to treat the primary medical disorder. The main medical disorders with associated sleep problems are listed in Box 33.10.

THE EFFECTS OF DRUGS AND ALCOHOL ON SLEEP

A wide variety of drugs used to treat medical conditions may impact upon sleep. Problems include sedation, initial insomnia, sleep fragmentation, reductions in REM sleep (or rebound on withdrawal), and associated nightmares (see Table 33.4). In this section we focus on the effects of drugs used in the treatment of psychiatric disorders and drugs of abuse, as sleep problems related to these drugs are more likely to present in psychiatric practice.

> **Box 33.10   Medical disorders with associated sleep disturbance**
>
> *Cardiovascular disease*
> - Nocturnal angina
> - Congestive cardiac failure
>
> *Respiratory disease*
> - Chronic obstructive pulmonary disease
> - Nocturnal asthma
>
> *Gastrointestinal disease*
> - Reflux oesophagitis
> - Peptic ulcer disease
>
> *Renal disease*
> - Uraemia due to chronic renal failure.
>
> *Endocrine disorders*
> - Acromegaly
> - Hypothyroidism
> - Hyperthyroidism
> - Diabetes mellitus
> - Addison's disease
> - Cushing's syndrome
>
> *Musculoskeletal disease*
> - Rheumatoid arthritis
> - Osteoarthritis
> - Spondyloarthritides
> - Fibromyalgia syndrome
>
> *Dermatological disease*
> - Due to pruritis, discomfort and pain
>
> *Haematological disease*
> - Sickle cell disease
> - Paroxysmal nocturnal haemoglobinuria
>
> *Neurological disorders*
> - Alzheimer's disease
> - Vascular dementia
> - Parkinson's disease
> - Prion disease (e.g. fatal familial insomnia)
> - Shy-Drager syndrome
> - Progressive supranuclear palsy
> - Olivopontocerebellar degeneration (OPCD)
> - Spinocerebellar degeneration
> - Huntington's chorea
> - Multiple sclerosis
> - Stroke
> - Brain tumours
> - Head trauma
> - Nocturnal epilepsy
> - Juvenile myoclonic epilepsy (Landau–Kleffner syndrome)
> - Headache (vascular, paroxysmal hemicrania, migraine, raised intracranial pressure, 'tension')
> - Infectious disease (sleeping sickness, HIV encephalopathy)
> - Neuromuscular disorders (myotonic dystrophy, myaesthenia gravis, motor neuron disease, poliomyelitis, polyneuropathy)

Drugs used in the treatment of psychiatric disorders

Antidepressants

Tricyclic antidepressants   In general, the sedating effects of tricyclic antidepressants tend to parallel their anticholinergic properties. Hence, the tertiary amines (amitriptyline, trimipramine, doxepin, imipramine, clomipramine) are the most sedating, and the secondary amines (nortriptyline, protriptyline, desipramine) are less so. There are immediate and profound effects on sleep architecture, with pronounced suppression of REM sleep

Table 33.4	The effects of drugs and alcohol on sleep
Drugs	Effects
Analgesics	• Generally sedative • High doses of NSAIDs may be alerting
Anticonvulsants	• Generally sedative • Lamotrigine may cause insomnia • Vigabatrin rarely very sedating
Antiemetics	• Generally sedative • Domperidone least sedative
Antihistamines • H1-antagonists • H2-antagonists	• Older, less selective drugs more sedating • May increase SWS and cause vivid dreams and nightmares
Antiparkinsonian drugs	• Levodopa may disturb sleep, with vivid dreams, nightmares and hallucinations • Ergot derivatives — sedating • Dopamine agonists — sedating (often dramatic) and hallucinations • Selegiline/amantadine — alerting
Bronchodilators	• Aminophylline, theophylline, pseudoephedrine — stimulant effects
Cardiovascular drugs	• ACE inhibitors, loop diuretics (spironolactone) — may be sedating • Beta-blockers (except propanolol) — initial insomnia, increased awakenings and nightmares • Methyldopa — daytime sedation and nightmares • Reserpine — sedation, lethargy and nightmares • Alpha-adrenoceptor agonists (clonidine) — insomnia and vivid dreams • Alpha-adrenoceptor antagonists (prazosin) — transient sedation • Calcium channel blockers (verapamil) — insomnia and nightmares
Other	• Digoxin toxicity — insomnia and nightmares • Muscle relaxants (baclofen) • Corticosteroids • Oral contraceptives • Chemotherapy agents • Thyroid hormones • Androgens (nandrolone) and anabolic steroids (stanozolol)
Poisoning	• Tend to present with drowsiness, hypersomnolence, sluggishness and irritability — e.g. arsenic, bismuth, mercury, copper, other heavy metals, carbon monoxide, vitamin A

Box 33.11	Sedative effects of antipsychotics	
Marked sedation	**Moderate sedation**	**Minimal sedation**
Chlorpromazine	Benperidol	Amisulpiride
Clozapine	Droperidol	Flupenthixol
Methotrimeprazine	Fluphenazine	Haloperidol
Pericyazine	Loxapine	Pimozide
	Olanzapine	Quetiapine
	Perphenazine	Risperidone
	Promazine	Sulpiride
	Thioridazine	Trifluoperazine
	Zuclopenthixol	Zotepine

ings. SSRIs have variable suppressing effects on REM sleep. Paroxetine, the SSRI with the most anticholinergic properties, may cause daytime sedation, and for this reason can be given at night.

Other antidepressants Tetracyclic antidepressants (maprotiline, mianserin) and trazodone (a triazolopyridine) also have marked sedating properties, although these are less related to their anticholinergic properties and may be due to their $5HT_2$ and histamine antagonism. They tend to increase SWS, but are less REM suppressant. These properties are shared by some of the newer antidepressants, such as nefazodone and mirtazepine. Reboxetine and bupropion tend to be more alerting and, like MAOIs, may be useful for 'atypical' depression, where hypersomnia is a particular problem. Venlafaxine behaves much like the SSRIs, and at higher doses insomnia may be a particular problem.

Mood stabilisers

Lithium Lithium tends to be mildly sedating, and studies of the effects of lithium on sleep architecture have shown that it suppresses REM sleep, increases REM latency and increases SWS.

Carbamazepine Drowsiness is a common complaint at the start of treatment or when the dose is being increased, but this is usually a transient effect. Carbamazepine, like lithium, has been shown to augment SWS and to suppress REM sleep.

Sodium valproate This is less sedative than carbamazepine, with only mild effects on sleep architecture in healthy controls; the only appreciable long-term effects are an increase in total sleep time, with a reduced number of arousals, and a reduction in sleep latency.

Antipsychotics

Most antipsychotics cause drowsiness and impaired performance. There is a great degree of variability even within groups of antipsychotics (Box 33.11). Subsequently, there are no particularly characteristic effects on sleep architecture, but most antipsychotics tend to reduce periods of wakefulness and increase the duration of SWS when given in therapeutic doses. The amount of REM sleep may be increased or decreased depending on the dose used. Equally, there tends to be a marked reduction in total sleep time and total REM sleep on cessation.

Benzodiazepines and associated hypnotics

Benzodiazepines and barbiturates have a characteristic influence on sleep architecture. They decrease sleep latency, increase total sleep time, reduce stage 1 sleep, REM sleep and SWS volumes, and increase the proportion of stage 2 sleep. This may be of

(particularly with clomipramine), increased SWS and increased stage 1 sleep.

Monoamine oxidase inhibitors (MAOIs) have a particular 'niche', due to their alerting effects in the treatment of hypersomnolence associated with 'atypical' depression and should be taken in the morning or early afternoon.

Selective serotonin reuptake inhibitors (SSRIs) Most SSRIs also have alerting effects, which may be due to their stimulating effects on $5HT_2$ receptors, and are usually taken in the morning. They can disrupt SWS and sometimes induce nocturnal myoclonus, which increases the frequency of nocturnal awaken-

benefit to patients whose sleep problems are related to a particular stage of sleep, but 'REM rebound' on discontinuation may lead to exacerbation of the underlying disorder, and tolerance to the beneficial hypnotic effects is common after long-term use. The 'newer' hypnotics, such as zopiclone and zolpidem, share the sleep-enhancing properties of the benzodiazepines, but are reported to have less influence on sleep architecture. Zopiclone may actually increase the amount of SWS.

Psychostimulant drugs

These drugs, used in the treatment of hypersomnia (particularly in narcolepsy), attention deficit hyperactivity disorder, and to suppress appetite, all tend to stimulate central transmission of catecholamines. Examples include: dexamphetamine, methylphenidate, methamphetamine, mazinol, pemoline and modafinil. They reduce total sleep time, decrease REM sleep and SWS, and increase sleep latency, with fragmentation of sleep due to frequent nocturnal awakenings. Cessation of these drugs, with the notable exception of modafinil, leads to increases in total sleep time and REM 'rebound'.

Alcohol and drugs of abuse

Alcohol

Alcohol most probably exerts its sedative effects through a combination of GABA facilitation and glutamate inhibition. The acute effects of alcohol lead to reduced sleep latency, increased total sleep time, increased SWS, mild suppression of REM sleep in the first half of the night, and subsequent increased REM sleep in the second half of the night, associated with sleep disruption, intense dreaming and even nightmares. Chronic effects of alcohol abuse include the loss of SWS, sleep disruption and significant insomnia. Withdrawal from alcohol is also associated with insomnia. Sleep architecture is disrupted, with increased sleep latency, reduced total sleep time, loss of SWS, increased REM density and/or amount. 'Delirium tremens', with marked agitation, confusion and hallucinations, is characterised by intense REM rebound.

Nicotine

Nicotine tends to cause initial insomnia, and may be associated with sleep disruption and increased REM sleep. Use of nicotine patches has been associated with vivid dreams and nightmares.

Cannabis

The hypnotic effects of cannabis are modulated by the cannabinoid-1 receptors in the brain and appear to be similar to the effects of benzodiazepines and alcohol, increasing SWS and suppressing REM sleep. Cessation may lead to problems of initial insomnia, sleep disruption and REM rebound.

Opiates

Although sleep is improved when opiates are used therapeutically for pain relief or in the treatment of restless legs, misuse is associated with generalised sleep disruption. Particular changes in sleep architecture include decreased sleep efficiency, decreased total sleep time, decreased SWS, and decreased REM sleep. Withdrawal symptoms include insomnia, with fragmentation of

sleep and disruption of normal sleep architecture, related to increased arousal and REM rebound.

Stimulants

This group encompasses a range of different types of compounds. The effects of amphetamine and some of its derivatives have been mentioned above, under 'Psychostimulant drugs', and similar alterations in sleep architecture are observed with cocaine, including reduced REM sleep and increased sleep and REM latency. Xanthines (caffeine, theophylline) also have similar effects, exerting their influence on sleep mechanisms through adenosine receptors, directly interfering with the generation of sleep (see the section on the biological basis of sleep, p. 772). The amphetamine derivatives fenfluramine and MDMA (3,4-methylene-dioxy-methamphetamine, 'Ecstasy') have a pharmacological action that is primarily serotonergic. This may lead to both daytime sedation and disturbed sleep (due to periods of drowsiness and wakefulness), as well as a reduced duration of REM sleep. SWS may be increased during the 'withdrawal' phase as a 'rebound' phenomenon.

FURTHER READING

Culebras A 1996 Clinical handbook of sleep disorders. Butterworth-Heinemann, Oxford
Kales A (ed) 1995 Pharmacology of sleep. In: Handbook of experimental pharmacology. Springer-Verlag, Berlin
Shneerson, J 2000 Handbook of sleep medicine. Blackwell Science, Oxford

REFERENCES

ASDA 1997 International Classification of Sleep Disorders, Revised: diagnostic and coding manual. American Sleep Disorders Association, Rochester, Minn
Bazire S 2001 Psychotropic drug directory. Quay Books, Mark Allen Publishing, London
Benedetti F, Barbini B, Campori E et al 1996 Dopamine agonist amineptine prevents the antidepressant effect of sleep deprivation. Psychiatry Research 65:179–184
Benedetti F, Zanardi R, Colombo C, Smeraldi E 1999 Worsening of delusional depression after sleep deprivation: case reports. Journal of Psychiatric Research 33:69–72
Berrettini W H 1980 Paranoid psychosis and sleep apnea syndrome. American Journal of Psychiatry 137:493–494
Billiard M, Guilleminault C, Dement W 1975 A menstruation-linked periodic hypersomnia: Kleine-Levin syndrome or new clinical entity? Neurology 25:436–443
Bliwise D 1993 Sleep in normal aging and dementia. Sleep 16:40–81
Bonkalo A 1974 Impulsive acts and confusional states during incomplete arousal from sleep. Psychiatry Quarterly 48:400–409
Broughton R, Billings R, Cartwright R et al 1994 Homicidal somnambulism: A case report. Sleep 17:253–264
Buchsbaum M, Gillin J, Wu J et al 1989 Regional cerebral glucose metabolic rate in human sleep assessed by positron emission tomography. Life Science 45:1349–1356
Buxton OM, Copinschi G, Van Onderbergen A et al 2000 A benzodiazepine hypnotic facilitates adaptation of circadian rhythms and sleep–wake homeostasis to an eight hour delay shift simulating westward jet lag. Sleep 23:915–927
Critchley M, Hoffman H 1942 The syndrome of periodic somnolence and morbid hunger (Kleine-Levin syndrome). British Medical Journal 1:137–139
Czeisler CA, Richardson GS, Coleman RM et al 1981 Chronotherapy: resetting the circadian clocks of patients with delayed sleep phase insomnia. Sleep 4:1–21

De Gennaro L, Ferrara M, Curcio G, Bertini M 2001 Visual search performance across 40 h of continuous wakefulness: Measures of speed and accuracy and relation with oculomotor performance. Physiology & Behavior 74:197–204

Devillieres P, Opitz M, Clervoy P, Stephany J 1996 [Delusion and sleep deprivation]. Encephale 22:229–231

Ebert D, Berger M 1998 Neurobiological similarities in antidepressant sleep deprivation and psychostimulant use: a psychostimulant theory of antidepressant sleep deprivation. Psychopharmacology (Berlin) 140:1–10

Ebert D, Feistel H, Kaschka W et al 1994 Single photon emission computerized tomography assessment of cerebral dopamine D2 receptor blockade in depression before and after sleep deprivation — preliminary results. Biological Psychiatry 35:880–885

Ebert D, Albert R, Hammon G 1996 Eye-blink rates and depression. Is the antidepressant effect of sleep deprivation mediated by the dopamine system? Neuropsychopharmacology 15:332–339

Gélineau J 1880 De la narcolepsie. Gazette Hôpital (Paris) 53:626

Gillin J C, Buchsbaum M, Wu J et al 2001 Sleep deprivation as a model experimental antidepressant treatment: findings from functional brain imaging. Depression & Anxiety 14:37–49

Harrison Y, Horne J A 1998 Sleep loss impairs short and novel language tasks having a prefrontal focus. Journal of Sleep Research 7:95–100

Harrison Y, Horne J A 2000a The impact of sleep deprivation on decision making: a review. Journal of Experimental Psychology Applied 6:236–249

Harrison Y, Horne J A 2000b Sleep loss and temporal memory. Quarterly Journal of Experimental Psychology A 53:271–279

Harrison Y, Horne J A, Rothwell A 2000 Prefrontal neuropsychological effects of sleep deprivation in young adults — a model for healthy aging? Sleep 23:1067–1073

Heinemann L G 1966 [Sleep deprivation for several days in the study of experimental psychosis. Psychopathology and EEG]. Archiv für Psychiatrie und Nervenkrankheiten 208:177–197

Heiss W-D, Pawlik G, Herholz K et al 1985 Regional cerebral glucose metabolism in man during wakefulness, sleep, and dreaming. Brain Research 327:362–366

Herxheimer A, Petrie K J 2002 Melatonin for the prevention and treatment of jet lag. Cochrane Database Systematic Review CD001520

Hobson J, McCarley R 1977 The brain as a dream state generator: An activation-synthesis hypothesis of the dream process. American Journal of Psychiatry 134:1335–1348

Hofle N, Paus T, Reutens D et al 1997 Regional cerebral blood flow changes as a function of delta and spindle activity during slow wave sleep in humans. Journal of Neuroscience 17:4800–4848

Horne J A 1988 Sleep loss and "divergent" thinking ability. Sleep 11:528–536

Horne J A 1993 Human sleep, sleep loss and behaviour: Implications for the prefrontal cortex and psychiatric disorder. British Journal of Psychiatry 162:413–419

Jaskowski P, Wlodarczyk D 1997 Effect of sleep deficit, knowledge of results, and stimulus quality on reaction time and response force. Perceptual & Motor Skills 84:563–572

Kadotani H, Faraco J, Mignot E 1998 Genetic studies in the sleep disorder narcolepsy. Genome Research 8:427–434

Kales A, Kales J 1970 Evaluation, diagnosis and treatment of clinical conditions related to sleep. Journal of the American Medical Association 213:2229–2235

Kales A, Soldatos C, Bixler E et al 1980 Hereditary factors in sleep walking and night terrors. British Journal of Psychiatry 137:111–118

Kaplan J, Dawson S, Vaughan T et al 1974 Effect of prolonged chlorpromazine administration on the sleep of chronic schizophrenics. Archives of General Psychiatry 31:62–66

Karni A, Tanne D, Rubenstein B S et al 1994 Dependence on REM sleep of overnight improvement of a perceptual skill. Science 265:679–682

Klawans H 1991 The sleeping killer. In: Trials of an expert witness. Little, Brown, Boston

Kleine W 1925 Periodische Schlafsucht. Monatsschrift für Psychiatrie und Neurologie 57:285–320

Kudriavtsev I A, Korolev I 1992 [Transient psychogenic psychoses in servicemen]. Zhurnal nevropatologii i psikhiatrii imeni S.S. Korsakova (Moscow) 92:72–76

Lauer C, Schreiber W, Pollmacher T et al 1997 Sleep in schizophrenia: a polysomnographic study on drug-naive patients. Neuropsychopharmacology 16:51–60

Lee S, Chiu H F, Chen C N 1989 Psychosis in sleep apnoea. Australia & New Zealand Journal of Psychiatry 23:571–573

Levin M 1936 Periodic somnolence and morbid hunger: a new syndrome. Brain 59:494–504

Lewy A J, Wehr T A, Goodwin F K et al 1980 Light suppresses melatonin secretion in humans. Science 210:1267–1269

Lin L, Faraco J, Li R et al 1999 The sleep disorder canine narcolepsy is caused by a mutation in the hypocretin (orexin) receptor 2 gene. Cell 98:365–376

Macquet P, Peters J, Aerts J et al 1996 Functional neuroanatomy of human rapid-eye-movement sleep and dreaming. Nature 383:163–166

Macquet P, Degueldre C, Delfiore G et al 1997 Functional neuroanatomy of human slow wave sleep. Journal of Neuroscience 17:2807–2812

May J, Kline P 1987 Measuring the effects upon cognitive abilities of sleep loss during continuous operations. British Journal of Psychology 78(Pt 4):443–455

McGuire B E, Basten C J, Ryan C J, Gallagher J 2000 Intensive care unit syndrome: a dangerous misnomer. Archives of Internal Medicine 160:906–909

Mieda M, Yanagisawa M 2002 Sleep, feeding and neuropeptides: roles of orexins and orexin receptors. Current Opinion in Neurobiology 12:339–345

Mignot E, Hayduk R, Black J et al 1997 HLA DQB1*0602 is associated with cataplexy in 509 narcoleptic patients. Sleep 20:1012–1020

Moldofsky H, Musisi S, Phillipson E A 1986 Treatment of a case of advanced sleep phase syndrome by phase advance chronotherapy. Sleep 9:61–65

Ohayon M, Priest R, Zulley J, Paive T 2002 Prevalence of narcolepsy symptomatology and diagnosis in the European population. Neurology 58:1826–1833

Pollak C P 1994 Regulation of sleep rate and circadian consolidation of sleep and wakefulness in an infant. Sleep 17:567–575

Rechtschaffen A 1998 Current perspectives on the function of sleep. Perspectives in Biology and Medicine 41:359–389

Rechtschaffen A, Kales A 1968 A manual of standardized terminology, techniques and scoring system for sleep stages of human subjects. US Government Printing Office Public Health Service, Washington DC

Reist C, Sokolski K N, Chen C C et al 1995 The effect of sleep deprivation on motor impairment and retinal adaptation in Parkinson's disease. Progress in Neuro-psychopharmacology & Biological Psychiatry 19:445–454

Roth B 1976 Narcolepsy and hypersomnia. Schweizer Archiv für Neurologie und Psychiatrie 119:31–41

Samkoff J S, Jacques C H 1991 A review of studies concerning effects of sleep deprivation and fatigue on residents' performance. Academic Medicine 66:687–693

Schenck C H, Mahowald M W 2002 REM sleep behavior disorder: clinical, developmental, and neuroscience perspectives 16 years after its formal identification in SLEEP. Sleep 25:120–138

Spadetta V, Caruso G 1968 [Sleep and dream deprivation]. Acta Neurologica(Napoli) 23:925–948

Sveinsson I S 1975 Postoperative psychosis after heart surgery. Journal of Thoracic & Cardiovascular Surgery 70:717–726

Terman M, Lewy A J, Dijk D J 1995 Light treatment for sleep disorders: consensus report. IV: Sleep phase and duration disturbances. Journal of Biological Rhythms 10:135–147

Thorpy M 2001 Current concepts in the etiology, diagnosis and treatment of narcolepsy. Sleep Medicine 2:5–17

van Kammen D, van Kammen W, Peters J 1988 Decreased slow-wave sleep and enlarged ventricles in schizophrenia. Neuropsychopharmacology 1:265–271

Vitiello M, Bliwise D, Prinz P 1992 Sleep in Alzheimer's disease and the sundown syndrome. Neurology 42:83–94

Vojtechovsky M, Skala J, Hort V 1969 [Experimental psychoses induced by sleep deprivation and hallucinogens in abstaining alcoholics]. Ceskoslovenska Psychiatrie 65:137–149

Wright J B 1993 Mania following sleep deprivation. British Journal of Psychiatry 163:679–680

Yoss R, Daly D 1957 Criteria for the diagnosis of the narcoleptic syndrome. Proceedings of the Staff of the Mayo Clinic 32:320

Zarcone V, Azumi K, Dement W et al 1975 REM phase deprivation and schizophrenia II. Archives of General Psychiatry 32:1431–1436

A1 | Mental health legislation and definitions

Lindsay D G Thomson

Definition	England & Wales Mental Health Act 1983	Northern Ireland Mental Health (NI) Order 1986	Scotland Mental Health (Scotland) Act 1984	Republic of Ireland Mental Treatment Act 1945
Mental disorder	Mental disorder means mental illness, arrested or incomplete development of mind, psychopathic disorder, and any other disorder or disability of mind	Mental disorder means mental illness, mental handicap and any other disorder or disability of mind	Mental disorder means mental illness or mental handicap however caused or manifested	—
Mental illness	Mental illness is not defined	Mental illness means a state of mind which affects a person's thinking, perceiving, emotion or judgement to the extent that he requires care or medical treatment in his own interests or the interests of other persons	Mental illness — not defined, but includes a mental disorder which is a persistent one manifested only by abnormally aggressive or seriously irresponsible conduct	—
Mental impairment	Mental impairment means a state of arrested or incomplete development of mind (not amounting to severe mental impairment) which includes significant impairment of intelligence and social functioning and is associated with abnormally aggressive or seriously irresponsible conduct on the part of the person concerned	—	Mental impairment means a state of arrested or incomplete development of mind, not amounting to severe mental impairment, which includes significant impairment of intelligence and social functioning and is associated with abnormally aggressive or seriously irresponsible conduct on the part of the person concerned	—
Severe mental impairment	Severe mental impairment means a state of arrested or incomplete development of mind which includes severe impairment of intelligence and social functioning and is associated with abnormally aggressive or seriously irresponsible conduct on the part of the person concerned	Severe mental impairment means a state of arrested or incomplete development of mind which includes severe impairment of intelligence and social functioning and is associated with abnormally aggressive or seriously irresponsible conduct on the part of the person concerned	Severe mental impairment means a state of arrested or incomplete development of mind which includes severe impairment of intelligence and social functioning and is associated with abnormally aggressive or seriously irresponsible conduct on the part of the person concerned	—

(continued)

Definition	England & Wales Mental Health Act 1983	Northern Ireland Mental Health (NI) Order 1986	Scotland Mental Health (Scotland) Act 1984	Republic of Ireland Mental Treatment Act 1945
Psychopathic disorder	Psychopathic disorder means a persistent disorder of disability of mind (whether or not including significant impairment of intelligence) which results in abnormally aggressive or seriously irresponsible conduct on the part of the person concerned	—	—	—
Mental handicap	—	Mental handicap means a state of arrested or incomplete development of mind which includes significant impairment of intelligence and social functioning	—	—
Severe mental handicap	—	Severe mental handicap means a state of arrested or incomplete development of mind which includes severe impairment of intelligence and social functioning	—	—
Exclusions	Persons suffering from mental disorder by reason only of promiscuity or other immoral conduct, sexual deviancy, or dependence on alcohol or drugs, are excluded	Persons suffering from mental disorder by reason only of personality disorder, promiscuity, or other immoral conduct, sexual deviancy, or dependence on alcohol or drugs, are excluded from detention on these grounds alone	Persons suffering from mental disorder by reason only of promiscuity or other immoral conduct, sexual deviancy, or dependence on alcohol or drugs, are excluded from detention on these grounds alone	—
Persons of unsound mind	—	—	—	A proper person to be taken charge of and detained under care and treatment who is unlikely to recover within 6 months of the date of examination
Temporary patient	—	—	—	A patient suffering from mental illness and believed to require for his recovery, not more than 6 months suitable treatment and who is unfit on account of his mental state for treatment as a voluntary patient; or an addict believed to require for his recovery at least 6 months preventive and curative treatment (continued)

Definition	England & Wales Mental Health Act 1983	Northern Ireland Mental Health (NI) Order 1986	Scotland Mental Health (Scotland) Act 1984	Republic of Ireland Mental Treatment Act 1945
Voluntary patient	—	—	—	A person who, acting by himself or in the case of a person less than 16 years of age by his parent or guardian submits himself voluntarily for treatment for illness of a mental or kindred nature
Addict	—	—	—	An addict is a person who: (1) by reason of his addiction to drugs or intoxicants is either dangerous to himself or others, or incapable of managing himself or his affairs, or of ordinary proper conduct; or (2) by reason of his addiction to drugs, intoxicants or perverted conduct is in serious danger of mental disorder

— Term not in Act/Order or undefined.

Mental Health (Scotland) Act 1984: Part V Compulsory Admission and Detention

Purpose	Section	Grounds for detention	Duration	Signatories / consent	Appeal
Emergency admission	24	• Mental disorder • Patient's health or safety / protection of others • Requires hospitalisation urgently	72 hours	One fully registered doctor / relative or Mental Health Officer if practicable	None
Emergency detention of patient in hospital	25(1)	• Mental disorder • Patient's health or safety / protection of others • Requires ongoing hospitalisation urgently	72 hours	One fully registered doctor / relative or Mental Health Officer if practicable	None
Emergency detention of patient in hospital: nurses' holding power	25(2)	• Mental disorder • Patient's health or safety / protection of others • Not practicable to secure immediate attendance of a doctor for the purpose of making an emergency recommendation	2 hours or until arrival of doctor with power to make an emergency recommendation	Nurse of the prescribed class	None
Short-term detention	26	• Mental disorder of a nature or degree to make hospital detention appropriate • Patient's health or safety / protection of others	28 days (further to S24 or S25(1))	Approved doctor / nearest relative or Mental Health Officer	To Sheriff or Mental Welfare Commission
Extension of short-term detention	26A	• Mental disorder • Detained under S.26 • Intention to lodge application for S.18	3 working days	Approved doctor / nearest relative or Mental Health Officer	To Sheriff or Mental Welfare Commission
Non-urgent admission or ongoing detention	18	• Mental disorder of a nature and degree which makes it appropriate to receive medical treatment in hospital; and (i) in the case where the mental disorder is a persistent one manifested only by abnormally aggressive or seriously irresponsible conduct such treatment is likely to alleviate or prevent a deterioration of his condition; or (ii) in the case where the mental disorder which he suffers is a mental handicap, the handicap comprises mental impairment (where such treatment is likely to alleviate or prevent a deterioration of his condition) or severe mental impairment; and • It is necessary for the patient's health or safety or for the protection of other people that he should receive such treatment and it cannot be provided unless he is detained	6 months, renewable for a further 6 months and subsequently yearly	Two doctors (one approved); application by nearest relative or Mental Health Officer; Sheriff's approval	To Mental Welfare Commission; To Sheriff if detention extended after 6 months

Detention can proceed from S.24 → S.26 (→S.26A) → S.18 but a S.24 or S.26 cannot be reapplied during this process. In a non-urgent situation a direct application is made to the Sheriff Court for a S.18. A section can be terminated at any stage by the Responsible Medical Officer, hospital managers or nearest relative (if not opposed by the RMO); or by a Sheriff or the Mental Welfare Commission following appeal.

Mental Health Act 1983: Part II Compulsory Admission and Detention					
Purpose	Section	Grounds for detention	Duration	Signatories / applicant	Appeal
Admission for assessment	2	• Mental disorder • Patient's health or safety / protection of others • Requires hospitalisation	28 days	2 doctors (one approved) / nearest relative or approved social worker applies	Mental Health Review Tribunal — application by patient
Admission for treatment	3	• Mental illness, (severe) mental impairment & psychopathic disorder makes hospital treatment appropriate — if psychopathic disorder or mental impairment, such treatment is likely to alleviate or prevent deterioration of his condition • Necessary for patient's health or safety or for protection of others and it cannot be provided unless detained	6 months	2 doctors (one approved) / nearest relative or approved social worker applies	Mental Health Review Tribunal — application by patient, nearest relative or by hospital managers
Emergency admission	4	• Mental disorder • Patient's health or safety, or protection of others • Requires urgent hospitalisation	72 hours	1 doctor / application by nearest relative or approved social worker	None
Emergency detention of patient in hospital	5(2)	• Liable to be detained in hospital in pursuance of an application for admission for assessment	72 hours	Doctor in charge or nominated deputy / same	None
Nurses' holding power	5(4)	• Mental disorder • Patient's health or safety / protection of others • Requires immediate restraint from leaving hospital • Not practicable to obtain doctor immediately for S.5(2)	6 hours	Nurse of the prescribed class / none	None

Detention can proceed from S.4 / S.5(2)→S.2→S.3 or commence with S.2 or S.3.

Detention can be terminated at any stage by the Responsible Medical Officer or by the Mental Health Review Tribunal

A draft Mental Health Bill for England and Wales was published in 2002. It does not appear in the Government's current legislative programme and has been met with considerable opposition. Its future is therefore uncertain.

Mental Health (Northern Ireland) Order 1986: Part II Compulsory Admission

Purpose	Article	Grounds for detention	Duration	Signatories / applicant	Appeal
Admission for assessment	4	• Mental disorder • Requires hospitalisation • Substantial likelihood of serious physical harm to self or others	7 days with possible extension to 14 days	1 doctor / nearest relative or approved social worker	Mental Health Review Tribunal
Assessment of patients already in hospital	7(2)	• Mental disorder • Requires ongoing hospitalisation • Substantial likelihood of serious physical harm to self or others	48 hours	Hospital doctor	None
Nurses' holding power	7(3)	• Mental disorder • Requires application for assessment • Not practicable to secure immediate attendance of doctor	6 hours	Nurse of the prescribed class	None
Detention for treatment	12	• Mental illness or severe mental impairment • Requires hospitalisation • Substantial likelihood of serious physical harm to self or others	6 months, renewable for a further 6 months and subsequently yearly	1 doctor approved by the Commission / nearest relative or approved social worker	Mental Health Review Tribunal

Detention can proceed from Article 7(3) if required→A.7(2) if required→A.4→A.12
Detention can be terminated at any stage by the Responsible Medical Officer, the Responsible Board, the nearest relative (if not opposed by the RMO), or by the Mental Health Review Tribunal following an appeal.

Mental Treatment Act 1945 Republic of Ireland: Compulsory Admission

Purpose	Section	Grounds for detention	Duration	Signatories / applicant	Appeal
Admission as voluntary patient	190 & 191		Must give 72 hours notice before taking own discharge	• Own application if aged over 16, or application of parent or guardian if less than 16, and • Recommendation by GP	None
Take charge of and detain under care and treatment	163 & 171	• Person of unsound mind	No limit	• Application by relative, social worker, or police, and • Recommendation by GP, and • Reception order by receiving consultant	• The High Court (habeas corpus) • The Minister for Health
Receive and detain for care and treatment	184	• Temporary patient	6 months, renewable every 6 months up to a maximum of 2 years	• Application by relative, social worker, any other, and • Recommendation by GP, and • Reception order by receiving consultant	• The High Court (habeas corpus) • The Minister for Health

Detention is terminated when the patient is discharged; or following a successful appeal.
There are some differences in the legislation for public and private patients.

Mental Health (Care and Treatment) (Scotland) Act 2003

This Act was passed by the Scottish Parliament in March 2003. Readers must be aware that the enactment of the provisions of the legislation will be gradual and that, in the interim, sections of the Mental Health (Scotland) Act 1984 will continue to apply.

Definitions

Term	Definition
Mental disorder	Mental disorder means any • Mental illness • Personality disorder or • Learning disability, however caused or manifested
Exclusions	A person is not mentally disordered by reason only of any of the following: • Sexual orientation • Sexual deviancy • Transsexualism • Transvestism • Dependence on, or use of, alcohol or drugs • Behaviour that causes, or is likely to cause, harassment, alarm or distress to any other person • Acting as no prudent person would act

Mental Health (Care and Treatment) (Scotland) Act 2003: Parts 5–7 Detention and Compulsory Treatment Orders — continued

Purpose	Section	Grounds	Duration	Signatories / consent	Revocation / Appeal
Emergency detention	36(1)	• Patient has a mental disorder • Patient has significantly impaired ability to make decisions about provision of medical treatment because of mental disorder • Matter of urgency to detain patient in hospital to determine what medical treatment requires to be provided • Significant risk to patient's health, safety or welfare; or to the safety of others • Undesirable delay in making arrangements for a short-term detention certificate	72 hours commencing at time of admission to hospital under the certificate, or at time of certification for pre-existing inpatients	One fully registered doctor / Mental Health Officer if practicable	An approved medical practitioner can revoke a certificate at the statutory post-certification medical examination No appeal
Nurses' power to detain pending medical examination	299	• Patient has a mental disorder • Necessary for the protection of the patient's health, safety or welfare; or the safety of others that the patient be immediately restrained from leaving the hospital • Not practicable to secure immediate medical examination • Necessary to carry out a medical examination to determine whether the granting of an emergency detention or short-term detention certificate is warranted	2 hours and can be extended by 1 hour if the doctor arrives after the expiry of the first hour of the holding period	Nurse of the prescribed class — usually Registered Mental Nurse	No appeal
Short-term detention in hospital	44(1)	• Patient has a mental disorder • Patient has significantly impaired ability to make decisions about provision of medical treatment because of mental disorder • Necessary to detain the patient in hospital to determine what medical treatment should be given, or to give medical treatment • Significant risk to patient's health, safety or welfare of patient; or to the safety of others • The granting of a short-term detention certificate is necessary	28 days	Approved medical practitioner / Mental Health Officer. Must consult named person if practicable	The RMO or Mental Welfare Commission can revoke the certificate The patient can appeal to the Mental Health Tribunal for Scotland

(continued)

Mental Health (Care and Treatment) (Scotland) Act 2003: Parts 5–7 Detention and Compulsory Treatment Orders

Purpose	Section	Grounds	Duration	Signatories / consent	Revocation / Appeal
Short-term detention: extension certificate	47(1)	• Patient is detained under short-term detention certificate • Patient has a mental disorder • Patient has significantly impaired ability to make decisions about provision of medical treatment because of mental disorder • Necessary to detain the patient in hospital to determine what medical treatment should be given, or to give medical treatment • Significant risk to health, safety or welfare of patient; or to the safety of others • An application should be made for a compulsory treatment order because of a change in the patient's mental health • Not reasonably practicable to apply for CTO before expiry of short-term detention certificate	3 working days from end of short-term detention certificate	Approved medical practitioner / Mental Health Officer if practicable	The RMO or Mental Welfare Commission can revoke the certificate The patient can appeal to the Mental Health Tribunal
Extension of short-term detention pending determination of application	68	• Patient detained under short-term detention certificate or an extension certificate. • Application for compulsory treatment order has been made • Determination of application is pending	5 working days	Automatic if grounds are satisfied	The Mental Health Tribunal must determine within the 5 days whether an interim compulsory treatment order should be made or, if not, it must determine the full application
Compulsory treatment order	64(4)	• Patient has a mental disorder • Medical treatment likely to prevent mental disorder worsening; or alleviate symptoms or effects of disorder; and such treatment is available • Significant risk to patient's health, safety or welfare; or to the safety of others without such medical treatment • Patient has significantly impaired ability to make decisions about provision of medical treatment because of mental disorder • The making of a compulsory treatment order is necessary	• 6 months • Renewable for a further 6 months and subsequently yearly • The care plan measures can be varied by application to the Tribunal	• 2 doctors (1 approved) • Application including proposed care plan by Mental Health officer • Mental Health Tribunal approval	Can be revoked by RMO or the Mental Welfare Commission To Mental Health Tribunal 3 months after making a CTO or once during each period of renewal

continued

Mental Health (Care and Treatment) (Scotland) Act 2003: Parts 5–7 Detention and Compulsory Treatment Orders

Purpose	Section	Grounds	Duration	Signatories/consent	Revocation/Appeal
Interim compulsory treatment order	65	• As for CTO except • The making of an interim CTO necessary	• 28 days • Maximum of 56 days in total for all interim measures	Determined by the Mental Health Tribunal for Scotland pending its determination of a CTO	Can be revoked by RMO, the Mental Welfare Commission, or automatically on granting of CTO

CTO, compulsory treatment order; RMO, Responsible Medical Officer.

Detention can proceed from an emergency certificate to a short-term certificate to a Compulsory Treatment Order. Alternatively, a short-term detention certificate can be granted immediately by an approved doctor with the consent of a Mental Health Officer. In a non-urgent situation an application can be made directly for a Compulsory Treatment Order. An emergency or short-term detention cannot be reapplied immediately.

Mental Treatment Act 2001 – Republic of Ireland

This Act has been passed by the Irish Parliament but has not yet been enacted. The Mental Treatment Act 1945 therefore contains the legislation currently in use.

Definitions

Term	Mental disorder	Mental illness	Severe dementia	Significant intellectual disability	Exclusions
Definition	Mental disorder means mental illness, severe dementia or significant intellectual disability	A state of mind which affects a person's thinking, perceiving, emotion or judgement and which seriously impairs the mental function of the person to the extent that he requires care or medical treatment in his interest or in the interest of other persons	A deterioration of the brain which significantly impairs the intellectual function of a person, thereby affecting thought, comprehension and memory, and which includes severe psychiatric or behavioural symptoms such as physical aggression	Means a state of arrested or incomplete development of mind which includes significant impairment of intelligence and social functioning and abnormally aggressive or seriously irresponsible conduct	Person suffering from a personality disorder, socially deviant, or addicted to drugs or intoxicants

Mental Health Act 2001 – Republic of Ireland: Part 2 – Involuntary Admission to approved centres

Purpose	Section	Grounds	Duration	Signatories / Applicant	Appeal
Admission Order	14	• Mental disorder • Impaired judgement — failure to admit would be likely to lead to a serious deterioration or prevent administration of appropriate treatment • Reception, detention and treatment would be likely to benefit or alleviate the condition of that person to a material extent	21 days	An *application* to a doctor for involuntary admission can be made by a relative, authorised officer of the Health Board, police officer or any other person over 18 with no financial interest in the admission or employment at the hospital concerned. Within 24 hours a *recommendation* for involuntary admission must be made by a doctor not on the staff of the hospital concerned or with a financial interest in the case. The receiving consultant psychiatrist has 24 hours to examine the patient and decide whether to make an *admission order*. The order is *reviewed* by a Mental Health Commission Tribunal within 21 days (or 35 days if ordered by Tribunal; or 49 days on application of patient)	To Circuit Court
Renewal Order	15	• Mental disorder • Impaired judgement — failure to admit would be likely to lead to a serious deterioration or prevent administration of appropriate treatment • Reception, detention and treatment would be likely to benefit or alleviate the condition of that person to a material extent	3 months, renewable for 6 months, then annually	• Responsible consultant psychiatrist • Reviewed by Mental Health Tribunal	To Circuit Court
Power to prevent voluntary patient leaving approved centre	23(1) – Adults	• Mental disorder • Impaired judgement — failure to admit would be likely to lead to a serious deterioration or prevent administration of appropriate treatment • Reception, detention and treatment would be likely to benefit or alleviate the condition of that person to a material extent	24 hours	Consultant psychiatrist, registered medical practitioner, or registered nurse on staff of approved centre	None

(continued)

Mental Health Act 2001 – Republic of Ireland: Part 2 – Involuntary Admission to approved centres — continued

Purpose	Section	Grounds	Duration	Signatories / Applicant	Appeal
Power to prevent voluntary patient leaving approved centre	23(1) – Child, i.e. under 18 unless married	• Mental disorder • Impaired judgement — failure to admit would be likely to lead to a serious deterioration or prevent administration of appropriate treatment • Reception, detention and treatment would be likely to benefit or alleviate the condition of that person to a material extent	Until reviewed under S. 25 at District Court within 3 days	• Consultant psychiatrist, registered medical practitioner, or registered nurse on staff of approved centre. • In custody of Health Board. Health Board shall, unless it returns the child to his / her parents, make an application under S.25	District Court within 3 days
Power to detain voluntary patients	24	• Mental disorder • Impaired judgement — failure to admit would be likely to lead to a serous deterioration or prevent administration of appropriate treatment • Reception, detention and treatment would be likely to benefit or alleviate the condition of that person to a material extent • Children (under 18 years unless married) are excluded	24 hours	Following a Section 23, the consultant psychiatrist responsible for the care and treatment of the patient must discharge him or obtain an examination by another consultant psychiatrist. If the second consultant psychiatrist is satisfied that the patient is suffering from a mental disorder he will issue a certificate and a responsible consultant shall make an admission order	None
Involuntary admission of children	25	• Mental disorder, and • Requires treatment which he is unlikely to receive unless an order is made under this section	21 days renewed by the Court for 3 months then renewed by the Court for 6 months, thereafter for periods not exceeding 6 months	• Health Board applies to District Court, and • Child has been examined by a consultant psychiatrist, or if parents do not consent to examination by psychiatrist or cannot be found, Health Board may apply to the Court without psychiatrist's examination. Court can then order a psychiatric examination	

Patient can be discharged by the responsible consultant psychiatrist if he becomes of the opinion that the patient is no longer suffering from a mental disorder, or by order of the Mental Health Commission.

A2 | Eponyms in psychiatry*

David M Semple

Alice in Wonderland syndrome The misperception of objects, which appear distorted, usually larger (macropsia) or smaller (micropsia) than they really are. This may be associated with a distorted sense of time and with visual hallucinations. Occurs most commonly in migraine, parietal lobe lesions and with hallucinogen intoxication.

Alper disease A rare degenerative disease of the brain, predominantly involving the grey matter. It is characterised by acute onset of severe convulsions leading to rapid intellectual and physical deterioration. Other characteristics are blindness, deafness, myoclonus, spasticity, choreoathetosis, cerebellar ataxia, growth retardation and terminal decortication. Manifests in early childhood and usually causes death within months. In its familial form, the disorder is transmitted as an autosomal recessive trait.

Alzheimer disease The commonest cause of dementia in late life. Pathological findings include generalised brain atrophy, with neurofibrillary tangles, senile plaques, and granulovacuolar degeneration in the hippocampal-pyramidal neurons, and deposition of type Aβ-amyloid protein in the cortex.

Angelman syndrome ('Happy puppet syndrome') Inherited congenital syndrome characterised by epilepsy, learning disability, 'puppet-like' movements and a happy disposition. Associated with deletions on chromosome 15 which may be maternally transmitted.

Anton syndrome Cortical blindness in which the patient lacks awareness of his condition, associated with persistent denial and confabulation. Classically associated with bilateral lesions of the occipital cortex, although this may not always be the case.

Asperger syndrome A developmental disorder, regarded as part of the autistic spectrum of disorders. Symptoms are similar to those of autism (see *Kanner syndrome*) without general intellectual decline and with normal language development.

Ballint syndrome A symptom complex comprising fixation (or apraxia) of gaze, optic ataxia (difficulty performing voluntary movements using visual guidance), constricted field of visual attention ('tunnel vision'), and the inability to recognise a whole picture despite recognising the individual parts (visual simultanagnosia). Usually caused by lesions of the bilateral superior parieto-occipital cortex.

Beard disease Obsolete term used for unexplained chronic, abnormal fatigue and lassitude, or 'nervous exhaustion'. Other associated symptoms included insomnia, back pain, nervousness, anxiety, depression, headache, difficulty in concentrating, reduced

sexual drive, and lack of appetite. The syndrome predominantly affected women in their 40s or 50s, and comparisons have been drawn with the current diagnosis of 'chronic fatigue syndrome'.

Bell mania An obsolete term for a 'pre-antipsychotic' syndrome in psychiatric patients, akin to 'neuroleptic malignant syndrome'. The clinical features include severe agitation, confusion, mutism, pyrexia, dehydration, delusions and hallucinations. Often fatal and essentially synonymous with *Stauder lethal catatonia*.

Binswanger disease A rare form of vascular dementia associated with multiple small infarcts. Usually presents in the 5th and 6th decades, and patients may have a history of hypertensive small vessel disease and raised plasma viscosity. CT and MRI reveal periventricular demyelination (including the external capsule), markedly enlarged ventricles, and subcortical infarcts.

Briquet syndrome (St Louis hysteria) Multiple somatisation disorder. Criteria for the diagnosis include: a history beginning before the age of 30, multiple physical symptoms (including pain, gastrointestinal symptoms, sexual symptoms, and psuedoneurological symptoms) severe enough to interfere with the patient's life and lead to contact with physicians, and a lack of any medical explanation despite appropriate investigations.

Broca aphasia Aphasia or impairment of expressive language, with preservation of comprehension, due to damage to the posterior part of the inferior frontal gyrus of the dominant hemisphere (Broca's language area, corresponding to Brodmann's areas 44 and 45).

Brueghel syndrome An idiopathic movement disorder, which comprises a particular subtype of *Meige syndrome* (blepharospasm and oromandibular dystonia), with extensive mandibular involvement as the main feature.

Capgras syndrome (L'illusion des sosies) The delusional belief that people, usually well known to the patient, have been replaced by other persons who appear to look exactly like them. Usually occurs in the context of a paranoid schizophrenic illness, but may also occur with other psychiatric disorders.

Charcot–Wilbrand syndrome A rare syndrome, following brain injury, particularly due to occlusion of the posterior cerebral artery of the dominant hemisphere, where there is visual agnosia, inability to revisualise images, and loss of all or part of dreaming. Sometimes associated with *Gerstmann syndrome*.

Charles–Bonnet syndrome Formed, complex, persistent, repetitive and stereotyped visual hallucinations, recognised by the patient as not real, without associated delusional ideas or hallucinations in other modalities. Most cases are reported in the elderly population and may be associated with visual impairment.

Clérambault–Kandinsky syndrome A term that is used in French diagnosis to describe a syndrome of 'mental automatism', similar

---

*The eponyms may be expressed in either the nominative (as here) or the possessive case (e.g. 'Alzheimer disease' or 'Alzheimer's disease').

to the Schneiderian concept of 'thought insertion' in schizophrenia. In this context, the syndrome includes all forms of psychosis in which thought insertion predominates, regardless of aetiology, and the prognosis is more varied than that of schizophrenia. 'Clérambault–Kandinsky syndrome' or 'De Clérambault–Kandinsky syndrome' are also used erroneously as synonyms for *De Clérambault syndrome* (erotomania — see below).

Cotard syndrome (Délire des negations)   A syndrome characterised by the presence of nihilistic delusional ideation. The patient may deny that he is alive, believe that part of his body is missing, or that the outside world no longer exists. The delusion tends to recur intermittently, rather than being chronic, and may be a feature of mood disorder, schizophrenia and organic disorders.

Couvade syndrome (Fathering syndrome, sympathetic pregnancy) A disorder that affects husbands either during their wives' pregnancies or at the time of delivery. The symptoms resemble those that pregnant women commonly suffer. Rarely other relatives, including children, may also be affected.

Creutzfeldt–Jakob disease   Rapidly progressive dementia associated with stiffness and weakness of the limbs, ataxia, myoclonus, characteristic triphasic waves on EEG, and diffuse spongiform degeneration of the brain. Although the majority of cases are sporadic, familial forms exist, with the remainder due to transmissible prions.

Crow type I and type II schizophrenia   A two-syndrome hypothesis of schizophrenia. Type I is characterised by acute onset, prominent positive symptoms (e.g. hallucinations, delusions and thought disorder), good premorbid adjustment, good treatment response, intact cognitive function, intact brain structure and probable underlying reversible neurochemical disturbance. Type II presents with insidious onset, prominent negative symptoms (e.g. affective flattening, poverty of speech and loss of drive), poor premorbid adjustment, poor treatment response, impaired cognitive function, structural brain abnormalities (e.g. ventricular enlargement) and presumed underlying pathology of irreversible neuronal loss.

Da Costa syndrome ('Soldier's heart', effort syndrome)   Original term for a syndrome characterised by palpitations, shortness of breath, subjective complaints of effort and discomfort on slight exertion, dizziness, shaking, sweating and insomnia. This constellation of symptoms has been compared to quite similar modern descriptions of anxiety and panic disorders, hyperventilation syndrome and chronic fatigue / neurasthenia.

Damocles syndrome   Used to describe the feelings of fragility and increased concern about illness and death, resulting in loss of self-confidence, and described originally in long-term survivors of cancer, but now applied to any 'fatal' diagnosis.

De Clérambault syndrome (erotomania)   A syndrome in which the delusional belief is held by the patient (almost invariably female) that a man, usually older, of higher status, famous, wealthy or in a professional relationship with the patient, is deeply in love with her.

De Lange syndrome (Cornelia de Lange syndrome, Amsterdam retardation)   Congenital form of learning disability associated with variable physical characteristics (e.g. small stature, microcephaly, low forehead, heavy eyebrows, depressed bridge of nose, flared nostrils, small mandible, low-set ears, limb / digit anomalies) and behavioural manifestations including self-injury, hyperactivity / sleeplessness and aggression.

Diogenes syndrome   A term applied when the hoarding of objects, usually of no practical use, leads to the neglect of one's home or environment. May be a behavioural manifestation of an organic disorder, schizophrenia, depressive disorder, obsessive–compulsive disorder, or reflect a reaction late in life to stress in a certain type of personality.

Down syndrome   Syndrome of learning disability usually caused by trisomy 21, although translocation and mosaic forms also occur. Characteristic features include slanting of the palpebral fissures, hyperextensible joints, brachycephalic skull with flattened occiput, ear anomalies, diastasis recti, high-arched palate, irregular teeth alignment, epicanthus, speckling of the iris, and heart murmurs. There is a clear association with early-onset Alzheimer disease.

Ekbom syndrome
1. *'Restless legs syndrome'*, consisting of an unpleasant sensation in the lower limbs that tends to be worse in the evening, or at night, and hence may interfere with sleep, causing insomnia. Aetiology is unknown but it may be familial and can be associated with iron deficiency, phenothiazines, barbiturate and benzodiazepine withdrawal, diabetes, uraemia, neuropathy, chronic respiratory disease and following cerebrovascular accident. It is also common in pregnancy, and fatigue, anxiety or stress may be associated exacerbating factors.
2. *'Delusional parasitosis'*, where the patient believes he is infested by parasites, associated with the extremely unpleasant sensation of worms, ants, bugs, mites or other small insects that are biting, crawling or creeping over or under, or burrowing into or out of, areas of the skin (often the outer rectal area). Most often seen in toxic psychoses caused by an organic agent such as alcohol, cocaine or morphine, but may also be a symptom in some patients with psychotic depression, schizophrenia or dementia. (See *Magnan sign.*)
3. *'Pisa syndrome'* or pleurothotonus. Tonic flexion of the trunk to one side which may be seen as a form of tardive dystonia, as a side-effect of antipsychotic medication, or as a symptom of Alzheimer disease.

Fahr syndrome   Idiopathic calcification of the basal ganglia leading to dementia with associated pyramidal, extrapyramidal and cerebellar signs. In some cases obsessive–compulsive, mood-related or psychotic symptoms are seen.

Frégoli phenomenon (or delusion)   A delusional belief that strangers are actually people, with whom the patient is familiar, in disguise. In this way the patient believes he is being pursued or persecuted.

Ganser syndrome   A syndrome with sudden onset and disappearance, characterised by 'approximate answers' (Ganser symptom), with clouding of consciousness ('twilight' state), memory disturbance, vorbereiden (talking at cross purposes) and dissociative symptoms. Originally described as a form of hysteria, but has been thought of as a factitious 'simulated' psychosis, schizophrenia or an acute psychotic reaction, and more recently a dissociative disorder.

Gardener–Diamond syndrome (psychogenic purpura)   A painful bruising syndrome, of presumed immunological pathogenesis, which occurs in association with psychological distress. It may be localised or extensive (e.g. a whole limb), may remit or recur in an unpredictable manner, and is seen more frequently in women than men.

Gélineau syndrome (also known as Friedmann disease) Narcolepsy. The association of daytime somnolence, cataplexy, sleep paralysis, and hypnagogic hallucinations.

Gerstmann syndrome   Finger agnosia, right–left disorientation, agraphia, and dyscalculia, said to be associated with dominant parietal lobe lesions.

Gerstmann–Sträussler–Scheinker disease   Familial form of Creutzfeldt–Jakob disease, caused by transmissible prions and affecting only those individuals with a specific autosomal dominant defect in chromosome 20.

Gilles de la Tourette syndrome   Multiple motor and verbal tic disorder, more frequently seen in boys than girls, associated with a family history (of perhaps less severe symptoms) and often comorbidity (obsessive–compulsive disorder, depression).

Gjessing syndrome   Periodic catatonia. Recurrent, fluctuating episodes of catatonic stupor or agitation, occurring in schizophrenia, and associated with variations in nitrogen metabolism.

Hakim–Adams syndrome   Normal-pressure hydrocephalus, leading to dementia with associated incontinence and gait disturbance, which may be reversible if treated promptly by surgical insertion of a shunt.

Hallervorden–Spatz syndrome   Progressive familial striatopallidal degeneration. Usually presenting in young adults with bilateral rigidity, speech problems, dementia, and sometimes associated with optic atrophy or hyperkinesis.

Hashimoto encephalitis   A treatable form of encephalitis secondary to autoimmune (Hashimoto) thyroiditis.

Heidenhain syndrome   A rare form of presenile dementia associated with cortical blindness, ataxia, dysarthria, athetotic movements, rigidity, and spongiform change in the cerebral cortex at postmortem. Thought to be a variant of Creutzfeldt–Jakob disease.

Heller syndrome   Also known as 'childhood disintegrative disorder' where there is loss of developmental milestones after the age of 2 in multiple areas of functioning.

Hoigne syndrome   An acute psychotic reaction to the intravenous injection of penicillin.

Hoover sign   Used to demonstrate feigned lower limb weakness absence of the 'normal' downward pressure usually exerted by the unaffected leg on attempting to lift (in the supine position) the affected leg, or hold it up against resistance.

Huntington disease   A heritable neuropsychiatric disorder, transmitted in an autosomal-dominant manner, due to a trinucleotide repeat located on the short arm of chromosome 4. The patient will usually present around the age of 35 with a progressive clinical picture including choreiform movements, dementia, psychiatric symptoms (behaviour disturbance, psychosis, depression), death within 15–20 years of onset, and associated with caudate atrophy.

Kahlbaum syndrome   Catatonia. A name given to abnormalities of movement and posture, including 'waxy flexibility', posturing and stupor, or excitement, agitation, stereotypies, hyperkinesia and impulsivity.

Kanner syndrome (autism)   A pervasive developmental disorder, with onset before the age of three years, characterised by abnormal functioning in the areas of social interaction, communication and behaviour (restricted, repetitive, stereotyped patterns of activities or interests). All levels of IQ may be seen, but the majority (about 75%) have significant learning disability.

Kleine–Levin syndrome   A rare syndrome occurring almost exclusively in male adolescents, characterised by periodic attacks of somnolence accompanied by excessive food intake, and a variety of psychiatric symptoms (e.g. confusion, irritability, restlessness, euphoria, hypersexuality, hallucinations, delusions and schizophreniform states). Attacks may occur every 3 to 6 months

and last from 2 to 3 days. Between attacks the patients recover completely, and the sleep periods usually disappear in adulthood.

Klinefelter syndrome   A genetic condition, where there is an extra sex chromosome (XXY pattern) and phenotypical male appearance, small testis and tall stature. Associated with mild learning disability and antisocial personality traits.

Klüver–Bucy syndrome   A syndrome, occasionally seen in dementia, particularly with the involvement of the fronto-temporal lobes, with clinical features that include visual agnosia (inability to recognise familiar people), emotional lability (particularly fear and rage reactions), increased sexual activity (with a disinhibited quality), bulimia and other eating disorders, hyperorality, hypermetamorphosis (excessive tendency to attend and react to visual stimuli) and memory disturbance.

Korsakoff syndrome   A syndrome characterised by a severe memory defect, particularly for recent events and new information (anterograde), for which the patient compensates by confabulation. Polyneuropathy may also be present, and other associated symptoms may include delirium, confusion, disorientation in time and place, impaired attention and concentration, anxiety, fear, depression, delusions and insomnia. It is caused by thiamine deficiency and shares underlying pathology with the more acute *Wernicke syndrome*.

Kozhevnikov syndrome   Progressive cognitive deterioration secondary to continuous partial epilepsy.

Kraepelin disease (Catatonia of Kraepelin)   A form of familial presenile dementia, regarded as analogous to Creutzfeldt–Jakob disease, but with very early onset of symptoms (late 20s / early 30s).

Kulenkampff–Tarnow syndrome   An acute dystonia of the face and neck, also known as neck–face syndrome or dyskinetic–hypertonic syndrome, that may be caused by antipsychotic medication.

Landau–Kleffner syndrome   Selective loss of language development in children as a result of continuous partial epilepsy.

Langfeldt psychosis   Psychosis without a deteriorating course.

Lesch–Nyhan syndrome   Congenital learning disability caused by a deletion of chromosome 26, leading to defective purine metabolism and associated clinically with self-injurious behaviour.

Lewy body dementia   Cortical dementia with the presence of diffuse Lewy bodies (intracytoplasmic inclusion bodies) in the cerebral cortex (particularly the temporal lobe, cingulate gyrus and insular cortex). Clinically similar to Alzheimer disease, with associated visual hallucinations, fluctuating conscious level, and sometimes parkinsonism. Patients may be very sensitive to the extrapyramidal side-effects of antipsychotic medication.

L'hermitte syndrome   Peduncular hallucinosis in which hallucinations appear bizarre (often Lilliputian) without other psychotic symptoms, due to lesions of the midbrain.

Lilliputian hallucinations   Microptic hallucinations with objects appearing to be of a much reduced scale. Reported in drug and alcohol intoxication, acute confusional states and with parietal/temporal lobe pathology.

Magnan sign   A crawling, illusory sensation of a foreign body under the skin, seen primarily in cases of cocaine addiction, but also described in alcohol and opiate withdrawal. (See also *Ekbom 2 syndrome*.)

Marchiafava–Bignami syndrome   Central necrosis of the corpus callosum, associated with alcoholism, presenting initially with agitation, confusion and ataxia. Later symptoms include apathy, inattention, akinetic mutism, hemiparesis or hemiplegia, seizures and, ultimately, death.

Marinescu reflex   The 'palmomental' reflex in which movement of the chin follows stroking of the palm. When present it is suggestive of frontal or diffuse brain injury.

Martin–Bell syndrome   Another name for fragile X-linked learning disability. The condition is due to trinucleotide repeats on the X chromosome and is associated with autism and attention-deficit hyperactivity disorder.

Meige syndrome   An idiopathic movement disorder characterised by blepharospasm and oromandibular dystonia. It may be confused with tardive dyskinesia and can occasionally occur as a side-effect of antipsychotic medication.

Morvan syndrome   A form of fibrillary chorea with involuntary muscle fibre activity, hyperhydrosis and insomnia, which if untreated may be fatal. Thought to be autoimmune mediated and can occur as a paraneoplastic syndrome.

Münchausen syndrome (Asher syndrome)   Multiple factitious disorder in which patients present, often dramatically, with a variety of physical (or psychiatric) complaints with the aim of being regarded as ill and given medical attention and treatment.

Münchausen syndrome by proxy (Polle syndrome, Meadow syndrome)   A form of child abuse, where parents (in most cases, the mother) deliberately invent or physically induce symptoms and signs in the child, leading to sometimes painful and often unnecessary physical examinations and treatments.

Myerson sign   The 'glabellar tap' reflex — failure to extinguish the 'blink reflex' after 4 taps on the forehead. A 'soft' neurological sign, indicating possible frontal, diffuse, or extrapyramidal disease.

Nevin–Jones disease   A form of subacute encephalopathy, characterised by blindness, paralysis, speech disorders, cerebellar symptoms, myoclonus and behavioural disorders, thought to be a variant of Creutzfeldt–Jakob disease.

Othello syndrome   Delusional jealousy where the patient is convinced that his partner is being unfaithful. May be a symptom of a number of disease processes, including schizophrenia, alcohol dependence, paranoid personality disorder and delusional disorder.

Parkinson disease (or syndrome)   A slowly progressive disease of the central nervous system, caused mainly by degeneration of the basal ganglia as a result of reduced production of dopamine in the substantia nigra. Characterised by a fine resting tremor, cogwheel rigidity, akinesia/bradykinesia, a festinating ('propulsive') gait, postural instability and immobile/mask-like facies. Parkinson syndrome refers to the occurrence of these 'extrapyramidal' signs secondary to another disease process or medication.

Pick disease   Dementia characterised by signs of severe frontal and temporal lobe dysfunction.

Pisa syndrome   See *Ekbom syndrome 3*.

Prader–Willi syndrome   Caused by a deletion of chromosome 15, this syndrome is characterised by learning disability, compulsive eating and self-mutilation.

Rasmussen syndrome   Unilateral brain atrophy, with continuous epilepsy, resulting in cognitive decline until the affected brain portion is removed.

Rett syndrome   An X-linked developmental disorder, mainly affecting girls, leading to severe learning disability. There is a profound loss of previously acquired cognitive and motor skills after the age of 5 months, with acquired microcephaly, ataxia, dyspraxia, stereotypical hand movements, growth retardation, and often epilepsy.

Russell sign   Skin abrasions, small lacerations, and callosities on the dorsum of the hand overlying the metacarpophalangeal and interphalangeal joints, found in patients with symptoms of bulimia. Caused by repeated contact of the incisors to the skin of the hand that occurs during self-induced vomiting.

Sanfilippo syndrome   Learning disability, due to a deletion of chromosome 12, characterised by aggressive behaviour and insomnia.

Smith–Magenis syndrome   Learning disability with characteristic severe self-injurious and 'self-hugging' behaviours.

Stauder lethal catatonia   See *Bell mania*. Another old term for a syndrome similar to that of 'neuroleptic malignant syndrome' described in the pre-antipsychotic era. Some commentators distinguished it from 'Bell mania', describing it as a form of hypokinetic catatonia (rather than Bell's 'agitated' form). Re-examination of Stauder's original case series does not, however, support this view, and the two syndromes are essentially synonymous.

Steele–Richardson–Olszewski disease   Form of dementia associated with characteristic ataxia, loss of vertical gaze (the ability to look up or down), and parkinsonism.

Strauss syndrome   Term formerly used for 'minimal brain damage syndrome'. Now replaced by 'attention-deficit hyperactivity disorder' with the cardinal features of impaired attention and overactivity.

Sydenham chorea   Movement disorder, often associated with obsessive–compulsive symptoms, following rheumatic fever. Recently the acronym PANDAS (Paediatric Autoimmune Neuropsychiatric Disorders Associated with Streptococcal infections) has been used.

Von Economo encephalitis (encephalitis lethargicans)   Of presumed viral aetiology, a syndrome that affected many individuals following an epidemic in the 1920s. Diverse chronic neurological symptoms, which often arose years later, included parkinsonism, lethargy, ophthalmoplegia and involuntary movements. Other psychiatric symptoms included associated depression, obsessive–compulsive symptoms, and behavioural disorders in children (similar to attention-deficit hyperactivity disorder.)

Von Recklinghausen disease (neurofibromatosis)   A disease characterised by café au lait spots (areas of increased skin pigmentation) and multiple, often soft, sessile, peripheral nerve tumours (neurofibromas / schwannomas). Other features include dysplastic changes of the skin, nervous system, bones, endocrine organs and blood vessels. Learning disability, epilepsy, hydrocephalus and other neuropsychiatric complications frequently occur. It is inherited as autosomal dominant, but half of cases are due to new mutations.

Waxman–Geschwind syndrome   In temporal lobe epilepsy, an interictal behavioural syndrome describing the association of hyposexuality, hyperreligiosity, hypergraphia and 'viscosity' (loss of social boundaries in normal conversation).

Wernicke aphasia   Loss of comprehension of spoken language, loss of ability to read (silently) and write, and distortion of articulate speech, without hearing loss. Speech may be fluent with natural language rhythm and prosody; however, it has neither understandable meaning nor syntax. Despite loss of comprehension, word memory is preserved and words are often chosen correctly. Alexia, agraphia, acalculia and paraphasia are frequently associated. Some patients may present as euphoric and / or paranoid. The disorder is due to cortical lesions in or near the posterior portion of the left first temporal convolution (superior temporal gyrus), known as the Wernicke area.

Wernicke encephalopathy   An encephalopathy syndrome classically characterised by the triad of ophthalmoplegia, ataxia and global confusion. Other features may include hypothermia, hypotension, coma, cardiovascular problems and peripheral neuropathies. Primarily due to thiamine deficiency secondary to alcoholism and/or starvation. Other less common aetiologies include self-induced starvation, protein-energy malnutrition resulting from inadequate diet or malabsorption, conditions associated with protracted vomiting (e.g. hyperemesis gravidarum in pregnancy), chronic renal failure, carbohydrate loading in the presence of marginal thiamine stores (feeding after starvation), transketolase function abnormalities, and beriberi (in infants and adults). There is a mortality rate of 10–20% for patients with Wernicke encephalopathy despite adequate treatment with thiamine replacement. Of those who survive, approximately 80% may develop symptoms of Korsakoff psychosis, with the typical features of retrograde and anterograde amnesia, decreased spontaneity and initiative, and confabulation. (See *Korsakoff psychosis*.)

Williams syndrome   Learning disability resulting from a deletion of chromosome 7 (which may include the gene for elastin)

and with the distinctive characteristics of growth retardation, 'elfin facies', a hoarse voice, premature wrinkling and sagging of the skin, and other vascular anomalies. Often patients have excellent verbal fluency, and cognitive deficits may be highly variable.

Wilson disease   A chronic disease of brain and liver with progressive neurological dysfunction, caused by a disturbance of copper metabolism. It is characterised by progressive degeneration of the basal ganglia of the brain, a brownish ring (Kayser–Fleischer ring) at the outer margin of the cornea caused by deposition of copper in the Descemet membrane, cirrhosis of the liver, splenomegaly, tremor, muscular rigidity, involuntary movements, spastic contractures, psychiatric disturbances and progressive weakness and emaciation. A rare, autosomal recessively inherited condition, it is caused by mutations or deletions of the ATP7B protein encoded on chromosome 13q14.3-q 21.1.

Wolfram syndrome   A rare autosomal recessive condition, caused by a chromosome 4 defect, characterised by juvenile onset diabetes mellitus and bilateral progressive optic atrophy. Other features may include diabetes insipidus and deafness, giving rise to the acronym 'DIDMOAD'. Diverse and serious psychiatric disorders are frequently seen, including severe depression, psychosis, 'organic brain syndrome' and impulsive verbal and physical aggression. Carriers of the gene also appear to have a high risk of psychiatric illness.

Index

Note: Page numbers followed by '*f*' and '*t 8*' refer to figures and tables/boxed material respectively